TEXTBOOK
OF PALLIATIVE
MEDICINE

TEXTBOOK OF PALLIATIVE MEDICINE

Edited by

Eduardo Bruera
Professor and Chair
Department of Palliative Care & Rehabilitation Medicine
The University of Texas MD Anderson Cancer Center
F.T. McGraw Chair in the Treatment of Cancer
Houston, Texas, USA

Irene Higginson
Cicely Saunders Institute
King's College London, London, UK

Charles F von Gunten
Ohiohealth, Columbus, Ohio, USA

Tatsuya Morita
Palliative and Supportive Care Division, Seirei Mikatahara Hospital
Hamamatsu, Japan

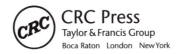

CRC Press
Taylor & Francis Group
Boca Raton London New York

CRC Press is an imprint of the
Taylor & Francis Group, an **informa** business

CRC Press
Taylor & Francis Group
6000 Broken Sound Parkway NW, Suite 300
Boca Raton, FL 33487-2742

Printed on acid-free paper
Version Date: 20160222

International Standard Book Number-13: 978-1-4987-7283-9 (Paperback)

Visit the Taylor & Francis Web site at
http://www.taylorandfrancis.com

and the CRC Press Web site at
http://www.crcpress.com

To Ed, Sofia, and Sebastian

Eduardo Bruera

To Kathleen and Leslie Higginson

Irene Higginson

Dedicated to the leadership, staff, and benefactors of OhioHealth for pursuing the vision of palliative care woven throughout a healthcare system dedicated to serving its community

Charles F. von Gunten

Dedicated to the memory of Doctor Satoshi Chihara, my first and best mentor

Tatsuya Morita

We would like to dedicate this book to the memory of the pioneers of palliative care, with gratefulness

Contents

Preface

Palliative medicine emerged in the United Kingdom during the 1960s as a response to the unmet needs of terminally ill patients and their families. This initially British movement became progressively a global movement. The original community-based services were followed by programs of increasing complexity in secondary and tertiary hospitals and comprehensive cancer centers. Educational initiatives became progressively more sophisticated, ultimately resulting in palliative medicine becoming a full medical specialty. Research into many of the complex problems faced by patients and families has provided a growing body of knowledge on how to conduct our clinical care, education, organization, and governance.

Our book has attempted to reflect the growth of our area of knowledge from a global perspective. Internationally recognized leaders have been asked to apply their first-hand knowledge in summarizing the principal issues in our discipline.

Palliative medicine covers a wide variety of subjects ranging from pharmacological interventions to historical, bioethical, and spiritual issues. This state-of-the-art book cohesively addresses the full range of disciplines regularly involved in palliative medicine. We have attempted to produce a scholarly but accessible text following a user-friendly format while respecting the needs of specific authors to deviate from the more traditional biomedical format when their area of content required them to do so.

We believe that this book will become a very useful resource for physicians, nurses, and other healthcare professionals involved in the clinical, academic, and administrative aspects of palliative care delivery worldwide.

Eduardo Bruera
Irene Higginson
Charles F. von Gunten
Tatsuya Morita

Editors

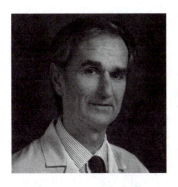

Eduardo D. Bruera, MD, earned his medical degree from the University of Rosario, in Argentina. He trained in medical oncology and relocated to the University of Alberta in Edmonton, Alberta, Canada, where he directed the clinical and academic palliative care programs until 1999. In 1999, Dr. Bruera relocated to The University of Texas MD Anderson Cancer Center, Houston, Texas, where he currently holds the F.T. McGraw Chair in the Treatment of Cancer and is the chair of the Department of Palliative Care and Rehabilitation Medicine. He is board-certified by the American Board of Internal Medicine and is certified in the subspecialty of Palliative Medicine by the American Board of Hospice and Palliative Medicine.

Dr. Bruera's main clinical interest is the care of the physical and psychosocial distress of patients with advanced cancer and the support of their families. He developed and led the Edmonton Regional and Palliative Care program for its first five years. This unique program provides access to palliative care to more than 80% of patients who die of cancer in the Edmonton region. He also developed and leads the Department of Palliative Care and Rehabilitation Medicine at The University of Texas MD Anderson Cancer Center since 1999.

Dr. Bruera has been interested in the development of palliative care programs internationally, particularly in the developing world where he helped in the establishment of numerous palliative care programs in the Latin American region, India, and different areas of Europe. Dr. Bruera acted as the president of the International Association of Hospice and Palliative Care for a period of four years ending in January 2006.

Over the last 20 years, Dr. Bruera has trained hundreds of physicians, nurses, and other health care professionals in the clinical delivery of palliative care. He established the first academic fellowship in palliative care at the University of Alberta in Canada and one of the first academic palliative care fellowships in the United States at The University of Texas MD Anderson Cancer Center.

Dr. Bruera has more than 1000 publications and has edited 30 books. He has given more than 900 major invited lectures.

Dr. Bruera has received a number of national and international awards including the American Cancer Society Lane Adams Quality of Life Award and the American Academy of Hospice and Palliative Medicine Lifetime Achievement Award. The Canadian Society of Palliative Care Physicians has established the "Eduardo Bruera Award" as a career award for palliative care specialists. He was also awarded the Vittorio Ventafridda Memorial Lectureship Award and the Hospice and Palliative Medicine Visionary Award from the American Academy of Hospice and Palliative Medicine in 2013.

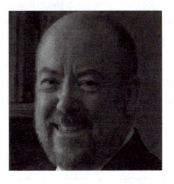

Dr. Charles F. von Gunten is the vice president, Medical Affairs, Hospice and Palliative Medicine for the OhioHealth System based in Columbus, Ohio. He is the founding chairman of the Test Committee for Hospice and Palliative Medicine of the American Board of Medical Specialties. He is editor-in-chief of the *Journal of Palliative Medicine*. He is co-principal for the Education for Physicians on End-of-life Care (EPEC) Project and its revision for oncology, EPEC-O. He received the Palliative Care Pioneer award from the American Cancer Society and the life-time achievement award from the American Academy for Hospice and Palliative Medicine in 2011, at the age of 54. In the same year he was named a "top doctor" in *U.S. News and World Report*. He is particularly interested in the integration of hospice and palliative care into health systems. He has published and spoken widely on the subjects of hospice, palliative medicine, and pain and symptom control.

Dr. von Gunten earned his BA with honors from Brown University in Providence, Rhode Island, in 1978. He then earned a PhD in biochemistry and an MD with honors from the University of Colorado Health Sciences Center in Denver, Colorado, in 1988. He subsequently pursued residency training in internal medicine, followed by subspecialty training in hematology/oncology at the McGaw Medical Center of Northwestern University in Chicago. After joining Northwestern's faculty, he directed programs in hospice and palliative care, education, and research. In 1999, he was recruited by the Institute for Palliative Medicine at San Diego Hospice, where he led the development of education and research programs as provost until 2012. He holds the academic rank of Clinical Professor of Medicine, University of California, San Diego.

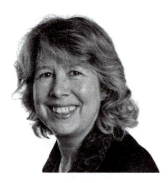

Irene J. Higginson, OBE, qualified in medicine from Nottingham University, Nottingham, United Kingdom and has worked in a wide range of medical and university positions, including radiotherapy and oncology, inpatient and home hospice care, and in various universities, as well as at the Department of Health (England). She is dual-trained in palliative medicine and public health medicine. She has developed and validated two outcome measures both freely available and used widely in palliative care: the Support Team Assessment Schedule and the Palliative Care Outcome Scale (see www.pos-pal.org). She is director of the Cicely Saunders Institute at King's College London, the world's first purpose-built institute of palliative care, integrating research, education, clinical services, and support and information. Professor Higginson is an NIHR senior investigator and was awarded the Fellowship of the Academy of Medical Sciences in 2013 for her contribution to the field. She has several active research programs, leads the MSc, diploma and certificate in palliative care, supervises several PhD students, and is active in teaching.

Professor Higginson has published over 400 articles in peer-reviewed journals, plus several books; her research interests and publications are in the following areas: quality of life and outcome measurements, evaluation of palliative care especially of new services and interventions, epidemiology, clinical audit, effectiveness, psychosocial care, symptom assessment, breathlessness, cachexia/anorexia, and elderly care. She plays an active role in the clinical service, including on call.

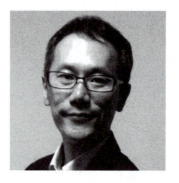

Tatsuya Morita, MD, is the vise president of the Seirei Mikatahara General Hospital and director of the Palliative and Supportive Care Division, Hamamatsu, Japan. He is one of the representative members of the Japanese Association of Palliative Medicine. He is member of the editorial boards of the *Journal of Pain and Symptom Management*, *Journal of Palliative Medicine*, and *Journal of Palliative Care*. He is also the associate editor of the *Japanese Journal of Clinical Oncology*, and is a clinical professor of medicine at Kyoto University.

Dr. Morita has conducted many government-granted research and educational activities, and published more than 200 scientific papers. His main research topics included delirium, palliative sedation, hydration, suffering, and care delivery. He has coordinated a variety of research groups, including epidemiology, symptom research, care delivery system, psycho-oncology, and rehabilitation.

After graduating from Kyoto University of Medicine in 1992, Dr. Morita completed a residency program in internal medicine at the Seirei Mikatahara General Hospital, an 800-bed general hospital located in the western area of the Shizuoka prefecture, Japan. He was a staff medical doctor of the Seirei Hospice, one of the oldest inpatient hospices (palliative care units) in Japan, and devoted most of his time to patient care in in-patient and home care settings from 1993 to 2002. In doing so, he leaned research methodology at the Psycho-Oncology Division of the National Cancer Center Research Institute East, Japan. He started a hospital palliative care program in 2002 as the head of Palliative Care Team as one of the pioneer activities in Japan.

Contributors

Rachel M. Adams
Assistant Professor of Medicine
Department of Geriatrics and Palliative Medicine
Icahn School of Medicine at Mount Sinai New York, New York

Carrie J. Aigner
Department of Pain Medicine
MD Anderson Cancer Center
The University of Texas
Houston, Texas

Tatsuo Akechi
Department of Psychiatry and Cognitive-Behavioral
    Medicine
Graduate School of Medical Sciences
Nagoya City University
Nagoya, Japan

Yesne Alici
Department of Psychiatry and Behavioral Sciences
Memorial Sloan-Kettering Cancer Center
New York, New York

Joseph Arthur
Department of Palliative Care and Rehabilitative Medicine
MD Anderson Cancer Center
The University of Texas
Houston, Texas

Rabia Atayee
Doris A. Howell Palliative Care Service
University of California, San Diego Medical Center
Moores Cancer Center
La Jolla, California

Ahsan Azhar
Department of Palliative Care and Rehabilitation Medicine
MD Anderson Cancer Center
The University of Texas
Houston, Texas

Anthony L. Back
Fred Hutchinson Cancer Research Center
University of Washington
Seattle, Washington

Kristian M. Bailey
Department of Cardiology
Royal Victoria Infirmary
Newcastle-upon-Tyne, United Kingdom

Dave Balachandran
MD Anderson Cancer Center
The University of Texas
Houston, Texas

Elizabeth A. Barnes
Department of Radiation Oncology
Odette Cancer Centre
University of Toronto
Toronto, Ontario, Canada

Claudia Bausewein
Department for Palliative Medicine
Munich University Hospital
Campus Großhadern
München, Germany

Julie Bayliss
Infection, Cancer and Immunity Unit
Great Ormond Street Hospital
London, United Kingdom

Estela Beale
Pediatrics – Patient Care
MD Anderson Cancer Center
The University of Texas
Houston, Texas

Robert Alan Bonakdar
Scripps Center for Integrative Medicine
La Jolla, California

Cara Bondly
Bruno Cancer Center
St. Vincent's Hospital
Birmingham, Alabama

Sara Booth
Macmillan Consultant in Palliative Medicine
Lead Clinician for Palliative Medicine
Cambridge Universities Foundation Trust
Cambridge, United Kingdom

Monica Bosco
Palliative Care Unit
Department of Oncology and Haematology
Ospedale G. Da Saliceto
Piacenza, Italy

Sue Boucher
International Children's Palliative Care Network
Bristol, United Kingdom

Kim Bower
Institute for Palliative Medicine
San Diego Hospice
San Diego, California

William Breitbart
Department of Psychiatry and Behavioral Sciences
Memorial Sloan-Kettering Cancer Center
and
Department of Psychiatry
Weill Medical College of Cornell University
and
Palliative & Supportive Care
International Psycho-Oncology Society
New York, New York

Eduardo Bruera
Section of Symptom Control and Palliative Care
Division of Cancer Medicine
Department of Palliative Care and Rehabilitative Medicine
MD Anderson Cancer Center
The University of Texas
Houston, Texas

Deanna Bryant
Department of Oncology
McMaster University
Hamilton, Ontario, Canada

Shirley H. Bush
Division of Palliative Care
Department of Medicine
University of Ottawa
and
Bruyère Research Institute
and
Department of Palliative Care
Bruyère Continuing Care
Ottawa, Ontario, Canada

Augusto T. Caraceni
Palliative Care, Pain Therapy and Rehabilitation Unit
Fondazione IRCCS
Istituto Nazionale dei Tumori
Milan, Italy

J. Brian Cassel
Data Analytic Services
Massey Cancer Center
Virginia Commonwealth University
Richmond, Virginia

Carlos Centeno
Clínica Universidad de Navarra
University of Navarra
Pamplona, Spain

Victor T. Chang
Section Hematology Oncology, Medical Service
VA New Jersey Health Care System
East Orange, New Jersey

and

Department of Medicine
Rutgers New Jersey Medical School
Newark, New Jersey

Nathan I. Cherny
Department of Oncology
Cancer Pain and Palliative Medicine Service
Shaare Zedek Medical Center
Jerusalem, Israel

Harvey Max Chochinov
Department of Psychiatry Faculty of Medicine
University of Manitoba
and
Manitoba Palliative Care Research Unit
CancerCare Manitoba
Manitoba, Canada

Edward Chow
Department of Radiation Oncology
Odette Cancer Centre
University of Toronto
Toronto, Ontario, Canada

Elizabeth J. Chuang
Division of Palliative Care
Department of Family and Social Medicine
Montefiore Medical Center
Albert Einstein College of Medicine
Bronx, New York

Alexie Cintron
Assistant Professor of Medicine
Baylor College of Medicine
and
Attending Physician in Palliative Medicine
Harris Health System
Houston, Texas

Josephine M. Clayton
HammondCare Palliative & Supportive Care Service
Greenwich Hospital
and
Sydney Medical School
University of Sydney
Sydney, New South Wales, Australia

Lorenzo Cohen
Department of General Oncology
MD Anderson Cancer Center
The University of Texas
Houston, Texas

S. Robin Cohen
Departments of Oncology and Medicine
McGill University
and
Lady Davis Institute
Jewish General Hospital
Montreal, Quebec, Canada

Massimo Costantini
Palliative Care Unit
Arcispedale Santa Maria Nuova
Istituto di Ricovero e Cura a Carattere Scientifico
Reggio Emilia, Italy

Kerry S. Courneya
Faculty of Physical Education & Recreation
University of Alberta
Edmonton, Alberta, Canada

Finella Craig
Paediatric Palliative Medicine
The Louis Dundas Centre
Great Ormond Street Hospital for Children NHS Foundation Trust
London, United Kingdom

J. Randall Curtis
Palliative Care Center of Excellence
and
Pulmonary and Critical Care Medicine
Harborview Medical Center
University of Washington
Seattle, Washington

Shalini Dalal
Department of Palliative Care and Rehabilitation Medicine
MD Anderson Cancer Center
The University of Texas
Houston, Texas

Mellar P. Davis
Department of Solid Tumor Oncology
The Harry R. Horvitz Center for Palliative Medicine
Cleveland Clinic Taussig Cancer Institute
and
College of Medicine
Case Western Reserve University
Cleveland, Ohio

Sara N. Davison
Division of Nephrology & Immunology
University of Alberta
Edmonton, Alberta, Canada

Maxine de la Cruz
Palliative Care and Rehabilitation Medicine
MD Anderson Cancer Center
The University of Texas
Houston, Texas

Liliana De Lima
International Association for Hospice and
    Palliative Care
Houston, Texas

Egidio Del Fabbro
Palliative Care Program
Virginia Commonwealth University
Richmond, Virginia

Marvin Omar Delgado-Guay
Department of Palliative Care and Rehabilitation Medicine
MD Anderson Cancer Center
The University of Texas
Houston, Texas

Mary Dev
Department of Social Work
MD Anderson Cancer Center
The University of Texas
Houston, Texas

Rony Dev
Department of Palliative Care and Rehabilitation Medicine
MD Anderson Cancer Center
The University of Texas
Houston, Texas

Travis DeVader
Department of Emergency Medicine
Department of Palliative Medicine
Stormont-Vail HealthCare
Topeka, Kansas

Alexandra M. Easson
Division of General Surgery
Mount Sinai Hospital
University of Toronto
and
Department of Surgical Oncology
Princess Margaret Hospital
Toronto, Ontario, Canada

Solvig Ekblad
Division of Social Medicine
Department of Public Health
Karolinska Institutet
and
Department of Learning, Informatics, Management and Ethics
Centre for Medical Education
Karolinska Institutet
Stockholm, Sweden

Badi El Osta
Department of Palliative Care and Rehabilitation Medicine
MD Anderson Cancer Center
The University of Texas
Houston, Texas

Linda Emanuel
The Buehler Center on Aging
Feinberg School of Medicine
Northwestern University
Chicago, Illinois

Bette Emery
Tertiary Palliative Care Unit
Grey Nuns Community Hospital
Edmonton, Alberta, Canada

Daniel Epner
Department of Palliative Care and Rehabilitation Medicine
MD Anderson Cancer Center
The University of Texas
Houston, Texas

Robin L. Fainsinger
Division of Palliative Care Medicine
Department of Oncology
University of Alberta
and
Grey Nuns Community Hospital
Health Services Centre
Edmonton, Alberta, Canada

Alysa Fairchild
Department of Radiation Oncology
Cross Cancer Institute
University of Alberta
Edmonton, Alberta, Canada

Lise Fillion
Department of Nursing Sciences
UniversitéLaval
Quebec City, Quebec, Canada

and

Department of Psychology
Université de Montreal
Montreal, Quebec, Canada

Ilora G. Finlay
Department of Palliative Medicine
Velindre Hospital
Whitchurch, United Kingdom

Michael Fisch
Department of General Oncology
MD Anderson Cancer Center
The University of Texas
Houston, Texas

Fabio Formaglio
Palliative Care and Pain Therapy Unit
Valtellina and Valchiavenna Hospitals
Morbegno, Italy

Kelley Fournier
Tertiary Palliative Care Unit
Grey Nuns Community Hospital
Health Services Centre
Edmonton, Alberta, Canada

Kathryn G. Froiland
Oncology Clinical Educator
Glaxo Smith Kline Inc.
Houston, Texas

Fabio Fulfaro
Operative Unit of Medical Oncology
University of Palermo
Palermo, Italy

Carl Johan Fürst
Palliativt Utvecklingscentrum
The Institute for Palliative Care
Lund University
Lund, Sweden

Flavio Fusco
Department of Primary and Community Care
Palliative Care Unit
ASL3 Genovese Medical Center
Genova, Italy

Bruno Gagnon
Department of Family Medicine and Emergency Medicine
Université Laval
Centre de recherche du Le Centre hospitalier universitaire de Québec,
Quebec City, Quebec, Canada

Pam Gamier
The Harry R. Horvitz Center for Palliative Medicine
The Cleveland Clinic Taussig Cancer Center
Cleveland, Ohio

Claudia Gamondi
Palliative Care Department
Oncology Institute of Southern Switzerland
Bellinzona, Switzerland

Pedro Garciarena
Neurology Department
Physicians Regional Hospitals
Naples, Florida

Sarah Gebauer
Anesthesiology and Palliative Care
University of New Mexico
Albuquerque, New Mexico

Hans Gerdes
Memorial Sloan-Kettering Cancer Center
Weill Medical College
Cornell University
New York, New York

Harumi Gomi
Center for Global Health
Mito Kyodo General Hospital
University of Tsukuba
Ibaraki, Japan

Christopher Green
Harper Cancer Research Institute
Indiana University School of Medicine
South Bend, Indiana

E. Iris Groeneveld
Cicely Saunders Institute
King's College London
London, United Kingdom

Erminia Guarneri
Scripps Center for Integrative Medicine
La Jolla, California

Ying Guo
MD Anderson Cancer Center
The University of Texas
Houston, Texas

Liz Gwyther
University of Cape Town
Cape Town, South Africa

Michelle L. Haney
Harper Cancer Research Institute
Indiana University School of Medicine
South Bend, Indiana

Richard Harding
Department of Palliative Care, Policy and Rehabilitation
Cicely Saunders Institute
King's College London
London, United Kingdom

Seiji Hattori
Cancer Pain Service/Palliative Care Center
The Cancer Institute Hospital of JFCR
Tokyo, Japan

Heather Herman
Doris A. Howell Palliative Care Service
University of California, San Diego Medical Center
and
Moores Cancer Center
La Jolla, California

Irene J. Higginson
Department of Palliative Care, Policy and
    Rehabilitation
Cicely Saunders Institute
King's College London
London, United Kingdom

Robert E. Hirschtick
Department of Medicine
Division of General Internal Medicine
Feinberg School of Medicine
Northwestern University
Chicago, Illinois

Winford E. (Dutch) Holland
Holland Management Consulting
Houston, Texas

Mary K. Hughes
Department of Psychiatry
MD Anderson Cancer Center
The University of Texas
Houston, Texas

David Hui
Department of Palliative Care & Rehabilitation Medicine
MD Anderson Cancer Center
The University of Texas
Houston, Texas

Jane M. Ingham
Faculty of Medicine
St. Vincent's Clinical School
The University of New South Wales
and
Sacred Heart Health Service
The Cunningham Centre for Palliative Care
Darlinghurst, New South Wales, Australia

Hiroshi Ishiguro
Outpatient Oncology Unit
Kyoto University Cancer Center
Kyoto University Hospital
Kyoto, Japan

Reena Jaiswal
Department of Psychiatry and Behavioral
    Sciences
Memorial Sloan-Kettering Cancer Center
New York, New York

Nora A. Janjan
MD Anderson Cancer Center
The University of Texas
Houston, Texas

Aminah Jatoi
Department of Oncology
Mayo Clinic
Rochester, Minnesota

Siri Beier Jensen
Section of Oral Medicine, Clinical Oral Physiology,
    Oral Pathology & Anatomy
School of Dentistry
Faculty of Health and Medical Sciences
University of Copenhagen
Copenhagen, Denmark

Stein Kaasa
Department of Oncology
Trondheim University Hospital
and
St. Olavs University Hospital
and
European Palliative Care Research Centre
and
The Faculty of Medicine
Norwegian University of Science and Technology
Trondheim, Norway

Louise Kashuba
Tertiary Palliative Care Unit
Grey Nuns Community Hospital
Edmonton, Alberta, Canada

Koji Kawai
Department of Urology
Institute of Clinical Medicine
University of Tsukuba
Tsukuba, Japan

Mark T. Kearney
Multidisciplinary Cardiovascular Research Centre
University of Leeds
Leeds, United Kingdom

Jeremy Keen
Highland Hospice
Inverness, United Kingdom

Luluel Khan
Department of Radiation Oncology
Odette Cancer Centre
University of Toronto
Toronto, Ontario, Canada

Kenneth L. Kirsh
Millennium Laboratories
San Diego, California

David W. Kissane
Department of Psychiatry
Monash University,
Melbourne, Victoria, Australia

and

Department of Psychiatry and Behavioral Sciences
Memorial Sloan-Kettering Cancer Center
New York, New York

Toshiyuki Kitano
Department of Haematology/Oncology
Kyoto University Hospital
Kyoto, Japan

Jonathan Koffman
Department of Palliative Care, Policy and Rehabilitation
Cicely Saunders Institute
King's College London
London, United Kingdom

Benedict Konzen
MD Anderson Cancer Center
The University of Texas
Houston, Texas

Ryo Kozu
Department of Rehabilitation Medicine
Nagasaki University Hospital
Nagasaki, Japan

Maia Kredentser
Department of Psychology
University of Manitoba
Winnipeg, Manitoba, Canada

Evgenia Krotova
Adult Palliative Care Services
Department of Medicine
Columbia University Medical Center
New York, New York

Geana Paula Kurita
Department of Oncology
Section of Palliative Medicine
and
Department of Neuroanaesthesiology
Multidisciplinary Pain Centre
Rigshospitalet Copenhagen University Hospital
Copenhagen, Denmark

Marco Lacerenza
Pain Medicine Center, Casa di Cura S. Pio X
Fondazione "Opera San Camillo"
Milan, Italy

Peter Lawlor
Bruyère Continuing Care
and
Division of Palliative Care
Department of Medicine
University of Ottawa
Ottawa, Ontario, Canada

Richard Lee
Integrative Medicine Center
MD Anderson Cancer Center
The University of Texas
Houston, Texas

David C. Leopold
Scripps Center for Integrative Medicine
La Jolla, California

Gabriel Lopez
Department of General Oncology
Integrative Medicine Program
MD Anderson Cancer Center
The University of Texas
Houston, Texas

Sonya S. Lowe
Department of Symptom Control and
    Palliative Care
Cross Cancer Institute
Edmonton, Alberta, Canada

David Lussier
Institut unversitaire de geriatrie de Montreal
University of Montreal

and

Division of Geriatric Medicine
and
Alan-Edwards Centre for Research on Pain
McGill University
Montreal, Quebec, Canada

Stephen Lutz
Department of Radiation Oncology
Blanchard Valley Regional Cancer Center
Findlay, Ohio

Joanne Lynn
Altarum Institute's Center for Elder Care and Advanced Illness
Washington, D.C.

Joseph Ma
Doris A. Howell Palliative Care Service
San Diego Medical Center
University of California
Moores Cancer Center
La Jolla, California

Rod MacLeod
University of Sydney
and
HammondCare
Greenwich Hospital
Greenwich, New South Wales, Australia

Karen Macmillan
Tertiary Palliative Care Unit
Grey Nuns Community Hospital
Edmonton, Alberta, Canada

Lisa Madlensky
Family Cancer Genetics Program
Moores Cancer Center
University of California, San Diego
La Jolla, California

Marco Maltoni
Palliative Care Unit
Azienda Unità Sanitaria Locale
Forlì, Italy

Paolo Marchettini
Pain Pathophysiology and Therapy
University of Southern Switzerland
Lugano, CH

and

Scientific Institute San Raffaele
and
Centro Diagnostico Italiano
Milano, Italy

Sue Marsden
Hospice North Shore
Auckland, New Zealand

Yoshiyuki Masuda
Department of Physical Medicine and Rehabilitation
Shizuoka Cancer Center
Shizuoka, Japan

Susan E. McClement
Faculty of Nursing
University of Manitoba
Winnipeg, Manitoba, Canada

Diane E. Meier
Center to Advance Palliative Care
and
Patty and Jay Baker Palliative Care National Center
Department of Geriatrics and Palliative Medicine
and
Department of Medicine Icahn School of Medicine at Mount Sinai
New Yor, New York

Sebastiano Mercadante
Anesthesia and Intensive Care Unit and Pain Relief and Palliative Care
    Unit
La Maddalena Cancer Center
and
Palliative Medicine
University of Palermo
Palermo, Italy

Kimberley Miller
Division of Psychiatry, Health & Disease
University of Toronto
and
Princess Margaret Hospital
University Health Network
Toronto, Ontario, Canada

William Mitchell
Doris A. Howell Palliative Care Service
University of California, San Diego Medical Center
Moores Cancer Center
La Jolla, California

Caterina Modonesi
Medical Oncology Unit
Padua, Italy

Sarah Mollart
St. Nicholas Hospice Care
Bury St. Edmunds, United Kingdom

Yukiko Mori
Department of Clinical Oncology
Kyoto University Hospital Cancer Center
Kyoto, Japan

Laura J. Morrison
Department of Internal Medicine
Section of Geriatrics
Yale Palliative Care Program
Yale University School of Medicine
Yale-New Haven Hospital
New Haven, Connecticut

Carolyn Mulroney
Blood and Marrow Transplant Program
University of California, San Diego Medical Center
Moores Cancer Center
La Jolla, California

Scott A. Murray
Primary Palliative Care Research Group
University of Edinburgh Medical School
Edinburgh, United Kingdom

Fliss E.M. Murtagh
Department of Palliative Care, Policy and Rehabilitation
Cicely Saunders Institute
King's College London
London, United Kingdon

Sarah Myers
Cincinnati Children's Hospital Medical Center
Cincinnati, Ohio

Rudolph M. Navari
Harper Cancer Research Institute
Indiana University
School of Medicine
South Bend, Indiana

Cheryl L. Nekolaichuk
Department of Oncology
University of Alberta
Edmonton, Alberta, Canada

Hans Neuenschwander
Palliative Care Departement
Oncology Institute of Southern Switzerland
Bellinzona, Switzerland

Linh My Thi Nguyen
Division of Geriatric and Palliative Medicine
Department of Internal Medicine
The University of Texas Health Science Center at Houston
    Medical School
and
Memorial Hermann-Texas Medical Center
Houston, Texas

Hiroyuki Nishiyama
Department of Urology
Institute of Clinical Medicine
University of Tsukuba
Tsukuba, Japan

Bill Noble
Academic Unit of Supportive Care
University of Sheffield
Sheffield, United Kingdom

Simon I.R. Noble
Department of Palliative Medicine
Velindre Hospital
Whitchurch, United Kingdom

Diane M. Novy
Department of Pain Medicine
MD Anderson Cancer Center
The University of Texas
Houston, Texas

Asao Ogawa
Psycho-Oncology Division
Research Center for Innovative Oncology
The National Cancer Center Hospital East
Chiba, Japan

Hitoshi Okamura
Institute of Biomedical & Health Sciences
Hiroshima University
Hiroshima, Japan

Regina Okhuysen-Cawley
Department of Pediatrics
MD Anderson Cancer Center
The University of Texas
Houston, Texas

Doreen Oneschuk
Department of Oncology
Division of Palliative Medicine
Edmonton, Alberta, Cananda

Steven D. Passik
Millennium Laboratories
San Diego, California

Sandra L. Pedraza
Department of Palliative Care and
    Rehabilitation Medicine
MD Anderson Cancer Center
The University of Texas
Houston, Texas

Jose Pereira
Bruyère Continuing Care
and
The Ottawa Hospital
and
Division of Palliative Care
Department of Medicine
University of Ottawa
Ottawa, Ontario, Canada

Hayley Pessin
Department of Psychiatry and Behavioral Sciences
Memorial Sloan-Kettering Cancer Center
New York, New York

Jane Phillips
School of Nursing
The University of Notre Dame Australia
Sydney, New South Wales, Australia

and

Sacred Heart Health Service
The Cunningham Centre for Palliative Care
St. Vincent's Hospital
Darlinghurst, New South Wales, Australia

Russell K. Portenoy
MJHS Institute for Innovation in Palliative Care
MJHS Hospice and Palliative Care
New York, New York

and

Albert Einstein College of Medicine
Bronx, New York

Julie R. Price
Louis Stokes Cleveland VA Medical Center
Cleveland, Ohio

Tammie Quest
Department of Emergency Medicine
and
Division of Geriatrics and Gerontology
Emory University School of Medicine
Atlanta, Georgia

Lukas Radbruch
Department of Palliative Medicine
University Hospital, Aachen
Aachen, Germany

Victoria H. Raveis
Psychosocial Research Unit on Health, Aging and the Community
New York University College of Dentistry
and
New York University Global Institute of Public Health
New York, New York

Suresh K. Reddy
Department of Palliative Care and Rehabilitation Medicine
Division of Cancer Medicine
MD Anderson Cancer Center
The University of Texas
Houston, Texas

Carla Ida Ripamonti
Supportive Care in Cancer Unit
Fondazione IRCCS
Istituto Nazionale dei Tumori
Milan, Italy

Nathan L. Roach
Harper Cancer Research Institute
Indiana University
School of Medicine
South Bend, Indiana

Graeme M. Rocker
Division of Respirology
QEII Health Sciences Centre
Dalhousie University
Halifax, Nova Scotia, Canada

Eric Roeland
Doris A. Howell Palliative Care Service
University of California, San Diego Medical Center
Moores Cancer Center
La Jolla, California

Álvaro Sanz
Medical Oncology
Hospital Universitario del Rio Hortega
Valladolid, Spain

Deborah P. Saunders
Department of Dental Oncology
North East Regional Cancer Center
Health Sciences North
and
Northern Ontario School of Medicine
Sudbury, Ontario, Canada

Richard Sawatzky
School of Nursing
Trinity Western University
Langley, British Columbia, Canada

and

CHEOS
Providence Health Care Research Institute
Vancouver, British Columbia, Canada

John F. Scott
The Ottawa Hospital
and
Division of Palliative Care
Department of Medicine
University of Ottawa
Ottawa, Ontario, Canada

Peter A. Selwyn
Department of Family and Social Medicine
Montefiore Medical Center
Albert Einstein College of Medicine
Bronx, New York

Hsien-Yeang Seow
Department of Oncology
McMaster University
Hamilton, Ontario, Canada

Ki Y. Shin
Department of Palliative Care and Rehabilitation Medicine
MD Anderson Cancer Center
The University of Texas
Houston, Texas

Per Sjøgren
Department of Oncology
Section of Palliative Medicine
Rigshospitalet Copenhagen University Hospital
and
Department of Clinical Medicine
Faculty of Health and Medical Sciences
University of Copenhagen
Copenhagen, Denmark

Thomas J. Smith
Sidney Kimmel Comprehensive Cancer Center
Johns Hopkins Medical Institutions
Baltimore, Maryland

Pasquale Spinelli
Division of Endoscopy
National Cancer Institute
Milan, Italy

Katie Stone
Department of Palliative Care, Policy and Rehabilitation
Cicely Saunders Institute
King's College London
London, United Kingdom

Paulina Taboada
Center for Bioethics
Department of Internal Medicine
Pontificia Universidad Católica de Chile Medical School
Santiago, Chile

Hisako Tajiri
Department of Physical Medicine and
    Rehabilitation
Shizuoka Cancer Center
Shizuoka, Japan

Akifumi Takaori-Kondo
Department of Haematology/Oncology
Kyoto University Hospital
Kyoto, Japan

Kimberson C. Tanco
Palliative Care and Rehabilitation Medicine
MD Anderson Cancer Center
The University of Texas
Houston, Texas

Silvia Tanzi
Palliative Care Unit
IRCCS Arcispedale Santa Maria Nuova
Reggio Emilia, Italy

Yoko Tarumi
Division of Palliative Care Medicine
Department of Oncology
University of Alberta
Edmonton, Alberta, Canada

Martin H.N. Tattersall
Department of Cancer Medicine
Sydney Medical School
University of Sydney
and
Sydney Cancer Centre
Royal Prince Alfred Hospital
Sydney, New South Wales, Australia

Katie Taylor
Hospice in the Weald Pembury
Kent, United Kingdom

Joan M. Teno
Center for Gerontology and Health Care Research
Brown University
Providence, Rhode Island

Jay R. Thomas
Comprehensive Care Program
HealthCare Partners
Arcadia, California

Tabitha Thomas
Arthur Rank House
Cambridge, United Kingdom

Kathryn Thornberry
Doris A. Howell Palliative Care Service
University of California, San Diego Medical Center
Moores Cancer Center
La Jolla, California

Andrew Thorns
University of Kent
East Kent Hospitals University Foundation Trust
Pilgrims Hospice, Margate
Kent, United Kingdom

Ivo W. Tremont-Lukats
Department of Neuro-Oncology
MD Anderson Cancer Center
The University of Texas
Houston, Texas

Satoru Tsuneto
Department of Multidisciplinary Cancer Treatment
Graduate School of Medicine
Kyoto University
Kyoto, Japan

James A. Tulsky
Duke Palliative Care
Duke University
Durham, North Carolina

Beth Tupala
Grey Nuns Community Hospital
Health Services Centre
Edmonton, Alberta, Canada

Yosuke Uchitomi
Department of Neuropsychiatry
Graduate School of Medicine, Dentistry and
Pharmaceutical Sciences
Okayama University
Okayama, Japan

Mary L.S. Vachon
Departments of Psychiatry and Public Health Science
University of Toronto
Toronto, Canada

Marieberta Vidal
Department of General Internal Medicine
Division of Internal Medicine
MD Anderson Cancer Center
The University of Texas
Houston, Texas

Charles F. von Gunten
Hospice and Palliative Care
OhioHealth Kobacker House
Columbus, Ohio

Jamie H. Von Roenn
Department of Medicine
Division of Hematology/Oncology
Feinberg School of Medicine
and
Robert H. Lurie Comprehensive
Cancer Center of Northwestern University
and
Palliative Care and Home Hospice Program
Northwestern Memorial Hospital
Chicago, Illinois

Rosemary Wade
Addenbrooke's Hospital
Cambridge, United Kingdom
and
West Suffolk Hospital
Bury St. Edmunds, United Kingdom

Tobias Walbert
Hermelin Brain Tumor Center
Department of Neurosurgery and
Department of Neurology
Henry Ford Health System
Detroit, Michigan

Paul W. Walker
Department of Palliative Care and Rehabilitation Medicine
Division of Cancer Medicine
MD Anderson Cancer Center
The University of Texas
Houston, Texas

Jen-Yu Wei
Division of Geriatric and Palliative Medicine
Department of Internal Medicine
University of Texas Health Science Center at Houston
Houston, Texas

Roberto Wenk
Programa Argentino de Medicina Paliativa
Fundación FEMEBA
Buenos Aires, Argentina

Batsheva Werman
Department of Oncology
Shaare Zedek Medical Center
Jerusalem, Israel

Michelle Winslow
Faculty of Medicine, Dentistry and Health
The School of Nursing and Midwifery
University of Sheffield
Sheffield, United Kingdom

Sriram Yennurajalingam
Department of Palliative Care and Rehabilitation Medicine
MD Anderson Cancer Center
The University of Texas at Houston
Houston, Texas

Joanne Young
Division of Respirology
Halifax, Nova Scotia, Canada

List of abbreviations

5-HT	5-Hydroxytryptamine
6MWT	6-Minute walk test (also 12MWT, 2 MWT)
ACE	Angiotensin-converting enzyme
ACTH	Adrenocorticotropic hormone
ADH	Antidiuretic hormone
ADL	Activities of daily living
AECOPD	Acute exacerbations of chronic obstructive pulmonary disease
AgRP	Agouti-related peptide
AGS	American Geriatrics Society
AHA	American Heart Association
AIDS	Acquired immune deficiency syndrome
ALCP	Latin American Association for Palliative Care (Asociación Latinoamericana de Cuidados Paliativos)
ALF	Assisted living facility
ALS	Amyotrophic lateral sclerosis
AMDA	American Medical Directors' Association
ANP	Advanced nurse practitioner
APCA	African Palliative Care Association
APHN	Asia Pacific Hospice Palliative Care Network
APM	Association of Palliative Medicine
AP–PC line	Anterior commissure–posterior commissure line
ARV	Antiretroviral (drug)
AS	Actual survival
ASCO	American Society of Clinical Oncology
AUC	Area under the curve
BDI	Beck Depression Inventory
BMI	Body mass index
BODE	Body mass index, the degree of airflow obstruction, dyspnea scores, and exercise capacity
BPI	Brief Pain Inventory
BSI	Bone scan index
BTS	British Thoracic Society
CACS	Cancer anorexia-cachexia syndrome
CAM	Confusion assessment method
CAM	Complementary and alternative medicine
CAPC	Center to Advance Palliative Care
CAPD	Chronic ambulatory peritoneal dialysis
CB	Cannabinoid (receptor)
CBT	Cognitive–behavioral therapy
CCOG	Cancer Care Ontario Guidelines
CDP	Complex decongestive physiotherapy
CES-D	Center for Epidemiologic Studies on Depression (scale)
CFS	Chronic fatigue syndrome
CGRP	Calcitonin gene-related peptide
CHF	Congestive heart failure
CHPCA	Canadian Hospice Palliative Care Association
CIHR	Canadian Institutes of Health Research
CIVI	Continuous intravenous infusion
CNS	Central nervous system
COPD	Chronic obstructive pulmonary disease
COREC	Central Office of Research Ethics Committees
COX–2	Cyclooxygenase 2
CPR	Cardiopulmonary resuscitation
CPS	Clinical Prediction of Survival
CRF	Cancer-related fatigue
CRF	Corticotrophin-releasing factor
CRH	Corticotrophin-releasing hormone
CRPS	Complex regional pain syndrome
CSF	Cerebrospinal fluid
CSI	Continuous subcutaneous infusion
CT	Computed tomography
CTZ	Chemoreceptor trigger zone
DIC	Disseminated intravascular coagulation
DLT	Decongestive lymphatic therapy
DNR	Do not resuscitate
DRG	Diagnosis-related group
DSM	*Diagnostic and Statistical Manual of Mental Disorders*
DSM-IV	*Diagnostic and Statistical Manual, 4th edition*
DVT	Deep vein thrombosis
EACA	ε-Aminocaproic acid
EAPC	European Association for Palliative Care
ECOG	Eastern Cooperative Oncology Group
EEG	Electroencephalogram
EFAT	Edmonton Functional Assessment Tool
EFPPEC	Educating Future Physicians in Palliative and End-of-Life Care Project
EORTC	European Organization for Research and Treatment of Cancer
EPA	Eicosapentaenoic acid
EPEC	Education in Palliative and End-of-life Care
ERCP	Endoscopic retrograde cholangiopancreatography
ERPCP	Edmonton Regional Palliative Care Program
ESAS	Edmonton Symptom Assessment Scale
ESRD	End-stage renal disease
ESS	Edmonton Staging Score
EUS	Endoscopic ultrasonography
FACIT-F	Functional Assessment for Chronic Illness Therapy–Fatigue
FAST	Functional Assessment Staging
FEV1	Forced expiratory volume in 1 second

FFGT	Family focused grief therapy	MMSQ	Mini-Mental State Questionnaire
FHSSA	Foundation for Hospices in Sub-Saharan Africa	MQOL	McGill Quality of Life Questionnaire
(F)NHTR	(febrile) Nonhemolytic transfusion reaction	MRCP	Magnetic resonance cholangiopancreatography
FQ	Fatigue Questionnaire	MRI	Magnetic resonance imaging
FVC	Forced vital capacity	MSAS	Memorial Symptom Assessment Scale
GABA	g-Aminobutyric acid	MSH	Melanocyte-stimulating hormone
GDS	Geriatric Depression Scale	MSKCC	Memorial Sloan-Kettering Cancer Center
GHQ	General Health Questionnaire	NCCAM	National Center for Complementary and Alternative Medicine
GMP	Good manufacturing practice		
HAART	Highly active antiretroviral therapy	NCCN	National Comprehensive Cancer Network
HADS	Hospital Anxiety Depression Scale	NCI	National Cancer Institute
HASA	Hospice Association of South Africa	NCSE	Nonconvulsive status epilepticus
HBI	Half-body irradiation	NF-kB	Nuclear factor kappa B
hCG	Human chorionic gonadotropin	NHO	National Hospice Organization
HCM	Hypercalcemia of malignancy	NHPCO	National Hospice and Palliative Care Organization
HDAT	Home Death Assessment Tool	NHS	National Health Service
HIV	Human immunodeficiency virus	NIPPV	Noninvasive positive pressure ventilation
HPCA	Hospice Palliative Care Association of South Africa	NIV	Noninvasive mechanical ventilation
HRQOL	Health-related quality of life	NMDA	N-methyl-D-aspartate
HRT	Hormone replacement therapy	NMS	Neuroleptic malignant syndrome
HU	Hounsfield Units	NNRTI	Nonnucleoside reverse transcriptase inhibitors
IADL	Instrumental activities of daily living	NNT	Number need to treat
IAHPC	International Association for Hospice and Palliative Care	NSCLC	Non-small-cell lung cancer
IARC	International Agency for Research on Cancer	NVR	Nausea, vomiting, and retching
ICC	Item-characteristic curve	NYHA	New York Heart Association
ICR	Institute of Cancer Research	OCCAM	Office of Cancer Complementary and Alternative Medicine
ICU	Intensive care unit		
ICV	Intracerebroventricular	OIN	Opioid-induced neurotoxicity
IL	Interleukin	OPG	Osteoprotegerin
IM	Intramuscular	OSI	Open Society Institute
IMRT	Intensity modulated radiation therapy	OTFC	Oral transmucosal fentanyl citrate
INCB	International Narcotics Control Board	PAC	Project advisory committee
IOELC	International Observatory in End-of-Life Care	PAINAD	Pain Assessment in Advanced Dementia
IPT	Interpersonal psychotherapy	PAMPFF	Programa Argentino de Medicina Paliativa–Fundacion FEMEBA
IRB	Institutional review board		
IRT	Item response theory	PaP	Palliative Prognostic (Score)
IT	Information technology	PCA	Patient-controlled analgesia
IV	Intravenous	PCCT	Palliative care consultation team
JCAHO	Joint Commission of the Accreditation of Healthcare Organizations	PCDH	Palliative care day hospitals
		PCIN	Patient-controlled intranasal
JCMHT	Joint Committee on Higher Medical Training	PCU	Palliative care unit
KPS	Karnofsky Performance Scale	PDCH	Palliative care day hospital
LAS	Lymphangioscintigraphy	PDIA	Project on Death in America
LMF	Lipid-mobilizing factor	PEAT	Palliative Education Assessment Tool for Medical Education
LOS	Length of stay		
LSP	Lumbosacral-plexopathy	PEP	Preexposure prophylaxis
M3G	Morphine-3-glucuronide	PHC	Palliative home care
M6G	Morphine-6-glucuronide	PHN	Postherpetic neuralgia
MAR	Medication administration record	PHPTH	Primary hyperparathyroidism
MBO	Malignant bowel obstruction	PI	Protease inhibitor
MC-R	Melanocortin receptor	PIF	Proteolysis-inducing factor
MD clinic	Multidisciplinary symptom control and palliative care clinic	POLST	Physician Orders for Life-Sustaining Treatment
MDAS	Memorial Delirium Assessment Scale	PPI	Palliative Prognostic Index
MDS	Minimum data set	PPS	Palliative Performance Score
MFI-20	Multidimensional Fatigue Inventory	PS	Performance status
MLD	Manual lymph drainage	PSQI	Pittsburgh Sleep Quality Index
MMSE	Mini-Mental State Examination	PTC	Percutaneous transhepatic cholangiography

PTH	Parathyroid hormone		SMWT	Self-paced minute walk test
PTHrP	Parathyroid hormone–related protein		SRE	Skeletal-related events
PVG/PAG	Periventricular gray/periaqueductal gray		SRT	Spinoreticular tract
QALY	Quality-adjusted life year		SSRI	Selective serotonin reuptake inhibitor
QELCC	Quality End-of-Life Care Coalition		STT	Spinothalamic tract
QI	Quality improvement		SUPPORT	Study to Understand Prognosis and Preferences for Outcomes and Treatments
QOL	Quality of life		SVCS	Superior vena cava syndrome
QTc	Rate-corrected QT		TCA	Tricyclic antidepressant
RANKL	Receptor activator of nuclear factor kB-ligand		THC	Tetrahydrocannabinol
RCT	Randomized Controlled Trial		TNF	Tumor necrosis factor
REC	Research Ethics Committee		TPCU	Tertiary palliative care unit
RSC	Research Steering Committee		TTS	Transdermal therapeutic system
RSCL	Rotterdam Symptom Checklist		VAS	Visual analog scale
RTOG	Radiation Therapy Oncology Group		VEGF	Vascular endothelial growth factor
SCEI	Simultaneous Care Educational Intervention		VNRS	Visual numerical rating scale
SCLC	Small cell lung cancer		VRS	Verbal rating scale
SDS	Symptom Distress Scale		WBRT	Whole-brain radiotherapy
SE	Status epilepticus		WHO	World Health Organization
SF-36	Medical Outcome Survey Short Form 36		ZAG	Zn-a2-glycoprotein
SLFC	Sublingual fentanyl citrate			

Reference annotation and evidence scores

REFERENCE ANNOTATION

The reference lists are annotated, where appropriate, to guide readers to primary articles, key review papers, and management guidelines, as follows:

●   Seminal primary article
◆   Key review paper
✱   First formal publication of a management guideline

We hope that this feature will render extensive lists of references more useful to the reader and will help encourage self-directed learning among both trainees and practicing physicians.

EVIDENCE SCORES

Supporting evidence has been graded in the main body of the text for each clinical intervention as follows:

***   Systematic review or meta-analysis
**   One or more well-designed randomized controlled trials
*   Nonrandomized controlled trials, cohort study, etc.

PART 1

The development of palliative medicine

Development of palliative medicine in the United Kingdom and Ireland

BILL NOBLE, MICHELLE WINSLOW

INTRODUCTION

Care of the dying has for centuries been an important part of a doctor's role, but the modern hospice movement and palliative medicine are relatively new and still defining themselves. Palliative medicine draws on the ancient ideas of holistic practice, prognostic concerns, and contemporary technology with its origins in established specialties. In the United Kingdom and Ireland, with their traditions of Christianity, charitable giving, and national health service (NHS), conditions were favorable for a few charismatic activists to set a course for the development of a new medical specialty. A new kind of service to care for the dying, freely available and funded from a variety of sources, developed throughout the twentieth century until it became firmly rooted in policy and British and Irish public expectations of statutory health care provision.

HISTORICAL CONTEXT

The original use of the term "hospice" referred to religious institutions run by religious orders in Europe. Care of the dying was integral to the activity of these early hospices, but it was not their focus; they were places where travelers could find refuge and shelter and where care was freely given to the sick and poor.

In Ireland in 1744, the Hospital for Incurables, a charitable initiative by the Dublin Charitable Musical Society, was established to offer care and shelter to the incurably ill and to remove *those miserable objects who were offensive to sight from the streets*. The building accommodated 21 patients but quickly proved inadequate for need; hence, a decade later, a purpose-built hospital was started for 84 patients and established new standards in institutional care.[1] The hospital still operates today, now known as The Royal Hospital.[2]

In the early nineteenth century, Mary Aikenhead, an Irishwoman and convert to Catholicism, created a new order of nuns, the Religious Sisters of Charity. In 1815, she began visiting Dublin's poor and sick in their own homes[3] and subsequently founded 13 houses around Ireland, their work ranging from missions to the poor, schools, orphanages, and a hospital.[4] In 1879, the order founded Our Lady's Hospice for the Dying in Dublin—a place where dying patients would receive spiritual and material comfort. The hospice was intended for dying patients who had been either refused admission to Dublin's crowded general hospitals or discharged home to die.[5,6] Our Lady's was opened with just 9 beds, increasing to 40 the following year, but overwhelmed with referrals, plans were made for a new 110 bedded hospice that was completed in 1888, largely through unexpected charitable donations; this still operates today as part of a complex of buildings run by Our Lady's Hospice.[7,8]

In 1904, a Protestant version of hospice called the Rest for the Dying, was founded in Dublin. The hospice was dedicated to the care of dying patients deemed unsuitable for treatment in general hospitals; it changed its name to the Gascoigne Home in 1962. Milford House was opened in Limerick in 1928, which had 9 beds for terminal care in 1977, and at Harold's Cross, a new 44-bedded unit was opened for palliative care in 1985; a homecare service and a purpose-built day centre followed in 1995.[9]

In England, in the late nineteenth century, homes dedicated to the care of the dying grew up in London, when major hospitals frequently excluded incurable patients from admission: the Friedenheim in 1885, the Hostel of God in 1891, and St. Luke's house in 1893. For the first time, the dying were seen as needing specialized care from qualified people in an institutional setting. These institutions required that a medical practitioner certify a patient to be dying before they could be admitted.

Around this time, ideas about *easy death* were under discussion. In 1887, William Munk, an English physician, published a detailed treatise entitled *Euthanasia: Or, Medical Treatment in Aid of an Easy Death*.[10] Munk uses the word "euthanasia" to describe helping the sufferer to a more comfortable death, rather than its modern sense of medical mercy killing.

Munk's book was favorably reviewed in a range of medical journals at the time (see, for example, *British Medical Journal* 1861; ii: 231–232; *British Medical Journal* 1884; i: 1155–1157; *Dublin Journal of Medical Science* 1884; 78: 38–39), and *The Lancet* printed a glowing account of *Euthanasia,* supporting Munk's argument and ideas about practice.[6] In 1888, it was also praised by William Osler,[11] physician-in-chief of Johns Hopkins Hospital, Baltimore, and professor of medicine at their planned school of medicine.[12] Although Munk was described as "the most influential Victorian writer on the care of the dying." *Euthanasia* remained the authoritative text on the medical care of the dying for the next 30 years,[13] but it had little influence on practice and was forgotten.

Clare Humphries highlights Christianity as an influence on the care of the dying and the development of hospices in England. Homes in the late nineteenth century had a strong Christian emphasis, and their religious underpinning continued as hospices evolved.[14] These institutions were small isolated pockets of reaction to wider changes that attempted to maintain a tradition of pastoral care. Yet they subsequently played a part in the founding of the modern hospice movement by recognizing the need for special institutional care for the dying. The foundation of the Home for the Compassion of Jesus in 1903 and the opening of St. Joseph's Hospice for the Dying in 1905[15] presaged the modern hospice movement and development of a systematized style of terminal care in the United Kingdom.

In 1952, a national survey by a joint committee of the Marie Curie Memorial and the Queen's Institute of District Nursing, chaired by the surgeon Ronald Raven, reported on data collected from 7050 cancer patients living at home. District nurses considered that 2195 (31%) were in severe distress. The report called for more residential and convalescent homes, better information, night nurses, home helps, and equipment.[16] In the 1960's, Marie Curie Memorial opened homes for terminally ill cancer patients and set up a national night nursing service.

In the late 1950s, St. Joseph's Hospice, Hackney, provided the context for Cicely Saunders early pain research.[15] Saunders advanced her clinical ideas there and developed a practice and philosophy of palliative care, which outlined the principles of preventing pain through detailed knowledge of available analgesia and administering regular pain relief. She identified the link between physical and mental pain and by 1964 had described her concept of *total pain,* a holistic concept of management focused on the individual patient, which recognizes the relationship between physical symptoms, mental distress, social problems, and emotional difficulties.[17] Cicely Saunders developed her work within a pioneering research milieu. Contemporaries who were involved in pain management in the United Kingdom and the United States included the psychologist Ronald Melzack, the University of Oregon; Henry Beecher, Harvard anesthiologist; Raymond Houde and Ada Rogers, Memorial Sloane Kettering;[18] and John Bonica,[19] who comprehensively discussed etiology, diagnosis, and treatment in his definitive work, *The Management of Pain* (1953). Mark Swerdlow, working in Manchester, was pioneering the use of anesthetic blocks in the nonsurgical management of difficult pain problems.[18]

In 1959, Margaret Bailey conducted a survey of patients with incurable lung cancer at the Brompton and Royal Marsden hospitals.[20] She had written earlier, "the fact of palliative treatment is not understood, and hospitals appear to be trying to cure all their patients and failing in a high proportion of cases." A report published in 1960 by Dr. H L Glyn Hughes described the care of the dying and recommended the developments of policy and service organization. At the time of the survey, two fifths of all deaths in the UK occurred in NHS hospitals. Hughes estimated that 270,000 people died each year outside NHS hospitals, who were in need of skilled terminal care. He also stressed the value of special terminal care beds in hospitals and recommended links to independent homes for the dying. John Hinton, a psychiatrist at the Maudsley Hospital in London, wrote a 1964 editorial in the *Journal of Chronic Diseases* calling for empirical research into better terminal care. "The large number of articles in which remembered experience is distilled into advice on the management of dying awesomely overshadows the few papers attempting to measure the degree of success or failure of treatment."[21]

Eric Wilkes, a rural general practitioner (GP) who later founded St. Luke's Hospice in Sheffield, in 1965 published in *The Lancet* on terminal cancer at home.[22] He wrote as follows: "There seems to be no valid reason why hospital provision for terminal care is so inadequate, or for the NHS to lean so heavily on the few Curie Foundation Homes and the devoted but over-worked religious institutions specialising in this work."[23]

Cicely Saunders planned her model of hospice care within this environment, emphasizing the need for regular opiates, including heroin and the Brompton Cocktail, a mixture that varied but often contained morphine, chlorpromazine, cocaine, syrup and gin, to treat pain, nausea, dyspnoea, anxiety, and drowsiness.

The growth of the modern hospice movement in the United Kingdom and Ireland is due to the work and commitment of a number of individuals; however, Cicely Saunders is the one who is generally acknowledged as the catalyst. In 1967, she opened St. Christopher's Hospice in Sydenham, and in its early days it was associated with major studies on pain control and the administration of strong opioids that were significant in the advancement of palliative care.[24] Their strategies for action in service delivery had strong emphasis on volunteer involvement and fund-raising. David Clark notes that within a decade of the inception of St. Christopher's, it was accepted that hospice principles could be practiced in specialist in-patient units, by home and day care services, and in hospital units where support teams brought new thinking about dying to acute medicine.[25]

Hospices proliferated throughout the 1970s and 1980s, funded by local charities. The first hospice outside London, St. Luke's Nursing Home, Sheffield, was started in 1971. Designed by the same architect as St. Christopher's, S.W.J. Smith, it shared many policies, including the involvement of volunteers. St. Luke's founder and medical director, Eric Wilkes, added the United Kingdom's first day hospice to the model. The facility was designed to provide weekly respite for carers of about 50 patients living at home, while also facilitating social interaction, medical review, physiotherapy, occupational therapy, and some aspects of personal care such as bathing and hair dressing. This feature was later replicated throughout the country.

RECOGNITION AND SPECIALIZATION

Around 10 new hospices were started every year during the 1980s,[24] and in a report on terminal care that came to be known as the *Wilkes Report*, Eric Wilkes expressed concern about this rapid and uncoordinated growth of hospices.[26] The theme was discussed in "No second chance: A discussion document for the Trent Regional Health Authority[27] on the development of terminal care services." The Trent Palliative Care Centre, a multidisciplinary unit for research, education, and service development attached to St. Luke's Hospice, was also initiated by Eric Wilkes. His vision was a network of regional centers researching and teaching the care of the dying, integrated with the NHS. In 1984, with the Duchess of Norfolk, Peter Quilliam, Dame Cicely Saunders and Eric Wilkes founded Help the Hospices, a national charity that was intended to give a collective voice to the many small organizations running new hospices throughout the United Kingdom.

In the United Kingdom, cancer charities have had a significant impact on palliative care development. The Macmillan organization, founded in 1912 by Douglas Macmillan, was originally known as the Society for the Prevention and Relief of Cancer. But as new charities, such as Marie Curie and Cancer BACKUP, emerged, branding became increasingly important, and the Society repeatedly changed its name and its emphasis.[28] The Marie Curie Memorial Foundation came into being in 1948; it created nursing homes, a domiciliary nursing service for patients with cancer, and a laboratory-based scientific research program. A shift was evident in the 1980s when the Marie Curie nursing homes began launching specialist palliative care centers and supporting educational and research activities. In recent years, the Marie Curie organization has been closely involved with the development of a national end-of-life strategy and has lobbied for a new legislation to support palliative care.[24]

In creating a network of care homes, the renamed Marie Curie Cancer Care succeeded with an initiative previously unsuccessful for Macmillan, the provision of specialist nurses. The Macmillan organization subsequently turned to providing "Macmillan nurses," who then became the centre of an effective fund-raising strategy. By the 1970s, Macmillan were supporting units in hospitals as well as funding nurse posts. A change of name to the Cancer Relief Macmillan Fund in 1984 was intended to modernize and strengthen the brand identity to retain a position in the public consciousness. The modern Macmillan charity works closely with the NHS, though the relationship has not been without its clashes. For example, Macmillan sought to avert charitable funds away from general cancer care budgets, while trying to avoid being confrontational or critical of NHS practices, to preserve their influence in cancer care policy.[28] In the 1970s, the organization underwent a period of substantial expansion and became

increasingly involved with palliative care and supporting training programs, creating specialist professional posts and academic positions, as well as supporting capital and service developments. Recently, the organization has switched focus to more direct support for people affected by cancer, as indicated in their change of name to Macmillan Cancer Support.[24]

As new hospices were opened, medical cover was mostly provided by GPs who were committed but who lacked the new skills in the care of the dying. In response, the Association for Palliative Medicine (APM) of Great Britain and Ireland was established in 1986 to support the development of specialty training while continuing to support GPs in their provision of palliative care.[29] The APM is an association of doctors who work in hospices and specialist palliative care units in hospitals, it now has around 1000 members from all over the United Kingdom and Ireland and includes doctors based overseas. Most UK medical practitioners active in clinical and academic palliative medicine, including interested GPs, have been members of the association. The APM was unique as it was the first medical organization of its kind in the world and arguably a catalyst for the growth of other professional associations in palliative care in Great Britain and the Republic of Ireland.[30] New associations for hospice physiotherapists, pharmacists, social workers, and others followed.

In 1987, the United Kingdom became the first country in the world to recognize palliative medicine as a medical specialty. Members of the APM, led by the first Chair, Dr. Derek Doyle, lobbied the Royal College of Physicians (RCP) and achieved specialty status remarkably quickly compared with other specialties. Shortly afterwards, a 4-year training program in the new discipline was established for senior registrars.[29] Since then has come the development of community palliative care services, hospital palliative care teams, and day-hospice units, forging new links between community, hospice, and hospital care and between the NHS and the voluntary sector.

Yet not all physicians were in favor of forming an association exclusively for medics. Some were against setting up a specialist society, concerned that it would further isolate palliative care doctors from mainstream medicine and that it would act as a barrier to good palliative care developed on a wider scale. There was a view at that time that it was the wrong moment to set up a specialty, partly because the public, as well as colleagues in other specialties, were not clear as to what palliative medicine was. Others were very wary of an association of doctors alone, fearing they would be seen as a narrow interest group within palliative care, lacking the influence that a larger multiprofessional body might wield.

In the context of the growth and spread of specialist palliative care services, the idea of a single body to speak on behalf of service providers was raised. Following the formation of the APM, many hospice groups were separately lobbying the Department of Health. However, Help the Hospices, led by the Duchess of Norfolk and Paul Rossi, then chief executive, agreed to step back from political lobbying in favor of a new body. With the support of Virginia Bottomley, the minister of health, he convened and chaired meetings between independent hospices, NHS units, and major charities, bringing them together in an umbrella organization. The National Council for

Hospice and Specialist Palliative Care Services was formed in 1991 with Jean Gaffin as its first director; its member organizations spanned across England, Wales, and Northern Ireland. Scotland was served by a separate organization, "The Scottish Partnership for Palliative Care," at that time.

A growing appreciation of end-of-life needs of adults brought the needs of children into focus. However, hospice services for children have more complex origins. The late 1970s saw the recognition of the need for palliative care for children. Helen House, the world's first children's hospice, was started in Oxfordshire in 1982, with an emphasis on respite rather than specialist medical support.[31] The development of hospice care for children is, however, a separate story; there are significant differences in approach due to the different circumstances of life-threatening illness in children. A major difference between adult and pediatric palliative care from the outset was its separation from the hospice and cancer model, treating children with all life-threatening diseases.[32]

By 2004, specialist palliative care services and hospices had been well established around the United Kingdom. However, their disease focus was cancer; palliative care was not generally available for other causes of death. In this environment, the National Council changed its name to The National Council for Palliative Care (NCPC) to extend its sphere of activity to represent palliative, end-of-life, and hospice care more broadly. Since 1995, the development of cancer services following the publication of the Calman-Hine report has given further impetus to specialist palliative care integrated with cancer services. In particular, this has led to a rapid and continuing expansion in consultant posts (Royal College of Physicians 2009).

RESEARCH

In the United Kingdom, the acquisition of knowledge in palliative care has undergone a transformation from the communication of personal views and subjectivity to rigorous scientific studies and objectivity in a relatively short period of time.[33]

Three studies in the 1950s and early 1960s (as discussed previously) were important to the emerging evidence base. The Marie Curie Memorial Foundation report highlighted suffering and deprivation among dying cancer patients; the Gulbenkian Foundation report found financial and staffing deficiencies in charitable homes and seriously inadequate conditions; and John Hinton's detailed work on dying patients in a London teaching hospital revealed physical and mental distress, augmented by unrelieved suffering and a lack of communication about prognosis.[34]

From the late 1950s, Cicely Saunders' research at St. Joseph's Hospice informed a modern strategy for hospice care. Central to Cicely Saunders' research were tape-recordings with patients about their illnesses and issues concerning them. Publications from St. Joseph's at the time show that her interest in pain was particularly concerned with prevention rather than alleviation, understanding of available analgesia, and recognizing the link between physical pain and mental distress.[35]

In 1960, papers on subjects related to palliative care were rare. However, by 2008, the situation had improved; Bennett, Davies, and Higginson identified 2800 publications categorized as end-of-life papers; 2400 on palliative care; 1500 on terminal care; 1050 referring to supportive care; and 800 publications on hospice.[36] The first specialist journal was *Palliative Medicine*, first published in 1987 and edited by Derek Doyle. Since then, papers on supportive care, palliative care, hospice, and end-of-life care have been published in increasing numbers, with research on terminal care becoming less common.

Since 2002, the National Cancer Research Institute (NCRI) has coordinated palliative care research in the United Kingdom, monitoring the investment in cancer research nationally to identify gaps and opportunities in research, in partnership with government, charity, and industry bodies. Through the initiative of "Supportive and Palliative Care (SuPaC) Collaboratives," two collaboratives were set up in 2006, "the Cancer Experiences Collaborative (CECo)" and the "COMPASS Collaborative," to bring together academic groups to build research capacity and transform the role of consumers in research.[37]

The Palliative Care Research Society (PCRS) focuses on research in any aspect of palliative care and facilitates dissemination; it works with academics and clinicians in research and educational activities to strengthen links between both. The PCRS is affiliated with the peer-reviewed journal *Progress in Palliative Care*.[38] Further scholarly journals for the dissemination of research in the United Kingdom based in palliative care are *Palliative Medicine*, *BMJ Supportive and Palliative Care*, and *International Journal of Palliative Nursing*. The Palliative Care Congress is the main palliative care event, jointly organized by the PCRS and the Association of Palliative Medicine.

The APM Scientific Committee seeks to advance the scientific profile of the palliative medicine specialty. The association is involved in developing evidence-based guidelines and protocols for palliative medical interventions and facilitating an ethical research culture, both in its own specialty and in work with others.[39] There are now several academic and clinical academic centers and departments in the United Kingdom, including the Cicely Saunders Institute at King's College London, the End of Life Observatory at the University of Lancaster, University College London and departments in Sheffield, Nottingham, Southampton, Liverpool, Cambridge, Manchester, Edinburgh, Bristol and Cardiff among others.

DEVELOPMENTS IN EDUCATION

In a relatively short period of time, teaching in palliative care has advanced from little or none to the provision of extensive programs of education in the United Kingdom. The early pioneering model of education centers attached to hospitals began a process in education that saw the formation of educational organizations on a national scale. Academic departments were created, and master's courses in palliative medicine and palliative care became established, notably at Cardiff University, King's College London, the University of Southampton, and the University of Sheffield.

In 2002, a survey of all schools offering clinical teaching in palliative care uncovered a huge variation in teaching provision. Specialist practitioners in palliative medicine were most frequently involved in teaching, with a decline of nonpractitioner input since the early 1980s. Courses comprised attitudes to death and dying and symptom relief in advanced illness, and a more integrated curriculum meant that learning could be applied in other contexts. In some places, patients were involved in teaching, and most included hospice participation.[40]

There is a view that many undergraduate students are being failed by their palliative care education during medical training through lack of meaningful contact with patients. A study in 2011 found that newly qualified doctors report learning on the job by "trial and error", seeking advice mainly from nursing staff and members of palliative care teams.[41]

There is widespread agreement that there are gaps in health-care professionals' palliative care knowledge that need filling. The end-of-life care strategy recognizes this and has identified priority areas for an expansion of education and training in communication skills, assessing needs and preferences, and advanced care planning and principles of symptom management.[42] A minority of educational initiatives have evaluated learning and its effect on practice and have found that successful courses contain participative and interactive learning strategies, interpersonal skills training, and case study discussion.[43] A significant educational gap is in the training of clinical nurse specialists. Currently, there is no formal specialist clinical training for nurses, who are expected to attend master's courses that offer theory but do not advance nurse practice.

Advanced communication skills training is open to nurses; this course has been developed in response to NICE Supportive and Palliative Care Guidance and intended for senior health-care professionals involved in cancer care delivery.[44]

CURRENT DEVELOPMENTS

The United Kingdom had relinquished its lead in palliative care policy by 2000, when the World Health Organization and the governments of Canada, Australia, and New Zealand developed policies for the coordination of palliative care services. However, the publication, in March 2004, of the National Institute for Clinical Excellence Guidance on Cancer Services, *Improving Supportive and Palliative Care for Adults with Cancer*, heralded a series of policies concerning palliative care.

Concerns about the uncoordinated expansion of palliative care in the Republic of Ireland and lack of integration with other health services in the country led to the formation of the National Advisory Committee on Palliative Care. The concern that palliative care was dependent on charitable giving led to a call for greater involvement of the health service, and the minister for health and children established the National Advisory Committee on Palliative Care in 1999.[45]

Professor Sir Mike Richards, national clinical director for cancer, a former oncologist and chair of palliative medicine, led the development of the NHS Cancer Plan that included

strategies concerning supportive and palliative care. Between 2004 and 2007, the NHS End of Life Care Programme promoted initiatives such as the Gold Standards Framework, the Liverpool Care Pathway, and the Preferred Place of Care. These were taken up by primary and secondary care services throughout the United Kingdom to a greater extent than anticipated. The Liverpool Care Pathway was withdrawn in 2013.[46]

Changes in health care have favored patient-focused care, and the organization of the care process in terms of quality, efficiency, and accessibility continues to be scrutinized by clinicians, policy makers, and health-care managers. A *care pathway* is a practice directed at a specific patient population; it is used in daily practice in palliative care and forms part of the patient's clinical documentation.[47] Pathways are a means to achieve continuous quality improvement; they have their origins in industrial processes and were first used in health care in the United States in the 1980s. In clinical settings, pathways are implemented as a method for monitoring processes and processing time to improve efficiency and to maintain or improve the quality of care. Today, clinical care pathways are used globally, though they still need to go some way before they are widely implemented.[48] In the United Kingdom, the Department of Health recommends the use of the Liverpool Care Pathway as the best practice model in end-of-life care.[42]

In October 2007, end-of-life care was identified as one of the only eight divisions of care in Lord Darzi's NHS next stage review, and for the first time, it explicitly included palliative care as a fundamental element of health service provision. Shortly afterward, the United Kingdom Department of Health Cancer Reform Strategy for England, building on the 2000 Cancer Plan, included a "National Cancer Survivorship Initiative," a partnership of charities, patients, and clinicians who will consider a range of approaches to improving the services and support available to cancer survivors. It has been suggested that treating the consequences of cancer treatment in this growing population of survivors represents a new challenge for supportive and palliative care services.[49]

In December 2007, the RCP, London, published its report, "Palliative care services: Meeting the needs of patients." This document comprised the views of the members of the APM, and it was supportive of the principles of palliative care for patients with all conditions, the role of physicians in delivering palliative care, and specialist palliative care services. The RCP describes the report thus: "The report is both philosophical and practical and will be relevant to all doctors and allied health-care professionals who wish to ensure that the needs of patients and their carers are properly met. It is essential reading for health-care planners, commissioners of palliative care services, and for providers of undergraduate and postgraduate education for all doctors."[50]

By 2007, throughout the United Kingdom and Ireland, the number of voluntary sector hospice and palliative care services had risen to 149. In addition, there were 10 Marie Curie Hospices, 6 Sue Ryder Homes, 62 NHS, and 4 Irish Health Board in-patient palliative care services, as well as 37 children's hospices.[51] In 2010, there were 220 in-patient hospices with 2500 beds, 417 home care support teams, and 307 hospital support teams.[52]

In July 2008, 60 years after the inception of the NHS and 40 years after the birth of the modern hospice movement, the United Kingdom Department of Health published the End of Life Care Strategy for England. It offered a *whole systems and care pathway approach* to improving care at the end of life. A national coalition, Dying Matters, was proposed *to raise the profile of end-of-life care and to change attitudes to death and dying in society.* It appeared that access to specialist palliative care services for every patient in need of referral was within the mainstream health service policy.

The APM of Great Britain and Ireland responded to this stream of policy initiatives and a variety of palliative care provisions by defining the role of doctors in palliative medicine in "Palliative Medicine in Supportive, Palliative and End of Life Care: A Strategy for 2008 to 2010":

> All doctors, whether general practitioners or specialists in any setting, hold clinical responsibility for the treatment of their patients and have a role in providing medical leadership in their patients' palliative care.
>
> The core role of the palliative medicine physician may be defined as the medical assessment of distress, symptom management and end of life care for patients with complex clinical needs due to advanced, progressive or life threatening disease.
>
> They provide medical leadership within palliative care services and hold clinical responsibility for the treatment of patients in their care. Areas of responsibility include ensuring good quality, efficiency and equitable access to services, advising on strategic planning including commissioning of services, and developing strategies for research, education and training in relation to specialist and generalist palliative care.[53]

There is scant provision of end-of-life care for patients with nonmalignant disease, yet the prevailing view is that access to palliative care should relate to need rather than diagnosis, encompassing the needs of patients with nonmalignant disease as reflected in the UK National Service Frameworks (NSFs).[54] Delivery and content of care for patients with chronic nonmalignant disease is under discussion in the specialty and represents a huge challenge in the future.

Considerations in nonmalignant palliative care focus on increased interdisciplinary communication to develop knowledge and understanding. Fallon and Foley see the evolution of palliative medicine as important in the UK culture; they call for evolution in research in nonmalignant areas and joint supervision between palliative care and relevant nonmalignant disease specialties.[55]

The organic growth of services outside the health service in England has resulted in a plethora of institutions with a variety of funding sources from NHS budgets to private sector health care providers and charitable giving to local and national organizations. An independent review of the means by which to pay for these services in future was commissioned by the Department of Health, and the Palliative Care Funding Review was published in July 2011. It set out a series of recommendations "designed to create a fair and transparent funding system for palliative care, which delivers better outcomes for patients and provides a better value for the NHS." In view of the lack of good-quality economic data available, it recommended that pilot site be set up in order to inform the design of set tariffs for commissioning palliative care services.

FUTURE OF PALLIATIVE MEDICINE IN THE UNITED KINGDOM AND IRELAND

Following the passage into the law of the Health and Social Care Bill in England 2012, the economic and political changes following the banking crisis of 2008, and the European debt crisis of 2011 and 2012, the extent to which strategic policy changes can be put into practice in the United Kingdom and Ireland is now uncertain. It may be unaffordable in the UK context of a rising death rate set to increase from 2013 by 25% in the following 18 years. In spite of half a century of palliative care in the United Kingdom and Ireland, the question of the cost of equitable and efficient palliative care services has not been addressed. In most voluntary sector hospice services, the cost of clinical care is not measured in relation to clinical activity, and these costs are not distinguished from the costs of management, fund-raising and extra services, such as complementary therapy, bereavement care, and kitchens that produce good-quality food.

The 2008 End of Life Care Strategy was based on the assumption that shifting end of life care into the community is what patients and families want, that it will save costs, and is achievable. Dying patients' needs tend to increase over time, as dependency increases, so early discharge out of secondary care has serious resource implications for primary care services, unlike in the case of postoperative or other elective care discharges. Latest indications are that the shift of place of death to the community is beginning to happen in the United Kingdom.[56] However, we do not have data on the cost of primary care activity related to palliative care in the community, and there are no comparative data available that would tell us whether primary care teams are more or less efficient than secondary care outreach teams doing terminal care.[57]

Although the United Kingdom was recently rated as leading the world in the *quality of death* ranking across 40 countries (Economist Intelligence Unit, 2010) possibly because of its early start in the field, the absolute burden of distress is still significant. For palliative care to become accessible for all, the view that its focus should be on public health seems to be finding a following.[58] However, all is not yet well in the care of individuals, and even in the hands of specialists, pain can still be difficult to treat when the disease or the individual does not respond to standard analgesic regimes. Other symptoms are less well controlled, and they also impact the quality of life in the increasing number of cancer survivors as well as patients at the end of life. It is possible that the projected upturn in palliative care activity will provide the spur for governments, charities, and industry research funders to promote clinical research that has for the last 50 years been so badly needed to improve practice.

CONCLUSION

In this chapter, we have attempted to describe the historical context of the late nineteenth and twentieth centuries in Ireland and the United Kingdom, which allowed ideas about a humane approach to the care of the dying to flourish. Religious orders and the support of charitable donation, together with the catalyst of the charismatic leadership of Cicely Saunders, transformed care of the dying from the sporadic activity in a few small institutions in the 1950s into the rapid expansion of voluntary hospices in the 1980s.

As analgesic usage evolved, largely outside the NHS, interested doctors came together in the APM of Great Britain and Ireland to debate and validate practice. The advent of national voluntary sector organizations supported the integration of the expanding sector with hospital services. The recognition of palliative medicine as a medical specialty in the United Kingdom in 1987 was instrumental in the rapid expansion of palliative care in the NHS. Palliative care–related training and education in the schools of medicine and nursing followed, and a few centers of research flourished from the 1990s onward. The advent of specialized learned journals and the financial support of national charities promoted academic activity, but there remains a relative shortage of clinical research and academic clinicians compared with other UK specialties.

The beginning of the twenty-first century saw major policy initiatives aimed at standardizing palliative care services in Ireland and in the United Kingdom. The current priorities influencing the policy and health service research are characterized by a public health approach to equitable access and efficient configuration of services in the mixed economy of palliative care services. European economic factors, public sector funding crises, and the reconfiguration of NHS commissioning in England may undermine the rational planning of the future supportive and palliative care provision.

Key learning points

- The earliest hospice in the British Isles was Our Lady's Hospice for the dying, founded in Dublin by Mary Aikenhead and her Religious Sisters of Charity in 1879.

- In the late 1950s, St. Joseph's Hospice provided the context for Cicely Saunders's early pain research.[15] By 1964, she had described *total pain*, a holistic concept that recognizes the link between physical symptoms, mental distress, social problems, and emotional difficulties.[17]

- Within a decade of St. Christopher's inception in 1967, hospice principles were utilized in specialist in-patient units, by home and day care services, and on hospital wards where support teams brought new thinking about dying to acute medicine.[25]

- The National Institute for Clinical Excellence Guidance on Cancer Services, *Improving Supportive and Palliative Care for Adults with Cancer*, heralded a series of UK policy documents

between 2004 and 2007; the NHS End of Life Care Programme promoted initiatives such as the Gold Standards Framework the Liverpool Care Pathway, and the Preferred Place of Care, culminating in the End of Life Care Strategy for England.

- Palliative medicine was recognized as a medical specialty in 1987 in the United Kingdom. In "Palliative Medicine in Supportive, Palliative & End of Life Care: A Strategy for 2008 to 2010," the APM of Great Britain and Ireland defined the role of doctors in palliative care: "All doctors, whether general practitioners or specialists in any setting, hold clinical responsibility for the treatment of their patients and have a role in providing medical leadership in their patients' palliative care. The core role of the palliative medicine physician may be defined as the medical assessment of distress, symptom management and end of life care for patients with complex clinical needs due to advanced, progressive or life threatening disease."

- The beginning of the twenty-first century saw major policy initiatives aimed at standardizing palliative care services in Ireland and the United Kingdom. The current priorities influencing the policy and health service research are characterized by a public health approach to equitable access and efficient configuration of services in the mixed economy of palliative care services.

REFERENCES

1   Kelly J., The emergence of scientific and institutional medical practice in Ireland 1650–1800. In Jones G. and Malcolm E (eds.) *Medicine, Diseases and the State in Ireland 1650–1940*. Cork University Press: Cork, Republic of Ireland, p. 28, 1999.

2   Healy T., *125 Years of Caring in Dublin 1879–2004*. Dublin, Ireland: A&A Farmer, 2004.

3   Winslow M. and Clark D., Partnerships in care. In: *St Joseph's Hospice, Hackney: A Century of Caring in East London*. Observatory Publications: Lancaster, U.K., Chapter 2, p. 25–26, 2005.

4   Healy T., *125 Years of Caring in Dublin: Our Lady's Hospice, Harold's Cross 1879–2004*. A&AFarmar: Dublin, Ireland, p. 9, 2004.

5   Lydon P., *A Catalogue of Records Retained by Hospices and Related Organisations in the UK and the Republic of Ireland*. University of Sheffield, EAHMH: Sheffield, U.K., p. 34, 1998.

6   Winslow M. and Clark D., Partnerships in care. In: *St Joseph's Hospice, Hackney: A Century of Caring in East London*. Observatory Publications: Lancaster, U.K., p. 26, 2005.

7   Winslow M. and Clark D., Partnerships in care. In: *St Joseph's Hospice, Hackney: A Century of Caring in East London*. Observatory Publications: Lancaster, U.K., p. 26, 2005.

8   Healy T., *125 Years of Caring in Dublin: Our Lady's Hospice, Harold's Cross 1879–2004*. A&AFarmar: Dublin, Ireland, p. 17, 2004.

9   O'Brien T. and Clark D., A national plan for palliative care - the Irish experience. In: Ling J. and O'Síoráin L., (ed.) Facing Death. Palliative Care in Ireland. Open University Press: Maidenhead, UK. p. 3–10, 2005.

10 Munk W., *Euthanasia: Or, Medical Treatment in Aid of an Easy Death*. Longmans, Green and Co.: London, U.K., 1887.

11 Cushing H., *The Life of Sir William Osler*. Oxford University Press: Oxford, U.K., 1940.

12   Johns Hopkins Medical Institutions, Medical Archives. Celebrating the Contribution of William Osler. http://www.medicalarchives.jhmi.edu/osler/biography.htm.

13   Jalland P., *Death in the Victorian Family*. Oxford University Press: Oxford, U.K., 1996.

14   Humphries C., "Waiting for the last summons": The establishment of the first hospices in England 1878–1914. *Mortality* 6: 146–166, 2001.

15   Winslow M. and Clark D., St Joseph's Hospice, Hackney: Documenting a centenary history. *Progress in Palliative Care* 14: 68–74, 2006.

16   Clark D., The development of Palliative Medicine in the UK and Ireland. In: Bruera E., Higginson I., Ripamonti C., and von Gunten C. (eds.) *Textbook of Palliative Medicine*. Hodder Arnold: London, U.K., 2006.

17   Winslow M. and Clark D., Partnerships in care. In: *St Joseph's Hospice, Hackney: A Century of Caring in East London*. Observatory Publications: Lancaster, U.K., pp. 43–71, 2005.

18   Meldrum M., A capsule history of pain management. *JAMA* 290: 2470–2475, 2003.

19   Seymour J. and Winslow M., Pain and palliative care: The emergence of new specialties. *Journal of Pain and Symptom Management* 29: 2–13, 2005.

20   Bailey M., A survey of the social needs of patients with incurable lung cancer. *Almoner* 11: 379–397, 1959.

21   Hinton J., Problems in the care of the dying. *Journal of Chronic Diseases* 17: 201–205, 1964.

22   Wilkes E., Cancer outside hospital. *Lancet* 20: 1379–1381, June 1964.

23   Wilkes E., Terminal cancer at home. *Lancet* i: 799–801, 1965.

24   Clark D., From margins to centre: A review of the history of palliative care in cancer. *Lancet Oncology* 8: 430–438, 2007.

25   Clark D., Small N., Wright M., Winslow M., and Hughes N., Hospice teamwork. In: *A Bit of Heaven for the Few: An Oral History of the Modern Hospice Movement in the United Kingdom*. Observatory Publications: Lancaster, U.K., 2005.

26   Working Group on Terminal Care [The Wilkes Report], *Report of the Working Group on Terminal Care*. DHSS: London, U.K., 1980.

27   *No Second Chance: A discussion document for the Trent Regional Health Authority on the Development of Terminal Care Services* (Trent Regional Health Authority 1987). Unpublished.

28   Rossi P., *Fighting Cancer with More Than Medicine: A History of Macmillan Cancer Support*. The History Press Ltd: Stroud, Gloucestershire, U.K., 2009.

29   Scott J. and Macdonald N., Education in palliative medicine. In Doyle D., Hanks G., and Macdonald, N (eds.) *Oxford Textbook of Palliative Medicine*. Oxford University Press, Oxford, U.K. 1993.

30   Clark D., Small N., Wright M., Winslow M., and Hughes N., Hospice growth and spread. In: *A Bit of Heaven for the Few: An Oral History of the Modern Hospice Movement in the United Kingdom*. Observatory Publications: Lancaster, U.K., 2005.

31   Hain R., Heckford E., and McCulloch R., Paediatric palliative medicine in the UK: Past, present, future. *Archives of Disease in Childhood* 97:381–384, Published online October 28, 2011.

32   Clark D., Small N., Wright M., Winslow M., and Hughes N., Hospice growth and spread. In: *A Bit of Heaven for the Few: An Oral History of the Modern Hospice Movement in the United Kingdom*. Observatory Publications: Lancaster, U.K., p. 62, 2005.

33   Charlton R. and Bevan M., Towards a pre-history of palliative care: A pilot study centred on medical education and practice in Birmingham c.1930–1970. http://www2.warwick.ac.uk/fac/arts/history/chm/research_teaching/archive/palliative/. Accessed June 15, 2012.

34   Saunders C., The evolution of palliative care. *Journal of the Royal Society of Medicine* 94: 430–432, 2001.

35   Winslow M. and Clark D., Partnerships in Care. In: *St Joseph's Hospice, Hackney: A century of caring in East London*. Observatory Publications: Lancaster, U.K., p. 47, 2005.

36   Bennett M., Davies E., and Higginson I., Delivering research in end-of-life care: Problems, pitfalls and future priorities. *Palliative Medicine* 24: 456–461, 2010.

37   See: National Cancer Research Institute, http://www.ncri.org.uk/

38   See: Palliative Care Research Society, http://www.pcrs.org.uk/aboutus.php

39   See: Association of Palliative Medicine Scientific Committee, http://www.apmonline.org/page.php?pageid=190

40   Field D. and Wee B., Preparation for palliative care: Teaching about death, dying and bereavement in UK medical schools 2000–2001. *Medical Education* 36: 561–567, 2001.

41   Gibbins J., McCoubrie R., and Forbes K., Why are newly qualified doctors unprepared to care for patients at the end of life? *Medical Education* 45: 389–399, 2011.

42   Department of Health, *End of life Care Strategy: Quality Markers and Measures for End of Life Care*. DH: London, U.K.

43   Pulsford D., Jackson G., O'Brien T., Yates S., and Duxbury J., UK Classroom-based and distance learning education and training courses in end-of-life care for health and social care staff: A systematic review. *Palliative Medicine* 27(3) p. 221–235, 2013.

44   See: Advanced Communication Skills Training for Senior Health Professionals in Cancer Care. http://www.the3ccancernet.org.uk/downloads/3CCN%20ACST%20Flyer%202009%202010.pdf.

45   Ling J. and O'Síoráin L., *Palliative Care in Ireland*. Open University Press: Maidenhead, U.K., 2005.

46   Hughes P., Bath P., Ahmed N., and Noble B., What progress has been made towards implementing national guidance on end of life care? A national survey of UK general practices. *Palliative Medicine* 24(1): 68–78, 2010.

47   Vanhaecht K., Massimiliano P., van Zelm R., and Sermeus W., An overview on the history and concept of care pathways as complex interventions. *International Journal of Care Pathways* 14: 117–123, 2010.

48   Vanhaecht K., Massimiliano P., van Zelm R., and Sermeus W., What about Care Pathways? In Ellershaw J. and Wilkinson S (eds.) *Care of the Dying: Pathways to Excellence*, 2nd edn. Oxford University Press: Oxford, U.K., 2011.

49   Maher J., Consequences of cancer treatment: A new challenge for supportive and palliative care. *BMJ Supportive & Palliative Care* 2(2): 82–83, 2012.

50   Royal College of Physicians Palliative care services: Meeting the needs of patients. Unpublished Report, 2007.

51   Wood J. and Clark D., The historical development of inpatient services within United Kingdom and Ireland adult voluntary hospices. *Palliative Medicine* 22: 293, 1–2, 2008.

52   Help The Hospices, Hospice and Palliative Care Directory 2011–2012. Help the Hospices, London, U.K. 2011. http://www.helpthehospices.org.uk/about-hospice-care/facts-figures.

53   Noble B., APM: Still much to be done to improve the delivery of care in the UK, *European Journal of Palliative Care* 16(1): 47–49, 2009.

54   NHS National End of Life Care Programme. *End of life care in long term neurological conditions: A framework for implementation*, 2010; NHS National End of Life Care Programme. *End of life care in heart failure: A framework for implementation*, 2010.

55   Fallon M. and Foley P., Rising to the challenge of palliative care for non-malignant disease. *Palliative Medicine* 26: 99–100, 2012.

56   Gomes B., Calanzani N., and Higginson I., Reversal of the British trends in place of death: Time series analysis 2004–2010. *Palliative Medicine* ol. 26(2): 102–107, 2012.

57   Cohen J. and Delien L.' (ed.) A Public Health Perspective on End of Life Care. In: A Public Health Perspective on End of Life Care. Oxford University Press: Oxford, U.K, p. 4–11.

58   Noble, B., Lansley's Monster is leaving the Laboratory. *BMJ Supportive & Palliative Care* 2(2): 80–81, 2012.

2

Development of palliative care in Europe

CARL JOHAN FÜRST, LUKAS RADBRUCH

EUROPE: DIVERSITY AND UNITY

Any description of the development of palliative care in Europe must first of all take into consideration the diversity and complexity of this continent. The World Health Organization (WHO) describes Europe as representing 53 different countries [1]. The Council of Europe, which is the oldest political European organization, has 47 member states with about 800 million citizens [2]. The European Union (EU) includes 27 nations, of which 17 make up the European monetary union [3]. Europeans speak more than 60 different official languages with three different alphabets [4]. Until the collapse around 1990 of the post-Second-World-War boundaries, Europe was separated in political, economical, and many other ways. The *iron curtain* was the border between the Soviet Union and its allies in Central and Eastern Europe (CEE) and the rest of Europe. The former communist countries and some former Soviet republics are now often referred to as CEE countries even though some of these countries are EU member states today. The Commonwealth of Independent States (CIS) is a loose organization of republics of the former Soviet Union. The many different political systems, historical pasts, cultures, religious beliefs, economies, and educational and health-care systems all naturally impact the development and current standing of palliative care.

Data from OECD and EU for the year 2010 are used in the succeeding text to give a sense of the differences in mortality rates in the different European countries and death related to cancer, ischemic heart disease, and stroke in some countries. The age-standardized death rates for all causes vary from 488 to 970/100,000 deaths in Europe (Switzerland as compared to Bulgaria) [5]. For cancer, the death rate (2010) varies from 98 in Cypriote women to 333 in Hungarian men. The death rates in lung cancer among women vary from <10/100,000 in Latvia and Portugal to 43 in Danish females. The lowest death rate for ischemic heart disease was found in French women, 19/100,000, and the highest in Lithuanian men, 429/100,000. For stroke, the age-standardized rate was 23/100,000 in French women and 214/100,000 in Bulgarian men. Different causes of death in EU countries in 2010 are displayed in Figure 2.1 [6].

In spite of all these differences, the overarching experience of Europe includes the many commonalities such as the common roots of history, regional similarities in languages, and relatively short distances. In regard to palliative care, there are both small and larger initiatives on political, academic, and other professional levels including those of the Council of Europe and the EU, with ambitions to cooperate internationally and to find common solutions and collaboration for the best of the patients and families.

In addition to the figures on differences in mortality rates, Europe faces a large and challenging demographic change with an increasing number of elderly people and a decrease in the available work force. The Eurostat forecast for EU countries for 2009–2060 implies an increase of the population ≥65 years of age from 17% to 30% (Figure 2.2) [7]. The old-age dependency ratio will increase from 28.4% to 58.5% [2]. This situation implies a range of challenges: changing epidemiology of disease, increasing age of caregivers, financial implications for the health-care systems, and the range of settings for care. It is estimated that the number of deaths outside of hospitals will increase. It is an enormous challenge for our societies to organize care for the ageing populations at home or in care homes with different levels of competencies [8,9]. To highlight this problem, the WHO Europe has published three illustrative booklets: *Better Palliative Care for Older People* [10], *The Solid Facts: Palliative Care* [11] in 2004, and *Palliative Care for Older People: Better Practices* in 2011 [7]. This series was supported by the Floriani Foundation in Milan and the Maruzza Foundation in Rome, the Open Society Institute (OSI), and the European Association for Palliative Care (EAPC).

HISTORICAL PIONEERS AND EARLY ADOPTERS

A historical perspective of palliative care in Europe includes the ancient guesthouses and hospices, often in the Alpine region, that gave shelter and care to pilgrims but also to incurable and dying patients. Jeanne Garnier was a predecessor of palliative care development in Europe when in 1842 in Lyon, France,

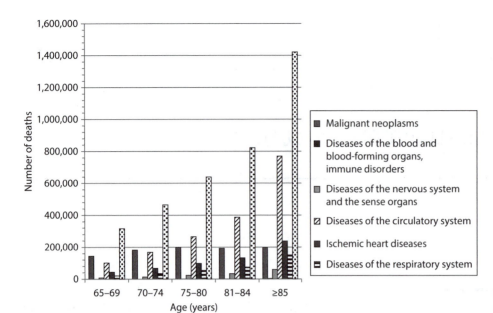

Figure 2.1 *Number of deaths by main disease-related causes in 27 EU countries, 2010.*

she started an association to care for incurable and dying patients until their death. She was a young widow and the mother of two children who died at a young age. A similar home for the dying opened in Paris in 1874 and the word hospice was used to describe the care setting. The founders organized themselves in an association called the sisters of Calvaire (Golgotha). At the same period, the efforts of Mary Aikenhead, superior of the Irish Sisters of Charity, led to the opening of St. Vincent's Hospital in Dublin in 1834. The modern development of palliative care in Europe was very much inspired by Dame Cicely Saunders and her UK colleagues at St. Christopher's Hospice in London (see Chapter 1). The founder of St. Luke's hospice in Sheffield, Erik Wilkes, seems to have been less known on the European continent in spite of his great influence in the United Kingdom [12]. The work by Swiss born Elisabeth Kübler-Ross who later came to work in the United States was a source of inspiration for many, particularly after the publication of her book *On Death and Dying* in 1969 [13]. Another important influence was the hospital-based palliative care unit in Montreal, Canada, led by Balfour Mount that opened in 1974. The term palliative care was used since hospice was associated with death by the French-speaking Canadians [14]. Palliative care services, home care, and inpatient hospices were set up in several European countries by pioneering professionals, volunteers, religious communities, and others. The first countries to have opened palliative care services include Poland in 1976, Sweden in 1977, France in 1978, Italy in 1980, Germany in 1983, Spain in 1984, and St. Petersburg in Russia in 1990 [15–20]. In the Netherlands, some of the Dutch nursing homes were early adopters of palliative care although the first hospice started in 1991 [21].

To a great extent, the development of palliative care was a reaction to what was experienced as the failure of modern medicine to care for the dying in the big hospitals. Humanitarian and Christian values in caring for the dying patient has been the foundation for many of the hospice and palliative care pioneers in the United Kingdom as well as in the rest of Europe.

The 1990 WHO definition of palliative care reflected the development of the field in Europe at that time, providing a holistic and humanistic definition based on clinical reality without a religious connotation [22,23] (Table 2.1).

The discussions that arose after the launch of the new and extended WHO definition in 2002 [24] reflected the discrepancy in perspective between the original hospice movement and the needs not only of those who are dying [25]. The new definition still focuses on care of the dying on one hand, and on the other hand, the broader spectrum of palliative care, including attitudes, assessments of need, and early interventions in patients where death is not anticipated in the near future. It also calls for palliative care in all settings: hospice, hospital, nursing home, or home.

The development of palliative care in Europe followed several paths, although all shared focus on alleviating suffering of the dying patient. Traditionally, most patients who received palliative care had a cancer diagnosis. Recent reports from, for example, the Swedish Palliative Care Registry confirm that this is still the case in that more than 90% of all deaths in hospice, palliative care units, and specialized palliative home care are due to cancer [26]. But to an increasing degree, palliative care services, as well as the referring physicians in Europe, open up to other groups of patients and to the needs of the patient and family rather than the diagnosis [27]. Multinational European professional interest groups have been formed to highlight the needs and professional challenges in caring for patients with specific needs, for example, older patients and children, for those with specific diagnoses such as neurological diseases and dementia, and for patients with intellectual disabilities [28].

Many European palliative care pioneers had a background in anesthesiology, pain management, and opioid pharmacology. The introduction of oral morphine solutions and opioids in subcutaneous syringe drivers made treatment of pain easier, even in nonhospital settings and in patients' homes [29].

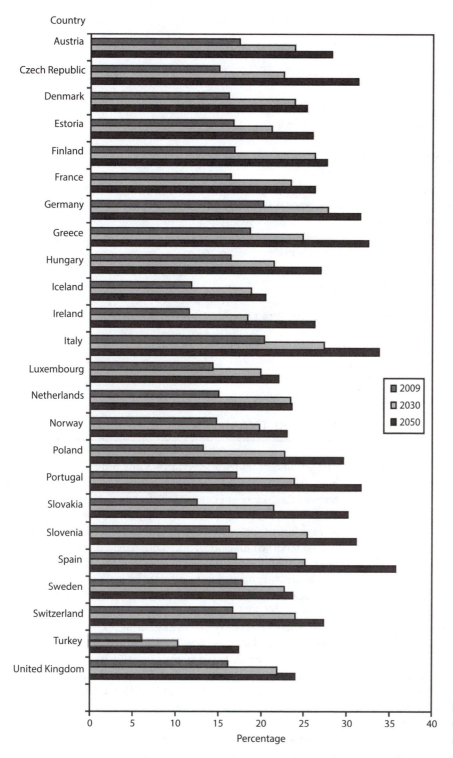

Figure 2.2 *Percentage of people aged 65 years and older in selected countries in the WHO European region in 2009 and projections for 2030 and 2050.*

Vittorio Ventafridda in Milan, with the support of Jan Stjernswärd at the WHO cancer unit and the Floriani Foundation and a number of renowned specialists in the field including Kathleen Foley, United States, and Robert Twycross, United Kingdom, produced the WHO pain ladder and strategy for pain relief. The WHO strategy was published in 1986 in the booklet entitled Pain Relief in Cancer [30], and it has had a remarkable impact on the management of pain and thereby on palliative care in general in Europe and worldwide.

Most European countries have publicly funded health-care systems in place, but much of the expansion of palliative care in Europe has taken place outside of these health-care systems. There are exceptions such as Spain, Italy, and the Scandinavian countries, where palliative care has been integrated in public health care but initially was very dependent on palliative care pioneers and specific funding initiatives. There is still a struggle, also in these countries, to reach sufficient coverage of palliative care through a full integration

Table 2.1 *Two crucial decades: Key milestones in palliative care development in Europe (1986–2008)*

1986	WHO cancer pain relief booklet
1987	Palliative medicine first issue of the journal
1987	EAPC founded
1988	Palliative medicine approved as a medical specialty in United Kingdom
1988	WHO collaborating center for palliative care in Oxford
1990	WHO definition of palliative care
1990	EAPC congress in Paris, first congress
1993	European Council adopt document on PC
1995	Barcelona declaration
1996	Chair in palliative medicine, St. Thomas' Hospital, London, United Kingdom, held by Professor Geoff Hanks
1996	EAPC Research Network
1996	EPCRN guidelines—Morphine in cancer pain: modes of administration
1999	Palliative medicine a specialty in Poland
2000	EAPC first research forum, Berlin
2002	New WHO definition of palliative care
2003	European Council recommendations on palliative care
2003	International observatory for palliative care
2008	WHO collaborating centers for palliative care approved in Catalonia and at the Cicely Saunders Institute, London

of palliative care in the health-care systems. Some see voluntarism and fund raising for hospice care as an important and integrated part of the hospice movement and of civil society. However, in some health-care models, there is little space for volunteers [31,32].

EUROPEAN DEVELOPMENT

A description and a map of palliative care delivery in Europe was produced in a collaborative project between the International Observatory for palliative care at the University of Lancaster, United Kingdom, then directed by David Clark, and the EAPC Task Force on the Development of Palliative Care in Europe, headed by Carlos Centeno in Navarra, Spain. Data were gathered on important aspects of palliative care such as current services, reimbursement and funding, opioid availability and consumption, coverage and palliative care work force, as well as on historical milestones and present challenges. The first edition was published in 2007 and a second and more detailed and developed version was published in 2013 [33,34]. The initiative has faced many challenges due to the different health-care systems and the absence of common definitions of care provision. To facilitate description, comparison, and benchmarking, EAPC has recently published a consensus document called the *EAPC white paper on standards and norms for hospice and palliative care in Europe* [35,36]. The document covers the most important and common concepts in palliative care, for example, what constitutes a hospice, a palliative care unit, a home care team, and specialized versus general palliative care.

NATIONAL EXAMPLES

Cicely Saunders visited Poland in 1978 and inspired the development of palliative home care and the opening of the first registered hospice, the Society of Friends of the Sick in Krakow in 1981 [19]. This development was parallel to the political solidarity movement before the collapse of the communist regime. Volunteers in Poland modelled development for both religious and secular services. In 1987, the first palliative care service within the national health structure opened in Poznan, led by Jacek Luczak who also established the Eastern and Central European Palliative Care Task Force (ECEPT) in 1989, aiming specifically to support the development of palliative care in Eastern and Central Europe. The objectives of ECEPT have now been integrated into the mandate of the EAPC. International courses in palliative care in Poznan were one outcome of academic links between Robert Twycross at his WHO collaborating center and the hospice, Sir Michel Sobell House, in Oxford, and Jacek Luczak at the Medical Academy in Poznan. In 2003, the palliative care service in Poznan as well as the pediatric palliative care services in Warsaw were nominated as beacons of palliative care development in an attempt to identify important services in Eastern and Central Europe [19]. Today, Poland has a large number of palliative care services with dominant hospices and home care teams. Other important and pioneering initiatives were the palliative care services in St. Petersburg, Russia; the hospice of hope, Casa Sperantei in Brasov, Romania; and the Hungarian Hospice Foundation in Budapest, Hungary. These units have all have a profound impact on the development of palliative care in this region in the years that followed.

The first Spanish palliative care services opened in 1984, and dedicated political support led to the WHO demonstration project on palliative care in Catalonia in 1990–1995 [37]. Xavier Gomez Batiste and the head of WHO cancer unit in Geneva, Jan Stjernswärd, initiated the project. The project was a successful demonstration of a large-scale public health-based implementation of palliative care, initially with a dominance of patients with cancer and AIDS but later including other patients in need of palliative care. The project was publicly planned and financed and aimed at an integration of palliative care into all parts of the health-care system. The program included revision of legislation governing the delivery of opioid analgesics, training of all health-care professionals in basic palliative care, development of a model for funding, integration into conventional health-care services, implementation of specialist palliative care services throughout the health-care system, and development of both professional standards and a monitoring and evaluation strategy. The WHO–Catalonian model has been described with positive outcomes in terms of coverage for both cancer and noncancer patients, increase in symptom control, and economical savings due to more adequate care and avoidance of futile treatment interventions in the final phase of life [38–40]. Today, palliative care is even well established in several other regions of Spain.

Again, St. Christopher's Hospice in London and St. Luke's Hospice in Sheffield inspired an initiative to implement palliative care in 1975 in a Dutch nursing home [21]. In the Netherlands, palliative medicine and the provision of palliative care has by and large been seen as a field for the general practitioner and not for specialists in palliative medicine, possibly reflected in the fact that the Netherlands is one of the European countries without a medical specialty in palliative medicine. Also, the Dutch nursing homes differ from those in many other countries in that there are specialized nursing home doctors.

The history and debate on euthanasia in the Netherlands and other European countries will not be covered in this chapter.

In France, the word hospice has never been generally used for palliative care services even though Hospices de Beaune or Hôtel-Dieu is one of the most well-known ancient hospices, founded in 1443. This is because in French, the word hospice means hospital and so adds confusion. Palliative care development has mainly taken place within the health-care system with a large number of mobile teams, hospital support teams, dedicated palliative care beds in hospitals, and palliative care inpatient units. Early adopters were, for example, Michelle Salamange in Paris and Rene Scherer in Grenoble, both of whom were founding members of the EAPC board [41].

The development in Germany has followed two different paths. The German hospice movement started as a social movement, which was much based on volunteers, fund raising and a limited medical input. In contrast, palliative care had closer links to the health-care system with a more medical perspective [34]. This may be reflected by the fact that Germany has both a large number of hospices and hospital teams. Today, nine medical faculties have chairs in palliative medicine.

A wider perspective

From a global perspective, palliative care is fairly well developed in many regions and nations of Europe and in some places, it is approaching integration into the health-care system (Figures 2.2 and 2.3). However, there are still large unmet needs even in those countries with the most developed specialized palliative care. This includes palliative care in hospitals, nursing homes, and community settings as well as the needs of specific groups such as the increasing number of migrants with cultural

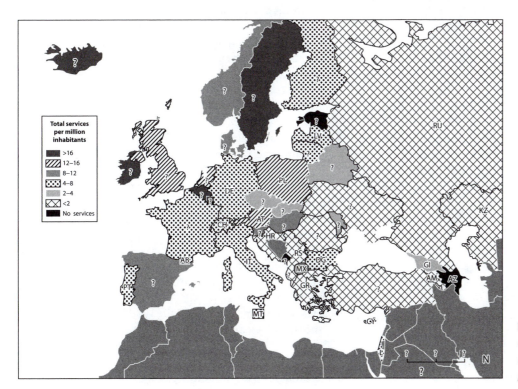

Figure 2.3 *Proportion of palliative care services in Europe per population. (From Centeno, C. et al.,. EAPC atlas of palliative care in Europe, 2013.)*

diversity found in most countries. The lack of an efficient collaboration and sometimes even competition between different care providers at different levels of care is another great challenge.

Opioid availability is still a problem in several countries, particularly in the eastern parts of Europe [42,43]. However, there are a several examples of model changes in the national legislation making most opioids available subsidized for patients. The change of legislation on controlled medicines in Romania can be taken as an example as well as legislation changes in, for example, Croatia, Czech Republic, Estonia, Georgia, Hungary, Latvia, Rumania, Serbia, and the Slovak Republic [44]. The EU seventh framework program supported project ATOME, which focuses on the promotion of opioid availability as described later in the chapter.

The financial, educational, and individual support for the development of palliative care in the CEE countries by the Open Society Institute and Foundation and particularly through the dedicated work by Kathleen Foley and Mary Callaway cannot be overestimated. This includes the Salzburg seminars that included courses on palliative care and country support to most CEE countries with Georgia, Hungary, Czech Republic, Romania, and Lithuania as examples [45].

EUROPEAN COLLABORATION

The EAPC was founded in December 1988, with Vittorio Ventafridda, Italy, and Derek Doyle, United Kingdom, as first chair and vice chair, respectively. The first board was multiprofessional with representation from Belgium, France, Italy, Spain, Sweden, Switzerland, and the United Kingdom [46]. The aim of EAPC was to increase awareness and to promote the development and dissemination of palliative care at scientific, clinical, and social levels. In 1992, the first national palliative care associations joined the EAPC collectively and in 2004, the EAPC became a federation with 49 associations from 31 countries. The first international congress of palliative care was organized by EAPC in Paris, France, in 1990. EAPC has since arranged biannual congresses in 12 European cities. Since 2000, there have been biannual EAPC research forums, the first one in Berlin, with a scientific focus and a smaller number of delegates. Much of the work in EAPC is channeled through task forces and interest groups that work on a specific topic for a limited time to produce a report or a recommendation or other suitable deliverables. Example of taskforces and working groups include those on standards and norms, ethics and spiritual care, different care settings, different patient groups, and family carers.

PUBLIC, PROFESSIONAL, AND POLITICAL AWARENESS

At the EAPC congress in Barcelona in 1995, the following declaration was launched as a vision for future policy work: "Based on inclusion of palliative care in national health care policies, the individual's right to pain relief and equitable availability of palliative care, governments should establish clear and immediate policies, implement specific services, educate health professionals and the public, ensure that necessary drugs are adequately available and simplify prescribing procedures" [47]. The declaration was signed by the leading officials of Catalonia, WHO, and EAPC.

The Poznan declaration of 1998 was signed by palliative care leaders from several eastern and central European countries attending the advanced course in palliative care in Poznan [48]. They subscribed to the aims of the ECEPT. These included a call for national policies, palliative care education, increased drug availability, a growth in palliative care services, and an increase in public awareness (Figure 2.4).

In 1999, the Parliamentary Assembly of the Council of Europe adopted a document on the *Protection of the human rights and dignity of the terminally ill and the dying* [49]. This document mentions and underlines the need for palliative care.

The Council of Europe released a second document in 2003 entitled *Recommendation REC 24 (2003) of the Committee of Ministers to member states on the organisation of palliative care*, which was approved and adopted by all ministers of health [50]. The expert group behind the recommendations was chaired by Tony O'Brien, Ireland. EAPC promoted the translation and dissemination of the recommendations in many different languages.

Also beyond Europe, EAPC was one of the driving forces behind the Korea declaration on hospice and palliative care in 2005 [51]. The main message, again to governments around the globe, was "palliative care as a human right," the integration of palliative care into health-care systems, national cancer control programs and AIDS strategies, and reinforcing the statements of the Barcelona declaration on a global level.

The Venice declaration was a collaborative initiative by EAPC and IAHPC at the EAPC Research Forum in Venice in 2006 in collaboration with all major international palliative organizations [52]. The main message was an agreement to work and collaborate together to support palliative care research in developing countries, to identify the research priorities in these countries, and to identify funders and help mobilize resources to support research in the developing world.

The Budapest commitments in 2007 was a call to EAPC associations and other relevant and interested organizations to identify and give priority to areas for improvement, set realistic goals, and work for their realization in their own countries [53,54]. Also, at the EAPC congress in Lisbon in 2011, a challenge was sent to governments to actually take on the previous policy statements with an emphasis on training professionals [55].

The Prague charter of 2013 is an appeal for governments to relieve suffering and ensure the right to palliative care [56]. It is a joint initiative between EAPC, International Association for Hospice & Palliative Care (IAHPC), Worldwide Palliative Care Alliance (WPCA), and Human Rights Watch (HRW).

Two major reports from the European Institutions have provided recommendations to governments and other stakeholders, one to the European Parliament (the Moreno report,

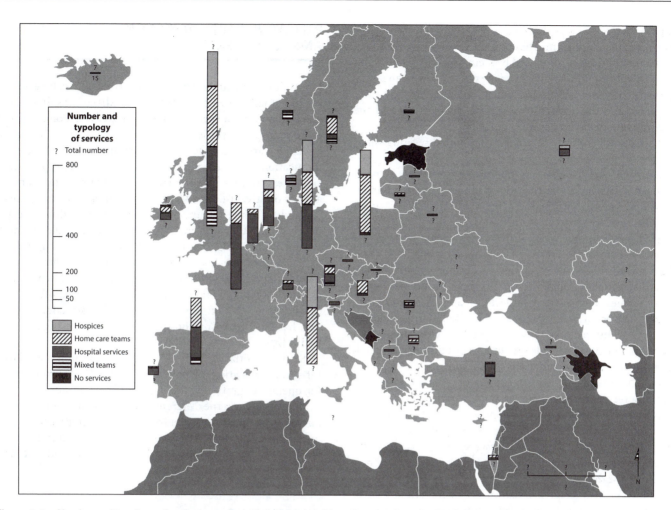

Figure 2.4 *Number and typology of palliative care services in Europe. (From Centeno, C. et al.,. EAPC atlas of palliative care in Europe, 2013.)*

based mostly on the work of the EAPC task force on development) and one to the parliamentary assembly of the Council of Europe (Wodarg report) [57,58].

There has been no formal evaluation of the effect of these initiatives to date. However, one can assume that the present general interest for palliative care in Europe has been preceded by the engaged professionals articulating the most important messages and political standpoints in the declarations and statements. The Budapest commitments were a more action-oriented program trying to engage people in goal-oriented improvement projects.

RESEARCH

EAPC research network

The European research network (EAPC-RN) was established within EAPC in 1996 and chaired by Franco de Conno, Italy [59].The initial outcomes of the research network were expert recommendations on different relevant topics within palliative care such as the use of morphine and other opioids and the management of pain, depression, and bowel obstruction. A further idea was to initiate multicenter

trials with a randomized controlled design, responding to the need for better scientific evidence on effective interventions for pain, other symptoms, and problems in the care of patients at the end of life. The EAPC research forums have been organized by the research network. The forums have had an increasing number of delegates and submitted scientific abstracts. Today, the research network works in close collaboration with the European Palliative Care Research Centre (PRC) in Trondheim, Norway, headed by Stein Kaasa. The research network has evolved continuously, also through research collaboratives funded by the framework programs of the EU such as the European Palliative Care Research Collaborative (EPCRC) and now reaches far beyond Europe with scientific studies in several areas of palliative care [60]. Important outcomes include the European cross-sectional study of palliative care patients, the European Pharmacogenetic Opioid Study (EPOS), and the work on clinical opioid guidelines [61–63].

European Union research funding

The EU through the European Commission (EU) regularly announces research calls for the health-care sector. One of the first projects, led by Ireland, was a European-wide audit of palliative care, supported in the 1990s through the Europe Against Cancer program. The sixth framework program supported the EPCRC in 2006. Led by Stein Kaasa in Trondheim, Norway, it brought together 11 centers in six European countries. EPCRC focused on assessment and treatment of pain, cachexia, and depression in cancer patients. This led to the development of evidence-based guidelines.

The seventh framework program supported several collaboratives focused on palliative care:

PRISMA was launched in 2008 with a total of 11 partners led by Richard Harding and Irene Higginson, London, United Kingdom, with main partners in Germany, Portugal, Italy, Spain, Norway, the Netherlands, Belgium, and Africa. It included European comparisons using tools such as the palliative care outcome scale (POS) and the Support Team Assessment Schedule (STAS) and examined cultural issues as well as patients' and clinicians' priorities for different care-related issues, such as place of death, treatment, and decision making. Over 26 peer-reviewed publications were generated from the group working on project PRISMA. Other important PRISMA outcomes included a survey on European research activities and recommendations for the future [64].

OPCARE9 was an EU 7th Framework–supported project focusing on the very last days and hours of life, more specifically on signs and symptoms of approaching death; end-of-life decisions; complementary comfort care; psychological and psychosocial support for patients, relatives, and caretakers; voluntary service; and development of the Liverpool Care Pathway (LCP) for the dying patient [65].

The ATOME project was launched in 2009 and aimed to improve access to opioids across Europe. A major focus of ATOME is to bring together experts from palliative care and harm reduction as well as government stakeholders, as the communication between these groups is a prerequisite to any change in the legislation [66].

The IMPACT project, launched in 2010, is a consortium of 12 research groups studying organization and implementation strategies for palliative care, specifically for patients with cancer or dementia [67].

The EURO-IMAPCT project was launched in 2011 with the aim to develop capacity in palliative and end-of-life care, to implement strategies for palliative care interventions, and to describe outcome and quality indicators for palliative care in a range of health-care settings. The project focuses on patients with cancer and with dementia. The project will also foster the development of research capacity by providing an international academic program for PhD students and has already published extensively [68].

The most recent addition is the INSUP-C project that started in 2013, evaluating models and concepts for integrative palliative care [69].

All projects have an underlying ambition to build networks and collaboration between researchers and research groups as well as to support and foster early career researchers.

EU funding of palliative care projects has been and remains important for the development of palliative care since national research funding for palliative care is scarce in many countries.

PALLIATIVE CARE: EDUCATION AND COMPETENCY

Many European universities but far from all include teaching in palliative medicine. Palliative medicine was first recognized as a medical specialty in the United Kingdom, where it is a 4-year specialist training program including the history of palliative care; most aspects of physical palliative care; communication with patient, family, and professionals; psychosocial care; attitudes, culture, language, religions, and spiritual aspects of care; ethics and legal frameworks; teamwork; learning and teaching; research; management; and clinical governance. Since then, several countries, for example, Ireland, Poland, Romania, Germany, and Malta, have followed, making palliative medicine a specialty, subspecialty, or other complementary specialty. Other countries are now following, such as Czech Republic, France, Slovenia, and Sweden (Table 2.2). Much of the work on European pre- and postgraduate curricula has been based on those from the United Kingdom and EAPC [70].

Several initiatives are aiming at common standards for nurse education in palliative care [71]. A problem for European integration is the different levels of nursing competencies between the different European countries. In many but far from all countries, nursing is a university degree and nursing schools include academic competent nurses being responsible for teaching as well as research and doctoral programs.

DISSEMINATION

The *European Journal of Palliative Care* (EJPC) is the official journal of EAPC and has been published since 1994. It includes articles on the latest development of palliative care and is an information channel for EAPC and for professionals working within palliative care throughout Europe and beyond. *Palliative Medicine* is the first European palliative care research journal that published its first issue in January 1987 and is the research journal of EAPC, publishing 8 issues yearly. *Journal of Supportive Care in Cancer* and more recently *BMJ Supportive and Palliative Care* and *The International Journal of Palliative Nursing* are also examples of European-based international peer-reviewed journals that extensively publish palliative care research. The official journal of the Multinational Association for Supportive Care in Cancer (MASCC) is *Supportive Care in Cancer* which publishes extensively, on palliative-care-related research since 2003.

The OSI founded an *EAPC-east* office for Eastern Europe in Stockholm in 2001 aimed at strengthening the networks of palliative care professionals in Eastern Europe. A monthly electronic newsletter was published as a major source of information on palliative care for Central European countries and CIS. This newsletter was adopted and further developed by the Hungarian Hospice Palliative Association with additional support from the EAPC, led by Katalin Hegedus as editor.

Table 2.2 *EU-funded projects: Objectives and outcome (2006 onward)*

Project acronym and leading institution	Objectives	Outcomes or aims for ongoing projects
EPCRC 2006–2010 Norwegian University of Science and Technology, Trondheim, Norway	*European Palliative Care Research Collaborative* Partners: Six European countries, United States, and Canada Focused on assessment and treatment of pain, cachexia, and depression in cancer patients	Systematic reviews on different aspects of assessment and management of pain, cachexia, and depression in cancer patients Multinational trial on opioid pharmacogenetics. Evidence-based guidelines on pain, depression, and cachexia.
PRISMA 2008–2011 Cicely Saunders Institute for Palliative Care, Kings College, London, United Kingdom 2008–2011 Cicely Saunders Institute for Palliative Care, Kings College, London, United Kingdom	*Reflecting the positive diversities of European priorities for research and measurement in end-of-life care* Partners: 12 partners in 9 countries European comparisons using tools such as the palliative care outcome scale (POS) and the Support Team Assessment Schedule (STAS) Cultural issues as well as patients' and clinicians' priorities in different care-related issues	New knowledge and European comparisons of measurement tools, patient, and public priorities for care and research. Guidance for clinicians on how to use tools in practice, and new short symptom version of the palliative care outcome scale (POS). Survey on European research activities recommendations for future research.
OPCARE9 2009–2011 Marie Curie Palliative Care Institute University of Liverpool, United Kingdom	*A European collaboration to optimize research and clinical care for patients in the last days of life* Partners: 9 core partners in Europe and two non-European nodes To explore, share, and collate current knowledge and practice in the following areas: Signs and symptoms of approaching death, end-of-life decisions, complementary comfort care, psychological and psychosocial support for patients, relatives, and caretakers, voluntary service and development of the Liverpool Care Pathway (LCP) for the dying patient	Recommendations on drugs for care of the dying patients. Description of difficult and important decisions at the end of life. Care issues in relation to the dying patient.
ATOME 2009—Universities of Bonn, Germany, and Lancaster, United Kingdom, and the WHO	*Access to opioid medication in Europe* Partners: 10 academic partners and public health organizations and 12 country teams Improve access to controlled medicines, e.g., opioids, in Europe Review and suggest changes for drug regulatory legislation in 12 countries in Europe Situational analysis for each country, looking into national legislation	Revision of WHO guideline on drugs Country workshops, national follow-up workshops. Analysis of legislation.
IMpAC T 2010- Radboud University Nijmegen Medical Centre The Netherlands	*IMplementation of quality indicators in PAlliative Care sTudy* Partners: 12 research groups in 12 European universities To develop optimal improvement strategies to improve the organization of palliative cancer and dementia care in Europe and to study factors influencing the effectiveness of the strategies.	Still in progress. Results presented to date include an integrative review on barriers and facilitators to implementing quality improvements in palliative care and changing palliative care: measuring and improving the organization of palliative dementia and cancer care.
EURO-IMPACT (2011–) Vrije Universiteit Brussel, Belgium	*European Intersectoral and Multidisciplinary Palliative Care Research Training* Partners: Five main collaborating countries Develop a multidisciplinary, multiprofessional, and intersectorial educational research framework in Europe aimed at monitoring and improving palliative care	Still in progress. Improving the capacity of researcher in the field. Bridge the gap between individual research institutes, multiple disciplines, and different sectors involved in palliative care research training in Europe. The group has presented findings to date widely at conferences and many publications are emerging.

Table 2.3 *European WHO collaborating centers for palliative care*

Cicely Saunders Institute, King's College, London	London	2008	United Kingdom	WHO Collaborating Centre for Palliative Care, Policy, and Rehabilitation
Institut Catala d'Oncologia, Departament de Salut	Barcelona	2008	Spain	WHO Collaborating Centre for Public Health Palliative Care Programmes
Churchill Hospital	Oxford	1988	United Kingdom	WHO Collaborating Centre for Palliative Care

The newsletter was made possible through a grant from Open Society Foundations and the newsletter is translated to Russian. The newsletter is today integrated in the new EAPC blog (www.eapcnet.wordpress.com). Similarly, Facebook and Twitter are being used increasingly for dissemination of information from, for example, EAPC.

There are three WHO collaborating centers for palliative care in Europe. Oxford was the first, established by Robert Twycross. The WHO collaborating center in Catalonia focuses on palliative care public health programs. The Cicely Saunders Institute in London, which was the first purpose-built institute for palliative care bringing together research, education, and clinical care, focuses on four main areas: developing and evaluating services and new models of care; focused clinical research into symptoms; development, validation, and dissemination in outcome measures; and research to improve living and dying in society, with research into culture, ageing, and home care (Table 2.3). The roles of the WHO collaborating centers are different, although with shared values and philosophies. The centers are placed at institutions such as research institutes, parts of universities, or academies, which are designated by the director general of WHO to carry out activities in support of the WHO's programs.

FUTURE DEVELOPMENT AND CHALLENGES: TO MEET THE NEEDS

The development of palliative care in Europe continues to remain uneven, uncoordinated, and in many countries poorly integrated into national health-care systems. Important factors are still the limited financial and staff resources, problems related to opioid availability, lack of public awareness and government recognition of palliative care, and lack of palliative care education and training programs as well as lack of research capacity. These challenges may be greater in some European countries but are recognized to a varying degree all over Europe. At the same time, there is an increasing political and public awareness of the needs of an ageing population, and the financial and human resources will be requested to meet these needs. The competencies—clinical, scientific, and political—now present within palliative care and also the experience and demands from patients, families, and the public are great resources with the potential to solve many of the problems and needs of European patients and their politicians (Tables 2.4 and 2.5).

Table 2.4 *Palliative medicine as a medical specialty (or sub-/branch specialty) in European countries*

	2005	2012 (certification or in process 2013)
United Kingdom	X	
Ireland	X	
Poland	X	
Romania	X	
Germany	X	
Malta	X	
France		X
Slovenia		X
Czech Republic		X
Norway		X
Denmark		(X)
Hungary		(X)
Slovenia		(X)
Spain		(X)
Sweden		(X)

Note: X, already established as a specialty.

Table 2.5 *Challenges for palliative care development in Europe*

Integration into health-care system and public funding
Expanding to include noncancer patients
Responding to a growing ageing population in a climate of economic uncertainty
Inclusion of palliative care in all relevant undergraduate and postgraduate curricula
Agree on common quality indicators and outcome measures, follow-up, and benchmark
Building research capacity and methods
Studies to build the evidence base underpinning and to improve palliative care practice

REFERENCES

1 WHO/Europe. April 30, 2013. Available from: http://www.euro.who.int/en/ countries.
2 Demography report 2010. Older, more numerous and diverse Europeans. European Commission. Directorate-General for Employment SAal, Unit D.4, Eurostat.; 2011 Contract No.: ISSN 1831-9440.
3 European Union. [cited June 2014]. Available from: www.europa.eu/ about-eu/countries/index_en.htm.

4   Ethnologue: Languages of the World. [cited June 2014]. http://www.ethnologue.com/region/Europe.

5   OECDiLibrary. [cited June 2014]. Available from: http://www.oecd-ilibrary.org/sites/9789264183896-en/01/03/index.html?itemId=/content/chapter/9789264183896-8-en

6   Eurostat. [cited June 2014]. Available from: http://epp.eurostat.ec.europa.eu/portal/page/portal/health/causes_death/data/database

7   Hall, S. Petkova, H. Tsouros, D. Costantini, M. Higginson, I. (ed.) *Better Palliative Care for Older People. Better Practices.* WHO: Copenhagen, Denmark, 2011.

8   Gomes B, Higginson IJ. Where people die (1974–2030): Past trends, future projections and implications for care. *Palliative Medicine.* January 2008;22(1):33–41. PubMed PMID: 18216075.

9   Simon ST, Gomes B, Koeskeroglu P, Higginson IJ, Bausewein C. Population, mortality and place of death in Germany (1950–2050)—Implications for end-of-life care in the future. *Public Health.* November 2012;126(11):937–946. PubMed PMID: 23041107.

10 Davies E, Higginson I. (eds.) *Better Palliative Care for Older People.* WHO: Copenhagen, Denmark, 2004.

11 Davies E, Higginson I. (eds.) *The Solid Facts. Palliative Care.* WHO: Copenhagen, Denmark, 2004.

12 Clark D. From margins to centre: A review of the history of palliative care in cancer. *The Lancet Oncology.* 2007;8(5):430–438.

13 Kübler-Ross E. *On Death and Dying: What the Dying Have to Teach Doctors, Nurses, Clergy, and Their Own Families.* Touchstone: New York, 1997.

14 A D. *A Moral Force: The Story of Dr. Balfour Mount.* Ottawa Citizen. A Moral Force: The Story of Dr. Balfour Mount. Ottawa Citizen. April 23, 2005. [cited June 2014]. Available from: http://www.canada.com/ottawacitizen/story.html?id=896d005a-fedd-4f50-a2d9-83a95fc56464, 2006 April 23, 2005.

15 Beck-Friis B, Strang P. The organization of hospital-based home care for terminally ill cancer patients: The Motala model. *Palliative Medicine.* 1993;7(2):93–100. PubMed PMID: 7505177.

16 De Conno F, Boffi R, Saita L, Ventafridda V. Eighteen years of home care: From assistance by phone to a complete service within the health care system. *Journal of Palliative Care.* 1998 Autumn;14(3):91–93. PubMed PMID: 9770929.

17 Gracia D, Nunez Olarte JM. Report from Spain. *Supportive Care in Cancer: Official Journal of the Multinational Association of Supportive Care in Cancer.* May 2000;8(3):169–174. PubMed PMID: 10789955.

18 Albrecht E. The development of hospice care in West Germany. *Journal of Palliative Care.* September 1989;5(3):42–44. PubMed PMID: 2795338.

19 Clark D, Wright M. *Transitions in End of Life Care.* Clark D, (ed.) Open University Press: Buckingham, U.K., 2003.

20 Serryn D, Hoeben N, Pigeotte H. *Les soins palliatifs en France.* Centre National de Ressources Soin Palliatif: Paris, France, 2012.

21 Baar F. Palliative care for the terminally ill in the Netherlands: The unique role of nursing homes. *EJPC.* 1999;6(5):169–172.

22 World Health Organization. RoaWEC. Cancer pain relief and palliative care. WHO Technical Report Series, No. 804, 1990.

23 Sepulveda C, Marlin A, Yoshida T, Ullrich A. Palliative care: The World Health Organization's global perspective. *Journal of Pain and Symptom Management.* 2002;24(2):91–96.

24 WHO definition of palliative care 2002. [cited June 2014]. Available from: http://www.who.int/cancer/palliative/definition/en/.

25 Doyle D. Proposal for a new name as well as having the new WHO definition of palliative care. *Palliative Medicine.* January 2003;17(1):9–10. PubMed PMID: 12597460.

26 Swedish Register of Palliative Care. [cited June 2014]. Available from: http://palliativ.se/wp-content/uploads/2014/03/SvenskaPalliatvregistret2014.pdf, p. 31.

27 Reitinger E, Froggatt K, Brazil K, Heimerl K, Hockley Jo, Kunz R Morbey, Parker D, Husebo B. Palliative care in long-term care settings for older people: Findings from an EAPC taskforce. *European Journal of Palliative Care.* 2013;20(5):251–253.

28 EAPC. Special interest groups. [cited June 2014]. Available from: http://www.eapcnet.eu/Themes/Specificgroups.aspx.

29 Innovation in pain management. The transcript of a Witness Seminar held by the Wellcome Trust Centre for the History of Medicine at UCL. London: The Trustee of the Wellcome Trust, 2004.

30 World Health Organization. *Cancer Pain Relief.* WHO: Geneva, Switzerland, 1996.

31 Suater S, Rasmussen BH. Volunteers in terminal care. *Omsorg.* 2012;27(1):25–28.

32 Smeding R, Mason S. The role of volunteers in palliative care. *European Journal of Palliative Care.* 2010;19(3):124–126.

33 Centeno C, Clark D, Lynch T. et al. *EAPC Atlas of Palliative Care in Europe.* EAPC Press: Milano, Italy, 2007, 336 p.

34 Centeno C, Lynch T, Donea O, Rocafort J, Clark D. EAPC atlas of palliative care in Europe 2013. Full Edition. Milan: EAPC Press; 2013.

35 Radbruch L, Payne S, Board of Directors of the EAPC. White Paper on standards and norms for hospice and palliative care in Europe: Part 1. Recommendations from the European Association for Palliative Care. *European Journal of Palliative Care.* 2009;16(6):278–288.

36 Radbruch L, Payne S, Board of Directors of the EAPC. White Paper on standards and norms for hospice and palliative care in Europe: Part 2. Recommendations from the European Association for Palliative Care. *European Journal of Palliative Care.* 2010;17(1):22–32.

37 Gomez-Batiste X, Fontanals MD, Roca J, Borras JM, Viladiu P, Stjernsward J et al. Catalonia WHO demonstration project on palliative care implementation 1990–1995: Results in 1995. *Journal of Pain and Symptom Management.* August 1996;12(2):73–78. PubMed PMID: 8754983.

38 Gomez-Batiste X, Porta J, Tuca A, Corrales E, Madrid F, Trelis J et al. Spain: The WHO demonstration project of palliative care implementation in Catalonia: Results at 10 Years (1991–2001). *Journal of Pain and Symptom Management.* August 2002;24(2):239–244. PubMed PMID: 12231156.

39 Gomez-Batiste X, Porta-Sales J, Pascual A, Nabal M, Espinosa J, Paz S et al. Catalonia WHO palliative care demonstration project at 15 Years (2005). *Journal of Pain and Symptom Management.* May 2007;33(5):584–590. PubMed PMID: 17482052.

40 Gomez-Batiste X, Caja C, Espinosa J, Bullich I, Martinez-Munoz M, Porta-Sales J et al. The Catalonia World Health Organization demonstration project for palliative care implementation: Quantitative and qualitative results at 20 years. *Journal of Pain and Symptom Management.* April 2012;43(4):783–794. PubMed PMID: 22265127.

41 Observatoire National de la Fin de Vie. [cited June 2014]. Available from: https://sites.google.com/site/observatoirenationalfindevie/.

42 Cherny N, Baselga J, de Conno F, Radbruch L. Formulary availability and regulatory barriers to accessibility of opioids for cancer pain in Europe: A report from the ESMO/EAPC Opioid Policy Initiative. *Annals of Oncology: Official Journal of the European Society for Medical Oncology/ESMO.* 2010;21:615–626.

43 Lynch T, Clark D, Centeno C, Rocafort J, Flores LA, Greenwood A et al. Barriers to the development of palliative care in the countries of Central and Eastern Europe and the commonwealth of Independent States. *Journal of Pain and Symptom Management.* 2009;37(3):305–315.

44 Mosoiu D, Ryan KM, Joranson DE, Garthwait JP. Reform of drug control policy for palliative care in Romania. *Lancet.* 2006;367(9528):2110–2117.

45 Levine, J. Callaway, M. Foley, K. Hepford, K. Silva, P. *Easing the Pain.* 2010; Open Society Foundations: New York.

46   EAPC. [cited June 2014]. Available from: http://www.eapcnet.eu/Corporate/AbouttheEAPC.aspx.

47   EAPC. [cited June 2014]. Available from: http://www.eapcnet.eu/Corporate/Events/EAPCpastcongresses/1995Barcelonareport.aspx.

48   Poznan Declaration 1998. *European Journal of Palliative Care.* 1999;6:61–63.

49   Council of Europe. Recommendation 1418 (1999)1. Protection of the human rights and dignity of the terminally ill and the dying. 1999.

50   Council of Europe. Recommendation. Rec(2003)24 of the Committee of Ministers to member states on the organisation of palliative care and explanatory memorandum (adopted by the Committee of Ministers 2003). 2003.

51   Korea declaration on hospice and palliative care 2005 [cited 2013]. Available from: http://www.coe.int/t/dg3/health/Source/KoreaDeclaration2005_en.pdf.

52   EACP and IAHPC Declaration of Venice. Adoption of a declaration to develop a global palliative care research initiative. *Progress in Palliative Care* 2006;14:215–217.

53   Radbruch L, Foley K, De Lima L, Praill D, Fürst CJ. The Budapest commitments: Setting the goals a joint initiative by the European Association for Palliative Care, the International Association for Hospice and Palliative Care and Help the Hospices. *Palliative Medicine.* 2007;21(4):269–271.

54   Fürst CJ, De Lima L, Praill D, Radbruch L. An update on the Budapest commitments. *European Journal of Palliative Care.* 2009;16(1):22–25.

55   Radbruch L, Payne S, de Lima L, Lohmann D. The Lisbon Challenge: acknowledging palliative care as a human right. *Journal of Palliative Medicine.* 2013;16(3):301–304.

56   Radbruch L, de Lima L, Lohmann D, Gwyther E, Payne S. The Prague charter: Urging governments to relieve suffering and ensure the right to palliative care. *Palliative Medicine.* 2013;27(2):101–102.

57   Martin-Moreno J, Meggan Harris M, Gorgojo L, Clark D, Normand C, Centeno C. Transforming research into action: A European Parliament report on palliative care. *Eurohealth.* 2009;15(2):22–25.

58   European Parliament, Social, Health and Family Affairs Committee 2008. Palliative care—A model for innovative health and social policy.

59   Kaasa S, Radbruch L. Palliative care research—Priorities and the way forward. *European Journal of Cancer.* May 2008;44(8):1175–1179. PubMed PMID: 18374560. Epub 2008/04/01. eng.

60   EPCRC. [cited June 2014]. Available from: www.epcrc.org.

61   Laugsand EA, Kaasa S, de Conno F, Hanks G, Klepstad P. Intensity and treatment of symptoms in 3,030 palliative care patients: A cross-sectional survey of the EAPC Research Network. *Journal of Opioid Management.* January–February 2009;5(1):11–21. PubMed PMID: 19344044. Epub 2009/04/07. eng.

62   Klepstad P, Fladvad T, Skorpen F, Bjordal K, Caraceni A, Dale O et al. Influence from genetic variability on opioid use for cancer pain: A European genetic association study of 2294 cancer pain patients. *Pain.* May 2011;152(5):1139–1145. PubMed PMID: 21398039. Epub 2011/03/15. eng.

63   Caraceni A, Hanks G, Kaasa S, Bennett M, European Palliative Care Research Collaborative (EPCRC), European Association for Palliative Care (EAPC). Use of opioid analgesics in the treatment of cancer pain: Evidence-based recommendations from the EAPC. *The Lancet Oncology.* 2012;13(2):58–68.

64   Daveson BA, Harding R, Derycke N, Vanden Berghe P, Edwards S, Higginson IJ. The PRISMA Symposium 4: How should Europe progress end-of-life and palliative clinical care research? Recommendations from the proceedings. *Journal of Pain and Symptom Management.* October 2011;42(4):511–516. PubMed PMID: 21963120. Epub 2011/10/04. eng.

65   Mason S, Ellershaw J. OPCARE9—Future directions for optimising the care of cancer patients in the last days of life. *European Journal of Pallivative Care.* 2012;19(4):181–184.

66   ATOME. Atome project. [cited June 2014]. Available from: www.atome-project.eu/.

67   IMPACT. [cited June 2014]. Avaliable from: www.impactpalliativecare.eu.

68   EURO IMPACT. [cited June 2014]. Available from: www.euro-impact.eu.

69   InSup-C. [cited June 2014]. Available from: www.insup-c.eu.

70   General Medical Council, UK. [cited June 2014]. Available from: www.gmc-uk.org/education/postgraduate.asp.

71   De Vlieger M, Gorchs N, Larkin P, Porchet F. Comment: Palliative nurse education—Towards a common language. *European Journal of Pallivative Care* 2204;11(4):135–138.

3

Development of palliative care in Canada

JOHN F. SCOTT, JOSE PEREIRA, PETER LAWLOR

It was in Canada that the early principles of hospice care were reshaped into what we now call palliative medicine. Dr. Balfour Mount coined the term "palliative care" and forged a unique model of care within the heart of academic medicine that combined the philosophy of American thanatology with the principles and techniques of St. Christopher's Hospice. This broadened, secularized model, which integrated palliative care into mainstream health care, became the template for international development of the field.

ORIGINS AND PRECURSORS

Most histories of Canadian palliative care pinpoint the simultaneous opening of two programs as the critical starting points in our development. A "terminal care unit" was opened at St. Boniface Hospital, Winnipeg, in December 1974, and a "palliative care unit" (PCU) at the Royal Victoria Hospital, Montreal, admitted its first patients in January 1975. Yet the full story is more lengthy, complex, and rich in detail. As documented by Wood and Clark [1], in the United Kingdom and Ireland, there exists a long history of care for the dying, incurable, and chronically ill in the tradition of precursor hospices, homes, and hospitals. While yet to be researched and written, this Canadian prepalliative care history would include the courageous work of the Recollets, Jesuits, Sisters of Charity (Grey Nuns), and other religious communities who developed most of Canadian health care from the seventeenth century. But it would also include the charitable homes that developed in the late nineteenth century and early twentieth century for patients with incurable illness, consciously modeled after the British and Irish examples [1].

MONTREAL

The modern history of palliative care, however, begins with the remarkable story of Dr. Balfour Mount [2,3]. In 1965, as a newly graduated physician, he was faced with a terminal prognosis from testicular cancer. In fact, he was referred for radical experimental therapy and survived his illness, eventually going on to become a surgical oncologist and full professor in urology at McGill University. In 1973, he participated in a panel discussing the 1969 book *On Death and Dying* by Elizabeth Kubler-Ross. This spurred him to undertake an exploratory study of the plight of the dying at his home base, the Royal Victoria Hospital, Montreal, perhaps the epitome of Canadian teaching hospitals at the time. The results of the study were explosive [4]. The extent of physical and psychological suffering was unexpected and the denial and neglect of the system demanded a solution. In searching for a response, Mount first turned to American thanatology. He became a friend and colleague of Kubler-Ross and the small cadre of academic psychologists, sociologists, lawyers, and physicians who formed an elite think tank, the International Work Group on Death, Dying, and Bereavement (usually known as IWG) [5]. Mount thrived on the academic dialogue, and eclecticism of these philosophers of the new death. Canadian palliative care, through Mount, always retained this larger perspective on death as it impacts the psyche, the culture, and the law. Yet he also recognized that the gaps in organization of care and the relief of symptoms were beyond the scope of thanatology. Kubler-Ross alerted him to the name Cicely Saunders and Mount made contact with her in 1973—setting up his first extended visit in early 1974. This began a relationship that was pivotal in the development of international palliative medicine as highlighted by the recent publication of Saunders' correspondence that includes many between Saunders and Mount [6]. He quickly recognized that St. Christopher's Hospice, London, demonstrated a set of principles and techniques that were revolutionary. Yet he also recognized that the model of care chosen by Saunders would need to be significantly reshaped to fit the needs and resources of Montreal and to fit the context of a teaching hospital. So, Mount forged a new model, founded on local need and direct research evidence but informed by both American thanatology and British hospice.

WINNIPEG

David Skelton also played a pivotal role in the shape of Canadian palliative care. This UK-trained geriatrician had heard Cicely Saunders' lecture and had participated in clinical rounds with her during his training prior to the opening of St. Christopher's Hospice. When he accepted a geriatrics post in Winnipeg, he developed an inpatient program at St. Boniface Hospital with both a short-term geriatrics unit and a "terminal care unit" [7]. In 1975, Dr. Paul Henteleff became medical director of the terminal care program changing its name to "palliative care" in light of Montreal developments [8]. Dr. Skelton went on to become chair of geriatric medicine in Edmonton where he was pivotal in the founding of a PCU at the Edmonton General Hospital.

CANADIAN MODEL OF "PALLIATIVE CARE"

In 1974, Mount proposed the term "palliative care" to designate a specific program and philosophy of care. His choice revealed a sensitivity to the bilingual culture of Montreal, since some francophones had warned him that "hospice" contained connotations of nursing homes for the indigent. Yet the key motivation arose from his background as an academic surgeon and his intuitive flare for communication. The surgical literature employed the adjective "palliative" sparingly for procedures, often quite demanding ones, aimed to mitigate or relieve pressure, bleeding, or obstruction in the context of tumor or disease that was incurable. When applied to health care, the etymology of the verb "to palliate" contained the sense of "to ease suffering, to abate the violence of pain or disease, and to cover, clothe, or shelter." Mount's genius lay in combining "palliative" with the words "care unit." In the culture of late-twentieth-century medicine, this name demanded attention, associating it with intensive care unit and coronary care unit. The PCU communicated a sense of intensity, urgency, specialized skill, and cutting-edge technology. The language was challenging and assertive: "not only must we stop hiding dying patients in the room at the end of the hall, but we challenge you to care for them in prime real estate at the heart of the tertiary hospital." Most importantly, "palliative" was novel. Despite its obscure usage in surgery, it was essentially a new title whose meaning could be shaped by its creator, and shaped it was. Mount was definitively the first to apply hospice principles in a hospital setting and the first to integrate them into a university.

Saunders, committed to shifting the culture of death, had chosen a monastic approach to addressing the neglect in terminal care. She created a "hospice," a pilgrim guest home, a safe place apart from the chaos of hospitals, NHS funding, and mainstream culture. In contrast, Mount saw "palliative care" as a frontal assault on the death-denying culture of medicine taking full aim at the core of its power, the teaching hospital. Mount was already an academic specialist in urological cancer and so he adopted this bold specialist mindset to the development of palliative care. He chose a completely integrated model, recognizing that success depended on it being embedded in the health-care system including its administrative and funding structures. Palliative care would need to be flexible, adaptable to a variety of health systems. It would need to be entirely secular although open to spirituality in its most inclusive sense. Although he initiated the approach in a teaching hospital and PCU, he continually stressed that palliative care could not be tied to a place. From its beginning, it was an idea, a discipline—not a type of facility. Most of his goals would be accomplished by leveraging knowledge through consultation, teaching, and research. While initially focused on terminally ill cancer patients, the setting of a teaching hospital, the prominent use of consultation, and Mount's strong connections with active oncology all led to involvement at earlier points in the disease than was possible in a hospice. This Canadian model made inevitable the future "upstreaming" and broadening of the scope of palliative care to earlier illness and non-cancer diagnoses, increasingly dominant themes in modern palliative medicine.

It is remarkable that within a few short years, Saunders and other key UK hospice leaders came to acknowledge that "palliative care," both its name and the scope of its meaning, was the appropriate term to designate the overall field and that "hospice" should be reserved for one dimension and form of palliative care. This shift in terminology, already evident in 1976, was essentially complete in 1986 when the World Health Organization (WHO) chose the term "palliative care" for their program [9].

Mount, in his lectures, films, conferences, and interviews, took the stories of hospice and palliative care and retold them in ways that captured the imaginations of the public, the politicians, and the leaders of medicine. In an era when the right to die and euthanasia could have completely dominated the story line, he kept winning people over to palliative care as the appropriate response. He de-emphasized the uniqueness of his creation and in fact used every opportunity to market the ideas of Saunders, Kubler-Ross, and other pioneers. Careful analysis, however, will demonstrate that, in fact, he reshaped their original messages and models, thereby shifting the direction of the international movement. The transition of hospice into palliative care, initiated in Canada in the 1970s, was a critical turning point in the history of the field.

SERVICES

In the past four decades, Canada has witnessed significant expansion in palliative care services but this development has been uneven and has lacked a systematic national approach. Today, Canada is a patchwork of services with many innovative regional models and world-renowned centers of excellence in both urban and rural jurisdictions, interspersed with areas in which there are significant gaps in access to services.

Public Funding: Canada has a health-care system with full public funding for all hospital and physician services and partial support for home care and outpatient pharmaceuticals.

While there are broad national health policies, the delivery of health care is a provincial responsibility and the resulting patchwork of 13 provincial and territorial budgets has led to regional discrepancies. With few exceptions, Canada's entire palliative care network of services has developed and is maintained through public funding. Some freestanding hospices have secured their capital funding through donations and some programs fundraise for a portion of their annual budget, but this is seldom as significant a proportion as in the United Kingdom. In Alberta, hospices are largely integrated within the provincial health-care system and funded largely through public health dollars. In Ontario, on the other hand, only about 40% of hospice budgets have been covered by the public system, contributing, in part, to the large number of cancer deaths in acute care hospitals: a province mean of 53% in 2009 [10].

Access: Canada has the second largest land mass in the world with a small population (35 million) spread over four and a half time zones across urban, rural, and remote regions, adding to regional disparity in access. The Economist Intelligence Unit report of 2010, *The Quality of Death*, ranks Canada as ninth in the world for availability of end-of-life care but fifth for the quality of the services that are available. Overall, it ranks Canada's Quality of Death Index as ninth with a score of 6.2 in comparison to the United Kingdom's first place with 7.9 [11]. While the methodology of this comparison is somewhat controversial, there is evidence that access is variable across provinces and territories and even among regions within provinces [12].

The Canadian Hospice Palliative Care Association (CHPCA) estimates that only 15%–30% of Canadians who require palliative care have access to it [13].

Regionalization: Several Canadian jurisdictions have been at the international forefront of approaching palliative care services from a broader, coordinated population basis. Early units such as Montreal's Royal Victoria Hospital, Toronto's Grace Hospital, and Ottawa's Elisabeth Bruyère Hospital were government funded as pilots with strict evaluation protocols. In Ottawa, the District Health Council formed a committee to plan palliative care services for the capital region in 1978, the first of many regional plans across Canada. Dr. Michael Downing spearheaded a new citywide Victoria Hospice, which began delivering services in 1984. In 1995, Dr. Eduardo Bruera created a comprehensive coordinated regional program in Edmonton, which remains a model for any metropolitan area [14]. These coordinated models have resulted in significant improvements in quality of care, access to health care, and reductions in health-care costs [15].

However, regionalization of services is still not universal in Canada. Provinces such as Alberta and British Columbia (BC) with regional health authorities in which one public entity is singularly responsible for providing all health services appear to have moved ahead in this area. In Ontario, where services are still provided by many different independent health service providers with no regional health authority, only one of the current 14 regions (Champlain Ottawa) have been able to establish a regional program.

Hospital Programs: Canada's trademark has been its strength in providing palliative care within an acute care hospital setting. The initial focus was the PCU model of Montreal and Winnipeg with considerable international interest in this approach of creating a specific ward for end-of-life care [16]. However, it is often not appreciated that much of the work in these seminal programs was consultation and education throughout the hospital and into the community including home care outreach components. Within a decade of the world's first such units in Winnipeg and Montreal, most major hospitals in Canada had some type of palliative care program, usually in the form of a consultation team, and many had designated beds in the form of a PCU. This rapid spread was remarkable in the absence of government policy or designated funding. This reflects a social/cultural movement much more than a rational policy-driven enhancement. In some provinces (such as Alberta), there continues to be an increase in the number of palliative care acute beds and hospices, while others such as Ontario are currently under pressure to decrease the number of beds within acute care hospitals because of the pressure to decrease health-care costs. There remains strong support for palliative care consultation models, and these have flourished, reaching levels of integration seldom seen in other jurisdictions (e.g., the palliative care program at Canada's largest hospital, the Ottawa Hospital, provided 3266 consultations in 2012). Almost all cancer centers in the country now have palliative and symptom management consult services and organizations. This includes Cancer Care Ontario, which oversees cancer care in Canada's most populous province and has made palliative care a priority with regional palliative care leads in each of the province's 14 regions. Cancer Care Ontario has pioneered a population-based systematic approach to screening for symptoms throughout all the province's outpatient cancer clinics using touch screen kiosk technology.

Community/Home Care: Most of the pioneer programs were hospital-focused and directed by hospital-oriented physicians. They reached out to their patients at home in the form of consultation or providing supplemental care alongside existing visiting home care resources. In 1980, under the direction of Dr. Michael Downing, a new program was launched in Victoria, BC, which included a small inpatient hospice but emphasized its home care program that covered the entire small city. This Victoria model has been adopted by most parts of the province of BC giving palliative care in that province a distinctive community orientation. Core government home care services in all provinces have needed to cope with huge demographic shifts. To decrease health-care institutional costs, there has been a rapid "downloading" of care into the community for acute, mental health, chronic, and palliative care. Despite the huge increase in home care budgets in Canada, the services available for an individual palliative care patient dying at home still vary considerably across provinces. Some jurisdictions have home nursing agencies specializing only in palliative care, while others are generalists. In addition to the regular home care program, many cities and some rural areas have independent palliative care or hospice programs that visit in the home to supplement the standard government service. There are serious gaps in primary care physician coverage across Canada. Many patients have no family physician and in some urban jurisdictions family physicians choose not to provide home visits or 24/7 coverage for their palliative care patients. To address this unmet need, some large cities have seen a cadre of physicians emerge who work full time in palliative home care. While some have palliative medicine training, there is a lack of standards and accountability.

Capacity building in the primary care sector to provide primary-level palliative care has been variable across the country. In some jurisdictions, including regional programs in Alberta (Edmonton, Calgary, and Chinook) and BC (Fraser Valley), the emphasis of the palliative care community teams has been on consultation support with occasional shared care, with the goal of increasing the number of primary care clinicians providing hospice palliative care. In Edmonton, for example, most of primary-level hospice palliative care is provided by family physicians with the support of a relatively small consultation team of five palliative care physicians and five nurses. In other urban areas, such as Toronto, palliative care physician teams have largely replaced primary physicians in providing primary-level palliative care. This model is arguably not sustainable. The reasons for this phenomenon are multifactorial but need to be addressed if future population needs are to be met.

Many regions have access to telephone advisory services and mobile teams of specialists in palliative medicine and palliative nursing who assess patients in their home or long-term care facility.

Given its geographic expanse, it is not surprising that innovative rural programs have emerged in Canada. One of the first was established in the late 1990s in the Lakeland Region in northeastern Alberta. This successful and innovative program closed however when regions amalgamated to form larger regions and no additional resources were allocated for palliative care. Since then, other successful rural programs have emerged in central (Calgary sector) and southern (Chinook sector) Alberta, the Truro region of Nova Scotia, and the Niagara region in southern Ontario [17], among others. Kelley et al. developed a framework for developing rural palliative care services and Pereira et al. developed training programs for rural-based family medicine residents [18,19]. Providing palliative care in remote regions such as communities in the far north and within the Arctic Circle remains a challenge.

Pediatric Palliative Care: Canada has been at the forefront of developing pediatric palliative care programs. The first was initiated in the mid-1990s in Halifax, Nova Scotia, by Dr. Gerri Frager. Since then, centers of excellence, in the form of pediatric hospices and home support programs, have opened in several large cities, including Montreal, Vancouver (Canuck House), Edmonton, Calgary, Winnipeg, Ottawa, and Toronto, among others.

Shifts in Terminology: "Palliative care" was the term used across Canada in the early years and remains the dominant term both for specific clinical services and for the academic field as a whole. It refers more broadly to care across the illness trajectory and to all disciplines and volunteers in the field. "Palliative medicine," in Canada, tends to be used to refer to specialist-level physicians in the field. "Hospice" began to be applied in BC in the mid-1980s and then more widely to programs of community-based terminal care, mainly residential freestanding facilities and community support programs. However, regional discrepancies in its usage continue to exist. By the 1990s, tension developed in some quarters between proponents of the broader approach of "palliative care," viewed by some as hospital-focused and interventionalist, and advocates of "hospice," which was more removed from mainstream medicine and limited to end-of-life care. In Ontario, separate associations developed for palliative care and hospice. The Canadian Palliative Care Association took a national and international lead in reconciling these two camps and advocating for a model in which both approaches were important elements on the same spectrum of care. This approach recognized that decision making and care plans could be different depending on where in the illness trajectory the patient found himself or herself to be: earlier in the illness versus at the end of life. To promote this emerging understanding, the national association changed its name in 2001 to CHPCA and today the inclusive term "hospice palliative care" is widely used in government and advocacy documents.

GOVERNMENT POLICY

In the Canadian constitution, health care is a provincial responsibility with considerable differences existing in day-to-day care across the 10 provinces and 3 territories. The federal government has had a history of maintaining broad overarching policy priorities in health, using its clout over funding distribution to the provinces to encourage national standards. However, more recent years have seen a greater distancing by the federal government on provincial health-care matters. For example, there are currently no federal-government-imposed standards on the provision of hospice palliative care.

From 1975 to 1985, many hospitals and community organizations began delivering palliative care without specific permission or policy from the government. They funded these from within their global budgets with minor supplementation from public donations. As the demand for more services and funding grew, provincial governments scrambled to develop responses, often feeling threatened by yet one more demand to increase costs in a system that was already straining. Several pilot projects were supported but governments were concerned to roll out a policy that would include a set of new PCUs across the country.

In 1983, the federal minister of health responded to the growing pressure for palliative care and the increased interest in euthanasia by focusing on the issue of unrelieved pain in cancer patients. An expert advisory committee was struck with Balfour Mount as vice-chair. While most committee members were academics with little exposure and some degree of antagonism to hospice/palliative care, the Saunders–Mount approach to pain management was adopted as the key recommendation [20]. A 40-page monograph on cancer pain management was commissioned and Health Canada distributed this to all physicians and health-care institutions in Canada in 1984 [21]. Translated for use in other countries, it became one of the templates for the WHO Pain Relief and Palliative Care Program launched in 1986.

The next step was for the palliative care community to organize and promote a vision that could be used in forming government policy. Regional and provincial organizations of palliative care began to form in the early 1980s (e.g., Ontario Palliative Care Association 1981). In 1987, a conference was held in Ottawa to begin a dialogue toward a national body, but it was not until 1991 that the Canadian Palliative Care Association was formed and another 3 years before they had a permanent office and staff in Ottawa. From the late 1980s, the palliative care community began to exercise pressure on the government by leveraging the public angst over unrelieved suffering in the dying and the looming issue of euthanasia.

In 1995, the Senate of Canada (the appointed upper house of parliament) formed a committee to study euthanasia and assisted suicide. Their report, *Of Life and Death*, failed to endorse euthanasia, which a number of senators on the committee had previously supported, but instead recommended strong actions to improve palliative care access, standards, and education [22]. Despite political rhetoric, no significant policy changes ensued. In 2000, a new senate committee chaired by the Honorable Sharon Carstairs reviewed the lack of progress since 1995 and called for action in their report *Quality End-of-Life Care: The Right of Every Canadian* [23]. In response, the Quality End-of-Life Care Coalition of Canada (QELCCC) was formed, an alliance of 30–40 national organizations who were committed to support the findings of this report [24]. Now it was not only the palliative care professionals and a few senators but a large consensus of national bodies who were demanding change. The prime minister responded dramatically by appointing Carstairs to the cabinet with special responsibility for palliative care. A National Secretariat on Palliative and End-of-Life Care (PELC) was established, which took the following concrete steps:

- Disability support payments for dying patients were streamlined.
- A new compassionate care benefit was established to allow family members to have support if they need to stop work to provide care for a gravely ill or dying relative.
- A national action plan for PELC began to be developed and a model was published in 2002 [25].
- Online directory of Canadian hospice and palliative care services.
- New education initiatives including support for Pallium Canada (see the following texts).
- A Canada Research Chair in Palliative Care established and awarded to Dr. Harvey Chochinov.
- In concert with the Canadian Council on Health Services Accreditation, an agreement was reached on standards of palliative care for all health-care facilities as well as volunteer organizations.

- The CHPCA also showed international leadership by developing national principles and norms for practice, using the concept of square of organization and square of care to guide the development of services and the provision of care. This model has been very influential within the country and has also been adopted and adapted internationally in several other countries.

Regretfully, a government change led to the end of the national secretariat in 2007. However, many of its accomplishments are maintained and even strengthened through other routes. In 2012, the government funded the QELCCC and the CHPCA to undertake a new wave of planning that will create a national framework or roadmap for palliative care in Canada. Their first report in draft form *The Way Forward* was released in 2013. The 2013 federal budget includes measures to expand the tax credits for family caregivers and to enhance palliative care education of frontline workers through Pallium Canada.

RESEARCH DEVELOPMENTS

Palliative care research in Canada has made a very substantive and important contribution to knowledge synthesis and policy development both nationally and internationally. Seminal studies, conducted in the 1990s, were largely based in specific single centers with highly motivated researchers such as Dr. Bruera in Edmonton [26–29]. These research projects, mostly in patients with cancer, were largely funded through relatively limited local sources, as major granting agencies often did not see the merits of palliative care research. In 1999, as part of the Canadian Strategy for Cancer Control (CSCC), the National Cancer Institute of Canada (NCIC), the Canadian Association of Provincial Cancer Agencies (CAPCA), Health Canada, and the Institute of Cancer Research (ICR) arm of the Canadian Institute of Health Research (CIHR) formed a research alliance to identify cancer research priorities. The identification of palliative care as a major research priority by this research alliance was a significant milestone and as such helped to change the landscape for palliative care research for much of the following decade [30].

As an initial step, the ICR capitalized on two CIHR-preapproved projects: a New Emerging Team (NET) project led by Dr. Pierre Allard from the University of Ottawa on end-of-life care for older persons and a Strategic Training Program grant led by Dr. Robin Cohen from McGill University, aiming to expose students and new researchers to palliative care and promote knowledge translation into clinical practice. The ICR linked with the CIHR Institute of Aging (IA) in equally funding the NET project and the NCIC in funding the Strategic Training Program, each project funded to $300,000 per year for 5 and 6 years, respectively [31].

In 2003, CIHR and 18 funding partners launched a major PELC research initiative [30]. The partnership included eight distinct CIHR Institutes, the CIHR Knowledge Translation Branch, and other agencies such as Heart and Stroke Foundation of Canada and thus gave impetus to PELC research not alone in the cancer domain but in other nonmalignant end-of-life conditions. In 2004, with the help of its various partners, CIHR announced $16.5 million in grants to support the PELC research initiative over a 6-year period. This remarkable development was aimed at meeting the many needs of the palliative research community, most notably interdisciplinary collaboration and infrastructural development. In addition to the previously funded NET and Strategic Training Program awards, the PELC in total funded 19 pilot projects, 10 NETs, and one career transition award. The NET grants supported a diverse array of projects such as palliative and end-of-life transitions, family caregiving, difficult pain, cancer-associated cachexia and anorexia, vulnerable populations, and improving communication and decision making.

Meanwhile, the national Health Canada Secretariat on PELC convened multiple stakeholders including palliative care researchers in 2002 as part of the Canadian Strategy on PELC [30]. A joint national palliative care research working group (RWG) was formed and co-chaired by ICR and Health Canada. The RWG supported the creation of a special review committee at CIHR, called the Palliative and End-of-Life Peer Review Committee (PLC). The PLC reviews PELC-related submissions to the CIHR Open Operating Grants competition, which is held twice yearly. The rationale for the creation of the PLC was to provide a more acceptable and informed review process for PELC research applications outside of the main CIHR PELC Initiative. The RWG contributed to the development and implementation of an online network of PELC researchers. This network is hosted through the Canadian Virtual Hospice website, which also includes PELC tools and resources. The RWG has also supported knowledge translation meetings.

A detailed impact assessment of the PELC Initiative was reported by CIHR in 2009 [30]. Perhaps the most striking impacts relate to simply bringing the research agenda in PELC more to the fore, increasing research productivity and capacity, the training of young investigators, the development of collaborative teams with integrated knowledge translation mechanisms to support the incorporation of research results into practice guidelines, the training of health-care professionals, and health-care policy development. Coinciding with the CIHR PELC Initiative, Canada has doubled its share of PELC publications between 2004 and 2009, sitting at 8%, which is almost twice Canada's overall global share of health research publications. This research productivity is heavily weighted toward the clinical as opposed to basic research. The U.K. National Cancer Institute have provided CIHR with a bibliometric study of 18 leading nations in relation to PELC studies predating the main thrust of the CIHR PELC Initiative: Canada was first ranked regarding the "clinicity" of studies, in that 85% of the papers were categorized as clinically oriented [30]. On a less enthusiastic note, the CIHR Open Operating Grants competitions have attracted less PELC applications than expected; this is despite the potential to be reviewed by the specially created PLC.

The international contribution of Canadian palliative care research warrants special recognition and a summary of the most noteworthy contributions. The contribution of Dr. Eduardo Bruera in the 1990s was immense and far reaching. For example, he developed the Edmonton Symptom Assessment System (ESAS) in 1991, initially as a series of nine visual analogs to rate symptom intensity, later modified to a numerical rating scale, and most recently revised and enhanced further as the revised ESAS or ESAS-r [32,33]. A recent bibliometric review determined that the original 1991 ESAS publication has been cited in over 300 publications [34]. The ESAS has undergone multiple translations and validations [35]. Dr. Bruera provided multiple elective research and clinical training elective for international visiting nurses and physicians, and in turn many of these are now leading international researchers in palliative care. Other notable Albertan research contributions relate to pain management and classification (Dr. Neil Hagen in Calgary and Drs. Robin Fainsinger and Cheryl Nekolaichuk in Edmonton), anorexia–cachexia (Dr. Vickie Baracos in Edmonton), and the economic analysis of health services delivery (Dr. Konrad Fassbender in Edmonton) [15,36,37].

Dr. Michael Downing and colleagues in Victoria developed the Palliative Performance Scale, which is now one of the most widely used performance measures internationally in palliative care settings [38]. The work of Dr. Harvey Chochinov and his colleagues in the Manitoba Palliative Care Research Unit is particularly well recognized internationally and he has collaborated with leading researchers globally. His work on dignity-conserving therapy is especially recognized [39]. Dr. Neil MacDonald of McGill University has published extensively on cancer-related cachexia and collaborated with many international researchers [40]. Dr. Ed Chow and colleagues in Sunnybrook Health Sciences, Toronto, has reported many studies on symptom control in relation to palliative radiation therapy [41]. The Canadian research contribution to knowledge synthesis on quality of life (Drs. Rodin and Zimmermann and colleagues at the University of Toronto and Dr. Robin Cohen and colleagues at McGill University) in its broadest context has been substantive [42,43]. Significant Canadian research contributions on delirium in palliative care have been made by groups in Laval, Ottawa, Montreal, and Edmonton [44–46]. Recognition should also be given to contributions from various other emerging or existing programs of research, including population-based symptom assessment [47], advanced care planning [48], health services research [17,18,49], spirituality [50], interprofessional education [51], and e-learning [52].

PROFESSIONAL EDUCATION

Since most of the pioneer programs in Canada were based in a teaching hospital, integration of palliative care into medical and nursing schools began early. Initially, this took the form of ad hoc lectures and elective rotations but designated time began to be established in some faculties of medicine by the mid-1980s.

In 1990, representatives from all 16 Canadian medical schools met under the leadership of Dr. Neil MacDonald to develop a palliative care curriculum in order to advance the teaching of the field at the undergraduate level. Published in 1991, the Canadian Palliative Care Curriculum is one of the world's first curricula for the field [53]. Becoming a national education committee of the new Canadian Society of Palliative Care Physicians, the group revised the curriculum in 1997 and published it with a *Case-Based Manual*, with each case illustrating a part of the curriculum [54]. For several years, every medical student in Canada received a copy of the manual and the committee kept deans informed on how their school compared with others in Canada in terms of curriculum uptake. A second national initiative entitled *Educating Future Physicians in Palliative and End-of-Life Care* (EFPPEC) was initiated by Drs. Larry Librach and José Pereira with the support of the Association of Faculties of Medicine of Canada and included many of the same goals as the earlier program. While continuing to compete with many priorities in the medical school curriculum, palliative medicine has been able to secure a foothold in almost all the schools—not only to teach the specifics of our discipline but also the overarching philosophy of medicine. Most crafters of medical education seek out palliative medicine for its capacity to demonstrate relevant examples of communication, ethics, goals of care, professionalism, interdisciplinary care, reflective practice, and whole person care.

In addition to the residency program for those aiming to be specialists in palliative medicine, there are compulsory or selective rotations (usually 4 weeks) for trainees in radiation oncology, general internal medicine, anesthesiology, neurology, family medicine, psychiatry, emergency medicine, and several subspecialties including medical oncology, geriatrics, and critical care. Increasingly, palliative care questions/scenarios are being included in the certification examinations of specialties, subspecialties, and family medicine.

There are several noteworthy education programs across the country for health professionals already in practice. These include the Pallium Project's Learning Essential Approaches to Palliative Care (LEAP), a 2-day interprofessional course for primary-level providers (physicians, nurses, and pharmacists), the McMaster and Victoria Hospice in-depth 5-day courses, and the de Souza Institute's training programs for nurses, among others. The precursor to the LEAP course was first developed in 2001 and LEAP currently is being delivered across the country. The Pallium Project is currently underway to renew the course and develop thematic courses ranging from LEAP Emergency Department and LEAP Chronic Illnesses, to LEAP Surgery and LEAP Oncology and LEAP Pediatrics.

SPECIALIZATION

It is ironic that Canada, perhaps the first country in which palliative care was embraced by academic medicine, has been one of the slowest to clarify the specialty status of this new discipline.

From 1990 to 1998, several palliative medicine training positions were developed on an ad hoc basis led by the pioneer fellowships in Ottawa (1990) and Edmonton (1991), but they lacked official recognition and linkage with one another. In 1992, several academic palliative care directors including Mount, MacDonald, and Scott, aided by John Seely, dean of medicine in Ottawa, agreed that formal specialization was critical [55]. The Royal College of Physicians and Surgeons of Canada (RCPSC), the body with responsibility for postgraduate training and specialty development, demanded that any new application arise from a national society of physicians who practice the new discipline. In 1993, the Canadian Society of Palliative Care Physicians was registered and a formal application for recognition was prepared. This outlined the urgent health-care need underlying the request, the history of Canadian leadership in the field internationally, the other jurisdictions who had granted specialty or subspecialty status to palliative medicine, the large number of academic posts and noncertified training programs in Canada, and the rapid growth in literature, journals, research, and conferences devoted to the field [56]. The 1994 application requested a 2-year subspecialty in palliative medicine with access from multiple specialties. The application was well received at the college and considered to be the strongest in many years. Medicine and surgery gave their approval and pediatrics was considering it when the politics of medicine stepped in to scuttle the proposal. Surprisingly, the College of Family Physicians of Canada (CFPC), who controls family medicine training, voiced strong opposition to the specialization proposal. They argued that palliative care was integral to the generalist vision of family medicine. Specialty development was claimed to be unnecessary and would compromise the role of primary care in caring for the dying [57]. Certainly, many of the palliative care leaders in Canada had been trained as family physicians but most of these recognized that family medicine did not have the desire or capacity to develop palliative medicine as a specific field. Behind these protests lay a series of other turf fights between the two accreditation colleges on emergency medicine, care of the elderly, and other areas in which family physicians focused their practice. The RCPSC, not wanting another conflict, refused to proceed in the face of family medicine opposition.

At this point, the diplomacy of John Seely was critical [58]. A compromise emerged with both colleges agreeing to a 1-year conjoint training program in palliative medicine with oversight by a unique conjoint advisory committee. The RCPSC designated palliative medicine as a subspecialty in the category accreditation without certification (AWC) based on it being an emerging discipline. The CFPC agreed to it as a year of additional training with no special designation (in 2012, a certificate of special competence was approved). From 1999 to 2010, this program trained 96 physicians at the 12 accredited universities [59].

In 2010, the RCPSC, responsible for all specialization in Canada, ruled that a formal specialization process was now required since the conjoint program was only acceptable on a temporary basis for an emerging discipline. In 2011, the Canadian Society of Palliative Care Physicians submitted a new application for a 2-year subspecialty in palliative medicine with access from multiple specialties. However, the controversy over entry criteria continued. Since family physicians comprise the largest group of palliative care physicians, the RCPSC was reluctant to approve a process of certification to which they had no access. On the other hand, the CFPC opposed using family medicine training as a base for RCPSC specialization, believing that its use as a 'stepping stone' would undermine development of comprehensive family medicine. Nonetheless, in October 2014, the RCPSC gave final approval to a 2-year subspecialty in palliative medicine with entry from the base specialties of medicine, pediatrics, anesthesiology, neurology and family medicine. This is the first time in Canada that family medicine certification will be accepted as an entry criteria for subspecialty training. There will also be a practice eligible route to challenge the subspecialty examination for certificants of either College who have practiced palliative medicine for at least 5 years.

What has been the impact of this lengthy delay? On one hand, it forced us into a unique and fruitful training partnership between specialists and generalists. On the other hand, it has probably slowed our momentum, blocking government funding, decreasing a research focus, and giving us a confusing patchwork of academic leadership. In the 17 medical schools in Canada, palliative medicine is a fully recognized division in only 8: 2 as a division of the department of medicine, 3 within a department of oncology, 3 under a department of family medicine, and 1 is a joint program under 3 departments. Most of the others have palliative care as a program or area of focus without formal designation. The tardiness in developing a specialty has left us without a secure academic home with few administrative champions and a relative dearth of scholarship opportunities. Nonetheless, many programs have stepped up to the challenge and overcome the obstacles through innovative alliances and new opportunities can be expected as a result of subspecialty approval.

NATIONAL INITIATIVES OF NOTE

- *International Congress on Palliative Care*
  Less than 2 years after opening, McGill hosted the first international meeting in the field—the International Congress on Care of the Terminally Ill, now called the International Congress on Palliative Care [60]. Meeting every 2 years since the first meeting in 1976 saw Mount bring Saunders, Kubler-Ross, and representatives from around the world to open a dialogue on this new field that he envisioned as wider than either American thanatology or British hospice. Historically, the congress has had a critical role in internationalizing palliative care. It has promoted a breadth of vision that allows all nations and cultures to translate palliative care principles into their own health-care system. The 2012 congress had 1300 delegates from 35 countries meeting over 5 days. The congress has been a canvas for the creativity of Mount incorporating art, music, poetry, film, dance, and all forms of cultural expression into the scientific format of a medical

conference. The congress successfully integrated sessions on psychosocial, spiritual, and cultural issues with those of basic and clinical science in such a way that physicians, nurses, social scientists, and volunteers all felt welcome.

- *Journal of Palliative Care*
  This "made in Canada" international journal published its first issue in 1985, one of the earliest and most influential publications in the field. Under the consistent guidance of a single editorial team (Dr. David Roy, Electa Baril), the journal has presented the best of Canadian palliative care work alongside many contributions from the international community. Historically, it was an important vehicle by which the Canadian terminology and model of palliative care was communicated globally.

- *Pallium Canada*
  The federal government first funded the Pallium Project in 2001 to improve the care of patients with advanced illness in rural and remote Canadian communities. Under the direction of Dr. Jose Pereira and Michael Aherne, the project broadened its focus in 2003 to primary care across Canada. Pallium began developing innovative educational programs [61]. It received $4 million dollars of funding from the primary care renewal envelope of Health Canada and produced 72 subprojects across the country, building palliative care capacity. These projects included the development of the LEAP courseware and a specialist-level palliative care chaplaincy program, the Pallium Palliative Pocketbook for primary health professionals, mapping out the competencies in palliative care using the DACUM method, an education program for care providers in first nations and aboriginal communities, telephone helplines across western provinces (BC, Alberta, Saskatchewan, and Manitoba), children's bereavement programs in Manitoba, materials for informal caregivers in the arctic regions, and monthly teleconferencing education programs for rural and remote communities [62]. In the federal budget of March 2013, Pallium was awarded new funding to provide training to frontline workers with a broadened community mandate to include long-term care, emergency, surgery, hospital, and noncancer diagnoses as well as using the new technologies of education, including apps, e-learning, and telemedicine.

- *Canadian Virtual Hospice*
  Launched in 2004, the Canadian Virtual Hospice (www.vitualhospice.ca) is an interactive network consisting of four website portals directed toward patients, family/friends, volunteers, and health-care providers with the aim to promote information exchange, communication, and mutual support. One may use a website for seeking specific information or as a two-way resource to share thoughts, ask questions, and learn from the experience of others. Led by Dr. Harvey Chochinov, it was initially supported by the federal secretariat on PELC.

- *Quality End-of-Life Care Coalition of Canada*
  In December 2000, the existing palliative care professional organizations formed a broader alliance with 30–40 national organizations with some stake or interest in the promotion of palliative care, with the CHPCA acting as the secretariat. The coalition has played a pivotal role in

all subsequent dealings with the government and in the interface with the public. Many of the accomplishments discussed earlier under government policy were possible because of the political support provided by such a strong alliance as illustrated by their documents: Blueprint for Action (2000), Dying for Care (2004), and The Way Forward (draft 2013). Even though the present government discontinued support for a national secretariat, it announced funding in 2013 for the coalition to develop strategies for community-oriented palliative care. The coalition continues to press for the full implementation of a national strategy on palliative care.

FUTURE TRENDS

The development of palliative care in Canada was driven by stories of unmet need and by the 1960s a shift in the culture of death. The future of palliative care will be shaped by the same two forces of demography and culture. The aging and immigration patterns predicted for the next two decades are similar to those of Western Europe with large proportionate increases in cancer, organ failure, and dementia. By 2041, one in four Canadians is expected to be over 65. The economy and health structures will struggle to cope with huge numbers, forcing new prognostic and cost-effectiveness boundaries. Simultaneously, the cultural angst of euthanasia forms an explosive, unpredictable backdrop to palliative care development. The federal parliament convincingly defeated a bill to legalize assisted suicide in 2010 by a vote of 226 to 59. Furthermore, a Parliamentary Committee on Palliative and Compassionate Care reported in 2011, voicing strong support for increased palliative care [63]. Nonetheless, several cases are now before the courts arguing for the right to assisted suicide and in June 2014, the province of Quebec enacted legislation to authorize euthanasia "medical aid in dying" which is expected to be challenged in the courts as a form of euthanasia that contravenes federal law. Much of the public media story is fueled by the fear of dying in distress and the life-affirming message, and symptom-relieving tools of palliative care are critically needed in this debate. While bureaucrats and most politicians agree that palliative care is the appropriate policy response, the cry for the right to die on demand often holds sway in the public forum.

The formal specialization of palliative medicine can be expected to initiate a period of expansion and clarification especially in academic circles. However, the salary support for specialist consultants and the funding of their training is far from secure in most provinces.

Canada's trademark facility, the PCU in an acute care setting, will see its role diminish. As demonstration/teaching units, they will remain invaluable, but proportionately more of the work will be done through consultants in hospital wards, clinics, homes, and long-term care facilities. Freed from the association with the tight prognostic boundaries of a unit's admission criteria, palliative care medicine can have a broader and earlier impact on all illness and on the culture of medicine

as a whole. There will always remain a strong instinct to create special places in which to protect, treasure, and listen to those close to death. Every regional plan must include sufficient hospice and PCU beds to care for those who have a clearly defined terminal illness and cannot be cared for at home or in their long-term care facility.

We look forward to policy at both federal and provincial levels that will ensure a strong and enduring national strategy for palliative care.

Key learning points

- The term "palliative care" was coined in Canada by Dr. Balfour Mount in 1974.

- The Canadian model of palliative care developed by Mount reshaped the Saunders UK model in several ways, becoming the template for further international development.

- Palliative care in Canada started in academic hospitals in the form of PCUs with outreach consultations to the community and other parts of the hospital.

- The pioneers in Canada were academic physicians, leading to early promotion of research and education initiatives.

- The development of palliative medicine as a subspecialty has been slower than in other countries, having met roadblocks in finding flexible entry criteria that do not exclude family physicians. Since 1999 the RCPSC has accredited palliative medicine as a subspecialty without certification and supported a one year conjoint residency for specialists and family physicians. In 2014 the RCPSC approved a 2 year subspecialty with certification which allows entry from multiple specialties including family medicine, as well as a practice eligible route to challenge the examination.

- Undergraduate medical education was promoted by the development of one of the first national palliative care curricula along with a case-based textbook (*Palliative Medicine: A Case-Based Manual*).

- Canada has a strong record of population-based planning for palliative care services and comprehensive regional programs (e.g., Edmonton, Victoria, Ottawa) that include community and hospitals.

- Productive, high-quality future research activity is dependent on sustaining the research capacity generated through CIHR's PELC Initiative: in particular, this will mean ongoing and even increased collaboration and sustained funding to support a clinically oriented cadre of researchers in PELC to have protected time and training to conduct research projects.

- The federal and provincial governments have supported many innovative initiatives but there remain serious gaps and regional disparities in access to palliative care (only 15%–30% of those who need palliative care have access to it).

REFERENCES

1   Wood J and Clark D. The historical development of inpatient services within United Kingdom and Ireland adult voluntary hospices. *Palliative Medicine* 2008;22:1–2

2   Hamilton J. Dr. Balfour Mount and the cruel irony of our care for the dying. *Canadian Medical Association Journal* 1995;153(3):334–336.

3   Duffy A. *A Moral Force: The Story of Dr. Balfour Mount.* The Ottawa Citizen. Ottawa, Ontario, Canada: Postmedia Network Inc., April 23 2005.

4   Mount BM, Jones A, and Patterson A. Death and dying: Attitudes in a teaching hospital. *Urology* 1974;4(6):741–748.

5   Mount BM. International group issues proposal for standards for care of terminally ill. *Canadian Medical Association Journal* 1979;120(10):1280–1282.

6   Clark D. *Cicely Saunders—Founder of the Hospice Movement. Selected Letters 1959–1999.* Oxford, U.K.: Oxford University Press, 2002.

7   Skelton D. The hospice movement: A human approach to palliative care. *Canadian Medical Association Journal* 1982;126(5):556–558.

8   Canadian Virtual Hospice. Paul Henteleff, take a bow. 2009. Available at http://www.virtualhospice.ca/en_US/Main+site+Navigation/Home/For+Professionals/Take+a+bow/Dr_+Paul+Henteleff.aspx. Accessed June 9th 2014.

9   World Health Organization. *Cancer Pain Relief.* Geneva, Switzerland: World Health Organization, 1986.

10 Cancer Quality Council of Ontario Report, 2012. http://www.csqi.on.ca/cms/one.aspx?portalId=258922&pageId=273637. Accessed June 9th 2014.

11 The Economist Intelligence Unit. The quality of death. Ranking end-of-life care across the world. 2010. Available at http://www.eiu.com/site_info.asp?info_name=qualityofdeath_lienfoundation&page=noads. Accessed June 9th 2014.

12 Sussman J, Barbera L, Bainbridge D, Howell S, Yang J, Husain A, Librach SL, Viola R, and Walker H. Health system characteristics of quality care delivery: A comparative case study examination of palliative care for cancer patients in four regions in Ontario, Canada. *Palliative Medicine* 2012;26(4):322–335.

13 Quality End-of-Life Care Coalition of Canada, Canadian Hospice Palliative Care Association. The way forward national framework: A roadmap for the integrated palliative approach to care. Draft—Spring 2013. Ottawa, Ontario, Canada: The Way Forward Integration Initiative, 2013.

14 Brenneis C and Bruera E. Models for the delivery of palliative care: The Canadian model. In: Bruera F and Portenoy R (eds.) *Topics in Palliative Care*, Vol. 5. New York: Oxford University Press, 2001.

15 Fassbender K, Fainsinger R, Brenneis C, Brown P, Braun T, and Jacobs P. Utilization and costs of the introduction of system-wide palliative care in Alberta, 1993–2000. *Palliative Medicine* 2005;19(7):513–520.

16 Mount BM. The problem of caring for the dying in a general hospital; the palliative care unit as a possible solution. *Canadian Medical Association Journal* 1976;115(2):119–121.

17 Marshall D, Howell D, Brazil K, Howard M, and Taniguchi A. Enhancing family physician capacity to deliver quality palliative home care: an end-of-life, shared-care model. *Canadian Family Physician* 2008;54(12)1703:e1–e7.

18 Kelley ML, Williams A, DeMiglio L, and Mettam H. Developing rural palliative care: Validating a conceptual model. *Rural & Remote Health* 2011;11(2):1717.

19 Pereira J, Palacios M, Collin T, Galloway L, Murray A, Violato C, and Lockyer J. The impact of a hybrid online and classroom-based course on palliative care competencies of family medicine residents. *Palliative Medicine* 2008;22(8):929–937.

20 Cancer pain: Report of the expert advisory committee on the management of severe chronic pain in cancer patients. Minister of Supply and Services Canada; 1984. Cat. No: H42-2/4-1984.

21 Scott J. Cancer pain: A monograph on the management of cancer pain. Minister of Supply and Services Canada; 1986. Cat. No.: H42-2/5-1984E.

22 Special senate committee on euthanasia and assisted suicide. Of life and death. Minister of Supply and Services Canada; 1995. Cat. No.: YC2-351/1-01E.

23 The Standing committee on Social Affairs, Science and Technology. Quality end-of-life care: The right of all Canadians: The final report. 2000. Available at http://www.parl.gc.ca/Content/SEN/Committee/362/upda/rep/repfinjun00-e.htm.

24 Quality End-of-Life Care Coalition of Canada. End of life care Canada: QELCCC Home. 2013. Available at http://www.qelccc.ca/. Accessed May 8, 2013.

25 Ferris F, Balfour H, Bowen K et al. *A Model to Guide Hospice Palliative Care.* Ottawa, Ontario, Canada: Canadian Hospice Palliative Care Association, 2002.

26 Bruera E, Neumann CM, Gagnon B, Brenneis C, Kneisler P, Selmser P, and Hanson J. Edmonton regional palliative care program: Impact on patterns of terminal cancer. *Canadian Medical Association Journal* 1999;161(3):290–293.

27 de Stoutz ND, Bruera E, and Suarez-Almazor M. Opioid rotation for toxicity reduction in terminal cancer patients. *Journal of Pain and Symptom Management* 1995;10(5):378–384.

28 Bruera E, Velasco-Leiva A, Spachynski K, Fainsinger R, Miller MJ, and MachEachern T. Use of the Edmonton Injector for parenteral opioid management of cancer pain: A study of 100 consecutive patients. *Journal of Pain and Symptom Management* 1993;18(8):525–528.

29 Bruera E, de Stoutz N, Velasco-Leiva A, Schoeller T, and Hanson J. Effects of oxygen on dyspnoea in hypoxaemic terminal cancer patients. *Lancet* 1993;342(8862):13–14.

30 Palliative and End-of-Life Care Initiative: Impact Assessment—Report http://www.cihr-irsc.gc.ca//41180.html.

31 A New Era in Canadian Palliative and End-of-Life Care Research http://www.cihr-irsc.gc.ca/e/27756.html.

32 Bruera E, Kuehn N, Miller MJ, Selmser P, and Macmillan K. The Edmonton Symptom Assessment System (ESAS): A simple method for the assessment of palliative care patients. *Journal of Palliative Care* 1991;7:6–9.

33 Watanabe SM, Nekolaichuk C, Beaumont C, Johnson L, Myers J, and Strasser F. A multi-centre comparison of two numerical versions of the Edmonton Symptom Assessment System in palliative care patients. *Journal of Pain and Symptom Management* 2011;41:456–468.

34 Cummings G, Biondo PD, Campbell D, Stiles C, Fainsinger R, Muise M, and Hagen N. Can the global uptake of palliative care innovations be improved? Insights from a bibliometric analysis of the Edmonton Symptom Assessment System. *Palliative Medicine* 2011;25(1):71–82.

35 Nekolaichuk C, Watanabe S, and Beaumont C. The Edmonton Symptom Assessment System: A 15-year retrospective review of validation studies (1991–2006). *Palliative Medicine* 2008;22(2):111–122.

36 Fainsinger RL, Nekolaichuk C, Lawlor P, Hagen N, Bercovitch M, Fisch M, Galloway L et al., An international multicentre validation study of a pain classification system for cancer patients. *European Journal of Cancer* 2010;46(16):2896–2904.

37 Prado CM, Lieffers JR, McCargar LJ, Reiman T, Sawyer MB, Martin L, and Baracos VE. Prevalence and clinical implications of sarcopenic obesity in patients with solid tumours of the respiratory and gastrointestinal tracts: A population-based study. *Lancet Oncology* 2008;9(7):629–635.

38 Downing M, Lau F, Lesperance M, Karlson N, Shaw J, Kuziemsky C, Bernard S. et al., Meta-analysis of survival prediction with Palliative Performance Scale. *Journal of Palliative Care* 2007;23(4):245–252.

39   Chochinov HM, Kristjanson LJ, Breitbart W, McClement S, Hack TF, Hassard, T, and Harlos M. Effect of dignity therapy on distress and end-of-life experience in terminally ill patients: A randomised controlled trial. *Lancet Oncology* August 2011;12(8):753–762.

40   MacDonald NE, Alexandra M, Mazurak VC, Dunn GP, and Baracos VE. Understanding and managing cancer cachexia. *Journal of the American College of Surgeons* July 2003;197(1):143–161.

41   Caissie A, Culleton S, Nguyen J, Zhang L, Zeng L, Holden L, Dennis K et al., EORTC QLQ-C15-PAL quality of life scores in patients with advanced cancer referred for palliative radiotherapy. *Supportive Care in Cancer* 2012;20(4):841–848.

42   Jones JM, McPherson CJ, Zimmermann C, Rodin G, Le LW, and Cohen SR. Assessing agreement between terminally ill cancer patients' reports of their quality of life and family caregiver and palliative care physician proxy ratings. *Journal of Pain & Symptom Management* 2011;42(3):354–365.

43   Cohen R, Leis AM, Kuhl D, Charbonneau C, Ritvo P, and Ashbury FD. QOLLTI-F: Measuring family carer quality of life. *Palliative Medicine* 2006;20(8):755–767.

44   Gagnon P, Allard P, Masse B, and DeSerres M. Delirium in terminal cancer: A prospective study using daily screening, early diagnosis, and continuous monitoring. *Journal of Pain and Symptom Management* 2000;19(6):412–426.

45   Gaudreau J-D, Gagnon P, Harel F, Roy M-A, and Tremblay A. Psychoactive medications and risk of delirium in hospitalized cancer patients. *Journal of Clinical Oncology* 2005;23(27):6712–6718.

46   Lawlor P, Gagnon B, Mancini I, and Pereira J. Occurrence, causes and outcome of delirium in patients with advanced cancer. *Archives of Internal Medicine* 2000;160:786–794.

47   Seow H, Barbera L, Sutradhar R, Howell D, Dudgeon D, Atzema C, Liu Y. et al., Trajectory of performance status and symptom scores for patients with cancer during the last six months of life. *Journal of Clinical Oncology* 2011;29(9):1151–1158.

48   Heyland DK, Barwich D, Pichora D, Dodek P, Lamontagne F, You JJ. et al. Failure to engage hospitalized elderly patients and their families in advance care planning. *JAMA Internal Medicine* 2013 (published online April 1 2013).

49   Seow H, Snyder CF, Mularski RA, Shugarman LR, Kutner JS, Lorenz KA, Wu AW, and Dy SM. A framework for assessing quality indicators for cancer care at the end of life. *Journal of Pain & Symptom Management* 2009;38(6):903–912.

50   Sinclair S and Chochinov HM. The role of chaplains within oncology interdisciplinary teams. *Current Opinion in Supportive and Palliative Care* 2012;6(2):259–268.

51   Luke R, Solomon P, Baptiste S, Hall P, Rukholm E, and Carter L. Online interprofessional health sciences education: From theory to practice. *Journal of Continuing Education in the Health Professions* 2009;29(3):161–167.

52   Pereira J and Murzyn T. Integrating the "New" with the "Traditional": An Innovative Educational Model. *Journal of Palliative Medicine* 2001;4(1):31–37.

53   MacDonald N, Mount B, Boston W, and Scott J. The Canadian palliative care undergraduate curriculum. *Journal of Cancer Education* 1993;8(3):197–201.

54   MacDonald N. (ed.) *Palliative Medicine—A Case-Based Manual.* Oxford, U.K.: Oxford University Press, 1998.

55   Scott J, MacDonald N, and Mount B. Palliative medicine education. In: Doyle D, MacDonald N, and Hanks G (eds.) *Oxford Textbook of Palliative Medicine.* Oxford, U.K.: Oxford University Press, 1993, pp. 1169–1199.

56   Mount BM, Scott JF, Bruera E, Cummings I, Dudgeon D, and MacDonald N. Palliative care—A passing fad? Understanding and responding to the signs of the times [editorial]. *Journal of Palliative Care* 1994;10(1):5–7.

57   Librach SL. Defining palliative care as a specialty could do more harm than good! *Journal of Palliative Care* 1988;4(1–2):23–24.

58   Seely JF, Scott JF, and Mount BM. The need for specialized training programs in palliative medicine. *Canadian Medical Association Journal* 1997;157(10):1395–1397.

59   Schroder C and Van Dijk J. Discussion paper: Postgraduate education for palliative medicine physicians. *Canadian Society of Palliative Care Physicians*; 2010.

60   Shephard DA. Principles and practice of palliative care. *Canadian Medical Association Journal* 1977;116(5):522–526.

61   Aherne M and Pereira J. A generative response to palliative service capacity in Canada: The Pallium project. *International Journal of Health Care Quality Assurance Incorporating Leadership in Health Services* 2005;18(1):iii–xxi.

62   Aherne M and Pereira JL. Learning and development dimensions of a Canadian primary health care capacity building project. *Leadership in Health Services* 2008;21(4):1751–1879.

63   Parliamentary Committee on Palliative and Compassionate Care. Not to be forgotten: Care of vulnerable Canadians. Ottawa: The Committee; 2011. Available at http://pcpcc-cpspsc.com/wp-content/uploads/2011/11ReportEN.pdf.

64   Assemblee nationale Quebec. Mourir dans la dignite [Rapport]. Quebec: Bibliothèque et Archives nationales du Québec; 2012. Available at http://www.assnat.qc.ca/fr/actualities-salle-presse/nouvelle/actualite-25939.html.

4

Development of palliative medicine in the United States

CHARLES F. VON GUNTEN

INTRODUCTION

The development of palliative medicine, the physician discipline working as part of the larger interdisciplinary field of palliative care, can be viewed in four distinct phases in the United States. The first phase lasted until the work of Dr. Kübler-Ross and Dr. Cicely Saunders became known. The second phase saw the development of hospice programs across the country. The third phase was characterized by the development of a distinct and officially recognized subspecialty of medicine. The fourth phase, in which we currently find ourselves, is the integration of the specialty within standard health care. Each of these phases is presented to the extent that their history is known either in the published literature or in the memories of those who experienced them. The focus is on the physician component of this history, which is the remit of this chapter. While seminal events in the development of hospice and palliative care in the United States are highlighted, we purposely do not fully describe the larger history and vast army of interdisciplinary pioneers due to space constraints.

EARLY HISTORY

In the United States, as elsewhere in the western world, dying was a routine part of life until the mid-twentieth century when it became medicalized [1]. Dr. William Osler reported on the first large series of dying patients during his time at the hospital he helped to found at Johns Hopkins Medical School in Baltimore, Maryland [2]. Interestingly, he found that the majority of deaths he observed were not painful. Osler is also reported to have said that morphine was *God's own medicine*. In his famous textbook *Principles and Practice of Medicine*, there is no specific mention of the care of the dying, though Cushing reports an anecdote involving Sir William's exceptionally sensitive care of a dying child [3].

Osler, who firmly based his practice in study of the history of medicine, was presumably referring to what little was written. A British monograph from 1701 refers to the curative and palliative uses of opium as a *noble panacea* [4]. In 1890, Dr. Herbert

Snow published a text on the palliative treatment of terminal cancer, with an appendix on the use of the opium pipe [5]. Yet while the term *palliate* appears in the title of a medical paper as early as 1802 in England [6], there was relatively little in the textbooks of medicine, or in formal medical training, to guide physicians in addressing the array of symptoms and issues associated with the care of the dying patient.

In 1935, Harvard physician Alfred Worcester published three lectures on *The Care of the Aged, the Dying and the Dead*, intending them to serve as outlines of what medical students should be taught because of the *unpardonable* shifting of care for the dying to nurses and sorrowing relatives [7]. The text was circulated during the early days of the hospice movement in the United States, in part because of its thorough clinical observations and procedural recommendations (referencing Sir Henry Halford, Sir William Temple, the Soeurs Augustines, and Florence Nightingale) and in part because of its specific injunctions that younger physicians not allow science to distract them from the arts of medical practice and the "indispensable qualifications of the physician: tact and courtesy...sympathy and devotion...(for) in the practice of our art it often matters little what medicine is given, but matters much that we give ourselves with our pills."

The care of the dying as a special or particular focus of activity was carried out in a small number of homes beginning in the nineteenth century, much like has been described in France, Ireland, Scotland, and England [8]. All of them had Christian roots. They were founded and run by religious orders devoted to the sick and dying as a demonstration of their faith. No particular physician component was identified. Rather, they appear to have been founded from a nursing perspective.

One early example in the United States is the Dominican Sisters of Hawthorne [9]. Rose Hawthorne, the daughter of the American novelist Nathaniel Hawthorne, took a 3-month nursing course at New York's Cancer Hospital, then moved into a three-room cold-water flat on New York City's Lower East Side, and began to nurse the poor with incurable cancer. Rose Hawthorne took the religious name Sister Alphonsa and founded a Roman Catholic order called the Dominican Congregation of St. Rose of Lima, later called the Servants of Relief for Incurable Cancer. In imitation of St. Rose of Lima, the order "strives to give their lives to prayer and compassionate service to Jesus, who comes to them in every patient." In 1901, Sister Alphonsa opened Rosary Hill Home in Hawthorne, New York (now the mother home of the order) as an inpatient facility to care for the dying [10]. The order is now called the Dominican Sisters of Hawthorne and operates six homes in five states [10]. True Ryndes, Adult Nurse Practitioner (ANP), a leader in the hospice movement in the United States, worked in their house in Fall River, Massachusetts, from 1971 to 1975.

Another example is Calvary Hospital in New York City. In 1899, a small group of widows began caring for destitute women with terminal diseases. They were inspired by the work of Madame Jeanne Garnier in Lyon, France, who founded several homes for the dying poor she called hospices or *Calvaires* beginning in 1842 [11]. These widows first worked out of their own homes, then in two town houses in Greenwich Village before moving to Bronx in 1915. The House of Calvary was renamed Calvary Hospital in 1969. Several Roman Catholic religious orders have served Calvary Hospital over the years, but the organization was never owned or run by a specific religious order [12].

This is not to say that physicians were unaware of the issues facing the dying during this period. However, in the United States, as elsewhere in Europe, the scientific method was introduced in the late nineteenth century as a way out of the fog of anecdote and quackery that passed for contemporary health care. Dr. William Osler, writing in the late nineteenth century, said "If all medicines were thrown in the ocean, it would be all the better for mankind and all the worse for the fish." The new idea was that human suffering stemmed from disease. If one could but understand the disease, the suffering would be stopped.

The Second World War marked the beginning of the U.S. federal government's unprecedented financial commitment to the expansion of medicine, medical research, and mental health services as well as to the construction and development of hospitals as the primary site of health care. In 1945, the research budget for the National Institute for Health was $180,000. In 1948, the National Institute for Health, advocating a categorical approach to research and treatment of disease, became the National Institutes for Health, with the creation of the National Heart Institute. Two years later, the budget had grown to $46.3 million [13]. The percentage of doctors describing themselves as full-time specialists grew from 24% in 1940 to 69% in 1966 [14]. As advances in medical science were made, the dispassionate, scientific, mechanistic approach to patient problems ironically fostered the unintended consequence where the patient was treated as a disassembled bystander bearing the disease. Patients who complied submissively with *the system* were deemed *good* patients, while those who sought a high degree of interactivity with their care providers and challenged routines, were often dubbed *problem patients*, deviant, and uncooperative [15]. Further, medicine adopted a near-sacred duty to combat all the known causes of death [16].

Organizational theorist William Starbuck has noted that organizations and their environments perform in a fashion described by scientists as *coevolution*, that is, "evolving simultaneously toward better fit for each other" [17]. Thus, it could be said that as the practice of medicine in the United States more greatly valued determinism and prediction in the postwar period, the environment changed, causing a need for compensatory medical care embodied in the palliative competencies of hospice care. Some long-time observers of this process have referred to this shift as "a return to good medicine" [18], a medicine that embraces the medical arts, along with appropriate and tailored use of therapeutics, as expressed in the twentieth century by physicians Alfred Worcester, Charles Aring, Eric Cassel, and Ira Byock [18–19]. While *good medicine* may sound trite, this evolutionary step heralded a shift in the meaning of the term *palliate*. Where palliative treatments were formerly advocated to *cloak* or *hide* symptoms, newer palliative approaches actually address the etiology of the symptoms and/or modify the disease, not addressing cure but the prospect of reduced symptom burden or longer life expectancy.

AFTER 1970

The success of the growing investment in medical research in the first half of the twentieth century produced unprecedented scientific discoveries and a change in the pattern of illness in the second. In the beginning of the twentieth century, Americans usually died of infectious diseases or trauma. This may explain why there was so little attention to it by physicians—it happened quickly. By the second half of the century, Americans were living longer and dying primarily of atherosclerotic diseases (myocardial infarctions, stroke, congestive heart failure) and cancer. Instead of death occurring quickly (in days), there was a new period of *dying* that occurred over weeks to years. The paradigm of the scientific method was developed to counter the causes of death of the early part of the century, such as pneumococcal pneumonia. From this point of view, the change in patterns of death without a change in the scientific method leads directly to the physician to perceive death as a medical failure. Suffering, with its physical, psychological, social, and spiritual components, was the result of the failure of the scientific method. Like most jests, the following statement, appearing in the medical literature in 1975, reflected an uncomfortable element of truth: "If only patients could leave their damaged physical vessels at the hospital for repair, while taking their social and emotional selves home" [20].

By the end of the 1960s, a lively discussion about American attitudes and practices related to death can be discerned [14]. For example, empirical research had demonstrated that patients with terminal illness did want to talk about death when they were given the opportunity to do so [21]. The publication of *On Death and Dying* by Dr. Elisabeth Kübler-Ross in 1969 capped this period with a fortuitous combination of media exposure and timely substance [22]. A remarkable feature of her work was that she interviewed real patients facing death in teaching sessions with other students in a manner similar to that used in teaching other medical subjects. More important, probably, was that Dr. Kübler-Ross was a highly effective speaker and was soon making personal appearances throughout the nation.

Another charismatic physician speaker in the United States at this period was Dr. Cicely Saunders. She founded St. Christopher's Hospice in a southern suburb of London England in 1967 as the culmination of nearly 20 years of direct observation of the care of terminally ill people. She had been publishing and speaking about her ideas about modern hospice care since the late 1950s. The work of Dr. Cicely Saunders and her colleagues at St. Christopher's Hospice in London reached the ears of many Americans like so many seeds on fertile ground—ground that was in part prepared by Dr. Kübler-Ross.

A particularly significant aspect of Kübler-Ross's presentations was the response of nurses [23], whom many credit, along with social workers and occasional lay persons, as the true force behind the hospice movement in the United States. The dialogue opened by Kübler-Ross helped to give recognition to what they had experienced and helped coalesce some of the anger they felt at how *modern* health care approached the care of the dying.

For a short but eventful period of time, death became the media's darling. This exaggerated attention was manifest in newspapers, magazines, television, and public presentations. Two early programs were established during this time.

In 1974, Florence Wald, then dean of the School of Nursing at Yale University in New Haven, Connecticut, led the founding of The Connecticut Hospice with the advice from Dr. Saunders [24] and two others. Dr. William Lamers, a psychiatrist who pioneered much of the early interactions between hospices and medical schools as medical director of one of the country's first hospice programs, Hospice of Marin, wrote "When we gathered in New Haven to talk about hospice care, Dr. Bal Mount of Montreal and I were the only two doctors there," crediting Dr. Mount, a urological surgeon from the Royal Victoria Hospital in Montreal, as "the true hospice pioneer on this continent" [25]. Dr. Sylvia Lack, a young physician who had just completed training in hospice medicine at St. Christopher's, was soon recruited to be the medical professional. Connecticut Hospice played a seminal role in the development of hospice care in the United States.

By contrast, in New York City, a consulting team began working throughout St. Luke's Hospital in 1974, the same year that Connecticut Hospice was founded. In contrast with Connecticut Hospice, this nurse-led team provided support only in the hospital for dying patients in a scattered-bed model [26]. It soon failed.

A grassroots *hospice movement* started in the United States at this time resulting in the founding of a large number of hospice programs. In contrast with the *flagship* program in New Haven, local circumstances varied greatly. Hospice advocates had to develop positive collaborations as *outsiders* to the established health-care system rather than as a part of the system itself. Advocates were united by a vision of care that was defined by a departure from the types of situations that had been increasingly criticized—the patient either subjected to invasive but useless medical care or virtually abandoned. Physicians who played notable local and national activist roles included Tom Licht (Wisconsin), Dan Hadlock (Florida), Bob Brown (Minnesota), and pediatric hematologist/oncologist

Doris Howell (Philadelphia and San Diego). Despite the roles that some physicians played, the hospice movement was perceived by the dominant medical system as antiphysician and countercultural. Those working in hospices at that time do not disown these perspectives, but remember it as a time that was more antipain and antisuffering than antiphysician.

In response to the enthusiasm but lack of consensus on common principles for hospice care in the United States, the Connecticut Hospice in New Haven sponsored a meeting for American and Canadian hospice advocates. From this meeting eventually emerged the National Hospice Organization (NHO). They developed a proposed set of standards and criteria that have been revised at least four times and expanded considerably since first developed [27].

National hospice study

The National Hospice Demonstration Project was a research study funded by the U.S. federal government to study hospice care in the United States [14]. The study aimed to select hospices from each of three models that had emerged in the United States: (1) hospital hospice programs, the majority of which had only a dedicated inpatient unit without a significant home care component, (2) home health agency hospice programs without a dedicated hospice inpatient unit, and (3) independent hospice programs exclusively serving terminally ill patients, with or without a special inpatient unit, staffed primarily by volunteers (professional and lay). The Health Care Financing Administration chose 26 existing hospice programs as demonstration projects out of 233 applicants in late 1979 and provided them with funding for their work. The chosen hospice programs were located in 16 states. A comparison sample of 14 hospice programs were chosen from among the three types as controls who did not receive federal demonstration project funding. The chosen hospices were not randomly selected. During the course of the National Hospice Study, 13,374 patients were admitted to participating demonstration and nondemonstration hospice programs between 1980 and 1982. Broadly, the study showed that patients who chose hospice care did not suffer any deprivation of care, often (although not always) required a lower level of expenditure, and were usually able to spend more time at home.

Medicare hospice benefit

Interestingly, the U.S. Congress enacted legislation in 1982 authorizing funding for hospice care to all beneficiaries of the federal health-care plan designed to cover the hospital needs of people over the age of 65 and those who are disabled. They did this while the National Hospice Study was still in progress. However, the findings were consulted in the subsequent development of the regulations that implemented the congressional action.

The standards and criteria that had been developed by the NHO received enough dissemination and favorable reaction in the U.S. Congress that they became part of the Medicare

Hospice Benefit. This broad source of funding led to rapid growth of hospice care in the United States. This federal funding led to the establishment of a hospice industry in the United States—a group of organizations that receive 85% of their funding under the terms of this federal legislation.

Hospice programs had to have a medical director—but, under Medicare guidelines, the role explicitly did not include direct patient care. The model was that the patient's primary care physician would continue to serve as the patient's physician with the support of the hospice team.

SUBSPECIALTY RECOGNITION

The path to formal recognition of the physician component of palliative care began to develop from physicians working either with hospice programs or from cancer programs. Kathleen Foley, MD, was an early pioneer [28]. As a neurologist at Memorial Sloan Kettering Cancer Hospital in New York, she both researched and advocated for better pain management as part of cancer care. Many of the physicians who trained with her as fellows in pain management have gone onto leadership roles in palliative medicine. For example, in 1987, Dr. T. Declan Walsh was recruited to the Cleveland Clinic to establish a palliative medicine program as part of the oncology division at the clinic. His program was unique in the United States in that it was a physician-led program that was hospital and health-care system based [29]. Dr. Walsh had received his training at St. Christopher's Hospice in London as well as Memorial Sloan Kettering in New York City. The program initially provided hospital consultation and outpatient clinic services.

Dr. Josefina Magno, founder and medical director of Hospice of Southeast Michigan, formed the International Hospice Institute in 1978 as a forum for education and dissemination of research findings [30]. It was also to be a forum for mutual support. In 1988, she instituted the Academy of Hospice Physicians comprised of 125 physicians who gathered in Estes Park, Colorado, at one of the meetings. The group subsequently became independent and changed its name to the American Academy of Hospice and Palliative Medicine. It has become the professional association for physicians practicing palliative medicine in the United States.

In 1993, Dr. David Weissman established a consultation service at the Medical College of Wisconsin in Milwaukee [31]. He subsequently described the elements of palliative medicine consultation [32]. That same year, Dr. Charles von Gunten established a consultation service at Northwestern Memorial Hospital in Chicago that was organizationally linked with a 10-bed acute palliative care unit and a hospice program. Their models led to rapid dissemination to other hospitals in the United States [33].

Progress toward a recognized specialty took an important step forward in 1997 when the Institute of Medicine (IOM), an independent and influential body that advises the U.S. Congress, highlighted deficiencies in the health-care system's approach to end-of-life care and called for the development

of professional expertise in palliative medicine in the United States to make this knowledge widely available in U.S. health care [34]. The IOM report recognized the benefits formal recognition of palliative medicine would confer [35].

A model for the physician role was described [36]. Primary palliative medicine is the responsibility of all physicians. This includes basic approaches to the relief of suffering and improving quality of life for the whole person and his or her family. Secondary palliative medicine is the responsibility of specialists and hospital or community-based palliative care or hospice programs. The role of the secondary specialist or program is to provide consultation and assist the managing service by taking over the care of the most challenging patients and families. Tertiary palliative medicine is the province of academic centers where new knowledge is created through research and new knowledge is disseminated through education. In addition, tertiary palliative medicine centers are likely to care for the most challenging cases.

The need for the specific skills of palliative medicine at the end of life was reinforced in concurring opinions from the U.S. Supreme Court that refused to recognize a constitutional right to assisted suicide [37]. The American College of Physicians and the American Board of Internal Medicine both called for general physician competency in the care of persons with terminal illness [38]. Efforts to introduce palliative medicine training into physician education followed [39–44].

Significant philanthropic funding spurred the development of palliative medicine. The Robert Wood Johnson Foundation, under the project direction of Rosemary Gibson and Victoria Weisfeld, invested U.S.$95 million between 1997 and 2004 in projects aimed to improve end-of-life care. The project that most influenced the physician component was the Education for Physicians on End-of-Life Care (EPEC) Project led by Linda Emanuel, MD, PhD, Frank D. Ferris, MD, and Charles F. von Gunten, MD, PhD. Initially developed in conjunction with the American Medical Association, the project convened leaders in the field to assemble a core curriculum in palliative medicine and disseminate it through a train-the-trainer dissemination model. The project was successful in reaching its educational targets [45]. But there were several unanticipated effects of the project. First, the AMA's imprimatur lent legitimacy to a cadre of EPEC trainers who felt encouraged to volunteer to teach the material at educational programs in their home institutions and advocate for curriculum change in their medical schools and residency programs. Second, in a survey of palliative medicine physicians, the majority said that the EPEC Project was their entry into the field [46].

The Robert Wood Johnson Foundation also sponsored the Center to Advance Palliative Care (CAPC), initially led by Christine Cassel, MD, and Diane Meier, MD. The focus of this national center was to advance palliative care in hospitals and health systems. Dr. Cassel had played an instrumental role in the recognition of geriatrics as a subspecialty 20 years earlier and held leadership positions in organized medicine in the United States.

Another major philanthropic spur was the Project on Death in America (PDIA). The Open Society Institute (funded by

George Soros) invested U.S.$45 million between 1994 and 2003 in a variety of projects to *change the culture of dying* in the United States. One of those projects, the PDIA Faculty Scholars' Program led by Susan D. Block, MD, aimed to develop academic leaders in palliative medicine in the nation's medical schools. By the conclusion of the U.S.$15 million project, the 89 PDIA Faculty Scholars had in turn been successful in attracting U.S.$115 million in grants and awards from federal and other funding sources. Many PDIA Scholars are now in leadership positions in the nation's medical schools, residency programs, and the committees that are shaping the specialty.

The combination of EPEC (a program of physician education), CAPC (a program to advance the practice of palliative medicine in hospitals and health systems), and the PDIA Scholars (a program to develop academic physician leaders) can be viewed as a strategy to stimulate an evolution in American health care more rapidly than it would otherwise take.

The strategy worked. In 2004, the American Board of Internal Medicine convened a summit of all member boards of the American Board of Medical Specialties to consider an application to formally recognize palliative medicine. Formal recognition followed in 2006 [47]. Unexpectedly, 10 members of the American Board of Medical Specialties agreed to cosponsor the subspecialty. This was the first time this has happened in the history or organized medicine in the United States: The American Board of Anesthesiology, the American Board of Emergency Medicine, the American Board of Family Medicine, the American Board of Internal Medicine, the American Board of Pediatrics, the American Board of Obstetrics and Gynecology, the American Board of Physical Medicine and Rehabilitation, the American Board of Psychiatry and Neurology, the American Board of Radiology (that includes radiation oncology), and The American Board of Surgery. Furthermore, members of the boards that do not cosponsor (such as the numerous subspecialty surgical boards) can petition through a cosponsoring board for a diplomate to be recognized (such as a member of the American board of Urology).

Also in 2006, the Accreditation Council for Graduate Medical Education established a 1-year training program for physicians training to be subspecialists in hospice and palliative medicine. Conceptually, the single approved pathway is open to any physician. However, some physicians like those from emergency medicine or pediatrics have been challenged to find a program that will accept a physician without training in standard adult medicine.

INTEGRATION INTO HEALTH CARE

In contrast with most countries of the world, the United States does not have a centrally planned health-care system; it has a health-care market. In general, innovations are driven by a business model and the decisions of independent hospitals rather than a response to a central directive with associated funding.

The CAPC at Mount Sinai Medical School in New York City developed both a sustained resource for individuals to advance the business case for palliative care in hospitals and health systems and a sustained social marketing effort to make hospitals and health systems want to hire palliative medicine physicians as part of palliative care programs. Their efforts drove the number of palliative care programs in hospitals to more than double [48]. Concomitantly, the number of hospice programs grew, the size of hospice programs increased, and more of them hired their own physicians. As a consequence, the demand for physician specialists in hospice and palliative medicine has outstripped supply.

The composition and minimum quality standards for hospice programs are driven by requirements for funding laid down in the Medicare Hospice Benefit—the funding source for 85% of all hospice care in the United States. There was no such standard for palliative care programs. Drawing on the experience of the Canadians [49], British, and Australians, a national consensus project for palliative care promoted U.S. standards that were adopted by the National Quality Forum and the Joint Commission for Accreditation of Hospitals and Health Care Systems [50]. Although voluntary, it is expected that with the passage of time, these standards will gradually make the isolated nurse, chaplain, or physician without training, experience, or interdisciplinary team to be regarded as a *palliative care service*.

Probably, the largest engine driving palliative medicine into U.S. health care will be the value proposition. Influential studies demonstrating that palliative care both improves quality and reduces cost for the care of the most ill (and most expensive) citizens are likely to drive palliative medicine from the margins to the center of the American health-care system [51,52].

The last element for palliative medicine to be well established in the United States is a stable platform in academic medicine. Academic faculty with adequate support for the development of integrated programs of clinical care, education, and research is essential for the field to grow and develop on a part with other medical disciplines. Sadly, the overall economic times in which this development in medicine has occurred, has limited the ability of the federal government to play its usual role in funding such a development. The political process needed to drive such federal funding is distracted by the larger mismatch between calls on the federal purse and sources of revenue to fund it.

The greatest challenge to the field of palliative medicine in the United States is now one of meeting the need that has been developed. As of 2012, there are about 5000 physicians working in specialist roles in palliative medicine. The need is projected to be 10,000–20,000 in response to the growing number of elderly with complex medical problems. Yet, as of 2012, fellowship programs train only about 200 physicians per year. It is unlikely that philanthropy will fund the needed additional training slots. While health systems might fund them, out of self-interest to meet the needs of a changing health-care system that moves away from a fee-for-service, volume-based model, that remains purely conjecture.

REFERENCES

1 Aries P. *Western Attitudes toward Death from the Middle Ages to the Present.* The Johns Hopkins University Press, Baltimore, MD, 1974, p. 76.

2 Hinohara S. Sir William Osler's philosophy on death. *Annals of Internal Medicine* 1993;118:638–642.

3 Cushing H. *The Life of Sir William Osler.* Oxford University Press, London, U.K., 1940.

4 Jones J. The mysteries of opium revealed. I. Gives an account of the name, make, choice, effects, etc., of opium. II. Proves all former opinions of its operations to be meer chimera's. III. Demonstrates what its true cause is; by which he easily and mechanically explains all (even its most mysterious) effects. IV. Shows its noxious principle, and how to separate it; there by rendering it a safe, and noble panacea; whereof, V. He shows the palliative and curative use. London, 1701 (monograph).

5 Snow HL. *The Palliative Treatment of Incurable Cancer; with an Appendix on the Use of the Opium-Pipe.* Churchill, London, U.K., 1890.

6 Reece R. The medical guide, for the use of the clergy, heads of families, and seminaries, and junior practitioners in medicine; comprising a complete modern dispensatory, and a practical treatise on the distinguishing symptoms, causes, prevention, cure, and palliation. London, 1802.

7 Starr P. *The Social Transformation of American Medicine.* Basic Books, New York, 1982, pp. 342–343.

8 Saunders C. History of hospice care. In: *Oxford Textbook of Palliative Medicine*, 2nd edn. edited by Derek Doyle, Geoffrey W. C. Hanks, and Neil MacDonald. New York, N.Y., Oxford University Press, 1999. Oxford University Press, New York, 1998.

9 http://www.eldritchpress.org/nh/rose.html. (Accessed October 4, 2004).

10 http://www.hawthorne-dominicans.org. (Accessed October 4, 2004).

11 Saunders C. Foreward. In: *Oxford Textbook of Palliative Medicine*, 2nd edn. edited by Derek Doyle, Geoffrey W. C. Hanks, and Neil MacDonald. New York, N.Y., Oxford University Press, 1999. Oxford University Press, New York, 1998, p. vi.

12 http://www.calvaryhospital.org. (Accessed October 4, 2004).

13 *The Social Transformation of American Medicine*, Basic Books, New York, 1982, pp. 358–359.

14 Mor V, Greer DS, and Kastenbaum R. The hospice experiment: An alternative in terminal care. In: *The Hospice Experiment.* Eds: Mor V, Greer D, and Kastenbaum R, Johns Hopkins University Press, Baltimore, MD, 1988, p. 6.

15 Raps CS, Peterson C, and Jonas M. Patient behavior in hospitals: Helplessness, reactance or both? *Journal of Personality and Social Psychology* 1982;42:1036–1041.

16 Callahan D. Death and the research imperative, *New England Journal of Medicine* March 2, 2000;342(9):654–656.

17 Starbuck WH Organizations and their environments, In: *Handbook of Industrial and Organizational Psychology.* Ed: Dunnette, MD, Rand, New York, , 1976, pp. 1069–1123.

18 Aring Charles D. *The Understanding Physician.* Wayne State University Press, Detroit, MI, 1971.

19 Cassell, EJ. *The Nature of Suffering and the Goals of Medicine.* Oxford University Press, New York, 1991.

20 Byock I, Caplan A, and Snyder L. Beyond symptom management-physician roles and responsibility in palliative care; for the American College of Physicians–American Society of Internal Medicine, End-of-Life Care Consensus Panel, 2001.

21 Lorber J. Good patients and problem patients: Conformity and deviance in a general hospital, *Journal of Health and Social Behavior* 1975;16:213–225.

22 Ptacek JT and Eberhardt TL. Breaking bad news. A review of the literature. *Journal of the American Medical Association* August 14, 1996;276(6):496–502.

23 Kuebler-Ross E. *On Death and Dying: What the Dying Have to Teach Doctors, Nurses, Clergy and Their Own Families.* MacMillan Publishing, Inc., New York, 1969.

24 Mor V, Greer DS, and Kastenbaum R. The hospice experiment: An alternative in terminal care. In: *The Hospice Experiment.* Eds: Mor V, Greer D, and Kastenbaum R, Johns Hopkins University Press, Baltimore, MD, 1988, P. 7.

25 Wald FS, Foster Z, and Wald JH. The hospice movement as a health care reform. *Nursing Outlook* 1980;28:173–178.

26 Personal Communication T Ryndes.

27 O'Neill WM, O'Connor P, and Latimer EJ. Hospital palliative care services: Three models in three countries. *Journal of Pain and Symptom Management* 1992;7:406–413.

28 *Hospice Standards.* National Hospice Organization, Arlington, VA, 1979.

29 Foley, K. Advancing palliative care in the United States. *Palliative Medicine* 2003;17:89–91.

30 Walsh TD. Continuing care in a medical center: The Cleveland Clinic Foundation palliative care service. *Journal of Pain and Symptom Management* 1990;5:273–278.

31 Holman GH and Forman WB. On the 10th anniversary of the organization of the American Academy of Hospice and Palliative Medicine (AAHPM): The first 10 years. *American Journal of Hospice and Palliative Care* July–August, 2001;18(4):275–278.

32 Weissman DE and Griffie J. Weissman Integration of palliative medicine at the Medical College of Wisconsin 1990–1996. *Journal of Pain and Symptom Management* March 1998;15(3):195–207.

33 Weissman DE. Consultation in palliative medicine. *Archives of Internal Medicine* Apr 14, 1997;157(7):733–737.

34 von Gunten CF and Martinez J. A program of hospice and palliative care in a private, non-profit U.S. teaching hospital. *Journal of Palliative Medicine* 1998;1(3):265–275.

35 Field MJ and Cassel CK, (Eds). Approaching death: Improving care at the end of life. National Academy Press, Washington, DC, 1997.

36 von Gunten CF. Secondary and tertiary palliative care in U.S. hospitals. *The Journal of the American Medical Association* 2002;287:875–881.

37 U.S. Supreme Court. No 95-1858, 96-110. Justice O'Connor, Justice Stevens concurring opinions.

38 American Board of Internal Medicine. *Caring for the Dying: Identification and Promotion of Physician Competency-Educational Resource Document.* American Board of Internal Medicine, Philadelphia, PA, 1996.

39 American Board of Internal Medicine. *Program Requirement for Residency Education in Internal Medicine.* American Board of Internal Medicine, Philadelphia, PA, 1998.

40 Billings JA and Block S. Palliative care in undergraduate medical education. *The Journal of the American Medical Association* 1997;278:733–743.

41 Block, SD, Bernier, GM, Crawley LM. et al. Incorporating palliative care into primary care education. *The Journal of General Internal Medicine* 1998;13:768–773.

42 Barnard D, Quill T, Hafferty F, Arnold R, Plumb J et al. Preparing the ground: Contributions of the pre-clinical years to medical education for care near the end-of-life. *Academic Medicine* 1999;74:499–505.

43 Meier DE, Morrison RS, and Cassel CK. Improving palliative care. *Annals of Internal Medicine* 1997;127:225–230.

44 Arnold, R. The challenges of integrating palliative care into postgraduate training. *Journal of Palliative Medicine* 2003;5:801–807.

45 Robinson K, Sutton S, von Gunten CF, Ferris FD, Molodyko N, Martinez J, and Emanuel LL. Assessment of the education for physicians on End-of-life Care (EPEC) project. *Journal of Palliative Medicine* 2004;7(5):637–645.

46 Cohen B and Salsberg, E. The supply, demand and use of palliative care physicians in the United States. A report prepared for the Bureau of HIV/AIDS, Health Resources and Services Administration. Center for Health Workforce Studies, School of Public Health, University at Albany, Albany, NY. September 2002. http://chws.albany.edu.

47 Von Gunten CF. Bedazzled by a home run. *Journal of Palliative Medicine* 2006;9:1036.

48 Morrison RS, Maroney-Galin C, Kralovec PD, and Meier DE. The growth of palliative care programs in United States hospitals. *Journal of Palliative Medicine* 2005;8:1127–1134.

49 West PJ, Ferris F, Balfour H, Bowen K, Farley J, Hardwick M, Lamontagne C, Lundy M, and Syme A. Not just any old standards...2002 Canadian Hospice Palliative Cae Association standards. *Canadian Oncology Nursing Journal* 2004;14:2:112–116.

50 Ferrell B, Connor SR, Cordes A, Dahlin CM, Fine PG, Hutton N, and Leenay M. The national agenda for quality palliative care: The National Consensus Project and the National Quality Forum. *Journal of Pain and Symptom Management* 2007;33:737–744.

51 Morrison RS, Penrod JD, Cassel JB, Caust-Ellenbogen M, Litke A, Spragens L, and Meier DE. Cost savings associated with U.S. hospital palliative care consultation programs. *Archives of Internal Medicine* 2008;168:1783–1790.

52 Kelley AS, Deb P, Du Q, Carlson A, and Morrison RS. Hospice enrollment saves money for Medicare and improves care quality across a number of different lengths-of-stay. *Health Affairs* 2013;32:552–561.

5

Development of palliative medicine in Latin America

ROBERTO WENK

THE REGION

The Latin American (LA) region with a total population of 572 million is made up of 20 different countries.[1] It is characterized by its heterogeneity: there are differences among countries in size, population, population density, natural resources, per capita income, resources assigned to the health, development, health systems, stages of demographic and epidemiological transition, etc.

The following figures help to display the differences:

- Area: Brazil 8,515,767 km^2 and El Salvador 21,040 km^2
- Population: Brazil 193,946,886 and Uruguay 3,286,314
- Population density: El Salvador 341.5/km^2 and Bolivia 9/km$^{2\,2}$
- Physician density: Cuba 6.39/1000 population and Colombia 1.35/1000 population
- Health expenditure (% of gross domestic income): Costa Rica 10.9% and Bolivia 4.8%[3]
- Human development index: medium 7, high 10, and very high 24

But certainly for the purpose of this chapter, one circumstance is common to the region: there are serious deficiencies in the way that most of the health systems care for patients with advanced incurable diseases.

NEED OF PALLIATIVE CARE

There is a growing need of palliative care (PC) in the region due to the increases of chronic diseases and the aging population.

LA countries are experiencing demographic transition from predominantly young societies to others, which are increasingly aging. Countries present an increased trend in life expectancy at birth, even if an important difference prevails in the region (62 years in Haiti, 79 years in Chile).[5] In 2011, people over 65 represented 10.7% of the population.[6]

Changes in lifestyle and increased risk factors have produced an increase in noncommunicable chronic diseases (NCDs). Approximately 46,904,000 > 69.3% = 1,859,255 persons die annually in LA (2010 world's crude death rate 8.2[7]). In 2009, NCDs were responsible for 69.3% of the deaths (3,364,500) in the South Cone region and Brazil: cardiovascular 41.9%, cancer 24.1%, respiratory 8.7%, digestive 7.2%, diabetes mellitus 6.2%, and others 11.9%.[8]

Sixty percent of all the patients (2,018,400) and 80% of the cancer patients (648,675) could have benefited from PC.[9] Since the treatment unit includes two responsible caregivers for each patient, more than 4 and 1.3 million, respectively, could have benefited from PC.

These data exhibit the current regional need of PC and predict its increase in the coming years with the current demographic and epidemiologic trends. Moreover, these data confirm that PC is and will continue to be the most cost effective and, in many cases, the only possible care option for many patients.

It is compulsory that the society be organized to increase its availability and accessibility to provide the care required by this group of patients and their families.

PALLIATIVE CARE

The development was erratic and without a definite pattern. It began in the early 1980s and had increasing intensity during the 1990s. The new century began with most countries having some activity in PC.

According to the classification of Wright et al. of countries according to PC development, 11 are in stage 3 (isolated provision of care), 6 in stage 4 (preliminary integration with standard health services), and 2 in step 4b (advanced integration with standard health services).[10]

PC is still not available to a significant and acceptable number of patients; regional receptiveness is not enough to meet the demands of PC. The main obstacles include inadequate health-care coverage, inefficient processes that fail to make opioids available and accessible, lack of expertise of health-care workers, and insufficient support from national health authorities.

To assess the existing PC, it is necessary to describe some interrelated issues that affect its availability and accessibility.

What Is Known at Present?

The following information is mostly based on the Latin American Atlas of Palliative Care (Atlas Latinoamericano de Cuidados Paliativos),[11] the first systematic study of PC in LA—most previous reports were based on partial information due to lack of regional data.[12–14] The beginning of the process of central collection and analysis of data is a big step forward in the efforts to disseminate PC.

For the purpose of this chapter, the term "service" includes individuals, teams, and units.[15]

Service Provision

Most of the regional health systems fail to provide proper care to patients with advanced, chronic life-threatening diseases.

In more than half of the countries, PC is not recognized as a discipline and is not included systematically in the free public or private health systems.

It is estimated that only 5%–10% of patients who need PC receive it, that over 90% of services are in large cities, and that most of them provide care to adult cancer patients. These facts make the situation certainly much worse for patients with non-oncological diseases, pediatric patients, or those residing in small cities or rural, remote, areas.

This failure in the provision of PC is due to both insufficient numbers of specific structures and trained health personnel.

In the region there are 922 PC services: 0.163 per 100,000 inhabitants ranging from 1,606 (Costa Rica) to 0.024 (Honduras). Chile has the highest number (277). Service distribution:

- By type of care: Home care (0.04 per 100,000 inhabitants), inpatient care (0.034 per 100,000 inhabitants), and multiple activities (0.033 per 100,000 inhabitants).
- By level of care: 523 (0.093 per 100,000 inhabitants) in the first level and 586 (0.104 per 100,000 inhabitants) in the second and third levels.

The number of day hospitals and volunteer personnel is low: 0.008 and 0.02 per 100,000 inhabitants, respectively.

There is still a lack of central information on the real number of services, their structures, the patients they serve, and the quality of the services they deliver. A common feature is that all struggle to operate adequately and sustain and increase their range of activities. Most of them have different funding sources such as the health system, NGOs, charity, or patients, who pay when possible. Many members work for free on a volunteer basis and most PC professionals earn fees with positions in other disciplines.[16]

Policy

There is a tendency to report insufficient support from the health authorities. Although this may be true, the following are new changes that reflect both policy developments and increasing commitment by health authorities to address PC:

- Three countries have a national PC law.
- Eight countries have PC programs, and in 2 countries, they are in the development/implementation stage.
- Sixteen countries have a national cancer program, and 13 of them include PC.
- All countries have first level of care programs, and 8 of them include PC.
- All countries have national HIV/AIDS programs, and 7 include PC.
- Five countries have government resources for the development of PC and 4 for research in PC.

In many instances, changes are still in paper: programs, laws, and decrees that promote and try to ensure that PC availability and accessibility are not met and fail to produce the desired changes.

Although transformation is smaller and slower than desired and required, the future is promising because of the willingness of the health authorities to modify the situation. This fact must be highlighted considering that many countries have not yet met other important health needs that require focus of the health authority.

Opioid Availability and Accessibility

Availability and accessibility of commercial, generic, and compound preparations of both weak and strong opioids are variable in countries, cities, and settings (i.e., public hospitals, social security systems, prepayments). But the regional consumption of opioid analgesics is persistently low.

Two indicators demonstrate this situation:

1. In 2010, the opioid consumption (morphine equivalent, mg per capita) in Argentina and Bolivia was 13.0 and 0.17, respectively. The Argentina consumption—higher in the region—was far below the Canada consumption (753.4).[17]
2. In 2006, in Argentina, the adequacy of consumption measure (ACM) (per capita consumption of opioids for adequate pain control for selected diseases) was 0.012; the standard ACM was 1.00.[18]

The main causes for this situation—although with differences between countries—are the following[19]:

1. Lack of knowledge and wrong attitudes about both pain and opioids
2. Restrictive policies and laws governing controlled drugs

3. Failures in systems to request and distribute controlled drugs
4. High costs of opioids and lack of coverage for opioid analgesics

The following are examples of how high prices of opioids (if not subsidized) compared with monthly incomes can limit their access and utilization (Argentina, March 2013):

- One 30 mg tablet costs ARS 5.8[20]; minimum monthly wage: ARS 2875 (617 USD).[21]
- Thirty days of treatment with an oral dose of 90 mg immediate-release morphine costs ARS 522.
- Accessibility: 5.5 working days—the number of days a worker receiving minimum wage would have to work to pay for 1 month of analgesic treatment.

Education

There is an increasing trend among health professionals to learn about PC and many universities offer PC mainly as optional subject. Also, some services include PC teaching in their activities.

In five countries, PC is officially accredited as a specialty and in seven as a subspecialty.

It is estimated that nearly 600 physicians are accredited in the region (mean 31.5, median 2) and 70% are in Mexico, Argentina, and Chile.

Sixty-five percent and forty-five percent of 60 faculties from 11 LA countries who participated in a regional workshop on PC education reported education for physician and nurse pregraduates and for first-level health-care professionals, respectively.

The information resulting from this meeting showed that education activity is intense in both the pre- and postgrad, with different updated educational strategies, contents, and methods, with online and/or face-to-face teaching, with or without guided clinical activity. The meeting demonstrated that the region has a growing need to understand and improve specific technical details of education. This is encouraging and prompts the requirement to define educational strategies to teach PC.

Professional Activity

- The Latin American Palliative Care Association (ALCP) (Asociación Latinoamericana de Cuidados Paliativos, http://www.cuidadospaliativos.org/) is a not-for-profit interdisciplinary scientific association created in 1991 with currently 302 members and a mailing list of 6,970. Its different working groups conduct scientific activities, international academic cooperation, and diffusion to the community.
- Eleven countries have a PC association; three countries have more than one.
- Eight countries have active research groups: Chile, Argentina, Mexico, Cuba, Colombia, Peru, Panama, and the Dominican Republic.

- Ten countries have at least one published treatment guideline.
- Five countries have a service directory.
- Brazil publishes a PC journal.
- Many countries develop collaborative activities for education and research among them and/or with regional or international institutions and organizations.

Advocacy

Different actions constantly take place to change the *what is* into a *what should be* regarding PC-related issues. They are run by different organizations and evolve within the political, professional, and social environment and their aim is to raise significant issues and to propose solutions:

- *PC indicators*
  Workshop developed by the International Association for Hospice and Palliative Care (IAHPC) in cooperation with the ALCP. Representatives of the IAHPC, the ALCP, and the Pan American Health Organization (PAHO) and experts in epidemiology, PC, health-care administration, and health-care systems met in Lima, Peru, in 2012 to develop a set of indicators applicable in all countries of the world. The proposed indicators are available in English at http://cuidadospaliativos.org/recursos/indicadores-de-cp
- *Latin American Atlas of Palliative Care*
  Developed by the ALCP in cooperation with the IAHPC, the European Association for Palliative Care (EAPC), the Sociedad Española de Cuidados Paliativos (SECPAL), and the University of Navarra (Spain). The funds were provided by the Open Society Foundations. This atlas presents a global vision of PC in 19 LA countries whose official language is either Spanish or Portuguese. Although the approach to gather data has limitations—the regional situation changes rapidly, there is an absence of data for some countries, and the data were reported by key persons in each country—this is the first systematic study that presents information on PC in LA. It is available in Spanish at http://www.cuidadospaliativos.org/article.php?id=62.
- *Integration of PC in health services*
  Developed by the PAHO in cooperation with the IAHPC. Health professionals leading PC; managers of chronic diseases, cancer, and PC programs; and health authorities meet to identify the main barriers and solutions to implement PC in their countries and to start projects for cooperation in the region.

Completed international workshops include the following:

- Honduras, 2011. Costa Rica, Dominican Republic, El Salvador, Guatemala, Honduras, Nicaragua, and Panama
- Uruguay, 2012. Argentina, Bolivia, Chile, Colombia, Paraguay, and Uruguay
- Availability and access to opioid medications in LA countries

Workshops developed by the IAHPC. The purpose is to identify, develop, and implement the steps and changes needed to ensure access to treatment with controlled medications to patients in need.

Completed workshops:

- Colombia, 2007. National workshop.
- Lima, 2010. International workshop (Peru, Mexico, Chile).
- Nicaragua, 2011. International workshop (Panama, Guatemala, Costa Rica, El Salvador, Honduras, Nicaragua).
- Chile, 2011. National workshop. Details of the activities and the outcomes in Chile, Colombia, Costa Rica, El Salvador, Guatemala, Honduras, Nicaragua, Panama, and Peru are available at http://hospicecare.com/about-iahpc/contributions-to-palliative-care/.
- PC education at the undergraduate and the first level of health care.

Regional workshop developed by the Programa Argentino de Medicina Paliativa-Fundación FEMEBA in cooperation with the IAHPC, the Universidad Austral (Argentina), the ALCP, and the Universidad de Navarra (Spain).

Sixty faculties from 11 countries met in November 2012 in Buenos Aires, Argentina. Topics were as follows: goals of the educational process, availability and training of faculty, teaching materials, operating costs, financing, fees, design, and quality control of the assessment tools.

The main conclusions of the activity are available in Spanish at http://cuidadospaliativos.org/comisiones/foro-educacion/home/.

DISCUSSION

A large percent of the LA population has inadequate access to PC. Problems such as limited number of services, lack of education, and inconsistent policies delay the integration of PC with the existing health systems.

In the last 30 years, a growing number of people, professional, and nonprofessional have been working trying to match the increasing need of PC. Their work aimed to homogenize and assure steady and adequate care in their workplaces. But both their activity and accomplishments exceeded the limits of their workplaces; they are also responsible for many inspiring key progresses:

- The poor sanitary situation of patients with advanced incurable diseases is perceived and acknowledged.
- There is growing regional evidence and conviction that PC is useful and that changes in systems of care are needed.
- There are a significant number of enthusiastic services that behave as reservoirs of interest and expertise in PC. They produce and share significant information that encourage and guide others during their development.
- Recognition that PC must be an integral part of every health-care professional's role is increasing—with specialists essential for education and for managing complex clinical situations.[22]

- It is recognized that PC should not be limited to cancer; it is slowly expanding to noncancer conditions.
- Pediatric PC is expanding.
- There is an increasing trend in PC education, with focus in quality.
- Quality care improvement is becoming a central issue.
- Many barriers to opioid availability and accessibility have been reduced.

The information given earlier may allow to venture that the sum of achieved goals is close to reaching (or reached) the critical mass needed to power the needed changes.

The scenario is hopeful.

With this concept in mind, which should be the main objectives to continue keeping in sight?

One already identified and always in the sight is the delay and slow speed of PC integration with mainstream medical practice and the health-care systems. Successful changes will require the recognition of PC as an essential component of care available and accessible for all who need it and the commitment to adopt policies and designate resources to make it possible.

Another problem ever evident is the lack of accurate clinical and financial data on PC: information is poor. The need for clinical and financial metrics and measurement systems is critical to set PC according to the local needs and resources.[23] Accurate specific information is crucial to join together the managerial, financial, and clinical factors that will allow and facilitate the required multilevel activities and approaches.

No changes will happen if the health authorities recognize the benefit of PC and decide to implement it without trained personnel, or vice versa, if trained personnel find unfunded services. Neither both members of the binomial do not have evidence of the cost-benefit ratio of the enterprise they are planning nor they are not sure about the best action to take in each of the possible scenarios: institutional or home care? specialist or primary PC?

There is a need to understand—and act accordingly—that objectives change with time, that all are interrelated, and that the PC community can influence them.

The process to accomplish the needed changes is complex, with different opportunities or difficulties related to widely varying levels of resources and interest in PC among health providers and authorities.

The region is in the right way, with its society organizing to provide adequate care to patients and their families.

REFERENCES

1   Latin America. Wikipedia. Internet. Accessed on March 7, 2013. Available at http://en.wikipedia.org/wiki/Latinoamerica.
2   Countries. Wikipedia. Internet. Accessed on March 7, 2013. Available at http://en.wikipedia.org/wiki/countries.
3   Central Intelligence Agency. The World Factbook. Internet. Accessed on June 23, 2014. Available at https://www.cia.gov/library/publications/the-world-factbook/index.html.

4   Wikipedia. Human development index. Internet. Accessed on March 10, 2013. Available at http://en.wikipedia.org/wiki/Human_Development_Index.

5   Life expectancy at birth, 2012. Pan American Health Organization. Internet. Accessed on March 14, 2013. Available at http://ais.paho.org/atlas/en/leb/atlas.html.

6   Population ages 65 and above (% of total). The World Bank. Internet. Accessed on March 10, 2013. Available at http://data.worldbank.org/indicator/SP.POP.65UP.TO.ZS.

7   Death rate, crude (per 1,000 people). The World Bank. Internet. Accessed on March 10, 2013. Available at http://search.worldbank.org/data?qterm=crude%20death%20rate&language=EN.

8   Mortality distribution by groups and subgroups of causes of deaths. Pan American Health Organization. Internet. Accessed on March 9, 2013. Available at http://new.paho.org/hq/index.php?option=com_content&view=article&id=5545&Itemid=2391&lang=en.

9   Stjernsward J, Foley KM, and Ferris FD. The public health strategy for palliative care. *Journal of Pain and Symptom Management* 2007; 33(5) :486–493.

10 Worldwide Palliative Care Alliance. Mapping levels of palliative care development: A global update 2011. Accessed on March 9, 2013. Available at http://www.thewpca.org/resources/.

11 Pastrana T, De Lima L, Wenk R, Eisenchlas J, Monti C, Rocafort J, and Centeno C. *Atlas de Cuidados Paliativos de Latinoamérica ALCP*, Primera edición. Houston, TX: IAHPC Press, 2012. Internet. Accessed on March 10, 2013. Available at http://www.cuidadospaliativos.org/article.php?id=62.

12 Wenk R and Bertolino M. Palliative care development in South America: A focus in Argentina. *Journal of Pain and Symptom Management* May 2007; 33(5):645–650.

13 Wenk R. The development of palliative medicine in Latin America. In: E. Bruera, I Higginson, C Ripamonti, and C Von Gunten (eds). *Textbook of Palliative Medicine*. London, U.K.: Hodder Arnold, 2006; pp. 36–41.

14 Wenk R, Mosoiu D, and Rajagopal MR. Cancer pain and palliative care in the developing world. In: E. Bruera and R.K. Portenoy (eds). *Cancer Pain, Assessment and Management*, 2nd edn. New York: Cambridge University Press, 2010; pp. 608–626.

15 Service. Wiktionary. Internet. Accessed on March 7, 2013. Available at http://es.wiktionary.org/wiki/servicio.

16 Wenk R. The state of development of palliative care in Argentina. *Progress in Palliative Care* 2012; 20(4), 208–211.

17 Pain & Policy Studies Group. University of Wisconsin. Opioid Consumption Data. Accessed on March 10, 2013. Available at http://www.painpolicy.wisc.edu/opioid-consumption-data.

18 Seya M, Susanne F, Achara O, Milani B, and Scholten W. A first comparison between the consumption of and the need for opioid analgesics at country, regional, and global levels. *Journal of Pain and Palliative Care Pharmacotherapy* 2011; 25:6–18.

19 Ryan K, De Lima L, and Maurer M. Disponibilidad de Opioides en Latinoamérica. P. Bonilla, L. De Lima, P. Díaz, M. Ximena Leon, and M. González (eds). *En: Uso de Opioides para el Tratamiento del Dolor: Manual para Latinoamérica*. Houston, TX: IAHPC Press, 2011. Internet. Accessed on March 9, 2013. Available at http://hospicecare.com/about-iahpc/publications/.

20 K@iros. Internet. Accessed on March 7, 2013. Available at http://ar.kairosweb.com/laboratorios/producto-neocalmans-8241.

21 Wikipedia. Salario mínimo. Internet. Accessed on March 7, 2013. Available at http://es.wikipedia.org/wiki/Salario_m%C3%ADnimo#Argentina.

22 Quill TE and Abernethy AP. Generalist plus specialist palliative care— Creating a more sustainable model. *N Engl J Med* 2013; 368:1173–1175. Accessed on March 20, 2013. Available at http://www.nejm.org/doi/full/10.1056/NEJMp1215620.

23 Diane E. Meier DE, and Beresford L. Health systems find opportunities and challenges in palliative care development. *Journal of Palliative Medicine* 2010; 13(4): 387–370.

6

Development of palliative medicine in Africa

LIZ GWYTHER, SUE BOUCHER, RICHARD HARDING

INTRODUCTION

There is a considerable burden of disease in Africa. Further, according to the World Bank Development Indices, Africa has more low-income countries than any other regions in the world [1]. Poverty, poor health infrastructure, and a high disease burden contribute to patients presenting for health care late in their illness and a strong need for palliative care. The African Palliative Care Association (APCA) estimated that "in 2009 22.5 million people in Sub-Saharan Africa were living with HIV/AIDS, representing 67% of the global disease burden, with 1.8 million new infections reported in that year alone" [2]. The improving access to antiretroviral medication has increased patients' life expectancy. However, low employment rates and disruptions to working opportunities mean that people living with HIV have additional socioeconomic needs added to the conventional palliative care physical, psychosocial, and spiritual needs. Africa also has a high burden of cancer, rudimentary cancer prevention programs, and experiences barriers to accessing cancer treatment. In 2007, there were more than 700,000 new cancer cases reported and nearly 600,000 cancer-related deaths in Africa. Of particular concern are childhood cancers. AfrOx reports that "in Africa, on average 5% of childhood cancers are cured, compared to nearly an 80% cure rate in the developed world" [3]. Cancer rates on the continent are expected to grow by 400% over the next 50 years. In addition, Africa is experiencing an increase in noncommunicable diseases. The NCD Alliance estimates that globally NCDs will increase by 17% in the next 10 years, in Africa by 27% [4].

HISTORICAL CONTEXT

Palliative care was first established in Africa through nongovernmental organizations (NGOs) responding to the need to care for patients with cancer and in particular to manage cancer pain. As charitable organizations relying on community financial support, these hospices started in communities that could afford to donate funds for hospice services. However, in response to patients' needs, the reach of hospice care expanded first in urban areas and then in rural areas to provide care to any patient requiring palliative care.

In many parts of Africa, hospice services were established by charismatic individuals, passionate and committed to the cause of developing hospice services. The UK influence, in particular the leadership and inspiration of Dame Cicely Saunders and St. Christopher's Hospice, was key to the development of hospice services.

In 1977, a young girl, Frances Butterfield, died in Zimbabwe, in severe pain from cancer. Her mother, Maureen, hearing about St. Christopher's Hospice in London, went there to see if she could prevent this suffering from continuing in Zimbabwe. This first move toward palliative care in Africa resulted in the opening of Island Hospice and Bereavement Service in Harare in 1979. Island Hospice was dedicated to home care and did not have an inpatient facility [5].

Dr. Christine Dare, a physiotherapist working at St. Christopher's Hospice in London, felt compelled to open a hospice in Cape Town, South Africa. She was advised by Cicely Saunders that she needed a medical degree to gain credibility in establishing palliative care. Christine enrolled in medical school in Cape Town and graduated in 1979, then started St. Luke's Hospice in 1980. Hospices in Johannesburg and Durban were also established between 1979 and 1982.

South African hospices were established to respond to the needs of cancer patients but responded effectively when faced with the devastation of the AIDS epidemic. The formal health system was slow to implement treatment for people living with HIV, due in part to political denialism that allowed a *run away* epidemic. Kath Defilippi, a professional nurse and manager of South Coast Hospice, KwaZulu-Natal, developed and implemented the Integrated Community-Based Home Care model of care. This approach used community members in the response to numbers of HIV patients who became sick and who died. The training and professional supervision of nonprofessional staff providing home-based care has been adopted throughout South Africa and has become an effective and cost-efficient method of care delivery suitable to a country with limited health resources [6]. The care is underpinned by clinical standards and an accreditation program for hospice services and also uses the APCA African Palliative care Outcome Scale (POS) [7,8] to audit quality of care in South African hospice services. Kath Defilippi was elected as the founding president of the APCA board of directors. She continues her innovative practices and was a member of the Hospice Palliative Care Association (HPCA) working group to develop guidelines for palliative care for TB patients [9].

A key figure in palliative care development in Africa is Dr. Anne Merriman. Dr. Merriman's work as a missionary sister doctor has taken her to Southeast Asia and to Africa. She introduced palliative care in Singapore in 1985, which became formalized and an accepted form of care with the founding of the Hospice Care Association in 1989, while she was a senior teaching fellow in the Department of Community, Occupational and Family Medicine (COFM) in the National University of Singapore. She returned to Africa as medical director of Nairobi Hospice in 1990.

Following a feasibility study to identify a suitable country for a model of palliative care appropriate to Africa among four proposed candidate African countries, Dr. Merriman established Hospice Africa Uganda (HAU) and started work in Kampala in 1993. Dr. Merriman was founding vice chair of the APCA and is still active at HAU heading the International Programmes, which are supporting new initiatives in Nigeria, Cameroon, Sierra Leone, Malawi, Ethiopia, and Zambia and working to establish a palliative care model for French-speaking countries in Africa. An early initiative was the training and support provided by HAU to teams in Tanzania, through ORCI (Ocean Road Cancer Institute) and PASADA (a comprehensive HIV/AIDS support organization under the Catholic Archdiocese) in Dar es Salaam.

BARRIERS TO PALLIATIVE CARE IN AFRICA

Barriers to the development of palliative care in Africa include competing priorities in a context of low resources, poverty, a high burden of disease, lack of understanding of palliative care by policy makers, and until recently legal barriers to access of opioid medication [10–12]. Health services in general are constrained by a shortage of health-care professionals both through limited resources to train health-care professionals and loss of health-care professionals to more affluent countries. Cultural barriers include the taboo of speaking about death as this would be seen to be *inviting death in* and issues of confidentiality and disclosure of diagnosis as well as a culture of not disclosing information about illness, especially HIV status to children. African countries have a high rate of maternal and child mortality. As reducing these rates is a designated UN Millennium Development Goal, they rightly receive high priority. It has been difficult to establish an indicator set for palliative care to measure palliative care delivery in a country, and although morphine consumption is a proxy measure, there is little incentive to implement programs that do not have clear reporting structures for implementation. The Wisconsin Pain & Policy Studies Group (PPSG) reports very low morphine consumption for Africa with only South Africa reporting morphine consumption above the global mean [13] (Figure 6.1).

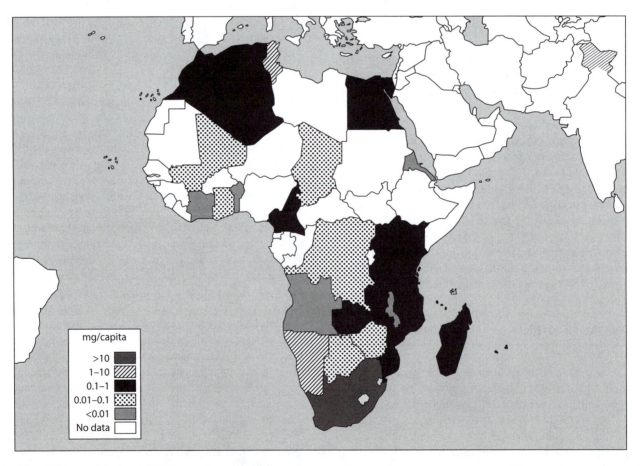

Figure 6.1 *Africa morphine map of 2010.*

A high proportion of the population in Africa consults *traditional healers* as their health carer, programs to collaborate with traditional healers are important, and training of traditional healers in the care of people living with HIV and in palliative care has been an important intervention [14].

ROLE OF THE WORLD HEALTH ORGANIZATION

In 2001, the World Health Organization (WHO) initiated a *community health approach to palliative care for HIV/AIDS and cancer patients in Africa project* in five African countries—Botswana, Ethiopia, Tanzania, Uganda, and Zimbabwe [15,16]. This project brought experience in Africa, in particular the Ugandan experience to four further countries by introducing country palliative care teams, research in situation analysis, and needs of patients and carers in the community with a view to persuading governments to support palliative care and to legalize procurement of essential drugs including morphine. The initiative was based on the WHO public health strategy for palliative care [17]. This strategy has four key components to integrate palliative care into a country's health system. These are (1) appropriate policies; (2) adequate drug availability; (3) education of policy makers, health-care workers, and the public; and (4) implementation of palliative care services at all levels of health-care and social support. This strategy has worked well as a framework to build and evaluate palliative care services in Africa.

African countries support the WHO definition of palliative care that "Palliative Care is an approach that improves the quality of life of patients and their families facing problems associated with life-threatening illness, through the prevention and relief of suffering, the early identification and impeccable assessment and treatment of pain and other problems, physical, psychosocial and spiritual" [18]. It has been important to have the authority of this definition in order to advocate for palliative care in a situation where influential funders have suggested developing definitions for palliative care to address specific diseases such as HIV. Dr. Merriman and palliative care practitioners in Africa are concerned that the trend to offer supportive care without pain and symptom control is lowering standards of care.

AFRICAN PALLIATIVE CARE ASSOCIATION

The APCA was developed from a meeting of palliative care trainers from five African countries (Kenya, South Africa, Tanzania, Uganda, and Zimbabwe) and international partners funded by the Diana, Princess of Wales Memorial Fund (DPOWMF) in 2002. This meeting was convened as a result of work on the WHO Five Country project. The outcome of the meeting was the election of a steering committee to establish a regional palliative care association and the Cape Town Declaration [19]. Kath Defilippi was elected as the chair of the steering committee and the founding chair of the APCA board of directors. This followed the official launch of the organization in June 2004 during its first annual general meeting and conference held in Arusha, Tanzania. Dr. Faith Mwangi-Powell was appointed as executive director of APCA and provided strong leadership to implement a strategy to reduce pain and suffering in Africa, finding *African solutions to African problems* [20]. APCA coordination of development activities for palliative care in Africa has built on earlier work of palliative care champions to take development efforts forward in a systematic way.

APCA has followed the WHO public health strategy to palliative care development in Africa, acting as a catalyst to facilitate meetings with government officials in review of health policies. APCA also works to support development of standalone palliative care policies working closely with governments and national HPCAs and local champions. This attention to health policies, attention to access to essential palliative care medication and training in palliative care, has been a successful approach in the integration of palliative care into country's health systems. International funders have supported and enabled APCA's activities such as opioid availability advocacy and strategy meetings funded by the Open Society Institute; meetings with the deans of universities to encourage palliative care training of medical and nursing students funded by the DPOWMF and PEPFAR; and policy review meetings. The U.S. Agency for International Development (USAID) has provided significant funding support initially for the 10 African countries supported through the PEPFAR grant and expanding to 14 countries. With cofunding, APCA has been active in 22 countries providing scholarships for palliative care training, facilitating advocacy and policy meetings, training in pain management and opioid use, and developing key materials to guide palliative care advocates and service providers. PEPFAR provided the seed funding for the development of APCA after the Arusha meeting in 2004 and maintained that support for palliative care development in Africa.

This focused activity has resulted in a growth in the provision of palliative care from services in 5 countries in 2002 to 22 countries in 2012. Important achievements include influencing the government in Ethiopia to develop policies for the use of opioids to ensure the access of morphine for pain relief. APCA supported the Rwandan government and Rwandan palliative care advocates to develop and launch a national palliative care strategy and palliative care policies and to adapt the APCA Standards for Providing Quality Palliative Care.

In Tanzania, 14 deans, principals, and senior lecturers from medical and nursing institutions were trained to facilitate integration of palliative care into health sciences curricula, and this has led to the establishment of a postgraduate diploma in palliative care in Tanzania.

APCA has produced a number of key resource documents including

- Palliative care core curriculum
- A framework for competencies for palliative care providers in Africa
- *APCA Standards for Providing Quality Palliative Care Across Africa*
- *Using Opioids to Manage Pain: A Pocket Guide for Health Professionals in Africa* [21]

APCA has a program to raise awareness and understanding about palliative care using traditional and social media to disseminate information about palliative care and partnering with human rights organizations to provide a voice for people with life-limiting illness and their families. In 2011, APCA appointed the Honorable Minister of Health for Swaziland Benedict N Xaba as an ambassador for palliative care in Africa.

NATIONAL ASSOCIATIONS

National HPCAs have been established in 15 African countries: Botswana, Cameroon, Cote d'Ivoire, Ethiopia, Ghana, Kenya, Malawi, Mozambique, Namibia, Nigeria, South Africa, Tanzania, Uganda, Zambia, and Zimbabwe. The role of the national association is that of advocacy for palliative care, supporting the government to integrate palliative care into all levels of health-care and social support, setting standards in palliative care, supporting palliative care services, and promoting quality palliative care. APCA has assisted in the establishment of national HPCAs and draws on the expertise of established national associations to assist in palliative care development in the region. The HPCA of South Africa was established in 1987 and has played a strong role in supporting and developing the hospice NGO sector in South Africa. In association with the Council for Health Services Accreditation of Southern Africa (COHSASA), HPCA developed standards of governance, management, and palliative care [22]. Through a facilitated mentorship process, HPCA staff assist and prepare member hospices for accreditation by COHSASA. This is the first example of NGO health-care accreditation in Africa. APCA's Institutional Self-Assessment Tool adapted from APCA standards audit has been used in hospitals in Africa to conduct assessment of hospital palliative care. The *Kenya Hospices and Palliative Care Association* (KEPHCA) has been particularly successful in integrating palliative care into hospitals in Kenya with good referral systems to local hospices. In addition, 17 medical and nursing schools have integrated palliative care into their curricula supported by KEHPCA. APCA, KEHPCA, and HPCA all have editions of ehospice, an initiative of the Worldwide Palliative Care Alliance using modern technology to disseminate news, views, and palliative care inspiration. APCA and national associations such as those of Kenya, Nigeria, and South Africa hold regular conferences to disseminate palliative care knowledge and research findings.

POLICY DEVELOPMENT

Uganda was the first country in Africa to include palliative care as an essential service as part of the 5-year strategic health plan. By 2000, the three priorities for a palliative care service in an African country were present in Uganda: drug availability, education, and government support.

Many countries have palliative care included in national cancer control programs [2]. Late presentation, inadequate diagnostic and treatment facilities, and poor availability of chemotherapy and radiotherapy all increase the need for palliative care and in particular adequate cancer pain control in Africa, so it is important to include palliative care in cancer control strategies [23]. Palliative care has also been included in national strategic plans for HIV, AIDS, and TB and in national strategic plans for noncommunicable diseases. Rwanda was the first country assisted by APCA to implement a stand-alone palliative care strategy, policies, and guidelines and this success has been followed by Swaziland and Mozambique. There have been some early initiatives in North Africa with discussions in Sudan and in Morocco, both of which countries have representatives on the current (2013) APCA board of directors.

DRUG AVAILABILITY

In 2004, the International Narcotics Control Board released a report prepared by the Wisconsin PPSG stating that approximately 84% of the total world consumption of morphine occurs in only 7 countries; that low- and middle-income countries—which host 80% of the world population, more than half of the world's cancer patients, and more than 95% of people living with HIV—account for just 6% of morphine consumption; and that 50 countries, including 32 countries in Africa, have almost no morphine distribution at all.

Several initiatives including individual meetings with drug control councils and government personnel have been implemented to address this humanitarian problem. Funded by the Open Society Institute, APCA held regional advocacy availability workshops bringing together government officials, palliative care professionals, health professionals including pharmacists, statutory bodies, and law enforcement personnel to discuss the need for opioid medication for clinical use and the measures to avoid diversion of medication and to prevent drug abuse. The WHO publication *Ensuring balance in national policies on controlled substances: Guidance on availability and accessibility of controlled medicines* has since been published and is a useful document to continue the advocacy for access to essential pain medication.

Two countries in Africa have passed laws allowing nurses with prescribing education to prescribe morphine. Palliative care advocates in South Africa have lobbied the government for nurse prescribing in South Africa, and legislation is pending on this matter. The Wisconsin PPSG reports show that only South Africa has opioid consumption above the global mean, and in 2010, the reported opioid consumption per capita for South Africa was 10.9 mg/capita compared with developed countries United Kingdom, United States, and Canada with opioid consumption between 40 and 60 mg/capita [13] (Figure 6.2). Human Rights Watch has been active in advocacy for access to essential pain medication worldwide and produced a comprehensive report on the plight of children suffering pain in Kenya [24]. HAU took a strong lead in reconstituting morphine powder in the hospice pharmacy to improve access to pain control, but there is still a long way to go to ensure that health-care

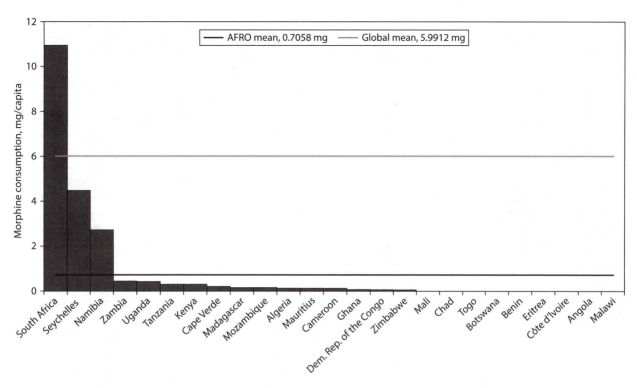

Figure 6.2 *AFRO morphine consumption of 2010. (From International Narcotics Control Board; World Health Organization population data by: Pain & Policy Studies Group, University of Wisconsin/WHO Collaborating Center, 2012.)*

professionals are trained in pain management and that there is appropriate access to essential pain medications in African countries. A report from Nigeria comments that opioid accessibility and affordability are challenging issues. APCA trained a Nigerian country opioids team between 2006 and 2008, and recently (2103), the UICC's Global Access to Pain Relief Initiative interacted with the Nigerian Federal Ministry of Health to bring back opioids to Nigeria a few months ago [25].

EDUCATION

In the early years, African hospices trained volunteers to assist in caring for patients or in providing bereavement care to families. Island Hospice and Bereavement Service has taken a strong lead in palliative care training in Africa as has HAU.

The HPCA in South Africa established a short course (8 months) in palliative care nursing in 1989 at the request of the South African Nursing Council. In 2000, HPCA received seed funding from the DPOWMF to develop a postgraduate medical degree course at the University of Cape Town (UCT). UCT Faculty of Health Sciences supported the course, and the UCT Department of Institutional Planning assisted in obtaining accreditation from the South African Qualifications Authority. The course was first offered in 2001, and with teaching support from Cardiff University, 21 doctors graduated with MPhil in palliative medicine. UCT also integrated palliative medicine teaching into the undergraduate medical curriculum and offers both a postgraduate diploma in palliative medicine

and a research degree, the MPhil in palliative medicine [26]. The programs have been realigned to include palliative care professionals from other health-care disciplines in addition to medicine. This was the only postgraduate palliative medicine training offered by an African university for about 10 years.

Wits Palliative Care, the Gauteng Centre of Excellence for Palliative Care at Chris Hani Baragwanath Hospital, provides training to medical students at the University of the Witwatersrand, as does Nelson Mandela Metropolitan University in KwaZulu-Natal. Palliative care is a required competency for family physicians in South Africa so is included in the training of family medicine registrars. The South African health minister's reengineering of primary health care plan [27] makes provision for a family physician in each district health team. This will increase the accessibility and availability of palliative care throughout the country.

In 2009, HAU's training department, the Institute of Hospice and Palliative Care in Africa (IHPCA), was accredited by the National Council for Higher Education in Uganda as an institution of higher learning. The IHPCA offers a number of courses including a diploma in clinical palliative care and a distance learning diploma in palliative care accredited by Makerere University.

Makerere University offers a 3-year degree program in palliative care, which is competency based and delivered by distance learning. This course began in 2009 with the first BSc graduates in January 2013 and has trained students from 10 countries across sub-Saharan Africa. A masters program in palliative care is now being developed at Makerere University. Training the future medical leaders is also important, and palliative care has been integrated into the curriculum of the undergraduate medical schools and many of the postgraduate courses in Makerere and Mbarara universities. A competency-based postgraduate curriculum was developed and implemented, during the second year of the 3-year postgraduate masters in internal medicine [28].

Mildmay in Uganda also offers diploma-level training in HIV/AIDS community palliative care, child counseling, and more recently children's palliative care (CPC) through innovative programs run in conjunction with Mbarara University of Science and Technology. Mildmay also runs a BSc in HIV/AIDS care and management with the University of Manchester, which contains a strong component of palliative care. In addition, there are a number of short courses and district-level trainings aimed at capacity building in the community setting and including groups such as faith leaders and traditional healers.

As discussed earlier, Tanzania has established a postgraduate diploma in palliative care presented by the International Medical and Technological University.

The DPOWMF also supported a focus on training for pediatric palliative care and supported this training in Malawi, Kenya, and South Africa.

PALLIATIVE CARE SERVICES

There are a number of models for the provision of palliative care in Africa. Initially, palliative care was provided by hospices in the nongovernmental sector, and palliative care is still most frequently provided by hospices. Within the NGO sector, home-based care has been the most common service model and the most appropriate for resource-poor settings. HPCA of South Africa has described an Integrated Community-Based Home Care model [6], which has strong referral links with other health and welfare partners and trained community-based carers who are supported and supervised by a palliative care professional nurse with access to an interdisciplinary team. In Uganda, Little Hospice Hoima was initiated as a demonstration project of an affordable service at the village level, and Mobile Hospice, Mbarara, offers mobile home-based palliative support through roadside clinics, as well as its initial goal of teaching palliative medicine at Uganda's second medical school [2].

Over the last 10 years, the move to integrate palliative care into hospitals and clinics in the formal health-care sector has made palliative care more accessible and available to patients in need of this care. Hospital palliative care is either provided by clinical staff such as oncologists trained in palliative care as part of their routine work (Kenyatta National Hospital, Nairobi) or by hospital palliative care teams (Wits Palliative Care, Chris Hani Baragwanath Hospital, Soweto; Mulago National Referral Hospital in Kampala, Uganda) or in standalone palliative care units (Settlers Hospital, Grahamstown). An innovative program, called the Abundant Life program and based on the UK Gold Standards Framework, was initiated at a district hospital in Cape Town, Victoria Hospital. Patients who would benefit from palliative care are identified during their hospital admission and referred to the Abundant Life program.

Once they are stable with optimal clinical management, they are discharged home but attend a support group at the hospital accompanied by a family member. They get to know and understand about their illness and maintaining optimal health and may be visited at home by the Abundant Life nurse if necessary. This program has reduced the number of hospital readmissions for patients with chronic illness and has reduced costs to the hospital and related costs for the patients [29].

Palliative care services in Africa have responded effectively in caring for people with HIV and those with TB and have taken an international lead in developing programs for patients with HIV and/or TB [9]. For example, research has demonstrated community- and home-based care for people with living HIV including symptom relief; supportive and palliative care is associated with better ART adherence, retention, and survival [30,31].

RESEARCH

In low- and middle-income countries where resources allocated to health are limited, the necessity to evaluate palliative care, and to ensure it is relevant and appropriate to local contexts, is essential [32]. Since the first review of African palliative care identified a wealth of clinical experience yet a dearth of evidence [9], there has been a growth of research activity to ensure that palliative care services are relevant, [14] effective [33–35], and based on local need [36,37]. Advances have been made in research methodology in African palliative care [38], but there is still comparatively little evidence in cancer compared to HIV populations [39] and an increasing need to respond appropriately to patients with drug-resistant TB [40,41]. In terms of ensuring that evidence reflects local epidemiology, sub-Saharan Africa faces the opposite challenge to high-income countries, in that cancer patients have less coverage and evidence than noncancer patients (i.e., the evidence base in HIV is much greater), although in common with high-income countries, there is comparatively little evidence to address the needs of organ failure patients.

The health economics of palliative care is a pressing concern globally [42], although little attention has been paid to costing palliative care in Africa. Exceptions are two South African costing studies conducted in hospital settings—one showing lower daily care costs for an outreach program [43] and one finding lower costs of care for a hospital-based program due to fewer admissions and increased home death [29]. The policy push for home death in high-income countries [44] demonstrates the importance of collecting local data to ensure relevance. Adapting the previous pan-European methodology from random-digit-dial recruitment to a street survey, data from Namibia found far lower preference for home death compared to Europe [45]. Recent data have also demonstrated the cultural challenges to practice that are adopted in the West—for example, advance care planning appears to be a challenging concept in the collectivist African setting compared to individualistic Western settings [46].

A notable achievement in African palliative care research has been the development [7] and validation [8] of the APCA African POS, which has been used in many settings to evaluate quality of care and to influence policy makers about the importance of palliative care [47]. It now forms a quality standard for South African Palliative Care Services [22], and measurement of patient outcomes now forms a central tenet in standards for the APCA [48]. The implementation of POS in Africa has enabled the generation of data to describe patient needs [36], audit and quality improvement studies [33], and now into randomized controlled trials [34]. This last example of a trial of palliative care for people on antiretroviral treatment is an example of how African palliative care has addressed the treatment/palliation of false dichotomy in HIV management [49]. In addition, in terms of sharing lessons learned from low- and middle-income countries, methods are being shared in quality improvement between Africa and India [50] (Table 6.1).

The African research agenda has focused greatly on drug availability [10], which has been a necessity due to the essential work on policy and legal aspects of pain relief in advanced disease. African palliative care advocates have also shown leadership in policy and legal research to identify existing global covenants to invoke a right to pain relief and palliative care [51].

This prior focus on drug availability has recently been balanced by a focus on understanding African patients' spiritual, communication, and information needs [52,53]. This has led to the validation of the "Spirit 8" measure of spiritual well-being [54].

In April 2012, APCA held a meeting of palliative care researchers from Africa and launched the African Palliative Care Research Network (APCRN) in partnership with the European Association for Palliative Care [55]. The aim of the APCRN is to develop collaborative relationships to generate and disseminate research-based palliative care evidence in Africa.

The UCT has a strong research program in the MPhil in palliative medicine, and family physicians are also conducting palliative care research. UCT is also initiating a PhD program for palliative care. In Uganda, research capacity has been built through an introduction to research module taught as part of the BSc curriculum, developing research agendas that link practice and quality outcomes, mentorship for new

researchers, and an innovative advanced research school run by a collaboration between Makerere University Palliative Care Unit, Edinburgh University, and HAU with significant international support. Doctoral and postdoctoral opportunities are more difficult to access, but this is crucial for academic leadership. Funding remains a significant challenge as it is difficult for young researchers in a relatively new specialty to establish the credibility for attracting grants. Developing collaborations in a country, regionally and internationally, is a way forward and also serves to extend the scope and reach of palliative care.

International support through King's College London (KCL) and the European Association for Palliative Care has been important in developing an evidence base for palliative care in Africa. Dr. Richard Harding has contributed significantly to research activities, and an important project was the validation of the APCA African POS [7].

DEVELOPMENT OF CHILDREN'S PALLIATIVE CARE IN AFRICA

Prior to the early 1990s, limited CPC provision could be found within adult services in Africa. In the mid-1990s, the devastation caused by HIV/AIDS provided the impetus for the emergence of services dedicated to looking after children such as the St. Nicholas Children's Hospice in Bloemfontein (now Sunflower House Children's Hospice) under Joan Marston, the Mohau Centre in Pretoria, and Cotlands in Johannesburg. In Uganda, HAU and Mildmay Uganda also saw the need to care for children.

In South Africa in 2003, hospital-based palliative care for children was introduced by Dr. Michelle Meiring, and in 2005, the DPOWMF provided for the development of the first curriculum for an introduction to CPC training course for professionals.

The support of the DPOWMF was to prove crucial to the development of CPC services in Africa as they went on to support the establishment of a pediatric palliative care portfolio within the management of the HPCA of South Africa, to which Joan Marston was appointed. This led to the rapid growth of child-centered services in this country over the next few years.

Table 6.1 *Use of APCA African POS*

POS user	Function of APCA APOS	Audience for APCA APOS	Outcome
HPCA	Quality of care audit at member hospices	Hospice management Report to funders Funding request	Improved patient care Sustainable funding
Hospices	Quality improvement programs	Hospice management Hospice staff	Improved patient care
Researchers	Identifying palliative care needs (broadly) Evaluating whether palliative care needs are met	Research site staff Policy makers Readers of scientific journals Conference delegates	Creating awareness of palliative care needs Influencing policy makers Identifying best practice that can be disseminated Identifying gaps in provision of care and education needs of health-care workers

In 2009, the DPOWMF funded the development and subsequent publication of the *Children's Palliative Care Textbook* for Africa [56], edited by Dr. Justin Amery and inspired by his experiences working at HAU. Another DPOWMF-funded project was the Beacon Centers of Excellence in South Africa, Uganda, and Tanzania—a 3-year project aimed at increasing care provision through the training of professionals. Centers of excellence were established at Mildmay, Uganda, and at Pasada in Tanzania and included a network of sites within South Africa. The fund was also instrumental in the development of the hospital-based Umodzi CPC service in Blantyre, Malawi. By 2012, similar services were made available in three additional hospitals in Malawi as a result of a 5-year project funded by the UK Department for International Development (DFID) through Help the Hospices and with technical support from the ICPCN.

Between 2011 and 2013, there have been developments in service provision and in the training of professionals in Kenya and Zambia, and introductory training has been provided for professionals in Sudan. Isolated services are also known to exist at present in Nigeria, Ethiopia, and Egypt.

Despite progress, the status of CPC remains precarious in Africa and is nonexistent in most countries on the continent. A recent review of evidence found very little data on children's needs, models of service, or outcomes [57], largely due to the lack of an outcome tool. A pediatric POS for Africa is currently in final stages of validation [58].

CONCLUSION

With a structured and systematic approach to palliative care development in Africa, there has been a substantial growth in palliative care services and evidence to underpin them. In the Worldwide Palliative Care Alliance report on mapping palliative care development [60], it is noted that "a regional analysis of palliative care development between 2006 and 2011 indicates that the most significant gains have been made in Africa." This has been largely due to the strategic leadership afforded by APCA and Dr. Faith Mwangi-Powell with support from funding partners. Further development will be influenced by the interaction with ministries of health, and it will be important to continue work in Francophone Africa and in North Africa. The evidence to date has focused on those countries where palliative care has greatest presence, that is, East and South Africa.

Future directions for African palliative care will need to address key challenges of how need can be met across settings—at home and in primary/secondary/tertiary care in the face of the aging population (as wealth grows and HIV treatment expands). Palliative care for those without an HIV diagnosis requires special effort, as currently the evidence of needs and outcomes is not available on which to base a clinical response, although essential service responses have been enacted [9]. In terms of lessons learned, future global palliative care research activity should be informed by the learning from provision with limited resources, and how high-income countries may learn to deliver quality services and least cost. The generalist/specialist debate may also be informed by low-/middle-income countries responding to a generalized HIV epidemic. Lastly, as global migration increases, the work to date on culturally appropriate palliative care development is increasingly relevant to all providers.

RELATED VIDEOS

Video 6.1, Jethro's Story (http://goo.gl/1SWWNr)
Video 6.2, Traditional Healers and Palliative Care Training (http://goo.gl/oJJC9f)
Video 6.3, Dr. Faith Mwangi (http://goo.gl/FPshaq)

REFERENCES

1   http://data.worldbank.org/data-catalog/world-development-indicators, accessed May 8, 2013.
2   http://africanpalliativecare.org/index.php?option=com_content&view=article&id=41&Itemid=26, accessed April 23, 2013.
3   http://www.afrox.org/26/london-declaration, accessed April 20, 2013.
4   http://www.ncdalliance.org/globalepidemic, accessed April 23, 2013.
5   Merriman A. The development of palliative medicine in Africa. In *Textbook of Palliative Medicine*. Eds. Bruera E, Higginson IJ, Ripamonti C, von Gunten C. Hodder Arnold, London, U.K., 2004.
6   Defilippi KM, Cameron S. Promoting the integration of quality palliative care—The South African Mentorship Program. *JPSM* 2007;**33**(5):552–557.
7   Powell RA, Downing J, Harding R et al. Development of the APCA African Palliative Outcome Scale. *J Pain Symptom Manage* 2007;**33**(2):229–232.
8   Harding R, Selman L, Agupio G et al. Validation of a core outcome measure for palliative care in Africa: The APCA African Palliative Outcome Scale. *Health Qual Life Outcomes* 2010;**8**. doi: 10.1186/1477-7525-8-10[published Online First: Epub Date].
9   http://www.hospicepalliativecaresa.co.za/pdf/patientcare/TB_Guidelines_2011.pdf, accessed May 8, 2013.
10 Harding R, Powell RA, Kiyange F et al. Provision of pain- and symptom-relieving drugs for HIV/AIDS in sub-Saharan Africa. *J Pain Symptom Manage* 2010;**40**(3):405–415. doi: 10.1016/j.jpainsymman.2009.12.025[published Online First: Epub Date].
11 Merriman A, Harding R. Pain control in the African context: The Ugandan introduction of affordable morphine to relieve suffering at the end of life. *Philos Ethics Humanit Med* 2010;**5**:10.
12 Logie DE, Harding R. An evaluation of a morphine public health programme for cancer and AIDS pain relief in Sub-Saharan Africa. *BMC Public Health* 2005;**5**:82.
13 http://www.painpolicy.wisc.edu/opioid-consumption-data, accessed April 30, 2013.
14 Graham N, Gwyther L, Tiso T et al. Traditional Healers' views of the required processes for a "Good Death" among Xhosa patients pre- and post-death. *J Pain Symptom Manage* 2012. doi: 10.1016/j.jpainsymman.2012.08.005 [published Online First: Epub Date].
15 Sepulveda C, Habiyambere V, Amandua J et al. Quality care at the end of life in Africa. *BMJ* 2003;**327**:209–213.

16   Olweny C, Sepulveda C, Merriman A et al. Desirable services and guide-lines for the treatment and palliative care of HIV disease patients with cancer in Africa: A World Health Organization consultation. *J Palliat Care* 2003;**19**:198–205.

17   Stjernsward J, Foley KM, Ferris FD. The public health strategy for pallia-tive care. *J Pain Symptom Manage* 2007;**33**(5):486–493.

18   http://www.who.int/cancer/palliative/definition/en/, accessed April 23, 2013.

19   Mpanga Sebuyira L, Mwangi-Powell F, Pereira J, Spence C. The Cape Town palliative care declaration: Home-grown solutions for sub-Saharan Africa. *J Palliat Med* June 2003;**6**(3):341–343.

20   http://africanpalliativecare.org/images/stories/pdf/ANNUAL_REPORT_FOR_WEB.pdf, accessed April 23, 2013.

21   http://www.africanpalliativecare.org/index.php?option=com_content&view=article&id=144&Itemid=79.

22   http://www.hpca.co.za/pdf/guidelinedocs/HPCA%20Standards.pdf, accessed April 30, 2013.

23   Harding R, Higginson IJ. Palliative care in Sub-Saharan Africa. *Lancet* 2005;**365**(9475): 1971–1977.

24   http://www.hrw.org/node/92939, accessed May 1, 2013.

25   Personal communication Dr. Folaju Oyebola.

26   Gwyther L, Rawlinson F. Palliative medicine teaching program at the University of Cape Town: Integrating palliative care principles into practice. *J Pain Symptom Manage* 2007;**33**:558–562.

27   Mayosi BM, Lawn JE, van Niekerk A, Bradshaw D, Abdool Karim S, Coovadia HM. Health in South Africa: Changes and challenges since 2009. *Lancet* 2012;**380**:2029–2043.

28   Personal correspondence Dr. Mhoira Leng, Prof Julia Downing.

29   DesRosiers T, Cupido C, Pitout E, van Niekerk L, Badri M, Gwyther L, Harding R. A hospital-based palliative service for patients suffer-ing from organ failure in sub-Saharan Africa reduces admissions and increases home death rates. *JPSM*. In Press.

30   Zachariah R, Teck R, Buhendwa L et al. Community support is associated with better antiretroviral treatment outcomes in a resource-limited rural district in Malawi. *Trans R Soc Trop Med Hyg* 2007;**101**:79–84.

31   Kabore I, Bloem J, Etheredge G, Obiero W, Wanless S, Doykos P, Ntsekhe P et al. The effect of community-based support services on clini-cal efficacy and health-related quality of life in HIV/AIDS patients in resource-limited settings in sub-Saharan Africa. *AIDS Patient Care STDS* September 2010;**24**(9):581–594.

32   Higginson IJ, Bruera E. Do we need palliative care audit in developing countries? *Palliat Med* 2002;**16**(6):546–547.

33   Harding R, Gwyther L, Mwangi-Powell F et al. How can we improve palliative care patient outcomes in low- and middle-income coun-tries? Successful outcomes research in sub-Saharan Africa. *J Pain Symptom Manage* 2010;**40**(1):23–26. doi: S0885-3924(10)00358-1 [pii]10.1016/j.jpainsymman.2010.04.007[published Online First: Epub Date].

34   Lowther K, Simms V, Selman L et al. Treatment outcomes in palliative care: The TOPCare study. A mixed methods phase III randomised con-trolled trial to assess the effectiveness of a nurse-led palliative care intervention for HIV positive patients on antiretroviral therapy. *BMC Infect Dis* 2012;**12**(1):288. doi: 1471-2334-12-288 [pii]10.1186/1471-2334-12-288[published Online First: Epub Date].

35   Harding R, Simms V, Alexander C et al. Can palliative care integrated within HIV outpatient settings improve pain and symptom control in a low-income country? A prospective, longitudinal, controlled intervention evaluation. *AIDS Care* 2012. doi: 10.1080/09540121.2012.736608[pub-lished Online First: Epub Date].

36   Harding R, Selman L, Agupio G et al. Intensity and correlates of mul-tidimensional problems in HIV patients receiving integrated palliative care in sub-Saharan Africa. *Sex Transm Infect* 2012;**88**(8):607–611. doi: 10.1136/sextrans-2011-050460[published Online First: Epub Date].

37   Delivering spiritual care in palliative care populations: Views and expe-riences of spiritual care providers in South Africa and Uganda. *African Palliative Care Association Conference*; 2010; Windhoek, Namibia.

38   Harding R, Powell RA, Downing J et al. Generating an African palliative care evidence base: The context, need, challenges, and strategies. *J Pain Symptom Manage* 2008;**36**(3):304–309.

39   Harding R, Selman S, Powell R et al. Research in palliative care: Improving advanced cancer care in Africa (Invited Review). *Lancet Oncol*. In Press.

40   Connor S, Foley K, Harding R et al. Declaration on palliative care and MDR/XDR-TB. *Int J Tuberc Lung Dis* 2012;**16**(6):712–7133 doi: 10.5588/ijtld.12.0267[published Online First: Epub Date].

41   Harding R, Foley KM, Connor SR et al. Palliative and end-of-life care in the global response to multidrug-resistant tuberculosis. *Lancet Infect Dis* 2012;**12**(8):643–646 doi: S1473-3099(12)70084-1 [pii]10.1016/S1473-3099(12)70084-1[published Online First: Epub Date].

42   Harding R, Gomes B, Foley KM et al. Research priorities in health economics and funding for palliative care: Views of an international think tank. *J Pain Symptom Manage* 2009;**38**(1):11–14 doi: S0885-3924(09)00496-5   [pii]10.1016/j.jpainsymman.2009.04.013[published Online First: Epub Date].

43   Hongoro C, Dinat N. A cost analysis of a hospital-based palliative care outreach program: Implications for expanding public sector palliative care in South Africa. *J Pain Symptom Manage* 2011;**41**(6):1015–1024 doi: 10.1016/j.jpainsymman.2010.08.014[published Online First: Epub Date].

44   Gomes B, Higginson IJ, Calanzani N et al. Preferences for place of death if faced with advanced cancer: A population survey in England, Flanders, Germany, Italy, the Netherlands, Portugal and Spain. *Ann Oncol* 2012 doi: 10.1093/annonc/mdr602[published Online First: Epub Date].

45   Powell RA, Namisango E, Gikaara N et al. Public priorities and preferences for end-of-life care in Namibia. *J Pain Symptom Manage* 2013. In Press.

46   Stanford J, Sandberg DM, Gwyther L, Harding R. Conversations worth having: The perceived relevance of advance care planning among teachers, hospice staff, and pastors in Knysna, South Africa. *J Palliat Med* 2013;**16**(7):762–767.

47   http://www.csi.kcl.ac.uk/files/Impact_of_APCA_POS.pdf, accessed May 8, 2013.

48   http://www.africanpalliativecare.org/images/stories/pdf/APCA_Standards.pdf, accessed July 14, 2013.

49   Selwyn P. Why should we care about palliative care for AIDS in the era of antiretroviral therapy? *Sex Transm Infect* 2005;**81**:2–3.

50   Selman L, Harding R. How can we improve outcomes for patients and families under palliative care? Implementing clinical audit for qual-ity improvement in resource limited settings. *Indian J Palliat Care* 2010;**16**(1):8–15 doi: 10.4103/0973-1075.63128[published Online First: Epub Date].

51   Brennan F. Palliative care as an international human right. *J Pain Symptom Manage* 2007;**33**(5):494–499.

52   Selman L, Higginson IJ, Agupio G et al. Meeting information needs of patients with incurable progressive disease and their families in South Africa and Uganda: Multicentre qualitative study. *BMJ* 2009;**338**:b1326.

53   Selman L, Harding R, Higginson I et al. Spiritual wellbeing in sub-Saharan Africa: The meaning and prevalence of 'feeling at peace'. *BMJ Support Palliat Care* 2011;**1**(A22) doi:10.1136/bmjspcare-2011-000020.66[published Online First: Epub Date].

54   Selman L, Siegert RJ, Higginson IJ et al. The "Spirit 8" successfully captured spiritual well-being in African palliative care: Factor and Rasch analysis. *J Clin Epidemiol* 2012;**65**(4):434–443 doi: 10.1016/j.jclinepi.2011.09.014[published Online First: Epub Date].

55   Powell RA, Harding R, Namisango E, Katabira E, Gwyther L, Radbruch L, Murray SA, El-Ansary M, Ajayi IO, Mwangi-Powell F. Palliative care research in Africa: An overview. *Eur J Palliat Care* 2013;**20**(4):162–165.

56   Amery J. (Ed.) *Children's Palliative Care in Africa.* Oxford University Press, Oxford, U.K., 2009.

57   Harding R, Albertyn R, Sherr L, Gwyther L. Paediatric palliative care in sub-Saharan Africa: A systematic appraisal. *JPSM.* In Press.

58   Downing J, Atieno M, Powell RA, Ali Z, Marston J, Meiring M, Ssengooba J, Williams S, Mwangi-Powell FN, Harding R, the APCA AIDSTAR Project Advisory Group. Development of a palliative care outcome measure for children in sub-Saharan Africa: Findings from early phase instrument development. *Eur J Palliat Care* 2012:**19**(6):292–295.

59   Lynch T, Connor S, Clark D. Mapping levels of palliative care development: A global update. *J Pain Symptom Manage* 2013;**45**:1094–1106.

Development of palliative care in Australia and New Zealand

JANE PHILLIPS, JANE M. INGHAM, ROD MACLEOD

INTRODUCTION

Similar to other parts of the developed world, the modern hospice and palliative care movements in Australia and New Zealand (NZ) have their genesis in the care of people with cancer. Over the past 30 years, palliative care in these countries has evolved rapidly and is increasingly inclusive of people with life-limiting illnesses other than cancer. As of 2012, there were approximately 226 services providing specialist palliative care to Australians with a variety of life-limiting illnesses [1] and 35 hospice services and 16 hospital palliative care services in NZ [2].

While the historical roots of care of the dying in Australia and NZ are linked to religious organizations, the modern palliative care movements in these countries emerged in the late 1970s, largely founded upon the pioneering work of Dame Cicely Saunders [3]. This development was largely driven by community concerns that people dying with advanced cancer were suffering needlessly [4]. Over the following two decades, a proliferation of organizations and specialist professional societies helped foster greater recognition of the need to provide better care to people facing a life-limiting illness and their families. By the turn of the century, palliative care in Australia and NZ was increasingly being shaped by national policy, government investment, and recognition of the need for evidence-based practice and a population-based approach to palliative care.

This chapter provides an insight into the rich history of palliative care in Australia and NZ and illustrates how national end-of-life policy in these countries is now being directed toward a more contemporary, needs-based model of care that focuses on needs rather than diagnosis; has the capacity to better meet the demands of an aging population, living longer with chronic conditions; acknowledges that palliation and treatment are equal and not separate; supports evidence-based practice; embeds palliative care across the entire health-care system, including rural and remote communities; and provides culturally sensitive care [5,6].

Australia

Despite its large land mass, Australia's population of nearly 23 million is largely urbanized with about 70% of people living in capital cities or metropolitan areas [7]. Australia is culturally diverse, with almost 400 different languages spoken and with 21% speaking a language other than English at home [8]. Indigenous Australians make up approximately 2.5% (517,174 people) of the total population [9]. This population comprises Aboriginal (90%), Torres Strait Islander (6%), and other peoples that identify with both cultural groups (4%) [9].

As a result of changing patterns of life, disease, and dying, Australians have one of the highest life expectancies at birth in the world, with the median age of death currently 80.9 years and rising [10]. Increased life expectancy has brought with it much higher rates of noncommunicable diseases, which currently account for more than 80% of the burden of disease and injury in Australia [5]. Many chronic illnesses can seriously affect a person's well-being and health-care needs, while others are more serious and life limiting [5]. It is estimated that at least half of the 144,000 annual deaths are anticipated [5] and that many of those who died and their families would have benefited from a palliative approach.

Australia is a federation of states and territories ("jurisdictions") with the responsibility for health care shared between these two tiers of government [11]. Since 1973, the Australian government's ("Commonwealth") universal health-care scheme ("Medicare") has been available to all permanent residents covering individual medical consultations, public hospital admissions, and access to subsidized pharmaceuticals. Australians can also elect to have private health-care coverage for hospital and ancillary health care. In essence, Australia has a publicly financed health insurance system with a privately financed option that complements health-care funding in some medical situations and offers an alternative in others. Many public hospitals in Australia are the major teaching institutions and centers of research excellence. The Commonwealth Government through the Australian Health-Care Agreements funds community-based primary and aged care services. As part of this agreement, the jurisdictions, which are responsible for hospital and ancillary services, are allocated funding according to local needs and priorities [12]. In 2009–2010, Australia spent 9.4% of its gross domestic product (GDP) on health, in contrast to the United States that spent 17.4% [13].

Aotearoa (New Zealand)

Aotearoa (NZ) is the largest of the Pacific Islands in the Oceania group lying some 1200 miles southeast of Australia. The population is comprised of Māori (14%–16%) indigenous people, settlers from the Pacific Islands (6%), and immigrants from Southeast Asian countries (11%), many who tend to die at a younger age compared to those of European descent who make up the majority of the population (67%) [14]. Māori comprise a larger proportion of the NZ population than other indigenous groups in Australia or the United States, and their different death and dying practices have influenced the development of palliative care in NZ [15].

In 2007, with a population nearing 4.4 million people, NZ had 27,257 deaths [16]. It is estimated that between 11,390 and 25,515 of the population who died would have benefited from palliative care [14]. Approximately 14,000 people received care and support from hospice organizations in 2011 [17]. Over the next 15 years, the NZ population is expected to increase by just over 19%, with the most significant increases in the over 65 age group (13.6%–21.2%) [16]. In 2009–2010, NZ spent 10.3% of its GDP on health, which is slightly more than the United Kingdom (9.8%) and slightly less than Canada (11.4%) [13]. With only one tier of government, health services in NZ are coordinated locally by the 20 District Health Boards organized around geographical areas of varying population sizes. These boards are responsible for providing or funding the provision of most health services in their district.

DEVELOPMENT OF PALLIATIVE CARE IN AUSTRALIA AND NEW ZEALAND

The context of palliative care development in Australia and NZ can be loosely categorized into the following three historical periods:

- *1838–1969*—Religious institutions caring for the dying, including the dying poor
- *1970–1999*—The modern palliative care movement
- *2000–onward*—A population health needs-based model of palliative care [18]

1838–1969: RELIGIOUS INSTITUTIONS CARING FOR THE DYING

Australia

The recorded history of care of the dying in Australia dates from modest beginnings toward the end of the nineteenth century [19]. This period is characterized by religious sponsorship

of designated institutions caring for the incurably ill and the dying poor in both Sydney and Melbourne, with a strong nursing focus [18]. In 1838, in response to a formal invitation to provide assistance to care for the cities' dying poor, the Irish "Sisters of Charity" sent five members to Sydney [20]. Similarly in Victoria, Melbourne City Mission was established during the chaos of the 1850s "gold rush" to care for the poor, who were often unwell and had flocked into the state hoping to make their fortune [19,20]. In 1885, the "Little Company of Mary" arrived in Sydney, establishing a community service providing prayer and succor for the dying within their own homes, support for the family, and a laying out service before opening a hospital in 1889 [18].

After half a century of caring for the incurably ill and dying poor in the community, the "Sisters of Charity" opened "St. Joseph's Consumptive Hospital" in Parramatta in 1886 and then "Sacred Heart Hospice" in Darlinghurst, New South Wales (NSW), in 1890 [21]. The pattern of religious orders establishing institutions for the dying poor continued into the early to mid-twentieth century, for example, with the "Sisters of Charity" opening St. Joseph's Hospice in Lismore, a rural community in NSW (1937); Caritas Christi Hospice, in Melbourne (1938); and Mt Olivet Hospital in Brisbane (1957) [22]. Over a period of 60 years, the Anglican Homes of Peace Sydney developed Eversleigh Hospice (1907), Neringah (1956), and Greenwich Hospitals (1966) [23] in Sydney. In the 1960s, the Little Company of Mary also embarked on a significant expansion program establishing Mary Potter Hospice in Adelaide, South Australia (SA) (1964), and Calvary Hospital in Sydney (1966) [18,24].

New Zealand

Similar to Australia, one of the striking elements of the development of NZ palliative care services is the significance of strong religious women with a commitment to caring for the sick and dying. The Daughters of Our Lady of Compassion opened St. Joseph's Home for Incurables in Wellington in 1900, along with the Little Company of Mary, who developed Calvary Hospital, Wellington (1929), and the Sisters of Mercy, who opened the Mater Misericordiae, Auckland (1952) [24].

1970–1999: THE MODERN PALLIATIVE CARE MOVEMENT

Dissatisfied families of patients with terminal cancer and several key clinicians began to publically express concerns about medical advances, which were leading to unnecessary suffering, which was the catalyst for the next iteration of development of care of the dying in Australia and NZ [25]. On the back of developments in the United Kingdom and Canada, the modern Australian and NZ palliative care movements slowly gained momentum from the early 1970s onward [19]. A combination of social action and key clinicians advocating for a model of care that was focused on promoting a better quality of life for people with advanced cancer resulted in the proliferation of new palliative care services, organizations, and professional societies in both countries during the latter part of the twenty-first century. These new services largely evolved organically, around existing hospices, acute care facilities, and community interests, and were not necessarily driven by strategic health services planning [26].

Australia

Prior to the allocation of the Commonwealth Medicare Incentives Program in the late 1980s, care of the dying was largely delivered in acute care hospitals and homes by individual clinicians and in "hospices" by religious and charitable organizations and volunteers. The delivery of palliative care was further strengthened with the establishment of the Commonwealth Palliative Care Program in 1993, providing additional funding to the states to support the expansion and/or establishment of palliative care services [27]. The balance between inpatient and community palliative care services and the extent to which they are integrated with existing health services has varied greatly between Australia's six states and two territories, with little jurisdictional or local planning to define this allocation [26]. An overview of some of the defining moments in the development of palliative care in these jurisdictions is provided in the following section.

NSW: Until the late 1970s, palliative care in NSW was predominantly focused on care of the dying and the dying poor within the established religious institutions in metropolitan Sydney. Similar to other parts of the developed world, by the 1980s, clinicians at several major teaching hospitals in Sydney, namely, Concord, Royal Prince Alfred, and St. Vincent's, had a growing interest in addressing the unmet needs of people dying within these acute hospitals [19]. Clinical leadership combined with local institutional support facilitated the appointment of palliative care medical specialists and palliative care clinical nurse consultants, who worked alongside acute care physicians and nurses to manage the needs of dying patients and their families [20].

Establishing home-based services proved to be more challenging in NSW, largely as a result of the states' historical focus on institutional care and the fact that no one domiciliary nursing service covered the sprawling metropolitan area. Consequently, there was limited state financial support and strategic direction in the early stages of palliative care development [19]. However, the availability of Commonwealth funding in the early 1980s facilitated the establishment of several clinical nurse consultant palliative care positions across regional NSW. In the absence of local palliative care physicians in these rural communities, many of these designated specialist palliative care nurses established strong primary care links and worked collaboratively with local generalist community nursing services to provide home-based palliative care [28]. During this period, the University of Newcastle appointed a chair in palliative medicine, thus fostering the development of a regional palliative care service servicing the Hunter River region of NSW [24]. Designated inpatient palliative care units were also being strengthened or established in several other regional centers, including Albury, Lismore, and Tamworth.

In the early 1980s, Sydney became the epicenter for Australia's HIV epidemic, with many services playing a pioneering role in caring for people dying from AIDS prior to the advent of anti-retroviral treatments [23]. This population challenged the traditional approach to hospice care as many people living with AIDS sought to combine palliative care and ongoing disease specific treatment, including participation in clinical trials. This tension ultimately fostered the stance that palliative care should be considered throughout a person's illness trajectory and served to promote the development of integrated models of care for adult and pediatric palliative care populations [23].

A pediatric palliative care program has operated at the Children's Hospital at Westmead since 1998, and Bear Cottage, a children's hospice in metropolitan Sydney, was established in 2001.

Victoria: Prior to 1980, palliative care in Victoria was only available in two separate and distinct inpatient units in Melbourne [28]. The Melbourne City Mission established a small inpatient palliative care unit within their nursing home in 1980 and the following year commenced a home care service extending palliative care to areas on the city fringes and into larger regional communities [18,20]. The allocation of the 1988 Medicare funding, which was aligned with state policy and funding, supported the establishment of regional palliative care services [28]. In 1994, geographically defined palliative care consortia were established by the state to help create networks to provide more regional development with service, education, and research linkages. These consortia include a hub and spoke model of provision of specialist support, with many metropolitan services providing medical outreach of a number of regional centers. By 1995, there were 18 metropolitan palliative care services and 27 rural services operating across Victoria, ensuring increased local palliative care access [28]. A pediatric palliative care program has operated at the Children's Hospital in Melbourne since 1984, with the "Very Special Kids House" (children's hospice) established in 1996 [18]. The release of the Victorian Palliative Care Strategic Framework (2011–2015) is evidence of Victoria's ongoing commitment to palliative care [29].

Queensland (QLD): Despite the establishment of Mt Olivet Hospital in Brisbane in 1957, it was not until 1982 that a medically directed hospice unit was established [19]. This development allowed for the expansion of palliative care into the community using the services of an established domiciliary nursing service to provide the UK Macmillan home nursing model of care [19]. The introduction of the 1988 Medicare funding allowed for an expansion of community palliative care services across Brisbane [20]. An integrated palliative care plan was developed for the Ipswich region, northwest of Brisbane, to ensure effective coordination of private and public palliative care services, with a general practitioner (GP) run hospice established in 1996 [30]. Private palliative care services were subsequently developed on the Gold Coast and in the regional centers of Mackay and much later in Toowoomba.

South Australia: In the 1980s, SA took the lead in a number of policy initiatives with the South Australian Health Commission accepting responsibility for the planning and coordination of palliative care services in the state with the release of the 1985 "Hospice Care Policy" [31]. The state also released a series of "natural death" acts [32], including the South Australian Consent to Medical Treatment and Palliative Care Act (1995), which acknowledges the importance of the terminally ill patient's wishes, in the form of an advanced directive or through a substitute decision maker [32]. In 1987, a chair in palliative medicine was established at Flinders University [33], helping to foster an innovative program of palliative care education [28]. In terms of service delivery, a palliative care team was established at Flinders Medical Centre, providing an inpatient and outreach service and utilizing hospital beds for the terminally ill at nearby Kalyra Hospital [19]. Other palliative care teams were subsequently established within the other three urban regions, each with a free-standing hospice or inpatient unit with informal linkages to smaller country units or services [28]. By the late 1980s, dedicated palliative care beds were also being established in Whyalla and Mt Gambier regional hospitals, with other regional centers setting up similar services concurrently [34].

Tasmania: In 1980, an inpatient palliative care unit was opened in Hobart Repatriation Hospital, and palliative care clinical nurse consultants were appointed to the palliative care team at Royal Hobart Hospital [20]. Despite palliative care services having started later in Tasmania than in other states, the early commitment of the government allowed for the establishment of a state-wide service, based in regional acute hospitals [19].

Western Australia (WA): The development of palliative care services in Perth has partially been shaped by an absence of established hospices and the existence of Silver Chain Nursing Association, a not-for-profit organization established in 1905, whose domiciliary nursing services by the 1980s cover the entire metropolitan area and a wide area of rural WA [35]. In 1981, the Cancer Foundation commissioned a hospice feasibility study, leading to two significant initiatives, namely, the establishment of a designated palliative care unit at Hollywood Repatriation Hospital [36] and a pilot study to test the feasibility and acceptability of an interdisciplinary community-based palliative care team, with strong primary care links [37]. The positive outcomes from this pilot led to Silver Chain being funded in 1985 to provide a 24 hour, 7 days per week, home-based palliative care service to cover the metropolitan area [36]. Around the same period, Bethesda, a small private hospital, provided the Cancer Foundation with access to a four-room facility as an inpatient palliative care unit [36]. A larger facility was deemed necessary, and after protracted negotiations, the 26-bed Cottage Hospice was opened in 1987 [36]. However, 19 years after opening, Cottage Hospice closed with its 26 hospice beds redistributed to Bethesda and several Perth outer metropolitan hospitals [38]. In the meantime, the St. John of God Murdoch Hospice (facility) was established in 1998 to service the community south of the city. Rural palliative care in WA is a combination of community care, with dedicated

palliative care beds available in several larger outer regional areas, including Albany and Bunbury.

Australian Capital Territory (ACT): Prior to 1984, GPs and community nurses provided end-of-life care to people in their own homes, including some limited after hours "call-out" care. Through the work of the ACT Hospice Society established in 1984 and the community nursing services, a small trial of home-based palliative care was undertaken in 1985, with cooperation of GPs and other medical specialists [39]. Funding obtained from the ACT government and the wider community maintained this service. After much planning, a hospice was opened in 1995 on the site of the old Canberra Hospital, where it operated for several years before the beds were relocated in 2001 to a purpose-built hospice "Clare Holland House" on the north shore of Lake Burley Griffin [39].

Northern Territory (NT): The NT occupies a vast area, which although sparsely populated is home to a large proportion of Australian Aboriginals. While the NT was one of the last Australian jurisdictions to fund palliative care, creating a Darwin-based palliative care team in 1993, it was the first jurisdiction in Australia to pass euthanasia legislation [40]. The Rights of the Terminally Ill Act (1995) was passed on May 25, 1995 and permitted both physician-assisted suicide and active voluntary euthanasia in certain circumstances [40]. Nine months later, this legislation was overturned by the Commonwealth, during which time seven terminally ill patients elected to have euthanasia [41]. In 2005, a decade after this legislation was repealed, a 12-bed hospice facility adjacent to Royal Darwin Hospital was opened [42]. This purpose-built facility was designed to address the needs of the local community, especially the needs of Aboriginal people and their families, many of whom live in remote isolated communities. In 1995, a palliative care team was established in Alice Springs to meet the needs of the remote Central Australian community. Territory Palliative Care now provides community specialist outreach services throughout the NT.

New Zealand

Philanthropic support fuelled the establishment of many of NZ's modern palliative care initiatives, including the Wellington and Hutt Valley Nurses Bureau in 1976, later became the Community Domiciliary Nursing Trust, enabling palliative care to be augmented into the home-based care provided by district nurses and other health workers [24], along with the NZ first modern hospices: Mary Potter Hospice, Wellington; St. Joseph's Hospice, Auckland; and Te Omanga Hospice, Lower Hutt, which opened within months of each other in 1979 [24]. These organizations evolved independently and largely outside of purposeful national policy planning.

In 1992, when the NZ Department of Health commissioned a study designed to provide an information base to build future hospice policy, several large palliative care organizations elected not to participate in the study [43]. Despite this limitation, it was apparent that a number of opportunities and challenges were to be faced by NZ hospices in the immediate future, including determining the relevant mix and level of services communities required, the need to enhance coordination within a fragmented service environment, recognition of the specialized skill requirements of hospice care, and sustaining strong community input to hospice organizations [43]. Hospice care was subsequently identified as an essential health service with a recommendation that regional health authorities fund related services. In January 1997, the National Health Committee commenced a project "Care of the Dying," providing clear specifications of the services, settings, and service providers required to care for palliative care populations [44]. It was not until 1999 that NZ's first specialist children's palliative care service was established [14].

Specialist organizations and professional societies

The development of palliative care in both Australia and NZ has been intrinsically intertwined with cancer care. Across Australia, the jurisdictionally based cancer councils or anticancer councils or foundations, as many were previously known prior to 1997, played a key role in lobbying for the establishment of local palliative care services and continue to work on a range of end-of-life care issues and activities. As palliative care evolved in Australia and NZ, there was scope and a need for a range of other nongovernment agencies and professional societies to develop, including those listed in the following.

Palliative Care Australia: This peak national body was established in 1991, having started out as the Australian Association of Hospice and Palliative Care, an umbrella organization representing the interests of the various state-based palliative care organizations [18]. Palliative Care Australia, in its various forms, has played a key role in shaping policy and informing health services reform. It was instrumental in developing the first "Standards for Hospice and Palliative Care Provision" in 1994 in partnership with the Australian Council on Health Standards [45] and a decade later "A guide to palliative care service development: a population-based approach" [6]. The latter document signaled a turning point for Australian palliative care by promoting a new way of conceptualizing palliative care from a public health perspective—an approach that continues to underpin national and jurisdictional policy.

Australian and New Zealand Society of Palliative Medicine (ANZSPM) and the Royal Australasian College of Physicians (RACP): Since its formal establishment in 1994, ANZSPM has played a key role in developing the credibility of palliative care medicine and the establishment of a recognized medical specialty [8]. A strategic collaboration between the ANZSPM and the RACP facilitated the establishment of a comprehensive training program in Australia and NZ and the establishment of two distinct specialist palliative medicine pathways, either via full specialist palliative medicine practice training conducted over 6 years by the RACP resulting in the award of a fellowship with credentialing in palliative medicine from the RACP, which has been available since 1991, or the Australasian Chapter of Palliative Medicine ("chapter") training program, which was approved by the college in 1999 [8]. In addition, in 2000, 218 doctors working in palliative medicine across Australia and NZ

became the foundation Fellows of the Australasian Chapter of Palliative Medicine (FAChPM). Having negotiated an identifiable specialty pathway into palliative medicine, securing access to appropriate reimbursement items became the organizations next priority [8]. This goal was achieved in NZ in 2001 after much negotiation and discussion, when palliative medicine was declared a specialty by the Medical Council of NZ, and in Australia in 2005, when palliative medicine was formally recognized as a specialty for reimbursement purposes, with relevant reimbursement items coming into effect in July 2006 [8].

During the same period, ANZSPM released a joint position statement in partnership with the Royal Australian and Royal New Zealand Colleges of General Practitioners and the Australian College of Rural and Remote Medicine acknowledging the essential role of GPs in palliative care delivery [8]. Since 2006, a Clinical Diploma in Palliative Medicine has been available to registered medical practitioners from an array of training backgrounds, who seek to increase their palliative care capabilities [8].

Sydney Institute of Palliative Medicine: The Sydney Institute of Palliative Medicine was created to provide opportunities for doctors without specialist training to accumulate palliative care experience and expertise [8]. It continues to provide educational opportunities for doctors seeking to gain experience in providing medical care in the inpatient, hospice, consultative, and community palliative care settings.

Palliative Care Nurses Association: The Palliative Care Nurses Association was formed in 2003 to promote excellence in palliative care nursing, through leadership, representation, and professional support. As a newly formed nongovernment organization, this association aims to foster the sustainability of the nursing workforce in palliative care; promote the professional development of nurses providing end-of-life care; provide opportunities for collaboration among members; facilitate knowledge, research, education, and policy in palliative care; promote palliative care nursing in a changing environment; and encourage participation in local, national, and international palliative care nursing activities.

Hospice New Zealand: Following consensus for the formation of a national hospice association for NZ in 1985, a conference and inaugural meeting was convened in May 1986 [46]. Hospice NZ was officially established, with its first objective being to "improve the quality of terminal and palliative care in New Zealand." It was also charged with negotiating with government and other national bodies for the good of the hospice movement in NZ, negotiating national policy affecting the future development of hospice programs and new hospices, and developing standards [46]. This organization continues to be actively involved in research and education; workforce development; establishing health-care standards; providing information and advice to hospices, stakeholders, and the general public; and helping and supporting hospices nationwide.

Palliative Care Council of New Zealand: To support the ongoing development of palliative care, Cancer Control New Zealand established the Palliative Care Council of NZ in 2008 [47].

This independent group provides expert advice to the minister of health and reports on NZ's performance in providing palliative and end-of-life care by reviewing data collected by the ministry of health on the activity of palliative care organizations and teams [47].

2000–ONWARD IN AUSTRALIA: A POPULATION HEALTH NEEDS–BASED MODEL OF PALLIATIVE CARE

By the late 1990s, the Australian government took a strategic approach to strengthen palliative care across the country, by funding national initiatives that aimed to build national policy, build the evidence base, support evidence-based practice, and build the capacity for services to focus on quality and effectiveness focusing on policy, practice, education, and research as detailed in the next section. In doing so, the Commonwealth encouraged the states to provide financial support for palliative care services. This occurred on a background of significant developments in palliative care alluded previously and also followed the passing and subsequent repeal of the Rights of the Terminally Ill Act (1995).

The Australian states and territories

Policy and planning: A population health approach is central to national and jurisdictional policy and planning in Australia and is reflected in the country's first National Palliative Care Strategy released in 2000 [48]. A population health approach captures the concepts of health promotion and provides a framework for needs-based planning and the foundation for the continued "individual approach" that is evident at the clinical level. A population health approach allows for the planning and integration of relevant services for palliative care in accordance with need. This approach is considerate of the needs of different population groups (i.e., pediatric, culturally and linguistically diverse background), conditions (i.e., cancer, end-stage heart failure), locations (i.e., regional, rural, and remote), and care settings (i.e., community, acute or aged care). It acknowledges the importance of fostering and supporting the ongoing provision of appropriate, high-quality end-of-life care that is largely provided by family, clinicians, and community workers through a palliative approach [5]. Promoting a palliative approach fosters an arrangement whereby specialist palliative care services focus on providing expert clinical advice to people with complex symptoms, provide direct care to a small number of people with more challenging care needs, and play an active role in supporting and building the capacity of other clinicians and services to provide a palliative approach to care [5].

The endorsement of the National Palliative Care Strategy (2000) by the Australian Health Ministers' Advisory Council (a "Commonwealth" body) and the allocation of funding provided opportunities to develop the systems and processes to enable the delivery of best evidence-based quality palliative care to more Australians, in accordance with need [48]. Over the following decade, the Commonwealth allocated funding

to support the expansion and strengthening of palliative care across Australia. These funds supported the state and territory governments' inpatient and community palliative care programs, as well as the National Palliative Care Program initiatives which aimed to increase (1) support for patients, families, and carers in the community; (2) access to palliative care medicines in the community; (3) workforce education, training, and support; and (4) research and quality improvement (Table 7.1) [48].

In addition to the National Palliative Care Strategy, four of the seven jurisdictions (states and territories) have a current palliative care plan, with NT and ACT plans having expired several years ago and the QLD plan awaiting ratification. Models of care are outlined in the WA and SA palliative care plans, with an emphasis on networking and developing palliative care partnerships [49,50], plus supplementary models of rural, pediatric, and adolescent palliative care [51,52].

Practice: The development of "CareSearch," an online resource designed to help those needing relevant and trustworthy palliative care information and resources, has been an important development aiming to ensure that more Australians, clinicians, and consumers have access to information about best evidence-based practice via a central hub (www.caresearch.com.au) [56]. This Commonwealth funded palliative care web-based resource seeks to capture and respond to the dynamic nature of the evidence and literature that supports palliative care practice, with the content evolving to meet identified needs.

Since 2000, the National Palliative Care Program has endeavored to promote greater awareness and collaboration between mainstream health-care services and Aboriginal community–controlled health services to ensure that the palliative care needs of Aboriginal and Torres Strait Islander peoples are appropriately addressed [54,71]. The National Indigenous Palliative Care Needs Study identified a range of issues to be addressed to ensure that palliative care is accessible to all indigenous Australians [54]. Several key documents and resources have emerged from this work, including a toolkit to better support specialist palliative care services to strengthen their links with local Aboriginal and Torres Strait Islander organizations and to provide culturally safe and culturally appropriate palliative care [71]. Palliative Care Australia was subsequently funded to developed multicultural palliative care guidelines to promote awareness and a commitment to deliver culturally safe palliative care [72].

Evidence-based guidelines for a palliative approach in residential aged care were developed in 2004 in response to the increasing recognition that that many older people in nursing homes often have unmet palliative care needs and could benefit from a palliative approach to care well before their final days or weeks of life. They provide aged care providers, GPs, and families with access to best evidence to assist decision making and to guide appropriate practice [57]. In 2011, these guidelines were adapted to support health professionals promote a palliative approach in community aged care settings [73].

In order to institute a more uniform palliative care system and to improve care outcomes, the Commonwealth also funded the establishment of the Palliative Care Outcomes Collaboration (PCOC) in 2006 to develop and support a

Table 7.1   *Overview of some of the achievements of Australia's National Palliative Care Program (1999–2010)*

Domain	Focus	Achievements
Support for patients, families, and carers in the community	Defining the need	Population-based identification of gaps in palliative care service provision [53]
		The National Indigenous Palliative Care Needs Study [54]
		Evaluation of palliative care needs of children [55]
	Evidence-based practice	Establishment of the Palliative Care Knowledge Network [56]
		Developed and disseminated *Guidelines for a Palliative Approach in Residential Aged Care* [57]
	Increasing access	National Rural Palliative Care Program: rounds 1 and 2 [58]
		Local Palliative Care Grants designed to support local health service and community groups to deliver palliative care [48]
		Caring Communities Program [59]
	Advance care planning	National Respecting Patient Choices Program [60]
Increased access to palliative care medicines in the community	Palliative medicines	Provision of palliative medicines on Pharmaceutical Benefits Scheme [61,62]
Workforce education, training, and support	Building capacity	National PCC4U [63]
		Evaluation education needs of GPs [64]
		PEPA [65]
Research and quality improvement	Research	Scoping study—Australia's Future in Palliative Care Research [66] NHMRC: • Doctoral research fellowships in palliative care • Programs of competitive investigator-driven research funding [67] PaCCSC, a multisite palliative care clinical trial network [68]
	Benchmarking	NSAP [69]
		PCOC [70]

national benchmarking system [74]. Currently, over 80% of people seen by Australian specialist palliative care services have point-of-care data collected related to service delivery from initial referral until their death [26]. This initiative compliments the "National Standards Assessment Program" (NSAP), also funded by the Commonwealth and led by Palliative Care Australia. NSAP aims to support palliative care services to move toward best practice by improving the quality of palliative care they provide through their existing quality improvement processes and accreditation cycles [69].

Responding to the challenges of evolving medical technologies capacity to prolonging life, the National Palliative Care Program funded a trial of the "Respecting Patient Choices Program©" in several jurisdictions [60]. This pilot served to foster an awareness of advance care planning, and there is increased discussion about advance care planning nationally with each jurisdiction taking initiatives in this area forward in differing ways.

Education: Building the palliative care capabilities of the existing and future health and aged care workforce underpins the delivery of best evidence-based palliative care [75]. The Palliative Care Curriculum for Undergraduates (PCC4U) program, funded as part of the National Palliative Care Program, aims to build undergraduate medical, nursing, and allied health trainees palliative care capabilities [76]. This online competency-based program is used in 39% of relevant university courses across Australia [76], with a concerted ongoing effort to increase uptake. For the existing health workforce, the Program of Experience in the Palliative Approach (PEPA) has funded a range of health workers (doctors, nurses, allied health professionals, and Aboriginal health workers) to gain short-term palliative care experience in a range of care settings and build a mentoring network between the specialist and nonspecialist workforce [65].

Research: Underpinning the national palliative care policy agenda was a commitment at the Commonwealth government level of the need to build the evidence base to inform palliative care practice as well as public policy and to establish national and international collaborations to undertake population-based research [25]. Building the research capacity of the palliative care community was identified as an important first step [48]. Having identified Australia's palliative care research priorities [66], $2 million was allocated by the Commonwealth in 2001 to the National Health and Medical Research Council (NHMRC) to establish the National Palliative Care Research Program to build the capacity of the palliative care research sector to be more competitive in securing general health and medical research funding [67].

On the back of this success, and having identified a need for good clinical data from well-conducted clinical trials designed to address efficacy, cost-effectiveness, and safety, the Commonwealth in June 2006 allocated $9.4 million to establish the Palliative Care Clinical Studies Collaborative (PaCCSC), a national multisite palliative care collaborative clinical studies group [62]. PaCCSC is conducting a range of palliative care randomized clinical trials across more than 12 sites in Australia and completed its first clinical trials in early 2011 [77], closely followed by the completion of the second randomized controlled trial in 2012 [78]. In addition to generating high-level palliative care evidence, PaCCSC has contributed significantly to building palliative care clinical trial expertise across more than a dozen specialist Australian palliative care services and has successfully generated additional competitive clinical research funding [79].

NEW ZEALAND'S NATIONAL RESPONSE

Prior to the development of the NZ's National Palliative Care Strategy in 2001, palliative care services had arisen in a variety of locations and evolved in the absence of a national planning strategy [44]. The ministry of health in partnership with the National Health Committee, Hospice NZ, and the Health Funding Authority developed the 2001 National Strategy with the agreed priorities being (1) assessment and care coordination, (2) clinical care, and (3) support care [44]. As a result of the ministry of health's leadership, 39 community-based hospice palliative care services and 16 inpatient palliative care services currently operate across NZ [14]. Supporting this work is a collaboratively developed national work plan encompassing a number of projects designed to facilitate more effective care provision within the sector [80].

Policy: Several initiatives have been undertaken in NZ to enable provision of palliative care in accordance with a population-based approach. The National Health Needs Assessment for Palliative Care used recognized methodologies to develop estimates of palliative care need on both a national and regional basis, provided an assessment of the services required to meet the identified need, and compared current service provision with determined need [14]. The first phase results emerging from this process will be instrumental in shaping services to address unmet needs over the coming decade [14]. The collaboration between government agencies and Hospice NZ is providing leadership to the sector that has been fragmented in past years. Although over a decade has passed since the publication of the original NZ National Strategy, there are many aspects of that document that are still relevant today, and the overall aim that "All people who are dying and their family/whānau who could benefit from palliative care have timely access to quality palliative care services that are culturally appropriate and are provided in a coordinated way" remains vital.

The National Service Plan for Adult Palliative Care provides clear expectations to planners, funders, providers, and the community to inform efficient and sustainable planning and funding decisions around palliative care service provision [80]. The current evaluation of Palliative Care Provision in Primary Care will assess the effectiveness of various palliative care programs currently in place and determine how these contribute to a nationally consistent approach to delivering palliative care in the primary care setting [80].

Practice: On a national basis, most NZ deaths occur in hospital settings (34%), followed by residential care (31%), and private residence (22%), with a smaller number occurring in a hospice inpatient unit (6%) [14]. A Hospital Palliative Care Service Capability Framework has been developed for use by individual hospital palliative care services to build a clear description of the services they offer and the staffing skills and experience needed to deliver these services [80]. Similarly, the Hospice Capability Project is being undertaken to develop a framework that can be used by individual hospices to build a clear description of the services they offer and of the staffing skills and experience needed to deliver these services [80].

Advance care planning in NZ has gained momentum in recent years, with advance care planning guidelines developed with ministry of health support, along with input from relevant clinical disciplines and an expert advisory group from the National Advance Care Planning Cooperative [81]. These guidelines reflect the NZ's Code of Health and Disability Services Consumers' Rights [81].

Various initiatives have been undertaken to address the palliative care needs of specific populations [80]. These initiatives acknowledge the Māori model of health: *te whare tapa whā* (four-sided house), with *wairua* (spiritual), *hinengaro* (thoughts and feelings), *tinana* (physical), and *whānau* (family and community aspects), as central to culturally appropriate and safe palliative care [15]. In recognition of the palliative care needs of the growing aged population, Hospice NZ has developed and implemented a *Fundamentals of Palliative Care* education program to be available for all residential aged care facilities over time and free distribution of the *Palliative Care Handbook* [82]. The current *Palliative Care Provision in Aged Residential Care* project aims to identify palliative care capacity in this care setting along with the palliative care aged care data gaps [80]. *The Guidance for Integrated Paediatric Palliative Care Services in New Zealand* aims to improve the integration of palliative care service delivery to children and young people in NZ. A summary document has the key recommendations of the guidance that district health board funders and planners can use as a quick reference guide [83].

The Hospice NZ Standards for Palliative Care supports quality management and improvement activities at a local, regional, and national level. Services use the information garnered from self-assessment and from peer review to address gaps, refine the delivery of care that does not meet standards, and replicate successes [80]. This activity aims to enable services to share and implement initiatives that will improve the extent to which they meet the standards as well as benchmarks [84].

Education: Despite the 1997 endorsement by medical school deans of the ANZSPM medical undergraduate curriculum for palliative care [85] and pressure from both students and faculty alike, NZ medical schools have been slow to acknowledge the development of the specialty, and thus, there is still often a lack of palliative care input into medical undergraduates' training and education [73]. The palliative medicine curriculum for advanced training in the specialty was developed by a team of fellows of the RACP over many months preceding its publication in 2005 and is now used in training of all fellows in palliative medicine throughout both Australia and NZ [86]. This curriculum outlines "the broad concepts, related learning objectives and the associated theoretical knowledge, clinical skills, attitudes and behaviours required and commonly used by palliative medicine physicians and paediatricians within Australia and New Zealand." It is intended that it is used in conjunction with the Professional Qualities Curriculum of the Royal Australian College of Physicians [86].

A National Professional Development Framework for Palliative Care Nursing in Aotearoa (NZ) details the competencies of nurses engaged in differing levels of palliative care delivery [87]. This framework provides competency indicators outlining the role expectations of nurses working in cancer control and palliative care [87]. There are also a small but increasing number of palliative care nurse practitioners scattered throughout the country.

Education for other health professionals is sparse, but as of the time of writing this chapter, some universities were responding to the importance of developing the emerging health workforce's palliative care capabilities, and postgraduate programs are now appearing with particular emphasis on the social work and counseling workforce. In addition, Health Workforce NZ has proposed that a Palliative Care Interdisciplinary Education/Training Board be established and tasked with prioritizing and progressing palliative care workforce's training needs [88].

Research: NZ's first, and only, chair in palliative care was established in 2003 through a partnership between South Link Health, the Otago Community Hospice, and the University of Otago, Dunedin School of Medicine. Funding for palliative care research in NZ is currently limited and not linked to national priorities, with many studies relying on small charitable trusts for funding.

CONCLUSION

Up to the mid-1990s, the configuration of Australian and NZ palliative care services was largely shaped by historical origins, number and location of palliative care beds, differing funding mechanisms, strength of local institutional support, and linkages with existing community nursing services. Building on the history of hospice and palliative care in these countries, strong professional and community advocacy has served to support and foster a shift to a more contemporary, nationally coordinated, needs-based, population health model that is now a clearly established priority for these countries.

Linking large metropolitan services with regional services to create clinical networks and developing innovative,

collaborative models of care are now seen as a "next step" to consider so as to enable access and equity for all, particularly for people with complex palliative care needs and those living outside the major metropolitan areas. There continues to be scope to more fully exploit the use of novel telecommunications technology to address unmet palliative care needs in less well-resourced communities and care settings. Building the palliative care capabilities of the health workforce is viewed in both countries as central to addressing the increasing burden of chronic disease. Ongoing investments in clinically relevant research and a commitment to translating evidence into practice in a timely manner are required to ensure that more people have access to best evidence-based palliative care. Achieving these outcomes will require responsive national and local policy–driven initiatives, an ongoing commitment to continue to build the evidence, an adequately equipped and supported health workforce, and a service culture that embraces change and innovation.

Key learning points

- Care of the dying in Australia and NZ has a documented history that dates back to the late 1880s, with religious organizations playing a key role in the early history.

- A number of key individuals, groups, and societies played a central role in establishing and continuing to shape the modern palliative care movement in Australia and NZ today.

- The release of Australia's first National Palliative Care Strategy in 2000, underpinned by a public health approach and supported by strategic funding of research, education, and practice initiatives aligned to national health policy, has strengthened palliative care delivery across this country.

- Many of Australia's recent national palliative care initiatives have attracted international attention for their innovative, collaborative approaches and potential to impact positively on the care provided to patients and their families, both nationally and internationally.

- NZ palliative care has benefited from a more coordinated approach since the release of its first Palliative Care Strategy in 2001, with continued opportunities to strengthen palliative care education and strategic research endeavors.

ACKNOWLEDGMENTS

The information contained in this chapter reflects a summation of information gleaned from various written materials. We gratefully acknowledge the assistance of our palliative care colleagues in various parts of Australia and New Zealand who provided feedback and directed us toward sources of information, notably David Currow (SA and NSW), Rita Evans (ACT), Peta Firns (WA), Ray Lowenthal (Tasmania), Fred Miguel (NT), Geoff Mitchell (QLD), Mary Schumacher (NZ), and Odette Spruyt (Victoria).

Professor Phillips' and Professor Ingham's work on this chapter was undertaken, in part, with funding support from the Cancer Institute NSW Academic Chairs Program. The views expressed herein are those of the authors and are not necessarily those of the Cancer Institute NSW.

REFERENCES

1   Australian Institute of Health and Welfare. *Palliative Care Services in Australia 2012*. Canberra, Australian Capital Territory, Australia: Australian Institute of Health and Welfare; 2012.

2   Central Region's Technical Advisory Services Limited. *Gap Analysis of Specialist Palliative Care in New Zealand: Providing a National Overview of Hospice and Hospital-Based Services*. Wellington, New Zealand: Ministry of Health; 2009.

3   Clark D. From margins to centre: A review of the history of palliative care in cancer. *The Lancet Oncology* 2007;**8**(5):430–438.

4   Maddocks I. A new society of palliative medicine. *Medical Journal of Australia* 1994;**160**(June):670.

5   Commonwealth of Australia. *Supporting Australians to Live Well at the End of Life: National Palliative Care Strategy 2010*. Barton, Australian Capital Territory, Australia: Commonwealth of Australia; 2010.

6   Palliative Care Australia. *A Guide to Palliative Care Service Development: A Population Based Approach*. Canberra, Australian Capital Territory, Australia: Palliative Care Australia; 2005.

7   Australian Bureau of Statistics. *Regional Population Growth, Australia 2010–2011*. Canberra, Australian Capital Territory, Australia: Australian Bureau of Statistics; 2012.

8   Cairns W. A short history of palliative medicine in Australia. *Cancer Forum* 2007;**31**(1):6–9.

9   Australian Institute of Health and Welfare. *The Health and Welfare of Australia's Aboriginal and Torres Strait Islander Peoples*. Canberra, Australian Capital Territory, Australia: Canberra Australian Institute of Health and Welfare; 2008.

10   Australian Bureau of Statistics. *Deaths, Australia 2010*. Canberra, Australian Capital Territory, Australia: ABS; 2011.

11   Gordon R, Eagar K, Currow D, Green J. Current funding and financing issues in the Australian hospice and palliative care sector. *Journal of Pain and Symptom Management* 2009;**38**(1):68.

12   Mitchell GK. Palliative care in Australia. *Ochsner Journal* Winter 2011;**11**(4):334–337.

13   Australian Institute of Health and Welfare. How much do we spend on health? Canberra, Australian Capital Territory, Australia; 2012; Available from: http://www.aihw.gov.au/australias-health/2012/spending-on-health/.

14   Palliative Care Council of New Zealand. *National Health Needs Assessment for Palliative Care Phase 1 Report: Assessment of Palliative Care Need*. Wellington, New Zealand: Palliative Care Council of New Zealand; June 2011.

15   Muircroft W, McKimm J, William L, Macleod RD. A New Zealand perspective on palliative care for Māori. *Journal of Palliative Care* 2010;**26**(1):54–58.

16   Ministry of Health. *Mortality and Demographic Data 2007*. Wellington, New Zealand: Ministry of Health; 2010.

17   Hospice NZ. About Hospice NZ—History. Wellington, New Zealand: Hospice NZ; 2012 [updated 2012; cited July 12, 2012]; Available from: http://www.hospice.org.nz/about-hospice-nz/history.

18   Harris RD, Finlay-Jones LM. Terminal care in Australia. *Hospice Journal: Physical, Psychosocial and Pastoral Care of the Dying* 1987;**3**(1):77–90.

19   Cavenagh JD, Gunz FW. Palliative hospice care in Australia. *Palliative Medicine* 1988;**2**(1):51–57.

20   Allen S, Chapman Y, O'Connor M, Francis K. The evolution of palliative care and the relevance to residential aged care: Understanding the past to inform the future. *Collegian: Journal of the Royal College of Nursing Australia* 2008;**15**(4):165–171.

21   Skewes EM. *This Little Gem: St Joseph's Hospital Auburn 1886-1986*. Auburn NSW: St Joseph's Hospital; 1986.

22   Skewes EM. *Life Comes to Newness: Mt Olivet Hospital, Brisbane*. Boolarong Publications, Brisbane, Australia; 1982.

23   Stuart-Harris R. The Sacred Heart Hospice: An Australian centre for palliative medicine. *Supportive Care in Cancer* 1995;**3**(5):280–284.

24   Lickiss JN. The development of palliative medicine in Australia/New Zealand. In: Bruera E, Higginson IJ, Von Gunten CF, Ripamonti C, eds. *Textbook of Palliative Medicine*. London, U.K.: Hodder Arnold; 2009, pp. 49–57.

25   Brooksbank M. Palliative care: Where have we come from and where are we going? *Pain* 2009;**144**(3):233–235.

26   Currow D, Allingham S, Bird S, Yates P, Lewis J, Dawber J et al. Referral patterns and proximity to palliative care inpatient services by level of socio-economic disadvantage. A national study using spatial analysis. *BMC Health Service Research* 2012;**12**(1):424.

27   Australian Government. Health and Family Services Portfolio Budget Statements 1997–1998. Canberra Australian Government, Department of Health and Ageing; 1997 [updated May 13, 1997; cited 2013 January 21, 2013]; Available from: http://www.health.gov.au/internet/main/publishing.nsf/Content/health-pubs-budget97-pbs-2-3bm.htm.

28   Sach J. *Palliative Care in Rural Australia*. Canberra, Australian Capital Territory, Australia: Commonwealth Department of Health and Family Services; 1996.

29   Victorian Government Department of Health. *Strengthening palliative pare: Policy and strategic directions 2011–2015*. Melbourne, Victoria, Australia: Department of Health; 2011.

30   Mitchell G, Price J. Developing palliative care services in regional areas. The Ipswich Palliative Care Network model. *Australian Family Physician* January 2001;**30**(1):59–62.

31   Hunt R, Bonett A, Roder D. Trends in the terminal care of cancer patients: South Australia, 1981–1990. *Australian and New Zealand Journal of Medicine* 1993;**23**(3):245–251.

32   Hunt RW. The hospice movement matures. *Medical Journal of Australia*. [Editorial]. 1996 April 15, 1996;**164**(8):452–453.

33   Kellehear A. *Death and Dying in Australia*. Melbourne, Victoria, Australia: South Melbourne; Oxford University Press; 2000.

34   Palliative Care Council SA. Palliative Care in South Australia. Adelaide, South Australia, Australia; 2012 [updated January 24, 2012; cited 2012 November 20, 2012]; Available from: http://www.pallcare.asn.au/about/history-of-palliative-care/palliative-care-in-south-australia.

35   Chetkovich J, Gare D. *A Chain of Care: A History of the Silver Chain Nursing Association, 1905-2005*. Fremantle, Western Australia, Australia: University of Notre Dame Australia Press; 2005.

36   Oliver B. "Outside the City Wall?": The hospice and palliative care movement in Western Australia. *Occasional Papers on Medical History Australia* 1991;**5**:134–137.

37   Allbrook DB. The hospice palliative care service of Western Australia. *World Medical Journal* November–December 1985;**32**(6):93.

38   Anon. *McGinty backs Cottage Hospice Review*. Post Newspapers, Shenton Park, Western Australia; 2005.

39   Billington A. *Recollections: Palliative care and ACT Hospice, 1984–2000*. Ainslie, ACT: A Billington; 2004.

40   Parliment of Australia Law and Public Administration Group. Research Paper 4: Active Voluntary Euthanasia. Canberra, Australian Capital Territory, Australia: Parliment of Australia; 1997 [cited October 20, 2012]; Available from: http://www.aph.gov.au/About_Parliament/Parliamentary_Departments/Parliamentary_Library/pubs/rp/RP9697/97rp4.

41   Kissane DW, Street A, Nitschke P. Seven deaths in Darwin: Case studies under the Rights of the Terminally III Act, Northern Territory, Australia. *The Lancet* 1998;**352**(9134):1097–1102.

42   Northern Territory Government Department of Health. Royal Darwin Hospital. Darwin, Northern Territory, Australia: Northern Territory Government Department of Health; 2012 [cited October 20, 2012]; Available from: http://www.health.nt.gov.au/Hospitals/Royal_Darwin_Hospital/index.aspx.

43   Barnett P, Smith K. *The organisation and funding of hospice care: An international and New Zealand view.* Health Research Services and Personal and Public Health Policy, Department of Health New Zealand; 1992.

44   Ministry of Health. *The New Zealand Palliative Care Strategy.* Wellington, New Zealand: Ministry of Health; 2001.

45   Ramadge J. Australian nursing practice and palliative care: Its origins, evolution and future. In: Ramadge J, ed. *Palliative Care in Australia.* Canberra, Australian Capital Territory, Australia: Royal College of Nursing; 2000.

46   Hospice New Zealand. History. Wellington, New Zealand: Hospice New Zealand; 2012 [cited October 20, 2012]; Available from: http://www.hospice.org.nz/about-hospice-nz/history.

47   Palliative Care Council of New Zealand. *Introducing the Palliative Care Council of New Zealand.* Wellington, New Zealand: Palliative Care Council; 2010.

48   Commonwealth Department of Health and Aged Care. *National Palliative Care Strategy: A National Framework for Palliative Care Service Development.* Canberra, Australia; Commonwealth Department of Health and Aged Care; 2000.

49   South Australia Health. *Palliative Care Services Plan 2009–2016.* Adelaide, South Australia, Australia: Government of South Australia; 2009 05–2009. (9780730899617 (pbk.)).

50   Department of Health Western Australia. *Palliative Care Model of Care.* Perth, Western Australia, Australia: WA Cancer & Palliative Care Network, Department of Health, Western Australian; 2008.

51   Department of Health Western Australia. *Rural Palliative Care Model in Western Australia.* Perth, Western Australia, Australia: WA Palliative Care & Cancer Network, Department of Health, Western Australia; October 2008.

52   Department of Health WA. *Paediatric and Adolescent Palliative Care Model of Care.* Perth, Western Australia, Australia: WA Palliative Care & Cancer Network; 2009 09–2009.

53   McNamara B, Rosenwax L. Factors affecting place of death in Western Australia. *Health and Place* 2007;**13**(2):356–367.

54   Australian Government. *National Indigenous Palliative Care Needs Study: Final Report.* Canberra, Australian Capital Territory, Australia: Department of Health and Ageing; 2003.

55   Healthcare Management Advisors Ltd. *Paediatric Palliative Care Service Model Review.* Canberra, Australian Capital Territory, Australia: Department of Health and Ageing; 2004.

56   Tieman J, Abernethy A, Fazekas B, Currow D. CareSearch: Finding and evaluating Australia's missing palliative care literature. *BMC Palliative Care* 2005;**4**(1):4.

57   Australian Department of Health and Ageing and National Health and Medical Research Council. *Guidelines for a Palliative Approach in Residential Aged Care—Enhanced Version.* Canberra, Australian Capital Territory, Australia; National Health and Medical Research Council; 2006.

58   Australian Divisions of General Practice. Rural palliative care program. Canberra, Australian Capital Territory, Australia; 2004 [http://www.adgp.com.au/site/index.cfm?display=683 December 1, 2006.].

59   Department of Health and Aged Care. The caring communities program. Canbera CareSearch; 2008 [cited October 11, 2012]; Available from: http://www.caresearch.com.au/caresearch/tabid/85/Default.aspx.

60   Respecting Patient Choices©. An Australian model of advance care planning. 2012 [cited 2013 January 21, 2013]; Available from: http://www.respectingpatientchoices.org.au/.

61   Department of Health and Ageing. Pharmaceutical benefits for palliative care. Canberra, Australian Capital Territory, Australia: Australian Government; 2012 [cited October 11, 2012]; Available from: http://www.pbs.gov.au/browse/palliative-care.

62   Rowett D, Ravenscroft PJ, Hardy J, Currow DC. Using national health policies to improve access to palliative care medications in the community. *Journal of Pain and Symptom Management* 2009;**37**(3):395–402.

63   Hegarty M, Currow D, Parker D, Turnbull B, Devery K, Canning DF et al. Palliative care in undergraduate curricula: Results of a national scoping study. *Focus on Health Professional Education* 2010;**12**(2):97–109.

64   Reymond L, Mitchell G, McGrath B, Welch D, Treston P, Israel F et al. *Research Study into the Educational Training and Support Needs of General Practitioners in Palliative Care.* Canberra, Australian Capital Territory, Australia: Australian Department of Health and Ageing; 2003.

65   Department of Health and Ageing. Program of experience in the palliative approach. Brisbane, Queensland, Australia; 2012 [cited 2012 November 19, 2012]; Available from: http://www.pepaeducation.com/.

66   Palliative Care Australia. *Australia's Future in Palliative Care research: A Collaborative Approach.* Canbera, Australian Capital Territory, Australia: Palliative Care Australia; 2000.

67   Currow DC, Tieman J. *Phase One of the National Palliative Care Research Program: Summary Paper.* Adelaide, South Australia, Australia: Flinders University; 2005.

68   CareSearch. Palliative care clinical studies collaborative,. Adelaide, South Australia, Australia: Flinders University; 2011 [updated March 30, 2012; cited October 11, 2012]; Available from: http://www.caresearch.com.au/caresearch/tabid/97/Default.aspx.

69   Palliative Care Australia. National Standards Assessment Program. Canbera Palliative Care Australia; 2012 [cited October 12, 2012]; Available from: http://www.palliativecare.org.au/Standards/NSAP.aspx.

70   Eagar K, Watters P, Currow DC, Aoun SM, Yates P. The Australian Palliative Care Outcomes Collaboration (PCOC)–measuring the quality and outcomes of palliative care on a routine basis. *Australian Health Review* 2010;**34**(2):186–192.

71   Australian Government. *Providing Culturally Appropriate Palliative Care: Aboriginal and Torres Strait Islander Resource Kit Project.* Canberra, Australian Capital Territory, Australia: Department of Health and Ageing; 2004.

72   Palliative Care Australia. Multilingual resources. Canberra, Australian Capital Territory, Australia; 2012 [cited November 19, 2012]; Available from: http://www.palliativecare.org.au/Default.aspx?tabid=2116.

73   Australian Government Department of Health and Ageing. *Guidelines for a Palliative Approach for Aged Care in the Community Setting—Best Practice Guidelines for the Australian Context.* Canberra, Australian Capital Territory, Australia: Australian Government Department of Health and Ageing; 2011.

74   Currow DC, Eagar K, Aoun S, Fildes D, Yates P, Kristjanson LJ. Is it feasible and desirable to collect voluntarily quality and outcome data nationally in palliative oncology care? *Journal of Clinical Oncology* 2008;**26**(23):3853–3859.

75   Ramjan JM, Costa CM, Hickman LD, Kearns M, Phillips JL. Integrating palliative care content into a nursing curriculum: The University of Notre Dame, Australia—Sydney experience. *Collegian* 2010;**17**(2):85–91.

76   Australian Government Department of Health and Ageing. Palliative Care Curriculum for Undergraduates (PCC4U). Brisbane, Queensland, Australia; 2012 [cited October 12, 2011]; Available from: http://www.pcc4ulearningresource.org/.

77   Hardy J, Quinn S, Fazekas B, Plummer J, Eckermann S, Agar M et al. Randomized, double-blind, placebo-controlled study to assess the efficacy and toxicity of subcutaneous ketamine in the management of cancer pain. *Journal of Clinical Oncology* September 10, 2012.

78   Currow DC, Clark K, Cartmill J, Pather S, Plummer J, Eckermann S et al. A multi-site, fixed dose, parallel arm, double-blind, placebo controlled, block randomised trial of the addition of infusional octreotide or placebo to regular ranitidine and dexamethasone for the evaluation of vomiting associated with bowel obstruction at the end of life. American Society of Clinical Oncology conference abstract TPS9153 in *Journal of Clinical Oncology* 30(15 Suppl 1):2012.

79   Lobb EA, Swetenham K, Agar M, Currow DC. A collateral benefit of research in palliative care. *Journal of Palliative Medicine* 2011;**14**(9):986–987.

80   Palliative Care Council of New Zealand, Hospice New Zealand, Ministry of Health. *Palliative Care: National Joint Programme.* Wellington, New Zealand: Ministry of Health; 2012.

81   Ministry of Health. *Advance Care Planning: A guide for the New Zealand health care workforce.* Wellington: Ministry of Health; 2011.

82   MacLeod RD, Vella-Brincat J, Macleod AD. *The Palliative Care Handbook* 6th edn. Wellington, New Zealand: Genesis Oncology Trust and Louisa and Patrick Emmett Murphy Trust; 2012.

83   Ministry of Health. *Guidance for Integrated Paediatric Palliative Care Services in New Zealand.* Wellington, New Zealand: Ministry of Health; 2012.

84   Hospice New Zealand. *Standards for Palliative Care: Quality Review Programme and Guide 2012.* Wellington, New Zealand: Hospice New Zealand; 2012.

85   Ashby M, Brooksbank M, Dunne P, MacLeod RD. *Australasian Undergraduate Medical Palliative Care Curriculum.* Melbourne, Victoria, Australia: ANZSPM; 1997.

86   Cairns W, Adler J, Agar M, Auret K, Brogan R, Brooksbank M et al. *Curriculum for the Training and Professional Development of Specialists in Palliative Medicine.* Sydney, New South Wales, Australia: Australasian Chapter of Palliative Medicine and Royal Australasian College of Physicians; 2005.

87   Ministry of Health. *A National Professional Development Framework for Palliative Care Nursing in Aotearoa New Zealand.* Wellington, New Zealand: Ministry of Health; 2008.

88   Health Workforce New Zealand. *Palliative Care Workforce Service Review.* Wellington, New Zealand: Health Workforce New Zealand; 2011.

8

Development of palliative medicine in Asia

SATORU TSUNETO

INTRODUCTION

Asia is the largest and most populous continent on Earth, covering 30% of its land area and hosting 60% of its population (4 billion people). The United Nations has recognized 48 nation states in Asia, which can be subdivided as follows: (1) Eastern Asia (five states), (2) Northern Asia (one state), (3) Central Asia (five states), (4) Southeastern Asia (11 states), (5) Southern Asia (nine states), and (6) Western Asia (17 states).

A wide diversity of races, languages, cultures, and religions, as well as political, economic, and health-care systems, exist within this region. Many countries are grappling with ways to provide basic health care in rapidly expanding and congested cities as well as in isolated rural areas where maternal and infant death rates are high. Infectious disease is still a major cause of illness, and the incidence of cancer is rising. Health-care professionals, especially nurses, often have relatively poor status and remuneration. In many Asian countries, traditional medicines are widely used, either instead of or concurrently with Western medicine.

There is also wide variation in the level of development of palliative care services. In some countries, including Hong Kong, Japan, Singapore, South Korea, and Taiwan, palliative care services are fairly well established with trained professional staffs and with partial or full government funding. However, in many countries, dedicated and committed individuals are struggling to establish credibility and find resources for both hospital-based and home care programs. The development of palliative care in Asia has been hampered by poverty, lack of resources, the need to address more urgent health-care needs, nondisclosure to terminally ill patients, and overprotective families when making treatment and care decisions concerning cultural, ethical, and professional issues [1].

APHN

The Asia Pacific Hospice Palliative Care Network (APHN) (www.aphn.org) was established in 2001 to promote a network of individuals and organizations actively involved in palliative care in the Asia-Pacific region [2,3]. The APHN promotes education and skills development, enhances awareness and communication, and fosters collaboration and research. The APHN is now having an increasing role in the conferences that are held biannually.

The APHN consists of members from Australia (Commonwealth of Australia), Bangladesh (People's Republic of Bangladesh), China (People's Republic of China), Hong Kong (Hong Kong, Special Administrative Region of the People's Republic of China), India (Republic of India), Indonesia (Republic of Indonesia), Japan, Macau (Macao, Special Administrative Region of the People's Republic of China), Malaysia, Mongolia, Myanmar (Republic of the Union of Myanmar), Nepal (Federal Democratic Republic of Nepal), New Zealand, Pakistan (Islamic Republic of Pakistan), Philippines (Republic of the Philippines), Singapore (Republic of Singapore), South Korea (Republic of Korea), Sri Lanka (Democratic Socialist Republic of Sri Lanka), Taiwan, Thailand (Kingdom of Thailand), and Vietnam (Socialist Republic of Vietnam).

PALLIATIVE CARE SERVICES IN THE FOUNDING SECTORS OF THE APHN

A sector is defined as a geographic region that may include one or more countries or part of a country. The APHN consists of the following 14 founding sectors: Australia, Hong Kong, India, Indonesia, Japan, Malaysia, Myanmar, New Zealand, Philippines, Singapore, South Korea, Taiwan, Thailand, and Vietnam. Here, I review the development of palliative care services in the 12 founding sectors of the APHN, excluding Australia and New Zealand (Table 8.1). These two countries are reviewed in Chapter 6.

Hong Kong

The first palliative care team in Hong Kong was formed in 1982 at Our Lady of Maryknoll Hospital. The Society for the Promotion of Hospice Care (http://www2.hospicecare.org.hk)

Table 8.1   *Palliative care development in the founding sectors of the Asia Pacific hospice palliative care network (excluding Australia and New Zealand)*

	Population (millions)	Death rate (deaths/1000 persons)	Cancer crude mortality rate (cancer deaths/population × 100,000)	Start year of specialist	Inpatient PCUs	Inpatient hospices' palliative care
Hong Kong	8	6.8	163	1982	10	3
India	1224	6.2	25	1986	35	24
Indonesia	239	6.3	74	1992	6	NA
Japan	126	9.5	280	1981	245	5
Malaysia	28	5.0	57	1991	20	2
Myanmar	47	9.7	NA	1998	0	2
Philippines	93	5.1	46	1991	8	1
Singapore	5	4.7	100	1985	0	4
South Korea	48	5.9	145	1988	34	6
Taiwan	23	6.8	174	1982	50	0
Thailand	69	7.3	84	1987	6	3
Vietnam	87	6.2	80	2000	6	1

was established in 1986. Six years later, they secured funding to open Bradbury Hospice, a 26-bed independent inpatient hospice in Shatin. The Hospital Authority of Hong Kong took over management of five hospice units in 1991, established six more in the next 3 years and took over Bradbury Hospice in 1995. This recognition of the role of the hospice in health care was a key milestone in the development of hospice care in Hong Kong.

In 2003, restructuring of health-care services into clusters resulted in the closure of Nam Long Hospital. Palliative care services from Nam Long Hospital were then transferred to Grantham Hospital. Efforts are now being made to form consultative teams in general hospitals, enhance liaisons with nursing homes, and encourage home care services. The Society for the Promotion of Hospice Care continues to play a major role in promoting public education and providing specialized professional training.

Professional organizations have been important in the development of palliative medicine in Hong Kong. In 1998, palliative medicine achieved specialty status under the Hong Kong College of Physicians (http://www.hkcp.org) [4]. This was largely due to the efforts of the Hong Kong Society of Palliative Medicine (http://www.hkspm.com.hk), the current academic body of palliative medicine specialists. Since 1997, the Hong Kong Hospice Nurses' Association (http://www.fmshk.com.hk/hkhna) has also been active in training and research. There are currently 13 inpatient palliative care services in Hong Kong. All except Bradbury Hospice are located in hospitals.

India

The first hospice in India, Shanti Avadna, opened in Mumbai in 1986. Subsequently, other independent hospices were built and some hospitals established pain clinics and home care services. The situation in India includes a shortage of resources, a majority of patients both being in the later stages of a disease when diagnosed and preferring to be cared for at home, and thus the model of care was adapted accordingly to focus on outpatient management of pain using trained volunteers for nursing and administrative duties, empowerment of families to provide care at home, and development of a network of clinics funded by the local community. Additionally, the Indian Association of Palliative Care (http://www.palliativecare.in), established in 1994, holds conferences in different states annually.

The Institute of Palliative Medicine (http://www.instituteofpalliativemedicine.org), a 40-bed inpatient facility that also provides accommodation for students and faculty, opened in Calicut (now Kozhikode) in 2003. Recently, India's health managers, clinicians, and policy makers have been actively involved in setting bench marks for palliative care practices, creating innovative models of care, developing trainers and training programs, and providing evidence-based clinical guidelines for the care of the dying [5]. In 2009, the Medical Council of India declared palliative medicine as an independent specialty. It is now a 3-year residential course equivalent in status to general medicine, general surgery, or pediatrics.

In the 16 states and union territories of India, 138 organizations currently provide palliative care services, and 83 of these (60%) are located in the southern Indian state of Kerala, where development in South Asia has largely been centered [6].

Indonesia

In Indonesia, palliative care services have been established in Surabaya and Jakarta since 1992. The establishment of the National Cancer Committee led to the National Cancer Control Program and ultimately to the Cancer Pain Relief and Palliative Care Program. The movement progressed from the establishment of committees and organization of scientific conferences to palliative care services that are provided in pilot health institutions. Although weak opioids had long been widely available in the country, oral morphine was not available until 1995, when it started to be used by some referral hospitals [7].

There are currently six centers providing palliative care in Indonesia: two in Jakarta; one in Surabaya; one in Denpasar, Bali; one in Yogyakarta; and one in Makassar, South Sulawesi. They provide hospital-based consultancy services with outpatient clinics and home care outreach. However, coverage is low and accessibility to opioids outside the hospitals continues to be a problem. The Indonesian Palliative Society (http://palliativeindonesia.org), established in 2000, continues to hold annual meetings.

Japan

In Japan, the first hospice was opened at Seirei Mikatahara Hospital in Hamamatsu in 1981. In 1989, a report published from a task force meeting of the Ministry of Health, Labour and Welfare for *Palliative care for terminally ill cancer patients* became the first standard guideline for palliative care focusing on terminally ill cancer patients. In 1990, the Japanese Ministry of Health, Labour and Welfare introduced reimbursement under health insurance for services provided by a specially equipped palliative care unit. As of 2012, 250 accredited palliative care units and hospices are actively operating in Japan. It is estimated that 9% of all cancer deaths occurred in palliative care units and hospices in 2011.

The Japanese Society for Palliative Medicine (http://www.jspm.ne.jp) was established in 1996 and as of 2012 consists of more than 10,000 members. In 2009, the Japanese Society for Palliative Medicine established a qualification system for obtaining a specialty in palliative medicine. Additionally, the Japan Nursing Association (http://www.nurse.or.jp) established an integrated training course for nurses majoring in palliative care and qualifying through examinations. In 2012, 327 oncology-certified nurse specialists and 1089 palliative-care-certified nurses were working as palliative care experts in Japan.

The Ministry of Health, Labour and Welfare introduced reimbursement under health insurance for hospital-based palliative care teams in 2002. In 2006, the Cancer Control Act was established, and the Basic Plan to Promote Cancer Control Programs, which included palliative care, in each prefecture was drawn up [8].

Malaysia

In Malaysia, home care programs were started by both Hospis Malaysia (http://www.hospismalaysia.org) in Kuala Lumpur and the National Cancer Society of Malaysia (http://www.cancer.org.my) in 1991. A palliative care unit was established at Queen Elizabeth II Hospital in Kota Kinabalu in 1995. A volunteer group (the Palliative Care Association of Kota Kinabalu) was formed to support patients who were discharged from the unit. The Malaysian government saw this close association between the government hospital and the nongovernmental organization providing home care in the community as a suitable model for palliative care in Malaysia [9].

In 1997, the Department of Health announced that by 2000, all government hospitals were to have at least a 6-bed palliative care unit or a palliative care team. Although attempts are being made to meet the need for palliative care in rural areas and introduce the principles of palliative care to rural health-care workers, most palliative care services are only available in urban areas.

The Malaysian Hospice Council (www.malaysianhospice-council.org) was set up as the coordinating body for hospice nongovernmental organizations in 1998. A forum for education and networking has been provided by an annual congress hosted by a different state each year. In 2003, Mount Miriam Hospital opened a palliative care facility. In 2004, the Hospice Association of Sandakan opened a day-care and training center. In 2006, palliative medicine became a subspecialty. Additionally, 20 government hospitals established facilities comprising 6- to 12-bed inpatient palliative care units. In Malaysia, at least 90 organizations currently provide 110 palliative care services. Among these providers, 22 nongovernmental organizations account for 33 of these services, 20 of which are home care programs [10].

Myanmar

The U Hla Tun Hospice (Cancer) Foundation (http://www.uhlatunhospicemyanmar.org) was founded in Myanmar in 1998. Two 40-bed independent inpatient hospices have been established by the foundation, one in Yangon and one in Mandalay. Another is planned to be built in Taunggyi. No further development of home care or hospital consultancy in Myanmar has been seen.

Philippines

The Philippine Cancer Society (http://www.philcancer.org.ph) founded the first hospice home care program in the Philippines and offered support to other interested groups in 1991. The first National Convention on Hospice Palliative Care was held in Manila in 1995. The formation of the National Hospice Palliative Care Council of the Philippines in 2004 was seen as an important step toward improved coordination of services and advocacy of palliative care in the Philippines. In 2007, palliative care services opened at both Far Eastern University–Nicanor Reyes Medical Foundation and The Medical City in Pasig. Palliative care concepts and principles are part of the curriculum in major medical and nursing schools and palliative care training programs are provided to health providers and volunteers [11]. Thirty-four organizations currently provide 108 palliative care services and compassionate care to the dying is provided by a wide range of these groups [12].

Singapore

In Singapore, the first hospice was established in 1985 at St. Joseph's Home. Subsequently, a volunteer hospice group began providing home care in 1987. Assisi Home and Hospice, owned by the Franciscan Missionaries of the Divine

Motherhood Sisters, allocated 12 beds for hospice care in 1988 and, 4 years later, underwent renovations and expanded to a 35-bed facility. An independent 40-bed inpatient hospice, Dover Park Hospice, opened in 1995 in a custom-built facility shared with the Hospice Care Association. The Singapore Hospice Council (http://www.singaporehospice.org.sg) was registered in 1995 as the umbrella body that incorporates all voluntary organizations providing hospice and palliative care [13].

In 1999, the establishment of a department of palliative medicine at the new National Cancer Centre Singapore (http://www.nccs.com.sg) marked another milestone in the development of palliative care in Singapore. This department provides consultancy and outpatient clinics for Singapore General Hospital, Kandang Kerbau Women's and Children's Hospital, and the National Cancer Centre. Palliative medicine was recognized as a medical subspecialty in 2006, and this paved the way for local training of palliative medicine specialists.

In 2008, The Lien Foundation made a timely and strategic decision to provide funding for support of education and research in palliative care. The Lien Center for Palliative Care was formed through a collaboration of four parties: the Lien Foundation, which served as the philanthropic donor; the Duke-NUS Graduate Medical School, which became the academic home for the center; the National Cancer Centre Singapore, which provided the policy guidance and support and the clinical setting for education and research; and SingHealth, which provided policy guidance and support at the cluster level. Palliative care in Singapore now includes four inpatient hospices with 125 beds, five home care services, two hospice day-care centers, and four major hospitals with consultative teams.

South Korea

The concept of hospice was introduced in South Korea as early as 1965, when an order of Catholic Sisters opened a service for dying patients in Seoul. The first hospice was established in 1988 at Seoul St. Mary's Hospital. The expansion was gradual until a World Health Organization Collaborating Centre for Hospice Palliative Care was established at the Catholic University of Korea College of Nursing in 1995. This center has had an important role in the training of professional hospice nurses. The following umbrella hospice organizations have been important in raising public and professional awareness: the Korean Hospice Association, established in 1991; the Korean Catholic Hospice Association, established in 1992; the Korean Society for Hospice and Palliative Care, established in 1998 (http://www.hospicecare.co.kr); and the Korean Buddhist Hospice Association, established in 2009.

The Korean government began to promote palliative care with its Cancer Control Plan since 2003. The Ministry of Health and Welfare Affairs established a policy that requires that its recognized palliative care centers be medically based, subsidize inpatient palliative care services with separate palliative care wards, have adequate human resources, and provide proper facilities and equipment. As a result of this initiative, the number of inpatient palliative care services increased from 15 to 40 between the years 2005 and 2010. Approximately 8%–10% of all patients with terminal cancer in Korea receive palliative care from these services. The government has proposed a per diem payment system for inpatient palliative care regardless of the actual medical treatment received. Constant monitoring of the quality of these services has become necessary. Furthermore, the Ministry of Health and Welfare Affairs funded the development of the Korean Terminal Cancer Patient Information System, which was created in order to provide national statistics and assist with evidence-based policy making [14]. Palliative care services should be extended to noncancer patients and under special circumstances such as the emergency room and the intensive care unit in the future [15].

Taiwan

The first inpatient hospice ward was opened in Mackay Memorial Hospital in Taiwan in 1990. By the year 2000, it had evolved into a custom-built 63-bed palliative care center complete with administrative offices, education facilities, and accommodation for students and faculty. The Taiwan government became involved in palliative care in 1995 and this led to the setting of standards for inpatient and home care and the development of guidelines for pain control.

National health insurance reimbursement was introduced in 2000 for services accredited by the Taiwan Academy of Hospice Palliative Medicine (http://www.hospicemed.org.tw) and the Department of Health. The following three religiously affiliated foundations have been important for the development of palliative care in Taiwan: the Hospice Foundation of Taiwan, established in 1990 (http://www.hospice.org.tw); the Catholic Sanipax Socio-Medical Service and Education Foundation, established in 1993 (http://www.kungtai.org.tw); and the Buddhist Lotus Hospice Care Foundation, established in 1994 (http://www.lotus.org.tw). The Taiwan Hospice Organization has also been a unifying body for hospice volunteers and professional staff since 1995. The Hospice Foundation of Taiwan has been providing education and training since 1990 and started a multidisciplinary program in 1993 that was revised in 1999. The Taiwan Academy of Hospice Palliative Medicine was established in 1999 and palliative medicine was accepted as a medical subspecialty in 2001. The majority of palliative care physicians have prior certification in family medicine.

The National Cancer Control Program launched in 2003 and has included the expansion of palliative care in its 5-year plan. In 2005, the cooperative care plan was initialized to deliver and extend hospice care in a medical model to terminal cancer patients in general wards; this led to patients now having choices between palliative care units, hospice home care services, and cooperative care plans. Since 2006, the expenses of the integrated delivery system of hospice care have been formally covered under national health insurance. The government also funds local nonprofit organizations that promote public education and hospice services [16]. By 2007, this had led to the establishment of a total of 556 palliative care beds in a combination of 35 hospitals, each having a consultation care team, 52 hospice home care teams, and 16 teaching hospitals accredited for palliative care training. The development of palliative care in Taiwan has considerably advanced the quality of end-of-life cancer care for both patients and their families.

Thailand

In Thailand, a home care program was set up as a demonstration model at the National Cancer Institute in Bangkok in 1996, and a 16-bed hospice was opened at the Mahavajiralongkorn Cancer Centre in Thanyaburi in 1998. The first palliative care conference was held in 2004 in the city of Hatyai, where a consultative team had already been operating since 1999 in Songklanagarind Hospital and where palliative medicine had been introduced into the undergraduate curriculum at the Songkla University Faculty of Medicine in 2001. Additionally, the Thai Hospice Palliative Care Club was founded in 2006 and the National Hospice Foundation of Thailand (http://www.chivantarak.org) was established in 2007. Currently, at least 13 organizations provide 40 palliative care services, mostly to inpatients. Eight of these organizations are government facilities, one is a private hospital, and two are faith-based institutions [17].

Vietnam

Funding in Vietnam has been provided by Volunteers International, a U.S.-based organization, since 1996. This organization provides support for professional education in Ho Chi Minh City, Hanoi, and Hue and enables doctors and nurses to visit palliative care programs in Australia and the United States. In 2005, Vietnam's Ministry of Health launched a palliative care initiative that based national palliative care program development on the public health strategy of the World Health Organization. A rapid situation analysis conducted in 2005 led to national guidelines on palliative care in 2006, radically improved opioid prescribing regulations in 2008, the training, using three curricula written especially for Vietnam, of more than 400 physicians in palliative care by early 2010, and the initiation of palliative care services in hospitals and the community [18]. Vietnam currently has six palliative care units and one hospice.

CHALLENGES FOR THE FUTURE

Palliative care services have become widespread in many Asian countries, especially in East and Southeast Asia in the past two or three decades. The practice of palliative care is expanding through services such as inpatient palliative care units, inpatient hospices, hospital-based palliative care teams, home care, and day care. Even though the need for palliative care services is becoming more widely accepted both by health-care professionals and the public, both the quality of services provided and the coverage of patients in need vary greatly, and the lack of manpower and funding continues to limit the scope of services in many Asian countries.

Additional challenges must be met in order to further develop palliative care in Asia [19–23]. First, palliative care services should be incorporated in health policies and health-care systems, including the management of cancer and other diseases, and the aims of palliative care plans should be equity, quality, and coverage of patients in need. Second, palliative care activities should be effectively publicized in order to disseminate and promote palliative care further, as a well-informed populace would lead to better decision making and a better understanding of palliative care. Third, palliative medicine has been accepted as a specialty in many countries, including Hong Kong, India, Japan, Singapore, Taiwan, and Malaysia, but further acceptance of palliative care as a specialty is required. Fourth, many countries are in the process of developing national strategies to enhance education and training of palliative care for undergraduate students, postgraduate physicians, and health-care professionals, and thus developing palliative care training programs for the next generation is essential. Lastly, a major challenge for the future is for palliative care to become a strong specialty in mainstream medical practice. Research is necessary in order to achieve this. Evidence-based medicine forms an essential part of medicine, and palliative care is not exempt from the need to prove that it is based on scientific evidence. Publication of research in English language journals from non-English-speaking countries such as Japan, South Korea, and Taiwan must continue to gradually increase.

Key learning points

- Palliative care services have become widespread in East and Southeast Asia in the past two or three decades.

- The APHN is promoting a network of individuals and organizations actively involved in palliative care in the Asia-Pacific region.

- The aims of palliative care plans should be equity, quality, and coverage of patients in need.

- Palliative care activities should be effectively publicized in order to disseminate and promote palliative care further.

- Palliative medicine has been accepted as a specialty in Hong Kong, India, Japan, Singapore, Taiwan, and Malaysia.

- It is essential to develop palliative care training programs for the next generation.

REFERENCES

1 Chin JJ, Ho CW, Arima H, Ozeki R, Heo DS, Gusmano MK, Berlinger N. Integration of palliative and supportive cancer care in Asia. *Lancet Oncol* 2012;13(5):445–446.

2 Goh CR. The Asia Pacific Hospice Palliative Care Network: A network for individuals and organizations. *J Pain Symptom Manage* 2002;24(2):128–133.

3 Goh CR. The Asia Pacific hospice Palliative Care Network: Supporting individuals and developing organizations. *J Pain Symptom Manage* 2007;33(5):563–567.

4   Chan KS. Two decades of palliative care. *Hong Kong Med J* 2002;8(6):465–466.

5   Loiselle CG, Sterling MM. Views on death and dying among health care workers in an Indian cancer care hospice: Balancing individual and collective perspectives. *Palliat Med* 2012;26(3):250–256.

6   McDermott E, Selman L, Wright M, Clark D. Hospice and palliative care development in India: A multimethod review of services and experiences. *J Pain Symptom Manage* 2008;35(6):583–593.

7   Al-Shahri M. The future of palliative care in the Islamic world. *West J Med* 2002;176(1):60–61.

8   Eguchi K. Development of palliative medicine for cancer patients in Japan: From isolated voluntary effort to integrated multidisciplinary network. *Jpn J Clin Oncol* 2010;40(9):870–875.

9   Lim G. Clinical oncology in Malaysia: 1914 to present. *Biomed Imaging Interv J* 2006;2(1):e18.

10 Wright M, Hamzah E, Phungrassami T, Bausa-Claudio A. *Hospice and Palliative Care in Southeast Asia: A Review of Developments and Challenges in Malaysia, Thailand and the Philippines.* New York: Oxford University Press, 2010:pp. 13–86.

11 Doorenbos AZ, Abaquin C, Perrin ME, Eaton L, Balabagno AO, Rue T, Ramos R. Supporting dignified dying in the Philippines. *Int J Palliat Nurs* 2011;17(3):125–130.

12 Wright M, Hamzah E, Phungrassami T, Bausa-Claudio A. *Hospice and Palliative Care in Southeast Asia: A Review of Developments and Challenges in Malaysia, Thailand and the Philippines.* New York: Oxford University Press, 2010:pp. 135–204.

13 Goh CR. Singapore: Status of cancer pain and palliative care. *J Pain Symptom Manage* 1996;12(2):130–132.

14 Choi JY, Shin DW, Kang J, Baek YJ, Mo HN, Nam BH, Seo WS, Park JH, Kim JH, Jung KT. Variations in process and outcome in inpatient palliative care services in Korea. *Support Care Cancer* 2012;20(3):539–547.

15 Kim HS, Kim BH. Palliative care in South Korea. In: Ferrell BR, Coyle N (Eds.), *Oxford Textbook of Palliative Nursing* (3rd edn.). New York: Oxford University Press, 2010:pp. 1339–1346.

16 Glass AP, Chen LK, Hwang E, Ono Y, Nahapetyan L. A cross-cultural comparison of hospice development in Japan, South Korea, and Taiwan. *J Cross Cult Gerontol* 2010;25(1):1–19.

17 Wright M, Hamzah E, Phungrassami T, Bausa-Claudio A. *Hospice and Palliative Care in Southeast Asia: A Review of Developments and Challenges in Malaysia, Thailand and the Philippines.* New York: Oxford University Press, 2010:pp. 87–133.

18 Krakauer EL, Cham NT, Khue LN. Vietnam's palliative care initiative: Successes and challenges in the first five years. *J Pain Symptom Manage* 2010;40(1):27–30.

19 Yamagishi A, Morita T, Miyashita M, Akizuki N, Kizawa Y, Shirahige Y, Akiyama M et al. Palliative care in Japan: Current status and a nationwide challenge to improve palliative care by the Cancer Control Act and the Outreach Palliative Care Trial of Integrated Regional Model (OPTIM) study. *Am J Hosp Palliat Care* 2008;25(5):412–418.

20 Miyashita M, Sanjo M, Morita T, Hirai K, Kizawa Y, Shima Y, Shimoyama N et al. Barriers to providing palliative care and priorities for future actions to advance palliative care in Japan: A nationwide expert opinion survey. *J Palliat Med* 2007;10(2):390–399.

21 Li J, Davis MP, Gamier P. Palliative medicine: Barriers and developments in mainland China. *Curr Oncol Rep* 2011;13(4):290–294.

22 Hirai K, Kudo T, Akiyama M, Matoba M, Shiozaki M, Yamaki T, Yamagishi A, Miyashita M, Morita T, Eguchi K. Public awareness, knowledge of availability, and readiness for cancer palliative care services: A population-based survey across four regions in Japan. *J Palliat Med* 2011;14(8):918–922.

23 O'Connor M, O'Brien AP, Griffiths D, Poon E, Chin J, Payne S, Nordin R. What is the meaning of palliative care in the Asia-Pacific region? *Asia Pac J Clin Oncol* 2010;6(3):197–202.

9

Palliative care as a public health issue

E. IRIS GROENEVELD, IRENE J. HIGGINSON

INTRODUCTION

Palliative care is an important public health issue due to aging societies, changes in population structures, and an increasing number of older people with complex needs and chronic illness. This requires a response that mobilizes communities, takes preventative measures, and increases access to services, broadening the focus of palliative care from patients and families to include a societal approach. This chapter provides an introduction to the core principles of public health and provides examples of public health solutions to challenges to palliative care development.

WHAT IS PUBLIC HEALTH?

The definition of public health as "the art and science of preventing disease, prolonging life and promoting health through the organized efforts of society," first introduced in England in 1988 [1], has been used by the World Health Organization (WHO) since [2]. Public health has further been interpreted as "...a collective action of State and Civil Society to protect and improve the health of individuals. It is a notion that goes beyond population or community-based interventions and includes the responsibility of ensuring access by citizens to quality healthcare. It does not approach public health as an academic discipline but rather as an interdisciplinary social practice" [3].

The key element that distinguishes public health from clinical care is being accomplished through social and political action, as opposed to action targeted at the individual or family level. Examples of public health include vaccination programs, smoking awareness campaigns, professional education, reform of public laws impacting on health (such as alcohol tax), and many other societal interventions.

The definition of what constitutes a public health issue has evolved with time. In its earliest western incarnation, after John Snow closed the famous London water pump and ended a cholera outbreak, public health's purview did not extend much beyond what is now considered basic infectious disease epidemiology. As, however, understanding of the determinants of

health has become more sophisticated, so has the perspective of public health practice. Disciplines of sociology, economics, psychology, nutrition, anthropology, and others are now considered by many to be important in understanding the health of individuals and, hence, populations and societies. The 1988 Acheson Report, commissioned by the UK Minister of Health to review and summarize health inequalities and to recommend priority areas for policy development and interventions to reduce them, noted that their work was based on a *socioeconomic model of health* that recognized that main determinants of health could be described as layers of environmental and social influence over the fixed individual constitutional factors. Similarly, the U.S. Institute of Medicine in their seminal report on the *Future of Public Health* defines health as a "public good" because "many aspects of human potential such as employment, social relationships, and political participation are contingent upon it" [4]. One area of action identified by this report was to adopt a population health approach that considers multiple determinants of health.

PUBLIC HEALTH APPROACH TO PALLIATIVE CARE

As a health issue that affects everyone, is amenable to population-based and public sector interventions, and has the potential to reduce suffering on a massive scale, palliative and end-of-life care is an important public health issue. The disciplines of palliative and supportive care, with their understanding of the interrelationships between physical, spiritual, emotional, and practical domains of human existence and suffering, fit quite comfortably into an approach to population health that recognizes multiple biopsychosocial determinants of health and enduring health problems. It has made this philosophy the cornerstone of clinical practice for decades.

Palliative care encompasses, but extends beyond, end-of-life care. WHO has defined palliative care as "...an approach which improves quality of life of patients and their families facing life-threatening illness through the prevention and relief of suffering by means of early identification and impeccable assessment and treatment of pain and other problems, physical, psychological and spiritual" [5]. A palliative approach then should be applied along all stages of serious illness regardless of the immediacy of death. To do otherwise can rightly be considered a failure to provide quality care. In this light, the public health mandate of palliative care becomes even larger and more complex: the target for palliative interventions is not just the result of a calculation based on incidence of death but, rather, on prevalence of life-threatening and serious disease in a defined population or geographic area [6].

PUBLIC HEALTH CHALLENGES IN PALLIATIVE AND SUPPORTIVE CARE

The size of the world's population in 2013 is expected to grow from 7.2 billion, by 1 billion in the next 12 years, to 9.6 billion in 2050. Most of the world population increase will be in the developing world. The population size of developed regions is expected to change minimally and would decline without migration from developing to more developed countries [7]. The World Bank estimates a 2011 crude death rate of 8.1 per 1000, equivalent to 58 million deaths. Assuming that each death affects at least 5 other people, end-of-life issues are estimated to affect at least 5% (1 in 20) of the world's population each year [8]. Noncommunicable diseases and the later more chronic phases of some communicable diseases (notably HIV/AIDS) are ever more prevalent, requiring symptom relief and emotional, social, and spiritual support. Thus, there is an increasing role for palliative and supportive care.

Inequities in distribution of burden of disease

Under the best and most stable of circumstances, provision of palliative care requires a wide range of human and fiscal resources. Trained medical professionals are necessary—as are informal caregivers, spiritual support, families, good nutrition, clean environments, good communication systems, access to medications, transportation, shelter, and, perhaps most important of all, peaceful societies.

The burden of illness requiring palliative care is disproportionately borne by the developing world—regions least able to mount an effective response. An important global trend that has affected the need for palliative care is the HIV/AIDS pandemic. Some 34 million people are now living with HIV/AIDS, of whom 69% live in sub-Saharan Africa (4.9% of the population). The Caribbean, Eastern Europe, and Central Asia are also heavily affected, with 1.0% of people infected. Although the prevalence of HIV in sub-Saharan is almost 25-fold that of Asia, almost 5 million people live with HIV in the combined regions of South, Southeast, and East Asia. Although the rate of new infections is continuing to decline and medication to slow disease progression is more available in many countries affected, the impact of HIV on societies remains profound [9].

Similarly, more than 60% of the world's cancer burden (numbers of cases and deaths) is now borne by less developed countries [10]. The 2008 World Cancer Report further documents that in wealthy countries, approximately 50% of patients with diagnosed cancer die compared with 80% of patients in the developing world. In wealthy countries, chronic infections (such as hepatitis B and C, human papillomavirus, and *Helicobacter pylori*) are implicated in 8% of all malignancies compared with 26% in the developing world [10]. Tobacco use also remains a global concern, killing nearly 6 million people a year. If current rates of use persist, it will rise to 8 million deaths annually, with 80% of these deaths in low- and middle-income countries [11]. Moreover, in both developing and developed countries, it is the poorest people who tend to smoke the most and who bear most of the disease burden [10].

Countries that shoulder the bulk of the world's disease burden and that have the greatest need for palliative care services are fiscally the least well equipped to act to provide it. The World Bank estimates that in 2010, 1.22 billion people consumed less than U.S.\$1.25 per day and 1.18 billion people consumed U.S.\$1.25–2 per day [12]. Variation in spending on health between the developed and developing regions of the world is dramatic: A 2010 analysis of expenditures showed that low-income countries spent an estimated U.S.\$28 per capita per year (5.3% GDP) on health, whereas high-income countries expended U.S.\$4828 per year (12.4% GDP). Importantly, the proportion of public contributions to total expenditure is much lower in low-income countries, while out-of-pocket expenses are much higher [13].

The implications of these global inequities are profound. Poverty correlates with disease and disease causes poverty—a vicious cycle resulting in higher and higher levels of suffering and morbidity. At a time when more health resources are needed than ever before, economies stand in danger of contracting as a result of the deterioration of their population's health and hence will become even less able to respond.

In developing regions of the world, a variety of trends can be expected to impact on the ability to deliver palliative care. The impact of the HIV/AIDS epidemic on family and, hence, social stability is significant. In 2009, it was estimated that there were 16.6 million children under the age of 18 who had been orphaned by AIDS, of whom nearly 90% (14.9 million) live in sub-Saharan Africa [14]. UNICEF estimates that there are over 132 million orphans (from all causes) in sub-Saharan Africa, Asia, Latin America, and the Caribbean in 2005 [15] facing uncertain futures with limited family support.

Social instability is exacerbated by trends in urbanization. Nearly 180,000 people are added to the world's cities each day, and it is expected that 70% of the world's population will live in urban areas by 2050 [16]. Urban environments may offer opportunities for health development, for example, through access to health care. On the other hand, urbanization concentrates health risks and introduces new hazards, for example, caused by a decrease in activity or disease outbreaks. Additionally, political instability and war in and of themselves cause suffering and hamper the ability of society to mobilize around human service needs like palliative and end-of-life care. Largely as a result of war and instability, there are now some 25 million internally displaced persons in the world and an additional 10.5 million refugees [17]. These populations are at high risk for disease, malnutrition, and death.

Population aging

Over the last two centuries, life expectancy has increased by 30–40 years in most developed countries. Until the 1920s, this gain in life expectancy could mostly be explained by improvements to infant and child health. Since the 1950s, however, life expectancy has continued to increase due to reduction in mortality at increasing age [18]. Due to the advancements in lifestyle (including safer work environments and improved diets) and health care, people are now able to live longer with their illnesses. As a consequence, more people are living with multiple disorders at the same time [19]. This will challenge palliative care services to respond to the needs of this elderly population with more complex and longer disease trajectories leading up to death [20].

Where increase in life expectancy and decreased fertility rates occur concurrently, the population group of older people will grow. United Nations (UN) projections show that population aging will affect high-income as well as low- and middle-income countries over the next decades. Work by the UN population division [21] compares 228 countries by age groups (0–24, 25–59, or 60+) in which strongest increase in population size will be experienced. It is shown that between 1950 and 1975, population change was dominated by increase in 0–24 year olds. In the period 1975–2015, change is dominant in the working-age population (25–59). After 2015, an increase in 60+ populations will be greatest in the majority of the world's countries.

The *total dependency ratio* illustrates the ratio of the number of children (under 15) and older persons (65+) to the number of people in working ages (15–64) per 100 population and is often used as a measure of social support needs. Projections up to 2050 show an increase in this ratio across continents (Europe, Northern America, Oceania, Latin America and the Caribbean, Asia, and Africa), which leaves relatively few to support a larger group [22]. In health financing systems that rely on (tax or insurance-based) contributions from the working population to supply for older persons, health systems will be under pressure to sustain.

While the number of deaths is expected to increase [23], the number of informal caregivers is expected to decrease. This is in part due to women, who have traditionally been relied on to care for people at the end of life, more frequently being in formal employment. Social changes such as smaller family size, dispersed families, and increased divorce rates have made informal carer availability less self-evident. In the United Kingdom, approximately 6 million people—10% of the population—served as unpaid caregivers for ill, frail, or disabled family member or friend [24]. A study of the economics of informal caregiving in the United Kingdom in 2011 valued it at £119 billion per year, which is considerably more than the total National Health Service (NHS) running costs in 2009–2010 [25]. This relative level of support cannot be relied on to continue in the face of demographic shifts. The cost to society

of supplanting these services will add to the already escalating demands on health resources.

PUBLIC HEALTH APPROACH TO SUSTAINING PALLIATIVE CARE

In practical terms, a public health approach to making it possible for everyone who needs quality palliative care to receive it, must involve a range of activities. WHO has identified three elements as necessary to further sustain palliative care [26]: governmental policy (establishing national policies, making sure that palliative care is harmonized with national health and social service agendas), education (of health professionals, the public, media, policy makers, and others), and ensuring access to pain medications. A public health approach would additionally emphasize the important role of research and development of a strong evidence base from which to build programs and policies. The responsibility for these activities will vary from society to society, but each in its own way is necessary. Political commitment is a prerequisite for effective action. This, in turn, depends upon the collective awareness and mobilization of civil society and includes individuals as well as organized groups. In all cases, sensitivity to various cultural perspectives and norms is essential.

Financing and reimbursement

Palliative care financing, in many counties, is characterized as having a mix of funding sources; in both the developed and developing world, most advances in palliative care and the hospice movement have begun in nongovernmental organizations and the private sector. Government funding has become available where the importance of increasing access to palliative care is recognized. Sustaining funding streams from each source requires strong leadership in coordination and collaboration.

Funding mechanisms for palliative care services can provide powerful levers to improve services but may at the same time prevent their development [27]. In the United States, for example, public resources only support Medicare hospice benefit for those who have been determined to have less than 6 months to live. This has had the effect of making integration of palliative care across earlier stages of illness difficult. In some countries, funding mechanisms have been used as a vector for introduction of routine outcome measurement. In Australia, for example, patient-level funding is determined by individual palliative care need, as measured by phase of illness and dependency score [28].

Consumer protection and quality assurance

Development of standards of care and exercise of oversight to ensure that they are met and applied equitably and consistently are important public health responsibilities. In some cases, such oversight is conducted through governmental associations. For example, in the United States, the hospice Medicare benefit also requires hospices to conduct comprehensive assessments of the quality of care provided [29]. In Uganda, the

Ministry of Health has established detailed specifications for implementing palliative care into the health-care system [30]. Recommendation of the European Association for Palliative Care to include outcome measurement to use outcome measures in clinical care, audit, training, and research has been endorsed by the European Commission [31]. Oversight is also conducted through private voluntary associations. For example, in the United States, the National Hospice and Palliative Care Organization has developed standards of care for hospice programs that have been widely promulgated [32].

Education

Educational efforts must be directed to the general public, media, policy makers, business leaders, and community leaders as well as to health professionals and others who come into contact with the sick. Public education is necessary to mobilize communities, prompt advocacy, offer hope, and make people aware that there are better ways to approach illness and death than is generally expected. In England, an initiative supported by the National Council for Palliative Care (NCPC) called Dying Matters has used various forms of media and outreach to focus on "to support changing knowledge, attitudes and behaviours towards death, dying and bereavement, and through this to make 'living and dying well' the norm" [33].

Important professional training initiatives are underway in many parts of the world. These range from the creation of academic departments and funded faculty positions in palliative care through distance-based learning programs to practical hands-on training in clinical settings. While there will always be a need for specialized palliative care training, it is important that palliative care education becomes part of the fundamental educational package offered to aspiring health professionals as palliative care is a complementary, not an alternative, therapy. The General Medical Council of the United Kingdom, for example, now demands all doctors to undertake end-of-life care training [34].

Ensuring access to essential medications

Crucial to the successful implementation of an effective palliative care program is to ensure that drugs are available to care for patients requiring palliative care, especially those used for pain management. It is estimated that 80% of the world's population have no or insufficient access to treatment of moderate to severe pain [35]. Access to pain medication, however, does not guarantee good pain management, as research suggests; older people (over 70), in particular, were shown to be less likely to be prescribed analgesics than younger people (under 50) [36]. Internationally, barriers to access to medications include failing to ensure drug supply systems, poor training of health workers, unnecessarily restrictive drug control, fear among health workers for legal sanctions, and high costs of treatment [37]. Although WHO and leading experts in palliative care have urged countries to develop comprehensive strategies, most countries do not have palliative care or pain treatment policies.

Case studies from Vietnam and Uganda, however, show that, even in low-resource settings, governments have taken steps to increase access to pain medication, for example, through training health-care staff in prescribing drugs or easing regulatory barriers [37]. Nongovernmental organizations, such as the Open Society Foundations, have contributed to this field of work by supporting local advocates for medical opioid availability [38].

Research

Clearly, tracking the scope of pain and suffering should be a vital concern that benefits public health and the public good. There is a clear need to develop an evidence base for policy and programs. Documenting chronic illness, pain, and symptoms and their management through epidemiologic and demographic and health surveys should be integral in both developed and developing countries. Research is needed to identify salient characteristics of successful palliative care programs. Studies must be performed that describe and analyze practice, policy, and advocacy to inform future developments and research for building programs that achieve the varied goals of palliative care—that is, achieving the best quality of life for patients and their families. To minimize risk of failure, it is important that new or expanding palliative care projects in developing countries understand both the successes and failures of existing programs [39]. Several issues recently identified as research topics for investigation include availability of pain-relieving drugs, pain and symptom control, access to services, education and training, identification of relevant needs and determination of outcomes for care at the community level, and evaluation of the impact of education of policy makers and program directors about palliative care [40]. Given the magnitude of palliative care required by people living in developing regions of the world, programs must also consider coverage and not simply strive to provide high-quality care to a few patients. End-of-life and palliative care research is currently allocated a minute proportion of research funding (e.g., 0.24% of cancer research funding in the United Kingdom and 1% in the United States). To ensure high-quality research outputs, investment in end-of-life care research is urgently needed [41].

CONCLUDING THOUGHTS: ADDRESSING PALLIATIVE CARE THROUGH AN EXPANDING PUBLIC HEALTH PARADIGM

Public health focuses on health promotion and prevention of disease and has often seen pain and suffering as removed from the public health paradigm, to be addressed by tertiary care in a biomedical/clinical model. Although WHO [42] and various scholars [43] have long argued a broadening of the concept of health that includes how well people are able to perform their daily tasks, only recently has daily functioning begun to be included routinely in the assessment of people's health status through measures of health-related quality of life. Simple measures have been tested and adapted for use in resource poor settings [44,45]. Investigators are going beyond the traditional paradigm that views health only in terms of adherence to or deviation from physical or biochemical markers. Instead, they are including in their assessment of health people's own reports of their sense of well-being and their ability to perform valued social roles [46,47]. Therefore, pain and suffering should be measured through epidemiological and social science methods as a critical health condition that should be tracked just as we track infectious diseases. By expanding the public health paradigm to include and promote palliative care, we further the goals of public health—prevention of disease and prolonging life in society. As life expectancy increases and medical advances are being made, people are living longer with chronic diseases. Therefore, an integrated model of palliative care has practical and pragmatic implications for public health universally. Marginalizing those in need of palliative care services to clinical specialists or ignoring them entirely creates a society in dire need of public health action and intervention.

REFERENCES

1 Acheson D. *Public Health in England*. London, U.K.: HMSO, 1988.
2 World Health Organization. Available from http://www.euro.who.int/en/what-we-do/health-topics/Health-systems/public-health-services.
3 PHPPO. Available from http://www.phppo.cdc.gov/dphsdr/whoccphp/documents/Instrument.doc.
4 National Academy of Sciences. *The Future of Public Health in the 21st Century*. Washington, DC: National Academies Press [Internet], 2003.
5 Sepulveda C, Marlin A, Yoshida T, Ullrich A. The World Health Organization's global perspective. *Journal of Pain and Symptom Management* 2002;24:91–96.
6 Murtagh F, Bausewein C, Verne J, Groeneveld E, Kaloki Y, Higginson I. How many people need palliative care? A study developing and comparing methods for population based estimates. *Palliative Medicine* January 2014;28(1):49–58.
7 United Nations, Department of Economic and Social Affairs, Population Division. World population prospects: The 2012 revision, Key findings and advance tables, 2013.
8 Singer PA, Bowman KW. Quality end-of-life care: A global perspective. *BMC Palliative Care* July 25, 2002;1(1):4. PubMed PMID: 12139768. Pubmed Central PMCID: 122082. Epub 2002/07/26. eng.
9 UNAIDS. UNAIDS report on the global AIDS epidemic 2012. Joint United Nations Programme on HIV/AIDS, 2012.
10 IARC. World cancer report. International Agency for Research on Cancer, 2008.
11 World Health Organization. WHO Report on the global tobacco epidemic, 2011: Executive summary. Geneva, Switzerland: World Health Organization, 2011.
12 The World Bank. Poverty 2013 [updated April 2013 June 17, 2013]. Available from http://web.worldbank.org/WBSITE/EXTERNAL/TOPICS/EXTPOVERTY/EXTPA/0,contentMDK:20040961~menuPK:435040~pagePK:148956~piPK:216618~theSitePK:430367~isCURL:Y,00.html.
13 World Health Organization. *World Health Statistics 2013*. Geneva, Switzerland: World Health Organization, 2013.
14 UNAIDS. UNAIDS report on the global AIDS epidemic 2010. Geneva, Switzerland: UNAIDS, 2010.
15 UNICEF. Orphans 2012 [updated May 25, 2012 June 18, 2013]. Available from: http://www.unicef.org/media/media_45290.html.
16 Urbanization and health. *Bulletin of the World Health Organization* 2010;88(4):241–320.
17 UNHCR. UNHCR Global Report 2012. 2012.
18 Christensen K, Doblhammer G, Rau R, Vaupel JW. Ageing populations: The challenges ahead. *The Lancet* 2009;374:1196–1208.
19 Barnett K, Mercer SW, Norbury M, Watt G, Wyke S, Guthrie B. Epidemiology of multimorbidity and implications for health care, research, and medical education: A cross-sectional study. *Lancet* July 7, 2012;380(9836):37–43. PubMed PMID: 22579043.
20 Hall S, Petkova H, Tsouros AD, Constantini M, Higginson IJ. *Palliative Care for Older People: Better Practices*. Copenhagen, Denmark: WHO Regional Office for Europe, 2011.
21 Lee R, Mason A, Cotlear D. *Some Economic Consequences of Global Aging*. Washington, DC: The World Bank, 2010.
22 United Nations DoEaSA, Population Division, World Population Ageing. 2009.
23 Simon ST, Gomes B, Koeskeroglu P, Higginson IJ, Bausewein C. Population, mortality and place of death in Germany (1950–2050)—Implications for end-of-life care in the future. *Public Health* November 2012;126(11):937–946. PubMed PMID: 23041107. Epub 2012/10/09. eng.
24 Office for National Statistics. 2011 Census—Unpaid care snapshot [June 18, 2013]. Available from http://www.ons.gov.uk/ons/guide-method/census/2011/carers-week/index.html.
25 Bruckner L, Yeandle S. *Valuing Carers 2011: Calculating the Value of Carers' Support*. Leeds, U.K.: Carers UK, University of Leeds, 2011.
26 World Health Organization. *National Cancer Control Programmes: Policies and Managerial Guidelines*. Geneva, Switzerland: World Health Organization, 1995.
27 Groeneveld EI, Bauswein C, Kaloki YE, Cassel JB, Higginson IJ, Murtagh F eds. Paying for palliative care services: Lessons from international experience. *13th World Congress of the European Association for Palliative Care*, Prague, Czech Republic, 2013.
28 Eagar K, Gordon R, Green J, Smith M. An Australian case mix classification for palliative care: Lessons and policy implications of a national study. *Palliative Medicine* April 2004;18(3):227–233. PubMed PMID: 15198135.
29 Code of Federal Regulations, Part 418—Hospice Care. (Revised 10/1/97), 1997.
30 Ministry of Health RoU. *National Sector Strategic Plan 2000/02–2004/05*. Kampala, Uganda: Ministry of Health, 2000.
31 Harding R, Simon ST, Benalia H, Downing J, Daveson BA, Higginson IJ et al. The PRISMA Symposium 1: Outcome tool use. Disharmony in European outcomes research for palliative and advanced disease care: Too many tools in practice. *Journal of Pain and Symptom Management* October 2011;42(4):493–500. PubMed PMID: 21963118.
32 National Hospice and Palliative Care Organization. *Standards of Practice for Hospice Programs*. Alexandria, VA: National Hospice and Palliative Care Organization, 2000.
33 Dying Matters. About Us [June 24, 2013]. Available from: http://dying-matters.org/overview/about-us.
34 General Medical Council. *Treatment and Care Towards the End of Life: Good Practice in Decision Making*. London, U.K.: General Medical Council, 2010.
35 World Health Organization. *Briefing Note: Access to Controlled Medications Programme*. Geneva, Switzerland: World Health Organization, 2008.
36 Gao W, Gulliford M, Higginson IJ. Prescription patterns of analgesics in the last 3 months of life: A retrospective analysis of 10202 lung cancer patients. *British Journal of Cancer* May 24, 2011;104(11):1704–1710. PubMed PMID: 21540860. Pubmed Central PMCID: 3111163. Epub 2011/05/05. eng.

37 Lohman D, Schleifer R, Amon JJ. Access to pain treatment as a human right. *BMC Medicine* 2010;8:8. PubMed PMID: 20089155. Pubmed Central PMCID: 2823656.

38 Open Society Foundations. [June 24, 2013]. Available from: http://www.opensocietyfoundations.org/topics/palliative-care.

39 Higginson IJ, Bruera E. Do we need palliative care audit in developing countries? *Palliative Medicine* November 2002;16(6):546–547. PubMed PMID: 12465706.

40 Harding R, Stewart K, Marconi K, O'Neill JF, Higginson IJ. Current HIV/AIDS end-of-life care in sub-Saharan Africa: A survey of models, services, challenges and priorities. *BMC Public Health* October 23, 2003;3:33. PubMed PMID: 14572317. Pubmed Central PMCID: 280683.

41 Sleeman KE, Gomes B, Higginson IJ. Research into end-of-life cancer care—Investment is needed. *Lancet* February 11, 2012;379(9815):519. PubMed PMID: 22325658. Epub 2012/02/14. eng.

42 World Health Organization. *The Constitution of the World Health Organization.* Geneva, Switzerland: World Health Organization, 1948.

43 Dubos RJ. *Man Adapting.* New Haven, CT: Yale University Press, 1965.

44 Harding R, Selman L, Agupio G, Dinat N, Downing J, Gwyther L et al. Validation of a core outcome measure for palliative care in Africa: The APCA African Palliative Outcome Scale. *Health and Quality of Life Outcomes* 2010;8:10. PubMed PMID: 20100332. Pubmed Central PMCID: 2825183.

45 Selman L, Harding R. How can we improve outcomes for patients and families under palliative care? Implementing clinical audit for quality improvement in resource limited settings. *Indian Journal of Palliative Care* January 2010;16(1):8–15. PubMed PMID: 20859465. Pubmed Central PMCID: 2936087.

46 Levine S. The changing terrains in medical sociology: Emergent concern with quality of life. *Journal of Health and Social Behavior* March 1987;28(1):1–6. PubMed PMID: 3571904.

47 Ware JE. *SF-36 Health Survey: Manual and Interpretation Guide.* Boston, MA: New England Medical Center, Health Institute, 1993.

10

Palliative care as a primary care issue

SCOTT A. MURRAY

SUMMARY

There is great potential for palliative and end-of-life care to be delivered accessibly and effectively in the community, especially by family doctors and community nurses. Primary care teams practicing a palliative care approach (see definitions in Box 10.1) can reach many more people than can specialists offering specialist palliative care to those referred to them. There is a need, therefore, for palliative care specialists and primary care teams to work together, using models of shared care. The quality of life for all people living with progressive life-threatening illnesses will be best improved for most people if specialists spend a major part of their time training and supporting generalists (both in hospitals and in the community) and providing clinical care to those with complex needs. This chapter highlights five areas and reasons why greater integration between palliative care and primary care (now called primary palliative care) is sensible in both resource-rich and resource-poor countries, and gives examples of how this is being successfully achieved in different countries.

PRIMARY PALLIATIVE CARE HAS A FIVEFOLD POTENTIAL TO DELIVER END–OF–LIFE CARE

The first potential is to *identify and treat people with any and all life-threatening illnesses*, taking palliative care beyond cancer from which only 25% of people now die. The second potential is to help people *earlier rather than later*, not just in the very terminal stage but from diagnosis of a life-threatening illness. The third potential is to care for all aspects of the person, *all dimensions*—physical, psychological, social, and spiritual—as good general practitioners already do. The fourth potential is to have reliably good end-of-life care available in *all community settings*: nursing homes and patients' homes. The fifth potential is making end-of-life care available for people in all nations, especially the *poorer countries*. Finally, primary care teams can support *family carers* in their time of caring and subsequent bereavement, as family carers are frequently cared for by the same primary care practice.

FIRST POTENTIAL OF PALLIATIVE CARE IN PRIMARY CARE: CARING FOR PEOPLE WITH ALL LIFE-THREATENING ILLNESSES

In economically developed countries, most people die after a longish period of disability at an average age of 78 with the top three categories of death now being cancer, organ failure, and frailty/dementia [1]. This can be illustrated by noting that a general practitioner in the United Kingdom, who has on average about 1800 patients on his or her registered list, has 20 deaths on average per year. Five of these deaths are from cancer, six from organ failure (such as chronic obstructive pulmonary disease, heart failure, liver failure, renal failure), and seven from frailty (either physical frailty or dementia). Only about 2 of the 20 are likely to die totally unexpectedly (Figure 10.1). So around 90% of deaths are not totally unexpected, and primary care staff have the opportunity to adopt a palliative care approach with most patients approaching death.

For these three main categories of dying, the implications for palliative care provision are quite different as the patients' needs are generally different. The cancer trajectory typically follows a generally predicable course with a short decline towards the end. Hospice care fits well with people dying with cancer and meets their needs [2]. Conversely, patients with organ failure may have a gradual decline over 2–5 years, but during that period, there are acute declines and frequently hospital admissions. Patients with organ failure may die suddenly at any time but, in contrast, are not *expected to die* in the next few months. Due largely to this prognostic uncertainty and various funding reasons, such patients rarely benefit from specialist palliative care. The frailty trajectory is variable and may last for many years from the onset of difficulties in activities of daily living. The needs of this group are for integrated

---

* Integration between Palliative Medicine and Primary Care can bring great benefit by extending the reach of palliative care to more people and earlier in their illnesses.

Box 10.1 Definitions used in this chapter

Key worker: Health or social care professional with responsibility for organizing the care of a particular patient.

Palliative care approach: An approach that generalist health and social care providers can adopt whereby they consider all dimensions of the patient experience and plan holistic care for the future as well as the present.

Primary palliative care: The practice of palliative care in primary care by general practitioners (family doctors) and community nurses.

Specialist palliative care: The provision of services whose core activity is the provision of palliative care. The main role of specialist palliative care is to manage patients with complex and demanding care needs while supporting and training generalist palliative care providers.

Surprise question: Name for a question that can be used to test clinical intuition about whether a patient is approaching end of life. "Would I be surprised if this patient died in the next 6–12 months?"

Terminal care: Care in the last days or week of life or *care in the dying phase.*

Transition in care: A change in setting or place of care or a change in focus of care from being largely curative to being more supportive and palliative.

clinical care and long-term support at home, carer support, and nursing care. In many countries, support for this group is inconsistent. Therefore, to reliably meet the end-of-life needs of all patients, we must provide multidimensional support to patients with all illnesses, and primary care is uniquely placed

to identify most patients with one or more advanced progressive illnesses. There is a challenge for specialist palliative care to redesign its services so that they are configured to meet the typical needs of people on the three archetypal trajectories, and extending and integrating with primary care is the obvious way to take this forward [3].

SECOND POTENTIAL OF PALLIATIVE CARE IN PRIMARY CARE: A PALLIATIVE CARE APPROACH FROM DIAGNOSIS OF A LIFE-THREATENING ILLNESS RATHER THAN TOWARDS THE END

With cancer, traditionally there was a period when a cure was attempted; then when cure was no longer possible, palliative care intervened. The new and better concept is that supportive and palliative care should start at diagnosis of a life-threatening illness and gradually increase while disease-modifying management may decrease (Figure 10.2). This model and understanding can be applied to all people with a progressive illness including organ failure and frailty [4,5]. As debility increases, from specific illnesses or general frailty, people can be considered for a palliative approach while continuing with disease-modifying treatment. Provision of palliative care should be triggered not by diagnosis, or even prognosis, but by need. Another specific trigger for consideration for a holistic palliative approach might be admission to a care home, as this is generally done to increase supportive care. Alternatively, another criterion could be the need of a certain number of hours of social care in the community.

In the organ failure and frailty trajectories, it has previously been more difficult to conceptualize and decide when a palliative care approach might be clinically appropriate. However,

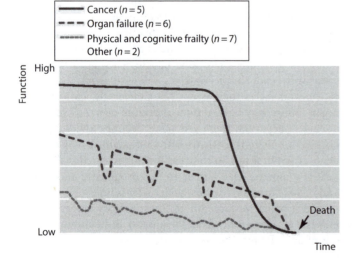

Number of deaths in each trajectory, out of the average 20 deaths each year per UK general practice list of 2000 patients

Legend:
— Cancer (*n* = 5)
- - - Organ failure (*n* = 6)
···· Physical and cognitive frailty (*n* = 7)
Other (*n* = 2)

Figure 10.1 *The three main trajectories of decline at the end of life. (From Murray SA and Sheikh A, BMJ 2008;336:958–959.)*

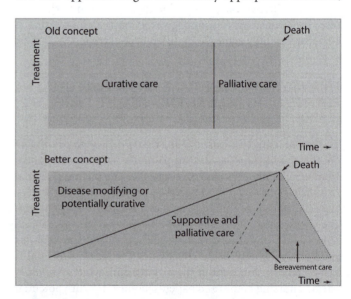

Figure 10.2 *Supportive and palliative care should start at diagnosis of life-threatening disease. (From Murray, S.A., Kendall, M., Boyd, K., and Sheikh, A., Illness trajectories and palliative care, BMJ, 330, 1007–1011, 2005, Copyright 2005, with permission from BMJ Publishing Group Ltd.)*

Function

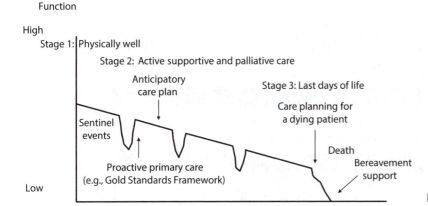

Figure 10.3   *Caring for people with organ failure: Three progressive stages in advanced illnesses.*

examining a typical organ failure trajectory, it is evident that events or triggers such as a hospital admission might be utilized to consider changing a chronic disease management approach dealing largely with physical concerns (stage 1) to a proactive, supportive, and palliative care approach (stage 2). Then when the patient reaches the last days of life, terminal care can be planned in stage 3, as illustrated in Figure 10.3. Alternatively, there might be clinical indicators such as breathlessness at rest to trigger stage 1 or even the *surprise question*. This question is where a physician asks himself or herself: "would I be surprised if this patient were to die in the next year?" If the answer is "no," this means that the patient is sufficiently at risk of dying for anticipatory care planning to be started *just in case*. Research has shown that patients can manage both preparation for death and hope for the future, as they tend to have dual, competing narratives in their mind [6].

Several tools have been developed for use in primary care to help doctors and community nurses identify patients as they transition to a point when a supportive and palliative care approach is beneficial. The current version of the Supportive and Palliative Care Indicator Tool (SPICT) is available for download from an open access website (http://www.spict.org.uk). SPICT can be used opportunistically at patient consultations or by scanning patient disease registers to identify such patients for a comprehensive needs assessment and a palliative care approach [7] (Figure 10.4).

Overzealous treatment later in the course of all these types of illnesses, in the very last days of life, can be prevented by diagnosing imminent death and caring for the patient and family using an *individualized*, holistic, end-of-life care plan. Some countries used a structured pathway for the last days/hours of life, but this is now being replaced with more flexible approaches to managing the individual needs of patients who are deteriorating and likely to die. This approach ensures that communication with patient and family is central, goals of care are clear, and treatments and tests that are not consistent with the agreed care goals or are of greater burden than benefit are stopped. Plans are made to manage any symptoms or problems that might develop, including as needed prescription of medications. Family, spiritual, religious, cultural, and other needs are considered and addressed.

THIRD POTENTIAL OF PALLIATIVE CARE IN PRIMARY CARE: MEETING ALL DIMENSIONS OF NEED (PHYSICAL, PSYCHOLOGICAL, SOCIAL, AND SPIRITUAL)

The biopsychosocial model of care that is a central tenet of palliative medicine is also a core concept in primary care. General practitioners are trained to identify, acknowledge, and deal with spiritual needs in people approaching the end of life. Family physicians are skilled at providing patient-centered care in the context of family and community and trained in person-centered communication. When the doctor–patient relationship is already established, as commonly happens in countries where primary care is strongly developed, the trust and mutual understanding that are essential to the therapeutic relationship are already present. Thus, when continuity of care over many years is already present, this can be built upon in primary care. This also helps patients receive support and care starting from the time of diagnosis of the potentially fatal illness, when psychological and existential distress may be especially acute [8,9].

It is now recognized in the United States and increasingly in Australia and the United Kingdom that everyone has spiritual needs when faced with serious life-threatening illness. An internationally accepted definition states, "spiritual needs are needs that relate to the meaning and purpose of life" [8]. People may or may not use religious vocabulary to express such needs. If the spiritual issue or need causes the person distress, it becomes *spiritual distress*. If such distress is upsetting the person, such as interfering with sleep or their ability to work, then this should be identified and addressed by someone because such distress also impinges on other areas: it makes pain more painful and anxiety less bearable and leads to increased health service utilization.

Work in the United Kingdom has confirmed that multidimensional distress can occur from diagnosis and that in lung cancer, social decline runs in parallel with the physical decline: "his old friends won't even take a cup of tea with me now I've got cancer" [8]. Our research also uncovered four times when distress can routinely be expected: at the time of diagnosis,

Supportive and Palliative Care
Indicators Tool (SPICT™)

Lothian

www.spict.org.uk

The SPICT™ is a guide to identifying people at risk of deteriorating and dying. Assessment of unmet supportive and palliative care needs may be appropriate.

Look for two or more general indicators of deteriorating health

- Performance status poor or deteriorating, with limited reversibility. (needs help with personal care, in bed or chair for 50% or more of the day).
- Two or more unplanned hospital admissions in the past 6 months.
- Weight loss (5%–10%) over the past 3–6 months and/or body mass index <20.
- Persistent, troublesome symptoms despite optimal treatment of any underlying condition(s).
- Lives in a nursing care home or NHS continuing care unit, or needs care to remain at home.
- Patient requests supportive and palliative care, or treatment withdrawal.

Look for any clinical indicators of advanced conditions

Cancer

Functional ability deteriorating due to progressive metastatic cancer.

Too frail for oncology treatment or treatment is for symptom control.

Dementia/ frailty

Unable to dress, walk, or eat without help.

Choosing to eat and drink less; difficulty maintaining nutrition.

Urinary and faecal incontinence.

No longer able to communicate using verbal language; little social interaction.

Fractured femur; multiple falls.

Recurrent febrile episodes or infections; aspiration pneumonia.

Neurological disease

Progressive deterioration in physical and/or cognitive function despite optimal therapy.

Speech problems with increasing difficulty communicating and/or progressive dysphagia.

Recurrent aspiration pneumonia; breathless or respiratory failure.

Heart/ vascular disease

NYHA Class III/IV heart failure, or extensive, untreatable coronary artery disease with:
- Breathlessness or chest pain at rest or on minimal exertion.

Severe, inoperable peripheral vascular disease.

Respiratory disease

Severe chronic lung disease with:
- Breathlessness at rest or on minimal exertion between exacerbations.

Needs long term oxygen therapy.

Has needed ventilation for respiratory failure or ventilation is contraindicated.

Kidney disease

Stage 4 or 5 chronic kidney disease (eGFR < 30 mL/min) with deteriorating health.

Kidney failure complicating other life limiting conditions or treatments.

Stopping dialysis.

Liver disease

Advanced cirrhosis with one or more complications in past year:
- Diuretic resistant ascites
- Hepatic encephalopathy
- Hepatorenal syndrome
- Bacterial peritonitis
- Recurrent variceal bleeds

Liver transplant is contraindicated.

Supportive and palliative care planning

- Review current treatment and medication so the patient receives optimal care.
- Consider referral for specialist assessment if symptoms or needs are complex and difficult to manage.
- Agree current and future care goals/ plan with the patient and family.
- Plan ahead if the patient is at risk of loss of capacity.
- Handover: care plan, agreed levels of intervention, CPR status.
- Coordinate care (e.g. with a primary care register).

SPICT™, November 2013

Figure 10.4 *SPICT™ (with permission). SPICT is available via an open access website to allow it to be revised and updated as required. Those wishing to use the SPICT are invited to register on the website (free of charge) so that they can access and download the latest version and receive notification of any updates (www.spict.org.uk).*

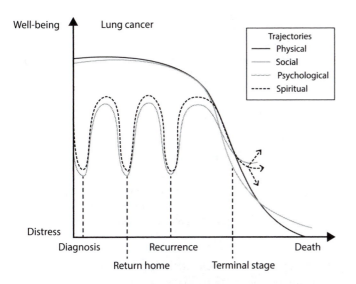

Figure 10.5 *Lung cancer—Physical, social, psychological, and spiritual trajectories from diagnosis to death.*

after initial treatment when the patient has returned from the hospital, at recurrence or disease progression, and then again in the terminal stage. Unsurprisingly, it was when someone was anxiously coming to a diagnosis that they were also thinking about the meaning and purpose of life. So it would appear that the spiritual trajectory in these patients with lung cancer was running in parallel with the psychological one. It appears that physical and social decline tend to run together as do the psychological and spiritual [8] (Figure 10.5).

Understanding multidimensional trajectories can help general practitioners address difficult questions such as "how long have I got," which patients sometimes ask early in the illness trajectory. A response could be "It's hard to know how long, but let me tell you what it might be like for you." If these patterns are then explained to patients and carers, they can then understand and feel empowered, knowing what the future may hold.

FOURTH POTENTIAL OF PALLIATIVE CARE IN PRIMARY CARE: MAKING A DIFFERENCE IN THE COMMUNITY

In many economically developed countries, only about 20%–25% of people die at home. However, it is believed that over 50% would prefer to die at home if possible. In the last decade, Professor Keri Thomas has pioneered in the United Kingdom the development of the Gold Standards Framework, which is used in over 80% of UK primary care teams. It gives a framework for general practitioners and community nurses to organize and coordinate care within their practices. In the United Kingdom, all patients in primary care are registered with a specific practice, so lists of all patients are available, and this framework is based on creating a register of all patients identified for supportive or palliative care within each practice. It highlights the *7Cs*, seven aspects that are vital for quality end-of-life care in the community: communication, coordination,

---

Box 10.2 Using two end-of-life care tools in nursing homes [11]

All seven private nursing care homes within one district in the United Kingdom undertook to implement, as a package, the Gold Standards Framework for Care Homes (GSFCH) and an adapted Liverpool Care Pathway for Care Homes (LCP). A community palliative care nurse specialist conducted an in-house training session every 2 weeks over 18 months and also supported the nursing home staff and visiting general practitioner more generally.

There was a highly statistically significant increase in use of do not attempt resuscitation (DNAR) documentation, advance care planning, and use of the LCP. An apparent reduction in unnecessary hospital admissions and a reduction in hospital deaths from 15% deaths prestudy to 8% deaths during the study were documented.

---

control of symptoms, continuity of care, continued learning, carer support, and care in the dying phase [10].

The three main steps of the Gold Standards Framework approach and indeed of primary palliative care are the following:

- Identify which patients would benefit from more support.
- Assess their current and future clinical and personal/family needs.
- Plan their future care.

This framework has been adapted for nursing care homes, and this is also associated with positive outcomes such as less hospital admissions in the last weeks of life and more frequent documentation of advance care plans and resuscitation status information [11–13] (see Box 10.2).

Other interventions that have improved palliative care in the community include community matrons as key workers for patients with frequent admissions and various interventions to improve collaboration between specialist palliative care and primary care such as case conferencing in Australia. Research in Canada has reported that an integrated model of palliative care services has resulted in a decline in emergency department visits. An evaluation of the Palliative Care Integration Project in Ontario, Canada, which was an attempt at creating an integrated set of networks, also revealed a decrease in emergency admissions and deaths in acute care.

FIFTH POTENTIAL OF PALLIATIVE CARE IN PRIMARY CARE: REACHING TO ALL IN NEED IN ECONOMICALLY POORER COUNTRIES AND LEARNING FROM THEM ABOUT BRINGING DEATH BACK TO LIFE

As primary care is the only level of care available to most people in less developed countries, its potential must be maximized and enhanced, ideally by international collaborations to let end-of-life care reach most people there.

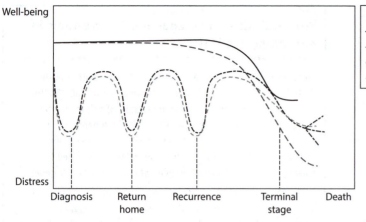

Figure 10.6 *Trajectories of physical, social, psychological, and spiritual well-being in family carers of patients with lung cancer, from diagnosis to death. (Copyright 2008 BMJ Publishing Group Ltd. With permission.)*

Having completed a study in Scotland of people dying with lung cancer, we took the opportunity to do a similar study with colleagues in Kenya [14]. We asked the same questions in Scotland and in Kenya to people at home "what are the main problems that you are facing just now?" and compared the findings.

In Scotland, the main issue that people would mention first was existential, leading to spiritual distress, whereas in Kenya, the main issue was that of physical suffering, especially pain. In Scotland, analgesia was effective and affordable, but in Kenya, it was unaffordable and largely unavailable. In Scotland, people felt anger in the face of the illness, whereas in Kenya, there was greater expression of acceptance. In Edinburgh, someone might say "I'll just keep it to myself," but in Kenya, there was community support and engagement, which was accepted by patients. In Scotland, the spiritual needs were evident but unmet, while in Kenya, patients were comforted and inspired by their belief in God. In Scotland, diagnosis brought active treatment, but in Kenya, it signalled waiting for death. This comparison indicates that communities in rural Africa can provide effective end-of-life care in all dimensions apart from the physical, whereas in the United Kingdom, nonphysical dimensions are less well met.

In Africa, only four countries have palliative care services integrated within their national health services, but most countries have vibrant communities where members visit the dying to comfort and support them practically. Economically developed countries can learn much from talking about death and dying and visiting people and supporting our friends and neighbors in the community at the end of life. In Australia, an exciting development known as *health promoting palliative care* is starting to address this. This calls for community involvement in end-of-life care and encourages people and the community to talk more openly and be more involved in many aspects of care at the end of life. This approach argues that if death and dying were brought more into the open, it would be much easier to plan for a good death.

The sixth potential of primary palliative care is for primary care teams to *support family carers* in their time of care and subsequent bereavement, as family carers are frequently cared for by the same primary care practice. Research has revealed that family carers of patients with lung cancer can experience a similar dynamic pattern of needs as the people they care for, so this must be acknowledged and addressed. (Figure 10.6) In the United Kingdom, general practitioners are encouraged to identify and keep registers of people who have a significant caring role and to assess their needs and support them.

FACILITATING FACTORS FOR STRONG PRIMARY PALLIATIVE CARE

Factors that facilitate palliative care in the community include a strong primary care system with large group practices with general practitioners and nurses working together. Such practices can proactively identify patients eligible for palliative care and provide multidisciplinary care to patients at home. There should be a reimbursement system that values home visits and adequate appointment durations, and integration with hospital and emergency care is vital to promote continuity of care and information throughout the 24 hours. Given adequate training, resources, and access to specialist support, family physicians can provide end-of-life care to most patients. Providing primary palliative care can help fast-track the extension of the palliative care approach to people with nonmalignant conditions.

CARING FOR ALL IN THE LAST YEAR OR PHASE OF LIFE

So palliative care can address many of its most pressing challenges through working with primary care. It can go beyond cancer and help people at the end of life no matter what the illness. We shouldn't palliate according to diagnosis or even prognosis but according to need. The second challenge primary palliative care can meet is to help earlier rather than later, when input is strategic and formative and when emotional needs are often acute. Thirdly, we can help patients with all dimensions of need in the community, going beyond the physical to the social, psychological, and spiritual. Fourthly, we can help more people live and then die where they want, often at home. Fifthly, we can assist resource-poor countries in setting up systems and training staff to meet substantial needs for good pain and symptom control in the community while learning from them how to talk more openly about dying and how to promote well-being in the face of death. Finally, palliative care in the community can take the lead in supporting family carers.

Key learning points

- There is great potential for palliative care to be delivered in the community, by family doctors and community nurses.

- Primary care teams can reach many more people with palliative care needs than can specialists.

- Palliative care specialists should strategically prioritize training and supporting hospital and community generalists and ideally provide clinical care to those with complex needs.

- Primary care is well placed to undertake palliative care for patients

  - With all life-threatening diseases
  - From early in the course of the illness
  - With all dimensions of need
  - In care homes and at home
  - In all countries, including resource poor
  - And also support family carers.

REFERENCES

1 Lunney JR, Lynn J, Foley DS, Lipson S, and Guralnik JM. Patterns of functional decline at the end-of-life. *JAMA* 2003;289:2387–2392.

2 Murray SA, Kendall M, Boyd K, and Sheikh A. Illness trajectories and palliative care. Clinical review. *BMJ* 2005;330:1007–1011.

3 Lynn J. Reliable comfort and meaningfulness. Making a difference campaign. *BMJ* 2008;336:958–959.

4 World Health Organization. *Palliative Care: The Solid Facts.* Copenhagen, Denmark: WHO, 2004.

5 Murray SA. Meeting the challenge of palliation beyond cancer. *European Journal of Palliative Care* 2008;15:213.

6 Murray SA, Boyd K, Kendall M, Worth A, Benton TF, and Clausen H. Dying of lung cancer or heart failure: Prospective qualitative interview study of patients and their carers in the community. *BMJ* 2002;325:929–932.

7 Boyd K and Murray SA. Recognising and managing key transitions in end of life care. *BMJ* 2010;341:649–652.

8 Murray SA, Kendall M, Grant E, Boyd K, Barclay S, Sheikh A. Patterns of social psychological and spiritual decline towards the end-of-life in lung cancer and heart failure. *JPSM* 2007; 34:393–402.

9 Cavers D, Hacking B, Erridge SE, Kendall M, Morris PG, and Murray SA. Social, psychological and existential well-being in patients with glioma and their caregivers: A qualitative study. *CMAJ* 2012, doi:10.1503/cmaj.111622.

10 The Gold Standards Framework. http://www.goldstandardsframework.org.uk/

11 Hockley J, Watson J, Oxenham D, and Murray SA. The integrated implementation of two end of life care tools in nursing care homes in the UK: An in-depth evaluation. *Palliative Medicine* July 27, 2010, doi: 10.1177/0269216310373162.

12 Badger F, Plumridge G, Hewison A, Shaw KL, Thomas K, and Clifford C. An evaluation of the impact of the Gold Standards Framework on collaboration in end-of-life care in nursing homes. A qualitative and quantitative evaluation. *International Journal of Nursing Studies* 2012;49(5):586–595.

13 Hall S, Goddard C, Stewart F, and Higginson IJ. Implementing a quality improvement programme in palliative care in care homes: A qualitative study. *BMC Geriatrics* 2011;11:31.

14 Murray SA, Grant E, Grant A, and Kendall M. Dying from cancer in developed and developing countries: Lessons from two qualitative interview studies of patients and their carers. *BMJ* 2003;326:368–372.

11

Future of palliative medicine

CHARLES F. VON GUNTEN, IRENE J. HIGGINSON

INTRODUCTION

A reliable forecast for the future requires a hard look at the present. Therefore, we will structure this chapter in three parts. First, we will broadly summarize the current state of palliative medicine in the world. Details of the development of palliative medicine in various parts of the world have been described in other chapters in this textbook. Second, we will summarize the case for a future that rests on a response to three features: the needs of patients and families, demographic changes, and the physician role in palliative medicine as a distinct subspecialty. Third, we will describe the challenges that palliative medicine must face in the future if it is to prosper.

PALLIATIVE MEDICINE NOW

The need for palliative care in the world is immense. Of 57 million deaths in 2008 worldwide, 36 million (63%) were from noncommunicable diseases. The vast majority will suffer from pain and other symptoms as well as psychosocial or spiritual problems that palliative care will address. Surely, the governments of the world will want to ensure that palliative medicine is part of the health system response to their public's needs [1].

The current state of that response around the world can be summarized as highly variable. Part of the issue is that there isn't a common language to describe palliative care services or the physician role [2]. Another is that each country has a different approach to the provision of health care for its citizens [3]. In some countries, the field is a recognized specialty or subspecialty with organized programs for clinical care, education, and research. In many others, a broad program of clinical care has emerged without the official recognition that grounds the discipline in the academic foundation of health care or the financing of health care. In the poorest nations, the most basic tools for the relief of suffering are unavailable.

One way to look at this is from an institutional change model. In such a model, an innovation (such as palliative medicine) is developed in one location (such as England) and then gradually spreads to other institutions as its merits become known. There is good evidence for this. From a handful of hospices worldwide in the 1970s and 1980s, the number of hospices and palliative care programs has grown to involve every continent of the world in more than one hundred countries. The total number of hospice or palliative care initiatives is in excess of 8000 and includes hospice inpatient units, hospital-based palliative care services, community-based teams, and day-care centers. In England and Wales, over 100,000 new patients were cared for by the 288 palliative home care teams in 2010, and 40,000 were cared for in one of the 193 inpatient hospice or palliative care units, with 2,881 beds. Of those cared for in inpatient hospices, just below 90% had cancer; of those cared for by home care teams, the proportion was around 86%, with 14% having conditions other than cancer. The mean length of stay in inpatient units was around 2 weeks. Just below half (44%) of patients who are admitted are discharged from inpatient care when their reasons for admission are addressed. This is usually to homes, where many receive ongoing support. In the same year, the number of cancer deaths in England was around 140,000, suggesting that around 65% of patients with cancer receive care from a palliative care/hospice home care team, and 18% die in a hospice [4].

In addition, over 85,000 new patients are seen by hospital palliative care teams each year; many of these go on to receive home care and/or hospice care. Hospital palliative care teams see more patients with noncancer conditions—on average, around 22% of patients are cared for, but this ranges from 0% to almost 50% [5]. In the United States, where hospice care is delivered by teams primarily in patient's homes, an estimated 1.1 million patients who died received hospice care in 2011 [6]. This corresponds with about 45% of all deaths in the United States. In contrast with England, 38% of patients served by hospice programs have cancer; the remainder die from heart disease, lung disease, or other conditions. The number of hospitals in the United States who report a palliative care team has increased to 66% [4].

Another way to look at the current state of affairs is from an economic point of view. Those countries that have most developed palliative care are comparatively wealthy countries where palliative care is paid for after other services are covered.

Even in countries where palliative care and hospice are widely developed, such as the United Kingdom, much remains to the charitable sector. In the United Kingdom, 75% of the inpatient hospices are managed by charities, with the National Health Service (NHS) covering on average 34% of their costs. In poorer countries where it hasn't yet developed, health-care funds are spent in other ways. In this world view, any money spent on palliative care in developing countries can be construed as a failure to provide the standard health care available in other countries. In other words, patients who can't get standard health care are given morphine in order to ease their otherwise preventable death.

Finally, the development of palliative medicine can be viewed from a public health point of view. An argument can be made that the most significant health-care developments of the past century relate to health promotion (e.g., nutrition), prevention (e.g., sanitation, smoking cessation), and palliation (e.g., pain relief). In this model, palliative medicine is a basic approach to health care that even the poorest countries can assure their citizens.

FUTURE OF PALLIATIVE MEDICINE

The future of palliative medicine rests on the responses to three features.

Meeting individual patient and family needs

People with serious chronic illness, and their families, experience a remarkably similar set of needs that are relatively independent of the specific disease or diseases from which they suffer. These can be categorized in the physical, psychological (emotional), social (practical), and spiritual (existential) domains. The prevalence of symptoms such as pain, breathlessness, and fatigue ranges from 50% to 80% [8]. Psychological conditions such as depression and anxiety affect both patient and family. The effect of the social domain, including family and community relationships and support, and the need for services can be provided. This includes the patient's and family's need for information and training. Finally, the spiritual or existential domain that involves the search for meaning is often affected by serious illness.

Fortunately, there is growing evidence that palliative care is an effective response to these needs. When pain and symptoms are controlled, information is shared, family and caregivers are supported, services are coordinated, and health-care outcomes are improved at a reasonable cost.

Responding to demographic changes

People in both the developed and developing world are aging. People live longer and the proportion of those living more than 65 years into very old age is also increasing rapidly. The pattern of disease from which these people die is now characterized by chronic progressive illnesses, including the frailty syndrome of advanced age. This means there will be more people needing health care toward the end of life.

At the same time there is a growth of people who need care, there is a decrease in the number of both formal and informal caregivers. Innovative ways of providing care are needed. One component of that plan is palliative care.

Developing a unique physician role

The development of the palliative medicine role within the multiprofessional teams who deliver palliative care within hospitals, inpatient units, nursing facilities, or patient's homes is a significant development of the past 50 years. The future of palliative medicine rests on the strength of the case for the field as a distinct specialty. The specialty of palliative medicine has moved from an emerging discipline to a recognized area of expertise in some parts of the world. It is formally recognized as a distinct specialty in Great Britain, Ireland, Australia, Canada, and the United States. We can expect similar recognition in other countries for the following reasons.

DISTINCT BODY OF KNOWLEDGE

A distinct body of scientific knowledge in palliative medicine has accumulated over the past 40 years [9]. The emergence of specialized journals, well-regarded textbooks, and formal curricula is an indicator. This textbook is but one repository. That knowledge is expressed in a variety of scientific and academic endeavors. For instance, the Cochrane Collaboration has a pain, palliative care, and supportive care review group that has produced over 80 reviews [10]. In 2004, the UK government published guidance from the National Institute of Clinical Excellence on supportive and palliative care in cancer [11]. The guidance had reviewed the evidence for the effectiveness of 13 areas of supportive and palliative care, including communication, information, psychological support, specialist palliative care, end-of-life care, and rehabilitation [12]. In 2013, the National Consensus Project for Quality Palliative Care published its third revision of the clinical practice guidelines for quality palliative care based on an extensive evidence review and consensus process with the major U.S. palliative care organizations [13]. Addressing the needs of policy makers, the World Health Organization's European Office produced an evidence-based guidance on palliative care in two complementary booklets. *Palliative Care: The Solid Facts* [14] dealt with general palliative care issues, future needs, and evidence, and *Better Palliative Care for Older People* [15] dealt with the need to address the demographic changes in society and take a public health approach to palliative care. Most recently, the National Institutes of Health in the United States is revisiting its landmark report from 1997 on the state of end-of-life care in the United States to see if there has been any progress [16].

The major skills central to palliative medicine are the assessment and management of physical, psychological, and spiritual suffering faced by patients with life-limiting illnesses and their families. Communication and teamwork are also critical skills in palliative medicine.

PUBLICATION OF SCHOLARLY RESEARCH

New knowledge is being discovered at an expanding rate. Research in the area of palliative medicine appears in at least nine international specialized peer-reviewed journals: *Journal of Palliative Care* (Canada), *Journal of Pain and Symptom Management* (including supportive and palliative care, United States), *Journal of Palliative Medicine* (United States), *Palliative Medicine* (United Kingdom), *American Journal of Hospice and Palliative Care* (United States), *Palliative and Supportive Care* (United States), *Progress in Palliative Care* (Australia), *BMC Palliative Care* (a web-based rapid publication from biomedcentral.com, an international group), *Supportive Care in Cancer* (Switzerland), and *European Journal of Palliative Care* (the United Kingdom). More than one curriculum for palliative medicine has been published [17–20]. Models to guide clinical palliative care have been disseminated [21], and a number of well-regarded textbooks are now available [22–24] of which the *Oxford Textbook of Palliative Care* is now in its third edition. In fact, the Oxford University Press now has a specific division for palliative care, with 2622 current offerings [25].

GRADUATE MEDICAL EDUCATION

New specialties are characterized by defined training programs that prepare the holder of an undergraduate medical degree for independent practice. In the United Kingdom, individuals begin the 4-year training program in palliative medicine once they have completed their medical degree and around 3 years of general medical posts, including hospital medicine. The Association for Palliative Medicine of Great Britain and Ireland has over 1000 physician members, of which 450 are in training, 100 are associate members registered in other medical specialties or general practice, and the rest are consultants (fully qualified) or associate specialists (completing a shorter program [26]). There is a national training program, with regionally organized advertising and monitoring. In the United States, there are 85 programs in operation with a total of 234 physicians in training [27].

PROFESSIONAL ASSOCIATION

New specialties are also characterized by professional associations. The American Academy of Hospice and Palliative Medicine (AAHPM) is the professional association for physicians in palliative medicine. AAHPM currently has 5000 physician members [27]. The Association for Palliative Medicine of Great Britain and Ireland has over 1000 members. The European Association for Palliative Care is a membership organization composed, in part, by members of the national associations of countries throughout western and central Europe. Similar associations have formed in Southeast Asia, Australia, Africa, South America, and most parts of the globe.

PRACTICE PATTERNS AND PROFESSIONAL ROLE

The 1997 Institute of Medicine report, *Approaching Death: Improving Care at the End of Life*, delineated a three-tiered structure for professional competence:

1. A basic level of competence in the care of the dying patient for all practitioners
2. An expected level of palliative and humanistic skills considerably beyond this basic level
3. A cadre of superlative professionals to develop and provide exemplary care for those approaching death, to guide others in the delivery of such care, and to generate new knowledge to improve care of the dying [28]

These three levels correspond to the primary, secondary, and tertiary levels around which medical care is commonly organized. Primary palliative care (a term used mainly in the United States; in the United Kingdom and much of the rest of Europe, the term used is *the palliative care approach*, or *generalist palliative care*, and here, primary palliative care refers to palliative care in the primary care setting, i.e., the community, organized by general practitioners and family doctors) is the responsibility of all physicians. This includes basic approaches to the relief of suffering and improving quality of life for the whole person and his or her family. Secondary (referred to also as specialist) palliative care is the responsibility of specialists and hospital or community-based palliative care or hospice programs. The role of the secondary specialist or program is to provide consultation and assist the managing service. Tertiary palliative care is the province of academic centers where new knowledge is created through research, and new knowledge is disseminated through education, as well as providing a clinical service.

The major competencies of the specialist level palliative medicine practitioner can be summarized under the broad patient-centered goals of

- Relief of symptom and suffering
- Promotion of quality of life for patients and families in the context of life-threatening illness
- Promotion of the development and growth possible at the end of life

While the knowledge domains and skills of palliative medicine overlap to some extent with the knowledge, attitudes, and skills that characterize other disciplines that care for patients with advanced illnesses, the specialty practice of palliative medicine is distinguished from other disciplines by its focus on the common features and symptoms associated with life-limiting disease. Palliative medicine reaches across many disease categories and organ systems to concentrate on relieving the burden of illness.

The palliative medicine specialist acquires and applies (1) a higher level of clinical expertise in addressing the multidimensional needs of patients with life-threatening illnesses, including a practical skill set in symptom control interventions, (2) a high level of expertise in both clinical and nonclinical issues related to death and dying, (3) a commitment to an interdisciplinary team approach, and (4) the strong focus on the patient and family as the unit of care. The specialist level competency required of practitioners in palliative medicine complements the core competency that should be maintained by other disciplines.

CHALLENGES FOR THE FUTURE

There are a number of challenges that confront the future of the field. These include the response of health-care policy makers, the definition of the boundaries of the specialty, and the training of the new physicians that are needed.

Health-care policy

The future of palliative medicine requires a social and political impetus that is beyond the scope of medicine and firmly in the sphere of government. For palliative medicine to prosper, health-care policy must place much greater emphasis on the care of people of all ages who are living with and dying from a range of serious chronic diseases. The structure of health care *as if* these prevalent illnesses are acute and curable must be changed. Therefore, publicly funded palliative care services as a core part of health care is needed; it cannot be an *add-on extra*. Those services must meet the needs in the rural and urban community dwelling public as well as in nursing homes and hospitals, including intensive care. Those services must be based on need rather than on specific diseases or prognosis. Finally, health-care policy must provide for the development of new knowledge through research. Despite the prevalence of palliative care need, national research budgets are paltry. Surely, we don't want to be using the same tools in 50 years that we have now. The example of Australia is particularly insightful here. In Australia, resourcing of palliative care has moved to a *needs-based* approach, with services receiving core funding and not having to rely on charitable income for the bulk of their day-to-day running costs. However, moving toward more core funding will bring with it a responsibility for specialist palliative care services to monitor and report their outcomes and to show the additional quality of care provided and complexity of patients and families cared for.

Professional boundaries

A significant issue that confronts the future of the field is whether it focuses on a condition (the dying patient) or relates to a broader set of competencies that can be integrated across the spectrum of serious and chronic illness. The roots of palliative medicine in hospice care for the dying would lend itself to the former. The experiences of hospital-based and outpatient office–based palliative medicine physicians suggest that the skills are more broadly applicable than just for the dying. Furthermore, good symptom management and psychosocial care require earlier palliative care intervention. Many patients and families should not have to wait until they are confirmed to be at the end of life to be offered the palliative care expertise

in symptom control or emotional, social, or spiritual support. New models of palliative care are exploring how it can be integrated with other specialties, so that patients can receive potentially life-extending treatment at the same time as symptom relief and psychosocial and spiritual support.

Palliative medicine is practiced within the context of a team. Some would say it cannot be practiced without a team. Yet, the broad interdisciplinary nature of palliative medicine makes it more challenging to define the boundaries of the specialty than for those with a disease focus (such as oncology), an organ focus (such as cardiology), or a technical skill (such as surgery). As with other fields, there are areas of overlap with other specialties and subspecialties. Delineating and negotiating those boundaries are an important aspect of the maturation of the discipline. There is little argument that palliative medicine is primarily a consulting specialty to the other primary disciplines. There is no agenda, expressed or implied, that all suffering and dying patients be cared for by physicians board certified in palliative medicine.

DEVELOPING NEW AND APPROPRIATE MODELS OF CARE IN RESPONSE TO THE DIFFERENT TRAJECTORIES OF ILLNESS AND DISEASES

Although the symptom and problem profile of patients with different chronic progressive conditions are similar, the trajectory of diseases is likely to vary. In addition, caring for older people, an increasing part of the palliative care population, has specific challenges—notably iatrogenic disease, multiple pathology, and difficulties in prognostication. The early models of palliative care may have to evolve to care for these patients. In particular, the model of consultation and palliative care offered for periods throughout the illness, rather than at a particular prognostic point, may have to develop. It will be a challenge for palliative medicine to develop and test such models of care while maintaining existing services. Some new models, such as short-term palliative care, are being developed and trialled. These test ways to offer palliative care earlier in the course of the illness, but in the short term, integrated with other services. Evidence to date is preliminary but suggests benefits. For example, a randomized trial of early palliative care in oncology for patients with lung cancer found quality of life and survival benefits [29]. Early palliative care for people severely affected by multiple sclerosis appeared to have benefits in terms of reduced caregiver burden and improved symptom control and lower overall costs, without worsening, and possibly improving, survival [30].

FUND-RAISING AND/OR REMAINING PART OF STATUTORY FUNDED CARE

Currently, much of palliative care is provided within the voluntary sector and not for profit organizations. These have a continued battle to raise funds to stand still—and provide a continued service to the community. The charitable sector is set to become more competitive in years to come and is subject to fluctuations in response to economic changes. Becoming part of the statutory sector or receiving increased statutory funds removes some of the freedom of previously voluntary units, although it provides more security. Achieving the right balance here can be a challenge, especially as national charity organizations in some countries (e.g., the charity commission in the United Kingdom) provide guidance that charities should not undertake tasks that should be provided by statutory services. Perhaps more and more, the role of charitable organizations will be to innovate and discover better treatments and ways to care, while they advocate for the statutory sector to pick up the funding of the services they have proven, through good research, as effective and cost effective.

Training

Another challenge to the field is to build enough capacity within training programs to train the next generation of specialists. The current interest in developing training programs is heartening, but financial resources are scarce and competition for them is strong. In England, palliative care posts go unfilled for want of trained specialists. In the United States, where the field is only emerging, a similar shortage is likely. There is no reason to think this won't be the case in other countries unless the field is recognized and sufficient capacity built into the nation's programs for training medical professionals. There is an inherent challenge here, because the field needs the best dedicated and bright clinicians who have undergone sufficient training. Therefore, a balance needs to be struck between filling posts and filling them with sufficiently experienced and qualified individuals who have the ability to deliver the services and development needed. Palliative medicine clinicians often find themselves in leadership roles and so have to not only provide clinical care but be versed in managing and motivating staff, strategically developing their services, and often negotiating contracts and teaching other doctors. Burnout is likely to be a problem in palliative care, especially if clinicians are isolated and asked to cover services 24 hours, without backup or peer support, as well as to deal with issues of staff management and service development. Equally, problems can arise in academic posts, where filling posts with individuals without sufficiently robust track records or from fields outside of palliative medicine can lead to loss of respect for the field or a distraction of effort away from palliative medicine patients.

Research

A major challenge for the future of palliative medicine is to become a strong specialty for the future. Knowledge has to be a central key to this. If the specialty is to make a real contribution to the future care of patients and families, then the evidence base for the treatment of many symptoms and problems needs to be improved. Unfortunately, research has been relatively

neglected in the past. There has been inadequate funding in all countries, a hesitancy on the part of some ethics committees and Institutional Review Boards (IRBs) to fully support research, and a reluctance of some staff, who entered the specialty because they felt it did not involve research. There are problems too because of the nature of research in palliative care, which is often difficult because of ethical concerns, the intangible nature of many aspects to be measured (e.g., fatigue, quality of life, quality of death), and the fact that patients are ill and difficult to interview. They may live for unpredictable times. Weighed against this, we should recognize that there have been enormous achievements in research in palliative medicine in the last decades, despite these problems and the lack of resources. This is a tribute to the few centers and individuals who are researching the field. In the future, an improved training in appraising and participating in research is needed for doctors and nurses entering the field. It is not expected that everyone will conduct research, but all will need to appraise it and may increasingly be part of large studies organized in tertiary centers.

SUMMARY

In summary, there can be a bright future for palliative medicine. There is a widespread need within society and this is set to increase in the future. There is now a body of good quality evidence that shows that palliative medicine within palliative care programs can meet the need. The challenge is clear. The field needs to grow to sufficient size to be a sustainable response. It also needs to develop mechanisms to meet the challenge of the changing population and in particular the increase in the elderly population and changed trajectory of illness; it needs to continually improve the calibre and skills of those in the field, through training, and to invest substantially in discovering and testing better methods of care and treatment.

Key learning points

- Palliative medicine is highly variable in the world.
- The evidence base supports the effectiveness of palliative care.
- The demographic changes in the world's populations (living longer with more chronic ultimately fatal disease) require expanded palliative care services.
- It is vital in the coming years that palliative care moves from being an add-on extra to become a core component of health care. To do this, it will have to become needs based and report its outcomes. The development of a unique palliative medicine role for the physician within multiprofessional teams is a phenomenon likely to develop in most countries.
- Expanding clinical services to meet the needs of patients and families will require modifications in patterns of care and new models of care and expansion of the numbers of trained physicians and other professionals needed to provide palliative care.

REFERENCES

1   Radbruch L, de Lima L, Lohmann D, Gwyther E, Payne S. The Prague Charter: Urging government to relieve suffering and ensure the right to palliative care. *Palliat Med* 2012:25:101–102.

2   von Gunten CF. Humpty-Dumpty syndrome. *Palliat Med* 2007:21:461–462.

3   Centeno C, Clark D, Lynch T, Racafort J, Praill D, De Lima L, Greenwood A, Flores LA, Brasch S, Giordano A et al. Facts and indicators on palliative care development in 52 countries of the WHO European region: Results of an EAPC Task Force. *Palliat Med* 2007:21:463–471.

● 4   National Council for Palliative Care: Minimum Data Set. *National Survey of Patient Activity Data for Specialist Palliative Care Services.* London, U.K.: National Council for Palliative Care, http://www.endoflifecare-intelligence.org.uk/resources/publications/patient_activity_data, 2013, pp. 51, (accessed September 7, 2013).

5   Palliative Care Information—U.K. http://www.helpthehospices.org.uk/about-hospice-care/facts-figures/, (accessed July 21, 2014).

6   NHPCO Facts and Figures: Hospice Care in America. 2012 addition. www.nhpco.org, (accessed March 28, 2013).

7   Center to Advance Palliative Care. www.capc.org/news-and-events/releases/08-27-12, (accessed April 3, 2013).

● 8   Solano JP, Gomez B, Higginson IJ. A comparison of symptom prevalence in far advanced cancer, AIDS, heart disease, chronic obstructive pulmonary disease (COPD) and renal disease. *JPSM* 2005:31:58–69.

9   von Gunten CF, Lupu D. Development of a medical subspecialty in palliative medicine: Progress report. *J Palliat Med* 2004:7(2):209–219.

◆ 10   http://onlinelibrary.wiley.com/cochranelibrary/search, (accessed April 3, 2013).

✳ 11   National Institute of Clinical Excellence (NICE). *Improving Supportive and Palliative Care for Adults with Cancer—The Manual.* 2004. London, U.K.: National Institute of Clinical Excellence.

◆ 12   Gysels M, Higginson IJ. *Improving Supportive and Palliative Care for Adults with Cancer: Research Evidence.* 2004. London, U.K.: National Institute of Clinical Excellence. www.nice.org.uk/pdf/csgsresearchevidence.pdf, (accessed September 7, 2013).

✳ 13   National Consensus Project for Quality Palliative Care. Clinical Practice Guidelines for Quality Palliative Care. http://www.nationalconsensusproject.org, (accessed April 3, 2013).

14   Davies E, Higginson IJ. *Palliative Care: The Solid Facts.* 2004. Denmark: World Health Organization.

15   Davies E, Higginson IJ. *Better Palliative Care for Older People.* 2004. Denmark: World Health Organization.

16   IOM End-of-Life Care. http://www.iom.edu/Activities/Aging/TransformingEndOfLife.aspx, (accessed July 21, 2014).

17   Billings JA, Block SD et al. Initial voluntary program standards for fellowship training in palliative medicine. *J Palliat Med* 2002:5(1):23–33.

◆ 18   Field MJ, Cassel CK, eds. *Approaching Death: Improving Care at the End of Life.* 1997. Washington, DC: National Academy Press, p. 208

◆ 19   Emanuel LL, von Gunten CF, Ferris FD, eds. *The Education for Physicians on End-of-life Care (EPEC) Curriculum.* 1999. www.epec.net., (accessed April 3, 2013).

20   Schonwetter RS, Hawke W, Knight CF, eds. *Hospice and Palliative Medicine Core Curriculum and Review Syllabus.* 1999. American Academy of Hospice and Palliative Medicine. Dubuque, IA: Kendall/Hunt Publishing Company.

21   Ferris F, Balfour H, Bowen K, Farley J, Hardwick M, Lamontagne C, Lundy M, Syme A, West P. A model to guide patient and family care. Based on nationally accepted principles and norms of practice. *J Pain Sympt Manage* 2002:24(2):106–123.

22   Berger AM, Portenoy RK, Weissman DE. *Principles and Practice of Palliative Care and Supportive Oncology.* 2002. Philadelphia, PA: Lippincott-Raven.

23   Doyle D, Hanks GW, MacDonald N, eds. *Oxford Textbook of Palliative Medicine.* 3rd edn. 2003. Oxford, England: Oxford University Press.

24   Portenoy RK, Bruera EB, eds. *Topics in Palliative Care, vol. 5.* 2001. New York: Oxford University Press.

25   Oxford University Press. http://www.oup.com/us/catalog/general/?queryField=keyword&query=palliative+medicine&view=usa&viewVeritySearchResults=true&ss=relevancy, (accessed April 4, 2013).

26   Association for Palliative Medicine, 2012 Accounts. Southampton, U.K.: Association of Palliative Medicine, 2013, (accessed September 7, 2013).

27   American Academy of Hospice and Palliative Medicine. www.AAHPM.org/fellowship/directory.html, (accessed April 4, 2013).

28   Field MJ, Cassel CK, eds. *Approaching Death: Improving Care at the End of Life.* 1997. Washington, DC: Institute of Medicine, National Academy Press.

29   Temel JS, Greer JA, Muzikansky A., Gallagher ER, Admane S, Jackson VA, Dahlin CM et al. Early palliative care for patients with metastatic non-small-cell lung cancer. *N Engl J Med* 2010a:363:733–742.

30   Higginson IJ, Mccrone P, Hart SR, Burman R, Silber E, Edmonds, PM. Is short-term palliative care cost-effective in multiple sclerosis? A randomized phase II trial. *J Pain Symptom Manage* 2009:38:816–826.

12

Palliative care and supportive care

EDUARDO BRUERA, DAVID HUI

INTRODUCTION

The development of palliative medicine in different regions of the world has been discussed in Chapters 1 through 7 of this book. In Chapter 1, David Clark discusses the origins of the modern hospice movement in the United Kingdom, and the other chapters discuss the progressive integration of these principles to other areas of the world.

Palliative care programs have three distinct characteristics:

- *Multidimensional assessment and management.* This includes the assessment and management of a large number of physical symptoms, psychosocial distress, and functional, spiritual, financial, and family concerns.
- *Interdisciplinary care.* This includes the pivotal role of a team including physicians, nurses, social workers, pastoral care, occupational therapy and physiotherapy, pharmacists, counselors, dieticians, and volunteers who work together in an integrated fashion for the delivery of care.
- *Emphasis on caring for patients and their families.* In the first palliative care programs, it was realized that the majority of physical and emotional care near the end of life is provided by the patient's family. Thus, programs were developed that aimed to support those families with counseling, education, respite, and bereavement care.

Physicians have had a major role in the development of palliative care programs in the United Kingdom and other areas of the world. They came from multiple specialties including family medicine, oncology, pain medicine, surgery, neurology, psychiatry, and geriatrics. These physicians are integrated with the other medical disciplines to establish palliative care teams in programs that were mostly based in the community.

During the first two decades of the development of palliative care, there was an impressive and global expansion of clinical programs. It soon became clear that some of the most seriously ill patients died in acute care hospitals and cancer centers, and palliative care programs progressively expanded from the community into major academic centers. The body of knowledge of palliative care started to progressively develop and the need for research became apparent. The growth in clinical programs, the variety of settings where palliative care was delivered, and the expanding body of knowledge and need for research led to the development of the specialty of palliative medicine.

PALLIATIVE MEDICINE AS AN EMERGING MEDICAL SPECIALTY

Dr. Cicely Saunders started the modern hospice movement in the 1960s at St. Christopher's Hospice in the United Kingdom, focusing on improving care for patients at the end of life. With increasing clinical knowledge and research, this has led to the establishment of a professional discipline with expertise in symptom management, psychosocial spiritual care, patient–clinician communication, complex healthcare decision making, and caregiver support.[1] In 1970s, Dr. Baulfor Mount in Canada coined the term *palliative care* to describe his hospice program in Canada, and this term has since gained worldwide acceptance.[2]

At the present time, palliative medicine has achieved specialty or subspecialty status in the United Kingdom (since 1987), the United States, Canada, and Australia. In addition, there are active efforts to establish palliative medicine as a subspecialty in many European countries and several countries in Latin America and Asia. The move towards accreditation is highly important because it allows palliative care practitioners to obtain standardized training and to be recognized for their expertise, clinical programs to set benchmarks for their operations, institutions and governments to allocate healthcare resources, and researchers to properly evaluate the structures, processes, and outcomes associated with palliative care services.

The only nation where the specialty of palliative medicine has existed long enough to allow for some evaluation of its impact is the United Kingdom, where physicians need to complete 4 years of specialty training to be qualified as palliative medicine consultants. Hospice and palliative medicine has become an accredited specialty in the United States since 2009, requiring physicians to complete a 1-year clinical fellowship program, with an optional second year focusing on research. The consensus among physician groups in most of the world is that the development of the specialty of palliative medicine is of great importance for the further development of the field, particularly in acute care institutions and universities.

ROLE OF SUPPORTIVE CARE

The term *supportive care* first emerged in the early 1990s and was defined by Page et al. as "the provision of the necessary services for those living with or affected by cancer to meet their informational, emotional, spiritual, social or physical need during their diagnostic treatment or follow-up phases encompassing issues of health promotion and prevention, survivorship, palliation and bereavement.... In other words, supportive care is anything one does for the patient that is not aimed directly at curing his disease but rather is focused at helping the patient and family get through the illness in the best possible condition. Clearly this type of help would need to be broad in scope and as varied as the individuals requiring it".[3] Others have used supportive care in a narrower sense to describe the management of treatment-related adverse effects, such as chemotherapy-induced nausea and vomiting, oral mucositis, peripheral neuropathy, and skin rash.[4] For instance, the Multinational Association of Supportive Care in Cancer has traditionally focused on the treatment of antineoplastic therapy–related adverse effects and has now expanded its scope to include palliative care domains such as psychosocial/spiritual care and communication, as well as survivorship care.

Given the significant overlap and confusion around the description of *supportive care*, *palliative care*, and *hospice care*,[5] we recently completed a systematic review to identify defining features for these three terms and developed a preliminary conceptual framework unifying these terms along the continuum of care (Figure 12.1).[4] *Hospice care* focuses on providing care

for patients at the end of life (i.e., last 6 months) predominately in the community setting. *Palliative care* includes not only hospice care services but also acute care programs in hospitals providing care for patients with advanced diseases. *Supportive care* is the most encompassing term that spans survivorship care services to bereavement programs for patients throughout the disease trajectory.

Given that supportive care includes palliative care, it is sometimes used interchangeably to describe palliative care programs or services. We recently surveyed oncologists and midlevel providers about their perception of *palliative care* and *supportive care*.[6] A majority of the respondents reported that *supportive care* was less likely to cause distress in patients and families compared to *palliative care* and that they were more likely to refer patients to a *supportive care* service. Based on this finding, we changed our program name to *supportive care* in 2007.[7] In a before and after name change comparison, we found that the name change to supportive care was associated with more inpatient referrals and earlier referrals in the outpatient setting.[8]

INTERDISCIPLINARY NATURE OF PALLIATIVE MEDICINE

Figure 12.2 illustrates the main disciplines involved in the palliative circle of care. Each of these disciplines is responsible for developing its own body of knowledge and for contributing to the integration of this body of knowledge with that of the other disciplines within the circle. The effective growth and interactions of these disciplines results in increased knowledge in palliative care, which in turn improves care for patients and families. In this theoretical model, palliative medicine is the medical component of the multidimensional and interdisciplinary domain known as palliative care.

Figure 12.3 shows that there are many important contributors to the body of knowledge of palliative medicine. These contributors have not only included subspecialties of medicine but a large contribution to the knowledge of medicine has also been made by disciplines such as nursing, rehabilitation, psychology, social work, pastoral care, and nutrition.[9] It is desirable to have representatives

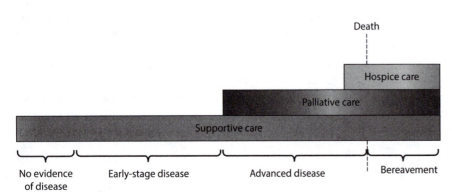

Figure 12.1 *Conceptual framework for supportive care, palliative care, and hospice care.*

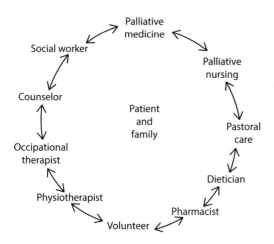

Figure 12.2 *Palliative circle of care.*

of these disciplines as part of the research and education in palliative care. It is likely that with the regular interaction as part of the palliative care circle, these disciplines will continue to influence the growth of palliative medicine in the future.

LEVELS OF PALLIATIVE MEDICINE

As palliative care matures into a professional discipline with specialized knowledge and skills, the practice of palliative care can be divided into three categories based on their level of involvement in clinical care, education, and research.[10] Box 12.1 summarizes the similarities and differences between primary, secondary, and tertiary palliative care. Palliative medicine specialists are not necessarily expected to see all patients with progressive, incurable diseases or their families. In most cases, the physician in charge of the primary care of the patient, either their family physicians (such as in Canada, the United Kingdom, and Australia[4]) or their primary specialists (such as in the United States,[11,12] most of continental Europe,[13] and the developing world[14]), can deliver the principles of palliative care assessment and management. These primary care physicians can access a number of other palliative care disciplines for the patient including nursing, social work, pastoral care, counseling, rehabilitation, or volunteer services. To ensure a high base level of primary palliative care delivery, we need to increase the intensity of palliative care training among medical students and postgraduate trainees.

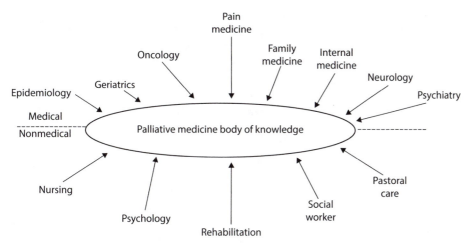

Figure 12.3 *Main medical and nonmedical disciplines that influenced the body of knowledge in palliative medicine.*

Box 12.1 Primary, secondary, and tertiary palliative care

	Primary palliative care	Secondary palliative care	Tertiary palliative care
Personnel	Primary care or specialists (e.g., oncologists, cardiologists)	Specialist palliative care teams	Specialist palliative care teams
Roles	Provision of primary care and basic palliative care	Provision of specialist palliative care as consultants	Provision of specialist palliative care and primary care
Settings	Community, hospitals, academic centers	Hospitals (palliative care clinics and palliative care inpatient consultations)	Academic centers (palliative care units)
Complexity of patient cases	+	++	+++
Involvement in palliative care education	–	+/–	+++
Involvement in palliative care research	–	+/–	+++

When patients present with physical or psychosocial distress that cannot be appropriately controlled by their primary care physician, involvement of secondary palliative care by specialized teams is advised. They can provide episodic care, such as consultations, or collaborative care by following up with the patient in an integrated manner with the primary physician.[15,16] The palliative medicine specialist will then be able to access all other members of the palliative care team as required.

A small percentage of patients are severely distressed, and this requires that the palliative medicine specialist becomes the primary care physician. This will take place both in the ambulatory care setting and particularly in palliative care units.[17–19] In many cases, the most important contribution of the palliative medicine specialist is to provide the sophisticated assessment and correct management plan that will help the team develop the most effective interventions. Tertiary palliative care specialists are not only active in the provision of complex care but also active in educating the next generation of clinicians and conducting palliative care research.[20]

These different levels of delivery of palliative care are not different from the role of other medical specialists in the management of different diseases. For example, it would not be reasonable to expect that cardiologists provide primary care to all patients with arterial hypertension or that endocrinologists provide primary care to all patients with type 2 diabetes. In most countries in the world, their own primary care physicians provide the majority of care for these patients. However, the specialist is available for consultation for a major proportion of these patients and for primary delivery of care in the most refractory situations.

The degree of use of the palliative medicine specialist as a consultant will be linked to the level of expertise of the primary physician. Some primary physicians will have acquired enough education and experience in palliative care to be able to resolve a large proportion of clinical problems, whereas others will have a much lower threshold for consultation. The best indicator for the appropriate utilization of palliative medicine specialty services will be the level of physical and psychosocial distress in patients and families in each institution and/or region.

Palliative medicine specialists are extremely important for undergraduate and postgraduate education.[21–24] They are also responsible for the continuing medical education of those primary care physicians already working in the community. The adoption of new assessments and pharmacological and non-pharmacological interventions by primary care physicians will heavily depend on the clinical and educational leadership of palliative medicine specialists in every community. Physicians adopt new diagnostic tests, medications, and procedures mostly as a result of the clinical leadership and education of those who have specialized in these specific areas of knowledge.

Finally, palliative medicine specialists are responsible for the development of the body of knowledge that will result in changes in the assessment and treatment of patients and families.[25] Although most physicians will use analgesics, antiemetics, and drugs for the management of delirium on a regular basis, there is a huge need for a small number of specialists with great dedication to the discovery of new assessments and treatments for pain, emesis, and delirium in palliative care.

Individuals who are fully focused on palliative care research will ensure that there is progress in this field.[26]

In summary, palliative medicine specialists are able to deliver clinical care to those patients and families with the most difficult problems, to educate colleagues about the appropriate delivery of palliative care, and to actively conduct research on new developments in assessment and management of clinical problems. Ideally, a significant proportion of palliative medicine specialists should operate within academically organized departments in medical schools. Such departments already exist in a number of universities in the United Kingdom, North America, and Europe. The university affiliation will allow palliative medicine specialists to have the necessary protected time for conducting academic activities, the possibility to influence the development of undergraduate and postgraduate curricula, and the possibility to establish research teams by interacting with experts in methodology, content, and biostatistics affiliated with different universities.

CONCLUSIONS

Since the establishment of the specialty of palliative medicine in the United Kingdom in 1987, similar efforts have been made in a number of countries. Palliative medicine specialists have been instrumental in the development of scientific organizations and meetings, peer-reviewed journals, and textbooks and in the development of a curriculum for the undergraduate and postgraduate teaching of palliative medicine for physicians. These specialists have also linked with other healthcare professionals and volunteers to maintain the multidimensional and interdisciplinary nature of palliative care.

The nature and content of the teaching curriculum, the financial viability of the different palliative specialist positions in different countries, and the overall body of knowledge are not completely defined for this young medical specialty. As palliative medicine is progressively adopted by acute care facilities and academic institutions, the need for palliative medicine specialists is likely to grow exponentially during the next decade in most parts of the world.

Key learning points

- Palliative care programs have three main characteristics: multidimensional assessment and management, interdisciplinary care, and emphasis on the patient and their families.
- Palliative medicine was initially established as a specialty in the United Kingdom in 1987.
- Palliative medicine specialists integrate with multiple other disciplines in the delivery of palliative care.
- Palliative medicine specialists provide clinical care in the most complex situations, graduate and postgraduate education, and research.

REFERENCES

1 Saunders C. Introduction: History and challenge. In: Saunders C, Sykes N, eds. *The Management of Terminal Malignant Disease*, London, Great Britain: Hodder and Stoughton, 1993: pp. 1–14.
2 Mount BM. The problem of caring for the dying in a general hospital; the palliative care unit as a possible solution. *CMAJ* 1976;115(2):119–121.
3 Page B. What is supportive care? *Can Oncol Nurs J* 1994;4:62–63.
4 Hui D, De La Cruz M, Mori M, Parsons HA, Kwon JH, Torres-Vigil I et al. Concepts and definitions for "supportive care," "best supportive care," "palliative care," and "hospice care" in the published literature, dictionaries, and textbooks. *Support Care Cancer* 2013;21(3):659–685.
5 Hui D, Mori M, Parsons H, Li ZJ, Damani S, Evans A et al. The lack of standard definitions in the supportive and palliative oncology literature. *J Pain Symptom Manage* 2012;43(3):582–592.
6 Fadul N, Elsayem A, Palmer JL, Del Fabbro E, Swint K, Li Z et al. Supportive versus palliative care: What's in a name? A survey of medical oncologists and midlevel providers at a comprehensive cancer center. *Cancer* 2009;115(9):2013–2021.
7 Bruera E, Hui D. Conceptual models for integrating palliative care at cancer centers. *J Palliat Med* 2012;15(11):1261–1269.
8 Dalal S, Palla S, Hui D, Nguyen L, Chacko R, Li Z et al. Association between a name change from palliative to supportive care and the timing of patient referrals at a comprehensive cancer center. *Oncologist* 2011;16(1):105–111.
9 Hui D, Parsons HA, Damani S, Fulton S, Liu J, Evans A et al. Quantity, design, and scope of the palliative oncology literature. *Oncologist* 2011;16:694–703.
10 von Gunten CF. Secondary and tertiary palliative care in U.S. hospitals. *JAMA* 2002;287(7):875–881.
11 Morrison RS, Meier DE. Clinical practice. Palliative care. *N Engl J Med* 2004;350(25):2582–2590.
12 White KR, Cochran CE, Patel UB. Hospital provision of end-of-life services: Who, what, and where? *Med Care* 2002;40(1):17–25.
13 Centeno C, Gomez-Sancho M. Models for the delivery of palliative care: The Spanish Model. In: Bruera E, Portenoy RK, eds. *Topics in Palliative Care*. Oxford, U.K.: Oxford University Press, 2001: pp. 25–38.
14 Wenk R, Bertolino M. Models for the delivery of palliative care: The Argentine Model. In: Bruera E, Portenoy RK, eds. *Topics in Palliative Care*. Oxford, U.K.: Oxford University Press, 2001: pp. 39–54.
15 Yennurajalingam S, Atkinson B, Masterson J, Hui D, Urbauer D, Tu SM et al. The impact of an outpatient palliative care consultation on symptom burden in advanced prostate cancer patients. *J Palliat Med* 2012;15(1):20–24.
16 Yennurajalingam S, Urbauer DL, Casper KL, Reyes-Gibby CC, Chacko R, Poulter V et al. Impact of a palliative care consultation team on cancer-related symptoms in advanced cancer patients referred to an outpatient supportive care clinic. *J Pain Symptom Manage* 2010;41(1):49–56.
17 Hui D, Elsayem A, Li Z, De La Cruz M, Palmer JL, Bruera E. Antineoplastic therapy use in patients with advanced cancer admitted to an acute palliative care unit at a comprehensive cancer center: A simultaneous care model. *Cancer* 2010;116(8):2036–2043.
18 Hui D, Elsayem A, Palla S, De La Cruz M, Li Z, Yennurajalingam S et al. Discharge outcomes and survival of patients with advanced cancer admitted to an acute palliative care unit at a comprehensive cancer center. *J Palliat Med* 2010;13(1):49–57.
19 Elsayem A, Swint K, Fisch MJ, Palmer JL, Reddy S, Walker P et al. Palliative care inpatient service in a comprehensive cancer center: Clinical and financial outcomes. *J Clin Oncol* 2004;22(10):2008–2014.
20 Hui D, Elsayem A, De la Cruz M, Berger A, Zhukovsky DS, Palla S et al. Availability and integration of palliative care at U.S. cancer centers. *JAMA* 2010;303(11):1054–1061.
21 LeGrand SB, Walsh D, Nelson KA, Davis MP. A syllabus for fellowship education in palliative medicine. *Am J Hosp Palliat Care* 2003;20(4):279–289.
22 Oneschuk D. Undergraduate medical palliative care education: A new Canadian perspective. *J Palliat Med* 2002;5(1):43–47.
23 Oneschuk D, Fainsinger R, Hanson J, Bruera E. Assessment and knowledge in palliative care in second year family medicine residents. *J Pain Symptom Manage* 1997;14(5):265–273.
24 Oneschuk D, Hanson J, Bruera E. An international survey of undergraduate medical education in palliative medicine. *J Pain Symptom Manage* 2000;20(3):174–179.
25 Bruera E, Hui D. Palliative care research: Lessons learned by our team over the last 25 years. *Palliat Med* 2013 Dec;27(10):939–51.
26 Rodgers EM. *Adoption of Innovation Theory: Diffusion of Innovation*, 4th edn. New York: Free Press, 1995.

Web Resources

Edmonton Regional Palliative Care Program: www.palliative.org
International Association of Hospice Care: www.hospicecare.com last, accessed June 3, 2014.

PART 2

Bioethics

13

Bioethical principles in palliative care

PAULINA TABOADA

INTRODUCTION

Ethical challenges in palliative medicine do not substantially differ from those encountered in other areas of medicine.[1-5] Nevertheless, the recognition of the needs of patients at the end of life demands some moral attitudes, skills, and knowledge that enable adequate decision-making in relation to the unique sources of suffering encountered in the dying and their relatives.[5]

> Simply stated, ethical issues in palliative care center around decisions which will enable us to satisfy the criteria for a peaceful death, dignified and assisted by a helpful society.
> Roy and MacDonald, p. 97[5]

Contemporary palliative care, in the international context, would extend this definition to include improving quality of life before death, not only the point of death. If the key ethical challenge in palliative medicine is having the practical wisdom to make adequate decisions that enable patients and their relatives to experience peace, dignity, and solidarity in the last phase of life and in the dying process, then identifying the criteria for adequate medical decision-making at the end of life becomes a central question. Are there such ethical criteria? Where can they be found? Is it possible to identify ethical principles that can be shared by people with different cultural, religious, ethnic, etc., sensibilities? Is it actually possible to introduce some order and rationality to ethical decision-making that seemingly pertain rather to the domain of the subjective and nonrational?

Answering these and other related philosophical questions goes far beyond the scope of this chapter. Thus, without denying their theoretical interest and difficulty, I shall rather adopt a practical approach and suggest that when dealing with concrete moral challenges in the care for terminally ill patients, it is helpful to apply a method for the systematization of ethical analysis and decision-making (Box 13.1).[6,7] In this context, I shall also offer a summary of the basic content and the inner logic of some relevant trends in contemporary

biomedical ethics (Box 13.2), comparing two of the most influential approaches, namely, "principlism"[8] (Box 13.3) and "personalism"[9] (Box 13.4). The former is the most widely used ethical framework in the Anglo-Saxon world, while the latter has been very influential in continental Europe and in some Latin American countries.

To conclude, I shall emphasize the importance of some fundamental moral attitudes and virtues that play a central role in orienting health-care professionals in the way in which these ethical principles ought to be applied, particularly in end-of-life care.[4,5,9] Indeed, I shall argue that two fundamental moral attitudes belong to the very essence of palliative medicine, namely, (1) an unconditional respect for human life and dignity even in situations of extreme weakness and vulnerability and (2) the acceptance of human finitude and death.[4,5,9] In addition, the virtues of truthfulness, prudence, and compassion also acquire a special relevance in the care for the dying.[10,11]

Systematizing the ethical analysis

Although health-care professionals tend to think that ethics consultations might be helpful, they often find it difficult to opportunely access ethics consultants when confronted with dilemmas in individual cases.[6,12,13] Some may not feel confident when dealing with ethical problems or may distrust their skills for a systematic analysis of the value conflicts that can arise between health professionals, families, and society in actual clinical decisions.

Our experience with ethics consultations suggests that having a method for the systematization of the ethical analysis of clinical cases is helpful in complex decision-making.[6,7] Indeed, several methods have been proposed over the years.[6,7,14-26] I shall briefly summarize here a method that involves eight different steps (Box 13.1).[6,7] Nevertheless, these various steps do not need to be understood and applied in a rigid manner but should rather serve as a reminder of the information that needs to be gathered and analyzed when solving ethical problems in clinical practice.

Box 13.1 Systematization of the ethical analysis of clinical cases

1. Identify the ethical problem and formulate the right question/s.
2. Refer to the ethical values/principles involved.
3. Collect and analyze the "ethically relevant" clinical information.
4. Inquire the patients' values and involve them in decision-making.
5. Review alternative courses of action.
6. Formulate an ethical solution.
7. Consider the best way of implementing the solution.
8. Reflect on the cases' lessons.

Box 13.2 Main trends in contemporary bioethics

- Hippocratic tradition
- Utilitarianism
- Libertarianism
- Kantian ethics
- Casuistry
- Relational and feminist ethics
- Virtue ethics
- Principlism
- Personalism

Box 13.3 Principles of biomedical ethics according to Principlism

- Nonmaleficence
- Beneficence
- Autonomy
- Justice

Box 13.4 Ethical principles according to Personalism

Primary principles

- Respect for human life and death
- Totality—Therapeutic principle
- Freedom and responsibility
- Sociability and subsidiarity

Secondary principles

- Double effect
- Therapeutic proportionality
- Truthfulness
- Prevention
- Nonabandonment

Identify the ethical problem and formulate the right question/s

A necessary—although not sufficient—condition to solve a problem is to adequately identify it. Indeed, if one has recognized a problem, one is able—among other things—to formulate the right questions. In the case of ethical problems in clinical settings, this might not be always easy. It is therefore important to make an intentional effort to formulate the ethical question/s as clearly as possible. Moreover, ethical question/s should be formulated in such a way that they can be actually answered (i.e., "operational questions"). Examples of "operationally" formulated ethical questions are the following: Are the family's requests to withhold the truth about diagnosis and prognosis to a patient ethically acceptable? Should a physician respect a family's request not to disclose to a patient the truth about his or her diagnosis and prognosis? Does a family have a right to make such a request? Do patients have a right not to know their diagnosis and/or prognosis?

Bernard Lo operationally defined an ethical problem in clinical settings as a difficulty in decision-making with regard to an individual case, for the resolution of which the mere technical information is not sufficient and one needs to refer to ethical principles that specify what should be done, in contradistinction to what can be (technically) done.[27]

In spite of some limitations of this definition, it has the merit of pointing to the fact that clinicians are confronted with ethical problems when they do not know whether they ought to do a medical intervention that can be actually done (at least from a merely technical point of view). Another contribution of the definition is the reference to the key to solve the problem: ethical principles or values. Nevertheless, the question arises: which ethical principles? Furthermore, an ethical problem commonly arises when two or more values or principles seem to confront—or do actually confront—with each other, and one is not certain which of them should have the priority. Hence, identifying the conflicting values or principles is a necessary step to solve the ethical problem. Nevertheless, to identify ethical principles is not enough in itself, as the solution to an ethical problem is the result of a prudential moral judgment, that is, a moral deliberation that takes into account the way in which general principles might be applied to a particular case, with its concrete circumstances.

Identify the ethical principles

Beneficence and nonmaleficence have traditionally been the leading principles of medical ethics.[8,9] They correspond to the so-called first principle of practical reason: do the good and avoid the bad (*bonum est faciendum, malum vitandum*).[28] With the influence of modern philosophy, the importance of the principles of respect for autonomy and justice was also acknowledged, especially in the context of pluralistic societies. So, today most health professionals are familiar with the so-called four principles of bioethics: autonomy, nonmaleficence, beneficence, and justice[8] (Box 13.3). In fact, these four principles are broadly used as "the" set of ethical principles that should guide medical decision-making. But this approach does actually correspond to one of the current trends of biomedical ethics: "principlism." Although certainly very influential, this approach has not been exempt from difficulties and strong criticisms.[28-44] Hence, a number of other approaches to medical ethics have been proposed.[9,28-44] Having a basic knowledge of these different trends and their potential contribution to medical decision-making is useful for health professionals. Thus, I shall come back to this point later.

Collect the ethically relevant clinical information

There is a corpus of clinical information that is relevant for the ethical analysis, for instance, the evidence-based certainty of the diagnosis and prognosis and the therapeutic options with their corresponding benefits, risks, and burdens. All these aspects are not "ethical information" but rather "technical" or "scientific information." Nevertheless, they are extremely relevant for the ethical analysis. Hence, this scientific and technical information needs to be carefully collected and analyzed, if one wants to perform an objectively founded ethical analysis of particular cases and not a merely theoretical discussion.

Inquire the patients' values and preferences and involve them in decision-making

Exploring the patients' values and preferences with regard to medical decision-making is required by the respect due to their dignity, freedom, and responsibility. Hence, the patients' capacity to actively participate in medical decision-making (competence) needs to be first established both in its cognitive and affective dimensions. If the patient is not competent, the right surrogate decision-maker has to be identified.

In addition, possible cultural differences with regard to medical decision-making should be inquired. There are cultures (e.g., Latin American countries; Middle eastern countries) in which the delegation of authority is culturally implicit so that the tendency is to inform the family about the diagnosis and plan of care, especially in the case of so-called bad news.[45-47] Not being aware of such cultural uses and sensibilities may cause irreversible damage to the physician–patient relationship as well as to the physician–family relationship. Nevertheless, the present trend toward globalization may result in a patient's appropriation of values different than the ones that are considered typical for his or her cultural background. Hence, one cannot just assume that a given patient will prefer one style over the other only because he or she belongs to a given culture

or ethnic group. Thus, one should always tactfully explore the values and preferences of the individual patient not only with regard to the concrete course of actions but also with regard to truth disclosure and decision-making styles.[2,8,10] Indeed, there are different styles of decision-making that can be—in principle—equally respectful of patient's autonomy. Thus, some patients may prefer a "patient-based" model, while others might choose a "family-based" style.[8,10] So, in order to respect the patients' decision-making style, as well as their personal values and preferences, it is mandatory to first explore them.[2]

Review alternative courses of action

The alternatives to be analyzed here do not refer to the therapeutic options but rather to possible courses of action with regard to the ethical question. For instance, if my question is whether it is ethically legitimate not to disclose the truth about the clinical situation to a patient at the family's request, then the alternatives can be, for instance, (1) to follow the family's request, (2) to disclose the truth against the family's wishes, and (3) to explore the patient's preferences with regard to communication and decision-making.

Sometimes, ethical problems seem to "dissolve" when one makes an intentional effort to open one's mind and seriously considers alternative paths of action than the ones one usually applies.

Suggest the ethical solution

After collecting and carefully analyzing all the necessary ethical, scientific, and technical information, one is usually in a better position to answer the ethical question, suggesting a solution to the problem and providing the foundations for this answer.

Consider the best way of implementing the suggested solution

For an action to be morally good, not only what I do and the reasons for doing it need to be good. Also, the way in which I do it is ethically relevant. Thus, to suggest a solution for ethical problems means not only to state what ought to be done and the reasons for doing it but also to provide some practical orientations with regard to the best way to do it (for instance, who, how, where, when). Indeed, classical ethics acknowledges the importance of the circumstances of an action.

Reflect on the cases' lessons

The exercise of systematically analyzing complex ethical problems in concrete clinical cases requires an intentional effort to deliberate about the way in which general ethical principles may orient our moral actions. This moral deliberation should be guided by the virtue of prudence, which is the practical wisdom about what ought to be done or avoided.[28,37] This practical wisdom is best acquired by the repeated exercise of being confronted to concrete ethical problems and learning from this experience.[14,22] Hence, to acquire the virtue of prudence, one should not miss the opportunity to learn from each concrete moral experience.

MAIN TRENDS IN CONTEMPORARY BIOETHICS

As already stated, different approaches to medical ethics have been proposed.[9,28–44] Having a basic knowledge of their potential contribution to medical decision-making is useful for health professionals. Thus, I shall briefly summarize the content of some of the main trends in contemporary bioethics (Box 13.2) and compare two very influential approaches, namely, "principlism"[8] (Box 13.3) and "personalism"[9](Box 13.4). The former is perhaps the most widely used ethical framework in the Anglo-Saxon world, while the latter has been developed mainly in continental Europe and in some Latin American countries, as previously said.[8,44,48–50]

Although a review of these different approaches may initially raise a sort of perplexity, a general knowledge of the different ethical frameworks used in medical ethics may actually help the readers identify their personal standpoint better. Moreover, it may also help them discover incoherencies in their ethical views, as we sometimes incorporate concepts without analyzing their foundations and concrete implications. So, while some ethical frameworks are compatible and complement each other, others are incompatible and exclude each other. Hence, one needs to take a standpoint. And one can best do so by contrasting the different positions with "reality" itself, that is, with the personal experience about how moral life actually functions and about the type of foundations we search for when we want to explain the reasons for our concrete behavior.

Hippocratic tradition

The Hippocratic tradition has dominated medical ethics for centuries.[8] It is usually said that Hippocrates taught that the first medical duty is "not to harm" (primum non nocere).[51] And from the duty of beneficence ("I will use treatment to help the sick according to my ability and judgement"), he deduced a number of secondary ethical principles contained in the Hippocratic Oath, such as confidentiality, integrity, and honesty to acknowledge the limits our knowledge.[8]

For centuries, the ethical values and principles contained in the Hippocratic Oath were applied to medical decision-making without any further questioning. Nevertheless, with the influence of modern philosophy, this way of approaching ethical considerations began to be regarded as excessively "paternalistic," as it does not give too much space to the respect due to patients' autonomy or to considerations of justice.

Utilitarianism

Jeremy Bentham[52] and John Stuart Mill[53] are the founders of Utilitarianism, an ethical trend that arose in England in the seventeenth century. Its main content is the idea that the

sole criterion that distinguishes good from bad actions is the "principle of utility," defined as the maximization of pleasure and the minimization of suffering for the greatest number. Although over the years different subtypes of utilitarianism have been proposed (e.g., hedonistic utilitarianism, preference utilitarianism, rule utilitarianism), all share the basic intuition that ethical deliberation is a calculus or balance aiming to maximize goods and minimize evils for the biggest number.[8]

Its application to medical decision-making results in conceiving the moral character of medical actions as the result of a balance between their good and bad consequences, with a view to the "greater good" or "lesser evil" that is actually possible to attain in a given situation.[8] In other words, the criterion for evaluating the moral rightness of an action is drawn from weighing the nonmoral or premoral goods that can be attained. Concrete medical behavior would be considered to be right or wrong according to whether it is capable of producing better conditions for all concerned. One of the most famous representatives of this trend in contemporary bioethics is the Australian Peter Singer.[54,55]

The clarity with which utilitarianism saw the moral relevance of taking into account the positive and negative foreseeable consequences of our actions is one of its biggest contributions. Indeed, the moment in which we balance the consequences of our actions is doubtless an important moment in moral reasoning. Nevertheless, an analysis of personal moral experience may show us that consequences are not the only aspect we take into consideration when deciding whether a concrete action is good or bad. Hence the popular saying, "the end does not justify the means." It seems that—besides the consequences—there are also other dimensions of our actions that have a key moral relevance in determining the ethical value of our actions.

Libertarianism

Stuart Mill[53] is the father of "libertarianism." He argued that society should permit individuals to live their lives according to their convictions, as long as they do not interfere with the expressions of liberty of others. Thus, Mill was concerned mainly about individuals' autonomy, which—according to him—requires both not interfering with and strengthening the expressions of individual liberty.[8]

A contemporary application of this conception to bioethics has been undertaken by HT Engelhardt.[53] The lack of moral consensus in contemporary pluralistic societies leads this author to propose his thesis about the "moral strangers in the public road" stating that—since we do not speak the same moral language nor can agree on ethical principles—the only solution for "public morality" is to establish "procedural guidelines" (rules of fair play) regarding the way in which we will come to a qualified "consensus." From this perspective, the only ethical principles for biomedical ethics are "permission" and "beneficence." The principle of permission entails both that (1) without the informed consent (permission) of the affected person, each action affecting them is illegitimate and (2) permission validates any type of action. On the other hand, the principle of beneficence holds that—in spite of the impossibility of having a common view regarding which is the good to be done or the evil to avoid—explicit social agreements (consensus) on what is considered as a benefit should be respected.

Kantian ethics

Kant proposed that ethics is mainly about "duties."[57] To act correctly is to act according to duty. The core of Kantian ethics is the trust in the capacity of human reason to discover what is our duty in a given situation. According to Kant, the key to discover our duty is the rule of "universalization": an action is right if one can wish that the maxim (general principle) that governs it can be applied by all others without entering into contradictions. Thus, analyzing the distinction between hypothetic (conditional) and categorical (unconditional) imperatives (commands), Kant concludes that only things that have value in themselves can ground "categorical imperatives." Indeed, hypothetic imperatives oblige only if one accepts the preestablished condition (e.g., if I want to go to Paris, I *ought* to buy a ticket; this implies that if I do not want to go to Paris, I do not have to buy a ticket). Contrarily, categorical imperatives oblige always, regardless of any condition (e.g., the person ought to be respected). This analysis leads him to the distinction between "things" and "persons." While things have a price (Preis), persons have a special type of value that he called "dignity" (Würde). For Kant, the source of the persons' dignity is their capacity to determine the ends of their actions for themselves, in other words, their capacity to give themselves the norms of their actions (autonomy). This insight leads him to conclude that the person themself is an end and can therefore never be used as a mere means for something else, as this would disrespect their capacity to choose the ends of her actions themself. Hence, Kant concludes that all our moral duties can be summarized in the imperative to treat humanity in oneself and in other human beings as end in themselves and never as mere means. Although Kant formulated his "categorical imperative" in at least four different ways, the most famous formulation is the one stating that the person shall always be treated as an end in themselves and never as a mere means.

Kantian ethics continues to be very influential up to our days. Thomas Nagel, for instance, has offered a contemporary interpretation of this type of ethical reasoning.[58] In bioethics, one can recognize the influence of the Kantian legacy in important international documents, such as the UNESCO's Universal Declaration on Bioethics and Human Rights, which begins (article 3) by stating that one ought to respect the person's dignity and fundamental rights.[59] Nevertheless, there are some important differences between the Kantian understanding of "autonomy" and the way in which some contemporary bioethicists understand this concept. Indeed, for Kant, the person's self-determination ought to be always conformed to the "categorical imperative." In other words, our capacity to choose is limited: one cannot choose whatever one wishes (inclination), but one has to choose actions that respect this universal norm (the "categorical imperative"). Contrarily,

some contemporary bioethicists have taken from Kant the idea of "self-determination" only, depriving it from the Kantian necessary link to the categorical imperative.

Casuistry

Casuistry is an alternative approach to ethical reasoning in contemporary medical ethics.[40] Unlike Kantian ethics, Casuistry suggests that—rather than analyzing abstract norms and principles—our common practical moral reasoning in paradigmatic cases is able to "generate" principles or norms. Hence, by analyzing our most immediate moral experiences, we are able to ground them in general rules that can serve as a basis from which a person can generalize to other, similar cases. Casuistry does not deny that ethical theories play a role, but it discusses them only when they are relevant to a case. In each case, the unique set of circumstances will require that practical judgment finds the optimal solution for all conflicting parties. Thus, if the circumstances of a case change or due to time or culture our perceptions become altered, the moral maxim applying to that case may change as well. Since case-based ethical reasoning is very similar to the method of case analysis used in traditional teaching on rounds in medical schools, this ethical trend has gained some influence in contemporary medical ethics.

Relational ethics

Relational and feminist ethics stresses the importance of taking into account the alternative ethical perspectives that arise from the different experiences of people according to their gender, culture, social roles, etc.[40-42] Alternative perspectives should have an uncompromised opportunity to compete with other ideas and values and thereby to establish themselves within the recognized ethical matrix.

Relational approaches to ethical analysis share the perspective that ethics must take seriously the interdependent, emotionally varied, and unequal relationships that shape our lives. Hence, abstract models are considered to be biased, insofar as they base ethical analysis in the concept of a generalized and abstract human being, without paying attention to particular attributes.[40-42] Accordingly, the proper way of finding the ethical solution for individual cases will be to discuss them in an adequately conformed ethics committee, that is, a committee in which different genders, social roles, and cultures are properly represented. Relational ethics calls attention to the idea that ethics arises out of community dialog and debate. Thus, the ethical solution will be reached by the consensus of the majority.

Virtue ethics

Traditional Aristotelian virtue ethics has been reformulated in contemporary medical ethics by Edmund Pellegrino and several others.[37,38] Virtue theory applied to medicine emphasizes physicians acquiring good traits of character more than learning about moral theories and principles. Ethical inquiry in particular cases asks about the way in which a good physician would act if he or she were confronted with a similar situation. Physicians should imitate the reasoning and empathy of good physicians, who are both knowledgeable and compassionate. And the central virtue in moral reasoning is prudence. But contrarily to the way in which prudence is usually understood in contemporary philosophy (i.e., rational self-interest), in virtue ethics, prudence is understood as the ability to be practically wise, that is, the capacity to make the right choice in particular case, in light of universal moral knowledge and principles. The prudent physician has a sense about what should be done and avoided and this moral sense shapes his or her medical decision-makings.

Principlism

Back in the 1970s, James Beauchamp and Tom Childress—from Georgetown University—proposed an approach to biomedical ethics known as "principlism."[8] This approach claims the existence of four sets or clusters of ethical principles that should function as guidelines for professional ethics. Quoting their words, "The four clusters are: (1) *respect for autonomy* (a norm of respecting the decision capacity of autonomous persons), (2) nonmaleficence (a norm of avoiding the causation of harm), (3) beneficence (a group of norms for providing benefits and balancing benefits against risks and costs) and (4) justice (a group of norms for distributing benefits, risks, and costs fairly)."[8]

Although this approach has been very successful in unifying a language to solve moral problems in medical settings, it has been also subject to strong criticisms over the past years.[29–44] In order to solve some of its difficulties, Diego Gracia has proposed a system in which the so-called principles of bioethics are placed in two levels following the classical ethical distinction between perfect and imperfect moral duties.[32–35] Perfect duties are moral minimums or negative prescriptions, which ought to be respected always. Nonmaleficence and justice belong to this category, according to Gracia. Imperfect duties are ethical maximums or positive prescriptions that allow different degrees of fulfillment. Among the latter, Gracia lists beneficence and autonomy. Gracia's version of principlism has been very influential in Spanish-speaking countries, both in Europe and in Latin America.

Personalism

Personalism is a philosophical trend that arose in Europe during the twentieth century.[28–30,60,61] Drawing from the insights of Aristotle, Aquinas, Kant, and phenomenological philosophy, this approach is characterized by a renewed discovery of the person's dignity. Hence, according to this perspective, it is not duty as duty, or law as law, or utility as utility, etc., that defines the content of moral obligations, as had been suggested by other major ethical trends. Personalism proposes rather that it is the dignity and the ontological structure of the person that defines the content of our moral duties.[44,48–50,60,61]

The core of moral reasoning is derived from the statement that the proper addressee for a moral subject is a concrete person. Hence, the most basic and fundamental norm of morality—called "personalist principle"—is that the person shall be affirmed because of their self and their dignity (*Persona est affirmanda propter seipsam et propter dignitatem suam*).[49,50] In other words, personalism holds that the clue for the resolution of ethical problems in medicine is to choose the path of actions that truly respect the dignity of each person as a person. This entails taking into account the way in which persons "are built" and function (the "ontological structure"). Sgreccia proposed an interesting way in which the "personalist principle" can be specified in a number of primary and secondary ethical principles, which can—in turn—be applied to medical decision-making, as we shall see later.[9]

WHICH ETHICAL PRINCIPLES FOR PALLIATIVE CARE?

After briefly describing some of the main trends in contemporary bioethics, I shall compare the content of the ethical principles proposed by two influential approaches to medical ethics, namely, "principlism" (Box 13.3) and "personalism" (Box 13.4). The interest of making such a comparison rests in the importance of being aware of the precise content and implications of the principles one uses to solve ethical problems in palliative medicine. Indeed, if one is not aware of that, one may use the principles incorrectly and/or conclude something that does not truly reflect the philosophy and goals of palliative medicine.

Principles of "principlist" bioethics

Most health-care professionals have heard about the so-called four principles of bioethics. Nevertheless, not all are aware of their original content and the general ethical framework proposed by Beauchamp and Childress, founders of this approach. Moreover, the content attributed to these principles in some medical textbooks does not necessarily coincide with the position of these two authors. Hence, I shall briefly summarize the proposal of the authors themselves (I shall do so following the fifth revised edition of their influential book *Principles of Biomedical Ethics*, which corrects some of the shortcomings of the previous editions).[8]

RESPECT FOR AUTONOMY

According to Beauchamp and Childress, autonomy is understood as "the capacity to act freely in accordance with a self-chosen plan and free from both controlling interference by others and from limitations"[8] (p. 58). Thus, the requirements for acting autonomously are—according to these authors—"to act (1) intentionally, (2) with understanding, and (3) without controlling influences that determine the actions"[8] (p. 59). Although such an understanding of autonomy corresponds to the libertarian view, the authors explicitly state that their aim is to construct a conception of respect for autonomy that is not excessively individualistic, not excessively founded in reason, and not unduly legalistic.

According to them, respect for patients' autonomy can be expressed as a negative obligation ("autonomous actions should not be subjected to controlling constraints by others") and also as a positive obligation ("we must respect individuals' views and rights as long as their thoughts and actions do not seriously harm other persons")[8] (p. 64). Specifying the concrete content of respect for autonomy, the authors explicitly state that they "concentrate on *autonomous choice* rather than general capacity of governance"[8] (p. 58). Hence, their main effort is to analyze a set of rules related to patients' competence, informed consent, and advanced directives.

Answering to criticisms, the authors state that within their set of principles, autonomy—although important—does not always have the priority, as it can sometimes be overridden by competing moral considerations. In fact, according to this approach, no principle has priority over the others. All of them are *prima facie*, that is, obligations that must be fulfilled unless they conflict—on a particular occasion—with an equal or stronger obligation. "Agents must then determine what they ought to do by finding an actual or overriding … obligation." Following David Ross, they understand ethical deliberation as the greatest balance of right and wrong.[8,62]

NONMALEFICENCE

The principle of nonmaleficence asserts the general obligation not to inflict harm on others. In an attempt to specify the concept of harm, the authors introduce the distinction between *injury* and *harm*. They suggest that a harmful action may not always be wrong or unjustified. So, they construct a narrower concept of harm understood as defeating or setting back someone's interest. Hence, according to them, harming is in general wrong, precisely because it sets back the interests of the person.

In this authors' view, the general principle of nonmaleficence supports several rules that serve to specify its content, such as "do not kill," "do not cause pain or suffering," and "do not cause offense"[8] (p. 117). Nevertheless, in the context of this ethical framework, both the general principle and its specification rules (including the "do not kill") are not absolute but can be overridden if "the greatest balance" of right and wrong results in such a decision. Hence, they argue—for example— "that sufficient moral reasons can exist in some cases to justify acts that intentionally hasten death"[8] (p. 144). Thus, principlism accepts that "active physician assistance for a narrow group of seriously ill and dying patients at their request can be morally justified"[8] (p. 144).

BENEFICENCE

Beauchamp and Childress remark that ethics requires not only respect of autonomy and avoidance of harming others but also contribution to their welfare. In this context, the authors examine two principles of beneficence: (1) *positive beneficence* and (2) *utility*[8] (p. 165). According to them, "positive beneficence

obliges us to help others further their important and legitimate interest" (p. 166). Hence, providing benefits is "acquiescing patient's wishes and choices"[8] (p. 165). On the other hand, "utility" requires the agents to produce the best overall results by balancing benefits and drawbacks. Hence, their analysis of beneficence focuses mainly on the "principle of utility" and in "balancing benefits, risks, and costs through analytical methods designed to implement the principle of utility in clinical care as an aid to decision-making"[8] (p. 165).

Once again, to specify the content of the general principle of beneficence, the authors mention some rules, such as "protect and defend the rights of others," "remove a condition that will cause harm to others," and "help persons with disabilities." But all these duties are considered *prima facie*, that is, obligations that must be fulfilled unless in a concrete situation in which they conflict with equal or stronger obligation.

With regard to medical decisions involving the moral valuing of lives, rather than referring to an "intrinsic value"— which has no place in their theory—they validate the use of "quality-adjusted life-years" (QALY) as a way of applying the principle of utility at the bedside. Nevertheless, they remark that the "principles of respect for autonomy and justice set limits on the uses of these techniques"[8] (p. 214).

JUSTICE

The concept of justice that Beauchamp and Childress have in mind is "distributive justice," understood as "fair, equitable, and appropriate distribution"[8] (p. 226). In an attempt to find suitable criteria for the just allocation of scarce medical resources, these authors analyze different theories of justice (such as egalitarian, communitarian, libertarian, and utilitarian theories). In the absence of consensus about the role of these competing theories in structuring a country's health-care system, they conclude that "society recognize an enforceable right to a decent minimum of health care within a framework for allocation that incorporates both utilitarian and egalitarian standards"[8] (p. 272).

In other words, according to the principlist approach, the concept of justice refers exclusively to "distributive justice," and the ethical criteria proposed for a just allocation of healthcare resources are the principles of "utility" and equity.

Summing up, the principlist approach to biomedical ethics is strongly influenced by the libertarian and utilitarian conceptions of ethics. In such a conception, autonomy plays a central role and is understood almost exclusively as the capacity to choose without having interference from illegitimate constraints. On the other hand, the "principle of utility" shapes the moral deliberation. Since no ethical principle is understood as absolute, each can be overridden if the "greatest balance" of right and wrong results in such a decision.

Principles of "personalist" bioethics

Elio Sgreccia has developed an interesting application of personalist philosophy to the field of biomedical ethics.[9] According to his approach, the "personalist principle" can be specified in the following primary ethical principles: (1) defense of human life, (2) totality or therapeutic principle, (3) freedom and responsibility, and (4) sociability and subsidiarity. Further secondary principles can be derived from these primary ones. The most relevant to palliative medicine are the principle of therapeutic proportionality and the principle of double effect.

PRINCIPLE OF RESPECT FOR HUMAN LIFE (AND DEATH)

According to this approach, life is conceived as the most basic human good and as a necessary condition—although not a sufficient one—for the achievement of other human goods, such as knowledge, the exercise of freedom, friendship, family, communication, and creativity. Moreover, the person's fulfillment and pursuit of vital goals are tightly linked with the actualization of these basic goods. Therefore, life is considered to be a morally relevant value that deserves a proper *value response*.[63] Under this perspective, health is not understood as a basic good but rather as an "instrumental good" that facilitates the fulfillment of other basic human goods and vital goals. Hence, there is moral duty to respect and promote human life and health. Actually this is seen as the most basic ethical imperative in relation to the self and to others.

Nevertheless, while this conception acknowledges a "negative" prescription that forbids taking innocent human life intentionally, it also acknowledges that the "positive" obligation to implement medical interventions in order to preserve and promote life and health has a limit, as we shall see later.

Indeed, under this perspective, it is accepted that persons have a "right to die with serenity and dignity," which is understood not as a right to hasten death but rather as a right to be assisted by others in the dying process, so that one can live one's life to the (natural) end.[9,44] In other words, it is stated that the human process of dying poses certain ethical demands to medical professionals as well as to the society as such. Palliative care is regarded as a concrete and active answer to these ethical demands.[64]

Although this approach asserts that intentionally hastening a person's death is always morally wrong, it does not necessarily exclude therapeutic interventions (such as the use of opioids or sedatives), which may under certain conditions shorten life. Indeed, with regard to the risk of shortening a patient's life, this approach emphasizes the importance of the distinction between intending and foreseeing. Thus, although the medical literature suggests that the risk of actually hastening a patient's death through the use of opioids and sedatives is not the rule but rather the exception,[65-68] this approach introduces the principle of double effect to justify the use of these drugs in those cases in which this risk may be certain.

- Principle of double effect in pain management and sedation

The traditional ethical principle of double effect sets the criteria for the justification of actions that have well-known, unavoidable, bad side effects.[69-75] In its application to palliative and end-of-life care, the principle of double effect provides that it can be morally good to shorten a patient's life as a foreseen but unintended side effect of an action undertaken for a good and proportionately grave reason (such as relieving severe, refractory symptoms), even if it is agreed that intentionally killing the patient or shortening the patient's life is always wrong. Nevertheless, the following conditions need to be simultaneously fulfilled:[28,69,70]

1. The action performed is not itself morally evil.
2. The good effect is not caused by the evil effect.
3. Only the good effects are directly intended; the bad effects are not intended but only tolerated (as unavoidable).
4. There is a due proportion between the good and bad effects.

Thus, the principle of double effect forbids the achievement of good ends by wrong means.

With regard to the moral justification of the use of opioids and sedatives at the end of life, two ethical problems need to be distinguished: (1) the negative effect of suppressing consciousness and (2) the risk of shortening a patient's life. The correct application of double effect relates only to the risk of hastening death, because that risk belongs to the sort of bad side effects that would be always morally wrong to intentionally pursue. On the contrary, the reduction of a person's awareness is not the type of effect that would always be morally wrong. In fact, the existence of a sufficiently grave reason—such as the need to alleviate severe and otherwise refractory symptoms at the end of life—would make it. Therefore, in such cases, the use of opioids or sedatives does not need to be justified by double effect reasoning but rather by the principle of proportionality in medical care (see section: "Principle of therapeutic proportionality", p. 112)[69-75]

It is important to emphasize here that there is a broad consensus among specialists in palliative care and pain management that when used appropriately, respiratory depression from opioid use is a rare side effect. Hence, the common belief that the use of opioids hastens death is not supported by the available empirical data. Indeed, Regnard et al. have produced evidence to show that when opioids are correctly prescribed, they do not hasten death.[76] If this is the case, there is no need to invoke the principle of double effect to justify their use. They argue that opioid dose requirements cannot be predicted. So, to avoid adverse effects, doses should always be titrated to the individual. In addition, the UK General Medical Council clearly distinguished between safe and dangerous prescribing of strong opioids. Thus, Regnard et al. conclude that there are no circumstances in which the prescription of a lethal dose of opioids is necessary to control suffering. Thus, the principle of double effect alert us against an unsafe prescribing of opioids, an abuse that can be eliminated by skilled palliative care clinicians (for clinical guidance on opioid prescribing, see Chapters 45 and 46).

PRINCIPLE OF TOTALITY (THERAPEUTIC PRINCIPLE)

In the context of biomedical ethics, more than speaking of "benefence"—which is an excessively broad concept—Sgreccia prefers to introduce the "principle of totality" or "therapeutic principle."[9,44] This principle specifies the conditions that medical interventions need to fulfill to be ethically validated. Since medical interventions may affect the person's physical integrity and sometimes even endanger the patient's life, their ethical legitimacy has to be grounded on some requirements: (1) The goal of the intervention has to be the protection of the whole person and her life; (2) the intervention must be directed to the sick part of the body or to the cause of the disease; (3) there must be no alternatives; (4) the expected benefits must be equal to or greater than the involved risks; and (5) the patient has to consent.[9,44]

Hence, this principle prohibits—for example—interventions resulting in mutilation of healthy parts of the human body or involving disproportionately grave risks or bad effects. Stating it in positive terms, it affirms the moral obligation to use available medical interventions directed to preserve life or restore health.

But this raises the question whether one could refuse medical interventions in spite of their potential benefits or accept treatments for which the risks are still high or not yet well known. In such situations, we are confronted with the question about the limits of our moral obligation to pursue health care. The ethical criterion that personalism applies to distinguish morally obligatory from nonobligatory medical interventions is the traditional moral distinction between "ordinary" and "extraordinary" means.[76–90] The content of this traditional distinction is presently better known as the principle of therapeutic proportionality.[81–83]

- Principle of therapeutic proportionality

This principle states the existence of a moral obligation to implement medical interventions that offer a reasonable hope of preserving life and restoring health and which are not the object of grave impossibility.[3,4,81–83] Conversely, it holds that there is no moral obligation to use medical interventions that do not offer a proportionate chance of preserving life or restoring health.

As stated earlier, this ethical principle is based on the traditional moral distinction between ordinary and extraordinary means. "Ordinary" means can be defined as all medicines, treatments, and operations that offer a reasonable hope of benefit and that can be obtained and used without excessive expense, pain, or other inconvenience.[77–83] "Extraordinary" means are all medicines, treatments, and operations that cannot be obtained or used without excessive expense, pain, or other inconvenience or that, if used, would not offer a reasonable hope of benefit.[77–83]

Accordingly, to verify whether a given medical intervention is morally mandatory, one has to carefully judge the utility of the intervention in the context of the patient's concrete circumstances. It is important to note that the utility/futility has to be referred to the patient's overall clinical evolution and not merely to some isolated physiological effects. Also the risks and burdens associated with the intervention should be carefully taken into account. But the notion of "burden" has to be understood in its widest sense, that is, physical, psychological, spiritual, humane, familial, social, and financial distress.[3,4]

Judgments about therapeutic proportionality are relative to an individual's unique situation.[77–83] This means that there is no predefined list of "ordinary/proportionate" or "extraordinary/disproportionate" medical interventions. Indeed, the moral judgment is not about the intervention as such but rather about the use of a certain intervention in a particular situation. Nevertheless, this does not mean that proportionality judgments are merely subjective. In fact, to be legitimate, these judgments need to be grounded in objective state of affairs regarding the clinical condition and the present state of medical art.

From a medical point of view, some of the elements that always need to be taken into account to judge the proportionality of a given intervention are: the certainty of the clinical diagnosis, the utility/futility of the intervention, the risks and side effects of the different therapeutic alternatives, and the accuracy of the prognosis. Evidence-based data become relevant, even though it is evident that a moral obligation cannot be sufficiently grounded on statistical probabilities.

According to Personalism, judgments about therapeutic proportionality are not the result of a mere cost/benefit equation.[91,92] Indeed, the way in which the different elements involved in therapeutic proportionality have to be weighted needs to be guided by the virtue of prudence (understood as practical moral wisdom).[80–83]

The moral relevance of proportionality judgments is that they allow one to draw the distinction between morally obligatory, optional, and illicit medical interventions. So, the implementation of interventions judged to be "proportionate" is morally obligatory. To omit them would represent either medical malpractice or a form of euthanasia (by omission). On the contrary, omitting disproportionate interventions might be morally obligatory or optional, according to the concrete circumstances.

PRINCIPLE OF FREEDOM AND RESPONSIBILITY

As already stated, respect for human dignity is the foundational ethical principle according to the Personalist conception. And the respect for human dignity is expressed both in the principle of respect for human life and in the principle of freedom and responsibility.[9,44] Nevertheless, it is very important to clarify the notion of freedom with which personalism operates. Drawing from Kant's conception, this approach acknowledges the importance of maintaining the essential link between the human capacity of self-determination and the power of human reason to discover what is objectively good for the person (the "truth about the good"). In other words, respect for the exercise of freedom is grounded in respect for the person and in the acknowledgment that as rational beings, we have the unique capability to make reasoned choices. Precisely because they are free, persons are morally accountable. So, the "personalist value" of human actions comes from the responsible exercise of freedom.[49,50] Hence, not allowing an individual to act freely and responsibly is a violation of his or her dignity as a person and thus a maleficent act.

This is the reason why Sgreccia prefers to speak about a "principle of freedom and responsibility" instead of "respect for autonomy."[9] With this wording, the author emphasizes the idea that freedom is best understood in its positive dimension (as the capacity to self-determination toward the good) rather than in its negative dimension (as a mere capacity to choose without having illegitimate constraints). Although both dimensions pertain to the notion of freedom, the former corresponds to its very essence, while the latter represents only an external condition for its exercise. Indeed, self-determination points to self-possession and self-governance as the proper structure of a person. Acknowledging the structure of self-determination of the person in their actions goes along with recognizing their responsibility for these actions.[49,50] Using Kant's expressions, the person can be blamed or prized for their free actions. The essential connection between freedom and responsibility becomes evident.

In order to be able to make reasoned decisions, patients need to have the necessary information. Hence, truthfulness in communication and participation in medical decision-making are practical rules derived from the principle of freedom and responsibility.

- Truthfulness in communication

According to Personalism, truth telling goes far beyond providing information.[9,44] Truth is not just the opposite of lies, not just the sum of correct statements, but a concrete manifestation of reciprocal respect in human relationships. Deception is harmful, because it does not acknowledge the person's right to know the truth. It therefore destroys the foundations of interpersonal relationships.

In the context of palliative medicine, it is not possible to offer good care without prior commitment to openness and honesty. Nevertheless, a frequent ethical challenge in palliative care is the question of truthfulness with terminally ill patients.[10,93–97] Reluctance to share the truth about diagnosis and/or prognosis with the patient is frequently associated with family pressures related to cultural backgrounds. While medical professionals usually consider truth disclosure to be part of their professional duty and a sign of respect for patients' dignity, in some cultures relatives regard truth disclosure as being harmful to the patient.

Usually, a family's request not to disclose the truth to the patient is based on the assumption that truth disclosure will induce serious anxiety and depression, causing real harm to the patient.[47] Indeed, detailed disclosure has been shown to increase anxiety in the short term.[96] Nevertheless, follow-up surveys reveal that the excess anxiety dissipates within a few weeks, whereas the effects of limited information on psychological adjustment may persist.[97] Evasion and lying isolate patients behind either a wall of words or a wall of silence that prevents a therapeutic sharing of their fears, anxieties, and other concerns.

PRINCIPLE OF SOCIABILITY AND SUBSIDIARITY

The person—as a social being—finds her fulfillment in relationships with others and in the contribution to the common good.[9,44,49,50] This implies that each person has a value not only as an individual but also as part of a community (social good). The principle of sociability states that each person that each person has a moral obligation to contribute to the common good. In the context of biomedical ethics, this means—for instance—that there is a moral obligation to promote healthy lifestyles, or to collaborate with the progress of medical knowledge through the contribution to clinical research, etc.[9,44] The other side of this responsibility is the person's right to get timely access to the medical interventions necessary to preserve life and restore health. Each of us and society as such have a moral obligation to provide assistance, especially to the most vulnerable (principle of subsidiarity).

No one will doubt that dying persons correspond to one of society's most vulnerable groups. Hence, these persons deserve our respect and competent assistance. If we accept the premise that the moral quality of an individual is expressed mainly in the way he or she treats the most vulnerable, then we may also accept the conclusion that future generations may deduce the moral character of today's societies by the way they treat the most vulnerable, among which are the dying, as previously stated. The sincerity of unconditional respect for human life and dignity is tested precisely in conditions of extreme vulnerability, weakness, and need. In such situations, also the value and meaning we attribute to pertaining to the human family is definitely expressed.[98]

Summing up, Personalism is grounded on key insights provided by Aristotle, Aquinas, Kant, and phenomenological philosophy. According to this approach, respect for human life and dignity are the central moral principles. This approach to biomedical ethics has an anthropological foundation that provides a specific content to ethical principles. Moreover, this conception proposes a hierarchy of moral principles that can be rationally grounded, as human life is the most basic of human goods that precedes and is a necessary condition for the achievement of all other human goods. In this context, respecting the person's freedom plays a central role as a concrete expression of respect for dignity. But freedom is understood as the capacity of self-determination to what is objectively good for the person and the common good. Under this perspective, moral deliberation in medical decision-making is understood as the ability to be practically wise, that is, as the capacity to make the right decision in particular cases by correctly applying general ethical principles to concrete situations. In other words, moral deliberation is guided by the virtue of prudence, which is the knowledge of what ought to be done and avoided in particular cases in light of general ethical principles.

Which principles of bioethics for palliative medicine?

The preceding summarized description of the content of some of the most influential ethical trends in contemporary biomedical ethics may raise certain perplexity. Which framework and ethical principles should be used? Some of these conceptions are complementary, but others are incompatible with each other.

My assumption when undertaking the effort of describing them was that a basic knowledge of the foundations and inner logic of these different ethical conceptions may help the readers to recognize their resonance or dissonance with "reality" itself. In other words, the reader would engage in a personal confrontation of these different trends with his or her personal experience about the way in which moral life actually "works." So, my invitation is to become aware of the type the arguments we actually search and consider valid to provide a solid foundation for our own moral decisions. The challenge is to try to be coherent and to provide consistent foundations for our ethical decision-making in concrete clinical cases. Unfortunately, my experience with ethical consultations shows that health professionals sometimes mix up the arguments from different ethical trends without necessarily realizing their incompatibility or their dissonance with their personal moral experience.

This (perhaps oversimplified) analysis of different ethical approaches to biomedical ethics seems to suggest that there is a certain coincidence or harmony between the Personalist conception and the philosophy and goals of palliative medicine. The World Health Organization's definition states that "Palliative Care affirms life and regards dying as a normal process, neither hastening nor postponing death."[64] This definition seems to correspond more to the principle of respect for human life and death as it is understood within the Personalist framework than with other approaches, especially inasmuch as here the so-called right to die with dignity is not simply conceived as a right to self-determination with regard to death but rather as a right to live one's life to the end and to be assisted by others in the dying process.[99–103]

Under this perspective, the dying process is understood to pose special ethical challenges to medical professionals as well as to society as such. The experience with palliative care patients shows that each patient is unique and unrepeatable. In spite of the similarities of clinical conditions, each individual has a specific constellation of symptoms, which in turn present themselves with different degrees of intensity in each case. Moreover, the personal experience with the disease, with the medical profession, with the family, with the friends, and with society differs as well, generating dissimilar psychological reactions among terminally ill patients.[99–103] Also the spiritual resources and the coping mechanisms vary according to their respective religious and cultural background. Dying persons have a right to receive integral and competent assistance at the end of life, addressing the different sources of suffering of the dying person and their relatives ("total pain").[99] Palliative medicine was originally conceived precisely as an active and competent answer to these ethical demands.

Fundamental moral attitudes and virtues relevant in palliative care

The peculiar needs and features of patients at the end of life demand from health-care workers—even more explicitly than in other areas of medicine—some fundamental moral attitudes and virtues. These attitudes are an unconditional respect for human life and dignity as well as the acceptance of human finitude. To discover what appropriate palliative care is, health professionals shall be dedicated to providing competent medical services with compassion and respect for human dignity[104] This statement summarizes three central virtues in the praxis of palliative care: medical expertise, compassion, and respect for human dignity—even in situations of extreme vulnerability and suffering. Indeed, these virtues are tightly interconnected. A genuinely compassionate attitude allows health-care professionals to identify the concrete way in which medical expertise has to be applied to truly respect the dignity of each person, especially in situations of extreme weakness and unavoidable death.

The term "compassion" is commonly understood as synonymous of pity. Nevertheless, it can be better defined as the virtue by which we have a sympathetic consciousness of sharing the distress and suffering of another person and on that basis are inclined to offer assistance in alleviating and/or living through that suffering.[104] Hence, there are two key elements in defining compassion: (1) an ability and willingness to enter into another's situation deeply enough to gain knowledge of the person's experience of suffering and (2) a virtue characterized by the desire to alleviate the person's suffering or, if that is not possible, to be supportive by living through it vicariously.[105,106] Compassion—understood as a moral virtue—entails the willingness to effectively alleviate a person's sufferings.[105,106] Hence, it demands unfolding the corresponding expertise or "know-how."

Human suffering at the end of life has different causes. Thus, medical interventions aimed at alleviating suffering in terminally ill patients cannot be narrowly understood as just those having the potential to produce certain physiological effects on the person's body. This is doubtless an important goal of end-of-life care, but the medical commitment toward a dying person goes far beyond the body. Indeed, a peculiar cause of human suffering at the end of life is the person's natural fear of imminent death, and health-care workers should develop a special sensitivity toward this aspect, permitting their patients to reflect on their moral duty to accept death and to receive the necessary psychological and spiritual assistance, if they want. This will require—among other things—the preservation of the patient's state of consciousness, as long as the clinical condition and the therapeutic goals allow it.

If compassion is primarily directed to the person in virtue of his or her sufferings and only secondarily to the sufferings, then we can draw another practical conclusion. In situations of extreme and prolonged suffering, a truly compassionate attitude will prevent a health-care provider from the temptation of accelerating death to alleviate their patient's sufferings. To end a person's life cannot be an act of true compassion, because such an act would eliminate the very object of compassion: the person. On the contrary, a compassionate attitude allows health-care providers to recognize the way in which their competent medical knowledge can be best used to palliate the person's sufferings in a way that truly respects each person's life and dignity, even in the events surrounding an unavoidable death.

CONCLUDING REMARKS

Summing up the topics I have revised in this chapter, I would remark that the ethics of palliative care centers around medical decision-making that enhances quality of life before death and enables a peaceful and dignified death. Systematizing the ethical analysis of complex clinical cases may help health-care professionals in difficult decision-making (see Box 13.1). A key step to solve complex ethical problems is the explicit reference to ethical principles. Nevertheless, in contemporary biomedical ethics, a variety of different trends coexist (see Box 13.2). Some of these conceptions are complementary, but others are incompatible with each other. Experience with ethical consultations suggests that health professionals sometimes mix up the arguments from different ethical trends without necessarily identifying their incompatibility. Thus, a basic knowledge of the foundations and inner logic of these different ethical conceptions may help professionals to identify the inner resonance or dissonance of these trends with their personal experience about the moral life.

Comparing the framework and content of the so-called four basic principles of principlist bioethics (nonmaleficence, beneficence, autonomy, and justice—see Box 13.3) with the principles of personalism (respect for human life and death, totality and therapeutic proportionality, freedom and responsibility, and sociability/subsidiarity—see Box 13.4), the latter seem to be more in harmony with the philosophy and goals of palliative medicine.

More important than the knowledge of ethical trends and principles are some fundamental moral attitudes and virtues that health-care professionals ought to express in the care for the dying (see Box 13.5). These are the virtues of prudence, compassion, and respect for human dignity even in situations of extreme vulnerability and suffering. They play a central role in orienting health-care professionals in the application of ethical principles to the resolution of complex ethical problems in end-of-life care.

Box 13.5 Fundamental moral attitudes and virtues in the care for the dying

1. Unconditional respect for human life and dignity
2. Acceptance of human vulnerability, finitude, and death
3. Prudence
4. Compassion
5. Truthfulness

Key learning points

Palliative care's ethics centers around decision-making that enhances quality of life during advanced disease and enables a peaceful and dignified death. Systematizing the ethical analysis of complex clinical cases helps in good decision-making (see Box 13.1). The reference to ethical principles is the key to solve ethical problems. Several trends have been proposed in contemporary bioethics (see Box 13.2). Comparing the framework and content of the so-called four basic principles of principlist bioethics (nonmaleficence, beneficence, autonomy, and justice—see Box 13.3) and the principles of personalism (respect for human life and death, totality and therapeutic proportionality, freedom and responsibility, and sociability/subsidiarity—see Box 13.4), the latter seem to be more in harmony with the philosophy and goals of palliative medicine. There are some fundamental moral attitudes and virtues that are essential in the care for the dying (see Box 13.5) and that play a central role in orienting health-care professionals in the application of ethical principles to the resolution of complex ethical problems in end-of-life care.

REFERENCES

1   Calman K. Ethical issues. Introduction. In: Doyle D, Geoffrey H, Cherny N, Calman K, eds. *Oxford Textbook of Palliative Care*, 3th edn. Oxford, U.K.: Oxford University Press, 2004: pp. 55–57.

2   Watson M, Lucas C, Hoy A, Wells J. Ethical issues. In: Watson M, Lucas C, Hoy A, Wells, J, eds. *Oxford Handbook of Palliative Care*, 2nd edn. Oxford, U.K.: Oxford University Press, 2009: pp. 1–16.

3   Taboada P. Ethical issues in palliative care. In: Bruera E, De Lima L, Wenk R, Farr W, eds. *Palliative Care in the Developing World. Principles and Practice*. Houston, TX: IAHPC Press, 2004: pp. 39–51.

4   Taboada P. Desafíos y principios éticos en Medicina Paliativa. In: Palma A, Taboada P, Nervi F, eds. *Medicina Paliativa y cuidados Continuos*. Santiago de Chile: Ediciones UC, 2010: pp. 41–52.

5   Roy D, MacDonald N. Ethical issues in palliative care. In: Doyle D, Hanks GW, MacDonald N, eds. *Oxford Textbook of Palliative Care*, 2nd edn. Oxford, U.K.: Oxford University Press, 1998: pp. 97–138.

6   Taboada P, López R. Análisis de problemas éticos frecuentes en Medicina Paliativa. *Ars Médica*. 2005; 11: 43–60.

7   Lavados M, Serani A. *Etica Clínica. Fundamentos y aplicaciones*. Santiago, Chile: Ediciones Universidad Católica, 1993.

8   Beauchamp T, Childress J. *Principles of Biomedical Ethics*, 5° Edición, New York: Oxford University Press, 2001.

9   Sgreccia E. *Manual de Bioética I Fundamentos y Ética Biomédica*, 4° Edición, Madrid, Spain: Biblioteca de Autores Cristianos, 2009.

10 Taboada P, Bruera E. Ethical decision-making on communication in palliative cancer care: A personalist approach. *Support Cancer Care*. 2001; 9: 335–343.

11 Taboada P. What is appropriate intensive care? In: Cherry M, Engelhardt HT, eds. *Allocating Scarce Medical Resources. Roman Catholic Perspectives*. Washington, DC: Georgetown University Press, 2002. pp. 53–73.

12 Kuuppelomäki M, Lauri S. Ethical dilemmas in the care of patients with incurable cancer. *Nursing Ethics*. 1998; 5(4): 283–293.

13   McClung JA et al. Evaluation of a medical ethics consultation service: Opinions of patients and health care providers. *American Journal of Medicine.* 1996; 100: 456–460.

14   Cottone R, Claus R. Ethical decision-making models: A review of the literature. *Journal of Counseling and Development.* 2000; 78: 275–283.

15   Jones T. Ethical decision making by individuals in organizations: An issue-contingent model. *Academy of Management Review.* 1991; 16 (2): 231–248.

16   Rest J. *Development in Judging Moral Issues.* Minneapolis, MN, EEUU: University of Minnesota Press, 1979.

17   Walker L. The model and the measure: An appraisal of the Minnesota approach to moral development. *Journal of Moral Education.* 2002; 31: 343–367.

18   Jonsen A, Siegler M, Winslade W. *Clinical Ethics: A Practical Approach to Ethical Decisions in Clinical Medicine.* New York, EEUU: McGraw-Hill, Health Professions Division, 1998.

19   Thomasma D, Marshal P. *Clinical Medical Ethics Cases and Readings.* Lanham, MD, EEUU: University Press of America, 1995.

20   Drane J. Métodos de Ética Clínica. *Boletín de la Oficina Sanitaria Panamericana.* 1990; 108: 415–425.

21   Gracia D. Bioética clínica. Bogotá, Colombia. Ed. El Búho, 1998.

22   Anguita V. La presentación de casos clínicos al Comité de Ética Hospitalaria [en línea]. Santiago: Centro de Ética, Universidad Alberto Hurtado [consulted in 2009]. Available online http://etica.uahurtado.cl/documentos/comite_hospitalario.pdf

23   McDevitt R, Giapponi C, Tromley C. A model of ethical decision making: The Integration of process and content. *Journal of Business Ethics.* 2007; 73: 219–229.

24   Whitter N, Williams S, Dewett T. Evaluating ethical decision-making models: A review and application. *Social and Business Review.* 2006; 1: 235–232

25   Janis I, Mann L. Decision making: A psychological analysis of conflict, choice, and commitment. New York, EEUU: The Free Press, 1977.

26   Lo B. *Resolving Ethical Dilemmas: A Guide for Clinicians.* Baltimore, MD, EEUU: Williams & Wilkins, 1995.

27   Lo B, Schroeder S. Frequency of ethical dilemmas in a medical inpatient service. *Archives of Internal Medicine.* 1981; 141: 1062–1064.

28   Gómez-Lobo A. *Los bienes humanos. Ética de la ley natural.* Mediterráneo, Santiago-Chile, 2006.

29   Clouser KD, Gert B. A critique of principlism. *Journal of Medicine and Philosophy.*. 1990; 15: 219–236.

30   Brody B. Philosophical critique of bioethics. *Journal of Medicine and Philosophy.* 1990; 15: 161–178.

31   DeGrazia D. Moving forward in bioethical theory: Theories, cases, and specified principlism. *Journal of Medicine and Philosophy.* 1992; 17: 511–539.

32   Gracia D. *Fundamentos de Bioética.* Madrid, Spain: Eudema, 1989.

33   Gracia D. *Fundamentación y Enseñanza de la Bioética.* Estudios de Bioética 1. Santa Fe de Bogotá: El Buho, 1998.

34   Gracia D. La deliberación moral: el método de la ética clínica. *Med Clin.* 2001; 117: 18–23.

35   Gracia D, Júdez J. Ética en la Práctica Clínica, Madrid, Spain: Triacastela, 2004.

36   Pellegrino E. The metamorphosis of medical ethics. A 30-year retrospective. *Journal of the American Medical Association.* 1993; 269: 9, 1158–1162.

37   Pellegrino E. Toward a virtue-based normative ethics for the health care professions. *Kennedy Institute of Ethics Journal.* 1995; 5: 253–277.

38   Pellegrino E. Virtue-based ethics: Natural and theological. In: Pellegrino ED, Thomasma D, eds. *The Christian Virtues in Medical Practice.* Washington, DC: Georgetown University Press, 1996: pp. 6–28.

39   MacIntyre A. *After Virtue: A Study in Moral Theory.* Notre Dame, France: University of Notre Dame Press, 1984.

40   Levi BH. Four approaches to doing ethics. *The Journal of Medicine and Philosophy.* 1996; *21*,1: 7–39.

41   Sherwin S. Feminist and medical ethics: Two different approaches to contextual ethics. *Hypatia.* 1989; 4(2): 52–72.

42   Waren V: Feminist directions in medical ethics. *Hypatia.* 1989; 4(2): 73–87.

43   León F. *Introducción a la Bioética,* Santiago de Chile: Diploma en Bioética PUC, 2010.

44   Di Pietro M. *Bioética, Educación y familia.* Santiago de Chile: Ediciones Universidad Católica, 2012.

45   Ali NS, Khalil HZ, Yousef W. A comparison of American and Egyptian cancer patient's attitudes and unmet needs. *Cancer Nursing.* 1993; 16: 193–203.

46   Pellegrino ED. Is truth telling to the patient a cultural artifact? *Journal of the American Medical Association.* 1992; 268(13): 1734–1735.

47   Levine C, Zuckermann C. The trouble with families: Toward an ethic of accommodation. *Annals of Internal Medicine.* 1999; 130: 148–152.

48   Spaemann R. Personen. *Der Unterschied zwischen Jemand und Etwas.* Stuttgart, Germany: Klett-Cotta, 1996.

49   Wojtyla K. *The Acting Person.* Dordrecht, the Netherlands: Reidel, 1980.

50   Wojtyla K. *Person and Community. Selected Essays.* [Transl. by Th. Sandok.] New York: Peter Lang, 1993.

51   Hippocratic Corpus. The art. In: Reiser SJ, Dick AJ, Curran WJ, eds. Ethics in medicine: Historical perspectives and contemporary concerns. Cambridge, MA: MIT Press, 1977.

52   Bentham J. An Introduction to the Principles of Morals and Legislation, Edited by Burns JH & Hart HLA, London: The Athlone Press, 1970.

53   Mill, S. On Liberty. In: *Collected Works of John Stuart Mill.* Vol. 18. Robson JM (ed.)Toronto: University of Toronto Press, 1977.

54   Singer P. *Practical Ethics.* 3rd edn. Cambridge, MA: Cambridge University Press, 2011.

55   Singer P. *One World. The Ethics of Globalization,* 2nd edn. Boston, MA: Yale University Press, 2004.

56   Engelhardt HT. *The Foundations of Bioethics,* 2nd edn. Oxford, U.K.: Oxford University Press, 1996.

57   Kant I. *Foundations of the Metaphysics of Morals.* [Transl. Beck, L.) Indianapolis, IN: Bobbs-Merrill Company, 1959.

58   Nagel T. *The View from Nowhere.* New York, 1986. Oxford University Press: Oxford, 1986.

59   UNESCO. Declaration on Bioethics and Human Rights. 2005. [consulted 05.06.2012]. Available online: http://www.unesco.org/new/en/social-and-human-sciences/themes/bioethics/bioethics-and-human-rights

60   Burgos JM. *Introducción al personalismo.* Madrid, Spain: Ediciones Palabra, 2012.

61   Burgos JM. El personalismo. Madrid, Spain: Ediciones Palabra, 2003.

62   Ross WD. *The Right and the Good.* Indianapolis, IN: Hackett Publishing Company, 1988.

63   Hildebrand D. *Moralia.* Regensburg, Germany: Kohlhammer, 1980.

64   World Health Organization. *Cancer Pain Relief and Palliative Care.* Report of a WHO Expert Committee. WHO Technical Report Series, No 804. Geneva, Switzerland: WHO, 1990.

65   Hawryluck LA, Harvey WR, Lemieux-Charles L, Singer PA. Consensus guidelines on analgesia and sedation in dying intensive care unit patients. *BMC Medical Ethics.* 2002; 3: 3. Available at http://www.biomedcentral.com/1472-6939/3/3

66   Cherny N, Radbruch L. European Association for Palliative Care (EAPC) recommended framework for the use of sedation in palliative care. *Palliative Medicine.* 2009; 23(7): 581–593.

67 Cherny N. Palliative sedation. In: Bruera E, Higginson I, Ripamonti C, von Gunten C, eds. *Textbook of Palliative Medicine.* London, U.K.: Hodder Arnold, 2006: pp. 976–987.

68 Claessens P, Menten J, Schotsmans P, Broeckaert B. Palliative sedation: A review of the research literature. *Journal of Pain and Symptom Management.* 2008; 36: 310–333.

69 Anscombe GEM. Medalist's Address: Action, Intention and 'Double Effect'. In: *The Doctrine of Double Effect.* Woodward PA (ed.) Notre Dame: University of Notre Dame Press, 2001, 50–66.

70 Boyle J. Medical ethics and double effect. The case of terminal sedation. *Theoretical Medicine and Bioethics.* 2004; 25: 53–54.

71 Boyle J. Toward understanding double effect. *Ethics.* 1980; 90: 527–538.

72 Cassell EJ, Rich BA. Intractable end-of-life suffering and the ethics of palliative sedation. *Pain Medicine.* 2010; 11: 435–438.

73 Jansen LA. Intractable end-of-life suffering and the ethics of palliative sedation: A commentary on cassell and rich. *Pain Medicine.* 2010; 11: 440–441.

74 Jansen LA, Sulmasy DP. Sedation, alimentation; hydration, and equivocation: Careful conversation about care at the end of life. *Annals of Internal Medicine.* 2002; 136: 845–849.

75 Fohr S. The double effect of pain medication: Separating myth from reality. *Journal of Palliative Medicine.* 1998; 1: 315–328.

76 Regnard C, George R, Grogan E, Harlow T, Hutchison S, Keen J, McGettrick S, Manson C, Murray SA, Robinson V, Stone P, Tallon C. So, farewell then, doctrine of double effect. *British Medical Journal.* 2011; 343 :d4512. doi: 10.1136/bmj.d4512.

77 Cronin D. Conserving human life. In: Smith R, ed. *Conserving Human Life.* Braintree, MA: Pope John Center, 1989: pp. 1–145.

78 Kelly G. *Medico-Moral Problems.* St. Louis, MO: Catholic Hospital Association, 1958.

79 Kelly G. The duty to preserve life. *Theological Studies.* 1951; 12: 550.

80 Wildes K. Conserving *Life and Conserving Means: Lead us not into Temptation.* In: *Philosophy and Medicine 51.* Dordrecht, the Netherlands: Kluwer Academic Publishers, 1995.

81 Calipari M. The principle of proportionality in therapy: Foundations and applications criteria. *NeuroRehabilitation.* 2004; 19 (4): 391–397.

82 Calipari M. Curarse y hacerse curar. Entre el abandono del paciente y el encarnizamiento terapéutico. Buenos Aires, Argentina: Educa, 2007.

83 Taboada P. Ordinary and extraordinary means of preserving life: The teaching of the moral tradition. In: Sgreccia E, Laffitte J. *Alongside the Incurably Sick and the Dying Person: Ethical and Practical Aspects.* Vatican City: Libreria Editrice Vaticana, 2009: pp. 117–142.

84 Sullivan S. The development and nature of the ordinary/extraordinary means distinction in the Roman Catholic tradition. *Bioethics.* 2007; 21 (7):386–397.

85 Guevin B. Ordinary, extraordinary, and artificial means of care. *National Catholic Bioethics Quarterly.* 2005 Autumn; 5 (3): 471–479.

86 Henke D. A history of ordinary and extraordinary means. *National Catholic Bioethics Quarterly.* 2005, Autumn; 5 (3): 555–575.

87 Mullooly J. Ordinary/extraordinary means and euthanasia. *Wisconsin Medical Journal.* 1987; 86 (3): 4–8.

88 Gillon R. Ordinary and extraordinary means. *British Medical Journal.* 1986; 25 (292): 259–261

89 Hickey JV, Fischer SA, Rachels J. "Ordinary" and "extraordinary" vary with the case. *Hastings Center Report.* 1983; 13 (5): 43–44.

90 (a) Devun, M. Extraordinary means in prolonging life. *Journal of the American Medical Association.* 1982; 248 (17): 2180; (b) Editorial: Ordinary and extraordinary means. *J Med Ethics.* 1981, 7 (2): 55–56.

91 Honnefelder L. Quality of life and human dignity: Meaning and limits of prolongation of life. In: Engelhardt HT, Cherry M, eds. *Allocating Scarce Medical Resources: Roman Catholic Perspectives.* Washington, DC: Georgetown University Press, 2002: pp. 140–153.

92 Schotsmans P. Equal care as the best care: A personalist approach. In: Engelhardt HT, Cherry M, eds. *Allocating Scarce Medical Resources: Roman Catholic Perspectives.* Washington, DC: Georgetown University Press, 2002: pp. 125–139.

93 Surbone A. Truth telling to the patient. *Journal of the American Medical Association.* 1992; 268: 1661–1662.

94 Simes RJ, Tattersal MHN, Coates AS et al. Randomized comparison of procedures for obtaining informed consent in clinical trials of treatment for cancer. *British Medical Journal.* 1986; 293: 1065–1068.

95 Fallowfield LJ, Baum M, Maguire GP. Addressing the psychological needs of the conservatively treated cancer patient: Discussion paper. *Journal of the Royal Society of Medicine.* 1987; 80: 995–997.

96 Devlen J, Maguire P, Phillips P, Crowther D. Psychological problems associated with diagnosis and treatment of lymphomas. II. Prospective Study. *British Medical Journal.* 1987; 295: 955–957.

97 Buttow N, Dunn S, Tattersall HN. Denial, misinformation, and the 'assault of truth'. In: Portenoy RK, Bruera E, eds. *Topics in Palliative Care,* Vol. 1. New York: Oxford University Press, 1997: pp. 263–278.

98 Markwell H. End-of-life: A Catholic view. *The Lancet.* 2005, 366: 1132–1135.

99 Saunders C. Foreword. In: Doyle D, Hanks GWC, MacDonald N, eds. *Oxford Textbook of Palliative Medicine.* Oxford, U.K.: Oxford University Press, 1998: pp. v–ix.

100 Blanco LG. *Muerte digna. Consideraciones bioético-jurídicas.* Buenos Aires, Argentina: Editorial Ad Hoc, 1997.

101 Laín Entralgo P. *Antropología Médica.* Barcelona: Salvat, 1958.

102 Kübler-Ross E. *Sobre la muerte y los moribundos.* Barcelona: Grijalbo, 1969.

103 Pieper J. Tod und Unsterblichkeit. In: Pieper J, ed. *Schriften zur philosophischen Anthropologie und Ethik: Grundstrukturen menschlicher Existenz.* Hamburg, Germany: Meiner Verlag, 1997: pp. 280–397.

104 American Medical Association. *Principles of Medical Ethics.* Chicago, IL: AMA, 1981.

105 Dougherty Ch, Purtilo R. Physicians' duty of compassion. *Cambridge Quarterly of Healthcare Ethics.* 1995; 4: 426–433.

106 Crespo M. El valor ético de la afectividad. Estudios de ética fenomenológica. Santiago, Chile: Ediciones Universidad Católica de Chile, 2012.

14

Ethics in the practice of palliative care

JAMES A. TULSKY

Excellent palliative care demands careful attention to diagnostic, prognostic, and therapeutic challenges. The palliative care clinician must demonstrate sensitivity to psychosocial and spiritual concerns and thoughtful, empathic communication with patients and families. Yet, even when these are done with superb skill, patients and providers may still meet ethical dilemmas along the journey through serious illness. Some dilemmas are subtle and, perhaps, not recognized. Others are easily apparent and may lead to conflict. This chapter will discuss several of the more common and vexing ethical issues that arise in the care of patients with advanced serious illness. These include truth telling, when and how to engage in advance care planning, requests for ineffective and unproven treatment, limitation of potentially beneficial treatments, and, finally, consideration of aggressive measures for treating terminal pain and suffering.

The following case raises each of these dilemmas. The case is not unusual and the problems are not profound. Yet, they are extremely common and reflect thorny issues that arise in the real daily practice of palliative care.

> S.K. is a 68-year-old retired, Korean born, university professor who was admitted to the hospital with pneumonia and chest pain. Chest CT revealed a 4 cm lesion obstructing the right upper bronchus and several rib lesions suspicious for malignancy. As the physician approached the patient's hospital room, he was pulled aside by Mr. K's son and daughter who wish to know the result of the CT scan. They request that the doctor not share the results with their father if it means he might have cancer.

DISCLOSURE AND TRUTH TELLING

Truth telling is fundamental to respectful patient care and a necessary component of informed consent. By fully including patients in all decision making, health-care providers honor patient autonomy. Truth telling also engenders trust in physicians and the profession and is desired by most patients. Surveys consistently show that most patients wish to receive as much information as possible,[1,2] perhaps as a way to cope with uncertainty.[3,4] In one typical survey of 2850 British patients, over 1000 of them receiving palliative care, nearly 90% stated they would like to be told most or all information about their illness.[5] Yet, patients also desire an individualized approach to receiving bad news and discussing prognosis that does not necessarily share all of the information at one time or in the same way.[6] In most Western societies, common practice is to answer patients' questions honestly and to share relevant information about their medical condition, prognosis, and therapeutic options, yet significant variation exists worldwide.[7,8]

Most patients prefer to participate in decision making but to receive a physician's advice regarding recommended options. Physicians must find the balance between conveying the ambiguity that clouds medical practice and helping patients find the best options for them. There are many good arguments for giving full information to patients.[5] Information allows patients to plan their futures and to make decisions. Lack of information may heighten their fear and anxiety, as the truth is often not as bad as what might be imagined, and they may lose the opportunity to achieve important goals prior to death. In addition, the secrecy and collusion necessary to withhold information may present a significant challenge to providers and families.

Nevertheless, even the most forthright physicians raise questions about the limits of disclosure. When patients don't ask, how much should health-care providers tell? For example, when starting a new medication, doctors rarely describe all of the possible side effects. They judge that this would not be helpful and, instead, mention only the most common, most serious, or most relevant side effects. Disclosure of serious diagnoses and their repercussions appears to be handled similarly. Physicians do not always share prognosis, and when they do, they tend to bias optimistically.[9]

Although withholding information or providing an overly optimistic assessment of illness may be deceptive, legitimate reasons for the practice also exist. Patients may find it too difficult to hear bad news or may consciously defer all decision making to their families. While such perspectives may challenge notions of patient autonomy, in fact, autonomy dictates that patients also have the right to not hear or to defer responsibility to others.

Cultural issues also play a role. In many societies, decision making is localized in the family and individual autonomy is not recognized. Blackhall surveyed members of four distinct ethnic groups in the United States and found widely disparate perspectives on whether a patient should be told a diagnosis of metastatic cancer. Only 47% of first-generation Korean Americans and 65% of first-generation Mexican Americans believed that patients should be told, whereas European Americans (87%) and African Americans (88%) were more likely to want to hear this news directly themselves.[10] In some cultures, the delivery of bad news may determine how patients confront illness and being told the wrong information can cause harm. For example, in Navajo society, the concept of *hozho* or living in beauty may be considered to be violated by statements that are viewed as negative.[11] Such observations imply that, in different cultures, personal autonomy carries different levels of importance. That said, patients' preferences are not simply a reflection of their ethnic background. In our case, we might expect that Mr. K has an approximately 50% likelihood of wanting the physician to honor his family's request and to tell the news only to them. However, there exists an equal likelihood that he would want to be told the news himself, and there are no identifiable predictors of such preferences.

In this context, some have argued for *necessary collusion*, or the need to delay disclosure of some specific prognostic information from patients to help maintain their hope.[12] This perspective does not advocate withholding information that is requested, but rather allowing the information to unfold only as requested or needed by the patient in a *measured series of forecasts*. This perspective appears to strike a common ground that protects those patients who do not want too much information. However, it also risks withholding information from those that would want it and makes assumptions about patients' needs or preferences that cannot be ascertained simply.

Therefore, a better resolution may be for the clinician to ask patients directly, "How much information are you interested in hearing about your illness?" Patients can declare clearly what they wish to hear and patients will receive only the amount of information they desire. Rather than waiting until the moment that more bad news presents itself, this question is well worth asking early in the care of any patient with serious illness and certainly at the time of conducting diagnostic and prognostic tests.

ADVANCE CARE PLANNING

> *Mr. K. was treated for his pneumonia and biopsy revealed non-small cell lung cancer, metastatic to rib. He received radiation to his lung and ribs and felt much better. He was seen six weeks later in his doctor's office, and the physician wonders whether this would be a good opportunity to begin advance care planning.*

Advance care planning is the process by which patients, together with their families and health-care providers, consider their values and goals and articulate preferences for future care.[13] Written advance directives formalize these preferences and include living wills or other statements of patient preferences, as well as durable powers of attorney for health care, which name health-care proxies. Do-not-attempt resuscitation (DNAR or DNR) orders are written by physicians to operationalize one specific set of preferences articulated by patients and their proxies. Advance care planning has been promoted widely in the United States and other countries, particularly in response to high-profile cases in which patients in a vegetative state have been kept alive despite a presumption that such treatment violated their preferences.[14]

Although it could refer simply to signing a form in a lawyer's or doctor's office, ideally, advance care planning creates an opportunity for patients to explore their own values, beliefs, and attitudes regarding quality of life and medical interventions, particularly as they think about the end of their lives. Patients may speak with loved ones, physicians, spiritual advisers, and others during the process. This reflective work can help patients make important decisions about issues that may come up even when they still have the capacity to make decisions. When a patient loses decision-making capacity, physicians and loved ones who have been involved in the advance care planning process may feel that they know the patient's goals and values better. This allows them to make medical decisions that are likely to be consistent with the patient's values and preferences.

Advance care planning accomplishes a variety of goals for patients and families.[15] First, patients may use the process to clarify their own values and to consider how these affect their feelings about care at the end of life. Second, patients can learn more about what they can expect as they face the end of life and about various options for life-sustaining treatment and palliative care. Third, they can gain a sense of control over their medical care and their future, obtaining reassurance that they will die in a manner that is consistent with their preferences. Finally, patients may increase the probability that loved ones and health-care providers will make decisions in accordance with their values and goals.

Advance care planning, or the process of naming a surrogate and discussing what is important in one's life given the presence of serious illness, may serve other goals, not directly related to medical treatments.[15] Patients may wish to relieve loved ones of the burden of decision making and to protect loved ones from having to watch a drawn-out dying process. Patients also may use the process to prepare themselves for death. Advance care planning may help one reflect more deeply about one's life, its meaning, and its goals. Patients may reflect on relationships with loved ones, *unfinished business*, and fears about future disability and loss of independence.

When the patient's illness has progressed to its final stages, health-care providers can use the groundwork from these earlier discussions to make specific plans about what is to be done when the inevitable worsening occurs. Among other things, the patient and the health-care providers can decide the following: Should an ambulance be called? Should the patient come to the hospital? Which life-prolonging treatments should be employed and which should be forgone?

Are there particular treatments aimed at symptomatic relief that should be employed?

Health-care providers have their own reasons for wanting to engage their patients in advance care planning.[15] First, clinicians may use these discussions to reassure patients that their wishes will be respected. This can enhance a sense of trust. Second, clinicians may hope that advance directives will help to decrease conflict among family members and between family members and the health-care team when the patient is seriously ill. Finally, they may hope that advance directives will assist them in making difficult decisions when the patient has lost decision-making capacity.

Physicians are often reluctant to raise the subject with their patients and often do so later than patients may desire.[16] They may be under time constraints. They may have never been trained to discuss this issue and are not sure how to introduce the topic. They may be worried that they will give patients the impression that they are *giving up* on them or that they think they will die soon. If they have focused in past discussions on interventions rather than patient values and goals, they may have found these discussions frustrating and unhelpful.

Time constraints are difficult to overcome. Physicians could dedicate visits to discussing advance directives; but insurance companies may not pay for such a visit, and many patients may not wish to make a separate trip to the doctor for this purpose. The use of booklets and other tools to introduce the concepts involved in advance care planning may help physicians efficiently use their time to answer specific questions patients may have and to guide patients through the process.[17,18] Enlisting nurses and social workers to help patients with the advance care planning process may also help. Finally, recent studies have demonstrated that showing videos about CPR, feeding tubes, and other interventions to patients prior to advance care planning discussions makes them significantly more likely to select less aggressive treatment options at the end of life.[19]

Although physicians are often worried that patients will be put off by a discussion about advance care plans, surveys show that most patients want to discuss these issues, early in the course of their disease, and that they think that the doctor should bring up the topic. Nevertheless, there will be some patients who are not ready to discuss advance directives. Health-care providers must be sensitive to these patients. Advance care planning is a process that should be offered to patients, not forced upon them.

The root cause of much of physicians' reluctance stems from lack of training in how to have these discussions. With training, physicians can feel more comfortable having these discussions, can learn how to deal with patients' emotional responses, and can have effective discussions that the physician will find truly helpful in caring for patients.[20,21]

Unfortunately, the impact of advance directives on actual resuscitation events remains unclear, with most of the older literature showing minimal effect.[22–29] This may be due to several causes. Discussions often do not occur or are not recorded in ways that may have a lasting effect.[30] Some of the barriers to successful implementation have been procedural when, for example, documents are not available when needed. More importantly, problems arise with deciding in advance about specific interventions,[31] the adequacy of communication,[32] the willingness of health-care providers to follow patient preferences,[27,30] and patient and family misunderstandings about the process. That said, a recent well-done randomized controlled trial of facilitated advance care planning led to a significantly higher rate of known and followed end-of-life care wishes for intervention group patients, with decreased anxiety, stress, and depression among their family members.[33] Furthermore, a new mechanism, often referred to as Physician Orders for Life-Sustaining Treatment (POLST) has been initiated in many U.S. states as a way of ensuring that patient preferences are enacted in practice.[34] POLST documents are actual medical orders, respected by emergency medical services and local health-care institutions, which implement a scope of treatment for a particular patient. Initial studies in small well-defined communities have shown promise.

Written advance directives are most likely to be useful when there is disagreement within a family, conflict between the family and health-care team, or when the patient assigns a non-traditional family member (e.g., friend or same-sex partner) as the surrogate. If the patient's preferences are known and understood by the family and team through an oral advance directive, in most states, the written document is superfluous.

Entering these conversations may feel awkward, but if they are viewed as conversations about hopes, fears, and goals rather than decisions for specific preferences, they may be easier to engage. For example, Mr. K. could be asked how he has been doing since his hospitalization. What was it like to learn of his diagnosis, and how does this make him feel about the future? The clinician can empathize with his emotions and ask about specific concerns he has looking forward. By careful exploration of patients' values, health-care providers can help patients discover their preferences. This expanded view of advance care planning allows people to think about their mortality and legacy. From such discussions, health-care providers can help patients consider specifically whether there are certain treatments that they might wish to forgo and to think about the circumstances under which they might forgo them.

REQUESTS FOR UNPROVEN OR INEFFECTIVE TREATMENT

Mr. K. chooses to undergo chemotherapy and receives carboplatin and gemcitabine. However, he experiences a significant decline in his renal function and his tumor progresses. He then tries pemetrexed but is hospitalized with neutropenia and fever and again has no response. Wishing to try something else, he is given erlotinib, but could not tolerate the diarrhea. At this point, his oncologist tells him that there are no more proven treatments left and that he would not suggest more treatment given his age and poor responses to previous agents. Mr. K asks "isn't there anymore chemotherapy? What about an experimental drug or laetrile?"

Desperate patients seek desperate measures. Mr. K. has exhausted the proven treatments for his cancer and, even though he has experienced significant side effects from his treatment, he does not want to die and is willing to consider other options. Such options generally fall into two categories, clinical trials of promising, but unproven therapies and alternative treatments generally considered ineffective by the mainstream medical community.

Phase I clinical trials are conducted to ascertain the safety of experimental therapies prior to testing for efficacy. Such studies are not meant to be therapeutic and, historically, approximately 5% of patients enrolled in such trials cancer agents achieve a response.[35,36] Nevertheless, most patients enroll with the intent of achieving therapeutic benefit.[37,38] Some have questioned whether this represents a failure of informed consent. Increasingly, it is recognized that patients choosing to enroll in phase I trials may have different values than those who do not enroll, and although they understand the prognostic data presented to them, they maintain a more optimistic perspective and believe that they will be the ones to gain benefit.[39,40] In fact, many now argue that hospice care and phase I trials ought to coexist simultaneously.[41,42]

In contrast, requests for alternative, ineffective treatments are viewed differently. While some may fall into a similar category as the agents used in established clinical trials, the majority are far less accepted and sometimes considered quackery. Although belief systems vary among patients and clinicians, the primary issue here is one of informed consent and trying to be sure that patients do not encounter more harm than good in reaching out to such treatments.

When receiving requests for unproven or ineffective therapy, physicians should counsel patients openly and not hesitate to give an opinion based upon their knowledge of the intervention and the patient's values. It is keenly important to acknowledge the patient's affect and recognize that requests for unproven or ineffective treatments are frequent proxies for patient distress and difficulty coping with impending death. A common pitfall is responding to such distress by offering more therapy rather than engaging the patient's emotional state. Similarly, others may tell patients that "we'll wait until you're stronger and can take the chemo then," knowing fully well that the patient will never meet such a goal. A more productive technique to use in this situation is the *wish* statement.[43] By letting patients know that "I wish I had more effective treatment to offer you," clinicians can both align themselves with patients, while implicitly acknowledging that this goal cannot be met.

In these settings, clinicians struggle to promote hope in the patient with advanced disease and to support a positive outlook.[1] Incorrectly, they fear that discussing death may distress patients.[9,44–47] As a result, doctors frequently convey overly optimistic prognoses or do not give this information at all.[48] Fearing the loss of hope, patients frequently cope by expressing denial and may be unwilling to hear what is said.[49] Not unexpectedly, patients with more optimistic assessments of their own prognosis are more likely to choose aggressive therapies at the end of life.[50,51] Yet, even more important, patients who have had no conversation about end-of-life issues at all are most likely to receive aggressive interventions prior to death.[52]

Physicians should recognize that it is not their job to *correct* the patient's hope for an unrealistic outcome.[53] Hope is the frame within which patients construct their future.[54] It may be a desire for a particular outcome or it may be, more broadly, trust or reliance. The key question is whether the patients' construction of hope is interfering with appropriate planning and behavior. Clinicians, at their best, can provide an empathic, reflective presence that will help patients to marshal and draw strength from their existing resources. Together, the physician and the patient can "hope for the best but prepare for the worst."[55] Helping the patient and family manage their hope and their resources in a realistic way may leave the family in the best possible shape after their loss.

LIMITATION OF TREATMENT

> Mr. K. became progressively more debilitated. He decided not to pursue unproven therapies and accepted a palliative approach to care, including a DNR order. He was spending an increasing percentage of his time in bed when he developed a fever and cough and stopped eating and drinking. His family wondered whether he was again suffering pneumonia and asked if he can receive antibiotics. In addition, they questioned whether a feeding tube should be placed or if an intravenous (IV) would be helpful.

Even when patients have elected to pursue a palliative approach to care, they and their care providers may struggle over the exact limitations of treatment. They may wonder whether treatments such as feeding tubes and IV fluids provide comfort and if their trade-off in treatment burden is worthwhile. Antibiotics are particularly interesting because they tend to be among the least refused of medical interventions.[56,57] Their use is high even in palliative care units, where they are administered to as many as 30%–40% of patients with comfort care plans.[58–60] The literature suggests that antibiotics can play a role in symptom relief, yet must be balanced against the burdens of needles, side effects, and cost.[58,59] In the case of Mr. K., pneumonia may be his terminal event, with or without the use of antibiotics. He and his family will need to decide whether IV antibiotics are worth a trip to the hospital or even whether it's worth trying to administer them at home intramuscularly or orally. His symptoms of cough and fever can be managed with antitussives and antipyretics—it is not clear if adding another few days or weeks to his life will meet his goals at this point. Such decisions become highly individualized with no correct answers.

Tube feeding has not shown a significant benefit for most patients with terminal illness.[61] Therefore, there is less controversy on medical grounds. In contrast, considerable debate exists as to the benefits of artificial hydration. Recent evidence suggests that subcutaneous hydration can alleviate common symptoms of terminal illness with minimal burden.[62]

Guidelines established by the European Association for Palliative Care recommend a three-step approach.[63] Step I includes assessing a variety of clinical factors, Step II involves an assessment of pros and cons to establish a well-defined goal of therapy and end point, and Step III requires periodic reevaluation of the decision.

OPTIONS OF LAST RESORT

> Mr. K's illness progressed and he was bedbound with fluctuating consciousness. He required large quantities of opioids for pain and dyspnea. The patient's daughter was concerned that the medication may hasten his death and was resisting the hospice nurse's suggestion to increase it further. Meanwhile, the son felt that his father had completed all he needed to do and was just lingering uncomfortably. He wanted to know how much longer he will continue to live and whether there was anything that can be done to stop the waiting.

One of the major barriers to aggressive symptom management at the end of life is the fear of hastening death. Many clinicians and family members are unsure where pain control stops and euthanasia begins. Moral clarity on these issues is critically important to ensure that no inappropriate boundaries are overridden and to give reassurance to ethical providers who are working hard to take the best care of patients.[64]

In situations such as Mr. K.'s, clinicians generally rely on the principle of double effect to justify their actions. This centuries-old ethical framework allows one to perform beneficial actions with potentially harmful consequences as long as four requirements are met.[65] The act itself must not be immoral; it must be undertaken only with the intention of achieving the possible good effect, without intending the possible bad effect even though it may be foreseen; it does not bring about the possible good effect by means of the possible bad effect; and, lastly, it is undertaken for a proportionately grave reason. Or, stated otherwise, the good effect must outweigh the bad effect. The principle of double effect has been very useful in medical practice generally and palliative care in particular because it helps many physicians overcome barriers to prescribing adequate pain relief and it provides a legal defense for opioid prescriptions at the end of life.[66] At the same time, it has also allowed the community to continue to reinforce prohibitions against directly and intentionally causing death.

Several problems exist with double effect.[67] It can be difficult to distinguish between intended and foreseen consequences, particularly regarding death at the end of life. Conscientious clinicians not sure of their actions may be tormented by the outcome. Furthermore, the principle of double effect prioritizes the absolute prohibition against patient death over patient autonomy. Advocates applaud the principle for exactly this reason. Yet those who wish to allow greater flexibility for ending patient suffering at the end of life find double effect to be

constraining. Finally, as discussed in the preceding chapter, because the skilled titration of opioids ought not increase the risk of death, some argue that double effect is not really a relevant consideration in these cases.[68] Others argue that when someone is known to be dying and the focus of care is a good dying, a somewhat shortened time to death is not a *bad effect*, and double effect doesn't hold.[69]

One practice, termed terminal or palliative sedation, links two acceptable acts in a controversial way. Patients are deeply sedated (perhaps double effect), yet receive no hydration or nutrition (withdrawal of life-sustaining therapy). This intervention is intended for dying patients with unbearable symptoms unresponsive to other therapies.[70] In the Netherlands, and perhaps elsewhere, the practice precedes a substantial number of deaths.[71] In the United States and most other countries, it still remains fairly rare. Because death is certain if sedation is not withdrawn, some people view this as a form of euthanasia, particularly those who believe in an absolute prohibition of hastening death.[72] Whatever the specific ethical justifications, there is a growing consensus in favor of the practice under appropriate circumstances, and it is legal in the United States and many other countries. Concerns remain about potential abuses,[73] yet the necessity of a team provides some safeguards.[74]

With regard to hastening death, other practices exist, and a detailed discussion of their history, merits, and risks is beyond the scope of this chapter. Briefly, these would include voluntary cessation of eating and drinking, assisted suicide, and euthanasia. Any competent patient who is approaching the end of life and confronting overwhelming suffering may choose to voluntarily stop eating and drinking.[64] This difficult and potentially unpleasant option takes tremendous conviction.[75] Nevertheless, some take advantage of this because it is legal in most jurisdictions and there is a growing ethical consensus in support of the practice. Furthermore, it does not require physician involvement, which removes a significant barrier.

In contrast to voluntarily stopping eating and drinking, which has received relatively little attention, physician-assisted suicide has been at the center of considerable controversy, including decisions by the U.S. Supreme Court. In the United States and many European nations, there is a majority public support for this practice,[76-78] yet considerable controversy exists over its appropriateness.[79,80] At the time of this writing, the practice is legal in three U.S. states, and in at least two European nations, although it is tacitly approved in others. The practice requires a competent patient, which is perceived as a safeguard to abuse, and somewhat distances the agency of physicians, which many prefer.

Euthanasia is the practice whereby someone other than the patient, usually a physician, administers a lethal agent to directly hasten a death. This practice is perceived differently in different countries.[81] In the United States, euthanasia is distinguished from physician-assisted suicide and no ethical consensus exists.[76] It is illegal everywhere and likely to be prosecuted. Whereas, in the Netherlands, Belgium, and some other countries, the public response to the two practices is fairly similar and more accepting. From a practical perspective, euthanasia does not require a competent patient, which has raised concerns about safeguards to abuses of vulnerable patients.[82]

The debate about assisted dying has played out in the press, courts, and legislatures. Yet, in the end, individual patients, families, and health-care providers confront real-life situations that must be resolved within the constraints of individual moral values and the law. As Mr. K lays dying, his daughter may be reassured knowing that aggressive use of opioids is entirely within the accepted standard of care as the intent is focused on controlling his pain and other symptoms. The son's position is also understandable. It is very difficult to sit at such a vigil and wait for a patient to die. In most settings, directly hastening his father's death will not be an option. Nevertheless, nothing more need to be done to extend his father's life, such as giving nutrition, hydration, or antibiotics. All efforts should be focused on the patient's comfort and helping the family find meaning during these last moments.

CONCLUSION

Ethical challenges lie in the paths of all patients, families, and health-care providers dealing with a life-limiting illness. At different points of an illness, these may range from truth telling to requests for assisted dying. Health-care providers must enter into such issues without assumptions about patient preferences and with an open mind to learn the underlying issues. Careful listening, clear thinking about the ethical issues at stake, and empathic communication will help resolve many such dilemmas.

Key learning points

- Truth telling engenders trust and is a central aspect of good palliative care, yet patients vary considerably in their preferences for information.

- Patients should be asked how much information they wish to receive early in the course of an illness so that their preferences can be known and honored.

- Advance care planning can serve multiple goals for patients, families, and health-care providers in addition to communicating preferences for future treatment.

- Patients value discussions of advance care planning, yet clinicians must initiate them.

- Recognize that requests for unproven or ineffective therapies may reflect patient distress and respond accordingly to their emotional state, not just the underlying question.

- When considering limiting therapies such as antibiotics and artificial nutrition or hydration, patients, families, and providers should assess clinical factors and the pros and cons of therapy and make a plan with well-defined end points.

REFERENCES

1 Butow PN, Dowsett S, Hagerty R, Tattersall MH. Communicating prognosis to patients with metastatic disease: What do they really want to know? *Support Care Cancer.* 2002; **10**(2): 161–168.
2 Ende J, Kazis L, Ash A, Moskowitz MA. Measuring patients' desire for autonomy: Decision making and information-seeking preferences among medical patients. *J Gen Intern Med.* 1989; **4**(1): 23–30.
3 Bruera E, Sweeney C, Calder K, Palmer L, Benisch-Tolley S. Patient preferences versus physician perceptions of treatment decisions in cancer care. *J Clin Oncol.* 2001; **19**(11): 2883–2885.
4 Heyland DK, Tranmer J, O'Callaghan CJ, Gafni A. The seriously ill hospitalized patient: Preferred role in end-of-life decision making? *J Crit Care.* 2003; **18**(1): 3–10.
5 Fallowfield LJ, Jenkins VA, Beveridge HA. Truth may hurt but deceit hurts more: Communication in palliative care. *Palliat Med.* 2002; **16**(4): 297–303.
6 Hagerty RG, Butow PN, Ellis PM, Lobb EA, Pendlebury SC, Leighl N et al. Communicating with realism and hope: Incurable cancer patients' views on the disclosure of prognosis. *J Clin Oncol.* 2005; **23**(6): 1278–1288.
7 Bruera E, Neumann CM, Mazzocato C, Stiefel F, Sala R. Attitudes and beliefs of palliative care physicians regarding communication with terminally ill cancer patients. *Palliat Med.* 2000; **14**(4): 287–298.
8 Peretti-Watel P, Bendiane MK, Obadia Y, Lapiana JM, Galinier A, Pegliasco H et al. Disclosure of prognosis to terminally ill patients: Attitudes and practices among French physicians. *J Palliat Med.* 2005; **8**(2): 280–290.
◆ 9 Christakis NA. *Death Foretold: Prophecy and Prognosis in Medical Care.* Chicago, IL: University of Chicago Press; 2000.
● 10 Blackhall LJ, Murphy ST, Frank G, Michel V, Azen S. Ethnicity and attitudes toward patient autonomy. *JAMA.* 1995; **274**(10): 820–825.
● 11 Carrese JA, Rhodes LA. Western bioethics on the Navajo reservation. Benefit or harm? *JAMA.* 1995; **274**(10): 826–829.
12 Helft PR. Necessary collusion: Prognostic communication with advanced cancer patients. *J Clin Oncol.* 2005; **23**(13): 3146–3150.
◆ 13 Sudore RL, Fried TR. Redefining the "planning" in advance care planning: Preparing for end-of-life decision making. *Ann Intern Med.* 2010; **153**(4): 256–261.
14 Lo B, Steinbrook R. Beyond the Cruzan case: The U.S. Supreme Court and medical practice. *Ann Intern Med.* 1991; **114**(10): 895–901.
15 Singer PA, Martin DK, Lavery JV, Thiel EC, Kelner M, Mendelssohn DC. Reconceptualizing advance care planning from the patient's perspective. *Arch Intern Med.* 1998; **158**(8): 879–884.
16 Johnston SC, Pfeifer MP, McNutt R. The discussion about advance directives. Patient and physician opinions regarding when and how it should be conducted. End of Life Study Group. *Arch Intern Med.* 1995; **155**(10): 1025–1030.
● 17 Hammes BJ, Rooney BL, Gundrum JD. A comparative, retrospective, observational study of the prevalence, availability, and specificity of advance care plans in a county that implemented an advance care planning microsystem. *J Am Geriatr Soc.* 2010; **58**(7): 1249–1255.
18 Au DH, Udris EM, Engelberg RA, Diehr PH, Bryson CL, Reinke LF et al. A randomized trial to improve communication about end-of-life care among patients with COPD. *Chest.* 2012; **141**(3): 726–735.
19 Volandes AE, Paasche-Orlow MK, Mitchell SL, El-Jawahri A, Davis AD, Barry MJ et al. Randomized controlled trial of a video decision support tool for cardiopulmonary resuscitation decision making in advanced cancer. *J Clin Oncol.* 2013; **31**(3): 380–386.

20 Back AL, Arnold RM, Baile WF, Fryer-Edwards KA, Alexander SC, Barley GE et al. Efficacy of communication skills training for giving bad news and discussing transitions to palliative care. *Arch Intern Med*. 2007; **167**(5): 453–460.

21 Fallowfield L, Jenkins V, Farewell V, Saul J, Duffy A, Eves R. Efficacy of a Cancer Research UK communication skills training model for oncologists: A randomised controlled trial. *Lancet*. 2002; **359**(9307): 650–656.

22 Baker DW, Einstadter D, Husak S, Cebul RD. Changes in the use of do-not-resuscitate orders after implementation of the Patient Self-Determination Act. *J Gen Intern Med*. 2003; **18**(5): 343–349.

23 Yates JL, Glick HR. The failed Patient Self-Determination Act and policy alternatives for the right to die. *J Aging Soc Policy*. 1997; **9**(4): 29–50.

● 24 Danis M, Southerland LI, Garrett JM, Smith JL, Hielema F, Pickard CG et al. A prospective study of advance directives for life-sustaining care. *N Engl J Med*. 1991; **324**(13): 882–888.

25 Ditto PH, Danks JH, Smucker WD, Bookwala J, Coppola KM, Dresser R et al. Advance directives as acts of communication: A randomized controlled trial. *Arch Intern Med*. 2001; **161**(3): 421–430.

◆ 26 Hanson L, Tulsky J, Danis M. Can clinical interventions change care at the end of life? *Ann Int Med*. 1997; **126**(5): 381–388.

● 27 SUPPORT Principal Investigators. A controlled trial to improve care for seriously ill hospitalized patients. The study to understand prognoses and preferences for outcomes and risks of treatments (SUPPORT). *JAMA*. 1995; **274**(20): 1591–1598.

28 Teno J, Lynn J, Wenger N, Phillips RS, Murphy DP, Connors AF, Jr. et al. Advance directives for seriously ill hospitalized patients: Effectiveness with the patient self-determination act and the SUPPORT intervention. SUPPORT Investigators. Study to Understand Prognoses and Preferences for Outcomes and Risks of Treatment. *J Am Geriatr Soc*. 1997; **45**(4): 500–507.

29 Molloy DW, Guyatt GH, Russo R, Goeree R, O'Brien BJ, Bedard M et al. Systematic implementation of an advance directive program in nursing homes: A randomized controlled trial. *JAMA*. 2000; **283**(11): 1437–1444.

30 Hofmann JC, Wenger NS, Davis RB, Teno J, Connors AF, Jr., Desbiens N et al. Patient preferences for communication with physicians about end-of-life decisions. SUPPORT Investigators. Study to Understand Prognoses and Preference for Outcomes and Risks of Treatment. *Ann Intern Med*. 1997; **127**(1): 1–12.

31 Brett AS. Limitations of listing specific medical interventions in advance directives. *JAMA*. 1991; **266**(6): 825–828.

● 32 Tulsky JA, Fischer GS, Rose MR, Arnold RM. Opening the black box: How do physicians communicate about advance directives? *Ann Intern Med*. 1998; **129**(6): 441–449.

33 Detering KM, Hancock AD, Reade MC, Silvester W. The impact of advance care planning on end of life care in elderly patients: Randomised controlled trial. *BMJ*. 2010; **340**: c1345.

● 34 Hickman SE, Nelson CA, Perrin NA, Moss AH, Hammes BJ, Tolle SW. A comparison of methods to communicate treatment preferences in nursing facilities: Traditional practices versus the physician orders for life-sustaining treatment program. *J Am Geriatr Soc*. 2010; **58**(7): 1241–1248.

35 Smith TL, Lee JJ, Kantarjian HM, Legha SS, Raber MN. Design and results of phase I cancer clinical trials: Three-year experience at M.D. Anderson Cancer Center. *J Clin Oncol*. 1996; **14**(1): 287–295.

36 Von Hoff DD, Turner J. Response rates, duration of response, and dose response effects in phase I studies of antineoplastics. *Invest New Drugs*. 1991; **9**(1): 115–122.

37 Daugherty C, Ratain MJ, Grochowski E, Stocking C, Kodish E, Mick R et al. Perceptions of cancer patients and their physicians involved in phase I trials. *J Clin Oncol*. 1995; **13**(5): 1062–1072.

38 Meropol NJ, Weinfurt KP, Burnett CB, Balshem A, Benson AB, 3rd, Castel L et al. Perceptions of patients and physicians regarding phase I cancer clinical trials: Implications for physician-patient communication. *J Clin Oncol*. 2003; **21**(13): 2589–2596.

39 Weinfurt KP, Sulmasy DP, Schulman KA, Meropol NJ. Patient expectations of benefit from phase I clinical trials: Linguistic considerations in diagnosing a therapeutic misconception. *Theor Med Bioeth*. 2003; **24**(4): 329–344.

◆ 40 Agrawal M, Emanuel EJ. Ethics of phase 1 oncology studies: Reexamining the arguments and data. *JAMA*. 2003; **290**(8): 1075–1082.

41 Byock I, Miles SH. Hospice benefits and phase I cancer trials. *Ann Intern Med*. 2003; **138**(4): 335–337.

42 Casarett DJ, Karlawish JH, Henry MI, Hirschman KB. Must patients with advanced cancer choose between a Phase I trial and hospice? *Cancer*. 2002; **95**(7): 1601–1604.

43 Quill TE, Arnold RM, Platt F. "I wish things were different": Expressing wishes in response to loss, futility, and unrealistic hopes. *Ann Intern Med*. 2001; **135**(7): 551–555.

44 Delvecchio MJ, Good BJ, Schaffer C, Lind SE. American oncology and the discourse on hope. *Cult Med Psychiatry*. 1990; **14**(1): 59–79.

45 Herth K. Fostering hope in terminally-ill people. *J Adv Nurs*. 1990; **15**(11): 1250–1259.

46 Koopmeiners L, Post-White J, Gutknecht S, Ceronsky C, Nickelson K, Drew D et al. How healthcare professionals contribute to hope in patients with cancer. *Oncol Nurs Forum*. 1997; **24**(9): 1507–1513.

47 Wenrich MD, Curtis JR, Shannon SE, Carline JD, Ambrozy DM, Ramsey PG. Communicating with dying patients within the spectrum of medical care from terminal diagnosis to death. *Arch Intern Med*. 2001; **161**(6): 868–874.

● 48 Lamont EB, Christakis NA. Prognostic disclosure to patients with cancer near the end of life. *Ann Intern Med*. 2001; **134**(12): 1096–1105.

49 Kreitler S. Denial in cancer patients. *Cancer Invest*. 1999; **17**(7): 514–534.

● 50 Murphy DJ, Burrows D, Santilli S, Kemp AW, Tenner S, Kreling B et al. The influence of the probability of survival on patients' preferences regarding cardiopulmonary resuscitation. *N Engl J Med*. 1994; **330**(8): 545–549.

● 51 Weeks JC, Cook EF, O'Day SJ, Peterson LM, Wenger N, Reding D et al. Relationship between cancer patients' predictions of prognosis and their treatment preferences. *JAMA*. 1998; **279**(21): 1709–1714.

● 52 Wright AA, Zhang B, Ray A, Mack JW, Trice E, Balboni T et al. Associations between end-of-life discussions, patient mental health, medical care near death, and caregiver bereavement adjustment. *JAMA*. 2008; **300**(14): 1665–1673.

53 Tulsky JA. Hope and hubris. *J Palliat Med*. 2002; **5**(3): 339–341.

◆ 54 Tulsky JA. Beyond advance directives: Importance of communication skills at the end of life. *JAMA*. 2005; **294**(3): 359–365.

55 Back AL, Arnold RM, Quill TE. Hope for the best, and prepare for the worst. *Ann Intern Med*. 2003; **138**(5): 439–443.

56 Ahronheim JC, Morrison RS, Baskin SA, Morris J, Meier DE. Treatment of the dying in the acute care hospital. Advanced dementia and metastatic cancer. *Arch Intern Med*. 1996; **156**(18): 2094–2100.

57 Ghusn HF, Teasdale TA, Skelly JR. Limiting treatment in nursing homes: Knowledge and attitudes of nursing home medical directors. *J Am Geriatr Soc*. 1995; **43**(10): 1131–1134.

58 Chen LK, Chou YC, Hsu PS, Tsai ST, Hwang SJ, Wu BY et al. Antibiotic prescription for fever episodes in hospice patients. *Support Care Cancer*. 2002; **10**(7): 538–541.

59 Clayton J, Fardell B, Hutton-Potts J, Webb D, Chye R. Parenteral antibiotics in a palliative care unit: Prospective analysis of current practice. *Palliat Med*. 2003; **17**(1): 44–48.

60 Pereira J, Watanabe S, Wolch G. A retrospective review of the frequency of infections and patterns of antibiotic utilization on a palliative care unit. *J Pain Symptom Manage*. 1998; **16**(6): 374–381.

61 Teno JM, Gozalo PL, Mitchell SL, Kuo S, Rhodes RL, Bynum JP et al. Does feeding tube insertion and its timing improve survival? *J Am Geriatr Soc*. 2012; **60**(10): 1918–1921.

62 Bruera E, Sala R, Rico MA, Moyano J, Centeno C, Willey J et al. Effects of parenteral hydration in terminally ill cancer patients: A preliminary study. *J Clin Oncol*. 2005; **23**(10): 2366–2371.

✳ 63 Bozzetti F, Amadori D, Bruera E, Cozzaglio L, Corli O, Filiberti A et al. Guidelines on artificial nutrition versus hydration in terminal cancer patients. European Association for Palliative Care. *Nutrition*. 1996; **12**(3): 163–167.

◆ 64 Quill TE, Lo B, Brock DW. Palliative options of last resort: A comparison of voluntarily stopping eating and drinking, terminal sedation, physician-assisted suicide, and voluntary active euthanasia. *JAMA*. 1997; **278**(23): 2099–2104.

65 Sulmasy DP, Pellegrino ED. The rule of double effect: Clearing up the double talk. *Arch Intern Med*. 1999; **159**(6): 545–50.

66 Meisel A, Snyder L, Quill T, American College of Physicians—American Society of Internal Medicine End-of-Life Care Consensus P. Seven legal barriers to end-of-life care: Myths, realities, and grains of truth. *JAMA*. 2000; **284**(19): 2495–2501.

67 Quill TE, Dresser R, Brock DW. The rule of double effect—A critique of its role in end-of-life decision making. *N Engl J Med*. 1997; **337**(24): 1768–1771.

68 Sykes N, Thorns A. The use of opioids and sedatives at the end of life. *Lancet Oncol*. 2003; **4**(5): 312–318.

69 Allmark P, Cobb M, Liddle BJ, Tod AM. Is the doctrine of double effect irrelevant in end-of-life decision making? *Nurs Philos*. 2010; **11**(3): 170–177.

70 Lo B, Rubenfeld G. Palliative sedation in dying patients: "We turn to it when everything else hasn't worked". *JAMA*. 2005; **294**(14): 1810–1816.

71 Rietjens JA, van der Heide A, Vrakking AM, Onwuteaka-Philipsen BD, van der Maas PJ, van der Wal G. Physician reports of terminal sedation without hydration or nutrition for patients nearing death in the Netherlands. *Ann Intern Med*. 2004; **141**(3): 178–185.

72 Jansen LA, Sulmasy DP. Sedation, alimentation, hydration, and equivocation: Careful conversation about care at the end of life. *Ann Intern Med*. 2002; **136**(11): 845–849.

73 Gillick MR. Terminal sedation: An acceptable exit strategy? *Ann Intern Med*. 2004; **141**(3): 236–237.

74 Sykes N, Thorns A. The use of opioids and sedatives at the end of life. *Lancet Oncol*. 2003; 4(5): 312–318.

75 Eddy DM. A piece of my mind. A conversation with my mother. *JAMA*. 1994; **272**(3): 179–181.

76 Blendon RJ, Szalay US, Knox RA. Should physicians aid their patients in dying? The public perspective. *JAMA*. 1992; **267**(19): 2658–2662.

77 Emanuel EJ, Fairclough DL, Emanuel LL. Attitudes and desires related to euthanasia and physician-assisted suicide among terminally ill patients and their caregivers. *JAMA*. 2000; **284**(19): 2460–2468.

● 78 van der Heide A, Deliens L, Faisst K, Nilstun T, Norup M, Paci E et al. End-of-life decision-making in six European countries: Descriptive study. *Lancet*. 2003; **362**(9381): 345–350.

79 Foley KM. Competent care for the dying instead of physician-assisted suicide. *N Engl J Med*. 1997; **336**(1): 54–58.

80 Quill TE, Lee BC, Nunn S. Palliative treatments of last resort: Choosing the least harmful alternative. University of Pennsylvania Center for Bioethics Assisted Suicide Consensus Panel. *Ann Intern Med*. 2000; **132**(6): 488–493.

81 Willems DL, Daniels ER, van der Wal G, van der Maas PJ, Emanuel EJ. Attitudes and practices concerning the end of life: A comparison between physicians from the United States and from The Netherlands. *Arch Intern Med*. 2000; **160**(1): 63–68.

82 Hendin H, Rutenfrans C, Zylicz Z. Physician-assisted suicide and euthanasia in the Netherlands. Lessons from the Dutch. *JAMA*. 1997; **277**(21): 1720–1722.

15

Dignity in palliative care

SUSAN E. McCLEMENT, HARVEY MAX CHOCHINOV, MAIA KREDENTSER

INTRODUCTION

The concept of dignity is of interest to researchers and palliative care clinicians alike. Researchers seek to carefully explicate the nature of dignity and evaluate interventions aimed at bolstering dignity for those living with life-limiting illnesses. Clinicians use research findings to inform the delivery of an evidence-based approach to patient care. As such, dignity needs to be examined and understood both in terms of empirical referents and its practical application in end-of-life care. Arriving at such an understanding is not without its challenges, however, and clinicians and researchers have several issues they must grapple with when notions of dignity in the provision of end-of-life care are invoked. The purpose of this chapter is to examine some of these issues. First, conceptual challenges identified in the literature related to the term dignity will be presented. Next, the salience of dignity in discussions regarding end-of-life care will be examined. Finally, empirical work examining the issue of dignity in end-of-life care will be presented, along with suggestions for future dignity-related research.

CONCEPTUAL CHALLENGES: DEFINING DIGNITY

The concept of dignity is ubiquitous, figuring prominently in discussions of bioethics, human rights documents, codes of research involving human subjects, patients' bill of rights, and decision making in end-of-life care [1–8]. Despite its widespread use, however, the term dignity is poorly understood, and consensus regarding both its meaning and utility in end-of-life discussions has yet to be realized [9–12]. The importance of conducting research into the construct of dignity was highlighted in the final report of a Special Committee of the Senate of Canada, mandated to explore the social, ethical, and legal aspects of euthanasia and assisted suicide [13]. This committee concluded that health professionals cannot fully understand requests for assisted death and fears about loss of dignity if the construct remains vaguely defined. Far more than an academic exercise, clarification of the concept of dignity is important because our understanding of it appears to guide

both health-care providers (HCPs) and the public about their approach to death and dying.

Dictionary definitions provide a starting point from which one can begin to understand what dignity means. The word dignity is derived from the Latin *dignitas* meaning "worthy" [14]. *Webster's Dictionary* defines dignity as "worth or excellence; nobility of manner; quality of commanding esteem, high office, or rank" [15]. Defined in this way, dignity evokes notions of worth, honor, and esteem [16]. It is not clear from these definitions what one is necessarily worthy of. There is a tacit suggestion that evaluations of dignity involve a comparative process; however, specification regarding who confers evaluations or judgments of being worthy or esteemed is not clear [12,17].

Synonyms for dignity include words like self-respect, self-esteem, poise, and pride [18], suggesting that the concept is a broad one encompassing several meanings. Such "umbrella" terms are typically difficult to define and operationalize [19]. Because the concept of dignity is not readily amenable to precise theoretical or operational definition, replacing it in favor of other concepts that appear to have greater definitional precision is tempting [20]. However, alternative concepts such as "autonomy" are imbued with ambiguity as well [7]. Mere word substitutions, then, will not produce the sought-after clarity.

One approach used to clarify the meaning of words is the process of concept analysis, a formal linguistic strategy that facilitates examination of the defining attributes or characteristics of a concept [19]. It is a process used to determine similarities and differences between concepts and create tentative theoretical and operational definitions [21]. Defining attributes identified in concept analyses of dignity include "an individual's ability to feel important and valuable in relation to others, communicate this to others, and be treated as such by others in contexts which are perceived as threatening" (p. 930) [17]. Characteristics of dignity identified by health professionals in a concept analysis conducted by Mairis [22] included notions of maintenance of self-respect and self-esteem and appreciation of what dignity means to the individual [22]. The theoretical definitions of these concept analyses suggest that dignity exists when individuals are able to exert control over their behavior, surroundings, and the way they are treated by others. Central to this definition is the capability of the person to be able to understand information and make decisions. This conceptual work also speaks to the dynamic, subjective, and interpersonal nature of dignity and the processes involved in maintaining positive self-regard amid threatening situations or circumstances.

Dignity, as defined by Justice Iacobucci of the Supreme Court of Canada, speaks of the self-respect and self-worth that individuals or groups feel, with a focus on physical and psychological integrity and empowerment [23]. It not only injects the notion of capacity for self-determination into the concept of dignity but also evokes what would appear to be critical attributes of dignity, such as autonomy, privacy, reputation, self-image, and intrinsic worth [22,23]. Such a broad range of alternative notions subsumed within this characterization of dignity, while capturing the complexity of the concept, makes definitional precision problematic. And like the theoretical definitions arising from the process of concept analyses of dignity, this characterization, while heuristic, lacks an empirical foundation.

What contributes to the ambiguity surrounding the term dignity? First, dignity seems to be closely intertwined with our ideas about autonomy, with both terms often referred to "in the same breath" [24]. The equating of human dignity with autonomy is not new and can be traced to the writings of eighteenth-century philosopher Immanuel Kant. Kant argued that human beings have an intrinsic worth—that is dignity—because they are rational agents capable of setting their own goals and making their own decisions. Following Kant's reasoning, the basic moral worth of every human being resides in the human capacity for rational choice [25,26]. The pervasive tendency to equate dignity with autonomy is troublesome, for it assumes that individuals lacking the capacity for autonomous thought also lack human dignity [27].

Some authors have attempted to affect the distinction between autonomy and dignity by examining the ways in which dignity is used in ordinary discourse. Pullman [7] asserts that the language of dignity embraces two distinct conceptualizations of the word. Basic dignity is the fundamental moral notion that speaks of the intrinsic worth of all human beings. In contrast, personal dignity refers to norms of dignity of the individual or subgroup of individuals [7]. Personal dignity is constructed through complex processes of social interaction and evaluation and is socially and individually referenced [7,12]. Moreover, given that considerations of what counts as dignified treatment or behavior are variable between individuals and across groups over time, personal dignity should be viewed as something that can be conferred (or eroded) by others [7].

Proulx and Jacelon's [28] contention that the concept of dignity is a dichotomy, consisting of both internal and external components, echoes Pullman's [7] assertion. Internal aspects of dignity speak of the inherent worth ascribed to all human beings, which is uniquely expressed in their life stories [28–30]. External aspects of dignity are connected to and vary with what matters to the individual person and include such factors as physical comfort, autonomy, meaningfulness, spirituality, and interpersonal connectedness. This later conceptualization

speaks of the subjective way in which individuals discern what is dignified for themselves and for others and the ways in which dignity is socially constructed [9].

IMPORTANCE OF THE NOTION OF DIGNITY

Confusion in the literature related to definitions of the term "dignity" has resulted in some authors characterizing the concept as "ambiguous," "euphemistic," "subterfuge-creating," "useless," and "cliché" [8,12,20,31]. While the concept of dignity currently enjoys neither definitional specificity nor consensual meaning [9,10], there does appear to be an agreement that dignity is foundational to the provision of quality end-of-life care [32]. Indeed, the link between providing palliative care and enabling patients to maintain their dignity is a perspective that Macklin [12] suggests proponents of palliative care are "wont to emphasize" (p. 214).

The philosophical grounding of palliative care within an acknowledgment of the inherent dignity of the individuals has been expressed in the literature [33], and dignity has been identified as one of five basic requirements that must be satisfied in caring for dying patients [34]. The basic tenets of palliative care, including symptom management, spiritual and psychological well-being, and care of the family unit may all be summarized under the goal of helping patients die with dignity [35–37]. When the preservation of dignity becomes the clear goal of palliation, care options expand well beyond the symptom management paradigm and encompass the physical, psychological, social, spiritual, and existential aspects of the patient's terminal experience [35]. Dignity is thus a relevant concept in discussions regarding care of the terminally ill, in that it provides an overarching framework that may guide the physician, patient, and family in discussing and defining the objectives of care at the end of life [38].

Considerations of helping patients to die with dignity are not, however, the sole purview of advocates of palliative care. Appeals to dignity are frequently invoked as the ultimate justification for euthanasia and assisted suicide. Ironically, both the hospice movement and the Hemlock Society invoke the ideal of dying with dignity in defense of their opposing perspectives [7,39–41]. For some, the notion of dignity is predicated on the notion that assisted death is consonant with, and the epitome of, respect for autonomy. This explains why in some circles the term "death with dignity" has become synonymous with the right to assisted suicide and euthanasia.[42] For others, however, such actions constitute the ultimate indignity [43].

That "loss of dignity" was the most common response of physicians when asked why their patients had selected euthanasia or some form of self-assisted suicide clearly underscores the importance of better understanding the concept of dignity in end-of-life care [44]. In a Dutch nationwide study on euthanasia and other medical decisions concerning the end of life, loss of dignity was cited by physicians in 57% of cases, followed by pain (46%), unworthy dying (46%), social dependency (33%), and tiredness of life (23%). Research conducted by Back et al. [45] examining physician-assisted suicide and euthanasia in Washington State found that physicians of 207 patients who expressed a preference for hastened death reported that a loss of dignity was a concern for 72% of these patients.

A study conducted by Seale and Addington-Hall [46] explored differences in preferences for hastened death between cancer patients and patients with cardiac disease, stroke, and respiratory disease. Approximately 25% of the "significant others" indicated that they would have preferred that the patient die sooner in his or her illness trajectory. Twenty-five percent of respondents also said that the patients themselves had expressed a desire for hastened death. Although these studies provide important insights into HCP and family member perspectives, they did not solicit input from patients directly concerning this issue. Therefore, our understanding regarding patient experiences is incomplete.

Research has been conducted examining the types of physical and psychological concerns that may prompt terminally ill individuals to desire a hastened death. There is some suggestion in the literature that severe pain can result in a heightened desire for death. In their study of terminally ill cancer patients, Chochinov et al. [47] found that 75% of patients who had a significant desire for early death experienced moderate to severe pain, compared with 46% of patients with mild or no pain. Similarly, Rosenfeld and associates' [48] research examining interest in physician-assisted suicide among terminally ill patients with acquired immune deficiency syndrome (AIDS) found that pain intensity contributed significantly to the prediction of desire for death in those patients with pain.

Evidence also exists that depression contributes significantly to a desire for death among terminally ill patients. In a review of literature pertaining to physical and psychological distress associated with a desire for early death, Chochinov and Wilson [49] concluded that clinical depression, poor pain control, and low social support are significantly related to desire for death and that the degree of distress in these individuals is frequently very high. In an examination of desire for death in terminally ill patients, it was found that 8.5% of patients reported at least a moderate desire for death that was consistent over time. Slightly more than half of the patients (55%) reported no desire for early death and 36% of patients reported intermittent desire for early death. Follow-up interviews 2 weeks later indicated that 4 out of 6 of the original 17 patients with at least a moderate desire for death had changed their minds. This finding demonstrates that even strong desires for early death can change over a relatively short period of time. Given that requests for euthanasia in the Netherlands are usually satisfied within 2 weeks of the patient's request, efforts to explicate the factors that contribute to a desire for early death must be a continued focus of research.

In their review of terminally ill patients' requests for hastened death, Block and Billings [50] emphasized the importance of detailing the clinical determinants and the meaning of the request for early death, so that the therapeutic options offered by care providers may be broadened. Variables considered important in shaping patients' decisions to hasten death include symptom control, social support, psychological distress, and the meaning of life and suffering. Clearly, the psychological context within which a fear of lost dignity is fostered needs to be understood empirically. Systematic examination and description of those factors identified by the patient as prompting requests for hastened death provide a solid foundation from which caregivers might implement dignity-preserving or dignity-bolstering interventions.

Central to the arguments for and against death-hastening measures are notions of what constitutes a "good death"— an experience within which notions of dignity appear to be embedded [51]. Emanuel and Emanuel [52] have examined the construct of a "good death," describing a detailed framework for this event. Though not empirically validated, these researchers synthesized the dying experience as a process with four critical components including fixed patient characteristics, mutable elements of the patient's experiences, interventions that are available, and overall outcome.

Steinhauser et al. [53] used a cross-section stratified random national survey to collect information from patients, families, and health-care practitioners, with an aim of identifying factors that were most important to them at the end of life. Factors identified by participants include pain and symptom management, preparation for death, decisions about treatment preferences, and being treated in a holistic fashion. Relevant strategies for addressing these factors were not identified in the study.

Turner et al. [54] sought to measure dignity in 50 terminally ill patients being cared for in an integrated palliative care service during the final 72 hours of life by focusing on symptom control, level of functioning, and negative events and situations that might compromise dignity. The limitations of this work include inconsistency and confusion regarding the ways in which these criteria were measured and sole reliance on HCP perspectives in assessing dignity.

There is consensus in the literature that dignity is a complex and multifaceted concept. However, it is only recently that the data informing definitions of dignity in the context of end-of-life care have included an emic or insider's perspective. A patient-centered approach to understanding dignity provides guidance to those caring for the dying regarding what constitutes dignity-enhancing or dignity-eroding actions, from those who are perhaps most qualified to speak about it—terminally ill patients themselves [39]. Examining dignity in end-of-life care from this perspective, and making what is tacit more explicit, reveals further dimensions of dignity and provides the foundation upon which empirically derived interventions aimed at bolstering dignity can be developed and evaluated.

EMPIRICAL WORK

The body of empirical literature examining the concept of dignity in end of life is increasing. Street and Kissane's [9*] discourse analysis of palliative patient and family case studies provides insights about how dying people feel about their bodies and the care they receive at the end of life. Results from their work help to further dimensionalize our understanding of dignity as it relates to the embodied experience of dying and the ways in which abjection of the body might serve as a source of shame for the terminally ill. Their findings regarding the reciprocal, relational nature of dignity serve as a poignant reminder that patient's perceptions of worth are greatly influenced by the ways in which care providers communicate with and care for them.

Enes [20*] conducted a phenomenological study examining the meaning of dignity from the perspectives of patients, relatives, and HCPs in a hospice inpatient unit in England. Thematic analysis arising from this work suggests that dignity concerns issues of relationship and belonging, having control, being human in terms of having rights and being worthy of respect, and maintaining the individual self. Patients, families, and HCPs, while in agreement regarding the various facets of dignity, placed their emphases differently. For example, whereas HCPs emphasized issues of control and privacy, relatives emphasized issues of relationship and humanity. These findings speak to the need for, and challenges inherent in, trying to balance the multiple needs of care recipients and providers.

Chochinov et al. have been engaged in a program of research using a combination of qualitative and quantitative research methods to arrive at an understanding of the concept of dignity from the perspective of the terminally ill patient and to identify various factors that support or erode a patient's sense of dignity [55*]. Inductive analysis of qualitative interviews conducted with 50 palliative cancer patients resulted in the generation of an empirically derived model of dignity in the terminally ill and direction regarding dignity-conserving care [56*] (Table 15.1).

The dignity model suggests that patient perceptions of dignity are related to and influenced by three major thematic areas:

1. Illness-related concerns, that is, those issues deriving from the illness that relate to one's level of independence and symptom experiences

2. The patient's dignity-conserving repertoire, that is, the personal approaches that individuals use to maintain their sense of dignity and the internally held views or perspectives of their inherent qualities

3. Social dignity inventory, that is, factors external to the patient that influence the quality of his or her interactions with others that may bolster or undermine the person's sense of dignity (Table 15.1)

Quantitative data were collected in conjunction with the qualitative work to examine how various demographic and disease-specific variables were related to the issue of dignity in the terminally ill. A cohort of just over 200 terminally ill cancer patients were asked to rate their sense of dignity and complete measures of psychological well-being. Nearly half of the patients in the sample indicated they experienced some, or occasional, dignity-related concerns. Compared with those patients whose dignity was intact, patients with significant dignity-related concerns reported that they had increased pain, decreased quality of life, and difficulty with bowel functioning and were dependent on others for bathing, dressing, and incontinence issues. These patients also reported a loss of will to live, increased desire for death, depression, hopelessness, and anxiety [35*]. The association between appearance (or the perception of how patients believe themselves to be seen or appreciated by others) and dignity leads to the assertion that "the reflection patients see of themselves in the eye of the beholder [care provider] needs to be one that is affirming of their sense of dignity" [57].

Factor analysis of these data revealed six primary factors, accounting for 40.5 percent of the variance. This factor solution includes distinct aspects of the dying patient's experience: pain, intimate dependence, hopelessness/depression, informal support network, formal support network, and quality of life [58*]. This factor structure supports the model of dignity in the terminally ill that arose from the qualitative work. Logistic regression analysis retaining those factors identified as being most malleable to palliative care intervention resulted in a

Table 15.1   *Model of dignity in the terminally ill: Summary of major categories, themes, and subthemes arising from qualitative work examining the construct of dignity from the perspective of the terminally ill*

Illness–related concerns	Dignity-conserving repertoire	Social dignity inventory
Symptom distress	Dignity-conserving perspectives	Social issues/relationship dynamics affecting dignity
Physical distress	Continuity of self	Privacy boundaries
Psychological distress	Role preservation	Social support
Medical uncertainty	Generativity/legacy	Burden to others
Death anxiety	Maintenance of pride	Aftermath concerns
	Hopefulness	
	Autonomy/control	
	Acceptance	
	Resilience/fighting spirit	
Level of independence	Dignity-conserving practices	
Cognitive acuity	Living in the moment	
Functional capacity	Maintaining normalcy	
	Seeking spiritual comfort	

highly significant two-factor solution that included hopelessness/depression and intimate dependency needs [58*].

Some may argue that the dignity model fails to resolve or dispel confusion around dignity's lack of definitional specificity. What every facet of the model has in common, however, is that each of the domains of concern identified within it has been raised by terminally ill individuals as having a bearing on their sense of dignity [32]. As such, the dignity model provides an empirically derived theoretical framework that aids our understanding of the notion of dignity in those nearing death. The model of dignity-conserving care offers a unique model of end-of-life care, which may lead to enhanced palliation and new possibilities in care of the dying. Practical clinical considerations as to how HCPs might begin to apply dignity-conserving care approaches in practice are outlined in Table 15.2.

In addition to enhancing our understanding of dignity in those approaching death and providing a foundation upon which to understand how a dying patient may experience a waning of their dignity, the dignity model also provides direction for how to construct dignity-enhancing interventions for patients nearing death [55]. One such approach is a brief psychotherapeutic intervention called dignity therapy.

Developed by Chochinov et al., dignity therapy is comprised of audio-recorded sessions that provide terminally ill patients the opportunity to speak of aspects of life they feel proudest of, things they feel are or were most meaningful, the personal history they would most want remembered, or words they might provide in the service of helping to look after their soon-to-be bereft loved ones. These sessions are transcribed and edited and the final document returned to the patient, thereby bolstering patients' sense of purpose, meaning, and worth. Engagement in this empathic, therapeutic process provides patients tangible evidence that their thoughts and words have—and will continue to have—value. The creation of a "generativity document" offers comfort in knowing that something of their essence will transcend beyond death itself. An international, randomized controlled trial of dignity therapy has shown significant benefits to patients marked by enhanced end-of-life experience. Patients who received dignity therapy and palliative care (as compared to those receiving client-centered therapy [an attentional control arm of the study] and standard palliative care or standard palliative care alone) were significantly more likely to agree that the intervention was helpful to them, improved their quality of life, and increased their sense of dignity.

Table 15.2 *Application of the dignity model to practice*

Illness-related concerns	Directions for practice
Symptom distress	
Physical distress	Baseline and ongoing assessment of physical and psychological symptoms
Psychological distress	
Medical uncertainty	Provision of timely, relevant information about the illness and plan of care
Death anxiety	Exploration of concerns associated with illness progression
Level of independence	
Cognitive acuity	Baseline and ongoing assessment of cognitive functioning
	Vigilance in detection and treatment of delirium
Functional capacity	Baseline and ongoing assessment of ability to carry out activities of daily living
	Referrals to occupational and physiotherapy as appropriate
	Provision of supports needed to maintain independence (e.g., walker, raised toilet seat)
	Involvement in decision making regarding plan of care, as desired by patient
Dignity-conserving repertoire	Directions for practice
Continuity of self	Communication with patient about those facets of life not affected by their disease
	Learning about the patient's biography, attending to those aspects of life that he or she values most
Role preservation	Exploration of roles important to the patient
	Facilitation of role enactment within limitations of patient's illness
Maintenance of pride	Discussion with patient about those aspects of their life that they are most proud of, ensure a professional demeanor in provision of care
Hopefulness	Talking with the patient about what is still possible, despite illness limitations
	Encouraging redefining of goals and expectations
Autonomy/control	Assessing the patient's perceived level of control and exploring preference regarding level of involvement in care decisions and planning
	Where possible, providing choices
Generativity/legacy	Facilitating life review or other activities that foster the sharing of memories that are meaningful to patient
Acceptance	Exploring the impact of the illness for the patient
	Appreciating the dynamism of the process of responding to a life-threatening illness
Resilience/fighting spirit	Identifying and promoting patient participation in those interactions/activities that are most meaningful, given limited life expectancy

Further, these patients also felt the intervention had helped or would be a help to their family and had changed or could change the way their family saw and appreciated them [59**].

Dignity therapy has also been used successfully in noncancer patient populations, with patients from diverse cultural groups, and those receiving care in the community as well as the hospital setting [60*,61**,62*,63*]. Chochinov et al. piloted dignity therapy with frail elderly residents of personal care homes. Twelve cognitively intact residents received the therapy, and 11 family member proxies of residents who were cognitively impaired participated on the residents' behalf. Common narrative themes emerged for the two groups, with the majority of both cognitively intact and impaired residents discussing the importance of relationships, sources of pride or accomplishment, and delights or joys. Thematic differences emerged between these two groups, with cognitively intact residents more likely to cite death/loss, formative experiences, and disappointments or regrets, while family member proxies of cognitively impaired residents more often cited the impact of illness, personal characteristics, and important roles. The majority of cognitively intact residents indicated that the therapy was helpful to them, and family members and HCPs of these residents who provided feedback echoed this sentiment and indicated that they would also recommend dignity therapy for other residents.

The majority of family members of cognitively impaired participants indicated that the dignity therapy document would help them and their family and would continue to be a source of comfort. The majority of both family members and HCPs of the cognitively impaired residents recommended it for other residents. For both cognitively intact and cognitively impaired residents, the majority of HCPs indicated that dignity therapy would help them provide care, changed how they appreciated the resident, and taught them new things about the resident [60*].

Regarding cross-cultural applications, empirical work examining the use of dignity therapy has been conducted in Denmark, China, Japan, Australia, Canada, the United States, Scotland, and England [59**,62*,64]. While in some instances the protocol had to be nuanced for cultural sensitivity (e.g., the notion of "pride" did not resonate among Danish study participants), dignity therapy is flexible and patient-guided, providing a framework that is easily adaptable.

The benefits of dignity therapy have been shown to extend to families of patient participants. McClement et al. [65*] reported positive effects on family members of patients who received dignity therapy. Patients who completed dignity therapy as part of a phase I clinical trial were asked to provide contact information for a family member who would receive their generativity document and who agreed to be contacted by researchers in the future. Of the 100 patients who completed dignity therapy, 60 family members provided feedback on the experience approximately 6 months to 1 year after the patient's death. Just over three-quarters of these family members reported that the generativity document helped them in their time of grief and would continue to be a comfort to them. Further, 95% of these family members said they would recommend dignity therapy to other families and patients.

FUTURE DIRECTIONS

The empirical work conducted to date examining the concept of dignity in end-of-life care is still evolving. What is clear, however, is that the conceptual challenges related to defining dignity are not easily solved. The multifaceted, dynamic, and subjective nature of the concept seems to preclude exploration of the dignity experience using narrow definitions[20]. This suggests the need for researchers to understand and apply dignity in specific contexts in which it can be "unpacked" [39].

There is increasing appreciation for the need of palliative care that is both culturally sensitive and addresses the needs of individuals living with life-limiting illnesses apart from cancer [66,67]. Future work could extend exploration of the concept of dignity from the perspective of diverse cultural groups and various specific vulnerable populations including the elderly and those with mental illness or disabilities. Continued exploration of the applications to those with nonmalignant conditions is essential for enhancing our understanding of this complex topic and would help explicate nuances of dignity and dignity-conserving care that may be disease- or group-specific.

Little is known regarding the impact of terminal illness on the perceptions and experience of dignity from the perspective of family members of the terminally ill. Family members who perceive deficits in their terminally ill relative's care experience changes in their own physical health and family functioning [68]. Therefore, research examining the provision of care appraised by a family that both erodes and supports patient dignity and the impact that such care has on family outcomes is needed.

It is likely that perceptions of dignity are shaped by a patient's specific needs, which in turn alter as the illness evolves [20]. This finding speaks to the dynamic nature of dignity and suggests that longitudinal work indexing patient experiences of dignity across the illness trajectory is warranted. Such longitudinal work may reveal differences in threats to dignity experienced in the early versus advanced stages of disease and help explicate a range of dignity-enhancing strategies that patients use over time.

CONCLUSION

Becker [69] asserts that a significant psychological factor affecting terminally ill people is the compromising of their perceived personal dignity. Palliative care has been characterized as care that "honours and protects those who are dying, and conveys by word and action that dignity resides in people" (p. 1) [70]. Indeed, the notions of dignity and palliative care are deeply intertwined, as are considerations of basic human rights and recognition of the inherent dignity of all people [71]. Thus, adequate palliative care and pain control that maintains such dignity at the end of life has been posited as a fundamental human right [72].

Those involved in care of the dying need to understand what dignity means to the recipients of care, bearing in mind the various issues subsumed within dignity-related concerns. Such understanding will arm HCPs with a range of patient-centered approaches and interventions, aimed at achieving humane care for individuals approaching the end of life.

Key learning points

- Dignity is a complex and multifaceted concept making it difficult to define and operationalize.

- Dignity is foundational to the provision of quality end-of-life care.

- Until recently, an understanding of dignity in end of life has largely been devoid of the voices of terminally ill patients.

- When the preservation of dignity becomes the clear goal of palliation, care options expand well beyond the symptom management paradigm and encompass the physical, psychological, social, spiritual, and existential aspects of the patient's terminal experience.

- A patient-centered approach to understanding dignity provides guidance to those caring for the dying regarding what constitutes dignity-enhancing or dignity-eroding actions.

REFERENCES

1 Sampio L. To die with dignity. *Social Science and Medicine.* 1992;35:433–441.
2 Badcott D. The basis and relevance of emotional dignity. *Medicine Health Care and Philosophy.* 2003;6:123–131.
3 Macklin R. Yet another guideline? The UNESCO draft. *Developing World Bioethics.* 2005;5:244–250.
4 Sullivan AD, Hedberg K, Fleming DW. Legalized physician-assisted suicide in Oregon: The second year. *New England Journal of Medicine.* 2000;342:598–604.
5 Leichtentritt RD, Rettig KD. Values underlying end-of-life decisions: A qualitative approach. *Health and Social Work.* 2001;26:150–159.
6 Stolberg SD. Human dignity and disease, disability, and suffering: A philosophical contribution to the euthanasia and assisted suicide debate. *Humane Medicine.* 1995;11:144–147.
7 Pullman D. Death, dignity, and moral nonsense. *Journal of Palliative Care.* 2004;20:171–178.
8 Lynch A. Death without dignity. *Annals of the Royal College of Physicians and Surgeons of Canada.* 1982;15:117–122.
● 9 Street A, Kissane DW. Constructions of dignity in end-of-life care. *Journal of Palliative Care.* 2001;17:93–101.
10 deRave L. Dignity and integrity at the end of life. *International Journal of Palliative Nursing.* 1996;2:71–76.
11 Coope CM. Death with dignity. *Hasting Centre Report.* 1997;27:37–38.
12 Macklin R. Reflections on the Human Dignity Symposium: Is dignity a useless concept? *Journal of Palliative Care.* 2004;20:212–216.
● 13 Senate of Canada. On Life and Death. A Report of the Special Senate Committee on Euthanasia and Assisted Suicide. Ottawa, Ontario, Canada: Minister of Supply and Services Canada; June 1995.
14 Sykes JB (ed). *The Oxford Concise Dictionary.* Oxford, U.K.: Clarendon Press; 1982.
15 Merriam-Webster. [March 12, 2012]; Available from: http://www.merriam- webster.com/dictionary/dignity
● 16 Chochinov HM. Dignity conserving care: A new model for palliative care. *JAMA.* 2002;287:2253–2260.
● 17 Haddock J. Toward further clarification of the concept of 'dignity'. *Journal of Advanced Nursing.* 1996;24:924–931.
18 Chapman RL. *Roget's International Thesaurus.* 4th edn. Toronto, Ontario, Canada: Fitzhenry & Whiteside; 1977.
19 Walker LO, Avant KC. *Strategies for Theory Construction in Nursing.* Norwalk, CT: Appleton & Lange; 1988.
20 Enes S. An exploration of dignity in palliative care. *Palliative Medicine.* 2003;17:263–269.
21 McCormack B. Intuition: Concept analysis and application to curriculum development. 1. Concept analysis. *Journal of Clinical Nursing.* 1992;1:339–344.
● 22 Mairis ED. Concept clarification in professional practice—Dignity. *Journal of Advanced Nursing.* 1994;19:947–953.
23 Downie J. Unilateral withholding and withdrawal of potentially life-sustaining treatment: A violation of dignity under the law. *Journal of Palliative Care.* 2004;20:143–149.
24 Pullman D. The ethics of autonomy and dignity in long-term care. *Canadian Journal of Aging.* 1999;18:26–46.
25 Rachels J. *The Elements of Moral Philosophy,* 2nd edn. New York: McGraw-Hill; 1993.
26 Grassian V. *Moral Reasoning: Ethical Theory and Some Contemporary Moral Problems,* 2nd edn. Englewood Cliffs, NJ: Prentice Hall; 1992.
27 Meyer MJ. Dignity, death and modern virtue. *American Philosophy Q.* 32:45–55.
28 Proulx K, Jacelon C. Dying with dignity: The good patient versus the good death. *American Journal of Hospice and Palliative Medicine.* 2004;21:116–120.
29 Holstein M. Reflections on death and dying. *Academic Medicine.* 1997;27:848–855.
30 Moody H. Why dignity in old age matters. *Journal of Gerontological Social Work.* 1998;29:13–38.
31 Caulfield T. Human cloning laws, human dignity and the poverty of the policy making dialogue. *BMC Medical Ethics.* 2003;4:E3.
32 Chochinov HM. Defending dignity. *Palliative & Supportive Care.* 2003;1:307–308.
33 Latimer E. Caring for seriously ill and dying patients: The philosophy and ethics. *Canadian Medical Association Journal.* 1991;144:859–864.
34 Geyman J. Dying and death of a family member. *Journal of Family Practice.* 1983;17:125–134.
● 35 Chochinov HM, Hack T, Hassard T, Kristjanson LJ, McClement S, Harlos M. Dignity in the terminally ill: A cross-sectional, cohort study. *The Lancet.* 2002;360(9350):2026–2030.
36 Ambiven M. Dying with dignity. *World Health Forum.* 1991;12:375–381.
37 Madan TN. Dying with dignity. *Social Science & Medicine.* 1992;35:425–432.
38 Quill TE. Perspectives on care at the close of life: Initiating end-of-life discussions with seriously ill patients: Addressing the 'elephant in the room'. *JAMA.* 2000;284:2502–2507.
39 McDonald M. Dignity at the end of our days: Personal, familial, and cultural location. *Journal of Palliative Care.* 2004;20:163–170.
40 Wanzer SH, Federman DD, Adelstein SJ et al. The physician's responsibility toward hopelessly ill patients. A second look. *New England Journal of Medicine.* 1989;320:844–889.
41 Wilson JK, Fox E, Kamakahi JJ. Who is fighting for the right to die? Older women's participation in the Hemlock Society. *Health Care Women International.* 1998;19:365–380.

42 Ganzini L, Nelson HJ, Lee MA et al. Oregon physicians' attitudes about and experiences with end-of-life care since the passage of the Oregon Death with Dignity Act. *JAMA.* 2001;285:2363–2369.

43 Simpson E. Harms to dignity, bioethics, and the scope of biolaw. *Journal of Palliative Care.* 2004;20:185–193.

● 44 Van der Mass PJ, van Delden JJM, Pijnenborg L, CWN L. Euthanasia and other medical decisions concerning the end of life. *Lancet.* 1991;338:669–674.

45 Back AL, Wallace JI, Starks HE, Pearlman RA. Physician-assisted suicide and euthanasia in Washington State. *JAMA: The Journal of the American Medical Association.* 1996;275(12):919–925.

46 Seale C, Addingtonhall J. Euthanasia—Why people want to die earlier. *Social Science & Medicine.* 1994;39(5):647–654.

● 47 Chochinov HM, Wilson KG, Enns M, Mowchun N, Lander S, Levitt M et al. Desire for death in the terminally ill. *American Journal of Psychiatry.* 1995;152(8):1185–1191.

48 Rosenfeld B, Krivo S, Breitbart W, Chochinov HM. Suicide, assisted suicide, and euthanasia in the terminally ill. In: Chochinov HM, Breitbart W, eds. *Handbook of Psychiatry in Palliative Medicine.* Oxford, U.K.: Oxford University Press; 2000. pp. 51–62.

49 Chochinov HM, Wilson KG. The euthanasia debate: Attitudes, practices and psychiatric considerations. *Canadian Journal of Psychiatry.* 1995;40(10):593–602.

50 Block SD, Billings JA. Patient Requests to Hasten Death: Evaluation and Management in Terminal Care. *Archives of Internal Medicine.* 1994;154(18):2039–2047.

51 Payne S, Langley-Evans A, Hillier R. Perceptions of a 'good' death: A comparative study of the views of hospice staff and patients. *Palliative Medicine.* 1996;10(4):307–312.

52 Emanuel EJ, Emanuel LL. The promise of a good death. *The Lancet.* 1998;351, Supplement 2(0):SII21–SII9.

53 Steinhauser KE, Christakis NA, Clipp EC, McNeilly M, McIntyre L, Tulsky JA. Factors considered important at the end of life by patients, family, physicians, and other care providers. *JAMA: The Journal of the American Medical Association.* 2000;284(19):2476–2482.

54 Turner K, Chye R, Aggarwal G, Philip J, Skeels A, Lickiss JN. Dignity in dying: A preliminary study of patients in the last three days of life. *Journal of Palliative Care.* 1996;12(2):7–13.

● 55 McClement S, Chochinov HM, Hack T, Kristjanson LJ, Harlos M. Dignity conserving care: Application of research findings to practice. *International Journal of Palliative Nursing.* 2004;10:173–179.

● 56 Chochinov HM, Hack T, McClement S, Kristjanson L, Harlos M. Dignity in the terminally ill: A developing empirical model. *Social Science & Medicine.* 2002;54(3):433–443.

57 Chochinov HM. Dignity and the eye of the beholder. *Journal of Clinical Oncology.* 2004;22(7):1336–1340.

● 58 Hack TF, Chochinov HM, Hassard T, Kristjanson LJ, McClement S, Harlos M. Defining dignity in terminally ill cancer patients: A factor-analytic approach. *Psycho-Oncology.* 2004;13(10):700–708.

● 59 Chochinov HM, Kristjanson LJ, Breitbart W, McClement S, Hack TF, Hassard T et al. Effect of dignity therapy on distress and end-of-life experience in terminally ill patients: A randomised controlled trial. *The Lancet Oncology.* 2011;12(8):753–762.

● 60 Chochinov HM, Cann B, Cullihall K, Kristjanson L, Harlos M, McClement SE et al. Dignity therapy: A feasibility study of elders in long-term care. *Palliative & Supportive Care.* 2012;10(01):3–15.

● 61 Hall S, Chochinov H, Harding R, Murray S, Richardson A, Higginson I. A Phase II randomised controlled trial assessing the feasibility, acceptability and potential effectiveness of Dignity Therapy for older people in care homes: Study protocol. *BMC Geriatrics.* 2009;9(1):9.

62 Houmann LJ, Rydahl-Hansen S, Chochinov HM, Kristjanson LJ, Groenvold M. Testing the feasibility of the Dignity Therapy interview: Adaptation for the Danish culture. *Palliative Care.* 2010;9:21–31.

● 63 Montross L, Winters, KD, Irwin SA. Dignity Therapy Implementation in a Community-Based Hospice Setting *Journal of Palliative Medicine.* 2011;14(6):729–734.

64 Chochinov HM. *Dignity Therapy: Final Words for Final Days.* New York: Oxford University Press; 2012.

65 McClement S, Chochinov HM, Hack T, Hassard T, Kristjanson LJ, Harlos M. Dignity therapy: Family member perspectives. *Journal of Palliative Medicine.* 2007;10(5):1076–1082.

66 Addington-Hall J, Higginson IJ, eds. *Palliative Care for Non-Cancer Patients.* Oxford, U.K.: Oxford University Press; 2001.

67 Pickett MC. Cultural awareness in the context of terminal illness. *Cancer Nursing* 1993;16(2):102–106.

68 Kristjanson LJ, Sloan JA, Dudgeon D, Adaskin E. Family members' perceptions of palliative cancer care: Predictors of family functioning and family members' health. *Journal of Palliative Care.* 1996;12(4):10–20.

69 Becker R. How will I cope?: Psychological aspects of advanced illness. In: Kinghorn S, Gamilin R, eds. *Palliative Nursing: Bringing Comfort and Hope.* Edinburgh, U.K.: Bailliere Tindall; 2001:79–94.

70 Field M, Cassell C, eds. *Approaching Death: Improving Care at the End of Life/Committee on Care at the End of Life.* Washington, DC: National Academy Press; 1997.

71 United Nations. The Universal Declaration of Human Rights; 1948.

72 Breitbart W. Palliative care as a human right. *Palliative & Supportive Care.* 2008;6(04):323–3325. http://www.un.org/en/documents/udhr/index.shtml

PART 3

Problems and challenges of global research

16

Transcultural palliative care

CARL JOHAN FÜRST, SOLVIG EKBLAD

TRANSCULTURAL PERSPECTIVES ON DEVELOPMENT OF PALLIATIVE CARE

Challenging assumptions based on one's own culture is essential to the development of knowledge and insight into others.[1]

There has been rapid development in palliative care in many countries during the past decades, as witnessed in clinical practice, organization, education, and research. This development has been diverse, depending on the local culture and traditions and the context of the care being delivered.[2–5] The many organizational models for end-of-life care around the world, both in the developing and developed countries, and the meaning of and terminology used in different countries and healthcare disciplines mirror some of these variations.[6,7] The World Health Organization (WHO) 2002 definition reflects a broadening concept of palliative care as compared with the previous WHO definition of 1990 but still does not specifically address cultural issues.[8–10]

Transcultural palliative care deals with the understanding and evaluation of cultural factors in advanced disease and end-of-life care. It takes into account the different cultural, religious, ethnic, and ethical value systems, and it bridges the gap between different cultural contexts by a more fulfilling communication between the care providers and patients and their families; it encompasses multiple perspectives.[11] For patients from immigrant and minority populations, transcultural palliative care takes a dual perspective of the norms of the prevailing dominant culture and of the minority group to which the patient belongs. This is relevant in palliative care services as well as in general health service in all parts of the world.

Models of palliative care, which have been developed in wealthier societies, are not easily transferred to societies where there is poverty, extended family structures, traditional medicine, and insufficient health infrastructure. There is a need to adjust to local social and culture contexts.[12,13] At the same time, spiritual care, which plays an essential part in the relief of suffering and pain, is just as important in developing countries where comfort and medical resources are limited.[14] In addition, it should be borne in mind that the basic needs and wishes of patients from ethnic minorities in palliative care are common to all human beings and independent of cultural background. Patients from ethnic minorities try to fit in with the dominant culture, which provides another argument against stereotypical cultural care not being appropriate.[15]

Thus, on the whole, transcultural palliative care includes knowledge of the practices and rites of different religions and cultures and is sensitive to the specific needs of foreign-born and minority groups. There are challenges in this regard, as evidence shows that those from minor ethnic groups can, in some instances, miss out on the best in palliative care.[16] One of the main findings from reflections from focus groups' interviews with hospice staff regarding cultural challenges in end-of-life care was that "to better understand other cultures it is important to raise awareness about the staff's own culture and to pay attention to culture especially in the context of the individual."[17]

In parallel with the development of palliative care, the world has experienced unrivalled advancements in medical technology and pharmacology, giving rise not only to hope for new possibilities but also to unrealistic expectations of cure and survival. Mobile phones being used in novel ways in low-resource countries that lack cancer care including patient follow-up and poor psychosocial support may help overcome some problems of poor communication in healthcare delivery.[18] Community volunteer workers in palliative care may play a main source of support and care for patients in developing countries.[19] Another factor that has influenced the development of palliative care has been the needs of patients with nonmalignant diseases.[9,20] Generally, the prevalence of chronic and life-threatening illnesses has increased due to the aging of populations in many developed countries. We are witnessing a change in social structures, toward smaller numbers of informal caregivers. Families look different, are becoming smaller, and are often dispersed and living at distance from each other. The pressures of a demanding society often influence the family structure and divorce rates are increasing in many countries. At the same time, societies and families have lost many of the rites and rituals that were often based on religion or historical traditions. In the past, these served as a support during life events such as dying and bereavement.

The acquired immune deficiency syndrome (AIDS) epidemic, in particular in the developing countries, especially has left large groups of children with little adult support and at risk for disease and early death. Grandmothers caring for their grandchildren orphaned by HIV/AIDS are an increasing concern in Africa.[21] At the same time, Western countries have witnessed increasing numbers of immigrants from developing countries, war-ravaged regions, and totalitarian regimes, putting new ethical demands on good-quality care at the end of life, when a flashback can come due to earlier life events.

CULTURAL COMPETENCE AND EFFECTIVE COMMUNICATION SKILLS

Culture is a process by which activities acquire moral and emotional meaning for individuals.[22] In the twenty-first century, human beings are interconnected globally in the virtual and physical worlds. From this, it follows that traditional definitions of culture are now challenged by globalization, which has led to differences within a cultural setting that may equal or exceed the dissimilarities between cultures.

In the literature, there are two main approaches to culture: the first generic approach identifies culture by location or language and views culture as unchanging and static. It does not pay much attention to the diversity within groups. The second approach emphasizes on individual caring needs within the cultural context.[23]

Cultural competence refers to a clinician's knowledge of various cultures and their ability to apply this knowledge to patient care.[24,25] This competence demands a dual stance: first the clinician's own perspective and then the perspective of the patient and family members. The issues that need to be dealt with by all palliative care clinicians irrespective of their background professions are illustrated by the example case in Box 16.1 and in the proposed assessment model (Box 16.2).

Box 16.1 Transcultural assessment

Sophia is 43 years old and a mother of three children between the ages of 12 and 19 years. She left Iraq with her husband and children 10 years ago. Sophia was diagnosed as having acute leukemia 2 years ago and has been through several chemotherapy regimens including a bone marrow transplant. She is newly admitted to your hospice from the hematology department. Her blood values and general weakness prevent further chemotherapy. She knows only a few words in your language. Her husband and his brother speak your language to some extent and try to act as interpreters. Mostly, they talk and answer on behalf of Sophia. Sophia is prescribed intravenous nutrition and blood platelets when required and is on intravenous antibiotics because of recent septicemia. Your impression is that Sophia is nearing death and is experiencing severe anxiety. The relatives are expecting a brief stay at the hospice before a new course of chemotherapy.

Questions
- How would you handle the situation?
- What more information do you need?
- Are there differences between the perspectives of the different professionals in the caring team?

Box 16.2 A transcultural assessment model: Attitudes, skills, and knowledge of transcultural palliative care

Attitudes—Issues to reflect upon
- Assumptions based on one's own culture and possible prejudices
- Your general standpoints on nutrition and fluids, personal care, drugs including smoking and alcohol, alternative treatments such as traditional medicine, anticancer treatment in end-of-life care
- Beliefs, attitudes, and values regarding diseases and prognosis, death customs and bereavement, patient-centered or authority-centered care, expectations of care by patient, family, and staff

Knowledge—Issues you need to know about
- Beliefs and practices related to illness and health; basic habits around dying, death, and bereavement in relation to the major religions
- Where to find *up-to-date information* on religious and cultural habits
- Biological variations, for example, genetic variation in susceptibility to disease
- Impact of earlier, untreated, traumatic life events during the terminal stage of life

Skills—Issues to be dealt with
- Social hierarchical structure, family patterns
- Identify adaptations already made by the patient
- Modification of emphasis in teaching, for example, targeting one of the parents or an elder family member to obtain accurate information and deliver education such as in home care
- Being supportive toward religious beliefs as well as toward profane attitudes
- Appropriately adapt communication and behavior according to family structures, communication patterns, and styles, based on cultural influences

Organizational issues:
- Space, for example, for patients and relatives to visit and pray if they wish
- Environmental factors, for example, food, presence of religious artifacts
- Contacts with religious representatives

The ability to communicate effectively gives the clinician an insight of the ethnic minority patient's immediate medical and psychosocial needs.

Barriers to cultural competence can be in relation to the clinicians and to health systems. The former barriers arise when clinicians lack knowledge of their patients' cultural practices and beliefs or when their beliefs differ from those of their patients and relatives. Those who expect their patients to respond as they themselves would to issues such as medical decision making, artificial nutrition and hydration, and death and mourning will be unprepared when patients respond differently. System-related barriers exist because most facilities have not been designed for cultural diversity, favoring instead a *one-size-fits-all* approach to care. For example, can a Buddhist family stay long enough with the dead body of a relative to allow for the spirit to leave by the open window?

Thus, culturally tailored care is an important quality factor,[26] but stereotypical cultural care may be inappropriate, since microcultural differences and individual diversifications within cultures are common. When needs are not obvious, it is necessary to specifically explore the cultural aspects of care, which may be different from the majority and dominant culture.

INDIVIDUAL AND FAMILY

At the end of life, and indeed at all points in palliative and supportive care, everyone should be treated with the same respect, independent of socioeconomic, educational, religious, cultural, language, and ethnic background. The fundamental ethical principle is the patient's right to live and die in the way he or she wants to, regardless of his or her condition, lifestyle, and beliefs. A culturally competent and ethical decision-making model is based on human rights and the use of ethical principles that include values and assumptions of the patients and their families, relatives, and significant others.

Patient autonomy is a key issue in the interface between the patient-centered care that is common in many Western societies and the cultures where the family and community have a more important role and function as advocates for the patient. In some cultures, the welfare of the community takes precedence over individual life, for example, Korean Americans and Mexican Americans have been shown to be more in favor of the family making decisions on end-of-life issues than African Americans and European Americans.[27] In reality, decisions are often made by consensus.[28]

It is common to use an empirical ethical analysis that is based on patient autonomy. Other common and relevant ethical principles of Western cultures include the concepts of nonmaleficence, beneficence, and justice. In European philosophy, there is sometimes a belief in absolute ethical principles that are the basis of morals. The two moral principles of nonmaleficence and justice are often seen as absolute.[2] Two other important principles are *sanctity of life* and *absence of suffering*.

BREAKING BAD NEWS, TO BE TRUTHFULLY INFORMED

I will always prefer not to know, or to know as little as possible. No human being knows when he is going to arrive in this world, therefore I believe that his natural state is also not to know when he will depart.[2]

The previous quotation illustrates the ethical dilemma of giving diagnostic and other medical information or requesting informed consent for a medical procedure from a patient who wishes to remain ignorant and how this challenges the physician to balance respect for the patient's attitude with information that could be beneficial. Truth telling or breaking bad news, as well as communication about impending death, has to be seen in this context.[29–31] The nature and the amount of information given to patients with cancer is still approached differently, depending on the country and culture.[32–35] An important ethical question from a transcultural perspective is: What ethical justification can support the withholding of information or the giving of information to patients about their terminal illness? Culturally competent communication about death and dying is increasingly important once biomedical intervention is shown to fail to cure.

In many cultures, families of the patients still generally prefer to receive the information first. They can then more or less filter the information to the patient. Their often-cited reasons for this include fear that the truth will cause the patient to lose hope, they need to protect the patient from bad news, and a strong religious belief.[36] However, effective communication about terminal prognosis allows patients and families to have a sense of control and purpose and gives a basis for a realistic hope.[37] A parallel to this is the parents' self-assumed duty to protect their child from knowing about a terminal prognosis. To carry out this family obligation, relatives should create a caring environment in which the patient does not have any unnecessary psychological burdens. Conflict occurs when the beliefs and wishes of family members differ from those of the patient, the clinical team members, or both. If the patient desires and is capable of understanding full disclosure, the ethical challenge for the physician is whether to respect the patient's wishes or to follow the cultural views of the family members, which may be different. The focus needs to be the quality of life of the patient,[38] and among the team's responsibilities is helping the family to understand the patient's need for information and help them to redefine hope so that it can prevail with a shift in content when life comes to an end.[39–41] And from a lonely patient's point of view: the new-coming seriously ill asylum seeker without relatives who wonder who will take care of his or her body after death. Will he or she become a burden and for whom? Is there anyone to trust?

Different cultures can also result in different symptoms and problems being interpreted differently. Comparing people from the Black Caribbean and white British-born communities, Koffman et al. found that although people from both groups identified pain as a *challenge* that needed to be mastered by the individual, other meanings differed. In particular, two further meanings of pain emerged from Black Caribbean patients' accounts: pain as a *test of faith* that referred to confirmation and strengthening of religious belief and pain as a *punishment* that was associated with wrongdoing. These meanings influenced the extent patients were able to accommodate their distress, suggesting a role for understanding the patient's cultural interpretation of pain.[42]

On the other hand, structures of social support offered in some communities and cultures may be particularly enhanced, or in other societies more limited.[43] And other aspects of preferences, for example the wish to be cared for at home and with the family may be more similar between communities.[44] These findings support the need for palliative care to make individualized assessments, rather than making too many cultural assumptions.

DIFFERENCES IN VIEWS WITHIN THE PROFESSIONAL CARING TEAM AND BETWEEN THE TEAM AND THE PATIENT AND FAMILY

Patients' needs may be expressed by themselves, by a family member, by another significant person (e.g., a religious leader or a friend), or by a member of staff. The medical, psychosocial, and spiritual needs must be recognized by the team and be thoroughly discussed. Frustration may occur in the team when views of the patient, family, significant other, and team differ with regard to acceptance of treatment, for example, of pain and other symptoms. Perceptions of the ethical challenges involved may differ and there may be difficulty in communication about the problems. The challenge is to understand each other's perceptions of the problem. If successful collaboration based on shared trust is to be achieved, which will include the participation and empowerment of patients and their families in decision making, the caring team needs to be sensitive to the unique values of each patient, be empathetic, and have the ability to communicate.

Patients and families may be used to a hierarchical healthcare system and may therefore have difficulties dealing with the democratic values of the palliative care team approach. Some male patients may get a feeling of degradation if seen by a female doctor and vice versa, for example, a female patient being seen by a male gynecologist.[45] Another issue can be the age of the doctor. Older patients may be critical of younger doctors and the doctors may have to demonstrate the required knowledge in order to be trusted. Furthermore, the patient may be anxious and feel fear by meeting a staff with a different sex or ethnic background. Some may want to stay in the hospital not to feel abandoned by healthcare while others prefer to stay at home for the last days of life and also to die there.

Access to a professional interpreter is an important right of patients. There may be some resistance on the part of the family members, who prefer to do the translation themselves. A professional interpreter can draw attention to unexpressed signals that may give important information to the staff, for example: Does the patient understand the questions? How does the patient formulate the answers? Are the answers direct? However, patients may be unwilling to talk about delicate matters through a professional interpreter, even when the interpreter is from the same country, region, or ethnic group as the patient. In spite of the fact that the interpreter will give assurance about professional secrecy, the patient or the family may not be fully trustful. The personal attitude and professionalism

Box 16.3 Issues causing moral distress in transcultural palliative care

- Communication: Breaking bad news; role of interpreter, patient/family, different team members
- Uncertainty: Role of doctor, role of medical treatment, *false hope*
- Scarce resources: Setting priorities for staff, medicine, hospice/hospital beds
- Competing values and hierarchical processes: Whose values and beliefs are the focus?

of the interpreter have a large influence on their ability to communicate and facilitate the meeting and professional supervision may sometimes be needed.[46–48]

Communication problems, hierarchical processes, uncertainty, cultural issues, scarce resources including staff and time limitation, and competing values are the usual causes for moral dilemmas in healthcare. Physicians and nurses responsible for making medical decisions in end-of-life care can experience moral distress. Every team will have different needs and difficulties when encountering suffering and trying to make the best possible decisions and handling the situation.[49] Some of these dilemmas are listed in Box 16.3.

RELIGION

The religious map in many countries has changed during the last decades. There is a profane wind in several countries and religious rites and traditions are getting less important. And yet traditional Christian values may still be dominant in that same society. Another large change is the growing number of Muslims, making Islam an important religion in several Western countries. Likewise, due to refugee immigration many Catholics and orthodox Christians have gone to the Lutheran countries of northern Europe. This broad map of patients' beliefs is just a background to the individual beliefs among healthcare staff who always have to respectfully meet the needs of their patients.

How a patient identifies himself or herself in terms of religious belief usually affects their perceptions of health and healthcare up to the end of their lives. Grief is influenced by the cultural meaning that every culture lends to death and loss.[25] The many different death rituals sometimes have a gender implication. For example, it is the Muslim norm that members of the same gender wash the deceased body.[50] A common spiritual belief in some religions is that the body must be as intact and unblemished as possible to facilitate the spirit's course through subsequent incarnations or rest. Box 16.4 gives a checklist of important culturally or religiously dependent practices and rituals.

With regard to the immediate handling of the body after death, health professionals need to respect the wishes and,

Box 16.4 Checklist of questions concerning cultural and religious practices and rituals (Individual preferences and concerns should always be considered.)

- *Fasting*: Christmas, before Easter, Ramadan, before funeral, fluids only

- *Dietary practices*: Vegetarian, flesh, meat, shellfish, no fermented, alcohol, kosher

- *Treatment*: Patient versus family, staff of same sex, no handshake, alternative treatment or approach, traditional medicine, shamanism

- *Professional interpreter*: Same sex, same religion, local dialect, trust

- *Autopsy*: Different levels of restriction, no organs taken

- *The dead body*: Rituals, washing, dressing, same sex, cremation, burial, time constraints, bury in home country or host country

if possible beforehand, gather information from relatives and significant others who the patient trust, such as a religious representative concerning restrictions on who (i.e., gender) will close the eyes and mouth of the deceased adult patient, straighten the legs, and, for example, for a Muslim patient, put the face and feet in a specific direction, taking into consideration the location of Mecca.[51] In addition, washing and shrouding procedures may also be related to religion and customs regarding death. If the patient had no relatives, usually the religious community will arrange the prescribed rituals if desired.

Organ transplantation, although uncommon in palliative oncology care situations, is another issue that may not be allowed due to religious beliefs and therefore it is always of importance that the family or a significant other of the deceased patient is given the information in a sensitive manner and accurately with due respect, that is, the family has a choice. In several religions, there is a custom to bury the deceased as soon as possible and cremation is usually avoided, for example, in Judaism and Islam.[46,52] This may become a problem if death occurs during a holiday in a foreign country, giving rise to anxiety among the relatives. Under such circumstances, a rapid release of the dead body prevents unnecessary and prolonged distress to the bereaved family and friends.[47] In Islam, as a sign of respect for the deceased, the grieving relatives will not eat until the funeral. In Islam, the woman's role is to mourn and the husband's duty is to protect his wife.

Bereavement is the objective state of having lost an important, significant person. Grief, on the other hand, is the emotional reaction following bereavement. Mourning is the behavioral reaction; reflections that a society expects will follow on bereavement. Family members may have more or less appropriate networks for support and sharing during the care and mourning process. An example of a supportive network is

the Jewish practice of *shiva*. The bereaved family stays at home for some days after the death. Family and friends bring food and help with the necessities of life. Such support may enhance the healing process for the family members.

Specific spiritual care recommendations, for example, for those from the Black Caribbean community, have been developed from empirical research. The report shows examples of good practice in spiritual care, including spiritual (rather than only religious) assessment, potential tools to aid this assessment, and the availably of appropriate support, including faith leads, patient support groups, counseling, and nonverbal therapies. It also considers in more detail the role of spiritual providers and their need for support. While these recommendations are focused on the Black Caribbean community, many are relevant to palliative and supportive care generally.[53]

VULNERABLE INDIVIDUALS

Asylum seekers and refugees with a past history of trauma are displaced from their homelands to new environments. It is hard to die as a stranger in a strange land. These patients have often lost their past and old ways of life, their friends, and their own people. So much is destroyed by war and, with the onset of palliative care, much of this will never be regained. To settle in the new host country, refugees need to make many changes, and old ways are not always helpful in the event of advanced disease. A life-threatening disease is likely to bring back suppressed memories of atrocities and of other terrible events. Unresolved traumatic life events may evolve into reactions of a psychiatric nature, such as psychoses, which need to be distinguished from the development of actual psychiatric disease and from expected reactions to trauma and crisis. Postmigration stress in refugee men in Sweden has been related to an increased risk for mortality in cardiovascular disease and of external causes.[54]

Survivors of the holocaust or concentration camps from the Second World War may have severe difficulties in coping at the end of life and may even develop psychotic symptoms. Also, dying prisoners who are confined or are undocumented migrants or who are not permitted to spend their last days in a hospice outside the prison need special attention. It is a challenge to bring competent palliative care to dying prisoners.[55]

It is a challenge in communication having to tell a pregnant mother from an ethnic minority, who is infected with HIV/AIDS, that she is at great risk of delivering a baby with life-limiting illness. With regard to the loss of a child, mourning is again related to culture and religious customs. Empowerment of the parents including psychological and spiritual support is of importance but is often neglected to prevent unnecessary suffering.[56] For example, an Islamic family may be reminded that children are innocent and pure and as such assured paradise.[57]

The cultural diversity among patients, family members, and staff is part of the modern European society. This gives rise to several challenges for all parties involved but is also a chance to enrichment on a personal level and to a deeper understanding of basic human values. There is a need for cultural awareness, self-knowledge, and cultural competence and communication skills in the palliative care team. Particularly since opposing ethical values and cultural norms can give rise to moral distress or conflict, transcultural assessment should be made following a proposed structural model. Quality indicators need to be developed and used. Research on almost all aspects of palliative care in this context should be given priority in order to increase the knowledge base and to include relevant transcultural aspects of palliative care in education and training for all staff categories.

Key learning points

- Transcultural aspects need to be included in palliative care.

- Cultural awareness, self-knowledge, and cultural competence are necessary tools for the palliative care team.

- Opposing ethical values and cultural norms may give rise to moral distress or conflict.

- Communication difficulties between staff, patient, and family or within the professional caring team need to be resolved.

- Transcultural assessment should be made following a proposed structural model.

- Transcultural aspects of palliative care should be included in education and training.

REFERENCES

1   Jensen R. Cross-cultural perspectives in palliative care. *J Pain Palliat Care Pharmacother* 2003; 17: 223–229.

2   Núñez Olarte JM, Guillén DG. Cultural issues and ethical dilemmas in palliative and end-of-life care in Spain. *Cancer Control* 2001; 8: 46–54.

3   Voltz R, Akabayashi A, Reese C et al. Organization and patients' perception of palliative care: A crosscultural comparison. *Palliat Med* 1997; 11: 351–357.

4   Clark D. The International Observatory on End of Life Care: A new initiative to support palliative care development around the world. *J Pain Palliat Care Pharmacother* 2003; 17: 231–238.

5   Clark, D. From margins to centre: A review of the history of palliative care in cancer. *Lancet Oncol* 2007; 8(5): 430–438.

6   Rajagopal MR, Venkateswaran C. Palliative care in India: Successes and limitations. *J Pain Palliat Care Pharmacother* 2003; 17: 121–128.

7   Harding R, Powell RA, Downing J et al. Generating an African palliative care evidence base: The context, need, challenges, and strategies. *J Pain Symptom Manage* 2008 September; 36(3): 304–309.

8   World Health Organization. *Cancer, Pain Relief and Palliative Care. Report of a WHO Expert Committee*. Geneva, Switzerland: World Health Organization, 1990.

9   World Health Organization. *National Cancer Control Programmes: Policies and Managerial Guidelines*, 2nd edn. Geneva, Switzerland: World Helath Organization, 2002.

10 Davis E, Higginson IJ, eds. *The Solid Facts. Palliative Care*. Copenhagen, Denmark: World Health Organization, Europe Region, 2004.

11 Somerville J. The paradox of_palliative care_nursing across cultural boundaries. *Int J Palliat Nurs* 2007; 13(12): 580–587. [Erratum in: *Int J Palliat Nurs* 2008 (1): 48.]

12 Clark D. Cultural considerations in planning palliative care and end of life care. *Palliat Med* 2012; 26(3): 195–196.

13 Gunaratnam Y. Intercultural palliative care: Do we need cultural competence? *Int J Palliat Nurs* 2007; 10: 470–477.

14 Lunn JS. Spiritual care in a multi-religious context. *J Pain Palliat Care Pharmacother* 2003; 17: 153–166.

15 Diver F, Molassiotis A, Weeks L. The palliative care needs of ethnic minority patients attending day-care centre: A qualitative study. *Int J Palliat Nurs* 2003; 9: 389–396.

16 Calanzani N, Koffman J, Higginson IJ. *Palliative and End of Life Care for Black, Asian and Minority Ethnic Groups in the UK*. London, U.K.: Marie Curie Cancer Care, 2013.

17 Abdullah SN. Towards an individualized client's care: Implication for education. The transcultural approach. *J Adv Nurs* 1995; 22: 715–720.

18 Odigie VI, Yusufu LM, Dawotola DA et al. The mobile phone as a tool in improving cancer_care_in Nigeria. *Psychooncology* 2012; 21: 332–335.

19 Jack BA, Kirton JA, Birakurataki J, Merriman A. The personal value of being a palliative care Community Volunteer Worker in Uganda: A qualitative study. *Palliat Med* 2012; 26: 753–759.

20 Davis E, Higginson IJ, eds. *Better Palliative Care for Older People*. Copenhagen, Denmark: World Health Organization, Europe Region, 2004.

21 Mudavanhu D. The psychosocial impact of rural grandmothers caring for their grandchildren orphaned by HIV/AIDS. Master of Science in Psychology, University of South Africa 2008. 2008.

22 Kleinman A. Culture and depression. *N Engl J Med* 2004; 351: 951–953.

23 Williamson M, Harrison L. Providing culturally appropriate care: A literature review. *Int J Nurs Studies* 2010; 47: 761–769.

24 Mazanec P, Tyler M. How ethnicity, age, and spirituality affect decisions when death is imminent. *Home Healthcare Nurse* 2004; 22: 317–326.

25 Huang Y, Yates P, Prior D. Factors influencing oncology nurses' approaches to accommodating cultural needs in palliative care. *J Clin Nurs* 2009; 18: 3421–3429.

26 Mystakidou K, Tsilika E, Parpa E et al. A Greek perspective on concepts of death and expression of grief, with implications for practice. *Int J Palliat Nurs* 2003; 9: 534–537.

27 Blackhall LJ, Murphy ST, Frank G et al. Ethnicity and attitudes toward patient autonomy. *JAMA* 1995; 274: 820–825.

28 Kagawa-Singer M. The cultural context of death rituals and mourning practices. *Oncol Nurs Forum* 1998; 25: 1752–1756.

29 Surbone A. Information, truth and communication. For an interpretation of truth telling practices throughout the world. *Ann N Y Acad Sci* 1997; 809: 7–16.

30 Butow PN, Tattershall MH, Goldstein D. Communication with cancer patients in culturally diverse societies. *Ann N Y Acad Sci* 1997; 809: 317–329.

31 Surbone A. Persisting differences in truth telling throughout the world. *Support Care Cancer* 2004; 12: 143–146.

32 Cherny N. Controversies in oncologist-patient communication: A nuanced approach to autonomy, culture and paternalism. *Oncology* 2012; 26: 37–41.

33 Ghavamzadeh A, Bahar B. Communication with the cancer patient in Iran. *Ann N Y Acad Sci* 1997; 809: 261–265.

34 Younge D, Moreau P, Ezzat A, Gray A. Communication with cancer patients in Saudi Arabia. *Ann N Y Acad Sci* 1997; 809: 309–316.

35 Mystakidou K, Parpa E, Tsilika E et al. Cancer information disclosure in different cultural contexts. *Support Care Cancer* 2004; 12: 147–154.

36 Ozdogan M, Samur M, Sat Bozcuk H et al. 'Do not tell': What factors affect relatives' attitudes to honest disclosure of diagnoses to cancer patients? *Support Care Cancer* 2004; 12: 497–502.

37 Hu W, Chiu T, Chuang R, Chen C. Solving family-related barriers to truthfulness in cases of terminal cancer in Taiwan. *Cancer Nurs* 2002; 25: 486–492.

38 Bozuk H, Erdogan V, Eken C et al. Does awareness of diagnosis make any difference to quality of life? *Support Care Cancer* 2002; 10: 51–57.

39 Fallowfield L. Truth sometimes hurts but deceit hurts more. *Ann N Y Acad Sci* 1997; 809: 525–536.

40 Sabbioni MEE. Informing cancer patients: Whose truth matters? *Ann N Y Acad Sci* 1997; 809: 508–513.

41 Kersten C, Cameron M, Oldenburg J. Truth in hope and hope in truth. *J Palliat Med* 2012; 15(1): 128–129.

42 Koffman J, Morgan M, Edmonds P, Speck P, Higginson IJ. Cultural meanings of pain: A qualitative study of Black Caribbean and White British patients with advanced cancer. *Palliat Med* 2008; 22(4): 350–359.

43 Koffman J, Morgan M, Edmonds P, Speck P, Higginson IJ. 'The greatest thing in the world is the family': The meaning of social support among Black Caribbean and White British patients living with advanced cancer. *Psychooncology* 2012; 21(4): 400–408.

44 Koffman J, Higginson IJ. Dying to be home? Preferred location of death of first-generation black Caribbean and native-born white patients in the United Kingdom. *J Palliat Med* 2004; 7(5): 628–636.

45 Rizk DE, El-Zubeir MA, Al-Dhaheri AM et al. Determinants of women's choice of their obstetrician and gynecologist provider in the UAE. *Acta Obstet Gynecol Scand* 2005; 84: 48–53.

46 Phelan M, Parkman S. How to do it: Work with an interpreter. *BMJ* 1995; 311: 555–557.

47 Kaufert JM, Putsch RW, Lavallee M. Experience of aboriginal health interpreters in mediation of conflicting values in end-of-life decision making. *Int J Circumpolar Health* 1998; 57(Suppl. 1): 43–48.

48 Mancuso L. Providing culturally sensitive palliative care. *Nursing* 2009; 39(5): 50–53.

49 Oberle K, Hughes D. Doctors' and nurses' perceptions of ethical problems in end-of-life decisions. *J Adv Nurs* 2001; 33: 707–715.

50 Lawrence P, Rozmus C. Culturally sensitive care of the Muslim patient. *J Transcult Nurs* 2001; 12: 228–233.

51 Gatrad R, Sheikh A. Palliative care for Muslims and issues after death. *Int J Palliat Nurs* 2002; 8: 594–597.

52 Bonura D, Fender M, Roesler M, Pacquiao D. Culturally congruent end-of-life care for Jewish patients and their families. *J Transcult Nurs* 2001; 12: 211–220.

53 Selman L, Harding R, Speck P et al. *Spiritual Care Recommendations for People from Black and Minority Ethnic (BME) Groups Receiving Palliative Care in the UK*. London, U.K.: Cicely Saunders Institute, 2010. http://www.csi.kcl.ac.uk/spiritual-care.html, access date June 2014.

54 Hollander A-C, Bruve D, Ekberg J et al. Longitudinal study of mortality among refugees in Sweden. *Int J Epidemiol* 2012; 41(4): 1153–61.

55 Lum K. Palliative care behind bars: The New Zealand prison hospice experience. *J Pain Palliat Care Pharmacother* 2003; 17: 131–138.

56 Davies B, Brenner P, Orloff S et al. Addressing spirituality in pediatric hospice and palliative care. *J Palliat Care* 2002; 18: 59–67.

57 Tarazi N. *The Child in Islam*. Bloomington, IN: ATP, 1995, pp. 84–87.

17

Palliative care: Global situation and initiatives

LILIANA DE LIMA

GLOBAL SITUATION

The World Health Organization (WHO) estimates that 55 million deaths occurred worldwide in 2011. Noncommunicable diseases (NCDs) were responsible for two-thirds of all deaths globally in that year, up from 60% in 2000. The four main NCDs are cardiovascular diseases, cancers, diabetes, and chronic lung diseases. In terms of number of deaths, 26 million (nearly 80%) of the 36 million of global NCD deaths in 2011 occurred in low- and middle-income countries. In terms of proportion of deaths that are due to NCDs, high-income countries have the highest proportion—87% of all deaths were caused by NCDs—followed by upper- to middle-income countries (81%). The proportions are lower in low-income countries (36%) and lower- to middle-income countries (56%). According to the data, the main causes of the total mortality for that year were the following [1]:

- Noncommunicable conditions, including cancers and cardiovascular diseases: 58.5%
- Communicable diseases, including AIDS, maternal and perinatal conditions, and nutritional deficiencies: 32.5%
- Intentional and unintentional injuries: 9%

In high-income countries, more than two-thirds of all people live beyond the age of 70 and predominantly die of chronic diseases: cardiovascular disease, chronic obstructive lung disease, cancers, diabetes, or dementia. Lung infection remains the only leading infectious cause of death. In middle-income countries, nearly half of all people live to the age of 70 and chronic diseases are the major killers, just as they are in high-income countries. Unlike in high-income countries, however, tuberculosis, HIV/AIDS, and road traffic accidents also are leading causes of death. In low-income countries, less than one in five of all people reach the age of 70, and more than a third of all deaths are among children under 15. People predominantly die of infectious diseases: lung infections, diarrheal diseases, HIV/AIDS, tuberculosis, and malaria. Complications of pregnancy and childbirth together continue to be the leading causes of death, claiming the lives of both infants and mothers.

In the last decade, infectious diseases such as malaria, dengue, tuberculosis, and cholera have caused over one-quarter of the cumulative deaths in developing nations. In addition, approximately 5% of the adult population is infected with the HIV virus in sub-Saharan Africa, and global AIDS deaths totaled 1.7 million during 2011 [2]. Cancer is among the major noncommunicable causes of death worldwide and accounted for 12.6% of the total deaths in 2011 [1]. The International Agency for Research on Cancer (IARC) projects that global cancer rates will increase by 50% from 10 million new cases worldwide in 2000 to 15 million new cases in 2020, primarily due to the aging of population and increases in smoking. Fifty percent of the world's new cancer cases and deaths occur in developing nations and approximately 80% of these cancer patients are already incurable at the time of diagnosis.

ACCESS TO PALLIATIVE CARE

Palliative care includes the management of symptoms and provision of spiritual and psychosocial support to patients and their families from the moment of diagnosis throughout the course of the disease. Palliative care can be provided simply and inexpensively in tertiary care facilities, community health centers, and at home. However, access to pain relief and palliative care services is often limited, even in developed countries due to a lack of political will, insufficient information and education, and overly restrictive laws and regulations on the use of opioids.

In 2006, the Worldwide Palliative Care Alliance (WPCA) commissioned a mapping project of the development of palliative care in the world. This resulted in a global report published in 2008 on palliative care development using four different levels based on the integration of palliative care services [3]. A new, updated, and more comprehensive report has recently been published that indicates that since the 2008 publication, there has been an increase in the number of countries of the world that have established one or more hospice or palliative care services. However, a slight increase has occurred in the total number of countries actively engaged in either delivering a hospice–palliative care service or developing the framework within which such a service can be delivered. Since 2006, a total of 21 countries (9%) moved from Groups 1 or 2 (no known activity/capacity building) into Groups 3 or 4 (some form of palliative care provision) [4].

ACCESS TO PAIN TREATMENT

For several years, morphine consumption has been used as an indicator of adequate access to pain relief, one of the cornerstones of palliative care. In 1986, the WHO and its Expert Committee on Cancer Pain Relief and Active Supportive Care developed the *WHO Analgesic Ladder* [5] for the relief of cancer pain. The method relies on the permanent availability of opioid analgesics, including morphine and codeine. The *WHO Ladder* has been widely disseminated throughout the world. Still, opioid analgesics are insufficiently available, especially in developing countries, and prescription of morphine is limited to a small percentage of physicians and is unavailable in many countries of the world. In recent years, as the number of opioid medications and formulations and the consumption of other opioids for the treatment of pain increased in these countries, there has been a tendency to monitor the consumption of all opioids, reported in morphine equivalence, as a more accurate measure of access to pain treatment. In that same trend, the recent WHO Action Plan for the Global Strategy for the Prevention and Control of Non-Communicable Diseases [6] includes a palliative care indicator, which is "Access to palliative care assessed by morphine-equivalent consumption of strong opioid analgesics (excluding methadone) per death from cancer." This indicator will require countries to monitor and report on a palliative care indicator based on the consumption of several opioids and not just morphine. The indicator has some limitations [7] but the international palliative care community welcomes the inclusion of a palliative care indicator in the global framework for the control, prevention, and treatment of NCDs.

The International Narcotics Control Board (INCB) collects the consumption data yearly from government reports [8] of all controlled medications, including morphine and other opioids. Good access to pain management is rather the exception than the rule: 5.5 billion people (83% of the world's population) live in countries with low to nonexistent access, 250 million (4%) have moderate access, and only 460 million people (7%) have adequate access [9]. According to Seya et al. [10], the world used 231 tons of morphine equivalents but the amount needed to meet the needs of all patients in pain would be over 1000 tons. Narcotic drugs such as morphine, fentanyl, and oxycodone are opioid analgesics effective for the treatment of moderate and severe pain. Data from 2009 show that more than 90% of the global consumption of these opioid analgesics occurred in Australia, Canada, New Zealand, the United States, and several European countries. This means that their availability was very limited in many countries and in entire regions. Although medical science has the capacity to provide relief for most forms of moderate to severe pain, over 80% of the world

population will have insufficient analgesia or no analgesia at all, if they suffer from such pain [11]. A recent report on availability and access to opioids for cancer pain treatment by the European Society for Medical Oncology (ESMO) in alliance with the European Association for Palliative Care (EAPC) reached similar conclusions [12].

In a study of advanced cancer care in Latin America, over 80% of the respondents reported either good or excellent availability of the main nonopioid analgesics and adjuvants in their practice settings. In contrast, the availability of both short- and long-acting opioid analgesics varied greatly across nations, by practice settings, and by specific medication [13]. The great majority of the countries reported difficulties in access and excessively strict regulations on the use of controlled substances.

The identification of a country's actual requirements for internationally controlled substances is a critical step in ensuring availability of opioids, and its importance was reiterated by the Commission on Narcotic Drugs in its resolution 54/6 [14] on promoting adequate availability of internationally controlled narcotic drugs and psychotropic substances for medical and scientific purposes while preventing their diversion and abuse. In the resolution, the commission encouraged INCB to continue its efforts, in cooperation with the WHO to develop guidelines to assist member states in estimating their medical and scientific requirements for internationally controlled narcotic drugs and psychotropic substances. In 2012, INCB and WHO published a set of guidelines to help governments establish the adequate estimate of controlled substances to meet the demand for medical and scientific needs [15].

In 2010, the EAPC in alliance with WHO developed the Access to Opioid Medication in Europe (ATOME) project, which aims to improve access to opioids across the region, particularly in Eastern Europe. By May 2012, key milestones of the ATOME project were successfully completed, such as the publication of the revised WHO policy guidelines *Ensuring Balance in National Policies on Controlled Substances* [16]. The guidelines provide guidance on policies and legislation with regard to availability, accessibility, affordability, and control of medicines regulated under the international drug control conventions to improve access to legitimate use while preventing diversion.

In a recent development that has global implications, the WHO included a list of essential medicines in pain and palliative care in the WHO Model List of Essential Medicines. The 18th edition of the model list includes morphine in all its available formulations for the management of pain, with oxycodone and hydromorphone as substitutes [17].

PALLIATIVE CARE AS A HUMAN RIGHT

Palliative care as a human right under the right to health

The right to health and freedom from torture and inhumane and degrading treatment is a fundamental part of our human rights and of our understanding of a life in dignity [18].

Internationally, it was first articulated in the 1946 Constitution of the WHO, whose preamble defines health as "a state of complete physical, mental and social well-being and not merely the absence of disease or infirmity" [19]. The preamble further states that "the enjoyment of the highest attainable standard of health is one of the fundamental rights of every human being without distinction of race, religion, political belief, economic or social condition."

In human rights instruments, the authoritative statement of the right to the highest attainable standard of physical and mental health can be found under article 12 in the 1966 International Covenant on Economic, Social and Cultural Rights (ICESCR) [20]:

> Article 12.1: The State Parties to the present Covenant recognize the right of everyone to the enjoyment of the highest attainable standard of physical and mental health.
>
> 2. The steps to be taken...to achieve the full realization of this right shall include those necessary for:
>
> ...d) The creation of conditions which would assure to all medical service and medical attention in the event of sickness.

In 2000, the committee overseeing the ICESCR issued a general comment on the right to health, stating what it saw as the *core obligations* of all signatory nations, irrespective of resources. They include obligations to ensure access to health facilities, goods, and services on a nondiscriminatory basis, to provide essential drugs as defined by the WHO, and to adopt and implement a national public health strategy. Interpreting this comment in the context of palliative care, this would oblige nations to ensure a universal access to services, the provision of basic medications for symptom control and terminal care, and the adoption and implementation of national palliative care policies [21]. In addition, the right to health and to treatment is also articulated in other international conventions [22]. As per these conventions, countries are obliged to take steps to ensure that patients have access to palliative care and pain treatment.

Most countries have acceded to at least one global or regional covenant or treaty confirming the right to health. After years of international discussions on human rights, many governments are moving towards practical implementation of their commitments. However, as indicated in the previous sections, the vast majority of patients with advanced, life-threatening conditions in the world are neglected by their health-care systems and providers. Given that many member states do not allocate any funds for palliative care in their national health budgets, palliative care services are not available. The national health systems do not have the facilities and the health-care providers do not have the knowledge nor skills to care for patients with advanced, life-threatening conditions, and whatever little palliative care patients can get is mostly provided only through expensive private, specialized consultation services or through clinics funded by charities. After a poor prognosis, many patients are sent home with *you are incurable and there is nothing else we can do for you.* Patients are neglected and abandoned in terrible situations, only because they do not respond to curative treatments any more.

It is a form of discrimination and denial of basic human right. In addition, in many countries, inexpensive opioids such as oral morphine are not available, while more expensive formulations and medications are. To raise awareness about this problem, Pallium India, the International Association for Hospice and Palliative Care (IAHPC), and the Pain and Policy Studies Group/the WHO Collaborating Center at the University of Wisconsin released the Morphine Manifesto [23] calling for an end to the unethical practice of promoting access to expensive opioid analgesics without also making available low-cost immediate-release oral morphine.

The right to palliative care and pain relief also implicates freedom from torture and cruel, inhuman, and degrading treatment. The UN Special Rapporteur on Torture, and Other Cruel, Inhuman or Degrading Treatment or Punishment has stated that "the de facto denial of access to pain relief, if it causes severe pain and suffering, constitutes cruel, inhuman or degrading treatment or punishment" [24]. In its recent report, the special rapporteur brought attention to critical obstacles that "unnecessarily impede access to morphine and adversely affect its availability" and issued the following recommendations to government:

- Adopt a human rights–based approach to drug control as a matter of priority to prevent the continuing violations of rights. Ensure that national drug control laws recognize the indispensable nature of narcotic and psychotropic drugs for the relief of pain and suffering; review national legislation and administrative procedures to guarantee adequate availability of those medicines for legitimate medical uses.
- Ensure full access to palliative care and overcome current regulatory, educational and attitudinal obstacles that restrict availability to essential palliative care medications, especially oral morphine. States should devise and implement policies that promote widespread understanding about the therapeutic usefulness of controlled substances and their rational use.
- Develop and integrate palliative care into the public health system by including it in all national health plans and policies, curricula and training programs and developing the necessary standards, guidelines and clinical protocols [18].

Based on the declarations, reports, and recommendations from international organizations [23,25–31] and human rights organizations [32–34], the palliative care obligations that member states have can be summarized as follows:

1. The creation and implementation of palliative care policies
2. Equity of access to services, without discrimination
3. Availability and affordability of essential medications, including opioids (especially oral solid immediate-release morphine)
4. The provision of palliative care at all levels of health care
5. The integration of palliative care education at all levels of the learning continuum from informal caregivers to health professionals

GLOBAL INITIATIVES AND RESOURCES

IAHPC: IAHPC is a global nonprofit, charity organization dedicated to the promotion and development of palliative care. The mission of IAHPC is to collaborate and work to improve the quality of life of patients with advanced life-threatening conditions and their families, by advancing hospice and palliative care programs, education, research, and favorable policies around the world. IAHPC focuses on advancing palliative care programs, education, research, and policies to improve the care provided to patients around the world. IAHPC supports programs, projects, and individuals around the world, especially in developing countries in Africa, Eastern Europe, Asia, and Latin America and on the identification of the essential components for palliative care provision, including a list of Essential Medicines for Palliative Care [35], a list of Essential Practices in Palliative Care [36], and an Opioid Essential Prescription Package [37]. More information at www.hospicecare.com.

International Children's Palliative Care Network (ICPCN): The ICPCN is a worldwide network of individuals and agencies working with children and young people with life-limiting and life-threatening conditions. The mission of ICPCN is to achieve the best quality of life and care for children and young people with life-limiting conditions, their families, and their carers worldwide, by raising awareness of children's palliative care, lobbying for the global development of children's palliative care services, and sharing expertise, skills, and knowledge. More information at http://www.icpcn.org/.

International Observatory on End of Life Care: The aim of the International Observatory on End of Life Care is to undertake high-quality research, clinical studies, evaluation, education, advocacy, and consultancy to improve palliative and end-of-life care for patients and family carers. More information at http://www.lancaster.ac.uk/shm/research/ioelc/.

International Palliative Care Family Carer Research Collaboration (IPCFRC): The purpose of the IPCFRC is to develop a strategic approach to palliative care research planning related to family carers of people requiring palliative care via establishing international partnerships and promoting information exchange. More information at http://centreforpallcare.org/index.php/research/ipcfcrc/.

International Palliative Care Leadership Development Initiative (LDI): The International Palliative Care LDI aims to grow global leaders and advance palliative care through skill building and mentorship of emerging palliative care physician leaders from around the world, including Africa, Central Asia, Eastern Europe, Latin America, the Middle East, and Southeast Asia. This initiative started at the Institute for Palliative Medicine at San Diego Hospice and is now housed in Ohio Health.

International Primary Palliative Care Network (IPPCN): The aim of IPPCN is to provide collegiate support to like-minded individuals, who are committed to see palliative care practiced as a core part of comprehensive primary care practice. This involves advocating for improved recognition of the role of primary care in the delivery of palliative care. The group also aims to encourage primary palliative care researchers to present their work and to explore the possibilities of international collaboration. IPPCN recognizes the vast need for palliative care in developing countries and hopes to assist local practitioners in these areas to develop sustainable and effective services. More information at http://www.uq.edu.au/primarypallcare/.

WPCA: The WPCA is a global action network focusing exclusively on hospice and palliative care development worldwide. Its members are national and regional hospice and palliative care organizations and affiliate organizations supporting hospice and palliative care. Its mission is to foster, promote, and influence the delivery of affordable, quality palliative care. WPCA coordinates several programs and activities, including the World Hospice and Palliative Care Day (also known as World Day), a unified day of action to celebrate and support hospice and palliative care around the world [38]. The first World Day was celebrated on October 8, 2005, and over the years it has become an annual global event. Activities take place worldwide and a collective global voice comprising of individuals and associations to raise awareness and understanding of the need and importance of hospice and palliative care. Each year, a different topic is selected and a report is published on that topic, to accompany the celebration. WPCA also manages the international edition of ehospice, a globally run news and information resource. More information at http://www.thewpca.org/.

REGIONAL ORGANIZATIONS

In addition to the global initiatives described earlier, there are several regional palliative care organizations whose aim is to help advance palliative care in their corresponding countries. All of them have developed successful programs, activities, and tools for governments, providers, and caregivers:

African Palliative Care Association (APCA): APCA works collaboratively with existing and potential providers of palliative care services to help expand service provision, governments, and policymakers to ensure that the optimum policy and regulatory framework exists for the development of palliative care across Africa. More information at http://www.africanpalliativecare.org/.

Asia Pacific Hospice Network (APHN): The mission of APHN is to promote access to quality hospice and palliative care for all in the Asia Pacific region. More information in http://aphn.org/.

European Association for Palliative Care (EAPC): The aim of the EAPC is to promote palliative care in Europe and to act as a focus for all of those who work, or have an interest, in the field of palliative care at the scientific, clinical, and social levels. More information at http://www.eapcnet.eu/Home.aspx.

Latin American Association for Palliative Care (Asociacion Latinoamericana de Cuidados Paliativos—ALCP): The mission of ALCP is to promote the development of palliative care in Latin America and the Caribbean, through communication and integration of all those interested in improving the quality of life of patients with advanced life-threatening diseases and their families. More information at http://www.cuidadospaliativos.org/.

CONCLUSION

The development of palliative care in the world has been an increasing trend in the last few decades. This has been largely the result of the commitment of extraordinary individuals and the financial support provided by generous donors and organizations. Many patients are now benefiting of hospice and palliative care services in developed countries, but services in developing countries are scarce and very fragile and more is needed to guarantee their permanence and survival.

Education needs to be incorporated in the undergraduate medical and nursing curricula in order to guarantee the provision of services by a large body of health-care providers, especially in developing countries. Services and medications need to be subsidized for those who are unable to pay and should be incorporated in the public health-care systems and reimbursement plans for providers.

More studies are needed on the status of palliative and hospice care services in the world and should be the focus of future research projects. Many organizations such as the ones described in this chapter have done an enormous effort and have had a large impact in the development of palliative care globally.

REFERENCES

1 The World Health Organization. The top 10 causes of death Fact sheet N°310. 2013. Available in http://who.int/mediacentre/factsheets/fs310/en/index.html, (accessed August 29, 2013).
2 WHO. 2013. Global Health Observatory Data Repository. Data on the size of the HIV/AIDS epidemic: Data by WHO region. Available in http://apps.who.int/gho/data/node.main.619?lang=en, (accessed September 5, 2013).
3 Wright M, Wood J, Lynch T, Clark D. Mapping levels of palliative care development: A global view. *J Pain Symptom Manage* 2008;35:469–485.
4 Lynch T, Connor S, Clark D. Mapping levels of palliative care development: A global update. *J Pain Symptom Manage* June 2013;45(6):1094–1106.
5 World Health Organization. Cancer pain relief and palliative care: Report of a WHO Expert Committee. (Technical Report Series No. 804), Geneva, Switzerland: WHO, 1990.
6 WHO. Draft comprehensive global monitoring framework and targets for the prevention and control of noncommunicable diseases. p. 6. Version dated March 15, 2013. Available at http://apps.who.int/gb/ebwha/pdf_files/WHA66/A66_8-en.pdf, (accessed September 1, 2013).
7 De Lima L, Wenk R, Krakauer E et al. Global framework for noncommunicable diseases: How can we monitor palliative care? *J Palliat Med* 2013 March;16(3):226–229.
8 International Narcotics Control Board. Availability of opiates for medical needs. Special Report prepared pursuant to Economic and Social Council Resolutions 1990/31 and 1991/43. Vienna, Austria: INCB, 1996.
9 World Health Organization Access to Controlled Medications Programme. Improving access to medications controlled under international drug conventions. Briefing note. 2012. Available from http://www.who.int/medicines/areas/quality_safety/ACMP_BrNote_Genrl_EN_Apr2012.pdf, (accessed September 3, 2013).
10 Seya MJ, Gelders SF, Achara OU, Milani B, Scholten WK. A first comparison between the consumption of and the need for opioid analgesics at country, regional, and global levels. *J Pain Palliat Care Pharmacother* 2011;25:6–18.
11 INCB. 2011. Availability of internationally controlled drugs: Ensuring adequate access for medical and scientific purpose. Available in http://www.incb.org/documents/Publications/AnnualReports/AR2010/Supplement-AR10_availability_English.pdf, (accessed September 9, 2013).
12 Cherny NI, Baselga J, De Conno F, Radbruch L. Formulary availability and regulatory barriers to accessibility of opioids for cancer pain in Europe: A report from the ESMO/EAPC opioid policy initiative. *Ann Oncol* 2010;21:615–626.
13 Torres I, Wang XS, Palos G, Gning I, Jones P, De Lima L, Mendoza TR, Cleeland CS. Advanced cancer care in Latin America and the Caribbean: A survey of healthcare professionals. Presented at the *American Public Health Association Conference*, Atlanta, GA. October 22, 2002.
14 United Nations Economic and Social Council. Commission on Narcotic Drugs Fifty-third session. Resolution 54/6. Implementation of the international drug control treaties: international cooperation to ensure the availability of narcotic drugs and psychotropic substances for medical and scientific purposes while preventing their diversion. Available in http://www.unodc.org/documents/commissions/CND-Uploads/CND-53-RelatedFiles/ECN72010_L6Rev1EV1051780.pdf, (accessed August 29, 2013).
15 INCB. 2015. Guidelines on estimating requirements for substances under international control. Available in http://www.incb.org/documents/Narcotic-Drugs/Guidelines/estimating_requirements/NAR_Guide_on_Estimating_EN_Ebook.pdf, (accessed August 20, 2013).
16 WHO. 2011. Ensuring balance in national policies on controlled substances, Guidance for Availability and Accessibility for Controlled Medicines. Available in several languages in http://www.who.int/medicines/areas/quality_safety/guide_nocp_sanend/en/, (accessed September 6, 2013).
17 World Health Organization (WHO). Model list of essential medicines. 2013. Available in http://www.who.int/medicines/publications/essentialmedicines/18th_EML_Final_web_8Jul13.pdf, (accessed July 22, 2013).
18 Human Rights Council. 22nd session Report of the Special Rapporteur on torture and other cruel, inhuman or degrading treatment or punishment. Available in http://www.ohchr.org/Documents/HRBodies/HRCouncil/RegularSession/Session22/A.HRC.22.53_English.pdf, (accessed August 13, 2013).
19 WHO. Constitution of the World Health Organization (July 1946). Available in http://apps.who.int/gb/bd/PDF/bd47/EN/constitution-en.pdf, (accessed September 6, 2013).
20 United Nations. International Covenant on Economic, Social and Cultural Rights (1966), Article 12. NY: UN, December 1966.
21 United Nations. Committee on Economic, Social and Cultural Rights, General Comment 14, The right to the highest attainable standard of health (Twenty-second session, 2000), NY: U.N. Doc. E/C.12/2000/4 (2000).
22 Universal Declaration of Human Rights, Article 25; Article 12 of the Convention on the Elimination of All Forms of Discrimination against Women; Article 24 of the Convention on the Rights of the Child; and Article 5(e)(iv) of the Convention on the Elimination of All Forms of Racial Discrimination.

23 Pallium India. The Morphine Manifesto. Available in http://palliumindia. org/manifesto/, (accessed September 6, 2013).

24 Human Rights Council. Report of the Special Rapporteur on torture and other cruel, inhuman or degrading treatment or punishment, Manfred Nowak, A/HRC/10/44, January 14, 2009. para. 72. Available in: http://www2.ohchr.org/english/bodies/hrcouncil/docs/10session/A. HRC.10.44AEV.pdf, (accessed August 4, 2013),

25 The palliative care trainers declaration of cape town November 13, 2002. *J Palliat Med* June 2003;6(3):339–340.

26 The Korea Declaration. Report of the second global summit of national hospice and palliative care associations, Seoul, March 2005. Available in   http://www.coe.int/t/dg3/health/Source/KoreaDeclaration2005_ en.pdf, (accessed September 2, 2013).

27 IAHPC and WPCA. Joint declaration for the recognition of access to pain treatment and palliative care as human rights IAHPC and WPCA. Available in http://hospicecare.com/about-iahpc/contributions-to- palliative-care/human-rights/, (accessed on April 18, 2013).

28 World Medical Association. World medical association resolu- tion on access to adequate pain treatment. http://www.wma.net/ en/30publications/10policies/p2/index.html, (accessed on April 19, 2013).

29 Pogge T. Montréal Statement on the Human Right to Essential Medicines. *Camb Q Healthc Ethics.* 2007 Winter;16(1):97–108.

30 International Framework for Palliative Care, European School of Oncology. 2004. Available in http://www.ejcancer.com/article/S0959- 8049%2804%2900497-6/abstract, (accessed April 19, 2013).

31 Radbruch L, De Lima L, Lohmann D, Gwyther E, Payne S. The Prague Charter: Urging governments to relieve suffering and ensure the right to palliative care. *Palliat Med* 2013;27:101, doi: 10.1177/0269216312473058.

32 Human Rights Watch. Please do not make us suffer anymore: Access to pain treatment as a human right. 2009. Available in http://www. hrw.org/reports/2009/03/02/please-do-not-make-us-suffer-any-more, (accessed September 2, 2013).

33 Human Rights Watch. Global state of pain treatment: Access to medi- cines and palliative care. HRW: New York, 2011. Available in http:// www.hrw.org/reports/2011/06/01/global-state-pain-treatment-0, (accessed September 5, 2013).

34 International Federation of Health and Human Rights Organization (IFHRO). Position statement on access to adequate pain treatment. 2011. Available in http://www.ifhhro.org/news-a-events/212-position-statement-on-access- to-adequate-pain-treatment, (accessed September 8, 2013).

35 De Lima L, Krakauer E, Lorenz K, Praill D, MacDonald N, Doyle D. Ensuring palliative medicine availability: The development of the IAHPC list of essential medicines for palliative care. *J Pain Symptom Manage* 2007 May;33(5):521–526.

36 De Lima L, Bennett MI, Murray SA, Hudson P, Doyle D, Bruera E, Granda- Cameron C, Strasser F, Downing J, Wenk R. International Association for Hospice and Palliative Care (IAHPC) list of essential practices in pallia- tive care. *J Pain Palliat Care Pharmacother* 2012 June;26(2):118–122. doi: 10.3109/15360288.2012.680010.

37 Vignaroli E, Bennett MI, Nekolaichuk C, De Lima L, Wenk R, Ripamonti CI, Bruera E. Strategic pain management: The identification and devel- opment of the IAHPC opioid essential prescription package. *J Palliat Med* 2012 February;15(2):186–191. doi: 10.1089/jpm.2011.0296 [Epub 2011 Oct 20].

38 World Hospice and Palliative Care Day. Retrieved from the internet August 30, 2013. Available in http://www.worldday.org/, (accessed August 30, 2013).

PART 4

Education

18

Undergraduate education in palliative medicine

DOREEN ONESCHUK

INTRODUCTION

In many countries, the incidence of advanced cancer and advanced chronic disease is rising as the population ages. Educators and health sciences students are increasingly realizing the importance of the need for the development and expansion of undergraduate education in the field of palliative and end-of-life care. While many countries and universities have commenced or improved upon their palliative care undergraduate teaching over the past 5–10 years, inconsistencies, variability, and deficiencies in the quantity and quality of undergraduate palliative medicine education continue to exist.

The first section of this chapter provides an update on the status of undergraduate palliative medicine education in North America, Western Europe, Australia and New Zealand, Japan, and India. The second section discusses educational factors to consider when initiating or looking to improve upon undergraduate palliative medicine educational programs.

CANADA

Educating Future Physicians in Palliative and End-of-Life Care (EFPPEC), a 5-year national project co-hosted by the Canadian Hospice Palliative Care Association (CHPCA) and the Association of Faculties of Medicine of Canada (AFMC), was completed in 2008. The overall goal of this project was to ensure that "by the year 2008, all undergraduate medical students and residents at Canada's 17 medical schools will be receiving effective training in palliative and end-of-life care and will graduate with competencies in these areas." EFPPEC supported the development of consensus-based palliative and end-of-life care common competencies for undergraduate trainees in medicine. The project involved working with palliative and end-of-life educators (champions and opinion leaders) across the country that collaborated in the development, implementation, integration, and evaluation of the education programs. Local interprofessional teams of educators from various disciplines facilitated the introduction of the curricula based on identified common competencies. An evaluation of the project showed that the incidence of specific learning objectives increased over the course of the project such that more schools had integrated specific learning objectives related to the six competencies into their curricula by the end of the project than they had been doing so at the beginning. At the conclusion of the project, 14 of the 17 medical schools completed inventories describing their curricula, and 13 were using the EFPPEC competencies. Progress in implementing palliative and end-of-life care in curriculum development was progressing more in the preclerkship than in the clerkship, with less success with student and curriculum evaluation.[1]

A follow-up 2011 survey of the 17 Canadian universities found that 10 of the universities offer less than 10 hours of training in their medical school, 1 school offers between 10 and 20 hours, and 6 schools offer more than 20 hours of training. The mean and median numbers of hours for all 17 schools were 14 and 7, respectively, with a range of 0–56 hours (personal communication in an e-mail from Serge Daneault, MD, PhD, Soinspalliatifs, Hopital Notre-Dame, Centre Hospitalier de l'Universitede Montreal in June 2012).

Funded by Health Canada, the Canadian Association for Schools of Nursing, in association with the CHPCA, is piloting models for integrating new palliative care competencies[2] into existing curricula and accreditation standards to improve undergraduate nursing education. A national repository of teaching and learning resources on palliative and end-of-life competencies is also being developed.[3]

Social work competencies in palliative and end-of-life care were also developed to be used at all levels of training.[4] A consultation process involved validation of the competencies, identification of strategies to implement them in the workplace, and incorporation into curriculum of schools of social work. A third phase of the project involved development and evaluation of model curricula based on the competencies that can be used for undergraduate, postgraduate, and continuing professional development education. Education learning modules have also been developed (www.chpca.net).[5]

UNITED STATES

Since 1996, many national accrediting organizations including the Liaison Committee on Medical Education (LCME), the Accreditation Council for Graduate Medical Education (ACGME), the National Board of Medical Examiners (NBME), and the American Board of Internal Medicine (ABIM) have mandated palliative medicine curricula for medical schools. Systematic reviews of palliative medicine curricula in medical schools document diverse, nonstandardized formats to incorporate palliative medicine principles and evidence-based data into the preclinical years.[6–9] Despite the requirements of the LCME for end-of-life care, the training that most medical students receive in this realm varies widely, is often disjointed and sporadic, and can leave students feeling unprepared.[10]

In a 2008 written survey, a brief update of Dickinson's 2006 report,[7] to deans of all 128 medical schools in the United States coupled with information obtained from the Curriculum Management and Information Tool (CurrMIT) national database of the Association of American Medical Colleges, found that of the 47/128 (37%) responding schools, "palliative and hospice care" is a required course in 30% of responding medical schools and a required rotation in 19%; 15% offer an elective course and 29% an elective rotation; and 53% integrate this subject into a required course. Most schools favor integrating subject material rather than creating new courses devoted to palliative care. At the time of this survey, there were no established guidelines to define what is encompassed by palliative care training and no mandated objectives and competencies on which to base an audit of an institution's curriculum.[11]

A more recent survey, published in 2011, revealed that between 1975 and 2010, the overall offerings in death and dying increased so that 100% of U.S. medical schools, from 2000 onwards, offered something on death and dying. A multidisciplinary team approach continued over the 35 years of the study.[12]

A study published in September 2000 found that the majority of nurse respondents felt that end-of-life content was important to basic nursing. However, 71% of respondents said their pain management education was inadequate, 62% rated their overall content on end-of-life care as inadequate, and 59% rated their education of management of other symptoms as inadequate. This study also found that less than 35% of nurses rated their grief/bereavement and spiritual support to patients at the end-of-life as effective.[13,14] A survey of senior nursing students completed at a major university in the fall of 2001 revealed that less than 5% of students had an end-of-life experience during their schooling. Nursing leaders from both the City of Hope National Medical Center and the Association of American Colleges of Nursing developed a comprehensive nursing education curriculum known as End-of-Life Nursing Education Consortium (ELNEC) for nursing faculty.[15] The purpose of the ELNEC, a Robert Wood Johnson Foundation funded project (2000–2004), was to develop and implement a comprehensive national effort to improve end-of-life care by nurses through a joint collaboration between the American Association of College of Nursing (AACN) and the City of Hope Cancer Center. Data from a 1-year follow-up of five

conferences convened for undergraduate faculty in schools of nursing revealed significant outcomes in a report of implementation in the nursing curriculum including an increase in the amount of content, perceived effectiveness of new graduates and of faculty expertise in end-of-life care, and a broad dissemination of all modules geographically.[14] Another study found a positive effect on nursing student attitudes toward care of the dying following use of the ELNEC education package.[13]

A descriptive study in which all accredited schools and colleges of pharmacy in the United States were queried regarding their level of curricular commitment to end-of-life care found that of the 60 schools who responded, 62% indicated end-of-life care education was provided in a didactic format, and 58% indicated that end-of-life care experiential clerkships were available. These data indicate that over half of U.S. pharmacy students receive some exposure to end-of-life care education. However, due to the already strained course load on current curricula, it was felt that clinical clerkship devoted solely to end-of-life care may not be feasible for many pharmacy programs. Revising the content or experiences of current clerkships already required was presented as a possible solution.[16]

To better address the end-of-life training needs of practitioners and students, including the development of end-of-life curricula, social work educators have published competencies that include a course set of practice knowledge, skills, and values that are applicable in various settings.[17,18]

UNITED KINGDOM

The Association for Palliative Medicine (APM) produced a previous undergraduate palliative medicine syllabus in 1992. The aim of this syllabus was to set standards in palliative medicine for undergraduate and postgraduate doctors. It is unclear how much this curriculum has been used because there is no published work on the use of the undergraduate document. All medical schools in the United Kingdom teach palliative medicine, but the amount and content is variable. The availability of academic departments or appropriately qualified academic staff varies considerably across the country.

A new APM consensus syllabus has been established that includes the following: basic principles, physical care, psychosocial care, cultural, language, religious and spiritual issues, ethics, and legal frameworks. Learning outcomes are categorized as essential or desirable. There is sufficient flexibility to allow all medical schools to ensure that their students achieve the essential learning outcomes by the time they graduate. The APM has subsequently endorsed the syllabus as a reference document to help in the development of undergraduate palliative medicine.[19]

The UK Department of Health has also recently highlighted the need to educate all health-care professionals to try and improve end-of-life care, and the third edition of the General Medical Council's *Tomorrow's Doctors* reiterates the need for students to be prepared to care for patients at the end of life.[20,21]

Nursing diploma students received a mean of 8 hours and degree students 12 hours of teaching and palliative care compared to the mean of 20 hours teaching offered to undergraduate medical students in the United Kingdom. Teaching was mainly theoretical and rarely formally assessed. Tutors identified the lack of suitably skilled staff to teach palliative care and a shortage of placement for nursing students within palliative care settings.[22,23]

EUROPE

In 2007, the European Association for Palliative Care Task Force on Medical Education published a Curriculum in Palliative Care for Undergraduate Medical Education (www.eapcnet.eu). However, a lack of palliative care education and training opportunities is the most frequently reported barrier to the development of palliative care in Western Europe. In Finland, Austria, Belgium, Greece, France, Italy, Norway, Luxemburg, and Turkey, it is reported that an insufficient focus on palliative care within both undergraduate and postgraduate medical education results in a lack of university curricula and training programs for health-care professionals and medical students. In Germany, it is reported that palliative care is not integrated into the obligatory syllabus for medical or nursing students, and the majority of medical universities do not have their own university palliative care unit.[22] It remained the responsibility of medical schools to offer courses in palliative care, and only a few of the 35 medical schools in Germany included mandatory courses. However, as a consequence of changes in the Medical Licensure Act of 2009, palliative care was required to become a mandatory part of undergraduate medical education for all schools in Germany by spring 2013.[24] Lack of palliative care education and training programs is reported as resulting in a dearth of research at the national level within Israel and also Iceland.[22] In Switzerland, the average number of mandatory hours of palliative care education is 10 hours. Most of the education occurs before the clinical years, and there are no mandatory clinical rotations. Three schools offer optional clinical rotations, but these are poorly attended. Although a number of domains are covered, ethics-related content predominates. Communication related to palliative care is largely limited to "breaking bad news." In two of the schools, the teaching is done primarily by palliative care physicians and nurses. In the others, it is done mostly by educators and other clinical specialties and ethics.[25] A survey administered to students during 2006–2008 found in Spain and Italy that some universities teach palliative care as part of other courses; in very few, it is taught as an elective course, but medical programs do not contain a required course on this subject.[26]

ARGENTINA

In Argentina, from approximately 2007, education on palliative care had not been made part of the undergraduate curriculum.[26] Nursing and medical undergraduate students at nursing and medicine schools in Buenos Aires and surrounding areas had a highly positive attitude toward terminally ill patients, even though some of them referred to the relationship

as arduous and in some cases they tended to avoid emotional involvement because they did not feel well trained. However, students unanimously were of the opinion that teaching about caring of terminally ill patients should be included in the curricula and that they would be well disposed to receive it.[27]

AUSTRALIA AND NEW ZEALAND

In 1997, the majority of schools in Australia endorsed the undergraduate medical palliative care curriculum of the Australia and New Zealand Society of Palliative Medicine (ANZSPM). An objective of the ANZSPM curriculum was to help standardize the coverage of core topics and address the processes of learning that might be adopted. A further objective was to "to promote a learning experience which permits students to develop the attitude, knowledge, and skill base required for them to participate in effective and compassionate palliative care."[28]

Subsequently, the Palliative Care Curriculum for Undergraduates project (PCC4U) (www.pcc4u.org) was developed. This is an initiative of the Australian Government Department of Health and Ageing through the National Palliative Care Program. There was an extension phase from July 2010 to June 2011 building on the achievements of previous phases that included promoting and sustaining the inclusion in all health-care training of the role of palliative care and its principles and practice in the care of people who are dying and supporting the inclusion of palliative care education as an integral part of all medical, nursing, and allied health undergraduate training and ongoing professional development. The PCC4U project supports the inclusion of palliative care through the provision of evidence-based student and facilitator learning resources, capacity building, and professional development activities. Graduate capabilities are based on four core capabilities identified as being integral for health professionals to provide a palliative approach to care for persons with a life-limiting illness. A PCC4U project update shows that current course implementation continues to demonstrate good uptake of PCC4U resources for most disciplines. There are peer-reviewed and evidence-based modules and topics designed so that they can be integrated into a variety of curriculum context and delivered via a range of flexible modes. New focus topics are also being designed.

Three of the six occupational therapy schools in Australia reported using the PCC4U Resource Kit in some manner. The main resources requested by the schools included occupational therapy–specific video footage, guest speakers with a lived experience of receiving palliative services or of working in the field, and case studies including the role of the occupational therapist in palliative care.[29]

JAPAN

A survey of members of the Japanese Society of Palliative Medicine and Hospice Palliative Care was done to identify barriers and future actions in the context of palliative care in Japan. One of the top three barriers was the need to "in undergraduate education, make palliative care a compulsory course." The latter relates to the following views: in undergraduate education for physicians, nurses, pharmacists, medical social workers, physical therapists, and occupational therapists, palliative care should be a compulsory course; the certification examination for each of these professional groups should contain questions relating to palliative care; and education on not only pain and symptom management but also psychosocial problems and communication skills should be provided in undergraduate courses.[30] Educational programs pertaining to palliative care for adults have already been developed in Japan.[31,32]

INDIA

There are few select medical schools in India that have palliative care in their undergraduate curricula. A study based on comparison of the level of awareness in palliative care concepts among medical students and interns found there was not much of an improvement, but rather a decline in some areas during internship suggesting that when medical students become interns, they need reinforcement of knowledge and more hands-on experience in palliative care. It was surmised that this occurred because the knowledge was theoretical and the trainees were not able to retain it due to lack of reinforcement in the clinical wards.[33]

FACTORS TO CONSIDER WHEN LOOKING TO INITIATE OR IMPROVE UPON UNDERGRADUATE EDUCATION IN PALLIATIVE MEDICINE

The ideal educational curriculum in palliative medicine for medical students during the clinical years has never been defined, but the authors of this article believe it should include five components: supervised experiential opportunities, communication practice and feedback, knowledge transfer, reflective time, and interdisciplinary participation.[34]

Death anxiety and limiting students seeing patients who are dying

Health-care students comment that caring for a dying patient can provoke anxiety, and educators, who may also share a feeling of emotional distress when being unable to provide curative treatment and needing to speak with patients and families, may be inclined to protect students from interacting and discussing issues associated with dying patients. However, while students cite this anxiety, at the same time, many realize the importance of acquiring the knowledge, skills, and attitude in providing care of terminally ill patients and welcome and encourage education in this area during their undergraduate teaching. Palliative medicine educational programs and placement experiences appear to be effective in reducing death anxiety.[35,36] For example, medical students, after participating as hospice volunteers, described positive outcomes of dealing with their discomfort around dying patients.[21,37] Faculty/schools should allow students to "see patients who are dying" with support available to those who may have strong emotional responses to some patients' deaths.[9]

Awareness of teaching and learning styles and methods

Identified competencies can be fulfilled by incorporating a number of different learning strategies such as small group work, didactic instruction, case simulations, role play, guest speakers, cross-discipline course exposure, and field experiences.[38]

Studies indicate that students prefer more interactive and mentored clinical and real-time experiences over didactic sessions and curricula for their end-of-life care training. More specific to communication training, students desire tools and experiences that highlight specific verbal and nonverbal strategies rather than prescriptive communication scripts. Students should be provided with sufficient time to practice communication skills, with the opportunity for feedback and debriefing following each encounter.[39,40] Actively engaging students and acknowledging and promoting experiential learning and self-reflective practices[6] are effective ways to educate students about communication[41] and have been associated with transformative educational learning and improved attitudes toward care of the dying.[9,13,42]

Role modeling is a preferred pedagogical approach for students. Observed interactions can emphasize the importance of relational and humanistic (compassionate) experiences with patients and families. However, to promote learning, these role model clinician–student interactions should be followed by a debriefing of the observed interactions.[40]

Clinicians should be aware that the "hidden curriculum" may lead to an impression of "detached concern" on behalf of the clinician that may leave students with the impression that compassion is more theoretical than practical. To improve skills and attitudes, faculty should promote a humanistic climate and model emotional support for terminally ill patients.[43]

Interprofessional education and palliative care

Palliative care is suitable as a focus for interprofessional education.[44] In an interprofessional education forum, students are introduced to the roles of different practitioners, the need for teamwork is highlighted, and a mutual respect among members of different professions is fostered.[45] Evaluation findings suggest that meaningful interprofessional education can be introduced effectively to students either prior to or while they are maturing in their professional roles.[46] Interprofessional team meetings can help students learn the value of interprofessional team functioning reinforcing the importance and functioning of the spectrum of health professionals necessary to provide comprehensive palliative care.[34]

FUTURE NEEDS AND DIRECTIONS

It is encouraging to see a greater number of countries having introduced or in the process of introducing palliative medicine into their undergraduate curricula and those countries currently offering undergraduate palliative medicine progressively expanding or developing new educational programs and initiatives. There is a global need to improve upon the quantity and quality of undergraduate palliative medicine education. There is no room for complacency in this area of medicine as patient numbers with advanced cancer and noncancer chronic diseases continue to grow.

Undergraduate palliative medicine education requires scrupulous curricular planning similar to other medical specialities. This should include the establishment of competencies, use of a mix of multiple teaching strategies, attention to student learning styles, a focus on interprofessional learning, and assessment and evaluation. Attention should be paid not only to instruction in knowledge but communication skills and other components of professionalism including compassion.

Key learning points

- More countries have or are introducing palliative medicine into undergraduate education.

- Deficiencies, variability, and inconsistencies exist globally in undergraduate palliative medicine education; however, a number of countries and programs with preexisting undergraduate education programs are developing and involving new initiatives that may improve this situation.

- Death anxiety is not uncommon in undergraduate education, although exposure to undergraduate palliative medicine educational experiences appears to lessen this anxiety.

- Educators are encouraged to use multiple teaching methods that promote experiential learning and student self-reflection.

- Students value role modeling as a pedagogical approach; role modeling in palliative care should include attention given to good communication techniques and other aspects of professionalism.

- Undergraduate palliative medicine education lends itself well to an interprofessional educational approach

REFERENCES

1   MacRury K, Byrne N. The EFPPEC Project Evaluation Report. Toronto, The Wilson Centre for Research in Education, University of Toronto, 2008. Canadian Partnership against Cancer. Competency-based education approaches in palliative and end-of-life care in cancer. Environmental Scan, March 2009. Available from: http://www.partnershipagainstcancer.ca/wp-content/uploads/3.2.2.7-PEOLC_Competency.pdf; http://www.afmc.ca/efppec, (accessed June 2, 2014).

2   Palliative and End-of-Life Care. Entry-to-practice competencies and indicators for registered nurses. CASN/ACESI, 2011. Available from http://www.casn.ca/vm/newvisual/attachments/856/Media/PEOLCCompetenciesandIndicatorsEn.pdf, (accessed June 2, 2014).

● 3   Vogel L. Nursing schools to teach new ways to cope with death. *Canadian Medical Association Journal.* 2011; **183(4)**: 418.

4   Bosma H, Johnston M, Cadell S et al. Canadian social work competencies for hospice palliative care: A framework to guide education and practice at the generalist and specialist levels, 2008. Available from http://www.chpca.net/media/7868/Social_Work_Competencies_July_2009.pdf, (accessed June 2, 2014).

5   Bosma H, Johnston M, Cadell S et al. Creating social work competencies for practice in hospice palliative care. *Palliative Medicine.* 2010; **24(1)**: 79–87.

◆ 6   Lloyd-Williams M, MacLeod RD. A systematic review of teaching and learning in palliative care within the medical undergraduate curriculum. *Medical Teacher.* 2004; **26(8)**: 683–690.

◆ 7   Dickinson GE. Teaching end-of-life issues in U.S. medical schools: 1975 to 2005. *American Journal of Hospice & Palliative Medicine.* 2006; **23**: 197–204.

◆ 8   Bickel-Swenson D. End-of-life training in U.S. medical schools: A systematic literature review. *Journal of Palliative Medicine.* 2007; **10**: 229–235.

◆ 9   Kitzes JA, Kalishman S, Kingsley DD et al. Palliative medicine death rounds: Small group learning on a vital subject. *American Journal of Hospice & Palliative Medicine.* 2009; **25(6)**: 483–491.

10   Radwany SM, Stovsky EJ, Frate DM et al. A four-year integrated curriculum in palliative care for medical undergraduates. *American Journal of Hospice & Palliative Medicine.* 2011; **28(8)**: 528–535.

11   Van Aalst-Cohen ES, Riggs R, Byock IR. Palliative care in medical school curricula: A survey of United States medical schools. *Journal of Palliative Medicine.* 2008; **11(9)**: 1200–1202.

12   Dickinson GE. Thirty-five years of end-of-life issues in U.S. medical schools. *American Journal of Hospice & Palliative Medicine.* 2011; **28(6)**: 412–417.

13   Mallory JL. The impact of a palliative care educational component on attitudes toward care of the dying in undergraduate nursing students. *Journal of Professional Nursing.* 2003; **19(5)**: 305–312.

14   Ferrell B, Virani R, Grant M. Analysis of end-of-life content in nursing textbooks. *Oncology Nursing Forum.* 1999; **26**: 869–876.

15   Norton C, Thacker A. Annie's song: A student's reflection on a memorable patient's end-of-life care. *American Journal of Hospice & Palliative Care.* 2004; **21(1)**: 67–68.

16   Herndon CM, Jackson II K, Fike DS, Woods T. End-of-life care education in United States pharmacy schools. *American Journal of Hospice & Palliative Care.* 2003; **20(5)**: 340–344.

17   Gwyther, L, Altilio, T, Blacker S et al. Social work competencies in palliative and end-of-life care. *Journal of Social Work in End-of-Life and Palliative Care.* 2005; **1(1)**: 87–120.

18   Simons K, Park-Lee E. Social work students' comfort with end-of-life care. *Journal of Social Work in End-of-Life & Palliative Care.* 2009; **5**: 34–48.

19   Paes P, Wee B. A Delphi study to develop the Association for Palliative Medicine consensus syllabus for undergraduate palliative medicine in Great Britain and Ireland. *Palliative Medicine.* 2008; **22**: 360–364.

20   General Medical Council. *Tomorrow's Doctors: Outcomes and Standards for Undergraduate Medical Education.* London, U.K.: GMC 2009. Available from: www.gmc-uk.org/guidance/ethical_guidance/end_of_life_care.asp, (accessed June 2, 2014).

● 21   Gibbins J, McCoubrie B, Forbes K. Why are newly qualified doctors unprepared to care for patients at the end of life? *Medical Education.* 2011; **45**: 389–399.

22 Lynch T, Clark D, Centeno C et al. Barriers to the development of palliative care in Western Europe. *Palliative Medicine*. 2010; **24(8)**: 812–819.

23 Lloyd-Williams M, Field D. Are undergraduate nurses taught palliative care during their training? *Nurse Education Today*. 2002; **22**: 589–592.

24 Weber M, Schmiedel S, Nauck F, Alt-Epping B. Knowledge and attitude of final-year medical students in Germany towards palliative care—An interinstitutional questionnaire-based study. *BMC Palliative Care*. 2011; **10**: 19.

25 Pereira J, Pautex S, Cantin B et al. Palliative care education in Swiss undergraduate medical curricula: A case of too little, too early. *Palliative Medicine*. 2008; **22**: 730–735.

26 Mutto EM, Cavazzoli C, Ballbe J et al. Teaching dying patient care in three universities in Argentina, Spain, and Italy. *Journal of Palliative Medicine*. 2009; **12(7)**: 603–607.

27 Mutto EM, Nelida M, Rabhansl MM, Villar MJ. A perspective of end-of-life care education in undergraduate medical and nursing students in Buenos Aires, Argentina. *Journal of Palliative Medicine*. 2012; **15(1)**: 93–98.

28 MacLeod RD, Robertson G. Teaching about living and dying: Medical undergraduate palliative care education in Wellington, New Zealand. *Education for Health*. 1999; **12(2)**: 185–192.

29 Meredith PJ. Has undergraduate education prepared occupational therapy students for possible practice in palliative care? *Australian Occupation Therapy Journal*. 2010; **57**: 224–232.

30 Miyashita M, Sanjo M, Morita T et al. Barriers to providing palliative care and priorities for future actions to advance palliative care in Japan: A nationwide expert opinion survey. *Journal of Palliative Medicine*. 2007; **10(2)**: 390–399.

31 Kato Y, Akiyama M, Itoh F, Ida H. A study investigating the need and impact of pediatric palliative care education on undergraduate medical students in Japan. *Journal of Palliative Medicine*. 2011; **14(5)**: 560–562.

32 Kizawa Y, Tsuneto S, Tamba K. Development of a consensus syllabus for undergraduate palliative medicine in Japan using a modified Delphi method. *Journal of Palliative Care*. 2010; **26(3)**: 227 (abstract from the 18th International Congress on Palliative Care).

33 Bharadwaj P, Vidyasagar MS, Kakria A, Tanvir Alam UA. Survey of palliative care concepts among medical interns in India. *Journal of Palliative Medicine*. 2007; **10(3)**: 654–657.

● 34 Weissman DE, Quill TE, Block SD. Missed opportunities in medical student education. *Journal of Palliative Medicine*. 2010; **13(5)**: 489–490.

35 Mason S, Ellershaw J. Death anxiety in fourth year medical undergraduates: Implications for palliative care. *Palliative Medicine*. 2000; **14(3)**: 246.

36 Mooney DC. Tactical reframing to reduce death in undergraduate nursing students. *American Journal of Hospice & Palliative Medicine*. 2005; **22(6)**: 427–432.

37 Shunkwiler SM, Broderick A, Stansfield RB, Rosenbaum M. Pilot of a hospice-based elective to learn comfort with dying patients in undergraduate medical education. *Journal of Palliative Medicine*. 2005; **8(2)**: 344–353.

38 Forrest C, Derrick C. Interdisciplinary education and end-of-life care: Creating new opportunities for social work, nursing, and clinical pastoral education students. *Journal of Social Work in End-of-Life & Palliative Care*. 2010; **6**: 91–116.

39 Billings ME, Engelberg R, Curtis JR et al. Determinants of medical students' perceived preparation to perform end-of-life care, quality of end-of-life care and education, and attitudes toward end-of-life care. *Journal of Palliative Medicine*. 2010; **13(3)**: 319–326.

40 Wittenberg-Lyles EM, Goldsmith J, Ragan SL, Sanchez-Reilly S. Medical students' views and ideas about palliative care communication training. *American Journal of Hospice & Palliative Medicine*. 2010; **27(1)**: 38–49.

41 Goldsmith J, Wittenberg-Lyles E, Shaunfield S, Sanchez-Reilly S. Palliative care communication curriculum: What can students learn from an unfolding case? *American Journal of Hospice & Palliative Medicine*. 2011; **28(4)**: 236–241.

42 De La Cruz S, White K, Johnson D, Aagaard E. End of life decisions: Using lectures, small groups and standardized patients to develop communication skills. *Journal of Palliative Care & Medicine*. 2012; **2(1)**: 1–4.

43 Branch WT, Jr., Kern D, Haidet P et al. The patient–physician relationship. Teaching the human dimensions of care in clinical settings. *Journal of the American Medical Association*. 2001; **286**: 1067–1074.

● 44 Wee B, Coles C, Mountford B, Sheldon F, Turner P. Palliative care: A suitable setting for undergraduate interprofessional education. *Palliative Medicine*. 2001; **15**: 487–492.

45 Latimer EJ, Deakin A, Ingram C et al. An interdisciplinary approach to a day-long palliative care course for undergraduate students. *Canadian Medical Association*. 1999; **61(6)**: 29–31.

46 Hall P, Weaver L, Fothergill-Bourbonnais F et al. Interprofessional education in palliative care: A pilot project using popular literature. *Journal of Interprofessional Education*. 2006; **20(1)**: 51–59.

19

Graduate education for nonspecialists

ILORA G. FINLAY, SIMON I.R. NOBLE

INTRODUCTION

Healthcare professionals are likely to be involved in the care of patients with life-threatening illness and who are facing death, soon after graduation. The proportion of graduates who embark on a career in specialist palliative care are small; yet, almost all chosen specialties will involve the management of patients with incurable disease. Palliative care expertise is recognized as an essential skill for trainee general practitioners/family physicians, and there is an increasing appreciation of the need for palliative care skills in specialties such as surgery, oncology, cardiology, respiratory medicine, rheumatology, care of the elderly, neurology, and nephrology. As medicine becomes more specialized, graduates may choose subspecialty interests within their field of practice. It is not uncommon to have a palliative care study for clinical specialties or within general/family practices, and as such, the last 10 years have seen an increasing need for graduate training in palliative care that is specific to the needs of a diverse range of practitioners.

In postgraduate learning, the focus switches from the need to pass examinations to the need to provide competent care for an individual patient. This drive to education from the need to learn is the most important feature of postgraduate education. Although terminology differs around the world, medical learning shares commonalities with respect to stages of training. After a period of school-based learning follows a period of apprenticeship. For those embarking on specialist training, this apprenticeship may continue for longer until a level of competency is achieved, enabling the individual to practice unsupervised. For the purposes of this chapter, the term "graduate education" refers to training that occurs following the initial apprenticeship, at the point of embarking on a specialist career in a particular field of medicine or surgery. In countries where fully qualified general or family practitioners have an interest in palliative medicine, the term "graduate education" would appropriately describe their ongoing learning.

DOMAINS OF LEARNING

A graduate program needs to focus around the four key domains in learning [1]:

1. Knowledge and understanding
2. Skills and competencies
3. Attitudes and professional behavior
4. Personal and professional development

Objective assessment of these competencies is easier in the first two domains (knowledge and understanding, and skills and competencies) than the others, although the importance of attitude and professional behavior should be an underpinning ethos in any graduate program. Different teaching methods cover different domains, so a mixture of methods is required. A didactic lecture may impart facts and increase "knowledge," but understanding does not develop until the application to and facts of the clinical scenario are explored and understood. Without understanding, cold "facts" may be applied inappropriately or even dangerously to a clinical situation. Similarly, communication skills training will not correct a poor underlying attitude to clinical practice; attitude difficulties may emerge during teaching sessions and must be separately addressed. While those embarking on a career in palliative medicine may recognize the need for learning methods such as role-play and reflective practice, those from other specialties may be unfamiliar with such techniques. It is not unusual for students to challenge learning styles they are unfamiliar with. Students used to didactic learning may struggle initially with reflection or self-directed learning, manifesting their concerns with attitudinal barriers. Before a change can occur, the learner needs to have insight into why their attitude appears appropriate, understand the fundamental reasons within themselves behind their behavior, and also inherently wish to change. Much work has been done on the way that people change behaviors [2]. Those who feel there is nothing wrong with their attitude or approach may have not even begun to contemplate the need to change. It is only by moving from this precontemplation stage toward contemplating that their attitude may be a barrier to effective practice that they can begin to address areas where change in behavior or lifestyle could improve their effectiveness. Many problems of team working are linked to attitudinal difficulties; course tutorials and small group work often reveal such difficulties. However, it may be the course administrative and secretarial staffs who are aware first of the student's aggressive or awkward approach.

Learning outcomes on a graduate program are driven by the core competencies that have to be attained and, therefore, are assessed by the end of the program. However, as graduate learning is usually driven by a powerful "need to learn," it is useful to allow the graduates to set their own learning needs and outcomes that they can specify as they go through a program and reflect on what they are learning [3]. This is particularly important for the graduate learner who is undertaking palliative care training for application within their own specialty. For example, the learning outcomes of a cardiologist are likely to be different to those of an oncologist, since they care for patients with different diseases, therapeutic options, and disease trajectories. A postgraduate program that allows the student to identify their own learning needs within their clinical framework allows for a more meaningful and successful learning process. Such learning outcomes, particularly when defined by the graduate, may not be easily assessed within the context of the graduate course itself. This will apply particularly to practical skills, such as draining a pleural effusion, although an imaginative curriculum will allow such assessment from the student's work place to be fed into the overall assessment on the graduate program.

Adult learning styles will determine how different graduates learn on a course [4]. Adults are more likely to learn if they wish to learn and they view the leaning to be purposeful. Adults learn much better when actively participating in learning rather than as passive listeners to a series of didactic lectures. Feedback on any work undertaken is essential, and adult learners should be encouraged at all times to be reflective in the way that they approach a topic.

Clear goals of learning, or learning outcomes, should state explicitly the skills and competencies that the learner is expected to be able to demonstrate.

REFLECTIVE PRACTICE

Reflective practice was described in the early 1930s, but the most celebrated description by Donald Schon has only become integrated into course design during the last two decades [5]. Reflection involves thinking about what we are doing, developing insight into our own approaches to a problem, analyzing the way that we tackle the problem, and looking critically at the outcome. It then involves reflecting on that process, paying particular attention to what will be learnt at the end of it. Questions that the learner might ask include the following:

- What features do I notice when I recognize this situation?
- What are the criteria by which I make this judgment?
- What procedures am I enacting when I perform this skill?
- How am I framing the problem that I am trying to solve?

The learner also needs to think about and draw on related knowledge and experiences to be able to criticize, restructure, and apply these principles for further learning. Schon calls this type of thinking *reflection-on-action*. This review of past experiences leads to a critical analysis of what led us to change our way of practice; sometimes reflection during the course of a process (*reflection-in-action*) involves modifications while dealing with a problem. It is very important that reflection is encouraged in a nonthreatening way so that the learner does not become demoralized. Although mistakes or unsatisfactory outcomes often provide the best stimuli for learning, such events need to be handled sensitively and appropriately. Much learning can be effectively undertaken by reflecting on ordinary situations as they arise, thereby building on good practice. This can be particularly important for the learner who lacks confidence. When mistakes have occurred, the learner should be encouraged to reflect on what they would do differently next time, rather than on what they did wrong.

In palliative care, the clinical situation is often extremely complex and many different ways of approaching the problem can have effective, or ineffective, outcomes. Emotionally charged situations can leave the palliative care learner feeling inadequate, upset, and sometimes with unrealistic expectations of himself or herself as a practitioner.

Greenwood has been particularly critical of Schon's module because it failed to recognize the importance of *reflection-before-action* [6]. In palliative care, such a reflective approach before acting integrates all previous experiences, with acquired knowledge and understanding, to empower the practitioner to behave differently to previously.

Boud defines reflection as "an important human activity in which people recapture their experience, think about it, mull it over and evaluate it" [7]. Here, the reflection focuses on the individual's experience, involving both cognition and feelings as the two are closely interrelated and interact. Feelings that may be "positive" or "negative" will prompt an individual to behave differently at the initial stage of reflecting, so Boud postulates that the individual encounters an experience, responds, and at the same time, starts to reflect. By returning later to recall what has happened, replaying the experience and re-evaluating, additional processes occur:

1. *Association*—Where new experiences relate to existing knowledge and understanding
2. *Integration*—Where the learner seeks relationship between the new information and what is already known
3. *Validation*—Where the learner determines validity of his/her feelings in response and the ideas that have resulted from it
4. *Appropriation*—Where the learner takes ownership of this knowledge and integrates it into long-term learning, to be used in future clinical practice

These reflective processes underpin changes in behavior. They can be very powerful and underpin many of the teaching methods used for teaching graduates; these will be dealt with later in the chapter.

ROLE OF A TUTOR IN A GRADUATE PROGRAM

For the purposes of this chapter, "a tutor" is defined as a person who facilitates the learning process. This term can be considered synonymous with mentor, teacher, or facilitator. All tutors need clear guidance about what is expected of them, and the time frame in which they are expected to be tutoring. They also need to be clear about the styles of tutoring that will encourage learners and styles that should be avoided as they lead to demoralization. Tutors need to be clear that they should operate within bounds of confidentiality, and explicitly explain to a student the issues that would be shared with the course organizers/course directors. Where students are being tutored in groups, confidentiality of the group discussions becomes important and each member of the group must be treated with respect. Each member should have time to participate, and care should be taken that no particular member of the group dominates. The most effective teaching occurs in a safe environment where the individual feels supported and good practice is reinforced. However sometimes, where individuals lack insight, the tutor may have to speak on a one-to-one basis with the student to help that student identify particular problems that they are having. Such difficult conversations should be held outside of the group setting.

Pendleton's method of feedback provides the useful set of rules by which feedback should be given [8]. It is a particularly useful feedback method in a small group setting but can be adapted for one-to-one feedback by replacing feedback from other learners with comments from the tutor themselves.

Pendleton's method

1. Asking the learner what they felt they did well or were particularly happy with.

2. Learner's/tutor's feedback on what they feel went well.

3. Asking the learner what they felt could be improved

4. Learner's/tutor's feedback on what they feel could be improved.

INDIVIDUAL STUDENT'S SITUATION

In selecting graduates for a training program, it is important to know what has motivated the student to come forward and wish to learn. Some may have been told in their appraisal that they must pursue a course to improve, while others may be motivated by their own, often bad, experience within their own friends or family, or a professional situation where they felt that their practice was substandard. Students have also come from a very wide range of clinical situations. While in Western Europe and the United States, libraries, journals, and Internet access abound, in many third world and developing

countries, there is limited access to journals in libraries, and Internet access is unreliable.

It is also important to know about the practice conditions of learners. While it can be useful for learners to be exposed to a wide range of ways of practicing, including some high-tech interventions, for those practicing in developing areas, most of their meaningful understanding and competency development will occur in relation to techniques and actions that they can instigate in their own work environment. Furthermore, there may be differences in access to drugs in common use in other countries as well as culture-specific spiritual and communication issues that may challenge Western palliative care service models.

REFLECTIVE CASE STUDY (PORTFOLIO LEARNING)

Reflective learning on an individual case can be a powerful teaching tool. The learner's everyday practice offers many stimuli for reflection as they go about their daily work, noting interesting or challenging situations as they occur. Many palliative care teams now use protected time for reflective practice in small groups. This can be successful within uniprofessional and interprofessional groups, provided it is conducted in a safe nonthreatening environment paying particular attention to confidentiality within the group. It can also be a powerful tool within the realms of team support and clinical supervision.

One of the most useful tools to capture and record reflection and personal development is portfolio learning. Portfolio learning is designed to provide a chronological record of the learning process of the student. The learning process is self-directed; the learner chooses the areas within a subject of particular interest. In the context of graduate education, this enables each learner to meet their own individual learning objectives. For example, a student who identifies a need to develop skills in the management of neuropathic pain can focus on this topic, while another colleague may concentrate on mouth care.

This style of learning varies greatly from the technical rational style encountered in most undergraduate schools. Those unaccustomed to this learning style will require gentle support and supervision. As reflective practice, portfolio, and problem-based learning become more widespread within undergraduate curricula, graduates become comfortable with this style of professional development. The beauty and simplicity of a reflective portfolio, which allows the learner to determine format, learning objectives, and emphasis to the learner, may be seen by some as too unstructured and challenging. Most physicians are new to the relative lack of prescribed formal structure in the portfolio. Depending upon the experience of the educational supervisor, even the method of presenting the portfolio can be relaxed if the reasons are clear. The learner should be encouraged to develop the portfolio in a similar way to an artist's portfolio, reflecting their freedom of creativity in presentation.

Most successful portfolios consist of the following elements that are interrelated and cross-referenced [9]:

- Factual case histories around which the learning usually occurs.
- References to diverse sources, e.g., textbook reading, literature search, lay press, conversations with colleagues.
- A record of the clinician's own decision-making processes including details of decisions made and how the learner arrived at the decision.
- Documentation as to how the learner felt at the time, sources of stress or doubts are as useful as the outcome since the personal feelings of the learner will influence how they were able to approach a problem.
- Ethical considerations.
- Illustrative items such as photographs, drawings, quotations, poetry etc, may clarify points being made. Care must be taken over anonymization and permission from the patient for such items to be used.
- Some form of indexing is important, so the learner and supervisor can follow the learning process and refer to specific items at a later date.

The self-directed learning portfolio acts as a tool for learning and as evidence to the supervisor that learning has taken place. The format of the portfolio can vary widely, allowing creative expression by the learner. Formative assessment between the supervisor and student, in an informal setting, is essential for learners to have feedback on their progress. It enables the supervisor to give constructive feedback to the student and provide support, especially to those new to the concept of portfolio learning. Summative assessment can help the student identify areas for future learning. Examples of marking schedules are given in the following; these are for guidance only as the learning process needs to be as flexible and adaptable as possible.

Summative portfolio mark schedule

Contextual description of case	5%
Biological issues of the case	5%
Individual issues of the case	5%
Team working	10%
Clarity of presentation	10%
Decision-making logic	20%
Attribution of evidence	20%
Critical analysis	15%
Index and discretionary marks	10%
Total	**100%**

Learners' guidance
Academic background 15%
- Display appropriate use of academic literature/research, other influences in learning.

Coverage of topic (total 40%)
Biology of the disease 10%
- The natural history of the disease
- Screening and diagnosis
- Staging and disease progression

Impact of disease 10%
- The psychological response to disease and the importance of honest communication
- The social impact of disease on patients and their families/carers
- The spiritual response to the diagnosis

Clinical management 10%
- Treatment options and how decisions are made
- Symptom control

Coordinated care 10%
- Multidisciplinary team working
- The response to loss and bereavement

Approach to patient and problems 10%
- Warmth
- Caring
- Empathy
- Respect
- Humanity

Holistic assessment and management (25%)

Communication and personal insight 10%
- Physical, psychological, social, and spiritual assessment
- The ability to engage and talk to a patient and their carers about their experience and develop a relationship with them
- Display insight into their own emotional reactions to difficult and sad situations

Patient responses 5%
- The identification of the patient's problems, hopes, and fears

Critical analysis of care 10%
- The process of evaluating the efficacy of care from both the medical and patient perspective
- Display evidence of clear critical analysis and synthesis of issues

Commitment 10%
- Throughout the course, the student should have displayed commitment to learning in tutorials and in self-directed learning time.

The supervisor will be aware that some factual clinical details of the portfolio cannot be verified or crosschecked, as the reader will not know patients or episodes described. However, it is better to base a leaning portfolio around real cases and events rather than a fabricated scenario, since the learner will gain more from *reflection-on-action* with which they have first-hand experience. The suggested marking schedules attribute only a small proportion of marks to the description of the case, awarding the majority of marks to evidence that learning has occurred.

Social and personal issues in the case history balance the biological evolution of the disease process. The marking scheme reflects the importance placed upon team working within palliative care, and the supervisor should actively encourage an appreciation of this if it is felt to be lacking in the portfolio.

For the graduate learners, a portfolio gives an excellent opportunity to focus experience. It can act as documentation of learning objectives, recording clinical situations commonly faced and areas of difficulty. For the supervisor, it helps to identify the topics requiring further experience or teaching. Often small group tutorials can be organized around subjects identified by several learners, all in a position to contribute in this environment with experiences to reflect upon and share.

Portfolio learning should be viewed as a dynamic, fluid learning process, which should ideally continue as long as the individual keeps learning. As all medical professionals become more accountable and are required to give evidence of continuing learning, the portfolio may become a more prominent educational tool within the whole of medicine, not just palliative care. The portfolio provides a unique opportunity for learning to occur in the wider context of the humanities. Relevant facets are incorporated and cross-referenced, giving validity to the learned experience described by others through art or literature.

COMMUNICATION SKILLS

The importance of communication skills is widely recognized in palliative care. Communication problems faced by graduates working in cancer medicine are not resolved by time and clinical experience [10], and there is strong evidence that training courses significantly improve key communication skills [11]. It seems insidious to allow any professional to graduate from a course in palliative care without having ascertained that they have developed the appropriate communication skills to deal with the complex difficulties that they will encounter in clinical practice.

Palliative care consultations are often the most challenging, since they may involve breaking bad news and talking about dying and loss [13,14]. Intrusive observation of such sensitive consultations, with recording devices or the presence of additional observers, may disrupt the flow of the consultation and hinder the patient's openness within discussions. Since the palliative care consultation is potentially difficult and may have wide ramifications if badly handled, the trainer must create a safe learning environment where the trainee can feel comfortable making mistakes without repercussions and protect potentially vulnerable patients. It necessarily follows that the use of real patients is not always appropriate.

Role–play

Role-play using either actors or colleagues as patients has long been established as a useful tool for developing communication skills [12]. It is best done as a small group of learners with one or more trained facilitators. It is important to keep the groups small enough to ensure that everyone has the opportunity to role-play in the time allocated. People are initially wary of role-play, since, for many, it is unlike any other training they may have encountered. Maintaining a small group will help them feel more comfortable in the process.

Role-play allows people to train for situations they rarely encounter, but when they do, they need to be ready. The skills for breaking bad news or dealing with anger are best learned prior to encountering these situations in practice. In the real world, one will not get a second opportunity to tackle a difficult consultation from scratch, over and over again. Role-play affords the learner this luxury.

There are several basic principles that should underpin any such learning session:

- Clearly established rules of role-play
- Strict adherence to confidentiality
- Safe environment
- Avoidance of role-playing situations that are potentially distressing for learners
- Option to call "time-out" at any point
- Opportunity for all learners to participate
- Nonconfrontational feedback
- Time for those involved to "come out of role" after a session
- Review of learning points and debrief at the end of each session

There are different ways that feedback can be given. Pendleton's method [8] is one of the safest ways to give feedback singly or involving other participants and has been discussed earlier in the chapter. This approach to feedback has the merit of first highlighting what was done well, thereby reinforcing good practice and offering positive suggestions for improvement. Those members of the group who are not role-playing should take an active part in the appraisal system, to observe and learn from peers. More recently, the Calgary-Cambridge approach to communication skills teaching has been developed as a facilitation tool [13,14]. It encourages a far more agenda-led approach to communication skills, encouraging learners to focus on those specific areas of the consultation they otherwise avoid due to a lack of confidence.

Over the past 5 years, the Cardiff course has developed a six-point tool kit to help learners during role-play [15]. It allows participants to *reflect-in-action* on techniques they may use to address specific challenges they face during the consultation.

"Cardiff six-point toolkit" (© Cardiff University)

1. Listening/use of silence
2. Reflection
3. Summarizing
4. Question style
5. Comfort
6. Language

The skills to facilitate such sessions sometimes need to be very sophisticated, so training is strongly recommended before embarking on this teaching style. Most learning of value will occur from the role-play itself and the feedback session, but summative assessment can highlight particular areas of weakness. Selected videotaped consultations can complement role-play. The following table illustrates a suggested marking scheme for the palliative care consultation. Marks are given in each section out of 10, 5 being the pass mark.

Cardiff course communication learning outcomes

At the end of the module, the students will be able to

- Demonstrate nonverbal ways of
  - Facilitating a patient feeling comfortable and safe
  - Opening up a communication
  - Helping a patient disclose their problems
- Demonstrate the use of open questions
- Demonstrate the use of focused questions
- Demonstrate the process of checking that a patient has understood information
- Apply the process of closure of a consultation
- Demonstrate a stepwise approach to breaking bad news
- Demonstrate respect of the patient and the patient's concerns
- List potential barriers to communication with patients, with patients' families, and with colleagues
- Suggest ways to overcome barriers to communication
- Reflect on their own communication style
- Analyze the processes they use in a consultation

TEACHING ETHICS

Ethical dilemmas abound in care of patients at the end of life. Ethical decision-making is never straightforward, so mastering reflection will help the learner function better within zones of indeterminate practice or as Schon [5] describes it as "the swamp." Ethical decision-making needs a sound understanding of the principles of autonomy, beneficence, nonmaleficence, and justice within the patient's clinical context [16]. Gillon has also highlighted the wide issues around each decision, which require the clinician to reflect on the "scope" of application of the decision-making process and its outcomes [17]. Although a formal lecture may appear useful to inform, the complex decision-making around each case requires ongoing reflection-in-action by both tutor and learner.

INFORMATION TECHNOLOGY AND INTERNET LEARNING

Progress within information technology (IT) has made a huge impact on the provision of healthcare across the world. The use of e-mail correspondence, computerized patient notes, digital storage of radiology, and patient information initiatives are becoming ubiquitous applications of IT development within several healthcare settings.

Distance learning postgraduate courses were traditionally organized as a correspondence course, with course packs delivered regularly and completed assignments duly returned. Such courses have moved toward web-based learning, where learners are able to access course packs online, with links to relevant articles. The benefits of web-based learning are clear, with reduction in stationary costs, administration time, and removal of the delay of postage, which for many distance learners can be considerable. More importantly, it allows professionals from diverse localities and cultures to learn alongside each other, sharing ideas and experiences under the supervision of a suitably qualified facilitator.

The benefits go far beyond those of administrative convenience; e-mail allows students direct access to tutors for guidance and submission of assignments and web-based chat rooms for students encourage informal sharing of ideas, avoiding the distance learner studying in isolation. As technology has improved and high-speed Internet facilities are more widely available, courses are able to offer greater resources online including video podcasts on core topics, copies of course lectures, and the opportunity for tutorials through videoconferencing [18,19].

Still in its infancy, learners tend to prefer face-to-face teaching to videoconferencing, especially for learning about sensitive subjects. However, research suggests that learning outcomes are similar for both modalities [20].

Almost all academic journals are available online, with many no longer available as paper copies. An increasing number of journals are now published according to open access agreements so that readers are not required to pay subscriptions. In addition to accessing online journals, the ubiquitous personal computer has accommodated the publication of major textbooks on CD-ROM.

Although there are clear opportunities for learning by the Internet and IT, it is important that these are focused appropriately and not instigated for the sake of progress. Videoconferencing may link learners across the globe but should never be considered as a complete alternative to traditional conferences, since opportunities to learn informally develop new ideas and network will be lost.

ORGANIZING A GRADUATE PROGRAM

Whenever a graduate program is organized, there are three distinct phases that need to be addressed: needs assessment, precourse planning, course delivery, and finally assessment after the course to allow modification and confirm that the course met its own aims and objectives. Overarching these three phases lies the need for a robust system of internal and external quality assurance (QA) to make sure that agreed standards are being met (or beaten) and that good practice is being shared. This is of the utmost importance for the following reasons:

- There are many postgraduate courses available and QA ensures the students have chosen a course that meets appropriate standards.
- QA confirms an agreed standard of training has been delivered by the organization.
- With several postgraduate courses becoming quotable qualifications, QA is essential to confirm the qualification is of sufficient standard required by medical governing bodies.
- It allows for the course to be flexible and develop over time, to reflect the changes in the specialty, market, and teaching resources.

Careful precourse planning is essential; fundamental decisions about the course must be made: in particular, the curriculum and format of the course. Planning should not be done by one individual in isolation but rather with the involvement of a committee of potential course tutors/facilitators. Once the course has been established, the committee should invite student representatives to contribute.

The curriculum, specific expected learning outcomes, and course delivery should take into account the needs of the learners and the resources available to meet them [21]. Graduates have different levels of palliative medicine knowledge and experience. Some may be general practitioners or specialists wishing to expand their palliative medicine skills, while others may be following a specialist career in palliative medicine. The number of learners intended on the course and their geographical location will have significant impact on resources and course delivery. Distance learning and web-based courses are more practical for a cohort of learners from a wide geographical distribution, but this will have resource implications.

Many countries have a core curriculum of learning needs and descriptors of competencies that need to be achieved during the course [22–26]. Several courses based upon these competencies have run successfully within the United Kingdom, with the Cardiff course training over 1000 postgraduates to diploma level within 20 years of activity. Although curricula that have been developed by national organizations can serve as "guideposts," they may not address the specific needs and culture of an individual [27]. Nevertheless, a survey of 263 clinicians from a wide variety of clinical, geographical, and cultural backgrounds suggests that the elements of such core curricula are of high relevance to their clinical practice [28]. Learners considered areas of particular importance to include communication skills, multiprofessional team working, and psychological aspects of care, subjects that lend themselves best to reflective practice and role-play.

Resource allocation and availability will affect the course format. Distance-learning courses require dedicated administrative staff and a cohort of course tutors. Some core competencies that cannot be facilitated or assessed by distance learning require face-to-face tutorials. Many distance-learning courses include residential weekends to address communication skills and allow group discussion on challenging topics; administrative staff salaries, teaching honoraria, and venue costs all need to be considered.

Delivering a course that encompasses a multiprofessional holistic patient-focused approach to care holds many challenges, especially since some of the core competencies and methods of assessment do not lend themselves well to the didactic exam-focused way in which many doctors are used to learning. It is likely that most will be new to reflective practice, portfolio learning, and using the humanities as a learning tool. Role-play in communication skills training is often met with trepidation usually manifest as resistance. The role of experienced, skilled facilitators/tutors cannot be underemphasized to provide the support and input inevitably required, particularly at the beginning of the course.

Any teaching program needs regular evaluation to ensure it is educationally effective. The course must respond to the changing and individual needs of participants, provide competent teaching in theory and practice, and enable students to make a difference in their clinical practice [29]. Structured feedback should be incorporated throughout the course, giving opportunities for learners and tutors alike to contribute to the continuing development of the venture. Feedback should be collated annually and reviewed by the planning committee, allowing time to act on areas in need of change. Student representatives should be encouraged to participate in this process and liaise directly with fellow learners.

CONCLUSION

As palliative care becomes widely recognized across other medical specialties, so too will be the need to increase the education opportunities available to graduate health care professionals. The special nature of palliative medicine with holistic, multiprofessional patient-centered care necessitates what some will find new learning techniques alien to the didactic method of training they are accustomed to. Communication skills, bereavement care, ethical decision-making, and spiritual care may be better learned by role-play and reflective practice. Distance-learning courses will facilitate the growing need for a geographically diverse group of professionals to learn together, particularly when facilitated by residential weekends and online access. With an inevitable increase in palliative care graduate programs aimed at the nonspecialist market, the need for robust QA becomes ever more important. The pursuit of delivering palliative care education to as many nonspecialists as possible should not compromise the importance of all palliative care education being of a high standard such that the training given to nonspecialists can be applied practically to the betterment of our patients.

REFERENCES

● 1 Beard RM, Hartley J. *Teaching and Learning in Higher Education.* Paul Chapman, London, 1984.

◆ 2 Prochaska JO, Velicer WF. The transtheoretical model of health behavior change. *Am J Health Promot* 1997; 12(1): 38–48.

◆ 3 Grant J. Learning needs assessment; assessing the need. *Br Med J* 2002; 324:156–159.

● 4 Knowles M. *Self Directed Learning.* New York: Association Press, 1988.

● 5 Schon D. *Educating the Reflective Practitioner: Towards a New Design for Teaching and Learning in the Professions.* San Francisco, CA: Jossey-Bass, 1987.

◆ 6 Greenwood J. The role of reflection in single and double loop learning. *J Adv Learn* 1998; 27; 1048–1053.

● 7 Boud D, Keogh R, Walker D. *Reflection: Turning Experience into Learning.* London, U.K.: Kogan Page, 1985.

● 8 Pendleton D, Schofield T et al. *The consultation: An Approach to Learning and Teaching.* Oxford, U.K.: Oxford University Press, 1984.

● 9 Finlay IG, Stott NCH, Marsh HM. Portfolio learning in palliative medicine. *Eur J Cancer Care* 1993; 2: 41–43.

● 10 Fallowfield L, Jenkins V, Farewell V, Saul J, Duffy A, Eves R. Efficacy of a Cancer Research UK communication skills training model for oncologists: A randomised controlled trial. *Lancet* 2002; 359(9307): 650–656.

*** 11 Fellowes D, Wilkinson S, Moore P. Communication skills training for health care professionals working with cancer patients, their families and/or carers. *Cochrane Database Syst Rev* 2004; (2): CD003751.

12 Finlay IG, Sarangi S. *Oral Medical Discourse, Communication Skills and Terminally Ill Patients. Encyclopaedia of Language and Linguistics,* 2nd edn, New York: Elsevier, 2005.

● 13 Mansfield F. Supervised role-play in the teaching of the process of consultation. *Med Educ* 1991; 25:485–490

● 14 Kurtz S, Silverman J, Draper J. *Teaching and Learning Communication Skills in Medicine.* Oxford, U.K.: Radcliffe Medical Press, 1988.

● 15 Noble SIR, Pease NJ, Finlay IG. Chapter 57: The United Kingdom general practitioner and palliative care model. In: *Handbook of Communication in Oncology and Palliative Care.* (eds.) Kissane DW, Bultz BD, Butow P, Finlay IG. Oxford, U.K.: Oxford University Press, 2010; 659–670.

● 16 Beauchamp TL, Childress JF. *Principles of Biomedical Ethics,* 3rd edn. New York: Oxford University Press, 1989.

● 17 Gillon R. Medical ethics: Four principles plus attention to scope. *BMJ* 1994; 309(6948): 184–188.

✳ 18 Regnard C. Using videoconferencing in palliative care. *Palliat Med* 2000; 14(6): 519–528.

✳ 19 Lynch J, Weaver L, Hall P, Langlois S, Stunt M, Schroder C, Bouvette M. Using telehealth technology to support CME in end-of-life care for community physicians in Ontario. *Telemed J E Health* 2004; 10(1): 103–107.

✳ 20 van Boxell P, Anderson K, Regnard C. The effectiveness of palliative care education delivered by videoconferencing compared with face-to-face delivery. *Palliat Med* 2003; 17(4): 344–358.

✳ 21 Ury WA, Arnold RM, Tulsky JA. Palliative care curriculum development: A model for a content and process-based approach. *J Palliat Med* 2002; 5(4): 539–548.

22 Association for Palliative Medicine. *Palliative Medicine Curriculum.* Southampton, U.K.: APM, 2002.

23 Irish Committee on Higher Medical Training. *Curriculum for Higher Specialist Training in Palliative Medicine.* Dublin, Ireland: RCPI, 1997.

24 Royal Australasian College of Physicians. *Requirements for Physician Training (Mango Book). Vocational Training in Palliative Medicine for 2003.* Sydney, New South Wales, Australia: RACP, 2002.

25 Hong Kong College of Physicians. *Guidelines for Higher Physician Training.* Hong Kong, China: HKCP, 2002.

26 LeGrand SB, Walsh D, Nelson KA, Davis MP. A syllabus for fellowship education in palliative medicine. *Am J Hosp Palliat Care* 2003; 20(4): 279–289.

✳ 27 Ury WA, Reznich CB, Weber CM. A needs assessment for a palliative care curriculum. *J Pain Symptom Manage* 2000; 20(6): 408–416.

✳ 28 Rawlinson F, Finlay I. Assessing education in palliative medicine: Development of a tool based on the Association for Palliative Medicine core curriculum. *Palliat Med* 2002; 16(1): 51–55.

✳ 29 Kenny LJ. An evaluation-based model for palliative care education: Making a difference to practice. *Int J Palliat Nurs* 2003; 9(5): 189–194.

20

Changing the norms of palliative care practice by changing the norms of education and quality improvement: A case example

LINDA EMANUEL

INTRODUCTION

Medical professionalism requires earnest adherence to optimal practices for patient care. Because of the potency of the medical armamentarium, the obligation to restrict medical practices to those that optimize patient care is a solemn duty.[1] Career-long learning and modification of practices in the light of new knowledge or new challenges are a necessary part of that duty.

In the past decades, medicine has generated hitherto unsurpassed capacities in symptom management and has garnered a welcome new focus on the patient's whole integrated experience and set of needs during serious illness. Medicine has also been launched on a process of reform in which organizations are accountable for cost and quality in new ways. Methods for altering practice to comply with these goals are blending with education efforts. The lost balance between the aim to cure and the need to ameliorate suffering that launched palliative care several decades ago must now be maintained and advanced in the challenges and opportunities of the present environment. The challenge to the profession to put out sufficiently effective palliative care education was taken on at a time when the norms of medical education were entrenched in dry didactic methods even though research had demonstrated their minimal impact on practices. This chapter traces the efforts of one project, as it coordinated its activities with that of other projects, to do its part among other key programs in overcoming not only this initial challenge but also the present day challenge.

ASSESSING THE CHALLENGE, SELECTING THE STRATEGY

The case-study project used here for illustrative purposes is the Education in Palliative and End-of-life Care (EPEC) project. How did this project assess its circumstances as it designed its strategy? How did it adapt to meet the changing environment of needs for palliative care?

Many studies have documented minimal impact on practices of carefully designed and implemented medical educational interventions.[2] More effective programs use multiple education methods and multiple interventions such as clinical reminders simultaneously.[3] Nonetheless, impact remained modest at best. Part of the problem is likely attributable to the fact that continuing medical education had become a ritualized process of information presentation. These forms of information delivery are not designed according to principles of adult education theory and are not much influenced by social science understandings of what can drive changes in social expectations and behavioral norms. A related, practical part of the problem was that palliative care was not accepted in mainstream practices, so that multimethod approaches such as clinical reminders and legislated requirements for advance care planning had little impact. The power of cultural norms had not been sufficiently addressed. Given the enormity of the challenge that palliative care needed to rise to and the inadequacy of education as a vehicle for an immediate change, the field faced the stark choice between becoming highly creative or plodding forward with too little and too late. Choosing the former, palliative care managed to bring about significant changes in a relatively short time, to the point that provided a model for other fields seeking to bring about changes in norms of practice. However, approaches to fully integrate and maintain accountable quality in palliative care have required that the field learn more from others again.

Starting out in the mid-1990s, the EPEC program took stock of what it could do best as one among other programs. It was situated, when it began, within a national physicians' organization serving all specialties that also had an international presence. So it chose as its mission to improve the skills of physicians from any discipline, and it aimed for a national and international scope. Aware that the focus on physicians might seem countercultural to the hospice and palliative care movement that emphasized the essential role of the interdisciplinary team, it nonetheless wanted to capitalize on its unique ability to reach physicians. It settled on a modified, single-wave train-the-trainer approach that would allow physician trainers to reach not only other physicians but nonphysician clinicians. Over time, its trainers have become multidisciplinary.

Other features informing the strategy of the EPEC project included the following. It would address the need to address norms among practicing clinicians, since it would take too long and may never work to rely on the gradual infiltration of change by incoming newly trained clinicians. A strategy was needed to address the need for changed practice norms: the knowledge was available but not applied in practice. Another issue that has evolved was initially the perception that palliative care was nonreimbursable and later the perception that palliative care might be a vehicle for saving needless costs. The question of which physicians to target came up early and has endured since there is a need for palliative care in virtually all the existing specialties in medicine. So the strategy for the project would have to allow for "uptake" within the cultures of these diverse specialties. Regarding geographical location, palliative care was needed globally, but the specific needs were different everywhere. Finally, the strategy would have to fit with the national nature of the organization from which the program was being launched, and still allow for local adaptations to meet all needs. More recently, two features emerged that influenced the evolving design. First, with the economic crisis starting in 2008 which dramatically limited national and regional in-person meetings, and with the advance of distance learning, it was imperative to allow electronic participation in the program. Second, with the successful integration of palliative care including disciplines focused on curative treatment, the need for training would grow.

SITUATING A PROGRAM WITHIN A BROADER STRATEGY, RELIANT ON SOCIAL CHANGE THEORY

What successes the EPEC program enjoyed were initially, in great part, made possible by the existence of a well-crafted and well-funded national strategy created by the staff and board of the Robert Wood Johnson Foundation. Their approach was driven by the awareness that even a well-designed program, if it is in a hostile larger social context, will be hard-pressed to succeed and even harder-pressed to sustain its impact after funding is over. Culture is all-powerful.

The Robert Wood Johnson Foundation invited a proposal to create what became the EPEC program as part of an overall, evolving strategy that included projects in nursing education (End-of-Life Nursing Education Consortium [ELNEC]), in training for physicians-in-residence (End of Life Physician Education Resource Center [EPERC]), in faculty development (provided by Harvard's Center for Palliative Care), to promote institutional palliative care programs (Center to Advance Palliative Care [CAPC]), to reach specific communities, for instance, the African-American community (APPEAL) and

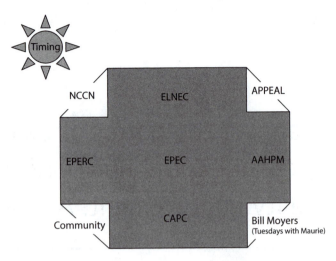

Figure 20.1 *Robert Wood Johnson Foundation strategic programming. AAHPM, American Academy of Hospice and Palliative Medicine; AHF, American Hospice Foundation; APPEAL, A Progressive Palliative Education Curriculum for Health Care for African-Americans at Life's End; CAPC, Center to Advance Palliative Care; CECC, Chicago End-of-Life Care Coalition; ELNEC, End-of-Life Nursing Education Consortium; EPEC, End-of-Life Care; EPERC, End of Life Physician Education Resource Center; NCCN, National Comprehensive Cancer Network.*

numerous projects for public education. Later on, when the time was right, support was also provided to the American Academy of Hospice and Palliative Medicine (AAHPM) to get it to a point where it could sustain specialty educational offerings. Reconstructed in retrospect, the strategy can be mapped approximately as in Figure 20.1.

Central to this strategy was a social marketing perspective for each major project that identified how to go about changing the social assumptions in the relevant sectors of society about end-of-life care. Significant involvement of consultative opinion from a social marketing group contributed importantly to the design of several of the major projects. In this fashion, the social taboos and other behaviors of denial that surrounded dying in America at the time were to be addressed and reversed to the point that a social movement could begin. The programs were also strongly encouraged to achieve programmatic self-sufficiency during their last stages of funding, so that their impact would be sustained after the end of grant funding. These strategies were coordinated with those of other funding agencies, including a "baton pass" to other agencies such as the American Cancer Society, and agencies at the National Institutes of Health such as the National Cancer Institute to sustain the growth that had been established. All were assisted by the publication of the Institute of Medicine report that called for panoramic improvements in care near the end of life.[4] Leaders had been successfully fostered and a Board of Hospice and Palliative Medicine had been established in association with the AAHPM, leading eventually to the recognition of palliative care by the American Board of Medical Specialties. Looking back on the decade between 1995 and 2005, the culture of society transformed from one in which death was denied, the dying were shunned, and those who cared for the dying were given minimal support in the practice of medicine to one in which palliative care became fashionable. It is widely accepted that dying is a matter for open discussion in society and palliative care is a type of service that patients and families demand. Medical institutions throughout the United States have palliative care services.

Most recently, a different type of cultural change has been the focus of programmatic design. With the exponential explosion of palliative care programs in every setting, quality control has come up for attention. Further, with the evolving era of accountable health care, physician's decisions are less dominant in the arena of factors that determine the environment of care while executive and administrative, nursing, and quality officer decisions have become more so. Other programs to bring about rapid change in practices have relied on legislated policy and transformative campaigns targeted at this latter group much more than at physicians. Palliative care programming design has focused on settings of care, specific disciplines, quality of care and data integration so that improvement and monitoring are inherent.

MAXIMIZING DISSEMINATION

Single-wave train-the-trainer strategy

The national and international scope for this project necessitated a highly effective dissemination strategy, especially given the expectation of modest funding. Effectiveness in bringing about a broad social change through the impact of one thought leader through a few opinion leaders to a large number of people who then institutionalize the new norms is a model that is new in medicine at the start of the program. However, the approach enjoyed enough success that a "tipping point" was reached much faster than expected.

The choice to use a single-wave train-the-trainer approach, which entails restricting the training of trainers to a carefully selected group of master facilitators, was driven by the need to have some quality control. The quality control was lodged in the selection of master facilitators who trained the trainers. These master facilitators were exemplar palliative care clinicians and educators who were all trained initially as trainers and were then given further advanced training in pedagogy and later quality improvement management skills and were included by invitation only if their early performance was outstanding. EPEC master facilitators, working with the EPEC program, are the only ones who can create EPEC trainers.

Four wheel drive: Leadership and professional grassroots buy-in

Attention to the social context and what would drive relatively rapid and sustainable social change was necessary. The platform from which the project was launched was, importantly, the most powerful, specialty federated, national medical association, the American Medical Association. It was launched with buy-in and input from leaders in the political and clinical spheres of medicine (front wheel drive).

The project chose to simultaneously involve clinicians at the grassroots level (rear wheel drive). An important mechanism for achieving buy-in at all of these diverse levels was to invite input into the project itself. The curriculum was drafted by a wide range of experts, and suggestions made by participants were taken very seriously in the production of the first edition of the curriculum. Suggestions are still taken at every conference and considered in every new edition of the curriculum.

The commitment of the hospice and palliative care fields to the interdisciplinary team drove a strong focus on how to be maximally inclusive. As the implementation of the project was tracked, it emerged that most EPEC trainers did indeed teach a full range of clinicians, so the targeting strategy seemed to have been effective.[5]

As the program developed, the emphasis was increasingly on leadership by active involvement at every level. Trainers were encouraged to come as interdisciplinary teams of two, three, or more, and the curriculum expanded to include practical palliative care improvement projects. Teams are now trained in quality improvement methods as applied to palliative care and tailored implementation of practice standards kits (TIPs kits) are provided or created and plans made for their use while still at the training course.[6]

Individual participants' investment

Additional features of the social and cultural context of individual motivation were also considered so that identification with and investment of the program content could be achieved. Curricular materials were made to be visually and technologically appealing; that is, the look-and-feel was designed to be meaningful and attractive, and the materials state of the art. Perhaps most important, permission was given to the EPEC trainer to modify the materials to suit his or her teaching style and his or her audience's needs. This allowed individual investment in and career advancement through this curriculum. Every trainer was able to look and be polished and effective in their initiatives when these materials were being used.

Widely applicable curriculum

In order to allow use of the curriculum by trainers in a wide range of settings, the curriculum was not only designed to cover core material that all practitioners need command of, but also designed in a modular format. Thus, a 16-module curriculum could be presented in full at a several day conference, over a longer time in periodic presentations or in part at individual seminars or presentations or as the guiding material for a practice improvement project.

Venues of discourse

Ultimately, the institutionalization process that moved the EPEC project from a one-time grant-funded project to an institution was inspired and shaped by its participants. Initial feedback made clear that the project was satisfying and appetite for collegial connection, so requests for list servs and ongoing advice as trainers conducted their own teaching were readily granted. Soon, trainers began to want to become members of the smaller group of master facilitators who were teaching the trainers. To allow for that, and later to allow for the quality improvement elements of the program, we instituted and continuously developed a professional development workshop. In this immersion course we first present and then provide intensive feedback as participants implement principles of education and quality improvement. Participants learn and master teaching and quality improvement skills using the most effective methods known to us. Participants in turn helped mold this part of the curriculum as well.

Virtual college of peer-to-peer constant improvement

The result of these developments was a transition to something much more than a train-the-trainer program. The project became virtually a college, complete with layers of training opportunities, certification, ways to advance up through the layers, educational materials, and venues for participant socialization. Like an oscillating quartz crystal that creates a perpetual standing wave, the virtual college generates an indefinitely sustainable, expanding wave of dissemination and implementation. Importantly, it developed largely, because the participants engaged in a community (the EPEC community as part of the palliative care community) in which the common goal of bringing palliative care to all who need it defined the culture and all participants were actively engaged in not only their own learning but in that of their peers. It became a peer-to-peer learning-teaching-implementing-leading community.

Tracking dissemination

The dissemination of EPEC teaching was estimated by an external group for a 1-year period between 1999 and 2000. They found that the *EPEC Curriculum* was well regarded and was perceived by most trainers to have provided great improvement in their knowledge of and ability to teach end-of-life care. More than 90% of trainers were actively using the *Curriculum* to teach; the 184 trainers in the study were estimated to have taught 120,000 professionals.[5] By extrapolation, it appears that by 2006, the EPEC project has probably reached about 1 million professionals. More recent estimates reach the multiple millions, although we note that reliable estimates have been hard to come by due to the amplification inherent in the design.

Partnership phase

The next step in dissemination demanded integration into all aspects of medical practice. This necessitated working with leaders in each area. By collaborating with respected clinicians in each specialty or discipline, and by working with specialty societies and with care provider institutions, the project made multiple curricular adaptations that had "entry" for the intended population. Adaptations for specific communities, such as Roman Catholics or the African American communities, and for specialties such as oncology, emergency medicine, and pediatrics already exist. The same model has been used for adaptations of EPEC in other countries and for other language groups.

Sustainable institution: A business model suitable for professional dissemination

To maintain programmatic integrity and reliable standards in the education associated with the project, the EPEC project retains the exclusive prerogative of creating EPEC trainers and owns the intellectual property on its materials. To continue the dissemination and accommodate adaptation to suit diverse audiences, automatic permission is granted to adapt the materials for educational, noncommercial purposes and a standard acknowledgment statement that users can apply to adapted material is provided. To allow for some cost recovery, teaching services are provided for a standard registration fee; costs for adaptation to new programs are covered by grants. The program is maintained within an academic medical institution on the same not-for-profit basis as other academic projects.

MAXIMIZING IMPACT

Change through education

Education theorists, led by Davis, Dixon, and others, describe different layers of learning, resulting in changes to norms of practice. First, attitudes are essential if suitable attention is to be given to the subject matter. Second, knowledge must be acquired. Third, skills that use the knowledge must be acquired. Fourth, behaviors that use the skills must be engaged. Fifth, the behaviors must have the intended outcome. Finally, changes must be brought about in society as a whole so that adjusted norms integrate and sustain the new behaviors and outcomes.[7]

Attitudes and knowledge change

To maximize the change in attitudes and knowledge, EPEC trainers must use the most effective educational methods and materials possible. Experts in adult education and physician education in particular emphasize the need for several features. Adult education theory notes that the human mind can only take in a modest number of facts at a time if the facts are to be retained and used. After a period of about 45 minutes, the human mind needs to take a break. Visual aids are most effective if the information presented is simple and to the point, with minimal distracting material. At the same time, if the information can be presented through multiple channels—say visual and auditory—that is helpful. For clinicians, time is precious, so learning must make good use of their time. Like other adult learners, clinicians are motivated to learn if they perceive a need. The use of data that identify need along with cases that illustrate a recognizable situation with human meaning in which clinical knowledge is needed can be very effective in generating the empathic feeling that, in turn, provides a teachable moment into which the curriculum can place its "just-in-time" learning. These and other points guided the design of the curricular materials for EPEC. The resulting materials used accessible language, presented information in simple units, and used slides with clear points using a minimum of words. The modules were all accompanied by a short video vignette or trigger tape that would provide the human meaning and recognizable, emotionally and intellectually engaging context for learning.

To provide for the layers of teaching and learning roles in the program's approach, materials were provided in the form of a participant's manual and a trainer's guide. As the curricular content grew, portions were designated as core or optional. For specialty societies where the cultural norm was for more complex information, that was provided and information was identified by its level of evidence.[8]

Over time, expectations of learners have changed with the altering electronic environment. Learners expect a useable concept to be delivered in 10 minutes or less, even 2 minutes. And well-designed materials can deliver this. Trainers are increasingly guided to use the smaller units and techniques embedded in the curriculum to deliver instantly available learning that can be provided to end-users at the clinical interface.

Behaviors, skills, and practice norms

Among the effective teaching methods, one used above others in the EPEC project was small-group role-play. The reason for this is that attitude and knowledge gains do not "stick" without the experience of their implementation. Both for delivering palliative care content and for training master facilitators how to create trainers, participants repeatedly try out their new skills in role-play and receive feed-back.

However, to cross the knowledge–practice chasm will take more than a wide dissemination of well-integrated attitude change, absorbed knowledge, and preliminarily practiced new skills. In noting a particularly successful, integrated program of education and practice change, Davis also underscores how complex it is to translate knowledge into practice.[9] Knowledge does not translate into practice change without suitable context and motivation.

The EPEC program has created training in how to engage implementation of new practices, using the methods of quality improvement. We anticipate that by linking learning to

behavioral accountability in this fashion, it may finally be possible to cross the boundaries between education and practice change.

Linking steps in education through normative changes: Use of program 'hinges'

By linking curriculum parts to intended portions of the cascade from attitude change through knowledge acquisition, skills attainment, behavior change, outcomes achievement, and establishment of norms, the EPEC program achieved what we called a hinged design. For every component of the curriculum, the program offered a guided pathway to its full integration into the norms of practice. This included starting with narratives to transform attitudes and create a teachable moment for uptake of information, exercises and settings in which to acquire and refine skills, and then tailored packages rehearsed and prepared in advance of returning to the institution with which to achieve the same among colleagues and behavior changes that yield the desired outcomes and become established as norms. These tailored packages (TIPS kits) are designed to have an evidence-driven/expert consensus–based clinical component (such as how to deliver difficult news, or how to assess palliative care needs in the emergency room setting, or how to select the right pain medication) linked to steps for its integration into a specific practice setting. These steps are the traditional steps for quality improvement, and include: project team formation, diagnosis of the barriers, intervention to integrate the practice with rapid cycles of measurement and adjustment until the outcome is achieved, spread beyond the pilot to all relevant areas, and sustainment through constant monitoring and repetition of the cycle as needed. This is illustrated in Figure 20.2.

MAXIMIZING EFFICIENCY

Long-term, sustainable change requires programs that are not only effective but also efficient and sustainable.

Investing in change agents and opinion leaders

One approach of the EPEC project, along with that of others such as the Ian Anderson Project in Canada,[11] has been to first use small-group learning for those who will become change agents or opinion leaders.

In the case of the EPEC project, immersion teaching to create trainers makes use of groups that are optimally sized at about 16 participants and are capped at 25. Although the cost of these immersion courses is large on a per-participant basis, when the trainers have reached their end-users, the cost can be calculated in terms of per-end-user, and the unit cost drops dramatically to about $10 per end-user, depending on the age of the program and other factors. Similarly, the "capital outlay" involved in producing a curriculum that is of high enough quality that it will

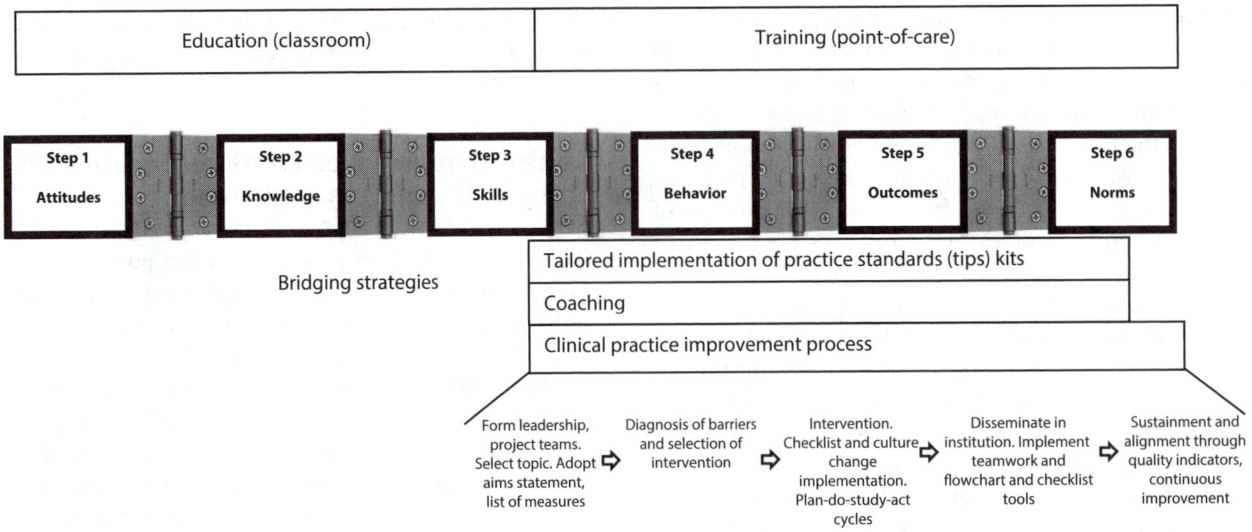

Figure 20.2 *Schema depicting the hinges design in which every curriculum component can be carried through to integration in care delivery settings.*

have enduring impact and wide appeal across disciplines and other social groupings is initially high. But the more the curriculum is used, the more the per-user unit cost drops.

Distance learning

Distance learning has been used in palliative care from early on. Among the first was one by Hospice Africa Uganda.[10] The Pallium Project made use of a similar paradigm, bringing educational opportunities to widely dispersed locations in Canada.[11]

The effectiveness of distance learning is now established, including for EPEC. Increasingly effective use of interactive methods in webinars allows peer mechanisms that might previously have been only effective only in face-to-face learning. Highly sophisticated versions of learning will also soon be available. Simulations of clinical images are already in use for surgical and other types of education. Additional developments are anticipated, including apps for specific situations or types of learning.

CONCLUSION

Medicine had become a victim of its own success by the time the hospice and palliative care movement decided to construct a different road to care in which comfort and quality of existence are emphasized. The challenges to the educational arm of this movement were many, and the power of traditional medical education was not sufficient for the task. By borrowing heavily from social change theory and adhering closely to proven but little used adult education practices and quality improvement methods, and by working as one among multiple coordinated projects, and in partnership with many groups, the EPEC project was able to contribute its part until eventually the integration of palliative care practices into medical norms was happening throughout medicine. Key features of

its design included its single-wave train-the-trainer structure with investment of intense education in a relatively small group of trainers; its modular, adaptable curriculum and emphasis on role play as a teaching method; its inclusion of quality improvement methods; and its use of a hinged design so that all curricular components could be brought from the classroom to practice, and its establishment of a self-perpetuating college like structure. However, the most important determinant of what impact it has had is probably the synthesis of many effective approaches and collaborations, all occurring in the setting of collaborative projects that could reset the cultural expectations of medicine and society at large.

ACKNOWLEDGMENTS

The learning that contributed to the educational and social change approaches identified in this chapter came from many people. Major contributors to the overall perspective include, but are not limited to the following. Charles von Gunten, Frank Ferris, Jeanne Martinez, Joyce Newman, Yvonne Steinert, Sharyn Sutton, Joshua Hauser, Michael Preodor, and Larry Librach, all contributed in major ways to the core EPEC project. Miles Sheehan, Richard Payne, Jamie von Roenn, Tammie Quest, Joan Teno, David Casarett, and Joanne Wolfe, all helped to pioneer adaptations of EPEC to specific groups in society or specialty groups in medicine. Kathryn Meshenberg brought management skills and essential patient perspective and Mike Meshenberg contributed the caregiver perspectives. Arthur Derse contributed legal expertise and experience in distance learning. RM Rajagopal, Vivek Khemka, Anne Merriman, Lydia Mpanga, and Ekie Kikule, all helped to pioneer palliative care collaborative or EPEC-adapted education in India, Africa, or both, building on excellent existing programs. David Weissman, Diane Meier, Betty Ferrel, and others contributed to the coordinated approach of the sibling programs that were funded by the Robert Wood Johnson Foundation. Rosemary Gibson and Vicky Weisfeld masterminded much of the coordinated approach at the Robert Wood Johnson Foundation. Kathy Foley, with the help of Mary Callaway, ran the Project on Death in America. All the master facilitators, many trainers, and many end-users of the EPEC project also contributed their suggestions. Michelle Grana, Elisa Roman, Emily Hagenmaier, Kami Chin, Sean Buchanon, Mark Yoon, Veronica Roman, Alexey Chamkin, Derek Jarvis, and Douglas Nichols have kept the program in excellent shape. Daniel Duffy appreciated the need for palliative care to be recognized by the ABMS and helped it to achieve specialty status. Not one single successful outcome of the effort to change the norms of education in palliative care could have been achieved without the extraordinary, collaborative approach of these and many other equally fine people.

Key learning points

- Didactic information transfer is a small component of education that, on its own, effects minimal practice change.

- The attitudinal and social context are strong determinants of practice, and educational interventions should include efforts to adjust both to the educational goals.

- Empathic consideration of the relevant situations stimulates attitudinal change and information intake. Use of trigger tapes can facilitate suitable emotional involvement.

- Dissemination programs are most effective if they invest heavily in small groups of opinion leaders and change agents.

  - Inclusion of quality improvement methods with education and dissemination methods allows for a hinged design in which all curriculum components can reach integration into practice norms.

- Education programs that seek enduring changes in practice norms must be sustained for many years.

REFERENCES

● 1 Wynia M, Latham S, Kao A et al. Physician professionalism in society. *N Engl J Med* 1999; 341: 1612–1615.

◆ 2 Davis DA, Thomson MA, Oxman AD, Haynes RB. Evidence for the effectiveness of CME. A review of 50 randomized controlled trials. *JAMA* 1992; 268: 1111–1117.

● 3 Tu K, Davis D. Can we alter physician behavior by educational methods? Lessons learned from studies of the management and follow-up of hypertension. *J Contin Educ Health Prof* 2002; 22: 11–22.

● 4 Field MJ, Cassel CK (eds.). *Approaching Death: Improving Care at the End of Life.* Washington, DC: Institute of Medicine, National Academy Press, 1997.

● 5 Robinson K, Sutton S, von Gunten CF et al. Assessment of the education for physicians on end-of-life Care (EPEC) curriculum. *J Palliat Med* 2004; 7: 637–645.

✱ 6 Emanuel LL, von Gunten CF, Ferris FD, eds. The Education for Physicians on End-of-life Care Curriculum. Chicago, IL: The EPEC Project, Northwestern University; 1999.

◆ 7 Davis D, Taylor-Vaisey AL. Two decades of Dixon: The question(s) of evaluating continuing education for the health professions. *J Contin Educ Health Prof* 1997; 17: 207–213.

● 8 Davis D. Clinical practice guidelines and the translation of knowledge: The science of continuing medical education. *Can Med Assoc J* 2000; 163: 1278–1279.

✱ 9 Anderson I. Continuing Education Program in End-of-life Care. University of Toronto. http://www.cme.utoronto.ca/endoflife/, (accessed June 2, 2014).

   10 Hospice Africa—Uganda. HYPERLINK "http://www.hospiceafrica.or.ug/index.php/home.html" www.hospiceafrica.or.ug/index.php/home.html, (accessed June 2, 2014).

   11 Kent H. Palliative Care: Project to improve end-of-life support in Western Canada. *Can Med Assoc J* 2004; 170: 1086.

PART 5

Research and audit

21

Challenges of research in palliative and supportive medicine

IRENE J. HIGGINSON

INTRODUCTION

All research, whatever the field, faces scientific, practical and ethical challenges. Palliative and supportive medicine are no exception.[1,2] Indeed, the challenges in palliative and supportive care are often greater than those experienced in other fields of medical research, because of the nature and complexity of the problems faced by patients and their families, the services they receive, the settings of care, and the way that patients' conditions can change dramatically in a short period of time. This is particularly so for palliative medicine and research among patients who are at the end of life.

There is often a web of challenges that the investigator has to face. As much as possible, problems should be anticipated and prepared for in advance to minimize their effects. But this is not always possible, and sometimes problems must be dealt with as they arise. Often it requires great courage, skill, and hard work to manage challenges that can occur during the course of a study and to minimize the effect these have on the quality of the findings. Many of the challenges described here apply equally to clinical audits, quality assurance, and total quality management projects.[3] An audit where the design is not appropriate, or a quality assurance review that collects information from a very biased sample of people, suffers from the same weaknesses and limitations as a research study with these problems.[4] The wealth of studies already conducted in palliative care and the evidence base to date demonstrate that successful research and audit are possible.[5,6]

SCIENTIFIC CHALLENGES

These are the most predictable challenges to be faced in any study and should be planned for in advance. Careful piloting of the methods can test possible solutions and may uncover further challenges that need to be planned for. A pilot will often consist of a small investigation, or series of investigations, to test specific components of study design and analysis. This may include, for example, testing the methods of recruitment to see how many patients can be recruited, testing the questionnaires to see how long they take and which are acceptable for patients, or the range of scores to calculate sample size. This next section works through the main steps in research, the challenges and possible ways to overcome them.

SETTING THE AIMS AND OBJECTIVES AND/OR HYPOTHESIS OR RESEARCH QUESTION

All research is driven by a question or idea that the investigator wants to answer or better understand. Focusing one's ideas on what is to be explored and what can be investigated in a study is an important step, requiring knowledge of clinical concerns, literature review (see Chapter 26), and self-discipline. It is better to decide to answer a question or explore an issue that can be achieved realistically within the resources and timescale available than to attempt to answer a whole multitude of questions that are very broad and cannot be covered within the scope of the study. Time spent refining the aims and objectives and then considering if these can be answered by the right study design is a fundamental step in any study (see also Chapter 23). When the design is one of grounded theory (in qualitative research), the process varies from those steps described above, but guidance is available.[7]

That said, it is important that the research question or aim builds on existing work and takes it further, rather than simply repeating earlier small studies. One of the many challenges within palliative care research is that there are many small studies that describe levels of need and problems, often repeatedly, without these being taken further to develop and test solutions to those problems.[8] This may be partly as a result of a lack of funding and capacity in the field, as sustainable funding and capacity are needed to ensure that research builds from one investigation to the next.[9] A further challenge is that many new interventions and services are complex, and even more simple interventions are offered to patients and/or their families with complex needs or circumstances. The new

MORECare (Methods Of Researching palliative and End of life Care) statement on the evaluation of interventions in palliative and end-of-life care proposes that a theoretical framework is developed to help both develop interventions and understand how it may be affecting outcomes.[10] This is an important step: a theoretical model will help to understand the potential benefits and harms of any intervention or new service or treatment, and also what components are key to its success.

STUDY DESIGN

Choosing the most appropriate design for a study's aims and objectives is then one of the most important decisions that any researcher can make.[11] Always the aims and research questions should lead the design. For example, there is no point attempting to test the efficacy of a new drug treatment by conducting a survey of patient's views of the drug. While such a survey might give interesting information about acceptability, side effects, actual use, and patient views, it will not give information about efficacy (i.e., whether the drug works better than the current best practice in controlled conditions). Chapter 23 outlines the different research designs and options for the researcher.

Certain study designs are problematic in palliative care, and perhaps the most often discussed is the randomized controlled trial. These have experienced such severe problems that the trial failed.[12] Nowadays, trials, especially crossover trials, for drug treatments in palliative care are more often used,[13,14] although there can be difficulties with recruitment, attrition, and measurement (see pages 178–81). However, trials of nondrug interventions often face additional difficulties in maintaining a difference between intervention and control and, because they are difficult to blind, can have problems of contamination and disappointment (if patients feel they are not receiving a service they wish to receive).[15–17] There is a growing body of literature showing that, although a well-conducted, randomized, controlled trial is the gold standard method in evaluative research, alternative, quasiexperimental, and observational methods can yield valuable results if their biases can be accounted for or controlled.[10,11,18,19]

Successful randomized trials have been conducted, for example, of communication skills training,[20] a nurse clinic for breathlessness,[21] community palliative care teams,[22,23] or early palliative care in lung cancer patients.[24–26] A broader range of trial methods have been developed including cluster randomized trials,[27–29] fast-track trials, wait-list-controlled trials (both of which need careful timing and are often possible only among patients with longer life expectancy),[30–37] and N of 1 trials.[38–40] Studying the designs of others, including those researching outside of palliative care, and their successes and failings can often provide useful guides.[41] In addition, once a design is chosen, there are now many statements that help guide their conduct and reporting. Examples include the CONSORT statement for randomized trials[42–45] and the STROBE statement for observational studies.[46–50]

Increasingly mixed-method study designs (combining quantitative and qualitative methods) are being used in health services and clinical research. These methods have much to offer palliative care.[10,51,52] The quantitative approaches can count numbers affected and provide external validity, whereas the qualitative methods can help to understand the more intangible aspects of symptoms, feelings, or treatment effects and provide internal validity.[53–59] A key in the mixed-method study is to plan in advance the way in which the methods will be combined. In the priority sequencing model, four ways of combining methods are described (see Table 21.1).[60] However, methods can also be combined simultaneously, using a nested or imbedded design, perhaps examining some aspects of the data in more depth. This combination should also be described in the analysis plan. The MORECare statement gives specific suggestions as to how the mixed methods may be combined and reported.[10]

SELECTION AND RECRUITMENT

Many studies in palliative care, whatever the design, can have problems with patient selection and recruitment. Selection (or sampling) bias occurs when the group of patients selected for or included in the study are different from the total population

Table 21.1 *Priority sequencing model offering four ways of combining qualitative and quantitative data in mixed-method studies depending on priority and sequencing*[60]

	Quantitative component is priority	Qualitative component is priority
Smaller component is preliminary.	1. Qualitative preliminary qual—QUANT Purposes: Smaller qualitative study helps guide the data collection in a principally quantitative study.	2. Quantitative preliminary quant—QUAL Purposes: Smaller quantitative study helps guide the data collection process in a principally qualitative study.
Smaller component is follow-up.	3. Qualitative follow-up QUANT—qual Purposes: Smaller qualitative study helps evaluate and interpret the results from a principally quantitative study.	4. Quantitative follow-up QUAL—quant Purposes: Smaller quantitative study helps evaluate and interpret results from a principally qualitative study.

of interest. For example, we might wish to study the management of pain in patients towards the end of life, but the way that we are able to recruit patients means that we exclude patients in the last week of life—because they could not participate in interviews or for some other reasons. There are many reasons why selection or sampling bias may occur; some of the common types and their effects are shown in Table 21.2. Chapter 22 considers the patient population in greater depth and the issues and problems of recruitment, including among disadvantaged groups.

Further recruiting patients who are often quite ill or carers who are distressed and/or bereaved can be difficult.[61] Many research studies assessing the efficacy of drug treatments have automatically excluded elderly people (even those over 65 years) and those with multiple pathologies because of the difficulties of recruiting individuals who are ill. In palliative care, excluding people in these categories would remove almost the entire sample, leading to considerable selection bias (see Table 21.2). However, recruiting ill or frail people into research studies requires skill, time, and energy. It involves winning the hearts of professionals who may refer patients to the study and interviewing patients and families in a way that makes them feel prepared to take part and continue to be involved.

Jordhoy et al. and others have written useful guidance on methods of improving recruitment,[1,62] including ensuring staff awareness and ensuring regular updates and feedback (see Chapter 26 for useful tips and Chapter 22 for more information on selecting the patient population). In palliative care, interviewers must be sensitive and flexible when attempting to recruit patients. There may need to be three or four visits to patients to secure one interview (because patients are ill, factors change, and patients may prefer the interviewer to come back at different time). In one study at King's College London, among patients with advanced cancer, in one instance, more than 10 contacts were required to secure a complete interview, despite the patient wishing to be involved in the study.[63] The MORECare statement gives suggestions as to how the recruitment can be optimized.[10]

Despite the difficulties of recruitment in palliative care, many patients in palliative and supportive care do wish to be involved in research, and to tell their story, particularly if they feel it may help others in their situation in the future. Equally, families, both contemporaneously and during bereavement, may wish to be involved. A recent systematic review found evidence in many countries and investigations that patients and families often welcome the opportunity to be involved. Including some open questions in any questionnaires, to allow the participant to "tell their story" or make comments as they wish, is recommended.[64,65] Also recommended is working with patients and families using the services and with clinicians to plan recruitment.[10]

A common challenge in palliative care is establishing suitable criteria for recruitment to the study. If prognosis is used, then past experiences suggest that patients may be referred too late for the study. In one instance, when patients with a prognosis of less than 1 year were to be referred for the study, one in four patients had died before the interviewer

could recruit them.[15] The criterion of the clinician "not being surprised if the patient had died within 1 year" has been suggested as likely to be more successful.[66] Validation work has suggested that this is a feasible and effective tool in cancer and some other conditions,[67-69] although it may not be acceptable in some cultures and there is variability in how different disciplines use it.[70] Prognostication is very difficult, but a range of estimated survival is more likely to be correct than any absolute assessment.[71] Further work is improving our prognostic assessments, by providing information on other relevant factors.[72] Other recruitment criteria, such as the nature of problems or functional assessment or a combination of these, may also be needed[1,73] (see Chapters 22 and 26). Careful piloting or preliminary qualitative work testing different approaches may shed light on the most effective strategies and methods for recruiting the research subjects and the information and updates needed for staff and subjects.

MEASUREMENT, INTERVIEWS, AND DATA COLLECTION

A constant challenge in palliative care research is to find measures that detect relevant changes and yet are suitable among very ill populations. This creates a tension between attempting to capture individual detail—by using long standardized measures or conducting qualitative interviews—and having short interviews, with short measures and/or short qualitative interviews. In the end, the researcher must balance the amount of information that can realistically, reliably, and validly be collected with the ideal needed. Often the plan of analysis is helpful here, as well as referring back to the aim, objectives, and/ or hypothesis of the research. The analysis plan helps to clarify how the data will be used, and this in turn clarifies what needs to be collected.

There are now many hundreds of quality-of-life instruments and a range of palliative outcome scales, which have been developed or validated specifically for palliative care. Chapter 24 provides more details of individual scales and outcome measurement. In addition, there are several books on quality-of-life assessment and reviews of the measures.[74-80] The European Community supported the project PRISMA that assessed potential outcome measures and measurement tools used in research and clinical practice.[81-83] It identified common tools but also a problem of too many different tools being used, with a lack of consistency.[82,84] Therefore, there is now every opportunity for researchers and clinician to use validated and tested scales. Only if a thorough systematic review reveals that no fully or partially suitable scale is available, should a new scale be developed. The MORECare statement makes recommendations of the key features required of outcome measures in research studies, their timing, and whether proxy or patient is used.[10,85]

Less frequently qualitative researchers publish their topic guides, which are generally developed for specific lines of

Table 21.2 *Common biases (i.e., systematic rather than random errors) that can be encountered in palliative care research*

Type of bias	Definition
Sampling bias	The inclusion of subjects that distort the nature of those that would have been chosen by chance.
—Selection bias	The selection of subjects that distort the nature of those that would have been chosen by chance, for example, selection by nurses or doctors or patients suitable for interview. There are many ways this can occur, but selection of any sample is likely to result in sample bias, especially in palliative care where patients may become too ill to contact, or may not be in contact with particular services from which patients are selected (e.g., clinic, hospital, primary care doctor), or may be excluded because staff feel they are too ill for interview.
—Nonresponse bias	The biasing of the sample due to the nature of those who do not respond being different to those who do respond. For example, relatives who are most distressed may (or may not) respond to a questionnaire.
—Attrition/dropout bias	The biasing of the sample due to subjects being lost to follow-up because they choose not to be involved in the study, or become too ill for interview, move away, or die. Some attrition bias is inevitable in palliative care.
—Missing data bias	The biasing of the responses due to some subjects not responding to some questions. For example, if the most distressed patients do not answer questions about depression. There is in effect a nonresponse by some of the sample to some of the questions.
Measurement bias	The collection of data or measurements that distort the nature of the data collected from its true state.
—Recall bias	The biasing of data collected because of inaccurate or varied recall, perhaps for some events more than others, or because of varied time (e.g., 1 year vs. 6 weeks) or events.
—Poor measurement tools, validity/reliability	The use of measurement tools that introduces bias because they are not valid or reliable in certain situations or among certain cultures.
—Digit preference bias	The use of measurement tools that introduces bias because respondents choose particular digits in their answers, for example, a scale of 1–100; most people tend to use numbers that end in 0 (10, 20, etc.).
—Observer/researcher's bias	The systematic error introduced by an expectation or belief on the part of the observer or researcher (this can be quite unconscious and is most common when researchers are not blinded to situations, although it can occur even then).
—Subject bias	The systematic error introduced by an expectation or belief on the part of the research subject (this can be quite unconscious and is most common when subjects are not blinded to situations, although it can occur even then).
—Hawthorne effect	The change in behavior made by people (e.g., staff or patients) when they know they are being studied. The effect was first noticed in the Hawthorne plant of Western Electric. Production increased not as a consequence of actual changes in working conditions introduced by the plant's management but because management demonstrated interest in such improvements.
Reporting bias	The reporting and publication of research findings in a way that distorts the dissemination of findings towards more positive or negative findings.
—Publication bias	The publication or nonpublication of research findings, depending on the nature and direction of the results. In general, positive studies are more often published than negative ones.
—Language bias	The publication of research findings in a particular language, depending on the nature and direction of the results. Research findings in some languages, particularly those in English, are more accessible.
—Funding bias	The reporting of research findings, depending on how the results accord with the aspirations of the funding body. Further, there may be a considerable hidden bias in the nature of research supported, whereby certain investigations are not funded.
—Selective outcome reporting bias	The selective reporting of some outcomes but not others, depending on the nature and direction of the research findings. For example, positive findings are reported, but a lot of negatives ones are not.
—Time-lag reporting bias	The delayed (or rapid) publication of research findings, depending on the nature and direction of the results.
—Developed-country bias	The publication of findings, depending on whether the authors were based in developed or in developing countries.

Note: Main categories of bias are shown in bold; subcategories/causes of this type of bias are shown in the table. Note that there are over 100 different types of biases that are known, but three main categories, sampling, measurement, and reporting, include most types.

enquiry. Such publication is useful, for conducted open qualitative interview is a highly skilled activity. Listening to the tapes of or reading or typing the transcripts of highly skilled qualitative interviews is very instructive.

In general, interviews should be kept as short as possible, and in some instances, the researcher should order the questions or scales so as to collect the more important information first. Missing data for some questions among some patients will be inevitable, and researchers should minimize this for the primary outcomes of their study. When patients become very tired or do not wish to continue interview, the data collection should be terminated, because collection will become unreliable if patients cannot concentrate. It may be necessary to return to complete the interview if the person is willing.

MISSING DATA AND ATTRITION

Missing data in palliative care studies are inevitable. Indeed, the recent MORECare statement reverses usual thinking about missing data and argues that a lack of missing data may mean that the study has not recruited the correct population. Missing data should be anticipated and planned for in advance. Data may be missing for individual questions (e.g., if the patient did not wish to answer a question or scale) or for individual subjects (e.g., if in a longitudinal study, patients may miss a follow-up interview because they are away or because of illness, or they may be lost to follow-up because they become too ill to participate in the study, or they die). The most important thing is to understand the reason for the missing data and in which subjects it occurs.[10,86]

Any missing data may bias the results (see Table 21.2). Therefore, missing data should never be ignored. In general, missing data should be classified and explored in three categories:

1. Data missing completely at random (i.e., there is no discernable pattern to the missing data with any variable in the data set).
2. Data missing at random (i.e., there is no relationship between the missingness of data and the outcome variables of interest, but there is a relationship with one of the other variables that does not appear to be related to the exposure or outcome variable). For example, in an evaluation of palliative day care, we found missingness was associated with whether patients had smoked or not, although there was no relationship with pain, symptoms, quality of life, hope, diagnosis, or any clinical variables.
3. Data missing not at random (i.e., the missingness of the data is associated with an important variable in the study, e.g., diagnosis, or very importantly one of the outcome variables, e.g., quality of life).

Because attrition is such a common problem in palliative care, the MORECare statement has also proposed a new classification for attrition in palliative care studies. This defines three main categories of attrition, depending on its cause[10,86]:

- Attrition due to death—ADD
- Attrition due to illness—ADI
- Attrition at random—AaR

The way that missing data due to attrition is managed will be different depending on its cause.[10,86]

The field of research into missing data and its effects is growing rapidly. New techniques are being developed (e.g., imputation and modeling) to handle missing data.[1,87,88] There is now even a website and group dedicated to understanding and advancing the handling of missing data (at www. missingdata.org.uk).

The old notion of just ignoring the missing data is now rarely acceptable, unless there is minimal missing data. Any analysis conducted with missing data excluded from the analysis is in effect assuming that those subjects with missing data will give the same results as those with complete data. Thus, there is an implicit imputation, even if the researcher has not formally carried it out. And even if data are missing completely at random, missing data will reduce the sample size and may mean that the study becomes underpowered. Missing data should always be reported and understood. In palliative care, the pattern of missing information can often say much about the sample and the subjects. If modeling or imputations are undertaken, then often several imputations are advisable, followed by a sensitivity analysis, to determine the effects of different approaches.

CLINICAL, ORGANIZATIONAL, AND PRACTICAL CHALLENGES

Challenges in this area can occur in all forms. There may be concerns among colleagues or reluctance to refer patients for studies in palliative care, both by specialists outside of palliative care and those within the field. This may be because of concerns about the nature of the questions or a belief that palliative care equates with end-of-life care, and so patients should only be included in studies when they are very close to death. Interviews may have to be organized around clinical treatments. Patients may not clearly distinguish between new services or interventions and the research interview, if both are introduced at the same time. The Hawthorne effect (see Table 21.2) is likely for a wide range of reasons.

In addition, there are many practical challenges to consider in a palliative care research project. There may be a need to travel to patients' homes to conduct interviews, and the nature of the home may make it difficult to ensure that patients and carers can be interviewed separately. Sometimes the only way to achieve separate patient and carer interviews is to have two interviewers, and even in some homes, this is not possible. Travel time and costs must be accounted for.

During the course of any study, things will change. New treatments or services may be introduced, which may require a change in the recruitment or inclusion criteria. Staff within the clinical service will change, which may mean there is a need to educate the new staff. Even the researchers on a study may leave because of being offered a post elsewhere, finding the work not as interesting as they thought or they may fall ill. A common problem in palliative care research is if the researcher suffers a personal bereavement and so begins to find interviewing difficult (see impact of research in the following paragraph). Senior investigators and research teams are often crucial here, they have seen this problem before, and there may be several individuals who can help out with the study or who can at least speak with the funding body and others to let them know what is happening.

The potential effects of interviews on those conducting them should also be considered in terms of safety and emotional effects. When interviewing patients in the community, the safety of interviewers, especially in more deprived and dangerous areas, should be considered. Community clinical services may provide useful information. Using mobile phones, keeping lists of places/people to be visited, agreeing buddies who will check whereabouts, and in difficult circumstances joint interviewing can be helpful. Conducting interviews, transcribing, and even analyzing data (including collected by post) can also be potentially distressing for researchers, particularly those who do not have clinical experience to make them aware of services that might be available for others. Often a system of support—even if mutual within a department—is helpful. At times of particular stress, for example, following a bereavement, as for clinical staff, it may be that the person should not conduct the interviews.

Using a project advisory group (PAG) can also be helpful. The PAG is usually comprised of relevant clinical investigations and, depending on the scale of the project, may be small (two or three individuals) or for complex projects may be large (involving several centers, representatives of the funding body, external experts, and users/patients). The PAG may be established by the funding body or by the investigators. It meets regularly and oversees the progress of the project and provides a forum to discuss challenges as they arise; monitor research ethics, governance, and progress; and consider the relevance of findings to patients, policy, and practice. For clinical trials, there are formal committees that need to be established to steer overall trial conduct and to monitor data quality and safety for participants. In smaller studies that are not trials of pharmacological treatments, these functions can be taken into the PAG role. Using external experts and patients/families or consumers is desirable in PAGs.

A final practical challenge is obtaining funding for the study. Many funding bodies do not see palliative care as a priority, and many scientific assessors on grant-awarding bodies are not aware of the specific outcome measures and methods needed. In Canada, a specific palliative care program has been established within the national research boards, which has international expert assessors. This is a good model for other countries, as only with specific programs dedicated to a field can the best studies be supported.

ANIMAL MODELS: ISSUES IN TRANSLATING FINDINGS TO PEOPLE

Often work with animal models involves the artificial inducement of the problem under study in the animals (e.g., the cancer is induced in the animal). Then the researchers measure parameters that they believe are sufficiently close to or reflect those of interest in humans. The animals are killed at a point when they are thought to be suffering. There are many challenges in animal model studies. Specific guidance exists in many countries as to the welfare of animals, and it is beyond the scope of this chapter to consider that here. Research using animal models requires a model sufficiently close to the situation experienced in humans to be developed in the animals. For example, to study hypertension, types of rats are bred specially to develop high blood pressure. To study problems in cancer, the cancer is often artificially induced. One of the apparent problems is being able, in animals, to induce sufficiently similar problems to those faced by humans and to find ways to measure them. Caution is therefore needed when extrapolating from animal studies to human beings. A further problem is that there are many concerns of palliative care, for example, symptoms such as breathlessness or fatigue; emotional, social, and spiritual worries; and issues related to the delivery of services, for which no relevant animal model can be developed.

ETHICAL ISSUES AND DEALING WITH INSTITUTIONAL REVIEW BOARDS

The ethical challenges in palliative care research are wide ranging, and for this reason, Chapter 25 deals with this subject in detail. Common ethical issues that can arise occur at the point of consent (ensuring that full information is given and the time taken for consent within the interview), during the interview, when researchers may uncover problems that they feel they need to act on, and dealing with distressed individuals. Nevertheless, it is arguably unethical to make decisions for patients about whether or not they should be given the option of being involved in research if they wish. The MORECare ethical work concluded that it is ethically desirable and in some instances may be unethical not to offer patients the opportunity to decide if they want to be involved in research.[64,65,89,90]

Institutional review boards (IRBs) or ethics committees will need to approve the research (and in many instances the audit) to be undertaken and will require detailed project information. They will cover not only research among patients but also staff surveys and any action that is not part of routine good clinical practice. Allowing sufficient time within a study for the review is essential. Ethical committees and IRBs vary in their approach and are often not familiar with palliative care and survey research and so may initially be reluctant to pass a study. Often considerable persistence and explanation is needed, although often their suggestions and advice improve the study. If in doubt about whether the study requires IRB approval, it is sensible to take advice from the chair of the committee. Chapter 24 provides further guidance.

INVOLVING USERS IN RESEARCH: CONSUMER COLLABORATION

There is a growing view, on the part of many patients, families, caregivers, and research investigators, that the involvement of patients and families/relevant others in research is helpful and good practice. Some charities that support research have user forums that help to decide on research priorities, questions, and the review of potential grants. For example, at King's College London, a study funded by the Multiple Sclerosis Society (United Kingdom) was reviewed by users as well as scientific experts during planning and was monitored by a PAG involving users, scientific experts, and clinicians. A user chaired our PAG. The notion of collaboration with users of services, patients, and families is especially helpful. Ideally, the research should be a collaboration of users, who bring their own knowledge of the condition and situation to the field. Increasingly, short job descriptions are developed to aid the role to be clear. National bodies, such as the UK National Institute for Health Research (NIHR), have also begun to recommend this approach and to establish and support user forums. For example, INVOLVE is a national advisory group that supports greater public involvement in NHS, public health, and social care research. It is funded by and part of the NIHR. It shares knowledge and learning on public involvement in research (see http://www.invo.org.uk, accessed 10 October, 2013).

However, there can be particular challenges in involving users in palliative care research and audit—patients are often quite ill, may need special facilities, and cannot be recruited in all circumstances. Increasingly, it is recognized that users involved in appraising research need some development or training, so that they can understand some of the concepts involved. This, and the course of a research study over 1–3 years, takes time. But it is completely unrealistic to expect palliative care patients to be involved for this period of time. Involving users who are not palliative care patients, for example, involving cured cancer patients, can be problematic, because these users—although very familiar with some of the problems in care—have not experienced the specific issues faced by palliative care patients. Other proxies, such as bereaved relatives, or representatives from relevant patient bodies and in some instances relevant clinicians may overcome this to some extent but bring other challenges. The ways to involve users in palliative care need more development and testing. The guide by Small provides a good introduction.[91]

REPORTING THE RESULTS

Many challenges can arise in the final stage in a research project—reporting the results (see Table 21.1 and Chapter 25). It can be difficult to write the paper up fully within the word limit required for many journals, and there is often a time lag between completing the study, analyzing the data, and finally getting the paper out. However, dissemination is an important part of all research, different audiences should be considered, and a dissemination strategy should be developed in the original protocol.

CONCLUSIONS

There are many challenges in conducting research in palliative care, which means that research in palliative care needs skills, training, effort, and links to those with expertise in dealing with such issues. Some of the challenges are similar to those in other fields (especially, e.g., psychiatry and health services research), whereas some challenges are especially unique (e.g., the problem of attrition and issues of involving users). There are growing numbers of units that are becoming skilled and experienced in conducting research in palliative care, which have sufficient expertise and infrastructure to begin to support others in their research training. In the future, bringing researchers, clinicians, and users together—through collaboratives, rotations,[92] and ideally institutes devoted to palliative care—will help to improve the infrastructure for researchers, especially new investigators. Successfully completed studies are rewarding, both for investigators and more importantly for patients and families. Research can begin to discover better, more effective, efficient, and humane ways of providing care and treatments to benefit patients and families.[93–95] But failed studies are demotivating for investigators and take valuable time from patients, families, and clinical staff.[96,97] Good research in palliative care can overcome many of the challenges, although there is a need to find better ways to deal with some of the problems of recruitment, attrition, outcome measurement, and missing data.

Key learning points

- Research in palliative care faces a complex web of scientific, practical, organizational, and clinical challenges.

- Many of these challenges are common to those faced in other fields, but some (e.g., attrition and missing data) are especially likely in palliative care.

- The MORECare statement gives a practical framework that can be used by those who are planning to conduct a research in palliative or supportive care to help ensure the best possible design.

- Scientific challenges include setting aims and objectives, study design, outcome measures, recruitment, follow-up, attrition, and dealing with missing data.

- Practical and other challenges include selling the project to others, interviewing patients in various settings and different contexts, managing changes in treatments and/or services and/or staff, ethical issues, and involving users.

- Many challenges can be avoided or their effects minimized by careful planning and piloting, developing a PAG, and working within or with units that possess relevant palliative care research expertise and skills.

- Research is important to palliative care, to develop the knowledge and discover improved treatments and care.

REFERENCES

1   Jordhøy MS, Kaasa S, Fayers P, Øvreness T, Underland G, Ahlner-Elmqvist M. Challenges in palliative care research; recruitment, attrition and compliance: Experience from a randomized controlled trial. *Palliat Med* 1999; 13:299–310.

2   Penrod JD, Morrison RS. Challenges for palliative care research. *J Palliat Med* 2004; 7(3):398–402.

3   Higginson I. *Clinical Audit in Palliative Care*. Oxford, U.K.: Radcliffe Medical Press; 1993.

4   Higginson I, McCarthy M. Evaluation of palliative care: Steps to quality assurance? *Palliat Med* 1989; 3:267–274.

5   Gysels M, Higginson IJ. *Improving Supportive and Palliative Care for Adults with Cancer: Research Evidence*. London, U.K.: National Institute of Clinical Excellence; 2004.

6   Harding R, Higginson IJ. What is the best way to help caregivers in cancer and palliative care? A systematic literature review of interventions and their effectiveness. *Palliat Med* 2002; 17(1):63–71.

7   Seale C. Classics revisited. Awareness of method: Re-reading glaser and strauss. *Mortality* 1999; 4:195–202.

8   Higginson IJ. It would be NICE to have more evidence? *Palliat Med* 2004; 18:85–86.

9   Evans CJ, Harding R, Higginson IJ. 'Best practice' in developing and evaluating palliative and end-of-life care services: A meta-synthesis of research methods for the MORECare project. *Palliat Med* 2013; 27:885–898.

10 Higginson IJ, Evans CJ, Grande G, Preston N, Morgan M, McCrone P et al. Evaluating complex interventions in end of life care: The MORECare statement on good practice generated by a synthesis of transparent expert consultations and systematic reviews. *BMC Med* 2013; 11:111.

11 Bausewein C, Higginson IJ. Appropriate methods to assess the effectiveness and efficacy of treatments or interventions to control cancer pain. *J Palliat Med* 2004; 7(3):423–430.

12 McWhinney IR, Bass MJ, Donner A. Evaluation of a palliative care service: Problems and pitfalls. *BMJ* 1994; 309:1340–1342.

13 Bruera E, de Stoutz N, Velasco Leiva A, Schoeller T, Hanson J. Effects of oxygen on dyspnoea in hypoxaemic terminal-cancer patients. *Lancet* 1993; 342(8862):13–14.

14 Sykes AJ, Kiltie AE, Stewart AL. Ondansetron versus a chlorpromazine and dexamethasone combination for the prevention of nausea and vomiting: A prospective, randomised study to assess efficacy, cost effectiveness and quality of life following single-fraction radiotherapy. *Support Care Cancer* 1997; 5(6):500–503.

15 Addington-Hall JM, MacDonald LD, Anderson HR, Chamberlain J, Freeling P, Bland JM et al. Randomised controlled trial of effects of co-ordinating care for terminally ill cancer patients. *BMJ* 1992; 305:1317–1322.

16 Grande GE, Todd CJ, Barclay SIG, Farquhar MC. A randomised controlled trial of a hospital at home service for the terminally ill. *Palliat Med* 2000; 14(5):375–385.

17 Hanks GW, Robbins M, Sharp D, Forbes K, Done K, Peters TJ et al. The imPaCT study: A randomised controlled trial to evaluate a hospital palliative care team. *Br J Cancer* 2002; 87:733–739.

18 Khaw K-T, Day N, Bingham S, Wareham N. Observational versus randomised trial evidence. *Lancet* 2004; 364:753–754.

19 McKee M, Britton A, Black N, McPherson K, Sanderson C, Bain C. Interpreting the evidence: Choosing between randomised and non-randomised studies. *BMJ* 1999; 319:312–315.

20 Fallowfield L, Jenkins V, Farewell V, Saul J, Duffy A, Eves R. Efficacy of a cancer research UK communication skills training model for oncologists: A randomised controlled trial. *Lancet* 2002; 359:650–656.

21 Bredin M, Corner J, Krishnasamy M, Plant H, Bailey C, A'Hern R. Multicentre randomised controlled trial of nursing intervention for breathlessness in patients with lung cancer. *BMJ* 1999; 318:901–904.

22 Zimmer JG, Groth Juncker A, McCusker J. Effects of a physician-led home care team on terminal care. *J Am Geriatr Soc* 1984; 32(4):288–292.

23 Zimmer JG, Groth Juncker A, McCusker J. A randomized controlled study of a home health care team. *Am J Public Health* 1985; 75(2):134–141.

24 Greer JA, Jackson VA, Meier DE, Temel JS. Early integration of palliative care services with standard oncology care for patients with advanced cancer. *CA Cancer J Clin* 2013; 63(5):349–363.

25 Greer JA, Pirl WF, Jackson VA, Muzikansky A, Lennes IT, Heist RS et al. Effect of early palliative care on chemotherapy use and end-of-life care in patients with metastatic non-small-cell lung cancer. *J Clin Oncol* 2012; 30(4):394–400.

26 Temel JS, Greer JA, Muzikansky A, Gallagher ER, Admane S, Jackson VA et al. Early palliative care for patients with metastatic non-small-cell lung cancer. *N Engl J Med* 2010; 363(8):733–742.

27 Fowell A, Russell I, Johnstone R, Finlay I, Russell D. Cluster randomisation or randomised consent as an appropriate methodology for trials in palliative care: A feasibility study [ISRCTN60243484]. *BMC Palliat Care* 2004; 3:1.

28 Torgerson DJ. Contamination in trials: Is cluster randomisation the answer? *BMJ* 2001; 322:355–357.

29 Costantini M, Ottonelli S, Canavacci L, Pellegrini F, Beccaro M. The effectiveness of the Liverpool care pathway in improving end of life care for dying cancer patients in hospital. A cluster randomised trial. *BMC Health Serv Res* 2011; 11:13.

30 Bausewein C, Jolley C, Reilly C, Lobo P, Kelly J, Bellas H et al. Development, effectiveness and cost-effectiveness of a new outpatient Breathlessness Support Service: Study protocol of a phase III fast-track randomised controlled trial. *BMC Pulm Med* 2012; 12:58.

31 Farquhar M, Higginson IJ, Booth S. Fast-track trials in palliative care: An alternative randomized controlled trial design. *J Palliat Med* 2009; 12(3):213.

32 Farquhar MC, Prevost AT, McCrone P, Higginson IJ, Gray J, Brafman-Kennedy B et al. Study protocol: Phase III single-blinded fast-track pragmatic randomised controlled trial of a complex intervention for breathlessness in advanced disease. *Trials* 2011; 12:130.

33 Farquhar MC, Higginson IJ, Fagan P, Booth S. The feasibility of a single-blinded fast-track pragmatic randomised controlled trial of a complex intervention for breathlessness in advanced disease. *BMC Palliat Care* 2009; 8:9.

34 Higginson IJ, Costantini M, Silber E, Burman R, Edmonds P. Evaluation of a new model of short-term palliative care for people severely affected with multiple sclerosis: A randomised fast-track trial to test timing of referral and how long the effect is maintained. *Postgrad Med J* 2011; 87(1033):769–775.

35 Higginson IJ, Booth S. The randomized fast-track trial in palliative care: Role, utility and ethics in the evaluation of interventions in palliative care? *Palliat Med* 2011; 25(8):741–747.

36 Edmonds P, Hart S, Wei G, Vivat B, Burman R, Silber E et al. Palliative care for people severely affected by multiple sclerosis: Evaluation of a novel palliative care service. *Mult Scler* 2010; 16(5):627–636.

● 37 Higginson IJ, McCrone P, Hart SR, Burman R, Silber E, Edmonds PM. Is short-term palliative care cost-effective in multiple sclerosis? A randomized phase II trial. *J Pain Symptom Manage* 2009; 38(6):816–826.

38 Bruera E, Schoeller T, MacEachern T. Symptomatic benefit of supplemental oxygen in hypoxemic patients with terminal cancer: The use of the N of 1 randomized controlled trial. *J Pain Symptom Manage* 1992; 7(6):365–368.

39 Hardy JR, Carmont SA, O'Shea A, Vora R, Schluter P, Nikles CJ et al. Pilot study to determine the optimal dose of methylphenidate for an n-of-1 trial for fatigue in patients with cancer. *J Palliat Med* 2010; 13(10):1193–1197.

40 Louly PG, Medeiros-Souza P, Santos-Neto L. N-of-1 double-blind, randomized controlled trial of tramadol to treat chronic cough. *Clin Ther* 2009; 31(5):1007–1013.

41 Kapo J, Casarett D. Working to improve palliative care trials. *J Palliat Med* 2004; 7(3):395–397.

42 Altman DG, Moher D, Schulz KF. Improving the reporting of randomised trials: The CONSORT Statement and beyond. *Stat Med* 2012; 31(25):2985–2997.

43 Campbell MK, Elbourne DR, Altman DG. CONSORT statement: Extension to cluster randomised trials. *BMJ* 2004; 328(7441):702–708.

44 Moher D, Schulz KF, Altman DG. The CONSORT statement: Revised recommendations for improving the quality of reports of parallel-group randomised trials. *Clin Oral Investig* 2003; 7(1):2–7.

45 Turner L, Shamseer L, Altman DG, Schulz KF, Moher D. Does use of the CONSORT Statement impact the completeness of reporting of randomised controlled trials published in medical journals? A cochrane review. *Syst Rev* 2012; 1:60.

46 Bastuji-Garin S, Sbidian E, Gaudy-Marqueste C, Ferrat E, Roujeau JC, Richard MA et al. Impact of STROBE statement publication on quality of observational study reporting: Interrupted time series versus before–after analysis. *PLoS One* 2013; 8(8):e64733.

47 Ebrahim S, Clarke M. STROBE: New standards for reporting observational epidemiology, a chance to improve. *Int J Epidemiol* 2007; 36(5):946–948.

48 Malta M, Cardoso LO, Bastos FI, Magnanini MM, Silva CM. STROBE initiative: Guidelines on reporting observational studies. *Rev Saude Publica* 2010; 44(3):559–565.

49 Nijsten T, Spuls P, Stern RS. STROBE: A Beacon for observational studies. *Arch Dermatol* 2008; 144(9):1200–1204.

50 von EE, Altman DG, Egger M, Pocock SJ, Gotzsche PC, Vandenbroucke JP. The Strengthening the Reporting of Observational Studies in Epidemiology (STROBE) statement: Guidelines for reporting observational studies. *J Clin Epidemiol* 2008; 61(4):344–349.

◆ 51 Seymour J. Combined qualitative and quantitative research designs. *Curr Opin Support Palliat Care* 2012; 6(4):514–524.

52 Farquhar MC, Ewing G, Booth S. Using mixed methods to develop and evaluate complex interventions in palliative care research. *Palliat Med* 2011; 25(8):748–757.

53 Corner J. In search of more complete answers to research questions: Quantitative versus qualitative research methods: Is there a way forward? *J Adv Nurs* 1991; 16:718–727.

54 Dale J, Shipman C, Lacock L, Davies M. Creating a shared vision of out of hours care: Using rapid appraisal methods to create an interagency, community oriented, approach to service development. *BMJ* 1996; 312:1206–1210.

55 Grande GE, Todd CJ, Barclay SI. Support needs in the last year of life: Patient and carer dilemmas. *Palliat Med* 1997; 11(3):202–208.

56 Kristjanson LJ, Atwood J, Degner LF. Validity and reliability of the family inventory of needs (FIN): Measuring the care needs of families of advanced cancer patients. *J Nurs Meas* 1995; 3:109–126.

57 Richardson A, Wilson Barnett J. A review of nursing research in cancer and palliative care. *J Nurs Meas* 1997:1–23.

58 Teno JM, Stevens M, Spernak S, Lynn J. Role of written advance directives in decision making: Insights from qualitative and quantitative data. *J Gen Intern Med* 1998; 13(7):439–446.

59 Wallen GR, Berger A. Mixed methods: In search of truth in palliative care medicine. *J Palliat Med* 2004; 7(3):403–404.

60 Tariq S, Woodman J. Using mixed methods in health research. *JRSM Short Rep* 2013; 4(6):2042533313479197.

61 Phipps E, Harris D, Braitman LE, Tester W, Madison-Thompson N, True G. Who enrolls in observational end of life research? Report from the cultural variations in approaches to end of life study. *J Palliat Med* 2005; 8(1):115–120.

62 Casarett D, Kassner CT, Kutner JS. Recruiting for research in hospice: Feasibility of a research screening protocol. *J Palliat Med* 2004; 7(6):854–860.

63 Shipman C, Hotopf M, Richardson A, Murray S, Koffman J, Harding R et al. The views of patients with advanced cancer regarding participation in serial questionnaire studies. *Palliat Med* 2008; 22(8):913–920.

● 64 Gysels M, Evans CJ, Lewis P, Speck P, Benalia H, Preston NJ et al. MORECare research methods guidance development: Recommendations for ethical issues in palliative and end-of-life care research. *Palliat Med* 2013; 27:908–917.

◆ 65 Gysels MH, Evans C, Higginson IJ. Patient, caregiver, health professional and researcher views and experiences of participating in research at the end of life: A critical interpretive synthesis of the literature. *BMC Med Res Methodol* 2012; 12:123.

66 Lynn J, Teno JM, Harrell FE, Jr. Accurate prognostications of death. Opportunities and challenges for clinicians. *West J Med* 1995; 163(3):250–257.

67 Johnson DC, Kutner JS, Armstrong JD. Would you be surprised if this patient died?: Preliminary exploration of first and second year residents' approach to care decisions in critically ill patients. *BMC Palliat Care* 2003; 2(1):1.

68 Moss AH, Lunney JR, Culp S, Auber M, Kurian S, Rogers J et al. Prognostic significance of the "surprise" question in cancer patients. *J Palliat Med* 2010; 13(7):837–840.

69 Moss AH, Ganjoo J, Sharma S, Gansor J, Senft S, Weaner B et al. Utility of the "surprise" question to identify dialysis patients with high mortality. *Clin J Am Soc Nephrol* 2008; 3(5):1379–1384.

70 Da Silva GM, Braun A, Stott D, Wellsted D, Farrington K. How robust is the 'Surprise Question' in predicting short-term mortality risk in haemodialysis Patients? *Nephron Clin Pract* 2013; 123(3–4):185–193.

71 Higginson IJ, Costantini M. Accuracy of prognosis estimates by four palliative care teams: A prospective cohort study. *BMC Palliat Care* 2002:1.

72 Vigano A, Donaldson N, Higginson IJ, Bruera E, Mahmud S, Suarez-Almazor M. Quality of life and survival prediction in terminal cancer patients. A multicenter study. *Cancer* 2004; 101:1090–1098.

73 Ling J, Hardy J, Penn K, Davis C. Evaluation of palliative care. Recruitment figures may be low [letter; comment]. *BMJ* 1995; 310(6972):125.

74 Bowling A. Choice of health indicator—The problem of measuring outcome. *Complem Med Res* 1988; 2:43–63.

75 Bowling A. *Measuring Disease*. Milton Keynes, U.K.: Open University Press; 1995.

76 Wilkin D, Hallam L, Doggett M. *Measures of Need and Outcome for Primary Health Care.* Oxford, U.K.: Oxford University Press; 1992.

77 Carr AJ, Higginson IJ, Robinson PG. *Quality of Life.* London, U.K.: BMJ Books; 2003.

78 Higginson IJ, Carr AJ. Measuring quality of life: Using quality of life measures in the clinical setting. *BMJ* 2001; 322:1297–1300.

79 Paci E, Miccinesi G, Toscani F, Tamburini M, Brunelli C, Costantini M et al. Quality of life assessment and outcome of palliative care. *J Pain Symptom Manage* 2001; 21:179–188.

80 Robinson PG, Carr AJ, Higginson IJ. How to choose a quality of life measure. In: Carr AJ, Higginson IJ, Robinson PG (eds.). *Quality of Life.* London, U.K.: BMJ Books; 2003. pp. 88–100.

81 Bausewein C, Simon ST, Benalia H, Downing J, Mwangi-Powell FN, Daveson BA et al. Implementing patient reported outcome measures (PROMs) in palliative care—Users' cry for help. *Health Qual Life Outcomes* 2011; 9:27.

82 Daveson BA, Simon ST, Benalia H, Downing J, Higginson IJ, Harding R et al. Are we heading in the same direction? European and African doctors' and nurses' views and experiences regarding outcome measurement in palliative care. *Palliat Med* 2012; 26(3):242–249.

83 Harding R, Higginson IJ. PRISMA: A pan-European co-ordinating action to advance the science in end-of-life cancer care. *Eur J Cancer* 2010; 46(9):1493–1501.

84 Harding R, Simon ST, Benalia H, Downing J, Daveson BA, Higginson IJ et al. The PRISMA Symposium 1: Outcome tool use. Disharmony in European outcomes research for palliative and advanced disease care: Too many tools in practice. *J Pain Symptom Manage* 2011; 42(4):493–500.

● 85 Evans CJ, Benalia H, Preston NJ, Grande G, Gysels M, Short V et al. The selection and use of outcome measures in palliative and end-of-life care research: The MORECare international consensus workshop. *J Pain Symptom Manage* 2013; 46:925–937.

● 86 Preston NJ, Fayers P, Walters SJ, Pilling M, Grande GE, Short V et al. Recommendations for managing missing data, attrition and response shift in palliative and end-of-life care research: Part of the MORECare research method guidance on statistical issues. *Palliat Med* 2013; 27:899–907.

87 Neymark N, Kiebert W, Torfs K, Davies L, Fayers P, Hillner B et al. Methodological and statistical issues of quality of life (QoL) and economic evaluation in cancer clinical trials: Report of a workshop. *Eur J Cancer* 1998; 34(9):1317–1333.

88 Robinson PG, Donaldson N. Longitudinal analysis of quality of life data. In: Carr AJ, Robinson PG, Higginson IJ (eds.). *Quality of Life.* London, U.K.: BMJ Books; 2003. pp. 101–112.

89 Gysels M, Shipman C, Higginson IJ. Is the qualitative research interview an acceptable medium for research with palliative care patients and carers? *BMC Med Ethics* 2008; 9:7.

◆ 90 Gysels M, Shipman C, Higginson IJ. "I will do it if it will help others:" Motivations among patients taking part in qualitative studies in palliative care. *J Pain Symptom Manage* 2008; 35(4):347–355.

91 Small N, Rhodes P. *Too Ill to Talk? User Involvement and Palliative Care.* London, U.K.: Routledge; 2000.

92 von Gunten CF, Von Roenn JH, Gradishar W, Weitzman S. A hospice/palliative medicine rotation for fellows training in hematology-oncology. *J Cancer Educ* 1995; 10(4):200–202.

93 Breitbart W, Bruera E, Chochinov H, Lynch M. Neuropsychiatric syndromes and psychological symptoms in patients with advanced cancer. *J Pain Symptom Manage* 1995; 10:131–141.

94 Corner J. Is there a research paradigm for palliative care? *Palliat Med* 1996; 10:201–208.

95 Ripamonti C. Management of dyspnea in advanced cancer patients [see comments]. *Support Care Cancer* 1999; 7(4):233–243.

96 Higginson I. Research degree supervision: Lottery or lifebelt. *Crit Public Health* 1990; 3:42–47.

97 Higginson I, Corner J. Postgraduate research training: The PhD and MD thesis. *Palliat Med* 1996; 10:113–118.

22

The population: Who are the subjects in palliative medicine research?

CLAUDIA BAUSEWEIN, FLISS E.M. MURTAGH

INTRODUCTION

Palliative care research has significantly increased over the last decade with a growing number of published studies [1]. Nevertheless, there is a continuous need for high-quality research to understand the changing concepts of palliative care, evaluate interventions, and increase the evidence base for palliative care [2]. The main focus of palliative care research is the patients, but there is also research interest in the needs and the situation of informal and professional caregivers, and the views and opinions of the general public regarding the issues of end-of-life care.

In general, the choice of the palliative care population is driven by the research question that impacts both methods and type of study. Considering the specific characteristics of participants is crucial when planning a study. These need to be determined through clear inclusion and exclusion criteria in preparing the study. But it is also a central responsibility of researchers to describe the characteristics of their research, including participants, in a way that helps clinicians to determine under what circumstances the findings can be applied to their patients [3], that is, to provide clinicians with some insight into the generalizability of the research findings. This is important as populations differ widely, and evidence derived in one population may or may not apply to other populations [3].

This chapter focuses on the challenge of defining the population to be studied and the specific characteristics of patients, carers, and the general population in the research context.

PATIENTS

Definitions of palliative care are often vague in describing the patient population. For example, the WHO defines, in the 1990 version, the patient population as "having a disease that is not responsive to curative treatment" [4], which is also used by the European Association for Palliative Care [5]. Later in 2002, the WHO defines the palliative care patient as "facing the problems associated with life-threatening disease" [4]. In consequence, there is some inconsistency as to how to define the palliative care patient population [6]. None of the definitions names a specific disease, but all include the improvement of physical, psychological, social, and spiritual needs.

Researchers and clinicians have, in some ways, redefined what characterizes a *palliative care patient*. In the early stages of palliative care, attention was focused on cancer patients near the end of life. More recently, however, there has been a shift to extending palliative care provision to patients with noncancer diagnoses and also acknowledging the need for and benefit derived from offering it to patients earlier in the disease trajectory [7]. Today, there is a strong drive for need, not diagnoses and/or prognoses, to be the most relevant factor in the provision of palliative care services [8]. However in research, depending on the research question, both diagnoses and prognoses may play an important role.

Diagnosis

Similar to the provision of palliative care to cancer patients, research studies focused either on specific cancer populations such as lung cancer [7] or on mixed populations across cancer entities [9,10]. With changing concepts and widening palliative care to all patients with chronic medical conditions, there was increasing interest in understanding the specific needs of individual patient groups, for example, patients with chronic kidney disease [11,12], chronic heart failure [13], or COPD [14], also in comparing these groups to cancer patients [15,16]. Studies focusing on one specific population give detailed information on this group but have limited generalizability to the whole palliative care population. In contrast, there might be considerable heterogeneity in studies with mixed patient groups, making findings harder to interpret. Furthermore, different conditions follow different disease trajectories [12,17], which has potential impact on patients' retention in the study and also the comparability of data as, for example, patients in cross-sectional studies may be at different stages in their disease trajectory. Ideally, the date of data collection should be related to a fixed point in the patients' disease trajectory, and commonly, death is used as the most obvious fixed point. However, this has the drawback of being identified only retrospectively and being often difficult to anticipate, even in the relatively late stages of illness.

Prognosis

Basing the definition of palliative care patients in research on prognoses raises other challenges. If inclusion criteria are confined to those with relatively poor prognoses, there is a risk of excluding a group of healthier patients whose inclusion would have improved the generalizability of the study results. In addition, if prognosis alone is used to define study eligibility, substantial inaccuracies must be overcome in the predictions of prognosis, even using the best available models as tools [18,19]. Physicians are not only reluctant to make prognostic estimates but also tend to overestimate life expectancy [18,20]. Compared to earlier in the disease trajectory, physicians can prognosticate slightly more accurately the closer a patient is to death, yet clinicians rarely can say with certainty whether an individual will likely live another day, week, or month [21]. Imprecision of prognosis also poses challenges for researchers as healthier patients with specific needs may be excluded and overestimation of survival time may lead to attrition and drop out if patients become too unwell.

The *surprise question* (Would you be surprised if the patient were to die in the next year?') that is often used in clinical practice to identify palliative care patients might also be too crude. Steinhauser et al. used an alternative approach, choosing clinical criteria associated with an estimated 50% 1-year survival for patients with, for example, stage IV cancer, NYHA stage III or IV congestive heart failure, and COPD with hypercapnia ($pCO_2 \geq 46$) and requirement of one emergency room visit or hospitalization within the previous year [21].

Need

In palliative care, support and interventions usually focus on patients' needs rather than diagnoses or prognoses alone. Therefore, many studies test the efficacy of interventions to improve symptoms such as pain or breathlessness and define the study population based on the presence of a specific symptom or symptom cluster. As many of these symptoms occur across conditions, these studies often include patients not only with one disease. For example, a number of studies into relief of breathlessness included patients with COPD, malignancies, and chronic heart failure [22,23]. This again introduces heterogeneity into the study. This can be overcome by stratifying the analysis by disease group, but if subanalysis is intended, the sample size of the subgroups needs to be high enough to allow meaningful results and conclusions. The overall prevalence of the symptom also needs to be considered as the recruitment of patients with a very common symptom such as pain or breathlessness will be much quicker compared with the recruitment of patients with rare symptoms such as itch or diarrhea. Differential prevalence, when a symptom is more common in one condition rather than another, may also need to be considered carefully, lest subgroups become very unbalanced.

Comorbidities

Increasingly, as populations in the developed countries age, palliative care patients have multiple comorbid conditions, rather than one single or predominant diagnosis. These changing patterns and combinations of multiple diseases have implications, not only for clinical care but also for research. Just as the primary diseases, and stage of disease, need to be carefully described in order that generalizability of evidence can be assessed, so too do the comorbidities (both the type and the severity of conditions). This ensures that the study population in palliative care studies is well characterized, enabling the assessment of relevance and generalizability, and this will become more important over the coming years, given the aging populations of developed countries.

Patients with cognitive impairment

In palliative care patients, high levels of cognitive impairment are frequently observed, particularly towards the end of life [24]. Cognitive impairment will comprise the patients' capacity to consent to participate in research. Level of impairment of capacity will vary, and it depends on the research question and inclusion and exclusion criteria whether participants with impaired capacity will be included in or excluded from a study. If participants with cognitive impairment are to be included, further detailed consideration of risks and benefits need to be considered, with greater effort to protect high risk patients [25]. Cognitive impairment may be difficult to identify in palliative care research because of varying cognitive function over time [26]. This is particularly important in longitudinal studies when patients are followed over time. Even if patients have the capacity to consent at the time of enrollment, they may not retain that capacity throughout the study [27]. In patients with greater risk of cognitive impairment, a formal assessment of capacity might be necessary. Specific tools have been developed to aid the assessment and decision about study inclusion [28,29].

During the last weeks and days of life, patients may not have the capacity to give consent to take part in a research study [30]. The following issues should be considered [30]: First, research risks and benefits must be reevaluated in the context of lack of capacity; how much risk is the individual participant exposed to by participating, and is the overall likely benefit of the research substantial? Second, the precise role of a proxy, such as a relative, in the consent process must be considered. Third, incapacity is variable and not always total: a participant may be able to give consent at some level, and it is important to include this within the consent process. Last, alternative consent procedures might be necessary, especially in the final days of life, such as the advanced consent suggested by Rees and Hardy [31].

Population-based research

So far, we have considered research that recruits participants (be they patients, carers, clinicians, or the public) into studies. However, another way of researching palliative care is to use existing large datasets to address epidemiological or population-based research questions. This can be done using death registration data [32,33] or other national or regional data sources such as healthcare utilization data [34], hospital episode statistics [35], or social care data [36], according to the research question. The advantages of such studies are the extent and inclusivity of the data available for inclusion, without the need for collecting primary data and all the resources this requires. It is also often possible for a complete dataset to be used; that is, the whole population is included, rather than a study sample. However, the secondary use of large datasets also has limitations; often, for instance, the data are collected for another reason than research and do not include the most relevant variables or extend as far as a researcher might hope. Large datasets are perhaps most useful when linked datasets are used, such as combined health and social care datasets [36] or combined acute hospital and community healthcare datasets [34]. Issues that arise in these studies include information governance (where unique patient identifiers are needed to link datasets) and the amount of missing data (some routinely collected data sources are detailed and complete, but many have large amounts of missing or questionable data). Some studies conducted in this way may be ecological studies (where the unit of analysis is the population) or at least use population-level, rather than individual-level, variables; it is important then that any inferences about the nature of individuals in this type of study are not assumed to apply at the individual level.

There is increasing interest in developing national or regional clinical datasets, which may then not only allow national benchmarking and quality improvement but also have the potential to support clinical research. An example is the Australian Palliative Care Outcomes Collaborative, which collects national outcomes data in palliative care (see http://www.pcoc.org.au/) and uses standardized validated clinical assessment tools. Although the focus to date has been on improving quality and outcomes, there is considerable potential for clinical research to be supported too.

FAMILY CARERS

In palliative care, the units of care is patients and their families. Although the specific characteristics and needs of family carers are increasingly in the focus of research, less than 10% of studies published in the palliative care literature targeted caregivers/family members as research topics [37]. There are still huge gaps in the understanding and knowledge of the caring experience [38,39]. Defining the informal carer population is

a challenge as every patient might have a number of caregivers that might not necessarily be related to family structures [39]. Also, they might not identify themselves as carers [39]. Research in family carers can be conducted during the patient's illness and postbereavement, after the death of the patient. Special considerations are necessary in each phase for family caregivers' involvement during research. During the patients' illness, caregiver burden is usually high. For some, involvement in research might add to the burden; for others, it might be a relief to have a voice and be able to share their experiences. When carers are approached via patients, patients often function as gatekeepers because they do not want to add more burden to their carers. To foster carers' autonomy, they should be given the choice directly whether they want to participate in research or not. When carers are approached after the death of the patient, for example, in a mortality follow-back survey, this can evoke distressing emotions to some, but some might find it a positive and useful experience [40]. There is debate about the best timing to approach bereaved carers, and time frames used vary from 3 to 9 months postbereavement [41,42].

PROFESSIONAL CARERS

A fair amount of palliative care research is conducted in health care professionals with about 20% of palliative care studies published in 2007 being conducted in this population [37]. Health care professionals either can provide specific information about the characteristics and care of their patients [43] or can be research objects themselves with the aim of improving competencies [44] or assessing their views and experiences on a specific topic such as outcome measurement [45].

GENERAL PUBLIC

Although not directly affected by palliative care, the general public comprises another potential research population as their opinion influences policy makers and they are potential future patients and carers. Studies can be specifically designed to approach the general public to study their views such as in a telephone survey where European citizens were asked about their preferences for end-of-life care [46] or acceptance of euthanasia [47]. Essential for the generalizability of these studies is the selection of a representative sample, for example, through probability sampling. A number of methods are available to ensure representativeness, such as simple random sampling, stratified random sampling, or cluster sampling.

CRITERIA FOR DESCRIPTION OF THE PALLIATIVE CARE POPULATION

In order to understand the population under study and to be able to judge the generalizability of the results, there is a need for explicit and clear description of key characteristics

Table 22.1   *Reporting of characteristics of study participants*

Domain	Subdomain	Measure
Individual participant's demographics (across groups)	Age	Mean (SD), median (range)
	Gender	Percentage
	Socioeconomic indices	A nationally accepted index
	Ethnicity	
Patients	Diagnoses	Cancer: Entity, stage; nonmalignant disease: type, stage
	Comorbidities	Charlson comorbidity index
	Performance status	Australian KPS or ECOG
		Number: Mean (SD), median (range)
	Symptoms: Physical, psychosocial, spiritual	Validated symptom measures, e.g., POS, MSAS, EORTC QLQ C30
		Validated symptom-specific measures
	Cognitive status	Mini-Mental State Examination (MMSE), MacArthur Competency Assessment Tool modified for clinical research (MacCAT-CR)
	Days from referral to death	Mean (SD), median (range)
	Prognosis	Validated prognostic index
Caregivers	Caregiver burden	Validated measure, e.g., Zarit Burden inventory
Health care professionals	Professional background	
	Experience in palliative care (years)	
General public	Marital status	
	Living arrangements	
	Urbanization levels	
	Religion/denomination	
	Financial situation	

Source: Currow, D.C. et al., *J. Pain Symptom Manage.*, 43(5), 902, 2012.

of the study sample. In a study coding characteristics of palliative care research, the most frequently reported subdomains were patient age, gender, diagnosis, and patient performance status [3]. Rarely reported subdomains included socioeconomic indices, ethnicity, and time from referral to death [3]. Overall, there was a significant underreporting of even basic patient demographic factors. Given wide local differences in the people referred to, and the structure of, palliative care services, the poor reporting of basic descriptive factors can be expected to complicate or impede the application of newly found knowledge in this field [3].

Currow et al. suggest that it is feasible to report standard study descriptors that can aid with evaluation of generalizability in supportive and palliative care [3]. Table 22.1 suggests a number of characteristics of study participants that should be included when reporting palliative care research.

To understand the sample of a study and put the results in context, reference to the wider population from which the sample is drawn is necessary. The sample is described as the numerator whereas the population is the denominator [48]. Researchers consistently fail to report information on the population they recruited their sample from, as demonstrated in a review of the published research literature where articles provided data only for people participating in the study; no article provided data for people referred to the service or for

the total population of people with life-limiting illnesses from whom the service population was drawn [3]. Demographic and clinical characteristics of the population are both important and necessary, in order to compare the sample with the population and understand substantial differences, which might constrain generalizability. In qualitative research, the sampling frame (population from which the qualitative study sample is drawn) is more often considered—in part because of the different intentions of sampling in qualitative research (to ensure diversity rather than representativeness, within the sample).

CONCLUSION

It is in the nature of palliative care for patients to have multiple symptoms and other problems, with diversity in the severity and interactions between these problems. Palliative care populations are therefore inherently heterogeneous. Although it can therefore be challenging to define the population for palliative care research, and some degree of heterogeneity cannot be avoided, the recommendations discussed earlier, if adopted, would help to markedly improve many existing or current studies. A balance is needed between narrower inclusion criteria, targeting more specific populations when appropriate, and broader inclusion criteria, to achieve successful recruitment (and reach required sample size) and to maintain the generalizability of findings. Careful consideration of the population to be targeted for any study, the use of detailed and well-justified inclusion and exclusion criteria, and thorough description of the study population (using criteria such as those proposed by Currow), including the denominator population, would all help to raise the standard of the increasing amount of palliative care research being undertaken.

The palliative care population includes many with whom it is challenging to undertake research; these include the very ill, those near the end of life, and those with limited capacity. There are methods by which these people can be included. As the population ages, we also need to ensure research is undertaken among older people and among those with complex, interacting comorbidities. A detailed, considered, and transparent approach, as suggested in this chapter, can go a long way toward addressing some of these diverse challenges.

REFERENCES

1 Tieman J, Sladek R, Currow D. Changes in the quantity and level of evidence of palliative and hospice care literature: The last century. *J Clin Oncol.* 2008;26(35):5679–5683.
2 Abernethy AP, Aziz NM, Basch E, Bull J, Cleeland CS, Currow DC et al. A strategy to advance the evidence base in palliative medicine: Formation of a palliative care research cooperative group. *J Palliat Med.* 2010;13(12):1407–1413.
3 Currow DC, Tieman JJ, Greene A, Zafar SY, Wheeler JL, Abernethy AP. Refining a checklist for reporting patient populations and service characteristics in hospice and palliative care research. *J Pain Symptom Manage.* 2012;43(5):902–910.
4 Sepulveda C, Marlin A, Yoshida T, Ullrich A. Palliative Care: The World Health Organization's global perspective. *J Pain Symptom Manage.* 2002;24(2):91–96.
5 Radbruch L, Payne S, EAPC BoDo. White Paper on standards and norms for hospice and palliative care in Europe. *Eur J Palliat Care.* 2009;16(16):278–289.
6 Van Mechelen W, Aertgeerts B, De Ceulaer K, Thoonsen B, Vermandere M, Warmenhoven F, et al. Defining the palliative care patient: A systematic review. *Palliat Med* 2013 Mar;27(3):197–208. First published on 6 February 2012, doi: 10.1177/0269216311435268.
7 Temel JS, Greer JA, Muzikansky A, Gallagher ER, Admane S, Jackson VA et al. Early palliative care for patients with metastatic non-small-cell lung cancer. *N Engl J Med.* 2010;363(8):733–742.
8 Department of Health. *End of Life Care Strategy.* London, U.K.: Department of Health 2008.
9 Teunissen SC, Wesker W, Kruitwagen C, de Haes HC, Voest EE, de Graeff A. Symptom prevalence in patients with incurable cancer: A systematic review. *J Pain Symptom Manage.* 2007;34(1):94–104.
10 Koffman J, Higginson IJ. Accounts of carers' satisfaction with health care at the end of life: A comparison of first generation black Caribbeans and white patients with advanced disease. *Palliat Med.* 2001;15(4):337–345.

11 Murtagh FE, Addington-Hall J, Edmonds P, Donohoe P, Carey I, Jenkins K et al. Symptoms in the month before death for stage 5 chronic kidney disease patients managed without dialysis. *J Pain Symptom Manage.* 2010;40(3):342–352.
12 Murtagh FE, Sheerin NS, Addington-Hall J, Higginson IJ. Trajectories of illness in stage 5 chronic kidney disease: A longitudinal study of patient symptoms and concerns in the last year of life. *Clin J Am Soc Nephrol.* [Multicenter Study Research Support, Non-U.S. Gov't]. 2011;6(7):1580–1590.
13 Blinderman CD, Homel P, Billings JA, Portenoy RK, Tennstedt SL. Symptom distress and quality of life in patients with advanced congestive heart failure. *J Pain Symptom Manage.* 2008;35(5):594–603.
14 Habraken JM, van der Wal WM, Ter Riet G, Weersink EJ, Toben F, Bindels PJ. Health-related quality of life and functional status in end-stage COPD: A longitudinal study. *Eur Respir J.* 2011;37(2):280–288.
15 Habraken JM, ter Riet G, Gore JM, Greenstone MA, Weersink EJ, Bindels PJ et al. Health-related quality of life in end-stage COPD and lung cancer patients. *J Pain Symptom Manage.* 2009;37(6):973–981.
16 Saini T, Murtagh FE, Dupont PJ, McKinnon PM, Hatfield P, Saunders Y. Comparative pilot study of symptoms and quality of life in cancer patients and patients with end stage renal disease. *Palliat Med.* 2006;20(6):631–636.
17 Lunney JR, Lynn J, Foley DJ, Lipson S, Guralnik JM. Patterns of functional decline at the end of life. *JAMA.* 2003;289(18):2387–2392.
18 Christakis NA, Lamont EB. Extent and determinants of error in doctors' prognoses in terminally ill patients: Prospective cohort study. *BMJ.* 2000;320(7233):469–472.
19 Teno JM, Harrell FE, Jr., Knaus W, Phillips RS, Wu AW, Connors A, Jr. et al. Prediction of survival for older hospitalized patients: The HELP survival model. Hospitalized Elderly Longitudinal Project. *J Am Geriatr Soc.* 2000;48(5 Suppl):S16–S24.
20 Lamont EB, Christakis NA. Prognostic disclosure to patients with cancer near the end of life. *Ann Intern Med.* 2001;134(12):1096–1105.
21 Steinhauser KE, Clipp EC, Hays JC, Olsen M, Arnold R, Christakis NA et al. Identifying, recruiting, and retaining seriously-ill patients and their caregivers in longitudinal research. *Palliat Med.* 2006;20(8):745–754.
22 Abernethy AP, Currow DC, Frith P, Fazekas BS, McHugh A, Bui C. Randomised, double blind, placebo controlled crossover trial of sustained release morphine for the management of refractory dyspnoea. *BMJ.* 2003;327(7414):523–528.
23 Abernethy AP, McDonald CF, Frith PA, Clark K, Herndon JE, 2nd, Marcello J et al. Effect of palliative oxygen versus room air in relief of breathlessness in patients with refractory dyspnoea: A double-blind, randomised controlled trial. *Lancet.* 2010;376(9743):784–793.
24 Pereira J, Hanson J, Bruera E. The frequency and clinical course of cognitive impairment in patients with terminal cancer. *Cancer.* 1997;79(4):835–842.
25 Casarett DJ. Assessing decision-making capacity in the setting of palliative care research. *J Pain Symptom Manage.* 2003;25(4):S6–S13.
26 Bruera E, Franco JJ, Maltoni M, Watanabe S, Suarez-Almazor M. Changing pattern of agitated impaired mental status in patients with advanced cancer: Association with cognitive monitoring, hydration, and opioid rotation. *J Pain Symptom Manage.* 1995;10(4):287–291.
27 Casarett D, Ferrell B, Kirschling J, Levetown M, Merriman MP, Ramey M et al. NHPCO Task Force Statement on the Ethics of Hospice Participation in Research. *J Palliat Med.* 2001;4(4):441–449.
28 Grisso T, Appelbaum PS, Hill-Fotouhi C. The MacCAT-T: A clinical tool to assess patients' capacities to make treatment decisions. *Psychiatr Serv.* 1997;48(11):1415–1419.
29 Folstein MF, Folstein SE, McHugh PR. "Mini-mental state". A practical method for grading the cognitive state of patients for the clinician. *J Psychiatr Res.* 1975;12(3):189–198.

30 Karlawish JH. Conducting research that involves subjects at the end of life who are unable to give consent. *J Pain Symptom Manage.* 2003;25(4):S14–S24.

31 Rees E, Hardy J. Novel consent process for research in dying patients unable to give consent. *BMJ.* 2003;327(7408):198.

32 Cohen J, Bilsen J, Miccinesi G, Lofmark R, Addington-Hall J, Kaasa S et al. Using death certificate data to study place of death in 9 European countries: Opportunities and weaknesses. *BMC Public Health.* 2007;7:283.

33 McNamara B, Rosenwax LK, Holman CD. A method for defining and estimating the palliative care population. *J Pain Symptom Manage.* 2006;32(1):5–12.

34 Dumont S, Jacobs P, Turcotte V, Anderson D, Harel F. The trajectory of palliative care costs over the last 5 months of life: A Canadian longitudinal study. *Palliat Med.* 2010;24(6):630–640.

35 Quinn MP, Cardwell CR, Rainey A, McNamee PT, Kee F, Maxwell AP et al. The impact of admissions for the management of end-stage renal disease on hospital bed occupancy. *Nephron.* 2009;113(4):c315–c320.

36 Bardsley M, Georghiou T, Chassin L, Lewis G, Steventon A, Dixon J. Overlap of hospital use and social care in older people in England. *J Health Serv Res Policy.* 2012 Jul;17(3):133–9. doi: 10.1258/jhsrp.2011.010171. Epub 2012 Feb 23.

37 Wheeler JL, Greene A, Tieman JJ, Abernethy AP, Currow DC. Key characteristics of palliative care studies reported in the specialized literature. *J Pain Symptom Manage.* 2012;43(6):987–992.

38 Payne S, Carers ETFoF. White Paper on improving support for family carers in palliative care: Part 2. *European Journal of Palliative Care.* 2010;17(5):286–290.

39 Grande G, Stajduhar K, Aoun S, Toye C, Funk L, Addington-Hall J et al. Supporting lay carers in end of life care: Current gaps and future priorities. *Palliat Med.* 2009;23(4):339–344.

40 Koffman J, Higginson IJ, Hall S, Riley J, McCrone P, Gomes B. Bereaved relatives' views about participating in cancer research. *Palliat Med.* 2012;26(4):379–383.

41 Addington-Hall J, McPherson C. After-death interviews with surrogates/bereaved family members: Some issues of validity. *J Pain Symptom Manage.* 2001;22(3):784–790.

42 Costantini M, Beccaro M, Merlo F. The last three months of life of Italian cancer patients. Methods, sample characteristics and response rate of the Italian Survey of the Dying of Cancer (ISDOC). *Palliat Med.* 2005;19(8):628–638.

43 Meeussen K, Van den Block L, Echteld M, Bossuyt N, Bilsen J, Van Casteren V et al. Advance care planning in Belgium and The Netherlands: A nationwide retrospective study via sentinel networks of general practitioners. *J Pain Symptom Manage.* 2011;42(4):565–577.

44 Shipman C, Burt J, Ream E, Beynon T, Richardson A, Addington-Hall J. Improving district nurses' confidence and knowledge in the principles and practice of palliative care. *J Adv Nurs.* 2008;63(5):494–505.

45 Bausewein C, Simon ST, Benalia H, Downing J, Mwangi-Powell FN, Daveson BA et al. Implementing patient reported outcome measures (PROMs) in palliative care—Users' cry for help. *Health Qual Life Outcomes.* 2011;9:27.

46 Gomes B, Higginson IJ, Calanzani N, Cohen J, Deliens L, Daveson BA et al. Preferences for place of death if faced with advanced cancer: A population survey in England, Flanders, Germany, Italy, the Netherlands, Portugal and Spain. *Ann Oncol.* 2012;23(8):2006–2015.

47 Cohen J, Marcoux I, Bilsen J, Deboosere P, van der Wal G, Deliens L. Trends in acceptance of euthanasia among the general public in 12 European countries (1981–1999). *Eur J Public Health.* 2006;16(6):663–669.

48 Teno JM, Coppola KM. For every numerator, you need a denominator: A simple statement but key to measuring the quality of care of the "dying". *J Pain Symptom Manage.* 1999;17(2):109–113.

23

Study designs in palliative medicine

MASSIMO COSTANTINI

> ... the question being asked determines the appropriate research architecture, strategy, and tactics to be used – not tradition, authority, experts, paradigms, or schools of thought.
>
> Sackett DL, Wenneberg JE 1997[1]

INTRODUCTION

The objectives of this chapter are to define, discuss, and compare study designs commonly used for quantitative research in palliative care. A specific area of the chapter will deal with study designs used in health services research, such as cluster trials, stepped wedge trials, and fast-track trials. Quantitative research uses the epidemiological approach to define and shape all the aspects of a study, including its design. Epidemiology is the study of disease and health in human populations.[2] In palliative medicine, we focus on at least two populations of interest: people at the end of their lives and their families. For both populations, "the disease" is a multidimensional problem involving suffering, dignity, care needs, and quality of life.[3]

Within these specific areas of interest, the general aims of epidemiologic research in palliative medicine are the following:

- *To describe* needs and problems of people at the end of their lives and their families in terms of frequency, risk factors (frequency within groups), and trends.
- *To explain* the causal relationships between the developing of one or more outcomes and one or more study factors or exposures. The outcome in palliative medicine is one or more components of the multidimensional concept of quality of life or other issues that, directly or indirectly, can help to better know and improve the quality of care. The study factors (the exposure) are the potential determinants of the outcome. These include characteristics of the subject, of the disease, or of the environment.
- *To assess the effectiveness of interventions* aimed at modifying the distribution of the problems in the population of interest by prevention of new occurrences, effective treatment of existing cases, or, in general terms, improving quality of life of affected persons.

High-quality research is required in order to achieve these aims, due to the unique challenges posed by studies focused on terminal patients. The choice of appropriate study design is probably the most important factor for the quality of a study. We can define a study design as the strategy adopted to describe a problem (in descriptive designs) or to test hypotheses and evaluate strengths of associations (in analytical and experimental designs). Each study design has a particular methodology and can investigate particular aims (Table 23.1).

Epidemiologic research makes use of observational, quasi-experimental, and experimental studies. In observational studies, there is no artificial manipulation of the study factors, and events and associations are described and analyzed as they naturally occur. Whenever there is an artificial manipulation of the study factor, the study is (1) experimental if the study factor is randomly allocated to study subjects or (2) quasi-experimental if the study factor is allocated without randomization.[2]

Any attempt to rank study designs according to their inherent value makes little sense, since it is the main objective that defines the most appropriate design for a specific study (Table 23.1).[1] This chapter seeks to help the researcher to identify the most appropriate design for answering a specific question.

STUDY DESIGNS

In all study designs, the investigator must be concerned with avoiding any effect or inference tending to produce results that depart systematically from true values. In other words, he or she should avoid any kind of bias at any stage of the study, from study design to publication of the results. More than 100 biases have been described.[4] A conceptually appealing classification identifies two general classes of systematic errors. The first, selection bias, includes any error that arises in the process of identifying the study population. The second, information bias, refers to any error in the measurement of information on exposure or outcome.

Table 23.1 *Types and general aims of the principal study designs*

Study design	Methodology	General aim
Cross-sectional	Observational	Descriptive–analytic
Retrospective cohort study	Observational	Analytic–descriptive
Prospective cohort study	Observational	Analytic–descriptive
Case–control	Observational	Analytic
Quasi-experimental	Experimental without randomization	Analytic
Experimental	Experimental with randomization	Analytic

Observational studies

There are three basic observational designs: cross-sectional, case–control, and cohort studies. The differences between them are related to the sampling frame and the time frame.

In a *cross-sectional study*, subjects are selected from the target population at a particular point in time, regardless of their exposure and disease, and the associations among variables are evaluated.[2] This type of study can be conducted at a specific point in time (e.g., of pain at a specific date), at a fixed point during the course of events (e.g., of pain at hospice admission), or in a specific time window (e.g., of pain during the last month of life).

In a *case–control study*, samples of subjects with (cases) and without (controls) a condition are identified and the groups compared with respect to prior exposure to one or more study factors.[2] The validity of this design depends on the ability to draw a valid sample of cases and controls from the target population. In palliative care, it is difficult to identify the whole population of palliative patients and to appropriately sample cases and controls (e.g., patients with and without a symptom). As a consequence, this design, seldom used in palliative care research, will not be discussed in this chapter. Of note, however, is that it is possible to nest a case–control study within a larger population-based study; see, for example, the QUALYCARE study that includes a nested case–control study of factors associated with the outcome of death at home or in hospital.[5]

In a *cohort study* (also called longitudinal study), samples of subjects with and without specific characteristics of exposure are followed forward in time from exposure to outcome, and the outcome in persons exposed to the study factor (exposed) is compared with the outcome in persons not exposed to the study factor (unexposed).[2] A cohort study can be done "prospectively," where the study population is identified at the time the study starts and then followed over a certain period to assess the outcome, or "retrospectively," where the study population of exposed and unexposed is identified in the past and the occurrence of the outcome is evaluated in the period elapsed from the time when exposure was assessed to the present.

The choice of a retrospective or prospective design is based essentially on logistic and scientific considerations. Retrospective studies require much less time and resources, because all events have already occurred when the study is initiated. In palliative care, retrospective cohort studies are difficult to perform because information on exposure or outcomes is usually not available retrospectively. The assessment of "hard outcomes," such as hospitalizations or place of death, or the availability of historical databases of routinely collected outcomes measures, such as the Palliative care Outcome Scale,[6] can make this approach feasible. Conversely, data collected for purposes other than research may be of questionable accuracy and reliability,[7] and information on potential confounders are often missing.

A specific design is the *after death approach*, where information is collected after the death of the patient from a proxy that was close to the patient during the period of observation. The proxy can be a family member who attended the patient during the last period of life[8] or a professional informed on some dimensions of end-of-life care received by the patient, for example, the GPs in the SENTI-MELC surveys.[9] This cross-sectional design—similar for some characteristics to a retrospective cohort design—has been used in a number of influential studies,[8–12] to estimate the multidimensional problems experienced by patients during their last period of life. The strength of this design lies in the possibility to evaluate a representative sample of patients with advanced and terminal disease, as the sample is built after deaths have occurred. This approach overcomes many of the problems of the studies performed directly on the patients, as it has been possible to generalize the results to the whole population of terminally ill patients. This approach has at least two weaknesses. First, the process of defining the cause of death is often unreliable, especially for elderly and noncancer patients, even when death certificates are used.[13] Second, the assessment of the outcomes from bereaved carers or from professionals, several months after patient's death, may result in a large distortion of the results.[14]

Experimental and quasi-experimental designs

In experimental and quasi-experimental designs, an intervention is deliberately introduced to observe its effects (the artificial manipulation of the study factor). The general aim of these designs is to study the efficacy (or the effectiveness) of the intervention. Random allocation of the intervention between groups of patients discriminates experimental (with randomization) from quasi-experimental (without randomization) studies.[2] All quasi-experimental and experimental studies are, by definition, prospective.

Quasi-experimental designs

A variety of quasi-experimental designs have been proposed: some are not very reliable, and others, more sophisticated, allow in some situation a strong causal inference.[15] The validity of the study design depends on the degree of control that the researcher has over several elements of the study design such as the assignment of the patients to different treatments, the measurement of the outcomes, the choice of comparison groups, or the application and the scheduling of the treatment.[15]

The uncontrolled before–after design is characterized by two measurement points: one before and one after the intervention, without any external control group. This study design is commonly used in health service research, for example, in phase 2 studies for assessing complex intervention.[16] This approach is considered inadequate to evaluate the causal relationship between the intervention and the outcomes.[17]

In the classical nonequivalent groups design, the two (or more) groups are identified from convenience (patients of different services, hospitals, health districts) or according to their voluntary behavior. The researcher can also compare the subjects of the experimental group with subjects who received a different intervention for the same condition at a different time, generally an earlier period (the so-called historical controls). In these studies, the control group is selected to be as similar as possible to the intervention groups for all characteristics but the intervention. Matching or stratifying for relevant characteristics or adjusting for baseline values of the outcomes can increase the comparability between groups.

These designs can prove severely biased when the subjects themselves determine the intervention they receive. People who choose a new therapy or to be followed by an experimental service are likely to be different for many characteristics related to the outcome of interest. Designs less amenable to selection bias are those in which the two groups are selected for factors not related to their preference for the intervention.

Experimental designs

In experimental studies, the population of units selected for the study is split into two (or more) groups using randomization. This procedure ensures that chance alone determines the groups to which each unit is assigned. Each group is assigned to a different intervention, and outcomes in the groups are compared to infer the relative effects of the intervention(s).

Randomization implies that the probability of receiving each of the possible interventions under study is the same for each unit being entered into the study. Notably, this probability does not need to be the same for all interventions being compared, and allocation ratios different from 1:1 can be chosen for various reasons (convenience, costs, organizational problems, etc.), although this may increase the required sample size. Randomization is a powerful tool that, if appropriately used, protects the study from the risk of selection bias. Note that randomization does not guarantee that the two groups are identical, even in large samples. However, it does guarantee that the distribution of known and unknown characteristics, in the two groups, is determined by chance alone.

Two experimental designs are commonly used in palliative care research: the parallel group design and the crossover design. In the parallel design, patients are randomly allocated to receive the intervention(s) of interest (the experimental group) and the best available treatment (the control group). Only if no effective treatment for the condition under study is available should the control group receive either a placebo or no treatment.[18] In a randomized crossover trial, patients are

randomly allocated to different sequences of treatments.[19] In the simplest design (AB/BA design), half of the patients are randomly allocated to receive treatment A followed by B and half to receive the treatment B followed by A.

Other study designs

In *randomized cluster trials*, the randomization unit is represented by the clusters (for instance, a GP, a ward, a service, a health district, each with their own clusters of patients and families).[20] This means that all the individuals belonging to that group will receive the same treatment and that different groups, at random, will receive different treatments. Cluster trials are a key tool in the process of evaluation of complex interventions that operate at a group level and that cannot be delivered to individuals. Two main types of cluster trial can be identified.[21] In the first type, the intervention involves the implementation of a program targeted to the health professionals, with the aim of finding a benefit for patients. The randomized cluster trial performed in Italy for assessing the effectiveness of the Liverpool Care Pathway is an example[22] (Figure 23.1). In the second type, the clusters are communities randomized to receive or not to receive the intervention. These "large field trials" are characterized by a relatively small number of clusters each enrolling a large number of subjects. The randomized cluster trial performed in Norway for assessing the effectiveness of a program aimed at enabling patients to spend more time at home and die there if they prefer is an example.[23] In cluster trials, observations on individuals of the same cluster tend to be correlated, and these studies require more participants to obtain equivalent statistical power. Cluster randomized trials are rather complex to design, to conduct, and to analyze. Specific statistical techniques to adjust for internal cluster correlation between individuals are needed.[20,21] A specific extension to cluster randomized trials have been developed for the CONSORT statements.[24]

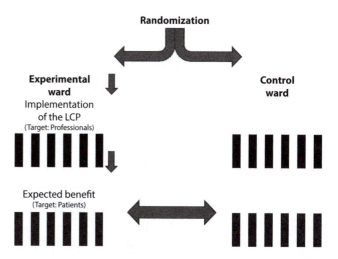

Figure 23.1 *The randomized cluster trial assessing the effectiveness of the Liverpool Care Pathway in 16 Italian general medicine wards. (Data from Shadish, W.R. et al., eds.,* Experimental and Quasi-Experimental Designs, *Houghton Mifflin Company, Boston, MA, 2002.)*

A promising study design is the stepped wedge design, where the intervention is implemented sequentially to the trial participants, usually clusters of individuals, over a number of time periods.[25] The order the clusters of individuals receive the intervention can be randomized. At the end of the study, all clusters have received the intervention. At each time period, outcomes are collected for all clusters, and a new cluster receives the intervention (Figure 23.2). As for cluster trials, clustering of observations should be taken into account in estimating the sample size and in analyzing the results.[25] This study design is advantageous when there are practical reasons that support the choice to implement the intervention in stages, avoiding some clusters not receiving the intervention at the end of the study.

Most recently in palliative care, the possibilities of performing randomized *fast-track trials* have been explored.[26] In this type of study, all individuals are offered the intervention, but they are randomized to either receive it immediately (the fast-track arm) or to receive the standard intervention (or no intervention) for a first period of time and then the intervention (the control arm) (Figure 23.3). The overlapping periods of evaluation of the outcomes in the two arms allow us to contrast the effectiveness of the intervention after the first period of time. At this point, the postintervention assessment (in the fast-track arm) is contrasted against the preintervention assessment (in the control arm). The main analysis is not different from that required for a classical parallel randomized trial. More complex statistical analyses are required to use the assessments of the second period of time for determining the long-term impact of the intervention and the interaction between time and intervention.[27]

STUDY AIMS

Descriptive studies

Descriptive studies describe "patterns of problems occurrence" in relation to variables such as person, place, and time. In palliative care, they have been used to describe the needs and problems encountered by patients and their families during the advanced and terminal phase of disease.[28]

Two basic designs are used: cross-sectional and longitudinal studies. The first design, regarded as primarily descriptive, provides a snapshot of the health experience of a population at a given time. The simplest design is relatively inexpensive and quick as compared to longitudinal studies. If well designed, the results from the study sample can be generalized to the population of interest. Moreover, it provides estimates of the prevalence of all factors measured. Studies describing the proportion of patients with severe pain among hospitalized patients,[29] or the prevalence of severe communication problems among patients followed by palliative care services,[30] are classical descriptive studies. The cross-sectional design is not well suited to study rare problems. It has an inherent bias (usually referred to as length biased sampling), since it overrepresents subjects with long duration of the problem.

Longitudinal studies represent the best way to describe the natural history of a disease, in terms of outcomes relevant for palliative care. The main advantage of a longitudinal design is that the individual development of the outcomes of interest over time can be studied. This approach is easy when the

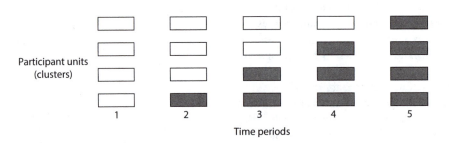

Figure 23.2 *The classical stepped wedge trial design. (Note: Grey cells are the intervention periods and blank cells are the control periods. Data on outcomes are collected in all cells from time 1 to time 5.)*

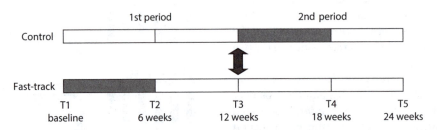

Figure 23.3 *The fast-track study design assessing the effectiveness of a new palliative care intervention for patients affected by multiple sclerosis. (Note: Grey cells are the intervention periods and blank cells are the control periods. Data on outcomes are collected at the five points. The effectiveness analysis was performed by comparing the outcomes at T3 (the gray arrow) adjusted for the baseline [T].) (Data from Higginson, I.J. et al.,* Postgrad. Med. J., *87, 769, 2011.)*

outcome variable is an irreversible endpoint. In palliative care, most outcomes should be measured in the same individual on different occasions and viewed in a dynamic prospective over time. To this purpose, a longitudinal design is the best choice, although statistical analysis of its results can be very complex.[31]

Apart from statistical problems, in longitudinal studies, researchers are to deal with a number of methodological issues, related to the validity of the results of their descriptive study. A descriptive study is valid inasmuch as it is able to describe what it intends to in the population from which the sample is drawn. Selection and information bias can compromise the ability of a study to provide information generalizable to the population of interest.[2]

Information bias is a particularly sensitive issue in palliative care, as it is difficult to measure without distortion of the "subjective point of view" of patients experiencing a progressive functional and cognitive decline. As far as selection bias is concerned, there is a theoretical and practical difficulty to identify the population of terminally ill patients of a specific geographic area. At least theoretically, cancer patients can be identified when they enter the terminal phase of disease and assessed when they are still alive. For most patients dying from noncancer diseases, there is uncertainty about the course of disease, and even theoretically, it is impossible to avoid any selection bias. Also for cancer patients, it is difficult to plan an unbiased population-based study (either cross-sectional or longitudinal) as these patients are followed by a number of health agencies in many different settings of care.

Analytical observational studies

Analytical studies are epidemiological investigations in which the association between a dependent variable (the outcome of interest) and one or more independent variables is evaluated, and possible cause–effect relationships are assessed. Although some implicit or explicit type of comparison exists in all study designs, analytical studies are primarily planned for determining if the frequency of an outcome is different for people exposed to a study factor (exposed) or not exposed to the factor (unexposed).

The presence of an association does not imply that the relationship between variables is one of cause and effect. We can speak of causal association only when an induced change in the quantity of the study factor results in a corresponding change in the quantity of the outcome. In theory, causality can be definitely demonstrated only through appropriately designed experiments. As a consequence, in observational studies, assessing whether the observed association (or the lack of one) represents a cause–effect relationship is a matter of determining the likelihood that alternative explanations could account for the observed results. In this process, at least three explanations should be considered:

- The observed association could be due to the play of chance.
- The association could be the result of a systematic error in the selection of the study subjects (selection bias) or in the assessment of exposure and/or the outcome (information bias).

- The association could be due to the effect of an extraneous factor associated with the study factor that independently affects the risk of outcome (confounding).

It is not possible to summarize in this chapter the long and often sophisticated discussions on the nature of causation and on the methods for identifying causal effects. On this topic, the Bradford Hill criteria (Hill) are very popular and seem to provide a road map through a complicated territory.[32,33] Although erroneously referred to as "causal criteria," they simply offer a systematic approach, neither necessary nor sufficient, to infer causation from a statistical association observed in epidemiological data.

A well-designed and conducted longitudinal study allows a valid inference about risk factors influencing the outcome(s) of interest. A number of variants of the basic design can be used, sometimes very difficult to design and analyze.[2] The most important weakness remains the unavoidable presence of a systematic distortion in the estimate of effect resulting from the manner in which subjects are selected for the study population (selection bias).

Studies to assess the effectiveness of an intervention

A fundamental objective of epidemiology in the area of palliative medicine is to produce knowledge that might be or is useful to prevent and control patients' and families' problems during the terminal phase of disease.

Although the randomized clinical trial represents the gold standard for the assessment of the effectiveness of an intervention, observational and quasi-experimental designs can provide, with different degree of feasibility, validity, and generalizability, useful information for establishing if (and to what extent) an intervention is effective both in clinical and in health services research. The feasibility of a trial depends on its acceptance by all the subjects involved into the research.[34]

Two criteria are used to assess the quality of a trial: internal and external validity. The internal validity implies an accurate measurement of the effect apart from random errors, but all studies, including randomized ones, are subject to some type of bias. The procedure used to allocate subjects to the different treatments is the major source of bias. In all nonrandomized studies, some selection bias is unavoidable, but in observational studies and in poorly designed quasi-experimental studies where little or no control is possible on allocation procedures, the risk of selection bias is very high.

Another major source of bias in palliative care studies derives from the patients effectively analyzed for the outcome. In randomized clinical trials, the principle of "intention to treat analysis" is recommended to preserve the internal validity. This approach should be extended, whenever is possible, to all effectiveness studies. According to the "intention to treat principle," all randomized (or registered) patients should be included in the analyses of results, independently of their effective eligibility, of the received treatment, of the adherence and compliance to the treatments, and of the compliance to the assessments procedures. In palliative care research, the attrition rate is usually high and the contamination of exposure (especially in health services research) frequent.

External validity refers to the generalizability and applicability of study results. In this regard, an important distinction is that between the efficacy and the effectiveness of an intervention, because it defines the general aim of the study.[35] Efficacy is the extent to which a specific intervention produces a beneficial result under ideal conditions. Effectiveness assesses the same beneficial effect in the field, estimating if it does what it is intended to do for a defined population. The studies require different study designs: explanatory for assessing the efficacy and pragmatic to assess the effectiveness of an intervention (Table 23.2).

Explanatory studies are aimed at providing the proof of principle that the intervention works (or does not work) under the most favorable conditions. On the other hand, pragmatic studies are interested in assessing the effectiveness of the intervention in a scenario as similar as possible to everyday practice.

In clinical research, explanatory randomized studies (both the crossover and the classical parallel design) on selected patients should be considered as the first option to assess the efficacy of a new intervention. Problems in recruitment could be overcome by implementing collaborative networks of high-quality palliative care units. For these studies, the internal validity is crucial, and also if the planned sample size is not attained, they can be combined with other studies in a systematic review.

When the clinical question becomes more pragmatic, and refers to the ability of the intervention to work in clinical everyday practice, the best design is often a quasi-experimental or an observational study. For health services research, the problems are more complicated. Most of the questions are intrinsically pragmatic, and pure randomized explanatory trials are very difficult to conceive. It is difficult to randomize selected series of patients, avoiding any contamination between the groups. To assess the effect of a service, a number of outcomes with their valid, reliable, and sensitive tools should be available and the best timing of the assessments clearly defined. Moreover, new activities are difficult to standardize, so that it is often difficult to be certain that the effect (or the lack of effect) is not due to the intrinsic quality of that specific team.

Table 23.2 *Differences between explanatory and pragmatic trials*

Explanatory design	Pragmatic design
(The aim is efficacy)	(The aim is effectiveness)
Selected patients	Patients as similar as possible to the common clinical practice
Sophisticated study protocol Intensive follow-up	Very simple study protocol Follow-up as in clinical practice
Multiple and complex end points	Simple end point (reflecting the benefit to the patient)
High-quality centers Minimal sample size	Generic centers Large sample size

CONCLUSIONS AND FUTURE PRIORITIES

In this chapter, the various study designs commonly used in palliative care research were reviewed and discussed in terms of feasibility, validity, and potential biases. Further methodological research is much needed in palliative care research and particularly in three critical areas:

- The validity of the "after death designs" and their ability to produce an accurate portrait of the care provided to dying patients[28]
- Advantages and disadvantages of quasi-experimental designs in palliative care research to assess the effectiveness of an intervention and the identification of the study designs that can provide a high level of internal validity
- The problems encountered in designing, conducting, and analyzing randomized cluster trials, stepped wedge trials, and the fast-track trials and their role in assessing complex interventions in palliative care

Key learning points

- As the design of a study is the strategy of answering a clinical or epidemiological question, it is the question that determines the appropriate study design.

- In studies regarded as primarily descriptive, selection and information bias (with a different degree according to the study design) can compromise the ability of the study to provide information generalizable to the population of interest.

- In analytical observational studies, the architecture of the study design should allow the researcher to assess if the observed associations represent cause–effect relationships or if alternative explanations could account for the observed results (chance, bias, and confounding).

- Studies aimed at assessing the efficacy or the effectiveness of an intervention require different study designs: explanatory for assessing the efficacy and pragmatic to assess the effectiveness.

- In clinical research, explanatory randomized studies should be the first option to assess the efficacy of a new intervention, followed by more pragmatic quasi-experimental or observational designs aimed at assessing the beneficial effect on the field. For health service research, the questions are often intrinsically pragmatic.

- Cluster randomized trials or alternative designs such as stepped wedge and fast-track trials have been shown to be feasible and valid options in palliative care research. These study designs should be considered as the first option for the assessment of the effectiveness of a complex intervention.

- The perfect study design for answering a specific question is not always feasible, and often the choice will be based on a compromise between feasibility, validity, and generalizability.

REFERENCES

● 1 Sackett DL, Wennberg JE. Choosing the best research design for each question. *BMJ*. 1997; **315**:1636.

2 Kleinbaum DG, Kupper LL, Morgenstern H. (eds.) *Epidemiologic Research*. New York: Van Nostrand Reinhold, 1982.

3 Davies E, Higginson IJ. (eds.) *Palliative Care. The Solid Facts*. Geneva, Switzerland: World Health Organization, 2004.

◆ 4 Sackett DL. Bias in analytic research. *J Chronic Dis* 1979; **32**:51–63.

5 Gomes B, McCrone P, Hall S, Koffman J, Higginson IJ. Variations in the quality and costs of end-of-life care, preferences and palliative outcomes for cancer patients by place of death: The QUALYCARE study. *BMC Cancer*. 2010;**10**:400. doi: 10.1186/1471-2407-10-400.

◆ 6 Bausewein C, Le Grice C, Simon S, Higginson IJ. The use of two common palliative outcome measures in clinical care and research: A systematic review of POS and STAS. *Palliat Med*. 2011; **25**(4):304–313.

7 Johnson JC, Kerse NM, Gottlieb G et al. Prospective versus retrospective methods of identifying patients with delirium. *J Am Geriatr Soc* 1992; **40**:316–319.

8 Costantini M, Beccaro M, Merlo F. The last 3 months of life of Italian cancer patients. Methods, sample characteristics and response rate of the Italian Survey of the Dying of Cancer (ISDOC). *Pall Med* 2005; **19**:628–638.

9 Van den Block L, Deschepper R, Bossuyt N et al. Care for patients in the last months of life: The Belgian Sentinel Network Monitoring End-of-Life Care study. *Arch Intern Med* 2008; **168**(16):1747–1754.

● 10 First national VOICES survey of bereaved people. London, U.K.: NHS Medical Directorate/End of Life Care, July 3, 2012. http://www.dh.gov.uk/health/files/2012/07/First-national-VOICES-survey-of-bereaved-people-key-findings-report-final.pdf (last accessed: April 5, 2013)

● 11 Cartwright A, Hockley L, Anderson JL. (eds.) *Life Before Death*. London, U.K.: Routledge and Kegan Paul, 1973.

12 Teno JM, Clarridge BR, Casey V et al. Family perspectives on end-of-life care at the last place of care. *JAMA* 2004; **291**:88–93.

13 Gau DW, Diehl AK. Disagreement among general practitioners regarding cause of death. *Br Med J* 1982; **284**:239–445.

● 14 McPherson CJ, Addington-Hall JM. Judging the quality of care at the end of life: Can proxies provide reliable information? *Soc Sci Med* 2003; **56**:95–109.

◆ 15 Shadish WR, Cook TD, Campbell DT. (eds.) *Experimental and Quasi-Experimental Designs*. Boston, MA: Houghton Mifflin Company, 2002.

16 Costantini M, Di Leo S, Beccaro M. Methodological issues in a before-after study design to evaluate the Liverpool Care Pathway for the Dying Patient in hospital. *Palliat Med* 2011;**25**:766–773.

17 Simon S, Higginson IJ. Evaluation of hospital palliative care teams: Strengths and weaknesses of the before-after study design and strategies to improve it. *Palliat Med* 2009; **23**(1):23–28.

18 Meinert CL, Tonascia S. (eds.) *Clinical Trials: Design, Conduct, and Analysis*. New York: Oxford University Press, 1986.

◆ 19 Senn S. (ed.) *Cross-Over Trials in Clinical Research*. London, U.K.: John Wiley & sons, Ltd, 2002.

● 20 Campbell MJ, Donner A, Elbourne D. Design and analysis of cluster randomized trials. *Stat Med* 2001; **20**:329–496.

21 Campbell MJ, Donner A, Klar N. Developments in cluster randomized trials and Statistics in Medicine. *Statist Med* 2007; **26**:2–19.

22 Costantini M, Ottonelli S, Canavacci L et al. The effectiveness of the Liverpool Care Pathway in improving end of life care for dying cancer patients in hospital. A cluster randomised trial. *BMC Health Services Res*. 2011; **11**:13.

23 Jordhøy MS, Fayers P, Saltnes T, Ahlner-Elmqvist M, Jannert M, Kaasa S. A palliative-care intervention and death at home: A cluster randomised trial. *Lancet* 2000; **356**: 888–893.

24 Campbell MK, Elbourne DR, Altman DG, for the CONSORT Group. CONSORT statement: Extension to cluster randomised trials. *BMJ* 2004; **328**:702–708.

25 Brown CA, Lilford RJ. The stepped wedge trial design: A systematic review. *BMC Med. Res Method*. 2006; **6**:54.

26 Farquhar M, Prevost AT, McCrone P et al. Study Protocol: Phase III single-blinded fast-track pragmatic randomised controlled trial of a complex intervention for breathlessness in advanced disease. *Trials* 2011; **12**:130.

27 Higginson IJ, Costantini M, Silber E, Burman R, Edmonds P. Evaluation of a new model of short-term palliative care for people severely affected with multiple sclerosis: A randomised fast-track trial to test timing of referral and how long the effect is maintained. *Postgrad Med J* 2011;**87**:769–775.

◆ 28 Higginson IJ. Palliative and terminal care. In: Stevens A, Raftery J. (eds.) *Health care Needs Assessment*. Oxon, U.K.: Radcliff Medical Press, 1997; 1–79.

29 Costantini M, Viterbori P, Flego G. Prevalence of pain in Italian hospitals: Results of a regional cross-sectional survey. *J Pain Symptom Manage* 2002; **23**:221–223.

30 Higginson IJ, Costantini M. Communication in end-of-life cancer care: A comparison of Team assessment in three European countries. *J Clin Oncol* 2002; **20**:3674–3682.

31 Twisk JWR. (ed.) *Applied Longitudinal Data Analysis for Epidemiology*. Cambridge, U.K.: Cambridge University Press, 2003.

32 Phillips CV, Goodman KJ. The missed lessons of Sir Austin Bradford Hill. *Epidemiol Perspect Innov*. 2004; **1**:3

● 33 Hill AB. The environment and disease: Association or causation? *Proc R Soc Med* 1965; **58**:295–300.

34 Cook AM, Finlay IG, Butler-Keating RJ. Recruiting into palliative care trials: Lessons learnt from a feasibility study. *Pall Med* 2002; **16**:163–165.

● 35 Schwartz D, Lellouch J. Explanatory and pragmatic attitudes in therapeutical trials. *J Chronic Dis* 1967; **20**:637–648.

24

Outcome measurement in palliative care

JOAN M. TENO

WHY MEASURE OUTCOMES?

Key to achieving excellence in palliative medicine is a process of self-reflection that measures the end results of care. To not know the outcomes of care is simply not an acceptable medical practice. Without knowledge of the outcomes of care, the quality of care will not be improved. Excellent quality of care is only achieved through a process of ongoing research that examines the outcomes of palliative care programs and medical treatments, audits that help to shape quality improvement efforts to change medical practice, and publicly reported quality indicators. Auditing the quality of care is not just applicable to industrial nations. Rather, program evaluation is important in developing nations with limited resources.[1] While outcome measures that examine new medications or other treatments are essential for the development of the evidence base of palliative medicine, the focus of this chapter will be on the use of measurement in health services research, quality improvement, and publicly reported quality indicators.

An outcome measure examines the "end results" of care. The "end results" are the impact of medical care on the dying person and/or family. For the seriously ill and aged, it is important for the measurement of the outcomes of care to acknowledge the important role of informal caregivers, usually close family members, and medical care must attend to the needs of both the seriously ill persons and those of their family. This view is ratified in the World Health Organization[2] definition of palliative medicine as achieving the best possible quality of life for dying patients and their families. Outcome measures are the ultimate judge of the quality of care. Achieving those outcomes is based on ensuring that processes of care are in place to achieve the desired outcomes. A process measure examines what health providers "do" for dying persons and their family. Often, process measures can be a proxy for outcome measures that can only be examined years later (e.g., the treatment of hypertension and prevention of strokes). Ultimately, the quality of care is based on the outcomes of care. However, a focus on achieving quality of care is to ensure that correct processes of care are undertaken for the right person at the right time.

A recent international European and African survey of clinicians identified reasons why staff wanted to use outcome measures. For those that used tools, most reported favorable outcome measurement experiences. For clinical purposes, the main advantage for doctors was assessment/screening and clinical decision making for nurses. For research, doctors were most influenced by a measure's comparability with national/international literature followed by its validation in palliative care. For nurses, validation in palliative care was followed by tool access.[3]

The natural reaction of staff to outcome measurement is fear that the results will be misinterpreted that they are providing inadequate care. Often, that is hardly the case. Outcome measurement should not be used to "punish" staff. The vast majority of people come to work every day to do the best possible job within the constraints of current health-care systems. It is important that the use of outcome measurement is not used to blame staff. Rather, outcomes are the result of complex interactions. It is important that the people assessing the quality of care approach the examinations of outcomes from this perspective. For example, a local hospice found that 80% of decedents were dying in the hospital as opposed to at home. One interpretation of these results is the staff are not doing their job in providing adequate supportive care that allows a person to die at home. In this particular example, a further exploration of semistructured interviews with the staff about the barriers to people dying at home revealed that all home deaths were being treated by the local authorities as potential homicide. Families had learned to avoid the embarrassment of having their loved ones' death be treated as a homicide investigation by insisting that the dying person was transferred to an acute care hospital. The solution is not blaming the staff but making changes to the system of care (e.g., developing an inpatient hospice unit and working with the police to change how expected home deaths are treated) to ensure that dying persons and their family are receiving medical care consistent with their needs and expectation. This is an important lesson. Achieving excellence in end-of-life care requires a critical examination of the systems and processes of care alongside the outcomes.

WHAT IS QUALITY OF CARE FOR SERIOUSLY ILL AND DYING PERSONS?

Having a serious illness that raises the possibility of mortality is unique and sentinels time of life, unlike any other time period. Consider the following two clinical cases and the implications for measuring the quality of care:

- A 45-year-old man presents with acute anterior wall myocardial infarction. One proposed measure of quality of care by the Center for Medicaid and Medicare Services, the branch of the U.S. government that oversees health-care services, is whether he is discharged with an aspirin.[4]
- For a person of the same age and gender with stage IV lung cancer, the development of quality indicators that examine both the outcomes and process of care is much more difficult. Not all persons will want active treatment. The vast majority of 45-year-olds without a contraindication to aspirin would want to take it given the evidence of its efficacy. Seriously ill persons with lung cancer are faced with important trade-offs where their preferences are important for measuring the outcomes of care.[4]

The importance of patient preferences is reflected in the Institute of Medicine's proposed definition of quality of care as "the degree in which health services for individuals and populations increase the likelihood of the *desired* health outcome and are consistent with current professional knowledge."[5] Over the past century, the majority of deaths have been from chronic, progressive illnesses, often involving a decision that weighs the quality versus quantity of life. There is an evolving consensus regarding what are the key goals and domains to examine the quality of care for seriously ill and/or dying persons. Table 24.1 outlines a synthesis of the goals and domains of high quality palliative care based on the U.S. National Consensus Project, Canadian Palliative Care Organization proposed key domains and processes of care, the National Quality Forum, A National Framework for Palliative and Hospice Care Quality,[5] and work by Teno et al.[6,7] As documented in Table 24.1, there are four C's key to a system perspective of examining the quality of care. High-quality palliative care is (1) competent care that is safe and the right care at the right time and right locus of care, (2) compassionate, (3) coordinated across health-care providers and settings of care, and (4) cost-effective.

To date, various sources of evidence have been used to formulate definitions of quality of medical care for the seriously ill and dying. Professional bodies that rely on expert opinion, such as the National Hospice and Palliative Care Organization[8] or the Canadian Palliative Care Organization, have proposed key domains and processes of care that define quality of palliative and/or hospice care. Newer proposed definitions of the quality of care have involved the input of consumers.[9,10] While there is agreement on many key domains, dying persons and their families provide a unique perspective that should be accounted for in definitions of quality of care. Based on experts and focus groups with dying persons and family members, Teno et al. have developed a model of quality medical care entitled patient-focused, family-centered medical care (see Table 24.1).[9]

Under this model, high-quality medical care is achieved when health-care providers

- Provide the desired physical comfort, symptom control and emotional, social and spiritual support
- Promote shared decision making, including advance care planning for future periods of impaired decision-making capacity
- Treat the dying person with dignity and respect
- Attend to the needs of the family for information and skills in providing care for the dying person
- Support the family at a time prior to and after the patient's death
- Listen to and respond promptly to quality concerns regarding the provision of care by that health care organization.
- Advocate for the best possible quality of life and quality of care for the dying patient
- Coordinate care across health care providers and settings of healthcare given the increasing fragmentation of the healthcare of the dying.

Over the past decade, a consensus has been emerging regarding what are the key domains to examine both the processes and outcomes of care. Future research is needed to link both structure and process measures to the key outcome measures (Table 24.1 proposes key structural and process of care that potentially are related to key outcomes). Such research will be critical as palliative medicine grows as a subspecialty recognized for scientific evidence base that identifies key processes of care and treatment that lead to improve outcomes.

WHAT ARE THE SOURCES OF INFORMATION TO JUDGE THE OUTCOMES OF CARE?

A key step in measuring the outcomes of care is the decision on what is the source of information to judge the outcomes of care. Each source has both advantages and limitations. Often, an audit will need to draw from multiple sources of information to provide a more comprehensive view of care of the seriously ill and dying. Among the available sources of information on the outcomes of the quality of care are as follows:

- The medical record either paper or electronic, e.g. one could examine whether patients in pain receive medications for pain
- Administrative data, e.g. site of death based on death certificate data, billing data regarding medical procedures or visit, etc.
- Staff reports of the outcomes of care, e.g. pain noted on the minimum data set (MDS)
- Interviews with dying persons and/or their families conducted prior to and after the patient's death
- Independent assessment of the quality of care performed by experts.

Each involves trade-offs of strengths, limitations, and financial costs.

Table 24.1 *Components of high-quality palliative care*

1. Competent care

Goal	Domain and supporting evidence from 30 existing guidelines	Structure	Process	Outcome	Example of measure from family evaluation of hospice care survey
Plan of care is based on goals, values, and needs of the patient and family.	Patient- and family-centered care (N = 21) (70%)[8,19,26–52] Shared decision making and advance care planning (N = 24) (80%)[2,8,26,28,32,34,35,38,50,53]	Qualified interdisciplinary staff with appropriate certification and excellent knowledge and assessment skills. Clear policy and procedures for documentation of goals of care.	Interdisciplinary assessment and care incorporates the goals and aligns the values and needs of the patient and family. Care plan is documented and updated. Continuity of care plan with health-care transitions.	The patient preferences and goals of care are honored. The patient and family felt their concerns and needs are addressed. Regularly reviewed, shared with the family and other health-care providers.	"At any time while [PATIENT] was under the care of hospice, did any hospice team member do anything with respect to end-of-life care that was inconsistent with [PATIENT'S] previously stated wishes?"
Screening, assessment, care planning, and monitoring of physical and emotional symptoms are done with the goal that the patient receives desired amelioration and emotional support.	Physical well-being (N = 30) (100%)[2,8,26–53] Psychological well-being (N = 28) (93%)[2,7,19,,21–43,45,46] Social well-being (N = 20) (67%)[7,19–21,23–26,36,38–41,46] Spirituality and transcendence (N = 21) (70%)[2,7,19–21,23,25–29,31,34,36–39,46] Grief (N = 19) (63%)[2,7,19–25,29–34,38,42,46]	Policy and procedures are in place for screening of symptoms and needs for emotional support, appropriate assessment, care planning, and monitoring of treatment plan. Qualified interdisciplinary team, including physician, nurse, social worker, pharmacist, and spiritual counselor that is available 24 hours a day, 7 days a week.	The patient screened for needs. Among those with a concern, an in-depth assessment is done utilizing standardized measurement tools. An individualized plan of care. Plan is monitored for whether it is achieving the patient and family goals. Relationship and involvement fostered with patients' clergy and religious advisors.	The patient receives their desired level of physical comfort and emotional support. The family receives their desired emotional support prior to and after the death of their loved one. The patient is able to connect with significant persons and bring closure to their life, if desired.	"How much medicine did [PATIENT] receive for [HIS/HER] pain? Would you say less than was wanted, just the right amount, or more than [HE/SHE] wanted?" "How much emotional support did the hospice team provide to you after [PATIENT'S] death? Would you say less than was wanted, the right amount, or more attention than you wanted?"
Practical and legal aspects of care are addressed.	Financial and practical aspects of care (N = 16) (53%)[2,7,19–20,22,24,26,30–32,35,37,,41,46]	Appropriate staff and referral sources to address the patient and family concerns. Policy and procedure for screening for these concerns.	Screened, assessed, and provided with appropriate services. Family handouts instructing in care.	The patient and family receive the needed support in the practical and legal aspects of the patient's care.	"Did staff provide too much, too little, or just enough support around practical issues of what might happen after [PATIENT'S] death?"
The family member is supported in the role as caregiver.	Caregiver well-being (N = 16) (53%)[2,19,,22,25–33,35,,40,43,46]	Staff with appropriate education in supporting caregiving.	Family handouts instructing in care.	The family receives the needed support in their caregiving role.	"How confident did you feel about doing what you needed to do in taking care of [PATIENT]? Would you say very confident, fairly confident, or not confident?"

(Continued)

Table 24.1 (Continued)   *Components of high-quality palliative care*

Goal	Domain and supporting evidence from 30 existing guidelines	Structure	Process	Outcome	Example of measure from family evaluation of hospice care survey
Care is culturally sensitive to spiritual beliefs, values, and customs of the patient and family.	Care that is patient- and family-centered	Staff trained in diversity and culture. Translators available 24 hours, 7 days a week.	Sensitive communication that respects the patient and family values and cultural traditions. Translator services utilized to ensure that language is not a barrier.	Care is consistent with the patient values and cultural customs.	"Did any member of the hospice team talk with you about your religious or spiritual beliefs?" "Did you have as much contact of that kind as you wanted?"
Recognize and appropriately manage the dying patient. Provide information and support to those who care for that dying person.	Multiple domains that included shared decision making, symptom management, and emotional support	Staff that are trained to appropriately recognize the patient as dying and educate the family about what to expect. Appropriate range of services, including the relationship of hospital-based palliative care service with hospice to ensure that the patient and family needs are met while the patient is dying.	The patient who is actively dying is recognized as such. The family is notified and educated on what to expect. For patient on hospital-based palliative care service, the patient and family are informed of the option of hospice care.	Medical record notes the patient is actively dying. The family is notified and receives age-appropriate education on what to expect while the patient is dying. Evidence-based symptom amelioration and emotional support provided to the patient and family.	"Did you or your family receive any information from the hospice team about what to expect while [PATIENT] was dying?" "Would you have wanted more information about what to expect while [PATIENT] was dying?"

2. Compassionate care

Goal	Domain and Evidence for that domain from existing guidelines	Structure	Process	Outcome	Example of measure from family evaluation of hospice care survey
The dying patient is treated with dignity and respect.	Personal dignity (N = 17) (57%)[2,19,22,25,27,29–33,35,42,44,47]	Appropriately trained staff	Assess patient's notions of self and values. Care for the patient in ways that promote and support the patient's concept of dignity and respect.	The patient and family are treated with dignity and respect.	"How often did the hospice team treat [PATIENT] with respect? Would you say always, usually, sometimes, or never?"

3. Coordinated care

Care coordination should occur across the disease trajectory, settings of care, and health-care providers.	Coordination and continuity of care (N = 21) (70%)[2,7,19–21,23–25,29–33,36–42,46]	Policy and processes are in place to ensure seamless transitions in the settings of care.	Timely communication of patient goals and plans of care when there is transition in health-care setting	Information continuity among staff such that new caregivers are aware of the goals of care, plan of care, and what they should monitor the patient for. An appropriate member of staff is seen as in charge of overall care.	"Was there any problem with hospice doctors or nurses not knowing enough about [PATIENT'S] medical history to provide the best possible care?" "While under the care of hospice, was there always one nurse who was identified as being in charge of [PATIENT'S] overall care?"

Source: Data from Surgeons ACo, Principles Guiding Care at the End of Life, www.facs.org/fellows_info/statements/; previously published in JAMA[6] which was adapted from the National Consensus Project[47] and National Quality Forum, *A National Framework and Preferred Practices for Palliative and Hospice Care Quality*[4] and Teno and colleagues.[8]

The medical record is a legal record that reflects health-care providers' documentation of the patient's condition and treatment decisions. The absence of documentation of a process of care in a chart audit of medical records does provide valuable information, given the legal standard that if it is not documented, it was not done. However, the medical record does reflect that bias of a health-care provider. For example, the documentation that discharged medications were reviewed with the patient and family may not indicate that the patient and family understood how properly to take the medications after discharge from the hospital.

Administrative data can range from information used for the purpose of billing to death certificate data. Similarly, these data sources reflect the perspective of the health-care providers. However, these data are often available at minimal costs and can provide important overall descriptive information for program planning. For example, aggregate death certificate data can provide important information on the site of death that can allow for examining changes in the location of death with time as well as differences among subpopulations such as leading cause of death, age groups, or ethnicity. This information, however, does not provide definitive information on the quality of care. It is important for tracking changes, and information on site of death can provide both hospice and palliative care programs with important information to strategize on where to provide services. For example, the state of Rhode Island, United States, went from twenty-fifth to second in the nation for nursing homes as the site of death.[11] This in itself may not indicate poor quality of care but provides important information for health-care providers regarding the importance of developing programs in nursing homes on care of the dying.

In the United States, all nursing homes are required to complete the Resident Assessment Instrument for every nursing home resident on admission, quarterly, and with significant changes in health status. Although the intent of this assessment is care planning, it represents an important source of information to examine some of the key domains. However, the important limitation similar to the other sources of data is ascertainment bias (e.g., pain is underreported when compared to an expert assessor of pain). Given the important role of patient preferences, surveys of dying persons and/or family provide an important source of information about the quality of care. There are important limitations of the typical satisfaction survey item that asks the respondent to rank a particular aspect of care on a scale from "excellent" to "poor." The distribution is often skewed given the reluctance of respondents to use "fair" or "poor." In addition, research has found that a respondent will rate that care is excellent despite reporting severe pain, reflecting the lowered expectations that the respondents have for the level of pain control that can be achieved among the dying. A third limitation is that the typical rating question does not provide information to guide improvement. Knowing that 85% of bereaved families rated an aspect of care as "very good" does not provide information that allows the health-care provider to improve. However, knowing that one in four people did not understand how to take their pain medications provides a target for improvement that has face validity. Such

information can provide information that raises awareness of the opportunity to improve.

In Europe and Africa, a European Community-funded network Preferred Reporting Items for Systematic Reviews and Meta-Analyses (PRISMA), working with the European Association for Palliative Care, the African Palliative Care Association, and various clinical and academic groups from different countries, has assessed and recommended ways forward in outcome measurement in research and practice.[12,13] Their work found that one of the major barriers to outcome use is the lack of training for staff and recommended that online resources should become freely available.[14] The main uses of outcome measures in these contexts were assessing patients' symptoms/needs, monitoring changes, evaluating care, and assessing family needs.[15] Further consensus work involving 32 professionals from 15 countries and 8 different professional backgrounds identified: (1) the need for standardization with improvement of existing Patient-reported outcomes measures (PROMs), for example, with a modular system and an optional item pool; (2) the aspects of further development with a multi-professional approach taking into account cultural sensitivity especially for translated versions; and (3) the need for guidance, training, and resources.[13]

WHAT TOOL SHOULD BE USED?

Key to selecting a measurement tool is to first clearly state the goals of measurement. Table 24.2 notes that the audience, focus of measurement, evidence base to justify the use of the measure, and psychometric properties vary based on the intended use of an outcome measure. A measure as part of an audit for a quality improvement–intended audience is the team working on improving the quality of care, and the focus of measurement is to provide information that will help select the target for improvement, raise awareness of the opportunity to improve, and monitor whether the quality improvement effort is achieving its stated goals. A measure for public reporting (or accountability) is held to higher standards given the focus is to provide consumers and payers with information to select health-care providers.[16] It is important that the chosen measure is under the control of that health-care institution and the psychometric properties have been validated across multiple settings of care. Detailed guidance on tool selection is included in the PRISMA guidance, which can be freely downloaded.[17]

The selection or development of the measurement tool should receive careful consideration. Too often, researchers and persons conducting an audit ignore the critical steps of ensuring the reliability and validity of the chosen or developed measures. Reliability examines the reproducibility of the measure. Two different nurses using the same chart abstraction tool getting different results would indicate a concern with the reliability of the tool. Achieving reliability is a key step, but not sufficient evidence of the validity of a measurement tool. A measurement tool is valid if there is evidence that it measures

Table 24.2 *Purpose of outcome measurements*

Purpose of measure

	Research	Improvement	Accountability
Main audience	Science community	Quality improvement team and clinical staff	Payers; public
Focus of measurement	Knowledge	Understanding care process	Comparison
Confidentiality	Very high	Very high	Purpose to compare groups
Evidence base to justify use of the measure	Builds off existing evidence to generate new knowledge	Important	Extremely important in that proposed domain ought to be under control of that institution
Importance of psychometric properties	Extremely important to that research effort	Important within that setting	Valid and responsive across multiple settings

Source: Adapted from Solberg et al.[11] and modified from *Journal of Pain and Symptom Management*,[48] Teno JM, Byock I, Field MJ. Research agenda for developing measures to examine quality of care and quality of life of patients diagnosed with life-limiting illness. White paper from the Conference on Excellent Care at the End of Life through fast-tracking Audit, Standards, and Teamwork (EXCELFAST), September 28–30, 1997, 75–82, Copyright 1999 with permission from The U.S. Cancer Pain Relief Committee.

the constructs that it purports to measure. Essentially, you are asking, "Is the tool measuring the 'truth'"? Often, there is not a "gold standard" to judge the validity of the measurement tool. In that situation, the measurement tool should present evidence of the content or face validity, construct, and potentially criterion validity if a "gold standard" exists.

The content validity essentially asks whether the measurement tool is examining the right constructs. To meet the goal of content validity, there should be evidence that the development of the measurement tool was based on a systematic review of the literature and involved experts in the field and that theoretical model informed the selection of items to include in the outcome measure. Construct validity tests whether known relationships hold with the measurement tool. For example, a survey that examines patient perceptions of the process of care regarding pain management should have at least a moderate correlation with the respondents' overall satisfaction with pain management. Criterion validity examines whether the measure is associated with an accepted "gold standard" or predicts future outcomes.

Over the past decade, there have been increasing numbers of measures to examine key outcome measures for the seriously ill or dying. Previously, a structured literature review was conducted by the staff at the Center to Improve Care of the Dying and Center for Gerontology and Healthcare Research[18] and updated by Lorenz et al.[19] for the National Institutes of Health conference on the State of the Science of End-of-Life Care in December 2004. Each key domain has several potential outcome measures with the majority of measures having psychometric properties reported. However, there are still two important areas for research. First, the responsiveness of measures is often not documented. Responsiveness examines the degree to which an intervention or historical event results in change in the outcome measure. For example, a change in policy regulation that limits access to opioids would be expected to result in different reports of bereaved family members regarding unmet needs for pain medications. Second, many of the instruments have been

developed and validated in a population of English-speaking people only. Future research needs to examine whether the same constructs hold in different cultures and, when appropriate, have the instrument translated into other languages.

More recently, the European Commission–funded network PRISMA conducted literature reviews, surveys of clinicians, and consensus workshops to assess the state of the art of outcome measures used in research and practice across Europe and Africa. One of the main challenges found in the PRISMA project was the large number of tools used only a few times or by a few people. For example, of the 311 European and African participants who completed an online survey, 99 tools in clinical care and audit and 94 in research were cited by less than 10 participants.[12] Further data revealed that respondents require the number of potential tools to be rationalized and that brief tools are favored.[12] PRISMA concluded that too often rather than use or adapt an existing measure, individuals would attempt to develop their own measure, without validation. However, the survey also identified that three outcome measures were commonly used by over one in four respondents for clinical practice and over one in 10 for research: the Karnofsky Performance Scale (KPS), followed by the Edmonton Symptom Assessment Scale (ESAS, available at www.cancercare.on.ca/common/pages/UserFile. aspx?fileId=13262) and the Palliative care Outcome Scale (POS, downloadable free from www.pos-pal.org). Measures were used twice as often in clinical practice as in research.[15] The group recommended that these should be developed further, with core and then add-on measures. In Africa, the main reason for not using outcome measures was a lack of guidance/training on using and analyzing measures, with 49% of 168 respondents saying that they would use the tools if this was provided. Forty percent of those using outcome measures in clinical practice used POS, and 80% used them to assess, evaluate, and monitor change. The POS was also the main tool used in research, with the principle criteria for use being validation in Africa, access to the tool, and time needed to complete it. Challenges to the use of tools were shortage of time and resources, lack of guidance and training for the professionals, poor health status of patients, and complexity of OM. Researchers also have problems analyzing outcome measurement data, which needs to be addressed in the future.[20]

Another common mistake in measurement is the attempt to examine every possible outcome. Rigorous data collection on a small number of items is far superior to any effort that collects a lot of items in a manner where there are concerns about the accuracy of the data collection. This can result in time-consuming data collection and raises important concerns in terms of respondent burden, especially when one is interviewing seriously ill or dying persons. Parsimony is important. Winnowing should be based on the goals of measurement and the realization that examining multiple outcomes raises the possibility that one outcome will be statistically significant based on chance alone. While time is one aspect of individual-respondent burden, a second concern is the number of subjects on which data collection occurs. The PRISMA network surveys and consensus found that clinicians and researchers mostly commonly wanted brief outcome measures with 8–10 questions.[12] All three most commonly used outcome measures in the PRISMA survey were 10 items or fewer. In order to see if the measures could be shortened further, PRISMA survey respondents were asked to rate the most important questions. Respondents prioritized brief measures that included physical and psychological domains.[3] The most favored questions were about pain, symptoms, and emotional and family aspects. There were no differences in the choice of the most important questions between doctors and nurses or between researchers and clinicians.[15]

For the purpose of a quality improvement effort, a small number of cases collected from a random sample can provide enough data to guide efforts to select targets for and monitor the rate of improvement. The sample size for research or accountability should be based on the effect size that is required to be able to measure the level of statistical significance and the probability that you want to be able to find that difference. Statistical software packages such as nQuery Advisor 4.0 (Statistical Solutions, United States) allow for estimation of the sample size with these three parameters.

WHOSE OUTCOMES ARE MEASURED?

A key specification of any proposed outcome measure is choosing a numerator (e.g., the number of people with a moderate or excruciating level of pain) and denominator (e.g., all people who are not comatose). At face value, this can seem quite simplistic. However, the difficulty is determining who should be counted among the "dying" or the denominator. This decision has important implications. Numerous studies have reported the limitation of physicians in prognostication[21] and that prognostic guidelines can be overly specific, but not sensitive.[22] Thus, careful consideration must be given to the specification of the sample. For the dying person, the last month of life often involves transitions in care and flare of symptoms such as pain

and dyspnea. Often, a dying person is not able to give interviews during the last month of life. One solution is the mortality follow-back survey that uses death certificates to determine the denominator and contact the next of kin. This represents an efficient data collection strategy with important, acknowledged limitations.[23] With this strategy, the denominator is clearly defined. However, family members more accurately report on factual information and their interactions with health-care providers. Those observations are valuable. Families are less accurate in reports of symptoms and other subjective patient outcomes.[24] This limitation needs to be acknowledged, but one should not ignore the perceptions of bereaved family members. Dame Cicely Saunders, the founder of the modern hospice movement, eloquently stated, "How people die remains in the memories of those who live on."[25]

The Institute of Medicine proposed overall dimensions to examine the quality of care: safe, effective, timely, patient centered, efficient, and equitable. To date, safety measures have focused on the safety concerns in acute care hospital. Careful thought needs to be given to adaptation of these measures to hospice and palliative care settings. For example, a safety measure that identifies medication errors is an important goal. Considering the example of a nurse who gives the wrong dosage of medication in an acute care hospital, no one would argue that this is an important safety concern for which a hospital should be held accountable. In contrast to the following situation in a hospice, a family caregiver of a hospice patient asks a neighbor to watch the patient while he or she does a quick errand. The neighbor mistakenly gives 10 times the amount of morphine. Is the hospital responsible for the actions of this next-door neighbor? A second concern with safety measures is at the close of life, patient preferences and disease trajectory may make some safety measures not applicable. For example, some medications may be appropriate for the dying patient, but their side effect profile raises concern in those persons not close to death. Patients may not choose certain treatments (e.g., tight control of diabetes) based on their preferences regarding care at this time of their life. As palliative medicine becomes part of integrated health-care system, careful consideration needs to be given to which safety and other system-wide measures developed in other settings of care are applicable to palliative care.

HOW DO YOU USE PROCESS AND OUTCOME MEASURES IN AN AUDIT?

Health-care providers often may view an audit as being equivalent to trying to speak a foreign language. A metaphor that may be helpful to think about the components of the key steps of an audit in terms of the routine history and physical exam. As part of routine history and physical exam (H and P), one asks a review of systems. A first key step in an audit is to use a measurement tool (e.g., a bereaved family survey) that will examine a number of domains of quality of care with the goal of identifying an opportunity to improve or in the metaphor of the routine H and P a symptom that you need to explore with further history, physical exam, and potentially laboratory tests that are needed to arrive at a diagnosis. Similarly, the next step after identifying an opportunity to improve based on bereaved family survey, is to collect more data to understand the key leverage process of care that would change the quality of care. Considering pain management in the acute care hospital, big key processes are as follows: (1) the patient is *screened* for pain (e.g., asking the patient to rate the pain on scale of 0–10); (2) among those screened positive, an *in-depth* assessment is done; (3) a *care plan* is formulated with both nonpharmacological and pharmacological treatments; and (4) finally, the effectiveness of that treatment is *monitored*. An abstraction of the medical record could examine each of these key processes of care. Once you arrive at a diagnosis or the key processes of care to improve, your next step is to come up with a care plan or potential intervention to change that key process of care that would alleviate pain. Often, this involves multiple small tests of interventions that are tested in plan, do, check, and study cycles that achieve your targeted measure of improvement in the outcome measure. Once you arrive at a satisfactory treatment plan, you would monitor the patient condition by screening their condition periodically. Similarly, one monitors the quality measure as part of your set of measures that you examine on a periodic basis. Further guidance on this is available in the PRISMA project outcome guidance.[17]

WHAT TO DO WITH CONFLICTING OUTCOME MEASURES?

Often a research effort involves examining multiple sources of data to evaluate an intervention, such as the palliative care team, or to conduct an audit of the quality of care that a hospice delivers. Sometimes the results are in conflict. In my experience, this is more likely in an audit or quality improvement effort. For example, an audit of nursing home pain management may use the MDS (i.e., an assessment form completed by nursing home staff), chart review (e.g., whether a complete pain assessment was done on admission to the nursing home), and interviews with cognitively intact nursing home residents regarding their observations of staff efforts in their pain management. Often, these results are in apparent conflict. For example, a nursing home could have a 10% prevalence of moderate pain, with the chart review indicating that only 30% of residents had a complete pain assessment done on admission and reporting that 45% of the nursing home residents had to wait too long for pain medications. The low prevalence of moderate pain seems in conflict with the other two results. However, this discrepancy is most likely explained by ascertainment bias, in that staff of the nursing home complete the MDS pain items and often they underreport the pain. The other two indicators provide tangible opportunities for improvement. The goal should be that 100% of the people should have a complete pain assessment on admission with as low as possible number of nursing home residents reporting they have to wait too long for pain medication.

CONCLUSION

Knowledge and use of outcome measure is an important tool for health-care providers with an interest in palliative and hospice medicine. Both process and outcome measures can provide important information to guide efforts to improve quality of care. Outcome measures are key to generating new scientific knowledge of the efficacy of medical treatments and interventions and to improving clinical care. A key step in the selection of a measurement tool is to be clear on the goals of measures including the proposed definition of the quality of care, the proposed source of data, and consideration of the bias and perspective of the source of data. The choice of measurement tools should be based on knowledge of the reliability and validity of the measure. The mistake of collecting information about every possible outcome should be avoided. Rather, a focused data collection effort on a small number of subjects can provide valuable information for quality improvement efforts. Guidance is now available to overcome some of the key barriers to outcome measurement use. It is recommended to use established validated short tools (which are freely available in the Internet) rather than invent new tools.

Key learning points

- Assessment of processes and outcomes is an important and essential part of examining the quality of palliative care in all settings.

- Consumer preferences are an important aspect of examining the quality of end-of-life care.

- Valid and reliable measures are needed whatever the purpose. Measures should also be responsive to change.

- Short and easy to use measures are available, especially the Edmonton Symptom Assessment Scale (ESAS) and the Palliative care Outcome Scale (POS). Both measures are short, well validated and used internationally in clinical practice and research.

- Free on-line guidance is available on how to select and implement outcome measures (http://www.csi.kcl.ac.uk/files/Guidance%20on%20Outcome%20Measurement%20in%20Palliative%20Care.pdf)

- Strengths and limitations of various sources of information need to be considered in the selection of measures and interpretation of results.

- Different purposes of measurement mean that different measures may need to be used.

- It is unwise and usually impractical to try to measure everything. Rather, a small amount of information collected on a random sample of subjects can guide quality improvement efforts. Clinicians favour outcome measures with 8–10 questions, and priority questions are concerned with pain, symptoms, emotional and family aspects.

REFERENCES

1   Higginson IJ, Bruera E. Do we need palliative care audit in developing countries? *Palliat Med. November 2002;16(6):546–547.*

2   Organization WH, ed. Cancer Pain Relief and Palliative Care: Report of a WHO Expert Committee. Geneva, Switzerland: World Health Organization; 1990. Technical Report Series No. 804.

3   Daveson BA, Simon ST, Benalia HH et al. Are we heading in the same direction? European and African doctors' and nurses' views and experiences regarding outcome measurement in palliative care. *Palliat Med.* April 2012;26(3):242–249.

4   Jencks SF, Cuerdon T, Burwen DR et al. Quality of medical care delivered to Medicare beneficiaries: A profile at state and national levels. *JAMA.* October 4, 2000;284(13):1670–1676.

5   National Quality Forum. A National Framework and Preferred Practices for Palliative and Hospice Care Quality, A Consensus Report. December 2006. Accessed July 1, 2014. http://www.qualityforum.org/publications/2006/12/A_National_Framework_and_Preferred_Practices_for_Palliative_and_Hospice_Care_Quality.aspx.

6   Teno JM, Casarett D, Spence C, Connor S. It is "too late" or is it? Bereaved family member perceptions of hospice referral when their family member was on hospice for seven days or less. *J Pain Symptom Manage.* 2012;43(4):732–738.

7   Teno JM, Connor SR. Referring a patient and family to high-quality palliative care at the close of life: "We met a new personality... with this level of compassion and empathy". *JAMA.* 2009;301(6):651–659.

8   Organization NH, ed. *A Pathway for Patients and Families Facing Terminal Illness: Self-Determined Life Closure, Safe Comfortable Dying and Effective Grieving.* Alexandria, VA: National Hospice Organization; 1997.

9   Teno JM, Casey VA, Welch L, Edgman-Levitan S. Patient-Focused, Family-Centered End-of-Life Medical Care: Views of the Guidelines and Bereaved Family Members. *J Pain Symptom Manage-Special Section on Measuring Quality of Care at Life's End II.* 2001;22(3):738–751.

10 Steinhauser KE, Clipp EC, McNeilly M, Christakis NA, McIntyre LM, Tulsky JA. In search of a good death: Observations of patients, families, and providers. *Ann Intern Med.* 2000;132(10): 825–832.

11 Teno JM. Facts on Dying: Brown Atlas Site of Death 1989–1997. 2004. http://www.chcr.brown.edu/dying/factsondying.htm. Published 2004. Accessed February 26, 2004.

12 Harding R, Simon ST, Benalia H et al. The PRISMA Symposium 1: Outcome tool use. Disharmony in European outcomes research for palliative and advanced disease care: Too many tools in practice. *J Pain Symptom Manage.* 2011;42(4):493–500.

13 Simon ST, Higginson IJ, Harding R et al. Enhancing patient-reported outcome measurement in research and practice of palliative and end-of-life care. *Support Care Cancer.* 2012;20(7):1573–1578.

14 Bausewein C, Simon ST, Benalia H et al. Implementing patient reported outcome measures (PROMs) in palliative care—Users' cry for help. *Health Qual Life Outcomes.* 2011;9:27.

15 Higginson IJ, Simon ST, Benalia H et al. Republished: Which questions of two commonly used multidimensional palliative care patient reported outcome measures are most useful? Results from the European and African PRISMA survey. *Postgrad Med J.* 2012;88(1042):451–457.

16 Solberg LI, Mosser G, McDonald S. The three faces of performance measurement: Improvement, accountability, and research. *Jt Comm J Qual Improv.* 1997;23(3):135–147.

17 Bausewein CD, Benalia, H, Simon, ST, Higginson IJ. Outcome measurement in palliative care: The essentials. London, U.K.: Cicely Saunders Institute; 2011: http://www.csi.kcl.ac.uk/files/Guidance%20on%20Outcome%20Measurement%20in%20Palliative%20Care.pdf. Accessed August 08, 2012.

18 Teno JM. *Toolkit of Instruments to Measure End of Life Care.* http://chcr.brown.edu/pcoc/toolkit.htm. Accessed January 18, 2001.

19 Lorenz K, Lynn J, Morton SC et al. End-of-Life Care and Outcomes. Summary. Evidence Report/Technology Assessment: Number 110, 2004; http://www.ahrq.gov/clinic/epcsums/eolsum.pdf. Accessed July 1, 2014.

20 Downing J, Simon ST, Mwangi-Powell FN et al. Outcomes 'out of africa': the selection and implementation of outcome measures for palliative care in Africa. *BMC Palliat Care.* 2012;11:1.

21 Teno JM, Coppola KM. For every numerator, you need a denominator: A simple statement but key to measuring the quality of care of the "dying". *J Pain Symptom Manage.* 1999;17(2):109–113.

22 Fox E, Landrum McNiff K, Zhong Z, Dawson NV, Wu AW, Lynn J. Evaluation of prognostic criteria for determining hospice eligibility in patients with advanced lung, heart, or liver disease. SUPPORT Investigators. Study to Understand Prognoses and Preferences for Outcomes and Risks of Treatments. *JAMA.* 1999;282(17):1638–1645.

23 Addington-Hall J, McPherson C. After-death interviews with surrogates/bereaved family members. some issues of validity. *J Pain Symptom Manage.* 2001;22(3):784–790.

24 McPherson C, Addington-Hall J. Judging the quality of care at the end of life: Can proxies provide reliable information. *Soc Sci Med.* 2003;56(1):95–109.

25 Saunders C. Pain and impending death. In: Wall PD, Melzack R, eds. *Textbook of Pain.* Edinburgh, U.K.: Churchill Livingstone; 1989: pp. 624–631.

26 Stewart AL, Teno J, Patrick DL, Lynn J. The concept of quality of life of dying persons in the context of health care. *J Pain Symptom Manage.* 1999;17(2):93–108.

27 Emanuel EJ, Emanuel LL. The promise of a good death. *Lancet.* 1998;351 (Suppl 2):SII21–SII29.

28 Association CPC. Palliative care: Towards a consensus in standardized principles of practice. In: Ferris FD, Cummings I, eds. Ottawa, Ontario, Canada: Canadian Palliative Care Association; 1995: pp. 53–54.

29 The care of dying patients: A position statement from the American Geriatrics Society. AGS Ethics Committee. *J Am Geriatr Soc.* 1995 May 1995;43(5):577–578.

30 ASCO. ASCO Special Article: Cancer care during the last phase of life. *J Clin Oncol.* 1998;16(5):1986–1996.

31 Carson NE. How to succeed in practice by really trying. Guidelines for the care of dying patients. *Aust Fam Physician.* 1983 Feb 1983;12(2):124–125.

32 Cherny NI, Coyle N, Foley KM. Guidelines in the care of the dying cancer patient. *Hematol Oncol Clin North Am.* 1996;10(1):261–286.

33 Donaldson MS, Field MJ. Measuring quality of care at the end of life. *Arch Intern Med.* 1998;158(2):121–128.

34 Keay TJ, Fredman L, Taler GA, Datta S, Levenson SA. Indicators of quality medical care for the terminally ill in nursing homes. *J Am Geriatr Soc.* 1994;42(8):853–860.

35 Latimer E. Caring for seriously ill and dying patients: The philosophy and ethics. *CMAJ.* 1991;144(7):859–864.

36 Latimer EJ, Dawson HR. Palliative care: Principles and practice. Section of Palliative Care, Ontario Medical Association [see comments]. *CMAJ.* 1993;148(6):933–936.

37 Lynn J. Measuring quality of care at the end of life: A statement of principles. *J Am Geriatr Soc.* 1997;45(4):526–527.

38 Focus on ethics. Care of the dying patient—Guidelines for nursing practice. *Nebr Nurse.* 1995;28(2):34.

39 Ruland CM, Moore SM. Theory construction based on standards of care: A proposed theory of the peaceful end of life. *Nurs Outlook.* 1998;46(4):169–175.

40 Saunders C. The philosophy of terminal cancer care. *Ann Acad Med Singapore.* 1987;16(1):151–154.

41 Singer PA, MacDonald N. Bioethics for clinicians: 15. Quality end-of-life care. *CMAJ.* 1998;159(2):159–162.

42 Wanzer SH, Federman DD, Adelstein SJ et al. The physician's responsibility toward hopelessly ill patients. A second look [see comments]. *N Engl J Med.* 1989 Mar 30 1989;320(13):844–849.

43 Committee VB, ed. *Ethical Issues in Long-Term Care.* VA National Headquarters, Washington, DC: National Center for Clinical Ethics; 1996.

44 Center TH, ed. *Guidelines on the Termination of Life-Sustaining Treatment and the Care of the Dying.* Bloomington, IN: Indiana University Press; 1987.

45 Cassel CK, Foley KM, eds. *Principles for Care of Patients at the End of Life: An Emerging Consensus among the Specialties of Medicine.* New York: Milbank Memorial Fund; 1999.

46 Task Force on Palliative Care. Last acts, A national coalition to improve care and caring at the end of life. Precepts of Palliative Care. December 1997. Accessed July 1, 2014. http://www.aacn.org/WD/Palliative/Docs/2001Precep.pdf.

47 Surgeons ACo. Principles Guiding Care at the End of Life. www.facs.org/fellows_info/statements/, accessed July 1, 2014.

48 Research AfHCPa, ed. *Clinical Practice Guidelines for the Management of Cancer Pain.*: AHCPR Publication No. 94–0592; 2001.

49 The American Medical Association, Eight "Elements of Quality Care for Patients in the Last Phase of Life"; subsequently published in the editorial "Caring to the End: Conscientious End-of-life Care Can Reduce Concerns about Care of the Terminally Ill," American Medical News (December 15, 1997). For more information, see the AMA Web site: http://www.ama-assn.org. Accessed July 1, 2014.

50 ANA Board of Directors. Position Statement of Registered Nurses Roles and Responsibilities in Providing Expert Care and Counseling at the End of Life. June 14, 2010. Accessed July 1, 2014. http://www.nursingworld.org/mainmenucategories/ethicsstandards/ethics-position-statements/etpain14426.pdf.

51 American Pain Society Taskforce on Pain S, and End of Life Care. Treatment of Pain at the End of Life: A Position Statement from the American Pain Society. www.ampainsoc.org/advocacy/treatment.htm.

52 Palliative care in neurology. The American Academy of Neurology Ethics and Humanities Subcommittee [see comments]. *Neurology.* 1996;46(3):870–872.

53 Life IOMCoCatEo, ed. *Approaching Death: Improving care at the End of Life.* Washington, DC: National Academy Press; 1997.

25

Ethics in palliative care research

JONATHAN KOFFMAN, KATIE STONE, FLISS E.M. MURTAGH

INTRODUCTION

Palliative care has, at its core, not only the discipline of rigorous symptom control but also the need for patient-centered communication, holistic care of the patients and their families, the consideration of advance directives, including patient preferences for place of care and death, and respect for spiritual and religious beliefs of patients and families.[1] Palliative care as a specialty remains unique in its contribution to patient and family care, but the fundamental ethical principles underpinning the conduct of medical research are identical to those in primary, secondary, and tertiary care. Where or how the research takes place should not affect the standards laid down in national and international guidelines such as the Declaration of Helsinki and the Belmont Report (as discussed later). However, the application of these guidelines, and their underlying principles, may have specific implications for particular types of research carried out in palliative care, and for the health and social care professionals involved. Given that palliative care is a relatively new specialty, the volume of research conducted is increasing. This includes exploration of disease groups and symptoms associated with advanced disease that are potentially amenable to palliative care intervention,[2-5] the context in which care is provided,[6-8] cost-effectiveness of service provision,[9] and provider effects, including how care is delivered and received by an increasingly diverse society.[10,11] The impact of the proliferation of "evidence-based guidelines" for managing advanced disease is also an all-pervading concern.[12] These areas, among others, were the subject of a recent National Institutes of Health State-of-the-Science Conference on End-of-Life Care.[13]

One of the most useful issues raised by the State-of-the-Science Conference summary statement were the ethical concerns associated with palliative and end-of-life research.[13] Expansion of research in palliative care requires more than merely transposing traditional clinical trials, methods of health services research, or epidemiological methodologies into the specialty. New methods and research approaches need to be developed and refined to explore the complex clinical, psychosocial, and service- and policy-related situations seen in palliative care. There has been some discussion of the theoretical and practical problems of research in palliative care and approaches to developing high-quality rigorous research[14-16] but less discussion of the ethical issues raised. Research in palliative care may raise different ethical questions to other specialties, including the nature of the study design, issues of consent, the balance of benefits versus the risks of involvement in research, what is considered a potential harm, and the importance of confidentiality. In this chapter, we apply the historical perspective of ethics in relation to medical research to palliative care, appraise international codes that guide ethical frameworks in research, describe a practical approach to research ethics, and discuss important ethical challenges when undertaking palliative care research. Box 25.1 defines some key terms.

HISTORICAL PERSPECTIVE ON RESEARCH ETHICS

There are historical reasons why the regulation of clinical and health research involving patients differs from the regulation of normal clinical practice. The horrific medical experiments conducted by a number of doctors under the Nazi regime led to the first internationally agreed guidelines on research involving people, the Nuremberg Code of 1947.[17] This consisted of 10 principles that were finally incorporated into the Declaration of Helsinki produced by the World Medical Association in 1964, an international body set up soon after the Second World War to represent doctors and funded by national medical associations. The Declaration has been revised no less than five times since 1964, the last being in 2000, and a further note of clarification was added in 2002[18] (see Box 25.2).

The Declaration has been significant in its influence in setting ethical standards for medical and human research.[19] However, the latest version has not been without its critics. In particular, disagreement has focused on clauses 29 and 30

Box 25.1 Key terms

- *Research* is defined as any form of disciplined inquiry that aims to contribute to a body of knowledge or theory.

- *Research ethics* refers to the moral principles guiding the research, from its inception to the completion and publication of results and beyond.

- *Human participants* (or subjects) are defined as including living human beings, human beings who have recently died (cadavers, human remains, and body parts), embryos and fetuses, human tissue and body fluids, and human data and records (such as, but not restricted to, medical, genetic, financial, personnel, criminal, or administrative records and test results including scholastic achievements).

Box 25.2 Extracts from the Declaration of Helsinki (2002) with particular considerations in palliative research (our italics)

1. The World Medical Association has developed the Declaration of Helsinki as a statement of ethical principles to provide guidance to physicians and other participants in medical research involving human subjects. Medical research involving human subjects includes research on identifiable human material or identifiable data.

5. In medical research on human subjects, considerations related to the well-being of the human subject should take precedence over the interests of science and society.

7. In current medical practice and in medical research, most prophylactic, diagnostic, and therapeutic procedures involve *risks and burdens*.

10. It is the duty of the physician in medical research to protect the life, health, privacy, and dignity of the human subject.

13. The design and performance of each experimental procedure involving human subjects should be clearly formulated in an experimental protocol. This protocol should be submitted for *consideration, comment, guidance*, and, where appropriate, *approval to a specially appointed ethical review committee, which must be independent of the investigator, the sponsor, or any other kind of undue influence.*

15. Medical research involving human subjects should be conducted only by scientifically qualified persons and under the supervision of a clinically competent medical person. *The responsibility for the human subject must always rest with a medically qualified person and never rest on the subject of the research, even though the subject has given consent.*

20. The subjects must be *volunteers and informed participants* in the research project.

29. The *benefits, risks, burdens*, and *effectiveness* of a new method should be tested against those of the best current prophylactic, diagnostic, and therapeutic methods. This does not exclude the use of placebo, or no treatment, in studies where no proven prophylactic, diagnostic, or therapeutic method exists.

30. At the conclusion of the study, every patient entered into the study should be assured of access to the *best proven prophylactic, diagnostic, and therapeutic methods identified by the study.*

Source: World Medical Association, *World Medical Association Declaration of Helsinki: Ethical Principles for Medical Research involving Human Subjects*, World Medical Association, Ferney-Voltaire, France, 2002.

(see Box 25.2), and concern has been voiced about the potential exploitation of research subjects in developing countries.[20] These clauses have also been criticized for being so crude and absolute that they may even be damaging to the very research subjects they are intended to protect by unintentionally limiting research in those countries.[21] This has serious implications for palliative care research, and particularly for research that takes place in developing countries. The reasons for this include increasing evidence that double standards are frequently adopted in the quality of clinical trials that could never pass ethical muster in the sponsoring country.[22]

The current version of the Declaration has also been criticized for its overly expansive remit. It now includes all forms of medical research.[23] It has, for example, changed its designation from "recommendations for doctors" to "ethical principles for everybody involved in research. Medical research, in general, and palliative care research, in particular, are frequently an interdisciplinary exercise, and there are times when research is either inadequately conceptualized or not addressed at all in the Declaration of Helsinki. The focus of the Declaration was originally, and still is, the *conduct of human experiments*: the frequent use of the term "experimentation" in the current version of the Declaration is just one manifestation of this. Doll states that the Declaration only really applies to "research in which patients are required to take drugs or have invasive procedures" (a relatively small part of palliative research) but that "even here, however, some of the principles show a lack of understanding of what their effects would be if rigidly applied."[23]

RESEARCH ETHICS COMMITTEES

The Declaration of Helsinki stipulates that any research involving human subjects should be reviewed by a properly constituted research ethics committee (REC) or institutional review board (IRB). As a result, many countries throughout the world now have strict regulations governing the formation and procedure of such bodies. The Netherlands, Belgium, and the United States have specific legislation in this area.[24–26] Until recently, the United Kingdom adhered to a regulatory system controlled by the government, but not by the legislation.[27] Following the implementation of the EU Clinical Trials

Directive in 2004, UK RECs now have a basis in law. Their accountability is also clearly defined: they are answerable to a Health Research Authority with the National Research Ethics Service (NRES) at its core.

Both RECs and IRBs are responsible for ensuring that they act independently within their institutions. They must be free from bias and undue influence from the institution in which they are located, from the researchers whose proposals they consider, and from the personal or financial interests of their members.[28] This independence is founded on its membership, on strict rules regarding conflict of interests, and on regular monitoring of and accountability for decisions made. The membership of an REC or IRB must ensure that it has the range of expertise and the breadth of experience necessary to provide competent and rigorous review of the research proposals submitted to it, and to do so from a position that is independent of both the researchers and the institution in which it is located. They should be multidisciplinary and consist of both men and women, as well as reflecting other aspects of diversity within society.[29] There must also be members who have broad experience of and expertise in the areas of research regularly reviewed and who have the confidence and esteem of the research community. This can be problematic with palliative care research given the limited number of ethics committee members who have experience of such research. End-of-life care is typically characterized by a focus on symptom control with minimum interference and intervention. Many RECs and IRBs are reluctant to approve studies in this group of patients. It has been suggested that this might be so because of the misconception that research studies may detract from the ethos of care, that studies are unlikely to be supported by previous good research in the field, and because of the perceived vulnerability of research participants. In addition, even when studies are approved, extensive gatekeeping by health professionals may create future barriers to recruitment.[30]

For all their good, RECS and IRBs are not without their critics. It has been stated that they are risk averse[31] and that they concentrate disproportionately on the information about a study that will be given to potential participants.[32] This includes the manner in which consent is recorded (the expectation is usually a signed consent form for each participant) and the justification and special procedures required for studies involving children, or mentally incompetent or otherwise vulnerable adults. However, given the emphasis on the production of information sheets for clinical trials or other research, there are still some participants who do not fully understand the information they have been given as part of the procedure to obtain consent for their participation.[33,34] As with research involving children or other vulnerable patients,[35,36] the closer scrutiny of research involving patients with advanced disease may necessitate that palliative care researchers need to invest more time, effort, and ingenuity in developing consent procedures to gain approval for their studies.[37] This may bring benefits in the protection of patients, and it may also result in fewer evaluated interventions and services for these groups.

PRACTICAL APPROACH TO RESEARCH ETHICS

Three broad areas of ethical concern outlined by Foster[38] have been identified in relation to research:

1. Duty of care to research participants
2. Respect for the rights and autonomy of research participants
3. The scientific validity of the research (without which no research can be ethically justified)

These areas approximate to different moral and philosophical traditions. Duty of care derives from duty-based deontological thinking, which acknowledges that there are rules of conduct that ought to be followed, not because of the ends that are likely to be achieved, but by the nature of those involved and their inherent responsibilities. Respect for rights derives from rights-based deontological traditions, which recognize the right of each person to self-determination and autonomy. Emphasis on the scientific validity of research draws on goal-based moral theory (consequentialism), which judges the moral worth according to predicted or actual outcomes. These different but complementary philosophical approaches have been used by Claire Foster to derive a framework for the consideration of research ethics,[38] and this can be a useful way to review any specific research project. Dilemmas or tensions that arise usually occur because of conflict between these different moral approaches; in palliative research, it is particularly important to recognize the reasons why conflict arises, understand the moral arguments in support of each approach, and then aim to achieve an acceptable balance between these different ethical demands.

These three broad areas of ethical concern can more simply be viewed as being based on key ethical principles,[39,40] and each principle should be applied in the context of any one research study (Table 25.1). But ethical considerations should be wider than just the single research study or group of studies. Allocation of research resources, cost-effectiveness (of both research and the interventions evaluated), population benefit (and harm), and overall public health must all be considered, and here, the concepts of justice and equity become important. The experience of individual research participants and the conduct of the researchers themselves are also important considerations, which introduce concepts of fidelity, trust, and truthfulness.

SPECIFIC ETHICAL CHALLENGES IN PALLIATIVE CARE RESEARCH

There has been extensive debate about whether research in palliative care raises ethical challenges unique to the specialty.[30,42] Particular ethical challenges in palliative research include research-related distress and the perceived vulnerability of participants; research burden for ill patients; consent and capacity issues; ensuring confidentiality and anonymity;

Table 25.1 *Ethical principles guiding medical research*

Ethical principles derived from[39] and [40]	Ethical principles derived from the Belmont Report[41]
Respect for autonomy: This implies self-rule but is probably better described as deliberated self-rule, a special attribute of all moral agents. If we have autonomy, we can make our own decisions on the basis of deliberation. In health care, respecting people's autonomy has many *prima facie* implications. It requires consulting people and obtaining their agreement before we do things to them.	*Respect for persons:* Incorporates at least two ethical convictions: first, those individuals should be treated as autonomous agents; second, persons with diminished autonomy are entitled to protection.
Beneficence: Whenever health care professionals try to help others, they inevitably risk harming them. Those who are committed to helping others must therefore consider the principles of beneficence and aim at producing net benefit over harm.	*Beneficence:* Persons are treated in an ethical manner not only by respecting their decisions and protecting them from harm but also by making efforts to secure their well-being. Such treatment falls under the principle of beneficence.
Nonmaleficence: An obligation not to inflict harm intentionally that is distinct from that of beneficence—an obligation to help others. In the codes of medical practice, the principle of nonmaleficence (*primum non nocere*) has been a fundamental tenet.	*Justice:* Who ought to receive the benefits of research and bear its burdens? This is a question of justice, in the sense of "fairness in distribution" or "what is deserved." An injustice occurs when some benefit to which a person is entitled is denied without good reason or when some burden is imposed unduly. Another way of conceiving the principle of justice is that equals ought to be treated equally.
Justice: This is often regarded as being synonymous with fairness and can be summarized as a moral obligation to act on the basis of fair adjudication between competing claims.	
Scope: There may be an agreement about substantive moral commitments and *prima facie* moral obligations of respect for autonomy, beneficence, nonmaleficence, and justice. Yet there still may be a disagreement about their scope of application, that is, about to whom we owe these moral obligations.	

and the methodological challenge of producing high-quality research, including the contribution of the randomized controlled trial (RCT).

Research-related distress and vulnerability of research participants

In Foster's ethical framework,[38] it is duty of care that requires that distress and vulnerability are given careful ethical consideration. It is often perceived that interviews, surveys, or questionnaires about end-of-life care may be distressing to those interviewed, whether patients or their unpaid informal caregivers. Indeed, patients with advanced disease often experience many distressing symptoms and are frequently fatigued, frail, depressed, and heavily dependent on others.[43-46] Questions therefore need to be raised regarding whether it is ethical to engage these patients in research at a time when they may wish to make use of their remaining time with their family and friends. Given that many of these patients will not stand to benefit directly from the research they are involved in, it could be argued that it is unreasonable and unethical for them to contribute their remaining time.[46] This concern is amplified when considering that patients with advanced disease, who may be experiencing many distressing symptoms, and who are functionally compromised, represent a captive audience who can be exploited.[48] Some have therefore argued that research involving dying patients as a result

of their vulnerability is ethically unacceptable.[49] Although some research bodies[50] have highlighted that special care should be taken where research participants are considered vulnerable, there is confusion about what this term implies and how it should be applied to research in general and palliative care in particular. Definitions of "vulnerable populations" vary, and they are usually identified as those with limited cognitive abilities or diminished autonomy.[51-53] Vulnerable populations, however, may possess autonomy but lack capacity to communicate opinions regarding participation in research. Moreover, this definition does not adequately engage with the context (social as well as medical) of research participants, which may create situations of vulnerability. Kipnis presents a more helpful definition of vulnerability as being a condition "intrinsic" or "situational" that puts some individuals at greater risk of being used in research in ethically inappropriate ways.[54] Within these two domains, Kipnis developed six caution areas intended to identify those considered vulnerable and advice on how researchers should manage them in research studies. The emphasis of this taxonomy is on conducting clinical trials. While each vulnerability category acts as a signal for researchers to initiate study safeguards, the taxonomy also serves as a checklist of criteria to potentially prevent the inclusion of these groups. This supports the principle of fairness, highlighted by the Belmont Report,[55] to exercise care among those who, historically, were selected inappropriately for research. However, there are also concerns about the unfair distribution of benefits of research. Protections that surround vulnerable populations may have unintended consequences. First, the principle of justice, often regarded as being synonymous with fairness, is compromised as they are denied the opportunity to contribute to the research process.[39] Second, being excluded from research potentially deprives them of the benefits and outcomes of being studied.[56] Therefore, medical advances may not be relevant to their needs or situation. These polarized positions should represent a concern for researchers and members of RECs since it is not always apparent what to do when confronted with those considered vulnerable or those who are not.

This delineation is important but fails to sufficiently protect those not considered to explicitly inhabit these groups. Recent research identifies tensions in this current understanding of vulnerability, which warrants further consideration.[57] First, interpretations of vulnerability need to take into consideration the relative importance of participants' individual and situational characteristics that can include the following: (1) communicative vulnerability, (2) institutional vulnerability, (3) deferential vulnerability, (4) medical vulnerability, and (5) social vulnerability. These are not exclusive categories, and importantly, researchers and RECs or IRBs should be aware that it is possible to populate more than one. Second, as with current debates about capacity[58] outlined in the 2005 UK Mental Capacity Act,[59] it is possible that vulnerability need not be viewed as a "once-and-for-all" label; participants can be vulnerable in certain circumstances and not in others. Third, the timing and location of research (institution or home) and, very importantly, the individual personality of participants may govern reactions or responses to the research, which may move them into areas associated with vulnerability. All these circumstances may create situations of caution where research should be viewed more flexibly and sensitively.

Most agree that it is unethical "not" to undertake palliative research, because the absence of research means patients cannot be provided with a high standard of evidence-based care. There is no doubt, however, that it is sensible to pay additional attention to the rights of palliative patients who take part in research and the ways in which those rights will be protected, in the same way that other vulnerable groups such as the elderly or cognitively impaired are considered. This approach has been adopted in a number of countries, with, for example, the Office of Human Research Protections in the United States classifying terminally ill patients as a "special class" for research purposes.[60] Incorporating the "user voice" is another way to protect the rights of vulnerable research participants and to ensure that the patient perspective influences research goals.[61]

It has been suggested that the patients who are cared for in the inpatient hospice setting may believe that refusing to participate in a study may result in their discharge. Some patients may be experiencing severe pain and rely on health care professionals to administer pain relief in addition to tending to intimate care needs. The patients' entirely appropriate reliance on health care professionals does not mean that it is ethical to ask them to participate in research, because they may well feel coerced into doing so or may be unwilling to give an honest appraisal of the care they have received.[62] Other evidence does not support this; on the contrary, many patients and their informal caregivers are very willing to participate in research.[63–65] The reasons that may account for this include altruism, defined as a desire to increase a third party's welfare.[65,66] Other important interrelated factors may involve gaining a sense of purpose from participation and finding the overall experience of being involved in research cathartic and helpful.[65–67]

Although postbereavement research has been shown to carry a small risk of distress, this has been shown to be much less than expected, and this distress was often outweighed by the benefits of open discussion.[68] Seamark et al. have also demonstrated low levels of distress in postbereavement interviews.[69]

Research burden: Balancing risk against benefit

The risks and benefits of research in palliative care are often hard to assess comprehensively because of the limited preexisting evidence. The frequent heterogeneity of study populations also makes weighing up risk and benefit difficult. In general, palliative research participants are likely to be at greater overall risk, because of their advanced disease and the nature of end-of-life care.

As previously mentioned, RECs and IRBs have tended to be reluctant to permit palliative patients to be burdened and many professionals "gatekeep" to protect patients from research because of perceptions about their frailty and distress,[64] which concur with the perception of this research group as vulnerable, as discussed earlier.

Consent and capacity

Informed consent and the patients' capacity to consent are prerequisites if any research in palliative care is going to be conducted. In order for consent to be valid, it must be informed, voluntary, and given by research participants with full decision-making capacity. However, the process of consent deserves additional consideration in palliative care research due to the perceived vulnerability of a population often seriously ill. Palliative care patients may have high levels of cognitive impairment and hence potentially impaired capacity,[70] creating ethical challenges regarding their inclusion. Previously, there has been little consideration or practical advice for palliative care research regarding the methodological challenges of informed consent[71]; however, an increased interest in more inclusive research to improve the acquisition of knowledge in palliative care is emerging.[72] With the introduction of the Mental Capacity Act 2005 in England and Wales, some clarification is given in terms of research guidance.

The England and Wales Mental Capacity Act (MCA) 2005 set out that participants who lack capacity must meet one of the following two requirements: the research has some chance of benefiting the person and the benefit must be in proportion to any burden caused by taking part; or the research would provide knowledge about the cause, treatment or care of people with the same, or similar impairing conditions.[73] The concepts outlined in the MCA were designed to inform the development of the best practice in the assessment of capacity and processes of consent, opening up the spectrum of research to include populations such as those receiving palliative care. An important question is how extensive and detailed assessment of decision-making capacity should be, which depends to a large extent on the level of capacity expected within a study population and the necessity to include participants who have limited mental capacity in the research. Literature informed from the discipline of psychiatry has highlighted the importance of both formal[74] (see Box 25.3) and informal[75] methods of capacity assessment and the impact these methodologies can have on research findings.[76]

Although there is still a comparative dearth of research involving palliative care patients, the introduction of the MCA aided a more inclusive approach enabling increased participation through adapted methodologies, such as advanced consent as suggested by Rees and Hardy.[37] Areas of contention still arise however, and several considerations are important.[77] First, ethical consideration of the research risks and benefits must be reevaluated in the context of lacking or limited capacity; how much risk is the individual participant exposed to by participating, and is the overall likely benefit of the research substantial? Second, the precise role of a proxy, such as a relative, in the consent process and whether, in heightened emotional states, they have full decision-making capacity themselves must be considered. Third, incapacity is variable and not always total: a participant may be able to give consent at some level, and it is important to include this in the consent process. Fourth, how to ethically tackle an individual's right to withdraw if he or she loses capacity during the course of the research.[37]

Confidentiality and anonymity

Most clinical or health research involves collecting patient data, which should always be kept confidential and anonymous. Palliative care research is no exception. A researcher could be found negligent if reasonable precautions were not taken to ensure that all the information gained during a study was not stored in a secure manner or if the identity of a research subject was compromised. Further more, information collected as part of a study should not be shared with a third party unless there is explicit consent of the research subject. This requirement is underpinned by the ethical principle of autonomy. In quantitative studies, these obligations are more straightforward, with the use of unique identifying codes in place of names. In qualitative research, however, the data collection process requires more prolonged face-to-face contact and makes the researcher–participant anonymity more challenging. Pseudonyms can be used in written reports and publications.

Box 25.3 The MacArthur Competency Assessment Tool modified for clinical research

The MacArthur Competency Assessment Tool Modified for Clinical Research (MacCAT-CR) consists of a series of scripted interview questions, divided into four sections that relate to four domains of decision-making capacity. The MacCAT-CR is scored on a scale of 0–2. Incorrect and correct responses are scored as 0 and 2, respectively. Responses that are difficult to interpret are scored as 1.

Understanding (total possible score 0-26)

The subject understands

- The purpose of the study is to test the effectiveness of a case-management intervention (2).
- The study lasts 1 year (2)
- The study requires two additional procedures (two questions) (4)
- The effectiveness of the intervention is unknown (2)
- Not all subjects will receive the intervention (2)
- Subjects who do not receive the intervention must complete surveys and undergo health evaluations (2)
- The intervention will be assigned at random (2)
- How the study results will benefit future patients (2)
- How subjects in the study may benefit (2)
- The study imposes two additional burdens (two questions) (4)
- Subjects can refuse to participate or can withdraw from the study without penalty (2)

Appreciation (total possible score 0-6)

The subject appreciates that he or she

- Would not be asked to be in the study solely for his or her personal benefit (2)
- Would not be assigned to receive the intervention or not based on his or her needs (2)
- Can refuse to participate or can withdraw from the study without penalty (2)

Reasoning (total possible score 0-8)

The subject is able to

- Describe two reasonable consequences of participating in the study (2)
- Compare the merits of participating versus not participating (2)
- Give two examples of the impact of participating on his or her everyday life (2)
- Express a choice that is consistent with the consequences that he or she has described (2)

Choice (total possible score 0-2)

- The subject is able to express a choice about whether or not to enroll (2)

Source: Reproduced from Grisso, T. et al., *Psychiatr. Serv.* 1997; 48: 1415–1419. With permission

Participant confidentiality can be further protected through the omission of identifying key contextual details and circumstances. However, the reality of small sample sizes and the detailed descriptions that accompany this information may be recognizable to some readers familiar with the setting.

Ethical challenges among disadvantaged patient or population groups

Ill health, chronic diseases, high levels of comorbidity, polypharmacy, cognitive impairment, and fatigue frequently challenge or prevent an individual's ability to consent and then participate in palliative care research. However, there are other patient- and population-related factors that may operate in isolation or in combination to further complicate this situation. These include very old patients, those with learning disabilities, and those from black and minority ethnic communities, to name just a few. It has been suggested that because of these difficulties, these groups may be excluded from the research.[78–83]

Older people represent a heterogeneous group where competency and capacity vary considerably. Indeed, many will have no problem with consent and will be able to participate in research. At a purely practical level, however, others may be excluded as a result of their inability to consent due to poor vision or hearing problems.[82,83] The type of research older people are invited to engage with also needs to be considered. It has been suggested that frail older people, who would probably not be competent enough to be included in a pharmaceutical trial because they may have difficulties understanding the extent of their involvement and possible implications for their health, may, however, still be eligible to participate in research if it involves noninvasive, semi-structured interviews, to discuss their experiences of advanced disease or service use.[84]

In the past, individuals with learning disabilities were sometimes chosen as research participants precisely because they were less capable of understanding what was being done to them and were less likely to object.[84] There are many different kinds and degrees of learning disability, and many patients, depending on the extent of the disability, will be able to consent on their own behalf.[85] Ensuring that the consent is indeed informed may be more difficult and require special skills in conveying the relevant information, but it should be attempted wherever at all possible. Even if a patient can give consent, it is always advisable to have the patient's relative as a witness to the consent process.

To date, there has been very little published research about engaging patients from black and minority ethnic communities and refugees in palliative care research.[80] Since these population groups have traditionally been socially excluded from the mainstream health services research, they have been referred to as "invisible" or "elusive" populations. Their notable absence and unheard voices in research therefore reflects their position on the periphery of the society.[86] Where they are identified and recruited, research considerations include those described

earlier. Heterogeneity will be evident, and naturally, many will be able to consent. Those who do not possess adequate language skills either may be excluded from the research or may have to rely upon family members or advocates to translate for them. Given the many sensitivities associated with palliative care, researchers need to be aware that confidentiality may become compromised, or in order to prevent this, the respondent, the family member, or advocate may distort realities to protect privacy.

Methodological challenges and the use of RCTs

The type of research methodology employed during palliative care research poses interesting ethical questions. While quantitative studies often place considerable time and energy demands on dying patients, participation in qualitative studies, which frequently explore issues in considerable detail, may create an emotional burden for patients and their families.[87] Qualitative interactions often become highly personal and interpersonal and, in that context, may be even more intrusive than quantitative approaches.[88] The researcher comes to know the interviewees in a more intimate manner. Interviews that raise issues such as terminal illness, suffering, and loss may bring research participants' feelings that may have been previously largely suppressed to the fore. These undisclosed problems may then be exposed with serious consequences. Johnson and Plant[89] and others[67] have reported that, in their interviews with cancer patients, participants sometimes reported they were emotionally troubled as a result of reminders of their diagnosis, experienced upset feelings in response to talking about their illness, and began to question if their condition might be more serious than they had assumed.

RCTs raise particular issues in palliative research. Traditionally, the RCT has been viewed as the gold standard for conducting clinical research.[90] Proponents of RCTs argue that where there is uncertainty, randomization minimizes the risks of exposure to unevaluated hazards. Although in select situations, RCTs have been successfully employed in palliative care research, for example, examining the management of pain,[91] breathlessness,[92] and the enhancement of advanced directives,[93] they are not without their problems[15] or ethical challenges.[94] Randomization can partially involve relinquishing individualized care and, for some patients, forgoing potential benefits to new treatment or care. McWhinney and colleagues endeavored to minimize the potential of the latter[95] during an evaluation of a palliative care home support team based in an inpatient unit. Patients in the study group received a service immediately, whereas those in the control group received the service a month later. The two groups were then compared after a period of one month using the measurement of symptom levels and patients' quality of life. The trial however failed. The reasons advanced for this included high rates of attrition due to death and low compliance rates due to very sick and weak patients. Knowing this, health professionals too may have been reluctant to cooperate with the study, discouraging the recruitment.

CONCLUSION

The ethical issues in palliative care research need to be understood in the context of the historical background of research ethics and the national and international frameworks, which already exist to inform ethical standards in research. Having said this, both impose some constraints on present day palliative research, having been developed primarily for research in different contexts. Imaginative and intelligent ways to refine existing research methodologies, develop new ones, and work with the vulnerabilities of palliative research participants need to be found. There are ways to respect patient autonomy, minimize harm, and reduce research burden. However these are not always easy to find, nor are they encouraged within existing structures for ethical review.

Key learning points

- Historically, research involving human subjects was not governed by guiding ethical principles. This had catastrophic consequences.

- International guidelines, notably the Declaration of Helsinki, relating to health research now advocate ethical review, and RECs and IRBs are almost a worldwide phenomenon.

- In many countries, RECs and IRBs now have a basis in law, their accountability is clearly defined, and their performance is regularly audited.

- Ethical regulation of medical research on humans provides essential reassurance that the risk of harm has been minimized for all participants.

- Palliative care research raises unique methodological and therefore ethical challenges. These include research-related distress and the perceived vulnerability of participants; research burden for ill patients; consent and capacity issues; ensuring confidentiality and anonymity; and the methodological challenge of producing high-quality research, including the contribution of the RCT.

REFERENCES

1   World Health Organization. *National Cancer Control Programmes: Policies and Managerial Guidelines*, 2nd edn. Geneva, Switzerland: World Health Organization, 2002.

2   Oneschuk D, Bruera E. The potential dangers of complementary therapy use in a patient with cancer. *J Palliat Care* 1999; 15: 49–52.

3   Lan LK, Chidgey J, Addington-Hall JM, Hotopf M. Depression in palliative care: A systematic review. Part 2 Treatment. *Palliat Med* 2002; 16: 279–284.

4   Ross JR, Saunders Y, Edmonds PM et al. Systematic review of the role of bisphosphonates in metastatic disease: Skeletal morbidity. *BMJ* 2005; 327: 469–472.

5   Jones B, Finlay I, Ray A, Simpson B. Is there still a role for open cordotomy in cancer pain management? *J Pain Symptom Manage* 2003; 25: 179–184.

6   Higginson IJ. It would be NICE to have more evidence? *Palliat Med* 2004; 18: 85–86.

7   Higginson IJ, Finlay IG, Goodwin DM et al. Is there evidence that palliative care teams alter end-of-life experiences of patients and their caregivers? *J Pain Symptom Manage* 2003; 25: 150–168.

8   Salisbury C, Bosanquet N, Wilkinson EK et al. The impact of different models of specialist palliative care on patient's quality of life: A systematic literature review. *Palliat Med* 1999; 13: 3–17.

9   Douglas HR, Normand CE, Higginson IJ et al; Palliative Day Care Project Group. Palliative day care: What does it cost to run a centre and does attendance affect use of other services? *Palliat Med* 2003; 17: 628–637.

10 Koffman J, Higginson IJ. Accounts of carers' satisfaction with health care at the end of life: A comparison of first generation black Caribbeans and white patients with advanced disease. *Palliat Med* 2001; 15: 337–345.

11 Tennstedt SL. Commentary on research design in end-of-life research: State of science. *Gerontologist* 2002; 42: 99–103.

12 Sackett DL, Rosenberg WM, Gray JA et al. Evidence based medicine: What it is and what it isn't [editorial]. *BMJ* 1996; 312: 71–72.

13 NIH Consensus Development Programme. National Institutes of Health State-of-the-Science conference on improving end-of-life care, Draft statement (December 6–8, 2004). Bethesda, MD: NIH Consensus Development Programme, 2005.

14 Kassa S, De Conno F. Palliative care research. *Eur J Cancer* 2001; 37: S153–S159.

15 Penrod JD, Morrison RS. Challenges in palliative care research. *J Palliat Med* 2004; 7: 398–402.

16 George LK. Research design in end-of-life research: State of science. *Gerontologist* 2002; 42: 86–98.

17 Vollman J, Winau R. Informed consent in human experimentation before the Nuremberg code. *BMJ* 1996; 313: 1445–1447.

18 World Medical Association. *World Medical Association Declaration of Helsinki: Ethical Principles for Medical Research involving Human Subjects*. Ferney-Voltaire, France: World Medical Association, 2002.

19 Human D, Fluss SS. *The World Medical Association's Declaration of Helsinki: Historical and Contemporary Perspectives*. Ferney-Voltaire, France: World Medical Association, 2001.

20 Guenter D, Esparza J, Macklin R. Ethical considerations in the internatir: HIV vaccine trials: Summary of a consultative process conducted by the joint United National Programme of HIV/AIDS (UNAIDS). *J Med Ethics* 2000; 26: 37–43.

21 Tollman SM. What are the effects of the fifth revision of the *Declaration of Helsinki*? Fair partnerships support ethical research. *BMJ* 2001; 323: 1417–1419.

22 Lurie P. Unethical trials of interventions to reduce perinatal transmission of the human immunodeficiency virus in developing countries. *N Engl J Med* 1997; 337: 853–856.

23 Doll R. What are the effects of the fifth revision of the *Declaration of Helsinki*? Research will be impeded. *BMJ* 2001; 323: 1421–1422.

24 Central Committee on Research Involving Human Subjects. EU Clinical Trial Directive in the Netherlands. Central Committee on Research Involving Human Subjects, 2005.

25 Ministere de la Same Publique et de 1'Environment. Arrete royal du 12 aout 1994 modifant 1'Arret6 royal du 23 Octobre 1964, fixant les normes auxelles les hospitaux et leurs services doivent repondre., Moniteur belge, 27 Septembre 1994. Belgium: Ministere de la Same Publique et de 1'Environment, 1994.

26 United States Department of Human and Human Services. Code of Federal Regulations Part 46. Protection of Human Subjects. United States Department of Human and Human Services, 2005.

27 Department of Health. Research Governance Framework for Health and Social Care. London, U.K.: Department of Health, 2005.

28 Economic and Social Research Council. *Research Ethics Framework*. London, U.K.: Economic and Social Research Council, 2005.

29 Gbolade BA. The recruitment and retention of members of black and other ethnic minority groups to NHS research ethics committees in the United Kingdom. *Res Ethics Rev* 2005; 1: 27–31.

30 Riley J, Ross JR. Research into care at the end of life. *Lancet* 2005; 365: 735–737.

31 Minnis HJ. Ethics review in research: Ethics committees are risk averse. *BMJ* 2004; 328: 710–711.

32 Boyce M. Observational study of 353 applications to London multicentre research ethics committee 1997–2000. *BMJ* 2002; 325: 1081.

33 Brown RF, Butow PN, Butt DG et al. Developing ethical strategies to assist oncologists in seeking informed consent to cancer clinical trials. *Soc Sci Med* 2004; 58: 379–390.

34 Gammelgaard A, Rossel P, Mortensen OS. Patients' perceptions of informed consent in acute myocardial infarction research: A Danish study. *Soc Sci Med* 2005; 58: 2313–2324.

35 Osborn DPJ, Fulford KWM. Psychiatric research: What ethical concerns do LRECs encounter? A postal survey. *J Med Ethics* 2003; 29: 55–56.

36 Glasziou P, Chalmers I. Ethics review roulette: What can we learn? *BMJ* 2004; 328: 121–122.

37 Rees E, Hardy J. Novel consent process for research in dying patients unable to give consent. *BMJ* 2003; 327: 198.

38 Foster C. *The Ethics of Medical Research on Humans*. Cambridge, U.K.: Cambridge University Press, 2001.

39 Beauchamp TL, Childress JF. *Principles of Biomedical Ethics*. Oxford, U.K.: Oxford University Press, 1989.

40 Gillon R. Medical ethics: Four principles plus attention to scope. *BMJ* 1994; 309: 184–188.

41 The National Commission for the Protection of Human Subjects of Biomedical and Behavioral Research. Belmont Report: Ethical Principles and Guidelines for the Protection of Human Subjects of Biomedical and Behavioral Research. Washington: The National Commission for the Protection of Human Subjects of Biomedical and Behavioral Research, 1979.

42 Casarett DJ, Knebel A, Helmers K. Ethical challenges of palliative care research. *J Pain Symptom Manage* 2003; 25: S3–S5.

43 Addington-Hall J, McCarthy M. Dying of cancer: Results of a national population-based investigation. *Palliat Med* 1995; 9: 295–305.

44 Lynn J, Teno JM, Phillips RS et al. Dying experience of older and seriously ill patients: Findings from the SUPPORT and HELP projects. *Ann Intern Med* 1997; 126: 97–106.

45 Koffman J, Higginson IJ, Donaldson N. Symptom severity in advanced cancer, assessed in two ethnic groups by interviews with bereaved family members and friends. *J R Soc Med* 2003; 96: 10–16.

46 Butters E, Higginson I, George R et al. Assessing the symptoms, anxiety and practical needs of HIV/AIDS patients receiving palliative care. *Qual Life Res* 1992; 1: 47–51.

47 Janssens R, Gordijn B. Clinical trials in palliative care: An ethical evaluation. *Patient Educ Couns* 2000; 41: 55–62.

48 Raudonis BM. Ethical considerations in qualitative research with hospice patients. *Qual Health Res* 1992; 2: 238–249.

49 De Raeve L. Ethical issues in palliative care research. *Palliat Med* 1994; 8: 298–305.

50 The British Sociological Association. Statement of Ethical Practice for the British Sociological Association. Internet. Durham, NC: The British Sociological Association, 2002.

51 Nickle PJ Vulnerable populations in research: The case of the seriously ill. *Theor Med Bioeth* 2006; 27: 245–264.

52 Quest T and Marco CA. Ethics seminars: Vulnerable populations in emergency medicine research. *Acad Emerg Med* 2003; 10(11); 1294–1298.

53 Slowther A-M. Determining best interests in patients who lack capacity to decide for themselves. *Clin Ethics* 2007; 2: 19–21.

54 Kipnis, K. *Vulnerability in Research Subjects: A Bioethical Taxonomy. Ethical and Policy Issues in Research Involving Human Research Participants*. Bethesda, MD: National Bioethics Advisory Commission; 2001:G1–G13

55 The National Commission for the Protection of Human subjects of Biomedical and Behavioral Research. *Belmont Report: Ethical Principles and Guidelines for the Protection of Human Subjects of Biomedical and Behavioral Research*. Washington, DC: The National Commission for the Protection of Human Subjects of Biomedical and Behavioral Research, 1979.

56 Eckstein S. Research involving vulnerable participants: Some ethical issues. In *Manual for Research Ethics Committees*, 6th edn. S. Eckstein, ed., Cambridge, U.K.: Cambridge University Press, pp. 105–109, 2003.

57 Koffman J, Morgan M, Edmonds P, Speck P, Higginson IJ. Vulnerability in palliative care research: Findings from a qualitative study of Black Caribbean and White British patients with advanced cancer. *J Med Ethics* 2009; 35(7): 440–444.

58 Chapman S. *The Mental Capacity Act in Practice: Guidance for End of Life Care*. London, U.K.: National Council for Palliative Care, 2008.

59 Office of Public Sector Information. Mental Capacity Act 2005. 2005.

60 Penslar RL. *Protecting Human Research Subjects: Institutional Review Board Guidebook*. Produced by The Poynter Center for the Study of Ethics and American Institutions, Indiana University, IN, for the United States Department of Health and Human Services, 2005.

61 Seymour J, Skilbeck J. Ethical considerations in researching user views. *Eur J Cancer Care (Engl)* 2002; 11: 215–219.

62 Addington-Hall J. Research sensitivities to palliative care patients. *Eur J Cancer Care* 2002; 11: 220–224.

63 Henderson M, Addington-Hall JM, Hotopf M. The willingness of palliative care patients to participate in research. *J Pain Symptom Manage* 2005; 29: 116–117.

64 Ross C, Cornbleet M. Attitudes of patients and staff to research in a specialist palliative care unit. *Palliat Med* 2003; 17: 491–497.

65 Emanuel EJ, Fairclough DL, Wolfe P, Emanuel LL. Talking with terminally ill patients and their caregivers about death, dying, and bereavement: Is it stressful? Is it helpful? *Arch Intern Med* 2004; 164: 1999–2004.

66 Batson CD. *The Altruism Question: Toward a Social and Psychological Answer*. Mahwah, NJ: Lawrence Erlbaum Associates Inc., 1991.

67 Davies EA, Hall SM, Clarke CR et al. Do research interviews cause distress or interfere in management? Experience from a study of cancer patients. *J R Coll Phys Lond* 1998; 32: 406–411.

68 Takesaka J, Crowley R, Casarett D. What is the risk of distress in palliative care survey research? *J Pain Symptom Manage* 2004; 28: 593–598.

69 Seamark DA, Gilbert J, Lawrence CJ, Williams S. Are postbereavement research interviews distressing to carers? Lessons learned from palliative care research. *Palliat Med* 2000; 14: 55–56.

70 Pereira J, Hanson J, Bruera E. The frequency and clinical course of cognitive impairment in patients with terminal cancer. *Cancer* 1997; 79: 835–842.

71 Casarett DJ. Assessing decision-making capacity in the setting of palliative care research. *J Pain Symptom Manage* 2003; 25: S6–S13.

72 Keeley PW. Improving the evidence base in palliative medicine: A moral imperative. *J Med Ethics* 2008; 34: 757–760

73 *Mental capacity Act* (2005) (c.9). London, U.K.: HMSO.

74 Grisso T, Appelbaum PS, Hill-Fotouhi C. The MacCAT-T: A clinical tool to assess patients' capacities to make decisions. *Psychiatr Serv* 1997; 48: 1415–1419.

75 Adamis D, Martin F, Treloar A. Capacity, consent, and selection bias in a study of delirium. *J Med Ethics* 2005; 31: 137–143.

76 Adamis D, Treloar A, Martin F, Macdonald A. Ethical research in delirium: Arguments for including decisionally incapacitated subjects. *Sci Eng Ethics* 2010; 16: 169–174.

77 Karlawish JHT. Conducting research that involves subjects at the end of life who are unable to give consent. *J Pain Symptom Manage* 2003; 25: S14–S24.

78 Regnard C, Mathews D, Gibson L, Clarke C. Difficulties in identifying distress and its causes in people with severe communication problems. *Int J Palliat Nurs* 2003; 9: 173–176.

79 Chouliara Z, Kearny N, Worth A, Stott D. Challenges in conducting research with hospitalized older people with cancer: Drawing from the experience of an ongoing interview-based project. *Eur J Cancer* 2004; 13: 409–415.

80 Gunaratnam Y. *Researching 'Race' and 'Ethnicity'*. London, U.K.: Sage, 2003.

81 Koffman J, Camps J. No way in: Including the excluded at the end of life. In: Payne S, Seymour J, Skilbeck J, Ingelton C, eds. *Palliative Care Nursing: Principles and Evidence for Practice*. Maidenhead, U.K.: Open University Press, 2004. 364–384.

82 Tuffrey-Wijne I. The palliative care needs of people with intellectual disabilities: A literature review. *Palliat Med* 2003; 17: 55–62.

83 Gregson BA, Smith M, Lecouturier N et al. Issues of recruitment and maintaining high response rates in a longitudinal study of older hospital patients in England–pathways through care study. *J Epidemiol Comm Health* 1997; 51: 541–548.

84 Dubler NN. Legal judgments and informed consent in geriatric research. *J Am Geriatr Soc* 1987; 35: 545–549.

85 Smith T. *Ethics in Medical Research*. Cambridge, U.K.: Cambridge University Press, 1999.

86 Koffman J, Higginson IJ. Rights, needs and social exclusion in palliative care. In: Faull C, Carter Y, Daniels L, eds. *Handbook of Palliative Care*. London, U.K.: Blackwell, 2005: pp. 43–60.

87 Dean RA, McClement SE. Palliative care research: Methodological and ethical challenges. *Int J Palliat Nurs* 2002; 8: 376–380.

88 Froggatt KA, Field D, Bailey C, Krishnasamy M. Qualitative research in palliative care 1990–1999: A descriptive review. *Int J Palliat Nurs* 2003; 9: 98–104.

89 Johnson B, Plant H. Collecting data from people with cancer and their families: What are the implications? In: de Raeve L, ed. *Nursing Research: An Ethical and Legal Appraisal*. London, U.K.: Bailliere Tindall, 1996: pp. 85–100.

90 Alderson P, Green S, Higgins JPT. *Cochrane Reviewers' Handbook*. Chichester, U.K.: John Wiley & Sons, 2004.

91 Rowbotham MC, Twilling L, Davies PS et al. Oral opioid therapy for chronic peripheral and central neuropathic pain. *N Engl J Med* 2003; 348: 1223–1232.

92 Bruera E, MacEachern T, Ripamonti C, Hanson J. Subcutaneous morphine for dyspnea in cancer patients. *Ann Intern Med* 2003; 119: 907.

93 Meier DE, Fuss BR, O'Rourke D et al. Marked improvement in recognition and completion of health care proxies. A randomized controlled trial of counseling by hospital representatives. *Arch Intern Med* 1996; 156: 1227–1232.

94 Snowdon C, Garcia J, Elbourne D. Making sense of randomization; responses of parents of critically ill babies to random allocation of treatment in a clinical trial. *Soc Sci Med* 1997; 45: 1337–1355.

95 McWhinney IR, Bass MJ, Donner A. Evaluation of a palliative care service: Problems and pitfalls. *BMJ* 1994; 309: 1340–1342.

26

Practical tips for successful research in palliative care

EDUARDO BRUERA, SRIRAM YENNURAJALINGAM

INTRODUCTION

Palliative medicine emerged in the United Kingdom during the 1960s as a response to the unmet needs of terminally ill patients and their families. The development of this movement in the United Kingdom has been addressed in Chapter 1. Chapters 2 through 7 have addressed the successful development of palliative medicine as a global discipline.

In most regions of the world, palliative care did not emerge as a result of main stream academia; instead, it emerged as a number of "bottom-up" approaches on the fringes of the existing health care movement. This relative isolation allowed palliative clinical programs to successfully interact with their communities and to develop the basic principles of the disciplines. However, this isolation also made it difficult for palliative medicine groups to interact with academic groups, including methodologists, biostatisticians, clinical trialists, epidemiologists, and other groups that are readily available to other content areas of health care.

Palliative medicine programs have a very strong clinical commitment and limited access to protected time for research and research training.[1-3] For this reason, our book has committed a considerable amount of space to chapters on the specific challenges of research, the patient population, the different research designs, outcomes, ethics in research, and the process of audit and quality improvement.

The purpose of this chapter is to discuss some practical issues that are not always available in methodology textbooks but that are crucial to the success of research projects in palliative care. Most of the tips included in this book are the result of difficulties encountered by our and other research teams in the process of establishing a research program.

SETTING FOR PALLIATIVE CARE RESEARCH

Choosing the appropriate setting is of great importance and one of the main reasons why research projects fail. Box 26.1 summarizes what is important about the setting where research will take place.

Appropriate understanding of the patient population requires not only the basic diagnosis and demographics but also many practical issues such as the level of literacy (several studies in the developing world could not be performed, because they required patients to complete questionnaires they were not able to read). The inclusion of minorities may be difficult in some areas of the United States unless Spanish versions of questionnaires are available. The average length of stay of patients in the specific setting or the average number of visits of patients to outpatient settings is very important to ensure that the study can be completed in time. In the case of studies on patients and families, it is important to know how many patients come accompanied by a relative and in how many cases, the relative lives with the patient. The percentage of patients unable to attend a scheduled outpatient visit ranges from 20% to 50% in most outpatient care settings, and this can have major impact on missing data for clinical studies. The ability of patients to communicate on the telephone for follow-up may be very useful in recovering some of this missing information. The availability of rooms where interviews can be conducted and discussing arrangements of the inpatient or outpatient areas needs to be appropriately planned prior to study initiation. Otherwise it may be impossible to keep a patient in an examining room for assessments or consent, and there may not be staff available for notification when a patient becomes eligible for a study.

The types of treatments are of great importance. In many clinical trials, there are criteria for eligibility including certain treatments. Appropriate understanding of these criteria will assist in determining how feasible a certain study is.

In two clinical trials in patients with dyspnea, patient accrual was extremely difficult, because although dyspnea is a very frequent symptom in palliative care settings, the clinical trials required patients to be able to complete self-assessment questionnaires with excellent cognitive status and comply with complex research designs.[4,5] As a consequence, a large number of patients were identified, but only a very small number were able to actually enter the clinical trial.

A clinical trial comparing methadone versus morphine as first-line opioid for cancer pain required simple assessments by patients with a very common pain problem. However, the main difficulty to admit and maintain patients on this study was the requirement for very frequent follow-up during the first week of treatment. Many of the centers were not able to conduct frequent assessments in the patients' home or admit the patients for a 1-week period.[6]

The idea for a study on the use of methylphenidate "as needed" for the management of cancer-related fatigue emerged from the comments of a colleague who had observed excellent response of patients to this modality of administration.[7] The idea for a clinical trial of donepezil on the management of sedation and fatigue emerged from a letter to the editor submitted by a clinician who had observed improvement among patients receiving opioids when treated with donepezil.[8,9]

A randomized controlled trial comparing methylphenidate "as needed" with placebo emerged from the result of the pilot study by the same group.[10]

These three examples emphasize the importance of publishing letters to the editor based on observations or pilot projects. This is one way in which colleagues can pick up important ideas from findings and translate into useful research projects.

RESEARCH IDEA

In palliative care, research ideas may emerge from a clinical observation, comments by colleagues, papers read in different journals, or previous research conducted by the group.

Clinical research is most successful when it is investigator driven since investigators who are highly committed to a certain domain will be much more motivated to spend a considerable amount of extra time in pursuing this research in addition to other clinical and educational responsibilities.

One of the most difficult processes is that of turning a research idea into a well-formulated hypothesis. Being able to frame the general idea into a very specific question is extremely important, because this will frame the whole methodology of the project. It is important for researchers to have a conversation with a mentor at a very early stage in the development of this early hypothesis. This will help them immediately identify how feasible the whole project may be.

LITERATURE SEARCH

It is very important to read good quality material, but it is not necessary to read all material on a given subject. The literature search should consist of a number of recent high quality

reviews of the area as well as a number of recent original papers on the subject under study. This quick review of the literature will rapidly demonstrate if the investigator's hypothesis has already been appropriately studied or if it would be justifiable to proceed with further research on the subject. If there have been only one or two brief reports or letters to the editor with a small number of cases, this suggests that there is probably strong justification for the study. If the investigator finds no reference at all, it is important to review if he/she is researching the correct literature on this subject.

The literature search is useful for three main purposes:

1. To provide an in-depth understanding of the content area where the investigator is planning to conduct his/her research
2. To be able to understand the methodology employed by other researchers
3. To understand the main outcomes conducted by previous researchers

As much as possible, the investigators should attempt to take advantage of previous knowledge and methodologies. This will save a great amount of time and also will increase the likelihood of publication of their findings since they can provide literature support for having followed a certain methodology.

The literature search is not only useful for justifying the project and applying to a research committee and/or granting agency. This literature search can per se become a major publication and be extremely helpful to other readers. For example, the literature search concerning survival estimation used for the design of a clinical trial was also very useful when published as a systematic review.[11,12]

DEFINING THE RIGHT OUTCOMES

In palliative care, outcomes are mostly subjective (i.e., symptom intensity, satisfaction with communication by patients and/or families, perceptions of quality of communication, etc.). These outcomes are much more likely to be subject to bias, and therefore, the nature of these outcomes will have a major impact on the methodology used by the investigator.

In the study of a specific problem such as cachexia, there may be a combination of outcomes highly unlikely to be influenced by patient or investigator bias such as body weight and other nutritional findings. Other groups that may have an intermediate risk of bias such as daily energy intake, and a third group that is highly subject to biases, such as anorexia, fatigue, etc. Similar statements could be made for other physical and psychosocial symptoms. The timing for modification of variables may also differ dramatically (e.g., anorexia or fatigue can be modified by an intervention in hours while body weight may require weeks).

It is important to use a methodological approach that will best address the most important question and to try to keep it very simple, since a likelihood of the completion of the study will be directly linked with the simplicity of the design.

One of the most common mistakes is to attempt to address too many outcomes or one main outcome that is beyond the reach of the research team.

In the case of cancer cachexia, clinical trials of megestrol acetate showed significant improvement in body weight but of limited clinical relevance when the main outcome was to successfully reverse cachexia.[13] On the other hand, when clinical trials were conducted using a very simple subjective outcome such as appetite, the same drug was found to be effective.[14,15]

ORGANIZING THE TEAM

The principal investigator will need to put together a research team. Box 26.2 summarizes the main components of the research team. The methodology expert will need to be an individual who may or may not work in the palliative care area but who is highly experienced in the use of the methodology for this research project, for example, an expert in surveys, clinical trials, and qualitative studies. This individual will have a major role in helping the team choose the different tools, the overall design, and refining the outcomes the principal investigator is currently considering.

The statistician should be approached very early in the process of considering the study. Even if the outcomes are likely to be mostly descriptive, the statistician may have a crucial role in assisting the team in the best use of the existing data. The role of the statistician will become more prominent as the study becomes more complex. One of the most important roles of the statistician is to assist the investigators in calculating the sample size they require. It may become clear early in the study that the number of patients required is too large for the setting where the investigator is planning to conduct the research. This will require the investigator to find a number of additional sites where data collection can take place. It is very important that this process takes place early in the research project so that the individuals responsible for the other sites can become part of the research team during the process of defining the study.

The principal investigator may certainly be a content expert. It is always very useful to have at least one more additional expert in the content under study. These experts are usually also familiar with many methodological issues, and they can make suggestions based on their personal experience and the connections they have with other content experts. For example, in a

Box 26.2 The research team

- Principal investigator
- Content expert
- Methodology expert
- Biostatistician
- Clinical expert
- Administrative expert

study on cachexia, a content expert may be aware of research being conducted by a colleague somewhere else and may be helpful in directly contacting this investigator for specific information about the rationale for a certain study or outcome.

The clinician experts include nurses, pharmacists, and other clinical colleagues. These individuals are essential for the success of any clinical study including trials, surveys, or qualitative studies. These individuals will be able to address many practical issues that are crucial for the success of the study. Clinical trials may be more apt to fail if patients receiving placebo are required to have multiple hospital visits, studies that require patients to take an excessive number of tablets, questionnaires that were too long and difficult to teach, and a number of practical aspects regarding the setting of care that the principal investigator and other experts did not completely understand.

It is important for the investigators to remember that the current access to global communication by low cost telephone and Internet allows teams to function quite well and in real time from multiple locations. It is important to understand if the local requirement of the institutional review board (IRB) puts some limitations on the participation by distance coinvestigators.

There are two very important items that need to be discussed very early in the process of planning the research:

1. *Authorship*—It is a very important issue to discuss in an open and friendly way the expectations of the different team members regarding authorship. It may be possible to designate expected first authors and senior authors for presentation, publication of the main paper, as well as other secondary publications that may result from the study. A frank discussion regarding the different roles of the investigators will help prevent misunderstandings and unnecessary stress on the participants. This is responsibility of the principal investigator.
2. *Financial issues*—It is very important to be open about any resources that may be obtained for conducting the study and how this will be distributed among the different participants. If an application is being made to a research granting agency or an industry sponsor, all details regarding the financial arrangements need to be disclosed before the application is submitted. This will maintain the friendly and open environment throughout the project and will ensure collaboration for future projects.

It is very important for the principal investigator to put together a successful research team. It is also important for the principal investigator to understand that it is his/her ultimate responsibility to write the proposal.

Palliative care is a content area, and researchers working in this area will need to use a variety of methodologies to better understand their areas of work. It is impossible for an investigator to become an expert on the methodology and biostatistics of all the different approaches. However, it should be expected that the principal investigator would have a basic understanding of methodologies and biostatistics to be able to appropriately communicate with these experts and be a resource for all areas of content.

WRITING THE PROTOCOL

The protocol should be written in all cases, including case series and retrospective reviews. The process of writing the protocol will help the research team clarify ideas and make sure that all aspects of the process are well outlined. The process of writing the protocol will clearly demonstrate to the team if they are attempting to address too many issues. In general, it is much more effective to address one aspect well rather than many aspects with a lower level of evidence. By its nature, palliative care research takes place with patients and families who are facing multiple problems, and therefore, the likelihood of our interventions may be at best only partially successful. Complex and lengthy studies have a very high chance of failure.

ADMINISTRATION OF THE STUDY

One of the main challenges is to maintain appropriate approval by the IRB. This may require the research team to make several modifications in their design, questionnaires, and consents. Understanding how the IRB operates, their main areas of expertise, and the wording they prefer to see in the research protocols and consent forms, can all prevent many problems.

It is important that at least one member of the research team is familiar with the operation of the IRB and is able to provide advice about the way the protocol and consent forms should be written. In case of doubt, it can be helpful to consult the chair of the IRB about specific aspects of the study before a full submission.

Once the study has been approved, it is very important to keep meeting regularly to see if there are any problems with the actual conduct of the study. Some of the most common problems include lack of patient accrual related to some of the eligibility criteria, missing data because of an excessively ambitious assessment method, patients who are unable to adhere to the study because of clinical and social issues, or unexpected side effects or distress by patients and families in the case of discussion of questionnaires.

It is important to make very early adjustments in the criteria for eligibility or methods since each adjustment needs to be submitted to the IRB for consideration and this will take a considerable amount of time.

It is also important to accept when studies just cannot be completed so that they can be completely rewritten in a more appropriate way.

PREPARATION OF THE MANUSCRIPT

While the input of the whole research team is very important at this stage, the principal investigator should write the initial draft of the manuscript. This will provide the necessary leadership for all the other experts to contribute. It is very important to write concise manuscripts summarizing the main

aspects of the study. If there is other information, this could be prepared as additional reports at scientific meetings or as additional publications.

During the last 10 years, there has been a major improvement in the number of peer-reviewed palliative medicine-related journals and in the number of scientific meetings where palliative medicine research can be published. It is very important to submit for publication all studies whether the results were encouraging or disappointing since this information can be invaluable to other researchers who are planning to conduct similar research.

It is very important to be flexible in responding to the comments from the reviewers and to take advantage of these reviews as a way of improving the manuscript even if the journal has decided to reject the manuscript. Consideration of the reviewer's comments will result in a better manuscript to be submitted to the next journal.

Young investigators frequently feel disheartened by devastating comments from reviewers. Journal editors should take appropriate steps to protect authors from vicious comments by reviewers protected by anonymity. Investigators should never decide to discard the manuscript without consulting with an experienced mentor who may help put some of the comments from the reviewer in perspective. It is important to remember that 100% of the manuscripts that are not resubmitted will not get published. Resubmission will result in a higher success rate than that one.

APPLYING FOR FUNDING

In many cases, the only way a research project can be conducted is after the research team applies for funding. This is time consuming and slow, but unfortunately, there is no other way to conduct successful research than establishing a research team and completing grant applications.

The methodology expert, biostatistician, and content expert will usually have considerable experience in grant writing and will be able to advise the investigator along the way.

Most of the time, it is most useful for the investigator to hold individual meetings with each of the members of the team as compared to lengthy meetings involving the whole team assembled together. It is important to understand that each of the experts has limited time and that the investigator should use this time in the way that is most conducive to writing a successful application.

In most cases, having some pilot data will be essential for writing a grant application. This short pilot study may need to be conducted with no access to funding. A number of organizations/universities provide bridge money for conducting brief pilot studies that will lead to major grant applications. These granting committees usually require very simple design outlines. The investigator may obtain considerable information about availability of philanthropic or bridge funding from the local research office of their university. It is important to arrange for a formal visit and consultation with the research director.

Box 26.3 summarizes a checklist of essential items to take into consideration while conducting a prospective clinical trial.

Box 26.3 Checklist for a successful completion of a research project

Research idea

- Is the research question valid? A review article on the topic may be helpful. Review the research idea and research objectives with your mentor or guide or peer or an informal survey; *Important to investigate if the research question is relevant and has a pressing need for further investigation.*

- Setting in which the study is conducted needs to specific? Prognosis should be clarified—Does the research objective fit the patient's trajectory of illness in question? *Few interventional studies are appropriate in patients with prognosis 7 days or less.*

- *Do the research objectives answer your research question?* Research objectives should be focused and may not be necessary to answer the entire research question.

- Are your research team and institution/s able to successfully complete the study and publish the results in a reasonable timeframe? *Most palliative care professionals have very limited dedicated time for prospective research project.*

- *Authorship and delegation of responsibilities resolved?* Most collaboration/mentorship relationships fail overtime due to lack of honest communication.

Study design and methods

Perhaps the most critical step that the success of a project really hinges on.

- *An initial feasibility study very helpful.* A pilot study will determine whether a larger study is necessary.

- Anticipated delays in accrual and attrition should be included in study design/sample size calculation. *Most intervention trials in palliative care may result in attrition of at least 25%.*

- *Short time frame is critical for successful completion of interventional clinical trials*—as it minimizes study burden and incorporates close monitoring and support for the patients on the study.

- Good performance status may be crucial to avoid attrition in intervention trials, *as majority of attrition is due to the deterioration of the patient's physical condition.*

- A proactive management of alleviating identified distress or symptoms should be included in the treatment plan once distress is identified or a patient is given placebo. *Survey studies should be limited in certain circumstances as it can "burn out" the research staff, as they are unable to intervene or relieve the distress expressed in the questionnaires; proposed treatment should be offered to all patients who received a placebo.*

Implementation

- Know that the approval by Clinical Scientific Board Review and Ethical Board Review, and funding are time consuming but critical for the sustenance of the research idea. *Most studies fail due to lack of resources (time and personnel).*

- *A study initiation and routine study accrual and data review meeting are essential for the vitality of study.* Poor ongoing study review may result in poor accrual, attrition, and inaccurate data as a result of a negative or inconclusive trial.

- *Present the study in local and national meeting to discuss concept and challenges.* Ongoing study review by peers may improve the chances of successful study completion.

- Always revise the protocol if there are issues such as slow accrual or dropouts. *This is as important as a well written protocol.*

Analysis and manuscript

- During the conduct of the study, review the data frequently to ensure data integrity and patient safety.

- Analyze data as stated in the protocol with the help of the research team (statistician)

- *Report positive and negative studies.* Reporting of negative studies is ethical and would help the science of palliative care advances faster.

- Principal investigator should supervise the analyses and is responsible for all aspects of manuscript writing and submission.

- *Identify and submit to the best journal for the topic.* You never know whether your result is of any interest to a given journal unless it is reviewed.

- *Respond to all comments of the reviewers promptly.* Always consider all constructive comments by reviewers; this will help you to improve your manuscript even if the journal rejects the paper. These changes will increase the likelihood of your paper to be accepted by the next journal you submit to.

Summary

- Research question should be thoroughly examined for relevance and priority.

- Research team should be well rounded and multidisciplinary. (Have a good mentor!)

- A pilot study, case report, or preliminary data are always critical to determine the feasibility of your project.

- Design should be sound and peer-reviewed. Keep it simple!!!

- Minimize dropouts in intervention trials by avoiding patients with (1) high symptom burden; (2) poor performance status.

CONCLUSIONS

Palliative medicine is a young specialty. A large number of aspects of this discipline are not well understood. Almost all clinicians are capable of making a meaningful contribution by publishing their observations, case series, retrospective studies, and other more sophisticated research designs.

Perhaps the most important tip for an investigator is to put together a research team that can collaborate in a friendly and effective manner. This will ensure not only that the research project is successful but also that the whole experience is highly enjoyable.

Key learning points

- Choosing appropriate setting for palliative care research is of great importance and is one of the reasons why research projects fail.

- Clinical research is most successful when it is investigator initiated.

- A thorough literature search is essential to complete prior to starting a research project, to take advantage of previous knowledge and methodologies.

- In palliative care research, the outcomes are mostly subjective (i.e., symptom intensity, etc.), and thus, it is essential for investigator to use a methodological approach that will address the most important question and keep the design of the study simple.

- Authorship and financial issues should be discussed early in the process of planning the research project.

- The research team should collaborate in a friendly and effective manner to ensure the success of the research project.

REFERENCES

1 Brenneis C., Bruera E. *Models for the Delivery of Palliative Care: The Canadian Model.* Topics in Palliative Care Volume 5; Oxford University Press, Oxford, U.K. 2001: pp. 3–23.
2 Clark D. *The Development of Palliative Care in the UK and Ireland.* Palliative Medicine. Edward Arnold Publishers Limited, London, U.K. 2005: In press.
3 Ryndes T. *The development of Palliative Medicine in the USA.* Palliative Medicine. Edward Arnold Publishers Limited, London, U.K. 2005: In press.
4 Bruera E., de Stoutz N., Velasco-Leiva A., Schoeller T. et al. Effects of oxygen on dyspnea in hyopoxaemic terminal-cancer patients. *Lancet,* 1993; 342(8862): 13–14.
5 Bruera E., MacEachern T., Ripamonti C., Hanson J. Subcutaneous morphine for dyspnea in cancer patients. *Ann Intern Med.* 1993; 119(9): 906–907.
6 Bruera E., Palmer JL, Bosnjak S, Rico M.A. et al. Methadone versus morphine as a first-line strong opioids for cancer pain: A randomized, double-blind study. *J Clin Oncol.* 2004; 22(1): 185–192.
7 Bruera E., Driver L., Barnes E.A., Willey J. et al. Patient-controlled methylphenidate for the management of fatigue in patients with advanced cancer: A preliminary report. *J Clin Oncol.* 2003; 21(23): 4439–4443.
8 Slatkin N., Rhiner M. Treatment of opioid-induced delirium with acetylcholinesterase inhibitors: A case report. *J Pain Symptom Manage.* 2004; 27(3): 268–273.
9 Bruera E., Strasser F., Shen L., Palmer J.L. et al. The effect of donepezil on sedation and other symptoms in patients receiving opioids for cancer pain: A pilot study. *J Pain Symptom Manage.* 2003; 26(5) 1049–1054.
10 Bruera E., Valero V., Driver L., Shen L. et al. Patient-controlled methylphenidate for cancer fatigue: A double-blind, randomized, placebo-controlled trial. *J Clin Oncol.* 2005. In press.
11 Vigano A., Donaldson N., Higginson I.J., Bruera E. Quality of life and survival prediction in terminal cancer patients: A multicenter study. *Cancer.* 2004; 101(5): 1090–1098.
12 Vigano A., Dorgan M., Buckingham J., Bruera E. et al. Survival prediction in terminal cancer patients: A systematic review of the medical literature. *Palliat Med.* 2000; 14(5): 363–374.
13 Maltoni M., Nanni O., Scarpi E., Rossi D. et al. High-dose progestins for the treatment of cancer anorexia-cachexia syndrome: A systematic review of randomized clinical trials. *Ann Oncol.* 2001; 12(3): 289–300.
14 Bruera E., Macmillan K., Kuehn N., Hanson J. et al. A controlled trial of megestrol acetate on appetite, caloric intake, nutritional status, and other symptoms in patients with advanced cancer. *Cancer.* 1990; 66(6): 1279–1282.
15 Bruera E., Ernst S., Hagen N., Spachynski K. et al. Effectiveness of megestrol acetate in patients with advanced cancer: A randomized, double-blind, crossover study. *Cancer Prev Control.* 1998; 2(2): 74–78.

27

Audit and quality improvement in palliative care research

HSIEN-YEANG SEOW, DEANNA BRYANT, SARAH MYERS, JOANNE LYNN

INTRODUCTION

High-quality care can mean better outcomes,[1] enhanced efficiency and patient safety,[2,3] and reduced disparities.[4,5] Traditionally, methods to improve the quality of care have aimed to use formal research to guide changes in practice and policy reform. Formal research is key to identifying more effective pharmaceuticals or procedures but less effective in guiding change in complex clinical practice and achieving improved outcomes at a rapid pace. In discerning how to deliver optimal care to a specific patient population without incurring unacceptable costs, quality improvement can be superior.

WHAT IS AUDIT AND QUALITY IMPROVEMENT?

Quality improvement (QI) is an empirical, goal-oriented method of improving the performance of a system.[6] Not a new concept by any means, QI as applied to healthcare dates back to the Crimean War in 1854, when Florence Nightingale began keeping statistical records to reform the hospital and sanitary administration within the British army.[7] In recent years, QI has become pervasive within the healthcare system. QI allows clinicians to assess whether they are doing the right thing, with the right patients, at the right time—and if not, to make needed changes quickly and with minimal disruption to the overall system of care.[8] These often occur in rapid cycles of change. Quality improvement models provide clinical teams with a structure for identifying areas ripe for improvement, strategies for identifying process improvements to test on a small scale, and tools for measuring progress toward reaching established goals. Generally, QI requires stating an aim, testing possible improvements, measuring success, and learning from the tests. Effective QI is an ongoing cycle that encourages ongoing organizational learning.[8–13] Quality improvement teams ideally begin by addressing discrete, narrow problems, but then expand their efforts in size and scope, moving from time-limited, focused tests of change to broad implementation of changes that their own data have proved to be effective.

Quality improvement methods rest on statistics originally developed by Shewhart[14] and are anchored in process control charting. Simple time series graphs of the performance of a production system illustrate trends and unusual occurrences, but formal process control charts add an important layer of insight about reliability of system performance and indicators of changes. With any particular production process, from generating well-functioning hips after replacement surgery to reducing medication errors in transitions from hospital to home, an ordinary pattern will have a central measure of performance and a variation around that mean. Deliberate improvements aim to do two things: to reduce the variation and to improve the mean. Reducing the variation is important, because a process that is reliable is much easier to manage than one that is more chaotic. The usual variation around the mean arises from sources that are "built in"—staff schedules, supply and disposition patterns, and so on. The usual variation is said to arise from "common cause," and the variation accepted as arising from common cause lies between a calculated "upper control limit" and "lower control limit." Variation that exceeds those limits or that lies on one side of the mean for a substantial series of sequential data points are very likely to arise from a new factor—deliberate or otherwise—and these variations are said to arise from "special causes," which require inquiry to establish a likely cause. There are simple rules and formulae for calculating upper and lower limits and for identifying special causes.[15] Thus, the key elements in tracking improvement are these: to measure one or more important indicators of the performance of the process repeatedly over time; to graph them and calculate means and upper and lower control limits, to seek to reduce common cause variation (narrowing upper and lower control limits), and to shift means toward improvement (as indicated by identifying special cause variation consistent with deliberate improvement efforts).

Audit is a related tool: "a continuous process whereby healthcare professionals review patient care against agreed standards and make changes, where necessary, to meet those standards."[16] The results of an audit identify deficiencies between current standards and what is actually happening. An audit can be as simple as reviewing a handful of hospital patient charts or as complex as a national review of administrative quality indicators. They evaluate clinical processes, organizations, or systems to ensure that the best practice is followed. Audit is commonly used to provide feedback for professional development and quality of practice.[17] It can be used as a tool to measure the quality of care, define standards and targets for good practice, and gather evidence about performance.[18] The results of the audit can inform future changes to address deficiencies and improve the quality of care. Audits can be formalized and centralized by a governmental body, such as the National Health Service in the United Kingdom. However, small organizations and teams can also embark upon and carry out audit efforts on their own initiative. Indeed, in the past several years, more and more healthcare organizations have been required to participate in audit and QI by payers or by their accrediting bodies. Audit and QI can apply to any size population from the quality of care for a few patients daily[19] (often called clinical QI or audit initiatives) to implementing guidelines across a nation.[20] Since minimal resources are needed to implement an audit, they can be used in many types of healthcare settings and in any healthcare system worldwide.[17,18,21] A systematic review of randomized trials of audit and feedback strategies found that audit and feedback can be an effective tool for increasing interprofessional collaboration, though effects are generally small to moderate.[17] Moreover, the review also found that use of audit and feedback is more likely to be effective when baseline adherence to recommended practice begins at a low level and when feedback is delivered more intensively.

AUDIT AND QUALITY IMPROVEMENT IN PALLIATIVE CARE

Over the past decade, a number of healthcare organizations began to incorporate formal and informal palliative care programs and services into their systems of care. However, in many nations, distinct palliative care programs are still relatively new in the healthcare system, with palliative care services having previously been a part of primary care, geriatrics, and hospice. This expanding field—with a growing number of standards and guidelines—continues to present tremendous opportunities for QI. The opportunities reach all aspects of palliative care, including advance care planning, symptom management, and continuity and coordination of care.

EXAMPLES FROM AROUND THE GLOBE

Quality improvement is applied to palliative care on large scale (e.g., national guidelines and care standards)[22–25] and small scale (e.g., clinical QI and audit initiatives).[19,26] The former is generally the purview of regulatory and oversight bodies and healthcare payers, both private and public. The latter often arises at the organizational level. A review of the experience of several countries and regions seeking to improve palliative care reveals a range of approaches in each domain. In the following,

we highlight some examples of such approaches from around the globe though we do not imply that these examples are superior to those not addressed here.

National guidelines and care standards

Many countries now have some experience using national guidelines and policies to improve palliative care, often in the form of accreditation. A global study for the World Health Organization (WHO) in 2000 identified 36 nationwide healthcare accreditation programs.[27] Starting with the Joint Commission in the United States in 1951, the number of programs around the world has doubled every 5 years since 1990.[28] The Joint Commission in the United States accredits healthcare organizations in compliance with their quality standards. Presently, nearly 16,000 healthcare providers—from small, rural clinics to expansive, complex healthcare networks—use Joint Commission standards to improve their quality performance and how they provide care.[29] In 2000, the Joint Commission added pain management standards that address assessment and management of pain, education around effective pain management to patients and families, and continuous organizational improvement.[30,31]

In 2004, the Joint Commission explicitly made advanced directives (addressing the patient's wishes related to end-of-life decisions) a part of the patient rights standards that hospitals and other healthcare organizations must adhere to.[32] And in September 2011, the Joint Commission created a certification program for palliative care[33] which aims to "recognize hospital inpatient programs that demonstrate exceptional patient and family-centered care and optimize the quality of life for patients (both adult and pediatric) with serious illness." Certified applicants must meet criteria related to program management; provision of care, treatment, and services; information management, and performance improvement.

Other efforts in the United States have aimed to develop and publish standards for the delivery of palliative care. In 2009, the National Consensus Project for Quality Palliative Care published the second edition of the Clinical Practice Guidelines for Quality Palliative Care.[34] This includes guidelines covering eight different domains, including structure and processes of care, social aspects of care, and ethical and legal aspects of care.

In the United Kingdom, the Department of Health in 2008 published its End of Life Care Strategy[35] targeting adults in England, which aimed to "provide people approaching the end of life with more choice about where they would like to live and die." The strategy offers a common national approach to develop quality standards of care delivered to people at the end of life. It focuses across the health and social care system and includes recommendations specific to various care settings, including acute care hospitals, primary care, long-term care homes, and ambulance services.[35] Supporting the national guidelines and standards work is the National Institute of Health and Clinical Excellence, which developed quality measures for every setting involved in end-of-life care, with sixteen standard measures made publicly available.[36] Achieving target rates on these measures affects payment. All quality markers are unified by the principle of being patient centered and are consistent with the holistic approach to care described in the strategy.

In Australia, the National Palliative Care Strategy was endorsed in 2010, culminating in a process which began in 1998 as a result of much national support.[37] The national strategy provides the framework for palliative care throughout Australia and serves as a guide for all policy decisions regarding palliative care policies and service delivery models across the country. The strategy addresses palliative care plans for a wide variety of health conditions and diseases for the health needs of the population as a whole. A key component of the strategy was the implementation and evaluation of palliative care interventions and quality improvement.[38] The four goal areas of the strategy are: awareness and understanding, appropriateness and effectiveness, leadership and governance, and capacity and capability. Additionally, the Council of Palliative Care Australia has developed three companion documents in response to the palliative care strategy, which outline the human resources required; standards of quality care with accompanying role expectation by providers; and a population-based plan for equitable, effective, and efficient service delivery.[38-40]

Palliative care programs are being introduced in the Middle East as well, and their experiences and outcomes are starting to be reported in the literature. A recent review of the establishment of these programs[41] highlights the challenges and opportunities associated with developing a system of palliative care across such a diverse geographic area. The authors state that in many Middle Eastern countries, palliative care "has not been fully or officially assimilated into the healthcare systems." Despite this, progress has been made, with only one of the 11 countries (Syria) reviewed by the authors lacking any known palliative care activity. Saudi Arabia, for example, opened a specialty palliative care unit in the early 1990s, which has grown to encompass an "intensive management unit, consultation services, outpatient clinics, and home healthcare programs." In many of the other countries reviewed, palliative care activities remain at a more nascent stage and many are provided by volunteers rather than being a formalized part of the healthcare system. In Iraq, which has been beset by war and political turmoil, there is one pain management center in Baghdad, but there are no "formal policies, guidelines, or practices for pain and there is low or no awareness among health professionals regarding the use of opioids." Qatar, a wealthy country in this region, established its first cancer-focused palliative care hospital in 2008[42] and is among the first to report on its design, processes, and outcomes. Al Kindi et al. (2012) reported on the experience of 223 patients receiving services at the hospital, showing that referrals have steadily increased since the opening of the hospital and length of stay (mean = 32 days) was long compared to similar hospitals around the world. They attribute this to cultural preferences regarding hospital care as well as the lack of other, less acute palliative care options for patients in this country. QI will be an essential component of these programs as they target interventions aimed at better meeting patients' needs.

Large-scale QI efforts have been implemented in some developing countries as well. In the early 2000s, the WHO was working with five African countries to improve the quality of life for patients with cancer and human immunodeficiency virus/acquired immune deficiency syndrome by developing palliative care programs with a community health approach.[43,44] Key to this collaboration program is its emphasis on developing palliative care services and standards and attempting to integrate them into existing health systems and national strategic plans for health and social services. For instance, the WHO has defined a minimum standard of care for HIV patients with cancer in Africa.[45] The initial phase of the project identified improved care for dying patients using palliative care as a national concern. Using data to guide reforms, the project collected information concerning target countries' health systems performance and also assessed needs and gaps in patient care.

In addition to the regional WHO work, the nations of Africa have begun to embrace quality improvement to enhance palliative care. For instance, the African Palliative Care Association was developed in 2004, with a mission to ensure palliative care is widely understood, integrated into health systems at all levels, and underpinned by evidence in order to reduce pain and suffering across Africa.[46] This mission is embedded into their national strategic palliative care plan for 2011–2020.[47] One main focus is to use evidence gathered within the continent of Africa to inform palliative care practice and quality. The association has developed several quality improvement tools such as a standards audit tool, pocket guides to manage pain, and the African Palliative Outcome Scale to measure palliative care outcomes.[48] In addition, the association hosted workshops throughout Africa to identify country-specific barriers to accessing pain medications for palliative care with an outcome of developing action plans to address these barriers.[49] Another example of national standards occurs in South Africa. The federal government funded a program to register traditional healers with mainstream medicine and to provide an integrated approach to palliative care that meets the cultural and linguistic needs of the population.[50]

Clinical QI and audit initiatives

In contrast with the national projects described earlier, many QI and audit initiatives have been implemented at the healthcare system and organization level. There are also many examples of individuals and grouped audit initiatives, and it is impossible to review them all. A large variety of individual topic based audits have led to improvements in practice for the management of individual symptoms, discharge planning, coordination, and education.[51-58] There has been the incorporation of outcome measures into clinical practice[51,59-61] (see also Chapter 24) and the use of these measures, for example, the Palliative care Outcome Scale (POS, see www.pos-pal.org), to help to audit care.

At a healthcare system scale, the Gold Standards Framework, widely used in the United Kingdom, aims to provide a "gold standard of care" for all people approaching the end of life. It gives frontline service providers a substantial set of skills and tools to (1) identify patients early, (2) assess their clinical and personal needs, and (3) plan for their needs by developing a plan of care.[62] Among many strategies to achieve improved care, it applies audit at a population level. As part of the Gold Standards Framework, providers proactively identify patients at the end of life; the patients are entered into a national registry, summarizing all patients who are receiving end-of-life care. This registry is then audited by region, physician practice, or care setting. Specifically, a web-based audit tool, the After Death Analysis, measures key quality markers, such as unscheduled hospital admissions, advanced care planning, place of death, and dying in the preferred place of death, for all patients identified as at the end of life.[63] Studies show that the Gold Standards Framework is a helpful process for improving interprofessional communication, palliative care knowledge among providers, out-of-hours protocols, and appropriate anticipatory prescribing.[64–66]

A case study using one QI model

The following case study describes a team's application of QI.

A hospital serves a substantial number of oncology patients through their clinical trials program. Although their remission rate is high, there are generally around 60 deaths per year in the hospital. Nurses are frustrated, because so many of these patients' families say that they would have preferred to die at home. Seeing an opportunity for improvement, a few colleagues express an interest in improving this outcome. Together, they analyze the potential causes of unwanted in-hospital deaths and determine that (1) no one is sure that staff are soliciting information about patients' preferred site of death, and (2) staff are uncomfortable with discussing this with patients who are pursuing aggressive cancer treatment.

First, the team develops a measurable aim: "Within two months, we will have documented site-of-death preference for 100 percent of relapsed acute leukemia patients, within 24 hours of admission." They start small by targeting only one segment of the oncology patient population. However, by setting an aim of 100% within 2 months, they alert their colleagues they want to change current clinical practice quickly. To achieve this, they test several different methods:

- Including a question regarding preferred site of death on the admission form
- Instituting a social worker visit within the first 24 hours of admission, during which site of death would be one topic of discussion
- Providing pamphlets regarding advance care planning in all patient rooms

To learn from their efforts, a nurse will review the chart of two patients in the target population each week to look for documentation of site of death preference, and the team will review the results. Over the next 2 months, the team test out their ideas with a small number of new patients. They quickly realize that the direct question asked on the admission form is well received, except when the patient is overwhelmingly ill at the time of admission. Having the question on the form does lead to an increase of

documented preferences in the medical record. They also learn that staff are still avoiding talks about preferred site of death. Based on these results, they continue the intervention, add role-playing about preferred site of death conversations for staff, and start expanding both to all new admissions. Later, they add a similar question to the discharge checklist, since most patients who leave will return. They also continue to review charts to track their effectiveness.

Within 2 months, 100% of acute leukemia patients have a site of death preference noted in their chart by the time of discharge, but just 80% within 24 hours of admission, since patients who came in very ill with a new relapse were unable to converse. In QI, changing the aim to accommodate learning is appropriate. Having achieved this process-oriented aim, the team sets an aim related to the actual outcome—increasing the number of patients for whom death occurs at their preferred site. Over the next several months, they set about testing changes and learning from their results.

In summary, the team identified a problem, stated an aim, tested ways to achieve their aim, measured their progress, and learned from their trials to modify current hospital practice and expand their efforts.

Examples at a regional level can be found in Ontario, Canada. The Provincial Palliative Care Integration Project began in 2006 to increase access to screening and improve processes and outcomes for cancer patients across Ontario.[67] To achieve this, the project specifically aimed to implement common tools for screening symptoms and functional performance status in regional cancer centers and in the community. Led by Cancer Care Ontario, the project used "rapid-cycle change" QI processes, measured data, and reported outcomes regularly. The results showed that across Ontario, they had increased screening uptake, improved symptom management, better integrated service provision, and increased access to palliative care services.[67,68]

Other examples of local collaborative QI efforts with a national impact come from the United States. For example, the RAND Palliative Care Policy Center partnered with over 200 healthcare provider organizations through QI collaboratives.[19,69] A collaborative consists of multiple healthcare organizations working together for up to 2 years to improve a specific clinical or operational area, under the guidance of a panel of national experts. Following the collaborative model, teams quickly learn from one another, promising ideas are easily disseminated among teams, and in turn, these teams spread proved interventions within their respective organizations. Past collaborations have made significant improvements in various palliative care areas such as pain, advanced care planning, and dyspnea around the country. In addition, other local QI efforts have led to wide dissemination of knowledge, tools, and resources. The Beth Israel Medical Center Division of Palliative Care and Pain Medicine in the United States developed a free online manual and toolkit based on its own QI learning.[70] The online manual includes tools such as an interdisciplinary plan of care and a documentation tool for daily assessments and interventions so that goals such as reducing unnecessary interventions and minimizing symptom distress can be achieved.

FUTURE OF QUALITY IMPROVEMENT

Despite documentation of some successes resulting from QI applied to palliative care, there is substantial room for continued improvement. Recent WHO Europe reports state that challenges in palliative care remain in integrating with health services; educating health professionals, policy makers and the public; implementing improvements; and prioritizing palliative care research.[71,72] Moreover, a qualitative study of palliative care in a developed (Scotland) and developing (Kenya) country demonstrates that dying patients in that developing country still lack access to analgesics, medical support, equipment and facilities, basic necessities, and relief from great physical suffering, whereas patients in the developed country on the whole do not.[73] The study also shows, however, that despite the availability of resources in the United Kingdom, people still have major areas of unmet need. Outlined in the following is a vision of the future of QI, building the case for its use as a widely adopted—and indeed sometimes required—method for change.

Building obligation and opportunities

All of those involved in the healthcare system—from the policy maker to each clinician—need to honor the obligation to provide the best possible quality of care. That obligation involves not accepting substandard care and making small improvements in everyday clinical practice guided by evidence that leads to large gains for patients over time. Financial incentives, such as performance linked to payment or accreditation, can help foster this obligation to improve quality of care.[74,75] Moreover, we need to develop more opportunities to utilize QI in everyday practice. For example, healthcare contracts should mandate audit and evaluation, a plan to implement research findings,[76–79] and forethought about the scalability, replicability, and spread of the intervention.[80] Quality improvement should be a part of the education of any healthcare provider.

Monitoring quality and responding

Quality must be continually monitored on a large scale, such as through tracking adherence to national quality standards as well as patient-centered outcomes. By doing so, the standards generate a feedback loop for quickly assessing which ideas are successful, which ones are not, and which require a mid-course correction.[23] Integrating technology into the monitoring process, such as pulling data directly from an electronic medical record where available so that the information is timely, meaningful, and actionable, is important. Furthermore, quality standards will help countries learn from each other through international comparisons,[81] alleviate the variation that exists among settings and geography,[82] fill in the missing gaps in knowledge as to which interventions are most effective in which settings, and help highlight the various factors for success.[83,84]

Publicizing benchmarks and supporting QI efforts

We need not only to monitor quality but also to publicize the results. Standards that are simple and transparent will help get the public involved as important advocates for change. Recognizing the exceptional facilities and revoking accreditation for those that fail to meet standards is key to validating the efforts. Lastly, we must provide support to QI through knowledge and finance, nurturing struggling facilities, and commitment to teaching the QI process, so that an environment exists that allows good ideas to succeed and spread.

Not long ago, discovering the latest drug or publishing the newest procedure in the professional literature was seen as sufficient to change clinical practice. No one believes that now. Deliberate, planned improvement activities are proving effective at changing practice. In order to build a care system that we can rely on and will serve us well at the end of life, we need to quickly acquire the skills that will allow us to learn from our current clinical practices, to improve upon it, and to disseminate the information broadly. Audit and QI can help us achieve that.

Key learning points

- Traditional methods to improve quality of care use formal research to guide improvement; however, these methods are less effective for introducing rapid change in clinical practice.

- Quality improvement and audit allow clinicians to assess whether they are doing the right thing, with the right patients, at the right time—and, if not, to make needed changes quickly. Effective QI is an ongoing cycle that encourages ongoing organizational learning.

- All aspects of palliative care, including advance care planning, symptom management, and continuity and coordination of care, present tremendous opportunities for QI.

- Many countries have begun using national guidelines and policies to improve palliative care, often in the form of accreditation, for example, Joint Commission in the United States.

- An example of QI beginning at the local health system level and growing to a national level is the "Gold Standards Framework" programs in the United Kingdom. The Gold Standards arose from general practitioner (family doctor) practices trying to improve care for those in the final year of life, more or less, and has since become mainstream in primary care (95% measure as competent at fundamentals) and is used in home care, nursing homes, and hospitals.

- Quality improvement has a growing role in improving palliative care. The future effectiveness of QI depends on several factors including building obligation and opportunities for QI; monitoring quality and responding; and publicizing benchmarks and supporting QI efforts.

REFERENCES

1   Institute of Medicine. *Crossing the Quality Chasm: A New Health System for the 21st Century.* Washington, DC: National Academies Press, 2001.

2   Kohn LT, Corrigan JM, Donaldson MS, eds. *To Err is Human: Building a Safer Health System.* Washington, DC: National Academies Press, 2000.

◆ 3   Chassin MR, Galvin RW. The urgent need to improve health care quality: Institute of Medicine National Roundtable on Health Care Quality. *JAMA* 1998; 11: 1000–1005.

4   Collins KS, Hughes DL, Doty MM et al. *Diverse Communities, Common Concerns: Addressing Health Care Quality for Minority Americans.* New York: The Commonwealth Fund, 2002.

5   Wennberg JE, Cooper M, eds. *The Dartmouth Atlas of Health Care in the United States.* Chicago, IL: American Hospital Publishing, 1998.

6   Nolan K, Nolan T. Learning from quality improvement in healthcare systems. In: Mitchell BM, Lynn J, eds. *Symptom Research: Methods and Opportunities.* [Online textbook] Washington, DC: National Institutes of Health, 2003. Available at: http://symptomresearch.nih.gov, (accessed August 2004).

7   Goldie SM. *Florence Nightingale: Letters from the Crimea 1854–1856.* Manchester, U.K.: Mandolin, 1997.

8   Higginson I. Clinical and organizational audit in palliative care. In: Doyle D, Hanks GWC, MacDonald N, eds. *Oxford Textbook of Palliative Medicine,* 2nd edn. New York: Oxford University Press, 1998; 163–170.

● 9   Lynn J, Nolan K, Kabcenell A et al. Reforming care for persons near the end of life: The promise of quality improvement. *Ann Intern Med* 2002; 2: 117–122.

10   Berwick DM. Developing and testing changes in delivery of care. *Ann Intern Med* 1998; 128: 651–656.

11   Langley G, Nolan K, Nolan T et al. *The Improvement Book.* San Francisco, CA: Jossey-Boss, 1996.

12   Shaw CD. *Medical Audit: A Hospital Handbook.* London, U.K: King's Fund Centre, 1989.

● 13   Institute for Healthcare Improvement. *Improvement Methods: How to Improve.* Available at: http://ihi.org/IHI/Topics/Improvement/ImprovementMethods/HowToImprove, (accessed September 2004).

14   Shewhart WA. *Economic Control of Quality of Manufactured Product.* Milwaukee, WI: ASQ Quality Press, 1931.

15   Wheeler DJ. *Understanding Variation.* Knoxville, TN: SPC Press, 1993.

16   Commission for Health Improvement. What is clinical audit? Available at: www.chi.gov.uk/eng/audit/about.shtml#00, (accessed September 2004).

17   Jamtvedt G, Young JM, Kristoffersen DT et al. Audit and feedback: Effects on professional practice and health care outcomes. *The Cochrane Library* 2006; 2.

18   Clinical Audit Support Centre. What is clinical audit? Available at: http://www.clinicalauditsupport.com/what_is_clinical_audit.html, (accessed May 2012).

● 19   Lynn J, Schuster JL, Kabcenell A. *Improving Care for the End of Life: A Sourcebook for Health Care Managers and Clinicians.* New York: Oxford Press, 2000.

✶ 20   National Institute for Clinical Excellence. *Improving Supportive and Palliative Care for Adults With Cancer: The Manual.* London, U.K.: National Institute for Clinical Excellence, 2004.

21   Tsaloglidou A. Does audit improve the quality of care? *Int J Caring Sci* 2009: 2(2): 65–72.

22   United Kingdom Parliament. *The NHS Plan: A Plan for Investment: A Plan for Reform.* CM; 4818-I. London, U.K.: The Stationery Office, 2000.

23   McGlynn EA, Cassel CK, Leatherman ST et al. Establishing national goals for quality improvement. *Med Care* 2003; 41(1 Suppl): I16–I29.

⇆ 24   National Committee for Quality Assurance. *The State of Health Care Quality 2003: Industry Trends and Analysis.* Washington, DC: NCQA Publications, 2003.

25   Department of Health. *NHS Performance Ratings: Acute Trusts, Specialist Trusts, Ambulance Trusts, Mental Health Trusts 2001/02.* 2002. Available at: www.performance.doh.gov.uk/performanceratings/2002/national.html (September 2004).

● 26   Bookbinder M, Romer AL. Raising the standard of care for imminently dying patients using quality improvement. *J Palliat Med* 2002; 5: 635–644.

27   International Society for Quality in Healthcare. *Global Review of Initiatives to Improve Quality in Health Care.* Geneva, Switzerland: World Health Organization, 2003.

28   Shaw CD. Evaluating accreditation. *Int J Qual Health Care* 2003; 15: 455–456.

29   Joint Commission on Accreditation of Healthcare Organizations. *Setting the Standard: The Joint Commission and Health Care Safety and Quality* [brochure]. Oakbrook Terrace, IL: Joint Commission on Accreditation of Healthcare Organizations, 2003.

✶ 30   Joint Commission on Accreditation of Healthcare Organizations. *Comprehensive Accreditation Manual for Hospitals.* Oakbrook Terrace, IL: Joint Commission on Accreditation of Healthcare Organizations, 2001.

✶ 31   Joint Commission of the Accreditation of Healthcare Organizations. *Improving the Quality of Pain Management Through Measurement and Action* [monograph]. Oakland Terrace, IL: Joint Commissions Resources Inc, 2003.

✶ 32   Joint Commission on Accreditation of Healthcare Organizations. *Ethics, Rights, and Responsibilities Standards for Hospitals.* Oakbrook Terrace, IL: Joint Commission on Accreditation of Healthcare Organizations, 2004.

33   Joint Commission. *Advanced Certification for Palliative Care Programs.* 2012. Available at: http://www.jointcommission.org/certification/palliative_care.aspx, (accessed May 2012).

34   National Consensus Project for Quality Palliative Care. *National Guidelines for Quality Palliative Care.* 2009. Available at: http://www.nationalconsensusproject.org/guideline.pdf, (accessed May 2012).

35   Department of Health. *End of Life Care Strategy.* July 2008. Available at: http://www.dh.gov.uk/prod_consum_dh/groups/dh_digitalassets/@dh/@en/documents/digitalasset/dh_086345.pdf, (accessed May 2012).

36   NICE. End of life care for adults quality standard. Available at: http://www.nice.org.uk/guidance/qualitystandards/endoflifecare/home.jsp, (accessed May 2012).

37   Common Wealth of Australia. *Supporting Australians to Live Well at the End of Life: National Palliative Care Strategy 2010.* Available at: http://www.health.gov.au/internet/main/publishing.nsf/Content/533C02453771A951CA256F190013683B/$File/NationalPalliativeCareStrategy.pdf, (accessed May 2012).

38   Palliative Care Australia. *A Guide to Palliative Care Service Development: A Population Based Approach.* February 2005. Available at: http://www.palliativecare.org.au/Portals/46/resources/PalliativeCareServiceDevelopment.pdf, (accessed May 2012).

39   Palliative Care Australia. *Palliative Care Service Provision in Australia: A Planning Guide.* September 2003. Available at: http://www.palliativecare.org.au/Portals/46/resources/PalliativeCareServiceProvision.pdf, (accessed May 2012).

40   Palliative Care Australia. *Standards for Providing Quality Palliative Care for all Australians.* May 2005. Available at: http://www.palliativecare.org.au/Portals/46/Standards%20for%20providing%20quality%20palliative%20care%20for%20all%20Australians.pdf, (accessed May 2012).

41   Abu Zeinah GF, Al-Kindi SG, Hassan AA. Middle east experience in palliative care. *Am J Hosp Palliat Care* 2012 [Epub ahead of print].

42   Al-Kindi SG, Abu Zeinah GF, Hassan AA. Pattern of hospitalization of patients with cancer in an acute palliative care setting: Qatar's experience. *Am J Hosp Palliat Care* 2012 [Epub ahead of print].

43   World Health Organization. *Africa Project on Palliative Care: Project Description*. 2003. Available at: www.who.int/cancer/palliative/projectproposal/en/, (accessed September 2004).

44   Sepulveda C, Habiyambere V, Amandua J et al. Quality care at the end of life in Africa. *BMJ* 2003; 327: 209–213.

45   Cecilia S. Minimum standard of care defined for HIV patients with cancer. *Bull World Health Organ* 2002; 80: 176.

46   African Palliative Care Association. About APCA. Available at: www.apca.org.ug, (accessed May 2012).

47   African Palliative Care Association. Strategic Plan. Available at: http://africanpalliativecare.org/images/stories/pdf/apca_sp.pdf, (accessed May 2012).

48   African Palliative Care Association. Tools and indicators. Available at: http://www.apca.org.ug/index.php?option = com_content&view = article&id = 135&Itemid = 41, (accessed May 2012).

49   Powell RA, Mugula R, Ddungu H et al. Advancing drug availability—Experiences from Africa. *J Pain Symptom Manage* 2010; 40(1): 9–12.

50   Harding R, Higgison I. Palliative care in Sub-Saharan Africa. *Lancet* 2005; 365: 1971–1977.

51   Stevens AM, Gwilliam B, A'hern R et al. Experience in the use of the palliative care outcome scale. *Support Care Cancer* 2005; 13: 1027–1034.

52   Moore S, Sherwin A. Improving patient access to healthcare professionals: A prospective audit evaluating the role of e-mail communication for patients with lung cancer. *Eur J Oncol Nurs* 2004; 8: 350–354.

53   Lloyd-Williams M, Payne S. Can multidisciplinary guidelines improve the palliation of symptoms in the terminal phase of dementia? *Int J Palliat Nurs* 2002; 8: 370–375.

54   Galvin J. An audit of pressure ulcer incidence in a palliative care setting. *Int J Palliat Nurs* 2002; 8: 214–221.

55   Rawlinson F, Finlay I. Assessing education in palliative medicine: Development of a tool based on the Association for Palliative Medicine core curriculum. *Palliat Med* 2002; 16: 51–55.

56   Lee L, White V, Ball J et al. An audit of oral care practice and staff knowledge in hospital palliative care. *Int J Palliat Nurs* 2001; 7: 395–400.

57   Neo SH, Loh EC, Koo WH. An audit of morphine prescribing in a hospice. *Singapore Med J* 2001; 42: 417–419.

♦ 58   Hearn J, Higginson IJ. Outcome measures in palliative care for advanced cancer patients: A review. *J Public Health Med.* 1997; 19: 193–199.

59   Higginson I. Clinical audit and organizational audit in palliative care. *Cancer Surv* 1994; 21: 233–245.

60   Dunckley M, Aspinal F, Addington-Hall JM et al. A research study to identify facilitators and barriers to outcome measure implementation. *Int J Palliat Nurs* 2005; 11: 218–225.

61   Hughes RA, Sinha A, Aspinal F et al. What is the potential for the use of clinical outcome measures to be computerised? Findings from a qualitative research study. *Int J Health Care Qual Assur Inc Leaders Health Serv* 2004; 17: 47–52.

62   The Gold Standards Framework. About GSF. Available at: http://www.goldstandardsframework.org.uk/, (accessed May 2012).

63   Thomas K, Clifford C. Measuring quality improvements in end-of-life care: The ADA audit tool. *Eur J Palliat Care* 2010; 17(5): 232–236.

64   Walshe C, Caress A, Chew-Graham C et al. Implementation and impact of the Gold Standards Framework in community palliative care: A qualitative study of three primary care trusts. *Palliat Med* 2008; 22: 736.

65   Dale J, Petrova M, Munday D et al. A national facilitation project to improve primary palliative care: Impact of the Gold Standards Framework on process and self-ratings of quality. *Qual Saf Health Care* 2009; 18: 174–180.

66   Munday D, Mahmood K, Dale J et al. Facilitating good process in primary palliative care: Does the Gold Standards Framework enable quality performance? *Fam Pract* 2007; 24 (5): 486–494.

67   Dudgeon D, King S, Howell D et al. Cancer Care Ontario's experience with implementation of routine physical and psychological symptom distress screening. *Psycho-Oncol* 2012; 21: 357–364.

68   Gilbert JE, Howell D, King S et al. Quality improvement in cancer symptom assessment and control: The Provincial Palliative Care Integration Project (PPCIP). *J Pain Symptom Manage* 2012; 43: 663–678.

● 69   Lynn J, Schall M, Milne C et al. Quality improvements in end of life care: Insights from two collaboratives. *Jt Comm J Qual Improv* 2000; 26: 254–267.

♦ 70   Beth Israel Continuum Health Partners Inc. Palliative Care for Advanced Disease (PCAD) Pathway: Unit Reference Manual [online manual]. Available at: www.stoppain.org/services_staff/pcad1.html, (accessed September 2004).

♦ 71   Davies E, Higginson IJ, eds. *The Solid Facts: Palliative Care.* Copenhagen, Denmark: World Health Organization Europe, 2004.

♦ 72   Davies E, Higginson IJ, eds. *Better Palliative Care for Older People.* Copenhagen, Denmark: World Health Organization Europe, 2004.

73   Murray SA, Grant E, Grant A, Kendall M. Dying from cancer in developed and developing countries: Lessons from two qualitative interview studies of patients and their carers. *BMJ* 2003; 326: 368.

74   The Leapfrog Group. *Rewarding Results Publications.* Available at: www.leapfroggroup.org/RewardingResults/pubs.htm, (accessed September 2004).

75   Bailit Health Purchasing and Sixth Man Consulting. *The Growing Case for Using Physician Incentives to Improve Health Care Quality.* Washington, DC: National Health Care Purchasing Institute, 2001.

76   Haines A, Jones R. Implementing findings of research. *BMJ* 1994; 308: 1488–1492.

77   Clancy C. Health services research: From galvanizing attention to creating action. *Health Serv Res* 2003; 38: 777–781.

⇆ 78   Ferlie EB, Shortell SM. Improving the quality of health care in the United Kingdom and the United States: A framework for change. *Milbank Q* 2001; 79: 281–315.

79   Stryer D, Clancy C. Boosting performance measure for measure. *BMJ* 2003; 326: 1278–1279.

80   Berwick DM. Lessons from developing nations on improving health care. *BMJ* 2004; 328: 1124–1129.

81   Marshall MN, Shekelle PG, McGlynn EA et al. Can health care quality indicators be transferred between countries? *Qual Saf Health Care* 2003; 12: 8–12.

♦ 82   Schuster MA, McGlynn EA, Brook RH. How good is the quality of health care in the United States? *Milbank Q* 1998; 76: 517–563.

♦ 83   Wilson T, Berwick DM, Cleary PD. What do collaborative improvement projects do? Experience from seven countries. *Jt Comm J Qual Saf* 2003; 29: 85–93.

84   Bradley EH, Webster TR, Baker D et al. *Translating Research into Practice: Speeding the Adoption of Innovative Health Care Programs* [issue brief]. New York: Commonwealth Fund, 2004.

PART 6

Organization and governance

28

Adoption of palliative care: The engineering of organizational change

WINFORD E. (DUTCH) HOLLAND

Imagine that you have just been named to the faculty of a distinguished medical institution. Further imagine that you have been asked by the director of the institution to "help us implement palliative care in our institution." What would you do? How would you do it? With whom would you work? Whom might you avoid? What missteps would you want to avoid?

Hopefully, many of the readers of this book will be asked exactly that question: "Can you help us implement palliative care?" The goal of this short chapter is to offer a framework for thinking about such an implementation as well as some practical tools that might be used to make such an implementation possible in a relatively short period of time.

The preceding two paragraphs are how our first version of this chapter started, some seven years ago. Since that time palliative care has continued to spread inside the medical community and inside M D Anderson Cancer Center, where our case study for this article originated. So this latest chapter will closely resemble the previous chapter while the case study at the end of the chapter has been updated to describe the continued success of PalCare at MDACC.

ELEMENTS OF THE FRAMEWORK

While most of us spend our time inside a large organization, we usually do not spend much time thinking about the organization. What is an organization? What is it made of? What do we mean when we talk about "changing the organization?" When we say that we want to implement palliative care in an organization, what does that mean?

The following three subject areas can form a framework for envisioning and then changing an organization and how it operates:

1. *The organization as a mechanical system.* A large organization can be thought of as a mechanical system made up of concrete "moving parts"—parts that can be altered to cause the organization to function in a different way, like delivering a new service such as palliative care to the institution's clients. As a metaphor, organizations can be thought of as "theater companies" performing in continuous "plays."
2. *The diffusion of innovation within a social organization.* Innovations—ideas that are new to an organization—diffuse through an institution in a patterned way over time, with some organization members far more inclined to adopt an innovation like palliative care than others.
3. *The role of leadership in creating change in an organization.* Leaders cause things to happen in an organization. Leaders take direct actions on the moving parts of an organization; they influence organization members to enable the organization to make changes like implementing palliative care on an institutional basis.

The following sections of this chapter will explore in more detail these three key framework ideas, providing both understanding and action steps that can be used to implement, or "engineer," an innovation in an institution in an effective and efficient way. The last section of the chapter will "pull it all together" to illustrate how the actions can be used for real-world implementation of palliative care.

ORGANIZATION AS MECHANICAL SYSTEM

Implementing a change, like the introduction of palliative care, requires us to know something about what an organization is from a structural or system point of view—the mechanics of organizations. In today's world of work, we must be able to do two things at the same time—to *use* the organization to get today's business done and *change* the organization so that we can be ready to do tomorrow's business.

Organizations as ongoing theatrical performances

We see an organization as an ongoing play, where organization members are the cast and crew doing a satisfying performance for clients/patients. Using the scenario of changing plays from "Romeo and Juliet" to "My Fair Lady" as an example of what happens in organizational change is a helpful framework for managers and employees to easily grasp the changes involved in moving a theater company from one performance to another—from learning new scripts to changing costumes and sets, all the way to the full dress rehearsal before opening.

Once this theater metaphor is learned, our students of change management can use it to understand why many changes they have seen go awry! More importantly, it becomes easy to understand the *single most important concept in organizational change—that organizations are structured, mechanical systems with concrete moving parts that must work and change together.* Translating the theater metaphor to organizations, students can see the four primary structural elements:

1. Vision, like the play's storyline and script
2. Work processes, like the roles in the play
3. Plant/equipment/tools, like costumes and sets
4. Performance agreements, like contracts for actors

While it is easy to comprehend the "work process—role" and the "plant/equipment/tools—props" connections, it does take some stretch to see that the "agreements for performance," like actor contracts, are an attribute of the organization and not the "employees—actors" themselves. In our experience, the most difficult part of organizational change for many companies is to understand the idea that change is designed to alter the roles that people play in the organization, not to alter people themselves. *Failure to grasp the idea that change hinges on altering roles* and subsequent performance agreements that we make with employees is the most common downfall of organizational change.

For an organization to change, all four mechanical attributes of the organization must change—in concert—or there will be no change (Figure 28.1). Vision alteration, work process alterations, plant/equipment/tools alterations as well as performance agreement changes are all done in a social setting. All the alterations have to be done by people who are involved and committed to (1) making the alterations and (2) working in the new organization after the alterations are made. Managing the people dynamics can be challenging, but it is doable as long as leaders of the change understand the mechanical things that must be done to achieve organizational change.

Five requirements for engineering change

As discussed, the way any organization works at a given point in time is the direct and inescapable result of the configuration of the firm's vision, work processes, physical plant, and performance system (agreements with employees and their competence to perform to those agreements). Just as in a mechanical system, the way the organization operates cannot change without a change in its key components.

Calling these needed alterations "requirements" allows us to see change as a true engineering challenge. These four alterations, along with disciplined project management, make up what we call the five requirements for engineering change. The critical part of organizational change is the unglamorous, detail-oriented, hard work of engineering.

Requirement one: Engineering and communicating the change vision

The first requirement of organizational change is to engineer a vision or picture of the organization's desired future that will be valid, complete, feasible, resourceable, and engaging. In this case, the detailed vision would picture the continued growth and success of the institution, showing palliative care as a core practice that serves patients and families well and at a decreased cost of serving those same patients in intensive care. Once detailed, the vision should be tested with members of the organization to ensure that it is an understandable picture of the desired future. To ensure that the organization is positioned to really hear and digest the vision, we construct a case for change that describes in some detail the potential consequences of keeping the organization exactly the way it is now.

An institution bent on implementing palliative care would be able to describe a time in the near future when such care was an integral part of the organization's services, providing a real alternative to end-of-life care in an intensive care facility. In addition, reasons for implementing palliative care, including benefits to patients and families, as well as institutional economics, should be clearly detailed.

Once the change vision and the case for palliative care are complete, the next step is to communicate with all organization members multiple times using multiple media. First and foremost would be direct communication by the CEO that explains why palliative care will be critical for the institution's continued success. The CEO's message can be picked up in today's

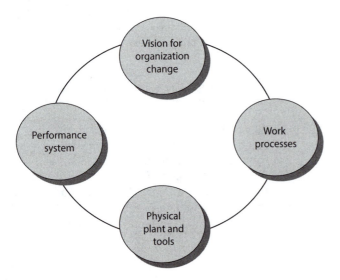

Figure 28.1 *Mechanical elements of an organization.*

world of communication: the institution's website as well as its internal communication programs. Palliative care brochures, signage, and even slogans, pins, and badges could complement the face-to-face communication of the vision.

Technically, this communication requirement is not complete until all management levels have worked through the vision and case for change and translated them into action terms for their level and function, as well as for their individual associates. The final step in this requirement is to test each employee's understanding of the translation of the palliative care vision for his/her job. Without this test, leaders of the change can hardly know if they are ready to move on to the next requirements of altering the other mechanical components of the organization.

Failure to communicate the palliative care vision and case for change would be like the director of a theater company who selects the next new play but who does not talk about the play, what it is, how it was selected, or about the future success of that play. Would you think that this director's approach would get their theater company off to a great start?

Requirements two through four: Engineering the organization's mechanical components

Requirements two through four call for the physical alteration of the institution's work processes, its physical plant/equipment/tools (PET), and the employee performance system. The first step in this alteration process is to create an inventory of the organization's current components—work processes, PET, and performance agreements with employees—to identify those elements that will not be in sync with the palliative care vision of the future organization. Once identified, each of the elements must be physically altered and tested. It is these alterations of the existing components, along with the addition of new work processes (e.g., billing procedures for palliative care), physical plant (e.g., dedicated palliative care beds), and performance agreements (e.g., job descriptions for personnel servicing palliative care beds) that will become the "stuff" of the changed organization that will include palliative care.

Development and negotiation of new performance agreements for all affected managers and employees is critical at this point to ensure they are signed up for palliative care in the institution. Organizations and theater companies alike deal with the reality that some employees, or actors, will *not* elect to sign up for the change. Completing these alterations is akin to the work that must get done in the theater company to ensure that the new play is translated into individual roles and scripts for the newly assigned cast, that the new costumes and sets have been constructed, and that the actors have been put under formal contract and rehearsed for the new play.

The final step in each of these three requirements is to systematically dismantle or remove those elements that will not be a part of the new organization's structure. Old work processes, procedures, tools, and equipment will need to be removed from the workplace to ensure they will not be used again. This dismantling includes the often-forgotten step of directly and formally canceling any agreements with managers and employees for performance in the old organization that did not contain palliative care. For example, we might want to verbally and in writing cancel the institutional procedure that assigned end-of-life patients to the intensive care unit or to that designated wing.

We want to cancel the agreements that our employee had for doing work the old way (without palliative care) now that they have already been signed up for doing work the new way (with palliative care as a main-stream service). This final dismantling is akin to the director removing all vestiges of the last play (old scripts, costumes, and props) to ensure that they will not be inadvertently used in the new production. Included in this dismantling step is the cancellation of any cast contracts that would have tied them to the old play.

Requirement five: Using project management to guide the engineering of change

Even though employees are clear on the vision that is to be implemented, they need day-by-day or week-by-week instructions or action plans to guide them through the many steps of organizational change (e.g., "Remember gang, this is the week for costume fittings; leads come in on Wednesday, dancers on Thursday"). Employees need an action plan that tells them "what to do on Monday morning…" to go forward with the coordinated implementation of the new vision.

These action plans must be a part of a critical path project management plan and master schedule that lays out all the engineering work to be done for the organizational change to embrace palliative care. Critical to the action planning requirement is the translation of action plans on a weekly or monthly basis for all involved managers and employees so that they are clear on their roles in (1) transitioning to the new organization and (2) playing new or altered roles in that new organization. Failure to keep action plans updated and communicated would be like the director who does not lay out and communicate detailed plans and schedules for reading the new roles, signing contracts, fitting new costumes, or rigging new props.

Project management of change is first and foremost a case of deciding exactly and precisely *what* alterations will be required in each of the components and then *how* the required alterations are to be made. The physical change piece is all about making the required alterations and ensuring that they were done … and done right.

The engineering challenge in this project management requirement is to ensure that all of the required modifications to vision, work processes, physical plant, and performance agreements have been done in a thorough, comprehensive manner. While it may be a technical challenge to keep track of all the needed alterations, particularly if the organization is large, it is technically not difficult to find out exactly where the organization is in organizational change.

Knowing where we are in engineering change to include palliative care is a matter of auditing the status of required alterations and dealing with the reality of what we find:

- Either work processes have been altered to include palliative care or they have not. New procedures that allow people to bill for palliative care have been written and distributed or they have not. The old processes and their supporting procedures that do not include palliative care have been dismantled/destroyed or they have not.
- Either new tools (beds devoted to palliative care) are assigned and working or they are not. Either the guidelines for operating the new palliative care suite have been written and distributed or they have not.
- And either the performance contract for each and every doctor, nurse, and administrator impacted by the introduction of palliative care has been altered and negotiated with each of them or it has not. Either each and every manager and employee has been trained on the new palliative care admission processes and new suite or they have not, and so on.

So ends this section of the framework that deals with the organization as a mechanical system, a system that can be literally engineered from one configuration to another. But organizations vary in their susceptibility to engineering, as explained in the next section.

DIFFUSION OF INNOVATION

While the mechanical approach to leading an organization change like the introduction of palliative care is simple and straightforward to describe, there are organizational situations in which it is an oversimplification. In professional organizations where there is a high degree of individual autonomy, another framework element has much to offer.

A major social study area for the last few decades has been the "diffusion of innovation"—the way and rate something new to an individual or organization gets adopted by the members of the organization. The basic idea is that an innovation spreads rather slowly across a social system, like a healthcare institution, by traveling from member to member. Key elements of the diffusion theory include:

1. *The innovation*—An idea or practice (like palliative care) that is perceived as new by individuals or the institution
2. *Communication channels*—The means by which messages about the innovation get from one individual to another (formal and informal communication between departments and members of the medical community)
3. *Time*—The relative time an innovation takes to be adopted by an individual or group
4. *Social system*—A set of interrelated units (departments) that are engaged in accomplishing a common goal (providing healthcare to patients—the institutional goal)

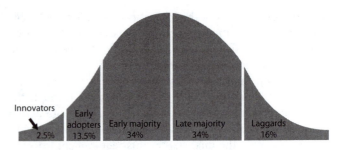

Figure 28.2 *Categories of adopters of innovations.*

In studying the diffusion process, researchers have been able to consistently identify individuals who have very different rates of adoption. The classic categories of adopters are as follows (Figure 28.2):

1. Innovators
2. Early adopters
3. Early majority
4. Late majority
5. Laggards

Researchers identified several characteristics dominant in innovators:

- Venturesome; desire for the rash, the daring, and the risky
- Ability to understand and apply complex technical knowledge
- Ability to cope with a high degree of uncertainty about an innovation

Characteristics identified in early adopters:

- Integrated part of the local social system
- Greatest degree of opinion leadership in most systems
- Serve as role model for other members or society
- Successful and respected by peers

Characteristics identified in the early majority:

- Interact frequently with peers
- Seldom hold positions of opinion leadership
- Deliberate before adopting a new idea
- Constitute one-third of the members of a system

Characteristics identified in the late majority:

- Are naturally cautious and skeptical
- Pressure from peers
- Economic necessity
- Constitute one-third of the members of a system

Characteristics identified in the laggards:

- Are isolates and possess no opinion leadership
- Point of reference in the past
- Suspicious of innovations
- Innovation–decision process is lengthy

The practical significance of these categories has not been lost on the advertising and sales communities who routinely take advantage of innovator categories. Change leaders can also take advantage of the research by treating different populations within their institutions differently.

For example, when an innovation like palliative care is first introduced into a department or institution, healthcare professionals produce an "adoption reaction." Thinking simply, about a third of the community is likely to have an open, even positive reaction, while another third might have a very closed or even negative reaction. A middle third might be observable as those professionals who lean no way or the other, as if waiting for the next act. In fact, this middle third is likely to be doing just that: waiting to see how the introduction goes.

From the point of view of the change leader(s), working with the three communities takes very different levels of energy and produces varying degrees of results:

- *First third (innovators and early adopters)*—Working with them is simple, straightforward, and positive. Reasonable suggestions about palliative care and its adoption are heard, evaluated, and frequently acted on.
- *Second third (majority adopters)*—Working with them is frequently frustrating, since they are less into "listening, trying, and evaluating ideas" than they are into "watching the success (or lack of success)" of the first third.
- *Third third (late majority and laggards)*—Working with this group is usually argumentative, frequently unfriendly, and sometimes downright nasty and unpleasant.

Change leaders assigned and/or committed to the implementation of palliative care have the choice of the populations they address. Diffusion of innovation research would suggest the tactic of working with the first third (innovators and early adopters) to gain as much implementation success as possible and then allowing nature to take its course as those in the first third do the job of influencing others through their own work and social channels.

LEADERSHIP IN ORGANIZATIONAL CHANGE

Organizational change does not happen without leadership … and lots of it! We have not seen success in change when the organization's leadership, at all levels, was unwilling to take responsibility for setting a direction or was lacking the courage and commitment needed to carry out that direction. Decisive leadership at the highest level of the organization is essential for successful change.

The leader who is unable or unwilling to pick a new future for the organization, describe that future in some detail, and then steer toward that future is destined to keep the organization right where it is. The bottom line is simple: organizational change takes leadership, from both the boss and his/her collaborators (Figure 28.3). The final word, however, is that the boss must be the one who brings the energy and excitement to organizational change along with the personal leadership to get collaborators on board.

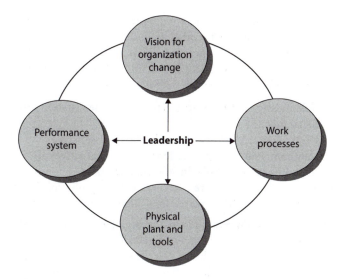

Figure 28.3 *Change leadership acts on the mechanical attributes of organizations.*

There are three critical sources of leadership that must be engaged for successful organizational change: the chief executive, key managers at the department level, and healthcare professionals. Each leadership source has a primary mission to accomplish in an organizational change to implement palliative care:

The *chief executive* is the "chief change officer" for the organization. Period. No one else in the organization has the authority and stroke to make change happen. No one else has the legal responsibility for the enterprise. No one else can be held accountable for the performance of the organization before, during, and after organizational change.

The chief executive's primary change mission is to *develop (or select) the desired future for the organization* and express it as the vision that includes palliative care, just like the director's job is to select a script that will result in a successful play. In addition, the executive must *resource with time, dollars and personal commitment the palliative care vision* as it is being implemented.

The chief executive must also *develop his/her own altered executive role* as it will need to be played for palliative care to become a reality. Actions speak louder than words, but we are talking about something more than that. What the chief executive does on a day-to-day, week-to-week, and month-to-month basis must routinely include the vision of palliative care if that vision is to become a reality (e.g., the CEO asks the controller to add "revenue from palliative care" to the document top management uses to hold their monthly revenue review; the zero will stand out like a sore thumb but make the CEO's expectation clear).

The *middle managers* serve as the organization's source of energy and initiative for altering work processes, altering the physical plant, and altering the performance management system to include palliative care. This category will likely include the organization's department directors as well as the palliative care leader(s) who have taken on primary responsibility for day-to-day operations as well as guiding the implementation effort.

The organization's middle managers are directly and personally responsible for completing the changes needed to get palliative care into operation. Their job is to be the "chief change communicator and director" for their part of the institution. Their primary change mission is threefold:

- Relentlessly communicate the palliative care vision to their department.
- Guide their department's healthcare professionals as they complete the organization's move to palliative care including professional education and training.
- Develop their own altered management and professional role as they will need to be played for palliative care to be a reality.

The *healthcare professionals* in the organization will do the majority of the change engineering needed to alter the organization's mechanical attributes. It is the workers who will physically do the detailed alternations needed in work processes and physical plant and develop the new organizational roles that enable palliative care. The primary change mission of the involved professionals must, however, be focused on the alteration and development of their own roles and skills needed for their success as a part of the palliative care vision.

Pulling it all together: A palliative care success story

Take for example, the introduction of palliative care at M D Anderson Cancer Center in Houston. The chief executive made the decision to move toward palliative care and hired a leading physician to come to Anderson and "run the show." Upon arrival, the newly appointed palliative care department head encountered stiff resistance and many logistical obstacles that were almost impossible to overcome. At the end of the first 18 months, progress in gaining acceptance of palliative care was very slow, and the third-third population of resisters (laggards) had made themselves heard all the way to the top. The situation was uncomfortable enough for the department head to say "that he felt like he had parachuted in behind enemy lines."

In an effort to move the ball, M D Anderson retained the services of a change consultant to work directly with the department head and his palliative care team of department member physicians and administrators. The steps taken included the following:

- Instruction of and consultation with the palliative care team in the change concepts that are described in this paper. The department head stated that the

consultations and training has "opened a window into the world of organizations" that allowed him to better see and understand the actions that he and his team needed to take.
- Decision of the palliative care team to "ignore the third-third detractors" and to find and work with "first-third" professionals only (i.e., working only with those who were relatively positive and eager to look at palliative care as a treatment alternative).
- Formation of a palliative care steering team made up of volunteer senior physicians/faculty members (all of whom were first third).
- Arranging an early meeting/workshop of the steering committee to hear directly from the MDACC chief executive. The chief executive explained to the steering team his reason for moving the institution toward palliative, his reasons for selecting the department head, and his vision of palliative care as a legitimate and important treatment modality for the institution.
- These key, friendly members helped establish a vision, mission, and strategic plan of action and not only provided extremely useful feedback but by the same process they were sold.
- The palliative care team and steering team worked directly with administrative officers of the institution to ensure that processes were in place to handle business and scheduling aspects of palliative care (i.e., to ensure money would start flowing).
- With a palliative vision and strategic in place, the department was able to launch communication and public relations programs, clinical education sessions, as well as consultations inside and outside MDACC.
- These programs initially focused on the first-third. As a result of positive acceptance by the first-third, members of the second-third began to sign up, and before long, the first two-thirds were chiding members of the third-third as "being behind the times."
- The result of this was the large growth in referrals to the palliative care program that have succeeded in fully establishing it as a viable clinical and financial program. Note the rapid rate of palliative care consultations in Table 28.1.
- The palliative care initiative has continued to increase in use and popularity, with consultations continuing to increase, while the number and cost of deaths in internal care continue to decline.

Table 28.1 *Impact of Palliative Care Services on overall hospital mortality in University of Texas M D Anderson Cancer Center, by Bruera et al.*

	1999	2000	2001	2002	2003	2004
Consultations prior to inpatient death under services other than palliative care service (PCS)	8	17	54	106	112	95
Inpatient death under primary care of the PCS	NA	NA	NA	54	123	169
Total number of patients accessing palliative care before death	8	17	54	160	235	264
Percent of patients accessing palliative care before death	1% (8/583)	3% (17/657)	8% (54/671)	24% (160/657)	35% (235/689)	35% (264/764)
Total number of palliative care inpatient visits (death and discharges)	800	1006	3396	5476	6489	6689

Blending the messages from the three framework elements is essential to effective change. The essential message of this chapter, therefore, is for leaders to

1. Take strong, aggressive, visible action ...
2. To work with "first-third" managers and professionals ...
3. To alter the mechanical attributes of the organization that will enact palliative care

In summary, key to the success of the effective and efficient introduction of palliative care will be the continuing partnership between the committed chief executive and leaders in the management cadre. Dedicated action in the engineering framework described in this chapter, along with huge doses of "blood, sweat, and tears," should lead to another palliative care success story. And there is one.

Palliative care success story continues ...

Palliative Care at MDACC had continued to grow at a rapid rate over the first 5 years, but in 2010, growth began to plateau. After checking and double checking what they had been doing to continue to attract new patients, the leader of palliative care and his direct reports held what could be called a "focus group" to talk about future growth. Invited attendees were several first third physicians (innovators and early adopters whose input led to a new hypothesis: that some physicians were not comfortable making a referral to palliative care lest they be seen as "giving up on the patient").

Information from the focus group energized the palliative care leadership to think through their approach again. They reached the conclusion that their brand needed to be altered from "palliative care and pain management" to "palliative care and rehabilitation medicine." They also changed the name of the facility they were using to The Supportive Care Center that "focuses on improving quality of life for MD Anderson Cancer Center patients and their families."

The palliative care team used the same change management approach they had used to stand up their initial practice, but now they knew what would work, and they were able to get all their needed change alterations underway in short order. They initiated a new communication plan focused on the supportive care center, they revised "processes, labels, buttons and badges" to include supportive care, they rethought their space

requirements, and added supportive care words to job descriptions of their healthcare professionals.

News of the re-branding spread like wildfire through the physician community and the physicians reacted accordingly. At year end 2011, palliative care's practice was up by a remarkable 41%. Dedicated leadership, passionate professionals, a proven road map for change, a lot of creative thinking, and energetic workers can move mountains as PalCare demonstrates.

Key learning points

1. The introduction of palliative care can be seen as a mechanical problem that can be engineered; organizational moving parts must be identified and altered.

2. Individuals have different rates of change acceptance. Plan to work with the most eager supporters of palliative care first.

3. Changing an organization's way of operating requires aggressive, visible, hands-on leadership. The boss must want and support palliative care.

4. Get the physical assets needed for palliative care in place early on so that the organization can see tangible organizational commitment.

5. Involvement of professionals must be done at every step of the way.

FURTHER READING

Davies S, *The Diffusion of Process Innovations*, Cambridge University Press, Cambridge, U.K., 1979.

Holland D, Rohe D, *Surviving and Thriving in Waves of Change for All Healthcare Leaders*, Xlibris Corporation, Bloomington, IL, 2012.

Holland D, Rohe D, *Successful Organizational Change: Completing Healthcare Projects on Target on Time and On Budget*, Xlibris Corporation, Bloomington, IL, 2012.

Holland WE, *Change Is the Rule: Practical Actions for Change: On Target, On Time, and On Budget*, Dearborn Trade Press, Chicago, IL, 2000.

Rogers EM, New product adoption and diffusion, *J Consumer Res*, 1976; 2: 290–301.

Rogers EM, *Diffusion of Innovations*, The Free Press, New York, 1972.

29

Principles of measuring the financial outcomes of specialist palliative care programs

J. BRIAN CASSEL, THOMAS J. SMITH

Of all the imperatives and outcomes for specialist palliative care (SPC) programs in hospitals, one would hope that financial issues would rank as among the least important. Surely the other motivations for SPC, and effects thereof—humanitarian, moral, ethical, clinical, to name a few—should be paramount. The hospice and palliative care innovators and paradigm shifters in the 1960s and 1970s responded to the unmet needs of patients, focusing on the relief of suffering and creating the ability to provide for a "good death" when death is inevitable and imminent. The primary motivation of these innovators was to reduce pain and suffering and, secondarily, to cease futile interventions that create more burden for the patient than benefits.[1] Be that as it may, measuring the financial impact of SPC may be crucial for ensuring sustained financial resources continue to be made available for training SPC professionals and sustaining SPC programs.[2,3]

FIRST PRINCIPLE: FINANCIAL OUTCOMES ARE A POSITIVE SECONDARY EFFECT OF PATIENT-CENTERED OUTCOMES

Outcomes for SPC may represent a variety of perspectives including patient, family, other care providers, the hospital, payers, and society. Improvement in the bio-psycho-social-spiritual experience for the patient is the central rationale for SPC involvement, and is the primary locus of outcomes to be measured. The word "primary" here has multiple meanings—it is most important; it is first to occur; and it is a necessary step in producing further positive outcomes. Secondary and tertiary outcomes ripple outward from this primary locus of impact (see Figure 29.1). This is not to say that all clinical effects (e.g., reduced pain) will automatically produce hospital-level financial and operational effects, but it is to say that financial outcomes are dependent upon clinical impact.

The first principle of measuring the financial impact of SPC, then, is to measure it as a consequence of patient-centered clinical and psycho-social-spiritual outcomes. Financial outcomes

are secondary effects of these, and therefore in practice, SPC program leaders should measure the patient-centered and social outcomes first, before turning to institutional outcomes such as lower costs or fewer ICU days.

SECOND PRINCIPLE: UNDERSTAND THE UTILIZATION AND CONTEXT

With responsibility for the small fraction of hospitalized patients who are SPC-appropriate diffused across all providers, disciplines, and cost centers, most hospital administrators will have little understanding of the nature of their care and the costs and reimbursement thereof. As a result, the SPC-appropriate population is almost entirely "under the radar" for administrative and clinical leaders in most institutions. Even the health services research that examines the high cost and high intensity of typical hospital care near the end of life[4-6] will not necessarily resonate with hospital administrators who are concerned about their own patients and providers. One of the critical differences that palliative care programs make, clinically, is to halt that diffusion of responsibility, and to provide accountability for the nature and cost of the care of such patients.

An analysis that can help to make the responsibility more salient is presented in Table 29.1.

The first two columns represent the SPC-relevant population as operationally defined as dying or being at high risk of death during that inpatient episode. These 10% of hospitalizations drive 26% of total bed days, 64% of ICU days, 33% of direct costs, and 100% of the losses incurred from limited Medicare reimbursement. In the United States, the vast majority of SPC cases are reimbursed by third-party payers,[8] which limit their payments per hospitalization prospectively.[9] Therefore, this kind of analysis can make the financial risk of "usual care" quite salient for hospital administrators. Similar approaches can be used in other countries and health systems where at least some information about costs and payments per

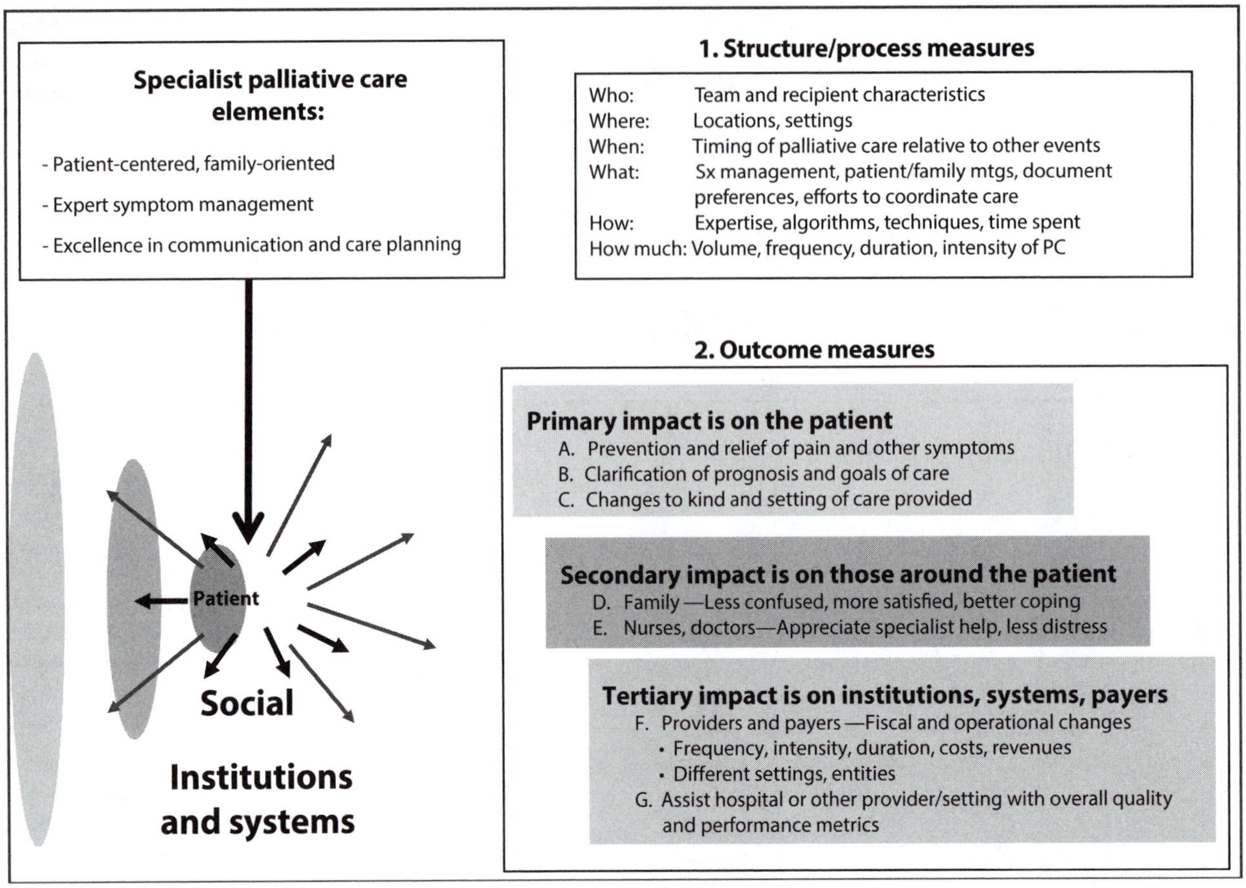

Figure 29.1 *The specialist palliative care measurement model. The primary and secondary outcomes, starting with the patient, ripple outward to others. The tertiary impact on institutions is a function of clinical impact. (Adapted from Cassel, J.B., Palliat. Med., 27(2), 103, 2013.)*

Table 29.1 *Hospitalizations of adults, FY2011, Virginia Commonwealth University Health System, categorized into three distinct groups, with the first two groups representing the SPC-relevant population*

All adult patients, all payers	Deaths	High-risk survivors	All other admits	Total
Cases	812	1,964	24,584	27,360
% of cases	3	7	90	100
Avg DRG weight (case-mix index)	4.03	4.12	1.53	1.79
% ICU days	20	44	36	100
% total days	6	20	75	100
Avg LOS	11.9	16.8	5.1	6.2
Direct cost/day	$3,064	$2,220	$1,683	$1,867
Direct cost/case	$36,335	$37,348	$8,628	$11,512
Direct cost/case (ratio)	4.2×	4.3×	1	
% cases with Medicare	49	52	30	33
All adult patients, who had Medicare as their primary payer	**Medicare deaths**	**Medicare high-risk survivors**	**All other Medicare admits**	**Total Medicare**
Medicare cases	396	1,030	7,469	8,895
% Medicare cases	4	12	84	100
Total costs/case	$52,948	$49,109	$15,413	$20,986
Reimbursed/case	$48,347	$44,256	$15,440	$20,242
Net margin (sum)	($1,822,204)	($4,998,219)	$197,960	($6,622,463)

Source: Adapted from Cassel et al., Measuring the intensity, cost, and duration of palliative care-relevant cases among all hospitalizations in three U.S. and UK hospitals, Research paper presented at American Academy of Hospice and Palliative Medicine, New Orleans, LA, 2013.

bed day can be measured or inferred. Delving into the baseline or status quo is important not only for eventual program evaluation, but also for program development in that it may help the nascent palliative care team better understand what they could change, and it may help administrators understand the costs of caring for this previously unknown or unrecognized patient population. Conducting and sharing financial analyses on the target population—dying or high-risk patients—may itself be an educational intervention for administrators and department chairs, whose attention may be drawn to that population for the very first time. From such analyses can come more strategic and comprehensive approaches to caring for this subpopulation scattered in all departments and units of a hospital.

This is a critical point for understanding why cost avoidance has been so important for the development and expansion of SPC programs in U.S. hospitals: cost-containment in the context of a fixed-price reimbursement structure has a direct effect on the hospital's net margin. It is that impact that is then balanced with the modest investment or subsidy that the SPC program needs, in order to show a budget-neutral program that greatly reduces pain and suffering for patients and families. This brings us to the third principle.

THIRD PRINCIPLE: RESEARCH HAS SHOWN THAT SPC REDUCES UTILIZATION AND COSTS

A variety of financial and operational outcomes have been measured in the past two decades including costs, length-of-stay, intensity of care (e.g., ICU days), revenues, and quality or performance metrics such as readmission rates and mortality rates. These have all been demonstrated or discussed as domains of interest in studies of SPC and related interventions. Higginson's early reviews[10,11] covered both SPC and related interventions that included utilization outcomes (e.g., bed days; costs) in studies dating from 1998. Smith's recent review[12] specifically on financial and economic outcomes covers 46 studies published from 2002 through 2011. The latter review found that, generally, SPC and similar interventions resulted in significantly lower healthcare costs, despite wide variation in cost measures, methodological quality, and type of intervention.

Research in the United States on cost and utilization outcomes has generally taken one of two approaches: a short-term effect (impact within the same hospitalization as the SPC encounter) and long-term effects (impact over weeks and months following SPC involvement, whether inpatient or community based). Short-term effects on direct costs have been demonstrated repeatedly.[8,13–16] Our first study[13] was one of the earliest U.S. studies to show that transfer to a palliative care unit was associated with within-patient significant reductions in the hospital's direct costs per day, and also compared to non-PCU deaths in the same hospital. White,[14] also from our program at VCU, showed that "usual care" for dying patients was not associated with a drop in direct costs in the final days, and that when SPC was involved, the greatest reduction in direct costs was for patients transferred from ICUs. Penrod[15] showed lower direct costs, and less ICU utilization, among SPC patients

in a military veterans (public) health system and used propensity scores to more rigorously match "usual care" patients to those that received SPC. Those three studies had two limitations: they were limited to patients who died during the index admission, and they were limited to single sites or health systems. The Morrison et al.[8] study of eight hospitals overcame both of those limitations while continuing the use of direct costs as the appropriate cost measure, and examining both survivors and decedents. For both survivors and decedents, both within-patient and between-patient analyses demonstrated significant reductions in direct costs, with the matching of SPC and "usual care" groups using propensity scores to minimize selection bias. Gade[17] overcame the limitations inherent in observational studies with a randomized controlled trial of inpatient SPC, but this study did not demonstrate short-term effects on costs or length of stay (within the index admission) for SPC recipients. Albanese[16] closely replicated the Smith[13] study and demonstrated significant reduction in direct costs for an inpatient SPC unit, especially for patients transferred from ICUs, for whom the cost reduction was almost five-fold greater than patients from acute units. Morrison[18] analyzed SPC impact but used total costs that include indirect costs. This is the wrong cost measure to use for such research, as it inflates the purported cost reduction attributed to SPC involvement.

Much of the research cited earlier is from observational and quasi-experimental studies. At least five true RCTs have been conducted on clinical SPC interventions that measured cost impact:

- Brumley[19] compared palliative home care (n = 145 followed for an average of 196 days) to usual home care (n = 152 followed for average of 242 days) for home-bound patients with chronic obstructive pulmonary disease (COPD), congestive heart failure (CHF), or cancer. SPC patients had greater satisfaction, were more likely to die at home, and had lower healthcare costs (net difference of US$7552 per patient) due to fewer ED visits and hospitalizations.
- Gade[17] compared inpatient SPC consultation (n = 275) to usual inpatient care (n = 237) among patients hospitalized with a life-limiting disease; utilization and costs were assessed across the 6 months following discharge. SPC patients had greater satisfaction, were re-admitted at the same rate as control patients but used ICU less if re-admitted to hospital, and had lower healthcare costs (net difference of US$6766 per patient) following discharge.
- Higginson[20] compared fast-tracked SPC (n = 25) to SPC delivered after a delay of 3 months (n = 21) for patients with severe multiple sclerosis. SPC was delivered in both home and community (clinic, hospital) settings. SPC patients' caregivers had lower ratings of burden, and lower total costs of care (net difference of £1789 per patient) after 12 weeks; those costs included both costs of formal healthcare as well as of informal caregiving.
- Temel randomized 151 non-small cell lung cancer patients to usual care versus usual care plus an interdisciplinary monthly palliative care (PC) team visit. Patients in the PC arm had more prognostic awareness, less depression and

anxiety, less aggressive end of life care, less intravenous chemotherapy in the last 60 days of life, lived 2.7 months longer[21] and cost several thousands of dollars less per person.

- Zimmermann randomized 24 Ontario oncology clinics to usual care, or usual care plus a palliative care team, with 461 randomized patients. By the third and fourth month, all the study endpoints favoured the group that had concurrent PC, including quality of life, spiritual well being, symptom severity and satisfaction with care. Data on cost has not been reported yet, but hospitalisations were not increased.[25]

These five RCTs of SPC are notable for a number of reasons. First, they were conducted using longitudinal assessments of healthcare costs in the 3–8 months following introduction of the SPC intervention (not just cost reduction during a hospitalization). They were conducted in the context of a non-fee-for-service system: a health maintenance organization for Brumley[19] and Gade,[17] and England's National Health Service for Higginson.[20] All three showed significant reductions in healthcare costs, owing primarily to a reduction in hospital costs.

These studies make the case that it is not inpatient SPC which by itself reduces later ED visits and hospitalizations, but rather the provision of home care or hospice which do so. Inpatient SPC teams by themselves can do little to manage symptoms or head-off emergencies for patients outside the hospital. This leads us to the fourth principle.

FOURTH PRINCIPLE: INPATIENT SPC REDUCES COSTS FOR HOSPITALS, WHILE OUTPATIENT SPC CAN AVOID THEM FOR PAYERS

For the most part, hospitals in the United States are reimbursed for inpatient care by government payers (Medicare, Medicaid) in such a way that reducing direct costs for a few days at the end of a long and costly admission will reduce the hospital's net loss, but will not affect the expenditures from the payers, which are prospectively determined and not affected by LOS or costs incurred. Thus, there is a financial incentive built into the inpatient payment model that has led hospitals to subsidize and support inpatient SPC teams, which help to improve patient care while reducing exposure to net losses for the costliest admissions. There is a financial incentive for entities to support the intervention of outpatient or community-based SPC and hospice involved earlier in the disease course,[21] but it is not necessarily an incentive for hospitals; it is however, one for third-party payers. Third-party payers do see less expenditure when there are fewer ED visits and hospitalizations and when symptoms and crises are managed at home, by outpatient visits, or in hospice instead.[22] Note that four U.S. studies that took a longer term measure of utilization and costs—Brumley[19,23] Gade,[17] and Enguidanos[24]—were all conducted in the context of a health maintenance organization

which sees hospitalizations as costs, and not as revenue opportunities. Similarly the Higginson RCT on multiple sclerosis[20] and most other non-U.S. studies take this longer term view, which makes sense in countries with government-based and government-funded health systems. In such settings, one does not need to parse direct and indirect costs (which are often not available in health systems outside of the United States), and can focus instead on the frequency, duration, and intensity of hospitalizations.[7]

CONCLUSIONS

Studies have demonstrated cost reduction for inpatient SPC and avoidance of hospitalizations for hospice and outpatient or community-based SPC. One can measure financial impact merely as a proxy for intensity of healthcare utilization, or as a crucial factor for garnering support for SPC programs and providers. Either way, one should always put financial analyses in the larger context of the primary and secondary outcomes that SPC achieves for patients and the individuals around them.

Key learning points

- SPC may reduce costs of care as a secondary effect of better patient care.
- SPC-relevant patients have high costs and long hospitalizations.
- Inpatient SPC reduces direct costs of care during those hospitalizations, and this can result in a substantial improvement in hospital financial outcomes and resource utilization.
- Outpatient, community-based SPC and hospice reduce costs for payers by reducing hospitalizations.

REFERENCES

1 Seymour JE. Looking back, looking forward: The evolution of palliative and end of life care in England. *Mortality* 2012;7(1).
2 Murray E. How advocates use health economic data and projections: The Irish experience. *J Pain Symptom Manage* 2009;38(1):97–104.
3 Cassel JB. The importance of following the money in the development and sustainability of palliative care. *Palliat Med* 2013;27(2):103–104.
4 Teno JM, Gozalo PL, Bynum JP, Leland NE, Miller SC, Morden NE, Scupp T, Goodman DC, Mor V. Change in end-of-life care for Medicare beneficiaries: Site of death, place of care, and health care transitions in 2000, 2005, and 2009. *JAMA* 2013;309(5):470–477.
5 Alemayehu B, Warner KE. The lifetime distribution of health care costs. *Health Serv Res* 2004;39(3):627–642.
6 Barnato AE, McClellan MB, Kagay CR, Garber AM. Trends in inpatient treatment intensity among Medicare beneficiaries at the end of life. *Health Serv Res* 2004;39:363–375.

7   Cassel, Kerr, Skoro, Shickle, Murtagh, Higginson, Adelfson, Meyers, Yanni. Measuring the intensity, cost and duration of palliative care-relevant cases among all hospitalizations in three U.S. and UK hospitals. Research paper presented at American Academy of Hospice and Palliative Medicine, New Orleans, LA, 2013.

8   Morrison JD, Penrod JB, Cassel M, Caust-Ellenbogen A, Litke L, Spragens DE. Meier for the Palliative Care Leadership Centers' Outcomes Group. Cost Savings Associated with Hospital-Based Palliative Care Consultation Programs. *Arch Intern Med* 2008;168(16):1783–1790.

9   Quinn K. New directions in Medicaid payment for hospital care. *Health Aff (Millwood)* 2008;27(1):269–280.

10 Higginson IJ, Evans CJ. What is the evidence that palliative care teams improve outcomes for cancer patients and their families? *Cancer J* 2010;16(5):423–435.

11 Higginson IJ, Finlay I, Goodwin DM, Hood K, Edwards AGK, Cook AM, Douglas H-R, Normand CE. Is there evidence that palliative care teams alter end-of-life experiences of patients and their caregivers? *J Pain Symptom Manage* 2003;25:150–168.

12 Smith S, Brick A, O'Hara S, Normand C. Evidence on the cost and cost-effectiveness of palliative care: A literature review. *Palliat Med* 2013 [epub ahead of print].

13 Smith TJ, Coyne P, Cassel JB, Penberthy L, Hopson A, Hager MA. A high volume specialist palliative care unit and team may reduce in-hospital end of life care cost. *J Palliat Med* 2003;6:699–705.

14 White KR, Stover KG, Cassel JB, Smith TJ. Non-clinical outcomes of hospital-based palliative care. *J Healthcare Manage* 2006;51(4):253–267.

15 Penrod JD, Deb P, Luhrs C, Dellenbaugh C, Zhu CW, Hochman T et al. Cost and utilization outcomes of patients receiving hospital-based PC consultation. *J Palliat Med* 2006;9:855–860.

16 Albanese TH, Radwany SM, Mason H, Gayomali C, Dieter K. Assessing the financial impact of an inpatient acute palliative care unit in a tertiary care teaching hospital. *J Palliat Med* 2013;16(3):289–294.

17 Gade G, Venohr I, Conner D, McGrady K, Beane J, Richardson RH et al. Impact of an inpatient palliative care team: A randomized control trial. *J Palliat Med* 2008;11:180–190.

18 Morrison RS, Dietrich J, Ladwig S, Quill T, Sacco J, Tangeman J, Meier DE. Palliative care consultation teams cut hospital costs for Medicaid beneficiaries. *Health Aff (Millwood)* 2011;30(3):454–463.

19 Brumley RD, Enguidanos S, Jamison P, Seitz R, Morgenstern N, Saito S et al. Increased satisfaction with care and lower costs: Results of a randomized trial of in-home palliative care. *J Am Geriatr Soc* 2007;55:993–1000.

20 Higginson IJ, McCrone P, Hart SR, Burman R, Silber E, Edmonds PM. Is short-term palliative care cost-effective in multiple sclerosis? A randomized phase II trial. *J Pain Symptom Manage* 2009;38(6):816–826.

21 Temel JS, Greer JA, Muzikansky A, Gallagher ER, Admane S, Jackson VA, Dahlin CM et al. Early palliative care for patients with metastatic non-small-cell lung cancer. *NEJM* 2010;363:733–742.

22 Kelley AS, Deb P, Du Q, Aldridge Carlson MD, Morrison RS. Hospice enrollment saves money for Medicare and improves care quality across a number of different lengths-of-stay. *Health Aff (Millwood)* 2013;32(3):552–561.

23 Brumley RD, Enguidanos S, Cherin DA. Effectiveness of a home-based palliative care program for end-of-life. *J Palliat Med* 2003;5:715–724.

24 Enguidanos S, Vesper E, Lorenz K. 30-Day readmissions among seriously ill older adults. *J Palliat Med* 2012;15(12):1356–1361.

25 Zimmermann C1, Swami N2, Krzyzanowska M3, Hannon B4, Leighl N3, Oza A3, Moore M3, Rydall A2, Rodin G5, Tannock I6, Donner A7, Lo C8. Early palliative care for patients with advanced cancer: A cluster-randomised controlled trial. *Lancet* 2014 May 17;383(9930):1721–30. doi: 10.1016/S0140-6736(13)62416-2. Epub 2014 Feb 19.

30

Organization and support of the interdisciplinary team

KAREN MACMILLAN, LOUISE KASHUBA, BETTE EMERY

INTRODUCTION

Palliative care encompasses the physical, psychosocial, and spiritual dimensions of the patient and family. Expertise of various healthcare professionals is necessary to manage their complex needs.[1–16] In this chapter, the interdisciplinary team will be explored. Team composition, communication and collaboration strategies, and support and leadership for interdisciplinary teams will be outlined. Areas of ongoing and required research will be identified. Future challenges in the organization and support of interdisciplinary teams will also be explored. Interdisciplinary teams can provide care and support in all settings; however, the focus will be on specialized palliative care units.

A common definition of terms provides a foundation upon which to build the ideas for organizational and support requirements for the interdisciplinary team. Multiprofessional teams have existed since the early 1900s in the interests of achieving efficiency by reducing cost and minimizing interventions.[10] Multiprofessional teams are either multidisciplinary or interdisciplinary. There is a notable distinction between multidisciplinary and interdisciplinary teams.[4,10,13,15,17] Multidisciplinary teams consist of independent healthcare professionals who conduct independent assessments, planning, and provision of care with little communication or coordination with other team members. In a multidisciplinary team, the physician traditionally prescribes the involvement of the other team members. Interdisciplinary teams, in contrast, function as collaborative units working together to establish common goals of care. The term "interdisciplinary" is often used interchangeably with the term "interprofessional." Automatic referral is assumed for each team member; the professional, along with the rest of the interdisciplinary team, determines the professional's involvement and the focus of interventions. In order to provide care, the interdisciplinary team uses skills of communication, problem solving, and goal setting to enhance the collaborative nature of interaction between team members.

INTERDISCIPLINARY TEAM: COMPOSITION

There are many publications on the value of interdisciplinary teams in palliative care; however, there is a paucity of research to support this belief.[5,18–20] Although palliative patients and their families report satisfaction with the interdisciplinary approach,[20,21] there is an absence of substantive research to fully describe the benefits.[5,18–20] Systematic literature reviews, meta-analysis, and meta-regression of published research on the effectiveness and impact of different models of palliative care teams have been inconclusive.[5,18–19,22–24] Inherent problems with all of these studies exist because of the vulnerability of the terminally ill patients being studied and the lack of comprehensive outcome measures. Nevertheless, even with the poor quality of the studies, there is evidence that palliative care teams have a positive effect on patient symptoms, length of stay, patient/family satisfaction, and costs.[6,7,9,20,25–27,32]

Interdisciplinary teams can ensure comprehensive coordinated care. This requires time and financial resources in order to be successful.[10,28,29] Some question the costs associated with multiple disciplines and caution about the effectiveness and efficiency of too large a team.[30] Yet others have demonstrated that developments of comprehensive interdisciplinary palliative care programs/teams are cost-effective in a variety of settings.[7,9,22] Again, there is limited research exploring team composition or team size based on patient caseloads.

Members of the interdisciplinary team may include the following:[3,6,7,12,13,24,31]

- Art therapists
- Dieticians
- Holistic health practitioners
- Music therapists
- Nurses
- Occupational therapists

- Pastoral/spiritual care
- Pharmacists
- Physicians
- Physiotherapists
- Psychiatrists
- Psychologists
- Recreation therapists
- Respiratory therapists
- Social workers
- Volunteers

Although all of these disciplines can add value to the patient and family experience, if resources are limited, choices must be made as to which disciplines will be part of the team. Many sources suggest a palliative care physician and a nurse as core members, with other team members added as determined by needs and resources.[32] The needs of the patient and family ultimately dictate which healthcare professionals are involved in their care. It is equally important that composition of the team reflects the needs of the patient group seen by the service. For example, a service that provides care for a large number of end-stage respiratory diseases might consider having a respiratory therapist as a permanent team member. Alternatively, if disciplines are not represented on the palliative care team, there needs to be a provision to consult them. Tracking the frequency of these referrals can support planning for team composition as programs expand and change.

INTERDISCIPLINARY COMMUNICATION AND COLLABORATION

Communication and collaboration are key aspects of any interdisciplinary team.[1,4,10,13,27,33] Each profession's education has unique vocabulary, similar problem-solving strategies, and similar world views.[4] Members of each specialty and discipline have a theoretical basis through which they interpret and address issues that arise in their work.[4] Team members must excel at their competencies, be secure in their own disciplines, and be able to uphold their ideas.[17] An essential assumption in the team approach is that the team itself functions well.[34] Successful contributing members of an interdisciplinary team require skills beyond those typically acquired in their discipline-specific programs.

Roles within an interdisciplinary team are less well defined than traditional roles of healthcare workers in other settings. As roles often blur, it is important that team members feel secure, thus avoiding being undermined by these overlapping roles.[35] Role blurring can be problematic if it is not well understood and can lead to under- or overutilization of team members.[35] These situations can lead to resentment, burnout, and team conflict. Poor communication is one of the major factors preventing effective interdisciplinary teamwork.[4] Exercises that clarify roles, professional competencies, perceptions, and expectations are valuable.[27,35] Many

Canadian postsecondary institutions support collaboration among students enrolled in health discipline faculties by offering interdisciplinary course work.[16,36] These courses are designed to promote shared understanding of roles and promote problem solving. Those new to a profession who have participated in these courses come to the practice setting better prepared to professionally collaborate.

Setting aside traditional roles is required to engage in creative dialog with each other. Ideally, each professional reviews the documentation completed by other team members, to clarify information, questions, and concerns prior to entering the patient's room. Patients should not have to repeatedly tell their stories if the team is effectively sharing information. This demonstrates courtesy and respect, as well as conserving the patient's energy. The use of plain language is important to enhance understanding and communication. It is recommended that all disciplines document in the same area of the health record. Documentation, including physician orders, must be supported by rationale to enhance understanding by all team members. Avoiding abbreviations enhances communication in documentation.

Team members must respect, value, understand, and trust each other's contributions.[13,15,37] Effective conflict resolution will foster team growth and maturation. Methods to reach consensus, resolve conflict, and effectively communicate are essential. While allowing for individual differences, bridges are built by striving to understand others' perspectives and ways of doing things. Formal staff debriefing is helpful when case circumstances are particularly traumatic or there have been multiple deaths in a short period of time. If care did not go well, a clinical postmortem can identify ways to improve in the future.

Care planning is ongoing, formally with interdisciplinary team conferencing, and more informally between meetings as the need arises. Daily "lightning rounds" provides an opportunity to share any immediate concern(s) for the day for the patient and allows care providers a common understanding all at the same time. Weekly team conference enhances coordination of care with assessment, planning, and evaluation of patient care. This is an appropriate time for team members to identify individual responsibilities related to tasks and interventions.

Patient/family conferences assist in directing care by updating medical information, formulating goals, and planning discharge. Not all members of the interdisciplinary team participate in a patient/family conference as having all of the professionals involved may overwhelm the patient and family. The goals of the patient/family conference and the patient needs will dictate which team members attend. To ensure a comprehensive picture, it is helpful to elicit pertinent input about the patient's level of functioning from team members not attending the conference. When there is conflict, a patient/family conference may help to problem-solve and/or support behavioral changes. Both team and patient/family conferences may serve as a forum to exchange ideas, share information, set shared goals, develop care plans, and solve problems.

SUPPORT FOR THE INTERDISCIPLINARY TEAM

Individual team members and the interdisciplinary team require support to ensure the success of the team.[35,38] Team members must be clinically competent in their discipline and be committed to improving their practice through ongoing education. There needs to be recognition that each member will be at a different stage in his or her professional and personal development. Team members are encouraged to be involved in discipline-specific professional development activities such as participating in special interest groups, courses and reading professional journals.[33] Completing an oral presentation for educational rounds and case reviews provides the team member a forum to present subjects relevant to their discipline and to other disciplines.[15] These represent only a few of the many possibilities for professionals working in palliative care. The intense nature of work in palliative care, as with most high-demand specialty areas, requires diverse opportunities to reflect, grow, and find balance.[38] Support is necessary at the group level as well as at the individual level coming from within the group itself as well as from administration.

Support requirements of an interdisciplinary team are greater than a sum of the needs of the individuals. Within the work environment, the development of supportive, collaborative relationships is fundamental.[4,33,35,39] Factors for coping are planned orientation, ongoing education, administrative support, and an environment conducive to team building.[24,39]

Planning a comprehensive orientation for new staff extends beyond the organization's corporate orientation. New team members must understand the roles of each discipline. When possible, a new team member overlaps with the team member they will replace. Time spent job shadowing prior to being independent allows scheduled time with a professional to answer questions and support the individual.[39] Well-established teams can be daunting; therefore strategies are required to integrate a new team member such as assigning a mentor can be used. Those in remote areas need mentors to call for consultation and support. New programs should consider partnering with successful programs, as this can provide them with a wealth of knowledge and support.

Keeping abreast of developments in a cutting-edge field can be challenging. A variety of palliative care texts, websites, professional peer-reviewed journals, and subscriptions to listservs are available as resources for information for professionals. Journal clubs and weekly rounds are a structured means of advancing knowledge. By sharing an article or presentation with peers, the individual professional has the opportunity to discuss ideas with their colleagues to glean their perspective. Workshops and conferences may be cost prohibitive. Distance learning, webinar, or video conferencing may be more economical. Often time is the limiting factor, rather than availability of options or resources.

Commitment from administration for time and education opportunities as well as acknowledgment of interdisciplinary and individual projects contributes to the success of the team.[2,29] Adequate space for meetings and individual offices or workspaces in close proximity to one another can enhance teamwork and collaboration.[40] Private designated space, allowing for counseling patients and families, may be required for team members.

LEADING INTERDISCIPLINARY TEAMS

Program management is an ideal structure, given the unique composition and needs of the palliative care interdisciplinary team. This is a management structure in which groups of professionals with skills and expertise care for a specific population of patients. Co-leaders may be necessary for managing the team. It is common that the leaders are a nurse and physician, although any discipline with management expertise, education, and skill could fill the nurse leader's role. The structure usually has physicians reporting to the physician leader and other disciplines reporting to the other co-leader (program manager). The physician leader engages the palliative physicians to ensure their accountability and responsibility as team members. The program manager has the same responsibilities with all other disciplines. The program manager is also responsible for management activities such as budget, finance, hiring, operations, and administration of the program. The co-leaders provide vision and direction for future planning, as well as drive and support change. Since team members report to the program manager, there needs to be a mechanism for managing professional issues that is specific to each discipline.[41,42] Support and guidance may be necessary from a professional peer as well as the program manager. In some organizations, professional practice leaders fulfill this role by collaborating with operational leaders and staff to provide clinical guidance, participate in and apply research as well as review or recommend changes in standards or practice. Informal leadership has a significant role in the palliative team as there may be a scarcity of experienced palliative care professionals as positions become available within the team. Experienced staff members assume the role of mentor to guide to new members of the team in the collaborative model of care and to support professional socialization of new professionals.

Clearly defined and established mission, purpose, standards of care, values and goals to guide and support the interdisciplinary team are foundational concepts.[2,24,40,43] The involvement of team members in articulating these concepts is essential as this supports team development and future strategic planning. Team building is an essential investment for the leader to initiate and support; functioning teams must have a clear sense of trust, efficacy, and team identity.[24,34,37] Strategic plans should be agreed upon by team members and revisited on a yearly basis. Consumer satisfaction surveys, outcome measurements, and program evaluations may also shape the program's future directions.[25] Outcome measures chosen must reflect the goals of the program.

Imbedding palliative care into the culture of an organization is significant for the long-term success of a palliative care program.[44] Ongoing collaboration with senior leadership from a position of proactive problem solving demonstrates flexibility and adaptability. Commitment and ongoing support by senior administration is key to successful program management models of care delivery.[6,24] Leaders must be clear on the direction of the program and able to make decisions in order to achieve the team's agreed-upon goals. The primary focus of the leaders is to serve the needs of the team, empower them in delivering care and advancing knowledge and skills in palliative care.[24,45,46]

One of the greatest barriers to an integrated team approach to end-of-life care is the structure of healthcare financing.[11] Physicians traditionally bill the healthcare system or the insurance company directly, whereas the program manager budgets for the other disciplines within the interdisciplinary team.[15] System reimbursements for physicians ought to address the importance of spending adequate time with the patient and family, the need for family meetings and team meetings, as well as the appropriate utilization of costly interventions in terminal care. The cost of the palliative care interdisciplinary team must be justified to senior administration. A database to collect information that quantifies time and tasks performed by each discipline in providing care to patients assists this process but can be time consuming. Team members must understand the significance of collecting and recording these data. This not only substantiates costs in the current program but also aids in projecting future resource requirements. Once the financial offsets are considered, the interdisciplinary approach to palliative care is a cost-effective program.[22] Leaders of palliative care interdisciplinary teams must be prepared to face the aforementioned administrative challenges by developing a strategic plan based on evidence and data analysis. Ensuring that the administrative needs of the program are addressed ultimately leads to a better functioning team that can more effectively provide care to the patient.

Even in health care systems that do not finance by physician billing, there can be barriers to the integrated team approach because of the different management structures that operate. Physician, nurse, social work, and chaplaincy may all be managed via different structures, lead individuals, and, in some instances, even different organizations. Sometimes these have different budgets. These different structures or organizations may have different priorities and systems that conflict with multidisciplinary working. Agreement and commitment at the management level is vital to ensure that team working can continue, but because palliative care is often a small specialty or concern, this does not always happen. [47]

FUTURE CHALLENGES

Palliative care professionals are positioned well to support the principles of patient-/family-centered care. There is growing collaboration with those providing care for noncancer patient populations. This broader perspective based on patient need rather than diagnosis supports those approaching end of life from a variety of chronic illnesses and aging. Teams will be

challenged by supporting the needs for those wishing to collaborate with them and the ongoing clinical demands of their work. Standard care pathway implementation and the empirical evaluation of implementation may be a key factor in ensuring palliative care bridges the gap in the noncancer populations.

In 2011, the first of the "baby boomer" cohort group reached age 65, marking the first wave of that generation reaching retirement age in North America. Every workplace and sector will face staff shortages as a result of this growing shift. The need for succession planning in palliative care is evident as this large cohort begins to retire from the clinical environment. Innovation in palliative care education delivery, recruitment and consultation services of the interdisciplinary team will support the needs of patients and their families as the workforce changes. Ongoing access to high-quality palliative care professionals and services must be maintained to support patient care, research, and education.

FUTURE DIRECTIONS IN RESEARCH

There are many unanswered questions related to interdisciplinary teams in palliative care.[4,19,48] Examples of possible research questions include:

- What outcomes need to be measured?
- What is the effectiveness of interdisciplinary teams?
- Do interdisciplinary teams provide more holistic and effective care?
- How is palliative care best delivered?
- How are interdisciplinary teams best organized?
- Which disciplines are essential to a palliative care team?
- What size and composition of interdisciplinary teams are most cost-effective?
- Are their subgroups that exist inside a team?
- What are the structural needs of the team?
- How to reduce compassion fatigue and moral distress?
- What are the impacts on staff satisfaction?

CONCLUSION

Successful teams value and support their members, have a commitment to improve communication, resolve disagreements, and provide services. Support for individuals within the team to pursue professional and personal growth is encouraged. A coordinated effort by administration and leadership is required to meet these needs. The investment by leaders to develop and build the team is essential in supporting the ongoing growth and success of the palliative care interdisciplinary team. Key factors for success of the palliative care interdisciplinary team are vision, leadership, and coordinated delivery of care, respectful interactions, professional development, and competence. Further and ongoing research is necessary to explore facets of the palliative care interdisciplinary team, its functioning, and effectiveness.

Key learning points

- The composition of the interdisciplinary team in palliative care is determined by the unique needs of the patient population being served.

- Effective role blurring is essential for the coordinated delivery of care.

- Concentrated efforts to hone communication and collaboration skills are needed to facilitate team growth.

- Commitment at all levels of leadership is required for the interdisciplinary teams in palliative care to succeed.

REFERENCES

1 Lickiss JN, Turner KS, Pollock ML. The interdisciplinary team. In: Doyle D, Hanks G, Cherney M, Calman K, eds. *Oxford Textbook of Palliative Medicine*, 3rd edn. Oxford, U.K.: Oxford University Press, 2004, pp. 42–46.

2 McCallin A. Interdisciplinary team leadership: A revisionist approach for an old problem? *J Nurs Manage* 2003; 11: 364–370.

3 Egan City KA, Labyak MJ. Hospice palliative care for the 21st century: A model for quality end-of-life care. In: Ferrell BR, Coyle N, eds. *Oxford Textbook of Palliative Nursing*. New York: Oxford University Press, 2010, pp. 13–52.

4 Hall P, Weaver L. Interdisciplinary education and teamwork: A long and winding road. *Med Educ* 2001; 35: 867–875.

5 Higginson IJ, Finlay IG, Goodwin DM et al. Is there evidence that palliative care teams alter end-of-life experiences of patients and their caregivers? *J Pain Symptom Manage* 2003; 25: 150–168.

6 Strasser F, Sweeney C, Willey J et al. Impact of a half-day multidisciplinary symptom control and palliative care outpatient clinic in a comprehensive cancer center on recommendations, symptom intensity, and patient satisfaction: A retrospective descriptive study. *J Pain Symptom Manage* 2004; 27: 481–491.

7 Bruera E, Michaud M, Vigano A. Multidisciplinary symptom control clinic in a cancer center: A retrospective study. *Support Care Cancer* 2001; 9: 162–168.

8 Hunt J, Keeley V, Cobb M et al. A new quality assurance package for hospital palliative care teams: The Trent Hospice Audit Group model. *Br J Cancer* 2004; 91: 248–253.

9 Bruera E, Sweeney C. The Development of palliative care at the University of Texas M.D. Anderson Cancer Center. *Support Care Cancer* 2001; 9: 330–334.

10 Fitzpatrick JJ. Building community: Developing skills for interprofessional health professions education and relationship-centered care. *J Nurse-Midwifery* 1998; 43: 61–65.

11 Billings JA. Vicissitudes of the clinician-patient relationship in end-of-life care: Recognizing the role for teams. *J Palliat Med* 2002; 5: 295–300.

12 Ahmedzai SH, Costa A, Blengini C et al. A new international framework for palliative care. *Eur J Cancer* 2004; 40: 2192–2200.

13 Crawford GB, Price SD. Palliative care. Team working: Palliative care as a model of interdisciplinary practice. *Med J Aust* 2003; 179(6 Suppl): S32–S34.

14 Kristjanson LJ, Toye C, Dawson S. New dimensions in palliative care: A palliative approach to neurodegenerative diseases and final illness in older people. *Med J Aust* 2003; 179(6 Suppl): S41–S43.

15 Bellamy A, Fiddian M, Nixon J. Case review: Promoting shared learning and collaborative practice. *International J of Palliat Nurs* 2006; 12(4): 158–162.

16 Hall P, Weaver L, Fothergill-Bourbonnais F, Amos S, Whiting N, Barnes P, Legault F. Interprofessional education in palliative care: A pilot project using popular literature. *J Interprofessional Care* 2006; 20 (1); 51–59.

17 Dyer JA. Multidisciplinary, interdisciplinary, and transdisciplinary educational models and nursing education. *Nurs Educ Perspect* 2003; 24: 186–188.

18 Higginson IJ, Finlay I, Goodwin DM et al. Do hospital-based palliative teams improve care for patients or families at the end of life? *J Pain Symptom Manage* 2002; 23: 96–106.

19 Teno JM. Palliative care teams: Self-reflection, past, present and future. *J Pain Symptom Manage* 2002; 23: 94–95.

20 Junger S, Pestinger F, Elsner F, Krumm N, Radbruch L. Criteria for successful multiprofessional cooperation in palliative care teams. *Palliat Med* 2007; 21: 347–354.

21 Oliver D, Porock D, Demiris G, Courtney K. Patient and family involvement in hospice interdisciplinary teams. *J Palliat Care* 2005; 47: 270–276.

22 Smith TJ, Coyne P, Cassel B et al. A high-volume specialist palliative care unit and team may reduce in-hospital end-of-life care costs. *J Palliat Med* 2003; 6: 699–705.

23 Zwarenstein M, Goldman J, Reeves S, Interprofessional collaboration; effects of practice-based interventions on professional practice and healthcare outcomes (review). *The Cochrane Collaboration.* 2009; 4: 1–29.

24 O'Connor M, Fisher C, Guilfoyle A. Interdisciplinary teams in palliative care; a critical reflection. *Int J Palliat Nurs* 2006; 12(3): 132–137.

25 Parkes CM, Parkes J. 'Hospice' versus 'hospital' care re-evaluation after 10 years as seen by surviving spouses. *Postgrad Med J* 1984; 60: 120–124.

26 Gomes et al. Effectiveness and cost-effectiveness of home-based palliative care services for adults with advanced illness and their caregivers. *Cochrane Database Syst Rev* 2013; 6: CD007760. doi: 10.1002/14651858. CD007760.pub2.

27 Higginson and Evans, What Is the Evidence That Palliative Care Teams Improve Outcomes for Cancer Patients and Their Families? *Cancer J* 2010; 16(5): 423–435. doi: 10.1097/PPO.0b013e3181f684e5.

28 MacDonald N. Palliative care and primary care. *J Palliat Care* 2002; 23: 58–59.

29 Mariano C. The case for interdisciplinary collaboration. *Nurs Outlook* 1989; 37: 285–288.

30 Wilson PR. Multidisciplinary ... transdisciplinary ... monodisciplinary ... where are we going? *Clin J Pain* 1996; 12: 253–254.

31 Sommers LS, Marton KI, Barbaccia JC, Randolph J. Physician, nurse, and social work collaboration in primary care for chronically ill seniors. *Arch Intern Med* 2000; 160: 1825–1833.

32 Stepans MB, Thompson CL, Buchanan ML. The role of the nurse on a transdisciplinary early intervention assessment team. *Public Health Nurs* 2002; 19: 238–245.

33 Davison G. Palliative care teams and the contingencies that impact them: From the teams. *Prog Palliate Care* 2006; 14(2): 55–61.

34 Malloch K, Porter-O'Grady T. Today's health care team and the role of the nurse leader. In: Pangman VC, Pangman C, eds. *Nursing Leadership from a Canadian Perspective.* Baltimore, MD: Lippincott Williams & Wilkins, 2010, pp. 226–250.

35 O'Connor M, Fischer C. Exploring the dynamics of interdisciplinary palliative care teams in providing psychosocial care: "Everybody thinks that everybody can do it and they can't". *J Palliat Med* 2011; 14(2) 191–196.

36 Smith DL, Meyer S, Wylie DM. Leadership for Teamwork and Collaboration. In: Hibberd JM, Smith DL, eds. Nursing Leadership and Management in Canada. Toronto, Ontario, Canada: Elsevier Canada, 2006, pp. 519–547.

37 Blacker S, Deveau C. Social work and interprofessional collaboration in palliative care. *Prog Palliat Care* 2010: 18(4): 237–243.

38 Maddix T, Pereira J. Reflecting on the work of palliative care. *J Palliat Med* 2001; 4: 373–377.

39 Dawson S. Interprofessional working: Communication, collaboration... perspiration! *Int J Palliat Nurs* 2007: 13(10): 502–505.

40 Robbins H, Finley M. Four myths about teams. In: *Why Teams Don't Work*. Available at: www.mfinley.com/articles/team-myths.htm, (accessed September 8, 2005).

41 VanDeVelde-Coke S. Restructuring health agencies: From hierarchies to programs. In: Hibberd JM, Smith DL, eds. *Nursing Management in Canada*. Toronto, Ontario, Canada: WB Saunders Company, 1999, pp. 135–155.

42 Tait A. Clinical governance in primary care: A literature review. *J Clin Nurs* 2004; 13: 723–730.

43 Vachon M. Staff burnout: Source, diagnosis, management and prevention. In: Bruera E, Portenoy R, eds. *Topics in Palliative Care.* New York: Oxford University Press, 1999, pp. 247–293.

44 Bruera E. The development of a palliative care culture. *J Palliat Care* 2004; 20(4): 316–319.

45 Mendes IA et al. The re-humanization of the executive nurse's job: A focus on the spiritual dimension. *Rev Latino-am Enfemangem* 2002; 10: 401–407.

46 Howatson-Jones IL. The servant leader. *Nurs Manage* 2004; 11: 20–25.

47 Speck P. *Teamwork in Palliative Care: Fulfilling or Frustrating.* Oxford, U.K.: Oxford University Press, 2006.

48 Higginson IJ, Finlay IG. Improving palliative care for cancer. *Lancet Oncol* 2003; 4: 73–74.

31

Population-based needs assessment for patient and family care

IRENE J. HIGGINSON, CHARLES F. VON GUNTEN

INTRODUCTION

As palliative care services develop across the globe, those planning and funding services for populations of people will seek to ensure that services are developed in a way to meet the needs of patients and families. This is a group of the population that is often least able to make their needs known—as Hinton said, "The dissatisfied dead cannot noise abroad their concerns." So it is often left to patient groups and professionals to advocate for them. Policy makers and planners responsible for the health care services to a population have to make decisions that involve a range of health services. One way to help to plan services is to undertake a population-based needs assessment. Therefore, to negotiate with planning officers, governments, and funders, and to develop services, those working in palliative medicine have to develop a good understanding of needs assessment.[1] This chapter explains the concepts of needs and shows various methods of needs assessment. It highlights some of the pitfalls and factors that should be considered in the different approaches. Needs assessment in this context takes as its starting point a community that requires palliative care, rather than individual patients.[2] It is concerned with how many people need what types of services, where, and when. The assessment of an individual patient can occasionally be described as a needs assessment,[3] but this is a component of assessment for direct clinical care planning and is not considered here.

WHAT IS NEED?

Contributions to the definitions of need come from the fields of sociology, epidemiology, health economics, and public health as well as from clinicians. Two main underpinning theories are used in palliative care—those of Bradshaw and Maslow.[2] Bradshaw outlined a "taxonomy of social need." This distinguished between felt need (what people want), expressed need (felt need turned into action), normative need (as defined by experts or professionals), and comparative need (arising where similar populations receive different service levels).[4] Raised within these distinctions are the questions of: who determines need (professional, politician, or public); what are the influences of education and media in raising awareness about health problems; and what are the cultural effects on need. Social and cultural factors have an enormous impact on levels of morbidity and on health and the expression of health need.

The theory of Abraham Maslow of motivation and the hierarchy of needs has been widely applied in social science and health care. It has also been adapted for palliative care by Zalenski and Raspa.[5] Their five levels of the hierarchy of needs adapted for palliative care are: (1) distressing symptoms, such as pain or breathlessness; (2) fears for physical safety, of dying or abandonment; (3) affection, love, and acceptance in the face of devastating illness; (4) esteem, respect, and appreciation for the person; (5) self-actualization and transcendence.

CONCEPTS OF NEED, SUPPLY, AND DEMAND IN HEALTH CARE

The preceding definitions of need do not take account of whether there is an effective remedy or treatment (i.e., supply) that can be provided for the problem experienced by the patient. Any assessment of the health needs of a community must take this into account. Thus, needs assessment includes both the health problem (whether felt, expressed, normative, or comparative—or a combination of these) and an effective, humane and accessible remedy or treatment for this problem.[6] The remedy can include prevention, treatment, rehabilitation, and palliation. The modern epidemiological approaches to needs assessment take account of both health need and effective treatment.[7]

Demand in health care is a function of expressed need, although economists would define it as: "What people would be willing to pay for in a market or might wish to use in a system

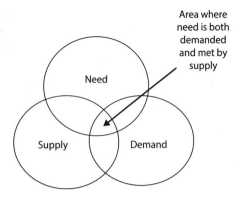

Figure 31.1   *Relationship between need, supply, and demand. Need ability to benefit from healthcare.*

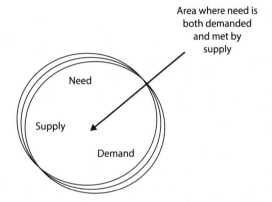

Figure 31.2   *Ideal relationship between need, supply, and demand.*

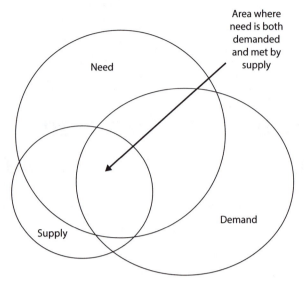

Figure 31.3   *Are the areas of need, supply, and demand of equal size? One hypothesis.*

of free health care."[5] Demand, therefore, is influenced by the nature of information available to patients and to communities, the social and educational backgrounds, the media, and the influence of doctors and nurses. Furthermore, for any patient or family, interpretation of information would be affected by the severity of his or her illness and his or her concern about that illness. The supply of health services has been influenced by historical patterns, political pressures, and pressures from health care professionals, public, the media, and patients.

Stevens and Raftery have argued that need for health care should be defined as: "the population's ability to benefit from health care."[7] They argue that need, supply, and demand partly overlap but also differ. Figure 31.1 demonstrates the differences and overlap, and shows eight different potential situations.[7] In the central area, need is both demanded and supplied. However, there may be supply where there is no need, there may be care demanded but not needed, and there may be demand and supply without need. The aim of a needs assessment in this context is to bring the circles to more closely overlap, as in Figure 31.2, so that need is demanded and supplied. This Stevens and Raftery hypothesis has one major flaw, however. It makes a rather simplistic assumption that need, demand, and supply are of equal size, and that reorganization of health care is a matter of lining up the need, demand, and supply. But, in reality, this is not likely to be the case. As part of the MSc in palliative care at King's College London, students from different countries report how they feel need, demand, and supply

are related and sized in their countries. Figure 31.3 shows one hypothesis, where supply is smaller than demand and need.

ALTERNATIVE APPROACHES TO NEEDS ASSESSMENT

Three main approaches to needs assessment have been developed.[2] These can be used independently or in combination. *A comparative needs assessment* contrasts the services received by a population in one area with those elsewhere. Thus, if one area has, for example, 40 hospice beds per million population, it might be seen as less well provided than an area with, say, 70 beds per million population. Figures 31.4 and 31.5 show examples of such a comparative assessment. However, such an assessment is clearly limited, as it does not take account of differences between the populations, nor of which model of care (more beds or more home nursing) is most effective for the population.

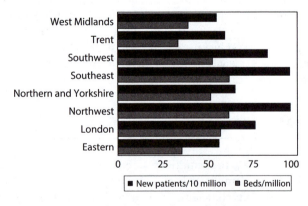

Figure 31.4   *An example of comparative needs assessment— comparing beds available. Beds per million population, new patients per 10 million population: Health regions in England (2000). (Redrawn with permission from Higginson, I., Palliative Care for Londoners, Department of Palliative Care and Policy, London, U.K., 2001.)*

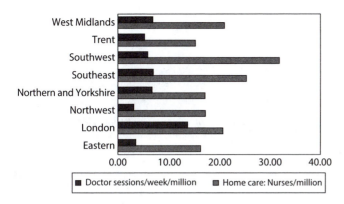

Figure 31.5 *An example of comparative needs assessment—comparing nurse and doctor sessions available. Home care nurses and doctor session per million population, England 2000. (Redrawn with permission from Higginson, I.,* Palliative Care for Londoners, *Department of Palliative Care and Policy, London, U.K., 2001.)*

The corporate approach to needs assessment is based on the demands, wishes, and alternative perspectives of interested parties including professionals, politicians, patients, and the public. A variety of interview schedules and tools in many areas of health care have been developed to aid this approach.[8] This approach commonly involves surveys of professionals[9–11] and may also survey the public, patients,[12] or a combination of views (e.g., professionals and public).[13] Perhaps the most comprehensive instrument is that developed by Currow et al., where 3027 randomly selected South Australians were surveyed on the need for, uptake rate of, and satisfaction with specialist palliative care services in 2000. One in three people surveyed (1069) indicated that someone "close to them" had died of a terminal illness in the preceding 5 years. Of those who identified that a palliative service had not been used (38%, 403), reasons cited included family/friends provided the care (34%, 136) and the service was not wanted (21%, 86). Respondents with higher income and those with cancer were more likely to report that a specialist palliative care service had been used.[14] Currow et al.'s approach utilized the views of proxies, that is, not directly the patients but bereaved carers or others. The corporate approach has the potential advantage of gaging the patient's (or their families') perspectives and capturing expressed need. However, surveying only professionals captures only normative need. And there is the added problem that expressed need is determined by individual's understanding of services, which is dependent on the provision of information about palliative care. Such information can be highly varied both within and between countries, and should be considered when interpreting a corporate needs assessment.

EPIDEMIOLOGICAL DATA–BASED NEEDS ASSESSMENT REVIEWS

The third approach to needs assessment is the epidemiologically based assessment. Epidemiological data have been applied in health care planning for many years.[6,15] Data on the incidence (the number of new cases arising in a given period) and

prevalence (the total number of cases existing at one time) of diseases, and demographic information on population structure and likely changes, were used by health care planners to determine the extent and impact of health problems. Epidemiological studies are also concerned with the quality of measurements, including the validity and reliability of tests. Population comparisons are usually more clearly made using rates rather than crude numbers, often giving age and sex specific rates or standardized according to the national population.

The epidemiological approach to needs assessment[9] combines elements of epidemiology and health economics and is a triangulation of three components: incidence and/or prevalence, health service effectiveness and cost-effectiveness, and information and views about existing services. Information allows funders and planners to determine the direction they wish to pursue in the future (see Figure 31.5).

Because any needs assessment will usually make incremental rather than dramatic changes to existing services and because there is little information on effectiveness and prevalence, it is usually recommended that this approach is combined with the more simple comparative and corporate approaches described earlier. The main components of the epidemiological based approach to needs assessment are shown in Table 31.1.

EPIDEMIOLOGICALLY BASED NEEDS ASSESSMENT FOR PALLIATIVE AND TERMINAL CARE

In several countries, epidemiologically (or population) based needs assessments have now been developed. These all provide standard definitions of palliative and end-of-life/terminal care and use national and local data on the incidence and prevalence of cancer, other diseases, and likely symptoms to estimate the numbers of patients and families needing palliative care. The absolute numbers of patients dying from cancer and other diseases likely to have a palliative period are available from government statistical departments in many countries. Applying the prevalence of symptoms to this population gives estimates of the range of problems and the size of population needing care.

Murtagh et al. recently identified and compared the main approaches to population-based needs assessment.[16] Three main approaches were identified:

1. Higginson used cause of death/symptom prevalence and, using pain prevalence, estimates that 60.28% (95% confidence interval = 60.20%–60.36%) of all deaths need palliative care (further information on this method is given on page 260 and at the original source[17]).
2. Rosenwax used the International Statistical Classification of Diseases and Related Health Problems-10th Revision (ICD-10) causes of death/hospital-use data,[18,19] and estimates that 37.01% (95% confidence interval = 36.94%–37.07%) to 96.61% (95% confidence interval = 96.58%–96.64%) of deaths need palliative care.
3. Gómez-Batiste used percentage of deaths plus chronic disease data, and estimates that 75% of deaths need palliative care.

Table 31.1   *Components of the epidemiological approach to needs assessment*

Component	Description
Statement of the context of the problem.	The problem in its context including labels attached to the disease or service, e.g., international classification of disease codes, health care resource groups (HRGs), etc. The context should relate the disease to the services it impinges upon.
Sub categories	A division of the health problem into categories that are of value to purchasing, planning, or providing health care. Often, this is based on severity or type of problem presenting. Conventional, medical subcategories sometimes do not help.
Prevalence and incidence	Prevalence and incidence data including that available for the subcategories described and/or need for treatment. It considers variations by age, sex, region, socioeconomic, and ethnic status.
Services available	Description of existing services defining the components, including the structures and processes as clearly as possible.
Effectiveness and cost-effectiveness of services	The efficacy (benefits achieved under study—usually ideal conditions), effectiveness (the benefit achieved in the real world), and efficiency (output or outcome of health care per unit of money expended). Efficacy is considered first, and the quality of the evidence is graded according to the strength of design of the studies. This is followed by a statement of the strength of recommendation to support or reject the use of the service or procedure based on the strength of the evidence.
Models of care and local assessment	Alternative models of providing services to meet patients needs. For example, one model might be orientated toward prevention, one toward treatment, and a third model, toward education of existing staff. An appraisal of the models and their application in different social, geographical, and health care settings is included.Here, local assessment of individual wishes or local data on the preferences/wishes of patients and families can be used. It may help to decide between the amounts of different models provided.
Outcomes, targets, information, and research	Outcome measures or targets which might prove useful in practice to monitor services plus other information and research needs.

Source: Zalenski, R.J. and Raspa, R., *J. Palliat. Med.*, 9(5), 1120, 2006.

Table 31.2   *Number of deaths in the population during 1 year for the most common causes*

Cause of death	Men	Women	Total
Neoplasms	1,460	1,340	2,800
Circulatory system	2,430	2,620	5,050
Respiratory system	600	630	1,230
Chronic liver and cirrhosis	30	30	60
Nervous system and sense organs**	90	90	180
Senile and presenile organic conditions	20	20	40
Endocrine, nutritional, metabolic, immunity	190	120	310
Total of these diseases	**4,820**	**4,850**	**9,670**
Total deaths from all causes	**5,360**	**5,640**	**11,000**

Total population = 1 million, estimate for developed country.
*Deaths in those aged under 28 days excluded.
**for breakdown of main groups (see Ref. 17).

In the original Higginson protocol, a standard population size is used, for example, 1 million people. Within such a population, if the age and gender mix is similar to that of a developed country, there are approximately 2800 cancer deaths per year and 6900 other deaths, some of which may have a period of advancing progressive disease, when palliative care would be appropriate.[17]

Table 31.2 shows the number of deaths within a population during 1 year for the most common causes, and Tables 31.3 and 31.4 show the likely prevalence of problems for patients with cancer or patients with progressive nonmalignant diseases. Any region or country would have their own actual data on the number of deaths, and it would be better to use these.

These prevalence data can then be contrasted with the numbers who are receiving different services in an area. For example, a needs assessment for the London region showed that in the over 7 million population, there were 15,780 deaths from cancer each year, and of these, it is estimated that 13,260 have pain. A total of 12,200 patients received hospital support each each year, and 11,700 home palliative care,[5] suggesting that there may be a reasonable but incomplete coverage (see Figure 31.6). However, the proportion of noncancer patients with symptoms and who received services was much smaller (see Figures 31.6 and 31.7), suggesting a need to develop services for these groups of patients.

Rosenwax et al. developed three estimates of the potential palliative care population, minimal, mid-range, and maximal, through focus groups, interviews, and the literature.[17,18] The minimal estimate was based on the underlying cause of death, with a restricted list, the mid-range incorporated hospital admission data, while the maximal estimate included all deaths except poisoning, injury, and maternal, neonatal, or perinatal deaths. These estimates were applied to the cohort of people who died in Western Australia between July 1, 2000 and December 31, 2002, by linking death records with hospital morbidity data through

Table 31.3   *Cancer patients: Prevalence of problems (per 1,000,000 population, developing country context[17])*

Symptom	% with symptom in last year of life*	Estimated number in each year
Pain	84	2357
Trouble with breathing	47	1318
Vomiting or feeling sick	51	1431
Sleeplessness	51	1431
Mental confusion	33	926
Depression	38	1065
Loss of appetite	71	1992
Constipation	47	1318
Bedsores	28	785
Loss of bladder control	37	1038
Loss of bowel control	25	701
Unpleasant smell	19	533
Severe family anxiety/worries**	33	930
Severe patient anxiety/worries**	25	700
Total deaths from cancer		2805

Note: Patients usually have several symptoms.

*Symptoms as per Cartwright and Seale study,[36,37] based on a random sample of deaths and using the reports of bereaved carers.

**Anxiety as per Field et al.,[38] Bennett et al.,[39] Higginson et al.,[40] Addington Hall et al.[41]

Table 31.4   *Patients with progressive nonmalignant disease: Prevalence of problems (per 1,000,000 population, developing country context[17])*

Symptom	% with symptom in last year of life*	Estimated number in each year
Pain	67	4599
Trouble with breathing	49	3363
Vomiting or feeling sick	27	1853
Sleeplessness	36	2471
Mental confusion	38	2608
Depression	36	2471
Loss of appetite	38	2608
Constipation	32	2196
Bedsores	14	961
Loss of bladder control	33	2265
Loss of bowel control	22	1510
Unpleasant smell	13	892
Severe family anxiety/worries**	33	2200
Severe patient anxiety/worries**	25	1600
Total deaths from other causes, excluding accidents, injury, and suicide, and causes very unlikely to have a palliative period		6864

Note: Patients usually have several symptoms.

*As per Cartwright and Seale study,[36,37] based on a random sample of deaths and using the reports of bereaved carers.

**Anxiety as per Field et al.,[38] Bennett et al.,[39] Higginson et al.,[40] Addington Hall et al.[41]

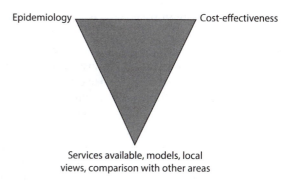

Figure 31.6   *The three main components of the "epidemiologically based" approach.*

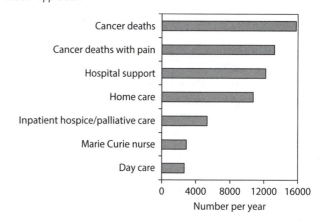

Figure 31.7   *Example 1 from Palliative Care for Londoners, 2001. Estimated yearly numbers of cancer deaths, cancer deaths with pain, and patients with cancer who receive different services in the London region. (Redrawn with permission from Higginson, I., Palliative Care for Londoners, Department of Palliative Care and Policy, London, U.K., 2001.[43])*

the Western Australian Data Linkage System. Rosenwax et al.'s estimate suggested that between 0.28% and 0.50% of people in the Western Australian population in any 1 year could potentially benefit from palliative care, many of whom die from conditions other than neoplasms. While neoplasms accounted for 59.5% of all underlying causes of deaths in the minimal estimate, heart failure (21.0%), renal failure (9.8%), chronic obstructive pulmonary disease (9.6%), Alzheimer's disease (4.0%), liver failure (3.2%), Parkinson's disease (1.3%), motor neurone disease (0.9%), HIV/AIDS (<0.01%), and Huntington's disease (<0.01%) accounted for other conditions in this estimate.[18,19]

Gomez-Bapiste et al. review the current causes of death. They conclude that in middle- to high-income countries, more than 75% of the population will die from chronic progressive diseases, and therefore, this should form the basis of the needs assessment. They argue that clinical status deteriorates progressively with frequent crises of needs, high social impact, and high use of costly healthcare resources. They argue that the challenges are to promote early and shared interventions, extended to all patients in need, in all settings of the social care and healthcare systems, to design and develop palliative care programs with a public health perspective.[20]

Murtagh et al. established an expert panel review of the three main approaches.[16] This identified changing practice (e.g., extension of palliative care to more noncancer conditions), changing patterns of hospital/home care and multiple, rather than single, causes of death as important. (Murtagh et al. therefore refined methods [using updated ICD-10 causes of death, underlying/contributory causes, and hospital use] to estimate the need for palliative care and developed an improved approach.)

A key change is that the ICD 10 codes can be more clearly specified. These are as outlined later, which expanded those used by both Higginson and Rosenwax, with the exception of Rosenwax's most extensive approach—which was all causes of death except poisoning, injury, and maternal, neonatal or perinatal deaths. Murtagh et al.'s proposed diseases to include were as follows:

- Malignant neoplasm C00–C97
- Heart disease, including cerebrovascular disease I00–I52, I60–I69
- Renal disease N17, N18, N28, I12, I13
- Liver disease K70–K77
- Respiratory disease J06–J18, J20–J22, J40–J47 & J96
- Neurodegenerative disease G10, G20, G35, G122, G903, G231
- Alzheimer's, dementia and senility F01, F03, G30, R54
- HIV/AIDS B20–B24

However, limiting those included to only these underlying causes of death may miss some who need palliative care. Therefore, the group tested applying not only underlying cause of death, but any mention of these conditions as contributing to the death. When only underlying cause of death was used, this suggested that a minimum of 63.03% (95% confidence interval = 62.95%–63.11%) of all deaths needed palliative care. However, if any mention was included, the data more closely reflected levels of need as suggested by hospital activity in the last months of life (as in the model developed by Rosenwax et al., but without needing this level of information). Simply including any death with these conditions as a primary or contributory cause of death gave lower and upper mid-range estimates between 69.10% (95% confidence interval = 69.02%–69.17%) and 81.87% (95% confidence interval = 81.81%–81.93%).

It seems therefore that simple death registration data using both underlying and contributory causes can give reliable estimates of the population-based need for palliative care, without needing symptom or hospital activity data. In high-income countries, 69%–82% of those who die need palliative care.[16] This has the advantage of not requiring data linkage, from hospital activity, an issue which proved problematic when attempting to use the Australian method of needs assessment in Canada. A further question exists as to whether people with these conditions would want palliative care. But the Australian survey suggested that less than 10% (86/1069) of people would not want palliative care services.[14]

INCORPORATING THE EVIDENCE BASE AND OTHER VIEWS

In addition to the data on prevalence of symptoms, an epidemiologically based needs assessment includes data on the effectiveness of different models of palliative care. Rather than attempt

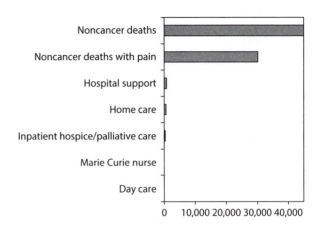

Figure 31.8 *Example 2 from Palliative Care for Londoners, 2001. Estimated yearly numbers of noncancer deaths, noncancer deaths with pain, and noncancer patients who receive different services in the London region. (Redrawn with permission from Higginson, I.,* Palliative Care for Londoners, *Department of Palliative Care and Policy, London, U.K., 2001.[43])*

new systematic literature reviews, a variety of high-quality systematic reviews and meta-analyses are available.[21–31] These show that specialist palliative care has benefits, particularly in terms of pain and symptom control and patient and carer satisfaction.[31,32] However, most evidence exists for specialist home care, and for inpatient palliative care, either with specialist beds in a freestanding unit or hospice, and/or advisory hospital teams, seeing patients on all wards, see Figure 31.8.[20] Other components of palliative care, including day care, outpatient services, and hospice at home, have not yet been well evaluated. This evidence has now been used in several countries to plan for services, and some evidence sources are available on the internet for free download for any group wishing to use it.[20,29] However, much of the evidence is drawn from developing countries and the evidence base in Africa and some other countries is now emerging.[33]

Gaps identified between the epidemiological information on need and the services currently provided can then be appraised against the evidence and any comparative or corporate data. The gaps may also suggest lines of enquiry in a survey of patient, carer, or professional views—for example, would they prefer more home care, hospital support or inpatient care developed. This then suggests options for the future development of palliative care services.

LIMITATIONS OF NEEDS ASSESSMENT

Although the approach provides a useful model for examining health needs, it is based on assumptions that limit its conclusions:

1. The overlapping circles of need, demand, and supply shown in Figure 31.1 imply that if only need, demand, and supply can be lined up, then need and demand will be satisfied by supply. If demand and need are larger than supply, they cannot be met completely, even if improved alignment is

of value. A needs assessment, where the supply of palliative care is limited, will lead to a demand for more resources, and health planners may not be prepared for this.

2. The data available to undertake the needs assessment are often limited. Epidemiological studies have often been more concerned with the etiology of diseases than the scope for benefit or need for services. For this reason, most of the epidemiological data are reliant on estimates from death registrations, and estimates of the prevalence of symptoms in selected populations. Death registrations may not be available and can be inaccurate, especially among older people, where there may also be multiple causes of death. Such data do not take account of the trajectory of illness and the time period that services are needed for. Thus, those undertaking the needs assessment must take these limitations into account when presenting the data.

3. Effectiveness and cost-effectiveness studies may be carried out in communities different from that where the service is concerned. For example, in palliative care, the well-designed randomized control trials occurred in the United States and not the United Kingdom. Thus, methods of needs assessment are needed for developing contexts and require some further development.

4. Effectiveness and cost-effectiveness are key components in an epidemiological approach. However, humanity, equity, acceptability, appropriateness, and accessibility are also essential in determining the quality of the service. However, it could be argued that without efficacy and effectiveness, these are of no value (one would not want a humane service which had no effectiveness or was even harmful). Nevertheless, these are important components of care and given that effectiveness data are often limited, excluding such components weakens the approach. A corporate assessment is often very useful in exploring aspects of appropriateness, acceptability, and humanity, while a comparative assessment may throw light on accessibility. These approaches can be combined with the epidemiologically based needs assessment.

5. The model of needs assessment for palliative care is currently focused more on adults and on using patients as the main determinant. More work is needed to develop needs assessments for children—although work is underway in Wales.[34] Equally, assessment of how well families are supported should be considered.[35]

CONCLUSIONS AND FUTURE ISSUES

The epidemiologically based needs assessment approach to planning palliative care services has emerged in the last decade. It has three main components: incidence and/or prevalence of a disease or condition, effectiveness and cost-effectiveness of services, and review of existing services. It can be combined with corporate and comparative approaches to needs assessment. This information is combined and culminates in recommendations for particular procedures or interventions based on

standard criteria for the quality of evidence and an appraisal of alternative models of care.

Because the approach is time-consuming and subject to limitations, some guidance is available, especially on the effectiveness of models of care and on incidence and prevalence guidance. However, there is a need to further develop approaches to needs assessment in developing countries and those where there is little palliative care. Ideally, a template is needed, which can be applied to different settings. Presentation of the data to local groups (statutory and voluntary and at public meetings) can help to facilitate discussion about where services should develop in the future.

Key learning points

- There are four main elements of needs—felt need, expressed need, normative need, and comparative need.

- Need, supply, and demand for services may not overlap.

- There are three common approaches to needs assessment, all of which have been used in palliative care.

- A comparative needs assessment determines need by a comparison of supply between areas.

- A corporate needs assessment determines needs by taking views from local stakeholders.

- Both of these approaches can tend to confirm the status quo, rather than identify groups who are missing out on care more fundamentally.

- An epidemiological approach to needs assessment examines the incidence and prevalence of problems, the effectiveness of services, and the services available and views on these.

- The most recent epidemiological approaches to needs assessment are based on underlying and contributing cause of death and suggest that between 69% and 82% of the population need palliative care.

- The epidemiological approach can be combined with the comparative and corporate approach.

REFERENCES

1 Clark D, Malson H, Small N, Daniel T, Mallett K. Needs assessment and palliative care: The views of providers. *J Public Health Med* 1997; 19:437–442.

2 Higginson IJ, Hart S, Koffman J, Selman L, Harding R. Needs assessments in palliative care: An appraisal of definitions and approaches used. *J Pain Symptom Manage* 2007; 33(5):500–505.

3 Osse BH, Vernooij MJ, Schade E, Grol RP. Towards a new clinical tool for needs assessment in the palliative care of cancer patients: The PNPC instrument. *J Pain Symptom Manage* 2004; 28(4):329–341.

4 Bradshaw JS. A taxonomy of social need. In: McLachlan G, ed. *Problems and Progress in Medical Care: Essays on Current Research.* Seventh series edn. Oxford, U.K.: Oxford University Press; 1972; 72–82.

5   Zalenski RJ, Raspa R. Maslow's hierarchy of needs: A framework for achieving human potential in hospice. *J Palliat Med* 2006; 9(5):1120–1127.

6   McCarthy M. *Epidemiology and Policies for Health Planning*. London, U.K.: King Edward's Hospital Fund for London; 1982.

7   Stevens A, Raftery J. Health care needs assessment. In: Stevens A, Raftery J, eds. *The Epidemiologically-Based Needs Assessment Reviews*. Oxford, U.K.: Radcliffe Medical Press; 1994, pp. 11–30.

8   Asadi-Lari M, Gray D. Health needs assessment tools: Progress and potential. *Int J Technol Assess Health Care* 2005; 21:288–297.

9   Shipman C, Addington-Hall J, Richardson A, Burt J, Ream E, Beynon T. Palliative care services in England: A survey of district nurses' views. *Br J Commun Nurs* 2005; 10(8):381–386.

10 Shirai Y, Kawa M, Miyashita M, Kazuma K. Nurses' perception of adequacy of care for leukemia patients with distress during the incurable phase and related factors. *Leukemia Res* 2005; 29:293–300.

11 Wotton K, Borbasi S, Redden M. When all else has failed: Nurses' perception of factors influencing palliative care for patients with end-stage heart failure. *J Cardiovasc Nurs* 2005; 20:18–25.

12 Skilbeck J, Mott L, Page H, Smith D, Hjelmeland-Ahmedzai S, Clark D. Palliative care in chronic obstructive airways disease: A needs assessment. *Palliat Med* 1998; 12:245–254.

13 Kwekkeboom K. A community needs assessment for palliative care services from a hospice organization. *J Palliat Med* 2005; 8:817–826.

14 Currow DC, Abernethy AP, Fazekas BS. Specialist palliative care needs of whole populations: A feasibility study using a novel approach. *Palliat Med* 2004; 18:239–247.

15 Knox D. *Epidemiology in Health Care Plannning*. Oxford, U.K.: Oxford University Press; 1979.

16 Murtagh FE, Bausewein C, Verne J, Groeneveld EI, Kaloki YE, Higginson IJ. How many people need palliative care? A study developing and comparing methods for population-based estimates. *Palliat Med* 2014 Jan; 28(1):49–58.

17 Higginson IJ. *Health Care Needs Assessment: Palliative and Terminal Care*. Stevens A and Raftery J (Series Eds). Health Care Needs Assessment. 2nd Series. Oxford: Radcliffe Medical Press. 1997.

18 McNamara B, Rosenwax LK, Holman CD. A method for defining and estimating the palliative care population. *J Pain Symptom Manage* 2006; 32(1):5–12.

19 Rosenwax LK, McNamara B, Blackmore AM, Holman CD. Estimating the size of a potential palliative care population. *Palliat Med* 2005; 19(7):556–562.

20 Gómez-Batiste X, Martínez-Muñoz M, Blay C, Espinosa J, Contel JC, Ledesma A. Identifying needs and improving palliative care of chronically ill patients: A community-oriented, population-based, public-health approach. *Curr Opin Support Palliat Care* 2012; 6(3):371–378.

21 Gysels M, Higginson IJ. *Improving Supportive and Palliative Care for Adults with Cancer: Research Evidence*. London, U.K.: National Institute of Clinical Excellence; 2004.

22 Davies E, Higginson IJ. Communication, information and support for adults with malignant cerebral glioma: A systematic literature review. *Support Care Cancer* 2003; 11:21–29.

23 Harding R, Higginson IJ. What is the best way to help caregivers in cancer and palliative care? A systematic review of interventions and their effectiveness. *Palliat Med* 2003; 17:63–74.

24 Finlay IG, Higginson IJ, Goodwin DM, Cook AM, Edwards AGK, Hood K. et al. Palliative care in hospital, hospice, at home: Results from a systematic review. *Ann Oncol* 2002; 13:257–264.

25 Goodwin DM, Higginson IJ, Edwards AGK, Finlay IG, Cook AM, Douglas H-R et al. An evaluation of systematic reviews of palliative care services. *J Palliat Care* 2002; 18:77–83.

26 Davies E, Higginson IJ. Systematic review of specialist palliative day care for adults with cancer. *Support Care Cancer* 2005; 13:607–627.

27 Gruenewald DA, Higginson IJ, Vivat B, Edmonds P, Burman RE. Quality of life measures for the palliative care of people severely affected by multiple sclerosis: A systematic review. *Multiple Sclerosis* 2004; 10:690–704.

28 Gysels M, Richardson A, Higginson IJ. Communication training for health professionals who care for patients with cancer: A systematic review of effectiveness. *Support Care Cancer* 12(10):692–700.

29 Gysels M, Higginson IJ, Richardson A. Communication training for health professionals who care for patients with cancer: A systematic review of training methods. *Support Care Cancer* 2005; 13:356–366.

30 Lorenz KA, Asch SM, Yano EM, Wang M, Rubenstein LV. Comparing strategies for United States veterans' mortality ascertainment. *Population Health Metrics* 2005; 3:2.

31 Harding R, Easterbrook PE, Karus D, Raveis VH, Higginson IJ, Marconi K. Does palliative care improve outcomes for patients with HIV/AIDS? A systematic review of the evidence. *Sex Transm Infect* 2004; 81(5):14.

32 Higginson IJ, Finlay IG, Goodwin DM, Hood K, Edwards AGK, Cook A et al. Is there evidence that palliative care teams alter end-of-life experiences of patients and their caregivers? *J Pain Symptom Manage* 2003; 25:150–168.

33 Hearn J, Feuer D, Higginson I, Sheldon T. Systematic reviews. *Palliat Med* 1999; 13:75–80.

34 Harding R, Higginson IJ. Palliative care in sub-Saharan Africa. *Lancet* 2005; 365:1971–1978.

35 Noyes J, Edwards RT, Hastings RP, Hain R, Totsika V, Bennett V et al. Evidence-based planning and costing palliative care services for children: Novel multi-method epidemiological and economic exemplar. *BMC Palliat Care* 2013; 12(1):18.

36 Ross L, Petersen MA, Johnsen AT, Lundstrom LH, Lund L, Groenvold M. Using mixed methods to assess how cancer patients' needs in relation to their relatives are met in the Danish health care system: A report from the population-based study "The Cancer Patient's World". *Support Care Cancer* 2012; 20(12):3211–3220.

37 Cartwright A. Changes in life and care in the year before death 1969–1987. *J Public Health Med* 1991; 13(2):81–87.

38 Seale C. A comparison of hospice and conventional care. *Soc Sci Med* 1991; 32:147–152.

39 Field D, Douglas C, Jagger C, Dand P. Terminal illness: Views of patients and their lay carers. *Palliat Med* 1995; 9(1):45–54.

40 Bennett M, Corcoran G. The impact on community palliative care services of a hospital palliative care team. *Palliat Med* 1994; 8(3):237–244.

41 Higginson IJ, Wade AM, McCarthy M. Effectiveness of two palliative support teams. *J Public Health Med* 1992; 14(1):50–56.

42 Addington-Hall JM, MacDonald L, Anderson H, Freeling P. Dying from cancer: The views of bereaved family and the friends about the experiences of terminally ill patients. *Palliat Med* 1991; 5:207–214.

43 Higginson I. *Palliative Care for Londoners*. London, U.K.: Department of Palliative Care and Policy, 2001.

32

Palliative care consult team

RACHEL M. ADAMS, ALEXIE CINTRON, DIANE E. MEIER

INTRODUCTION

Many people with chronic and debilitating diseases are living longer lives, but 9150 spend substantial amounts of time in the hospital, often needs unmet by the traditional health care system. A large body of evidence demonstrates inadequately treated pain and other symptoms,[1,2] significant psychological distress experienced by patients and their families,[3] and lack of communication with doctors about achievable goals for care.[1] While many wish to die with dignity at home, studies have found that the majority of people die, at great cost, in acute care centers.[5,6] Health care systems facing rising and unsustainable costs for the care of the sickest and most vulnerable patients.[4] Patients with serious illness need access to expert symptom management, communication and decision-making support, and care coordination. The palliative care consultation team (PCCT) aims to improve hospital care for patients living with serious illness.

Palliative care and hospice

Palliative care (PC) is an interdisciplinary medical specialty focused on relieving suffering and improving quality of life for patients with serious illnesses and their families.[7] In the United States, hospice is a type of PC supported by a federal insurance benefit, which is limited to persons at the end of life with a prognosis of 6 months or less with the caveat that they agree to forego curative or life-prolonging treatments. Hospice exists as a U.S. government–sponsored benefit under the Medicare and Medicaid and private insurance programs.[8] Unlike hospice, palliative care is accessible to patients at every stage of illness independent of life expectancy. Ideally, it is offered at the time of diagnosis and in conjunction with other appropriate medical treatments, including those given with the intent of cure.

PC is now defined by primary, secondary, and tertiary levels of focus. Primary-level PC should be within the domain of all treating clinicians and should address pain and symptom management as well as communication about care priorities and advance directives. Trained PC specialists provide secondary PC for more complex cases. Tertiary PC includes research and teaching in addition to specialist level care.[9,10] The development and implementation of PC practices has been proven to effectively elicit and identify patient wishes and also to effectively implement changes in the care plan directed by these wishes. Research, which will be further discussed later in this chapter, has shown that PC improves patient satisfaction, symptom management, and coordination of care and helps decrease the need for emergency hospitalization and emergency department (ED) visits. In some populations, PC and hospice may also be associated with life prolongation.[11–15] Reduced health care spending is an epiphenomenon, not the intent, of the better quality of care associated with PC.

Palliative care internationally

International availability of PC services in hospitals has grown rapidly over the last decade, but access is widely variable across regions. Currently, 58% of countries in the world offer some form of PC, but numbers of hospice–PC services in a country may range anywhere from 2 in Cambodia to 686 in Japan by estimates from 2011. PC is more developed in many parts of Western Europe and North America but is still patchy in the degree of its dispersion in these regions. There is a notable palliative presence in Uganda, but it is less prevalent in other regions of Africa. In some countries, including Canada, England, and, to some degree, the United States, PC has increasingly been integrated into health care delivery models.[16]

In nearly all regions, there remains a palliative work force shortage and need for further program development.

Models of delivery

A fully integrated PC program includes an inpatient consultation service, a geographic inpatient unit, and an outpatient practice. Historically, PC has largely been limited to two types of delivery models: home hospice care for dying patients and hospital-based PC consultation for inpatients with serious illness. Evolving hospital PC programs structure a variety of personnel resources, including medical and nursing specialists, social workers, and chaplains, into coordinated teams that function not only within consult services but also increasingly in dedicated inpatient units, outpatient clinics, or other delivery systems and community partnerships appropriate to each institution's needs.[7] As the model of hospital-based PC spreads internationally, studies continue to show that it has applicability across diverse cultural settings.[17,18]

PC need persists in community settings, including outpatient, nursing home, and home-based PC. Without access to community PC, patients who are not candidates for hospice must resort to hospitalization when family caregivers are overwhelmed with the burden of care or when they have uncontrolled symptoms like pain, nausea, and vomiting. In the U.S., development of PC in the community setting has been limited by lack of reimbursement, but this may change with recent changes in health care payment models.[19]

Delivery and payment model changes

Many health systems identify PC implementation as a way to improve quality care metrics. In many countries, hospitals increasingly recognize PC as a needed and beneficial service from the perspectives of both quality of care and cost.[9] PC is positioned to become standard of care for patients with high symptom burden related to chronic life-threatening illness.

Palliative care consult team

The in-hospital PCCT constitutes the dominant form of service delivery outside of hospices and home care. Because the PCCT has the ability to reach patients throughout the hospital and allows outreach to other clinicians, it serves as a natural first point of program development.[20] This chapter will focus primarily on how the inpatient PCCT works; how it can benefit patients, families, and clinicians, and what strategies can be adopted for starting a new palliative consult team or expanding an existing one. The team's goal is to assess the physical, psychological, social, spiritual, and cultural needs of patients with serious illness. How is a team structured? Why do providers request a PC consultation? What strategies have been employed to improve access to PC services? What is the effectiveness of hospital PC teams?

STRUCTURE OF THE PALLIATIVE CONSULT TEAM

As described in the National Consensus Project Clinical Practice Guidelines to Quality Palliative Care (http://www.nationalconsensusproject.org), PC is optimally delivered through an interdisciplinary group consisting of at least a physician, a nurse, and a social worker with appropriate training and education in PC.[21] Many programs conduct a daily interdisciplinary team meeting where each patient's case is discussed from multiple team member perspectives.[22] Due to fiscal constraints, especially in smaller hospitals, the full team model may be difficult to achieve, and teams vary in size and personnel depending on an institution's capacity and needs. Some programs have a solo practitioner model run by a physician or advanced nurse practitioner who works in conjunction with the hospital's social work and pastoral care departments to provide the necessary services.[23] Larger programs may incorporate additional disciplines, including clergy, rehabilitation professionals, psychologists, and psychiatrists. Some programs are also expanding to incorporate massage, art, and music therapists, who offer valuable nonmedical treatment options.

Palliative team members should have skills and training in complex medical evaluation, pain and symptom management, professional-to-patient and family and professional-to-professional communication, addressing difficult decisions about goals of care, sophisticated discharge planning, and bereavement support.[24]

Reasons for PC consultation

Most institutions report pain and symptom management or help in clarifying goals for care as the primary reason for PC consultation.[24–29] Other common consultation triggers include neuropsychiatric issues (delirium, confusion, and sedation), constipation, dyspnea, and nausea and vomiting.[25,26] Consultation may also be requested for discharge planning, organization of care plans, and end-of-life discussions. The PCCT provides psychosocial, spiritual, and bereavement support.[24] PC consultation usually makes three to four recommendations per patient,[27,28] and these recommendations are usually implemented.[28,29]

Teams may have difficulty eliciting the reason for the consultation from the primary (or generalist) team, which can occur when palliative support is needed for communication difficulties, complex family and professional dynamics, and assistance in coordination of care. Dealing with many care providers can be confusing for patients and their families. The PCCT may be called upon to ease frustration, rebuild patient and family trust in the health care team, and expedite care by facilitating conversations among provider team members.

Strategies for increasing PC consultations

PC needs often go unrecognized and unaddressed in all care settings. The number of problems identified by the PCCT tends to be higher than those initially reported by the primary care provider.[25,27] Research also showed that consults typically occur late in a disease process and that patients would benefit from earlier PC involvement.[30,31]

Various strategies can be employed to increase numbers and timing of palliative consults. Historically, palliative consults could only be ordered by attending physicians, but to

Table 32.1 *Criteria for a palliative care assessment*

A Potentially life-limiting or life-threatening condition and...

Primary criteria

- The surprise question: You would not be surprised if the patient died within 12 months
- Frequent admissions (e.g., more than one admission for the same condition within several months)
- *Difficult to control physical or psychological symptoms*: Moderate-severe symptoms for more than 24–48 h
- *Complex care requirements*: Functional dependency, complex home support for ventilator/antibiotics/feedings, family inability to meet needs
- *Functional decline*: Feeding intolerance, weight loss, or failure to thrive
- *Disagreements or uncertainty among the patient, staff, and/or family concerning the following*: Major medical treatment decisions, resuscitation preferences, use of nonoral feeding, or hydration

Source: Modified from Weissman, D.E. and Meier, D.E., *J. Palliat. Med.*, 14(1), 17, 2011.

increase outreach, many institutions now encourage patients, families, or any other member of the medical team who identifies a palliative need to initiate a consult, seeking the attending physician's assent.[7] Some hospitals trigger consults automatically when a patient meets checklist criteria. Checklists that identify criteria indicating need for a palliative assessment are included in guidelines from the Center to Advance Palliative Care (CAPC). Palliative consults may be triggered based on the type of disease, stage of disease, uncontrolled symptoms, functional impairment, caregiver exhaustion, repeated hospitalizations or ED visits, or psychosocial needs (Table 32.1).[31] The CAPC-IPAL website (http://www.capc.org/ipal/project) describes checklists to trigger PC involvement in particular settings, including intensive care units and emergency rooms, and for high-risk patient populations, including patients with advanced cancer.[32]

Budgeting time, resources, and billing

The consultation process is time-consuming. One study reported that the median time spent in consultation was 60 minutes by the PC fellow and 30 minutes by the PC attending physician.[33] Another study reported that an initial consult of over 2 hours was common.[29] Moreover, the total time spent in consultation and follow up—including review of the medical record, interviewing and examining the patient, meeting with the family, and having discussions with the attending physician, nurse, social worker, or other member of the primary care team—often exceeds 5 hours.[29] The process can therefore take several visits over several days. Most consultation time is spent eliciting and giving information and providing counseling.[28,34] Because the work is so time-intensive, many programs find that billing for time is the most profitable.[35]

Case load

Recommendations from established programs suggest that a maximum caseload for an individual palliative physician or advanced practice nurse would consist of no more than four *new* cases per day and an average daily census of no more than 15 patients. Service volumes above these thresholds are too high to allow the intensive and repeated communication with patients, families, and health professionals that are necessary to improve care quality for complex and vulnerable patients.

CONSULTATION PROCESS

The goal of a consult may vary depending on the needs of the patient and the concerns of the consulting team. General guidelines for a PC assessment may begin with identifying distressing symptoms, social and spiritual concerns, assessment of the patient's and the family's understanding of a disease, and identification of person-centered goals of care (Table 32.2). Tools have been developed to aid teams in their work, for example, the support team assessment schedule (STAS), used widely by services to aid the assessment and measurement of the outcomes of hospital-based teams.[36–40] A primary (generalist) palliative assessment should be achievable for any physician or other health care professional, but when symptoms are

Table 32.2 *Primary (generalist) palliative care assessment components*

Pain/symptom assessment
- Are there distressing physical or psychological symptoms?

Social/spiritual assessment
- Are there significant social or spiritual concerns affecting daily life?

Understanding of illness/prognosis and treatment options
- Does the patient/family/surrogate understand the current illness, prognostic trajectory, and treatment options?

Identification of patient-centered goals of care
- What are the goals of care as identified by the patient/family/surrogate?
- Are treatment options matched to informed patient-centered goals?
- Has the patient participated in an advanced care planning process?
- Has the patient completed an advance care planning document?

Transition of care postdischarge
- What are the key considerations for a safe and sustainable transition from one setting to another?

Source: Adapted from Weissman, D.E. and Meier, D.E., *J. Palliat. Med.*, 14(1), 17, 2011.

difficult to treat or psychosocial issues are very complex, a formal consultation is recommended. The concepts detailed in this section are practiced in many centers, and a new service may consider modeling itself after a preexisting one.[41]

Assessing and treating symptoms

When patients are uncomfortable, the first priority for a palliative consult is to diagnose the cause of the symptoms and to prescribe appropriate treatment. Studies show that involvement of a PCCT can improve symptoms including pain, fatigue, dyspnea, nausea and vomiting, and constipation for patients suffering from advanced disease.[22,40,42]

In treating a patient's symptoms, validated assessment instruments should be used whenever possible as they serve two important functions:

1 Track symptom changes to guide clinical approach
2 Provide metrics of program quality for the team, for hospital administration, and/or for use in research

Commonly used scales include the Memorial Symptom Assessment Scale and the Edmonton Symptom Assessment Scale, both of which are available on the National Palliative Care Research Center website (www.npcrc.org).[43] Versions of these scales may be incorporated into a progress note template. As pain is one of the most frequent palliative symptoms, pain management pocket cards are a useful tool for clinicians in assessing pain and selecting appropriate analgesics. They also serve to help educate other clinicians and students about pain management. Details of pain management are shown in Part 8.

Establishing goals of care and family meetings

Discussions of goals of care may cover a broad range of topics including decisions about treatment options and their pros and cons, advance care planning in preparation for future likely decisions, executing a Do Not Resuscitate (DNR) order, assignment of health care proxy (HCP), disposition planning, or any other quality of life issue for the patient/family. Primary teams may also request assistance for communicating difficult news to the patient and family. Many patients wish to involve family in these discussions. Often, goals of care discussions require a family meeting with participants including the patient, the patient's family, representatives of the PCCT, and the primary teams. Depending on the topic of the meeting, relevant participants may also include representatives from other medical consultation services, nursing, social work, and/or chaplaincy. PCCT has been shown to effectively solicit goals of care in as many as 85% of patients seen. The most commonly cited goals of care were

- Improved symptom control
- Return home
- Receipt of hospice care
- No further hospital admissions
- A comfortable death[33]

PCCTs have also been effective in increasing discussions of advance directives, including discussion about a DNR order[15,28,33] and designation of an HCP.[28]

Any discussion of goals of care should begin by eliciting the patient's and family's understanding of the disease and its treatment as well as their opinions about what they hope to achieve through medical care, what matters most to them, and what their perspective is on an acceptable quality of life for the patient. It is critical to determine the patient's or family's desire for information, before discussing prognosis, or treatment options. Some prefer to defer decision-making to a family member, clergy, or a physician and may not wish to know the truth or the details about an illness. Those who want to know will tell you so. While this type of decision varies person to person, evidence does suggest that many people do want to know their prognosis.[44] Surrogate decision makers, such as health care proxies or other legal representatives, are encouraged to make decisions according to their understanding of what the patient himself or herself would want if they were able to decide. With the patient's permission, the team will involve family and elicit their understanding of the disease and its treatment and provide support and education about the patient's distress and symptom management, practical needs, and plans for the future. An appropriate plan of care and discharge plan should take into account family support systems, including their physical, emotional, and financial resources, and should be consistent with the established goals of care. A short video on 10 key steps to effective communication in PC is available at www.capc.org/capc-resources/capc-videos.

Clear communication facilitated by palliative teams not only clarifies patients' wishes but also modifies the care plans to better align with what matters most to the patient and family.

PC consultation outcomes:

PC consultation has been show to decrease

- Use of acute care beds[45]
- Length of intensive care unit (ICU) stays[46]
- ICU admissions[15]
- Hospital readmissions[47]

Significantly, patients have decreased length of ICU stay without significant difference in mortality or length of hospital stay.[48] When a PC team is involved, there is decreased use of nonbeneficial treatments in the ICU.[46]

Facilitating communication among providers

Throughout the consultation process, the PCCT maintains a close working relationship with the primary care team. This begins with good communication regarding the reason for requesting the consultation in the first place, the outcomes of the PCCT assessment, and recommendations made, paying particular attention to responsiveness to the original reasons for the consultation. A concerted effort should be made to establish personal contact in person or by telephone with the primary service rather than rely solely on communication by notes in the medical chart. While the primary care service generally decides whether or not to implement the consult team's recommendations, the PCCT can seek permission from the primary service to implement certain interventions promptly in order to avoid symptom distress from delays in communication.[28] The consult team should encourage participation from the primary service at family meetings (especially important in teaching hospitals) and should educate all staff on the team regarding the particular aspects of the patient's management and care plan.

The PCCT may also need to play a role in coordinating communication among multiple providers, in an effort to decrease fragmentation of care and conflicting understanding about the goals of such care. In addition to discussions with the primary team, discussions with other consultants are also beneficial in an effort to align and assure consistent decisions, messages, and communication from all providers to each other and to the patient and family. Interaction with, and engagement of, nursing and support staff is key to the success of the consult. The consult team should encourage participation from nursing and support staff in the formulation of the patient's care plan, educate the nursing and support staff about PC management issues specific to their patient, and provide the staff with bedside support regarding difficult patient situations and treatment decisions.

Referrals to outpatient PC and hospice

At the time of discharge, PCCT care coordination and transition support may involve enrolling patients in outpatient or home-based PC, house call programs, certified home health agencies, long-term care and rehabilitation facilities, or, for those with a short (weeks to a few months) prognosis, hospice. Patients may first be introduced to PC in the inpatient setting, but ensuring that they have ongoing access to PC after discharge from the hospital is predicated on the availability of greater outpatient PC support. The United States has a robust model for home care of patients at the end of life in the form of hospice, but only patients with a prognosis of less than 6 months who are willing to forgo insurance coverage for life-prolonging treatment are hospice eligible. For the large number of persons with a serious chronic illness who are not predictably dying or are not dying soon, the gap in access to community-based PC is a major driver of unnecessary ED and hospital utilization.

Hence, a huge need remains for outpatient and community PC services based on need, not prognosis.[9] Many patients who are not eligible for or do not wish to enroll in hospice are symptomatic from their diseases and wish to avoid unnecessary hospitalization for predictable events such as pain crisis, which may be safely and effectively managed at home with the right support.[49] The health care system at large faces challenges in identifying patients at risk for readmission and implementing safeguards to prevent this occurrence. Some palliative programs have taken the initiative of hiring dedicated personnel to follow up with patients postdischarge.[50] A few home-based PC programs do exist and appear efficacious in improving the quality of care. A randomized trial of comparing home-based

PC with usual care showed improved satisfaction with care, reduction in emergency department visits, decreased risk of hospital admission at the end of life, and significantly lower costs of care.[51] In another study, this type of planning saved U.S.\$4855 over 6 months following discharge and improved patient and provider satisfaction scores without any change in mortality.[15]

IMPACT OF PALLIATIVE CARE CONSULT TEAM SUPPORT ON PATIENT SATISFACTION AND COST

Patient and family satisfaction

Patients who receive PCCT report increased satisfaction with their care experience [15] and so do their families.[52] Relatives of patients receiving PC consultation were more likely to report that doctors listened to them (100% versus 86%) and that they received the right amount of information regarding the patients' condition (100% versus 85%) and were informed as to how the patients' pain would be managed (100% versus 60%) compared with families not receiving PC.[28] PC improves families' perceptions of a patient's quality of care, and the earlier the PC is involved, the more pronounced the effect. Improved perception of care has been attributed to the emotional, psychosocial, and spiritual support provided by the PCCT.[53,54] While most of these studies are small, and the subject matter does not lend itself well to randomized controlled trials, in meta-analyses, involvement of PC does appear to have a beneficial impact for patients and families.[55,56]

Decreasing costs of care

The effect of streamlining care plans, identifying what patients and families want, and improving communication between care teams decreases inappropriate health care dollar spending. Cost reduction occurs when treatment plans align with the patient-oriented goals of care. Inpatient PC consultation has been shown to significantly decrease the cost of hospitalization by an average of U.S.\$2659 per patient per admission.[57] Currently, PC is estimated to affect approximately 1.5% of hospital discharges, saving 1.2 billion per year in hospital costs in the United States. PC is still reaching only a fraction of patients who could benefit. A study in Australia estimated that 35% of patients admitted to the hospital had palliative goals[58] and numbers were similar in a study in Norway.[59] In the United States, it is estimated that if capacity expanded to reach 6% of discharges, PC could potentially save over four billion dollars annually.[9,60]

RESOURCES FOR BUILDING A PC PROGRAM

PC programs that have been successful at developing funded interdisciplinary teams have done so by creating strong business cases that demonstrate significant improvement in both quality of care and cost savings to hospitals.[19] The CAPC (www.capc.org) has created a number of resources to help in the process of founding or expanding a PC program within the hospital infrastructure. CAPC's mission is to increase the availability of quality PC services in hospitals and other health care settings for people with serious illnesses, their families, and caregivers.

Developing a program requires a collection and analysis of metrics that define program success. Metrics provide important data about the impact of a program to ensure high quality care, and to demonstrate effectiveness necessary to ensure sustainability and growth. Quality outcomes are also vital for demonstrating the worth of the program to the hospital at large. Consensus statements from CAPC detail operational features for hospital palliative programs,[20] consult service metrics,[61] clinical care and customer satisfaction metrics,[62] and features that identify patients in need of palliative assessment.[31]

A good starting place for programs that are either new or looking to expand their services in the hospital is the CAPC publication, A *Guide to Building a Hospital-Based PC Program.* The guide outlines how to build a business case for a program, what administrative building blocks are needed, what metric to collect, and how to illustrate the relevance of PC for key audiences, including administrators, clinicians, patients and families, and philanthropic donors.[63]

ADDITIONAL RESOURCES

In addition to CAPC, a number of other U.S. organizations create guidelines for the U.S. delivery of PC, provide support for practitioners, and promote research and education. This section will provide a brief overview of the National Consensus Project for Quality Palliative Care, the American Academy for Hospice and Palliative Medicine (AAHPM), the Hospice and Palliative Nurses Association (HPNA), and the National Palliative Care Research Center (NPCRC).

The National Consensus Project for Quality Palliative Care (http://www.nationalconsensusproject.org) is a collaborative effort of five national PC organizations, with a mission of creating consensus guidelines for quality PC in the United States. As part of its mission, it encourages standardization of care structures and processes both within and across care settings in the interest of consistent quality, continuity, and reliability of care. In 2013, *the Clinical Practice Guidelines for Quality Palliative Care* was released in a third edition.[64]

AAHPM (http://www.aahpm.org) is the professional organization for approximately 5000 U.S. physicians specializing in hospice and palliative medicine. It is dedicated to advancing hospice and palliative medicine and improving the care of patients with life-threatening illness and plays a role in health policy advocacy. It regularly releases position statements on important PC topics and has helped define key palliative and hospice medicine issues. It offers a curriculum for physicians in the field including the UNIPAC textbooks. AAHPM hosts a wide range of special interest groups and a national annual scientific meeting.[65]

HPNA (http://www.hpna.org) is a professional organization for nurses specializing in hospice and palliative medicine. It offers educational materials and online materials for all levels of nursing in the field. Similar to AAHPM, HPNA is also committed to health care advocacy and lobby on behalf of palliative and hospice teams and patients and regularly develops position statements on important PC and hospice topics. It is an important source of support for palliative nursing research.[66] It hosts an annual conference associated with the AAHPM conference.

NPCRC (www.npcrc.org) was formed to develop the evidence base for clinical practice and models of care for the seriously ill. As part of its mission, it works to establish priorities for PC research, develop a new generation of successful researchers in PC, and coordinate and support studies focused on improving care for patients living with serious illness and their families.[67]

FUTURE DIRECTIONS FOR PC

Workforce shortages

While the spread of PC has expanded dramatically in the last 10 years, there are still many regions that lack PC services, and a PC workforce shortage persists in the United States and internationally. The need for PC is only growing in the United States with the growth and aging of the population. There is currently only one palliative physician for 1200 persons living with a serious or life-threatening illness.[68] PC fellowship training programs have increased in number but cannot produce enough physicians to meet the need. Expansion of the workforce requires additional training tracks for MDs and enhanced utilization of non-MD practitioners such as advanced practice nurses. Historically, the U.S. fee-for-service system has only provided physician and advanced practice nursing reimbursement, without support for other members of the interdisciplinary team. Finding ways to educate all clinicians in core PC competencies and lobbying for further reimbursement of non-MD clinicians are two ways in which the work force may expand.[69]

Reimbursement systems and development of community-based programs

The expansion of palliative support in the outpatient and home-based settings is predicated on changes in reimbursement models. Reimbursement systems have played a key role in how PC has developed in the United States and how it will continue to develop. Despite the lack of reimbursement for full team support, the hospital interdisciplinary team model has succeeded because it is a cost-saving intervention for hospitals. Hospitals are paid a lump sum for each admission according to admission diagnosis (diagnosis-related group payment), and PC involvement decreases costs, thereby increasing the hospital's profit margin. The same incentives have not traditionally existed in the outpatient setting. Recent changes in U.S. health care payment models, specifically the passage of the 2010 Patient Protection and Affordable Care Act, contain a number of provisions for fiscal and quality incentives that may prompt further development of community and home-based PC services. Under new payment models, hospitals are penalized for unnecessary readmissions and excess hospital mortality. New delivery and payment models such as accountable care organizations, patient-centered medical Homes, and bundled payment strategies place providers at varying levels of financial risk and create incentives to deliver the right care, as opposed to past incentives that rewarded volume, not quality. These changes may encourage generalists to offer primary PC and may also encourage the development of dedicated outpatient and home-based palliative programs. To ensure the ongoing growth of PC services in the new health care climate, further work will need to develop clinical and fiscal metrics of PC services to align with these new and rapidly spreading health care delivery and payment models.[19]

CONCLUSION

The PC consult team helps improve symptom management and quality of life for patients with serious illness and their families. The consult team has been the dominant model for palliative service delivery in hospitals. Through its success in supporting medical teams to develop care plans aligned with what matters most to patients and families, it has been proven to improve quality of care, leading to decreases in hospital and health system costs. PC is quickly becoming standard of care for patients with serious illness.

REFERENCES

1 SUPPORT Principal Investigators et al. A controlled trial to improve care for seriously ill hospitalized patients. The study to understand prognoses and preferences for outcomes and risks of treatments (SUPPORT). JAMA. 1995;274(20):1591–1598.
2 Desbiens NA, Wu AW. Pain and suffering in seriously ill hospitalized patients. J Am Geriatr Soc. 2000;48(5 Suppl):S183–S186.
3 Wright AA, Keating NL, Balboni TA, Matulonis UA, Block SD, Prigerson HG. Place of death: Correlations with quality of life of patients with cancer and predictors of bereaved caregivers' mental health. J Clin Oncol. 2010;28(29):4457–4464. doi: 10.1200/JCO.2009.26.3863; 10.1200/JCO.2009.26.3863.
4 Hoover DR, Crystal S, Kumar R, Sambamoorthi U, Cantor JC. Medical expenditures during the last year of life: Findings from the 1992–1996 medicare current beneficiary survey. Health Serv Res. 2002;37(6):1625–1642.
5 Gomes B, Calanzani N, Gysels M, Hall S, Higginson IJ. Heterogeneity and changes in preferences for dying at home: A systematic review. BMC Palliat Care. 2013;12:7-684X-12-7. doi: 10.1186/1472-684X-12-7; 10.1186/1472-684X-12-7.
6 Bruera E, Russell N, Sweeney C, Fisch M, Palmer JL. Place of death and its predictors for local patients registered at a comprehensive cancer center. J Clin Oncol. 2002;20(8):2127–2133.
7 Meier DE, Spragens LH, Sutton S. A Guide to Building a Hospital-Based Palliative Care Program. New York: Center to Advance Palliative Care; 2004.
8 Connor SR. U.S. hospice benefits. J Pain Symptom Manage. 2009;38(1):105–109. doi: 10.1016/j.jpainsymman.2009.04.012; 10.1016/j.jpainsymman.2009.04.012.
9 Meier DE. Increased access to palliative care and hospice services: Opportunities to improve value in health care. Milbank Q. 2011;89(3):343–380. doi: 10.1111/j.1468-0009.2011.00632.x; 10.1111/j.1468-0009.2011.00632.x.
10 von Gunten CF. Secondary and tertiary palliative care in U.S. hospitals. JAMA. 2002;287(7):875–881.
11 Temel JS, Greer JA, Muzikansky A et al. Early palliative care for patients with metastatic non-small-cell lung cancer. N Engl J Med. 2010;363(8):733–742. doi: 10.1056/NEJMoa1000678; 10.1056/NEJMoa1000678.
12 Connor SR. Development of hospice and palliative care in the United States. Omega (Westport). 2007;56(1):89–99.
13 Bakitas M, Lyons KD, Hegel MT et al. Effects of a palliative care intervention on clinical outcomes in patients with advanced cancer: The project ENABLE II randomized controlled trial. JAMA. 2009;302(7):741–749. doi: 10.1001/jama.2009.1198; 10.1001/jama.2009.1198.
14 Brumley R, Enguidanos S, Jamison P et al. Increased satisfaction with care and lower costs: Results of a randomized trial of in-home palliative care. J Am Geriatr Soc. 2007;55(7):993–1000. doi: 10.1111/j.1532-5415.2007.01234.x.
15 Gade G, Venohr I, Conner D et al. Impact of an inpatient palliative care team: A randomized control trial. J Palliat Med. 2008;11(2):180–190. doi: 10.1089/jpm.2007.0055; 10.1089/jpm.2007.0055.
16 Lynch T, Connor S, Clark D. Mapping levels of palliative care development: A global update. J Pain Symptom Manage. 2013;45(6):1094–1106. doi: 10.1016/j.jpainsymman.2012.05.011; 10.1016/j.jpainsymman.2012.05.011.
17 Kao CY, Hu WY, Chiu TY, Chen CY. Effects of the hospital-based palliative care team on the care for cancer patients: An evaluation study. Int J Nurs Stud. 2013. doi: 10.1016/j.ijnurstu.2013.05.008; 10.1016/j.ijnurstu.2013.05.008.
18 de Santiago A, Portela MA, Ramos L et al. A new palliative care consultation team at the oncology department of a university hospital: An assessment of initial efficiency and effectiveness. Support Care Cancer. 2012;20(9):2199–2203. doi: 10.1007/s00520-012-1476-x; 10.1007/s00520-012-1476-x.
19 Morrison RS. Models of palliative care delivery in the United States. Curr Opin Support Palliat Care. 2013;7(2):201–206. doi: 10.1097/SPC.0b013e32836103e5; 10.1097/SPC.0b013e32836103e5.
20 Weissman DE, Meier DE. Operational features for hospital palliative care programs: Consensus recommendations. J Palliat Med. 2008;11(9):1189–1194. doi: 10.1089/jpm.2008.0149; 10.1089/jpm.2008.0149.
21 Clinical Practice Guidelines for Quality Palliative Care, 3rd edn. http://www.nationalconsensusproject.org/GuidelinesTOC.pdf. Accessed June 10, 2013.
22 Elsayem A, Swint K, Fisch MJ et al. Palliative care inpatient service in a comprehensive cancer center: Clinical and financial outcomes. J Clin Oncol. 2004;22(10):2008–2014. doi: 10.1200/JCO.2004.11.003.
23 Center to Advance Palliative Care. Program model options chart. http://www.capc.org/building-a-hospital-based-palliative-care-program/designing/characteristics/program-model-chart/document_view. Accessed 9/10, 2013.
24 National Consensus Project for Quality Palliative Care. Clinical Practice Guidelines for Quality Palliative Care. 3rd edn., Pittsburg, PA: 2013.

25 Braiteh F, El Osta B, Palmer JL, Reddy SK, Bruera E. Characteristics, findings, and outcomes of palliative care inpatient consultations at a comprehensive cancer center. *J Palliat Med.* 2007;10(4):948–955. doi: 10.1089/jpm.2006.0257.

26 Potter J, Hami F, Bryan T, Quigley C. Symptoms in 400 patients referred to palliative care services: Prevalence and patterns. *Palliat Med.* 2003;17(4):310–314.

27 Virik K, Glare P. Profile and evaluation of a palliative medicine consultation service within a tertiary teaching hospital in Sydney, Australia. *J Pain Symptom Manage.* 2002;23(1):17–25.

28 Manfredi PL, Morrison RS, Morris J, Goldhirsch SL, Carter JM, Meier DE. Palliative care consultations: How do they impact the care of hospitalized patients? *J Pain Symptom Manage.* 2000;20(3):166–173.

29 Warren SC, Emmett MK. Palliative care consultation in West Virginia. *W V Med J.* 2002;98(3):94–99.

30 Olden AM, Holloway R, Ladwig S, Quill TE, van Wijngaarden E. Palliative care needs and symptom patterns of hospitalized elders referred for consultation. *J Pain Symptom Manage.* 2011;42(3):410–418. doi: 10.1016/j.jpainsymman.2010.12.005; 10.1016/j.jpainsymman.2010.12.005.

31 Weissman DE, Meier DE. Identifying patients in need of a palliative care assessment in the hospital setting: A consensus report from the center to advance palliative care. *J Palliat Med.* 2011;14(1):17–23. doi: 10.1089/jpm.2010.0347; 10.1089/jpm.2010.0347.

32 Center to Advance Palliative Care. Get palliative care: For clinicians. http://www.getpalliativecare.org/resources/clinicians/. Accessed July 3, 2013.

33 Homsi J, Walsh D, Nelson KA et al. The impact of a palliative medicine consultation service in medical oncology. *Support Care Cancer.* 2002;10(4):337–342. doi: 10.1007/s00520-002-0341-8.

34 von Gunten CF, Camden B, Neely KJ, Franz G, Martinez J. Prospective evaluation of referrals to a hospice/palliative medicine consultation service. *J Palliat Med.* 1998;1(1):45–53. doi: 10.1089/jpm.1998.1.45.

35 Sophocles A. Time is of the essence: Coding on the basis of time for physician services. *Fam Pract Manag.* 2003;10(6):27–31.

36 Nakajima N, Hata Y, Onishi H, Ishida M. The evaluation of the relationship between the level of disclosure of cancer in terminally ill patients with cancer and the quality of terminal care in these patients and their families using the support team assessment schedule. *Am J Hosp Palliat Care.* 2013;30(4):370–376. doi: 10.1177/1049909112452466; 10.1177/1049909112452466.

37 Bausewein C, Le Grice C, Simon S, Higginson I, PRISMA. The use of two common palliative outcome measures in clinical care and research: A systematic review of POS and STAS. *Palliat Med.* 2011;25(4):304–313. doi: 10.1177/0269216310395984; 10.1177/0269216310395984.

38 Chan WC, Epstein I. Researching "good death" in a Hong Kong palliative care program: A clinical data-mining study. *Omega (Westport).* 2011;64(3):203–222.

39 Sasahara T, Miyashita M, Umeda M et al. Multiple evaluation of a hospital-based palliative care consultation team in a university hospital: Activities, patient outcome, and referring staff's view. *Palliat Support Care.* 2010;8(1):49–57. doi: 10.1017/S1478951509990708; 10.1017/S1478951509990708.

40 Edmonds PM, Stuttaford JM, Penny J, Lynch AM, Chamberlain J. Do hospital palliative care teams improve symptom control? Use of a modified STAS as an evaluation tool. *Palliat Med.* 1998;12(5):345–351.

41 Bruera E, Hui D. Conceptual models for integrating palliative care at cancer centers. *J Palliat Med.* 2012;15(11):1261–1269. doi: 10.1089/jpm.2012.0147; 10.1089/jpm.2012.0147.

42 Hanson LC, Usher B, Spragens L, Bernard S. Clinical and economic impact of palliative care consultation. *J Pain Symptom Manage.* 2008;35(4):340–346. doi: 10.1016/j.jpainsymman.2007.06.008; 10.1016/j.jpainsymman.2007.06.008.

43 National Palliative Care Research Center. Pain and symptom management. http://www.npcrc.org/resources/resources_show.htm?doc_id=376168. Accessed September 10, 2013.

44 Harding R, Simms V, Calanzani N et al. If you had less than a year to live, would you want to know? A seven-country European population survey of public preferences for disclosure of poor prognosis. *Psychooncology.* 2013. doi: 10.1002/pon.3283; 10.1002/pon.3283.

45 Back AL, Li YF, Sales AE. Impact of palliative care case management on resource use by patients dying of cancer at a veterans affairs medical center. *J Palliat Med.* 2005;8(1):26–35. doi: 10.1089/jpm.2005.8.26.

46 Campbell ML, Guzman JA. Impact of a proactive approach to improve end-of-life care in a medical ICU. *Chest.* 2003;123(1):266–271.

47 Nelson C, Chand P, Sortais J, Oloimooja J, Rembert G. Inpatient palliative care consults and the probability of hospital readmission. *Perm J.* 2011;15(2):48–51.

48 Norton SA, Hogan LA, Holloway RG, Temkin-Greener H, Buckley MJ, Quill TE. Proactive palliative care in the medical intensive care unit: Effects on length of stay for selected high-risk patients. *Crit Care Med.* 2007;35(6):1530–1535. doi: 10.1097/01.CCM.0000266533.06543.0C.

49 Enguidanos S, Vesper E, Lorenz K. 30-Day readmissions among seriously ill older adults. *J Palliat Med.* 2012;15(12):1356–1361. doi: 10.1089/jpm.2012.0259; 10.1089/jpm.2012.0259.

50 Meier DE, Beresford L. Palliative care's challenge: Facilitating transitions of care. *J Palliat Med.* 2008;11(3):416–421. doi: 10.1089/jpm.2008.9956; 10.1089/jpm.2008.9956.

51 Brumley R, Enguidanos S, Jamison P et al. Increased satisfaction with care and lower costs: Results of a randomized trial of in-home palliative care. *J Am Geriatr Soc.* 2007;55(7):993–1000. doi: 10.1111/j.1532-5415.2007.01234.x.

52 Gelfman LP, Meier DE, Morrison RS. Does palliative care improve quality? A survey of bereaved family members. *J Pain Symptom Manage.* 2008;36(1):22–28. doi: 10.1016/j.jpainsymman.2007.09.008; 10.1016/j.jpainsymman.2007.09.008.

53 Casarett D, Pickard A, Bailey FA et al. Do palliative consultations improve patient outcomes? *J Am Geriatr Soc.* 2008;56(4):593–599. doi: 10.1111/j.1532-5415.2007.01610.x; 10.1111/j.1532-5415.2007.01610.x.

54 Casarett D, Johnson M, Smith D, Richardson D. The optimal delivery of palliative care: A national comparison of the outcomes of consultation teams vs inpatient units. *Arch Intern Med.* 2011;171(7):649–655. doi: 10.1001/archinternmed.2011.87; 10.1001/archinternmed.2011.87.

55 Simon S, Higginson IJ. Evaluation of hospital palliative care teams: Strengths and weaknesses of the before-after study design and strategies to improve it. *Palliat Med.* 2009;23(1):23–28. doi: 10.1177/0269216308098802; 10.1177/0269216308098802.

56 Higginson IJ, Finlay I, Goodwin DM et al. Do hospital-based palliative teams improve care for patients or families at the end of life? *J Pain Symptom Manage.* 2002;23(2):96–106.

57 Morrison RS, Penrod JD, Cassel JB et al. Cost savings associated with U.S. hospital palliative care consultation programs. *Arch Intern Med.* 2008;168(16):1783–1790. doi: 10.1001/archinte.168.16.1783; 10.1001/archinte.168.16.1783.

58 To TH, Greene AG, Agar MR, Currow DC. A point prevalence survey of hospital inpatients to define the proportion with palliation as the primary goal of care and the need for specialist palliative care. *Intern Med J.* 2011;41(5):430–433. doi: 10.1111/j.1445-5994.2011.02484.x; 10.1111/j.1445-5994.2011.02484.x.

59   Sigurdardottir KR, Haugen DF. Prevalence of distressing symptoms in hospitalised patients on medical wards: A cross-sectional study. *BMC Palliat Care*. 2008;7:16-684X-7-16. doi: 10.1186/1472-684X-7-16; 10.1186/1472-684X-7-16.

60   Smith S, Brick A, O'Hara S, Normand C. Evidence on the cost and cost-effectiveness of palliative care: A literature review. *Palliat Med*. 2013. doi: 10.1177/0269216313493466.

61   Weissman DE, Meier DE, Spragens LH. Center to Advance Palliative Care. Palliative care consultation service metrics: Consensus recommendations. *J Palliat Med*. 2008;11(10):1294–1298. doi: 10.1089/jpm.2008.0178; 10.1089/jpm.2008.0178.

62   Weissman DE, Morrison RS, Meier DE. Center to Advance Palliative Care. Palliative care clinical care and customer satisfaction metrics consensus recommendations. *J Palliat Med*. 2010;13(2):179–184. doi: 10.1089/jpm.2009.0270; 10.1089/jpm.2009.0270.

63   Center to Advance Palliative Care (CAPC). *A Guide to Building a Hospital-Based Palliative Program*. New York: 2004.

64   National Consensus Project. http://www.nationalconsensusproject.org/. Accessed September 10, 2013.

65   American Academy of Hospice and Palliative Medicine. www.aahpm.org. Accessed September 10, 2013.

66   Hospice and Palliative Care Nurses Association. http://www.hpna.org/Default2.aspx. Accessed September 10, 2013.

67   National Palliative Care Research Center. http://www.npcrc.org/. Accessed September 10, 2013.

68   Center to Advance Palliative Care. A state-by-state report card on access to palliative care in our nation's hospitals. http://www.capc.org/reportcard/recommendations. Accessed July 5, 2013.

69   Lupu D, American Academy of Hospice and Palliative Medicine Workforce Task Force. Estimate of current hospice and palliative medicine physician workforce shortage. *J Pain Symptom Manage*. 2010;40(6):899–911. doi: 10.1016/j.jpainsymman.2010.07.004; 10.1016/j.jpainsymman.2010.07.004.

33

Models of palliative care delivery

BADI EL OSTA, EDUARDO BRUERA

INTRODUCTION

Palliative care delivery has changed considerably during the last 30 years. During the second half of the past century in North America, care of terminally ill patients moved from the home, where most patients state that they would prefer to die,[1] to hospitals, where medical technology shifted the focus to prolonging life and avoiding death.

After a brief presentation of the different settings of palliative care delivery discussed elsewhere in this book, this chapter will attempt to provide an integrated vision for palliative care programs capable of delivering high rates of access and seamless care to patients in the palliative stages of their illness and to their families.

PATIENT AND FAMILY NEEDS

Palliative care is appropriate at every stage of the disease whether or not the patient is seeking curative treatment. By introducing palliative care earlier in the disease process, it becomes possible for health care professionals to detect subtle shifts that take place and help the patient and his family to adapt to the disease progression, redefine the goals of care and reframe hope. Therefore, understanding patient and family needs and expectations is very important for the patient's care. Lack of addressing their needs and expectations adequately leads to further distress and conflicts between patients, family members, and health care workers.[2]

Terminally ill patients develop a number of devastating physical and psychological symptoms[3] that imply the need for access to a multidisciplinary palliative care service in order to achieve better symptom control and psychosocial and spiritual support until death (Table 33.1). Patients need to have good symptom control in order to improve the quality of life.[4] Among symptoms at the end of life, fatigue was reported to be the most common symptom[3,4] and pain, depression, and anxiety were reported to be the most distressing for advanced cancer patients.[3]

Patients expect to be treated with dignity and respect and not as a *disease*, and they also appreciate physicians who listen

to them and allow them to express their personal concerns and feelings.[5] Most patients expect truth telling from their physician in an honest, timely, and sensitive manner as well as the continuity of care and ability to participate in their plan of care, especially when more than one option is available.[5] They need interdisciplinary help while coping with the physical, financial, psychosocial, and spiritual impact of their disease. Finally, most terminally ill patients seek to live the remainder of their life as fully as possible until death overtakes them, rather than marking time, waiting to die.[5]

Assisting families in meeting their needs will also lead to an improvement in the patient's care. Informational needs were identified as the most important among other needs.[6] Given et al. identified three types of needs for family members of a dying person[7]: need for information regarding the disease; need for assistance with how to structure care activities; continued guidance to alleviate stressors, burden, and associated depression.

Families should be provided with clear information about physical care and comfort measures, what to expect and how to manage symptoms as the disease progresses, treatments and their side effects, the patient's emotional response, and community resources. Families need assistance in monitoring and reporting symptoms, nutritional considerations, transportation, coordination of care, financial concerns, and coping with escalation of care as the patient's disease status declines without forgetting their psychosocial needs as well as the respite care.

In conclusion, the interdisciplinary approach of the patient and family needs leads to improvement of the patient's care and avoidance of a vicious circle of severe burnout and conflicts between the patient, the family, and the medical team. Effective communication secures the trusting partnership and help to ease their burden.[4]

INTERDISCIPLINARY CARE

Palliative care has been very successful in borrowing ideas and techniques from other disciplines in healthcare, in order to meet the patients' and families' needs during the terminal illness trajectory. The timely referral to each discipline allows its members to carry out baseline assessment, monitor changes, and apply appropriate interventions that meet the physical, psychosocial, and spiritual needs of the patients and their families.

The main disciplines involved in palliative care are occupational therapy, physical therapy, music therapy, speech therapy, nutrition, pharmacy, clinical psychology (counselor), social work, and chaplaincy.[8]

In some settings (e.g., acute care hospitals), these disciplines are readily available. Therefore, outpatient facilities, inpatient hospices, acute palliative care units, and day hospitals (DHs) should ideally take place geographically within acute care facilities that already have these healthcare professionals available. Otherwise, if outpatient centers, inpatient hospices, and DHs operate somewhere else, it may be necessary to make the appropriate transportation arrangements to allow the different disciplines to see the patients in case these facilities do not have their own interdisciplinary team (IDT).

Interdisciplinary care may be very difficult, if not impossible, to conduct at home or in a nursing home (NH) because of the cost of transportation of all the different disciplines to the patient's location. However, the possibility of video interactive techniques for the access to social worker, counselor, pastoral care, and other members of the IDT will be a promising way to stay in touch with the patients and their families. These techniques have been used in psychiatry for various purposes.[9,10] Studies need to be done in palliative care telemedicine to assess cost effectiveness of these techniques, as well as patients' and families' satisfaction.

The best level of palliative care delivery consists of having multiple disciplines involved in each setting to provide care that meets the needs of patients and families. The following paragraphs discuss the different settings of palliative care and their integration into a seamless network that every patient can access.

DIFFERENT SETTINGS FOR PALLIATIVE CARE DELIVERY

Home

While most patients die in the hospital or a nursing home, surveys indicate that more than 70% of people would prefer to die at home.[11] Despite the existence of different models internationally, palliative home care (PHC) provides patients the possibility of a quality of life and death at home if it is the preferred place to spend his or her last days. This setting has its own advantages and limitations and can be challenging as well as rewarding for the patient and the family. Wenk and DeLima have discussed these issues in depth in another chapter.

At home, most patients have more autonomy, privacy, and freedom, and they also feel safer at home than anywhere else.[12] The family can potentially anticipate the loss, have a better bereavement, and familiarize with death by learning that death is a normal stage of life.[12] Care at home at the end of life can also reduce the cost of care: it prevents unnecessary

admissions to acute hospital and skilled nursing facilities and avoids an unnecessary use of the emergency department by having nurses (backed up by a palliative care specialist) on call 24 hours/day, 7 days/week to provide a rapid response to changes in symptoms in the last days of life.[13]

On the other hand, care at home may be difficult or impossible if the patient does not wish so, lives alone or far away, cannot afford the care expenses, or needs higher skilled care; if his family is physically or emotionally tired, cannot deal with uncontrolled symptom, or cannot provide him with 24 hours care; or if the home does not meet the minimal comfort needs.[14]

When providing PHC, the team should be able to get early referrals, have access to an inpatient hospice unit for possible direct admission, provide medications and home's equipment for the patient, be able to assess and control symptoms using universal tools, and document visits and phone calls on the patient's chart.

The responsible caregiver (RC) is the member of the family who is in better condition (health, relation, proximity, and available time) to carry out and coordinate the care.[15] The education of the RC must be done progressively, with simple verbal, written, and audio- and/or video-taped instructions about how to administer medications; evaluate symptoms, diet, hydration, hygiene and evacuation, and position and dressing changes; organize family tasks; and recognize death. To prevent frequent hospitalization, the RC needs support with the guarantee of the best possible symptom control, the availability of the team and access to easy admissions 24/7, establishing a caring plan and a schedule of activities, anticipating the changes that can occur in the patient's condition, reducing doubts and uncertainty, and providing material resources.

Usually, one month of care should include approximately two medical visits per week, two nursing visits per week, two psychology/counseling interviews for the patient and two for the family per month, and the provision of oral and parenteral opioids analgesic. When the patient's condition is stable, medical and nursing visits can occur once weekly; in the terminal phase, one or more visits are needed per day. However, available services can vary dramatically in different areas of the world, particularly regarding access to medical care.

Volunteer collaboration increases both team activity and interaction with the community.[16] After their selection and training, the volunteers can help in evaluating patients at home or on the phone, educate RC, offer practical support (housekeeping, transport, etc.), and provide company for the patient and family.

The home hospice service enables patients to live at home in the last days of life. The demand for such services is expected to increase in the future because of the aging population.[17] This rapidly growing concept can be a source of ethical dilemmas.[18] It is very important to have a complete discussion with the patient and family regarding the choices and wishes of where to receive end-of-life care and get into an agreement within some principles with the possibility of changing choices at any time[19]: patients and families should be aware that PHC does neither medicalize nor technify the dying process, and PHC should not be an intrusion to the privacy of their home, nor should it disturb the family life.[1]

Finally, it is unclear whether PHC produces savings by the reduction of the expenses of both fragmented care and the use of high-tech interventions; however, in many cases, the burden of cost shifts from the health care system to the caregiver.[12] Because nonprofessional caregiving is crucial to effective end-of-life care for patients who wish to die at home, early recognition of family distress, validation of their role, and effective communication by physicians may ease their burden and avoid physical illness, emotional distress, financial hardship, and early mortality in the caregivers.[20] If PHC is promoted and implemented, resources should be minimized for medications and maximized for RC funding.

Outpatient centers

Patients with advanced cancer often develop devastating physical, psychosocial, and existential distress[21–25] associated with the disease or its treatment.[21,23,24] These symptoms cannot be controlled appropriately[22] in a standard setting based on a physician/nurse team with a waiting area and small private examining rooms, which do not allow interactions between the members of different disciplines. Therefore, the multidisciplinary symptom control and palliative care (MD) clinics were developed to unify members from different disciplines in a team that combines their assessments and formulates a plan of care[22,23] that meets the needs of patients and families in the same visit and at the same place. The MD clinic helps patients and their families to avoid the distress generated by the visits to several offices located in different areas of a tertiary hospital and by the waiting time before each appointment in order to receive a multidisciplinary assessment and management.

In an effort to understand one of the main problems of palliative care programs, that of late access to palliative care, El Osta et al. reviewed 2868 consecutive patients who had their first palliative care referral during a 30-month period.[99] The growth increased 20%, which was significantly higher than institution, thereby suggesting there was relative growth in the program. However, during the period of observation, the median time between first palliative care and death was 42 days (48 days for solid and 14 days for liquid tumors). The period of advanced cancer diagnosis by medical oncologists to death was 250 days, suggesting that there were considerable opportunities for earlier referral. One of the possible reasons of delay in advanced cancer diagnosis to palliative care is the naming of the service. For this reason, we conducted an anonymous survey on a random sample of 100 medical oncologists and 100 oncology midlevel providers with the response rate of 70% in each group.[100] Clinicians were likely to refer almost 90% patients with incurable cancer to both services. However, patients in the earlier stage of the disease, including those receiving active treatments or recently diagnosed, were twice as likely to be referred to a program supportive care to as compared to one named palliative care. In this survey, the name was a barrier to

referral, and clinicians reported the name palliative care as a four times barrier for referrals compared with supportive care 23% vs. 3%). In addition, 44% of clinicians reported palliative care to decrease the hope of the patient and family.

For these reasons, our outpatient palliative care program is named supportive care center. This center is operated by board-certified palliative care specialists in all cases, and it delivers a full range of supportive and palliative care services to patients at all stages of their disease trajectory. An assessment and outcome that Dalal et al. conducted comparing 6-month pre- and postname changes, we observed an increase at the time of first referral to palliative care to D in the outpatient center (1.7 months earlier referrals with median referral increased from 5.2 to 6.9 months).[101] Perhaps, more surprising was an overall 41% increase in referrals of both inpatients and outpatients after adjusting for the institutional growth. These findings suggest that change in name allowed the oncologists who were reluctant to refer patients due to the name palliative care to refer more of their patients to both outpatient and inpatient services after the name was changed to supportive care.

In their retrospective study,[21] Strasser et al. compared the assessment of 138 consecutive patients with advanced cancer referred to the MD clinic and 77 patients referred to a traditional pain and symptom management clinic. The two groups were similar in tumor type, demographics, and symptom burden. Patients of both clinics were evaluated using the same tools: Edmonton Symptom Assessment System[26] (ESAS), CAGE questionnaire,[27] and Mini-Mental State Questionnaire[28] (MMSQ). In addition to a physician and a nurse, the patient was assessed by a social worker, physical and occupational therapist, pharmacist, clinical nutritionist, pastoral care worker, and psychiatric nurse practitioner. The MD clinic had no waiting area, and patients had their own private rooms with a full-sized bed and a bathroom. After the patient's evaluation, the multidisciplinary team would discuss the assessment, interventions, and recommendations in a team conference. The patient as well as his oncologist and primary care physician would receive a handwritten and audio-taped[29] form of the team conference. A follow-up visit would be scheduled within 1–2 weeks of initial assessment[21] and monthly thereafter; otherwise, follow-ups would be provided per patient or family needs at the MD[21] or over the phone.[22] Patients from the MD clinic received a total of 1066 nonphysician recommendations (median 4 per patients, range 0–37) in a 5 hours assessment. In 83 patients interviewed after the MD clinic visit, satisfaction was rated as excellent in the following areas: caring team members, adequate assessment, treatment plan, useful recommendations, and time spent.

In contrast, the duration of the pain and symptom management clinic assessment, done only by a physician and a nurse, was 30–45 min. There were no nonphysician recommendations given; instead, eight patients were referred to specialists in psychiatry, three to rehabilitation, and three to social work.[21]

In conclusion, the interventions of a interdisciplinary half-day symptom control and palliative care clinic can result in the reduction of the physical and psychosocial distress of patients with advanced cancer,[21,22] high number of physician and non-physician specific care recommendations,[21] and high levels of patient satisfaction.[21,22]

There are some specific characteristics of successful outpatient palliative care delivery:

1. *Just-in-time access*: Patients need to access these consult programs without lengthy appointments or waiting time. It is important to encourage a *drop-in* approach.
2. *Physical facility*: The rooms need to have enough space for a full size bed since palliative care patients are frequently severely symptomatic and cannot tolerate long period on examining tables. These rooms also need enough space for families to be able to sit comfortably with the patient. Privacy is important for different discussions that take place.
3. *Availability of team members*: A successful outpatient palliative care program requires rapid access to different disciplines. Physicians and nurses are generally ineffective in identifying problems that require interdisciplinary interventions.[22] Therefore, palliative care patients and families should ideally be provided access to as many disciplines as possible during the course of an initial outpatient consultation. Further follow-up may not be required by all disciplines.

Few studies evaluated the outcomes of the outpatient palliative care consult on the treatment of cancer pain at the first follow-up visit.

Yennu et al.[102] reviewed 1612 consecutive cancer patients whose symptoms were evaluated at the outpatient palliative care center between January 2003 and December 2010 at the first referral (or baseline) and at the first follow-up visits in order to determine the pain intensity changes after the palliative care intervention. The median of the first follow-up visit from baseline was 15 days. They found that 462 (29%) patients had no-to-mild pain intensity, 511 (32%) patients had moderate pain intensity (4–6), and 639 (39%) patients had severe pain intensity (7 or above) at baseline ESAS. A total of 728 (45%) patients had their pain improved at the first follow-up (at least 2 points or at least 30% intensity reduction from the baseline), among them, 228 (31%) patients still reported pain scores of 4 or above at the first follow-up. Among the patients with no-to-mild pain intensity, 147 (32%) had worse pain at the first follow-up visit.

Using the same patient database, Kang et al.[103] showed that patients with no-to-mild symptom intensity at baseline ESAS had worse symptoms at the first follow-up. Whereas patients with moderate-to-severe symptom intensity at baseline ESAS had a significant improvement of their symptoms at the first follow-up. Of note, the latter patients still had symptom intensity rated 4 or above on ESAS at the first follow-up.

Both authors concluded that various strategies such as earlier first visit follow-up and the implementation of telephone calls and interactive voice response (IVR) are needed for earlier assessment and treatment in order to optimize cancer-related symptom control in patients with advanced cancer.

Day hospital

DHs were originally developed for the geriatric population[30] in response to a lack of continuity of care between acute hospitalization and long-term placement[31] and with the idea of lowering the cost of care.[32–37] Later on, DHs extended to other specialties,[38] including palliative care.

Day care hospitals vary in funding, facilities, and staff.[39] They are mainly funded by the private sector.[39–56] One third is attached to inpatient units, another third is attached to inpatient units with home care teams, and the last third is attached to a home care team alone or freestanding.[39,46] Palliative Care Day Hospitals (PCDHs) are usually open 3–5 days a week and are mainly led and managed by nurses.[39,46,56] The DH staff are specialized in palliative care and include physicians, bedside and clinical nurses, psychologists, social workers, physical and occupational therapists, chiropodists, dieticians, chaplains, managers, aromatherapists, hairdressers, and volunteers. A mixture of hospital bedrooms with private washrooms, clinic-type rooms, interview rooms, treatment rooms, and specific rooms with special research equipment is ideal. Sufficient space for patients and family members should be provided, such as a waiting room, a kitchen, a private meeting room, etc. A unified, well-planned central working area for the staff increases the efficiency of communication and should not replace separate offices to allow team members to perform their charting and telephonic communications. It is essential to plan a lounge area within the DH setting for the staff to rest while remaining accessible to respond to the needs of patients and families during their resting time.

PCDH provides palliative care assessment and management to patients with severe symptoms, existential distress, and difficult family situation, regardless of their prognosis. It assumes a consult role for patients who are not in terminal phase of their illness and a treating physician role with terminal patients with complex palliative care issues. It also provides family meetings, advanced care planning, including clarification of code status, emergency consults within 48 hours, and specialized services to special populations (i.e., patients with lymphedema, wound care, methadone clinic, etc.). PCDH coordinates referrals to other palliative care services and allows access to other disciplines available in a tertiary care hospital such as anesthesiologists, surgeons, oncologists, radio-oncologists, skin care nurses, etc. PCDH should improve links between specialized services of the hospital, promote links with home care services and hospices through adequate referral, respond to home *crisis* by giving support to home-based palliative care teams and by coordinating admissions to the DH or the inpatient unit to prevent terminally ill patients' visits to the emergency room, provide phone consultations to physicians and nurses in the community regarding complex issues, and develop protocols of care with community services. The DH setting has been discussed in depth by Gagnon in Chapter 35.

Fifteen papers reported data from 12 observational studies of day care, 11 from the United Kingdom[41–56] and 1 from the United States,[40] and provided some information on the structure, process, and outcomes of day care. Many qualitative studies found that most patients were highly satisfied and valued the social contact[41,44,50,52–55] and the opportunity to take part in activities that day care provided. Caregivers' opinions were sought in one study:[55] the majority found care *excellent* or *good* and were *greatly helped* by their day off. However, further studies are needed to provide the conclusive evidence of improved symptom control, mainly pain[41,43–55] and quality of life in PCDH, as well evidence-based standards of care.[39]

The three settings discussed earlier, home care programs, outpatient centers, and DHs are part of the palliative care services available to patients who are still staying at home. In these settings, bus rounds[57,58] would be a useful mechanism for unifying criteria and sharing strategies for patient care as well as promoting continuing patient-based education in palliative care for physicians, nurses, and medical students in the community. They were highly satisfactory from participants' perspective,[58] and the overall cost was low.[57]

Consult teams in acute care facilities

Consult teams in acute care facilities act as a bridge between the *palliative* and *active* models[59,60] of care by providing access to palliative care services at a time when the patient is still receiving active treatment.

In a retrospective study,[59] Jenkins et al. reviewed the charts of 100 consecutive cancer patients who had been referred to a palliative care consult team within a tertiary acute care hospital during a 6-month period. The palliative care consult team consisted of a physician and a nurse trained in palliative care and available on a full-time basis. Demographic characteristics, including reason for admission and disease status upon admission, length of stay, length of time from consult to discharge, admission location, and code status on admission and discharge were recorded. Symptom acuity, cognitive status, and risk for substance abuse were evaluated, respectively, using the ESAS,[26] CAGE[27] questionnaire, and MMSQ.[28]. Medications before and after the consult were compared to the recommended medications; compliance of the primary team with the consult team recommendations was assessed. Five patients were not palliative at the time of the consult. Only 46/95 (48%) were known to have untreatable cancer at the time of their admission. The CAGE questionnaire for alcoholism and the MMSQ were abnormal in 19/78 (24%) and 40/91 (44%), respectively. The most intense symptoms, as measured by the 100 mm scales of the ESAS were fatigue (72 ± 24), appetite (60 ± 32), and well-being (50 ± 29). Eighty-nine of the ninety-five patients were living at home prior to admission and 34/95 (36%) were able to return home. The median length of time between consultation and discharge was 6 days[59] (5 days in a recent study[61] carried out by O'Mahony et al.). Twenty patients died during hospitalization, 23 were transferred to a palliative care unit, and the remaining 18 were discharged to another hospital or long-term care facility. Two-thirds of the patients were on dimenhydrinate as antiemetic by their primary team, 4% of the patients had neuroleptics ordered before the consult compared with 19% for whom neuroleptics were recommended, 22% of the patients were not prescribed opioids, and 54% were prescribed opioids on an as-needed basis. The patients' physician complied with the palliative care consult team's recommendations in 122/137 cases (89%).

Hospitalization of terminally ill patients is a pivotal time in their disease course. In this study,[59] 52% learned that they were palliative during this hospitalization. The consult team was able to rapidly assess and treat patients, verify a terminal diagnosis, and ensure that medical options have been exhausted. By providing alternative palliative care resources and placement options, the consult team helped in reducing the number of patients admitted to the hospital for social reasons,[59] hospital charges,[61] length of stay,[59,61] and interunit transfers.[61] Using the tools cited earlier,[26–28] the consult team was able to help the primary team in detecting the missed delirium in about half of the patients and assessing and managing cancer pain as well as opioid side effects and other symptoms related to the cancer more effectively. The high rate of adherence to the consult team's recommendations[59,61] suggests that the primary team was able to incorporate palliative care approaches into the management of acute patients. Higher adherence rate (>90%) was reported in a recent study carried out by O'Mahony et al. after evaluating data regarding 592 consecutive patients seen by their palliative care consult team during a 16-month period.[61]

Palliative care units

A tertiary palliative care unit (TPCU) is a distinct type of palliative care unit, designated for terminally ill patients who require intensive involvement of a specialist IDT able to manage their complex problems. Von Gunten defined it as an academic medical center where specialist knowledge for the most complex cases is practiced, researched, and taught.[62]

Given the physical, psychosocial, and spiritual nature of the TPCU patient population complexity, the ideal location for such a unit is in an acute care hospital that offers a full range of diagnostic and interventional procedures, support services, specialty, and subspecialty consultation. The TPCU staffing includes palliative care specialists, nurse practitioners, registered nurses, research nurses, licensed practical nurses, nursing attendants, a chaplain, a social worker, a physical therapist, an occupational therapist, a pharmacist, a clinical dietician, a palliative care counselor, a clerk, and volunteers. The optimal unit size for staffing efficiency is 16–24 beds and the minimum size is 10–12 beds.[63] Wantanabe has discussed in depth this setting in a later chapter.

One example of TPCU is the Edmonton Regional Palliative Care Program (ERPCP) PCU in Canada.[64] The ERPCP is a publicly funded program that provides a comprehensive range of palliative care services, including home care and specialist consultation in the community, long-term care, hospices, ambulatory care, and acute care settings. Its TPCU is located in an acute care teaching hospital, and it has 14 beds. Amenities include a patient smoking room, a family lounge, a kitchenette, a quiet room, and a conference room. Family members may stay overnight if they wish, and pets are allowed. Referrals are screened after a direct patient assessment by the palliative care consultants. Such patients are referred for acute symptom control, emotional and family distress, difficult discharge planning, and rehabilitation. As discussed in Chapter 37, the TPCU is intended to be a short-term place of care until symptoms have stabilized sufficiently to allow discharge of the patient to another palliative care setting: the expected length of stay is less than 2 weeks. The goal of admission and its temporary nature should be discussed with the patients and their families. Most patients are asked to agree electively to a *do-not-resuscitate* status prior to admission. Discussing *do-not-resuscitate* status is a valuable opportunity to clarify the patient's and family's understanding of the illness, prognosis, and goals of care.[65] The tools used daily for assessment are ESAS,[26] CAGE questionnaire,[27] MMSQ,[28] Edmonton Staging System (ESS) for cancer pain,[66] Edmonton Labeled Visual Information System[67] (ELVIS), Edmonton Functional Assessment Tool[68] (EFAT), palliative performance score[69] (PPS), and constipation score.[70] A family conference coordinated by the social worker and attended by the team, the patient, family members and friends whom the patient wishes to involve is often advisable to clarify goals and establish plans of care and further discharge to a more appropriate palliative care setting that will satisfy their needs. Patients have the option not to be present at the family conference.

For those patients who are discharged home, clear and timely communication with community health care providers (e.g., primary care physician, home care manager, and pharmacist) is critical. Transfer to a hospice may pose a difficult transition for the patients and their families because of their need to adjust to a new environment and staff and most importantly because they may view hospice as a lower level of care and feel a sense of abandonment.[71] These concerns may be alleviated by explaining to them that the fact that the patient does not require treatment in a TPCU is a positive outcome and that the option of coming back is possible if the symptoms exacerbate and the patient decides so.

The TPCU provides an excellent environment for research in which all the IDT's medical members are expected to participate. Since patients are under direct care of the medical team, the process of screening and recruiting them for studies becomes easier. The TPCU of the ERPCP receives undergraduate and postgraduate medical trainees from the University of Alberta on a regular basis. Clinical teaching is enhanced by journal club,[72] held three mornings a week, during which time relevant articles to palliative care are presented and discussed. Other educational activities include tests taken before and after the residents' PCU rotation,[69] seminars, weekly grand rounds, and presentations from other specialists sharing their expertise as applied directly or indirectly to palliative care.

In order to determine the optimal setting of palliative care delivery, Casarett et al.[104] conducted a nationwide telephone survey with one family member of each of the 5901 patients who died in one of the 77 Veterans Administration (VA) medical centers that offered palliative care consultation services and dedicated palliative care units between July 1, 2008, and December 31, 2009. The survey consisted of one global rating item and nine core rating items describing the patient's care in the last month of life. Families of patients who received care in palliative care units were more likely to report excellent care than the ones who received a palliative care consultation (adjusted proportions: 63% vs. 53%; OR, 1.52; 95% CI, 1.25–1.85; $P < 0.001$). The authors found that care received in palliative care units offered more improvements in care through communication, providing physical, emotional, and spiritual support than those achieved with the palliative care consultations during the last month of life.

Inpatient hospices

Hospice is a model designed to provide care at the end of life. The goal of hospice is to palliate the suffering at the end of life by addressing the emotional, social, physical, and spiritual needs of the patient and their family. The inpatient hospice care is the highest level of care within a hospice program. It is designated to control physical suffering and support family and patients when such care is not manageable at home.

Described in depth by Keen in another chapter, the majority of inpatient hospices is staffed by at least one full-time physician trained in palliative medicine, nurses, physiotherapists, occupational therapists, social workers, and chaplains and offers bereavement support services. In addition to providing inpatient end-stage care, patients are admitted for symptom control, rehabilitation, and sometimes respite care.

Statistically, five independent factors were found to predict inpatient hospice care: pain in the last year of life, constipation, breast cancer, being under 85 year of age, and being dependent on others for help with the activities of daily living for between one and six months before death.[73] Hinton demonstrated a higher rate of admission from patients receiving PHC over those that were living alone or with unfit relatives and those with breast cancer.[74] One study of data relating to cancer deaths showed that patients accessing palliative care services were significantly younger and had longer survival times from diagnosis.[75] An analysis of place of death of cancer patients demonstrated an increased likelihood of dying in a hospice if they lived close by.[76]

In the United States, cancer diagnosis accounted for 46% of hospice admissions during 2004 while noncancer diseases accounted for 64%: end-stage heart disease and dementia were the most two common terminal illnesses.[77] Medicare, through Part A, limits inpatient hospice care reimbursement ($491.19/day in 2000).[78] The length of stay per hospice admission was 4–5, days and the median length of stay in 2004 was 22 days.[77] In the United Kingdom, the average length of stay in inpatient hospice was 13.5 days,[79] compared with Canada, where the average length of stay was 44 days, and the median length of stay was 22 days.[80] The principal problems triggering admission were anorexia, weakness, and drowsiness.[3]

There is little good quality research measuring the contribution that inpatient hospice care makes to patient care. However, the studies at St. Christopher's Hospice comparing hospice and hospital care from the viewpoint of the surviving spouse found a consistent impression of a better social and psychological environment within the hospice compared with the hospital.[81,82]

Consult teams in nursing homes

More than 25% of Americans die in a nursing home (NH).[83] Considerable evidence indicates that NH residents do not receive optimal end-of-life care,[84,85] their pain is undertreated,[86] and they are often transferred to an acute care setting to receive aggressive rather than palliative treatment in the last weeks of life.[87,88] Therefore, families express dissatisfaction with the end-of-life care that their loved ones receive in NHs.[89] Hospice care may improve the quality of end-of-life care for NH residents, but it is underutilized by this population, in part because physicians are not aware of their patients' preferences.[84]

Casarett et al. carried out a randomized controlled trial of 205 NH residents and their surrogate decision makers in 3 U.S. NHs to determine whether it is possible to increase hospice utilization and improve the quality of end-of-life care by identifying residents whose goals and preferences are consistent with hospice care.[84] A structured interview identified NH residents whose goals for care, treatment preferences, and palliative care needs made them appropriate for hospice care. Of the 205 NH residents, 107 were randomly assigned to receive the intervention, and 98 received usual care. Intervention residents were more likely than usual care residents to enroll in hospice within 30 days (21/107 [20%] vs. 1/98 [1%]; $P < 0.001$ [Fisher exact test]) and to enroll in hospice during the follow-up period (27/207 [25%] vs. 6/98 [6%]; $P < 0.001$). Intervention residents had fewer acute care admissions (mean: 0.28 vs. 0.49; $P = 0.04$ [Wilcoxon rank sum test]) and spent fewer days in an acute care setting (mean: 1.2 vs. 3.0; $P = 0.03$ [Wilcoxon rank sum test]). Families of intervention residents rated the resident's care more highly than did families of usual care residents (mean on a scale of 1–5: 4.1 vs. 2.5; $P = 0.04$ [Wilcoxon rank sum test]).

In conclusion, by increasing early access to hospice care in an NH setting by a simple and prompt communication

intervention, pain will be better controlled, inappropriate medications as well as physical restraint use and acute hospital's admissions will decrease, and families' satisfaction of end-of-life care will increase.[84]

INTEGRATION OF CARE

Figure 33.1 summarizes the different components of palliative care delivery. The most important aspect of this model is the different arrows connecting the different settings of care. The flow of patients needs to be seamless, and this is facilitated by using compatible assessment tools, similar treatment and counseling protocols, and frequent communication among the different teams, using videoconferencing, regular teaching rounds, or bus rounds. However, the different settings do not need to have a unified ownership or administrative structure to be able to meet the goal of seamless patient and family care.

During the past several decades, terminally ill patients were increasingly dying in acute care setting.[90-92] With the recent changes in health care, there is greater emphasis on providing care at home and supporting families to enable more home deaths.[92,93] Since home death may not be simple, practical, or desirable in every family situation,[92-96] there is a need for an objective way to assess the viability of a home death in each family situation.

Cantwell et al. were able to formulate a new tool called the Home Death Assessment Tool (HDAT) as a result of a cohort study[14] conducted to describe the relative role of predictors of home death in palliative care patients with advanced cancer. They created a simple questionnaire of five questions to assess the viability of a home death: patients' and caregivers' desire for a home death, physician's support for a home death, presence of more than one caregiver, patients' environment, and sufficient financial resources. Ninety questionnaires were administered by home care coordinators, and a follow-up questionnaire was administered to record the place of death. Of the 73 patients, 34 (47%) died at home and 39 (53%) died in a hospital or a hospice.

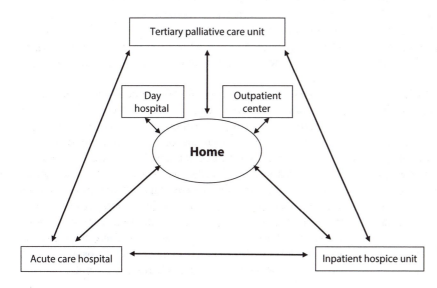

Figure 33.1 *Home as the center of palliative care delivery.*

Logistic regression identified a desire for home death by both the patient and the caregiver as the main predictive factor for a home death. The presence of more than one caregiver was also predictive of home death. The financial resources in a private health care system, can determine also the feasibility of death at home. However, the physician's support for a home death and the patient's environment were not significant predictors of home death in Cantwell's study.

The HDAT was highly specific in identifying patients who were not going to die at home but was not sensitive in identifying those who would die at home. It was used to guide the care coordinator in planning a home death and to increase the understanding among patient, family, and professional caregivers of what is required for successful palliative care delivery at home.[14] If there are fewer than three positive answers, the home care coordinator should explore a different setting as a care plan.

Home death is not universal and has its limitations. Decreased support, symptom distress, and inability of the PHC and caregivers to meet patients' needs make peaceful death at home impossible. Also, patients and caregivers can change their minds about their desire for a home death as their circumstances change.[14,96,97] In these cases, the patient has to be moved to a higher skilled setting. The role of a DH team in this case is very important: it assures support to the PHC team and responds to home crisis within 48 hours, provides optimal care if possible, or helps coordinating the patient's disposition to the appropriate setting (specialized clinics, TPCUs, acute care hospitals, and inpatient hospice units).

There are no systematic reviews of the effectiveness of palliative day care and no randomized controlled trials comparing this care with other settings.[39] There are no studies of referral into day care or the cost of this care.[39] Planned to provide a leadership role in promoting links between a tertiary care hospital and community services, the DH should be for patients with terminal illness who are still receiving active treatment and for patients in their terminal phase who need rapid access to palliative care.

Inpatient care can be delivered, in decreasing order of patient and family distress, at the TPCU, by consult teams in acute care hospitals and hospices. In a review of admission data for all patients discharged from the ERPCP from November 1, 1997, to October 31, 1998, patients with high symptom distress, positive screening for alcoholism, and poor prognostic indicators of cancer pain (Edmonton Staging Score or ESS[66] > 0/5) were referred to TPCU, while those with a lower level of distress, negative screening for alcoholism, and better prognostic indicators (ESS = 0) were treated in acute care hospitals, hospices, and the community.[3]

The availability of a palliative care consult team allows patients access to palliative care at an early stage of their illness, when they are still receiving active treatment and when they are still candidates for cardiopulmonary resuscitation.[59] It has reduced significantly hospital charges[61] as well as length of stay,[59,61] interunit transfers,[61] and admissions for social reasons.[59]

In the United States, admissions to inpatient hospice are limited to a median of approximately 5 days. This length of stay is related to the need to deliver 80% of hospice care at home. Since the median length of inpatient hospice stay in the United States during 2004 was 22 days,[77] the median inpatient hospice stay per admission is approximately 5 days (20% of the yearly total stay). This duration is relatively short compared with Canada or the United Kingdom where its average is 44[80] and 13.5[79] days, respectively. Therefore, admission to hospice in the United States may not be able to meet the patients' and families' needs, and referrals to higher skilled setting would be the appropriate choice so patients can spend more time at home after discharge from a TPCU, for example, and avoid recurrent admissions to inpatient hospice.

The availability and degree of integration of palliative care at U.S. cancer centers vary widely between NCI and non-NCI designated cancer centers despite the significant increase in the number of palliative care programs in the past decade. Hui et al.[105] conducted a survey of 71 NCI and 71 non-NCI designated cancer centers between June and October 2009. NCI-designated cancer centers were significantly more likely to have a palliative care program (98% vs. 78%; $P = 0.002$), at least one palliative care physician (92% vs. 74%; $P = 0.04$), an inpatient palliative care consultation team (92% vs. 56%; $P < 0.001$), and an outpatient palliative care clinic (59% vs. 22%; $P < 0.001$). Few centers had dedicated palliative care beds (23%) or an institution-operated hospice (37%). The median (interquartile range) reported durations from referral to death were 7 (4–16), 7 (5–10), and 90 (30–120) days for inpatient consultation teams, inpatient units, and outpatient clinics, respectively. Executives were supportive of stronger integration and increasing palliative care resources. This integration requires acting at different levels of palliative care delivery and education: educating patients, families, and referring oncologists on the benefits of palliative care and simultaneous care; increasing the availability of outpatient palliative care clinics will enhance earlier referral to palliative care; increasing the availability of PCU will improve symptom control and emotional suffering at the end of life; encouraging oncologists to participate regularly in family conferences and palliative care educational rounds and similarly encouraging palliative care specialists to attend tumor boards will increase earlier referral to palliative care; enhancing the education of medical oncology fellows in core competencies related to palliative care can prompt more timely referrals to palliative care; dedicating more resources toward research in the models of palliative care integration and clinical outcomes.

In the outpatient setting, the MD clinic allows a better integration of care between a cancer center and community-based physicians and nurses. It also allows patients access to multiple disciplines that are not available outside tertiary centers.[22]

Home is considered the center of palliative care delivery since most patients and their families prefer to stay at home as long as possible,[1] and during all the early stages of the illness, patients receive all their care while residing at home. From home, patient can be moved to an acute care hospital (e.g., patient develops hematemesis), to a TPCU (e.g., control of severe symptoms or psychosocial distress), or even to an inpatient hospice unit in case the RC becomes ill or needs a respite. Of note, patients can also be transferred from one setting to another within this model based on their needs as well as their family needs (e.g., after controlling an acute exacerbation of a right arm pain in a TPCU, a patient can be moved to an inpatient hospice unit while awaiting his caregiver to recover from a severe flu; the same or a different patient can be transferred from an inpatient hospice unit to an acute care hospital after a hip fracture secondary to a fall from his bed; again, the same or a different patient can be transferred from a surgery floor to a TPCU if he develops a delirium that the surgeon cannot manage appropriately). In any of these settings, the discharge plan would be directed, if practical and desirable, toward returning the patient home to spend his last days surrounded by his loved ones.

The two main issues in deciding the setting of care are the level of distress and available support. The patient's distress may be physical, psychosocial, or spiritual and can be measured with the ESAS,[26] the MDAS (104), the McGill Quality of Life Questionnaire[98] (MQOL), the EFAT,[68] the PPS,[69] the constipation score,[70] and others. The level of support can be determined by the structure and function of the family, financial status, medical insurance, and overall physical condition of the home.

If there is worsening of the physical and the psychosocial distress, the patient has to be transferred to an acute care hospital where he/she will have access to many disciplines (e.g., consult teams or TPCU). Once the distress is controlled, the patient can be moved to the community or home if they have good social and financial support. Otherwise, a transfer to an inpatient hospice unit would be more appropriate. If the distress could not be alleviated or the support could not be provided, the patient would not be able to return home and might die in an acute care hospital or in the inpatient hospice unit (Figure 33.2).

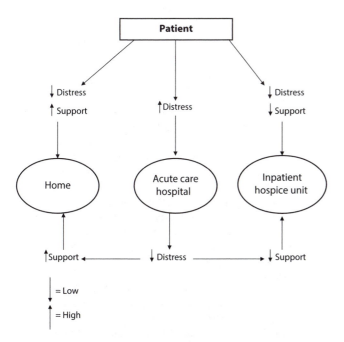

Figure 33.2 *Matching palliative care services to the patient and family needs.*

The Memorial Delirium Assessment Scale (MDAS) is a widely used and validated screening tool for delirium in cancer patients. In a pilot study conducted by Fadul et al.,[106] thirty-one palliative care health professionals obtained the correct diagnosis of delirium in 90%–100% of the time on three simulated patients' scenarios after they received a training session on the MDAS. The authors concluded that MDAS provided an accurate test to diagnose delirium once palliative care health professionals were trained on how to use it. Further research in the palliative care clinical setting is needed to further confirm these results. MDAS has replaced MMSQ and is being used by our palliative care providers as a tool to diagnose delirium.

Fadul et al.[100] conducted a survey among a random sample of 100 medical oncologists and 100 midlevel providers at a comprehensive cancer center to determine whether a perceived association between the name palliative care and hospice was a barrier to early patient referral. Seventy percent of each group of providers responded. More participants preferred the name *supportive care* (80, 57%) compared with *palliative care* (27, 19%, P < 0.0001). They stated that the name change to *supportive care* would increase the likelihood of patient referral on active primary (79% vs. 45%, P < 0.0001) and advanced cancer (89% vs. 69%, P < 0.0001) treatments. The name *palliative care* compared with *supportive care* was perceived more frequently by these providers as a barrier to referrals (23% vs. 6%, P < 0.0001), decreasing hope (44% vs. 11%, P < 0.0001), and causing distress (33% vs. 3%, P < 0.0001) in patients and families. Future research is needed to study the perception of cancer patients and their families in regard to the service name change from *palliative care* to *supportive care*.

After the implementation of the name change at our cancer center, Dalal et al.[101] conducted a retrospective chart review of 4701 consecutive new palliative consults where 1950 (41%) were referred prior to the name change and 2751 (59%) thereafter. The authors found that the name change was associated with 41% overall growth in referrals after adjusting for the institutional growth; these referrals were mainly inpatient referrals (733 vs. 1451 patients, P < 0.001). In the outpatient setting, the name change was associated with referrals being made 1.7 months earlier (5.2 vs. 6.9 months, hazard ratio [HR] 0.82, P < 0.001), a shorter duration from hospital registration to palliative care consultation (median, 9.2 vs. 13.2 months, HR 0.85, P < 0.001), and a 1.5 month longer overall survival duration from palliative care consultation (median 6.2 vs. 4.7 months, HR 1.21, P < 0.001). Outpatient supportive care centers facilitated earlier access to our services at our cancer center, and we believe they should be established in more cancer centers.

In summary, palliative care services should match the needs of patients and families. These services can be provided in an inpatient or outpatient setting. The inpatient care can be delivered in TPCUs, acute care hospitals, and the inpatient hospice units. Outpatient care can be delivered at home, in DHs, in NHs, or in MD clinics.

No single palliative care program needs to have all these components. These settings can be owned by one institution or can have different owners to integrate palliative care delivery.

Most importantly, every palliative care patient should be able to have access to any of these settings in a seamless way appropriate to their needs.

To reach a seamless network for the delivery of care, palliative care programs should have resources: agreement between different settings, bus rounds, common assessment tools, common treatment guidelines, and regular communication (audiovisual: patient care and education).

CONCLUSION

In more than 30 years since the inception of the modern hospice movement, a number of clinical programs have emerged. These programs have demonstrated their value in a number of specific patient populations.

One of the greater challenges has been to make it possible for patients in different regimen of the world to access the system that is most appropriate to their needs (i.e., home care and day hospital as compared to inpatient hospice or inpatient acute care facility). In addition, a setting that is appropriate for a patient at a certain time, that is, a patient's comfort at home with home care, may be inappropriate when there is complete family burnout or severe aggravation of symptoms distress.

One of the greatest challenges is to have seamless care so that patients at any given time are able to receive palliative care in the setting that is most appropriate to their needs. There has been significant progress in recognizing that the different settings described in this chapter are complementary rather than competitive. There is still considerable need for research on the best way to integrate these different programs into a seamless network.

Key learning points

- Place of death
- Patient and family needs
- Symptom distress observed in terminally ill patients
- IDT
- Outpatient palliative care settings
- Inpatient palliative care settings
- Integration of different settings into a seamless network

REFERENCES

1 Lattimer, EJ. Ethical decision-making in the care of the dying and its application to clinical practice. *J Pain Symptom Manage* 1991; **6**: 329–336.

2 Neuenschwander H, Bruera E, Cavalli F. Matching the clinical function and symptom status with the expectations of patients with advanced cancer, their families, and health care workers. *Support Care Cancer* 1997; **5**(3): 252–256.

◆ 3 Bruera E, Neumann C, BrenneisC, Quan H. Frequency of symptom distress and poor prognostic indicators in palliative cancer patients admitted to a tertiary palliative care unit, hospices, and acute care hospitals. *J Palliat Care* 2000; **16**(3): 16–21.

4 McMillan SC, Small BJ. Symptom distress and quality of life in patients with cancer newly admitted to hospice home care. *Oncol Nurs Forum* 2002; **29**(10): 1421–1428.

5 Farber SJ, Egnew TR, Herman-Bertsch JL, Taylor TR, Guldin GE. Issues in end-of-life care: Patient, caregiver, and clinician perceptions. *J Palliat Med* 2003;**6**(1): 19–31.

6 Tringali CA. The needs of family members of cancer patients. *Oncol Nurs Forum* 1986; **13**(4): 65–70.

7 Given BA, Given CW, Kozachik S. Family support in advanced cancer. *CA: Cancer J Clin* 2001; **51**: 213–231.

8 Doyle D, Hanks G, Cherny N, Calman K, *Oxford Textbook of Palliative Medicine*, 3rd ed, Oxford University Press, New York, NY, 2004 15, pp. 1033–1084.

9 Pesamaa L, Ebeling H, Kuusimaki ML, Winblad I, Isohanni M, Moilanen I. Videoconferencing in child and adolescent telepsychiatry: A systematic review of the literature. *J Telemed Telecare* 2004; **10**(4): 187–192.

◆ 10 Kuulasma A, Wahlberg KE, Kuusimaki ML. Videoconferencing in family therapy: A review. *J Telemed Telecare*.

11 Solloway M, LaFrance S, Bakitas M, Gerken M. A chart review of seven hundred eighty-two deaths in hospitals, nursing homes, and hospice/home care. *J Palliat Med* 2005; **8**(4): 789–796.

12 Wilkinson J. Ethical issues in palliative care. In: Doyle D, Hanks GWC, MacDonald C. (Ed.) *Oxford Textbook of Palliative Medicine.* New York: Oxford Medical Publications; 1993.

13 von Gunten CF, Martinez J. A program of hospice and palliative care in a private, nonprofit U.S. Teaching Hospital. *J Palliat Med* 1998; **1**(3): 256–276.

◆ 14 Cantwell P, Turco S, Brenneis C, Hanson J, Neumann CM, Bruera E. Predictors of home death in palliative care cancer patients. *J Palliat Care* 2000; **16**(1): 23–28.

15 Neale, B. Informal care & community care. In Clark, D. (Ed.) *The Future for Palliative Care: Issues of Policy and Practice.* Buckingham, U.K.: Open University Press; 1993, pp. 52–67.

16 Claxton-Oldfield S, Jefferies J, Fawcet C, Wasylkiw L, Claxton-Oldfiel J. Palliative care volunteers: Why do they do it? *J Palliat Care* 2004; **20**(2): 78–84.

17 Tyrera F, Exley C. Receiving care at home at end of life: Characteristics of patients receiving hospice at home care. *Fam Pract* 2005; **22**(6): 644–646.

18 Randall F, Downie RS. *Palliative Care Ethics, a Companion for All Specialties.* New York: Oxford Medical Publications. 1999. ISBN 0-19-263068-7.

19 Van Eys J. The ethics of palliative care. *J Palliat Care* 1991; **7**(3): 27–32.

20 Fleming DA. The burden of caregiving at the end-of-life. *Mo Med* 2003; **100**(1): 82–86.

◆ 21 Strasser F, Sweeney C, Willey J, Benisch-Tolley S, Palmer JL, Bruera E. Impact of a half-day multidisciplinary symptom control and palliative care outpatient clinic in a comprehensive cancer center on recommendations, symptom intensity, and patient satisfaction: A retrospective descriptive study. *J Pain Symptom Manage* 2004; **27**(6): 481–491.

◆ 22 Bruera E, Michaud M, Vigano A, Neumann CM, Watanabe S, Hanson J. Multidisciplinary symptom control clinic in a cancer center: A retrospective study. *Support Care Cancer* 2001; **9**(3): 162–168.

23 Walsh D, Donnelly S, Rybicki L. The symptoms of advanced cancer: Relationship to age, gender, and performance status in 1,000 patients. *Support Care Cancer* 2000; **8**: 175–179.

24 Vainio A, Auvinen A. Prevalence of symptoms among patients with advanced cancer: An international collaborative study. Symptom Prevalence Group. *J Pain Symptom Manage* 1996; **12**: 3–10.

25 Bruera E. Symptom control in patients with cancer. *J Psychosoc Oncol* 1990; **8**: 47–73.

◆ 26 Bruera E, Kuehn N, Miller MJ, Selmser P, Macmillan K. The Edmonton Symptom Assessment System (ESAS): A simple method for the assessment of palliative care patients. *J Palliat Care* 1991; **7**: 6–9.

◆ 27 Ewing J. Detecting alcoholism: The CAGE Questionnaire. *JAMA* 1984; **252**: 1905–1907.

◆ 28 Folstein MF, Folstein S, McHugh PR. "Minimental state": A practical method for grading the cognitive state of patients for the clinician. *J Psych Res* 1975; **12**: 189–198.

◆ 29 Bruera E, Pituskin E, Calder K, Neumann CM, Hanson J. The addition of an audiocassette recording of a consultation to written recommendations for patients with advanced cancer: A randomized, controlled trial. *Cancer* 1999; **86**(11): 2420–2425.

30 Evans LK, Forciea MA, Yurkow J, Sochalski J. The geriatric day hospital. In: Katz PR, Kane RL, Mezey MD (Eds.) *Emerging Systems in Long-Term Care.* New York: Springer Publishing Company, Inc.; 1999, pp. 67–87.

31 Densen PM. *Tracing the Elderly Through the Health Care System: An Update.* AHCPR 91–11 ed. Rockville, MD: Department of Health and Human Services, 1991.

32 Dekker R, Drost EA, Groothoff JW, Arendzen JH, van Gijn JC, Eisma WH. Effects of day-hospital rehabilitation in stroke patients: A review of randomized clinical trials. *Scand J Rehabil Med* 1998; **30**(2): 87–94.

33 Mor V, Stalker MZ, Gralla R, Scher HI, Cimma C, Park D et al. Day hospital as an alternative to inpatient care for cancer patients: A random assignment trial. *J Clin Epidemiol* 1988; **41**(8): 771–785.

34 Rogge R. Diabetic day hospital in Wiesbaden: Education and treatment under everyday conditions during job and leisure time. *Medizinische Welt* 2000; **51**(7–8): 219–222.

35 Wisseler HM, Lautenschlager J, Leichner-Hennig R, Henrich H. Rheumatological day clinic in the Auerbach Clinic Dr. Vetter—Beginnings and initial experiences. *Aktuelle Rheumatol* 2003; **28**(1): 30–35.

36 Gill HS, Walter DB. The day hospital model of care for patients with medical and rehabilitative needs. *Hosp Technol Ser* 1996; **15**(17): 1–14.

37 Capomolla S, Febo O, Ceresa M, Caporotondi A, Guazzotti G, La Rovere M et al. Cost/utility ratio in chronic heart failure: Comparison between heart failure management program delivered by day-hospital and usual care. *J Am Coll Cardiol* 2002; **40**(7): 1259–1266.

38 Biem HJ, Cotton D, McNeil S, Boechler A, Gudmundson D. Day medicine: An urgent internal medicine clinic and medical procedures suite. *Healthc Manage Forum* 2003; **16**(1): 17–23.

39 Davies E, Higginson IJ. Systematic review of specialist palliative day-care for adults with cancer. *Support Care Cancer.* 2005 Aug; **13**(8): 607–27.

40 Thompson B. Hospice day care. *Am J Hosp Care* 1990; **7**(1): 28–30.

41 Wilkes E, Crowther AGO, Greaves CWKH. A different kind of day hospital—For patients with preterminal cancer and chronic disease. *BMJ* 1978; **2**: 1053–1056.

42 Cockburn M, Twine J. A different kind of day unit. *Nurs Times* 1982; **78**: 1410–1411.

43 Sharma K, Oliver D, Blatchford G, Higginbottom P, Kahn V. Medical care in hospice day care. *J Palliat Care* 1993; **9**: 42–43.

44 Edwards A, Livingston H, Daley A. Does hospice day care need doctors? *Palliat Care Today* 1997; **6**:36–37.

45 Kennett CE. Participation in a creative arts project can foster hope in hospice day care. *Palliat Med* 2000; **4**: 419–425.

46 Copp G, Richardson A, McDaid P, Marshall-Searson DA. A telephone survey of the provision of palliative day care services. *Palliat Med* 1998; **12**: 161–170.

47 Higginson IJ, Hearn J, Myers K, Naysmith A. Palliative day care: What do services do? *Palliat Med* 2000; **14**: 277–286.

48 Faulkner A, Higginson IJ, Heulwen E, Egerton H, Power M, Sykes N, Wilkes E. Hospice day care: A qualitative study. Help the Hospices and Trent Palliative Care, Sheffield, 1993.

49 Langley-Evans A, Payne S. Light-hearted death talk in a palliative day care context. *J Adv Nurs* 1987; **26**:1091–1097.

50 Douglas H-R, Higginson, IJ, Myers K, Normand CE. Assessing structure, process and outcome in palliative day care: A pilot for a multicentre trial. *Health Soc Care Commun* 2000; **8**(5):336–344.

51 Hopkinson JB, Hallet CE. Patients' perceptions of hospice day care: A phenomenological study. *Int J Nurs Stud* 2001; **38**:117–125.

52 Lee L. Inter-professional working in hospice day care and the patients' experience of the service. *Int J Palliat Nurs* 2000; **8**:389–400.

53 Goodwin DM, Higginson IJ, Myers K, Douglas H-R, Normand CE. What is palliative day care? A patient perspective of five UK services. *Support Care Cancer* 2002; **10**: 556–562.

54 Goodwin DM, Higginson IJ, Myers K, Douglas H-R, Norman CE. Effectiveness of palliative day care in improving pain, symptom control and quality of life. *J Pain Symptom Manage* 2003; **25**(3): 202–212.

55 Mays N, Pope C. Rigour and qualitative research. *BMJ* 1995; **311**:109–112.

56 Mays N, Pope C. Assessing quality in qualitative research. *BMJ* 2000; **320**:50–52.

◆ 57 Bruera E, Fornells H, Perez E, Tattangelo M, Neumann C. Bus rounds for medical congresses on palliative care. *Support Care Cancer* 1998; **6**:529–532.

∗ 58 Bruera E, Selmser P, Pereira J, Brenneis C. Bus rounds for palliative care education in the community. *Can Med Assoc J* 1997; **157**: 729–732.

59 Jenkins CA, Schulz M, Hanson J, Bruera E. Demographic, symptom, and medication profiles of cancer patients seen by a palliative care consult team in a tertiary referral hospital. *J Pain Symptom Manage* 2000; **19**(3): 174–184.

60 Fins JJ, Miller FG. A proposal to restructure hospital care for dying patients. *N Engl J Med* 1996; **334**: 1740–1742.

◆ 61 O'Mahony S, Blank AE, Zallman L, Selwyn PA. The benefits of a hospital-based inpatient palliative care consultation service: Preliminary outcome data. *J Palliat Med* 2005; **8**(5): 1033–1039.

62 von Gunten CF. Secondary and tertiary palliative care in U.S. hospitals. *JAMA* 2002; **287**: 875–881.

◆ 63 von Gunten CF, Ferris FD, Portenoy R, Glachen M. (eds.) *CAPC Manual: Everything You Wanted to Know About Developing a Palliative Care Program but Were Afraid to Ask.* 2001. Available at: http://www.capcmssm.org.

64 Brenneis C, Bruera E. Models for the delivery of palliative care: The Canadian model. In: Bruera E, Portenoy RK. (Eds.) *Topics in Palliative Care, Volume 5.* New York: Oxford University Press; 2001, pp. 3–23.

65 von Gunten CF. Discussing do-not-resuscitate status. *J Clin Oncol* 2001; **19**: 1576–1581.

66 Bruera E, Schoeller T, Wenk R et al. A prospective multicenter assessment of the Edmonton Staging System for cancer pain. *J Pain Symptom Manage* 1995; **10**: 348–355.

◆ 67 Walker P, Nordell C, Neumann CM, Bruera E. Impact of the Edmonton Labeled Visual Information System on physician recall of metastatic cancer patient histories: A randomized controlled trial. *J Pain Symptom Manage* 2001; **21**: 4–11.

68 Kaasa T, Loomis J, Gillis K et al. The Edmonton Functional Assessment Tool: Preliminary development and evaluation for use in palliative care. *J Pain Symptom Manage* 1997; **13**: 10–19.

69 Oneschuk D, Fainsinger R, Hanson J, Bruera E. Assessment and knowledge in palliative care in second year family medicine residents. *J Pain Symptom Manage* 1998; **14**: 265–273.

◆ 70 Bruera E, Suarez-Almazor M, Velasco A et al. The assessment of constipation in terminal cancer patients admitted to a palliative care unit: A retrospective review. *J Pain Symptom Manage* 1994; **9**: 515–519.

71 Maccabee J. The effect of transfer from a palliative care unit to nursing homes—Are patients' and relatives' needs met? *Palliat Med* 1994; **8**: 211–214.

72 Mazuryk M, Daeninck P, Neumann CM, Bruera E. Daily journal club: An education tool in palliative care. *Palliat Med* 2002; **16**: 57–61.

73 Addington-Hall J, Altmann D, McCarthy M. Which terminally ill cancer patients receive hospice in-patient care? *Soc Sci Med* 1998; **46**: 1011–1016.

74 Hinton J. Which patients with terminal cancer are admitted from home care? *Palliat Med* 1994; **8**: 197–210.

75 Gray JD, Forster DP. Factors associated with the utilization of specialist palliative care services: A population based study. *J.Public Health Med* 1997; **19**: 464–469. 1997.

76 Gatrell AC, Harman J, Francis BJ, Thomas C, Morris SM, McIllmurray M. Place of death: Analysis of cancer deaths in part of North West England. *J Public Health Med* 2003; **25**: 53–58.

◆ 77 National Hospice and Palliative Care Organization. Hospice facts and figures 2004. www.nhpco.org. Accessed November 19, 2005.

78 Elsayem A, Driver L, Bruera E. *Hospice Services. The M.D. Anderson Symptom Control and palliative Care Handbook*, 2nd edn., 2003, 19, pp. 131–136.

79 Bradshaw PJ. Characteristics of clients referred to home, hospice and hospital palliative care services in Western Australia. *Palliat Med* 1993; **7**: 101–107.

80 Regional palliative Care Program. Annual Report April 1, 1996 to March 31, 1997. *Capital Health Authority.* Edmonton, Alberta, 1997.

81 Parkes CM, Parkes J. 'Hospice' versus 'hospital' care—Re-evaluation after 10 years as seen by surviving spouses. *Postgrad Med J* 1984; **60**: 120–124.

82 Seale C, Kelly M. A comparison of hospice and hospital care for people who die: Views of the surviving spouse. *Palliat Med* 1997; **11**: 93–100.

83 Teno J. *The Brown Atlas of Dying in the United States: 1989–2001.* Available at: http://www.chcr.brown.edu/dying/brownsodinfo.htm. Accessed November 23, 2004.

84 Casarett D, Karlawish J, Morales K, Crowley R, Mirsch T, Asch DA. Improving the use of hospice services in nursing homes: A randomized controlled trial. *JAMA* 2005; **294**(2): 211–217.

85 Rice KN, Coleman EA, Fish R, Levy C, Kutner JS. Factors influencing models of end-of-life care in nursing homes: Results of a survey of nursing home administrators. *J Palliat Med* 2004; **7**(5): 668–675.

86 Bernabei R, Gambassi G, Lapane K et al. Management of pain in elderly patients with cancer. *JAMA* 1998; **279**: 1877–1882.

87 Levy CR, Fish R, Kramer AM. Site of death in the hospital versus nursing home of Medicare skilled nursing facility residents admitted under Medicare's Part A Benefit. *J Am Geriatr Soc* 2004; **52**: 1247–1254.

88 Miller SC, Gozalo P, Mor V. Hospice enrollment and hospitalization of dying nursing home patients. *Am J Med* 2001; **111**: 38–44.

89 Teno J, Clarridge B, Casey V et al. Family perspectives on end-of-life care at the last place of care. *JAMA* 2004; **291**: 88–93.

90 Thorpe G. Enabling more dying people to remain at home. *J Palliat Care.* 2000; **16**(1): 23–28.

91 Mount BM, Ajemian I. the palliative care service integration in a general hospital. In: Ajemian I, Mount BM (Eds). *The R.V.H. Manual on Palliative/Hospice Care.* New York: Arno Press; 1980, pp. 269–280.

92 Stajduhar KI, Davies B. Death at home: Challenges for families and directions for the future. *J Palliat Care* 1998; **14**(3): 8–14.

93 McWhinney IR, Bass MJ, Orr V. Factors associated with location of death (home or hospital) of patients referred to a palliative care team. *CMAJ* 1995; **152**(3): 361–367.

94 StephanyTM. Place of death: Home or hospital. *Home Healthcare Nurse.* 1992; **10**(3): 62.

95 Dudgeon DJ, Kristjanson L. Home versus hospital death: Assessment of preferences and clinical challenges. *CMAJ* 1995; **152**(3): 337–340.

96 Doyle D. Domiciliary palliative care. In: Doyle D, Hanks G, MacDonalds C (Eds). *Oxford Textbook of Palliative Medicine.* New York: Oxford University Press Inc.; 1998, pp. 957–963.

97 Hinton J. Can home care maintain an acceptable quality of life for patients with terminal cancer and their relatives? *Palliat Med* 1994; **8**(3): 183–196.

◆ 98 Cohen SR, Mount BM, Bruera E, Provost M, Rowe J, Tong K. Validity of the McGill quality of life questionnaire in the palliative care setting: A multi-centre Canadian study demonstrating the importance of the existential domain. *Palliat Med* 1997; **11**: 3–23.

◆ 99 Osta BE, Palmer JL, Paraskevopoulos T, Pei BL, Roberts LE, Poulter VA, Chacko R, Bruera E. Interval between first palliative care consult and death in patients diagnosed with advanced cancer at a comprehensive cancer center. *J Palliat Med* 2008; **11**(1): 51–57.

◆100 Fadul N, Elsayem A, Palmer JL, Del Fabbro E, Swint K, Li Z, Poulter V, Bruera E. Supportive verus palliative care: What's in a name?: A survey of medical oncologists and midlevel providers at a comprehensive cancer center. *Cancer* 2009; **115**(9): 2013–2021.

◆101 Dalal S, Palla S, Hui D, Nguyen L, Chacko R, Li Z, Fadul N, Scott C, Thornton V, Coldman B, Amin Y, Bruera E. Association between a name change from palliative to supportive care and the timing of patient referrals at a comprehensive cancer center. *Oncologist* 2011; **16**(1): 105–111.

◆102 Yennurajalingam S, Kang JH, Hui D, Kang DH, Kim SH, Bruera E. Clinical response to an outpatient palliative care consultation in patients with advanced cancer and cancer pain. *J Pain Symptom Manage* 2012; **44**(3): 340–350.

◆103 Kang JH, Kwon JH, Hui D, Yennurajalingam S, Bruera E. Changes in symptom intensity among cancer patients receiving outpatient palliative care. *J Pain Symptom Manage* 2013; **46**(5): 652–660.

◆104 Casarett D, Johnson M, Smith D, Richardson D. The optimal delivery of palliative care: A national comparison of the outcomes of consultation teams vs inpatient units. *Ach Intern Med* 2011; **171**(7): 649–655.

◆105 Hui D, Elsayem A, De la Cruz M, Berger A, Zhukovsky DS, Palla S, Evans A, Fadul N, Palmer JL, Bruera E. Availability and Integration of pallilative care at U.S. cancer centers. *JAMA* 2010; **303**(11): 1054–1061.

◆106 Fadul N, Kaur G, Zhang T, Palmer JL, Bruera E. Evaluation of the memorial delirium assessment scale (MDAS) for the screening of delirium by means of simulated cases by palliative care health professionals. *Support Care Cancer* 2007; **15**(11): 1271–1276.

34

Palliative home care

ROBERTO WENK

INTRODUCTION

Palliative care is a specialized medical care for people with life-threatening diseases. It is focused on providing patients with relief from the symptoms and stresses of a serious illness—whatever the diagnosis. The goal is to improve the quality of life for both the patient and the family.[1]

Palliative care needs to be available to patients and families in all settings where they receive care, including outpatient clinics, acute and long-term care facilities, and homes.

When palliative care is provided at home, every patient has the possibility to receive good quality care in their home; it is an option for patients who wish to be cared for at home when they meet at least the following conditions: healthcare services available, needs that can be fulfilled at home, and home where care can be provided and the family collaborates.[2]

WHAT IS ALREADY KNOWN?

Palliative home care (PHC) is defined as an array of health and social support coordinated services provided to patients in their own home or residence that may prevent, delay, or be a substitute for temporary or long-term institutional care.[3] The target group is patients with life-threatening diseases, and care is provided by an interdisciplinary healthcare professional team.[4]

PHC is common today in many areas of the world, with a rising trend in the future in response to the growing need of palliative care due to the increase of chronic diseases and the aging population and also in response to the ever-increasing costs of inpatient care.[5]

Extensive research on the effectiveness of PHC provides evidence of its benefits in helping patients to be cared for at home with effective symptom control without impacting on caregiver grief.[6]

The overall perception is that PHC outcomes are positive in two main different areas:

The patient. A systematic review of numerous studies provides evidence that the majority of people in high-income countries prefer to be cared for and die at home (this was reported in 75% of 130 studies) and that around four-fifths of patients did not change preference as their illness progressed. This trend in preferences is determined by the quality of available options to stay at home.[7] There is also evidence that PHC is more effective than usual care in relieving the patients' symptoms.[6] The concept that remaining at home is the best alternative in order to maintain his/her quality of life[8] is valid.

The society and the healthcare system. Different studies report decreased admission to hospital, reduction of inpatient hospital days, less fragmented care, and fewer high-tech interventions.[9–11]

The following are the advantages of PHC related with the patients' and the family's (persons with biologic, legal or social relationship with the patient, for the purpose of this chapter) safety, independence, and psychological well-being[12]:

1. Familiarity with the setting.
2. Autonomy. The patient stays with the family and decides his/her activity, rest, and diet. He/she maintains some roles.
3. Privacy. The patient is not exposed to the interference, at times unnecessary and undesired, of medical activities, nor is he/she exposed to the suffering of other patients.
4. Protection and quietness. The patient is less exposed to therapeutic procedures, which at times are futile, with lesser risk of hospital-acquired infections.
5. Better bereavement outcomes. The family can anticipate the loss.
6. Less discomfort with the notion of death. The death of a relative happening in the place where the life was shared is a way to learn that the death is a normal nonaberrant stage of life.

Effective PHC is determined by demographic, medical, psycho-social, and sanitary factors unique to each patient and family.[13] Results of studies that include more than 1.5 million cancer patients from 13 different countries, mostly from the United Kingdom, the United States, Australia, and Canada, provide evidence that issues that make PHC possible can be grouped in the following[14]:

- Factors related to illness: Long length of disease and low functional status; low expectation of sudden clinical changes
- Demographic variables: Good social conditions and good income
- Personal variables: Patients' preferences and agreement between the preferences of patients and carers for PHC; historical trends
- Environmental factors: Healthcare services including PHC; use and adequacy of home care
- Social support: Living with relatives, extended family support, and being married

Certainly, some circumstances may make PHC impossible:

1. Patients live in distant or rural areas.[15]
2. Patients live alone, with no family or friends willing or able to provide care.
3. Family tired, older carers, physically or emotionally weak, or dysfunctional.
4. Home unsuitable and unable to be adapted (e.g., no kitchen, running water, indoor toilets, electricity, and accessible bed/bathroom/toilet).

WHAT STILL NEEDS TO BE KNOWN?

PHC has grown significantly during the last few years and will continue to grow even more in the future. It has been taken for granted worldwide. In many middle-income and low-income countries, it has been idealized as the *gold standard*,[16] and it is progressively adopted but research about its practice does not yet exist.

The next section includes comments based on observations in Argentina, a country where PHC is progressively more available to families and patients that need it.

The comments are based on the analysis of some dynamic interrelated issues that should be considered to optimize this new process that makes possible the transition from palliative care delivered almost exclusively in institutions to palliative care provided in the patient's home. The comments may be applicable to other countries where PHC is in the same stage of development: they may be useful to identify benefits and confront problems.

The following questions guide the analysis:

Does PHC occur only when the patient loses autonomy?

PHC is introduced to provide an additional service to the institutional care when the patient diminishes his/her mobility with the service provided by the healthcare personnel. Although the participation of licensed medical personnel makes a difference with the definition of home care, it may be

possible—and necessary—to consider that PHC starts in the ambulatory stage before the patient loses his/her mobility.

PHC may be understood differently under the concept that both components of the unit of care—patient and family—have needs that are domains of the palliative care model.

The mobile patient with a life-threatening disease may have symptoms and attends the outpatient palliative care clinic or primary caregiver office for their adequate control; controlled symptoms reduce the physical and psychological burdens of patient care and are a key component to the success of home care.[17–19]

The family that has a central caring role with sometimes long-term increases in emotional and technical duties[20,21] and may become the main focus of care.[22] Negative effects on families may be important.

After the initial diagnosis and/or an inpatient treatment—two key transition points—cancer patients and families often experience heights and depths of stress and uncertainty.[23,24] They are particularly vulnerable when in the home and sometimes, they feel they are *in limbo*.[25]

Families often follow patterns of suffering that parallels that of patients and in some cases limit their ability to care.[26,27] They may experience negative emotions and develop crisis and psychological disorders,[28] such as considerable reduction of activities, and economic hardship as a result of an increase in expenses, and reduction of income associated with caregiving.[29]

Patients and families at this stage of conserved mobility require proactive management and support—domains of palliative care—to minimize the risk of predictable suffering.[30,31]

Actually, care with this inclusive concept of PHC is not yet provided in this stage of ambulatory care.

Are the three levels of care recognized?

According to a conceptual model based on the needs of a palliative care patient,[32] almost two-thirds of the patients do not require access to specialist palliative care. Instead, their needs are met either through their own resources or with the support of primary care providers (i.e., generalist physicians and nurses); the remaining third of the patients need palliative care services because their condition requires the participation of skilled practitioners, in partnership with primary care providers. This model requires integration of both generalist and specialist services that are offered across primary, secondary, and tertiary care settings.[33]

PHC teams are involved mostly in specialized home care. Primary care professionals should also be involved in basic-level PHC.

The central role of primary care providers in the home setting is acknowledged as a key component to improving access to palliative care.[34] Two requisites are central to this assumption: primary care providers have basic expertise in palliative care,[35] and while a solo practitioner can provide palliative care, he/she cannot work in isolation.[36] They need support from interdisciplinary palliative care team specialists to support their ability to provide PHC.

This shared care model in palliative care that enables the needs of patients to be met early in the trajectory of life-threatening illness can occur only with strengthened interprofessional cooperation.[37]

The need of cooperation between health professionals is bigger if individuals or teams belong to different organizations; it demands knowledge and acceptance of each other's abilities, qualities, and roles in the delivery of care.[38]

Actually, this kind of shared care with interprofessional cooperation is still lacking.

Is the importance of outpatient consultation and telephone support enough recognized?

Patients with life-threatening diseases may be cared as outpatients for a variable time. They and their families can have early access to palliative care services in the ambulatory care setting[39]; outpatient clinics expand availability and access to palliative care.[40]

Outpatient consultation may be in institutional, specialist, or primary care offices; outpatient palliative care can be either basic or specialized.[41]

Patients receiving palliative care require frequent medication adjustments and education to ensure that they and their families understand the care plan. Routine assessments of patients and families are essential to the success of PHC: there is always the need to improve and adjust the services provided.

The activity should be performed in places strategically and conveniently located, easily accessible with proper operation: short time of appointment, attention on time, and consultation with sufficient duration to discuss and address all the concerns.

The outpatient activity can be reinforced with scheduled or on-demand communication with patients and families via telephone (hotline?) and/or through e-mail.

There are often crises, either real or perceived, that may occur outside of normal working hours and may result in the feeling of responsibility in isolation. Many reports show that telephone support solves most of the issues identified by patients and families.[42,43]

Both the organized outpatient activity and the telephone support can help the patients to receive timely appropriate interventions for troubling symptoms.

Actually, the value and benefits of any of both adjuvants for PHC are still fully recognized.

Is there adequate communication between the professionals involved? Is the activity coordinated?

As the disease progresses, it is necessary that health personnel involved in the care of the patient have complete updated information of the situation; this knowledge is key to delivering effective PHC[44,45] with adequate planning and distribution of tasks. To achieve this goal, a network with adequate communication between the participating health personnel is essential.

Communication within the network must be easy and should develop with acknowledgment of the following issues:

- Trust and mutual respect, both personally and professionally, are the foundations for cooperation.
- Prejudice and lack of respect are barriers to cooperation; incompetence, reluctance to establish teamwork, or lack of enthusiasm about palliative care are causes of disrespect.
- Personal contact with each other breaks down prejudices and facilitates cooperation.

Communication is necessary to coordinate care and thus to improve the delivery of PHC. Information exchange and coordination could be facilitated by a webpage with the following:

- Disease information: Diagnosis, treatment and side effects, prognosis, and therapeutic plan.
- Professional judgments about the patient's levels of needs, that is, basic or specialized palliative care.
- What had been said to the patient and the relatives?
- Changes in need that occur during the disease trajectory.
- Professional contact information.
- Practical information about palliative care issues.

Actually, the value of the preceding things is still poorly recognized; in most cases, health care personnel involved in the palliative care of a patient do not share information on the ongoing caring process.

CONCLUSIONS

The transition process happens and facilitates the passage from one stage of a disease to another or from one treatment to another.[46] Transitions are difficult because they generate changes, positive or negative, that produce stress on the patient and the family. During this process, the fragmentation of the healthcare system with poorly coordinated care may become evident.

PHC may be considered an umbrella activity that comprises many issues related to care activities that need to be identified, defined, understood, and changed to optimize the transition process. As the field of PHC is wide and its future demand is great and will be greater, it is necessary to distinguish the diversity of factors that can promote or impede PHC to act accordingly to both increase its benefits and reduce its disadvantages.

Research is also needed to elucidate how these factors interact with each other and with the health system.

Application of this approach may enable healthcare providers to focus on the issue of inadequately relieved suffering and articulate treatment methods that encompass the needs of patients and families.

PHC is a central area of palliative care. Adequate care of the patient at his/her home has much to do with his/her well-being and quality of life.

REFERENCES

1   Center to advance Palliative Care. Defining palliative care. Internet. Accessed on April 1, 2013. Available at http://www.capc.org/building-a-hospital-based-palliative-care-program/case/definingpc.
2   Field MJ and Cassel CK (eds.), Committee on Care at the End of Life, Division of Health Care Services, Institute of Medicine. *Approaching Death: Improving Care at the End of Life.* Washington, DC: National Academy Press, 1997. ISBN 0-309-06372-8.

3   Knight S and Tjassing H. Health care moves to the home. *World Health* 1994; 4: 413–444.

4   Home care. Wikipedia. Internet. Accessed on March 30, 2013. Available at http://en.wikipedia.org/wiki/Home_care.

5   Medpac. Hospital inpatient and outpatient services. Internet. Accessed on April 5, 2013. Available at http://www.medpac.gov/chapters/Mar12_Ch03.pdf.

6   Gomes B, Calanzani N, Curiale V, McCrone P, and Higginson IJ. Effectiveness and cost-effectiveness of home palliative care services for adults with advanced illness and their caregivers. *Cochrane Database of Systematic Reviews* 2013; 6: 25. Art.No.:CD007760. DOI: 10.1002/14651858.CD007760.

7   Gomes B, Calanzani N, Gysels M, Hall S, and Higginson IJ. Heterogeneity and changes in preferences for dying at home: A systematic review. *BMC Palliative Care.* 12:7; 1–13. Accessed on May 24, 2013. Available at http://www.biomedcentral.com/1472-684X/12/7.

8   Singer PA and Bowman KW. Quality care at the end of life. *BMJ* 2002; 324: 1291–1292.

9   Robbins MA. The economics of palliative medicine. In: D. Doyle, G.W.C. Hanks, and N. MacDonald (eds). *Oxford Textbook of Palliative Medicine.* 2nd edn. Oxford, U.K.: Oxford University Press, 1997.

10 Thome B, Dykes A, and Hallberg I. Home care with regard to definition, care recipients, content and outcome: Systematic literature review. *Journal of Clinical Nursing* 2003; 12(6): 860–872.

11 Wenk R and Bertolino M. Direct medical costs of an Argentinian domiciliary palliative care model. *Journal of Pain and Symptom Management* 2000; 20: 162–164.

12 Stajduhar K and Davies B. Death at home: Challenges for families and directions for the future. *Journal of Palliative Care* 1998; 14(3): 8–14.

13 Wenk R. Palliative home care. In: E. Bruera, I Higginson, C Ripamonti, and C Von Gunten (eds). *Textbook of Palliative Medicine.* London, U.K.: Hodder Arnold, 2006; pp. 277–284.

14 Gomes B and Higginson IJ. Factors influencing death at home in terminally ill patients with cancer: Systematic review. *BMJ* 2006; 332: 1012.1. Accessed on May 24, 2013. Available at http://www.bmj.com/content/332/7540/515.

15 Buehler JA and Lee HJ. Exploration of home care resources for rural families with cancer. *Cancer Nursing* 1992; 15(4): 299–308.

16 Devlin M and McIlfatrick S. Providing palliative and end-of-life care in the community: The role of the home-care worker. *International Journal of Palliative Nursing* 2009; 15(11): 526–532.

17 Coyle N, Cherny NI, and Portenoy RK. Subcutaneous opioid infusions at home. *Oncology* (Huntingt) 1994; 8(4): 21–27; discussion 31–32, 37.

18 Ferrell BR, Cohen MZ, Rhiner M et al. Pain as a metaphor for illness. Part II: Family caregivers' management of pain. *Oncology Nursing Forum* 1991; 18(8): 1315–1321.

19 Ferrell BR, Rhiner M, Cohen MZ et al. Pain as a metaphor for illness. Part I: Impact of cancer pain on family caregivers. *Oncology Nursing Forum* 1991; 18(8): 1303–1309.

20 Cameron JI, Franche RL, Cheung AM et al. Lifestyle interference and emotional distress in family caregivers of advanced cancer patients. *Cancer* 2002; 94(2): 521–527.

21 Maloney CH and Preston F. An overview of home care for patients with cancer. *Oncology Nursing Forum* 1992; 19(1): 75–80.

22 Glajchen M. Role of the family caregivers in cancer pain management. *Journal of Pain and Symptom Management* 2003; 26: 644–654.

23 Grov EK and Eklund ML. Reactions of primary caregivers of frail older people and people with cancer in the palliative phase living at home. *Journal of Advanced Nursing* 2008; 63(6): 576–585.

24 Ingunn Hunstad I and Svindseth MF. Challenges in home-based palliative care in Norway: A qualitative study of spouses' experiences. *International Journal of Palliative Nursing* 2011; 17(8): 398–404.

25 Brogaard T et al. Who is the key worker in palliative home care? Views of patients, relatives and primary care professionals. *Scandinavian Journal of Primary Health Care* 2011; 29: 150–156.

26 Murray A et al. Archetypal trajectories of social, psychological, and spiritual wellbeing and distress in family care givers of patients with lung cancer: Secondary analysis of serial qualitative interviews. *BMJ* 2010; 304: c2581.

27 Wenk R and Monti C. El sufrimiento de los cuidadores responsables. *Med Pal* 2006; 13: 64–68.

28 Vachon M. Psychosocial needs of patients and families. *Journal of Palliative Care* 1998; 14(3): 49–56.

29 Kinsella G, Cooper B, Picton C, and Murtagh D. A review of the measurement of caregiver and family burden in palliative care. *Journal of Palliative Care* 1998; 14(2): 37–45.

30 Payne S and Hudson P. EAPC Task Force on Family Carers: Aims and objectives. *European Journal of Palliative Care* 2009; 16(2): 77–81.

31 Grande G and Ewing G, on behalf of the National Forum for Hospice at Home. Informal career bereavement outcome: Relation to quality of life support and achievement of preferred place of death. *Palliative Medicine* 2009; 23: 248.

32 Pallipedia. Population and needs-based planning for care at the end of life. Accessed on April 1, 2013. Available at http://pallipedia.org/term.php?id=525.

33 Genet N, Boerma N, Kroneman M, Hutchinson A, and Saltman R (eds.), World Health Organization. *Home Care across Europe Current Structure and Future Challenges.* Copenhagen, Denmark: EurHOMap, 2012. Stichting NIVEL. Accessed on May 24, 2013. Available at http://www.nivel.nl/en/home-care.

34 Howell D. Comprehensive palliative home care: A need for integrated models of primary and specialist care. *International Journal of Palliative Nursing* 2007; 3(2): 54–55.

35 De Lima L, Bennett MI, Murray SA, Hudson P, Doyle D, Bruera E, Granda-Cameron C, Strasser F, Downing J, and Wenk R. International Association for Hospice and Palliative Care (IAHPC) List of Essential Practices in Palliative Care. *Journal of Pain and Palliative Care Pharmacotherapy* June 2012; 26(2): 118–122.

36 Emanuel L et al. Integrating palliative care into disease management guidelines. *Journal of Palliative Medicine* 2004; 7(6): 774–782.

37 Neergaard MA et al. Shared care in basic level palliative home care: Organizational and interpersonal challenges. *Journal of Palliative Medicine* 2010; 13(9): 1071–1077.

38 Groot MM, Vernooij-Dassen MJ, Crul BJ, and Grol RP. General practitioners (GPs) and palliative care: Perceived tasks and barriers in daily practice. *Palliative Medicine* 2005; 19: 111–118.

39 Jane Griffith J, Lyman J, and Blackhall L. Providing palliative care in the ambulatory care setting. *Clinical Journal of Oncology Nursing* 2010; 14(2): 171–175.

40 Rabow MR et al. Patient perceptions of an outpatient palliative care intervention: "It had been on my mind before, but I did not know how to start talking about death". *Journal of Pain and Symptom Management* 2008; 36(1): 11–21.

41 Oliver D. The development of an interdisciplinary outpatient clinic in specialist palliative care. *International Journal of Palliative Nursing* 2004; 10(9): 446–448.

42 Phillips JL et al. Supporting patients and their caregivers after-hours at the end of life: The role of telephone support. *Journal of Pain and Symptom Management* 2008; 36(1): 11–21.

43 Rabow MW et al. Patient perceptions of an outpatient palliative care intervention: "It had been on my mind before, but I did not know how to start talking about death". *Journal of Pain and Symptom Management* 2003; 26(5): 1010–1015.

44 McMillan SC and Small BJ. Symptom distress and quality of life in patients with cancer newly admitted to hospice home care. *Oncology Nursing Forum* 2002; 29(10): 1421–1428.

45 Costantini M, Higginson IJ, Boni L et al. Effect of a palliative home care team on hospital admissions among patients with advanced cancer. *Palliative Medicine* 2003; 17(4): 315–321.

46 Transitional Care Planning. National Cancer Institute. Internet. Accessed on April 3, 2013. Available at http://www.cancer.gov/cancertopics/pdq/supportivecare/transitionalcare/HealthProfessional.

35

Palliative day-care centers and day hospitals

BRUNO GAGNON

INTRODUCTION

Provision of palliative care services has been in constant evolution since the initiation of the modern hospice movement in 1960. At first, emphasis was placed on inpatient beds in hospices or in hospital settings. Rapidly, home care services, often in association with hospice settings, were developed to take palliative care expertise into the home and to allow the terminally ill to remain at home until death, if at all possible and if desirable. The first palliative care day-care center, inspired by the experience of day-care services provided to the elderly and psychiatric patients, opened in 1975 at St. Luke's hospice in Sheffield, United Kingdom, to support patients with preterminal cancer and chronic disease.[1] This experience was reproduced extensively in the United Kingdom and elsewhere around the world in countries such as the United States, Australia, Japan, and several European countries.[2]

Davies and Higginson[3] systematically reviewed the literature on specialist palliative day-care centers. Fifteen articles were found suitable to provide information on service structure and care processes. Day-care centers were defined on a *social*, *social and medical*, or exclusively *medical* model. Most are led by nurses and complemented by a mix of other healthcare professionals including physicians, physiotherapists, occupational therapists, social workers, and non-health-care services available at a varying degree in each specific specialist palliative day-care center. These day-care programs may be attached to an inpatient hospice with or without home care services or be free-standing day-care centers. This close relationship with inpatient hospices often means that most patients of specialist palliative day-care centers are already receiving other forms of palliative care. This systematic review also suggests that the services offered by specialist palliative day-care centers are not based on previous need assessment. In general, these centers offer, among other health-care services, pain and symptom control through assessments, investigation and prescription of medication, wound care, and physiotherapy interventions. Other services such as occupational therapy, social work, chiropody, dietary advice, and music therapy tend to depend on available resources. Such variation in services greatly limits the possibility of establishing a clear definition of palliative care (PC) day centers and assessing their value in the care of the dying.

NEED FOR PALLIATIVE DAY HOSPITALS

Palliative care should be accessible to all cancer patients[4] as there is growing evidence that proper symptom management and psychological and existential support can be contributory in cancer control.[5] Furthermore, a recent control trial on the utility of early PC in advanced lung cancer clearly demonstrated an improvement in quality of life and even suggested increased survival.[6]

The concept of the day hospital was originally developed for the geriatric population. In 1951, the first geriatric day hospital was opened in Oxford, England,[7] in response to a lack of continuity of care between acute hospitalization and long-term placement.[8] By 1995, more than 400 day hospitals were implemented in the United Kingdom.[9] Hospital based, these facilities operate 5 days a week; however, patients visit only two to three times a week and service duration is usually up to 12 weeks.[10] This type of center has been defined as "an outpatient facility where frail older patients can receive sub-acute or acute medical, nursing, social and/or rehabilitative services over any portion of a full day, with return visits as necessary."[11] However, in the United States, although standard day hospitals do exist,[12,13] the Collaborative Assessment and Rehabilitation for Elders Program established a community-based center offering similar services to the day hospitals.[14] This initiative challenges the definition of the day hospital based on its location as similar services could be provided in the community.

The geriatric day hospital, by offering services centered on rehabilitation, aims at improving physical, mental, and social function of the elderly with the objective of prolonging survival, decreasing hospital admissions, institutionalization, and dependency.[15] However, concerns have been raised about the superiority in efficiency and overall cost of this type of center in comparison with other forms of comprehensive medical care.[15] In brief, geriatric day hospitals focus on rehabilitating the elderly or more specific populations such as poststroke individuals and those with dementia or Alzheimer's disease, while improving clinical and health service utilization outcomes. Even though the efficiency of this model of care has been put into question, its long existence seems to support its value.

During the same period, the concept of day hospital has also been developed for patients with mental illnesses. Psychiatric day hospitals are defined as hospital-based day-care centers providing "diagnostic and treatment services to acutely ill patients who would otherwise be treated in traditional psychiatric inpatients units."[16] Psychiatric day hospitals usually offer services and care on a daily basis; however, a recent survey of five European countries found no consistent profile of structure and procedural features.[17] Furthermore, the desire to manage patients within lower cost settings has led to the extension of day hospitals to other medical illnesses such as orthopedic surgery, laparoscopic surgery, stroke,[18] cancer,[19] diabetes mellitus,[20] rheumatological diseases,[21] chronic obstructive pulmonary disease (COPD),[22] congestive heart failure (HF),[23] and other illnesses.[24] Cost-effectiveness remains the major issue for most day-hospital initiatives. Interestingly, day hospitals have also been established for the management of pain crises related to sickle cell anemia with successful pain management and possible reduction of hospital admissions.[25,26]

PALLIATIVE CARE DAY HOSPITAL

General characteristics

The palliative care day hospital (PCDH), taking advantage of the experience from day hospitals, could be considered as a novel way to deliver earlier palliative care services to patients with advanced cancer. Based on a medical model, physicians and other health professionals provide their expertise to patients who, too often, are still receiving active oncology treatments and may otherwise lack access to specialized palliative care, such as complex interventions necessitating the hospital setting. A PCDH was inaugurated in 1998 at the Montreal General Hospital in Montreal, Canada. After 6 years of operation, we reviewed our experience using a Delphi method. Twenty-one members of our team participated in the review process, which included eight physicians, five nurses, two clinical nurses, two administrators, a psychologist, a pastoral person, a patient assistant, and a clerk.

Mandate

From the beginning, the PCDH was planned to provide a leadership role in promoting links between a tertiary care hospital and community services. Box 35.1 enumerates the different

---

Box 35.1　Mandates and roles of the palliative care day hospital

- The day hospital provides palliative care services to patients with life-threatening illnesses, primarily cancer; due to the complexity of their symptoms and/or their psychosocial context, these patients could not be appropriately cared for without being hospitalized. Patients may still be receiving palliative chemotherapy and can be candidates for complex medical/surgical interventions to improve quality of life.

- The day hospital provides specialized palliative care that is not available in the community or in other institutions. The goal of the day hospital is to improve the quality of life of patients and to support their families while allowing them to remain at home as long as possible.

- The day hospital works as a coordination center between hospital services, including inpatient palliative care services, and community-based services such as home care services and hospices to improve continuity of care and access to appropriate services according to patients' specific needs.

- The day hospital, as part of the McGill Palliative Care Division, promotes academic excellence by participating in teaching and research.

---

mandates assumed by the PCDH. Special emphasis was made to be all inclusive for patients in need of palliative care interventions during the whole disease trajectory from diagnosis to the terminal phase of their illness. At the present time, patients with a cancer diagnosis are mainly, but not exclusively, referred to the PCDH, as part of an initiative promoted in close collaboration with the oncology services. The PCDH offers services to patients who could not access such comprehensive palliative care without hospitalization due to the complexity of their clinical situation and their limited physical tolerance and to less sick patients with difficult pain or other symptoms who then can receive, in a relaxed setting, specialized palliative care not available in the community. The PCDH rapidly evolved as a communication center between community services and tertiary hospital services. Being situated in a university teaching facility, the PCDH contributes to the development of academic excellence in palliative care through teaching and research.

Box 35.2 describes in more detail the specific roles assumed by the PCDH. The team acts as a consultant to primary physicians by providing optimal palliative care assessment and specialized interventions. However, the reality of limited resources in the community, especially of physicians making home visits,[27] and the complexity of the clinical presentation warrant that the team should assume a more direct role in caring for this very sick population. The clinical condition of patients with advanced cancer can change drastically in a very short time and may mandate rapid interventions to adjust the plan of care. The PCDH can respond to such changes and provide support to the community by ensuring good

Box 35.2 Roles of the palliative care day hospital

Patient care

- Should provide optimal palliative care to patients with severe symptoms, existential distress, and difficult family situations, regardless of their prognosis

- Should assume a consultation role for patients who are not in the terminal phase of their illness

- Should assume treating physician role with terminally ill patients only in special situations: complexity of palliative care issues to supplement lack of resources in the community

- Should coordinate referrals to other palliative care services: pastoral, psychology, etc.

- Should organize advance care planning including clarification of code status

- Should provide emergency consultations within 48 hours

- Should coordinate special investigation and interventions to patients in the terminal phase of their illness and, in coordination with other hospital outpatient services, to patients receiving active treatment

- Should provide specialized services to special populations, for example, patients with lymphedema or severe anorexia–cachexia syndrome

Coordination of services

- Should improve links between specialized services of the hospital, especially oncology services and community resources

- Should promote links with home care services and hospices through adequate referral

- Should respond to a home *crisis* by giving support to home-based palliative care teams and by coordinating admission to the day hospital or the inpatient unit so as to prevent, if at all possible, visits to the emergency room by terminally ill patients

- Should provide phone consultations to physicians and nurses in the community regarding complex issues

- Should develop protocols of care with community services

Education

- Should educate colleagues in other disciplines within the hospital about day hospital mandates, resources available in the community, and the process to link patients and family with community resources

- Should promote palliative care through teaching within the institution, in the community, and at national and international congresses

- Should offer training sessions to physicians, nurses, social workers, and other specialized caregivers

- Should participate in teaching medical students, residents, fellows, and students of other health-care disciplines

Research

- Should provide equivalent care to all palliative care patients including those participating in research

- Should collect baseline clinical and sociodemographic data for research purposes

coordination by communicating through phone calls with hospital and community services, by offering emergency visits to the day hospital and to other services within the hospital, and by coordinating admission to palliative care inpatient units. This coordination effort is an important component of the PCDH role and provides an important benefit to patients and caregivers.

Figure 35.1 illustrates the different links and the possible movement of patients between the places of care. While it was originally thought that most referrals to the PCDH would originate from community services for patients in need of specialized palliative care not available in the community, the experience demonstrated that most referrals came from other outpatient services within the hospital, such as oncology, radio oncology, and surgical clinics. Such a pattern of referrals is explained by the fact that cancer patients receive care mainly through outpatient hospital services and minimal input from community services until they reach the terminal phase of their illness.[27] A possible explanation is that patients with cancer retain overall good physical function until late in the disease progression [28,29] and are therefore able to be cared for in outpatient clinics by cancer specialists. Therefore, the PCDH naturally evolved into an evaluation, stabilization, and referral facility, within the hospital, for patients needing palliative care. Since they are located within the hospital, the PCDH team members have access to entire patient charts, previous investigations, and the technical support

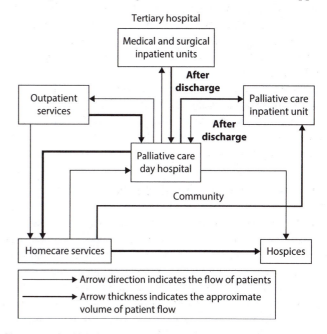

Figure 35.1 *Links between the PCDH and other services.*

needed to rapidly assess and stabilize patients and to provide community services with a complete palliative care evaluation and advanced care plan. Nonetheless, the PCDH continues to provide valuable support to patients whose care has been assumed by community resources by providing ongoing reevaluation for complex situations and by offering specialized interventions.

The team members of the PCDH are all specialized in palliative care; they assume a leadership role in education and in research. Because the population of patients seen at the PCDH includes a spectrum of clinical conditions from the early diagnosis to the terminal phase of the illness within the same day, it is an ideal setting for teaching and research. Research with this population of patients is challenging due to the complexity and instability of the patients' clinical situations. The PCDH provides a secure setting to patients with advanced disease, allowing them to contribute to the development of knowledge of palliative care by participating in research activities. Such participation offers these patients, whose disease has often removed their social role, a sense that they are still contributing members of society.

Palliative care multidisciplinary team

The basic team consists of physicians, bedside nurses, and a clinical nurse specialist in palliative care. Depending on the specific needs of individual patients, other members of the palliative care team such as a psychologist, social worker, physiotherapist, dietician, pharmacist, and pastoral care person will be involved in the care of the patient. Depending on the acuity of the clinical situation and resources available in the community, a given patient may be evaluated on the same day or at a later date by the members of the extended PCDH team or referred to services available in the community. The unit clerk, patient attendee, and the volunteers who provide an attentive ear and a helping hand during the patient's stay in the unit are also important elements of the team. Creating an environment wherein patients can interact with staff and other patients is considered a significant aspect of the therapeutic benefits of palliative care.[30]

The PCDH makes it possible to access valuable highly specialized expertise available in a tertiary care hospital such as anesthesiologists, surgeons, oncologists, radio oncologists, psychiatrists, skin care nurses, stomal therapy nurses, and other medical specialist.

Day-to-day functioning of the day hospital

The daily functioning of the PCDH is based on a model of care delivered by a primary team composed of a bedside nurse and a physician. Box 35.3 presents their respective roles. As patients may be referred to the PCDH at any point along their illness trajectory, it is essential that the palliative care physician, if necessary, communicates with the treating physician to clarify the exact diagnosis and prognosis in order to determine the level of involvement by the palliative care team and the need for follow-up. In some instances, palliative care interventions

---

Box 35.3 Roles of the primary team members

Roles of the day-hospital physicians

- To take a complete history that including the assessment of pain and other important symptoms, and to perform a physical examination
- To document diagnosis and prognosis
- To establish the priority of palliative care interventions: investigation, medication and therapeutic interventions, and referrals, in collaboration with the bedside nurse to other team members
- To clarify the level of care and resuscitation status
- In collaboration with other team members, to establish advanced care planning: follow-up, admission, referral to hospice, etc.
- To call and to run family meetings
- To communicate information to treating physician
- To respond to phone consultations from the community related to medical issues

Roles of bedside nurse

- To evaluate the basic palliative care nursing including documentation of symptoms, performance status, cognitive testing, basic psychosocial assessment, drug profile, and specific care issues such as catheter, wounds, and stoma
- To establish a nursing care plan
- To teach patient and caregivers about proper use of medications, especially related to symptom management and any other care issues
- To provide support to patients and families facing the palliative course of a disease
- To coordinate the involvement of the other team members from the PCDH or from the community
- To take an active role in the running of family meetings
- To organize and to coordinate care between the hospital and the community services to ensure continuum of care
- To assure support to community nurses

---

are limited in time until optimization of symptom control before returning the patient to the treating physician. In most instances, the PCDH initiates care for patients receiving palliative oncology treatments and gradually assumes a growing role until assuming full care. This process involves a constant communication effort in order to prevent confusion of roles and undue suffering of the patients and their caregivers. A challenging aspect of this process is the determination of level of care and resuscitation status. The treating physician has the primary responsibility in determining this important aspect of care. In most situations, the PCDH team is called to help patients and their families to understand the meaning of a palliative care approach. By establishing a concrete advanced care plan and by calling a family meeting, it is usually possible to have a smooth process that provides patients and caregivers with a sense of security and control over the situation. However, the PCDH team is at times confronted with distressed patients and family members who may not have fully understood the meaning of the information provided by the treating physicians. In these circumstances, it is useful to invite the treating physician to participate with the team in the family meeting. This approach has been extremely beneficial to this group of patients and has also revealed itself as a powerful tool to teach other specialists about the communication of bad news.

In view of better efficiency, the role of the bedside nurse is based on the concept of case management of the patient and family in relation to the environment. A thorough biological, psychological, social, and existential evaluation of the patient is carried out by the nurse. As most patients present with complex clinical situations, the use of specific tools like the Edmonton Symptom Assessment Scale[31] (ESAS) to document symptom profiles, the Palliative care Outcome Scale (POS, www.pos-pal.org) to document palliative problems, the Palliative Performance Scale[32] to evaluate the physical performance status, Folstein's mini–mental status examination[33] to screen for cognitive deficits, and a locally developed semistructured nursing interview assures completeness of the evaluation in a timely fashion. This basic evaluation is also a therapeutic intervention that allows patients and caregivers the opportunity to freely express their needs and concerns, often for the first time, and by this very process to develop a trustful relationship with the palliative care team. It is an invaluable part of the service offered by the PCDH.

After the initial assessment has been performed by the nurse and the physician, the clinical situation of the patient is discussed in order to establish the plan for that day regarding further investigations, therapeutic interventions, and referrals to other team members. The stay in the PCDH offers a comfortable environment for patients and families and an opportunity for observation. As the day progresses, it is not rare that hidden issues are voiced by patients and family members as they develop trust in the team members. Usually, patients are first in need of symptom control before advanced care planning begins. The PCDH offers access to multiple services (see Box 35.4) that allow rapid management of distressing symptoms without the need for multiple visits. After the symptoms are managed optimally, usually accomplished within one to three visits to the PCDH, patients and family caregivers, and occasionally professional caregivers from the community, are called for a family meeting. This advanced care plan includes provision of home care services, recommendations to follow in case of difficulties with symptom management or emergency situations, and steps to follow when death occurs. Of special mention, this plan includes, in case care could not be provided at home until death, a referral to a hospice or tertiary palliative care unit for patients with complex syndromes necessitating specialized care.

During this process or after patients have been referred either to the treating oncologist, if still receiving active treatments, or to the community resources for terminal care, the

---

Box 35.4 Services offered at the day hospital

Clinical services

1. Thorough palliative care assessment

2. Diagnostic tests including radiological imaging tests

3. Coordination and administration of treatments available in tertiary hospital:
   - Blood transfusions
   - Abdominal paracentesis, thoracocentesis, etc.
   - Anesthetic interventions
   - Radiotherapy for symptom control
   - Wound and stoma care

4. Teaching to patients and family caregivers:
   - Pain medication and other care issues
   - Community services available
   - Solutions to special distressing situations like major bleeding events (38)

5. Family meeting

6. Palliative care counseling services:
   - Psychologist
   - Pastoral care
   - Nutrition
   - Physiotherapy and ergotherapy

Specialized clinics

- Lymphedema clinic
- Cancer nutrition and rehabilitation clinic
- Cancer-related cognitive failure clinic
- Neuropathic cancer pain/methadone clinic

PCDH remains a support resource through phone calls or emergency visits. In certain situations, especially with patients in severe pain or distressing situations, or when community resources are insufficient, the PCDH assures regular follow-up until death in collaboration with the community health-care providers.

Physical setting

Because the PCDH serves patients with a wide range of clinical conditions from bed bound to fully ambulated, from specific single issues such as weight loss or lymphedema, to multiple palliative care issues, the physical setting should be variable. Our experience shows that a mixture of hospital bedrooms with private washrooms, clinic type rooms, interview rooms, treatment rooms, and specific rooms with special research equipment is ideal. The exact number is determined by the volume of daily visits. Sufficient space for patients and family members to relax should be provided such as a waiting room and kitchen. A specific meeting room for family meetings and private discussions is essential to ensure privacy. A unified, but well-thought-out, well-planned central working area for the staff increases efficiency of communication but should not replace separate offices to allow team members to perform their charting and telephone communication. Finally, it is essential to plan a lounge area within the day-hospital setting for the staff to rest while remaining accessible to patients and family members.

Instrumental in allowing palliative care research

The PCDH has become over the years an important setting to enable research with this fragile population. Thorough palliative care assessments and optimal symptom management assure that only patients with sufficiently stable conditions are offered the opportunity to participate in research protocols. Furthermore, accessing patients and family members with palliative care needs earlier on during the illness trajectory has made it feasible to study ongoing changes in quality of life over a longer time frame, as well as the occurrence of early cognitive failure, the value of nutritional and rehabilitation interventions when anorexia–cachexia is only beginning, new drugs for the treatment of cancer pain that require patients with longer survivals, etc. The PCDH physical setting and organization provide a supervised environment sometimes needed in specific research protocols. The establishment of specialized clinics (see Box 35.4) within the PCDH has allowed the development of expertise in specific fields of research.

Palliative care day hospital in numbers

In 1999, after 9 months of operation, we reviewed 154 new consecutive referrals to the PCDH over a period of 8 months.[34] Table 35.1 gives the characteristics of the patients at the initial PCDH visit. The reduced representation of patients with breast cancer is explained by the limited number of women treated in our hospital. As expected, the majority of patients had advanced disease but we were agreeably surprised by the number of patients with regional disease in need of symptom control. While some patients were followed up from the palliative care inpatient services, the great majority (77%) were new referrals to palliative care. The symptom profile as measured by the ESAS was characterized by fatigue, loss of appetite, and decreased well-being, for which 50% of patients scored their level of distress as moderate to severe (>40 on a visual analog scale from 0 mm = no symptom to 100 mm = worst symptom). Pain remained quite prevalent at 69% with 35% of these patients expressing moderate-to-severe pain. In fact, most of these patients needed some opioid adjustments: initiation (15%), increase (20%), or switch to other opioids (12%). Table 35.2 provides a summary of the follow-up of these patients. These 154 patients were seen 469 times. For 12% of patients, a same-day admission to the palliative care inpatient unit was necessary at their first visit. For the majority of patients (74%), one to three visits were sufficient to optimize their comfort and to arrange community-based care. However, 26% of patients

Table 35.1 *Characteristics of the patients at the initial day-hospital visit (N = 154)*

		Percent
Age in years (mean ± SD)	65.6 ± 12	
Sex, M/F	93/61	60/40
Primary cancer diagnosis		
Lung	36	23
Genitourinary	45	29
Gastrointestinal	45	29
Breast	9	6
Others	19	12
Extent of cancer		
Metastatic	112	73
Locoregional	42	27
Referral source		
New consults to palliative care, follow-up from palliative care	118	77
Inpatient consultation service	36	23
Symptom profile prevalence (out of 144 patients)		
Pain	99	69
Decreased level of activity	127	88
Nausea	51	35
Depressive mood	73	51
Anxiety	98	68
Drowsiness	86	60
Loss of appetite	117	81
Shortness of breath	74	51
Decrease in well-being	125	87
Type of pain medication		
None	25	16
Acetaminophen or nonsteroidal anti-inflammatory drugs	21	14
Codeine ± acetaminophen	25	16
Oxycodone	4	3
Morphine	45	29
Hydromorphone	17	11
Fentanyl patch	11	7
Others	6	4
Morphine equivalent daily dose in mg (mean ± SD)	118 ± 80	

needed four or more visits to be cared for by the PCDH team. This group of patients is composed of patients with difficult symptoms or psychosocial issues and of patients without access to a family physician in the community. During this period, the specialized clinics (see Box 35.4) were not yet organized. With these new specialized clinics, patients with more than three visits to the PCDH should represent a higher proportion of the PCDH workload. The majority of patients were seen 2–3 months before death.

The cost of the PCDH has not been fully evaluated. In Quebec, physicians working in such settings are paid a fixed salary. The nurses and other team members are paid by the

Table 35.2 *Characteristics of the follow-up of the day-hospital patients*

	N	Percent
Total number of day-hospital visits	469	100
Number of direct admissions to the palliative care inpatient service	58	12
Number of day-hospital visits per patient		
1	54	35
2	39	25
3	21	14
4–7	24	16
8 or more	16	10
Patient follow-up at the end of the chart review		
Number of patients still alive	33	21
Lost to follow up	25	16
Number of patients deceased	96	62
Place of death (96 deaths)		
Home	21	22
Acute palliative care unit	33	34
Hospice	20	21
Hospital beds	22	23
Length of follow-up for deceased patients' median (10th and 90th percentiles)		54 (15, 125)

budget allocated for palliative care services. Transportation from home to the PCDH hospital is usually covered by the patients or their families. For patients 65 years and older, ambulance transportation is usually paid by social programs. The return transportation from the PCDH to home by ambulance or adapted transportation, if necessary, is covered by the hospital.

Is the PCDH cost-effective? This remains to be determined as it has not been decided which outcomes should be used. For example, even if the majority of patients are still referred late in their illness trajectory, what is the exact value of earlier symptom management, especially through our specialized clinics? From a health service research perspective, among other benefits, enhanced communication between the cancer center and the community-based services would need to be evaluated: (1) the value of rapid referral back to the specialized palliative care based at the PCDH could be difficult to quantify; (2) the continuum of care from specialized oncology services and hospital-based palliative care to home care services should be established; (3) the prevention of emergency room visits should be quantified; and (4) a reduction in the utilization of inpatient beds could lead to cost saving but should be supported by evidence of good quality of care at home. Of note, the closest similar experience available has been the one of multidisciplinary symptom control clinics based within cancer centers. Two similar clinics, one in Canada and another in the United States, were partially evaluated and were found to be effective in improving symptom control and patient satisfaction.[35,36] However, cost-effectiveness was not evaluated. Other research has found that day-care attendance might substitute home nursing and primary care for patients who attend.[37] However,

when a more *social model* of day care was evaluated, its use did not affect other services received.[38] Douglas et al. proposed that rather than using conventional methods to assess cost-effectiveness in day care, the choice experiment method might be appropriate. In this approach, patients select their favored choices. In their study, involving 79 day-care patients across four centers in the United Kingdom, access to specialist therapies was three times as important as medical support and twice as important as staying all day.[39] This approach may be fruitful in determining what aspects of day-care patients value most.

EVALUATING OUTCOMES OF PALLIATIVE CARE DAY HOSPITAL AND DAY-CARE CENTERS

Stevens et al.[40] reviewed all studies evaluating outcomes and the impact of quality of life on attendees to palliative day-care centers from 1980 to 2009. The authors divided the results of their review into two broad categories of studies: (1) perceptions of attendees and stakeholders and (2) investigating outcomes using validated outcome measures. The former category, using qualitative methodologies, evaluated the effects of various services such as rehabilitation care/physiotherapy approaches, complementary therapies, support groups, and creative arts on subjects' experience of these services. Overall, attendees felt that the services offered by these facilities were beneficial. They identified the possibility to be with other people with cancer, in a supportive and caring environment, as one of the most valuable aspects of day centers. Access to medical care and therapies was considered as having an impact on psychological well-being, self-worth and self-esteem, and decreasing social isolation. Within the latter category, the authors identified three randomized clinical trials[41–43] with sample sizes varying between 26 and 46 subjects testing the effects of reflexology, multisensory environment, and aromatherapy, respectively, using various patient reported outcomes to test their efficacy. Unfortunately, the three studies found no significant effects. In their review, they also presented the results of the largest study comparing (nonrandomized) 120 day-care patients with 53 patients in conventional services in five different regions in the south of the United Kingdom. The study found few differences in overall quality of life over time.[44] A recent comparative study suggested that day-care attendance may improve hope compared to existing services.[45] Overall despite a long tradition of day-care centers, little evidence supports its value in improving quality of life, except for improving overall well-being of family caregivers.

Other than the small number of well-designed studies, other reasons may also explain the limited number of positive outcomes found in the literature. Experience from the geriatric day hospital whose primary goal is rehabilitation could provide some possible explanations. In an attempt to explore the differences in standards of care between geriatric day hospitals and day centers, Reilly et al.[46] carried out a survey of 75 day centers. While day hospitals were found to have higher standards in assessment and rehabilitation of patients and promoting caregiver involvement, day-care centers offered services mostly to older people with dementia, and their staff received more specific training to care for their patients. These day hospitals are clearly distinct from day-care centers. No study looking at the difference between PC day hospitals and day-care centers has been carried out at this time. However, the different types of day-care services offered by these centers vary greatly between day-care centers and within centers over time.[3] Such reality renders any attempt to evaluate the impact of health outcomes by these centers quite challenging. Furthermore, concerns have been raised about the superiority in efficiency and the overall cost of these centers in comparison with other forms of comprehensive medical care. A Cochrane review in 2009[15] concluded that geriatric day hospitals were significantly superior to other forms of comprehensive care in preventing death, *poor* outcome and deterioration, and a trend in reducing hospital cost. Unfortunately, secondary outcomes on QoL and caregiver distress were minimally evaluated in these trials, and relevant conclusions could not be drawn. Recently, an attempt is being made to determine the clinical characteristics of elderly patients who could benefit the most from the services offered by geriatric day hospitals. Desrosiers and colleagues[47] found that the improvement made by participants was different depending on the underlying pathology causing their functional deficits. Stroke patients along with individuals afflicted by neurological diseases and musculoskeletal conditions or who underwent amputations were found to improve the most. Participants with cognitive deficits or psychopathological disorders experienced improvement mainly in well-being as well as a decrease in caregiver burden. Dasgupta et al.[48] documented an improvement mainly in participants with cardiac diseases or depression, while those with dementia benefited the least. Pereira et al.[49] found that the 6 min walk test was the best predictor of improvement. Such attempts to identify the characteristics of participants who could benefit the most from attending PC day-care centers would be helpful to determine admission criteria for these types of centers. Reviews of effectiveness on various forms of care services offered to people with psychiatric illnesses suggest other avenues for further research on the benefits of PC day hospitals and day-care centers. A Cochrane review in 2011[50] on the psychiatric care of 10 clinical trials found that acute psychiatric day hospitals were providing similar levels of care as acute inpatient care. Another Cochrane review in 2009[51] suggests that psychiatric day hospitals, despite limited data, may decrease the readmission rate of people with schizophrenia. Both of these reviews provide further avenues of research on the efficacy of PC day hospitals and day centers in improving the care of people with terminal illnesses.

Furthermore, cost-effectiveness has been tested in other chronic and terminal illnesses. In stroke recovery where multiple trials have been carried out, the lack of a standardized definition of the concept of day-hospital rehabilitation has made it impossible to fully demonstrate the effectiveness in hastening functional recovery and reducing outpatient visits among older stroke patients without additional costs.[18] A randomized trial comparing the effectiveness of a day-hospital program to usual care in 234 patients with congestive HF demonstrated reduction in morbidity and mortality with a cost/utility ratio for the integration of the day-hospital management of U.S.$19,462 (95% CI U.S.$13,904 to $34,048).[23] These examples could serve as guidance to further evaluate the cost benefits of PC hospitals and day-care centers. While it would be inappropriate to expect day-care centers to serve every individual that could benefit since generally a significant part of their costs are covered by the private sector, it is required that PC day hospitals demonstrate their cost-effectiveness, justifying the funding received from health-care authorities. However, this may reveal itself difficult as there are no clear definitions of PC day hospitals and day-care centers.

From another perspective, Patrick et al.[53,54] had proposed a model to evaluate the quality of dying and death (QODD). Contrary to quality of life, which refers to "perceptions of their position in life in the context of particular culture and values systems, and in relation to their personal goals, expectations, standards and concerns,"[55] QODD is defined as "the degree to which a person's preferences for dying and the moment of death agree with the observations of how the person actually died, as reported by others."[53] QODD is based on patient factors, structure and process of care, and outcomes of care. QODD measures six conceptual domains with corresponding items: (1) symptoms and personal care, (2) preparation for death, (3) moment of death, (4) family, (5) treatment preferences, and (6) whole person concerns. Their model of QODD could provide another dimension in evaluating the impact of PC day centers on patients' outcomes. Furthermore, this model could serve in defining the role that a specific day center wants to assume and to use the appropriate outcome measures adapted to estimate the effects of their interventions. Using this taxonomy, for example, a specific day center may focus on addressing the needs of the family and the whole person concerns, and not providing services in relation to symptom control. By clarifying its role, the day-care centers could elaborate well-defined criteria of admission and provide patients and family members with a set of goals that could be accomplished by attending the day center. In this case, this day center should select a population with optimal symptom control and be in close contact with other settings where symptoms could be optimally managed in a timely fashion. When the time comes to evaluate the efficacy and efficiency of the day services, specific outcomes should aim to measure the degree to which the attendees were properly selected in regard to symptom control at admission, whether an adequate process was in place to monitor symptoms and proceed with the appropriate referral, and whether the attendees found meaning and the family members felt supported. In contrast, other centers such as PC day hospitals, aim to improve access to palliative care for all people with cancer. They do so by providing optimal symptom control, facilitating coordination of care with psychosocial and home care services, preparing patients for acceptance of their terminal condition, and guiding in the decision of preferred place of death, all with appropriate family and caregiver support. Moreover, proper evaluation of the benefits of PC day hospitals should determine the extent to which all people within the entrapment area served by these services receive appropriate care through the use of rigorous epidemiological study designs.[52] While it would be inappropriate to expect day-care centers to serve every individual that could benefit (since generally a significant part of their costs are covered by the private sector), it is highly desirable for PC hospitals to do so and to obtain appropriate funding from health-care authorities.

PROVIDING PALLIATIVE CARE TO PEOPLE WITH OTHER TERMINAL ILLNESSES

Similar to people with cancer, people with COPD experience intense physical and psychological symptoms and family–social needs, are equally expecting open communication about prognosis, and are also wishing to die home.[56] It is evident that people with COPD necessitate access to PC. A similar situation exists in people with HF. Lemond and Allen[57] suggest in their review that people with HF, as the disease progresses, enter into a *storm* of factors supporting the need for hospice care. They also argue that the illness trajectory of HF, which includes multiple acute deteriorations and recuperations, renders the determination of prognosis quite challenging and often prevents timely referral to hospices. The same is true about people with COPD as both diseases share similar illness trajectories.[28] However, they also propose that optimal symptom control and other PC interventions, such as advanced care planning, could and should be offered as soon as dyspnea, pain, depression, and other symptoms are present regardless of life expectancy. Following the model suggested by Rocker et al.,[58] they propose a step-by-step approach for symptom control. Nonetheless, the access to PC remains quite limited for people with COPD and HF. Interestingly, day hospitals for people with respiratory diseases[59] and HF[23,60,61] were recently developed. Respiratory day hospitals aim at preventing hospital admissions and emergency room visits by readily providing access to acute respiratory care. Freimark et al.[61] describe a congestive HF day hospital designed to provide ongoing care of patients with HF resistant to oral medication in the form of close clinical monitoring and therapeutic medical interventions including intravenous treatments. Two other congestive HF day hospitals are described as providing ongoing supervision of clinical conditions, rehabilitation, and education for people with HF.[23,60] Unfortunately, none of the aforementioned day hospitals have health professionals trained in PC or describe specific protocols for managing PC issues. These settings offer great opportunities for the integration of PC with mainstream medical care and could act as coordination centers with PC home services and hospices.

CONCLUSION

Assuring access to optimal care for patients in need of palliative care remains a challenge. The creation of day hospitals within tertiary hospitals or cancer centers is a valuable option for patients with advanced cancer who are still receiving active care and for those in the terminal phase of their illness who need rapid access to palliative care due to their deteriorating medical condition. Furthermore, the existing day hospitals for other advanced, life-threatening illnesses, such as COPD, congestive HF, and neurological degenerative diseases, provide opportunities to provide palliative care to a large proportion of people who unfortunately remain as the forgotten dying of our medical system.

Key learning points

- Access to optimal palliative care remains limited to very few.
- Day-care centers have been successful at increasing services in the community.
- A PCDH can increase access to palliative care, especially earlier on in the illness trajectory.
- The PCDH links the tertiary care center with community resources.
- The PCDH provides access to specialized palliative care techniques.
- The PCDH offers an ideal setting for end-of-life clinical research.
- Day hospitals serving people with terminal pulmonary and cardiac conditions offer opportunities for PC involvement.
- Research on the efficiency of day-care centers and PCDH remains challenging.

REFERENCES

1 Wilkes E, Crowther AG, Greaves CW. A different kind of day hospital—For patients with preterminal cancer and chronic disease. *British Medical Journal.* 1978; **2**: 1053–1056.
2 Clark D, ten Have H, Janssens R. Common threads? Palliative care service developments in seven European countries. *Palliative Medicine.* 2000; **14**: 479–490.
3 Davies E, Higginson IJ. Systematic review of specialist palliative daycare for adults with cancer. *Supportive Care in Cancer.* 2005; **13**: 607–627.
4 MacDonald N. Palliative care—An essential component of cancer control. *Canadian Medical Association Journal.* 1998; **158**: 1709–1716.
5 MacDonald N. Palliative care—The fourth phase of cancer prevention. *Cancer Detection and Prevention.* 1991; **15**: 253–255.
6 Temel JS, Greer JA, Muzikansky A et al. Early palliative care for patients with metastatic non-small cell lung cancer. *New England Journal of Medicine.* 2010; **363**: 733–742.
7 Evans LK, Forciea MA, Yurkow J, Sochalski J. The geriatric day hospital. In: Katz PR, Kane RL, Mezey MD (eds). *Emerging Systems in Long-Term Care.* New York: Springer Publishing Company Inc, 1999: pp. 67–87.

8   Densen PM. *Tracing the Elderly through the Health Care System: An Update.* Rockville, MD: Department of Health and Human Services, 1991. AHCPR 91-11.

9   Brocklehurst J. Geriatric day hospitals. *Age and Ageing.* 1995; **24**: 89–90.

10 Brocklehurst JC. The development and present status of day hospitals. *Age and Ageing.* 1979; **8**(suppl): 76–79.

11 Siu AL, Morishita L, Blaustein J. Comprehensive geriatric assessment in a day hospital. *Journal of the American Geriatric Society.* 1994; **42**: 1094–1099.

12 Cummings V, Kerner JF, Arones S, Steinbock C. Day hospital service in rehabilitation medicine: An evaluation. *Archives of Physical Medicine and Rehabilitation.* 1985; **66**: 86–91.

13 Lorenz EJ, Hamill CM, Oliver RC. The day hospital: An alternative to institutional care. *Journal of the American Geriatric Society.* 1974; **22**: 316–320.

14 Eng C, Pedulla J, Eleazer GP, McCann R, Fox N. Program of All-inclusive Care for the Elderly (PACE): An innovative model of integrated geriatric care and financing. *Journal of the American Geriatric Society.* 1997; **45**: 223–232.

15 Forster A, Young J, Lambley R, Langhorne P. Medical day hospital care for the elderly versus alternative forms of care. *Cochrane Database of Systematic Reviews* 2008. Art. No.: CD001730.

16 Rosie JS. Partial hospitalization: A review of recent literature. *Hospital & Community Psychiatry.* 1987; **38**: 1291–1299.

17 Kallert TW, Glockner M, Priebe S et al. A comparison of psychiatric day hospitals in five European countries: Implications of their diversity for day hospital research. *Social Psychiatry and Psychiatric Epidemiology.* 2004; **39**: 777–788.

18 Dekker R, Drost EA, Groothoff JW et al. Effects of day-hospital rehabilitation in stroke patients: A review of randomized clinical trials. *Scandinavian Journal of Rehabilitation Medicine.* 1998; **30**: 87–94.

19 Mor V, Stalker MZ, Gralla R et al. Day hospital as an alternative to inpatient care for cancer patients: A random assignment trial. *Journal of Clinical Epidemiology.* 1988; **41**: 771–785.

20 Rogge R. Diabetic day hospital in Wiesbaden: Education and treatment under everyday conditions during job and leisure time. *Medizinische Welt.* **51**, 219–222 (2000).

21 Wisseler HM, Lautenschlager J, Leichner-Hennig R, Henrich H. Rheumatological day clinic in the Auerbach Clinic Dr. Vetter—Beginnings and initial experiences. *Aktuelle Rheumatologie.* 2003; **28**: 30–35.

22 Gill HS, Walter DB. The day hospital model of care for patients with medical and rehabilitative needs. *Hospital Technology Series.* 1996; **15**: 1–14.

23 Capomolla S, Febo O, Ceresa M et al. Cost/utility ratio in chronic heart failure: Comparison between heart failure management program delivered by day-hospital and usual care. *Journal of the American College of Cardiology.* 2002; **40**: 1259–1266.

24 Biem HJ, Cotton D, McNeil S, Boechler A, Gudmundson D. Day medicine: An urgent internal medicine clinic and medical procedures suite. *Healthcare Management Forum.* 2003; **16**: 17–23.

25 Benjamin LJ, Swinson GI, Nagel RL. Sickle cell anemia day hospital: An approach for the management of uncomplicated painful crises. *Blood.* 2000; **95**: 1130–1136.

26 Wright J, Bareford D, Wright C et al. Day case management of sickle pain: 3 Years experience in a UK sickle cell unit. *British Journal of Haematology.* 2004; **126**: 878–880.

27 Gagnon B, Mayo NE, Hanley JA, MacDonald N. Pattern of care at the end of life: Does age make a difference in what happens to women with breast cancer? *Journal of Clinical Oncology.* 2004; **22**: 3458–3465.

28 Teno JM, Weitzen S, Fennell ML, Mor V. Dying trajectory in the last year of life: Does cancer trajectory fit other diseases? *Journal of Palliative Medicine.* 2001; **4**: 457–464.

29 Lunney JR, Lynn J, Foley DJ, Lipson S, Guralnik JM. Patterns of functional decline at the end of life. *Journal of the American Medical Association.* 2003; **289**: 2387–2392.

30 Langley-Evans A, Payne S. Light-hearted death talk in a palliative day care context. *Journal of Advanced Nursing.* 1997; **26**: 1091–1097.

31 Bruera E, Kuehn N, Miller MJ, Selmser P, Macmillan K. The Edmonton Symptom Assessment System (ESAS): A simple method for the assessment of palliative care patients. *Journal of Palliative Care.* 1991; **7**: 6–9.

32 Anderson F, Downing GM, Hill J, Casorso L, Lerch N. Palliative performance scale (PPS): A new tool. *Journal of Palliative Care.* 1996; **12**: 5–11.

33 Folstein MF, Folstein SE, Mchugh PR. Mini-mental state—Practical method for grading cognitive state of patients for clinician. *Journal of Psychiatric Research.* 1975; **12**: 189–198.

34 Schreier G, Gagnon B, Lawlor K. The McGill University Health Center Palliative Care Day Hospital: A Unique Approach. Poster presented at Palliative Care Conference—Palliative Care in Different Cultures, Jerusalem, Israel, March 2000.

35 Bruera E, Michaud M, Vigano A et al. Multidisciplinary symptom control clinic in a cancer center: A retrospective study. *Supportive Care in Cancer.* 2001; **9**: 162–168.

36 Strasser F, Sweeney C, Willey J. Impact of a half-day multidisciplinary symptom control and palliative care outpatient clinic in a comprehensive cancer center on recommendations, symptom intensity, and patient satisfaction: A retrospective descriptive study. *Journal of Pain and Symptom Management.* 2004; **27**: 481–491.

37 Douglas HR, Normand CE, Higginson IJ et al. Palliative day care: What does it cost to run a centre and does attendance affect use of other services? *Palliative Medicine.* 2003; **17**: 628–637.

38 Higginson IJ, Gao W, Amesbury B et al. Does a social model of hospice day care affect advanced cancer patients' use of other health and social services? A prospective quasi-experimental trial. *Supportive Care in Cancer.* 2010; **18**: 627–637.

39 Douglas HR, Normand CE, Higginson IJ et al. A new approach to eliciting patients' preferences for palliative day care: The choice experiment method. *Journal of Pain and Symptom Management.* 2005; **29**: 435–545.

40 Stevens E, Martin CR, White CA. The outcomes of palliative care day services: A systematic review. *Palliative Medicine.* 2011; **25**: 153–169.

41 Ross CS, Hamilton J, Macrae G et al. A pilot study to evaluate the effect of reflexology on mood and symptom rating of advanced cancer patients. *Palliative Medicine.* 2002; **16**: 544–545.

42 Schofield P, Payne S. A pilot study into the use of a multisensory environment (Snoezelen) within a palliative day-care setting. *International Journal of Palliative Nursing.* 2003; **9**: 124.

43 Schofield P. Snoezelen within a palliative care day setting: A randomised controlled trial investigating the potential. *International Journal on Disability and Human Development.* 2011; **8**: 59–66.

44 Goodwin DM, Higginson IJ, Myers K et al. Effectiveness of palliative day care in improving pain, symptom control, and quality of life. *Journal of Pain and Symptom Management.* 2003; **25**: 202–212.

45 Guy MP, Higginson IJ, Amesbury BD. The effect of palliative daycare on hope: A comparison of daycare patients with two control groups. *Journal of Palliative Care.* 2011; **27**: 216.

46 Reilly S, Venables D, Hughes J, Challis D, Abendstern M. Standards of care in day hospitals and day centres: A comparison of services for older people with dementia. *International Journal of Geriatric Psychiatry.* 2006; **21**: 460–468.

47 Desrosiers J, Hebert R, Payette H et al. Geriatric day hospital: Who improves the most? *Canadian Journal on Aging.* 2004; **23**: 217–229.

48 Dasgupta M, Clarke NC, Brymer CD. Characteristics of patients who made gains at a geriatric day hospital. *Archives of Gerontology and Geriatrics.* 2005; **40**: 173–184.

49 Pereira SR, Chiu W, Turner A et al. How can we improve targeting of frail elderly patients to a geriatric day-hospital rehabilitation program? *BMC Geriatrics.* 2010; **10**: 82.

50 Marshall M, Crowther R, Sledge WH et al. Day hospital versus admission for acute psychiatric disorders. *Cochrane Database of Systematic Reviews 2011.* Art. No.: CD004026.

51 Shek E, Stein AT, Shansis FM et al. Day hospital versus outpatient care for people with schizophrenia. *Cochrane Database of Systematic Reviews 2009.* Art. No.: CD003240.

52 Costantini M, Beccaro M. Health services research on end-of-life care. *Current Opinion in Supportive and Palliative Care.* 2009; **3**: 190–194.

53 Patrick DL, Engelberg RA, Curtis JR. Evaluating the quality of dying and death. *Journal of Pain and Symptom Management.* 2001; **22**: 717–726.

54 Stewart AL, Teno J, Patrick DL, Lynn J. The concept of quality of life of dying persons in the context of health care. *Journal of Pain and Symptom Management.* 1999; **17**: 93–108.

55 Diehr P, Lafferty WE, Patrick DL et al. Quality of life at the end of life. *Health and Quality of Life Outcomes.* 2007; **5**: 51.

56 Habraken JM, Willems DL, de Kort SJ, Bindels PJ. Health care needs in end-stage COPD: A structured literature review. *Patient Education and Counseling.* 2007; **68**: 121–130.

57 Lemond L, Allen LA. Palliative care and hospice in advanced heart failure. *Progress in Cardiovascular Diseases.* 2011; **54**: 168–178.

58 Rocker G, Horton R, Currow D et al. Palliation of dyspnoea in advanced COPD: Revisiting a role for opioids. *Thorax.* 2009; **64**: 910–915.

59 Schwartzman K, Duquette G, Zaoude M et al. Respiratory day hospital: A novel approach to acute respiratory care. *Canadian Medical Association Journal.* 2001; **165**: 1067–1071.

60 Racine-Morel A, Deroche S, Bonnin C et al. Heart failure patient management: Evolution, organization, application on a local scale. *Annales de Cardiologie et d'Angeiologie. (Paris.)* 2006; **55**: 352–357.

61 Freimark D, Arad M, Matetzky S et al. An advanced chronic heart failure day care service: A 5 year single-center experience. *Israel Medical Association Journal.* 2009; **11**: 419–425.

36

Inpatient hospices

JEREMY KEEN

INPATIENT HOSPICES

Evolution of inpatient hospices

The lineage of modern, freestanding, inpatient hospices is usually traced back to the medieval hospices that were initially *guest-houses* (from the Latin *hospitium*) run by religious orders for journeying pilgrims. These hospices inevitably became involved in the care of sick and dying travellers hoping for miraculous cures at the shrines to which they were heading. It is interesting to note that the words hospice, hospital, and hospitality are derived from the Latin *hospes*, which, over time, has had different meanings as either *guest/stranger* or *host*. This reflects the intimate relationship between carer and the *cared-for* and was integral to the aspirations of the modern hospice movement.

The history of hospice evolution is punctuated by the influence of a series of remarkable individuals, mostly women, mostly with a religious conviction, who have sought to offer hospitality to the dying. Jeanne Garnier formed L'Association des Dames du Calvaire in Lyon, in 1842, and opened a home for the dying the following year. The development of hospice and palliative care in Paris and New York can trace its lineage directly back to Jeanne Garnier and this first establishment in Lyon.

As superior of the Irish Sisters of Charity, Mary Aikenhead was instrumental in the opening of St. Vincent's Hospital, Dublin, in 1834. Fulfilling her long-held ambition, the convent where she spent her final years became Our Lady's Hospice for the Dying in 1879. The Sisters of Charity opened St. Joseph's Hospice in East London in 1905, and other hospices were to follow in Australia, Canada, and Scotland. During the period between 1879 and 1905, four other institutions opened in London specifically for the care of the *dying poor,* but did not call themselves hospices. According to one commentator, this close association with workhouses for the poor would, later in the twentieth century, lead to the early rejection of the concept of inpatient hospice care by the French and Belgian medical profession[1] and was possibly influential in the coining of an alternative term, *palliative care,* when first introduced in French-speaking Quebec.

St. Luke's Home for the Dying Poor, opened in 1893, was the only institution established by a doctor, and its organization of services and delivery of care was most closely linked to that developed in modern hospices. Although St. Luke's employed lay nursing staff rather than those drawn from religious orders, as in the other establishments, the emphasis was still firmly on spiritual care. Dr. Howard Barrett the founder of St. Luke's wrote:

> It is much if we can render the last weeks and months less destitute of comfort, less tortured by pain. It is far more if through any instrumentality of ours some become humble followers of Christ.

Interested readers are directed to an excellent review of the development of hospices in the period 1878–1914.[2]

The influence of St. Luke's on the development of the *modern hospice* is due in no small part to the time spent in St. Luke's by Dame Cicely Saunders as a volunteer nurse. When planning St. Christopher's Hospice, Dr. Saunders stated:

> The name hospice, 'a resting place for travellers or pilgrims,' was chosen because this will be something between a hospital and a home, with the skills of one and the hospitality, warmth, and the time of the other.

She sought to capture the core value of hospitality in hospice but recognized that this was not enough on its own to ensure the optimal relief of suffering. Her vision for the model, upon which so many hospices in the United Kingdom and elsewhere are based, very much included aspirations toward research and the application of best evidence as an integral part of the provision of care.

After St. Christopher's opened in 1967, there was a steady growth in the number of hospices opening in the United Kingdom, and internationally, a growth in the *hospice movement* that has developed and adapted the philosophy of hospice care more often in a community setting rather than in freestanding institutions caring for inpatients called *hospices*. Having spent time in St. Christopher's, Dr. Balfour Mount sought to introduce the principles of hospice care into the general hospital and established a *palliative care* consultation service in Montreal in 1975.

The rate at which new freestanding inpatient hospices (for adults) opened in the United Kingdom reached a peak during the late 1980s and early 1990s with the majority resulting from local community enthusiasm and support rather than NHS planning.[3] There have been very few new inpatient hospices opened since the mid-1990s. All independent hospices in the United Kingdom now tender their services to the NHS and in so doing receive contributions approximating to one-third of their total budget. The UK government is committed to increasing its contribution to hospice care provided by the independent sector but with *strings attached* to ensure equity of access regardless of, for example, diagnosis or ethnicity.[4]

In the United Kingdom, the freestanding hospices have traditionally been the principal focus of inpatient palliative care, research, and education. However, since the recognition of palliative medicine as a specialty by the Royal College of Physicians in 1987 and the proliferation of hospital-based services and academic departments of palliative medicine and care, the focus, particularly in terms of research, has tended to shift towards the teaching hospital. This has allowed a break from the perceived constraints of the hospices, by promoting specialist palliative care for patients regardless of diagnosis and exploring *supportive care* for patients at earlier stages of a disease process.[5,6]

The acceptance of palliative care as a speciality within mainstream hospital care has led to questioning of the validity of hospices as separate institutions for the dying.[7] They were famously described as being "too good to be true and too small to be useful"[8] and institutions that simply provided, to quote a general surgeon at a national meeting, "designer deaths." At the same time, as voices outside the discipline were beginning to question hospice care, warnings were being issued from within the ranks.[9–11] Although the future of palliative and supportive care within acute hospital services seems to be assured, authors have continued to echo Professor David Clark's question: "Whither the Hospices?"[12] Perhaps the evidence of the wishes of those facing the end of their lives is the most pertinent with a recent report from the United Kingdom demonstrating that while 47% of individuals noted their preferred place of death to be their own home, 33% would prefer to die in a freestanding hospice with only 1% wishing to die in an acute hospital.[13] This same report demonstrated an increasing preference for death in a hospice with increasing age, although nationally, the elderly have been shown to be the least likely of those expressing a wish to die in a hospice to actually do so.[14] Internationally, the picture is similar. A recent study of the preferences for place of care at the end of life, expressed by currently healthy individuals, showed national variation with 9.9% of interviewees in Belgium to 35.7% in Portugal wishing to die in a hospice or palliative care unit.[15] The same study reported that 29% of interviewees in the United Kingdom wished to die in a hospice, which, interestingly, is close to the figure of 33% of those actually coming to the end of their lives found in the study quoted earlier.

The development of hospices outside the auspices of the NHS has facilitated the introduction and development of new models of care with an emphasis on a holistic approach dependent on true interdisciplinary team working. Features of these approaches, even the associated *symbiotic niceness* behavior as recognized and defined by one study,[16] are now found within mainstream medicine, but equally, increasing technology and issues of clinical governance have found their way back into the hospices. As the systems of care come closer together, there is a danger that for hospice care at least, the original concepts become lost in a drift toward medicalization and bureaucracy. However, the maintenance of independent institutions brings with it the danger of inequitable delivery of services and a lack of coordination in efforts to improve the delivery of care.[17,18]

As hospices struggle with their changing role in patient care, perhaps their origins will provide a key to their further evolution. The rate of development in knowledge of symptom control has not been matched by the development (or rediscovery?) of psychological and spiritual care. Now perhaps, as at no other time in history, the spiritual needs of those suffering life-shortening illnesses, who have little in the way of personal religious terms of reference or the distraction of overriding physical symptoms, are becoming obvious. To use the relative freedoms of independent institutions to maintain excellence in symptom control but also to address other aspects of suffering in a novel and creative fashion may be a way forward. This may begin to ease the tensions of some of those working in hospices who feel they have become part of *just another specialty*.[11]

Who is admitted to a hospice?

Figures for 2009–2010 show that approximately 45,300 people in the United Kingdom were admitted as an inpatient to a hospice for the first time.[19] Hospices had a total of 51,900 inpatient admissions with an estimated 30,000 people dying during their stay and a mean length of admission of 14 days. In England and Wales, 5.2% of all deaths occurred in *freestanding* hospices.[20] The age distribution of individuals admitted to inpatient hospices in the United Kingdom is compared to that for those admitted to hospice programs in the United States in Figure 36.1. Those entering hospice programs in the United States tend to be older with 38.9% of admissions in 2009–2010 being over the age of 85 compared to only 12.5% in England and Wales.[19,21] Of deaths occurring in inpatient hospices in England and Wales, 91% were certified to be primarily due to malignancy, which demonstrated a modest (4%) increase in the proportion of individuals admitted with a principal diagnosis other than cancer over the preceding 5 years. This is in contrast with a significant increase, over the same time period, in the numbers of individuals with nonmalignant diagnoses seen by palliative care specialists as outpatients or in-hospital consultations (Figure 36.2). However, cancer is still the primary diagnosis of the vast majority of individuals seen which contrasts with equivalent data from, for example, the United States where

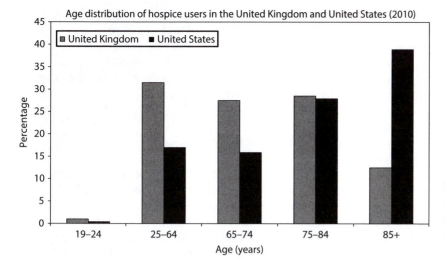

Figure 36.1 *A comparison of the age distribution of individuals admitted to UK inpatient hospices (31,923) and of the total of those admitted to hospice programs in the United States (1.58 million people) during a 12-month period in 2009/2010.*

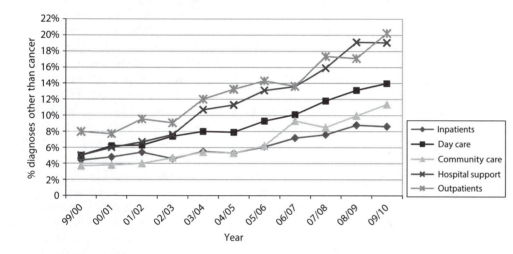

Figure 36.2 *Growth in proportion of individuals with diagnoses other than cancer referred to different elements of the hospice and palliative care services in the United Kingdom. (From National Survey of Patient Activity Data for Specialist Palliative Care Services, MDS Full Report for the year 2009–2010, The National Council for Palliative Care.)*

the percentage of individuals admitted to hospice programs with nonmalignant diagnoses rose from 24% in 1992 to 64% in 2010.[21] Data from England and Wales over the period of 2008–2010 demonstrate that 17.3% of all cancer deaths occur in freestanding hospices compared with 26.8% at home and 42.9% in NHS hospitals.[19] In the United Kingdom, since 2004, there has been a reversal of the progressive reduction in proportion of deaths occurring at home noted since 1974, with a slight increase in home deaths, particularly from malignancy.[22] This comes long after a similar reversal of the trend away from home deaths in the United States (since the mid-1980s) and Canada (since the mid-1990s).[23] The proportion of deaths in inpatient hospices has increased marginally since 2004 with the swing in numbers of deaths being from acute hospitals to the home and these being largely deaths from cancer. One wonders if the relatively uncertain trajectory of nonmalignant life-threatening illnesses may make it more likely that death occurs in an institution, particularly if such illnesses are, in the United Kingdom at least, poorly catered for by intensive community palliative care programs. Clearly, diagnosis is not the only factor influencing place of

death, and Higginson, who has published extensively on the trends in place of death, noted that the overall proportion of deaths at home had variations dependent upon several social and geographical parameters.[24*]

The relative underrepresentation of individuals from ethnic backgrounds other than *White, British* among those admitted to Hospice has long caused concern in the United Kingdom. One study reported in 2001 that an individual of Asian ethnicity with cancer was only half as likely to die in a hospice in the United Kingdom as a similar individual of non-Asian background.[25] However, the latest figures for the United Kingdom suggest a gradual increase in the population from ethnic minority groups referred for community hospice care with 6% of all referrals coming from such groups in 2009/2010 (8% of the total UK population comprises ethnic minorities).[19]

Douglas in his oft-quoted *personal view* in the *British Medical Journal* accused the independent hospice movement of being inefficient in that it provided *deluxe* care for a favored minority.[8] A review of data generated by the Regional Study of Care of the Dying sought to address the issue of which cancer patients, dying in 1990, received inpatient hospice care.[26*] Statistically, five factors were found to independently predict hospice inpatient care: having pain in the last year of life, having constipation, being dependent on others for help with activities of daily living for between 1 and 6 months before death, having breast cancer, and being under 85 years of age. Hinton demonstrated a higher rate of admission to an inpatient hospice from patients receiving palliative home care in those that were living alone or with unfit relatives and those with breast cancer.[27] Patients and relatives felt that the principal problems triggering admission were most frequently weakness, pain, depression, and anxiety. A further study of data relating to cancer deaths in 1991 compared those who had accessed any palliative care service, including home care, with those who had not.[28*] The group accessing palliative care services was significantly younger, had longer survival times from diagnosis, and tended to have been referred from certain general practices. A systematic review of access and referral to specialist palliative care found a lack of standardized criteria to guide referral.[29***] There are no national referral guidelines in the United Kingdom, but most areas will have locally based guidance.[30]

Although general practitioner referral patterns may contribute to a recognized inequity of access to palliative care across the United Kingdom,[5,31*] geographical and historical factors are likely to be more important. An analysis of place of death of cancer patients in the North West England demonstrated an increased likelihood of dying in a hospice if they lived close by.[32] Wood et al. have suggested a method of analyzing the provision of inpatient hospice care to a geographical region with particular reference to estimated level of demand, ease of accessibility in terms of *drive time*, and levels of material deprivation.[33] In so doing, the group was able to define an area within their region in which there was potential high demand, poor access, and high levels of deprivation and which therefore merited a discussion of additional inpatient hospice provision. A recent national review using similar methodology offers powerful data for future planning of services and resource allocation.[34] Studies of the significance of place and palliative care, carried out in British Columbia, have added extra dimensions to the question of patterns of access to inpatient palliative care services with particular reference to rural communities.[35] For example, the aesthetics of the available inpatient environment was found to be a significant factor determining choice for admission particularly if this involved significant travel from a remote community.

The issue of the provision of inpatient hospice care for those with diagnoses other than cancer has been debated for many years now. Although many working within hospices would agree with the principle of broadening the diagnostic criteria for admission and have been actively encouraged to do so by the UK government, the hospice inpatient population has only very recently started to show evidence of a small change. This inertia has likely been a result of a perceived (and in some areas real) lack of skills and expertise among hospice staff for the assessment of patients with nonmalignant diagnoses for admission and ongoing clinical management. There is, in addition, an ongoing perception that if their doors were opened to all with a *life-limiting* illness, the hospices would be overwhelmed

by referrals, with inpatient beds taken up by the frail elderly or younger individuals with long-term conditions. There has been no convincing argument or evidence put forward to support this view, and with referral patterns beginning to change, there has been no suggestion that inpatient services are struggling with numbers of referrals.

What do hospices provide?

In 1994, Walter in his book *The Revival of Death* describes his impression of visiting a hospice near London, United Kingdom: "I felt as I was ushered to a reproduction period armchair in the peach wall-papered and thickly carpeted waiting area that I was walking into a Laura Ashley showroom—soft, feminine, traditional and almost aristocratic, and unlike any hospital I knew of."[36] Julia Lawton, reporting her observational study, sent ripples through the hospice movement when she described hospices as *nonplaces* where unbounded bodies (i.e., with discharge or incontinence) could be sequestered for the protection of society.[37] In a more recent study, commissioned by the European Parliament, a freestanding hospice was described as "a place which cultivates harmony and peace and transcends the title of 'healthcare resource' to act as an active element in patient care."[38] Clearly, while the early inpatient hospices modelled themselves very much on St. Christopher's, the evolution over the past 45 years of a specialty that continues to struggle to define itself has produced a wide variation in the models of care practiced. There is no doubt that, in the United Kingdom at least, many hospices do retain elements that could be described as Christian, middle class, and feminine. However, rigorous national standards of health, safety, and infection control, in addition to a tendency towards medicalization of care (encouraged by both physicians and nurses) and a secularization of society, has had an impact on the environment to be found in hospices (Box 36.1).

The majority of inpatient, freestanding hospices in the United Kingdom are staffed by at least one full-time physician trained

---

Box 36.1   Inpatient hospices in the United Kingdom: Service provision 2009/2010

- Total number of adult hospices and palliative care units—220
- Beds per million population (adults)—51
- Beds per hospice (mean)—14.8
- Most common size—10 beds
- Mean length of stay—13.5 days
- Average discharge rate—49%
- Total inpatient admissions 2009/2010—51,900
- Total new inpatient admissions 2009/2010—45,300

Source: From National Survey of Patient Activity Data for Specialist Palliative Care Services, MDS Full Report for the year 2009–2010, The National Council for Palliative Care; National End of Life Care Intelligence Network, http://www.endoflifecare-intelligence.org.uk/end_of_life_care_profiles, accessed May 26, 2012.

in palliative medicine, nurses, physiotherapists, occupational therapists, social workers, and chaplains. Luxurious staffing levels in comparison to acute hospitals ensure that perhaps the most important aspect of care delivered to patients is the carer's time. In addition to providing inpatient end-stage care, hospices accept admissions for symptom control, rehabilitation, and often but not always, respite care. Most inpatient hospices will also provide day care and run multidisciplinary outpatient services for general palliative care needs and increasingly symptom-specific clinics for the management of, for example, lymphedema and breathlessness. In the independent hospices particularly, both inpatients and day patients may be able to access complementary therapies and, in some units, art and music therapy. The majority of hospices offer bereavement support services. The hospice and its staff will also act as a resource for the community providing advice and education to health-care workers and carers, and practical support in terms of equipment loans. The gathering of interdisciplinary professional expertise under one roof with ready access to those who are living with life-shortening illness and often experiencing the most complex of problems provides extraordinary potential for research. However, although this was certainly part of Dame Cicely Saunders' vision for the work of hospices, it is probably fair to say this potential has not been fully realized. The freestanding hospice should, therefore, act as a center of excellence, a community focal point, and a resource and inspiration for palliative and end-of-life care. Although St. Christopher's Hospice is the outstanding example of the potential of such a focal point, there are many stories of the influence of a freestanding hospice on the local community and culture. The role of Casa Sperantei (*House of Hope*) on the development of palliative care in Romania and in the whole of Southeastern Europe serves as one remarkable example of the power of a hospice to evoke change in people and their governments.[39] However, the development of Casa Sperantei would not have been possible without substantial funding from out-of-country charitable sources, based principally in the United Kingdom. The prohibitive ongoing cost of running a freestanding inpatient unit has been a significant factor in the decision to focus on home care and hospital consultation services as the major component of new palliative care initiatives in resource-poor countries (e.g., in Sub-Saharan Africa[40]).

Are hospices successful?

An editorial published in one of the most established journals of palliative medicine in 2012, 45 years after St. Christopher's opened its doors, described measurement tools that capture the quality of palliative care as remaining as elusive as Lewis Carroll's Snark.[41] Peer-reviewed literature supporting the care afforded by hospices is sparse, certainly in terms of strictly controlled studies of sound methodology. Despite this, however, the independent local hospices, which provide 69% of available hospice beds in the United Kingdom, continue to find funds (in the United Kingdom, over £1 million a day is donated to charitable hospices) from charitable giving and operate large armies of volunteers (in the United Kingdom, over 100,000

people are registered as volunteers for freestanding charitable hospices). A survey of 2000 members of the public drawn randomly from the population in the United Kingdom asked participants to rank 12 different areas of health care in order of priority.[42] Interestingly, "special care and pain relief for people who are dying" was ranked second overall to "treatments for children with life-threatening diseases" coming above such services as hip replacements, transplant surgery, community nursing, and psychiatric services. The area of care ranked as the lowest priority was care for those over 75 years of age with acute life-threatening illness. Although numbers of freestanding hospices in the United Kingdom have remained static over the last decade, a large proportion have raised significant funds from the public for renovation and rebuilding projects. Elsewhere in Europe, while countries such as France and Spain continue to employ a model of palliative care based in the community and acute hospitals, the numbers of freestanding inpatient hospices in Germany continue to increase year on year.[43]

The measurement of the influence of hospice care upon an individual patient's illness experience is both a personal (for the hospice worker) and institutional problem. The early studies by Parkes in St. Christopher's Hospice that attempted to illustrate some of the differences between the experience of inpatient hospice care and that of inpatient acute hospital care reported very positive opinions in favor of the inpatient hospice.[44*] However, a methodology that relies on retrospective carer interviews has been questioned.[45] When Parkes repeated his study 10 years later, it is of interest to note the relatively minor perceived difference between hospital and hospice care, particularly in terms of symptom control. A similar observation was made in a later study of the perceptions of surviving spouses.[46*] These observations were somewhat discouraging of further attempts at evaluation of a service that remains in a continuing battle for financial support. The focus for evaluation of inpatient hospice care shifted toward satisfying nationally approved standards of care, against which the institutions are independently assessed, that are for the most part derived from easily measurable components of service provision. However, a more recent study, returning to the principles of the early St. Christopher's studies, has again attempted to look at the opinions of surviving family members in a comparison of their experiences of care in acute hospitals and a freestanding inpatient hospice.[47*] Using a modified version of the Views of Informal Carers—Evaluation of Services (VOICES) questionnaire,[48] all respondents reported a greater satisfaction with care given in the inpatient hospice. Statistically, significant differences were noted in 8 out of 13 variables including reports of better medical, nursing, and personal care in which the individual's dignity was upheld, better pain control and better communication from medical and nursing staff. While carers' views are important and helpful, it is interesting that for a movement that has supposedly been the epitome of patient-centered care, so very little has been published in peer-reviewed literature of patients' experiences of life in inpatient hospices. Data from a UK national patient survey performed in 2010 showed, for example, that 83% of patients felt that staff *always* explained what they were doing and 74% were *very satisfied* with their involvement in care planning.[49*]

However, only 52% felt that they had had an opportunity to discuss their future care up until the end of life. Satisfaction with the care and environment of an inpatient hospice could be inferred from a recently published study from New Zealand.[50*] The authors reported an increased likelihood of an individual dying in an inpatient hospice if they had previously experienced an episode of inpatient respite care despite good access to comprehensive palliative home care services. The authors of an Australian study summarize the patients' perceptions of an inpatient hospice as having the "potential to create an environment without the trauma of potential uncontrolled pain and distress; to help ease the transition between life and death without the burden on family and friends."[51*] The potential of the hospice environment to help maintain a patient's sense of control was also a dominant theme in the interviews. However, there was a tension evident between the sense of control afforded by being able to relieve the burden of care from relatives at home and the loss of control ceded to the clinical team and also to the hospice culture in which there was a perceived pressure to approach death in a particular, open, and *cheerful* manner.

Needham and Newbury attempted to give an evaluation of inpatient hospice care by assessing outcomes in terms of the achievement of individual goals set at the start of an admission by the patient, main carer, and hospice staff.[52*] Interestingly, the authors report a trend toward patients' and carers' goals of admission being more specific and functional compared with those of the staff that were more symptom or problem oriented. However, the large majority of goals evaluated from the three different perspectives were at least partially achieved in those patients discharged from hospice, with evaluations by carers and family of those dying proving difficult to obtain. More goals set by the staff were at least partially achieved than those goals set by patients or their main carers. This may reflect more realistic goal setting, optimistic assessments, or possibly the relatively poor ability to identify a patient's *goals* demonstrated in an earlier study of hospice nurses.[53*] A very recent study conducted in an Australian inpatient hospice noted a continuing difficulty in proxy assessment with relatively poor correlation between symptom scores of patients and their nurses, particularly for symptoms such as fatigue and appetite that often are very difficult for care staff to influence.[54*] Perhaps, the words of Dame Cicely Saunders from over 30 years ago still need to be heeded:

> No patient will thank you for much handholding or sympathetic counselling unless the things he or she perceives as the basics at that moment are attended to first.[55]

The early studies at St. Christopher's Hospice comparing inpatient hospice and inpatient acute hospital care from the viewpoint of the surviving spouse found a consistent impression of a better social and psychological environment within the hospice compared to the hospital.[44*,46*]

A more recent study of patient and carer satisfaction suggested a greater influence on *satisfaction with care* from perceived quality of life within a hospice than from the presence of physical symptoms.[56*] This, as the authors observe, may reflect the general improvement in physical symptom control, delivered by better informed nonspecialists in palliative care,

now occurring before admission to hospice. If a person receiving palliative care is to be aided to *live until he dies at his own maximum potential,*[57] then this should indeed be reflected in a wish within hospices to seek to maximize an individual's quality of life. However, a systematic review could find no evidence that inpatient hospices improve patients' quality of life[58***] but remarked on the lack of good quality research. A more recent single Canadian study did suggest that quality of life improves after admission but recognized its limitations with a mere 12% of patients able to complete the study tool on admission, and only 8% of admissions were able to complete a follow up interview after one week.[59*] The study used the McGill questionnaire and was able to show improvements in physical, psychological, and existential domains. Earlier work by the same author demonstrated the importance of the *meaningful existence* subscale of the McGill questionnaire in determining overall quality of life in palliative care.[60] The close link between spiritual care at the end of life, provided by both the medical and pastoral care teams, and overall perceived quality of life has been confirmed in one recent study.[61*] Improving, or at least maintaining, quality of life through the preservation of a meaningful existence by, for example, the maintenance of dignity and personhood[62,63] may become an increasing focus of research and development in the care delivered in inpatient hospices in the future.

CONCLUSIONS

The modern hospice movement and the specialty of palliative care have revolutionized the approach to the care of those living and dying with incurable illness. Freestanding inpatient hospices modelled on St. Christopher's Hospice are now to be found in all parts of the world, although it is hospice as a philosophy of care, in the community or acute hospital, which has been developed most widely.

Inpatient hospices have proven over the centuries to be institutions that have been visionary in terms of providing for gaps in the provision of care for others. The early medieval hospices spawned hospitals and later the modern hospices, which very much maintained the central ethos of providing hospitality for the stranger with the spiritual dimension of care as critical to this process. The *modern* inpatient hospice in the United Kingdom, with independence in terms of resources and management structure, enjoyed space for the development of true holistic care and the new specialty of palliative care. The control of physical symptoms in the first phase of modern hospice development proved to be of overriding importance, and necessarily so because, just as during the care of any individual patient, one cannot properly address psychological and spiritual issues in a setting of uncontrolled physical symptoms. However, with a slowing of the rate of new developments in physical symptom control, and with the aid of comprehensive education programs, often run by the hospices, clinicians other than specialists in palliative care are now generally able to provide a very good level of symptom control. Initially attracted into hospice work by these early major advancements in palliative care, many individual clinicians in the United Kingdom are now finding themselves having to critically examine their role in hospice care. This may be particularly pertinent for practitioners who are hospice-based, rather than hospital- or community-based, specialists in palliative care.

A recent observational study noted that, in one freestanding hospice, despite good levels of staffing, patients were left alone for significant amounts of time and reminded us that the power of *being with* is fundamental to hospice care and hospitality.[64] Increasing bureaucracy and the attendant administrative tasks are partly accountable for a recent study showing that nurses in inpatient hospices in the United Kingdom spend, on average, only 45% of their time in direct patient care.[65] Has care in hospices become so medicalized and regulated that a carer's time is so consumed by medical interventions and paper (or keyboard) work that the focus and driving force of a hospice, it's patients, and their families have been sidelined? Have hospices, by becoming specialist palliative care units, taken on too broad a spectrum of patients (in terms of diagnosis and prognosis) so that those who are dying and physically *comfortable* are not afforded as much time as others? Do hospice staff feel relatively helpless when faced with patient's significant emotional and spiritual difficulties unmasked by good physical symptom control? In response to questions such as these, there have been calls for *hospice care* and *palliative care* in the United Kingdom to proceed as distinct specialties,[66] in a somewhat similar fashion to the evolution of end-of-life care in North America and parts of Europe.

The debate over the role and future of hospices has been ongoing since the early 1980s perhaps, in part, for reasons summed up eloquently by Torrens[67] as quoted by Small[68]:

Early on it was clear who the villains and the heroes were, where the challenges lay, what were the pitfalls to be avoided. There was the good work and it was easy to devote one's life….I think now we have passed that stage and ahead lie many diverse paths, many confusions of a subtler nature.

Now, nearly 30 years later, perhaps, it is finally time for the hospices to admit their weaknesses, as well as their strengths, and to realize their opportunities. The hospices do have the space, time, and expertise to critically push forward psychological and spiritual care accompanied by good-quality evaluative research. The acknowledgment of the existential dimension to suffering has always been fundamental to any definition of what hospices do, and many authors have tried to explore the approaches that can be taken within hospices and in palliative care. However, it is only now that, in general terms, patients have a relative freedom from physical symptoms and the hospices are mature enough to seriously explore these issues. If history is anything to go by, this would only be good news for the hospitals and health care of tomorrow.

Key learning points

- Modern inpatient hospices evolved from institutions for the dying where spiritual care was paramount.

- There has been a phenomenal spread of the hospice movement and palliative care principally through the influence of the activity of early individual hospice practitioners.

- Significant developments in palliative and now supportive care are increasingly centered on the provision of care in mainstream hospitals and home care in the community.

- The value and role of inpatient hospice care have been questioned by the health-care professions, but not by the lay public.

- There is little good quality research measuring the contribution inpatient hospice care makes to patient care.

- Recent research into the maintenance of personhood and dignity with an emphasis on the spiritual and psychological aspects of care may point the way to major areas of influence that inpatient hospices may have on the palliative and general medical care of the future.

REFERENCES

1 Palouzie A-M. Aspects of the European dying process. *Ser. Sci. Med.* 1985; **20**: 851–853.

2 Humphreys C. "Waiting for the last summons": The establishment of the first hospices in England 1878–1914. *Mortality* 2001; **6**: 146–166.

3 Clark D, Neale B, Heather P. Contracting for palliative care. *Soc. Sci. Med.* 1995; **40**:1193–1202.

4 HM Government UK. Government response to house of commons health committee report on palliative care. Fourth report of session 2003–4. 2004. London, U.K.: HMSO.

5 NICE. *Supportive and Palliative Care for People with Cancer.* London, U.K.: National Institute for Clinical Excellence and King's College, 2004.

6 Cherny NI, Catane R, Kosmodis P. ESMO takes a stand on supportive and palliative care. *Ann. Oncol* 2003; **14**: 1335–1337.

7 Seale CF. What happens in hospices: A review of research evidence. *Soc. Sci. Med.* 1989; **28**: 551–559.

8 Douglas C. For all the saints. *BMJ* 1992; **304**: 479.

9 James N, Field D. The routinization of hospice: Charisma and bureaucratization. *Soc. Sci. Med.* 1992; **34**: 1363–1375.

10 Scott JF. Palliative care 2000: What's stopping us? *J. Palliat. Care* 1992; **8**: 5–8.

11 Kearney M. Palliative medicine—Just another specialty? *Palliat. Med.* 1992; **6**: 39–46.

12 Clark D. Whither the Hospices? In Clark D, ed. *The future for Palliative Care: Issues of Policy and Practice.* London, U.K.: Open University Press, 1993: pp. 167–177.

13 National End of Life Intelligence Network. *What Do We Know Now That We Didn't Know a Year Ago?* England: NHS, 2011.

14 Gomes B, Calanzani N, Higginson IJ. *Local Preferences and Place of Death in Regions within England 2010.* London, U.K.: Cicely Saunders Institute, 2011.

15 Gomes B, Higginson IJ, Calanzani N et al. Preferences for place of death if faced with advanced cancer: A population survey in England, Flanders, Germany, Italy, the Netherlands, Portugal and Spain. *Ann. Oncol.* 2012; **23**:2006–2015.

16 Li S. 'Symbiotic niceness': Constructing a therapeutic relationship in psychosocial palliative care. *Soc. Sci. Med.* 2004; 58: 2571–2583.

17 Bradshaw PJ. Characteristics of clients referred to home, hospice and hospital palliative care services in Western Australia. *Palliat. Med.* 1993; **7**: 101–107.

18 Payne S. To supplant, supplement or support? Organisational issues for hospices. *Soc. Sci. Med.* 1998; **46**: 1495–1504.

19 National Survey of Patient Activity Data for Specialist Palliative Care Services. MDS Full Report for the year 2009–2010. The National Council for Palliative Care.

20 National End of Life Care Intelligence Network. http://www. endoflifecare-intelligence.org.uk/end_of_life_care_profiles. Accessed May 26, 2012.

21 NHPCO. *Facts and Figures: Hospice Care in America.* Alexandria, VA: National Hospice and Palliative Care Organisation, 2011.

22 Gomes B, Calanzani N, Higginson IJ. Reversal of the British trends in place of death: Time series analysis 2004–2010 *Palliat. Med.* 2012; **26**:102–107

23 Wilson DM, Truman CD, Thomas R et al.. The rapidly changing location of death in Canada, 1994–2004. *Soc. Sci. Med.* 2009; **68**: 1752–1758.

24 Higginson IJ, Jarman B, Astin P, Dolan S. Do social factors affect where patients die: An analysis of 10 years of cancer deaths in England. *J. Public Health Med.* 1999; **21**: 22–28.

25 Silcocks PBS, Rashid A, Culley L, Smith L. Inequality even in terminal illness? [abstract]. *Eur J Cancer* 2001; **37**(Suppl 2):S1–S126.

● 26 Addington-Hall J, Altmann D, McCarthy M. Which terminally ill cancer patients receive hospice in-patient care? *Soc. Sci. Med.* 1998; **46**: 1011–1016.

27 Hinton J. Which patients with terminal cancer are admitted from home care? *Palliat. Med.* 1994; **8**: 197–210.

28 Gray JD, Forster DP. Factors associated with the utilization of specialist palliative care services: A population based study. *J.Public Health Med.* 1997; **19**: 464–469.

29 Ahmed N, Bestall JC, Ahmedzai SH et al. Systematic review of the problems and issues of accessing specialist palliative care by patients, carers and health and social care professionals. *Palliat. Med.* 2004; **18**: 525–542.

✳ 30 Bennett M, Adam J, Alison D et al. Leeds eligibility criteria for specialist palliative care services. *Palliat. Med.* 2000; **14**: 157–158.

31 Shipman C, Addington-Hall J, Barclay S et al. How and why do GPs use specialist palliative care services? *Palliat. Med.* 2002; **16**: 241–246

32 Gatrell AC, Harman J, Francis BJ et al. Place of death: Analysis of cancer deaths in part of North West England. *J. Public Health Med.* 2003; **25**: 53–58.

33 Wood DJ, Clark D, Gatrell AC. Equity of access to adult hospice inpatient care within north-west England. *Palliat. Med.* 2004; **18**: 543–549.

34 GatrellAC, WoodDJ. Variation in geographic access to specialist inpatient hospices in England and Wales. *HealthPlace.* 2012; **18**: 832–840.

35 Castleden H, Crooks VA, Schuurman N, Hanlon N. "It's not necessarily the distance on the map...": Using place as an analytic tool to elucidate geographic issues central to rural palliative care. *Health Place.* 2010; **16**: 284–290.

36 Walter T. *The Revival of Death.* London, U.K.: Routledge, 1994: pp. 87–90

37 Lawton J. Contemporary hospice care: The sequestration of the unbounded body and 'dirty dying'. *Sociol Health Illness.* 1998; **20**: 121–143.

38 Martin-Moreno JM, Harris M, Gorgojo L et al. *Palliative Care in the European Union.* Brussels, Belgium: European Parliament, Policy Department, Economic and Scientific Policy, 2008.

39 Economist Intelligence Unit. *The Quality of Death: Ranking End-of-Life Care across the World.* London, U.K.: Economist Intelligence Unit, July 2010

40 Merriman A, Heller KS. Hospice Uganda-A model palliative care initiative in Africa: An interview with Anne Merriman. *Innovations in End-of-Life Care.* 2002; **4**, www.edc.org/lastacts.

41 Dy SM, Lupu D, Seow H. Progress towards systems of quality measurement that capture the essence of good palliative care. *Palliat. Med.* 2012; **26**: 291–293.

42 Bowling A. Health care rationing: The public's debate. *BMJ* 1996; **312**: 670–674.

43 Wegweiser Hospiz- und Palliativmedizin und DHPV-Datenbank, 2011.

44 Parkes CM, Parkes J. 'Hospice' versus 'hospital' care—Re-evaluation after 10 years as seen by surviving spouses. *Postgrad. Med. J.* 1984; **60**: 120–124.

45 Hinton J. How reliable are relatives' retrospective reports of terminal illness? Patients and relatives' accounts compared. *Soc. Sci. Med.* 1996; **43**: 1229–1236.

46 Seale C, Kelly M. A comparison of hospice and hospital care for people who die: Views of the surviving spouse. *Palliat. Med.* 1997; **11**: 93–100.

47 Addington-Hall JM, O'Callaghan AC. A comparison of the quality of care provided to cancer patients in the UK in the last three months of life in in-patient hospices compared with hospitals, from the perspective of bereaved relatives: Results from a survey using the VOICES questionnaire. *Palliat. Med.* 2009; **23**: 190–197.

48 Addington-Hall J, Walker L, Jones C et al. A randomised controlled trial of postal versus interviewer administration of a questionnaire measuring satisfaction with and use of services received in the year before death. *J. Epidemiol. Commun.Health* 1998; **52**: 802–807.

49 Centre for Health Service Studies, University of Kent: Results of the 2010/2011 Hospice Patient Survey, General Report. Commissioned by Help the Hospices.

50 Taylor EJ, Ensor B, Stanley J. Place of death related to demographic factors for hospice patients in Wellington, Aotearoa New Zealand. *Palliat. Med.* 2012; **26**: 342–349.

51 Broom A, Cavenagh J. On the meanings and experiences of living and dying in an Australian hospice. *Health* 2011; **15**: 96–111.

52 Needham PR, Newbury J. Goal setting as a measure of outcome in palliative care. *Palliat. Med.* 2004; **18**: 444–451.

53 Heaven CM, Maguire P. Disclosure of concerns by hospice patients and their identification by nurses. *Palliat. Med.* 1997; **11**: 283–290.

54 ToTH, OngWY, Rawlings D et al. The disparity between patient and nurse symptom rating in a hospice population. *J. Palliat. Med.* 2012; **15**: 542–547.

55 Saunders C. The Hospice: Its meaning to patients and their physicians. *Hosp. Pract.* 1981; **16**: 94.

56 Tierney RM, Horton SM, Hannan TJ, Tierney WM. Relationships between symptom relief, quality of life, and satisfaction with hospice care. *Palliat. Med.* 1998; **12**: 333–344.

57 Saunders C. Foreward. In Doyle D, Hanks G, MacDonald N eds. *Oxford Textbook of Palliative Medicine.* Oxford, U.K.: Oxford University Press, 1998.

58 Salisbury C, Bosanquet N, Wilkinson EK et al. The impact of different models of specialist palliative care on patients' quality of life: A systematic literature review. *Palliat. Med.* 1999; **13**: 3–17.

59 Cohen SR, Boston P, Mount BM, Porterfield P. Changes in quality of life following admission to palliative care units. *Palliat. Med.* 2001; **15**: 363–371.

60 Cohen SR, Mount BM, Strobel MG, Bui F. The McGill Quality of Life Questionnaire: A measure of quality of life appropriate for people with advanced disease. A preliminary study of validity and acceptability. *Palliat. Med.* 1995; **9**: 207–219.

61 Balboni TA, Paulk MA, Balboni MJ et al. Provision of spiritual care to patients with advanced cancer: Associations with medical care and quality of life near death. *J. Clin. Oncol.* 2010; **28**: 445–452.

62 Chochinov HM. Dignity-conserving care—A new model for palliative care: Helping the patient feel valued. *JAMA* 2002; **287**: 2253–2260.

63 Kabel A, Roberts D. Professionals' perceptions of maintaining personhood in hospice care. *Int. J. Palliat. Nurs.* 2003; **9**: 283–289.

64 Haraldsdottir E. The constraints of the ordinary: 'Being with' in the context of end-of-life nursing care. *Int. J. Palliat. Nurs.* 2011; **17**: 245–250.

65 Roberts D, Hurst K. Evaluating palliative care ward staffing using bed occupancy, patient dependency, staff activity, service quality and cost data *Palliat. Med.* 2013; 27: 123–130.

66 Biswas B. The Medicalization of Dying: A nurse's view. In Clark D ed. *The Future for Palliative Care: Issues of Policy and Practice.* Open University Press, Buckingham, 1993: pp. 132–139.

67 Torrens P. Achievement, failure and the future: Hospice analyzed. In Saunders C, Summers DH, Teller N eds. *Hospice: The Living Idea.* London, U.K.: Edward Arnold, 1981: pp. 187–194.

68 Small N. HIV/AIDS: Lessons for policy and practice. In Clark D ed. *The Future for Palliative Care: Issues of Policy and Practice.* London, U.K.: Open University Press, 1993: pp. 80–97.

37

Palliative care unit

KAREN MACMILLAN, KELLEY FOURNIER, BETH TUPALA

INTRODUCTION

The term *palliative care unit* (PCU) usually applies to a group of beds designated for the care of patients with terminal illness, located in an acute care hospital. Various models of PCUs are possible, depending on local needs, resources, system characteristics, and philosophies of care. In some countries, these are also called hospices within hospitals, but the term PCU is more widespread and therefore is adopted in this chapter. Potential options in the design of a PCU are listed in Table 37.1, each of which presents advantages and disadvantages.[1,2] Reasons for admission to a PCU may include symptom control, end-of-life care, respite care, special treatment and investigations, and rehabilitation.[4] However, the availability of diagnostics, procedures, support services, and consultants in an acute care hospital makes PCUs particularly suited to the care of patients with problems of a complex nature.

A tertiary palliative care unit (TPCU) is a distinct type of PCU, defined as an "academic centre where specialist knowledge for the most complex cases is practiced, researched and taught."[1,5] The purpose of this chapter is to describe and discuss the role, structure, and operation of a TPCU, using the authors' unit in Edmonton, Canada, as an example to provide detailed information on staffing and processes. The final section considers the wider international context and evidence.

CONTEXT

The TPCU in Edmonton is an integral component of the Alberta Health Services, Edmonton Zone Palliative Care Program (EZPCP).[5,6] This publicly funded program provides a comprehensive range of palliative care services, including home care and specialist consultation in the community, long-term care, ambulatory care, and acute care settings. It also supports designated units in long-term care facilities (i.e., hospices) for patients who have a life expectancy of 3–4 months or less.

The TPCU is located in an acute care teaching hospital. It consists of 20 private and semiprivate rooms in a dedicated geographical area. Amenities include a family lounge with kitchenette, a laundry room, a quiet room, and a conference room. Family members may stay overnight if they wish, and pets are allowed.

PATIENT SELECTION

Admission criteria for the TPCU are listed in Box 37.1. The role of the TPCU is to provide care for the subset of patients who have the most complex problems and who require the intensive involvement of a specialist interdisciplinary or interprofessional team. The problems may be in the physical, psychological, social, or spiritual domains. Although no limitations are placed around diagnosis, the vast majority of patients have cancer as their primary illness. Unlike the hospice setting, life expectancy is not specified. However, the TPCU is intended as a temporary place of care until symptoms have stabilized sufficiently to allow discharge to another setting. Patients are asked to agree to a *do-not-resuscitate* status prior to admission; the pros and cons of this policy will be reviewed later in this chapter.

Referrals to the EZPCP are screened by the palliative care consultants covering the various settings. The consultant determines, after direct assessment of the patient, whether or not a referral to the TPCU is indicated. The goals of admission to the TPCU and the temporary nature of the admission are discussed with the patient and family. The consultant is also responsible for confirming and documenting that the patient accepts a do-not-resuscitate status and has discussed their preferred goals of care designation, which is reviewed later in this chapter.

Once admission has been agreed upon, the patient's health records are forwarded to the TPCU. The referrals are triaged to determine priority. Patients are usually scheduled for admission on weekday mornings. This allows sufficient time for a comprehensive assessment and discussion of the goals and plan of care with the patient and family. However, admissions for problems requiring urgent intervention can be accommodated 24 hours a day, 7 days a week.

Table 37.1　*Options in the design of PCUs*

	Design element	Options
Location	Inside main hospital	Outside main hospital
Admission policy	Open (any physician)	Closed (specialist only)
Visiting hours	Open	Limited
Source of admissions	Direct from home	In-hospital transfer only
Range of procedures, tests,	Unlimited	Limited therapies
Do-not-resuscitate status	Required	Not required

Source: von Gunten, C.F., *JAMA*, 287, 875, 2002.

Box 37.1　Admission criteria for the TPCU, Edmonton, Canada

Intensive, interdisciplinary intervention required for severe symptom problems for which management has not been successful.

Symptoms require ongoing monitoring/assessment.
When stable, patient will be discharged to the most appropriate care setting.
Average length of stay is 34 weeks; exceptions are expected.
Age 18+.
Accepts DNR status.

STAFFING

Staffing of the TPCU is described in Table 37.2. The patients are admitted under the care of physicians who are specialists in palliative medicine, one of whom also assumes the medical administrative responsibilities. The nurses function in a team nursing model and work 8 hour shifts. The complexity of the patient population necessitates the inclusion of a chaplain, social worker, psychologist, physical therapist, occupational therapist, music therapist, pharmacist, and dietician as core members of the team. The program manager is responsible for the organizational administrative responsibilities of the TPCU, including the triage process for admissions to the unit. The clinical educator supports the team's educational needs. The unit clerks, secretaries, and volunteers play an essential supporting role.

Other hospital support services, such as respiratory therapy, are often involved. The TPCU has a formal arrangement with an anesthesiology service at another acute care hospital for support for procedures such as spinal administration of analgesics. Patients may also be referred to the regional cancer center for palliative oncological therapies. Other specialists may be accessed from within the hospital as needed.

Table 37.2　*Staffing of the TPCU at Edmonton, Canada*

Type of staff	Full-time equivalent
Registered nurses	14.3 (3 per shift)
Licensed practical nurses	8.4 (3–4 per shift)
Nursing attendants	8.4 (2 per night shift)
Physicians	2.5
Chaplain	1.0
Social worker	1.0
Physical therapist	0.6
Occupational therapist	0.5
Music therapist	0.7
Dietician	0.2
Pharmacist	0.2
Clinical educator	1.0
Program manager	1.0
Unit clerks	1.7
Secretaries	1.6

ASSESSMENT

The tools routinely employed on the TPCU are listed in Table 37.3. Many were developed on the TPCU itself.[7-14] The tools have been adopted in all the settings of the EZPCP.

The Edmonton Symptom Assessment System Revised (ESAS-r) is a validated tool for measuring the intensity of common symptoms in palliative care patients.[7] Besides providing important clinical information on a daily basis, it has been successfully utilized for audit and research purposes.[9] The mini-mental state examination[16] is used because cognitive failure is an extremely common and potentially distressing complication in palliative care patients, but one that is easily missed without the use of a screening tool.[17] Identification of a history of alcohol abuse with an instrument such as the CAGE questionnaire[18] is important because of this condition's underdiagnosis and association with poor pain outcomes.[18b,19] The Edmonton Classification System for Cancer Pain (ECS-CP) is a clinician-rated assessment tool for classification of five pain features—mechanism of pain, incident pain, psychological distress, addictive behavior, and cognitive function. It is a standardized, comprehensive, and simple approach, which is used to improve clinical assessments and management of cancer pain. The assessment informs resource allocation decisions in clinical programs through early identification of patients with complex pain syndromes. It improves communication in the interdisciplinary team members. It is a valuable tool for accurately predicting the complexity of pain management.[13] As constipation is a frequent problem in this patient population, the constipation score is used to objectively quantify and locate stool, based on a plain abdominal radiograph.[20,21] The type, total dose, and route of opioid are recorded daily to track patient progress. The Palliative Performance Scale version 2 (PPSv2) describes functional status.[22]

Table 37.3 *Assessment tools used on the TPCU at Edmonton, Canada*

Tool	Domain measured	Team member responsible	Frequency
ESAS-r[5]	Intensity of common symptoms	Nurse	Daily
Folstein mini-mental state examination[11]	Cognition	Physician	On admission and weekly
CAGE questionnaire[13]	History of alcoholism	Physician	On admission
ECS-CP[7]	Prognosis for achieving pain control	Physician	On admission
Constipation score[15] of retained stool	Quantity and location	Physician	On admission and as needed
Morphine equivalent daily dose	Type, dose, and route of opioid	Physician	Daily
Palliative Performance Scale version 2[17]	Performance status	Physician	On admission and weekly

WARD ROUTINE

At the beginning of the day, the nurses' observations of the patients during the previous two shifts are relayed to the medical and interdisciplinary teams. The physicians then spend the morning assessing the patients and negotiating a plan of care for the day. Interaction with the team occurs on an ongoing basis. A team conference is held once a week during which the admissions of the previous week are discussed in detail and a comprehensive management plan is formulated. The progress of the other patients is also reviewed, and plans are adjusted accordingly.

While discussions with patients and families take place throughout the course of admission, a designated family conference is often advisable to clarify goals and establish plans of care. The conference is coordinated by the social worker and attended by the team, the patient, and all family members whom the patient wishes to involve.

DISCHARGE PLANNING

Approximately 20% of the patients admitted to the TPCU are eventually discharged to other settings compared to 50% in 2002; this represents the increasing complexity of patients admitted to the TPCU and the inability to manage these patients in other settings. Some may be able to return home. Usually a discharge home is preceded by a family conference that includes the home care case manager. It is important that the patient and family understand who will be responsible for care once the discharge has taken place. The primary roles of the family physician and the home care case manager are therefore emphasized. If the success of the discharge is in question, a trial discharge is recommended, whereby the patient's bed on the TPCU is retained for a few days in case the patient needs to return. Once the patient has been discharged, a medical summary is immediately entered into our health systems database for review electronically by the family physician, and a copy is faxed to the home care office. Patients whose symptoms have stabilized but who are unable to return home may be transferred to a hospice.

A significant number of patients remain on the TPCU until death. Some cannot be discharged because of progressive deterioration, whereas others have ongoing needs that cannot be met in any other setting. For example, hospices do not have the resources required to manage spinal analgesics, total parenteral nutrition, or complex respiratory care.

EDUCATION AND RESEARCH

All members of the team are expected to participate in education and research. Most of the physicians have appointments in the Division of Palliative Care Medicine of the Department of Oncology, University of Alberta.

The TPCU receives undergraduate and postgraduate medical trainees from the University of Alberta on a regular basis. A total of four residents and fellows may be accommodated at a given time. Family medicine residents undertake a mandatory 2-week palliative medicine rotation on the TPCU. An analysis of multiple-choice-question examinations given to family medicine residents at the beginning and the end of their palliative care rotations demonstrated a significant improvement in knowledge.[23] Oncology residents also spend part of their compulsory 4-week palliative medicine rotation on the TPCU. Residents in the 1-year palliative medicine program spend 6 months on the TPCU. Elective rotations are open to residents from other programs and to medical students. Learners from other disciplines such as nursing and social work are also welcome. The TPCU has a long history of training palliative care specialists from across Canada and around the world.

Clinical teaching is complemented by journal club, held three mornings per week, during which time articles with relevance to palliative care are presented and discussed. A survey revealed that a majority of trainees found this activity to be of value for education, clinical practice, and development of critical appraisal skills.[24] Other educational activities include seminars and weekly program-wide rounds, which incorporate medical, interdisciplinary, and research topics. Presenters from other specialties are invited to share their expertise as applied directly or indirectly to palliative care, thus fostering the exchange of knowledge between different health-care fields.

Funding for research on the TPCU is derived from a variety of sources. The priority given to this activity is reflected in the numerous examples of innovations in symptom assessment and treatment developed in this setting.[4–15,25–27]

OUTCOMES

Patients on the TPCU are significantly younger and have significantly higher frequency of positive CAGE scores, poor prognosis for achieving good pain control, and severe symptoms. This suggests that patients were being appropriately selected for admission to this setting.

In 2011, the total number of patients admitted to the TPCU represented 7% of all patients seen by the EZPCP compared to 17% in 2002.[29] Median length of stay was 19 days and bed occupancy was 83% compared to 91% in 2002. Eighty-two percent of patients died on the TPCU, while 14% and 3% were discharged to the home and hospice settings, respectively. The changes in these outcomes are related to an increase of beds on the TPCU from 14 to 20 and the additional consult services available throughout the zone. With increased specialists and expertise, many complex symptoms can be managed in other care settings, decreasing the need for admission to a tertiary-level setting. The annual budget for the TPCU is approximately $4,750,000, of which 85% is used to fund salaries (excluding physician salaries, which are paid from a separate source). Another 8% is directed toward drugs, while the remainder is allocated for supplies.

DISCUSSION AND THE WIDER INTERNATIONAL CONTEXT

TPCUs fulfill a unique clinical role in the continuum of care for patients with terminal illness. They are designed to care for patients with the most complex problems of a physical, psychological, social, or spiritual nature. In a comprehensive, integrated palliative care program, approximately 10% of patients would be appropriate for admission to such a unit.

Given the complexity of the patient population, the ideal location for such a unit is in an acute care hospital that offers a full range of diagnostic and interventional procedures (e.g., magnetic resonance imaging [MRI], endoscopy), support services (e.g., respiratory therapy), and specialty and subspecialty consultation (e.g., anesthesiology, surgery, internal medicine, psychiatry). For units that admit cancer patients predominantly, access to oncological consultation and therapy is essential. Indeed, it is possible for such units to be situated in cancer centers, although access for patients with diagnoses other than cancer may be limited. In the opinion of some administrators, the optimal unit size for staffing efficiency is 16–24 beds and the minimum size is 10–12 beds.[30]

The issue of requiring a do-not-resuscitate status for admission to a PCU is controversial. This policy is based on the finding that the chance of success of cardiopulmonary resuscitation, defined as survival to discharge from hospital, is nil in patients with metastatic cancer.[31] Agreement on this issue prior to admission lessens the chance of subsequent confusion about the overall goals of care. Furthermore, patients and families are spared the distress of experiencing or witnessing a resuscitation attempt. However, this policy may pose a barrier to care for those patients who could benefit from the unit's services but are not willing to accept a do-not-resuscitate status. Moreover, some palliative care specialists perceive that selected patients may be appropriate for resuscitation, depending on prognosis, quality of life, and the patient's wishes.[32] Whatever decision is made regarding policy, discussion of do-not-resuscitate status presents a valuable opportunity to clarify the patient's and family's understanding of the illness and prognosis, as well as goals of care.[33]

In order that the limited resources of the TPCU may be used for the appropriate patients, a process for screening referrals is required. Direct assessment of the patient by a palliative care consultant is preferred. Besides determining whether or not the patient's concerns warrant admission to this specialized setting, the consultant is able to prepare the patient and family for the type of care that will be provided on the unit. Meticulous communication between the referring and receiving teams is important for continuity of care and to minimize unnecessary duplication of assessments.

Given the complex nature of the patients' problems, a specialist interdisciplinary team is required. The team should comprise members who together can address the breadth of concerns of the patients and families referred to the TPCU. Consultants from other specialties also make a significant contribution to the care of patients on a TPCU.

A disciplined approach to assessment and documentation of patient and family concerns is essential for achieving the goals of admission. First, it is a fundamental step in identifying and characterizing the patient's issues. Second, it allows for tracking of the patient's course over time and outcomes of interventions. Third, it facilitates communication of the patient's situation to the various care providers involved. Finally, the data collected may be used for program management, quality assurance, and research. As much as possible, the tools should be validated, easy to understand, not burdensome to complete, and clinically useful. Also, they should capture the multidimensional nature of patients' concerns. Ideally, the same tools should be used in all associated health-care settings, as the use of a common language facilitates transfer of care between settings and allows for comparisons to be made among settings.[28,29] The acuity and complexity of the patients admitted to the TPCU necessitate frequent assessment, rapid adjustment of therapies, timely communication between team members, and careful coordination of efforts. The patient and family must be recognized as being central to the team.

In order that the TPCU beds remain readily accessible to patients requiring admission, an effective and proactive discharge planning process is required. Options for discharge depend on local resources. For those patients who are discharged home, clear and timely communication with community health-care providers (e.g., primary care physician, home care manager, pharmacist) is critical. Transfer to a hospice often poses a difficult transition for the patients and families, not only because of their need to adjust to a new environment and staff, but also because they may view hospice as a lower level of care and feel a sense of abandonment.[34] These concerns may be alleviated by noting that the fact that the patient no longer requires management on the TPCU is a positive outcome, providing reassurance that the patient's needs can be adequately met in hospice, and arranging for families to tour the hospice. Depending on the resources available outside the TPCU, there may also be patients who stay despite stable symptoms because their needs cannot be met in any other setting. Some of these patients may remain on the TPCU for a prolonged period of time.

As a setting for the management of the most complex cases, the TPCU has an inherent mandate to transfer its knowledge to others as well as to advance the state of that knowledge. These roles are facilitated by locating the unit in a teaching hospital and by appointing the staff to faculty positions in the university. The TPCU presents a number of advantages as a learning environment. It provides learners with the opportunity to be exposed to a broad range of problems in palliative care, to follow patients closely, to gain experience dealing with distressed families, and to work with an interdisciplinary team, all under the direct supervision of experts in the field. The potential disadvantage is that the patients and problems encountered on the TPCU are highly selected and not necessarily representative of those encountered in other practice settings. Also, the interventions performed on the TPCU may not be transferable to other settings because of resource limitations. The TPCU provides an environment that is well suited to the conduct of research. Since the patients are under the direct care of the team, the process of screening and recruiting for studies may be simpler. If the study involves medically complex interventions or monitoring, then this may be most readily achieved in an acute care setting such as the TPCU. However, patients on a TPCU have a greater degree of symptom distress and therefore may not be well enough to participate in studies. In addition, the results may not be generalizable to other palliative patient populations. Nonetheless, many patients admitted to PCUs are willing to consider participation in clinical trials.[35]

A number of publications have reported variable symptom outcomes in patients admitted to individual PCUs.[9,36-39] Generalizability of the data is uncertain, in part because the characteristics of these units are diverse or incompletely described. A prospective, multicenter study demonstrated that admission to PCUs resulted in significant improvements in the physical, psychological, and existential domains of quality of life.[40]

The economic impact of PCUs has also been described. In a report from a 23-bed PCU in a comprehensive cancer center, costs were shown to exceed revenues if length of stay was greater than 10 days. Also, cost was inversely proportional to patient census.[41] Analysis from a palliative care inpatient service in another comprehensive cancer center revealed that mean daily charges were 38% lower than in the rest of the hospital.[39] Both units are characterized by intensive interdisciplinary symptom management and discharge planning, high patient volumes, short lengths of stay, and low mortality rates. Economic outcomes have been described for a different model of PCU, located in an acute care facility but providing terminal care for patients with a variety of diagnoses. Charges

and costs were 66% lower for days on the unit, compared with days in hospital prior to transfer to the unit, and almost 60% lower for patients who died on the unit versus matched controls who died elsewhere in the hospital.[42] Economic issues are of course influenced by the funding mechanisms particular to each health-care system. For example, in the United States, the distinction between acute palliative care services and hospice services is essential for reimbursement purposes.[39]

CONCLUSION

By providing specialist interdisciplinary care for the most complex patients, TPCUs fulfill a unique and leading role in clinical care, education, and research within palliative care programs, health-care systems, and academic centers. Further study is needed to clarify the impact of such units on clinical, economic, and academic outcomes.

Key learning points

- Different models of PCUs in acute care hospitals are possible.
- A PCU admits patients with the most complex problems.
- The key roles of a PCU are clinical care, education, and research.
- Effective use of a PCU requires a process for selecting appropriate patients and for discharging them.
- Successful management of these patients requires a specialist interdisciplinary team and access to diagnostic and interventional procedures, support services, and consultants.
- A disciplined approach to assessment and documentation is essential for achieving the goals of admission.

REFERENCES

1 von Gunten CF. Secondary and tertiary palliative care in U.S. hospitals. *JAMA* 2002; 287: 875–881.
2 Smith T, Coyne P, Cassel J. Practical guidelines for developing new palliative care services: Resource management. *Ann Oncol* 2012; 23(suppl 3):70–75.
3 Elsayem A, Calderon B, Camarines E, Lopez G, Bruera E, Fadul N. A month in an acute palliative care unit: Clinical interventions and financial outcomes. *Am J Hospice Palliat Med* 2012; 28(8): 550–555.
4 Heedman P, Starkhammar H. Patterns of referral to a palliative care unit: An indicator of different attitudes toward the dying patient? *J Palliat Med* 2002; 5: 101–106.
5 Brenneis C, Bruera E. Models for the delivery of palliative care: The Canadian model. In: Bruera E, Portenoy RK, eds. *Topics in Palliative Care*, Vol. 5. New York: Oxford University Press, 2001: pp. 3–23.
6 Fainsinger R, Brenneis C, Fassbender K. Edmonton, Canada: A regional model of palliative care development. *J Pain and Symptom Manage* 2007; 33(5): 634–639.

7   Bruera E, Kuehn N, Miller MJ et al. The Edmonton symptom assessment system (ESAS): A simple method for the assessment of palliative care patients. *J Palliat Care* 1991; 7: 6–9

8   Watanabe SM, Nekolaichuk C, Beaumont C, Johnson L, Myers J, Strasser F. A multi-centre comparison of two numerical versions of the Edmonton Symptom Assessment System in palliative care patients. *J Pain Symptom Manage* 2011; 41:456–468.

9   Bruera E, Kuehn N, Miller MJ, Selmser P, Macmillan K. The Edmonton symptom assessment system (ESAS): A simple method for the assessment of palliative care patients. *J Palliat Care* 1991; 7:6–9

10   Bruera E, Sweeney C, Willey J et al. Perception of discomfort by relatives and nurses in unresponsive terminally ill patients with cancer: A prospective study. *J Pain Symptom Manage* 2003; 26: 818–26.

11   Bruera E, Schoeller T, Wenk R et al. A prospective multicenter assessment of the Edmonton Staging System for cancer pain. *J Pain Symptom Manage* 1995; 10: 348–355.

12   Fainsinger R, Nekolaichuk C, Lawlor P, Neumann C. *Edmonton Classification System for Cancer Pain Administration Manual.* 2010. Retrieved June 27, 2012 from http://www.palliative.org/PC/ClinicalInfo/AssessmentTools/Edmonton%20Classification%20System%20for%20Cancer%20Pain%20(ECS-CP)%20Manual%20Sept10-final.pdf

13   Fainsinger RL, Nekolaichuk C, Lawlor P, et al. An International Multicentre Validation Study of a Pain Classification System for Cancer Patients. *Euro J of Cancer* 2010; 46(16): 2865–2866.

14   Walker P, Nordell C, Neumann CM, Bruera E. Impact of the Edmonton Labeled Visual Information System on physician recall of metastatic cancer patient histories: A randomized controlled trial. *J Pain Symptom Manage* 2001; 21: 4–11.

15   Dudgeon DJ, Harlos M, Clinch JJ. The Edmonton symptom assessment scale (ESAS) as an audit tool. *J Palliat Care* 1999; 15: 14–19.

16   Folstein MF, Folstein S, McHugh PR. 'Mini-mental state': A practical method for grading the cognitive state of patients for the clinician. *J Psych Res* 1975; 12: 189–198.

17   Bruera E, Miller L, McCallion J et al. Cognitive failure in patients with terminal cancer: A prospective study. *J Pain Symptom Manage* 1992; 7: 192–195.

18   (a) Ewing J. Detecting alcoholism: The CAGE questionnaire. *JAMA* 1984; 252: 1905–1907; (b) Parsons H, Delgado-Guay M, Osta B, Chacko R, Poulter V, Palmer J, Bruera E. Alcoholism screening in patients with advanced cancer: Impact on symptom burden and opioid use. *J Palliat Care* 2008; 11(7): 964–968.

19   Bruera E, Moyano J, Seifert L et al. The frequency of alcoholism among patients with pain due to terminal cancer. *J Pain Symptom Manage* 1995; 10: 599–603.

20   Starreveld JS, Pols MA, Van Wijk HJ et al. The plain abdominal radiograph in the assessment of constipation. *Z Gastroenterol* 1990; 28: 335–338.

21   Bruera E, Suarez-Almazor M, Velasco A et al. The assessment of constipation in terminal cancer patients admitted to a palliative care unit: A retrospective review. *J Pain Symptom Manage* 1994; 9: 515–519.

22   Anderson F, Downing GM, Hill J et al. Palliative performance scale (PPS): A new tool. *J Palliat Care* 1996; 12: 5–11.

23   Oneschuk D, Fainsinger R, Hanson J, Bruera E. Assessment and knowledge in palliative care in second year family medicine residents. *J Pain Symptom Manage* 1998; 14: 265–273.

24   Mazuryk M, Daeninck P, Neumann CM, Bruera E. Daily journal club: An education tool in palliative care. *Palliat Med* 2002; 16: 57–61.

25   Bruera E, Fainsinger R, MacEachern T, Hanson J. The use of methylphenidate in patients with incident cancer pain receiving regular opiates. A preliminary report. *Pain* 1992; 50: 75–77.

26   Bruera E, de Stoutz N, Velasco-Leiva et al. The effects of oxygen on the intensity of dyspnea in hypoxemic terminal cancer patients. *Lancet* 1993; 342: 13–14.

27   de Stoutz ND, Bruera E, Suarez-Almazor M. Opioid rotation (OR) for toxicity reduction in terminal cancer patients. *J Pain Symptom Manage* 1995; 10: 378–384.

28   Bruera E, Neumann C, Brenneis C, Quan H. Frequency of symptom distress and poor prognostic indicators in palliative cancer patients admitted to a tertiary palliative care unit, hospices, and acute care hospitals. *J Palliat Care* 2000; 16: 16–21.

29   *Regional Palliative Care Program Annual Report April 1, 2002–March 31, 2003 and April 1, 2003–March 31, 2004.* 2005. Available at: www.palliative.org, (accessed September 7, 2005).

30   von Gunten CF, Ferris FD, Portenoy R, Glachen M, eds. *CAPC Manual: Everything You Wanted to Know About Developing a Palliative Care Program but Were Afraid to Ask,* 2001. Available at www.capcmssm.org, (accessed September 7, 2005).

31   Faber-Langendoen K. Resuscitation of patients with metastatic cancer. Is transient benefit still futile? *Arch Intern Med* 1991; 151: 235–239.

32   Thorns AR, Ellershaw JE. A survey of nursing and medical staff views on the use of cardiopulmonary resuscitation in the hospice. *Palliat Med* 1999; 13: 225–232.

33   von Gunten CF. Discussing do-not-resuscitate status. *J Clin Oncol* 2001; 19: 1576–1581.

34   Maccabee J. The effect of transfer from a palliative care unit to nursing homes—Are patients' and relatives' needs met? *Palliat Med* 1994; 8: 211–214.

35   Ross C, Cornbleet M. Attitudes of patients and staff to research in a specialist palliative care unit. *Palliat Med* 2003; 17: 491–497.

36   Rees E, Hardy J, Ling J et al. The use of the Edmonton symptom assessment scale (ESAS) within a palliative care unit in the UK. *Palliat Med* 1998; 12: 75–82.

37   Lo RSK, Ding A, Chung TK, Woo J. Prospective study of symptom control in 133 cases of palliative care inpatients in Shatin Hospital. *Palliat Med* 1999; 13: 335–340.

38   Mancini I, Lossignol D, Obiols M et al. Supportive and palliative care: Experience at the Institute Jules Bordet. *Support Care Cancer* 2002; 10: 3–7.

39   Elsayem A, Swint K, Fisch M et al. Palliative care inpatient service in a comprehensive cancer center: Clinical and financial outcomes. *J Clin Oncol* 2004; 22: 2008–2014.

40   Cohen SR, Boston P, Mount BM, Porterfield P. Changes in quality of life following admission to palliative care units. *Palliat Med* 2001; 15: 363–371.

41   Davis MP, Walsh D, Nelson KA et al. The business of palliative medicine—Part 2: The economics of acute inpatient palliative medicine. *Am J Hospice Palliat Care* 2002; 19: 89–95.

42   Smith TJ, Coyne P, Cassel B et al. A high-volume specialist palliative care unit and team may reduce in-hospital end-of-life care costs. *J Palliat Med* 2003; 6: 699–705.

PART 7

Overview of assessment

38

Multidimensional patient assessment

MARVIN OMAR DELGADO-GUAY, EDUARDO BRUERA

INTRODUCTION

Supportive and palliative care aims to decrease symptom burden and alleviate psychosocial distress in patients and families. There has been significant growth of supportive and palliative care services and increasing international awareness of the role of supportive and palliative care for patients with advanced illness and their caregivers.[1–3]

Studies have showed that supportive and palliative care is associated with improved symptom control, mood, and better quality of life (QOL), in the context of an appropriate health resource use, increased patient and caregiver satisfaction, health-care savings, and possibly even better survival.[4–10]

A patient's experience of advanced illness is complex: from suffering physical symptoms to coping, financial concerns, caregiver burden, social and family changes, and spiritual concerns (Figure 38.1). Suffering is a state of distress that occurs when the intactness or integrity of the person is threatened or disrupted. Much of this suffering is often left unaddressed when health care is focused on the disease rather than the person with the disease.[11]

These issues should be managed through an interdisciplinary approach, with the focus of care being the patient and the family rather than the disease. Physicians must work together with many other professionals, such as nurses, psychologists, chaplains, occupational therapists, physical therapists, nutritionists, social workers, pharmacists, and volunteers, to provide care and support.[12] This enables a multidimensional evaluation that includes assessment of the patient's clinical and psychosocial characteristics, identification of specific prognostic factors related to symptoms, and the patient's self-reported symptom burden (Figure 38.2).

This chapter aims to bring together and summarize the different components of multidimensional bedside clinical assessment in supportive and palliative care and its importance for symptom control, QOL, and decision making. The type of assessment tool and the intensity of assessment will vary according to the patient population (e.g., cancer patients, geriatric patients), the setting (palliative care unit, outpatients, home, etc.), and a variety of issues related to the team composition, culture, etc. The reader is referred to specific chapters in this book for a more comprehensive assessment and the use of specific tools for each particular symptom.

DISTRESSING SYMPTOMS

Symptoms are inherently subjective. They are perceptions, usually expressed by language.[13] Patient self-report is the primary source of information of symptom presence and severity.

The physical and psychological symptoms experienced by patients with advanced-stage cancer are not uncommon, yet these issues are frequently addressed improperly in the conventional care setting.[13–15] Communication between clinicians and caregivers and pain management continue to be less than adequate during the process of dying. One group reported that only 54% of 357 ovarian cancer patients with pain received high-intensity analgesic medication near their time of death,[16] suggesting that there is room for improvement in the care of ovarian cancer patients at the end of life.

Improving communication with caregivers will allow clinicians to inform, educate, and identify areas of distress that they might encounter during the care of their patient.[17,18] This approach empowers patients and their families to exercise their decision-making options and self-control while balancing the benefits and risks of treatments, with the goal of improved QOL near its end.

For clinicians, the interaction with patients facing life-threatening illness can be a rewarding experience, although it remains one of the most challenging aspects of their work. Formal training about communication remains low during residency or fellowship and even specialist received few proper training about communication with these patients with different cultural and ethnic background.[19–21] The benefit of good communication on patient care and outcomes is unequivocal, whereas deficiencies in communication are associated with medical errors and a negative patient experience.[22]

It is always important to prepare oneself for the encounter, try to create a supportive environment, use appropriate nonverbal behaviors, and express empathy.[23]

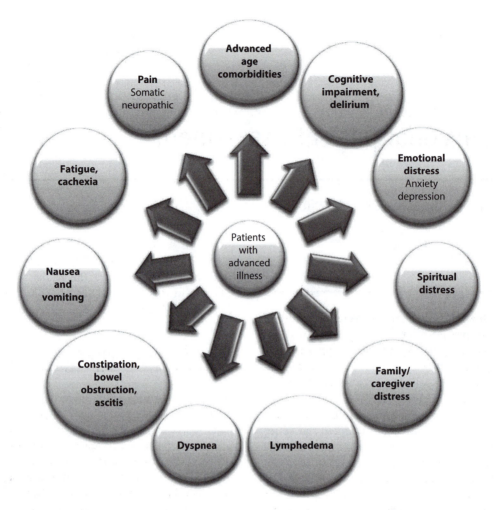

Figure 38.1 *Multiple distressing symptoms, factors, and complications that affect the QOL in patients with advanced illness.*

Communication is frequently difficult in advanced and terminally ill patients because of delirium or severe sedation due to drugs, metabolic abnormalities, infections, brain metastases, etc.[24] Proxies may be considered as an alternative or complementary source of information, especially during end-of-life care.[25] However, numerous studies have demonstrated that observer and patient assessments are not highly correlated and that the accuracy of a clinician's assessment cannot be assumed.[26–28]

Health-care providers often underestimate the severity of pain and other symptoms.[25,29] In studies of patients with terminal cancer assessed by health-care workers as compared with the patients, agreement was higher for physical than psychological and cognitive symptoms, there was a greater agreement on absence rather than on the presence of a symptom,[24] and the variation in symptom scores was minimal when at least two individuals contributed in the assessment.[30]

Data about concordance of patient proxies' reports suggest that a patient's and their family members' reports of patient pain and performance status were highly correlated, although family members consistently reported more pain and disability.[27] Another study that assessed patients and their spouse caregivers suggests that caregivers agree with patients on objective measures

with observable referents (e.g., ability to dress independently) but disagree with subjective aspects of patients' functioning (e.g., depression, fear of future, and confidence in treatment).[28]

FREQUENCY OF SYMPTOMS

Patients with advanced illnesses have an extraordinarily high frequency of physical and psychological complaints that impact on QOL. Symptoms may vary with age, sex, primary tumor, and extent of disease.[31] In different studies[32–33] conducted in cancer patients referred to a palliative medicine program both as inpatients or outpatients, the median number of symptoms per patient was 11 (range 1–27). The 10 most prevalent symptoms were pain, lack of energy, dry mouth, dyspnea, feeling drowsy, anorexia, insomnia, feeling sad, constipation, and greater than 10% weight loss. The frequency of these 10 symptoms ranged from 50% to 84%. The most common symptoms were also the most severe. Gastrointestinal symptoms were also common in nongastrointestinal primary site cancers. Specific symptoms were influenced by age, sex, or performance status. For example, males had more dysphagia, hoarseness, 10% weight loss, and sleep problems;

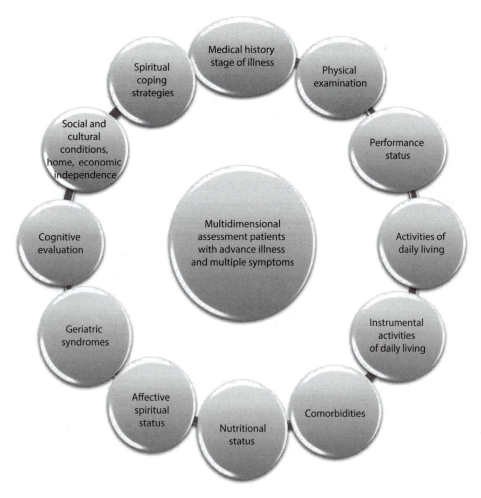

Figure 38.2 *Multidimensional approach to evaluate patients with advanced illness and with multiple distressful symptoms.*

females had more early satiety, nausea, vomiting, and anxiety. In a sample of 504 outpatients with acquired immunodeficiency syndrome (AIDS), multiple symptoms (mean of 16) with higher symptom distress was observed. The most prevalent symptoms were worrying, fatigue, sadness, and pain. Patients with intravenous drug use as an HIV transmission factor reported more symptoms and higher overall and physical symptom distress.[34]

MULTIDIMENSIONAL ASSESSMENT

It is always important to perform a comprehensive and multidimensional assessment in all patients with advanced illness with multiple symptoms.[35–37] Production of a symptom is the process by which nociception occurs. There are three steps in the experience of symptoms: production, perception, and expression. In the case of cancer pain, for example, J-receptor stimulation in the lung results in the production of dyspnea or the afferent stimulus from the gastrointestinal tract or central nervous system results in the production of nausea. Production can be significantly different in one individual to another and in different areas within the same individual (e.g., some patients have multiple bone metastases of which only one hurts). Perception

is the process by which the symptom reaches the brain cortex. This can also differ significantly from one individual to another (in the case of pain, endorphins or descending inhibitory pathways can significantly confound the intensity of the pain perceived). Unfortunately, these two stages cannot be measured. Finally, the expression of the distress is the only measurable part of the experience and is a target of therapy. However, this stage can also vary from one individual to another due to beliefs about the symptom experience, intrapsychic factors such as depression or somatization, and even cultural factors.[35,38–40]

In summary, although it is important to measure the intensity of a certain symptom such as pain, fatigue, or nausea, it is important to recognize that this intensity of expression does not have the same unidimensional value of, for example, blood glucose in of the control of diabetes or blood pressure in the control of arterial hypertension. Interpreting the intensity of pain expression as being only the expression of nociception would deny that in addition to variability in nociception, there is a great variability in both perception and expression. Rather, symptom expression should be interpreted as a multidimensional construct. In a given patient, a score of 8 out of 10 in pain intensity could be the result of nociception plus a certain level of somatization, coping chemically, and mild delirium. The multidimensional assessment should help in the recognition of the contribution of

Table 38.1　*Multidimensional assessment of patients with advanced illness in the supportive and palliative care setting*

Multidimensional assessment of patients with advanced illness	
Dimension assessment	
a. History	Stage of the cancer/illness
	Recent chemotherapy and/or radiotherapy or other therapy
	Self-rated symptoms scales
	Characteristics, intensity, location, aggravating factors of distressful symptoms
b. Performance status	Karnofsky performance scale or Eastern Cooperative Oncology Group scale scores
c. Activities of daily living (ADL) and instrumental activities of daily living (IADL)	Assessment of *ADL* (bathing, dressing and undressing, eating, transferring from bed to chair and back, voluntarily control urinary and fecal discharge, using the toilet, and walking)
	Assessment of *IADL* (light housework, preparing meals, taking medications, shopping for groceries or clothes, using the telephone, and managing money)
d. Assessment of distressful symptoms (pain, fatigue, anorexia, nausea, dyspnea, insomnia, drowsiness, constipation)	Edmonton symptom assessment system (ESAS)
	Abdominal x-ray to assess constipation vs. bowel obstruction (consider abdominal CT scan)
e. Assessment of psychosocial symptoms: anxiety/depression	Anxiety/depression (ESAS)
	Identification of mood disorder during interview
f. Family/caregiver's distress	Assessment for family/caregiver distress during the interview
	Sociocultural and financial issues evaluation
g. Assessment of delirium	Memorial delirium assessment scale (MDAS)
	mini–mental state examination (MMSE)
	Confusion assessment method (CAM)
h. Assessment of spiritual distress/spiritual pain	Spiritual assessment: SPIRITual History, FICA
	Self-rated spiritual pain (pain deep in the soul/being that is not physical)
	Identification of spiritual distress during interview
i. Assessment for chemical coping	CAGE questionnaire
j. Evaluation of medications and possible interactions (polypharmacy)	
k. Physical examination	

the different dimensions to the patient's symptom expression and thereby assist in the planning of care. A purely unidimensional interpretation of intensity of pain would result in assuming that 100% success can be achieved with the simple use of higher and higher doses of analgesics. This simplistic approach could result in massive doses of opioids, opioid-related toxicity, and excessive reliance on pharmacologic, as compared with nonpharmacologic, approaches to symptom control. A number of tools (Table 38.1) can be used to assess the contribution of different dimensions of the patient's symptom expression.[35,38–40]

DISEASE STATUS

Good symptom assessment precedes effective symptom treatment. Symptom assessment is very important because symptoms directly affect patient distress, QOL, and survival.[13] Symptoms can be related to disease, treatment, concurrent comorbid illnesses, or a combination of all three.[13,41] The early stages of cancer are associated with considerable symptomatology, and the symptom burden (symptoms and their interference with life) increases with cancer stage, possibly reflecting tumor burden.[41–43] One important point to consider is that symptom burden decreases patient QOL.[13,44] QOL is a multidimensional construct with specific emotional, physical, and social aspects.[45–47] The presence of symptoms affects, but does not necessarily determine, QOL.[13]

An initial step in the multidimensional assessment of the patient seen by the supportive and palliative care team involves a complete medical history that reviews the disease diagnosis (cancer, AIDS, end-stage chronic obstructive pulmonary disease, congestive heart failure, or renal disease, etc.), the chronology of disease-related events, previous and current therapies, and all relevant medical, surgical, and psychiatric problems. A detailed history includes current and prior use of prescription and nonprescription drugs, "alternative" medical therapies, drug allergies, and previous adverse reactions. The patient should be questioned about prior treatment modalities for each symptom and their perceived efficacy. Symptom assessment must include a thorough physical examination and review of the available laboratory and imaging data. Specific imaging, laboratory tests, or specialist referral may be appropriate to understand the pathophysiology of symptoms and their relationship to the disease.[13,42]

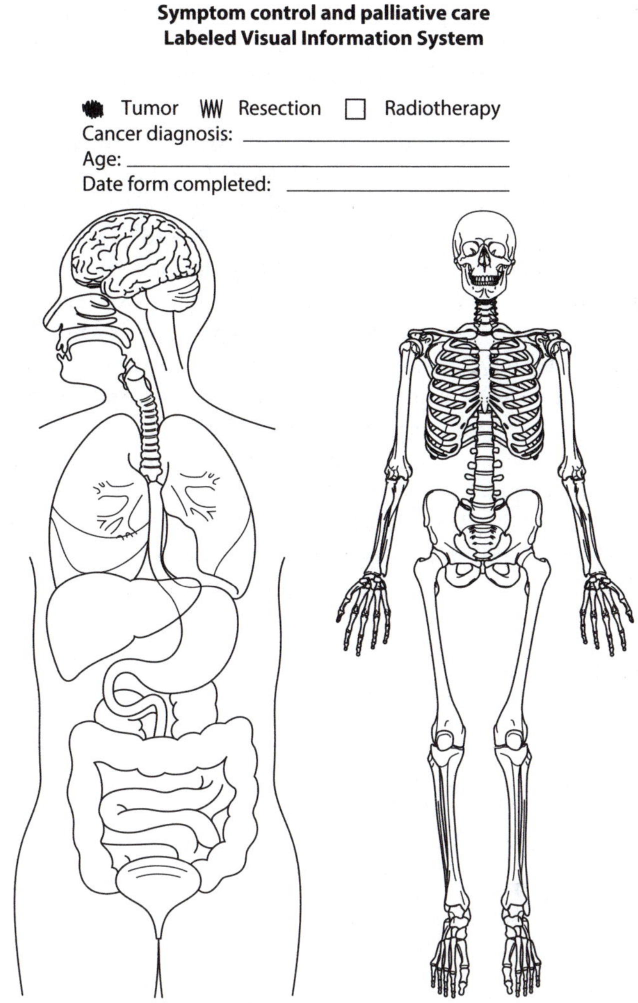

**Symptom control and palliative care
Labeled Visual Information System**

◆ Tumor 〜 Resection ☐ Radiotherapy

Cancer diagnosis: _____

Age: _____

Date form completed: _____

Figure 38.3 *ELVIS.*

The Edmonton Labeled Visual Information System (ELVIS)[48] is a pictorial representation that has been developed and tested to improve the physician's ability to comprehend and remember the basic details of the patient's disease status and prior treatments (Figure 38.3). This instrument is a simple one-page line diagram that is used to graphically document the extent of disease in advanced cancer. It consists of two figures, of which one is used to document visceral and soft-tissue disease and the second, portraying the skeleton, is used to document bony disease. The diagrams are simple and require the user to draw in, as necessary, sex-specific organs such as breasts, ovaries, the uterus, or testes, as well as other structures that have not been included. White space is provided to add labels to the visual representations and to document type and date of different treatments.

Supportive and palliative care specialists need to be knowledgeable about the natural history and treatment of patients referred to their care. This allows for the appropriate recognition of patients referred to the supportive and palliative care team who might significantly benefit from disease-modifying therapy, or occasionally even curative therapy. For example, a patient with advanced testicular cancer or Hodgkin disease may be severely

symptomatic and appropriate for a palliative care referral. However, this patient should also immediately be referred to an oncologist because there is potentially curative therapy available. Similarly, a patient with opportunistic symptomatic infections related to AIDS with no history of previous triple antiviral therapy should be treated by the palliative care team in coordination with an AIDS specialist.

ASSESSMENT TOOLS

In the process of instrument selection, the physician must carefully consider the goals of assessment and the practicality and acceptability of the assessment instrument by the patient with advanced illness. Assessment tools allow for the identification of many more symptoms than do simple unstructured evaluations.[49,50]

Simple assessment tools are the most appropriate for patients with advanced illnesses. These patients may be weak and experiencing symptoms that make it difficult to complete a time-consuming and complex assessment tool.

Assessment tools are useful not only to diagnose and evaluate the intensity of the symptoms but also to monitor the effectiveness of therapy and to screen for side effects of medications. They play a role in the early identification of poor prognostic factors that can hamper the management of the symptoms of advanced illness. Assessment tools should be used regularly, especially when patients experience new symptoms, an increase in the intensity of preexisting symptoms, or when therapy changes. The results should be documented in the patient's chart to ensure accuracy in the monitoring of the symptoms.

Efficient symptom-assessment instruments include the Edmonton symptom assessment system (ESAS), the memorial symptom assessment scale (MSAS), the Rotterdam symptom checklist[51] (RSCL), and the symptom distress scale (SDS).

The ESAS[52-56] is used to assess 10 common symptoms (pain, fatigue, nausea, depression, anxiety, drowsiness, shortness of breath, appetite, sleep problems, and feeling of well-being) experienced by patients with cancer or chronic illness over the past 24 hours. In this scale, the patient rates the intensity of symptoms on a 0 to 10 numerical scale, with 0 representing "no symptom" and 10 representing the "worst possible symptom." It was developed in 1991 to evaluate the intensity of the most frequent physical and psychological symptoms in cancer patients receiving palliative care and was rapidly adopted by many cancer and supportive and palliative care programs (Figure 38.4a).[57] It is widely used in supportive and palliative care research. Its ease of use and visual representation make it an effective and practical bedside tool[56,57] that allows the health-care provider to track symptoms over time with regard to intensity, duration, and responsiveness to therapy.

There have been independent validations of this tool in palliative care and cancer patients by a number of different authors and in a variety of different languages: for example, in English, [49,58-62] Italian,[63] French,[64] German,[65] Spanish,[66]

Korean,[67] and Thai.[68] Two recent reviews on ESAS studies have found limited psychometric evidence that supports the need for further validation studies.[69,70]

Based on concerns raised in the literature,[61,70–72] and the findings of the think-aloud study, a revised version of the ESAS, the ESAS-r, was created. The ESAS-r retains the core elements of the ESAS (nine common symptoms, option of adding a 10th symptom, 11-point numerical rating scales), with key revisions focusing on the following: (1) Symptom assessment time frame, specified as "now." (2) Terminology: brief definitions have been added to some symptoms, and "appetite" has been changed to "lack of appetite" to express the concept as a symptom. (3) Item order: related symptoms (e.g., tiredness and drowsiness, nausea and appetite, depression and anxiety) are grouped together, and "well-being" is now the ninth symptom at the end of the instrument. (4) Format: horizontal lines over the numbers have been removed (Figure 38.4b).[73]

The ESAS has been validated against a widely used scale, the hospital anxiety and depression scale (HADS), for assessing the presence of depression and anxiety in advanced cancer patients.[74] The ideal cutoff point of ESAS of 2 out of 10 is sensitive for the presence of depression and anxiety in patients in the palliative care setting.

The MSAS, a lengthier assessment tool, is mostly used for research purposes. With the MSAS, patients rate the frequency, severity, and distress associated with 32 physical and psychological symptoms.[75] There is a short-form MSAS[76] (MSAS-SF) that captures the patient-rated distress associated with 26 physical symptoms and the frequency of 4 psychological symptoms. Another tool that can be completed in 2–4 min and contains both QOL and survival information is the condensed MSAS (CMSAS),[77] which provides equivalent information that approximates to the original 32 items. The symptoms identified by Chang et al.[77] are also included in other widely used clinical symptom-assessment instruments, such as the ESAS, RSCL, and SDS. This report is also one of the first to demonstrate that scales from a shorter instrument can be predictive of survival and that there is a core of symptoms that provide

Figure 38.4 ESAS (a).

(Continued)

Edmonton Symptom Assessment System: (revised version) (ESAS-R)

Please circle the number that best describes how you feel NOW:

No Pain	0 1 2 3 4 5 6 7 8 9 10	Worst Possible Pain
NoTiredness (*Tiredness = Lack of energy*)	0 1 2 3 4 5 6 7 8 9 10	Worst Possible Tiredness
No drowsiness (*Drowsiness = Feeling sleepy*)	0 1 2 3 4 5 6 7 8 9 10	Worst Possible Drowsiness
No Nausea	0 1 2 3 4 5 6 7 8 9 10	Worst Possible Nausea
No Lack of Appetite	0 1 2 3 4 5 6 7 8 9 10	Worst Possible Lack of Appetite
No Shortness of Breath	0 1 2 3 4 5 6 7 8 9 10	Worst Possible Shortness of Breath
No Depression (*Depression = Feeling sad*)	0 1 2 3 4 5 6 7 8 9 10	Worst Possible Depression
No Anxiety (*Anxiety = Feeling nervous*)	0 1 2 3 4 5 6 7 8 9 10	Worst Possible Anxiety
Best Wellbeing (*Wellbeing = how you feel overall*)	0 1 2 3 4 5 6 7 8 9 10	Worst Possible Wellbeing
No _____ Other Problem (for example constipation)	0 1 2 3 4 5 6 7 8 9 10	Worst Possible _____

Patient's Name _____

Date _____   Time _____

Completed by (check one):
☐ Patient
☐ Family caregiver
☐ Health care professional caregiver
☐ Caregiver-assisted

(b)   BODY DIAGRAM ON REVERSE SIDE

Figure 38.4 (*Continued*) *ESAS-r (b).*

most of the information about health, QOL, and survival. The SDS is a patient-rated instrument that assesses the intensity, frequency, and distress level associated with nine physical and two psychological symptoms.[78,79] It is important to recognize that the research instruments may differ from those used for clinical practice.[77]

ASSESSMENT OF DELIRIUM AND COGNITIVE IMPAIRMENT

The presence of cognitive impairment, whether as a result of delirium or dementia, presents a major impediment in the assessment of symptoms in patients with advanced disease.[80] Delirium is an important source of distress to patients, family members, and caregivers. Patient assessment becomes difficult, communication of patients with caregivers and

family members is impaired, the patient's expression of their symptoms is usually increased, and they are usually unable to participate in their own care.[81] The frequency of delirium in patients with advanced cancer varies from 28% to 40% on admission.[82,83] Eventually, up to 83% of patients develop delirium in their final days, and 10%–30% of them may require palliative terminal sedation.[84,85] In some studies, delirium was not detected in 22%–50% of the cases.[86]

The diagnosis of delirium is made on the basis of acute onset, fluctuation in course, reduced sensorium, attention deficit, and cognitive and perceptual disturbance, which occurs in the presence of an underlying organic derangement.[81,87]

Historically, the mini–mental state examination (MMSE)[88] was used in multiple studies on cognitive failure in cancer patients with delirium.[89,90] However, it only assesses cognitive function, and because of its high rates of false negatives and false positives, individual scores should be interpreted with caution and followed by more detailed assessments.[91] For example, two delirious patients with an MMSE score of 14 of 30 can range from being completely lethargic to completely agitated and unmanageable.

Different tools have been developed and validated for screening or monitoring the course of delirium, such as the memorial delirium assessment scale[92,93] (MDAS), the delirium rating scale,[94,95] and the confusion assessment method[96,97] (CAM). The MDAS is a 10-item, 4-point, clinician-rated instrument (possible range, 0–30). It was originally designed to measure severity but can be used as a diagnostic tool. It has been validated in inpatient palliative care settings with a sensitivity of 97% and a specificity of 95% at a cutoff score of 7.

Based on the level of psychomotor activity, there are three subtypes of delirium: hyperactive, hypoactive, and mixed, which is the most frequent form of presentation.[98,99] Misdiagnoses of hypoactive delirium as depression or agitated delirium as anxiety disorder is not unusual. The emotional lability, disinhibition, and psychomotor agitation components of delirium are frequently interpreted as worsening pain by relatives, and sometimes by medical and nursing staff,[100] especially in the absence of any objective cognitive testing. Fainsinger et al.[101] described a "destructive triangle" created as a result of the family's misinterpretation of the patient's delirium as pain and their consequent desire for nursing and the physician's efforts to "do something." The doctor may be placed under pressure to relieve the patient and family's distress. This emotional overload may lead to an increase in the opioid dose and aggravate the agitation, in particular when the opioid is already implicated as a precipitant.[102]

Delirium can result in misinterpretation of symptoms and emotion expression and conflict between the patient's family and health-care professionals or even among different health-care professionals with regard to the patient's behavior. Once the diagnosis of delirium has been confirmed by a thorough medical assessment, it is important to appropriately inform the different disciplines in the team about the presence of this syndrome because a number of pharmacologic, rehabilitation, and counseling interventions may be inappropriate in patients with severe cognitive failure or delirium. Education for the family will also be important to help them understand the inhibited expression of physical or emotional distress in a cognitively impaired or delirious patient.

A multidimensional assessment in this setting will lead to cognitive testing and the recognition of delirium. This assessment may result in more appropriate interventions, such as opioid rotation or dose reduction and prescription of a neuroleptic for the symptomatic treatment of delirium.[103]

ASSESSMENT OF PHYSICAL FUNCTION

The majority of patients with advanced and terminal illness have impaired ability to perform everyday functions during the various stages of the disease. Functional status is an independent predictor of survival.[104] It is also essential for planning the setting of care, which can be the home, hospice, or acute service.

The Karnofsky performance scale[105] (KPS) and the Eastern Cooperative Oncology Group[106] (ECOG) have been used widely in the assessment of physical function in cancer patients. The KPS is considered a "gold standard" for assessment of functional status in cancer patients.[107,108] However, in patients with advanced cancer in palliative care setting assessments, these instruments tend to generate clustering of scores at the extreme end of impairment. Consequently, newer instruments such as the Edmonton Functional Assessment Tool[109] (EFAT) and the palliative performance scale[110] (PPS) have been developed. The EFAT includes domains such as pain, mental alertness, sensory function, communication, and respiratory function, in addition to domains that more directly reflect physical function, such as balance, mobility, wheelchair mobility, activity, activities of daily living, and dependence performance status. This information can give physicians prognostic information about the patient. For example, a bedridden patient with severe pain due to a pathological hip fracture has a much better potential for recovery than a patient bedridden due to cachexia and delirium. A revised version of the EFAT has recently been validated.[111] The PPS is essentially a modification of the KPS and assesses ambulation, activity, self-care, intake, and conscious level.[112]

An objective assessment of physical functioning constitutes part of the multidimensional symptom assessment in palliative care. Impairment in physical functioning and distressing physical symptoms such as pain have the potential to adversely affect psychosocial function.[113,114] Physical and occupational therapy assessments may reveal deficits and suggest interventions that can be essential to maintaining functional capacity, ensuring patient safety, conserving energy, and decreasing fatigue. A speech therapy assessment can provide valuable information regarding swallowing function, while a nutritional assessment by a dietician can aid in determining caloric intake.

The assessment of physical function in supportive care and palliative care will allow for the identification of simple measures such as special wheelchairs, ramps if there are steps in the home, bathroom supplies, a trapeze for bed mobility, or the need for a formal rehabilitation approach. On the other hand, in some cases, decreased function may be associated with conditions such as severe incidental pain, delirium, dyspnea with minimal efforts, or irreversible neurological damage and in these cases appropriate adaptation to the loss in function, and patient and family education will be the most appropriate course of action. Therefore, the assessment of physical function needs to be integrated with an understanding of the underlying disease status, symptom control, and psychosocial distress.

ASSESSMENT OF PSYCHOLOGICAL DISTRESS

The perception of different symptoms, such as pain or fatigue, may be accentuated by the emotional or psychological distress of the patient. Psychological distress impairs the patient's capacity for pleasure, meaning, and connection; erodes QOL; amplifies pain and other symptoms;[115] reduces the patient's ability to do the emotional work of separating and saying good-bye; and causes anguish and worry among family members and friends. Finally, psychological distress, particularly depression, is a major risk for suicide and for requests to hasten death.[116] On the other hand, severe undertreated physical distress leads to severe psychological distress. Untreated or undertreated pain, nausea, dyspnea, or other uncomfortable physical symptoms can profoundly disturb mood and sleep and make it impossible for patients to relate appropriately to their family and their health-care professionals.

A psychological assessment should be done to evaluate mainly mood and coping. It is important for a team's members to become familiar with each of these areas and to recognize when there are issues that need further assessment and/or intervention by another health-care discipline. Medical staff often fails to recognize and address psychological distress, and this impacts negatively on QOL.[115,116]

Patients with advanced and terminal diseases have a variety of ways of coping with their diagnosis, including fear, anger, avoidance, denial, intellectualization, intense grieving, and existential questioning. The distinction is often difficult to make between the normal psychological burden that exists in relation to physical and psychological distress and certain aspects of psychopathology such as somatization, anxiety, adjustment disorder, and depression.[117] In addition, physical symptoms of depression (such as fatigue, anorexia, sleep disturbance) may be attributable to the disease itself.

Numerous factors act as barriers to recognition and treatment of psychological symptoms. Both patients and clinicians believe that psychological distress is a normal feature of the dying process and fail to differentiate natural, existential distress from clinical depression. Physicians lack clinical knowledge and skills to identify depression, anxiety, and delirium, especially in terminally ill patients where the diagnostic clues are confounded by coexisting medical illness and appropriate sadness. Patients and clinicians often avoid exploration of psychological issues because of time constraints and concerns that such exploration will cause further distress. Physicians are reluctant to prescribe psychotropic agents, which can have additional adverse effects, and therefore may hesitate to diagnose a condition that they feel they cannot treat successfully. Finally, when caring for dying patients, physicians may feel a sense of hopelessness that can lead to therapeutic nihilism.[114,118]

MOOD DISORDERS

Mood disorders are among the most prevalent and important of the psychiatric illnesses.[119,120] Depression coexists with a number of physical symptoms in patients with advanced cancer. Its frequency varies widely, but it is considered to be present in approximately 25% of these patients. [120–125] In a recent meta-analysis, it was reported that the prevalence of adjustment disorder alone was 15.4% and of anxiety disorders 9.8%, while the prevalence of all types of depression combined was of 24.6%, depression or adjustment disorder 24.7%, and all types of mood disorder 29.0%.[126] Also, it was reported that

the prevalence of depression diagnosed by the Diagnostic and Statistical Manual of Mental Disorders (DSM) or International Classification of Diseases (ICD) criteria was 16.3%; for DSM-defined major depression, it was 14.9%; and for DSM-defined minor depression, it was 19.2%. The prevalence of adjustment disorder was 19.4%, anxiety 10.3%, and dysthymia 2.7%. Combination diagnoses were common; all types of depression occurred in 20.7% of patients, depression or adjustment disorder in 31.6%, and any mood disorder in 38.2%.[126]

Mood disorders in medically ill patients are underdiagnosed and are therefore undertreated. [123–127] To improve the accuracy of screening for depression, several self-reporting tools have been created that are easy to administer without extensive training.[128] Lloyd-Williams et al.[128] showed the association between depression and physical symptoms in patients with advanced cancer using a seven-item verbal rating scale.

The clinical interview is the gold standard for diagnosis of depression.[129,130] Chochinov et al.[131] found that the single question "Are you depressed?" provides a sensitive and specific assessment of depression in terminally ill patients. Another useful question is: "Have you often been bothered by having little interest or pleasure in doing things?" The first question targets mood, while the latter is an indicator of anhedonia.[132] A patient who responds affirmatively to any of these questions is likely to receive a diagnosis after a comprehensive interview.[133,134]

HADS[135,136] is a brief, self-administered, widely used screening tool to measure psychological distress in patients. It is sensitive to change, both during the course of disease and in response to medical and psychological interventions. HADS consists of 14 items on two subscales (7 for anxiety and 7 for depression). Ratings are made on 4-point scales representing the degree of distress during the previous week. The two scales are then scored separately. A score of 7 or less indicates noncases, 8–10 doubtful cases, and 11+ definite cases for anxiety and/or depression (with ranges of 0–21 for each subscale). Also, a one-third cutoff of the range (a score of 14–15) has been proposed as the indicator for severe disorder. In different studies,[135,136] HADS showed good reliability and validity in assessing symptom severity, anxiety disorders, and depression in somatic, psychiatric, and primary care patients and even in the general population.

Patients who are at increased risk for developing psychiatric complications are those with low performance status, those receiving certain cancer treatments, and those with uncontrolled physical symptoms, functional limitations, lack of social support, and past history of psychiatric disorder and substance abuse or family history of depression or suicide.[137,138] Clinicians always should remain vigilant for mood complications, not just depression.

SOMATIZATION

Somatization is broadly defined as the somatic manifestation of psychological distress. This should be distinguished from the "somatization disorder" in the somatoform disorders section of DSM-IV.[139] Somatoform disorders are rare in cancer patients and have a restrictive set of criteria.[140,141] Somatization is closely related to depression, anxiety, personality disorders, and cognitive impairment.[142,144] Patients who somatize will have a tendency to express pain intensity as higher, will have poorly defined etiology after appropriate investigations, will describe pain "all over the body," and derive little benefit (but often toxicity) from pharmacological treatment.[145] In addition to a history of affective disorder, a history of functional somatic syndromes[146] (e.g., chronic pelvic pain, irritable bowel syndrome, fibromyalgia, tension headache, chronic fatigue syndrome) and the simultaneous presence of multiple highly intense symptoms (high ESAS scores in multiple domains) are all signs suggestive of somatization. Because of the absence of a gold standard, the diagnosis of somatization is made based on a number of repeated observations and after extensive discussion with the patient and family.[147]

Patients who somatize frequently express increased symptom intensity associated with stressors, and many patients are unaware of this coping mechanism. It is important to recognize that in most palliative care patients, somatization consists of the increased expression of a symptom for which there is a clear pathophysiological mechanism, rather than the expression of symptoms for which there is no demonstrable pathophysiology, as is the case for somatoform disorders.

CHEMICAL COPING

Patients who have a past or active history of substance abuse present a special problem for symptom management. Their history of abuse reflects maladaptive coping strategies, which frequently lead to excessive expression of symptomatology. Several studies suggest that patients who cope chemically tend to express a higher degree of symptoms.[148–150] In patients with pain, this is often misinterpreted as nociception and may lead to an escalation of opioids and opioid-induced neurotoxicity.[151]

Patients who have a history of alcohol or drug use are susceptible to addiction when prescribed with opioid analgesics,[152] whereas in patients without such a history, the use of opioids to control cancer pain very rarely results in abuse or addiction. The frequency of addictive disorders in the United States ranges from 3% to 16% with the higher rates reflecting prevalence of alcoholism.[153,154] In cancer patients, frequency of alcoholism rises in up to 28% of patients.[155,156]

Alcoholism is strongly linked with other addictive substances, including tobacco and illicit drugs,[157] and the aberrant use of these substances to help cope with life stressors is defined as chemical coping.[158] A history of chemical coping is an independent poor prognostic factor for pain control using opioid analgesia.[159]

The CAGE[160] alcohol questionnaire is frequently used as a brief screening tool for detection of alcohol abuse. A positive screen for alcohol abuse and dependence is made with two positive answers of the four questions with an average sensitivity of 0.71 and specificity of 0.90.[161] A positive screen should be followed by a proper diagnostic evaluation using standard clinical criteria. The questions refer to lifetime experience and not to any specific or limited time frames in the patient's history. To improve the validity of the CAGE results, the questionnaire should be completed as part of the initial assessment, in particular before asking the patients about amounts of alcohol or drugs ingested.

The 14-item Screener and Opioid Assessment for Patients with Pain (SOAPP)[162] was created as a promising brief self-report measure to capture important information in order to identify which chronic pain patients may be at risk for problems with long-term opioid medication. Each of the items are rated from 0 = "never" to 4 = "very often." A cutoff score of 8 of 56 or higher indicates a high risk of opioid abuse. The SOAPP revealed five factors labeled (1) history of substance abuse, (2) legal problems, (3) craving medication, (4) heavy smoking, and (5) mood swings.[163]

It has been reported that tobacco use was associated with higher opioid use.[164] Also, patients who had a history of tobacco abuse had more severe symptoms of pain and dyspnea and were more likely to be prescribed strong opioids before palliative care consultation.[164]

Relative to the general population, individuals who smoke are four times more likely to be addicted to alcohol, and alcoholic patients are three times more likely to be dependent on nicotine.[165] In addition, patients with a history of opioid addiction reportedly had a threefold or greater increased frequency of tobacco use.[166] Despite alcohol and nicotine have different mechanisms of action, recent research suggests that both drugs may share the ability to modulate the endogenous opioid system.[167] A history of abuse of either alcohol or tobacco may indicate an individual's predisposition to chemical coping.

Cancer patients are living longer, and those with chronic pain may be treated with opioids for prolonged periods. In the past, assessment of risk factors for addiction may have been overlooked in patients with cancer, because it was believed they had a short life expectancy. Identifying patients who are at risk for chemical coping has important clinical implications, including the need for close monitoring of opioid use, consideration for early referral to pain specialists or palliative care physicians, and management by an interdisciplinary team to avoid inappropriate escalation, neurotoxicity, and side effects of strong opioids. Before prescribing pain medications, clinicians need to carefully screen for behaviors that place patients at risk for addiction or chemical coping, including past history of alcohol, prescription drug, or nonprescription drug abuse.[168]

SPIRITUAL ASSESSMENT

Spirituality is recognized as a factor that contributes to health in many people and is an important component in the care of patients with life-threatening illnesses, such as cancer and congestive heart failure.[169–172] Spiritual and religious beliefs can affect the way patients cope with their illnesses creating distress and worsening the burden of the illness.[169,173–177] Spirituality is a dimension of personhood and a part of our being and religion is a construct of human making, which enables the conceptualization and expression of spirituality.[178,179] A key goal of supportive and palliative care services is to alleviate patient suffering. Suffering is a biopsychosocial, multidimensional construct that includes physical, emotional, as well as spiritual pain. The spirituality and religiosity field is important to consider when we evaluate patients with advanced and terminal illness, because it can influence coping strategies and QOL. The presence of spiritual pain can be an important component of the patients with chronic or acute pain and other physical and psychological symptoms.[180] Spirituality can be defined as "the aspect of humanity that refers to the way individuals seek and express meaning and purpose and the way they experience their connectedness to the moment, to self, to others, to nature, and to the significant or sacred."[169] The spirituality is a dimension of personhood and a part of our being, while religion is a construct of human making, which enables the conceptualization and expression of spirituality;[179] this encompasses structured belief systems that address spiritual issues, often with a code of ethical behavior and philosophy.[181]

Spiritual needs should be met in an individualized reciprocal process. Patients like conversations that allow them to set the pace and agenda. Patients selected simple questions such as "What principles do you live by?" "Do you have a personal faith?" and "Have you ever prayed about your situation?" as useful ways to start discussions. Most importantly is that attention to religious/spiritual issues has been shown to have a significant influence on several important indicators of quality care. Several studies have documented the positive relationship between meeting spiritual needs and patient satisfaction.[182,183] Several other findings suggest that attention to spiritual needs improves QOL[4] and reduces use of aggressive care at the end of life.[184]

Spiritual assessment is a conversation in which the patient is encouraged to tell and explore their spiritual story. As in spiritual screening, there are several options in the literature for taking a spiritual history. It is to be patient centered and guided by the extent to which the patient chooses to disclose his or her spiritual needs. There are several tools available for taking a spiritual history, including the systems of belief inventory-15R,[185] brief measure of religious coping,[186] functional assessment of chronic illness therapy–spiritual well-being,[187,188] SPIRITual History,[189] HOPE,[190] and FICA (faith, importance, community, address in care) Spiritual History.[191] Some of these instruments are intended primarily for research, whereas the others have been used primarily in the clinical setting for nonchaplain clinicians.

The SPIRITual History tool,[189] with the acronym SPIRIT, six domains are explored: S for spiritual belief system, P for personal spirituality, I for integration with a spiritual community, R for ritualized practices and restrictions, I for implications for medical care, and T for terminal events planning. The six domains include 22 items that may be covered in as little as 10 or 15 minutes or integrated into general interviewing over several appointments.

The FICA tool developed at the George Washington Institute for Spirituality and Health (Table 38.2) has been tested and

Table 38.2 *FICA tool for spiritual assessment*

FICA Tool	
F—Faith, belief, meaning	QuestionsDo you consider yourself spiritual or religious?Do you have spiritual beliefs that help you cope with stress?What gives your life meaning?
I—Importance and influence	What importance does your faith or belief have in your life?On a scale of 0 (not important) to 5 (very important), how would you rate the importance of faith/belief in your life?Have your beliefs influenced you in how you handle stress?What role do your beliefs plan in your health-care decision making?
C—Community	Are you a part of a spiritual or religious community?Is this of support to you and how?Is there a group of people you really love or who are important to you?
A—Address in care	How would you like your health-care provider to use this information about your spirituality as they care for you?

validated.[191] It is recommended that it be incorporated into the social history section of the overall history and physical. In incorporating this area into a history, providers should be conscious of not imposing their own beliefs on the patient or trying to answer any questions or concerns that the patient may have in this area. Such questions and concerns should be referred to a professional chaplain. They also should be clear that this process does not oblige them to discuss their own beliefs and practices. The main goal of this process is to understand the role of spiritual and religious beliefs and practices in the patient's life and the role they play in coping with illness. As in the screening, a basic goal of the history is to diagnose spiritual distress, which should be referred to the professional chaplain.[192,193] Through active listening, a relationship between the patients and the professional chaplain is established. The chaplain then extracts themes and issues from the story to explore further with the patient. These themes might include meaning, making God as judge versus God as comforter, grief, despair, and forgiveness. This assessment should result in a spiritual care plan that is fully integrated into the patient's and family's total plan of care, which should be communicated to the rest of the treatment team.[193]

FAMILY/CAREGIVER ASSESSMENT

Chronic illness from advanced disease impacts on all the family members. The distress created with the knowledge of a limited life span and the patients' relationship with their world and with their families/caregivers change. The patient's role/roles within the family, as a provider, a caregiver, a parent, a spouse, or a sexual partner, may be challenged. Therefore, the particular issues and needs of family members, in addition to the patient, must also be assessed.[194] Although the family is traditionally defined by individuals of blood relationship, a broader definition of family/caregiver is most appropriate, best defined as those individuals considered as family by the patient.[195,196]

The family/caregiver assessment is particularly important for patients who will receive care at home. The willingness of the family to deliver care at home is the most important predictor of a home death.[197] Family members will be involved in all aspects of patient care at home including hygiene, repositioning, and administration of multiple medications. Knowledge of the family's structure and function will help clinicians organize medications and other aspects of care.

Furthermore, because care will be provided by family members in the home setting, the family should also be consulted and educated about the diagnosis, treatment options, the illness trajectory, symptom burden and treatment, and caregiving.[198]

A genogram or family tree facilitates the understanding of a particular family's structure and dynamics. It helps to identify the family structure in a clear and comprehensive way. It highlights relationships and strengths and weaknesses and can often clarify some of the family norms around disease/illness and coping. Family communication patterns, roles, and coping methods are components of family functioning affected by the cancer. For example, family members frequently do not share their thoughts or concerns with one another in an effort to protect each other. These "conspiracies of silence" may complicate coping, and they should be diagnosed and treated.[199]

Caring for a person with cancer is demanding and overwhelming and can be a stressful experience that may erode the physical and psychological health of the caregiver.[200] For example, caregivers who provide 24 hours day care often experience cumulative sleep disruption, and fatigue is common.[201] Also, caregivers of patients with cancer-related pain report even higher levels of depression, tension, and mood disturbances than caregivers of pain-free patients.[202,203] Therefore, to address and manage these issues, these patients should be managed together with psychologists and social workers, and this is important to reduce the psychological distress of caregivers. The patient–family unit is expected to make decisions about treatment options, goals of care, advance directives, and finances. The importance of advance care planning for the patient and family is stressed and this is best addressed early in the course of illness and frequently reassessed. Early discussions regarding prognosis, likely course of the disease and events to anticipate and clarifying advanced directives all can serve to mitigate subsequent dilemmas and increase control and lessen angst.

Ultimately, the level of family care available will be the main defining factor in discharging a patient back to the community or to an institution. Family meetings should be conducted in the majority of cases when a palliative care team discharges a patient home.

Involvement of family caregivers is essential for optimal treatment of cancer patients at the end of life, especially in ensuring treatment compliance, continuity of care, and social support.[204] For example, family members who fear drug addiction or respiratory depression may undermedicate a patient even though the patient is experiencing unrelieved pain.

Other more structured tools to evaluate family/caregiver distress involve the Zarit Burden Interview[205] and the brief symptom inventory (BSI).[206]

In the Zarit Burden Interview,[205] "caregiver burden" is an all-encompassing term to describe the physical, emotional, and financial toll of providing care. It is the most widely referenced scale in studies of caregiver burden and has been demonstrated to have high internal consistency (Cronbach's α = 0.94).

The BSI and its short form[206] provide an overview of a caregiver's symptoms and their intensity at a specific point in time. The BSI is an 18-item self-reported symptom inventory designed to reflect the psychological symptom patterns of psychiatric and medical patients and nonpatients. This inventory reports profiles of nine primary symptom dimensions and three global indices of distress. Each item is rated on a 5-point scale of distress ranging from 0 ("not at all") to 4 ("extremely"). The depression and anxiety subscales of the BSI are well established. The approximate completion time for these items is 5 min. The internal consistency estimates of these two subscales are 0.85 (depression) and 0.81 (anxiety). Estimates of the construct validity of these subscales also are satisfactory.

SOCIAL, FINANCIAL, AND CULTURAL ASSESSMENT

A number of socioeconomic factors have great influence on the expression of symptoms, psychosocial distress, family dynamics, and even overall access to health-care professionals and medications. Socioeconomic status is one of the main predictors of home death,[207] and it is particularly important in countries where there is no universal access to health care such as the United States. However, socioeconomic status can also be an independent predictor of home death in other countries. The appropriate assessment of social and cultural needs will provide for better counseling, better planning of the site of care, enhanced communication, and even better adherence to pharmacological therapy. Culturally competent communication skills are necessary in health-care settings so that quality of care is promoted and the opportunities for distress are minimized. For example, patients with limited coverage for medications may not be able to afford some expensive opioid analgesics or antibiotics and it may be preferable to prescribe less expensive medications to ensure adherence to the treatment. Even patients with adequate insurance incur substantial burdens related to uncovered services such as transportation or home care, lost salaries and work, household modifications, and alternative treatments.[208]

One of the less frequently explored effects of cancer is its impact on personal finances and the contribution of financial-related distress to overall suffering and QOL has. Financial issues has been recently found to be the second most frequent source of distress identified by cancer patients in a community cancer center context (22%).[209]

A substantial proportion of patients and families experience adverse financial events during this period, probably due to the increased direct out-of-pocket expenses related to cancer diagnosis and to loss of income secondary to functional status decline, among others.[210]

The assessment of the impact of financial distress on QOL in patients with advanced cancer and the identification of possible associations and explanations is of paramount importance. Developing tools and strategies to correctly assess these domains will help us better understand what is happening to our patients and identify possible interventions to ease their suffering and improve their QOL.

In some cases, a simple social assessment will reveal that patients may benefit from a disabled parking sign, application for benefits, preparation of a will or funeral arrangements, or assistance with financial planning. These issues can greatly improve the QOL for the patients and their communication with health-care professionals and their family.

CONCLUSION

For the patients, the presence of multiple symptoms and the distress they cause are linked to the disease experience. In clinical practice, patients present with multiple symptoms requiring simultaneous assessment and management. Our primary goal is to improve QOL for both the advanced-illness patients and the family/caregiver, and we offer treatments to relieve symptoms, pain, and distress. In order to treat advanced-illness patients, we first listen and seek to understand their symptom experience and the psychological and spiritual sources of suffering. Our communication with these patients and caregivers can bring peace and healing and warranty a quality of care and satisfaction through all the illness process. It is very important to have an effective strategy that requires a multidimensional assessment of and a specific plan for each patient, with an interdisciplinary approach, respecting the treatment goals and the patient's wishes.

REFERENCES

1   Hui D, Elsayem A, De la Cruz M et al. Availability and integration of palliative care at U.S. cancer centers. *JAMA* 2010; 303(11):1054–1061.

2   Byock I, Twohig JS, Merriman M, Collins K. Promoting excellence in end-of-life care: A report on innovative models of palliative care. *J Palliat Med* 2006; 9(1):137–151.

3   Yennurajalingam S, Atkinson B, Masterson J, Hui D, Urbauer D, Tu SM, Bruera E. The impact of an outpatient palliative care consultation on symptom burden in advanced prostate cancer patients. *J Palliat Med* 2012; 15:20–23.

4   Casarett D, Pickard A, Bailey FA et al. Do palliative consultations improve patient outcomes? *J Am Geriatr Soc* 2008; 56(4):593–599.

5   El-Jawahri A, Greer JA, Temel JS. Does palliative care improve outcomes for patients with incurable illness? A review of the evidence. *J Support Oncol* 2011; 9(3):87–94.

6   Higginson IJ, Evans CJ. What is the evidence that palliative care teams improve outcomes for cancer patients and their families? *Cancer J* 2010; 16(5):423–435.

7   Lorenz KA, Lynn J, Dy SM et al. Evidence for improving palliative care at the end of life: A systematic review. *Ann Intern Med* 2008; 148(2):147–159.

8   Hearn J, Higginson IJ. Do specialist palliative care teams improve outcomes for cancer patients? A systematic literature review. *Palliat Med* 1998; 12(5):317–332.

9   Zimmermann C, Riechelmann R, Krzyzanowska M, Rodin G, Tannock I. Effectiveness of specialized palliative care: A systematic review. *JAMA* 2008; 299(14):1698–1709.

10 Temel JS, Greer JA, Muzikansky A et al. Early palliative care for patients with metastatic non-small-cell lung cancer. *N Engl J Med* 2010; 363(8):733–742.

11 Cassell EJ. Diagnosing suffering: A perspective. *Ann Intern Med* 1999; 131: 31–34.

12 Muir JC, McDonagh A, Gooding N. Multidimensional patient assessment. In: Berger D, Portenoy RK, Weissman DE, eds. *Principles and Practice of Palliative Care and Supportive Oncology*, 2nd edn. Philadelphia, PA: Lippincott Williams & Wilkins, 2002, pp. 653–660.

13 Kirkova J, Davis MP, Walsh D et al. Cancer symptom assessment instruments: A systematic review. *J Clin Oncol* 2006; 24:1459–1473 (erratum in: *J Clin Oncol* 2006;24:2973).

14 Bruera E, Neumann C, Brenneis C, Quan H. Frequency of symptom distress and poor prognostic indicators in palliative cancer patients admitted to a tertiary palliative care unit, hospices, and acute care hospitals. *J Palliat Care* 2000; 16:16–21.

15 Nelson JE, Meier D, Oei EJ et al. Self-reported symptom experience of critically ill cancer patients receiving intensive care. *Crit Care Med* 2001; 29:277–282.

16 Rolnick SJ, Jackson J, Nelson WW et al. Pain management in the last six months of life among women who died of ovarian cancer. *J Pain Symptom Manage* 2007; 33:24–31.

17 Ash DA, Hansen-Flaschen J, Lanken P. Decisions to limit or continue life-sustaining treatment by critical care physician in the United States. Conflicts between physicians' practices and patients' wishes. *Am J Respir Crit Care Med* 1995;151:288–292.

18 Solomon MZ, O'Donnell L, Jennings B et al. Decision near the end of life: Professional views of life-sustaining treatments. *Am J Public Health* 1993;83:14–23.

19 Baile WF, Glober GA, Lenzi R, Beale EA, Kudelka AP. Discussing disease progression and end-of-life decisions. *Oncology* (Williston Park) 1999;13:1021–1031.

20 Pauls MA, Ackroyd-Stolarz S. Identifying bioethics learning needs: A survey of Canadian emergency medicine residents. *Acad Emerg Med* 2006;13:645–652.

21 Sise MJ, Sise CB, Sack DI, Goerhing M. Surgeons' attitudes about communicating with patients and their families. *Curr Surg* 2006;63:213–218.

22 Barclay JS, Blackhall LJ, Tulsky JA. Communication strategies and cultural issues in the delivery of bad news. *J Palliat Med* 2007;10:958–977.

23 Keating NL, Gandhi TK, Orav EJ, Bates DW, Ayanian JZ. Patient characteristics and experiences associated with trust in specialist physicians. *Arch Intern Med* 2004;164:1015–1020.

24 Zhukovsky DS, Abdullah O, Richardson M et al. Clinical evaluation in advanced cancer. *Semin Oncol* 2000;27:14–23.

25 Brunelli C, Constantini M, Di Guilio P et al. Quality of life evaluation: When do terminal cancer patients and health care providers agree? *J Pain Symptom Manage* 1998;15:149–150.

26 Grossman SA, Sheidler VR, Swedeen K et al. Correlation of patient and caregiver ratings of cancer pain. *J Pain Symptom Manage* 1991;6:53–57.

27 Elliott BA, Elliott TE, Murray DM et al. Patients and family members: The role of knowledge and attitude in cancer pain. *J Pain Symptom Manage* 1996;12:209–220.

28 Clipp EC, George LK. Patients with cancer and their spouse caregivers. Perceptions of illness experience. *Cancer* 1992;69:1074–1079.

29 Nekolaichuk CL, Bruera E, Spachynski K et al. A comparison of patient and proxy symptom assessments in advanced cancer patients. *Palliat Med* 1999;13:311–323.

30 Nekolaichuk CL, Maguire TO, Suarez-Almazor M et al. Assessing the reliability of patient, nurse, and family caregiver symptom ratings in hospitalized advanced cancer patients. *J Clin Oncol* 1999;17:3621–3630.

31 Komurcu S, Nelson KA, Walsh D et al. Common symptoms in advanced cancer. *Semin Oncol* 2000;27:24–33.

32 Walsh D, Donnelly S, Rybicki L. The symptoms of advanced cancer: Relationship to age, gender, and performance status in 1,000 patients. *Support Care Cancer* 2000;8:175–179.

33 Chang VT, Hwang SS, Feuerman M et al. Symptom and quality of life survey of medical oncology patients at a veterans affairs medical center: A role for symptom assessment. *Cancer* 2000;88:1175–1183.

34 Vogl D, Rosenfeld B, Breitbart W et al. Symptom prevalence, characteristics, and distress in AIDS outpatients. *J Pain Symptom Manage* 1999;18:253–262.

35 Delgado-Guay MO, Bruera E. Management of pain in the older person with cancer. Part 1. *Oncology* 2008;22:56–61.

36 Basso U, Monfardinin S. Multidimensional geriatric evaluation in elderly cancer patients: A practical approach. *Eur J Cancer Care* 2004;13:424–433.

37 Hurria A, Lachs M, Cohen H et al. Geriatric assessment for oncologists: Rationale and future directions. *Crit Rev Oncol/Hematol* 2006;59:211–217.

38 Bruera E. Patient assessment in palliative cancer care. *Cancer Treat Rev* 1996;22(Suppl A):3–12.

39 Kim HN, Bruera E, Jenkins R. Symptom control and palliative care. In: Cavalli F, Hansen HH, Kaye SB, eds. *Textbook of Medical Oncology*. Boca Raton, FL: Taylor & Francis, 2004, pp. 353–370.

40 Bruera E, Kim HN. Cancer pain. *JAMA* 2003;290:2476–2479.

41 Coyle N, Adelhardt J, Foley K et al. Character of terminal illness in the advanced cancer patient: Pain and other symptoms during the last four weeks of life. *J Pain Symptom Manage* 1990;5:83–93.

42 Corner J, Hopkinson J, Fitzsimmons D et al. Is late diagnosis of lung cancer inevitable? Interview study of patients' recollections of symptoms before diagnosis. *Thorax* 2005;60:314–319.

43 Cleeland C, Reyes-Gibby C. When is it justified to treat symptoms? Measuring symptom burden. *Oncology* 2002;16:64–70.

44 Cleeland C, Mendoza T, Wang X et al. Assessing symptom distress in cancer patients: The M. D. Anderson Symptom Inventory. *Cancer* 2000;89:1634–1646.

45 Portenoy R, Thaler H, Kornblith A et al. Symptom prevalence, characteristics and distress in a cancer population. *Qual Life Res* 1994;3:183–189.

46 Bruley D. Beyond reliability and validity: Analysis of selected quality of life instruments for use in palliative care. *J Palliat Med* 1999;2:299–390.

47 Veikova G, Stark D, Selby P. Quality of life instruments in oncology. *Eur J Cancer* 1999;35:1571–1580.

48 Walker P, Nordell C, Neumann CM et al. Impact of the edmonton labeled visual information system on physician recall of metastatic cancer patient histories. A randomized controlled trial. *J Pain Symptom Manage* 2001;21:4–11.

49 Stromgren A, Goldschmidt D, Groenvold M et al. Self-assessment in cancer patients referred to palliative care: A study of feasibility and symptom epidemiology. *Cancer* 2002;94:512–520.

50 Stromgren A, Groenvold M, Pedersen L, Olsen A, Spile M, Sjogren P. Does the medical record cover the symptoms experienced by cancer patients receiving palliative care? A comparison of the record and patient self-rating. *J Pain Symptom Manage* 2001;21:89–96.

51 De Haes JC, van Knippenberg FC, Neijt JP. Measuring psychological and physical distress in cancer patients: Structure and application of the Rotterdam Symptom Checklist. *Br J Cancer* 1990;62:1034–1038.

52 Watanabe SM, Nekolaichuk CL, Beaumont C. The Edmonton Symptom Assessment System, a proposed tool for distress screening in cancer patients: Development and refinement. *Psycho-Oncology* 2012;21:977–985.

53 Bruera E., Kuehn N., Miller M.J., Selmser P., Macmillan K. The Edmonton Symptom Assessment System (ESAS): A simple method for the assessment of palliative care patients. *J Palliat Care* 1991;7:6–9.

54 Porzio G, Ricevuto E, Aielli F et al. The supportive care task force at the University of L'Aquila: 2-years experience. *Support Care Cancer* 2005;13:351–355.

55 Rees E, Hardy J, Ling J, Broadley K, A'Hern R. The use of Edmonton Symptom Scale (ESAS) within a palliative care unit in the UK. *Palliat Med* 1998;15:213–214.

56 Stromgren AS, Groenvold M, Peterson MA et al. Pain characteristics and treatment outcome for advanced cancer patients during the first week of specialized palliative care. *J Pain Symptom Manage* 2004;27:104–113.

57 Philip J, Smith W, Craft P, Lickiss N. Concurrent validity of the modified Edmonton Symptom Assessment Scale (ESAS) with the Rotterdam Symptom Checklist and the Brief Pain Inventory. *Support Care Cancer* 1998;6:539–541.

58 Osterlind J. Establishing ESAS in daily Care. Poster communication in abstract book of the 8th EAPC Congress, 2003. The Hague, Netherlands.

59 Chang V, Hwang S, Feuerman M. Validation of the edmonton symptom assessment scale. *Cancer* 2000;88(9):2164–2171.

60 Rees E, Jardy J, Ling J, Broadley K, A'Hern R. The use of the Edmonton Symptom Assessment Scale (ESAS) within a palliative care unit in the UK. *Palliat Med* 1998;12:75–82.

61 Watanabe S, Nekolaichuk C, Beaumont C, Mawani A. The edmonton symptom assessment system—What do patients think? *Support Care Cancer* 2009;17:675–683.

62 Nekolaichuk C, Maguire P, Suarez-Almanzor M, Rogers W, Bruera E. Assessing the reliability of patient, nurse, and family caregiver symptom rating in hospitalized advanced cancer patient. *J Clin Oncol* 1999;11:3621–3630.

63 Moro C, Brunelli C, Miccinesi G et al. Edmonton symptom assessment scale: Italian validation in two palliative care settings. *Support Care Cancer* 2005;14:30–37.

64 Pautex S, Berger A, Catelain C, Hermann F, Zulian G. Symptom assessment in elderly cancer patients receiving palliative care. *Crit Rev Oncol Haematol* 2003;47:281–286.

65 Stiel S, Matthes ME, Bertram L et al. Validation of the new version of the minimal documentation system (MIDOS) for patients in palliative care: The German version of the Edmonton Symptom Assessment Scale (ESAS). *Schmerz* 2010;24(6):596–604.

66 Carvajal A, Centeno C, Watson R, Bruera E. A comprehensive study of psychometric properties of the Edmonton Symptom Assessment System (ESAS) in Spanish advanced cancer patients. *Eur J Cancer* 2011;47:1863–1872.

67 Kwon JH, Nam SH, Koh S et al. Validation of edmonton symptom assessment system in Korean patients with cancer. *J Pain Symptom Manage* 2013;46:947–956. http://dx.doi.org/10.1016/j.jpainsymman.2013.01.012

68 Jaturapatporn D. Validity and cross-cultural adaptation of the Thai version of the edmonton symptom assessment scale (ESAS). *Palliat Med* 2008;22:448.

69 Richardson L, Jones W. A review of the reliability and validity of the edmonton symptom assessment system. *Curr Oncol* 2009;16:53–64.

70 Nekolaichuck C, Wataneabe S, Beaumont C. The edmonton symptom assessment system: A 15 year retrospective review of validation studies (1991–2006). *Palliat Med* 2008;222:111–122.

71 Watanabe S, McKinnon S, Macmillan K et al. Palliative care nurses' perception of the Edmonton Symptom Assessment Scale: A pilot survey. *Int J Palliat Nurs* 2006;12:111–114.

72 Garyali A, Palmer JL, Yennurajalingam S et al. Errors in symptom intensity self-assessment by patients receiving outpatient palliative care. *J Palliat Med* 2006;9:1059–1065.

73 Watanabe SM, Nekolaichuk C, Beaumont C, Johnson L, Myers J, Strasser F. A multi-centre validation study of two numerical versions of the Edmonton Symptom Assessment System in palliative care patients. *J Pain Symptom Manage* 2011;41:456–468.

74 Vignaroli E, Pace E, Willey J, Palmer L, Zhang T, Bruera E. The Edmonton Symptom Assessment System as a screening tool for depression and anxiety. *J Palliat Med* 2006;9:296–303.

75 Portenoy R, Thaler H, Kornblith A et al. The Memorial Symptom Assessment Scale: An instrument for the evaluation of symptom prevalence, characteristics and distress. *Eur J Cancer* 1994;30A:1326–1336.

76 Chang V, Hwang S, Feuerman M, Kasimis B, Thaler H. The Memorial Symptom Assessment Scale Short Form (MSAS-SF). Validity and reliability. *Cancer* 2000;89:1163–1171.

77 Chang V, Hwang S, Kasimis B, Thaler H. Shorter symptom assessment instruments: The Condensed Memorial Symptom Assessment Scale (CMSAS). *Cancer Invest* 2004;22:526–536.

78 McCorkle R., Young K. Development of a symptom distress scale. *Cancer Nurs* 1978;1:373–378.

79 McCorkle R., Quint-Benoliel J. Symptom distress, current concerns and mood disturbance after diagnosis of life-threatening disease. *Soc Sci Med* 1983;17:431–438.

80 Ingham J, Breitbart W. Epidemiology and clinical features of delirium. In: Portenoy RK, Bruera E, eds. *Topics in Palliative Care*, Vol. 1. New York: Oxford University Press, 1997, pp. 7–19.

81 Centeno C, Sanz A, Bruera E. Delirium in advanced cancer patients. *Palliat Med* 2004;18:184–194.

82 Lawlor PG, Gagnon B, Mancini IL et al. Occurrence, causes, and outcome of delirium in patients with advanced cancer: A prospective study. *Arch Intern Med* 2000;160:786–794.

83 Minagawa H, Uchitomi Y, Yamawaki S et al. Psychiatric morbidity in terminally ill cancer patients. A prospective study. *Cancer* 1996;78:1131–1137.

84 Bruera E, Miller L, McCallion J et al. Cognitive failure in patients with terminal cancer: A prospective study. *J Pain Symptom Manage* 1992;7:192–195.

85 Morita T, Tei Y, Tsunoda J et al. Underlying pathologies and their associations with clinical features in terminal delirium of cancer patients. *J Pain Symptom Manage* 2001;22:997–1006.

86 Inouye SK. The dilemma of delirium: Clinical and research controversies regarding diagnosis and evaluation of delirium in hospitalized elderly medical patients. *Am J Med* 1994;97:278–288.

87 American Psychiatric Association. *Diagnostic and Statistical Manual of Mental Disorders.* 4th edn, text revision. Washington, DC: American Psychiatric Association; 2000.

88 Folstein MF, Folstein SE, McHugh PR. 'Mini-mental state'. A practical method for grading the cognitive state of patients for the clinician. *J Psychiatr Res* 1975;12:189–198.

89 Bruera E, Franco JJ, Maltoni M et al. Changing pattern of agitated impaired mental status in patients with advanced cancer: Association with cognitive monitoring, hydration, and opioid rotation. *J Pain Symptom Manage* 1995;10:287–291.

90 Breitbart W, Marotta R, Platt MM et al. A double-blind trial of haloperidol, chlorpromazine, and lorazepam in the treatment of delirium in hospitalized AIDS patients. *Am J Psychiatry* 1996;153:231–237.

91 Hjermstad M, Loge JH, Kaasa S. Methods for assessment of cognitive failure and delirium in palliative care patients: Implications for practice and research. *Palliat Med* 2004;18:494–506.

92 Breitbart W, Rosenfeld B, Roth A et al. The Memorial Delirium Assessment Scale. *J Pain Symptom Manage* 1997;13:128–137.

93 Lawlor PG, Nekolaichuk C, Gagnon B, Mancini IL, Pereira JL, Bruera ED. Clinical utility, factor analysis, and further validation of the Memorial Delirium Assessment Scale in patients with advanced cancer: Assessing delirium in advanced cancer. *Cancer* 2000;88(12):2859–2867.

94 Trzepacz PT, Baker RW, Greenhouse J. A symptom rating scale for delirium. *Psychiatry Res* 1988;23:89–97.

95 Gagnon P, Allard P, Masse B et al. Delirium in terminal cancer: A prospective study using daily screening, early diagnosis, and continuous monitoring. *J Pain Symptom Manage* 2000;19:412–426.

96 Inouye SK, van Dyck CH, Alessi CA et al. Clarifying confusion: The confusion assessment method. A new method for detection of delirium. *Ann Intern Med* 1990;113:941–948.

97 Fabbri RM, Moreira MA, Garrido R et al. Validity and reliability of the Portuguese version of the Confusion Assessment Method (CAM) for the detection of delirium in the elderly. *Arq Neuropsiquiatr* 2001;59(2-A):175–179.

98 Ross CA, Peyser CE, Shapiro I et al. Delirium: Phenomenologic and etiologic subtypes. *Int Psychogeriatr* 1991;3:135–147.

99 Liptzin B, Levkoff SE. An empirical study of delirium subtypes. *Br J Psychiatry* 1992;161:843–845.

100 Coyle N, Breitbart W, Weaver S et al. Delirium as a contributing factor to 'crescendo' pain: Three case reports. *J Pain Symptom Manage* 1994;9:44–47.

101 Fainsinger RL, Tapper M, Bruera E. A perspective on the management of delirium in terminally ill patients on a palliative care unit. *J Palliat Care* 1993;9:4–8.

102 Lawlor P, Walker P, Bruera E et al. Severe opioid toxicity and somatization of psychosocial distress in a cancer patient with a background of chemical dependence. *J Pain Symptom Manage* 1997;13:356–361.

103 Lawlor PG. Multidimensional assessment: Pain and palliative care. In: Bruera E, Portenoy RK, eds. *Cancer Pain*. New York: Cambridge University Press, 2003, pp. 67–88.

104 Vigano A, Dorgan M, Buckingham J, et al. Survival prediction in terminal cancer patients: A systematic review of the medical literature. *Palliat Med* 2000;14:363–374.

105 Yates JW, Chalmer B, McKegney FP. Evaluation of patients with advanced cancer using the Karnofsky performance status. *Cancer* 1980;45:2220–2224.

106 Osoba D, MacDonald N. Principles governing the use of cancer chemotherapy in palliative care. In: Doyle D, Hanks GWC, MacDonald N, eds. *Oxford Textbook of Palliative Medicine*, 2nd edn. Oxford: Oxford University Press, 1998, pp. 249–267.

107 Conill C, Verger E, Salamero M. Performance status assessment in cancer patients. *Cancer* 1990;65:1864–1866.

108 Mor V, Laliberte L, Morris JN et al. The Karnofsky Performance Status Scale. An examination of its reliability and validity in a research setting. *Cancer* 1984;53:2002–2007.

109 Kaasa T, Loomis J, Gillis K et al. The Edmonton Functional Assessment Tool: Preliminary development and evaluation for use in palliative care. *J Pain Symptom Manage* 1997;13:10–19.

110 Anderson F, Downing GM, Hill J et al. Palliative performance scale (PPS): A new tool. *J Palliat Care* 1996;12:5–11.

111 Kaasa T, Wessel J. The Edmonton Functional Assessment Tool: Further development and validation for use in palliative care. *J Palliat Care* 2001;17:5–11.

112 Virik K, Glare P. Validation of the palliative performance scale for inpatients admitted to a palliative care unit in Sydney, Australia. *J Pain Symptom Manage* 2002;23:455–457.

113 Portenoy RK, Payne D, Jacobsen P. Breakthrough pain: Characteristics and impact in patients with cancer pain. *Pain* 1999;81:129–134.

114 Walsh D, Rybicki L, Nelson KA et al. Symptoms and prognosis in advanced cancer. *Support Care Cancer* 2002;10:385–388.

115 Breitbart W, Bruera E, Chochinov H et al. Neuropsychiatric syndromes and psychological symptoms in patients with advanced cancer. *J Pain Symptom Manage* 1995;10:131–41.

116 Chochinov HM, Wilson KG, Enns M et al. Desire for death in the terminally ill. *Am J Psychiatry* 1995;152:1185–1191.

117 Block SD. Assessing and managing depression in the terminally ill patient. ACP-ASIM End-of-Life Care Consensus Panel. American College of Physicians–American Society of Internal Medicine. *Ann Intern Med* 2000;132:209–218.

118 Block SD, Billings JA. Patient requests to hasten death. Evaluation and management in terminal care. *Arch Intern Med* 1994;154:2039–2047.

119 Massie MJ. Prevalence of depression in patients with cancer. *J Natl Cancer Inst Monogr* 2004;32:57–71

120 Block S. Assessing and managing depression in the terminally ill patient. *Ann Intern Med* 2000;32:209–218.

121 Hotopf M, Chidgey J, Addington-Hall J, Lan Ly K. Depression in advanced disease: A systematic review. Part 1: Prevalence and case finding. *Palliat Med* 2002;16:81–97.

122 Massie MJ, Gagnon P, Holland JC. Depression and suicide in patients with cancer. *J Pain Symptom Manage* 1994;9:325–340.

123 Radbruch L, Nauck F, Ostgathe C et al. What are the problems in palliative care? Results from a representative survey. *Support Care Cancer* 2003;11:442–445.

124 Ng K, von Guten C. Symptoms and attitudes of 100 consecutive patients admitted to an acute hospice/palliative care unit. *J Pain Symptom Manage* 1998;16:307–316.

125 Reuben D, Mor V, Hiris J. Clinical symptoms and length of survival in patients with terminal cancer. *Arch Intern Med* 1998;148:1586–1591.

126 Mitchell AJ, Chan M, Bhatti H, Halton M, Grassi L, er Johansen C, Meader N. Prevalence of depression, anxiety, and adjustment disorder in oncological, haematological, and palliative-care settings: A meta-analysis of 94 interview-based studies. *Lancet Oncol* 2011;12:160–174

127 Kurtz M, Kurtz J, Stommel M, Given C, Given B. Physical functioning and depression among older persons with cancer. *Cancer Practice* 2001;9:11–18.

128 Lloyd-Williams M, Dennis M, Taylor F. A prospective study to determine the association between physical symptoms and depression in patients with advanced cancer. *Palliat Med* 2004;18:558–563.

129 Koenig HG, Cohen HJ, Blazer DG et al. A brief depression scale for use in the medically ill. *Int J Psychiatry Med* 1992;22:183–195.

130 Gerety MB, Williams JW Jr, Mulrow CD et al. Performance of case-finding tools for depression in the nursing home: Influence of clinical and functional characteristics and selection of optimal threshold scores. *J Am Geriatr Soc* 1994;42:1103–1109.

131 Chochinov HM, Wilson KG, Enns M et al. 'Are you depressed?' Screening for depression in the terminally ill. *Am J Psychiatry* 1997;154:674–676.

132 Fisch MJ. Depression. In: Elsayem A, Driver L, Bruera E, eds. *The MD Anderson Symptom Control and Palliative Care Handbook*, 2nd edn. Houston, TX: The University of Texas-Houston Health Science Center, 2002, pp. 91–96.

133 Lloyd-Williams M, Spiller J, Ward J. Which depression screening tools should be used in palliative care? *Palliat Med* 2003;17:40–43.

134 Whooley MA, Avins AL, Miranda J et al. Case-finding instruments for depression. Two questions are as good as many. *J Gen Intern Med* 1997;12:439–445.

135 Johnston M, Pollard B, Hennessey P. Construct validation of the hospital anxiety and depression scale with clinical populations. *J Psychosomatic Res* 2000;48:579–584.

136 Bjelland I, Dahl AA, Haug TT, Neckelmann D. The validity of the Hospital Anxiety and Depression Scale: An updated literature review. *J Psychosom Res* 2002;52:69–77.

137 Grassi L, Malacarne P, Maestri A et al. Depression, psychosocial variables and occurrence of life events among patients with cancer. *J Affect Disord* 1997;44:21–30.

138 Breitbart W. Identifying patients at risk for, and treatment of major psychiatric complications of cancer. *Support Care Cancer* 1995;3:45–60.

139 American Psychiatric Association. Somatoform disorder. In: *Diagnostic and Statistical Manual of Mental Disorders*, 4th edn. Washington, DC: American Psychiatric Association, 1994, pp. 445–465.

140 Gureje O, Simon GE, Ustun TB et al. Somatization in cross-cultural perspective: A World Health Organization study in primary care. *Am J Psychiatry* 1997;154:989–995.

141 Lipowski ZJ. Somatization: The concept and its clinical application. *Am J Psychiatry* 1988;145:1358–1368.

142 Simon GE, VonKorff M, Piccinelli M et al. An international study of the relation between somatic symptoms and depression. *N Engl J Med* 1999;341:1329–1335.

143 Chaturvedi SK, Maguire GP. Persistent somatization in cancer: A controlled follow-up study. *J Psychosom Res* 1998;45:249–256.

144 Chaturvedi SK, Hopwood P, Maguire P. Non-organic somatic symptoms in cancer. *Eur J Cancer* 1993;29A:1006–1008.

145 Robinson K, Bruera E. The management of pain in patients with advanced cancer: The importance of multidimensional assessments. *J Palliat Care* 1995;11:51–53.

146 Wessely S, White PD. There is only one functional somatic syndrome. *Br J Psychiatry* 2004;185:95–96.

147 Daeninck PJ, Bruera E. Opioid use in cancer pain. Is a more liberal approach enhancing toxicity? *Acta Anaesthesiol Scand* 1999;43:924–938.

148 Parsons HA, Delgado-Guay MO, El Osta B et al. Alcoholism screening in patients with advanced cancer: Impact on symptom burden and opioid use. *J Palliat Med.* 2008;11:964–968.

149 Lawlor P, Walker P, Bruera E, Mitchell S. Sever opioid toxicity and somatization of psychosocial distress in a cancer patient with a background of chemical dependence. *J Pain Symptom Manage* 1997;6:356–361.

150 Gonzales GR, Coyle N. Treatment of cancer pain in a former opioid abuser: Fears of the patient and staff and their influence on care. *J Pain Symptom Manage.* 1992;4:246–249. (Original Article 4556 Cancer October 1, 2011.)

151 Liptzin B, Levkoff SE. An empirical study of delirium subtypes. *Br J Psychiatry* 1992;161:843–845.

152 Simoni-Wastila L, Strickler G. Risk factors associated with problem use of prescription drugs. *Am J Public Health* 2004;94:266–268.

153 O'Connor PG, Schottenfeld RS. Patients with alcohol problems. *N Engl J Med* 1998;338:592–602.

154 Nedeljkovic SS, Wasan A, Jamison RN. Assessment of efficacy of long-term opioid therapy in pain patients with substance abuse potential. *Clin J Pain* 2002;18(Suppl):39e51.

155 Braiteh F, El Osta B, Palmer JL, Reddy SK, Bruera E. Characteristics, findings, and outcomes of palliative care inpatient consultations at a comprehensive cancer center. *J Palliat Med.* 2007;10:948–955.

156 Bruera E, Moyano J, Seifert L, Fainsinger RL, Hanson J, Suarez-Almazor M. The frequency of alcoholism among patients with pain due to terminal cancer. *J Pain Symptom Manage.* 1995;10:599–603.

157 WHO Expert Committee on Problems Related to Alcohol Consumption. Alcohol availability and consumption in the world. In: World Health Organization, ed. *WHO Technical Report Series* 944. Geneva, Switzerland: World Health Organization; 2007:9–19.

158 Strasser F, Walker P, Bruera E. Palliative pain management: When both pain and suffering hurt. *J Palliat Care.* 2005;2:69–79.

159 Fainsinger RL, Nekolaichuk CL, Lawlor PG et al. A multicenter study of the revised Edmonton Staging System for classifying cancer pain in advanced cancer patients. *J Pain Symptom Manage.* 2005 Mar;29(3):224–237.

160 Ewing JA. Detecting alcoholism. The CAGE questionnaire. *JAMA* 1984;252:1905–1907.

161 Dhalla S, Kopec JA. The CAGE questionnaire for alcohol misuse: A review of reliability and validity studies. *Clin Invest Med* 2007;30(1):33–41.

162 Butler SF, Budman SH, Fernandez K et al. Validation of a screener and opioid assessment measure for patients with chronic pain. *Pain* 2004;112:65–75.

163 Akbik H, Butler SF, Budman SH et al. Validation and clinical application of the Screener and Opioid Assessment for Patients with Pain (SOAPP). *J Pain Symptom Manage* 2006 Sep;32(3):287–293.

164 Dev R, Parsons HA, Palla S et al. Undocumented alcoholism and its correlation with tobacco and illegal drug use in advanced cancer patients. *Cancer* 2011 Oct 1;117(19):4551–4556.

165 Grant BF, Hasin DS, Chou SP et al. Nicotine dependence and psychiatric disorders in the United States: Results from the national epidemiologic survey on alcohol and related conditions. *Arch Gen Psychiatry* 2004;61:1107–1115.

166 Clemmy P, Brooner R, Chutuape MA et al. Smoking habits and attitudes in a methadone maintenance treatment population. *Drug Alcohol Depend* 1997;44:123–132.

167 Drews E, Zimmer A. Modulation of alcohol and nicotine responses through the endogenous opioid system. *Prog Neurobiol* 2010;90:1–15.

168 Passik SD. Issues in long-term opioid therapy: Unmet needs, risks, and solutions. *Mayo Clin Proc* 2009;84:593–601.

169 Puchalski C, Ferrel B, Virani R et al. Improving the quality of spiritual care as a dimension of palliative care: The report of the consensus conference. *J Palliat Med* 2009;10:885–904.

170 Puchalski C, Dorff R, Hendi I. Spirituality, religion, and healing in palliative care. *Clin Geriatr Med* 2004;20:689–714.

171 The National Consensus Project for Quality Palliative Care Clinical Practice Guidelines for Quality Palliative Care 3rd edition 2013. http://www.nationalconsensusproject.org/. Accessed May 2013.

172 National Cancer Institute: Spirituality in cancer care. 2012. http://www.nci.nih.gov/cancertopics/pdq/supportivecare/spirituality/. Accessed May 2013.

173 Pargament KI, Koenig HG, Tarakeshwar N, Hahn J. Religious coping methods as predictors of psychological, physical and spiritual outcomes among medically ill elderly patients: A two year longitudinal study. *J Health Psychol* 2004;9:713–730.

174 Hinshaw D. Spiritual issues at the end of life. *Clin Fam Practice* 2004;6:423–440.

175 Balboni T, Vanderwerker L, Block S et al. Religiousness and spiritual support among advanced cancer patients and associations with end-of-life treatment preferences and quality of life. *J Clin Oncol* 2007;25:550–560.

176 Puchalski C. Spirituality in health: The role of spirituality in critical care. *Crit Care Clin* 2004;20:487–504.

177 Chochinov H, Cann B. Interventions to enhance the spiritual aspects of dying. *J Palliat Med* 2005;8:S103–S115.

178 Puchalski C, Romer A. Taking a spiritual history allows clinicians to understand patients more fully. *J Palliat Med* 2000;3:129–137.

179 Kearney M, Mount B. Spiritual care of the dying patient. In: Chochinov H, Breitbart W (eds), *Handbook of Psychiatry in Palliative Medicine.* New York: Oxford University Press, 2000, pp. 357–373.

180 Delgado-Guay MO, Hui D, Parsons HA, Govan K, De la Cruz M, Thorney S, Bruera E. Spirituality, religiosity, and spiritual pain in advanced cancer patients. *J Pain Symptom Manage* 2011 June; 41(6):986–994.

181 Rousseau P. Spirituality and the dying patient. *J Clin Oncol* 2000;18:2000–2002.

182 Williams JA, Meltzer D, Arora V, Chung G, Curlin FA. Attention to inpatients' religious and spiritual concerns: Predictors and association with patient satisfaction. *J Gen Intern Med* 2011;26(11):1265–1271.

183 Astrow AB, Wexler A, Texeira K, He MK, Sulmasy DP. Is failure to meet spiritual needs associated with cancer patients' perceptions of quality of care and their satisfaction with care? *J Clin Oncol* 2007;25(36):5753–5757.

184 Balboni TA, Paulk ME, Balboni MJ, Phelps AC, Loggers ET, Wright AA, Block SD, Lewis EF, Peteet JR, Prigerson HG. Provision of spiritual care to patients with advanced cancer: Associations with medical care and quality of life near death. *J Clin Oncol* 2010;28(3):445–452.

185 Holland JC, Kash KM, Passik S et al. A brief spiritual beliefs inventory for use in quality of life re- search in life-threatening illness. *Psychooncology* 1998;7:460–469.

186 Pargament KI, Smith BW, Koenig HG, Perez L. Patterns of positive and negative religious coping with major life stressors. *J Sci Study Relig* 1998;37:710–724.

187 Brady MJ, Peterman AH, Fitchett G, Mo M, Cella D. A case for including spirituality in quality of life measurement in oncology. *Psychooncology* 1999;8:417–428.

188 Cella DF, Tulsky DS, Gray G et al. The functional assessment of cancer therapy scale: Development and validation of the general measure. *J Clin Oncol* 1993;11:570–579.

189 Maugans TA. The SPIRITual history. *Arch Fam Med* 1996;5:11–16.

190 Anandarajah G, Hight E. Spirituality and medical practice: Using the HOPE questions as a practical tool for spiritual assessment. *Am Fam Physician* 2001;63:81–89.

191 Borneman T, Ferrell B, Puchalski C. Evaluation of the FICA tool for spiritual assessment. *J Pain Symptom Manag* 2010;20(2):163–173.

192 Fitchett G, Canada AL. The role of religion/spirituality in coping with cancer: Evidence, assessment, and intervention. In: Holland JC, ed. *Psycho-Oncology*, 2nd edn. New York: Oxford University Press, 2010, pp. 440–446.

193 Handzo, G. Spiritual care for palliative patients. *Curr Probl Cancer* 2011;35(6):365–371.

194 Vachon ML. Psychosocial needs of patients and families. *J Palliat Care* 1998;14:49–56.

195 Ferrell BR, Ferrell BA, Rhiner M et al. Family factors influencing cancer pain management. *Postgrad Med J* 1991;67(Suppl 2):S64–S69.

196 Panke JT, Ferrell BR. Emotional problems in the family. In: Doyle D, Hanks G, Cherny N, Calman K, eds. *Oxford Textbook of Palliative Medicine*, 3rd edn. Oxford: Oxford University Press, 2004, pp. 985–992.

197 Cantwell P, Turco S, Brenneis C et al. Predictors of home death in palliative care cancer patients. *J Palliat Care* 2000;16:23–28.

198 Teno JM, Nelson HL, Lynn J. Advance care planning. Priorities for ethical and empirical research. *Hastings Cent Rep* 1994;24:S32–S36.

199 Kristjanson LJ. The family as a unit of treatment. In: Portenoy RK, Bruera E, eds. *Topics in Palliative Care*. Vol. 1. Oxford: Oxford University Press, 1997, pp. 245–262.

200 Glajchen M. The emerging role and needs of family caregivers in cancer care. *J Support Oncol* 2004;2:145–155.

201 Schulz R, Beach SR. Caregiving as a risk factor for mortality: The care-giver health effects study. *JAMA* 1999;282:2215–2219.

202 Miaskowski C, Kragness L, Dibble S et al. Differences in mood states, health status, and caregiver strain between family caregivers of oncology outpatients with and without cancer-related pain. *J Pain Symptom Manage* 1997;13:138–147.

203 Haley WE, LaMonde LA, Han B et al. Family caregiving in hospice: Effects on psychological and health functioning among spousal caregivers of hospice patients with lung cancer or dementia. *Hosp J* 2001;15:1–18.

204 Warner JE. Involvement of families in pain control of terminally ill patients. *Hosp J* 1992;8:155–170.

205 Zarit S, Reever K, Bach-Peterson J. Relatives of the impaired elderly: Correlates of feelings of burden. *Gerontologist* 1980;20:649–655.

206 Derogatis LR, Melisaratos N. The Brief Symptom Inventory: An introductory report. *Psychol Med* 1983;13:595–605.

207 Higginson I, Webb D, Lessof L. Reducing hospital beds for patients with advanced cancer. *Lancet* 1994;344:409.

208 Covinsky KE, Goldman L, Cook EF et al. The impact of serious illness on patients' families. SUPPORT Investigators. Study to Understand Prognoses and Preferences for Outcomes and Risks of Treatment. *JAMA* 1994;272:1839–1844.

209 Kendall, J. et al. What do 1281 distress screeners tell us about cancer patients in a community cancer center? *Psychooncology* 2011; 20(6):594–600.

210 Stommel, M, Given CW, Given BA, The cost of cancer home care to families. *Cancer* 1993;71(5):1867–1874.

39

Tools for pain and symptom assessment

VICTOR T. CHANG

INTRODUCTION

The field of symptom assessment, and the variety of tools available for pain and symptom assessment, has expanded dramatically. The importance of symptoms was recognized by the convening of a NIH symposium to discuss the target symptoms of fatigue, pain, and depression.[1] All palliative care personnel assess and manage pain and symptoms.[2] Symptom tools provide an organized approach to symptom assessment. While both symptom and quality of life tools emphasize patient-rated outcomes, symptom tools differ from quality of life instruments in emphasis on symptoms rather than general physical, social, or emotional well-being. This distinction is becoming blurred as symptom subscales are developed for specific diseases and therapies, especially in the Functional Assessment Cancer Therapy (FACIT) and European Organization for Research Treatment Cancer (EORTC) family of quality of life instruments. The purpose of this chapter is to provide a brief background and describe some of the more well-known symptom assessment instruments. The vivid and unusual descriptions provided by patients in clinical encounters are not routinely captured by these tools.

FUNDAMENTALS OF SYMPTOM MEASUREMENT AND ASSESSMENT TOOLS

Biological underpinnings

Best understood for pain, the perceived intensity of a sensory stimulus is proportional to the rate of firing by sensory nerves, and the number of nerves that send impulses. Sensory impulses reach the cerebral cortex where they may be recognized and trigger evaluative (severity), affective (unpleasantness or distress), and behavioral (agitation) responses.

Theoretical underpinnings of symptom instruments

CLINIMETRICS

Clinimetrics focuses on the quality of measurements in clinical medicine.[3] Descriptive statements (mensuration) are combined to express a numerical summary (quantification).[4] The descriptive statements are chosen on the basis of clinical relevance, usually by clinicians, and can be eclectic with a variety of symptoms, physical findings, and laboratory findings. An example is the Apgar score, where five items (heart rate, skin color, respiratory effort, muscle tone, reflex irritability) are combined to form a score to describe the condition of a newborn infant.[5]

PSYCHOMETRICS

The degree to which a respondent agrees with items (statements) allows an inference about whether the respondent has a particular, otherwise, unmeasurable psychological state (latent trait), such as pain, anxiety, or depression. Another analogy is the blind men describing an elephant. Each blind man is an item, and the latent trait is the elephant. The extent of agreement between items commonly determined with Likert scales, (e.g., not at all, a little bit, somewhat, quite a bit, very much). The intraclass correlation coefficient (Cronbach's alpha) is a measure of self-consistency between the statements; alpha levels of 0.70 or greater are considered acceptable. Factor analyses and other statistical techniques are used to analyze the collection of statements to see whether they measure one factor, and are therefore unidimensional, or a more than one factor. Longer instruments with more items are preferred to minimize variation and maximize the Cronbach's alpha.

ITEM RESPONSE THEORY

Item response theory (IRT). In this very simplified explanation, IRT starts with the concept of item difficulty, the percentage of respondents who respond correctly to a test item. Similar to psychometrics, IRT estimates a latent trait. The correspondence between the item difficulty and the latent trait is described by the item-characteristic curve (ICC), which is usually sigmoid shaped. Easier items are on the left of the trait scale, and more difficult items on the right. IRT models estimate the difficulty parameter for each item from questionnaire data, where the difficulty parameter is the trait level needed to answer the item correctly 50% of the time. The different kinds of IRT models differ in the numbers and types of parameters used to describe the ICC. The attractiveness of this approach lies in its ability to recognize that different items are different, and versatility through the availability of item banks. Potential improvements in symptom assessment include shorter questionnaires, computerized adaptive testing, and comparisons of different instruments. Questionnaires will not be as dependent on the population being tested. This is an area that is being realized in the revision of existing instruments, and the implementation of the National Institutes of Health Patient Reported Outcome Management Information System (PROMIS) website (www.nihpromis.org) with an assessment center to aid clinical trials,[6] a collaborative effort by the European Association for Palliative Care,[7] and the development of patient-rated outcome version of the common clinical toxicity criteria; more developments are anticipated in the future.[8–10]

Properties of symptom assessment instruments

This section presents basic information on common terms used in discussing instruments. Symptom instruments rely upon patient's ratings and descriptions of symptoms. For more detailed discussions, the reader is referred to.[11–14]

VALIDITY AND RELIABILITY

Validity means that the instrument measures what it claims to measure. Measures of validity include face validity (items that are easy to understand), content validity, criterion validity, and construct validity. Content validity asks how the items in the instrument represent the symptom that the instrument is trying to measure. For example, a pain instrument might include a rating of pain severity.[15] Criterion validity is shown by correlation with other accepted measures of the symptom in question. Criterion validity can be demonstrated by expected agreement (convergent validity) or expected disagreement (divergent validity). Because symptoms are not directly observable, a construct is a definition of what is being measured, such as the symptom, by a group of related observations. Construct validity is an assessment of how well the construct, and the symptom instrument based on the construct, measures the symptom.[16,17] In construct validity, the relationships between these observations are tested to see if they are present as expected.

More recently, the concept of validity has been extended to consider the patient population and clinical setting studied with an instrument, and whether an instrument, or a group of instruments are appropriate for a palliative care population.[18,19] Validation of instruments used in an electronic format represents another new area of research.[20]

Reliability implies freedom from error and is defined as the true variance divided by the true variance and variance from repeated administration of the instrument. Reliability can be measured by the degree of reproducibility (test–retest) and self-consistency (Cronbach's alpha).[21]

RESPONSIVENESS

Responsiveness of the instrument to changes has received increased attention, along with the notion of minimal clinically significant difference. Measures of clinically significant difference are important for sample size estimation in trials designed to improve symptom control or quality of life. They also illustrate the transformation of symptom instruments into outcome measures. Much of the work to date has been done with quality of life measures, where the minimal clinically important difference has been defined as "the smallest difference in score in the domain of interest which patients perceive as beneficial and which would mandate, in the absence of troublesome side effects and excessive cost, a change in the patient's management."[22]

Anchor-based and distribution-based methods have been used to define clinically important differences.[23] Anchor-based methods use established clinical criteria or patient ratings as ways to anchor interpretations of difference scores. An example is the performance status rating. Distribution-based methods rely upon the statistical aspects of the score distributions.[24] A half of the standard deviation may be a good approximation of the minimally important difference (MID).[25] Recent recommendations have been to use multiple approaches and to base the MID on patient-based and clinical anchors.[26]

It has been suggested that instruments that are designed to evaluate the patient at a point in time may not be the optimal instruments for measuring changes because of the large number of items.[27] An alternative approach has been the transition rating, a single item where the patient is asked to rate the change he or she perceives in the target measure. This can be expressed as a percentage, as a seven-point Likert scale ranging from very much worse to very much better, to visual analog scales. Likert and VAS approaches were equivalent in one study.[28] While the ability of the patient to remember his previous symptom status has been questioned, this approach is quick, sensitive, and corresponds to the usual clinical conversation between the patient and the health care provider. The minimum difference has been estimated at 0.5 on a seven-point scale. The magnitude of the transition score is correlated with the pretreatment score.[29]

SCALES

Nominal scales have items that cannot be combined. Ordinal scales have graded categorical responses. Numerical scales ask the respondent to assign a number. Numerical scales can be an interval scale, where the difference between the numerical values is a number (e.g., weight), or a ratio scale, which contains a true zero. The type of scale determines the kinds of data analysis to be done.

DIMENSIONS

Symptoms have dimensions. A medical history will ask about the presence of a symptom, exacerbating and alleviating events, temporal variation, descriptors, and relief. A palliative symptom history can additionally include severity, frequency, duration, distress, effect on function, and associated meanings for the patient. Many of these terms are self-explanatory.

It remains an open question as to how many dimensions are needed. Is one dimension enough? Severity tends to be the most dimension most commonly used, followed by distress. However, symptoms are not always categorized easily by one dimension. In speaking with a patient who has breakthrough bone pain, he/she may have difficulty deciding whether the severity or frequency or both are important. This has led to interest in the use of multidimensional symptom instruments, such as the memorial symptom assessment scale (MSAS).

To summarize, potentially important dimensions of a symptom include frequency, severity, distress, duration, and associated meanings.

TYPES OF RESPONSE CATEGORIES

Visual analog scales—The symptom of interest is represented by a straight line 10 cm long. Anchors are no symptom on one end, and worst on the other end. The patient marks off with a straight line the severity of the symptom. Horizontal and vertical VAS scales have been described. Visual analog scales are one of the oldest forms of symptom assessment approaches, and have the advantage of providing a continuous variable for subsequent analyses.[30] VAS scales have been used for many symptoms. Disadvantages include a tendency for the marks to bunch up in the middle, and physical problems completing the form in patients with impaired eyesight and/or motor disability. Mechanical VAS scales have been described, where patients move a marker along the line.

Numerical rating scale—Patients are asked to rate the symptom on a numerical scale, such as 0–5 or 0–10. However, not all patients are able to express themselves numerically. In one study, 10% of hospice patients were unable to use a numerical rating scale for pain.[31]

Categorical rating scales—Patients are asked to categorize the symptom by severity or other attributes. The simplest is a dichotomous response, yes/no. These categories often are none, a little bit, somewhat, quite a bit, and very much in the Likert version. Other categories have also been described. This presents an alternative for patients who cannot give numerical values.

Ranking—Patients are asked to rank symptoms in order of priority. This provides a different way of characterizing symptoms, and may help the interviewer set priorities for symptom control. Patients in palliative care may have many severe symptoms and may have difficulty ranking symptoms.

Pictorial approaches—Best known examples include the FACES design for children[32] and the use of symbols such as fire to characterize intensity. These approaches are appropriate in populations where the ability to read may be a barrier.

Descriptors—Patients select from a list of adjectives to capture qualitative aspects of the symptoms.

Cutpoints—Where the response is given as a numerical value, the cutpoint helps to identify a threshold number where the interpretation or clinical importance of the rating changes. Usually, a cutpoint is where severity of the symptom changes markedly from mild to moderate, or moderate becomes severe.[33] Cutpoints for pain, fatigue, and additional symptoms have been derived on the basis of interference caused by the symptom with daily activities.[34]

SINGLE SYMPTOM VERSUS MULTISYMPTOM INSTRUMENTS

Many instruments are devoted to information about one symptom. Because palliative care patients may have multiple symptoms, instruments that assess multiple symptoms have been developed. A related question is how many symptoms should be routinely covered? By the time patients reach palliative care status, patient stamina can last for 5–10 questions at most. Many symptoms—pain, tiredness, nausea, difficulty sleeping, drowsiness, dry mouth, shortness of breath, and sadness—are common to most of the multisymptom instruments.

SPECIFIC SYMPTOM INSTRUMENTS

A very large number of instruments have been developed. This section presents information on many widely used instruments, but there are few, if any standard instruments.

Appetite

Visual analog scale, a 10 cm line, where the left represented no appetite and the right anchor was 100% appetite[35].

The *North Central Cancer Treatment Group* patient questionnaire[36] has seven items and a VAS score for quality of life.

The *functional assessment of appetite cancer therapy.*[37] Subscale has 12 items rated on a Likert score.

Constipation

The *constipation assessment scale* is a validated eight-item scale for the assessment of constipation in cancer patients.[38]

Delirium

The *confusion assessment method*[39,40] is based upon DSM-III criteria and nonpsychiatrist clinicians can use an algorithm of four items—acute onset and fluctuating course, inattention, either altered level of consciousness or disorganized thinking. The CAM has been translated into German,[41] Korean,[42] and

Portuguese,[43] and versions have been developed for adult ICU (the CAM-ICU)[44] and pediatric ICU patients.[45]

The *delirium rating scale*[46] is a ten-item instrument with clinician rated symptoms. The delirium rating scale has been translated into Japanese[47] and validated for adolescents.[48] A revised longer 16-item version has been developed with improved sensitivity and specificity.[49] The DRS-98 has been translated into Chinese,[50] Dutch,[51] Japanese,[52] Korean,[53] and Portuguese[54] and studied in the pediatric population.[55]

The *memorial delirium assessment scale*[56] (MDAS) is a ten-item tool, which can be used for diagnosis, severity, and repeated assessments. A cutoff score of 13 is diagnostic, and a cutoff score of 7 has been proposed for advanced cancer patients in a palliative care setting.[57] The MDAS has been translated into Italian[58] and Japanese[59] and studied in an intensive care unit[60] and at a tertiary referral center.[61]

The *mini mental status exam*[62] was originally developed as a screening test for dementia, and has been used as a screen for other cognitive dysfunction. Norms should be adjusted for age and educational level.[63,64] The instrument has been translated into Chinese,[65] French,[66] Gujarati,[67] Hebrew,[68] Hindi,[69] Japanese,[70] Korean,[71] Sinhalese,[72] and Spanish[73] and shorter versions developed with IRT approaches.[74,75]

Other special situations include hepatic encephalopathy in patients with advanced liver disease.[76]

In a comparison of 12 different delirium tools, the CAM was felt to be the best diagnostic tool and the delirium rating scale best for screening symptom severity. The CAM-ICU was recommended for ICU patients and the MDAS for cancer patients.[77] A recent systematic review also supported use of the CAM.[78]

Depression

Depression instruments have served primarily as screening instruments, and for epidemiologic surveys.

Single-item *visual analog scales* have correlated well with depression tools.[79]

Screening questions—Single[80] and two question screens[81] have been validated. In one literature review of depression screening tools for use in a palliative care population, the authors concluded that the single questions "Are you depressed" had the highest sensitivity and specificity, and identified cutoff values of 20 for the hospital anxiety and depression scale, and 13 for the Edinburgh postnatal depression scale.[82] This still remains an area for further study.

The *Beck depression inventory*[83] is a 21-item instrument where the patient rates the severity of attitudes and symptoms over a 1-week period. In 1996, the Beck depression inventory II was released to conform to the DSM IV criteria[84]. The Beck depression inventory has been translated into modern standard Arabic,[85] Chinese,[86] German,[87] Greek,[88] Icelandic,[89] Japanese,[90] Persian,[91] Russian,[92] and Spanish.[93]

The *Center for Epidemiologic Studies on Depression*[94] is a validated instrument with 20 items and asks for patient-rated frequency and has been studied in cancer patients. The CES-D

has been translated into Brazilian Portuguese,[95] Chinese,[96] Greek,[97] Italian,[98] Japanese,[99] Spanish,[100] and Turkish.[101] A 10-item version has been introduced[102].

The *geriatric depression scale*[103] is a 30-item instrument, which can be administered by telephone[104] and has been translated into Chinese,[105] Hindi,[106] Spanish,[107] Swedish,[108] and Turkish.[109] A geriatric depression scale short form with 15 items has been validated[110] and translated into Arabic,[111] Danish,[112] French,[113] Greek,[114] Korean,[115,116] Persian,[117] and Spanish.[118] IRT analysis led to a seven-item version for Asian patients[119]. A shorter five-item version has been reported[120] and translated into Chinese.[121] The GDS may not be valid in patients with moderate to severe dementia.

The *Hamilton depression rating scale*[122] is a 17-item severity rated scale and is widely used in trials of antidepressants. It has been translated into Chinese[123] and Turkish.[124] A six-item version has been developed.[125] This instrument has been validated in advanced cancer patients.[126]

The *hospital anxiety depression scale* (HADS) is a validated instrument that has two subscales.[127] Patients rate frequency of symptoms for 14 items, 7 related to anxiety and 7 for depression. The HADS is widely used in Europe, and has been translated into Arabic,[128] Chinese,[129] French,[130] German,[131,132] Hungarian,[133] Japanese,[134] Malayalam,[135] Maltese,[136] Persian,[137] and Spanish.[138]

The *Zung* self-rating depression scale is a 20-item instrument.[139] The Zung scale has been translated into Arabic,[140] Chinese,[141] Czech,[142] Dutch,[143] Finnish,[144] Greek,[145] studied in India,[146] and Spanish.[147] A shorter 12-item version has been translated into Dutch.[148] Both have been validated in ambulatory cancer patients.[149,150]

The PHQ 9 is a criterion-based instrument that has been widely used in general medicine settings as a screening tool for depression.[151,152] The PHQ-9 has been translated into Chinese,[153] Korean,[154] and Thai,[155] and implemented in India[156] and Kenya.[157] It has been used to screen for depression in cardiac[158] and palliative care populations.[159] A two-item version, the PHQ2, has also been developed.[160]

An area of ongoing interest is the applicability of these tools in palliative care patients. The cutoff points have not been derived for palliative care patients, and that the patient's self report may be influenced by stress and the desire to be socially acceptable.[161]

Dysphagia

Most studies have used an ordinal scale for measuring dysphagia in five categories, no symptoms, can take solids, can take soft food, can take liquids, cannot swallow at all. Many studies do not specify whether this is patient rated or observer rated. The EORTC and the FACIT have each introduced modules for malignant dysphagia.[162,163]

Dyspnea

The *Borg scale* measures symptoms with a vertical scale from zero to ten anchored by descriptive words, and requires an exertional test.[164]

A visual analog scale is a validated measure of dyspnea,[165] as is a numeric rating scale.[166]

The *chronic respiratory questionnaire*[167] and the *St. George's respiratory questionnaire*[168] are quality of life instruments for patients with Chronic Obstructive Pulmonary Disease (COPD), with an emphasis on dyspnea. The chronic respiratory questionnaire has 20 items and has been translated into Arabic (Moroccan),[169] Chinese,[170] German,[171] Japanese,[172] Portuguese,[173] and Spanish.[174] A shorter version of the chronic respiratory questionnaire has been developed.[175]

The *St. George's respiratory questionnaire* has 50 items and has been translated into American English,[176] Chinese (Cantonese),[177] Chinese (Mandarin),[178] French,[179] Japanese, Persian,[180] Polish,[181] Portuguese,[173] Spanish,[182] and Swedish.[183] The minimal important difference for the St. George's is estimated at 4 on a scale of 0–100.[184]

Descriptions of many other instruments can be found in the following reviews.[185–188]

Fatigue

To date, most measures of fatigue have been based on cancer-related fatigue.

A *single item* of distress from fatigue correlated well with responses to the brief fatigue inventory and the FACIT Fatigue model.[189]

The *numeric rating scale* (0–10) has been studied as part of the brief fatigue inventory. A cutoff for worst fatigue of three or usual fatigue of two separates mild from moderate fatigue.[190]

The *brief fatigue inventory*[191] assesses fatigue severity and interference with a numeric rating scale. It has been translated into Chinese,[192,193] Filipino,[194] Italian,[195] German,[196] Greek,[197] Japanese,[198] and Korean.[199]

The *piper revised fatigue scale*[200] contains 22 items and four subscales: behavioral/severity, affective meaning, sensory, and cognitive/mood. It has been translated into Chinese,[201] Dutch,[202] French,[203] Italian,[204,205] and Swedish.[206]

The *FACIT fatigue module*[207] is a 13-item subscale with Likert responses that has been used for epidemiologic purposes and as an outcome measure in clinical trials.

Readers are referred to articles for more detailed reviews.[208–211]

Nausea

The development of a solid accepted methodology for measuring chemotherapy-related nausea and vomiting, and response has helped advance the field of palliating chemotherapy-related emesis. Nausea is measured with a VAS and vomiting is quantitated as the number of episodes per 24 hours period.[212]

Pain

VAS scale—A mark of more than 30 mm is more than mild pain.[213] A clinically significant change was estimated at 13 mm for patients with initial VAS scores of 34 and 28 mm for patients with initial VAS scores greater than 67.[214]

Numerical rating scale of 0–10—Analysis of pain severity in a multinational sample suggests that 1–4 may be mild pain, 5–6 moderate pain, and 7–10 severe pain.[215] Changes in severity of two may correspond to a minimally clinically significant difference.[216,217] Pain reports on numerical scales and VAS are comparable.[218]

The *brief pain inventory*[219] and the brief pain inventory short form is a widely used validated pain instrument. The instrument contains a body diagram, NRS ratings of pain severity, relief, and interference with function. The BPI has been translated into Chinese,[220,221] German,[222] Greek,[223] Hindi,[224] Italian,[225] Japanese,[226] Norwegian,[227] Spanish,[228] and additional languages.[229]

The *McGill pain questionnaire*[230] has a present pain intensity item, and 20 sets of descriptors to assess for sensory, affective, and evaluative components of pain. It has been translated into Amharic,[231] Arabic,[232] Brazilian Portuguese,[233] Chinese,[234] Danish,[235,236] Dutch,[237] Finnish,[238] Flemish, French,[239] German,[240,241] Greek,[242] Italian, Japanese,[243,244] Norwegian,[245] Polish, Slovak,[246] Spanish.[247,248] The McGill short form has 17 items: present pain intensity, pain severity VAS, and ratings of 15 descriptors.[249] It has been translated into Czech,[250] Greek,[251] Persian,[252] Swedish,[253] and Turkish.[254]

The *memorial pain assessment card*[255] has one item for each of the dimensions of severity, mood, relief, and a set of descriptors, and has been translated into Spanish.[256,257]

Neuropathic pain scales have been developed where patients rate the presence and severity of pain descriptors. The purpose of these research scales has been to screen for neuropathic pain, or to provide a fuller measurement.[258] These include the *neuropathic pain scale*,[259] the *Leeds assessment of neuropathic signs and symptoms*,[260] (translated into Arabic,[261] Spanish,[262] and Turkish[263]) and the *neuropathic pain questionnaire*.[264]

An important new area for oncologists is the recognition of chemotherapy-related peripheral neuropathy. Two instruments are widely used in studies, the *EORTC chemotherapy-induced peripheral neuropathy scale*,[265] and the *FACT neurotoxicity subscale*.[266]

Breakthrough pain continues to be assessed with the *breakthrough pain questionnaire*,[267] and a pediatric version has been developed.[268] No standard instrument exists.[269]

MULTIPLE SYMPTOM INSTRUMENTS

Originally developed for cancer patients, these instruments are being studied and adapted for patients with other advanced illnesses. This section provides some of the more widely used instruments; readers are referred to Kirkova for a more detailed review.[270]

Symptom distress scale

The symptom distress scale (SDS) introduced the concept of distress to symptom assessment.[271] The SDS has 13 items, with 11 symptoms; pain and nausea are each assessed twice. Variations include the adapted symptom distress scale[272] and the symptom experience scale.[273] The adapted symptom distress scale has 31 items for 14 symptoms, and includes symptom occurrence. The SDS has been translated into Chinese,[274] Dutch, Italian,[275] Korean,[276] Spanish, and Swedish.[277] The SDS has been studied in patients receiving cancer chemotherapy, home care,[275] and a variety of other settings.

Edmonton symptom assessment scale

The *Edmonton symptom assessment scale*[278] (ESAS) is a nine-item validated VAS scale with eight symptoms and a well-being item[279,280,281]; a newer version, the ESAS r, with a numerical rating scale and brief definitions of symptoms has been recently unveiled.[282] French,[283] Italian,[284] Norwegian,[285] Spanish,[286] Thai,[287] Flemish,[288] and German[289] versions have been developed. The ESAS has been studied in multiple settings, including hospice, palliative care consultation teams,[290] home care,[291] quality improvement,[390] and the Intensive Care Unit[292].

MD Anderson symptom inventory

The *MD Anderson symptom inventory*[293] was derived from hierarchical cluster analysis on patient responses. A core number of 14 items accounted for 64% of the variance in symptom distress. Patients are asked to rate the severity of 13 symptoms and 6 interference items with a numeric rating scale. It has been translated into Arabic,[294] Chinese,[295] French,[296] Japanese,[297] and Russian.[298]

Memorial symptom assessment scale

The MSAS is a validated patient-rated instrument in which patients rate symptom severity, distress, and frequency for 32 highly prevalent physical and psychological symptoms.[299,300] Each symptom is rated on a Likert scale and scored from 0 to 4 ranging from "no symptom" to "very much." The MSAS subscales include: the global distress index (GDI), the physical symptom distress (PHYS), the psychological symptom distress (PSYCH). In the MSAS Short Form, patients rate symptom distress for physical symptoms and symptom frequency for psychological symptoms.[301] In the condensed MSAS, the number of items has been reduced to 14.[302] The MSAS has been used in cancer chemotherapy,[303] hospital settings,[304] hospice,[305] intensive care unit,[306] patients with hematologic malignancies,[307] heart failure,[308] chronic obstructive pulmonary disease,[309] chronic renal disease,[310] and in longitudinal studies.[311] The minimal CSD has been estimated for the MSAS Short Form.[312] A caregiver version[313] and a children's version have been developed.[314] There are translated versions in Arabic (Lebanese),[315] Chinese,[316,317] Turkish,[318] Arabic (Israeli), Dutch, English, French, German, Hebrew, Italian, Polish, Spanish, and Turkish.[319]

Rotterdam symptom checklist

The *Rotterdam symptom checklist*[320] is a validated 34-item instrument where patients rate distress. A physical and a psychological symptom subscale are described. It has been translated into French,[321] Italian,[322] Spanish,[323] and Turkish.[324] A modified version has been validated in an American population of cancer patients.[325] This instrument has been used extensively in European cancer chemotherapy trials and symptom intervention studies.

APPLICATIONS OF SYMPTOM INSTRUMENTS

Epidemiology and descriptive studies—Symptom surveys with the ESAS, MSAS, and other instruments have established that multiple symptoms are highly prevalent. Descriptive longitudinal studies with symptom instruments are now being reported.[311,326,327]

Improvement of Symptom recognition—Surveys of symptom data concurrently gathered with the symptom tools show that routine symptom assessment by doctors and nurses often misses significant data.[328-331] There is a growing consensus that the use of symptom instruments is feasible and contributes important information.

Clinical Trials—Symptom instruments have been used as outcome measures of clinical trials (see section on responsiveness)

Patient-rated adverse events—The National Cancer Institute has incorporated patient-reported symptoms as part of the toxicity assessment for clinical trials.[332]

Drug labeling indications—The Food and Drug Administration and the European Medicine Agency have provided guidance for industry on the role of symptom assessment measurements in pharmaceutical trials.[333,334]

Patient prioritization—One British study used data from a symptom checklist to suggest that patients with lung cancer or brain tumors should be high priority for specialist palliative care.[335] Another British study found differences in symptom patterns by service component of patients referred to a hospice inpatient service, a community team, an NHS hospital support team, and an outpatient service, suggesting that different symptom management strategies may be needed for different patient groups.[336]

Prognosis—Patient ratings of symptoms can add prognostic information. In studies of patients with cancer, individual symptoms as well as combinations of symptoms provide prognostic information in addition to that provided by the Karnofsky performance score.[337] Physical symptoms may carry more of the prognostic information.[338]

Symptom clusters—Factor analyses with the MSAS, Rotterdam symptom check list, and the Canberra symptom scorecard[339] have shown two major groups of symptoms—physical and psychological symptoms. The use of multisymptom instruments is a logical step in establishing the presence of these clusters.[340]

Symptom burden—Patient ratings of symptom severity and interference have enabled measurements of symptom burden, a concept that is easy to understand and clinically useful.[341,342]

Quality of care—Tools may also be important to the program as evidence for the quality of care given, where the act of symptom assessment is taken as the process. In this concept, tools may be important as a way of evaluating the structure of the program.[343] More recently, symptom assessment has become an integral part of quality of care standards by many organizations within the United States, including the National Quality Forum.[344]

Treatment Outcome—Tools can serve by recording the outcomes of symptom management.

Symptom monitoring—The combination of symptom tools and new computerized technology has led to the concept of symptom monitoring.[345] A symptom monitoring program could cover more areas of patient concern, identify symptoms before they become severe, complement measures of tumor response, and assist in clinical decision making.

Studying the relationship of symptoms to other concepts—Studying the relationship of symptoms to other aspects of palliative care, such as spirituality[346] and dignity.[347]

SPECIAL POPULATIONS

In patients who are unable to communicate, the ascertainment of symptoms becomes more difficult. This is especially true for the pediatric, geriatric, and intensive care unit populations. One approach has been the development of behavioral measures of pain, which can be recorded by observers.

For pediatric patients, behavioral scales include the FLACC,[348] and for demented patients, the PainAD[349] and pain assessment for the dementing elderly.[350] Pain behaviors have been described for ICU patients.[351]

More recent recommendations have included a hierarchy of approaches, whereby findings with these and other instruments are combined with other clinical data.[352]

PRACTICAL ISSUES

The selection of tools for pain and symptom assessment reflects a balance, as elsewhere, between what is possible and what is desirable. These considerations include the nature of the organization, and the uses to which the information from the tool will be put.

Research and practical tools

The difference between research and practical tools lies in their purpose and function. Most instruments in use started out as research tools to better describe symptom(s). As such, these reflected concepts about the symptom, tended to be longer, studied healthier patients, were administered by research personnel. These studies have provided many insights into symptom epidemiology and their relationship to other aspects of patient experience, and demonstrated feasibility. In the clinical context, pragmatism is emphasized, and time and personnel are limited. As instruments are converted from research to

clinical application, there is then an evolutionary pressure for the development of shorter and simpler instruments that can be rapidly administered and interpreted.

Research	Practical
Comprehensive	Screening
Based upon specific theories	Empirical
Longer	Shorter
Wide choice of answers	Yes/No
Specific	Global
Multiple item	Single item
Patient rated	Observer rated

Patient stamina is decisive. Many terminally ill patients may be unable to answer more than a handful of questions. In one study of patients with terminal cancer at an American hospital, only half were able to complete one of the three instruments offered—the McGill pain questionnaire, the memorial pain assessment card, or the faces pain rating scale.[353] In a study of hospice inpatients, only 30 out of 71 patients with pain were available to participate in a study where they were asked to answer a six-item questionnaire about pain, with each item scaled from 0 to 10. The ratings were completed without difficulty and showed good reproducibility after 1 hour.[354]

Availability of instruments

In addition to the time honored practice of contacting the developers of an instrument or finding the journal, many instruments may be viewed on websites. These include the American Thoracic Society web page (www.atsqol.org), the Center to Advance Palliative Care (www.capc.org), the International Hospice Association (www.hospicecare.com), the MAPI Research Institute (www.mapi-research-inst.com, www.qolid.org), the Regional Palliative Care Program in Edmonton, Alberta (www.palliative.org), the Robert Wood Johnson Promoting Excellence in End of Life Care (www.promotingexcellence.org), and the Toolkit of instruments to measure end-of-life care (www.chcr.brown.edu/pcoc/Physical.htm).

Another source for symptom items can be quality of life instruments, such as the FACT system,[355] the EORTC QLQ-C30,[356] and the RAI-PC[357] which have developed disease-related modules. The first two have been translated into many languages and have symptom items. More recently, PROMIS and pro-CTCAE items have become available and may be helpful.

Choosing an instrument

Criteria for an ideal pain instrument, as listed by Chapman and Syralja, apply for symptom instruments in general. These criteria include (1) minimal patient burden, (2) understandable by patients, (3) produce a wide range of scores, (4) sensitive to interventions, (5) demonstrate appropriate reliability and validity, and (6) availability of appropriate norms.

Their principles of selection are equally applicable. These ultimately depend on the needs of the clinician and limitations of the patient population. The principles include (1) defining the goal of assessment (complexity of problem and information required), (2) deciding which dimensions are appropriate for the problem at hand (severity, behavior, and function), (3) selecting subparts of instruments most suitable, (4) considering the development of a clinical database—layout to be suitable for analyses, (5) considering automated data collection, (6) avoiding too much data, (7) being sure the test instruments fit the patient population, and (8) taking care to collect responses to all items on the forms.[358]

For newer palliative care programs, selecting a short and easily available tool is a good starting point after assessing initial goals. For research purposes, the instrument is guided by the underlying scientific question and the type of measurement needed. For pharmaceutical trials, current recommendations are influenced by regulatory guidelines.[359] These include developing a model of how components of patient-reported outcomes are expected to change, and selection of tools accordingly.[360]

Sometimes the question arises as to when a new tool is needed. Despite the large number already developed, for a particular research question, there may not be an available instrument. Depending upon the circumstances and resources available, one may take a standard instrument with additional items,[15] adapt an instrument from another field, or start afresh.[361,362]

Caregivers and patients ratings

Ideally, patients should be the source of information about symptoms, but become unable near the end of life. The role of caregivers or other proxies in symptom assessment has been an area of ongoing research and studied with symptom scales.[363–366]

Mode of administration

Tools were originally completed by the patient, or an interviewer, and it is helpful to check the patient's understanding of the items.[367] For pencil and paper instruments, checking the forms for missing items after a patient has finished can save time. Tools can now be completed by the patient in a variety of ways including pen and paper, telephone, computer, internet, interactive voice response, touch tablet,[368] and other modalities. Much recent research has been on the feasibility of obtaining symptom data by different forms of electronic interface.[369] The flexibility of modern information technology will enable symptom assessment on a large scale and in new ways.[370]

Translation of instruments

Even within the same language, symptoms and aspects of symptoms may be difficult to describe for the purposes of a symptom questionnaire (e.g., British vs American English).

These problems are magnified further when translations are attempted as different connotations may be associated with the symptom or the items in the second language.[371] However, it may be easier to translate an instrument than to develop one.

If the reader would like to translate an instrument, it is advisable to work with the group that developed the original instrument. The instrument is translated into the new language, then back-translated into the original language by a second team, and then retranslated into the new language by a third team. After each translation, the instrument is reviewed again.[372] Newer guidelines have been developed[373] including manuals[374,375] and the subject recently reviewed.[376,377]

Validation

In a new population, or with a new language, the tool should be validated. A representative sample of at least 40 patients should complete the tool, a reference tool known to be valid, and have their performance status and demographic data recorded. Practical aspects, such as ease of administration and comprehension, should also be recorded. These data can then be analyzed for validity.[16] For instruments to be used in multinational trials, a sample size of 200 patients has been recommended.[378]

Implementation of tools

Many palliative care professionals are not familiar with symptom instruments.[379] Principles of implementation by Higginson[380] are applicable to symptom tools. These include

1. Measures that form a part of treatment planning and evaluation are more likely to influence clinical decision making than monitoring alone.
2. Are the symptoms relevant?
3. How long does it take to complete?
4. Will it measure differences?
5. Who will use the measures?
6. Involve staff and patients.
7. Plan and begin training in both the use of the measure and associated clinical skills. I would add that a plan of action for symptom control should be in place or no improvements will result.

Subsequent experience has led to additional emphasis on understanding the purpose and context of implementation, and attention to how the data will be gathered and reported.[381] The perspective of symptom assessment implementation as a modification, and requiring the support, of a health care system will be increasingly relevant.[382]

UNEXPLORED AREAS/FUTURE DIRECTIONS

With the increasing importance of symptom assessment and other patient-reported outcomes for clinical use, health services research, and intervention trials, and the availability of newer methodologies and modes of administration, symptom assessment will be an active area for the foreseeable future.

An emerging area will be deciding what kind of symptom assessment, and instrument, and method of administration is most applicable for palliative care patients. A second area is the implementation of symptom assessment into the field of palliative medicine, and into general medical practice. A third area will be finding where IRT-developed approaches fit into the general world of symptom assessment instruments. A fourth area will be how the large scale of symptom data acquisition made possible by informatics will affect symptom analysis and management. A fifth area may be reconciling the different demands put upon symptom instruments as the result of more stringent development criteria, different applications (e.g., screening vs clinical trial), and different populations. A sixth area will be whether the number of instruments continues to increase, or some form of consolidation starts to take place. A seventh area is whether the distinction between quality of life and symptom assessment remains. An eighth area to follow will be to what extent instruments originally designed for advanced cancer patients can be used in patients with other advanced illnesses.

PROPOSE AN IDEAL TOOL PACKAGE WITH GOOD PSYCHOMETRIC PROPERTIES AND MINIMAL OVERLAP

How is it done at certain centers?

MD Anderson[383]: ESAS, mini-mental status exam, CAGE questionnaire,[384] Morphine equivalent daily dose, Functional Impairment Measure[385]

Institut Jules Bordet[386]: Mini-mental status exam, MDAS, Edmonton functional assessment tool,[387] ESAS

University of Cologne[388]: Mini-mental status exam, brief pain inventory, medical outcome study short form-12[389]

Duke University[390]: FACT G, FACIT F, MDASI

Ontario Province Palliative Care Improvement Project[382]: ESAS

How to select a tool

No instrument is perfect and the package depends upon the local needs of the patients (types of disease and prevalence of symptoms) and resources available to the staff (manpower, time) and purpose (research or practice or screening).

Areas of practical interest at intake include the ability of the patient to make decisions, the presence of key symptoms, and a performance status rating. Additional instruments can be added depending upon the interest of the group. At follow-up, we need to screen for new symptoms, and determine if older symptoms have changed.

If the reader is planning to set up a palliative care program, it is better to select an available validated instrument (or module) and add items than to pick and choose items from different

tools. The reader may wish to try out different tools on a few patients to see which one works best in terms of comprehension and ease of administration.

Possible combinations are presented in the following:

	Better KPS Research	Worse KPS (KPS < 50%) Practice/Screening
Symptoms	RSCL, MSAS	ESAS, CMSAS, SDS, MDASI
Pain	BPI, McGill SF	Numeric Rating Scale
Depression	HADS	Screening questions PHQ 9
Noncommunicative	PAINAD	PAINAD
Mental Status	CAM	CAM
		MDAS

SUMMARY

Many validated and reliable tools are available for many symptoms, as well as for multiple symptoms. Responsiveness is being established.

The usefulness and validity of these tools in different populations continues to require further study.

The items of the symptom instruments selected should be perceived as useful, easy to understand, easy to answer, and easy to interpret. Follow-up plans for symptom treatment should be developed.

Symptom tools are versatile in their applications.

The choice of symptom tools depends on the priorities set by the palliative care staff and the stamina of the patients.

Application of these instruments to clinical care is the next challenge.

REFERENCES

1 Patrick DL, Ferketich SL, Frame PS et al. National Institutes of Health State-of-the-Science Panel. National Institutes of Health State-of-the-Science Conference Statement: Symptom Management in Cancer: Pain, Depression, and Fatigue, July 15–17, 2002. *J Natl Cancer Inst* 2003;**95**:1110–1117.

2 National Consensus Project. *Clinical Practice Guidelines for Quality Palliative Care.* New York: National Consensus Project for Quality Palliative Care. www.nationalconsensusproject.org. 3rd edition, 2013, accessed June 9, 2014.

3 de Vet HCW, Terwee CB, and Bouter LM. Current challenges in clinimetrics. *J Clin Epidemiol* 2003;**56**:1137–1141.

4 Feinstein AR. *Clinical Epidemiology.* Philadelphia, PA: WB Saunders Co., 1985.

5 Feinstein AR. Multi-item "instruments" vs Virgina Apgar's principles of clinimetrics. *Arch Intern Med* 1999;**159**:125–128.

6 Cella D, Riley W, Stone A et al.; PROMIS Cooperative Group. The patient-reported outcomes measurement information system (PROMIS) developed and tested its first wave of adult self-reported health outcome item banks: 2005–2008. *J Clin Epidemiol* 2010;**63**:1179–1194.

7 Kaasa S, Loge JH, Fayers P, Caraceni A, Strasser F, Hjermstad MJ, Higginson I, Radbruch L, and Haugen DF. Symptom assessment in palliative care: A need for international collaboration. *J Clin Oncol* 2008;**26**:3867–3873.

8 Hays RD, Morales LS, and Reise SP. Item response theory and health outcomes measurement in the 21st century. *Med Care* 2000;**38**(9 Suppl. 2):28–42.

● 9 Hambleton RK and Swaminathan H. *Item Response Theory: Principles and Applications.* Norwell, MA: Kluwer Academic Publishers, 1985.

10 Embretson SE and Reise SP. *Item Response Theory for Psychologists.* Mahwah, NJ: Lawrence Erlbaum Associates, 2000.

11 Streiner DL and Norman GR. Health measurement scales. *A Practical Guide to Their Development and Use*, 4th edn. New York: Oxford University Press, 2008.

12 Educational Research Association, American Psychological Association, and National Council on Measurement in Education. *Standards for Educational and Psychological Testing.* Washington, DC: American Educational Research Association, 1999.

13 Sloan JA, Halyard MY, Frost MH, Dueck AC, Teschendorf B, Rothman ML; Mayo/FDA Patient-Reported Outcomes Consensus Meeting Group. The Mayo Clinic manuscript series relative to the discussion, dissemination, and operationalization of the food and drug administration guidance on patient-reported outcomes. *Value Health* 2007;**10**:S59–S63.

14 Mokkink LB, Terwee CB, Patrick DL et al. The COSMIN study reached international consensus on taxonomy, terminology, and definitions of measurement properties for health-related patient-reported outcomes. *J Clin Epidemiol* 2010;**63**:737–745.

15 Rothman M, Burke L, Erickson P, Leidy NK, Patrick DL, and Petrie CD. Use of existing patient-reported outcome (PRO) instruments and their modification: The ISPOR good research practices for evaluating and documenting content validity for the use of existing instruments and their modification PRO task force report. *Value Health* 2009;**12**(8):1075–1083.

16 Jensen MP. Questionnaire validation: A brief guide for readers of the research literature. *Clin J Pain* 2003;**19**:345–352.

17 Jensen MP and Karoly P. Self-report scales and procedures for assessing pain in adults. In Turk DC, Melzack R (eds.), *Handbook of Pain Assessment*, 2nd edn. New York: The Guilford Press, 2001, p. 15.

18 Hjermstad MJ, Gibbins J, Haugen DF et al.; EPCRC, European Palliative Care Research Collaborative. Pain assessment tools in palliative care: An urgent need for consensus. *Palliat Med* 2008;**22**:895–903.

19 Nelson CJ, Cho C, Berk AR et al. Are gold standard depression measures appropriate for use in geriatric cancer patients? A systematic evaluation of self-report depression instruments used with geriatric, cancer, and geriatric cancer samples. *J Clin Oncol* 2010;**28**:348–356.

● 20 Coons SJ, Gwaltney CJ, Hays RD, Lundy JJ, Sloan JA, Revicki DA, Lenderking WR, Cella D, Basch E; ISPOR ePRO Task Force. Recommendations on evidence needed to support measurement equivalence between electronic and paper-based patient-reported outcome (PRO) measures: ISPOR ePRO good research practices task force report. *Value Health* 2009;**12**(4):419–429.

21 Pickering RM. Statistical aspects of measurement. *Palliat Med* 2002;**16**:359–364.

22 Jaeschke R, Singer J, and Guyatt GH. Measurement of health status: Ascertaining the minimal clinically important difference. *Control Clin Trials* 1989;**10**:407–415.

◆ 23 Guyatt GH, Osoba D, Wu AW et al. Methods to explain the clinical significane of health status measures. *Mayo Clin Proc* 2002;**77**:371–383.

◆ 24 Sprangers MA, Moinpour CM, Moynihan TJ et al. Assessing meaningful change in quality of life over time: A users' guide for clinicians. *Mayo Clin Proc* 2002;**77**:561–571.

● 25 Norman GR, Sloan JA, and Wyrwich KW. Interpretation of changes in health-related quality of life: The remarkable universality of half a standard deviation. *Med Care* 2003;**41**:582–592.

◆ 26 Revicki D, Hays R, Cella D et al. Recommended methods for determining responsiveness and minimally important differences for patient reported outcomes. *J Clin Epidemiol* 2008;**61**:102–109.

27 Kirshner B and Guyatt G. A methodological framework for assessing health indices. *J Chronic Dis* 1985;**38**:27–36.

28 Guyatt GH, Townsend M, Berman LB, and Keller JL. A comparison of Likert and visual analogue scales for measuring change in function. *J Chronic Dis* 1987;**40**:1129–1133.

29 Guyatt GH, Norman GR, Juniper EF, and Griffith LE. A critical look at transition ratings. *J Clin Epidemiol* 2002;**55**:900–908.

30 McCormack HM, Horne DJ, and Sheather S. Clinical applications of visual analogue scales. A critical review. *Psychol Med* 1988;**18**:1007–1019.

31 Sze FK, Chung TK, Wong E et al. Pain in chinese cancer patients under palliative care. *Palliat Med* 1998;**12**:271–277.

32 Bieri D, Reeve RA, Champion GD et al. The faces pain scale for the self-assessment of the severity of pain experienced by children: Development, initial validation, and preliminary investigation for ratio scale properties. *Pain* 1990;**41**:139–150.

● 33 Serlin RC, Mendoza TR, Nakamura Y, Edwards KR, and Cleeland CS. When is cancer pain mild, moderate or severe? Grading pain severity by its interference with function. *Pain* 1995;**61**:277–284.

34 Jeon S, Given CW, Sikorskii A, and Given B. Do interference-based cut-points differentiate mild, moderate, and severe levels of 16 cancer-related symptoms over time? *J Pain Symptom Manage* 2009;**37**:220–232.

35 Coates A, Dillenbeck CF, McNeil DR et al. On the receiving end—II. Linear analogue self-assessment (LASA) in evaluation of aspects of the quality of life of cancer patients receiving therapy. *Eur J Cancer Clin Oncol* 1983;**19**:1633–1637.

36 Loprinzi CL, Sloan JA, and Rowland KM, Jr. Methodologic issues regarding cancer anorexia/cachexia trials. In Portenoy RK, Bruera E (eds.), *Research and Palliative Care: Methodologies and Outcomes.* New York: Oxford University Press, 2003, pp. 25–40.

37 Ribaudo JM, Cella D, Hahn EA et al. Re-validation and shortening of the functional assessment of anorexia/cachexia therapy (FAACT). *Qual Life Res* 2000;**9**:1137–1146.

● 38 McMillan SC and Williams FA. Validity and reliability of the constipation assessment scale. *Cancer Nurs* 1989;**12**:183–188.

● 39 Inouye SK, van Dyck CG, Alessi CA et al. Clarifying confusion: The confusion assessment method. *Ann Intern Med* 1990;**113**:941–948.

40 Wei LA, Fearing MA, Sternberg EJ, and Inouye SK. The confusion assessment method: A systematic review of current usage. *J Am Geriatr Soc* 2008;**56**:823–830.

41 Hestermann U, Backenstrass M, Gekle I et al. Validation of a German version of the confusion assessment method for delirium detection in a sample of acute geriatric patients with a high prevalence of dementia. *Psychopathology* 2009;**42**:270–276.

42 Heo EY, Lee BJ, Hahm BJ et al. Translation and validation of the Korean confusion assessment method for the intensive care unit. *BMC Psychiatry* 2011;**11**:94.

43 Fabbri RM, Moreira MA, Garrido R, and Almeida OP. Validity and reliability of the Portuguese version of the confusion assessment method (CAM) for the detection of delirium in the elderly. *Arq Neuropsiquiatr* 2001;**59**(2-A):175–179.

44 Ely EW, Inouye SK, Bernard GR et al. Delirium in mechanically ventilated patients: Validity and reliability of the confusion assessment method for the intensive care unit (CAM-ICU). *JAMA* 2001;**286**:2703–2710.

45 Smith HA, Boyd J, Fuchs DC et al. Diagnosing delirium in criti-
    cally ill children: Validity and reliability of the pediatric confu-
    sion assessment method for the intensive care unit. *Crit Care Med*
    2011;**39**:150–157.

● 46 Trzepacz PT, Baker RW, and Greenhouse J. A symptom rating scale
        for delirium. *Psychiat Res* 1988;**1**:89–97.

47 Isse K, Uchiyama M, Tanaka K et al. Delirium: Clinical find-
    ings and its neuro-psychological etiology. *Rinsyo seisin yakuri*
    1998;**1**:1231–1242.

48 Turkel SB, Braslow K, Tavare CH, and Trzapacz PT. The delir-
    ium rating scale in children and adolescents. *Psychosomatics*
    2003;**44**:126–129.

● 49 Trzepacz PT, Mittal D, Torres R et al. Validation of the delirium rat-
        ing scale-revised-98: Comparison with the delirium rating scale
        and the cognitive test for delirium. *J Neuropsychiat Clin Neurosci*
        2001;**13**:229–242.

50 Huang MC, Lee CH, Lai YC et al. Chinese version of the delirium
    rating scale-revised-98: Reliability and validity. *Compr Psychiatry*
    2009;**50**:81–85.

51 de Rooij SE, van Munster BC, Korevaar JC, Casteelen G, Schuurmans
    MJ, van der Mast RC, and Levi M. Delirium subtype identification
    and the validation of the delirium rating scale-revised-98 (Dutch
    version) in hospitalized elderly patients. *Int J Geriatr Psychiatry*
    2006;**21**:876–882.

52 Kato M, Kishi Y, Okuyama T et al. Japanese version of the delir-
    ium rating scale, revised-98 (DRS-R98-J): Reliability and validity.
    Psychosomatics 2010;**51**:425–431.

53 Lee Y, Ryu J, Lee J et al. Korean version of the delirium rating
    scale-revised-98: Reliability and validity. *Psychiatry Investig*
    2011;**8**:30–8.

54 de Negreiros DP, da Silva Meleiro AM, Furlanetto LM, and Trzepacz
    PT. Portuguese version of the delirium rating scale-revised-98:
    Reliability and validity. *Int J Geriatr Psychiatry* 2008;**23**:472–477.

55 Janssen NJ, Tan EY, Staal M et al. On the utility of diagnostic instru-
    ments for pediatric delirium in critical illness: An evaluation of the
    pediatric anesthesia emergence delirium scale, the delirium rating
    scale 88, and the delirium rating scale-revised (R-98). *Intensive
    Care Med* 2011;**37**:1331–1337.

● 56 Breitbart W, Rosenfeld B, Roth A et al. The memorial delirium
        assessment scale. *J Pain Symptom Manage* 1997;**13**:128–137.

57 Lawlor PG, Nekolaichuk C, Gagnon B et al. Clinical utility, factor
    analysis, and further validation of the memorial delirium assess-
    ment scale in patients with advanced cancer: Assessing delirium in
    advanced cancer. *Cancer* 2000;**88**:2859–2867.

58 Grassi L, Caraceni A, Beltrami E et al. Assessing delirium in can-
    cer patients: The Italian versions of the delirium rating scale and
    the memorial delirium assessment scale. *J Pain Symptom Manage*
    2001;**21**:59–68.

59 Matsuoka Y, Miyake Y, Arakaki H et al. Clinical utility and valida-
    tion of the Japanese version of the memorial delirium assessment
    scale in a psychogeriatric inpatient setting. *Gen Hosp Psychiatry*
    2001;**23**:36–40.

60 Shyamsundar G, Raghuthaman G, Rajkumar AP, and Jacob KS.
    Validation of memorial delirium assessment scale. *J Crit Care*
    2009;**24**:530–534.

61 Fadul N, Kaur G, Zhang T, Palmer JL, and Bruera E. Evaluation of
    the memorial delirium assessment scale (MDAS) for the screening
    of delirium by means of simulated cases by palliative care health
    professionals. *Support Care Cancer* 2007;**15**:1271–1276.

● 62 Folstein ME, Folstein SE, and McHugh PR. Mini-mental state. A
        practical method for grading the cognitive state of patients for the
        clinician. *J Psychiatr Res* 1975;**12**:189–198.

63 Crum RM, Anthony JC, Bassett SS, and Folstein MF. Population-
    based norms for the mini-mental state examination by age and
    educational level. *JAMA* 1993;**269**:2386–2391.

64 Dufouil C, Clayton D, Brayne C et al. Population norms for the MMSE
    in the very old: Estimates based on longitudinal data. Mini-mental
    state examination. *Neurology* 2000;**55**:1609–1613.

65 Xu G, Meyer JS, Huang Y et al. Adapting mini-mental status exami-
    nation for dementia screening among illiterate or minimally edu-
    cated elderly Chinese. *Int J Geriatr Psychiatry* 2003;**18**:609–616.

66 Derouesne C, Poitreneau J, Hugunot L et al. Mini-mental state
    examination: A useful method for the evaluation of the cognitive
    status of patients by the clinician. Consensual french version. *Presse
    Med* 1999;**28**:1141–1148.

67 Lindesay J, Jagger C, Mlynkik-Szmid A et al. The mini-mental state
    examination (MMSE) in an elderly immigrant Gujarati population in
    the United Kingdom. *Int J Geriatr Psychiatry* 1997;**12**:1155–1167.

68 Werner P, Heinik J, Mendel A et al. Examining the reliability and
    validity of the Hebrew version of the mini mental state examina-
    tion. *Aging (Milano)* 1999;**11**:329–334.

69 Khurana V, Gambhir IS, and Kishore D. Evaluation of delir-
    ium in elderly: A hospital-based study. *Geriatr Gerontol Int*
    2011;**11**:467–473.

70 Mori E, Mitani Y, and Yamadori A, Usefulness of a Japanese version
    of the mini-mental state in neurological patients. *Shinkeishinrigaku*
    1985;**1**:82–90.

71 Jeong SK, Cho KH, and Kim JM. The usefulness of the Korean version
    of modified mini-mental state examination (MMSE) for dementia
    screening in community dwelling elderly people. *BMC Public Health*
    2004;**4**:31.

72 De Silva HA and Gunatilake SB. Mini mental state examination in
    sinhalese: A sensitive test to screen for dementia in Sri Lanka. *Int J
    Geriatr Psychiatry* 2002;**17**:134–139.

73 Lobo A, Saz P, Marcos G, Dia JL et al. Revalidation and standardiza-
    tion of the cognition mini-exam (first Spanish version of the mini-
    mental status examination) in the general geriatric population. *Med
    Clin (Barc)* 1999;**112**:767–774.

74 Fayers PM, Hjermstad MJ, Ranhoff AH et al. Which mini-mental
    state exam items can be used to screen for delirium and cognitive
    impairment? *J Pain Symptom Manage* 2005;**30**:41–50.

75 Lou MF, Dai YT, Huang GS, Yu PJ. Identifying the most effi-
    cient items from the mini-mental state examination for cogni-
    tive function assessment in older Taiwanese patients. *J Clin Nurs*
    2007;**16**:502–508.

76 Sakamoto M, Perry W, Hilsabeck RC et al. Assessment and use-
    fulness of clinical scales for semiquantification of overt hepatic
    encephalopathy. *Clin Liver Dis* 2012;**16**:27–42.

77 Schuurmans MJ, Deschamps PI, Markham SW, and Shortridge-
    Baggett LM. The measurement of delirium: Review of scales. *Res
    Theory Nurs Pract* 2003;**17**:207–224.

◆ 78 Wong CL, Holroyd-Leduc J, Simel DL, and Straus SE. Does this
        patient have delirium?: Value of bedside instruments. *JAMA*
        2010;**304**:779–786.

79 Chochinov HM. Depression in the terminally ill: Prevalence and
    measurement issues. In Portenoy RK, Bruera E (eds.), *Issues in
    Palliative Care Research*. New York: Oxford University Press, 2003,
    pp. 189–202.

80 Chochinov HM, Wilson KG, Enns M, and Lander S. Are you depressed?
    Screening for depression in the terminally ill. *Am J Psychiatry*
    1997;**154**:674–676.

81 Whooley MA, Avins AL, Miranda J, and Browner WS. Case-finding
    instruments for depression. Two questions are as good as many. *J Gen
    Intern Med* 1997;**12**:439–445.

82   Lloyd-Williams M, Spiller J, and Ward J. Which depression screening tools should be used in palliative care? *Palliat Med* 2003;**17**:40–43.

● 83   Beck AT. An inventory for measuring depression. *Arch Gen Psychiatry* 1961;**4**:53–61.

84   Beck AT, Steer RA, and Brown GK. *The Psychological Corporation.* San Antonio, TX: BDI–Fast Screen for Medical Patients.

85   Abdel-Khalek AM. Internal consistency of an Arabic adaptation of the beck depression inventory in four Arab countries. *Psychol Rep* 1998;**82**:264–266.

86   Zhang Y, Wei L, Gos L et al. Applicability of the Chinese beck depression inventory. *Compr Psychiatry* 1988;**29**:484–489.

87   Kühner C, Bürger C, Keller F, and Hautzinger M. Reliability and validity of the revised beck depression inventory (BDI-II). Results from German samples. *Nervenarzt* 2007;**78**:651–656 (in German).

88   Mystakidou K, Tsilika E, Parpa E et al. Beck depression inventory: Exploring its psychometric properties in a palliative care population of advanced cancer patients. *Eur J Cancer Care Engl* 2007;**16**:244–250.

89   Arnarson TO, Olason DT, Smári J, and Sigurethsson JF. The beck depression inventory second edition (BDI-II): Psychometric properties in Icelandic student and patient populations. *Nord J Psychiatry* 2008;**62**:360–365.

90   Kojima M, Furukawa TA, Takahashi H et al. Cross-cultural validation of the beck depression inventory-II in Japan. *Psychiatry Res* 2002;**110**:291–299.

91   Ghassemzadeh H, Mojtabai R, Karamghadiri N, and Ebrahimkhani N. Psychometric properties of a Persian-language version of the beck depression inventory-second edition: BDI-II-PERSIAN. *Depress Anxiety* 2005;**21**:185–192.

92   Andriushchenko AV, Drobizhev MIu, and Dobrovol'skii AV. A comparative validation of the scale CES-D, BDI, and HADS(d) in diagnosis of depressive disorders in general practice. *Zh Nevrol Psikhiatr Im S S Korsakova* 2003;**103**:11–18.

93   Penley JA, Wiebe JS, Nwosu A. Psychometric properties of the Spanish beck depression inventory-II in a medical sample. *Psychol Assess* 2003;**15**:569–577.

● 94   Radloff LS. The CES-D scale: A self-report depression scale for research in the general population. *Appl Psychol Meas* 1977;**1**:385–401.

95   Da Silveria DX and Jorge MR. Reliability and factor structure of the Brazilian version of the center for epidemiologic studies depression. *Psychol Rep* 1998;**82**:211–214.

96   Rankin SH, Galbraith ME, and Johnson S. Reliability and validity data for a Chinese translation of the center for epidemiological studies-depression. *Psychol Rep* 1993;**73**(3 Pt 2):1291–1298.

97   Fountoulakis K, Iacovides A, Kleanthous S et al. Reliability, validity and psychometric properties of the Greek translation of the center for epidemiological studies-depression (CES-D) scale. *BMC Psychiatry* 2001;**1**:3. Epub 2001 June 20.

98   Fava GA. Assessing depressive symptoms across cultures: Italian validation of the CES-D self-rating scale. *J Clin Psychol* 1983;**39**:249–251.

99   Furukawa T, Hirai T, Kitamura T, and Takahashi K. Application of the center for epidemiologic studies depression scale among first-visit psychiatric patients: A new approach to improve its performance. *J Affect Disord* 1997;**46**:1–13.

100 Soler J, Perez-Sola V, Puigdemont D et al. Validation study of the center for epidemiological studies-depression of a Spanish population of patients with affective disorders. *Actas Luso Esp Neurol Psiquiatr Cienc Afines* 1997;**25**:243–249.

101 Spijker J, van der Wurff FB, Poort EC et al. Depression in first generation labour migrants in Western Europe: The utility of the center for epidemiologic studies depression scale (CES-D). *Int J Geriatr Psychiatry* 2004;**19**:538–544.

102 Irwin M, Artin KH, and Oxman MN. Screening for depression in the older adult. Criterion validity of the 10-item center for epidemiological studies depression scale (CES-D). *Arch Intern Med* 1999;**159**:1701–1704.

● 103 Yesavage JA, Brink TL, Rose TL et al. Development and validation of a geriatric depression screening scale: A preliminary report. *J Psychiatr Res* 1982–1983;**17**:37–49.

104 Burke WJ, Roccaforte WH, Wengel SP et al. The reliability and validity of the geriatric depression rating scale administered by telephone. *J Am Geriatr Soc* 1995;**43**:674–679.

105 Chan AC. Clinical validation of the geriatric depression scale (GDS): Chinese version. *J Ageing Health* 1996;**8**:238–253.

106 Ganguli M, Dube S, Johnston JM et al. Depressive symptoms, cognitive impairment and functional impairment in a rural elderly population in India: A Hindi version of the geriatric depression scale (GDS-H). *Int J Geriatr Psychiatry* 1999;**14**:807–820.

107 Fernandez-San Martin, Andrade C, Molina J et al. Validation of the Spanish version of the geriatric depression scale (GDS) in primary care. *Int J Geriatr Psychiatry* 2002;**17**:279–287.

108 Gottfries GG, Noltorp S, and Norgaard N. Experience with a Swedish version of the geriatric depression scale in primary care centres. *Int J Geriatr Psychiatry* 1997;**12**:1029–1034.

109 Ertan T and Eker E. Reliability, validity, and factor structure of the geriatric depression scale in Turkish elderly: Are there different factor structures for different cultures? *Int Psychogeriatr* 2000;**12**:163–172.

110 Lesher EL and Berryhill JS. Validation of the geriatric depression scale short form among inpatients. *J Clin Psychol* 1994;**50**:256–260.

111 Chaaya M, Sibai AM, Roueiheb ZE et al. Validation of the Arabic version of the short geriatric depression scale (GDS-15). *Int Psychogeriatr* 2008;**20**:571–581.

112 Djernes JK, Kvist E, Olesen F, Munk-Jørgensen P, and Gulmann NC. Validation of a Danish translation of geriatric depression scale-15 as a screening tool for depression among frail elderly living at home. *Ugeskr Laeger* 2004;**166**:905–909.

113 Clement JP, Nassif RF, Leger JM, and Marchan F. Development and contribution to the validation of a brief French version of the Yesavage geriatric depression scale. *Encephale* 1997;**23**:91–99.

114 Fountoulakis KN, Tsolaki M, Iacovides A et al. The validation of the short form of the geriatric depression scale (GDS) in Greece. *Aging* 1999;**11**:367–372.

115 Jang Y, Small BJ, and Haley WE. Cross-cultural comparability of the geriatric depression scale: Comparison between older Koreans and older Americans. *Aging Ment Health* 2001;**5**:31–37.

116 Bae JN and Cho MJ. Development of the Korean version of the geriatric depression scale and its short form among elderly psychiatric patients. *J Psychosom Res* 2004;**57**:297–305.

117 Malakouti SK, Fatollahi P, Mirabzadeh A, Salavati M, and Zandi T. Reliability, validity and factor structure of the GDS-15 in Iranian elderly. *Int J Geriatr Psychiatry* 2006;**21**:588–593.

118 Baker FM and Espino DV. A Spanish version of the geriatric depression scale in Mexican-American elders. *Int J Geriatr Psychiatry* 1997;**12**:21–25.

119 Broekman BF, Niti M, Nyunt MS et al. Validation of a brief seven-item response bias-free geriatric depression scale. *Am J Geriatr Psychiatry* 2011;**19**:589–596.

120 Hoyl MT, Alessi CA, Harker JO et al. Development and testing of a five-item version of the geriatric depression scale. *J Am Geriatr Soc* 1999;**47**:873–878.

121 Cheng ST and Chan AC. A brief version of the geriatric depression scale for the Chinese. *Psychol Assess* 2004;**16**:182–186.

● 122 Hamilton M. Development of a rating scale for primary depressive illness. *Br J Soc Clin Psychol* 1967;**6**:278–296.

123 Zheng YP, Zhao JP, Phillips M et al. Validity and reliability of the Chinese Hamilton depression rating scale. *Br J Psychiatry* 1988;**152**:660–664.

124 Akdemir A, Türkçapar MH, Orsel SD et al. Reliability and validity of the Turkish version of the Hamilton depression rating scale. *Compr Psychiatry* 2001;**42**:161–165.

125 O'Sullivan RL, Fava M, Agustin C et al. Sensitivity of the six-item Hamilton depression rating scale. *Acta Psychiatr Scand* 1997;**95**:379–384.

126 Olden M, Rosenfeld B, Pessin H, and Breitbart W. Measuring depression at the end of life: Is the Hamilton depression rating scale a valid instrument? *Assessment* 2009;**16**:43–54.

● 127 Zigmond A and Snaith RP. The hospital anxiety depression scale. *Acta Psychiatric Scand* 1983;**67**:367–370.

128 El-Rufaie OE and Absood GH. Retesting the validity of the Arabic version of the hospital anxiety and depression (HAD) scale in primary health care. *Soc Psychiatry Psychiatr Epidemiol* 1995;**30**:26–31.

129 Leung CM, Wing YK, Kwong PK et al. Validation of the Chinese-Cantonese version of the hospital anxiety and depression scale and comparison with the Hamilton rating scale of depression. *Acta Psychiatr Scand* 1999;**100**:456–461.

130 Lépine JP, Godchau M, Brun P et al. Evaluation de l'anxiété et de la dépression chez des patients hospitalisés en médecine interne. *Ann Medico-Psychol* 1985;**143**:175–189.

131 Herrmann C, Scholz KH, and Kreuzer H. Psychologic screening of patients of a cardiologic acute care clinic with the German version of the hospital anxiety and depression scale. *Psychother Psychosom Med Psychol* 1991;**41**:83–92.

132 Hinz A and Schwarz R. Anxiety and depression in the general population: Normal values in the hospital anxiety and depression scale. *Psychother Psychosom Med Psychol* 2001;**51**:193–200.

133 Muszbek K, Szekely A, Balogh EM et al. Validation of the Hungarian translation of hospital anxiety and depression scale. *Qual Life Res* 2006;**15**:761–766.

134 Higashi A, Yashiro H, Kiyota K et al. Validation of the hospital anxiety and depression scale in a gastro-intestinal clinic. *Nippon Shokakibyo Gakkai Zasshi* 1996;**93**:884–892.

135 Thomas BC, Devi N, Sarita GP, Rita K, Ramdas K, Hussain BM, Rejnish R, and Pandey M. Reliability and validity of the Malayalam hospital anxiety and depression scale (HADS) in cancer patients. *Indian J Med Res* 2005;**122**:395–399.

136 Baldacchino DR, Bowman GS, and Buhagiar A. Reliability testing of the hospital anxiety and depression (HAD) scale in the English, Maltese and back-translation versions. *Int J Nurs Stud* 2002;**39**:207–214.

137 Montazeri A, Vahdaninia M, Ebrahimi M, and Jarvandi S. The hospital anxiety and depression scale (HADS): Translation and validation study of the Iranian version. *Health Qual Life Outcomes* 2003;**1**:14.

138 Quintana JM, Padierna A, Esteban C et al. Evaluation of the psychometric characteristics of the Spanish version of the hospital anxiety and depression scale. *Acta Psychiatr Scand* 2003;**107**:216–221.

● 139 Zung WWK. A self-rating depression scale. *Arch Gen Psychiatry* 1965;**12**:63–70.

140 Kirkby R, Al Saif A, and El-din Mohamed G. Validation of an Arabic translation of the Zung self-rating depression scale. *Ann Saudi Med* 2005;**25**:205–208.

141 Lee HC, Chiu HF, Wing YK et al. The Zung self-rating depression scale: Screening for depression among the Hong Kong Chinese elderly. *J Geriatr Psychiatry Neurol* 1994;**7**:216–220.

142 Kozeny J. Psychometric properties of the Zung self-rating depression scale. *Act Nerv Super (Praha)* 1987;**29**:279–284.

143 Van Marwijk HW, van der Zwan AA, Mulder JD Jr. The family physician and depression in the elderly. A pilot study of prevalence of depressive symptoms and depression in the elderly in 2 family practices. *Tijdschr Gerontol Geriatr* 1991;**22**:129–133.

144 Kivela SL and Pahkala K. Sex and age differences of factor pattern and reliability of the Zung self-rating depression scale in a Finnish elderly population. *Psychol Rep* 1986;**59**(2 Pt 1):589–597.

145 Fountoulakis KN, Iacovides A, Samolis S et al. Reliability, validity and psychometric properties of the Greek translation of the Zung depression rating scale. *BMC Psychiatry* 2001;**1**:6. Epub 2001 October 20.

146 Master RS and Zung WW. Depressive symptoms in patients and normal subjects in India. *Arch Gen Psychiatry* 1977;**34**:972–974.

147 Martinez KG, Guiot HM, Casas-Dolz I et al. Applicability of the Zung self-rating depression scale in a general Puerto Rican population. *P R Health Sci J* 2003;**22**:179–185.

148 Gosker CE, Berger H, and Deelman BG. Depression in independently living elderly, a study with the Zung-12. *Tijdschr Gerontol Geriatr* 1994;**25**:157–162.

149 Dugan W, McDonald MV, Passik SD et al. Use of the Zung self rating depression scale in cancer patients: Feasibility as a screening tool. *Psychooncology* 1998;**7**:483–493.

150 Sela RA. Screening for depression in palliative cancer patients attending a pain and symptom control clinic. *Palliat Support Care* 2007;**5**:207–217.

● 151 Kroenke K, Spitzer RL, and Williams JB. The PHQ-9: Validity of a brief depression severity measure. *J Gen Intern Med* 2001;**16**:606–613.

152 Kroenke K, Spitzer RL, Williams JB, and Löwe B. The patient health questionnaire somatic, anxiety, and depressive symptom scales: A systematic review. *Gen Hosp Psychiatry* 2010;**32**:345–359.

153 Yeung A, Fung F, Yu SC et al. Validation of the patient health questionnaire-9 for depression screening among Chinese Americans. *Compr Psychiatry* 2008;**49**(2):211–217.

154 Han C, Jo SA, Kwak JH et al. Validation of the patient health questionnaire-9 Korean version in the elderly population: The Ansan geriatric study. *Compr Psychiatry* 2008;**49**:218–223.

155 Lotrakul M, Sumrithe S, and Saipanish R. Reliability and validity of the Thai version of the PHQ-9. *BMC Psychiatry* 2008;**8**:46.

156 Poongothai S, Pradeepa R, Ganesan A, and Mohan V. Reliability and validity of a modified PHQ-9 item inventory (PHQ-12) as a screening instrument for assessing depression in Asian Indians (CURES-65). *J Assoc Phys India* 2009;**57**:147–152.

157 Monahan PO, Shacham E, Reece M et al. Validity/reliability of PHQ-9 and PHQ-2 depression scales among adults living with HIV/AIDS in western Kenya. *J Gen Intern Med* 2009;**24**:189–197.

158 Stafford L, Berk M, and Jackson HJ. Validity of the hospital anxiety and depression scale and patient health questionnaire-9 to screen for depression in patients with coronary artery disease. *Gen Hosp Psychiatry* 2007;**29**:417–424.

159 Rayner L, Lee W, Price A et al. The clinical epidemiology of depression in palliative care and the predictive value of somatic symptoms: Cross-sectional survey with four-week follow-up. *Palliat Med* 2011;**25**:229–241.

160 Gilbody S, Richards D, Brealey S, and Hewitt C. Screening for depression in medical settings with the patient health questionnaire (PHQ): A diagnostic meta-analysis. *J Gen Intern Med* 2007;**22**:1596–1602.

◆ 161 Stiefel F, Trill MD, Berney A et al. Depression in palliative care: A pragmatic report from the expert working group of the European association for palliative care. *Support Care Cancer* 2001;**9**:477–488.

● 162 Blazeby JM, Conroy T, Hammerlid E et al. European organisation for research and treatment of cancer gastrointestinal and quality of life groups. Clinical and psychometric validation of an

EORTC questionnaire module, the EORTC QLQ-OES18, to assess quality of life in patients with oesophageal cancer. *Eur J Cancer* 2003;**39**:1384–1394.

● 163 Darling G, Eton DT, Sulman J et al. Validation of the functional assessment of cancer therapy esophageal cancer subscale. *Cancer* 2006;**107**:854–863.

164 Borg G. *Borg's Perceived Exertion and Pain Scales.* Champaign, IL: Human Kinetics, 1998.

165 Gift AG. Validation of a vertical visual analogue scale as a measure of clinical dyspnea. *Rehabil Nurs* 1989;**14**:323–325.

166 Gift AG and Narsavage G. Validity of the numeric scale as a measure of dyspnea. *Am J Crit Care* 1998;**7**:200–204.

● 167 Williams JE, Singh SJ, Sewell L et al. Development of a self-reported chronic respiratory questionnaire (CRQ-SR). *Thorax* 2001;**56**:954–959.

● 168 Jones PW, Quirk FH, Baveystock CM, and Littlejohns P. A self-complete measure of health status for chronic airflow limitation. The St. George's respiratory questionnaire. *Am Rev Respir Dis* 1992;**145**:1321–1327.

169 El Rhazi K, Nejjari C, Benjelloun MC et al. Validation of the St. George's respiratory questionnaire in patients with COPD or asthma in Morocco. *Int J Tuberc Lung Dis* 2006;**10**:1273–1278.

170 Meng NH, Chen FN, Lo SF, and Cheng WE. Reliability and validity of the Taiwan (Mandarin Chinese) version of the chronic respiratory questionnaire. *Qual Life Res* 2011;**20**:1745–1751.

171 Puhan MA, Behnke M, Frey M et al. Self-administration and interviewer-administration of the German chronic respiratory questionnaire: Instrument development and assessment of validity and reliability in two randomized studies. *Health Qual Life Outcomes* 2004;**2**:1. www.hqlo.com/content/2/1/1.

172 Hajiro T, Nishimura K, Tsukino M et al. Analysis of clinical methods used to evaluate dyspnea in patients with chronic obstructive pulmonary disease. *Am J Respir Crit Care Med* 1998;**158**:1185–1189.

173 Moreira GL, Pitta F, Ramos D, Nascimento CS, Barzon D, Kovelis D, Colange AL, Brunetto AF, and Ramos EM. Portuguese-language version of the chronic respiratory questionnaire: A validity and reproducibility study. *J Bras Pneumol* 2009;**35**:737–744.

174 Guell R, Casan P, Sangenis M et al. Quality of life in patients with chronic respiratory disease: Spanish version of the chronic respiratory questionnaire (CRQ). *Eur Respir J* 1998;**11**:55–60.

● 175 Tsai CL, Hodder RV, Page JH, Cydulka RK, Rowe BH, and Camargo CA Jr. The short-form chronic respiratory disease questionnaire was a valid, reliable, and responsive quality-of-life instrument in acute exacerbations of chronic obstructive pulmonary disease. *J Clin Epidemiol* 2008;**61**:489–497.

176 Barr JT, Schumacher GE, Freeman S et al. American translation, modification, and validation of the St. George's respiratory questionnaire. *Clin Ther* 2000;**22**:1121–1145.

177 Chan SL, Chan-Yeung MM, Ooi GC et al. Validation of the Hong Kong Chinese version of the St. George respiratory questionnaire in patients with bronchiectasis. *Chest* 2002;**122**:2030–2037.

178 Xu W, Collet JP, Shapiro S et al. Validation and clinical interpretation of the St. George's respiratory questionnaire among COPD patients, China. *Int J Tuberc Lung Dis* 2009;**13**:181–189.

179 Bouchet C, Guillemin F, Hoang T et al. Validation of the St. George's questionnaire for measuring the quality of life in patients with chronic obstructive pulmonary disease. *Rev Mal Respir* 1996;**13**:43–46.

180 Fallah TS, Cheraghvandi A, Marashian M et al. Measurement of the validity and reliability2 of the persian translation of the Saint George respiratory questionnaire for patients with chronic obstructive pulmonary disease. *Open Respir Med J* 2009;**3**:107–111.

181 Kuzniar T, Patkowski J, Liebert J et al. Validation of the polish version of St. George's respiratory questionnaire in patients with bronchial asthma. *Pneumonol Algerol Pol* 1999;**67**:497–503.

182 Ferrer M, Alonso J, Prieto L et al. Validity and reliability of the St. George's respiratory questionnaire after adaptation to a different language and culture: The Spanish example. *Eur Respir J* 1996;**9**:1160–1166.

183 Engstrom CP, Persson LO, Larsson S, and Sullivan M. Reliability and validity of a Swedish version of the St. George's respiratory questionnaire. *Eur Respir J* 1998;**11**:61–66.

184 Schunemann HJ, Griffith L, Jaeschke R et al. Evaluation of the minimal important difference for the feeling thermometer and the St. George's respiratory questionnaire in patients with chronic airflow obstruction. *J Clin Epidemiol* 2003;**56**:1170–1176.

185 Van der Molen B. Dyspnoea: A study of measurement instruments for the assessment of dyspnea and their application for patients with advanced cancer. *J Adv Nurs* 1995;**22**:948–956.

186 Mancini I and Body JJ. Assessment of dyspnea in advanced cancer patients. *Support Care Cancer* 1999;**7**:229–232.

187 Dorman S, Byrne A, and Edwards A. Which measurement scales should we use to measure breathlessness in palliative care? A systematic review. *Palliat Med* 2007;**21**:177–191.

188 Bausewein C, Booth S, and Higginson IJ. Measurement of dyspnoea in the clinical rather than the research setting. *Curr Opin Support Palliat Care* 2008;**2**:95–99.

189 Hwang SS, Chang VT, and Kasimis BS. A comparison of three fatigue measures in veterans with cancer. *Cancer Investig* 2003;**21**:363–373.

190 Hwang SS, Chang VT, Cogswell J, and Kasimis BS. Clinical relevance of fatigue levels in cancer patients at a Veterans Administration Medical Center. *Cancer* 2002;**94**:2481–2489.

● 191 Mendoza TR, Wang XS, Cleeland CS et al. The rapid assessment of fatigue severity in cancer patients: Use of the brief fatigue inventory. *Cancer* 1999;**85**:1186–1196.

192 Wang XS, Hao XS, Wang Y et al. Validation study of the Chinese version of the brief fatigue inventory (BFI-C). *J Pain Symptom Manage* 2004;**27**:322–332.

193 Lin CC, Chang AP, Chen ML et al. Validation of the Taiwanese version of the brief fatigue inventory. *J Pain Symptom Manage* 2006;**32**:52–59.

194 Mendoza TR, Laudico AV, Wang XS et al. Assessment of fatigue in cancer patients and community dwellers: Validation study of the Filipino version of the brief fatigue inventory. *Oncology* 2010;**79**:112–117.

195 Catania G, Bell C, and Ottonelli S. Cancer-related fatigue in Italian cancer patients: Validation of the Italian version of the brief fatigue inventory (BFI). *Support Care Cancer* 2013;**21**(2):413–419. Epub 2012 July 13.

196 Radbruch L, Sabatowski R, Eisner F et al. Validation of the German version of the brief fatigue inventory. *J Pain Symptom Manage* 2003;**25**:449–458.

197 Mystakidou K, Tsilika E, Parpa E et al. Psychometric properties of the brief fatigue inventory in Greek patients with advanced cancer. *J Pain Symptom Manage* 2008;**36**:367–373.

198 Okuyama T, Wang XS, Akechi T et al. Validation of the Japanese version of the brief fatigue inventory. *J Pain Symptom Manage* 2003;**25**:106–117.

199 Yun YH, Wang XS, Lee JS et al. Validation study of the Korean version of the brief fatigue inventory. *J Pain Symptom Manage* 2005;**29**:165–172.

● 200 Piper BF, Dibble SL, Dodd MJ et al. The revised piper fatigue scale: Psychometric evaluation in women with breast cancer. *Oncol Nurs Forum* 1998;**25**:677–684.

201 So WK, Dodgson J, and Tai JW. Fatigue and quality of life among Chinese patients with hematologic malignancy after bone marrow transplantation. *Cancer Nurs* 2003;**26**:211–219.

202 Dagnelie PC, Pijls-Johannesma MC, Pijpe A et al. Psychometric properties of the revised piper fatigue scale in Dutch cancer patients were satisfactory. *J Clin Epidemiol* 2006;**59**:642–649.

203 Gledhill JA, Rodary C, Mahe C, and Lizet C. French validation of the piper fatigue scale. *Rech Soins Infirm* 2002;**68**:50–65.

204 Giacalone A, Polesel J, De Paoli A et al. Assessing cancer-related fatigue: The psychometric properties of the revised piper fatigue scale in Italian cancer inpatients. *Support Care Cancer* 2010;**18**(9):1191–1197.

205 Annunziata MA, Muzzatti B, Mella S et al. The revised piper fatigue scale (PFS-R) for Italian cancer patients: A validation study. *Tumori* 2010;**96**:276–281.

206 Ostlund U, Gustavsson P, and Fürst CJ. Translation and cultural adaptation of the piper fatigue scale for use in Sweden. *Eur J Oncol Nurs* 2007;**11**:133–140.

● 207 Yellen SB, Cella DF, Webster K et al. Measuring fatigue and other anemia-related symptoms with the functional assessment of cancer therapy (FACT) measurement system. *J Pain Symptom Manage* 1997;**13**:63–74.

208 Minton O and Stone P. A systematic review of the scales used for the measurement of cancer-related fatigue (CRF). *Ann Oncol* 2009;**20**:17–25.

209 Whitehead L. The measurement of fatigue in chronic illness: A systematic review of unidimensional and multidimensional fatigue measures. *J Pain Symptom Manage* 2009;**37**:107–128.

210 Agasi-Idenburg C, Velthuis M, and Wittink H. Quality criteria and user-friendliness in self-reported questionnaires on cancer-related fatigue: A review. *J Clin Epidemiol* 2010;**63**:705–711.

211 Seyidova-Khoshknabi D, Davis MP, and Walsh D. Review article: A systematic review of cancer-related fatigue measurement questionnaires. *Am J Hosp Palliat Care* 2011;**28**:119–129.

◆ 212 Hesketh PJ, Gralla RJ, duBois A et al. Methodology of antiemetic trials: Response assessment, evaluation of new agents and definition of chemotherapy emetogenicity. *Support Care Cancer* 1998;**6**:221–227.

213 Collins SL, Moore RA, and McQuay HJ. The visual analogue pain intensity scale: What is moderate pain in millimeters? *Pain* 1997;**72**:95–97.

214 Bird SB and Dickson EW. Clinically significant changes in pain along the visual analog scale. *Ann Emerg Med* 2001;**38**:639–643.

● 215 Serlin RC, Mendoza TR, Nakamura Y et al. When is cancer pain mild moderate or severe? Grading pain severity by its interference with function. *Pain* 1995;**61**:277–284.

● 216 Farrar JT, Young JP Jr, LaMoreaux L et al. Clinical importance of changes in chronic pain intensity measured on an 11-point numerical pain rating scale. *Pain* 2001;**94**:149–158.

217 Farrar JT, Berlin JA, and Strom BL. Clinically important changes in acute pain outcome measures: A validation study. *J Pain Symptom Manage* 2003;**25**:406–411.

◆ 218 Hjermstad MJ, Fayers PM, Haugen DF et al. European palliative care research collaborative (EPCRC). Studies comparing numerical rating scales, verbal rating scales, and visual analogue scales for assessment of pain intensity in adults: A systematic literature review. *J Pain Symptom Manage* 2011;**41**:1073–1093.

● 219 Daut RL, Cleeland CS, and Flanery RC. Development of the Wisconsin brief pain questionnaire to assess pain in cancer and other diseases. *Pain* 1983;**17**:197–210.

220 Wang XS, Mendoza TR, Gao SZ, and Cleeland CS. The Chinese version of the brief pain inventory (BPI-C): Its development and use in a study of cancer pain. *Pain* 1996;**67**:407–416.

221 Ger LP, Ho ST, Sun WZ et al. Validation of the brief pain inventory in a Taiwanese population. *J Pain Symptom Manage* 1999;**18**:316–322.

222 Radbruch L, Loick G, Kiencke P et al. Validation of the German version of the brief pain inventory. *J Pain Symptom Manage* 1999;**18**:180–187.

223 Mystakidou K, Mendoza T, Tsilika E et al. Greek brief pain inventory: Validation and utility in cancer pain. *Oncology* 2001;**60**:35–42.

224 Saxena A, Mendoza T, and Cleeland CS. The assessment of cancer pain in north India: The validation of the Hindi brief pain inventory—BPI-H. *J Pain Symptom Manage* 1999;**17**:27–41.

225 Caraceni A, Mendoza TR, Mencaglia E et al. A validation study of an Italian version of the brief pain inventory (Breve Questionario per la Valutazione del Dolore). *Pain* 1996;**65**:87–92.

226 Uki J, Mendoza T, Cleeland C, Nakamura Y, and Takeda F. A brief cancer pain assessment tool in Japanese: The utility of the Japanese brief pain inventory BPI-J. *J Pain Symptom Manage* 1998;**16**:364–373.

227 Klepstad P, Loge JH, Borchgrevink PC et al. The Norwegian brief pain inventory questionnaire: Translation and validation in cancer pain patients. *J Pain Symptom Manage* 2002;**24**:517–525.

228 Badia X, Muriel C, Gracia A et al. Validation of the Spanish version of the brief pain inventory in patients with oncological pain. *Med Clin (Barc)* 2003;**120**:52–59.

229 http://www3.mdanderson.org/depts/symptomresearch/, accessed June 9, 2014.

● 230 Melzack R. The McGill pain questionnaire: Major properties and scoring methods. *Pain* 1975;**1**:277–299.

231 Aboud FE, Hiwot MG, Arega A et al. The McGill pain questionnaire in Amharic: Zwai health center patients' reports on the experience of pain. *Ethiop Med J* 2003;**41**:45–61.

232 Harrison A. Arabic pain words. *Pain* 1988;**32**:239–250.

233 Varoli FK and Pedrazzi V. Adapted version of the McGill pain questionnaire to Brazilian Portuguese. *Braz Dent J* 2006;**17**:328–335.

234 Hui YL and Chen AC. Analysis of headache in a Chinese patient population. *Ma Zui Xue Za Zhi* 1989;**27**:13–18.

235 Drewes AM, Helweg-Larsen S, Petersen P et al. McGill pain questionnaire translated into Danish: Experimental and clinical findings. *Clin J Pain* 1993;**9**:80–87.

236 Perkins FM, Werner MU, Persson F et al. Development and validation of a brief, descriptive Danish pain questionnaire (BDDPQ). *Acta Anesthesiol Scand* 2004;**48**:486–490.

237 van der Kloot WA, Oostendorp RA, van der Meij J, and van den Heuvel J. The Dutch version of the McGill pain questionnaire: A reliable pain questionnaire. *Ned Tijdschr Geneeskd* 1995;**139**:669–673.

238 Ketovuori H and Pontinen PJ. A pain vocabulary in Finnish—The Finnish pain questionnaire. *Pain* 1981;**11**:247–253.

239 Boureau F, Luu M, and Doubrere JF. Comparative study of the validity of four French McGill pain questionnaire (MPQ) versions. *Pain* 1992;**50**:59–65.

240 Kiss I, Muller H, and Able M. The McGill pain questionnaire—German version. A study on cancer pain. *Pain* 1987;**29**:195–207.

241 Stein C and Mendl G. The German counterpart to McGill pain questionnaire. *Pain* 1988;**32**:251–255.

242 Mystakidou K, Parpa E, Tsilika E et al. Greek McGill pain questionnaire: Validation and utility in cancer patients. *J Pain Symptom Manage* 2002;**24**:379–387.

243 Hasegawa M, Hattori S, Mishima M et al. The McGill pain questionnaire, Japanese version, reconsidered: Confirming the theoretical structure. *Pain Res Manage* 2001;**6**:173–180.

244 Satow A, Nakatani K, and Taniguchi S. Japanese version of the MPQ and pentagon profile illustrated perceptual characteristics of pain. *Pain* 1989;**37**:125–126.

245 Strand LI and Ljunggren AE. Different approximations of the McGill pain questionnaire in the Norwegian language: A discussion of content validity. *J Adv Nurs* 1997;**26**:772–779.

246 Bartko D, Kondas M, and Janco S. Quantification of pain in neurology. The Slovak version of the McGill-Melzack pain questionnaire. *Cesk Neurol Neurochir* 1984;**47**:113–121.

247 Escalante A, Lichtenstein MJ, Rios N, and Hazuda HP. Measuring chronic rheumatic pain in Mexican Americans: Cross cultural adaptation of the McGill pain questionnaire. *J Clin Epidemiol* 1996;**49**:1389–1399.

248 Lazaro C, Caseras X, Whizar-Lugo VM et al. Psychometric properties of a Spanish version of the McGill pain questionnaire in several Spanish-speaking countries. *Clin J Pain* 2001;**17**:365–374.

● 249 Melzack R. The McGill short form pain questionnaire. *Pain* 1987;**30**:191–197.

250 Solcova I, Jakoubek B, Sykora J, and Hnik P. Characterization of vertebrogenic pain using the short form of the McGill pain questionnaire. *Cas Lek Cesk* 1990;**129**:1611–1614.

251 Georgoudis G, Oldham JA, and Watson PJ. The development and validation of a Greek version of the short form McGill pain questionnaire. *Eur J Pain* 2000;**4**:275–281.

252 Adelmanesh F, Arvantaj A, Rashki H et al. Results from the translation and adaptation of the Iranian short-form McGill pain questionnaire (I-SF-MPQ): Preliminary evidence of its reliability, construct validity and sensitivity in an Iranian pain population. *Sports Med Arthrosc Rehabil Ther Technol* 2011;**3**:27.

253 Burckhardt CS and Bjelle A. A Swedish version of the short-form McGill pain questionnaire. *Scand J Rheumatol* 1994;**23**:77–81.

254 Yakut Y, Yakut E, Bayar K, and Uygur F. Reliability and validity of the Turkish version short-form McGill pain questionnaire in patients with rheumatoid arthritis. *Clin Rheumatol* 2007;**26**:1083–1087.

● 255 Fishman B, Pasternak S, Wallenstein SL, Houde RW, Holland JC, and Foley KM. The memorial pain assessment card. A valid instrument for the evaluation of cancer pain. *Cancer* 1987;**60**:1151–1158.

256 Contreras J, Valcárcel F, Dómine M, and Escobar Y. Sensivity to change of the Spanish validated memorial pain assessment card in cancer patients. *Clin Transl Oncol* 2008;**10**:654–659.

257 Escobar Y, Domine M, Contreras J, and Valcárcel F. Linguistic adaptation and validation of the Spanish version of the memorial pain assessment card (MPAC). *Clin Transl Oncol* 2009;**11**:376–381.

◆ 258 Bouhassira D and Attal N. Diagnosis and assessment of neuropathic pain: The saga of clinical tools. *Pain* 2011;**152**(3 Suppl.):S74–S83.

259 Galer BS and Jensen MP. Development and preliminary validation of a pain measure specific to neuropathic pain: The neuropathic pain scale. *Neurology* 1997;**48**:332–338.

260 Bennett M. The LANSS pain scale: The Leeds assessment of neuropathic symptoms and signs. *Pain* 2001;**92**:147–157.

261 Elzahaf RA, Tashani OA, Unsworth BA, and Johnson MI. Translation and linguistic validation of the self-completed Leeds assessment of neuropathic symptoms and signs (S-LANSS) scale for use in a Libyan population. *Pain Pract* 2013;13(3):198–205. Epub 2012 June 22.

262 Pérez C, Gálvez R, Insausti J et al.; Group for the study of Spanish validation of LANSS. Linguistic adaptation and Spanish validation of the LANSS (Leeds assessment of neuropathic symptoms and signs) scale for the diagnosis of neuropathic pain. *Med Clin (Barc)* 2006;**127**:485–491.

263 Koc R and Erdemoglu AK. Validity and reliability of the Turkish self-administered Leeds assessment of neuropathic symptoms and signs (S-LANSS) questionnaire. *Pain Med* 2010;**11**:1107–1114.

264 Krause SJ and Backonja MM. Development of a neuropathic pain questionnaire. *Clin J Pain* 2003;**19**:306–314.

265 Postma TJ, Aaronson NK, Heimans JJ et al. EORTC quality of life group. The development of an EORTC quality of life questionnaire to assess chemotherapy-induced peripheral neuropathy: The QLQ-CIPN20. *Eur J Cancer* 2005;**41**:1135–1139.

266 Huang HQ, Brady MF, Cella D, and Fleming G. Validation and reduction of FACT/GOG-Ntx subscale for platinum/paclitaxel-induced neurologic symptoms: A gynecologic oncology group study. *Int J Gynecol Cancer* 2007;**17**:387–393.

● 267 Portenoy RK, Payne D, and Jacobsen P. Breakthrough pain: Characteristics and impact in patients with cancer pain. *Pain* 1999;**81**:129–134.

268 Friedrichsdorf SJ, Finney D, Bergin M et al. Breakthrough pain in children with cancer. *J Pain Symptom Manage* 2007;**34**:209–216.

269 Cavaletti G, Frigeni B, Lanzani F et al. Chemotherapy-induced peripheral neurotoxicity assessment: A critical revision of the currently available tools. *Eur J Cancer* 2010;**46**:479–494.

270 Kirkova J, Davis MP, Walsh D et al. Cancer symptom assessment instruments: A systematic review. *J Clin Oncol* 2006;**24**:1459–1473.

● 271 McCorkle R and Young K. Development of a symptom distress scale. *Cancer Nurs* 1978;**1**:373–378.

272 Rhodes VA, McDanies RW, Homan SS et al. An instrument to measure symptom experience. Symptom occurrence and symptom distress. *Cancer Nurs* 2000;**23**:49–54.

273 Samarel N, Leddy SK, Greco K et al. Development and testing of the symptom experience scale. *J Pain Symptom Manage* 1996;**12**:221–228.

274 Lai YH, Chang JT, Keefe FJ et al. Symptom distress, catastrophic thinking, and hope in nasopharyngeal carcinoma patients. *Cancer Nurs* 2003;**26**:485–493.

275 Peruselli C, Camporesi E, Colombo AM, Cucci M, Mazzoni G, and Pac E. Quality-of-life assessment in a home care program for advanced cancer patients: A study using the symptom distress scale. *J Pain Symptom Manage* 1993;**8**:306–311.

276 Oh EG. Symptom experience in Korean adults with lung cancer. *J Pain Symptom Manage* 2004;**28**:133–139.

277 Tishelman C, Degner LF, and Mueller B. Measuring symptom distress in patients with lung cancer. A pilot study of experienced intensity and importance of symptoms. *Cancer Nurs* 2000;**23**:82–90.

● 278 Bruera E, Kuehn N, Miller MJ, Selmser P, and Macmillan K. The Edmonton symptom assessment system (ESAS): A simple method for the assessment of palliative care patients. *J Palliat Care* 1991;**7**:6–9.

279 Philip J, Smith WB, Craft P, and Lickiss N. Concurrent validity of the modified Edmonton symptom assessment system with the Rotterdam symptom checklist and the brief pain inventory. *Support Care Cancer* 1998;**6**:539–541.

280 Chang VT, Hwang SS, and Feuerman M. Validation of the Edmonton symptom assessment scale. *Cancer* 2000;**88**:2164–2171.

◆ 281 Nekolaichuk C, Watanabe S, and Beaumont C. The Edmonton symptom assessment system: A 15-year retrospective review of validation studies (1991–2006). *Palliat Med* 2008;**22**:111–122.

● 282 Watanabe SM, Nekolaichuk C, Beaumont C et al. A multicenter study comparing two numerical versions of the Edmonton symptom assessment system in palliative care patients. *J Pain Symptom Manage* 2011;**41**:456–468.

283 Pautex S, Berger A, Chatelain C et al. Symptom assessment in elderly cancer patients receiving palliative care. *Crit Rev Oncol Hematol* 2002;**47**:281–286.

284 Moro C, Brunelli C, Miccinesi G et al. Edmonton symptom assessment scale: Italian validation in two palliative care settings. *Support Care Cancer* 2006;**14**:30–37.

285 Bergh I, Aass N, Haugen DF, Kaasa S, Hjermstad MJ. Symptom assessment in palliative medicine. *Tidsskr Nor Laegeforen.* 2012;132:18–9.

286 Carvajal A, Centeno C, Watson R, and Bruera E. A comprehensive study of psychometric properties of the Edmonton symptom assessment system (ESAS) in Spanish advanced cancer patients. *Eur J Cancer* 2011;**47**:1863–1872.

287 Chinda M, Jaturapatporn D, Kirshen AJ, and Udomsubpayakul U. Reliability and validity of a Thai version of the Edmonton symptom assessment scale (ESAS-Thai). *J Pain Symptom Manage* 2011;**42**:954–960.

288 Claessens P, Menten J, Schotsmans P, and Broeckaert B. Development and validation of a modified version of the Edmonton symptom assessment scale in a Flemish palliative care population. *Am J Hosp Palliat Care* 2011;**28**:475–482.

289 Stiel S, Matthes ME, Bertram L et al. Validation of the new version of the minimal documentation system (MIDOS) for patients in palliative care: The German version of the Edmonton symptom assessment scale (ESAS). *Schmerz* 2010;**24**:596–604.

290 Jenkins CA, Schulz M, Hanson J, and Bruera E. Demographic, symptom, and medication profiles of cancer patients seen by a palliative care consult team in a tertiary referral hospital. *J Pain Symptom Manage* 2000;**19**:174–184.

291 Heedman PA and Strang P. Pain and pain alleviation in hospital-based home care: Demographic, biological and treatment factors. *Support Care Cancer* 2003;**11**:35–40.

292 Nelson JE, Meier DE, Oei EJ et al. Self-reported symptom experience of critically ill cancer patients receiving intensive care. *Crit Care Med* 2001;**29**:277–282.

● 293 Cleeland CS, Mendoza TR, Wang XS et al. Assessing symptom distress in cancer patients: The MD Anderson symptom inventory. *Cancer* 2000;**89**:1634–1646.

294 Nejmi M, Wang XS, Mendoza TR et al. Validation and application of the Arabic version of the MD Anderson symptom inventory in Moroccan patients with cancer. *J Pain Symptom Manage* 2010;**40**:75–86.

295 Wang XS, Wang Y, Guo H et al. Chinese version of the MD Anderson symptom inventory: Validation and application of symptom measurement in cancer patients. *Cancer* 2004;**101**:1890–1901.

296 Guirimand F, Buyck JF, Lauwers-Allot E et al. Cancer-related symptom assessment in France: Validation of the French MD Anderson symptom inventory. *J Pain Symptom Manage* 2010;**39**:721–733.

297 Okuyama T, Wang XS, Akechi T et al. Japanese version of the MD Anderson symptom inventory: A validation study. *J Pain Symptom Manage* 2003;**26**:1093–1104.

298 Ivanova MO, Ionova TI, Kalyadina SA et al. Cancer-related symptom assessment in Russia: Validation and utility of the Russian MD Anderson symptom inventory. *J Pain Symptom Manage* 2005;**30**:443–453.

● 299 Portenoy RK, Thaler HT, Kornblith AB et al. The memorial symptom assessment scale: An instrument for the evaluation of symptom prevalence, characteristics and distress. *Eur J Cancer* 1994;**30A**:1326–1336.

300 Chang VT, Hwang SS, Thaler HT et al. The memorial symptom assessment scale. *Expert Rev Pharmacoeconomics Outcomes Res* 2004;**4**:171–178.

301 Chang VT, Hwang SS, Feuerman M et al. The memorial symptom assessment scale short form (MSAS-SF). *Cancer* 2000;**89**:1162–1171.

302 Chang VT, Hwang SS, Kasimis BS, and Thaler HT. Shorter symptom assessment instruments: The condensed memorial symptom assessment scale (CMSAS). *Cancer Invest* 2004;**22**:526–536.

303 Spichiger E, Müller-Fröhlich C, Denhaerynck K et al. Prevalence of symptoms, with a focus on fatigue, and changes of symptoms over three months in outpatients receiving cancer chemotherapy. *Swiss Med Wkly* 2011;**141**:w13303.

304 Tranmer JE, Heyland D, Dudgeon D et al. Measuring the symptom experience of seriously ill cancer and noncancer hospitalized patients near the end of life with the memorial symptom assessment scale. *J Pain Symptom Manage* 2003;**25**:420–429.

305 McMillan SC and Small BJ. Symptom distress and quality of life in patients with cancer newly admitted to hospice home care. *Oncol Nurs Forum* 2002;**29**:1421–1428.

306 Nelson JE, Meier DE, Litke A et al. The symptom burden of chronic critical illness. *Crit Care Med* 2004;**32**:1527–1534.

307 Manitta V, Zordan R, Cole-Sinclair M et al. The symptom burden of patients with hematological malignancy: A cross-sectional observational study. *J Pain Symptom Manage* 2011;**42**:432–442.

308 Blinderman CD, Homel P, Billings JA et al. Symptom distress and quality of life in patients with advanced congestive heart failure. *J Pain Symptom Manage* 2008;**35**:594–603.

309 Blinderman CD, Homel P, Billings JA et al. Symptom distress and quality of life in patients with advanced chronic obstructive pulmonary disease. *J Pain Symptom Manage* 2009;**38**:115–123.

310 Murtagh FE, Addington-Hall JM, Edmonds PM et al. Symptoms in advanced renal disease: A cross-sectional survey of symptom prevalence in stage 5 chronic kidney disease managed without dialysis. *J Palliat Med* 2007;**10**:1266–1276.

311 Hwang SS, Chang VT, Fairclough DL et al. Longitudinal quality of life in advanced cancer patients: Pilot study results from a VA medical cancer center. *J Pain Symptom Manage* 2003;**25**:225–235.

312 Chang VT, Hwang SS, Alejandro Y et al. Clinically significant differences (CSD) in the memorial symptom assessment scale short form (MSAS-SF). *Proc ASCO* 2004;**23**:792, Abstract 8269.

313 Lobchuk MM. The memorial symptom assessment scale: Modified for use in understanding family caregivers' perceptions of cancer patients' symptom experiences. *J Pain Symptom Manage* 2003;**26**:644–654.

314 Collins JJ, Byrnes ME, Dunkel IJ et al. The measurement of symptoms in children with cancer. *J Pain Symptom Manage* 2000;**19**:363–377.

315 Abu-Saad Huijer H, Abboud S, and Doumit M. Symptom prevalence and management of cancer patients in Lebanon. *J Pain Symptom Manage* 2013;**44**(3):386–399. Epub 2012 June 22.

316 Cheng KK, Wong EM, Ling WM et al. Measuring the symptom experience of Chinese cancer patients: A validation of the Chinese version of the memorial symptom assessment scale. *J Pain Symptom Manage* 2009;**37**:44–57.

317 Lam WW, Law CC, Fu YT et al. New insights in symptom assessment: The Chinese versions of the memorial symptom assessment scale short form (MSAS-SF) and the condensed MSAS (CMSAS). *J Pain Symptom Manage* 2008;**36**:584–595.

318 Yildirim Y, Tokem Y, and Bozkurt N. Reliability and validity of the Turkish version of the memorial symptom assessment scale in cancer patients. *Asian Pac J Cancer Prev* 2011;**12**:3389–3396.

319 http://www.mapi-institute.com/questionnaires-and-translation, accessed August 12, 2012.

● 320 De Haes JCJM, van Knippenburg FCE, and Nejit JP. Measuring psychological and physical distress in cancer patients: Structure and application of the Rotterdam symptom checklist. *Br J Cancer* 1990;**62**:1034–1038.

321 Tchen N, Soubeyran P, Eghbali H et al. Quality of life in patients with aggressive non-Hodgkin's lymphoma. Validation of the medical outcomes study short form 20 and the Rotterdam symptom checklist in older patients. *Crit Rev Oncol Hematol* 2002;**43**:219–226.

322 Paci E. Assessment of validity and clinical application of an Italian version of the Rotterdam symptom checklist. *Qual Life Res* 1992;**1**:129–134.

323 Agra Y and Badia X. Evaluation of psychometric properties of the Spanish version of the Rotterdam symptom checklist to assess quality of life of cancer patients. *Rev Esp Salud Publica* 1999;**73**:35–44.

324 Can G, Durna Z, and Aydiner A. Assessment of fatigue in and care needs of Turkish women with breast cancer. *Cancer Nurs* 2004;**27**:153–161.

325 Stein KD, Denniston M, Baker F et al. Validation of a modified Rotterdam symptom checklist form with cancer patients in the United States. *J Pain Symptom Manage* 2003;**26**:975–989.

326 Huang HY, Wilkie DJ, Chapman CR, and Ting LL. Pain trajectory of Taiwanese with nasopharyngeal carcinoma over the course of radiation therapy. *J Pain Symptom Manage* 2003;**25**:247–255.

327 Cella D, Pulliam J, Fuchs H et al. Evaluation of pain associated with oral mucositis during the acute period after administration of high-dose chemotherapy. *Cancer* 2003;**98**:406–412.

328 Stromgren AS, Groenvold M, Pedersen L et al. Does the medical record cover the symptoms experienced by cancer patients in palliative care? A comparison of medical records against patient self rating. *J Pain Symptom Manage* 2001;**21**:191–198.

329 Stromgren AS, Gorenvold M, Sorenson A, and Andersen L. Symptom recognition in advanced cancer. A comparison of nursing records against patient self rating. *Acta Aneasthesiol Scand* 2001;**45**:1080–1085.

● 330 Homsi J, Walsh D, Rivera N et al. Symptom evaluation in palliative medicine: Patient report vs systematic assessment. *Support Care Cancer* 2006;**14**:444–453.

331 White C, McMullan D, and Doyle J. Now that you mention it, doctor …: Symptom reporting and the need for systematic questioning in a specialist palliative care unit. *J Palliat Med* 2009;**12**:447–450.

● 332 Dueck AC, Mendoza TR, Mitchell SA et al. Validity and reliability of the patient-reported outcomes version of the common terminology criteria for adverse events (PRO-CTCAE). *J Clin Oncol* 2012;**30**(Suppl.), Abstract 9047.

333 U.S. Department of Health and Human Services Food and Drug Administration, Center for Drug Evaluation and Research, Center for Biologics Evaluation and Research, and Center for Devices and Radiological Health. Guidance for industry patient-reported outcome measures: Use in medical product development to support labeling claims, 2009. http://ppurl.access.gpo.gov/GPO/LPS113414; http://www.fda.gov/download/Drugs/GuidanceCompliance Regulatory/Information/Guidances/UCM071975.pdf; http://www.ispor.org/work-paper/FDA%20PRO%20Guidance.pdf, accessed August 10, 2012.

334 Bottomley A, Jones D, and Claassens L. Patient-reported outcomes: Assessment and current perspectives of the guidelines of the food and drug administration and the reflection paper of the European medicines agency. *Eur J Cancer* 2009;**45**:347–353.

335 Lidstone V, Butters E, Seed PT et al. Symptoms and concerns amongst cancer outpatients: Identifying the need for specialist palliative care. *Palliat Med* 2003;**17**:588–595.

336 Potter J, Hami F, Bryan T, and Quigley C. Symptoms in 400 patients referred to palliative care services: Prevalence and patterns. *Palliat Med* 2003;**17**:310–314.

337 Chang, VT. The value of symptoms in prognosis of cancer patients, In Bruera E, Portenoy RK (eds.), *Topics in Palliative Care*. New York: Oxford University Press, 2000, Vol. 4, pp. 23–54.

338 Vigano A, Donaldson N, Higginson IJ et al. Quality of life and survival prediction in terminal cancer patients. *Cancer* 2004;**101**:1090–1098.

339 Barresi MJ, Shadbolt B, Byrne D et al. The development of the Canberra symptom scorecard: A tool to monitor the physical symptoms of patients with advanced tumors. *BMC Cancer* 2003;**3**:32.

340 Paice JA. Assessment of symptom clusters in patients with cancer. *J Natl Cancer Inst Monogr* 2004;**32**:98–102.

341 Bausewein C, Booth S, Gysels M et al. Understanding breathlessness: Cross-sectional comparison of symptom burden and palliative care needs in chronic obstructive pulmonary disease and cancer. *J Palliat Med* 2010;**13**:1109–1118.

342 Cleeland CS. Symptom burden: Multiple symptoms and their impact as patient-reported outcomes. *J Natl Cancer Inst Monogr* 2007;**37**:16–21.

343 Dudgeon DJ, Harlos M, and Clinch JJ. The Edmonton symptom assessment scale (ESAS) as an audit tool. *J Palliat Care* 1999;**15**:14–19.

◆344 Ferrell B, Connor SR, Cordes A et al. National consensus project for quality palliative care task force members. The national agenda for quality palliative care: The national consensus project and the national quality forum. *J Pain Symptom Manage* 2007;**33**:737–744.

345 Soni M, Cella D, Masters G et al. The validity and clinical utility of symptom monitoring in advanced lung cancer: A literature review. *Clin Lung Cancer* 2002;**4**:153–160.

346 Nelson CJ, Rosenfeld B, Brietbart W, and Galietta M. Spirituality, religion and depression in the terminally ill. *Psychosomatics* 2002;**43**:213–220.

347 Chochinov HM, Hack T, Hassard T et al. Dignity in the terminally ill: A cross-sectional, cohort study. *Lancet* 2002;**360**:2026–2030.

348 Merkel SI, Voepel-Lewis T, Shayevitz JR, Malviya S. The FLACC: A behavioral scale for scoring postoperative pain in young children. *Pediatr Nurs* 1997;**23**:293–297.

● 349 Warden V, Hurley AC, and Volicer L. Development and psychometric validation of the pain assessment in advanced dementia (PAINAD) scale. *J Am Dir Assoc* 2003;**4**:9–15.

350 Villanueva MR, Smith TL, Erickson JS et al. Pain assessment for the dementing elderly (PADE): Reliability and validity of a new measure. *J Am Med Dir Assoc* 2003;**4**:1–8.

351 Puntillo KA, Morris AB, Thompson CL et al. Pain behaviors observed during six common procedures: Results from Thunder project II. *Crit Care Med* 2004;**32**:421–427.

◆352 Herr K, Coyne PJ, McCaffery M et al. Pain assessment in the patient unable to self-report: Position statement with clinical practice recommendations. *Pain Manage Nurs* 2011;**12**:230–250.

353 Shannon MM, Ryan MA, D'Agostino N, and Brescia FJ. Assessment of pain in advanced cancer patients. *J Pain Symptom Manage* 1995;**10**:274–278.

354 Costello P, Wiseman J, Douglas I et al. Assessing hospice inpatients with pain using numerical rating scales. *Palliat Med* 2001;**15**:257–258.

355 Webster K, Cella D, and Yost K. The functional assessment of chronic illness therapy (FACIT) measurement system: Properties, applications, and interpretation. Review. *Health Qual Life Outcomes* 2003;**1**:79. www.hqlo.com/content/1/1/79.

356 Aaronson NK, Ahmedzai S, Bergman B et al. The European organization for research and treatment of cancer QLQ-C30: A quality of life instrument for use in international clinical trials in oncology. *J Natl Cancer Inst* 1993;**85**:365–376.

357 Steel K, Ljunggren G, Topinkova E et al. The RAI-PC: An instrument for palliative care in all settings. *Am J Hosp Palliat Care* 2003;**20**:211–219.

358 Chapman CR. Syralja measurement of pain. In Loeser JD (ed.), *Bonica's Management of Pain*, 3rd edn. New York: Lippincott Williams and Wilkins, 2001, pp. 310–328.

359 U.S. Department of Health and Human Services Food and Drug Administration, Center for Drug Evaluation and Research, Center for Biologics Evaluation and Research, and Center for Devices and Radiological Health. Guidance for industry patient-reported outcome measures: Use in medical product development to support labeling claims, 2009. http://ppurl.access.gpo.gov/GPO/LPS113414; http://www.fda.gov/download/Drugs/GuidanceCompliance Regulatory/Information/Guidances/UCM071975.pdf.

360 Snyder CF, Watson ME, Jackson JD et al.; Mayo/FDA Patient-Reported Outcomes Consensus Meeting Group. Patient-reported outcome instrument selection: Designing a measurement strategy. *Value Health* 2007;**10**(Suppl. 2):S76–S85.

361 American Educational Research Association, American Psychological Association, and National Council on Measurement in Education. *Standards for Educational and Psychological Testing.* Washington, DC: American Educational Research Association, 1999.

362 Johnson C, Aaronson N, Blazeby JM et al. European Organization for Research and Treatment of Cancer Quality of Life Group. Guidelines for developing questionnaire modules. 4th edn. http://groups.eortc.be/qol/sites/default/files/archives/guidelines_for_developing_questionnaire-_final.pdf. 2011, accessed August 10, 2012.

363 Lobchuk MM and Degner LF. Symptom experiences: Perceptual accuracy between advanced-stage cancer patients and family caregivers in the home care setting. *J Clin Oncol* 2002;**20**:3495–3507.

364 Nekolaichuk CL, Maguire TO, Suarez-Almazor M et al. Assessing the reliability of patient, nurse, and family caregiver symptom ratings in hospitalized advanced cancer patients. *J Clin Oncol* 1999;**17**:3621–3630.

365 Kutner JS, Bryant LL, Beaty BL, and Fairclough DL. Symptom distress and quality-of-life assessment at the end of life: The role of proxy response. *J Pain Symptom Manage* 2006;**32**:300–310.

366 Molassiotis A, Zheng Y, Denton-Cardew L, Swindell R, and Brunton L. Symptoms experienced by cancer patients during the first year from diagnosis: Patient and informal caregiver ratings and agreement. *Palliat Support Care* 2010;**8**:313–324.

367 Garyali A, Palmer JL, Yennurajalingam S et al. Errors in symptom intensity self-assessment by patients receiving outpatient palliative care. *J Palliat Med* 2006;**9**:1059–1065.

368 Abernethy A, Herndon JE II, Wheeler JL et al. Improving health care efficiency and quality using tablet personal computers to collect research quality patient reported data. *Health Serv Res* 2008;**43**:1975–1991.

◆369 Gwaltney CJ, Shields AL, and Shiffman S. Equivalence of electronic and paper-and pencil administration of patient-reported outcome measures: A meta-analytic review. *Value Health* 2008;**11**:322–333.

370 Bennett AV, Jensen RE, and Basch E. Electronic patient-reported outcome systems in oncology clinical practice. *CA Cancer J Clin* 2012;**62**(5):337–347. doi: 10.3322/caac.21150.

371 Shun SC, Beck SL, Frost CJ, and Berry PH. Assessing cultural appropriateness of three translated cancer-related fatigue instruments. *Cancer Nurs* 2007;**30**:E1–E9.

●372 Guillemin F, Bombardier C, and Beaton D. Cross-cultural adaptation of health-related quality of life measures: Literature review and proposed guidelines. *J Clin Epidemiol* 1993;**46**:1417–1432.

373 Hilton A and Skrutkowski M. Translating instruments into other languages: Development and testing processes. *Cancer Nurs* 2002;**25**(1):1–7.

374 Dewof L, Koller M, Velikova V et al. *EORTC Quality of Life Group: Translation Procedure,* 3rd edn. Brussels, Belgium: EORTC, 2009. http://groups.eortc.be/qol/downloads/translation_manual_2009.pdf, accessed August 10, 2012.

375 Acquadro C, Conway K, Giroudet C, Mear I (eds.). *Linguistic Validation Manual for Health Assessments,* 2nd edn. Lyon, France: MAPI Institute, 2012.

376 Wild D, Grove A, Martin M, Eremenco S et al. ISPOR task force for translation and cultural adaptation. Principles of good practice for the translation and cultural adaptation process for patient-reported outcomes (PRO) measures: Report of the ISPOR task force for translation and cultural adaptation. *Value Health* 2005;**8**:94–104.

377 Acquadro C, Conway K, Hareendran A et al. Literature review of methods to translate health-related quality of life questionnaires for use in multinational clinical trials. *Value Health* 2008;**11**:509–521.

378 Frost MH, Reeve BB, Liepa AM et al.; Mayo/FDA Patient-Reported Outcomes Consensus Meeting Group. What is sufficient evidence for there liability and validity of patient-reported outcome measures? *Value Health* 2007;**10**(Suppl. 2):S94–S105.

379 Bausewein C, Simon ST, Benalia H et al.; PRISMA. Implementing patient reported outcome measures (PROMs) in palliative care-users' cry for help. *Health Qual Life Outcomes* 2011;**9**:27.

380 Higginson IJ and Carr AJ. Using quality of life measures in the clinical setting. *BMJ* 2001;**322**:1297–1300.

381 Snyder CF, Aaronson NK, Choucair AK, Elliott TE, Greenhalgh J, Halyard MY, Hess R, Miller DM, Reeve BB, Santana M. Implementing patient-reported outcomes assessment in clinical practice: A review of the options and considerations. *Qual Life Res.* 2012 Oct;21(8):1305–14.

382 Gilbert JE, Howell D, King S et al. Quality improvement in cancer symptom assessment and control: The provincial palliative care integration project (PPCIP). *J Pain Symptom Manage* 2012;**43**:663–678.

383 Bruera E and Sweeney C. The development of palliative care at the University of Texas MD Anderson Cancer Center. *Support Care Cancer* 2001;**9**:330–334.

384 Ewing JA. Detecting alcoholism: The CAGE questionnaire. *JAMA* 1984;**252**:1905–1907.

385 Keith RA, Granger CV, Hamilton BB, and Sherman FS. The functional independence measure; a new tool for rehabilitation. In Eisenberg MG, Grzesiak RC (eds.), *Advances in Clinical Rehabilitation.* New York: Springer, 1987, Vol. 2, pp. 6–18.

386 Mancini I, Lossignol D, Obiols M et al. Supportive and palliative care: Experience at the Institut Jules Bordet. *Support Care Cancer* 2001;**10**:3–7.

387 Kaasa T, Loomis J, Gillis K, Bruera E, and Hanson J. The Edmonton functional assessment tool: Preliminary development and evaluation for use in palliative care. *J Pain Symptom Manage* 1997;**13**:10–19.

388 Radbruch L, Sabatowski R, Loick G et al. Cognitive impairment and its influence on pain and symptom assessment in a palliative care unit: Development of a minimal documentation system. *Palliat Med* 2000;**14**:266–276.

389 Ware J Jr, Kosinski M, and Keller SD. A 12-item short form health survey: Construction of scales and preliminary tests of reliability and validity. *Med Care* 1996;**34**:220–233.

390 Abernethy AP, Zafar SY, Uronis H et al. Validation of the patient care monitor (Version 2.0): A review of system assessment instrument for cancer patients. *J Pain Symptom Manage* 2010;**40**:545–558.

40

Quality of life assessment in palliative care

S. ROBIN COHEN, RICHARD SAWATZKY

INTRODUCTION

The ultimate goal of palliative care is to optimize the quality of life (QOL) of people living with a life-threatening illness and that of their families. Assessment of QOL is therefore necessary if we are to provide the best care possible and ensure that we are eliminating unnecessary suffering. In this chapter, we hope to clarify the concept of QOL at the end of life, identify the questions that you must ask yourself before deciding how to best assess QOL in your particular situation, and discuss the foundations of QOL instrument validation.

WHAT IS QOL?

The WHO QOL working group defined QOL as "individuals' perceptions of their position in life in the context of the culture and value systems in which they live and in relation to their goals, expectations, standards and concerns" [1]. Although this definition is much argued about across and within disciplines, there is general agreement that QOL is a perception. How else can we explain that we may have two people in similar physical situations and close to death, but one judges their QOL to be good and cherishes each day while the other feels that life is not worth living? Health-care professions consider QOL an important outcome in many situations. However, a careful look at many of the QOL instruments used in health-care reveals that health, which the WHO defines as "a state of complete physical, mental and social well-being, and not merely the absence of disease" [2], rather than QOL is being measured [3].

The term health-related QOL, which we and others consider a misnomer [3,4], was developed to broaden the prevalent focus on physical health at the time to also include physical and social functioning, as well as mental health, *and/or* to exclude from concern domains perceived as unrelated to health care, such as spirituality and life satisfaction. Whatever the reason for developing the concept of health-related QOL, it involves limiting the concept of QOL to certain aspects of the person whose QOL we want to assess. Whole person care is more than simply caring for all aspects of a person; it is also the recognition and understanding

that all aspects of the person are interrelated, affecting one another. For this reason, we believe that the concept of health-related QOL was created for the convenience of health-care researchers with good intentions, but it is not a construct that has a match in reality. We cannot separate the physical, psychologic, and social aspects of the person from other essential parts, such as existential well-being or spirituality. Furthermore, good QOL is not simply the absence of problems, as it is often defined in health-related QOL measures. QOL is determined by the evaluation of both the positive and negative aspects of one's life and the value or weight you put on each aspect [4–7]. The complexity of the concept of QOL, including but not limited to the fact that QOL is a perception of one's position in life and that contexts, goals, and expectations create that perception, means that QOL is created by *the interaction of external circumstances with who the person is*. This complexity has implications for optimizing QOL and measuring it. A few examples are given in the following:

- *QOL is the discrepancy or gap between a person's expectations and their actual situation* [5,8,9]. This provides us with two means of improving QOL (or decreasing the gap): we can improve the actual situation (e.g., reduce pain) and we can decrease expectations where we cannot improve the actual situation (e.g., desire to retain full physical functional status).
- *Response shift or adaptation* [5]. People have an amazing capacity to adapt to new and even difficult circumstances. This is a powerful way of coping with a difficult situation which is in large part out of your control. Response shift here refers to the situation in which the frame of reference, by which people appraise their QOL (or other patient-reported outcomes), changes over time. People may have (1) changed their internal standards (called recalibration), (2) focused on areas in which they are doing better and deemphasized the importance of areas in which they are not doing well (called reprioritization), or (3) changed what areas they call to mind when they answer "How is your QOL?" (called reconceptualization) [5]. There is much evidence for this response shift in people with a life-threatening illness, both early in the disease trajectory and at more advanced phases [10–12].

Several studies have shown that ignoring response shift could lead to the inability to detect treatment effects on patient-reported outcomes, such as QOL [13]. If we are truly interested in subjective well-being and recognize QOL as a perception, then the fact that response shift or adaptation is affecting our assessment of QOL is not a problem. Response shift could be viewed as a therapeutic outcome. However, when we are determining the effect of an intervention on QOL, then if there is differential response shift in two groups we are comparing, it is often important to know how response shift or adaptation is affecting our assessment of QOL. If the group that received the intervention improves a lot and therefore does not experience a response shift (there is no need to adapt, as the situation has improved), but the group that did not get the intervention had a large response shift over the month that the intervention was being given to the other group (e.g., they deemphasized the importance of the area in which they were not doing well), the two groups may assess their QOL as similar. In the case of the intervention group, it will be because the situation has improved. In the case of the control group, it will be because they have changed their expectations or evaluation of the situation. Both are coping well, but this will hide the effectiveness of the intervention. Supporting this idea of differential response shift, Kvam et al. [14] found that response shift plays a greater role in evaluating QOL when the condition of people with multiple myeloma deteriorates than when it improves.

Clearly the possibility of response shift must be taken into account when using QOL assessments in empirical studies and informing clinical practice. Although further study is needed, significant progress has been made during the past decade to establish reliable statistical and research design approaches to detect, measure, and accommodate response shift in QOL assessment and to identify people who experience response shift [5]. However, this needs to be done with care as each method has advantages and drawbacks. Items that directly measure change (e.g., "Has your social life changed for better or worse?" with responses ranging from "a lot worse" to "a lot better") have been used to help interpret changes in scores on standardized QOL measures. However, response shift has also been shown to affect these direct measures of change and in different ways depending on whether there is improvement or deterioration [15]. Other approaches to response shift detection rely on statistical methods, including structural equation modelling [16]. The choice of method can lead to different results and interpretations. Although the research on response shift detection is in development, palliative care practitioners and researchers need to be aware of the phenomenon and take into account that longitudinal QOL difference scores cannot always be taken at face value.

Individual differences in the meaning and interpretation of QOL appraisals. Whereas response shift pertains to a change in the meaning of QOL within individuals over time, differences in the meaning of QOL can also be present between individuals or groups. Such sources of population heterogeneity may be the result of cultural, developmental, gender or personality differences, or because of differences in health and illness experiences or life circumstances. People from different cultural backgrounds and with different life experiences may not interpret the questions that we use to assess

QOL in the same way. If ignored, these differences could distort the comparison of QOL scores between individuals or different groups of people. A variety of approaches have been used to identify and accommodate these sources of heterogeneity in patient-reported outcomes and QOL assessment in non-palliative contexts of care [17,18]. Although significant advances have been made, we need to better understand the various factors that influence how people, particularly in contexts of palliative care, interpret and respond to questions about their QOL so as to be able to accurately interpret observed differences in QOL assessments between individuals and groups with different backgrounds and life experiences. When assessing QOL in palliative care contexts, it is important to recognize that different people may not ascribe the same meaning and interpretation to the questions used in QOL assessment instruments.

STANDARDIZED VERSUS INDIVIDUALIZED MEASURES

Standardized measures of QOL have fixed questions and fixed response options. Depending on the questionnaire, answers can be combined to obtain either a score for overall QOL, separate scores for different domains contributing to QOL, or both. Standardized measures can also include items asking people to rate the importance to them of various items or domains. Weighting the responses by the importance assigned to each area or question by each participant has not seemed to change the results when studying the QOL of groups of people, and it therefore is rarely used as it adds to participant burden [19,20]. In contrast, individualized QOL measures, such as the Schedule for the Evaluation of Individual Quality of Life (SEIQoL) [21], ask each person to name the areas of their life that are most important to their QOL, how satisfied they are in these areas, and the relative importance of each area named.

Which is best? It depends on the purpose of QOL assessment. While there are individual differences in the meaning and interpretation of QOL assessments, there appears to be sufficient commonality among people in the domains that are generally considered to be important in QOL assessment. For example, most people want to be physically comfortable, be neither depressed nor anxious, be comfortable with their place in the world, etc. Differences in aspects of QOL that are relevant to particular disease populations can be accommodated using standardized disease-specific QOL measures. Nonetheless, standardized measures remain limited in the extent to which they accurately represent individuals' perspectives of their QOL. Individualized measures may therefore be more informative if the purpose is to obtain a measure of an individual's QOL from his or her point of view. However, individualized measures are limited in the extent to which the QOL scores of an individual can be meaningfully compared with those of other people. Thus, to inform clinical practice, some combination of standardized measures (to obtain accurate comparisons with a reference group) and individualized measures (to better understand the meaning of QOL from an individual's point of view) may be most beneficial.

The utilization of QOL measures, some of which are composed of long lists of questions, has been constrained by the time and energy required by people to complete them. Recent methodological advances, including item response theory, item banking, and computerized adaptive testing, are increasingly being utilized to tailor QOL assessments to individuals, thereby reducing the number of items. Computerized adaptive tests involve administering items based on an individual's responses to previous items such that accurate assessment can be achieved while administering just a few items. Thus, different items from a common pool of items (an item bank) are administered to different people to produce a standardized and yet individualized measure. Computerized adaptive tests thus have the advantage achieving accurate assessments with reduced response burden by exposing individuals fewer items and by avoiding items that are not relevant or applicable given responses to prior items. Although further research is needed to validate computerized systems, they provide a promising approach to facilitate the utilization of QOL assessment instruments with the least burden to respondents [22].

HOW CAN QOL MEASURES SUPPORT CLINICAL PRACTICE?

The clinical usefulness of measures of QOL and health status has been tested in many different health-care settings [23,24]. Despite variation in population and QOL instrument used, giving clinicians the results of a QOL or health status measure completed by their patient just prior to their appointment has been reported to improve clinician–patient communication [25*]; make the clinician aware of patient problems of which they were otherwise unaware, especially psychological problems [26**]; and change the care plan [26**,27*]. The worse or more complex the patient's condition, the more useful this assessment is for communication and management [28*]. Contrary to clinicians' expectations, interviews in which the instrument information is considered do not take more time [26**,29**]. In palliative care, use of QOL measures in practice aids in detecting patient problems [27] and enhances collaboration among staff [25*].

HOW DO YOU MEASURE QOL?

Here are some questions you must answer in order to decide how best to assess QOL for your purpose:

- *Am I interested in QOL or rather in a specific contributor to QOL?* If the latter is true (e.g., symptoms), choose a measure of that contributor rather than of QOL (although if you also expect overall QOL to be affected or QOL in several domains to be affected, you may decide to make these secondary measures).

- *What level of QOL information do I need?* You may only want an answer to the question: how is your QOL? However, for many purposes, more detailed information is required, and you will want to know in what domains the person is doing well and in what domains they are doing poorly. This is especially important in palliative care, where there is an inevitable decline in some areas such as physical well-being, but there may be improvement in others such as relationships or existential well-being. If you only measure overall QOL over time, it may remain steady despite large changes in different domains. In this case, you would select either an instrument that has well-established subscales for different domains (standardized measure with psychometrically sound subscales) or one that allows the person to name the domains important to their QOL and rate their status in each one (individualized measure).

- *Am I interested in comparing groups of people?* If yes, do these people have the same disease or different diseases? If you are comparing groups of people with different diseases, do the contributors to QOL differ at the level at which you want to measure QOL? If not, you can use a standardized measure. If the contributors to QOL differ for the two groups at the level you are measuring, the content of a standardized measure will not be equally valid for both groups, and an individualized measure is required for validity. If the contributors to QOL are the same for both groups, do you need to compare at the level of domains (in which case you will need a standardized measure) or at the level of overall QOL (in which case you can choose either an individualized or a standardized measure)?

- *Do I need information regarding everyone in the group, or is it acceptable to have only information regarding people capable of completing a questionnaire?* If you are in the camp that agrees that QOL is subjective, then it is clear that the person whose QOL is being measured is the best person to rate their own QOL. However, the physical or cognitive status of many palliative care patients precludes them being able to participate in rating their QOL. In this case, proxy measures may be considered. Ideally, someone who knows the patient well will rate the patient's QOL on his or her behalf. This may be a member of the staff or the family. However, proxy measures are known to differ from the patient's own ratings, and the difference tends to be greatest for areas that are less concrete (such as existential well-being) and where the patient is doing poorly. Many studies have been conducted regarding proxy measures, and the results are inconsistent [30–32]. There is no perfect solution in palliative care. You will have to balance the limitations of using proxy measures against the limitation of assessing only those who are well enough to complete a questionnaire.

- *How do I interpret a change in scores?* What amount of change in the scale is clinically meaningful to the patient? A statistically significant difference in scores between groups or over time is not necessarily an important one. Some researchers suggest relying on statistically determined measures of the minimal clinically important difference, which appears to be similar across many QOL studies with different populations and represents about 0.2–0.5 standard deviations or 5%–10% of the scale range [33]. Others suggest that anchor-based approaches are more appropriate for determining minimally important differences [34]. The ideal is to put the change in scores into a clinically meaningful context (e.g., an improvement in score of 25% or 2 points on psychological subscale X corresponds to the difference between someone who is clinically depressed and someone who is not really enjoying every day but is not depressed). Sometimes relevant information about score interpretation is available for the instrument you are using. For example, the difference in score between bad, average, and good days is known for the McGill Quality of Life Questionnaire (MQOL) [35]. However, if you expect a more subtle change due to your intervention or difference between groups, you may need to be creative and think of ways of asking the person completing the questionnaire to in some way directly rate the importance of the change or indicate what it means clinically (e.g., if measuring physical functioning, what can you do now that you could not do before?) [36–39]. In addition, in some circumstances, response shift must be taken into account.

- *Do I want to assess QOL to help a particular patient or family caregiver?* If so, do I just want an initial assessment, periodic assessments, or do I want to track change in QOL over time? Will the answers to a formal assessment be useful (e.g. the scores), or should I use the QOL instrument as a guide for what to ask, without focusing on the numbers generated? For clinical purposes, QOL measures cannot replace a good, thorough clinical interview. However, QOL measures are helpful as an initial interview guide or to flag areas that need further attention [27,40–42]. Although several studies suggest that QOL measures are useful in clinical practice, much work needs to be done to address barriers to its use in this way [43].
- *How much can I expect my participants to do?* Can they complete the questionnaires on their own—do they have the strength, concentration, sight, and reading skills? Or does someone need to read the questions to them? Or is it too long even if read to them? You may want to consider using a short-form or a computerized adaptive test specifically designed to reduce response burden when collecting QOL data. However, further research is needed for such abbreviated instruments to be developed and validated for use in palliative care.
- *Will response shift (adaptation) interfere with my interpretation of the answer, or is the extent to which it occurs irrelevant to my question?* If a response shift may greatly influence your conclusions, ideally you would plan some way of measuring the degree of response shift to help you interpret your data [5]. Including a change question, or "then-test," may be helpful, but it is important to consider that the same factors that cause response shift may also influence individuals' interpretations and responses to the change question. The then-test may also be influenced by

recall bias. Other statistical methods may be required to reliably detect and adjust for response shift if the purpose is to obtain an accurate evaluation of change in QOL over time (e.g., intervention research).

- *If assessing over time, how will I use the data from the different times of data collection? How will I handle the inevitable missing data?* There are many established ways of dealing with data missing completely at random. However, in palliative care, most of our missing data are *not* missing at random: usually data are missing because the patient has become too ill to respond or has died or the patient's deterioration means that the family caregiver no longer has time to complete the questionnaire. There is no perfect solution, but it is an active area of investigation [44]. If you are conducting a study, we suggest you check the recent literature for new publications on the topic.
- *What time-frame should the questions refer to?* It is important that your questions clearly indicate the time period that people are to consider when answering. QOL measures developed for the general population often refer to the past month, while those that are disease-specific often use a time-frame of the past week. Cohen feels that, because QOL often changes so rapidly near the end of life, a 2-day time-frame is better.

FOUNDATIONS OF QUALITY OF LIFE ASSESSMENT VALIDATION

Meaningful QOL assessment requires that we understand people's responses to the questions or items that comprise QOL instruments. That is, the use of individual's responses to questions for QOL assessment requires that we understand how these responses relate to the construct (e.g., overall QOL or a particular domain) that we wish to measure. Zumbo [45] discusses four foundational elements of assessment validation theory for establishing such an understanding: validity, psychometrics, utility, and social consequences.

Construct validity

Any assessment of QOL needs to have construct validity: you need to be assessing QOL, and not some other construct (such as health status). To what extent can you legitimately make inferences about people's QOL based on their responses that are used as assessment indicators of QOL? This includes establishing the various domains that comprise QOL, the "why" and "how" of individual's responses to questions for the assessment of QOL, and understanding the factors that explain QOL (antecedents) and those that are influenced by it (consequences). There is no complete agreement in the literature as to which domains are relevant to the QOL of palliative care patients, but there is a general consensus that QOL comprises at least the physical, psychological, social/relationship, and existential/spiritual domains [46,47]. Other domains such as cognitive functioning [48,49], environment [48], and communication have been found to be important in some but not all studies [46,48]. The experts as to what content is most relevant to QOL are members of the groups of people whose QOL is to be measured (e.g., patients, family caregivers for their own QOL). Consequently, when assessing QOL in different cultures, validity needs to be established for each culture that differs in ways related to QOL and what is important to it. It is not enough to know that the translation of the scale or interview is accurate and embraces the same concepts; it is necessary to be sure that the interview or questionnaire includes all the relevant content and only relevant content.

Psychometrics

An important component of establishing assessment validation involves the use of statistics to examine the statistical relationships between QOL and its assessment indicators. This includes the use of factor analysis techniques to determine the dimensional structure of a set of assessment indicators (e.g., to create subscales) and evaluation of the indicators' trustworthiness (test–retest and internal consistency reliability) [50]. In addition, modern statistical approaches, such as item response theory and latent variable mixture modelling, are increasingly used to establish assessment scales and evaluate the extent to which assessment properties might be different for different groups of people. A foundational principle is that psychometric evaluation in one population may not be directly applicable to another (e.g., people from a different culture or age group) and should ideally be reexamined.

Utility

QOL instruments have been created for a variety of purposes. Some instruments are specifically designed to evaluate changes in QOL in different groups (e.g., for use in clinical trials). Other instruments are more appropriate for measuring QOL of larger populations (e.g., for epidemiological studies). Instruments have also been developed for purposes of economic analysis. And some instruments are particularly appropriate for use in clinical practice (e.g., to monitor treatment effectiveness or identify particular areas of needs). Instruments are typically developed to maximize the usefulness (utility) and accuracy (sensitivity and specificity) for the particular purpose(s) for which it was developed. When using a QOL instrument, it is therefore important to determine whether this is the most appropriate instrument for your intended purpose.

Any assessment of QOL needs to be acceptable to the person whose QOL is being assessed. The questions must not be distressing. They may raise important feelings and even bring tears, but if these appear to be a welcome opening by the person to discuss important issues with the assessor, then we do not consider it distressing, provided they are given the opportunity to discuss these issues. We and others have informally noted that many palliative care patients find QOL assessments therapeutic. A formal study demonstrates this to be true for family caregivers as well [51]. The instrument must also be within the limits of the strength and other capabilities (e.g., reading, or else the opportunity to have it read aloud) of the person whose QOL is being assessed.

Social consequences

The use of assessment instruments can have both intended and unintended consequences [52]. QOL instruments are typically meant to make visible some aspects of QOL from the respondent's point of view so that this information can be used to inform practice, policy, and research. However, the selection of QOL domains that are made visible could have unintended consequences. For example, some QOL instruments include a subscale measuring existential or spiritual domains, whereas others do not. If existential or spiritual domains are important for an individual, then excluding an assessment of this domain could have detrimental consequences. Clinicians may not adequately take existential or spiritual well-being into account when such needs are not made visible. Conversely, instruments that reveal complex existential or spiritual needs may cause clinicians to address these needs without having adequate expertise to do so. As another example, some instruments may reveal aspects of QOL that are important in particular cultural groups. This could lead to the needs of other cultural groups being underrepresented. These types of social consequences must be taken into account when using QOL instruments. Another unintended consequence could occur when people who have experienced response shift are inadvertently penalized for not demonstrating a decline in QOL scores over time, for example, by not being offered an intervention that would alleviate a problem (e.g., pain) so that they don't have to adjust to it.

MEASURING QOL THROUGHOUT THE DISEASE TRAJECTORY

Since palliative care is appropriate from diagnosis on, ideally we would have QOL assessment instruments that are valid throughout the disease trajectory. However, instrument properties such as construct validity and ability to complete the instrument may vary along the trajectory, due to response shift and deteriorating physical status as the disease progresses. For example, women with a recurrence of breast cancer describe their experience and concerns now that the cancer has recurred as quite different from what they were when they were first diagnosed and thought that they could be cured. They describe different kinds of adaptations needed and a reprioritizing of various aspects of their life. They also now grieve for an anticipated future that won't be lived and experience anxiety about the dying process [12]. However, other studies suggest that while a reprioritization may occur at different disease stages, physical, psychological, social, and spiritual/existential well-being are contributors to QOL at all stages (although they may not be so named) [49,53,54]. It may be that there is more interindividual variability in what is important to QOL than there is across disease stages.

Many instruments used at earlier stages of the disease and into long-term survivorship tend to focus primarily (although not always exclusively) on physical symptoms and functioning [55,56]. Those commonly used further along the disease trajectory tend to measure the social and spiritual/existential domains as well. Instruments commonly used earlier in the disease trajectory tend to be longer than those used at later stages, when the patient's capacity to complete the questionnaires becomes a central concern. Few studies have tried to follow patients throughout the disease trajectory, in part because the research questions of interest at different phases tend to differ and in part because of feasibility issues. Another issue that will require study is whether a change in scores has the same meaning at different stages of the disease trajectory. There is evidence that differences in scores are larger when there is deterioration than when there is improvement in QOL [15,35,38].

One solution to the problems of reprioritization and length of the instrument might be to use an individualized measure of QOL, as the domains will always be important to the respondent. However, when the goal includes assessment of change in one or more particular domains over time, individualized measures cannot be used since the advantage that allows the instrument to account for reprioritization also means that the domains measured may shift over time.

QOL ASSESSMENT TOOLS

A full review of QOL instruments is beyond the scope of this chapter. Reviews and compendiums of QOL instruments in the palliative care setting are available [57,58]. All instruments to date have some limitations. In the following, we briefly mention a few instruments that have been most commonly used for the assessment of the QOL of patients and family caregivers in palliative care.

Patient QOL

The MQOL [59,60] is the most widely used QOL instrument for studies of people near the end of life and was developed specifically for people with a life-threatening illness. The European Organization for the Research and Treatment of Cancer Quality of Life Questionnaire–Cancer, 30 items (EORTC QLQ-C30) [56], and Functional Assessment of Cancer Therapy–General (FACT-G, later called FACIT-G) [53] are widely used in studies of people undergoing anticancer treatment, the population for which they were designed. In palliative care studies of the outcome of interventions aimed at physical symptom management, they are the most often used QOL instruments, often with add-on modules for different cancer sites or diseases. To make them more suitable for palliative care, the EORTC has developed a short form

(EORTC PAL) [61] and an add-on module has been developed for the FACT to create the FACIT-PAL [62], although neither has yet been widely used. While standardized QOL instruments developed for people at the end of life measure the existential/spiritual domain, with MQOL having a validated existential well-being subscale, instruments developed for use primarily with people undergoing anticancer treatment often do not. Because of the increasing recognition of the spiritual domain as important to QOL, modules measuring this aspect of QOL have been developed for the FACIT [63] and the EORTC has developed a stand-alone measure [64]. The FACIT spirituality module is being used fairly frequently for research where spirituality is an important outcome, on its own or in conjunction with the FACIT-G. QUAL-E is another QOL instrument developed for people at the end of life [65]. The individualized QOL instrument Schedule for Evaluation of Individualized Quality of Life–Direct Weighting (SEIQoL-DW) [66] can be used for patients or family caregivers. Interest in QOL assessment for people with end-stage diseases other than cancer is more recent. Most use the SF-36 [67], even though it is a health status measure, or disease-specific measures, although MQOL has been used for some, especially ALS [68].

Since palliative care is much less developed for life-threatening illnesses other than cancer, there is a concomitant relative lack of QOL studies in those areas, although these are increasing. Unfortunately, the same mistake regarding content validity is often made as when studies of "QOL" in cancer first began; the tendency to focus mainly on physical symptoms and functioning or health [67], rather than the broader concept of QOL, is being repeated with assessment of QOL for some other diseases (e.g., COPD, heart failure [55,69]). Fortunately, there are exceptions [68,70]. We hope that a careful evaluation of the construct validity of QOL measures for all life-threatening illnesses will be carried out in the near future.

Family caregiver QOL

There has been much less research regarding the QOL of family caregivers. The Caregiver Quality of Life–Cancer instrument [71], Caregiver Quality of Life Index [72], and Quality of Life in Life-Threatening Illness–Caregiver [73] have all been developed to measure the QOL of family caregivers of people at the end of life. More experience in their use is needed to understand their strengths and weaknesses.

TO KEEP IN MIND WHEN INTERPRETING QOL SCORES

Just as with many medical tests, there are conditions that may invalidate QOL scores even from well-developed instruments or make them difficult to interpret. These cautions apply especially if QOL scores are being used to inform care plans, but also for research:

- Items may not be interpreted as intended and different people may not interpret items in the same way.
- Construct validity is an important consideration as different instruments may not be measuring the same QOL construct (e.g., some instruments might focus predominantly on symptoms and functioning, whereas others include questions pertaining to a broader understanding of QOL).
- Although some instruments use items that need to be reverse scored (i.e., the best QOL is not always at the same end of the rating scale, in order to avoid the respondent developing a habit of checking off the same answer without carefully considering the item), this can be confusing, resulting in the wrong answer being selected. This is likely especially true when fatigue or medication decreases cognitive acuity.
- Response shift needs to be considered.

If possible when there are scores that are counterintuitive, it is best to speak with the respondent to determine their understanding of the item and their intended answer. Studies can be designed as mixed-methods studies, with a qualitative component intended to inform interpretation of the QOL instrument scores.

THE FUTURE

Despite the need to interpret QOL scores carefully, QOL assessment has brought renewed focus in health care to what is important to people whose QOL is in jeopardy. We look forward to a future where patients and family caregivers will be understood and described not only in terms of their disease and symptom status but also in terms of their QOL. Only then can palliative care really be addressing whole person care.

Key learning points

- Improving QOL is the main goal of palliative care; therefore, assessing it is critical if we want to understand the extent to which we are achieving our goals.

- QOL assessment provides an assessment of the whole person. QOL is a perception. It is not a specific set of external circumstances, but rather the interaction of the person with external and internal circumstances

- The "best" way of assessing QOL will depend on your purpose in assessing it.

- There is no perfect way to assess QOL in palliative care. Choose the best way, or combination of ways, and be aware of its strengths and limitations.

REFERENCES

1 WHO. The World Health Organization Quality of Life Assessment (WHOQOL): Position paper from the World Health Organization. *Social Science & Medicine.* 1995;41(10):1403–140

2 WHO. WHO definition of health. [cited 2012 May 29]; Available from http://www.who.int/about/definition/en/print.html

3 Michalos AC. Social indicators research and health-related quality of life research. *Social Indicators Research.* 2004;65(1):27–72.

4 Hunt SM. The problem of quality of life. *Quality of Life Research.* 1997;6(3).

5 Schwartz CE. Applications of response shift theory and methods to participation measurement: A brief history of a young field. *Archives of Physical Medicine and Rehabilitation.* 2010;91(9 Suppl.):S38–S43.

6 Sprangers MAG, Schwartz CE. Integrating response shift into health-related quality of life research: A theoretical model. *Social Science & Medicine.* 1999;48(11):1507–1515.

7 Folkman S. Positive psychological states and coping with severe stress. *Social Science & Medicine.* 1997;45(8):1207–1221. [Epub 1997/09/25.]

8 Cantril H. *The Pattern of Human Concerns.* New Brunswick, NJ, Rutgers U P; 1966.

9 Campbell A, Converse PE, Rodgers WL. *The Quality of American Life: Perceptions, Evaluations, and Satisfactions.* New York: Russell Sage Foundation; 1976.

10 Kreitler S, Chaitchik S, Rapoport Y, Kreitler H, Algor R. Life satisfaction and health in cancer patients, orthopedic patients and healthy individuals. *Social Science & Medicine.* 1993;36(4):547–556.

11 Neuman HB, Park J, Fuzesi S, Temple LK. Rectal cancer patients' quality of life with a temporary stoma: Shifting perspectives. *Diseases of the Colon & Rectum.* 2012;55(11):1117–1124. [Epub 2012/10/10.]

12 Kenne Sarenmalm E, Thoren-Jonsson AL, Gaston-Johansson F, Ohlen J. Making sense of living under the shadow of death: Adjusting to a recurrent breast cancer illness. *Quality Health Research.* 2009;19(8):1116–1130. [Epub 2009/07/30.]

13 Schwartz C, Bode R, Repucci N, Becker J, Sprangers M, Fayers P. The clinical significance of adaptation to changing health: A meta-analysis of response shift. *Quality of Life Research.* 2006;15(9):1533–1550.

14 Kvam AK, Wisloff F, Fayers PM. Minimal important differences and response shift in health-related quality of life; a longitudinal study in patients with multiple myeloma. *Health & Quality of Life Outcomes.* 2010;8:79.

15 Taminiau-Bloem EF, Van Zuuren FJ, Visser MR, Tishelman C, Schwartz CE, Koeneman MA et al. Opening the black box of cancer patients' quality-of-life change assessments: A think-aloud study examining the cognitive processes underlying responses to transition items. *Psychology & Health.* 2011;26(11):1414–1428. [Epub 2011/07/09.]

◆ 16 Schwartz CE, Ahmed S, Sawatzky R, Sajobi T, Mayo N, Finkelstein J et al. Guidelines for secondary analysis in search of response shift. *Quality of Life Research.* 2013;22(10):2663–2673.

17 Sawatzky R, Ratner P, Johnson J, Kopec J, Zumbo B. Sample heterogeneity and the measurement structure of the multidimensional students' life satisfaction scale. *Social Indicators Research.* 2009;94(2):273–296.

18 Sawatzky R, Ratner P, Kopec J, Zumbo B. Latent variable mixture models: A promising approach for the validation of patient reported outcomes. *Quality of Life Research.* 2012;21(4):637–650.

19 Skevington SM, O'Connell KA. Can we identify the poorest quality of life? Assessing the importance of quality of life using the WHOQOL-100. *Quality of Life Research.* 2004;13(1):23–34.

20 Cella D. The Functional Assessment of Cancer Therapy-Anemia (FACT-An) Scale: A new tool for the assessment of outcomes in cancer anemia and fatigue. *Seminars in Hematology.* 1997;34(3 Suppl. 2):13–19.

21 McGee HM, O'Boyle CA, Hickey A, O'Malley K, Joyce C. Assessing the quality of life of the individual: The SEIQoL with a healthy and a gastroenterology unit population. *Psychological Medicine.* 1991;21(03):749–759.

22 Garcia SF, Cella D, Clauser SB, Flynn KE, Lad T, Lai J-S et al. Standardizing patient-reported outcomes assessment in cancer clinical trials: A patient-reported outcomes measurement information system initiative. *Journal of Clinical Oncology.* 2007;25(32):5106–5112.

23 Greenhalgh J. The applications of PROs in clinical practice: What are they, do they work, and why? *Quality of Life Research.* 2009;18(1):115–123. [Epub 2008/12/24.]

24 Valderas JM, Alonso J. Patient reported outcome measures: A model-based classification system for research and clinical practice. *Quality of Life Research.* 2008;17(9):1125–1135. [Epub 2008/10/07.]

25 Schwartz CE, Merriman MP, Reed G, Byock I. Evaluation of the Missoula-VITAS Quality of Life Index—Revised: Research tool or clinical tool? *Journal of Palliative Medicine.* 2005;8(1):121–135.

26 Velikova G, Booth L, Smith AB, Brown PM, Lynch P, Brown JM et al. Measuring quality of life in routine oncology practice improves communication and patient well-being: A randomized controlled trial. *Journal of Clinical Oncology.* 2004;22(4):714–724.

27 Eischens MJ, Elliott BA, Elliott TE. Two hospice quality of life surveys: A comparison. *American Journal of Hospice and Palliative Medicine.* 1998;15(3):143–148.

28 Wagner AK, Ehrenberg BL, Tran TA, Bungay KM, Cynn DJ, Rogers WH. Patient-based health status measurement in clinical practice: A study of its impact on epilepsy patients' care. *Quality of Life Research.* 1997;6(4):329–341.

29 Detmar SB, Muller MJ, Schornagel JH, Wever LDV, Aaronson NK. Health-related quality-of-life assessments and patient-physician communication: A randomized controlled trial. *Journal of the American Medical Association.* 2002;288(23):3027–3034.

30 Jones JM, McPherson CJ, Zimmermann C, Rodin G, Le LW, Cohen SR. Assessing agreement between terminally ill cancer patients' reports of their quality of life and family caregiver and palliative care physician proxy ratings. *Journal of Pain and Symptom Management.* 2011;42(3):354–365.

31 Horton R. Differences in assessment of symptoms and quality of life between patients with advanced cancer and their specialist palliative care nurses in a home care setting. *Palliative Medicine.* 2002;16(6):488–494.

32 McPherson CJ, Addington-Hall JM. Judging the quality of care at the end of life: Can proxies provide reliable information? *Social Science & Medicine.* 2003;56(1):95–109.

33 Norman GR, Sloan JA, Wyrwich KW. Interpretation of changes in health-related quality of life: The remarkable universality of half a standard deviation. *Medical Care.* 2003;41(5):582–592.

34 Hays RD, Farivar SS, Liu H. Approaches and recommendations for estimating minimally important differences for health-related quality of life measures. *COPD.* 2005;2(1):63–67. [Epub 2006/12/02.]

35 Cohen SR, Mount BM. Living with cancer: "Good" days and "bad" days—What produces them? *Cancer.* 2000;89(8):1854–1865.

36 Osoba D, Rodrigues G, Myles J, Zee B, Pater J. Interpreting the significance of changes in health-related quality-of-life scores. *Journal of Clinical Oncology.* 1998;16(1):139–144.

37 Cella D, Bullinger M, Scott C, Barofsky I. Group vs individual approaches to understanding the clinical significance of differences or changes in quality of life. *Mayo Clinic Proceedings.* 2002;77(4):384–392.

38 Cella D, Hahn EA, Dineen K. Meaningful change in cancer-specific quality of life scores: Differences between improvement and worsening. *Quality of Life Research.* 2002;11(3):207–221.

39 Guyatt GHGH, Osoba DD, Wu AWAW, Wyrwich KWKW, Norman GRGR. Methods to explain the clinical significance of health status measures. *Mayo Clinic Proceedings.* 2002;77(4):371–383.

40 Finlay IG, Pratheepawanit N, Salek MS. Monitoring self-reported quality-of-life among patients attending a palliative medicine outpatient clinic. *Palliative Medicine.* 2003;17(1):83–84.

41 Higginson IJ, Alison JC. Measuring quality of life: Using quality of life measures in the clinical setting. *British Medical Journal.* 2001;322(7297):1297–1300.

42 Hughes R, Aspinal F, Addington-Hall J, Chidgey J, Drescher U, Dunckley M et al. Professionals' views and experiences of using outcome measures in palliative care. *International Journal of Palliative Nursing.* 2003;9(6):234–238.

43 Hughes R, Aspinal F, Addington-Hall JM, Dunckley M, Faull C, Higginson I. It just didn't work: The realities of quality assessment in the English health care context. *International Journal of Nursing Studies.* 2004;41(7):705–712.

44 Fairclough DL. *Design and Analysis of Quality of Life Studies in Clinical Trials.* Boca Raton, FL: Chapman & Hall; 2010.

45 Zumbo BD. Validity as contextualized and pragmatic explanation, and its implications for validation practice. In: Lissitz RW (ed.). *The Concept of Validity: Revisions, New Directions and Applications.* Charlotte, NC: Information Age Publishing; 2009. pp. 65–82.

46 Cohen SR. Assessing quality of life in palliative care. In: Portenoy R, Bruera E (eds.). *Issues in Palliative Care Research.* New York: Oxford University Press; 2003. pp. 231–241.

47 Ferrans CE. Definitions and conceptual models of quality of life. In: Lipscomb J, Gotay CC, Snyder C (eds.). *Outcomes Assessment in Cancer: Measures, Methods, and Applications.* Cambridge, NY: Cambridge University Press; 2005. pp. 14–30.

48 Cohen SR, Leis A. What determines the quality of life of terminally ill patients from their own perspective? *Journal of Palliative Care.* 2002;18(1):48–58.

49 Padilla G, Ferrell B, Grant M, Rhiner M. Defining the content domain of quality of life for cancer patients with pain. *Cancer Nursing.* 1990;13(2):108.

50 Fayers P, Machin D. *Quality of Life: The Assessment, Analysis and Interpretation of Patient-Reported Outcomes.* Chichester, U.K.: John Wiley & Sons; 2007.

51 Hudson P. The experience of research participation for family caregivers of palliative care cancer patients. *International Journal of Palliative Nursing.* 2003;9(3):120–123.

52 Messick S. Validity of psychological assessment: Validation of inferences from persons' responses and performances as scientific inquiry into score meaning. *American Psychologist.* 1995;50(9):741–749.

53 Cella DF, Tulsky DS, Gray G, Sarafian B, Linn E, Bonomi A et al. The Functional Assessment of Cancer Therapy scale: Development and validation of the general measure. *Journal of Clinical Oncology.* 1993;11(3):570–579. [Epub 1993/03/01.]

54 Ferrell B, Grant M, Funk B, Garcia N, Otis-Green S, Schaffner M. Quality of life in breast cancer. *Cancer Practice.* 1996;4(6):331.

55 Habraken JM, van der Wal WM, Ter Riet G, Weersink EJ, Toben F, Bindels PJ. Health-related quality of life and functional status in end-stage COPD: A longitudinal study. *European Respiratory Journal.* 2011;37(2):280–288.

56 Aaronson NK, Ahmedzai S, Bergman B, Bullinger M, Cull A, Duez NJ et al. The European Organization for Research and Treatment of Cancer QLQ-C30: A quality-of-life instrument for use in international clinical trials in oncology. *Journal of the National Cancer Institute.* 1993;85(5):365–376.

57 Albers G, Echteld MA, de Vet HC, Onwuteaka-Philipsen BD, van der Linden MH, Deliens L. Evaluation of quality-of-life measures for use in palliative care: A systematic review. *Palliative Medicine.* 2010;24(1):17–37.

58 Research Trust M. Patient-reported outcomes and quality of life instruments database. MAPI Research Trust; 2012 [cited 2012 June 4]; Available from: www.proqolid.org

59 Cohen SR, Mount BM, Bruera E, Provost M, Rowe J, Tong K. Validity of the McGill Quality of Life Questionnaire in the palliative care setting: A multi-centre Canadian study demonstrating the importance of the existential domain. *Palliative Medicine.* 1997;11(1):3–20.

60 Cohen SR, Mount BM, Tomas JJN, Mount LF. Existential well-being is an important determinant of quality of life: Evidence from the McGill Quality of Life Questionnaire. *Cancer.* 1996;77(3):576–586.

61 Groenvold M, Petersen MA, Aaronson NK, Arraras JI, Blazeby JM, Bottomley A et al. The development of the EORTC QLQ-C15-PAL: A shortened questionnaire for cancer patients in palliative care. *European Journal of Cancer.* 2006;42(1):55–64.

62 Greisinger AJ, Lorimor RJ, Aday LA, Winn RJ, Baile WF. Terminally ill cancer patients. Their most important concerns. *Cancer Practice.* 1997;5(3):147–154.

63 Peterman AH, Fitchett G, Brady MJ, Hernandez L, Cella D. Measuring spiritual well-being in people with cancer: The functional assessment of chronic illness therapy—Spiritual Well-being Scale (FACIT-Sp). *Annals of Behavioral Medicine.* 2002;24(1):49–58.

64 Vivat B, Young T, Efficace F, Sigurdadottir V, Arraras JI, Asgeirsdottir GH et al. Cross-cultural development of the EORTC QLQ-SWB36: A stand-alone measure of spiritual wellbeing for palliative care patients with cancer. *Palliative Medicine.* 2013;27(5):457–469. [Epub 2012/07/31.]

65 Steinhauser KE, Bosworth HB, Clipp EC, McNeilly M, Christakis NA, Parker J et al. Initial assessment of a new instrument to measure quality of life at the end of life. *Journal of Palliative Medicine.* 2002;5(6):829–841.

66 Waldron D, O'Boyle CA, Kearney M, Moriarty M, Carney D. Quality-of-life measurement in advanced cancer: Assessing the individual. *Journal of Clinical Oncology.* 1999;17(11):3603–3611.

67 Ware JE, Jr., Sherbourne CD. The MOS 36-Item Short-Form Health Survey (SF-36): I. Conceptual framework and item selection. *Medical Care.* 1992;30(6):473–483.

68 Robbins RA, Simmons Z, Bremer BA, Walsh SM, Fischer S. Quality of life in ALS is maintained as physical function declines. *Neurology.* 2001;56(4):442–444.

69 Mulligan K, Mehta PA, Fteropoulli T, Dubrey SW, McIntyre HF, McDonagh TA et al. Newly diagnosed heart failure: Change in quality of life, mood, and illness beliefs in the first 6 months after diagnosis. *British Journal of Health Psychology.* 2012;17(3):447–462.

70 Grady KL, de Leon CFM, Kozak AT, Cursio JF, Richardson D, Avery E et al. Does self-management counseling in patients with heart failure improve quality of life? Findings from the Heart Failure Adherence and Retention Trial (HART). *Quality of life Research.* 2014;23(1):31–38.

71 Weitzner MA, Jacobsen PB, Wagner H, Friedland J, Cox C. The Caregiver Quality of Life Index—Cancer (CQOLC) scale: Development and validation of an instrument to measure quality of life of the family caregiver of patients with cancer. *Quality of Life Research.* 1999;8(1):55–63.

72 McMillan SC, Mahon M. The impact of hospice services on the quality of life of primary caregivers. *Oncology Nursing Forum.* 1994;21(7):1189–1195.

73 Cohen SR, Leis AM, Kuhl D, Charbonneau C, Ritvo P, Ashbury FD. QOLLTI-F: Measuring family carer quality of life. Palliat Med. December 2006;20(8):755–67.

PART **8**

Pain

41

Pathophysiology of chronic pain

SEBASTIANO MERCADANTE

INTRODUCTION

Cancer pain is a complex issue. It is initially a signal of ongoing injury associated with the onset or recrudescence of disease or may be caused by some diagnostic procedures. Commonly it subsides after oncological treatments. In different stages of disease, however, the causes cannot be adequately eliminated, and symptoms persist. At this point, cancer pain serves no biological purpose of alerting the organism to the presence of harmful stimuli but assumes the status of a chronic disease and is characterized by alterations in mood and pain behavior. The differences between acute and chronic pain include peripheral responses of the organism and central nervous system modifications induced by the chronic afferent volley of nociceptor activity [1].

In the presence of damage of tissues, peripheral nerves transmit this information from the body tissues to the spinal cord, from where neurons relay the information to the brain and simultaneously trigger reflexes that withdraw the body part involved in the painful stimulus. The higher brain centers organize the appropriate behaviors that restore health by protecting and facilitating the healing of the damaged body site. Pain tends to diminish as healing progresses. Thus, in healthy individuals, pain serves highly adaptive, survival-oriented purposes. However, pain can occur as a consequence of dysfunction of the peripheral or central nervous system, or prolonged and intense stimuli from damaged tissues.

The clinical picture of cancer pain varies depending on the pathophysiological mechanism, which further depends on the characteristics and progression of disease and the preferential sites of metastases. Traditionally, the pain related to malignant disease has been classified as nociceptive-inflammatory (somatic and visceral) and neuropathic. Somatic and visceral pains involve direct activation of nociceptors, and these pains are often a complication of infiltration of tissue by tumor or tissue injury as a consequence of oncological treatments. Neuropathic pain may be a complication of injury to the peripheral or central nervous system. This type of pain is often poorly tolerated and difficult to control. In the chronic pain situation that occurs following the injury, infection, or inflammation of peripheral nerves, sensory processing in the affected body region is grossly abnormal. Environmental stimuli that would not normally result in the sensation of pain now do so, and painful stimuli elicit exaggerated perceptions of pain. Finally, pain is frequently spontaneous; that is, no stimulus can be identified to account for the pain.

Although nociceptive and neuropathic pains depend on separate peripheral mechanisms, they are both significantly influenced by changes in the central nervous system function. It is now clear that cancer pain is a more complex entity, particularly regarding the response to analgesics, where numerous factors play a role. However, it remains unclear whether cancer pain is a unique type of pain or merely a subtype of inflammatory or neuropathic pain, as in cancer pain models there are changes in transmitters commonly produced in either neuropathic or inflammatory pain state [2].

PHYSIOPATHOLOGY OF NOCICEPTIVE PAIN

No specific histological structure acts as a nociceptive receptor. Primary afferent sensory neurons are the gateway by which sensory information from peripheral tissues is transmitted. Aδ and C nociceptors have been clearly identified in fibers innervating somatic structures, but not in the viscera, where the situation is even more complicated. In cutaneous tissue, thermal, mechanical, and chemical stimuli that induce tissue damage activate unmyelinated polymodal transducers attached to Ad and C fibers. Nearly all large-diameter myelinated A and B fibers normally conduct non-noxious stimuli. In contrast, most small-diameter sensory fibers (unmyelinated C fibers and finely myelinated Ad fibers) are specialized sensory neurons, the main function of which is to detect and convert environmental stimuli, chemical or physical, into electrochemical signals that are transmitted to the central nervous system. As the intensity of the stimulus increases, high-threshold receptors are involved. Various chemicals are released into damaged tissue cells. Sustained stimuli or damage to the nerve can alter the profile of several peptides such as substance P contained within primary afferents. Substance P is able to induce the production of nitric oxide (NO), a vasodilator, and the degranulation of mast cells with further vasodilation and subsequent extravasation and release of bradykinin. Bradykinin is a powerful algogenic substance, which also sensitizes nociceptors by means of prostaglandin E_2. Other substances such as cytokines are released after the tissue damage under the influence of bradykinin. These substances have an important role in the inflammatory process. Although prostaglandins are weak algogens, they have a major role in the sensitization of nociceptors to other substances. The concerted effects of these mediators at the site of tissue damage underlie peripheral hyperalgesia, which accounts for much of the peripheral sensitization of nociceptors [3].

Thus, a repeated and intense stimulus induces the release of several inflammatory mediators that reduce the threshold for activation, increase the response to a given stimulus, or induce the appearance of spontaneous activity. This sensitization of nociceptors is responsible for some features of hyperalgesia. Many inactive receptors may become excitable in the condition of inflammation and are recruited to amplify the stimuli in these circumstances. Sensory neurons may change their phenotype. Substance P, for example, binds and activates the neurokinin-1 receptor, which is expressed by a subset of spinal cord neurons. Of interest, inflammation is able to unmask opioid receptors peripherally. Primary hyperalgesia involves increased sensitivity to noxious stimulation at the site of the injury and is mediated by peripheral mechanisms, whereas secondary hyperalgesia extends beyond the site of the injury and is related to central activity or sensitization. The latter is characterized by a prolonged excitation of dorsal horn cells, resulting in an expansion of receptive fields of dorsal horn neurons. As a consequence of such sensitization, the expression of c-*fos* in the superficial dorsal horn increases. Peripheral nerve injury leads to the abnormal expression of receptors and channels that may result in ectopic discharges from neurons.

After injury to somatic, visceral, and neural structures, there may be an alteration in the response of the autonomic nervous system, which may react by novel sprouting of sympathetic efferents and formation of rings around dorsal root ganglia. Central neural mechanisms are also involved, leading to a constellation of peripheral vasomotor and sudomotor changes [4]. Immune system cells, including macrophages, neutrophils, and T cells, either in the tumor mass or produced as a reaction, sensitize or directly excite primary afferent neurons. Local acidosis produced by cancer cells can activate or express further nociceptors. Moreover, tumor necrosis factors and inflammatory cells are able to express opioid receptors, which may influence the response to opioids by initial sequestration first and then by the release of NO, known as hyperalgesic agent (see the following text) [5].

VISCERAL PAIN

The viscera have a complex peripheral nervous system, and different neurophysiological understandings of visceral pain have been reported. Unlike their cutaneous counterparts, visceral nociceptors do not appear to be a simple acute warning system. Many viscera are innervated by receptors that do not evoke conscious perception. Visceral nociceptors, however, have a wide range of responses and may be activated in the presence of inflammation or tissue injury. Therefore, visceral afferents are considered polymodal, providing excitatory responses to different stimuli, including inflammation, stretching, and distension. Two distinct classes of nociceptive sensory receptors that innervate internal organs have been proposed:

1. High-threshold receptors—mostly mechanical, activated by stimuli within the noxious range
2. Low-threshold receptors—activated in the range of stimulation intensity from innocuous to noxious.

According to this theory, high-threshold receptors contribute to the peripheral encoding of noxious events in the viscera. Other prolonged and intense stimuli, such as hypoxia or tissue inflammation, result in the sensitization of these receptors and bring into play previously silent receptors, normally unresponsive to innocuous stimuli. The activity of afferents and the excitability of dorsal horn neurons are increased with repeated or persistent stimuli due to the process of sensibilization of afferents, which occurs secondary to local release of chemical substances in damaged or ischemic tissues. A critical level of preceding activity in the afferents is required to induce the facilitation of dorsal horn neuronal responses via central mechanisms [6].

Neurons that transmit visceral sensory information to the spinal cord have cell bodies that reside in the dorsal root ganglia. These primary afferents travel through the paravertebral ganglia and the prevertebral ganglia and have sensory endings in the viscera themselves. These afferents occur in conjunction with motor fibers of parasympathetic and sympathetic nervous system. Most visceral afferents have relatively slow conduction velocities.

Visceral pain tends to be diffuse because of the absence of a separate visceral sensory pathway and a low proportion of visceral afferent nerve fibers compared with those of somatic origin. Thus, neurological mechanisms of visceral pain differ from those involved in somatic pain. The nature of pain referred is not clearly defined. Some spinal neurons are involved in the localization of pain and project it to the brain, whereas another group of neurons has short ascending projections with collaterals into multiple spinal segments. The activation of visceral efferents should lead to changes in the excitability of multiple spinal units, including those responsible for somatic nociceptive sensory pathways, or direct activation of neurons receiving both visceral and somatic inputs. Alternatively, the brain may misinterpret the activity in the viscero-somatic neurons. Convergent receptive fields are generally described as multidermatomal, centered in the dermatome corresponding to the spinal segment stimulated, and are significantly larger than the receptive fields of spinal neurons receiving only somatic input [7,8]. These observations explain why visceral pain is difficult to localize and is often referred to other areas of the body. Pain originating from any viscus cannot be easily differentiated from the pain originating in another viscus, although some visceral pains are associated with specific etiologies, such as in the case of pancreatic pain or peptic ulcer pain.

Mechanic stimuli, such as torsion or traction of mesentery, distension of hollow organs, stretch of serosal and mucosal surfaces, and compression of some organs, produce pain in humans. These conditions are frequently observed in cancer patients with abdominal diseases and intraperitoneal masses. Human studies have revealed that pain is produced when the intraluminal pressure of hollow organs is maintained above certain pressure thresholds. Obstruction or inflammation within the biliary tract or pancreatic duct induces pain directly related to the increased intraluminal pressure with consequent inflammation and the release of pain-producing substances. Capsular stretch of liver due to cancer growth produces pain. Distension or traction on the gallbladder leads to deep epigastric pain, inspiratory distress, and vomiting. Spontaneous spasm of the sphincter of Oddi or that induced by morphine on the one hand leads to an increase in pain sensation, resulting in a paradoxical opioid-induced pain. On the other hand, morphine and other opioids may counterbalance this effect, increasing the pressure threshold necessary to produce the sensation of pain due to the distension of the biliary system [9].

Renal colic is usually secondary to ureteral obstruction and subsequent distension of the ureter and renal pelvis. This may be seen in circumstances in which an abdominal–pelvic mass compresses or invades the ureters, as often occurs in gynecological cancers. The pain is reported to be directly related to the compression of the urinary bladder. Bladder distension may also activate the mechanisms related to the phenomenon of counterirritation. Better localization of stimulus occurs when the disease extends to a somatically innervated structure such as the parietal peritoneum. Thus, initially, visceral pain is poorly localized and dull because of the wide divergence of visceral afferents in the spinal cord. Poorly localized visceral pain becomes localized as visceral afferent input increases due to the spinal facilitation or activation of visceral nociceptors. The greatest localization occurs when somatic structures such as the peritoneum become involved [10].

BONE PAIN

Many common tumors (breast and prostate, thyroid, kidney, and lung) have a strong predilection to simultaneously metastasize to multiple bones [11]. Animal models have shown a dramatic proliferation and hypertrophy of osteoclasts, as well as bone destruction, and a disruption of bone homeostasis. Osteoclast-mediated bone remodeling results in a robust production of extracellular protons, which are known potent activation of nociceptors. Two acid-sensing ion channels are expressed by nociceptors, such as vanilloid 1 (TRPV1) and acid-sensing ion channel 3 (ASIC-3), in the acid microenvironment. As inflammatory and immune cells invade the tumor, these cells also release further protons to produce a local acidosis [12].

Simultaneously, changes in spinal cord neurochemistry develop, including an upregulation of C-fos immunoreactive neurons, dynorphin, and a reactive appearance of astrocytes. These phenomena were correlated with ongoing and movement-evoked pain behaviors increase in severity with time. Of interest, the response to opioids was 10-fold less than in animals with an inflammatory model determining the same level of pain intensity, suggesting a state of spinal hyperexcitation with a lower pain threshold. These data suggest that bone cancer pain may have both an inflammatory and a neuropathic component [13]. Tumor-induced pain is usually described as dull in character, constant, and gradually increasing in intensity with time. Bone cancer pain results from a combination of background pain at rest, spontaneous pain at rest, and breakthrough pain, incident in nature, as a consequence of non-noxious movement of mechanical load.

CHRONIC PAIN AND PLASTIC CHANGES OF THE CENTRAL NERVOUS SYSTEM

Chronic pain, regardless the initial etiology, produces important changes in the central nervous system. A prolonged stimulus from the periphery through the stimulation of either nociceptors or ectopic firing after neural damage leads to repetitive activation of C fibers. This results in an augmentation of activity in dorsal horn wide dynamic range neurons and a strong increase in the magnitude of the responses evoked by subsequent stimuli. Thus, increased input from injured neurons, ectopic nerve action potentials, and sensitization of nociceptors by the peripheral nerves produce tonic input to the spinal cord.

Central sensitization and a windup phenomenon at the spinal and supraspinal levels have been described to explain the pathophysiological background of chronic pain conditions due to persistent peripheral stimuli or nerve injury [14]. The existence of peripheral hyperalgesia has a bearing on the induction of central hypersensitivity in the spinal cord. The enhanced release of substance P and other neurokinins may provide the mechanisms by which the N-methyl-D-aspartate (NMDA) receptor for the excitatory amino acids becomes more easily activated. These transmitters cooperate to activate spinal cord neurons. The release of peptides such as substance P into the spinal cord on afferent stimulation removes the magnesium block of the channel of the NMDA receptor and thus allows glutamate to activate the NMDA receptor in the range of persistent pain states [3]. The ion channel for the NMDA receptor allows vast amounts of calcium to enter into the neurons, resulting in an amplification of the response underlying central hyperalgesia. The repetition of a constant intensity C fiber stimulus induces the phenomenon of windup, that is, the switch from a low level of pain-related activity to a high level without any change in the inputs arriving from the peripheral nerves. This results in the prolongation and amplification of nociceptive activity even after the cessation of the peripheral input.

The activation of such receptors is involved in the development and maintenance of injury-induced central hyperactive states by initiating a variety of intracellular processes. These principally consist of an increase in the concentration of intracellular calcium, activation of protein kinase C (PKC), and the calcium–calmodulin-mediated production of NO, leading to neuronal excitability in a complex manner. It has been suggested that feedback by NO increases the release of C fiber transmitters, further enhancing pain transmission. PKC translocation and NO production may enhance postsynaptic neuronal excitability, leading to the development of hyperactive states. Furthermore, PKC and NO may activate presynaptic NMDA receptors localized on primary afferent fibers by removing the magnesium blockade of the NMDA receptor. In so doing, even small amounts of excitatory amino acid ligands may allow the opening of calcium channels, with further activation of a second pool of PKC (Figure 41.1). Increases in intracellular calcium and activation of PKC also result in c-*fos* expression in postsynaptic dorsal horn neurons as well as in supraspinal areas. This is considered to be a third messenger, probably involved in encoding a variety of cellular responses that are responsible for the neural changes associated with hyperalgesia [15]. This has been demonstrated by similar time courses of c-*fos* expression and the development of hyperalgesia [16]. Whereas the entry of calcium can also

activate phospholipases and lead to the spinal production of prostanoids, persistent activation of excitatory amino acid receptors within the spinal cord may contribute to central hyperexcitability. This is because irreversible morphological changes may occur with the loss of function of spinal cord inhibitory interneurons. These excitotoxic processes may result in disinhibition phenomena, reinforcing the central hyperactivity state [17].

Peripheral nerve injury also results in a number of dorsal horn effects, such as changes in the distribution and density of a-amino-3-hydroxy-5-methyl-4-isoxazole propionic acid receptors (better known as AMPA), release of neurotrophins, sprouting of central terminals, and loss of inhibitory neurons containing g-aminobutyric acid.[3] Mechanisms of normal synaptic transmission and intense and prolonged activation are shown in Figures 41.2 and 41.3. Similar mechanisms are presumably operating at the supraspinal level, although available data are less clear. Pain activates brain structures, such as the periaqueductal gray matter of the midbrain (which is involved in blood pressure regulation, respiration, vasomotor control, and metabolic homeostasis) and the thalamus (which is a major relay in the transmission of nociceptive information). Prolonged activation of these structures can have a strong impact on psychological function, also inducing complex cognitive responses.

DESCENDING MODULATION OF NOCICEPTION

Brainstem descending pathways constitute a major mechanism for modulating nociceptive transmission at the spinal level. The rostral ventromedial medulla (RVM) includes the nucleus raphe magnus and adjacent lateral reticular formation. A biphasic descending modulation of nociception has been postulated,

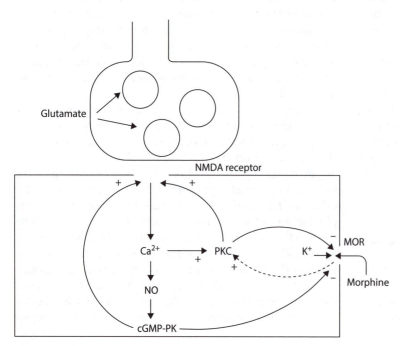

Figure 41.1 *Activation of NMDA receptors increases intracellular Ca²⁺ concentration and subsequent intracellular activation of PKC and NO. Substrate phosphorylation by PKC or NO-mediated protein kinase may produce the enhanced activity of glutamate receptor–Ca²⁺ complex, with the development of hyperactive states. PKC and NO-mediated protein kinase actions may produce uncoupling of G-protein with mu opioid receptor (MOR), thus reducing morphine antinociception.*

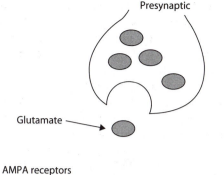

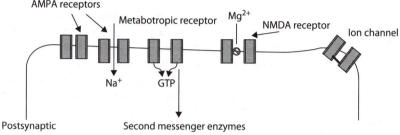

Figure 41.2 *Normal synaptic transmission: Presynaptic activation produces the exocytosis of glutamate, which binds to postsynaptic receptors: (i) AMPA receptors, leading to the opening of Na$^+$ and K$^+$ channels and resulting in depolarization; (ii) metabotropic receptors, causing the binding of GTP to G-proteins and activation of second messengers (PKC, adenyl cyclase); and (iii) NMDA receptors, potentially opening ion channels. Mg^{2+} blocks the ion flux.*

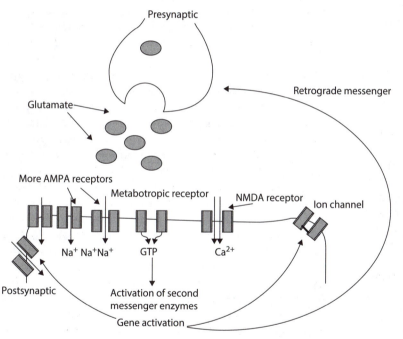

Figure 41.3 *Intense and prolonged activation causes an abnormal release of glutamate. More AMPA receptors are activated, limiting the Mg^{2+} block on NMDA receptors. Ca^{2+} ions flow through these channels, interacting with the second messenger enzymes, resulting in more availability of AMPA receptors, as a consequence of gene activation. Phosphorylation of ion channels makes the cell more excitable. Retrograde messengers also act on presynaptic nerve terminals, causing the release of more glutamate.*

through the activation of facilitation and inhibition of nociceptive processes, consequent to activation of two types of cell group, *on-cell* and *off-cell*, respectively. Descending pathways are activated by tissue injury to counteract the cascade of events that ultimately contribute to the development of inflammatory hyperalgesia. Opioidergic circuits are involved in descending inhibition of nociception, increasing the activity of the antinociception-inhibiting *off-cells*, and decreasing the activity of the nociceptive-facilitating *on-cells* of the RVM. Studies suggest that descending serotonergic and noradrenergic pathways differently suppress the responses of spinal neurons [18]. The organization and functional significance of the facilitatory network is less known and is possibly involved in pronociceptive

mechanisms. For example, prolonged administration of opioids induces neuroplastic changes, resulting in the enhanced ability of cholecystokinin (CCK) to excite facilitatory pathways from the RVM, and/or upregulation of dynorphin levels, evoking the release of excitatory transmitters from primary afferents (see below) [19]. Ventrolateral periaqueductal gray matter could be one of the sites where the repeated administration of opioids induces opioid tolerance. There is evidence that endogenous or exogenous opioids lead to an enhancement of CCK activity, which in turn attenuates the antinociceptive effect of opioids and may be one of the mechanisms responsible for opioid tolerance [20]. The dynamic plasticity of descending pathways may render the system vulnerable and lead to pathological consequences.

CHRONIC PAIN STATES AND OPIOID ACTIVITY

Opioids inhibit or block the excitation of dorsal horn cells by depressing firing through both presynaptic and postsynaptic inhibitory effects in the spinal cord [21]. The physiological targets of both exogenous and endogenous opioids are receptors coupled to G-proteins: m, d, and k receptors. The acute effects of the opioids include inhibition of cAMP formation, activation of inward K^+ channels, and inhibition of voltage-gated Ca channels. These lead to presynaptic hyperpolarization, inhibition of excitatory neurotransmitter release, and activation of descending antinociceptive pathways [22]. Opioid receptors undergo adaptations such as desensitization, downregulation, and internalization in response to agonist treatment. The reduction in receptor function is hypothesized to contribute to opioid tolerance. Opioid receptors are desensitized on the cell surface through a phosphorylation process. On the other hand, receptor internalization is now believed to contribute to resensitization through a dephosphorylation during endosomal stages [23]. An inverse relation between tolerance liability and m-opioid receptor endocytosis has been shown. On the other hand, the loss of response to opioid agonists upon long-term treatment seems to be the result of two partially overlapping processes: the gradual loss of inhibitory opioid signal transduction and an increase in excitatory signaling [24]. Chronic opioid agonist treatment simultaneously desensitizes the inhibitory effects of the opioids and augments the stimulatory signaling, possibly through a time-dependent alteration of the specificity of opioid–G-protein coupling. The supersensitivity of neurons to the excitatory effects of opioids seems to be to a GM1 ganglioside–mediated conversion of the opioid receptors from an inhibitory (Gi coupled) to an excitatory (Gs coupled) mode [25]. These changes cause a compensatory increase in cellular cAMP formation, due to an increased activity of PKC. This superactivation is manifested by an apparent desensitization of the inhibitory opioid signaling.

Clinically, it seems that opioids differ in their capability of inducing such molecular events, although the degree and the time course of tolerance are influenced by several factors, including dosing schedules and routes of administration, and humoral factors associated with the disease [26].

Several factors common to neuropathic pain and tolerance have been found, although some central changes at spinal cord level typically present in neuropathic pain states are not found with chronic exposure to morphine. Activation of spinal cord NMDA receptors, PKC activation, and NO production are biochemical steps equally capable of leading to a state of hyperalgesia or the development of morphine tolerance [16,21]. Substrate phosphorylation by PKC and NO may result either in enduring enhancement of synaptic activity at spinal cord level [27] and decreasing the mu-receptor activity, uncoupling of G-protein with the m receptor or facilitating its desensibilization [28,29]. Thus, the reduction of morphine analgesia induced by nerve injury may share a mechanism similar to that of morphine tolerance. Reduction of morphine antinociception occurs after hyperalgesia induced by nerve injury in the absence of daily exposure to morphine [16], as nerve injury would produce a reduction of morphine nociception prior to exposure to morphine itself. In other terms, it is possible that a sort of tolerance and/or hyperalgesia develops before exposure to morphine, and a neuropathic pain state may be equivalent to that of the development of morphine tolerance or facilitating hyperalgesia with a consequent pronociceptive effect [16,30]. This is consistent with the clinical observation of increased opioid requirements in patients with neuropathic pain [31,32]. However, these neuroplastic changes may be distinct, and divergent intracellular events may take place, as the expression of hyperalgesia is not necessarily associated with the expression of tolerance and vice versa. A single dose of MK-801, an inhibitor of NMDA receptors, has been shown to reduce hyperalgesia but not to enhance morphine antinociception [16,28].

Descending facilitation at RVM level has been reported. This pronociceptive activity has been found to be associated with increases in the expression of dynorphin in the spinal dorsal horn, which promotes the release of excitatory transmitters from primary afferent neurons [33]. Prolonged opioid treatment not only results in a loss of opioid antinociceptive efficacy but also leads to activation of a pronociceptive system characterized by a reduction of nociceptive threshold. [34]. Thus, it has been suggested that the concurrent expression of hyperalgesia during chronic opioid administration (OIH) counteracts antinociception, producing an impression of tolerance due to compensatory neuronal hyperactivity. In the periphery vanilloid receptors and chitokines appear to be involved in OIH. Central OIH pathways may be mediated by opioid receptors, NMDA receptors, 5HT3 receptors in descending pathways, and cholecystokinin in the RVM. Opioid receptors may be involved in several ways [35]. One mechanism could be an increased release of dynorphin and an increased expression of opioid receptors in the excitatory Gs-coupled state, as opposed to the Gi/Go-coupled state. The descending spinal facilitation opioid-mediated by *on-cells* may also contribute to OIH. There are controversies regarding the role of the diffuse noxious inhibitory control, which should be reduced by exogenous opioids, suppressing the antinociceptive pathways normally mediated by endogenous opioids [36].

As it becomes clear that chronic pain, particularly cancer pain, is able to specifically modify the response of the central nervous system, recent data indicate a close relation between cancer disease and its metabolic and immunological consequences, and plastic changes of the central nervous system associated with the concomitant chronic administration of opioids, which require better knowledge of molecular events underlying such mechanisms. An integrated approach that takes into account information from both experimental work and the bedside is recommended.

Key learning points

- The clinical picture of cancer pain varies depending on the pathophysiological mechanism, which further depends on the characteristics and progression of disease, and the preferential sites of metastases. Although the pain related to malignant disease can be classified as nociceptive-inflammatory and neuropathic, they are both significantly influenced by changes in the central nervous system function.

- It is now clear that cancer pain is a more complex entity, particularly regarding the response to analgesics, where numerous factors play a role.

- Central sensitization and a windup phenomenon at the spinal and supraspinal level have been described to explain the pathophysiological background of chronic pain conditions.

- Brainstem descending pathways constitute a major mechanism for modulating nociceptive transmission at the spinal level. The dynamic plasticity of descending pathways may render the system vulnerable and lead to pathological consequences.

- Opioids produce inhibition or block excitation of dorsal horn cells within the spinal cord. Repeated administration of opioids produces a decrease in analgesia, an effect termed "tolerance."

- There are several common factors in neuropathic pain and tolerance.

- Prolonged opioid treatment not only results in a loss of opioid antinociceptive efficacy but also leads to activation of a pronociceptive system characterized by a reduction of nociceptive threshold.

REFERENCES

1   Porreca F. Nociceptors, the spinal dorsal horn, and descending modulation. In: *Pain 2010*. IASP press, Seattle 2010; pp. 3–12.
2   Dickenson A, Bee L. Neurobiological mechanism of neuropathic pain and its treatment. In: *Pain 2010*. J. Mogil ed. IASP press, Seattle 2010; pp. 271–282.
3   Besson JM. The neurobiology of pain. *Lancet* 1999;353:1610–1615.
4   Siddall PJ, Cousins MJ. Persistent pain as a disease entity: Implications for clinical management. *Anesth Analg* 2004;99:510–520.
5   Friedman R. Pain at the cellular level: The role of the cytokine tumor necrosis factor. *Reg Anesth Pain Med* 2000;25:110–112.
6   Ness TJ, Gebhart GF. Visceral pain: A review of experimental studies. *Pain* 1990;41:167–234.
7   Cervero F, Laird JMA. Visceral pain. *Lancet* 1999;353:2145–2148.
8   Giamberardino MA. Recent and forgotten aspects of visceral pain. *Eur J Pain* 1999;3:77–92.
9   Mercadante S. Neoplasm-induced pain. In: *Neurobiology of Disease*. S. Gilman ed. Elsevier, San Diego, CA 2006; pp. 1007–1020.
10 Mercadante S. Abdominal pain. In: *Gastrointestinal Symptoms*. C. Ripamonti & E. Bruera eds. Oxford University Press, New York 2002; pp. 223–234.
11 Mercadante S. Management of bone pain. In: *Handbook of Cancer-Induced Bone Disease*. R. Coleman, P. Abrahamsson, P. Hadji eds. Bioscientifica 2010; pp. 145–160.
12 Jemenez-Andrade JM, Mantyh W, Bloom A, Ferng A, Geffre C, Mantyh P. Bone cancer pain. *Ann N Y Acad Sci* 2010;1198:173–181.
13 Luger N, Mach D, Sevcik M, Mantyh P. Bone cancer pain: From model to mechanism to therapy. *J Pain Symptom Manage* 2005;29: S32–S46.
14 Woolf CJ, Thompson SW. The induction and maintenance of central sensitization is dependent on N-methyl-D-aspartic acid receptor activation: Implications for the treatment of post-injury pain hypersensitivity states. *Pain* 1991;44:293–299.
15 Coderre TJ, Katz J, Vaccarino AL, Melzack R. Contribution of central neuroplasticity to pathological pain: Review of clinical and experimental evidence. *Pain* 1993;52:259–285.
16 Mao J, Price D, Mayer DJ. Experimental mononeuropathy reduces the antinociceptive effects of morphine: Implications for common intracellular mechanisms involved in morphine tolerance and neuropathic pain. *Pain* 1995;61:353–364.
17 Dubner R. Neuronal plasticity and pain following peripheral tissue inflammation and nerve injury. In: *Pain Research and Clinical Management, Vol. 4, Proceedings of the Sixth World Congress on Pain*. Bond MR, Charlton JE, Woolf CJ, eds. Elsevier, Amsterdam, the Netherlands, 1991; pp. 263–276.
18 Ren K, Zhuo M, Willis W. Multiplicity and plasticity of descending modulation of nociception: Implications for persistent pain. In: *Proceedings of the Ninth World Congress on Pain*. Devor M, Rowbotham M, Wiesenfeld-Hallin Z, eds. IASP Press, Seattle, WA, 2000; pp. 387–400.
19 Ossipov M, Lai J, Vanderah T, Porreca F. Induction of pain facilitation by sustained opioid exposure: Relationship to opioid antinociceptive tolerance. *Life Sci* 2003;73:783–800.
20 Tortorici V, Nogueira L, Salas R, Vanegas H. Involvement of local cholecystokinin in the tolerance induced by morphine microinjections into the periaqueductal gray of rats. *Pain* 2003;102:9–16.
21 Mayer DJ, Mao J, Price DD. The development of morphine tolerance and dependence is associated with translocation of protein kinase C. *Pain* 1995;61:365–374.
22 Varga EV, Yamamura Hi, Rubenzik et al. Molecular mechanisms of excitatory signaling upon chronic opioid agonist treatment. *Life Sci* 2003;74:299–311.
23 He L, Fong J, von Zastrow M, Whistler JL. Regulation of opioid receptor trafficking and morphine tolerance by receptor oligomerization. *Cell* 2002;25:271–282.
24 Ueda H, Inoue M, Mizuno K. New approaches to study the development of morphine tolerance and dependence. *Life Sci* 2003;74:313–320.
25 Crain SM, Shen KF. Antagonists of excitatory opioid receptor functions enhance morphine's analgesic potency and attenuate opioid tolerance/dependence liability. *Pain* 2000;84:121–131.
26 Mercadante S, Portenoy RK. Opioid poorly responsive cancer pain. Part 2. Basic mechanisms that could shift dose-response for analgesia. *J Pain Symptom Manage* 2001;21:255–264.
27 Chen L, Huang LYM. Protein kinase C reduces Mg^{2+} block of NMDA-receptor channels as a mechanism of modulation. *Nature* 1992;356:521–523.
28 Trujillo KA, Akil H. Inhibition of morphine tolerance and dependence by the NMDA receptor antagonist MK-801. *Science* 1991;251:85–87.
29 Collin E, Cesselin F. Neurobiological mechanisms of opioid tolerance and dependence. *Clin Pharmacol* 1991;14:465–488.
30 Basbaum AI. Insights into the development of opioid tolerance. *Pain* 1995;61:349–352.
31 Portenoy RK, Foley KM, Inturrisi CE. The nature of opioid responsiveness and its implications for neuropathic pain: New hypothesis derived from studies of opioid infusions. *Pain* 1990;43:273–286.

32 Mercadante S, Dardanoni G, Salvaggio L et al. Monitoring of opioid therapy in advanced cancer patients. *J Pain Symptom Manage*
1997;13:204–212.

33 Vanderah TW, Ossipov MH, Lai J et al. Mechanisms of opioid-induced
pain and antinociceptive tolerance: Descending facilitation and spinal
dynorphin. *Pain* 2001;92:5–9.

34 Mao J. Opioid-induced abnormal pain sensitivity: Implications in clinical opioid therapy. *Pain* 2002;100:213–217.

35 Colvin LA, Fallon MT. Opioid-induced hyperalgesia: A clinical challenge.
Br J Anaesth 2010;104:125–127.

36 Chu LF, Angst MS, Clarck D. Opioid-induced hyperalgesia in humans:
Molecular mechanisms and clinical considerations. *Clin J Pain*
2008;24:479–496.

42

Causes and mechanisms of pain in palliative care patients

MARIEBERTA VIDAL, SURESH K. REDDY

INTRODUCTION

Pain due to cancer is one of the most common symptoms experienced by palliative care patients, as shown by many studies in this patient population.[1-3] The consequences of undertreatment of pain are daunting, yet pain is underdiagnosed and undertreated for many reasons.[4,5] One of the main reasons for undertreatment of pain in patients with cancer continues to be a lack of appropriate pain assessment.[6,7] In cancer, pain is predominantly caused by the tumor and its consequences. Other reasons include treatment side effects and coexisting pain conditions[3,8] (Box 42.1). In noncancer situations, pain may result from chronic degenerative disorders of the spine and joints[9-11]: central pain because of spinal cord injury and neuropathic pain due to metabolic, infective, and other causes[12-14] (Box 42.2).

Pain results from the activation of nociceptors by a variety of chemical mediators released from damaged cells. The mediators include potassium, serotonin, bradykinin, and histamine and are usually associated with the redness and swelling of inflammation. In addition, cells may be sensitized by other substances such prostaglandins, leukotrienes, and substance P. Sensitization can extend to areas away from the original damage, resulting in hypersensitivity of the area.

Cancer pain can occur after activation of peripheral nociceptors (somatic and visceral "nociceptive" pain) or by direct injury to peripheral or central nervous structures (neuropathic or "deafferentation" pain). In addition, both nociceptive and neuropathic pain may be modified by the involvement of the sympathetic nervous system, resulting in sympathetically maintained pain (SMP) or complex regional pain syndrome type 1 (CRPS). Each of these painful states has somewhat unique clinical characteristics that may aid in its identification and directed treatment. A key step, therefore, in the evaluation of a cancer patient with pain is to elicit a careful history of the quality, nature, and location of perceived pain, as the descriptors may provide valuable clues to the etiology of the complaint.

Somatic pain results from the involvement of bone and muscle structures. Metastatic bone disease is the most common pain syndrome in patients with cancer. Myelinated and unmyelinated afferent fibers are present in bone, and their density is greatest in the periosteum. Prostaglandins play a multifactorial role in the etiology of bone pain. Prostaglandin concentrations are increased at sites of bone metastasis.[15] In addition, prostaglandins are now known to mediate osteolytic and osteoclastic metastatic bone changes. Prostaglandin E_2 is known to sensitize nociceptors and produce hyperalgesia. These observations have resulted in steroidal and nonsteroidal anti-inflammatory drugs (NSAIDs) as important therapy for metastatic bone pain. Reports suggest that NSAIDs are uniquely effective.[16]

Visceral pain is also common in patients with cancer, and presumably results from stretching or distending or from the production of an inflammatory response and the release of analgesic substances in the vicinity of nociceptors. Visceral pain is commonly referred to cutaneous sites, which can mislead the examiner, particularly since those cutaneous sites may be tender to palpation. This property likely results from convergence of visceral and somatic afferent information onto common neuronal pools in the dorsal horn of the spinal cord.[17] Neuropathic pain from neural injury such as brachial plexus infiltration by tumor is often severe. The pain is described as paroxysms of burning or electric-shock-like sensations, which may result, at least in part, from spontaneous discharges in the peripheral and central nervous systems.

Somatic, visceral, and deafferentation pain may be modified by the sympathetic nervous system. Sympathetically maintained pain is often suspected when pain is severe in intensity (even after relatively trivial tissue insults) and described as burning in quality, with associated features of allodynia, hyperpathia, brawny edema, and osteoporosis.[18] Several mechanisms involving both peripheral and central nervous systems have been postulated to

Box 42.1 Common clinical pain syndromes and their causes

Tumor pain

- Bone pain due to metastasis (somatic pain) from breast, prostate, and other cancers
- Plexopathy pain (neuropathic pain) due to Pancoast tumor/pelvic tumor
- Abdominal pain (visceral pain) due to pancreatic cancer and liver metastasis
- Chest wall pain due to mesothelioma (somatic and neuropathic pain)

Cancer treatment pain

- Postchemotherapy pain syndromes
- Peripheral neuropathy due to cisplatin and paclitaxel

Postirradiation pain syndromes

- Chronic throat pain due to radiation-induced mucositis
- Chronic abdominal pain due to radiation-induced enteritis in fistulas
- Radiation-induced plexopathy pain

Postsurgical pain syndromes

- Postmastectomy pain syndrome
- Postradical neck dissection pain syndrome
- Phantom limb pain syndrome

Noncancer pain

- Chronic low back pain due to degenerative process in the spine
- Pain secondary to osteoarthritis and rheumatoid arthritis
- Migraine headaches

Box 42.2 Noncancer pain syndromes

Headache

- Migraine
- Tension-type headache
- Cluster headache
- Miscellaneous

Facial pain

- Trigeminal neuralgia
- Temporomandibular joint pain
- Glossopharyngeal neuralgia
- PHN
- Myofascial pain syndromes

Neck pain

- Diskogenic radicular pain
- Whiplash injury pain syndrome
- Cervicogenic pain
- Facet joint pain syndrome

Thoracic pain syndromes

- Costochondritis
- Intercostal neuralgia
- PHN
- Facet joint pain syndrome
- Chronic shoulder pain: Frozen shoulder; rotator cuff tear

Abdominal pain

- Chronic pancreatitis
- Chronic peptic ulcer disease
- Postcholecystectomy syndrome
- Crohn disease
- Irritable bowel syndrome

Pelvic pain

- Chronic interstitial cystitis
- Chronic testicular pain
- Chronic prostatitis pain
- Chronic pelvic pain from inflammatory pelvic disease
- Endometriosis-related pain syndromes

Low back and lower extremity pain

- Central pain
- Lumbosacral spine disease: Myofascial; diskogenic; osteoporotic; facet joint pain syndrome
- Peripheral vascular disease and ischemic pain syndrome
- Dorsal tunnel syndrome
- CRPS
- Phantom limb pain

explain SMP. For example, one peripheral mechanism may be the development of ephaptic connections at sites of tissue injury such that efferent sympathetic impulses produce activation of afferent nociceptive pathways. Others have postulated that traumatic injury to peripheral tissues may produce sensitization of spinal cord nociceptive neurons, which may then be secondarily activated by efferent sympathetic activity.

It is common for patients with cancer to present with mixtures of the pain types described earlier. Furthermore, the pattern of pain intensity is often not constant, but rather includes episodes of pain exacerbations on a background of continuous pain, called "breakthrough" pain (see Chapter 54).[19]

SPECIFIC PAIN SYNDROMES IN PATIENTS WITH CANCER

There are several specific pain syndromes that may present difficult diagnostic and therapeutic problems, of which the palliative care specialist needs to be aware during the evaluation of

Medical diseases causing pain

- Chronic fatigue syndrome
- Sickle cell disease
- Peripheral neuropathy pain (e.g., diabetes)
- Rheumatoid arthritis, multiple sclerosis, osteoarthritis

HIV/AIDS pain syndromes

- Headache (e.g., cryptococcal meningitis)
- Oral cavity pain secondary to candidiasis, herpes simplex, or Kaposi sarcoma
- Chest pain secondary to candidal esophagitis
- Chronic abdominal pain from infections such as cryptosporidiosis, CMV, cholecystitis, pancreatitis
- Pain syndromes related to Kaposi sarcoma
- Neuropathic pain syndromes (e.g., predominantly sensory neuropathy, myelopathy, radicular pain from Guillain–Barré syndrome)

the cancer patient with pain.[20] The characteristic clinical features of these syndromes are summarized in Box 42.3 and discussed in the following. Please note that notable but short-lived pain syndromes, such as mucositis, that complicate chemotherapy and radiation therapy, and the acute pain associated with diagnostic and therapeutic procedures, such as bone marrow aspiration, are not included in Box 42.3.

TUMOR HEMORRHAGE

Tumor hemorrhage can present as an acute pain syndrome in cancer patients and might need urgent treatment. This syndrome is common in hepatocellular carcinoma, presenting usually with severe RUQ pain and it could be a potential life-threatening complication when the tumor ruptures. Another example is an ovarian cancer causing bleeding inside the tumor leading to severe flank pain.[21,22] Other intra-abdominal malignancies can also present with acute bleeding into the tumor causing pain.

TUMOR INFILTRATION OF BONE

Pain from invasion of bone by either primary or metastatic tumor is the most common cause of pain in patients with cancer. Several important pain syndromes are often misdiagnosed because physicians are unfamiliar with the characteristic signs and symptoms, and plain x-rays of the involved areas may show normal findings.

The pathophysiology of metastatic bone pain is poorly understood. Although most patients with bone metastasis report pain, a large proportion of patients with radiographic

Box 42.3 Clinical characteristics of intractable pain syndromes

- Tumor-related infiltration of bone—Acute and chronic nociceptive pain.
- Skull-base metastasis—Severe head pain (usually referred to vertex or occiput) with associated cranial nerve deficits. Bone scan and plain films of the skull may show normal findings.
- Vertebral metastasis—Significant risk of associated spinal cord compression. Of patients with back pain and vertebral body metastasis, 30% will eventually develop epidural spinal cord compression, and pain alone may precede root or spinal cord signs by many months.
- Pelvis and long bones—Risk of pathological fracture with weight-bearing activities; orthopedic consultation helpful.
- Tumor-related infiltration of nerve—Acute and chronic neuropathic pain.
- Brachial/lumbosacral plexopathy—May occur by contiguous spread of tumor or by hematogenous dissemination; radiographic studies helpful to distinguish from radiation-induced plexopathy.
- Spinal cord compression—Neurological emergency requiring prompt treatment with corticosteroids, radiation therapy, and/or surgery.
- Meningeal carcinomatosis—Headache and meningeal signs. Causes significant pain in about 15% of patients.
- Visceral tumor infiltration—Acute and chronic visceral pain that is poorly localized and widely referred. Common examples include pancreatic carcinoma, liver metastasis, and pleural effusion.
- Therapy-related postsurgical pain—Chronic pain that persists well beyond healing of the incision and may or may not be associated with recurrent disease.
- After thoracotomy—May be associated with recurrent tumor or may occur as a chronic intercostals neuralgia.
- After mastectomy—Occurs in 5% of women; more common in women undergoing modified radical procedure with axillary dissection; intercostal brachioradial neuralgia is one cause.
- After radical neck surgery—Mechanisms unclear; chronic infection may play a role.
- After amputation—Stump pain and phantom phenomena are common; role of preventive analgesic and anesthetic therapies is under investigation.

evidence of disease deny pain. This has been best studied in breast cancer,[23] but is also true in prostate cancer. Tumor growth in bone may produce pain by several mechanisms:

- Relatively rapid growth causing expansion of the marrow space and increased interosseal pressure (beyond 50 mmHg). In theory, this may activate mechanoreceptive nociceptors in bone. In addition, elevation or invasion of the periosteum may also activate nociceptors that innervate this structure.

- Weakening of the bone leading to fractures.
- Edema and inflammation associated with tumor growth in bone may liberate chemical mediators that activate nociceptors.
- Recent data regarding mechanisms of bone destruction emphasize that osteoclasts may be stimulated by a number of humoral factors associated with tumors. For example, carcinomas may secrete prostaglandins,[15] which would have the dual role of activating osteoclasts and sensitizing nociceptors. These observations have provided a rationale for the use of corticosteroids and NSAIDs for the management of metastatic bone pain.[24]

Metastatic bone pain is often associated with neurological dysfunction because of the close anatomical relations between the brain and cranial nerves and the skull vault, and the spinal cord and its roots and the vertebral column. Therefore, characteristic clinical syndromes may be identified by the site of bony involvement, the coexistence of mechanical instability secondary to fractures, and neurological dysfunction caused by tumor infiltration of contiguous neurological structures. Bone metastasis to the hip and pelvis often produces local pain that is exacerbated by movement, especially when weight bearing. In addition to palliative radiotherapy, this type of "incident pain" may require specific orthopedic interventions.

Spread of cancer to the vertebral bodies and calvarium, especially the base of the skull, often produces distinctive neurological syndromes. These are important to recognize early because prompt initiation of antitumor treatments, especially radiation, may avoid neurological impairment. For example, local and radicular back or neck pain is the predominant symptom in epidural spinal cord compression, complicating vertebral body metastasis in these locations. Pain may be the only symptom of impending spinal cord compression, and often precedes motor weakness and bowel or bladder incontinence by days or weeks. The spinal cord is compromised by growth of the tumor in an anterior direction from the vertebral body. Irreversible spinal cord injury may occur when the vascular supply is compromised as a result of severe compression. Thoracic spine vertebral body metastases often produce bilateral radicular pain and sensory symptoms (a "band-like" squeezing sensation across the upper abdomen or chest) because of the close proximity of the thoracic nerve roots to the vertebral body. On the other hand, metastases in the cervical or lumbar spine may produce unilateral pain and sensory loss as the vertebral bodies are wider in these areas and lateral extension of the tumor may compress only one root at the time.

Skull metastasis

Spread of tumor to the calvarium may produce neurological symptoms by two mechanisms. Metastases to the skull vault, which grow to compress the sagittal sinus may produce a syndrome of severe headache with associated papilledema and seizures caused by elevation in the intracranial pressure (ICP). If untreated, focal neurological deficits may

occur secondary to venous infarction of the brain. The cause of metastatic sagittal sinus occlusion is usually obvious, and is easily confirmed by magnetic resonance imaging (MRI) of the brain. The gadolinium-enhanced MRI will not only demonstrate the tumor metastasis, but will also demonstrate the blood clot in the sagittal sinus. It is noteworthy that non-metastatic sagittal sinus occlusion may also occur in prostate cancer as a complication of a hypercoagulable state induced by diethylstilbestrol treatment.

Tumor metastasis to the base of the skull may also produce distinct neurological syndromes.[25] Bone metastasis to this portion of the skull often produces severe headache referred to the top of the head or the occiput. Also, single or multiple cranial nerve palsies usually accompany basal skull metastasis. For example, clival metastasis often compresses the hypoglossal nerve, producing unilateral weakness of the tongue and deviation of the tongue to the side of the lesion when protruded from the mouth. Bone metastasis to the middle cranial fossa may compress and infiltrate the facial nerve, producing ipsilateral weakness of the upper and lower face. Tumor invasion of the jugular foramen will produce severe head pain with associated dysphagia, dysphonia, and hoarseness caused by dysfunction of the glossopharyngeal and vagal nerves, which exit the skull base through this foramen. Involvement of foramen ovale may result in compression of trigeminal nerve leading to facial pain.

Small lesions at the skull base may not be visible on plain x-rays or bone scans. It is mandatory that computed tomography (CT) scans with bone windows and 5 mm sections are done to demonstrate the tumor. It is sometimes necessary to do MRI scans of the base of the skull when CT scans are negative.[20]* Radiation therapy directed to the base of the skull is the preferred treatment. Again, prompt recognition of these syndromes and aggressive treatment is indicated to prevent irreversible cranial nerve palsies that often produce devastating neurological impairments.

Cervical spine metastasis

Metastatic disease involving the odontoid process of the axis (first cervical vertebral body) results in a pathological fracture. Secondary subluxation occurs and results in spinal cord or brainstem compression. The symptoms are usually severe neck pain radiating to the posterior aspect of the skull to the vertex, exacerbated by movement. The diagnostic evaluation may require MRI, as plain x-rays and bone scans may not show the problem. Imaging procedures must be carried out carefully to ensure spinal stability.

Pain in C5–C6 is characterized by a constant dull aching pain radiating bilaterally to both shoulders with tenderness to percussion over the spinous process. Radicular pain in a C7–C8 distribution occurs most commonly unilaterally in the posterior arm, elbow, and ulnar aspect of the hand. Paresthesias and numbness in the fourth and fifth fingers, progressive hand and triceps weakness are the neurological signs. Horner syndrome suggests paraspinal involvement. The diagnostic evaluation must be done carefully. Plain x-rays are often negative since this area is visualized poorly in these, and CT or preferably MRI scans are necessary to define metastatic disease.

Thoracic spine metastasis

The onset of back pain in association with band-like tightening across the chest or upper abdominal or radicular arm or leg pain may be the first sign of impending spinal cord compression. Motor and sensory loss occurs later, and autonomic disturbances producing bladder and bowel incontinence occur later still. Thus, the evaluation of the patient should begin at the onset of pain for the best chance to preserve motor and sphincteric function. This should include plain x-rays of the entire spine, focused on the symptomatic area, and an MRI. This is necessary because there is about a 15% incidence of another epidural lesion.[26] Corticosteroid therapy should be started even before the radiological evaluation, since this may decrease pain and protect the spinal cord from further compression caused by edema from the tumor or radiotherapy. Even if metastatic disease is found on plain spine films, the MRI should be done to define the extent of tumor invasion in the epidural space because this will influence the size of the radiation therapy ports and will determine the dose and duration of corticosteroid therapy. If anterior vertebral body subluxation has occurred and there is bony compression of the spinal cord, surgical decompression is indicated should the patient's medical condition permit. This is usually followed by radiation therapy. Surgery is usually not attempted as a primary modality of treatment because the results of radiation therapy and corticosteroid treatment are usually equal to surgical decompression.[26] This is especially true if a simple posterior decompressive laminectomy is done. However, if patients have recurrent spinal cord compression in a previously irradiated port, then an anterior spinal approach with removal of tumor from the vertebral body, decompression of tumor from the spinal canal, and restructuring of the vertebral body with methyl methacrylate should be considered.[27]

Lumbar spine and sacral metastasis

Dull and aching mid-back pain exacerbated by lying or sitting and relieved by standing is the usual presenting complaint of L1 metastasis. Pain may be referred to the hip, both paraspinal lumbosacral areas, and to the sacroiliac joint or superior iliac crest. Aching pain in the low back or coccygeal region exacerbated by lying or sitting, relieved by walking, is the common complaint with sacral metastases. Associated symptoms include perianal sensory loss, bowel and bladder dysfunction, and impotence.

Local invasion of tumor from the pelvis into the sacrum may produce the syndrome of perineal pain, which is often difficult to manage. This syndrome is characterized by local pain in the buttocks and perirectal area, which is often accentuated by pressure on the perineal region such as that caused by sitting or lying prone. In its most extreme form, the patient cannot sit to eat meals or lie flat to sleep, and may spend much of their time standing. Because of the critical role of the parasympathetic sacral innervation to normal bladder and rectal sphincter function, continence is impaired early in the course of this syndrome, perhaps even before significant weakness can be discerned in the legs.

Carcinomatous meningitis

Cancer arising outside the nervous system can metastasize to the CNS, including the meninges. Leptomeningeal disease occurs in approximate 5% of cancers. When meningeal disease presents as a late complication of malignant disease, the general prognosis is poor. The patients can present with different pain syndromes including headaches, cranial neuropathies, back pain, and radiculopathies. These particular symptoms are produced by the tendency of malignant cells in the cerebrospinal fluid (CSF) to congregate in specific sites like in the base of skull producing cranial neuropathies, obstruction of CSF flow, and raised ICP. They can also accumulate in the base of spine producing back pain, leg weakness, radiculopathies, bowel/bladder disturbance.[28,29]

TUMOR INFILTRATION OR TRAUMA TO PERIPHERAL NERVE, PLEXUS, ROOT, AND SPINAL CORD

These syndromes present with radicular pain in the neck, chest, or trunk and the differential diagnosis includes tumor infiltration of the peripheral nerves, and surgical injury, partial, complete or secondary to direct surgical interruption or traction, and nerve compression secondary to musculoskeletal imbalance, diabetic peripheral neuropathy, acute herpes zoster, and postherpetic neuralgia (PHN).

Pain is characterized by constant burning pain with hypoesthesia and dysesthesia in an area of sensory loss. The most common causes are tumor compression in the para-vertebral or retroperitoneal area or in association with metastatic tumor in rib causing intercostal nerve infiltration. Pain is usually the first sign of tumor infiltration of nerve and presents as either a local, radicular, or referred pain. Local and radicular pain is seen with tumor infiltration or compression of nerve peripheral to the paraspinal region, whereas referred pain with or without a radicular component is seen with tumor infiltration of the paraspinal region and more proximal areas. Associated autonomic dysfunction causing loss of sweating and loss of axonal flair response to pin scratch can help define the site of the nerve compression or infiltration. The pain is characterized initially by a dull, aching sensation with tenderness to percussion in the distribution of the nerve. Mild paresthesia or dysesthesia can occur as the next sensory symptom followed by the late appearance of motor symptoms and signs.

As tumor invades the perineurium or compresses nerve externally, the nature of the pain changes to a burning, dysesthetic sensation. A careful neurological examination followed by a CT scan to define the site of nerve compression is the diagnostic procedure of choice. Electromyography (EMG) can help to define the site of nerve involvement, but it is not diagnostic. Rib erosion and retroperitoneal and paraspinal soft tissue masses are the most common associated findings. In patients with paraspinal tumor, MRI scanning is often necessary to exclude epidural extension. Antitumor therapy is the first-line therapy when possible, but interim pain management with analgesics is almost always necessary. Steroids may provide a useful diagnostic test, and provide both anti-inflammatory and antitumor effects, or may act to reduce local swelling, and secondarily to relieve pain.

Brachial plexopathy

Brachial plexopathy in patients with cancer may occur by metastatic spread of tumor to the plexus or radiation injury producing transient sensory and motor symptoms. More prolonged neurological dysfunction may result from previous radiation therapy to a port which has included the plexus, involvement of the plexus by radiation-induced tumor such as malignant schwannoma or fibrosarcoma, and trauma to the plexus during surgery and anesthesia.

Tumor infiltration and radiation injury are the most common causes.[30] A review of 100 cases suggested that there are reliable clinical signs and symptoms to distinguish metastatic plexopathy from radiation injury. The characteristics of the pain are quite different and a useful distinguishing clinical sign.[30] MRI has been advocated as a better means to image the brachial plexus,[31] and may be a useful means to diagnose metastatic brachial plexopathy. Rarely biopsy of the brachial plexus may be necessary to distinguish from radiation fibrosis versus a recurrent tumor or a new primary tumor.[32] However, biopsy is not always definitive.

Metastases to the brachial plexus most commonly involve the lower cords of the brachial plexus, giving rise to neurological signs and symptoms in the distribution of the C8, T1 roots. In contrast, radiation plexopathy most commonly involves the upper cords of the plexus, predominantly in the distribution of the C5–C7 roots. Severe pain is most commonly associated with metastatic plexopathy, and Horner syndrome is more commonly associated with metastatic plexopathy than radiation plexopathy. A significant number of patients with metastatic plexopathy show epidural extension of disease. A primary tumor of the lung, the presence of Horner syndrome, or involvement of the whole plexus should alert the physician to the possibility of epidural extension and warrants immediate MRI. Neither a negative surgical biopsy nor observation for several years for other metastases rules out recurrence of tumor or a new primary tumor.[32]

Brachial plexopathy in Pancoast tumors

Brachial plexopathy in Pancoast tumor, as described by Kanner et al.[33] is an integral part of the disease. Pain in the distribution of C8–T1 is an early sign and is part of the clinical diagnosis of Pancoast syndrome. Pain is the most reliable sign to follow as it closely reflects progression of disease and may be the only sign of epidural cord compression. Plain x-rays and bone scans are not reliable diagnostic tests for this disorder, and MRI yields the most important diagnostic information. As many as 50% of patients develop epidural cord compression, with pain being the earliest and most consistent clinical symptom. In patients who present with Pancoast syndrome and involvement of the brachial plexus, the initial diagnostic workup should include MRI to determine the extent of tumor infiltration. Initial antitumor surgery should be directed at radial removal of all the local tumor and secondary treatment with external radiation therapy and brachytherapy.[34]

The Pancoast syndrome is commonly misdiagnosed and confused with cervical disk disease, which appears in less than 5% of patients in a C8–Tl distribution.

Lumbosacral plexopathy

Lumbosacral plexus tumor infiltration most commonly occurs in genitourinary, gynecological, and colonic cancers. Pain varies with the site of plexus involvement. Radicular pain occurs in L1–L3 distribution (i.e., anterior thigh and groin) or down the posterior aspect of the leg to the heel when in an L5–S1 distribution. In some instances, there is only referred pain without local pain over the plexus. Common referred points are the anterior thigh, knee, and lateral aspect of the calf. These areas are commonly painful, but the origin of the pain is in the plexus. Pain is the earliest symptom, followed later by complaints of paresthesia, numbness, and dysesthesia leading to motor and sensory loss.

Jaeckle et al.[35] have described the clinical symptoms and natural history of this disorder in a review of 85 patients with lumbosacral plexopathy. In this study, the pain was noted to be of three types: local in 72 of 85 patients, radicular in 72 of 85 patients, and referred in 37 of 85 patients. Local pain in the sacrum or sciatic notch occurred in 59% of patients followed by low back pain in 27% and pain in the groin or lower abdominal quadrant in 21%. Pain referred pain to the hip or flank occurred in patients with upper plexus lesions, whereas pain in the ankle or the foot occurred in patients with a lower plexopathy. Typically, the pain precedes objective sensory, motor, and autonomic signs for weeks to months, with a mean of 3 months. Also, initially, the CT scan may be negative. Unilateral and bilateral plexopathy with significant motor weakness is commonly associated with epidural extension, and both CT and MRI are necessary to define the extent of tumor infiltration and/or epidural compression. Plain x-rays are not often helpful because the lumbosacral plexus lies within the substance of the psoas muscle and is not radio-dense.

Pain occurs in 40% of patients with leptomeningeal metastases[36] and is of two types:

1. Headache with or without neck stiffness
2. Back pain localized to the low back and buttock regions

There may be associated confusion, delirium, cranial nerve palsies, radiculopathy, and myelopathy. Diagnostic workup should include MRI, with contrast to determine enhancement in the basal subarachnoid cisterns and to rule out hydrocephalus; MRI to rule out bulk disease on nerve roots which might require focal radiation therapy; and a lumbar puncture to determine CSF glucose, protein, cell count, cytology, and biochemical markers.

PAIN SYNDROMES ASSOCIATED WITH CANCER THERAPY

This category includes those clinical pain syndromes that occur in the course of or subsequent to treatment of cancer patients with the common modalities of surgery, chemotherapy, or radiation therapy.

Postsurgical injury to peripheral nerves

Four distinct pain syndromes involving the peripheral nerves occur following surgery in patients with cancer.

POSTTHORACOTOMY PAIN

This pain occurs in the distribution of an intercostal nerve following surgical interruption or injury. The intercostal neurovascular bundle courses along a groove in the inferior border of the rib. Traction on the ribs and rib resection are the common causes of nerve injury during a surgical procedure on the chest. Kanner et al.[33] prospectively followed 126 consecutive patients undergoing thoracotomy and defined several groups of patients. In the majority (79 patients), immediate postoperative pain was reduced at approximately 2 months, but in 13 of the 79 patients, recurrence of the pain occurred. Recurrence of tumor in the distribution of the intercostal nerves was the cause of recurrent pain. The immediate postoperative pain is characterized by an aching sensation in the distribution of the incision with sensory loss with or without autonomic changes. There is often exquisite point tenderness at the most medial and apical point of the scar with a specific trigger point. In another group (20 of the 126 patients), pain persisted following the thoracotomy and increased in intensity during the follow-up period. In this group of patients, local recurrence of disease and/or infection was the most common cause of increasing pain. In the third group, 18 of the 126 patients had stable or decreasing pain that resolved over time and did not represent a difficult management problem.

Thus, persistent or recurrent pain in the distribution of the thoracotomy scar in patients with cancer is commonly associated with recurrent tumor. However, a small number of patients will have a traumatic neuroma at the site of their previous thoracotomy scar, but this should not be the initial consideration in evaluating such cancer patients.

POSTMASTECTOMY PAIN

Postmastectomy pain occurs in the posterior arm, axilla, and anterior chest wall following any surgical procedure on the breast from lumpectomy to radical mastectomy.[37] It may be more likely to occur from axillary dissection and lymph node dissection.[38] There is marked anatomical variation in the size and distribution of the intercostal brachial nerve accounting for its variable appearance of this syndrome in patients undergoing mastectomy.[37] The pain results from interruption of the intercostal brachial nerve, a cutaneous sensory branch of T1–T2. The pain may occur immediately following the surgical procedure but as late as 6 months following surgery. It is characterized as a tight, constricting, burning pain in the posterior aspect of the arm and axilla radiating across the anterior chest wall. The pain is exacerbated by the movement of the arm and relieved by the immobilization of the arm. Patients often posture the arm in a flexed position close to the chest wall and are at risk to develop a frozen shoulder syndrome if adequate pain and postsurgical rehabilitation are not implemented early on.

Approximately 5% of women undergoing surgical procedures on the breast develop the syndrome. The nature of the pain and the clinical symptomatology should readily distinguish it from tumor infiltration of the brachial plexus. The syndrome appears to occur more commonly in patients with postoperative complications who are at risk for local fibrosis in and about the nerve following surgery, following wound infection or seroma. Typically, a trigger point in the axilla or on the anterior chest wall may be found and this is usually the site of the traumatic neuroma. Breast reconstruction does not alter the tight, constricting sensation in the anterior chest wall that is associated with this syndrome.

AFTER RADICAL NECK SURGERY

Prospective studies of pain after radical neck dissection are lacking. In any patient in whom the pain occurs late, that is, several months following the surgical procedure, and particularly any pain occurring several years following the surgical procedure, reevaluation is necessary to exclude recurrence of tumor.

POSTAMPUTATION PAIN

Loss of a body part is often followed by psychological adjustment, which may include a grief reaction.[39] The physiological phenomena of nonpainful and painful phantom sensations referred to the missing part, pain in the scar region after limb amputation, and involuntary motor activity also occur. Many patients note more sensations in the distal phantom limb or in the nipple of the phantom breast. A phantom visceral organ may be associated with functional sensations, for example, the urge to urinate or defecate.

There are a few reports on the course of postamputation pain in malignant disease. In a study of 17 patients with cancer who underwent forequarter amputation, none of the seven survivors had pain, requiring the use of analgesics after an average of 69 months follow-up.[40] Larger surveys of postmastectomy patients reveal that at least 10% experience chronic phantom breast pain, more than is generally believed.[41] Increasing pain in the cancer amputee may signify disease progression or recurrence.[42,43]

Chemotherapy-related pain syndromes

Painful dysesthesias follow treatment with several chemotherapeutic agents, in particular, the vinca alkaloid drugs such as vincristine and vinblastine. Cisplatin and taxol are also toxic to peripheral nerve.[44,45] These agents produce a symmetrical polyneuropathy as a result of a subacute with chronic axonopathy. Pain is usually localized to the hands and feet, and is characterized as burning pain exacerbated by superficial stimuli, which improves as the drug is withdrawn. Aseptic necrosis of the humeral and more commonly femoral head is a known complication of chronic steroid therapy.[46] Pain in the shoulder and knee or leg is the common presenting complaint, with x-ray changes occurring several weeks to months after the onset of pain. The bone scan and MRI are the most useful diagnostic procedure.

PHN[47] can be thought of as a postchemotherapy pain syndrome since immunocompromised patients are at risk for acute zoster infection or a recurrence of latent zoster. Persisting pain after healing of the cutaneous eruption of herpes zoster infection has generally three components:

1. A continuous burning pain in the area of sensory loss
2. Painful dysesthesias
3. Intermittent shock-like pain

Older patients are at greater risk of this complication.

Postradiation therapy pain

These syndromes are becoming less common as the sophistication with which radiation therapy portals are planned decreases the likelihood of radiation overdose to tissues and spares surrounding normal tissues. Nonetheless, radiation fibrosis of peripheral neural structures such as the brachial and lumbar plexus still occurs, and radionecrosis of bone is occasionally seen.

Radiation fibrosis of the brachial plexus was discussed previously. Pain occurring in the leg from radiation fibrosis of the lumbar plexus is characterized by the late onset of pain in the course of progressive motor and sensory changes in the leg.[48,49] Lymphedema, a previous history of radiation therapy, myokymia on EMG, and x-ray changes demonstrating radiation necrosis of bone may help to establish this diagnosis.

Pain is an early symptom in 15% of patients with radiation myelopathy.[50,51] Some patients may have the Lhermitte sign, signifying transient demyelination in the posterior columns, which does not necessarily predict the development of myelopathy. Pain may be localized to the area of spinal cord damage or may be a referred pain with dysesthesias below the level of injury. The neurological symptoms and signs often start as Brown–Séquard syndrome, a lateral hemisection of the cord, such that pain and temperature sensation are lost contralateral to the side of weakness. Position and vibration sensation are lost ipsilateral to the side of weakness. The incidence of myelopathy increases with increasing radiation exposure and approaches 50% with 1500 ret exposure. The latency from completion of radiation to the onset of symptoms of myelopathy ranges from 5 to 30 months, with an average of 14 months in most series.

A painful enlarging mass in an area of previous irradiation suggests a radiation-induced peripheral nerve tumor.[52-55] In one study, seven of nine patients who developed radiation-induced nerve tumors presented with pain and progressive neurological deficit with a palpable mass involving the brachial of lumbar plexus; these nine patients developed their tumors 4–20 years following radiation therapy. Neurofibromatosis is associated with an increased risk for the development of radiation-induced peripheral nerve tumors.[52]

NONCANCER PAIN SYNDROMES AND MECHANISMS

Like cancer pain syndromes, noncancer pain syndromes may be nociceptive or neuropathic in nature. Internists and family physicians deal with common degenerative, musculoskeletal pain syndromes along with specialist assessment as indicated. Palliative care specialists are likely to encounter pain in patients with human immunodeficiency virus (HIV) infection/acquired immune deficiency syndrome (AIDS).

Human immunodeficiency virus and pain

Pain is a common symptom in HIV and AIDS patients. With the increasing burden of this disease in Africa and Asia, palliative care specialists are likely to encounter these pain syndromes. Pain syndromes encountered in HIV and AIDS are diverse in nature and etiology. The most common pain syndromes include painful sensory peripheral neuropathy, pain due to extensive Kaposi sarcoma, headache, oral and pharyngeal pain, abdominal pain, chest pain, arthralgias and myalgias, and painful dermatological conditions.[56-61] Hewitt and colleagues in 1997 demonstrated that although pains of a neuropathic nature (e.g., polyneuropathies, radiculopathies) certainly comprise a large proportion of pain syndromes encountered in AIDS patients, pains of a somatic and/or visceral nature are also common clinical problems.[60] The etiology of pain syndromes seen in HIV disease can be categorized into three types:

1. Those directly related to HIV infection or consequences of immunosuppression
2. Those due to AIDS therapies
3. Those unrelated to AIDS or AIDS therapies

In studies to date, approximately 45% of pain syndromes encountered are directly related to HIV infection or consequences of immunosuppression; 15%–30% are due to therapies for HIV- or AIDS-related conditions and to diagnostic procedures; and the remaining 25%–40% are unrelated to HIV or its therapies.[58,60]

Oropharyngeal pain

Oral cavity and throat pain is common, accounting for approximately 20% of the pain syndromes encountered in one study.[62] Common sources of oral cavity pain are candidiasis, necrotizing gingivitis, and dental abscesses and ulcerations caused by herpes simplex virus (HSV), cytomegalovirus (CMV), Epstein–Barr virus (EBV), atypical and typical mycobacterial infection (MAI), cryptococcal infection, or histoplasmosis. Frequently no infectious agent can be identified and painful recurrent aphthous ulcers (RAU) are encountered.[63]

Esophageal pain

Many HIV/AIDS patients experience dysphagia or odynophagia, most commonly caused by esophageal candidiasis. Ulcerative esophagitis is usually a result of CMV infection but can be idiopathic. Infectious causes of esophagitis include HIV, papovavirus, HSV, EBV, *Mycobacterium*, *Cryptosporidium*, and *Pneumocystis carinii*. Kaposi sarcoma and lymphoma have both been reported to invade the esophagus, resulting in dysphagia, pain, and ulceration.[63] Nonsteroidal medications as well as zidovudine and zalcitabine have been implicated in esophagitis.

Abdominal pain

The abdomen is the primary site of pain in 12%–25% of patients with HIV disease.[64] Infectious causes of abdominal pain predominate, and include cryptosporidiosis, *Shigella*, *Salmonella*, and *Campylobacter enteritis*, CMV ileitis, and (MAI. Perforation of the small and large intestine secondary to CMV infection has been described.[65] Repeated intussusception of the small intestine has been seen in association with *Campylobacter* infection.[66] Lymphoma in the gastrointestinal tract can present with abdominal pain and intestinal obstruction.[63,66] Other causes of abdominal pain in HIV-positive patients[63] include ileus, organomegaly, spontaneous aseptic peritonitis, toxic shock, herpes zoster, and Fitzhugh–Curtis syndrome (perihepatitis in association with tubal gonococcal or chlamydia infection).

Many antiretroviral agents are responsible for gastrointestinal symptoms, but lactic acidosis, a rare but serious complication of some highly active antiretroviral therapy (HAART) regimens, can present with abdominal pain.[67] Didanosine, zalcitabine, and stavudine can cause pancreatitis, whereas patients taking indinavir are at increased risk for nephrolithiasis. Cholecystitis is a painful condition that may occur in HIV-infected patients as a result of opportunistic infection.[68] CMV and *Cryptosporidium* are the most common infectious agents. Drug-induced hepatic toxicities as well as viral hepatitis as coinfection may lead to abdominal pain. Pancreatitis is an extremely painful condition often related to adverse effects of HIV-related therapies such as didanosine, stavudine, and dideoxycytidine.[69] Intravenous pentamidine is also associated with pancreatitis. Other causes of pancreatitis include CMV infection, MAI, cryptococcal lymphoma, and Kaposi sarcoma.

Anorectal pain

Perirectal abscesses, CMV proctitis, fissure-in-ano, and human papilloma virus and HSV infection often cause painful anorectal syndromes.

Chest pain syndromes

Chest pain is a common complaint in patients with HIV disease, comprising approximately 13% of the pain syndromes encountered in a sample of ambulatory AIDS patients.[60] The index of suspicion for coronary artery disease, even in young patients with no other risk factors, must be high if the patient is being treated with HAART. In immunosuppressed patients, infectious causes of chest pain should be considered, particularly in the presence of fever and some localizing sign such as dysphagia, dyspnea, or cough. Infectious causes of chest pain include *Pneumocystis* pneumonia, esophagitis (CMV, candidiasis), pleuritis/pericarditis, and PHN.

Opportunistic cancers, Kaposi's or lymphoma invading the esophagus, pericardium, chest wall, lung, and pleura may also be sources of chest pain. Rarely, pulmonary embolus or bacterial endocarditis may be the cause of chest pain.

Neurological pain syndromes

Pain syndromes originating in the nervous system include headache, painful peripheral neuropathies, radiculopathies, and myelopathies. The HIV is highly neurotropic, invading central and peripheral nervous system structures early in the course of HIV disease. Consequently, many complications of HIV/AIDS and opportunistic infections result in neurological pain, and many commonly used HIV/AIDS medications can also be implicated in neurological pain. Rarely, cerebrovascular events (e.g., thalamic stroke) occurring in hypercoagulable states can result in central pain syndromes.

HEADACHE

Headache is extremely common in the HIV/AIDS patient and can pose a diagnostic dilemma for providers in that the underlying cause may range from benign stress and tension to life-threatening central nervous system infection.[63] The differential diagnosis of headache in patients with HIV disease includes:

- HIV encephalitis and atypical aseptic meningitis
- Opportunistic infections of the nervous system
- AIDS-related central nervous system neoplasms
- Sinusitis
- Tension
- Migraine
- Headache induced by medication (particularly azathioprine [AZT])

Toxoplasmosis and cryptococcal meningitis are the two most commonly encountered opportunistic infections of the central nervous system that cause headaches in patients with HIV disease. More benign causes of headache in the patient with HIV disease include AZT-induced headache, tension headache, migraine with or without aura, and unclassifiable or idiopathic headache.[70]

NEUROPATHIES

Neuropathic pain occurs in about 40% of AIDS patients.[58,60] The most common painful neuropathy seen is the predominantly sensory neuropathy (PSN) of AIDS. However, other potentially painful neuropathies in HIV/AIDS patients can have other viral and nonviral causes or may be caused by demyelination leading to Guillain–Barré syndrome, nutritional deficiencies, alcohol, and HIV therapies.[71] Predominantly symmetrical sensory neuropathy of AIDS is the most frequently encountered neuropathy. This is typically a late manifestation, occurring most often in patients with an AIDS-defining illness.[72] The prevalence of this neuropathy in hospice populations ranges from 19% to 26%.[73,74] The predominant symptom in about 60% of patients is pain in the soles of the feet. Paresthesia is frequent and usually involves the dorsum of the feet and soles. Most patients have signs of peripheral neuropathy and, although the signs progress, the symptoms often remain confined to the feet.[75,76] Although patients' complaints are predominantly sensory, electrophysiological studies demonstrate both sensory and motor involvement.

Rheumatological pain syndromes

In studies conducted by the Memorial Sloan-Kettering group, over 50% of pain syndromes were classified as rheumatological in nature including various forms of arthritis, arthropathy, arthralgias, myositis, and myalgias.[60]

The most frequently reported arthritis is a reactive arthritis or Reiter's syndrome.[77–81] Acute HIV infection may present with a polyarthralgia in association with a mononucleosis-like illness. There is also a syndrome of acute severe and intermittent articular pain, often referred to as HIV-associated painful articular syndrome, which commonly affects the large joints of the lower limbs and shoulders.

Psoriasis and psoriatic arthritis have been reported in patients with HIV infection.[82] Septic arthritis has been reported in patients with HIV disease, including arthritis due to bacterial infections and infections with *Cryptococcus neoformans* and *Sporothrix schenckii*.[77,78]

OPIOID-INDUCED HYPERALGESIA

Opioid-induced hyperalgesia is a state of nociceptive sensitization that is caused by exposure to opioids. It is characterized by a paradoxical response when a patient receiving opioids for the treatment of pain may actually become more sensitive to certain painful stimuli and, in some cases, experience pain from ordinarily nonpainful stimuli (allodynia). The phenomenon of opioid-induced hyperalgesia, linked to the development of analgesic tolerance, has been clearly demonstrated in animal models, and has relevance in the clinical setting.[83,84] Patients who demonstrate a loss of opioid effect in the absence of progressive illness (i.e., develop analgesic tolerance), or develop a syndrome of worsening or more diffuse pain during a period of aggressive opioid escalation, may be demonstrating opioid-induced hyperalgesia. Clinicians should be aware of this phenomenon, which often occurs when moaning that arises from delirium at the end of life is mistaken for pain, and extra boluses of opioids are given. All patients with worsening or more diffuse pain during a period of aggressive opioid escalation should be evaluated for delirium and opioid-induced hyperalgesia. When suspected, it is reasonable to consider opioid rotation, or the use of a nonopioid strategy for pain control.

CALCIPHYLAXIS

Calciphylaxis is a rare and serious disorder characterized by systemic medial calcification of the arterioles that leads to ischemia and subcutaneous necrosis.[85] Calciphylaxis most commonly occurs in patients with end-stage renal disease (ESRD) who are on hemodialysis or who have recently received a renal transplant. Calciphylaxis should be suspected in patients with skin lesions characterized by painful, nonulcerating subcutaneous nodules or plaques, nonhealing ulcers, and/or necrosis, which are most commonly present in the thigh and areas of increased adiposity.[86,87] Ulceration carries a mortality of greater than 80%. There should be an aggressive program of wound care and adequate pain control, avoidance of local tissue trauma.

ACKNOWLEDGMENTS

Thanks to Katja Sullivan and Ben Petties, Jr., for their help in the preparation of this manuscript.

Key learning points

- Pain is the most common symptom for which palliative care specialists are consulted.

- Cancer pain is the most common pain encountered, but pain syndromes due to HIV/AIDS are on the rise in Africa and Asia.

- Pain is classified into nociceptive and neuropathic in broad terms, but the majority are mixed.

- Pain in cancer is caused by tumor, treatment, or as coexisting chronic pain.

- Tumor size may not correlate with pain intensity.

- There are well-defined pain syndromes described in the literature based on the cause and the location.

- Metastatic bone pain is often associated with neurological deficit due to close proximity between skull and cranial nerves, and spinal cord and its roots with vertebral column.

- Not all bony metastatic sites hurt.

- Detailed history with emphasis on neurological examination will lead to early diagnosis of spinal cord compression.

- Suspect epidural disease with new onset neck, upper or lower back pain.

- Critical assessment of pain syndrome helps with optimal pain management, avoiding erroneous polypharmacy.

- A new pain or a sudden change in intensity of existing pain in cancer patient is invariably due to recurrence.

- Headache should always raise suspicion for base of skull metastasis or leptomeningeal disease.

- Exclude constipation as the cause of increased abdominal pain.

- Exclude infection as the cause of intractable pain, especially in head and neck cancers.

- Pain syndromes in HIV/AIDS often follow similar pattern as cancer. But neuropathic pain, and rheumatic and musculoskeletal pain syndromes predominate, with high incidence of psychosomatic issues.

- Delirium can masquerade as pain.

- Generalized body pains may be a sign of somatization.

REFERENCES

1 Twycross RG, Fairfield S. Pain in far-advanced cancer. *Pain* 1982;14:303–310.
2 Levin DN, Cleeland CS, Dar R. Public attitudes toward cancer pain. *Cancer* 1985;56:2337–2339.
3 Portenoy RK. Cancer pain. Epidemiology and syndromes. *Cancer* 1989;63:2298–2307.
4 Cleeland CS. Pain control: Public and physicians' attitudes. *Advances in Pain Research and Therapy* 1989:81–89.
5 Von Roenn JH, Cleeland CS, Gonin R, Hatfield AK, Pandya KJ. Physician attitudes and practice in cancer pain management. A survey from the Eastern Cooperative Oncology Group. *Annals of Internal Medicine* 1993;119:121–126.
6 Cleeland CS. Undertreatment of cancer pain in elderly patients. *JAMA* 1998;279:1914–1915.
7 Cleeland CS, Gonin R, Hatfield AK et al. Pain and its treatment in outpatients with metastatic cancer. *The New England Journal of Medicine* 1994;330:592–596.
8 Foley KM. The treatment of cancer pain. *The New England Journal of Medicine* 1985;313:84–95.
9 Weiner DK, Sakamoto S, Perera S, Breuer P. Chronic low back pain in older adults: Prevalence, reliability, and validity of physical examination findings. *Journal of the American Geriatrics Society* 2006;54:11–20.
10 Pinals RS. Mechanisms of joint destruction, pain and disability in osteoarthritis. *Drugs* 1996;52(Suppl 3):14–20.
11 Hardin JG. Complications of cervical arthritis. *Postgraduate Medicine* 1992;91:309–315, 318.
12 Yezierski RP. Spinal cord injury: A model of central neuropathic pain. *Neuro-Signals* 2005;14:182–193.
13 Woolf CJ, Mannion RJ. Neuropathic pain: Aetiology, symptoms, mechanisms, and management. *Lancet* 1999;353:1959–1964.
14 Dworkin RH, Backonja M, Rowbotham MC et al. Advances in neuropathic pain: Diagnosis, mechanisms, and treatment recommendations. *Archives of Neurology* 2003;60:1524–1534.
15 Galasko CS. Mechanisms of bone destruction in the development of skeletal metastases. *Nature* 1976;263:507–508.
16 Stambaugh J, Drew J. A double-blind parallel evaluation of the efficacy and safety of a single dose of ketoprofen in cancer pain. *Journal of Clinical Pharmacology* 1988;28:S34–S39.
17 Milne RJ, Foreman RD, Giesler GJ, Jr., Willis WD. Convergence of cutaneous and pelvic visceral nociceptive inputs onto primate spinothalamic neurons. *Pain* 1981;11:163–183.
18 Payne R. Neuropathic pain syndromes, with special reference to causalgia and reflex sympathetic dystrophy. *The Clinical Journal of Pain* 1989;2.
19 Portenoy RK, Hagen NA. Breakthrough pain: Definition, prevalence and characteristics. *Pain* 1990;41:273–281.
20 Kelly JB, Payne R. Pain syndromes in the cancer patient. *Neurologic Clinics* 1991;9:937–953.
21 Dewar GA, Griffin SM, Ku KW, Lau WY, Li AK. Management of bleeding liver tumours in Hong Kong. *The British Journal of Surgery* 1991;78:463–466.
22 Srivastava DN, Gandhi D, Julka PK, Tandon RK. Gastrointestinal hemorrhage in hepatocellular carcinoma: Management with transheptic arterioembolization. *Abdominal Imaging* 2000;25:380–384.
23 Front D, Schneck SO, Frankel A, Robinson E. Bone metastases and bone pain in breast cancer. Are they closely associated? *JAMA* 1979;242:1747–1748.
24 Levick S, Jacobs C, Loukas DF, Gordon DH, Meyskens FL, Uhm K. Naproxen sodium in treatment of bone pain due to metastatic cancer. *Pain* 1988;35:253–258.
25 Greenberg HS, Deck MD, Vikram B, Chu FC, Posner JB. Metastasis to the base of the skull: Clinical findings in 43 patients. *Neurology* 1981;31:530–537.
26 TN B, SG W. Epidural spinal cord compression: Diagnosis and treatment. *Contemporary Neurology Series* 1990;33.
27 Sundaresan N, DiGiacinto GV, Krol G, Hughes JE. Spondylectomy for malignant tumors of the spine. *Journal of Clinical Oncology* 1989;7:1485–1491.

28 Kaplan JG, DeSouza TG, Farkash A et al. Leptomeningeal metastases: Comparison of clinical features and laboratory data of solid tumors, lymphomas and leukemias. *Journal of Neuro-Oncology* 1990;9:225–229.

29 Kesari S, Batchelor TT. Leptomeningeal metastases. *Neurologic Clinics* 2003;21:25–66.

30 Kori SH, Foley KM, Posner JB. Brachial plexus lesions in patients with cancer: 100 cases. *Neurology* 1981;31:45–50.

31 Blair DN, Rapoport S, Sostman HD, Blair OC. Normal brachial plexus: MR imaging. *Radiology* 1987;165:763–767.

32 Payne R, Foley KM. Exploration of the brachial plexus in patients with cancer. *Neurology* 1986;36.

33 Kanner RM, Martini N, Foley KM. Incidence of pain and other clinical manifestations of superior pulmonary sulcus (Pancoast's tumors). *Advances in Pain Research and Therapy* 1982;4.

34 Sundaresan N, Hilaris BS, Martini N. The combined neurosurgical-thoracic management of superior sulcus tumors. *Journal of Clinical Oncology* 1987;5:1739–1745.

35 Jaeckle KA, Young DF, Foley KM. The natural history of lumbosacral plexopathy in cancer. *Neurology* 1985;35:8–15.

36 Wasserstrom WR, Glass JP, Posner JB. Diagnosis and treatment of leptomeningeal metastases from solid tumors: Experience with 90 patients. *Cancer* 1982;49:759–772.

37 Watson CP, Evans RJ, Watt VR. The post-mastectomy pain syndrome and the effect of topical capsaicin. *Pain* 1989;38:177–186.

38 Vecht CJ, Van de Brand HJ, Wajer OJ. Post-axillary dissection pain in breast cancer due to a lesion of the intercostobrachial nerve. *Pain* 1989;38:171–176.

39 Bradway JK, Malone JM, Racy J, Leal JM, Poole J. Psychological adaptation to amputation: An overview. *Orthotics and Prosthetics* 1984;38:46–50.

40 Steinke NM, Ostgard SE, Jensen OM, Nordentoft AM, Sneppen O. Thoraco-scapular amputation in sarcomas of the shoulder girdle. *Ugeskrift for Laeger* 1991;153:2555–2557.

41 Kroner K, Krebs B, Skov J, Jorgensen HS. Immediate and long-term phantom breast syndrome after mastectomy: Incidence, clinical characteristics and relationship to pre-mastectomy breast pain. *Pain* 1989;36:327–334.

42 Sugarbaker PH, Weiss CM, Davidson DD, Roth YF. Increasing phantom limb pain as a symptom of cancer recurrence. *Cancer* 1984;54:373–375.

43 Boas RA, Schug SA, Acland RH. Perineal pain after rectal amputation: A 5-year follow-up. *Pain* 1993;52:67–70.

44 Young DF, Posner JB. Nervous system toxicity of chemotherapeutic agents. *Handbook of Clinical Neurology.* Amsterdam, the Netherlands, 1969;91.

45 Asbury AK, Bird SJ. Disorders of peripheral nerve. *Diseases of the Nervous System: Clinical Neurobiology* 1992;1.

46 Ihde DC, DeVita VT. Osteonecrosis of the femoral head in patients with lymphoma treated with intermittent combination chemotherapy (including corticosteroids). *Cancer* 1975;36:1585–1588.

47 Loeser JD. Herpes zoster and postherpetic neuralgia. *Pain* 1986;25:149–164.

48 Thomas JE, Cascino TL, Earle JD. Differential diagnosis between radiation and tumor plexopathy of the pelvis. *Neurology* 1985;35:1–7.

49 Aho K, Sainio K. Late irradiation-induced lesions of the lumbosacral plexus. *Neurology* 1983;33:953–955.

50 Jellinger K, Sturm KW. Delayed radiation myelopathy in man. Report of twelve necropsy cases. *Journal of the Neurological Sciences* 1971;14:389–408.

51 Palmer JJ. Radiation myelopathy. *Brain* 1972;95:109–122.

52 Foley KM, Woodruff JM, Ellis FT, Posner JB. Radiation-induced malignant and atypical peripheral nerve sheath tumors. *Annals of Neurology* 1980;7:311–318.

53 Ducatman BS, Scheithauer BW. Postirradiation neurofibrosarcoma. *Cancer* 1983;51:1028–1033.

54 Thomas JE, Piepgras DG, Scheithauer B, Onofrio BM, Shives TC. Neurogenic tumors of the sciatic nerve. A clinicopathologic study of 35 cases. *Mayo Clinic Proceedings* 1983;58:640–647.

55 Powers SK, Norman D, Edwards MS. Computerized tomography of peripheral nerve lesions. *Journal of Neurosurgery* 1983;59:131–136.

56 Penfold J, Clark AJ. Pain syndromes in HIV infection. *Canadian Journal of Anaesthesia Journal Canadien D'anesthesie* 1992;39:724–730.

57 Katz N. Neuropathic pain in cancer and AIDS. *The Clinical Journal of Pain* 2000;16:S41–S48.

58 Wesselmann U. Pain syndromes in AIDS. *Der Anaesthesist* 1996;45:1004–1014.

59 Verma S, Estanislao L, Simpson D. HIV-associated neuropathic pain: Epidemiology, pathophysiology and management. *CNS Drugs* 2005;19:325–334.

60 Hewitt DJ, McDonald M, Portenoy RK, Rosenfeld B, Passik S, Breitbart W. Pain syndromes and etiologies in ambulatory AIDS patients. *Pain* 1997;70:117–123.

61 Lebovits AH, Lefkowitz M, McCarthy D et al. The prevalence and management of pain in patients with AIDS: A review of 134 cases. *The Clinical Journal of Pain* 1989;5:245–248.

62 Singer EJ, Zorilla C, Fahy-Chandon B, Chi S, Syndulko K, Tourtellotte WW. Painful symptoms reported by ambulatory HIV-infected men in a longitudinal study. *Pain* 1993;54:15–19.

63 Breckman B. Stoma management. *Oxford Textbook of Palliative Medicine* 2004, pp. 843–894.

64 Barone SE, Gunold BS, Nealson TF. Abdominal pain in patients with acquired immune deficiency syndrome. *Annals of Surgery* 1986;204:619–623.

65 Balthazar EJ, Reich CB, Pachter HL. The significance of small bowel intussusception in acquired immune deficiency syndrome. *The American Journal of Gastroenterology* 1986;81:1073–1075.

66 Davidson T, Allen-Mersh TG, Miles AJ et al. Emergency laparotomy in patients with AIDS. *The British Journal of Surgery* 1991;78:924–926.

67 Cello JP. Acquired immunodeficiency syndrome cholangiopathy: Spectrum of disease. *The American Journal of Medicine* 1989;86:539–546.

68 Richman DD, Fischl MA, Grieco MH et al. The toxicity of azidothymidine (AZT) in the treatment of patients with AIDS and AIDS-related complex. A double-blind, placebo-controlled trial. *The New England Journal of Medicine* 1987;317:192–197.

69 Guo JJ, Jang R, Louder A, Cluxton RJ. Acute pancreatitis associated with different combination therapies in patients infected with human immunodeficiency virus. *Pharmacotherapy* 2005;25:1044–1054.

70 Evers S, Wibbeke B, Reichelt D, Suhr B, Brilla R, Husstedt I. The impact of HIV infection on primary headache. Unexpected findings from retrospective, cross-sectional, and prospective analyses. *Pain* 2000;85:191–200.

71 Griffin JW, Wesselingh SL, Griffin DE, Glass JD, McArthur JC. Peripheral nerve disorders in HIV infection. Similarities and contrasts with CNS disorders. *Research Publications—Association for Research in Nervous and Mental Disease* 1994;72:159–182.

72 Lange DJ, Britton CB, Younger DS, Hays AP. The neuromuscular manifestations of human immunodeficiency virus infections. *Archives of Neurology* 1988;45:1084–1088.

73 Parry GJ. Peripheral neuropathies associated with human immunodeficiency virus infection. *Annals of Neurology* 1988;23(Suppl):S49–S53.

74 Dalakas MC, Pezeshkpour GH. Neuromuscular diseases associated with human immunodeficiency virus infection. *Annals of Neurology* 1988;23(Suppl):S38–S48.

75 Fuller GN, Jacobs JM, Guiloff RJ. Association of painful peripheral neuropathy in AIDS with cytomegalovirus infection. *Lancet* 1989;2:937–941.

76   Harrison RH, Seng-jaw S, Weiss H. A mixed model for factors predictive of pain in AIDS patients with herpes zoster. *Journal of Pain and Symptom Management* 1999;17:410–417.

77   Espinoza LR, Aguilar JL, Berman A, Gutierrez F, Vasey FB, Germain BF. Rheumatic manifestations associated with human immunodeficiency virus infection. *Arthritis and Rheumatism* 1989;32:1615–1622.

78   Kaye BR. Rheumatologic manifestations of infection with human immunodeficiency virus (HIV). *Annals of Internal Medicine* 1989;111:158–167.

79   Rynes RI, Goldenberg DL, DiGiacomo R, Olson R, Hussain M, Veazey J. Acquired immunodeficiency syndrome-associated arthritis. *The American Journal of Medicine* 1988;84:810–816.

80   Dalakas MC, Pezeshkpour GH, Gravell M, Sever JL. Polymyositis associated with AIDS retrovirus. *JAMA* 1986;256:2381–2383.

81   Watts RA, Hoffbrand BI, Paton DF, Davis JC. Pyomyositis associated with human immunodeficiency virus infection. *British Medical Journal* (Clinical research ed) 1987;294:1524–1525.

82   Johnson TM, Duvic M, Rapini RP, Rios A. AIDS exacerbates psoriasis. *The New England Journal of Medicine* 1985;313:1415.

83   Chu LF, Angst MS, Clark D. Opioid-induced hyperalgesia in humans: Molecular mechanisms and clinical considerations. *The Clinical Journal of Pain* 2008;24:479–496.

84   Silverman SM. Opioid induced hyperalgesia: Clinical implications for the pain practitioner. *Pain Physician* 2009;12:679–684.

85   Adrogue HJ, Frazier MR, Zeluff B, Suki WN. Systemic calciphylaxis revisited. *American Journal of Nephrology* 1981;1:177–183.

86   Kent RB, III, Lyerly RT. Systemic calciphylaxis. *Southern Medical Journal* 1994;87:278–281.

87   Janigan DT, Hirsch DJ, Klassen GA, MacDonald AS. Calcified subcutaneous arterioles with infarcts of the subcutis and skin ("calciphylaxis") in chronic renal failure. *American Journal of Kidney Diseases* 2000;35:588–597.

43

Opioid analgesics

GEANA PAULA KURITA, STEIN KAASA, PER SJØGREN

INTRODUCTION

Derivates of the opium poppy (*Papaver somniferum*) have a long history as pain-relieving agents. The main constituent, the alkaloid called morphine, was isolated by Sertürner in 1803 and was later shown to be almost completely responsible for the analgesic effects. Today, morphine is still in many countries the most widely used opioid and remains the "gold standard" when effects of other opioid analgesics are to be compared.

The concept of a specific opioid receptor was established in the middle of the twentieth century based on the stereospecificity and availability of selective antagonists to the analgesic actions.[1,2] In the 1970s, opioid receptors were recognized as specific biochemical structures and the evidence for the existence of multiple receptors was established.[3–5] Based on their activities in vivo, opioids are now classified according to their sensitivity and selectivity in receptor-binding studies, and it is now agreed that there are three main types of opioid receptors, μ (mu), δ (delta), and κ (kappa). In 1994, a fourth opioid receptor called the nociceptin/orphanin FQ (N/OFQ) receptor was discovered, which mediates pronociceptive effects instead of analgesia.[6] Morphine as well as other opioids exert their analgesic action by a specific interaction with one or more subclasses of the three most important opioid receptors: μ, δ, and κ. Genes encoding for these receptors have been cloned. Based on their different pharmacologies, a number of subclasses have been described: μ_1 and μ_2, d_1 and δ_2, and κ_{1-3}. Evidence for multiple μ-receptors came from binding studies that showed biphasic binding properties of μ-agonists.[7] The μ-agonists' mechanism of action is complex, resulting in subtle pharmacological differences among them and with unpredictable differences in their potency, effectiveness, and tolerability among patients. Highly selective μ-agonists do not bind to a single receptor. Rather, they interact with a large number of μ-receptor subtypes with different activation profiles for the various drugs. Thus, μ-receptor-based drugs are not all the same and it may be possible to utilize these differences for enhanced pain control in a clinical setting.[8] In the recent years, a growing number of candidate-gene studies searching for associations between genes and efficacy or side effects of opioids have emerged. Until now, the clinical and genetic complexity of response to opioids has resulted in limited clinical applicability.[9]

Clinically, differences were observed as patients who did not tolerate one μ-agonist could be switched to another, which was easily tolerated. Also incomplete cross-tolerance was observed in connection with "rotation" from one μ-agonist to another: far lower doses than predicted of the new drug were necessary to control pain.[10,11] Most of the clinically relevant opioids are relatively selective for the μ-receptor, reflecting their similarity with morphine at least within normal dose ranges (Table 43.1). However, higher doses used to overcome development of tolerance may result in interaction with additional receptor subtypes and result in changes in their pharmacological profile.

Opioids act by inhibiting the ascending nociceptive signal transmission from the dorsal horn in the spinal cord. The periaqueductal gray region is a major anatomical locus for opioid activation of descending inhibitory pathways to the spinal cord and is thus an important site for μ-receptor-mediated analgesia. Furthermore, opioid receptors have also been demonstrated in inflamed tissue in terminals of peripheral nerves in animals as well as in humans.[12]

In this chapter, the most widely used and clinically relevant opioid analgesics in palliative care are described.

MORPHINE

Morphine is the most thoroughly investigated opioid drug, and it is recommended as a first-line opioid in major cancer relief guidelines.[13,14] It is a pure opioid agonist with affinity primarily to the μ-receptors and to a lesser degree to the δ- and κ-receptors (see Table 43.1). Morphine can be administered by the oral, rectal, intravenous, intramuscular, subcutaneous, epidural, intrathecal, and intracerebroventricular routes.

Absorption

After oral administration, morphine is almost completely absorbed from the gastrointestinal tract.[15] The rate of absorption from the gut depends on the pharmaceutical formulation.

Table 43.1 *Primary receptor binding and pharmacologic data of important opioids in palliative medicine*

Opioid	Pathways	Bioavailability average (%)	Major metabolites	Metabolism/ excretion	Safety in renal failure
Morphine	μ-Receptor agonist	25	M3G3 M6G[a]	Hepatic/renal	Not safe
Methadone	μ-Receptor agonist	80	Pyrrolidine[b]	Hepatic/fecal	Safe
Oxycodone	μ-Receptor agonist	60	Oxymorphone[a] Nororxycodone[b]	Hepatic/renal	Uncertain
Oxymorphone	μ-Receptor agonist	10	Oxymorphone-3-glucuronide[c] 6-OH-oxymorphone[a]	Hepatic/renal	Uncertain
Fentanyl	μ-Receptor ago-nist	90	Phenylacetic acid[b] Norfentanyl[b] p-Hydroxy(phenethyl)fentanyl[a]	Hepatic/renal/fecal	Safe
Buprenorphine	μ-Receptor agonist κ-Receptor antagonist	50	Norbuprenorphine[b]	Hepatic/renal	Safe

M6G, morphine-6-glucuronide; M3G, morphine-3-glucuronide.

[a] Active.

[b] Inactive.

[c] Uncertain.

Immediate-release morphine tablets reach their maximum plasma concentrations within an average of 60–70 min and sustained-release morphine tablets designed for twice or thrice daily administration within an average of 140–200 min.[16,17]

Pharmacokinetics

About 20%–38% of morphine is bound to plasma proteins, primarily albumin.[18] The mean volume of distribution varies between 2.1 and 4.0 L/kg in cancer patients and healthy individuals, decreasing to half the value in elderly individuals.[19–21] In cancer patients and healthy individuals, mean elimination half-life varies between 1.6 and 3.4 hours and mean systemic plasma clearance between 9 and 33 mL/kg/min.[20–22]

Extensive first-pass metabolism after oral morphine administration results in a low and variable bioavailability between 19% and 47%[21,23] (see Table 43.1). The two most important metabolites quantitatively and qualitatively are morphine-3-glucuronide (M3G) and morphine-6-glucuronide (M6G) (see Table 43.1). M3G has no analgesic effect; however, it has been reported to antagonize morphine analgesia and produce side effects, while M6G has been reported to produce higher analgesic effect than morphine. Regardless of the route of administration, approximately 44%–55% of a morphine dose is converted into M3G, 9%–10% to M6G, and 8%–10% is excreted in the urine unchanged.[21] The major pathway for morphine metabolism is conjugation with the cosubstrate uridine-diphosphate (UDP)-glucuronic acid. The process is catalyzed by UDP glucuronyltransferase (UDPGT) and takes place mainly in the liver, although a part takes place in the kidneys, gut, and brain[23,24] (see Table 43.1). UDPGTs are a multienzyme family, and it has been demonstrated that the UGT2B7 is likely to be the major isoform responsible for morphine glucuronidation

in humans, capable of catalyzing the glucuronidation process at the 3- as well as 6-positions.[25] The presence of other metabolic isoenzymes involved in the large glucuronidation at the 3-position in vitro has been suggested (UGT1A1), but in vivo UGT2B7 isoenzyme seems to be the primary metabolic enzyme for morphine.[26] During long-term treatment, neither dose level nor treatment length seems to influence glucuronidation of morphine.[27] The capability to glucuronidate morphine varies among individuals, and studies have proposed that polymorphisms of UGT2B7 may be responsible for such variability.[28,29] In humans, UGT2B7 haplotype 4 was associated with increasing enzyme activity and gene expression with effects on the biotransformation of UGT2B7 substrates[28]; however, another study conducted with patients with cancer did not show considerable variations in glucuronide-to-morphine ratios associated with polymorphism related to this enzyme.[30]

Elimination

During the process of glucuronidation, morphine is made more hydrophilic, and the enhanced water solubility eases its excretion via the kidneys (see Table 43.1). The role of the kidneys in the excretion process has been demonstrated in a study of patients with renal failure given intravenous morphine. Subsequent plasma concentrations of M3G and M6G were observed to be several fold greater in these patients than in a control group with normal renal function.[31] The clearance of the metabolites is significantly correlated to the creatinine clearance.[32] As a consequence of the accumulation of M3G and M6G in patients with renal impairment, toxic effects of morphine metabolites may be expected[33,34] (see Table 43.1). There exist few clinical trials regarding morphine treatment of cancer patients with renal impairment and the outcomes regarding toxicity are inconsistent.[35]

Pharmacokinetics of M6G and M3G

In healthy volunteers, the plasma protein binding of M3G and M6G has been found to be low, 15% and 11%, respectively. Formation of the metabolites takes time, and T_{max} for M6G and M3G occurs later than for morphine. After long-term administration of morphine to cancer patients, the cerebrospinal fluid (CSF) and plasma ratios for M3G and M6G range between 0.08 and 0.18 and 0.07 and 0.15, respectively.[36,37]

M6G and analgesia

Animal studies demonstrated that, although M6G and morphine were almost equally potent after peripheral administration, the analgesic potency of M6G was 100-fold higher than morphine after intracerebroventricular injection. These pharmacological data suggest that the brain penetration of M6G is significantly attenuated relative to that of morphine.[38] A study using transcortical microdialysis in rat brain cells showed that systemically administered morphine entered brain cells, whereas M6G crossed the blood–brain barrier extremely slowly and was trapped in the extracellular fluid. A high concentration of M6G in this limited space in the brain may account for the durable availability of M6G to opioid receptors.[39] Another explanation for the prolonged analgesia elicited by systemically administered M6G compared with morphine was a threefold slower rate of elimination of M6G than morphine from the mouse brain.[40]

Intravenous M6G has analgesic effects in cancer patients; however, its potency compared with morphine has not been established in humans.[41] A critical clinical issue is the role and contribution of M6G to the analgesic action seen after long-term morphine administration. In this respect, controversy exists as a few clinical studies have found evidence for M6G being a contributor to the analgesic action observed after morphine administration,[42,43] whereas other clinical studies have not been able to demonstrate this.[27,37,44,45] In general, these studies are confounded by a multitude of other factors that influence patients' perception of pain, including psychological factors and varying responses to morphine administration due to different pain mechanisms and opioid receptor properties, concentration of opioids at the target sites, variability of nonspecific endogenous opioids, and varying plasma sampling times for determining M6G/morphine.

M3G: Antagonism of antinociception and neurotoxicity

M3G appears to have no μ-agonist properties and therefore to be devoid of analgesic activity. In some studies, subcutaneous or intracerebroventricular administration of M3G prior to or after the administration of morphine or M6G has been shown to reduce the antinociceptive response of the two analgesic agents.[46,47] In contrast, other studies in rodents have not found any influence of M3G on morphine analgesia.[48,49] Apart from its possible role as an antianalgesic, M3G and high-dose morphine have also been associated with "morphine-induced neurotoxicity" such as generalized hyperalgesia/allodynia and myoclonus.[50] Several studies in rodents have found that M3G and high-dose morphine administered by the intracerebroventricular[51] as well as the intrathecal routes produce symptoms of sensory and motor excitation.[52,53]

Clinically, the symptoms of hyperalgesia, allodynia, and myoclonus have mostly been observed in cancer patients treated with high doses of morphine administered by several different routes,[54,55] although these side effects have also been associated with other opioids.[56,57] High plasma levels of morphine and M3G as well as accumulation of M3G relative to morphine or M6G may be associated with these symptoms. A study has shown that although M3G does not cross the blood–brain barrier with the same ease as morphine, the mean steady-state M3G concentration in the CSF is approximately twofold higher than the respective CSF morphine concentration following long-term morphine treatment.[50] Opioid switching or rotation, whereby a structurally dissimilar opioid (e.g., methadone [open-chain opioid analgesic] or fentanyl [anilinopiperidine opioid analgesic]) is substituted for a benzomorphan opioid, such as morphine (or hydromorphone), will also result in the clearance of M3G from the brain tissue, giving a time-dependent resolution of the neuroexcitatory behaviors while maintaining analgesia with methadone or fentanyl.[58]

In a study with healthy volunteers, M3G was administered in small intravenous doses. In these doses, neurotoxicity did not occur.[59]

Clinical aspects

An update[60] of a Cochrane review[61] on the use of oral morphine concluded that it is an effective analgesic with frequent adverse effects that did not result in higher rate of treatment discontinuation than other opioids and that morphine has similar effects as oxycodone and hydromorphone in cancer patients. According to recent guidelines, morphine represents a first-choice opioid together with other frequently used opioids like oxycodone and hydromorphone.[14] Recent studies in patients with cancer have demonstrated that a variety of genetic polymorphisms may be responsible for pain relief variability[62,63]; however, the literature is still sparse. The largest cross-sectional study conducted to analyze the influence of genetic variability on opioid mechanisms did not show any association between 112 single nucleotide polymorphisms in 25 candidate genes for opioid actions and the efficacy of commonly used opioids, including morphine.[9]

METHADONE

Methadone is increasingly being considered as a second-choice drug alternative to morphine in cancer pain treatment. It is a long-acting μ-receptor agonist, with pharmacological properties qualitatively similar to those of morphine (see Table 43.1). Earlier reports of severe toxicity of methadone have given rise to misconceptions and render its effective use in cancer pain difficult.[64,65] With better understanding of the pharmaco-kinetics of methadone, it has subsequently been found to be a safe, effective, and cheap alternative to other opioids when prescribed by physicians experienced in its use. Methadone is administered by the oral, rectal, and intravenous routes. Methadone is not suitable for subcutaneous administration because of the high frequency of local reactions.[66]

Absorption

Methadone is a synthetic opioid with an almost complete absorption when administered orally and rectally.[67] Its oral bioavailability is generally high and considered to be higher than that of other oral opioids such as morphine; it is in the region of 80% and ranges from 41% to 99%[68,69] (see Table 43.1). It is a lipophilic drug and is subject to considerable tissue distribution.[70] The peripheral tissue reservoir sustains plasma concentrations during long-term treatment.[71] Methadone is extensively metabolized through P450 system in the liver to inactive metabolites via N-demethylation[72] (see Table 43.1). In most countries, methadone is used in a racemic mixture of S- and R-enantiomers, although the latter form has significantly longer elimination half-life, larger volume of distribution, slower clearance, and more analgesic potency.[73,74]

Pharmacokinetics

Methadone is characterized by a rapid and extensive distribution phase (half-life, 2–3 hours) followed by a slow elimination phase (b-half-life, 15–60 hours). After oral administration, measurable concentrations appear in plasma after 30 min.[70] There is a large inter-individual variation of the elimination phase, which can be the reason for accumulation and potential toxicity.[75]

Elimination

Methadone is mainly excreted by the fecal route, and only a minor part is eliminated in the urine (see Table 43.1). Renal clearance is enhanced by lowering the urinary pH.[76] As the elimination is primarily via feces, significant accumulation is not likely in renal failure (see Table 43.1).

Clinical aspects

In recent years, methadone has been used extensively for opioid switching or rotation. In cancer patients, when switching for uncontrolled pain and opioid-induced toxicity, significant improvements have been reported in pain intensity and a number of toxicities.[77] Recent reviews did not identify randomized controlled trials which support the practice of opioid switching. The uncontrolled trials analyzed in the reviews involving 679 patients showed that opioid switching to manage uncontrolled pain is more frequent when side effects limit dose increase than when side effects are tolerable. The successful rates of switching range from 40% to 80%, and the most common switch is

from other pure agonists to methadone.[8,78] A major problem encountered when switching to methadone from another opioid is the huge interindividual variations in the equianalgesic ratio of methadone to other opioids.

Methadone becomes relatively more potent with increasing prior exposure to other opioids and can be up to 10 times more potent in patients given daily doses >500 mg of morphine than in patients given daily doses <100 mg of morphine.[79] Some mechanisms for the dynamic equipotency relations can be hypothesized: (1) incomplete cross-tolerance of opioid receptors, (2) N-methyl-D-aspartate (NMDA) receptor antagonism, and (3) elimination of active metabolites. In addition, of course, combinations of these mechanisms may be in play. Regarding the NMDA receptor antagonism methadone may possess a dual effect on opioid receptors and NMDA receptors, which clinically may be advantageous to other opioids in decreasing the development of tolerance and increasing analgesia in neuropathic pain conditions. However, methadone has only been found to be a relatively potent NMDA inhibitor in in vitro studies.[80] A Cochrane review of methadone in cancer patients based on nine RCTs involving active opioid comparators did not support the notion that methadone should be advantageous in neuropathic pain conditions.[81]

OXYCODONE

Oxycodone (14-hydroxy-7,8-dihydrocodeinone) has become the most commonly used opioid in the United States and can be administered by the oral, rectal, and intravenous routes. It is a μ-receptor agonist, but a part of its antinociceptive effects may be mediated by the κ-receptors (see Table 43.1). Its metabolite oxymorphone (14-hydroxydihydromorphinone) is a powerful analgesic, and currently, semisynthetic immediate- and sustained-release formulations have been developed and designed, aiming to increase analgesic efficacy and reduce side effects. It can be administered by oral, rectal, subcutaneous, and intravenous routes.

Absorption

Oral oxycodone bioavailability in humans is about 60% (range 50%–87%)[82,83] (see Table 43.1). Oxycodone is subject to extensive hepatic first-pass effects. Oxycodone is metabolized by the liver to the active metabolite, oxymorphone, and to the inactive, but quantitatively most prevalent metabolite, noroxycodone[84] (see Table 43.1). Oral bioavailability of oxymorphone in humans is approximately 10%,[85] and it is highly metabolized in the liver into oxymorphone-3-glucuronide and 6-OH-oxymorphone.[86]

Pharmacokinetics

T_{max} of oxycodone is approximately 1 hour and the mean half-life after single-dose is 3.5–5.65 hours.[83,87] The half-life is not influenced by the route of administration.[83] Oxycodone's physicochemical properties, liposolubility, and protein binding are similar to morphine.[87] Controlled-release oxycodone is absorbed in a biexponential fashion, with a rapid mean half-life of 37 min and a slow phase of 6.2 hours. T_{max} is 3.2 6 2.2 hours.[88]

Oxymorphone plasma concentrations reach T_{max} at 0.5 hour after single-dose administration,[86,89] and the half-life ranges from 7.2 to 9.4 hours.[86] Its structure is related to hydromorphone, and it is more lipophilic than morphine, facilitating rapid access to brain and spinal cord.[90,91] The sustained-release formulation maintains the plasma level for 12 hours.[88]

Elimination

Oxycodone and its metabolites are mainly excreted via the kidneys. Oxycodone elimination is prolonged with renal failure and in end-stage liver disease[92,93] (see Table 43.1). Oxymorphone accumulates with renal failure, and there is little information regarding the effects of hepatic insufficiency.[94]

Clinical aspects

Oral equianalgesic ratios of oxycodone to morphine have varied from 1:1 to 1:2, 2:3, and 3:4 as a result of significant interindividual differences in oral bioavailability and unequal non-cross-tolerance, and sex differences in the metabolism of oxycodone.[95-97] Women seem to eliminate oxycodone 25% more slowly than men.[98]

Equianalgesic dose ratio of sustained-release morphine to sustained-release oxymorphone is 1.8:1 and of sustained-release oxycodone to sustained-release oxymorphone is 1.2:1.[85] A recent multicenter cross-sectional study in cancer patients has showed that plasma concentrations of oxycodone and its metabolites were not associated with pain intensity, nausea, tiredness, and cognitive dysfunction.[99]

ROLE OF TRANSDERMAL OPIOIDS

Transdermal fentanyl and buprenorphine delivery systems enable slow increase of drug plasma levels with very long apparent half-lives (several days) and a long latent period before pharmacological steady states are reached.[100] The use of these preparations as first-choice strong opioids or as alternatives to weak opioids has been debated. For patients unable to swallow, they are an effective, noninvasive means of opioid delivery. Titration must be done according to the apparent drug half-life—that is, every 3 days with the use of immediate-release opioids in the stabilizing phase. Thus, transdermal fentanyl and buprenorphine are alternatives to oral opioids.[14]

FENTANYL

Fentanyl is a synthetic phenyl piperidine derivative and a chemical congener of the reversed ester of meperidine. It has selective high affinity for the m-receptor, where it acts as a pure agonist[101] (see Table 43.1). Fentanyl has a short duration of action and is therefore administered continuously by the transdermal, subcutaneous, or spinal routes or used on demand by the intravenous and transmucosal routes. The transdermal therapeutic system (TTS) was designed to release fentanyl at a constant rate of 72 hours and has gained enormous popularity in Western countries for the treatment of cancer pain.

Recent marketed nasal and buccal delivery devices of fentanyl show a rapid onset with a clinical meaningful response rate in approximate 20%–50% with the patient after 10 min and in 50%–90% after 30 min.[14]

Absorption

A mean bioavailability of 92% (range 57%–146%) has been reported for TTS fentanyl, although marked interindividual variation is apparent[102] (see Table 43.1). Although fentanyl has been detected in the blood 1–2 hours after initial application of TTS, considerable delays (17–48 hours) between patch application and occurrence of C_{max} were also apparent. The delay has been attributed to depot accumulation of the drug in the skin under the TTS before diffusion into the systemic circulation. Steady-state concentrations are achieved after application of the second patch.[103]

Pharmacokinetics

Fentanyl is predominantly metabolized in the liver and produces phenylacetic acid, norfentanyl, and small amounts of the active metabolite, p-hydroxy(phenethyl)fentanyl[103] (see Table 43.1). It is highly lipid soluble, which facilitates rapid transfer across the blood–brain barrier and into the central nervous system (CNS). This is reflected in the half-life for equilibration between the plasma and the CSF of approximately 5 min.[104]

Elimination

Renal elimination of fentanyl is prolonged after transdermal application compared with intravenous administration (see Table 43.1). Elimination half-life values of 13–25 hours have been reported after TTS.[103]

Clinical aspects

The relative analgesic potency of intravenous fentanyl to morphine from single-dose studies is approximately 1:100, and the transdermal fentanyl to oral morphine during long-term administration is 1:150.[104,105] Two major difficulties have been identified with the transdermal route: a delay of 12–24 hours occurs in obtaining steady-state plasma concentrations and a prolonged period of continued fentanyl effect following removal of the patch.[106] In cancer patients, the continuous subcutaneous route provides some advantages over the extensively described transdermal route in patients with unstable pain, requiring rapid dose escalation or reduction. Furthermore, on demand, doses can be administered by the very same route for breakthrough pain.[104] Recently, oral transmucosal fentanyl citrate has been formulated as buccal as well as intranasal administration for breakthrough pain to achieve analgesic action within minutes.[107,108]

Breakthrough pain (e.g., incident pain) can be effectively managed with oral, immediate-release opioids or alternatively with buccal or intranasal fentanyl preparations. In some cases, the buccal or intranasal fenanyl preparations are preferable to immediate-release oral opioids because of more-rapid onset of action and shorter duration of effect.[14]

BUPRENORPHINE

Buprenorphine is a semisynthetic opioid derived from thebaine, a natural opium alkaloid structurally similar to morphine. It has a potent analgesic effect due to agonist activity and a high binding affinity for μ-opioid receptors. In addition, an antagonistic activity can be seen on the k-receptor. Buprenorphine is an opioid with a potency 25–30 times that of morphine.[109] The high analgesic potency of buprenorphine and its high lipophilicity and low molecular weight make it ideal for transdermal delivery systems.[110] There is consensus that buprenorphine, acting as a full μ-agonist, has no ceiling effect except for respiratory depression.[111] Efficacy is dose-related, and the duration of sublingual or parenteral analgesia is long, approximately 6–8 hours. However, the transdermal application may be relevant in cancer pain and this administration form is exclusively mentioned in the following.

Absorption

Delivered transdermally, buprenorphine has a similar time of onset as transdermal fentanyl but a longer duration of action (up to 7 days). Therefore, this formulation of the buprenorphine patch can be changed twice weekly on fixed days.[112]

Pharmacokinetics

Approximately one-third of buprenorphine is metabolized predominantly by cytochrome P450 3A4 in the liver, yielding the active metabolite norbuprenorphine—about 40 times less potent.[112] Nevertheless, the contribution of norbuprenorphine to the central clinical effect of burprenorphine is questionable as norbuprenorphine is less lipophilic and thereby does not readily cross the blood–brain barrier.[112]

Elimination

In case of hepatic impairment, the half-life of the drug is prolonged, but because of the low activity of the metabolites, this is of low clinical relevance. Nevertheless, careful monitoring of patients with hepatic impairment is recommended. In cases of renal impairment, no clinically important accumulation of metabolites has been observed; therefore, a dose reduction is not necessary.[112]

Clinical aspects

A systematic review of transdermal fentanyl and buprenorphine for moderate to severe cancer pain[113] includes the results of one meta-analysis of four RCTs that compared oral morphine with fentanyl or buprenorphine.[114] No significant differences in efficacy emerged between either transdermal preparation and other opioids, but a difference in favor of transdermal preparations was seen for constipation and patients' preferences.

LONG–TERM CONSEQUENCES OF OPIOID TREATMENT

Apart from providing analgesia and other potentially desired effects, opioids also induce traditional side effects (nausea, sedation, constipation, itching, etc.). However, long-term opioid treatment may also have other consequences that should be considered in palliative care including physical dependence, tolerance, opioid induced hyperalgesia, addiction and abuse, and suppression of immune and reproductive systems.

Physical dependence

Physical dependence is a pharmacological phenomenon and the expected consequence of use of opioids. It is defined by the appearance of withdrawal symptoms when the opioid dose is reduced or abruptly discontinued during long-term treatment and/or there is decreasing blood level of opioid, but may also occur within few days of continuous use of opioids.[115,116] Noradrenergic mechanisms, overactivity of the locus ceruleus, and possibly other unknown mechanisms are involved in the physical expression of withdrawal symptoms.[117,118] Withdrawal symptoms may include various physiological and psychological signs such as sweating, diarrhea, tremors, anxiety, irritability, lacrimation, rhinorrhoea, nausea/vomiting, and disturbed sleep. Also pain or increased pain is common, often described as abdominal spasms, muscle pain, and bone pain.[116]

Intermittent withdrawal phenomena, breakthrough withdrawal symptoms, or on-off phenomena, which may appear as increased pain, are common in patients using short-acting opioids on demand.[119] Opioid withdrawal can, to some extent, be prevented by gradually tapering off the opioid until complete discontinuation.

Tolerance

Pharmacologically, tolerance may develop with the repeated use of opioids and is characterized by the necessity of increased doses in order to maintain the drug effects. Tolerance results from adaptive mechanisms at the cellular, synaptic, and network levels, where adaptations due to homeostatic mechanisms tend to restore normal function in spite of the continued perturbations produced by opioid agonists. Some major research concepts for the explaining and treating opioid tolerance have appeared in recent years.

The first is the determination of cellular responses by the agonist–receptor complex but not by activated receptor alone. When this concept is applied to opioid tolerance, it implies that different opioids that work on the same receptor may induce different cell responses to cause tolerance. This theory may explain the well-known asymmetric cross-tolerance between drugs that activate the same receptor, but have different intrinsic activities (e.g., a patient who develops morphine tolerance may have good analgesic effects from sufentanil) and a commonly used technique of opioid rotation for patients requiring chronic opioid use.[120] Along this line, different β-arrestins have been found to mediate cell responses after different opioids, which are all μ-receptor agonists. Thus, β-arrestins may be intracellular targets for modifying cell responses such as tolerance induced by individual opioids. The second concept is that receptor internalization and recycling reduce opioid tolerance. If this is proved to be true in humans, one simple way to reduce opioid tolerance in clinical practice would be to combine morphine with a subanalgesic dose of an opioid with high intrinsic efficacy (these opioids usually induce receptor internalization). The development of drugs that induce receptor internalization, but do not activate opioid receptors, may be another useful approach to reduce morphine tolerance.[121] The third concept is that morphine exposure results in a strong upregulation of spinal microglia.[122,123] Alpha2-adrenoreceptor agonists (e.g., clonidine) and NMDA antagonists (e.g., ketamine or dextromethorphan) can minimize tolerance development. In addition, opioid rotation and multimodal analgesia are other alternative approaches.[124]

Opioid-induced hyperalgesia

Opioid-induced hyperalgesia (OIH) is broadly defined as a state of nociceptive sensitization caused by an exposure to opioids. The condition is characterized by a paradoxical response whereby a patient receiving opioids for the treatment of pain might actually become more sensitive to certain painful stimuli. The type of pain experienced by an individual might be the same as the underlying pain or different from the original underlying pain, and typically, OIH produces diffuse pain, less defined in quality, which extends to the areas of distribution, than the preexisting pain. Thus, the original pain type may be amplified, combined with a state of more generalized hyperalgesia/allodynia resembling neuropathic pain. However, there still exists no generally accepted operational definition of OIH among researchers in human clinical trials; hyperalgesia is defined either as decrease in pain threshold or pain tolerance after chronic opioid exposure. In the beginning of the 1990s, OIH was primarily described in patients with advanced cancer receiving high doses of opioids for prolonged periods,[55] but recent studies indicate that OIH may be much more prevalent and clinical relevant, as observed in different populations treated with opioids.[125–127]

OIH has been reliably demonstrated to exist in the preclinical literature, and it is most often in this context defined as a decrease in pain threshold due to opioid exposure. The NMDA-receptor activation seems to be crucial for the development of OIH, and opioid receptors may not exclusively be involved in the development of OIH. From the first anecdotal reports on OIH, a dose reduction or switching to other opioids has been suggested as an effective remedy in cancer patients. The switching has not only abolished the OIH, but also substantially reduced other opioid toxicities. The beneficial rotation to methadone has most frequently been explained by the assumption that methadone has a weak NMDA receptor antagonism, which could explain the effect.[128,129] The potential involvement of the NMDA receptors in generation of OIH has promoted the use of more specific NMDA-receptor-blocking agents. The most powerful available of these is ketamine, which has been used to reduce OIH in humans.[130,131]

Addiction

Addiction is a phenomenon distinct from physical dependence and tolerance.[132] Addiction in the context of opioid therapy for pain constitutes a constellation of maladaptive behaviors including loss of control over use, preoccupation with opioid use despite adequate pain relief and continued use of the drugs despite apparent obvious adverse consequences due to their use.[133] Other suggestive signs of addiction may be unwillingness to terminate opioid treatment even if other treatment possibilities are offered, preference for short-acting opioids used on demand, and not being interested in other treatment possibilities. Addiction differs from pseudo-addiction and abuse. Pseudo-addictive condition is a result of undertreated pain, in which the patient becomes focused on getting or hoarding analgesics or even illicit drugs in order to obtain pain relief. Usually, the abnormal behavior is resolved when pain is effectively treated.[133] Abuse refers to the condition in which the medication is used for a pain indication but in a way that may cause harm to self or others. Abuse may or may not be associated with physical dependency or addiction.

Addiction is anticipated to have a complex etiology including genetic, psychological, social, and cultural influences, and drug exposure.[134–136] Neurobiologically, addiction is believed to be related to dopaminergic phenomena in the limbic reward center and changes in related systems that reinforce pleasant effects of several substances, which stimulate drug craving and compulsive use in vulnerable individuals.[137]

The factors that promote addiction in some people are not fully understood, although it is known that individuals with a family history of alcoholism or drug addiction or persons with a prior history of addiction have some increased risk of addiction or of relapse to addiction in association with therapeutic use of opioids.[138]

There are few studies regarding the prevalence of opioid addiction in patients with cancer. In these studies, the definition terms for evaluation of addiction and diagnostic criteria are not clearly specified, but they indicate that addiction varies from 0% to 7.7%. ICD-10[139] and Portenoy's criteria[140] may be appropriate instruments to assess addiction in chronic pain patients treated with opioids.[141]

Immune system

Opioids have for years been known to influence the immune system, and recently, experimental studies have added new knowledge to the literature.[142–144] Opioids may have detrimental immunomodulatory effects on nearly all measurable parts of the system. Earlier studies showed that opioids can suppress lymphocyte proliferation,[145,146] trafficking,[147] natural killer cell activity,[148] antibody production,[149] and the overall number of circulating leukocytes.[150] Animal studies indicate that short-term opioid treatment has fewer adverse effects than long-term exposure, and that abrupt withdrawal may enhance the immunosuppression.[151] Also different opioids seem to act differently on the immune system, as exemplified through methadone, which may be less suppressive than morphine.[152,153]

There is little evidence of effects of opioids on the immune system in humans; however, experimental studies in vitro and in animals have demonstrated differences in neuroimmunomodulation according to the different opioid receptors. Some reports suggest that a synthetic agonist of μ-opioid receptors (enkephalin DAGO) can modulate the production of IgM- and IgG-AFC,[154] and macrophage function[155]; ligands for δ-receptor (enkephalin DPDPE) can stimulate proliferation of murine T-lymphocytes[156] and inhibit macrophage function[155]; and specific agonist of κ-opioid receptors (amide decapeptide rimorphine) can decrease IgM-AFC.[157]

An enhanced sensitivity to viral and bacterial infections is seen in drug abusers, and there is evidence regarding mechanisms of increasing susceptibility to immunodeficiency virus in monkeys adapted to morphine dependence[158] and bacterial infections in mice during opioid withdrawal that suggest shortened survival and high bacterial load.[159] However, these findings need to be revisited in future human studies.[160]

Reproductive system

Abs et al.[161] found among patients treated with opioids intrathecally decreased libido or impotence in almost all the men and significantly lowered serum testosterone levels. Decreased libido was present in about 70% of women receiving opioids, and all premenopausal females developed amenorrhea or an irregular menstrual cycle. Serum luteinizing hormone, estradiol, and progesterone levels were significantly lower in the opioid-treated group than among the controls. Finch et al.[162] and Roberts et al.[163] have also found decreased libido and testosterone levels in men, and it can be concluded that opioids administered intrathecally may induce hypogonadotropic hypogonadism, which is of clinical importance for the majority of men and in premenopausal women. A study in men on methadone or buprenorphine maintenance treatment (MMT, BMT) investigated the prevalence and etiology of hypogonadism. Men on MMT had high prevalence of hypogonadotrophic hypogonadism, whereas the extent of hormonal changes associated with buprenorphine needs to

be explored further in larger studies.[164] Other studies have indicated that a differential effect of gender on bone mineral density might be explained in part by differences in gonadal function during long-term opioid therapy. A study of individuals in MMT indicated that low levels of testosterone are associated with accelerated bone loss particularly in men,[165] but hypogonadism has also been reported in women during treatment with oral opioids.[166] In summary, these findings may suggest that individuals receiving long-term methadone and maybe other opioids are at increased risk of osteoporosis and physicians should consider evaluating the skeletal health of such individuals, including the estimation of absolute fracture risk. Controlled longitudinal studies of bone mineral density and bone turnover are indicated to define the timing and pace of the bone loss. Furthermore, future studies of hypogonadism in opioid-treated individuals should examine the potential benefits of dose reduction, choice of opioid medication, and sex hormone replacement therapy.

SUMMARY

This chapter discussed the history and recent evidence regarding opioid receptors along with clinical observations of individual responses and incomplete cross-tolerance to different opioids. The up-to-date pharmacology of the most commonly used strong opioids—morphine, methadone, oxycodone/oxymorphone, fentanyl, and buprenorphine—has been reviewed. Important clinical issues associated with long-term administration of these drugs are highlighted.

Key learning points

- Morphine is the most thoroughly investigated opioid drug; however, new and puzzling aspects of its metabolism are still unclear.

- Although M6G undoubtedly possesses analgesic effects, its contribution to clinical analgesia is unknown. M3G may be involved in the development of antagonism of antinociception as well as opioid-induced neurotoxicity.

- Methadone is increasingly being considered as a second-choice drug alternative to morphine and has interesting properties when switching to it from other opioids. Methadone seems to become relatively more potent with increasing exposure to other opioids.

- Oxycodone has become the most commonly used opioid in the United States, although its pharmacology at therapeutic dose levels seems to be closely related to that of morphine.

- The fentanyl patch is increasingly popular; however, in dynamic pain states, titrating may be difficult.

- The clinical relevance of the buprenorphine patch in palliative medicine has to be further investigated.

- Long-term opioid treatment has other consequences than the "classic" side effects and opioid-induced neurotoxicity. In palliative medicine physical dependence, tolerance, opioid induced hyperalgesia and addiction should also be considered as they may be related to poor treatment outcomes.

- New knowledge concerning the potential influence of long-term administration of opioids on the immune and reproductive systems is emerging.

REFERENCES

1 Beckett AH, Casy AF. Synthetic analgesics: Stereochemical considerations. J Pharm Pharmacol 1954; 6: 986–1001.
2 Portoghese PS. Stereochemical factors and receptor interactions associated with narcotic analgesics. J Pharm Sci 1966; 55: 865–887.
3 Terenius L. Specific uptake of narcotic analgesics by subcellular fractions of the guinea-pig ileum. Acta Pharmacol Toxicol 1972; 31: 50–55.
4 Terenius L. Characteristics of the 'receptor' for narcotic analgesics in synaptic plasma membrane from rat brain. Acta Pharmacol Toxicol 1973; 33: 377–384.
5 Martin WR, Eades CG, Thompson JA et al. The effects of morphine and nalorphine-like drugs in the non-dependent and morphine-dependent chronic spinal dog. J Pharmacol Exp Ther 1976; 197: 517–532.
6 Mollereau C, Parmentier M, Mailleux P et al. ORL1, a novel member of the opioid receptor family. Cloning, functional expression and localization. FEBS Lett 1994; 341: 33–38.
7 Pasternak GW. Pharmacological mechanisms of opioid analgesics. Clin Neuropharmacol 1993; 16: 1–18.
8 Dale O, Moksnes K, Kaasa S. European Palliative Care Research Collaborative pain guidelines: Opioid switching to improve analgesia or reduce side effects. A systematic review. Palliat Med 2011; 25: 494–503.
9 Klepstad P, Fladvad T, Skorpen F, Bjordal K, Caraceni A, Dale O, Davies A et al. Influence from genetic variability on opioid use for cancer pain: A European genetic association study of 2294 cancer pain patients. Pain 2011; 152: 1139–1145.
10 Crews JC, Sweney NJ, Denson DD. Clinical efficacy of methadone in patients refractory to other mu-receptor agonist analgesics for management of terminal cancer pain. Case presentations and discussion of incomplete cross-tolerance among opioid agonist analgesics. Cancer 1993; 72: 2266–2272.
11 Pasternak GW. Preclinical pharmacology and opioid combinations. Pain Med 2012; 13 (Suppl 1):S4–S11.
12 Stein C, Pflüger M, Yassouridis A, Hoelzl J, Lehrberger K, Welte C, Hasssan AHS. No tolerance to peripheral morphine analgesia in presence of opioid expression in inflamed synovia. J Clin Invest 1996; 98: 793–799.
13 World Health Organization. Cancer Pain Relief and Palliative Care. Geneva, Switzerland: World Health Organization, 1996.
14 Caraceni A, Hanks G, Kaasa S, Bennett MI, Brunelli C, Cherny N, Dale O et al. Use of opioid analgesics in the treatment of cancer pain: Evidence-based recommendations from the EAPC. Lancet Oncol 2012; 13: 58–68.
15 Brunk SF, Delle M. Morphine metabolism in man. Clin Pharmacol Ther 1974; 16: 51–57.
16 Poulain P, Hoskin PJ, Hanks GW et al. Relative bioavailability of controlled release morphine tablets (MST Continus) in cancer patients. Br J Anaesth 1988; 61: 569–574.
17 Christrup LL, Sjogren P, Jensen N-H et al. Steady-state kinetics and dynamics of morphine in cancer patients. Is sedation related to the absorption rate of morphine? J Pain Symptom Manage 1999; 18: 164–173.
18 Olsen GD. Morphine binding to human plasma proteins. Clin Pharmacol Ther 1975; 17: 31–35.
19 Owen JA, Sitar DS, Berger L et al. Age-related morphine kinetics. Clin Pharmacol Ther 1983; 34: 364–368.
20 Säwe J, Kager L, Svensson J-O, Rane A. Oral morphine in cancer patients: In vivo kinetics and in vitro hepatic glucuronidation. Br J Clin Pharmacol 1985; 19: 495–501.
21 Osborne R, Joel S, Trew D, Slevin M. Morphine and metabolite behavior after different routes of morphine administration: Demonstration of the importance of the active metabolite morphine-6-glucuronide. Clin Pharmacol Ther 1990; 47: 12–19.
22 Crotty B, Watson KJR, Desmond PV, Mashford ML, Wood LJ, Colman J, Dudley FJ. Hepatic extraction of morphine is impaired in cirrhosis. Eur J Clin Pharmacol 1989; 36: 501–506.
23 Wahlström A, Pacifici GM, Lindstrom B, Hammar L, Rane A. Human liver morphine UDP-glucuronyl transferase enantioselectivity and inhibition by opioid congeners and oxazepam. Br J Pharmacol 1988; 94: 864–870.
24 King CD, Rios GR, Assouline JA, Tephly TR. Expression of UDP-glucuronosyltransferases (UGTs) 2B7 and 1A6 in the human brain and identification of 5-hydroxytryptamine as a substrate. Arch Biochem Biophys 1999; 365: 156–162.
25 Coffman BL, Rios GR, King CD, Tephly TR. Human UGT2B7 catalyzes morphine glucuronidation. Drug Met Disp 1997; 25: 1–4.
26 Stone AN, Mackenzie PI, Galetin A, Houston JB, Miners JO. Isoform selectivity and kinetics of morphine 3- and 6-glucuronidation by human udp-glucuronosyltransferases: Evidence for atypical glucuronidation kinetics by UGT2B7. Drug Metab Dispos 2003; 31: 1086–1089.
27 Andersen G, Sjogren P, Hansen SH et al. Pharmacological consequences of long-term morphine treatment in patients with cancer and chronic non-malignant pain. Eur J Pain 2004; 8: 263–271.
28 Innocenti F, Liu W, Fackenthal D, Ramírez J, Chen P, Ye X, Wu X, Zhang W, Mirkov S, Das S, Cook E Jr, Ratain MJ. Single nucleotide polymorphism discovery and functional assessment of variation in the UDP-glucuronosyltransferase 2B7 gene. Pharmacogenet Genomics 2008; 18: 683–697.
29 Di YM, Chan E, Wei MQ, Liu JP, Zhou SF. Prediction of deleterious non-synonymous single-nucleotide polymorphisms of human uridine diphosphate glucuronosyltransferase genes. AAPS J 2009; 11: 469–480.
30 Holthe M, Klepstad P, Zahlsen K, Borchgrevink PC, Hagen L, Dale O, Kaasa S, Krokan HE, Skorpen F. Morphine glucuronide-to-morphine plasma ratios are unaffected by the UGT2B7 H268Y and UGT1A1*28 polymorphisms in cancer patients on chronic morphine therapy. Eur J Clin Pharmacol 2002; 58: 353–356.
31 Osborne R, Joel S, Grebenik K et al. The pharmacokinetics of morphine and morphine glucuronides in kidney failure. Clin Pharmacol Ther 1993; 54: 158–167.
32 Klepstad P, Dale O, Kaasa S et al. Influences on serum concentrations of morphine, M6G and M3G during routine clinical drug monitoring: A prospective survey in 300 adult cancer patients. Acta Anaesthesiol Scand 2003; 47: 725–731.
33 Hasselström J, Berg U, Löfgren A, Säwe J. Long lasting respiratory depression induced by morphine-6-glucuronide? Br J Clin Pharmac 1989; 27: 515–518.

34   Bodd E, Jacobsen D, Lund E et al. Morphine-6-glucuronide might mediate the prolonged opioid effect of morphine in acute renal failure. *Human Exp Toxicol* 1990; 9: 317–321.

35   King S, Forbes K, Hanks GW, Ferro CJ, Chambers EJ. A systematic review of the use of opioid medication for those with moderate to severe cancer pain and renal impairment: A European Palliative Care Research Collaborative opioid guidelines project. *Palliat Med* 2011; 25: 525–552.

36   Van Dongen RTM, Crul BJP, Koopman-Kimenai PM, Vree TB. Morphine and morphine-glucuronide concentrations in plasma and CSF during long-term administration of oral morphine. *Br J Clin Pharmacol* 1994; 38: 271–273.

37   Goucke CR, Hackett LP, Ilett KF. Concentrations of morphine, morphine-6-glucuronide and morphine-3-glucuronide in serum and cerebrospinal fluid following morphine administration to patients with morphine-resistant pain. *Pain* 1994; 56: 145–149.

38   Wu D, Kang YS, Bickel U, Pardridge WM. Blood-Brain Barrier permeability to morphine-6-glucuronide is markedly reduced compared with morphine. *Drug Met Disp* 1997; 25: 768–771.

39   Stain-Texier F, Boschi G, Sandouk P, Scherrmann JM. Elevated concentrations of morphine 6-beta-D-glucuronide in brain extracellular fluid despite low blood-brain barrier permeability. *Br J Pharmacol* 1999; 128: 917–924.

40   Frances B, Gout R, Monsarrat B, Cros J, Zajac J-M. Further evidence that morphine-6b-glucuronide is a more potent opioid agonist than morphine. *J Pharmacol Exp Ther* 1992; 262: 25–31.

41   Osborne R, Thomsen P, Joel S et al. The analgesic effect of morphine-6-glucuronide. *Br J Clin Pharmacol* 1992; 34: 130–138.

42   Dennis GC, Soni D, Dehkordi O et al. Analgesic responses to intrathecal morphine in relation to CSF concentrations of morphine-3b-glucuronide and morphine-6,beta-glucuronide. *Life Sci* 1999; 64: 1725–1736.

43   Klepstad P, Kaasa S, Borchgrevink PC. Start of oral morphine to cancer patients: Effective serum morphine concentrations and contribution from morphine-6-glucuronide to the analgesia produced by morphine. *Eur J Clin Pharmacol* 2000; 55: 713–719.

44   Quigley C, Joel S, Patel N et al. Plasma concentrations of morphine, morphine-6-glucuronide and their relationship with analgesia and side effects in patients with cancer-related pain. *Palliat Med* 2003; 17: 185–190.

45   Klepstad P, Borchgrevink PC, Dale O et al. Routine drug monitoring of serum concentrations of morphine, morphine-3-glucuronide and morphine-6-glucuronide do not predict clinical observations in cancer patients. *Palliat Med* 2003; 17: 679–687.

46   Smith MT, Watt JA, Cramond T. Morphine-3-glucuronide—A potent antagonist of morphine analgesia. *Life Sci* 1990; 47: 579–585.

47   Gong Q-L, Hedner J, Björkman R, Hedner T. Morphine-3-glucuronide may functionally antagonize morphine-6-glucuronide induced antinociception and ventilatory depression in the rat. *Pain* 1992; 48: 249–255.

48   Hewett K, Dickenson AH, McQuay HJ. Lack of effect of morphine-3-glucuronide on the spinal antinociceptive actions of morphine in the rat: An electrophysiological study. *Pain* 1993; 53: 59–63.

49   Quellet DM-C, Pollack GM. Effect of prior morphine-3-glucuronide exposure on morphine disposition and antinociception. *Biochem Pharmacol* 1997; 53: 1451–1457.

50   Smith MT. Neuroexcitatory effects of morphine and hydro-morphine: Evidence implicating the 3-glucuronide metabolites. *Clin Exp Pharmacol Physiol* 2000; 27: 524–528.

51   Barlett SE, Cramond T, Smith MT. The excitatory effects of morphine-3-glucuronide are attenuated by LY274614, a competitive NMDA receptor antagonist, and by midazolam, an agonist at the benzodiazepine site on the GABAA receptor complex. *Life Sci* 1994; 54: 687–694.

52   Yaksh TL, Harty GJ, Onofrio BM. High doses of spinal morphine produce a nonopiate receptor-mediated hyperesthesia: Clinical and theoretic implications. *Anesthesiology* 1986; 64: 590–597.

53   Yaksh TL, Harty GJ. Pharmacology of the allodynia in rats evoked by high dose intrathecal morphine. *J Pharmacol Exp Ther* 1988; 244: 501–507.

54   Rozan JP, Kahn CH, Warfield CA. Epidural and intravenous opioid-induced neuroexcitation. *Anesthesiology* 1995; 83: 860–863.

55   Sjøgren P, Jonsson T, Jensen NH, Drenck NE, Jensen TS. Hyperalgesia and myoclonus in terminal cancer patients treated with continuous intravenous morphine. *Pain* 1993; 55: 93–97.

56   Kaiko RF, Foley KM, Grabinski PY et al. Central nervous system excitatory effects of mepiridine in cancer patients. *Ann Neurol* 1983; 13: 180–185.

57   Bruera E, Pereira J. Acute neuropsychiatric findings in a patient receiving fentanyl for cancer pain. *Pain* 1997; 69: 199–201.

58   Sjogren P, Jensen NH, Jensen TS. Disappearance of morphine-induced hyperalgesia after discontinuing or substituting morphine with other opioid agonists. *Pain* 1994; 59: 313–316.

59   Penson TP, Joel SP, Clark S et al. Limited phase 1 study of morphine-3-glucuronide. *J Pharm Sci* 2001; 90: 1810–1816.

60   Wiffen PJ, McQuay HJ. Oral morphine for cancer pain. *Cochrane Database Syst Rev* October 17, 2007:CD003868.

61   Caraceni A, Pigni A, Brunelli C. Is oral morphine still the first choice opioid for moderate to severe cancer pain? A systematic review within the European Palliative Care Research Collaborative guidelines project. *Palliat Med* 2011; 25: 402–409.

62   Sai K, Itoda M, Saito Y, Kurose K, Katori N, Kaniwa N, Komamura K et al. Genetic variations and haplotype structures of the ABCB1 gene in a Japanese population: An expanded haplotype block covering the distal promoter region, and associated ethnic differences. *Ann Hum Genet* 2006; 70(Pt 5): 605–622.

63   Campa D, Gioia A, Tomei A, Poli P, Barale R. Association of ABCB1/MDR1 and OPRM1 gene polymorphisms with morphine pain relief. *Clin Pharmacol Ther* 2008; 83: 559–566.

64   Symonds P. Methadone and the elderly. *Br Med J* 1977; 1: 512.

65   Hunt G, Bruera E. Respiratory depression in a patient receiving oral methadone for cancer pain. *J Pain Symptom Manage* 1995; 10: 636–648.

66   Bruera E, Fainsinger R, Moore M et al. Local toxicity with subcutaneous methadone. Experience of two centers. *Pain* 1991; 45: 141–143.

67   Fainsinger R, Schoeller T, Bruera E. Methadone in the management of cancer pain: A review. *Pain* 1993; 52: 137–147.

68   Nilsson MI, Meresaar U, Anggard E. Clinical pharmacokinetics of methadone. *Acta Anaesthesiol Scand* 1982; 74 (Suppl): S66–S69.

69   Gourlay GK, Cherry DA, Cousins MJ. A comparative study of the efficacy and pharmacokinetics of oral methadone and morphine in the treatment of severe pain in patients with cancer. *Pain* 1986; 25: 297–312.

70   Säwe J. High-dose morphine and methadone in cancer patients. Clinical pharmacokinetic considerations of oral treatment. *Clin Pharmacokinet* 1986; 11: 87–106.

71   Dole VP, Kreek MJ. Methadone plasma levels: Sustained by a reservoir of drug in tissue. *Proc Natl Acad Sci USA* 1973; 70: 10.

72   Inturrisi CE, Colbum WA, Kaiko RF et al. Pharmacokinetics and pharmacodynamics of methadone in patients with chronic pain. *Clin Pharmacol Ther* 1987; 41: 392–401.

73   Kristensen K, Christensen CB, Christrup L. The mu1, mu 2, delta, kappa opioid receptor binding profiles of methadone stereoisomers and morphine. *Life Sci* 1995; 56: 45–50.

74   Kristensen K, Blemmer T, Angelo HR et al. Stereoselective pharmacokinetics of methadone in chronic pain patients. *Ther Drug Monitor* 1996; 18: 221–227.

75 Plummer JL, Gourlay GK, Cherry DA, Cousins MJ. Estimation of methadone clearance: Application in management of cancer pain. *Pain* 1988; 33: 313–322.

76 Ripamonti C, Zecca E, Bruera E. An update on the clinical use of methadone for cancer pain. *Pain* 1997; 70: 109–115.

77 Bruera E, Sweeney C. Methadone use in cancer patients with pain: A review. *J Palliat Med* 2002; 5: 127–138.

78 Quigley C. Opioid switching to improve pain relief and drug tolerability. *Cochrane Database Syst Rev* 2004; 3: CD004847.

79 Ripamonti C, De Conno F, Groff L et al. Equianalgesic dose/ratio between methadone and other opioid agonists in cancer pain: Comparison of two clinical experiences. *Ann Oncol* 1998; 9: 79–83.

80 Ebert B, Andersen S, Krogsgaard-larsen P. Ketobemidone, methadone and pethidine are non-competitive N-methyl-D-aspartate (NMDA) antagonists in the rat cortex and spinal cord. *Neurosci Lett* 1995; 187: 165–168.

81 Nicholson AB. Methadone for cancer pain. Review. Update in: *Cochrane Database Syst Rev* 2007; 4: CD003971.

82 Kalso E, Vainio A. Morphine and oxycodone hydrochloride in the management of cancer pain. *Clin Pharmacol Ther* 1990; 47: 639–646.

83 Leow KP, Smith MT, Williams B et al. Single-dose and steady-state pharmacokinetics and pharmacodynamics of oxycodone in patients with cancer. *Clin Pharmacol Ther* 1992; 52: 487–495.

84 Heiskanen T, Olkkola KT, Kalso E. Effects of blocking CYP2D6 on the pharmacokinetics and pharmacodynamics of oxycodone. *Clin Pharmacol Ther* 1998; 64: 603–611.

85 Sloan P, Slatkin N, Ahdieh H. Effectiveness and safety of oral extended-release oxymorphone for the treatment of cancer pain: A pilot study. *Support Care Cancer* 2005; 13: 57–65.

86 Adams MP, Ahdieh H. Single- and multiple-dose pharmacokinetic and dose-proportionality study of oxymorphone immediate-release tablets. *Drugs R D* 2005; 6: 91–99.

87 Poyhia R, Seppala R, Olkkola KT, Kalso E. The pharmacokinetics and metabolism of oxycodone after intramuscular and oral administration to healthy subjects. *Br J Clin Pharmacol* 1992; 33: 617–621.

88 Mandema JW, Kaiko RF, Oshlak B et al. Characterization and validation of a pharmacokinetic model or controlled-release oxycodone. *Br J Clin Pharmacol* 1996; 42: 747–756.

89 Gimbel JS, Walker D, Ma T, Ahdieh H. Efficacy and safety of oxymorphone immediate release for the treatment of mild to moderate pain after ambulatory orthopedic surgery: Results of a randomized, double-blind, placebo-controlled trial. *Arch Phys Med Rehabil* 2005; 86: 2284–2289.

90 Sinatra RS, Hyde NH, Harrison DM. Oxymorphone revisited. *Semin Anesth* 1988; 7: 208–215.

91 Matsumoto AK. Oral extended-release oxymorphone: A new choice for chronic pain relief. *Expert Opin Pharmacother.* 2007; 8: 1515–1527.

92 Kirvela M, Lindgren L, Seppala T, Olkkola KT. The pharmacokinetics of oxycodone in uremic patients undergoing renal transplantation. *J Clin Anesth* 1996; 8: 13–18.

93 Tallgren M, Olkkola KT, Seppala T et al. Pharmacokinetics and ventilatory effects of oxycodone before and after liver transplantation. *Clin Pharmacol Ther* 1997; 61: 655–661.

94 Prommer E. Oxymorphone: A review. *Support Care Cancer* 2006; 14: 109–115.

95 Heiskanen T, Kalso E. Controlled-release oxycodone and morphine in cancer related pain. *Pain* 1997; 73: 37–45.

96 Zhukovsky DS, Walsh D, Doona M. The relative potency between high dose oral oxycodone and morphine: A case illustration. *J Pain Symptom Manage* 1999; 18: 53–55.

97 Hanks GW, Conno F, Cherny N et al. Expert Working Group of the Research Network of the European Association for Palliative Care. Morphine and alternative opioids in cancer pain: The EAPC recommendations. *Br J Cancer* 2001; 84: 587–593.

98 Kaiko RF, Benziger DP, Fitzmartin RD et al. Pharmacokinetic-pharmacodynamic relationship of controlled-release oxycodone. *Clin Pharmacol Ther* 1996; 59: 52–61.

99 Andreassen TN, Klepstad P, Davies A, Bjordal K, Lundström S, Kaasa S, Dale O. Is oxycodone efficacy reflected in serum concentrations? A multicenter, cross-sectional study in 456 adult cancer patients. *J Med Econ* 2012; 15: 87–95.

100 Gourlay GK. Treatment of cancer pain with transdermal fentanyl. *Lancet Oncol* 2001; 2: 165–172.

101 Villiger JW, Ray LJ, Taylor KM. Characteristics of fentanyl binding to the opiate receptor. *Neuropharmacology* 1983; 22: 447–452.

102 Varvel JR, Sharfer SL, Hwang SS et al. Absorption characteristics of transdermally administered fentanyl. *Anesthesiology* 1989; 70: 928–934.

103 Jeal W, Benfield P. Transdermal fentanyl. *Drugs* 1997; 53: 109–138.

104 Paix A, Cloeman A, Lees J et al. Subcutaneous fentanyl and sufentanil infusion substitution for morphine intolerance in cancer pain management. *Pain* 1995; 63: 263–269.

105 Sloan PA, Moulin DE, Hays H. A clinical evaluation of Transdermal Therapeutic System Fentanyl for the treatment of cancer pain. *J Pain Symptom Manage* 1998; 16: 102–111.

106 Miser AW, Narang PK, Dothage JA et al. Transdermal fentanyl for pain control in patients with cancer. *Pain* 1989; 37: 15–21.

107 Zeppetella G. Nebulized and intranasal fentanyl in the management of cancer-related breakthrough pain. *Palliat Med* 2000; 14: 57–58.

108 Streisand JB, Varvel JR, Stanski DR et al. Absorption and bioavailability of transmucosal fentanylcitrate. *Anesthesiology* 1991; 75: 223–229.

109 Sorge J, Sittl R. Transdermal buprenorphine in the treatment of chronic pain: Results of a phase III, multicenter, randomized, double-blind, placebo-controlled study. *Clin Ther* 2004; 26: 1808–1820.

110 Sittl R, Griessinger N, Likar R. Analgesic efficacy and tolerability of transdermal buprenorphine in patients with inadequately controlled chronic pain related to cancer and other disorders: A multicenter, randomized, doubleblind, placebo-controlled trial. *Clin Ther* 2003; 25: 150–168.

111 Pergolizzi J, Aloisi AM, Dahan A et al. Current knowledge of buprenorphine and its unique pharmacological profile. *Pain Pract* 2010; 10: 428–450.

112 Kress HG. Clinical update on the pharmacology, efficacy and safety of transdermal buprenorphine. *Eur J Pain* 2009; 13: 219–230.

113 Tassinari D, Drudi F, Rosati M, Maltoni M. Transdermal opioids as front line treatment of moderate to severe cancer pain: A systemic review. *Palliat Med* 2011; 25: 478–487.

114 Tassinari D, Sartori S, Tamburini E et al. Adverse effects of transdermal opiates treating moderate-severe cancer pain in comparison to long-acting morphine: A meta-analysis and systematic review of the literature. *J Palliat Med* 2008; 11: 492–501.

115 Way WL. Basic mechanisms in narcotic tolerance and physical dependence. *Ann N Y Acad Sci* 1978; 311: 61–68.

116 Jaffe J. Opiates: Clinical aspects. In: Lowinson JH, Ruiz P, Millman RG, eds. *Substance Abuse. A Comprehensive Textbook.* Baltimore, MD: Williams and Wilkens, 1992: 186–194.

117 Rasmussen K. The role of the locus coeruleus and N-methyl-D-aspartic acid (NMDA) and AMPA receptors in opiate withdrawal. *Neuropsychopharmacology* 1995; 13: 295–300.

118 Camí J, Farré M. Drug addiction. *N Engl J Med* 2003; 349: 975–986.

119 Savage SR. Addiction in the treatment of pain: Significance, recognition and treatment. *J Pain Symptom Manage* 1993; 8: 265–278.

120 Ballantyne JC, Mao J. Opioid therapy for chronic pain. *N Engl J Med* 2003; 349: 1943–1953.

121 Finn AK, Whistler JL. Endocytosis of the mu opioid receptor reduces tolerance and a cellular hallmark of opiate withdrawal. *Neuron* 2001; 32: 829–839.

122 Horvath RJ, Romero-Sandoval EA, De Leo JA. Inhibition of microglial P2X4 receptors attenuates morphine tolerance, Iba1, GFAP and
mu opioid receptor protein expression while enhancing perivascular
microglial ED2. *Pain* 2010; 150: 401–413.

123 Zhou D, Chen ML, Zhang YQ et al. Involvement of spinal microglial
P2X7 receptor in generation of tolerance to morphine analgesia in
rats. *J Neurosci.* 2010; 30: 8042–8047.

124 Raith K, Hochhaus G. Drugs used in the treatment of opioid tolerance
and physical dependence: A review. *Int J Clin Pharmacol Ther* 2004; 42:
191–203.

125 Doverty M, White JM, Somogyi AA, Bochner F, Ali R, Ling W.
Hyperalgesic responses in methadone maintenance patients. *Pain*
2001; 90: 91–96.

126 Guignard B, Bossard AE, Coste C et al. Acute opioid tolerance:
Intraoperative remifentanil increases postoperative pain and morphine requirement. *Anesthesiology* 2000; 93: 409–417.

127 Chu LF, Clark DJ, Angst MS. Opioid tolerance and hyperalgesia in
chronic pain patients after one month of oral morphine therapy: A
preliminary prospective study. *J Pain* 2006; 7: 43–48.

128 Blackburn D, Somerville E, Squire J. Methadone: An alternative conversion regime. *Eur J Pall Care* 2002; 9: 93–96.

129 Axelrod DJ, Reville B. Using methadone to treat opioid-induced hyperalgesia and refractory pain. *J Opioid Manage* 2007; 3: 113–114.

130 Koppert W, Sitti R, Scheuber K, Alsheimer M, Schmelz M, Schüttler
J. Differential modulation of remifentanil-induced analgesia and
postinfusion hyperalgesia by s-ketamine and clonidine in humans.
Anesthesiology 2003; 99: 152–159.

131 Forero M, Chan PSL, Restrepo-Garces CE. Successful reversal of hyper-
algesia/myoclonus complex with low-dose ketamine infusion. *Pain
Pract* 2012; 12: 154–158.

132 Savage SR, Joranson DE, Covington EC, Schnoll SH, Heit HA, Gilson AM.
Definitions related to the medical use of opioids: Evolution towards
universal agreement. *J Pain Symptom Manage* 2003; 26: 655–667.

133 American Society of Addiction Medicine. Definitions Related to the
Use of Opioids for the Treatment of Pain: Consensus Statement of
the American Academy of Pain Medicine, the American Pain Society,
and the American Society of Addiction Medicine. 2001. http://www.
asam.org/docs/publicy-policy-statements/1opioid-definitions-con-
sensus-2-011.pdf?sfvrsn = 0, (accessed in May 30, 2012).

134 Enoch MA, Goldman D. The genetics of alcoholism and alcohol abuse.
Curr Psychiatry Rep 2001; 3: 144–151.

135 Savage SR. Assessment for addiction in pain-treatment settings. *Clin J
Pain* 2002; 18: S28–S38.

136 Lin SW, Anthenelli RM. Determinants of substance abuse and depen-
dence. In: Lowinson JH, Ruiz P, Milman RB, Langrod JG, eds. *Substance
Abuse. A Comprehensive Textbook.* Philadelphia, PA: Lippincott
Williams and Wilkins; 2005. pp. 33–120.

137 Gardner EL. Brain-reward mechanisms. In: Lowinson JH, Ruiz P, Milman
RB, Langrod JG, eds. *Substance Abuse. A Comprehensive Textbook.*
Philadelphia, PA: Lippincott Williams and Wilkins; 2005. pp. 48–97.

138 Halikas J. Craving. In: Lowinson JH, Ruiz P, Millman RG, Langrod JG,
eds. *Substance Abuse. A Comprehensive Textbook.* Baltimore, MD:
Williams and Wilkins; 1997. pp. 85–90.

139 World Health Organization. ICD-10 Version: 2010. http://apps.who.int/
classifications/icd10/browse/2010/en. (Accessed in June 8, 2014).

140 Portenoy RK. Chronic opioid therapy in nonmalignant pain. *J Pain
Symptom Manage* 1990; 5(1 Suppl): S46–S62.

141 Højsted J, Sjøgren P. Addiction to opioids in chronic pain patients: A
literature review. *Eur J Pain* 2007; 11: 490–518.

142 Sacerdote P, Limiroli E, Gaspani L. Experimental evidence for immunomodulatory effects of opioids. *Adv Exp Med Biol* 2003; 521: 106–116.

143 Devoino LV, Al'perina EL, Gevorgyan MM, Cheido MA. Involvement of
dopamine D1 and D2 receptors in the rat nucleus accumbens in immu-
nostimulation. *Neurosci Behav Physiol* 2007; 37: 147–151.

144 Nelson CJ, Schneider GM, Lysle DT. Involvement of central mu- but not
delta- or kappa-opioid receptors in immunomodulation. *Brain Behav
Immun* 2000; 14: 170–184.

145 Bryant HU, Bernton EW, Holaday JW. Immunosuppressive effects of
chronic morphine treatment in mice. *Life Sci* 1987; 41: 1731–1738.

146 Fecho K, Maslonek KA, Dykstra LA, Lysle DT. Mechanisms whereby
macrophage-derived nitrous oxide is involved in morphine-induced
suppression of splenic lymphocyte proliferation. *J Pharmacol Exp Ther*
1995; 272: 477–483.

147 Flores LR, Wahl SM, Bayer BM. Mechanisms of morphine-induced
immunosuppression: Effect of acute morphine administration on lymphocyte trafficking. *J Pharmacol Exp Ther* 1995; 272: 1246–1251.

148 Yakota T, Uehara K, Nomota Y. Intrathecal morphine suppresses NK
cell activity following abdominal surgery. *Can J Anaesth* 2000; 47:
303–308.

149 Bussierre JL, Adler MW, Rogers TJ, Eisenstein TK. Cytokine reversal of
morphine-induced suppression of the antibody response. *J Pharmacol
Exp Ther* 1993; 264: 591–597.

150 Fecho K, Lysle DT. Heroin-induced alterations in leukocyte numbers
and apoptosis in the rat spleen. *Cell Immunol* 2000; 202: 113–123.

151 Rahim RT, Adler MW, Meissler JJ Jr. et al. Abrupt or precipitated withdrawal from morphine induces immunosuppression. *J Neuroimmunol*
2002; 127: 88–95.

152 Sacerdote P, Manfredi B, Mantegazza P, Panerai AE. Antinociceptive
and immunosuppressive effects of opiate drugs: A structure related
study. *Br J Pharmacol* 1997; 121: 834–840.

153 De Waal EJ, Van Der Laan JW, Van Loveren H. Effects of prolonged
exposure to morphine and methadone on in vivo parameters of
immune function in rats. *Toxicology* 1998; 129: 201–210.

154 Taub DD, Eisenstein TK, Geller EB, Adler MW, Rogers TJ.
Immunomodulatory activity of mu- and kappa-selective opioid agonists. *Proc Natl Acad Sci USA* 1991; 88: 360–364.

155 Szabo I, Rojavin M, Bussiere JL, Eisenstein TK, Adler MW, Rogers TJ.
Suppression of peritoneal macrophage phagocytosis of Candida albicans by opioids. *J Pharmacol Exp Ther* 1993; 267: 703–706.

156 Kowalski J. Immunomodulatory action of class mu-, delta- and kappa-
opioid receptor agonists in mice. *Neuropeptides.* 1998; 32: 301–306.

157 Idova GV, Alperina EL, Cheido MA. Contribution of brain dopamine, serotonin and opioid receptors in the mechanisms of neuroimmunomodulation: Evidence from pharmacological analysis. *Int
Immunopharmacol* 2012; 12: 618–625.

158 Kumar R, Torres C, Yamamura Y, Rodriguez I, Martinez M, Staprans
S, Donahoe RM, Kraiselburd E, Stephens EB, Kumar A. Modulation by
morphine of viral set point in rhesus macaques infected with simian
immunodeficiency virus and simian-human immunodeficiency virus.
J Virol 2004; 78: 11425–11428.

159 Wang J, Barke RA, Charboneau R, Schwendener R, Roy S. Morphine
induces defects in early response of alveolar macrophages to
Streptococcus pneumoniae by modulating TLR9-NF-kappa B signaling. *J Immunol* 2008; 180: 3594–3600.

160 Roy S, Ninkovic J, Banerjee S, Charboneau RG, Das S, Dutta R,
Kirchner VA, Koodie L, Ma J, Meng J, Barke RA. Opioid drug abuse
and modulation of immune function: Consequences in the susceptibility to opportunistic infections. *J Neuroimmune Pharmacol* 2011;
6: 442–465.

161 Abs R, Verhelst J, Maeyaert J et al. Endocrine consequences of long-
term intrathecal administration of opioids. *J Clin Endocrinol Metab*
2000; 85: 2215–2222.

162   Finch PM, Roberts LJ, Price L et al. Hypogonadism in patients treated with intrathecal morphine. *Clin J Pain* 2000; 16: 251–254.

163   Roberts LJ, Finch PM, Bhagat CI, Price LM. Sex hormone suppression by intrathecal opioids: A prospective study. *Clin J Pain* 2002; 18: 144–148.

164   Hallinan R, Byrne A, Agho K, McMahon CG, Tynan P, Attia J. Hypogonadism in men receiving methadone and buprenorphine maintenance treatment. *Int J Androl* 2009; 32: 131–139.

165   Grey A, Rix-Trott K, Horne A, Gamble G, Bolland M, Reid IR. Decreased bone density in men on methadone maintenance therapy. *Addiction* 2011; 106: 349–354.

166   Daniell HW. Opioid endocrinopathy in women consuming prescribed sustained-action opioids for control of nonmalignant pain. *J Pain* 2008; 9: 28–36.

44

Assessment and management of opioid side effects

SHALINI DALAL

INTRODUCTION

Opioids are the cornerstone of pain management in the palliative care setting. Successful pain management with opioids requires that adequate analgesia be achieved without excessive side effects. Approximately 10%–30% of patients treated with opioids do not have a successful outcome due to either excessive side effects and inadequate pain relief or a combination of both.[1] All opioids have potential for side effects (Table 44.1), which may compel some patients to decrease or discontinue opioids. The most common include constipation, nausea, and sedation, while dose limiting side effects typically involve the central nervous system (CNS) and include cognitive impairment, delirium, and myoclonus. In recent years with the increased long-term use of opioids such as in the chronic nonmalignant pain situation, effects of prolonged use on the endocrine, particularly on sex hormones, and the immune system are being increasingly recognized and researched. The clinical importance of these effects for palliative care patients is not yet clear.

The concept of individualizing analgesic therapy to the patient's pain syndrome with close monitoring of treatment outcomes (pain relief, side effects of treatments) and changing clinical circumstances is fundamental to achieving success with pain management. Depending on these assessments, opioids are titrated or switched to another to maintain a favorable balance between efficacy and side effects.[1] Further, some opioids may be better suited than others among vulnerable patients, such as the elderly or terminal cancer patients, who may already have, or be at increased risk for impaired renal and hepatic functions. Assessment of hydration status and renal functions plays an important role when using opioids in palliative care patients.

Greater compliance is likely if clinicians educate patients/family of anticipated side effects, and discuss plans for management. Side effects may be limited by using appropriate opioid doses, coadministration of adjuvant analgesics if indicated, and use of medications to prevent/manage expected side effects.

OPIOID-MEDIATED GASTROINTESTINAL SIDE EFFECTS

The etiology of opioid-induced gastrointestinal (GI) effects is multifactorial and predominantly mediated by three opioid receptors, mu-, delta-, and kappa-, which are widely distributed in the myenteric and submucosal neurons throughout the GI tract.[2–4] Opioids modify GI function by interacting with these opioid receptors, thereby reducing neuronal excitability and neurotransmitter (acetylcholine) release, with an overall inhibitory effect on motility and secretion.[2–6] Major physiological effects include inhibition of gastric emptying and increased gastric acid secretion; delayed colonic transit, increased colonic tone/segmentation, increased colonic absorption, and decreased secretion; increased pyloric and anorectal tone; and increased gall bladder contraction with decreased secretion, and spasm of sphincter of Oddi.[3,4] The inhibitory effect on colonic secretions also appears to involve complex mechanisms involving 5-HT2 receptors, α2-adrenoreceptors, and noradrenaline release.[7] These effects may result in a myriad of GI symptoms that include early satiety, nausea and emesis, abdominal bloating and cramping, and constipation (passage of hard stool, infrequent stool, straining during bowel movement, and incomplete evacuation). In addition, opioid-induced gallbladder effects may result in biliary pain and delayed digestion. This constellation of opioid-induced GI symptoms is referred to as opioid-induced bowel dysfunction (OBD),[3] of which constipation is the most frequently reported and distressing symptom in patients taking opioids.[8]

Constipation

Constipation is the most common side effect of opioid use[9] and should be anticipated, monitored, and treated throughout the duration of opioid therapy. In the noncancer setting, approximately 40% of chronic opioid users for pain management develop constipation.[8] This frequency is higher in patients with advanced illness such as cancer, where more

Table 44.1 *Opioid side-effects*

Gastrointestinal	Respiratory/Cardiac
• Nausea	• Respiratory depression
• Constipation	• Non-cardiogenic pulmonary
Central nervous system	edema
• Sedation	**Autonomic**
• Opioid induced neurotoxicity	• Dry mouth
• *severe sedation*	• Urinary retention
• *delirium*	**Endocrine**
• *hallucinations*	• Hypogonadism
• *myoclonus and seizures*	• Hypopituitarism
• *hyperalgesia and allodynia*	**Immune**
Cutaneous	
• Pruritis	
• Sweating	

Table 44.2 *Prevention and management of opioid induced constipation*

Non-specific measures:
- Maintaining adequate hydration
- Maintaining ambulatory status
- Diet rich in fruit and vegetables, fiber
- Availability of privacy during defecation
- Opioid sparing regimens

Therapeutic measures:
- Laxatives: E.g. sennosides, bisacodyl, poly
- Rectal suppositories, enemas
- Prokinetic agents: E.g. metoclopramide
- Peripherally restricted opioid receptor antagonists: E.g. Methylnaltrexone (parenteral administration)
- Manual disimpaction

than 90% of patients on opioids develop constipation.[9,10] Often dismissed as a trivial side effect, constipation can adversely impact patient's quality of life, and make patients avoid or reduce the opioid dose, resulting in decreased analgesic benefits. Untreated and severe constipation can lead to partial or complete bowel obstruction with attendant issues of severe morbidity. Unlike many of the other opioid side effects such as nausea and sedation which may occur on opioid initiation, constipation usually does not improve over time, and majority of patients will require therapy. Frequently several other factors predisposing to constipation coexist in palliative care patients, such as autonomic failure, metabolic disorders (such as uremia, hypercalcemia), neurological lesions, prolonged immobility, dehydration, or other medications (such as anticholinergics, antacids, or antidepressants). The etiology of constipation in the palliative care setting is discussed in detail in Chapter 59.

Assessment and management of constipation

Assessment should include a history of the frequency and difficulty of defecation and consideration of other possible contributors. Physical examination should include palpation of the abdomen and a rectal examination may be needed. Occasionally, an abdominal x-ray may be required if the history is unclear.[11,12] Constipation-specific instruments that assess the impact and severity of the condition include the Patient Assessment of Constipation Quality of Life (PAC-QOL) and the Patient Assessment of Constipation Symptoms (PAC-SYM) questionnaires. The PAC-QOL and PAC-SYM instruments have been shown to be reliable, valid, and responsive measures of constipation and opioid-induced constipation respectively,[13,14] and predominantly used in research setting.

All patients receiving opioids should be counseled about opioid-induced constipation and have an individualized bowel regimen plan in place. This may include a combination of measures, as illustrated in Table 44.2. Therapeutic interventions include the administration of oral laxatives,

suppositories, rectal enemas, peripherally restricted opioid receptor antagonists, and manual disimpaction. Oral laxatives include bulk agents, osmotic agents, contact cathartics, lubricants, and prokinetic agents.

Lower doses of opioids, or weaker opioids such as codeine, are just as likely to cause constipation, and clinicians should therefore base laxative prescribing and titration on bowel function rather than opioid type and dose.[15] There is no single correct approach to laxative prescribing in palliative care. Although there are various recommendations in the literature on initiating patients on a bowel regimen, the most important point to remember is that regimens should be individualized and titrated to response. One approach to constipation prevention and management is presented in Table 44.3.

While there are no studies revealing the superiority of one approach over the other, the most common treatment the palliative care setting is the use of a bowel stimulant such as senna, with or without a stool softener. Additionally, milk of magnesium oral concentrate, polyethylene glycol, or lactulose may be initiated and titrated until a large bowel movement occurs. Bisacodyl suppository, a milk-and-molasses enema, or a fleet enema may be required. Bulk-forming laxatives should be avoided in patients unable to maintain adequate fluid intake. Nondrug approaches, such as increasing fluid intake and increasing physical activity, should be implemented if feasible, but are seldom sufficient by itself.

Occasionally, it may be required to switch opioids. There is preliminary evidence to suggest that transdermal fentanyl may be less constipating than morphine and oxymorphone.[16,17] In a retrospective study of laxative use, laxative doses needed were significantly lower with methadone than with equianalgesic doses of morphine or hydromorphone.[18] Tapentadol, a mu-opioid receptor agonist that also inhibits norepinephrine reuptake, has been shown to have a more favorable GI side-effect profile than oxycodone in several studies.[19–21]

Two peripherally restricted opioid receptor antagonists, methylnaltrexone and alvimopam, do not cross the blood–brain barrier at therapeutic doses and selectively counteract opioid-inducing constipating effects without reversal of

Table 44.3 *Suggested approach for the prevention and management of opioid induced constipation and nausea*

Side Effect	Prevention	Management

Constipation	Unless there are existing alterations in bowel patterns such as bowel obstruction or diarrhea, all patients receiving opioids should be started on laxative bowel regimen and receive education for bowel management.
	
	1. Stimulant laxative +/– stool softener:Eg: Senna 8.6 plus Docusate 50mg
	2. Ensure adequate fluids, dietary fiber and exercise if feasible.
	3. Prune juice following by warm beverage may be considered.
		1. Assess potential cause that can cause constipation (such as recent opioid dose increase, use of other constipating medications, new bowel obstruction)
		2. Increase Senna and/or docusate tablets and add 1 or both of the following:
		  a. Milk of Magnesia oral concentrate: 10 mL PO every 2–4 times daily
		  b. Polyethylene glycol: 17 grams in 8 ounce beverage once daily
		  c. Lactulose 15–30 cc every 4–6 hours
		3. If no response to above, do digital rectal examination (DRE) to rule out low impaction. Continue above steps AND
		• **If impacted:** disimpact manually if stool is soft. If not, soften with mineral oil fleets enema before disimpaction. Follow up with milk of molasses enemas until clear with no formed stools.
		• Consider use of rescue analgesics before disimpaction.
		• **If not impacted** on rectal examination, patient may still have higher level impaction, and if history is appropriate consider abdominal imaging and/or administer milk of molasses enema along with magnesium citrate 8 oz PO.
		
		Please note: DRE, manual disimpaction, & enemas may be contraindicated in several circumstances such as presence of colitis, neutropenia, thrombocytopenia or coagulopathy.

Nausea and Vomiting	Titrate opioid dose slowly and steadily. Make antiemetics available with opioid prescription. Metoclopramide 10 mg PO For patients at high risk of nausea consider around the clock regimen for 5 days and then change to PRN.	Investigate for other causes of nausea (e.g. constipation , bowel obstruction, chemotherapyor other medications) and treat per guideline. Initiate around the clock antiemetic regimen . Example Metoclopramide 5 to 10 mg PO, IV, or subcutaneously around the clock every 4–6 hours. Add or increase non-opioid or adjuvant medications for additional pain relief so that opioid dose can be reduced. If analgesia is satisfactory, reduce opioid dose by 25% Consider opioid rotation if nausea remains refractory

analgesia. Methylnaltrexone, a quaternary ammonium derivative of naltrexone, has been investigated in several clinical studies, including two phase III studies of patients with advanced illness.[22–25] In the study by Thomas et al.,[24] 133 patients with terminal illness (cancer or other end-stage disease) on opioids for 2 or more weeks with opioid-induced constipation despite the use of laxatives for 3 or more days received methylnaltrexone (at 0.15 mg/kg) or placebo subcutaneously (s.c.) every other day for 2 weeks. Methylnaltrexone was found to be superior (p < 0.0001) to placebo on the primary outcomes of laxation (defecation) within 4 hours after the first dose (48% vs 16%), and laxation within 4 hours after two or more of the first four doses (52% vs 9%). For those who responded to methylnaltrexone, the median time to laxation was 30 min. Methylnaltrexone was well tolerated, with transient abdominal cramping and flatulence being the most common adverse events. Methylnaltrexone for s.c. use has been approved by regulatory agencies in United States, Canada, and the European

Union for the management of opioid-induced constipation in patients with late-stage, advanced illness who are receiving chronic opioid therapy.[26] The usual dosing schedule is one dose every other day, as needed, but no more frequently than one dose in a 24 hours period. The recommended dose of methylnaltrexone is 8 mg for patients weighing 38–62 kg or 12 mg for patients weighing 62–114 kg. Patients whose weight falls outside of these ranges should be dosed at 0.15 mg/kg.

Alvimopan is an orally administered peripherally restricted mu-opioid receptor antagonist approved for short-term use in hospitalized patients for the management of postoperative ileus in patients undergoing bowel resection. It is not approved for management of opioid-induced constipation. While several studies in chronic noncancer pain patients have suggested benefit,[27,28] a recent double-blind, placebo-controlled trial conducted over 12 weeks in 485 patients with noncancer pain found no statistically significant difference in the proportion of patients with spontaneous bowel movements (primary outcome) between the three groups: alvimopan 0.5 mg once daily (63%), alvimopan 0.5 mg twice daily (63%), or placebo (56%, p > 0.05).[29]

Naloxone, a peripherally acting opioid antagonist with low systemic bioavailability (<3%) following oral administration, acts almost exclusively on opioid receptors in the GI tract.[4] Combining opioids with naloxone is emerging as a promising approach for managing opioid-induced constipation. Several studies in the noncancer pain population including three randomized, placebo-controlled phase III trials,[30–35] have demonstrated beneficial effects of combined oxycodone–naloxone tablets as compared to oxycodone alone. In cancer patients, a recent randomized, double-blind, active-controlled, double-dummy, parallel-group study[36] of 185 patients were randomized to receive up to 120mg/day of combined oxycodone–naloxone prn or oxycodone prn alone over 4 weeks. After 4 weeks, the combination group provided superior bowel function (as measured by bowel function index) and 20% lower laxative intake, as compared to oxycodone alone, without compromising analgesic efficacy or safety.

Tegaserod is a promotility agent, which acts as an agonist at serotonin type 4 (5-HT4) receptors in the GI tract. It normalizes impaired motility in the GI tract, inhibits visceral sensitivity, and stimulates intestinal secretion. Tegaserod is approved by the Food and Drug Administration (FDA) for short-term treatment only of constipation-predominant irritable bowel syndrome in patients below 65 years of age. Its use in palliative care patients has not been investigated.

NAUSEA

The exact prevalence of opioid-induced nausea is not known, but estimated to be approximately 25%.[37] Nausea with or without vomiting usually occurs when patients are initiated on opioids for the first time or when the dose is substantially increased. In most patients, this responds well to antiemetic medication and disappears spontaneously within 3 or 4 days.[38] Occasionally, patients experience chronic and severe nausea; this may be more likely in those receiving higher doses of opioids, or when there are other contributing etiologies for nausea.

Opioids cause nausea by a number of mechanisms, including stimulation of the chemoreceptor trigger zone and vomiting center, and increasing the sensitivity of the vestibular center.[39] In addition, opioids reduce GI motility causing gastroparesis and constipation that may also contribute to nausea. Chronic nausea has been associated with accumulation of active morphine metabolites such as morphine-6-glucuronide, which can occur with higher doses of opioids or in the presence of renal insufficiency.[40] Although not as well defined as the other neuronal inputs, the cortex has direct input into the vomiting center through several types of neuroreceptors. A patient may remember unpleasant feelings of nausea associated with past opioid therapy. When presented with the sight, smell, or even anticipation of taking an opioid again, a strong nausea reflex may result.

Assessment and management of opioid-induced nausea

As there are many potential causes of nausea and vomiting in patients receiving palliative care, it is important to search for and treat potential contributing factors in addition to opioid use. It is recommended that antiemetic medication be available to all patients who commence opioid therapy or when there is a significant dose increase. A number of different antiemetic medications can be used to effectively to treat opioid-induced nausea and vomiting in palliative care patients, such as dopamine antagonists metoclopromide and haloperidol.[41–43]

As a prokinetic agent, metoclopramide may also help in symptoms of early satiety and constipation. In cases of persistent or refractory nausea, opioid rotation should be considered. Persistent nausea should always trigger a search for coexisting contributors such as constipation, metabolic alterations (hypercalcemia), other emetogenic therapies, and brain metastasis. For the management of opioid-induced nausea, a recent systematic review concluded that there is limited evidence to prioritize between symptomatic treatment and opioid adjustments (opioid rotation or route change) in cancer patients.[44]

SEDATION

Sedation is common following opioid initiation or significant dose increase and usually resolves after few days. Providing reassurance to the patient/family is usually sufficient. However, in the presence of comorbidities such as dementia, metabolic encephalopathy, brain metastases, or other sedating medications, sedation is more likely to persist. Management should involve treatment of reversible causes of sedation, and discontinuation of other sedating medications. If pain is well controlled, the opioid dose may be reduced. Opioid rotation and/or addition of a psychostimulant may be appropriate if sedation is refractory. Excessive sedation may also be a feature of opioid-induced neurotoxicity, discussed later in greater detail.

Psychostimulants may be helpful in patients who have persistent sedation, and allow for continued use of opioids and even opioid dose increase when sedation is a dose-limiting factor.[45–50] Psychostimulants should not be prescribed in patients with known psychiatric disorders, or if they are exhibiting delirium, hallucinations, or paranoid behaviors. They are also relatively contraindicated with a history of substance abuse or hypertension. The best type and dose of psychostimulant for the treatment of opioid-induced sedation has not been determined. Methylphenidate has been the most extensively studied of the group for this indication and is usually commenced at a dose of 5 mg twice daily. A beneficial effect is usually evident within 2 days of treatment, and the dose can be increased to 10 mg twice daily. Morning and noon administration are recommended in an attempt to minimize potential sleep disturbance. Donepezil, a cholinesterase inhibitor, was found in an open-label study to reduce sedation and fatigue with cancer pain and opioid-induced sedation.[49] A retrospective study of 40 patients receiving opioids (mainly for cancer pain) also found a reduction in sedation with donepezil treatment in majority (73%) patients[50]; however, tolerance to donepezil was reported to occur in approximately 116 patients.

Driving and opioids

Opioids have the potential to interfere with driving ability by impairing psychomotor skills and/or cognitive function. An evidence-based review of driving-related skills in opioid-dependent/tolerant patients concluded that the majority of studies found no evidence of impaired driving-related skills.[51] However, the review grouped three different populations of patients on opioids together: former addicts on maintenance programs, patients with chronic nonmalignant pain, and patients with chronic cancer pain. The majority of studies reviewed were carried out in the former population, and there was some lack of consistency in the findings of studies in cancer patients.

In palliative care populations, the situation is more complicated. The underlying disease as well as other medications and treatments may contribute to the impairment of skills that are considered to be important for driving. A number of studies looking at cognitive function and psychomotor abilities have been carried out in cancer patients receiving opioids.[52–56] In some studies, when compared with healthy controls, cancer patients receiving opioids have been found to have delayed continuous reaction times.[54,56] However, in studies comparing cancer patients receiving stable opioid doses with those not receiving opioids, there appears to be some evidence that both populations are similar in terms of psychomotor and cognitive skills.[52,53] When both these groups were compared to healthy controls, some deficits were found.[52] A study looking at the influence of opioid use, pain, and performance status on neurophysiological function found that both pain and performance status appeared to affect neurophysiological tests; long-term use opioids did not in itself appear to negatively affect these tests.[55] Controlled studies of actual driving ability in cancer patients on opioids have not been carried out. Further research is needed in this area.

In general, cancer patients receiving opioids should be advised that their ability to drive may be compromised and that they should not drive if they feel drowsy or sedated. In addition, patients should be advised to avoid driving for 4–5 days after initiation of opioid medication or after a dose increase. They should also be informed that other medications used to treat symptoms can cause sedation and to check with their physician before driving if in doubt. Advising a patient to do a driving test may be appropriate if there is concern about a patient's driving ability and they are anxious to continue driving.

OPIOID-INDUCED NEUROTOXICITY

Opioid-induced neurotoxicity (OIN) refers to a constellation of neuropsychiatric symptoms such as excessive sedation, cognitive impairment, delirium, hallucinations, myoclonus,

Table 44.4 *Risk factors for opioid induced neurotoxicity*

- Large doses of opioids
- Extended period of treatment with opioids
- Rapid opioid dose escalation
- Dehydration
- Renal failure
- Underlying delirium or dementia
- Infection
- Concomitant use of other psychoactive drugs (e.g. benzodiazepines)
- Older age

seizures, and hyperalgesia.[57–59] In some situations, these symptoms may be indistinguishable from those of disease progression or inadequate analgesic control and lead to further escalation in opioid dose, resulting in a vicious cycle that may further worsen OIN. If any of these symptoms are present in a patient taking opioids, OIN should be suspected. Risk factors for OIN are presented in Table 44.4. Terminally ill patients are especially at risk for OIN due to the high prevalence of cognitive decline due to their disease, use of psychoactive medication, dehydration, and renal and metabolic impairments in these patients. Individual features of OIN are discussed further. These can be present alone or in any combination.

Cognitive impairment and delirium

Impaired cognition and delirium is frequently present in terminally ill patients, is usually progressive, and is a cause of immense distress to patients and families.[60–64] Clinical features of delirium are presented in Table 44.5. Although restlessness and agitation is the most commonly recognized feature of delirium, it is not essential to its diagnosis. The two essential component of delirium diagnosis are disordered attention (arousal) and cognition, in contrast to dementia which does not have alteration in attention or arousal.

Delirium has multiple contributing etiologies such as end-organ failure, dehydration, and the accumulation of toxic opioid metabolites.[60,65,66] Opioid use is a major contributor to delirium in frail terminally ill patients who may have renal

Table 44.5 *Clinical features of delirium*

- Disorientation to time, place or person
- Memory impairment
- Reduced attention, easy distractibility
- Altered arousal
- Increased or decreased psychomotor activity
- Restlessness, anxiety, irritability
- Disturbance of sleep-wake cycle
- Affective symptoms (sadness, anger, emotional lability, euphoria)
- Altered perceptions (misperceptions, delusions, hallucinations)
- Disorganized thinking
- Myoclonus
- Acute onset and fluctuation during the course of the day

failure or impaired fluid intake.[66,67] Nonagitated or hypoactive delirium is often missed by healthcare professionals when no objective testing is performed.[68,69]

Hallucinations

In OIN, hallucinations are typically visual in nature, although tactile hallucinations are not uncommon. Auditory hallucinations may also occur. The overall prevalence of hallucinations in the palliative care setting is unknown. The prevalence of visual hallucinations has been reported as 1%[70] while more recent work has reported the figure to be nearer 50%.[71] Hallucinations are commonly associated with cognitive impairment but are occasionally seen in patients who have not experienced cognitive impairment.[72]

Myoclonus and seizures

Myoclonus is a sudden, shock-like involuntary movement or twitching caused by active muscular contractions, which may involve a whole muscle or may be limited to a small number of muscle fibers.[73] It has been postulated that generalized myoclonus is a type of tonic-clonic seizure.[74] Myoclonus is one of the more frequently observed features of OIN, and if present, there should be a high index of suspicion for the diagnosis. It has been described following administration of most commonly used opioids but is more common with opioids that have active metabolites such as morphine,[75,76] hydromorphone,[77,78] and meperidine.[79,80] However, myoclonus has also been described with fentanyl[74,75] and methadone. It has been proposed that myoclonus results from accumulation of neurotoxic opioid metabolites.[77] Myoclonus may occur more commonly in patients who have impaired renal functions.

Hyperalgesia and allodynia

Abnormally heightened pain sensations can occur with the use of opioids. These are characterized by a lowering of the pain threshold (hyperalgesia) and pain elicited by normally innocuous stimulation (allodynia).[81] Hyperalgesia may present as an exaggerated nociceptive response to a painful stimulus or as a worsening of the underlying pain syndrome, termed paradoxical pain.[82] This paradoxical pain may be misinterpreted by clinicians and the opioid dose increased further, resulting in worsening OIN. Opioid-induced hyperalgesia and allodynia should be suspected when pain increases despite opioid escalation, presence of pain all over, and increased sensitivity to touch. Mechanisms involved include increase in excitatory nonanalgesic opioid metabolites and N-methyl-D-aspartate (NMDA) activation.[81,83]

Mechanism of opioid-induced neurotoxicity

The precise mechanism of OIN is not fully understood, but likely to involve multiple mechanisms. The accumulation of neuro-excitatory opioid metabolites has been postulated to be the main underlying cause of the opioid-induced toxicity. These effects are not mediated via the mu-receptor, and therefore, mu-receptor antagonists are not usually useful unless there is excessive sedation from accumulation of the parent drug. Another important proposed mechanism is CNS sensitization due to opioid activation of the NMDA receptors in the CNS that can initiate an imbalance between the excitatory and inhibitory neurons, resulting in aberrant nerve activity.[84,85]

Morphine, hydromorphone, and fentanyl have all been found to cause agitation, myoclonus, hyperalgesia, and tonic-clonic seizures in animals when administered systemically or intrathecally.[85,86] Morphine followed by hydromorphine have received the most scrutiny. Both are both metabolized to active metabolites that are devoid of analgesic properties, morphine-3-glucuronide (M3G) and hydromorphone-3-glucuronide, (H3G), respectively, have been postulated to be responsible for some of the neuro-excitatory effects.[87,88] These metabolites are usually eliminated by the kidneys and usually do not accumulate to produce toxicity. However, in the presence of renal impairment, or rapidly escalating high doses, these can accumulate and result in manifestations of OIN such as myoclonus, hallucinations, allodynia, and hyperalgesia. However, there is also conflicting reports where M3G failed to produce excitatory and antianalgesic effects in rats.[89] In a phase I study of healthy volunteers, M3G did not elicit any clinical effects when given alone.[90] The possibility of interindividual variation in metabolism of opioids and the impact of renal functioning on metabolite elimination are likely some of the many factors responsible for conflicting findings. Further research is required to gain a better understanding of the pathophysiology of OIN.

Assessment of OIN

Numerous risk factors predispose patients to the development of OIN, which are summarized in Table 44.4 and Figure 44.1. A detailed medication history should include the dose/duration of opioid therapy, the onset of OIN features in relation to opioid initiation or dose increase, the use of psychoactive medications (e.g., benzodiazepines, tricyclic antidepressants) or drugs that may impair renal function. Examination should look for signs of infection, dehydration, and jerking movements should be noted. Cognitive function should be assessed as a matter of routine. It is important to enquire specifically about hallucinations. A number of tools exist to assess cognitive function.[62] Although no gold standard tool has been identified, the mini-mental state examination[91] has been widely used in this population.[92] Other tools include the memorial delirium assessment scale (MDAS)[93] and the delirium rating scale (DRS).[94] Delirium assessment is covered in more detail in Chapter 70. If OIN is suspected and appropriate for the clinical circumstance, blood should be sent for biochemical and hematological analysis to exclude for infection, renal failure, or hypercalcemia.

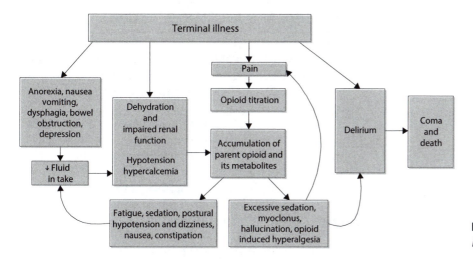

Figure 44.1 *Potential contributors for opioid-induced neurotoxicity/delirium in terminal illness.*

Management of OIN

OIN is frequently managed by correction of identifiable and reversible factors contributing to OIN, hydration, opioid rotation, and symptomatic medications directed toward controlling patient distress (Table 44.6).

Dose reduction or discontinuation of opioids may usually not be an option for management of OIN due to the presence of uncontrolled pain or dyspnea. Opioid rotation, the term used for substituting one opioid for another, is usually preferred and allows for the reduction of neurotoxicity symptoms while simultaneously retaining or improving analgesia.[1,58,60,91,92] However, opioid rotation has not been systematically studied in randomized controlled trials, and this evidence is mainly from observational or uncontrolled trials.[93]

For the management of specific OIN symptoms, haloperidol is considered first-line therapy for patients who have agitated delirium because of its efficacy and low incidence of cardiovascular and anticholinergic side effects. Chlorpromazine can be used if sedation is required, although hypotension may be a concern. Benzodiazepines are best reserved for refractory situations, as in some patients, it may paradoxically worsen delirium.

Preliminary studies conducted in advanced cancer suggest that hydration intervention may help in delirium prevention, or

Table 44.6 *Key approaches to management of opioid induced neurotoxicity*

- Maintaining adequate hydration (oral or parenteral)
- Treat reversible causes as clinically appropriate for the setting (such as antibiotics for infection, bisphosphonates for hypercalcemia)
- Opioid rotation. Opioid reduction may be considered if patient reports no pain.
- Use of adjuvant analgesics (e.g. NSAIDs or anticonvulsants) if appropriate
- Discontinuation of psychoactive or sedating medications.
- Symptomatic treatment (e.g. haloperidol for hallucinations or agitation)
- Reassurance and explanation

its reversal when delirium is attributed to dehydration or opioid toxicities.[94-96] By switching opioids and providing hydration, the parent opioid and its toxic metabolites are allowed to be excreted. Once OIN has been recognized and treated, steps must be taken to reduce the risk of further episodes.

RESPIRATORY DEPRESSION

Respiratory depression is a potentially fatal side effect of opioids. It primarily occurs in opioid-naïve patients who are administered high doses of opioid. Fortunately, tolerance to respiratory depressing opioid effects develops within days of opioid use, and is extremely rare in patients on chronic opioids. Majority of studies have been conducted in the postoperative setting, where the incidence of clinically recognized and relevant respiratory depression is about 1%–2% in postoperative patients receiving opioids.[97-99] However, close monitoring in patients who are at high risk of respiratory depression is advised such as patients with morbid obesity, sleep apnea, advanced age, and those with multiple comorbidities.[100] In rare circumstances, respiratory depression has been observed in opioid-tolerant patients such as when there is sudden reduction of opioid requirements following a successful neurolytic block resulting in reduced pain,[101] or following opioid rotation to methadone where the equianalgesic conversion ratio may not be certain,[102] or in the presence of renal failure due to the buildup of morphine metabolites.[103] Therefore, it is important to reevaluate opioid dosing requirements in the palliative care patient where any of these scenarios may occur.

The management of respiratory depression involves reducing or omitting the next regular opioid dose, or stopping an infusion temporarily, to allow plasma levels to reduce with a plan to recommence the infusion at a lower dose. Naloxone, a nonselective competitive opioid antagonist,[104] should be administered in patients with symptomatic respiratory depression in a diluted solution, and in small increments to avoid symptoms of opioid withdrawal. It is administered parenterally due to its low bioavailability with oral administration. Opioid-induced sedation in the absence of respiratory

Table 44.7 *Management of opioid-induced respiratory depression*

Management of opioid-induced respiratory depression
1. Discontinue opioid (E.g. stop opioid infusion if ongoing)
2. Provide supplemental oxygen
3. Dilute 1 ml ampoule of naloxone (E.g. 0.4 mg/ml) with 9 ml of saline.*
4. Give 0.5–1 ml of above diluted mixture either IV or SC and repeat**every 1–2 minutes until the respiratory rate increases to above 8-10/minute
5. The aim is for partial opioid reversal but not a complete reversal
6. Additional small amounts can be given at appropriate intervals to maintain an adequate respiratory rate
7. If no change with naloxone, there may be other causes for respiratory depression

*Giving the complete ampoule will result in an acute withdrawal from the opioid and cause immediate reversal of analgesia.
**Repeat doses are required due to the short half-live of naloxone.

depression is not an indication for using naloxone. Naloxone in these patients can result in opioid withdrawal syndrome and severe pain.[105] Naloxone is indicated only if there is significant respiratory depression, that is, a respiratory rate of less than 8 breaths/min, and if the patient is barely arousable and/or cyanosed. Table 44.7 summarizes the use of naloxone in opioid-induced respiratory depression. Naloxone has a shorter half-life than most opioids; therefore, it is important to observe patients carefully over a period of hours. Additional administration of naloxone may be required if the respiratory rate falls or clinical status changes. One must take care to distinguish opioid-induced respiratory depression from respiratory changes at the very end of life, which are to be expected and need no intervention. Research into new treatments/and or approaches to prevent opioid respiratory depression without affecting analgesia are ongoing with agents such as serotinine agonists, ampakines, and the antibiotic minocycline.[100]

OPIOID-INDUCED BLADDER DYSFUNCTION

Opioid-induced bladder dysfunction (difficulty voiding or urinary retention) is recognized as a side effect of opioid therapy but has not been well researched in the palliative care setting. Two studies conducted in the postoperative setting reported prevalence estimates of approximately 4% for urinary retention requiring catheterization, and 18% of urinary retention.[106,107] The mechanism of urinary retention is still not completely understood but is likely due to opioid-induced decreased detrusor muscle tone and force of contraction, decreased sensation of bladder fullness and urge to void, and inhibition of the voiding reflex. These effects likely involve both central and peripheral opioid effects,[108–110] and shown to be reversed by naloxone.[111] A more recent study demonstrated reversal of opioid-induced bladder changes by the peripherally restricted opioid antagonist methylnaltrexone.[112]

PRURITUS AND ALLERGIC REACTIONS

Hypersensitivity reactions to opioids are rare. Patients may report being "allergic" to opioids, and it is important to distinguish between "true" immune-mediated reactions (rare) and reactions that mimic an immune allergic response (nonallergic or pseudoallergy). Patients often consider side effects (e.g., nausea, sedation) to be an allergy; hence, it is important to check what problems a specific opioid has caused for an individual patient.

The prevalence, severity, and pathophysiology of opioid-induced pruritus depend on the type of opioid, dosage, and route of administration. Pruritus (itching) occurs in 2%–10% of patients treated with systemic opioids, is usually mild, and self-limited. The frequency of pruritus increases with increasing opioid dosages.[113] The likely mechanism involves direct mast cell degranulation, with histamine release causing local itching and a typical weal and flare response. While all opioids may cause direct histamine release, morphine, codeine, and meperidine are more potent offenders than others. Histamine release also may be associated with vasodilation, which is more common in volume depleted patients. This is not a contraindication to opioid use, and an alternative opioid may be well tolerated. Antihistaminics may be added for use on as needed basis.

Neuroaxially administered opioids, especially morphine, have higher pruritus risk, and appears not to be mediated via histamine, but via mu-opioid receptors.[114–118] Pruritus invoked by intrathecal morphine is of longer duration and is difficult to treat.[119] Treatment options remain a challenge, and much of the research has emerged from surgical patients who received neuro-axial opioids, and have looked at agents as prophylaxis rather than treatment.[116] Naloxone and naltrexone, both mu-opioid receptor antagonists, have demonstrated anti-pruritic effects, but their usage is limited by decreased analgesic effects.[119–121] Nalbuphine, a mixed opioid-receptor agonist-antagonist, was shown to be effective without compromising analgesia, but its usage is limited due to its sedating effects.[122–124] Serotonin (5-HT3) receptor antagonists (ondasetron, dolasetron) have demonstrated mixed results with respect to their effectiveness in pruritus management, with some studies suggesting benefit,[125–128] and others that do not.[129–131] Dopamine D2-receptor agonists, droperidol and alizapride, have demonstrated some benefit in the management of pruritus prophylaxis.[132,133]

Type 1 hypersensitivity reactions are IgE mediated, resulting in the immediate systemic release of potent mediators that result in hypotension, bronchospasm, angiodema, hives, and vascular collapse. Fortunately, these events are extremely rare with opioid use. Emergent management with epinephrine, steroids, and histamine blockers is instituted. Patients with prior IgE-mediated allergic reaction should not be re-challenged with the offending opioid. For both these immune-mediated reactions, an allergist may be consulted to identify appropriate alternatives. Opioids from an alternative chemical class may also be considered.

OPIOID–INDUCED ENDOCRINE AND IMMUNE EFFECTS

Evidence is emerging that opioids have potential effects on the functioning of endocrine and immune systems. The most commonly reported effects are suppression of gonadal function and immune suppression.

Opioid effects on Gonadal Hormones and Sexual Function: A growing number of studies conducted in the settings of opioid addiction (e.g., heroin abuse), opioid addiction treatment (such as methadone maintenance programs), and the use of opioids for the management of chronic noncancer pain have demonstrated that opioids suppress gonadal hormone secretion in men and women.[134–145] Potential symptoms of opioid-induced hypogonadism include loss of libido, infertility, fatigue, depression, anxiety, loss of muscle strength/mass, osteoporosis, and compression fractures, in both men and women; impotence in men; and menstrual irregularities and galactorrhea in women.

Several of these studies suggest that the effect of opioids is rapid, dose dependent, and reversible on discontinuation of opioids. In the study by Mendleson et al., total testosterone levels declined within 7–9 hours of single oral dose of 30–80 mg of methadone, suggesting a rapid decline in testosterone levels within hours of opioid ingestion.[137] Among subjects with heroin abuse, one study demonstrated normalization of testosterone levels 1 month after cessation of heroin use.[139] Another study showed a dose–response effect, in that subjects on lower doses of methadone (10–60 mg/day) had no evidence of testosterone level suppression, whereas patients on higher doses (80–150 mg/day) did.[137] One case series described amenorrhea and galactorrhea in female heroin addicts.[140]

In men with nonmalignant chronic pain, a case controlled observational study found chronic opioid therapy to be associated with a dose-dependent decline in total testosterone levels in 74% of opioid users.[145] In this study, of the men who reported normal erectile function before opioid use, 87% of men who reported normal erectile function prior to opioid initiation reported either severe erectile dysfunction or diminished libido after starting opioids.

In women with nonmalignant pain treated with sustained-action oral or transdermal opioids,[146] low levels of FSH and LH, estradiol, and adrenal androgens (testosterone and dehydroepiandrosterone sulfate [DHEAS]) production has been demonstrated.

A recent prospective study conducted in men and women attending a pain clinic for chronic nonmalignant pain demonstrated males to have lower free testosterone (FT) and prolactin levels in opioid users, and in women lower FT. In both groups, there was no relationship between symptoms of sexual dysfunction and abnormal hormone levels or opioid use.[147]

A single preliminary study conducted in men with opioid addiction has suggested that burprenorphine may not have the same gonadal suppressive effects as methadone.[141] In this study, those treated with buprenorphine (n = 17) had significantly higher testosterone and a significantly lower frequency of sexual dysfunction compared with patients treated with

methadone (n = 37), and did not differ from healthy controls (n = 51).

There are no prospective studies that have evaluated the effects of opioids on gonadal hormones or sexual functions in the palliative care patients. Among male cancer survivors without evidence of disease, and on opioids for chronic pain, a cross-sectional study (n = 20) demonstrated abnormally low testosterone levels.[148] In a follow-up case control study, 18 (90%) of 20 patients who were taking more than 200 mg of morphine daily or equivalent opioids for chronic pain exhibited abnormally low testosterone levels, compared with 40% in the matched control group (n = 20).[149] Median testosterone and luteinizing hormone levels were significantly lower in the opioid group and were associated with sexual dysfunction, anxiety, depression, and overall decreased QoL.

Among patients with advanced cancer, a retrospective chart review demonstrated that chronic use of even lower doses of opioids (morphine 30 mg or more) was associated with low testosterone levels in men.[150] Prospective studies are needed to better characterize the effect of opioids on gonadal hormones and sexual function in cancer patients.

Opioid effects on immune function

In animal experiments and opioid addicts, chronic opioid use has been shown to induce immune suppression and increase the rate of infection.[151] In vitro studies demonstrate alterations in several immune parameters, induced by the direct effects of morphine and other opioids on immune cells. These include impaired chemotaxis, phagocytosis and intracellular killing of neutrophils and monocytes, reduced effector cell responses in B and T cells, as well as increased apoptosis in lymphocytes and phagocytic cells. Currently, the mechanisms that modulate these changes are not well understood. It has been suggested that opioid interaction with opioid receptors in the CNS and endocrine axis (HPA and sympathetic nervous system), as well as its direct interaction with opioid receptors on immune cells are likely involved. The immunomodulatory effects of morphine are attenuated significantly in mu-opioid receptor knockout mice.

Current evidence suggests that not all opioids have the same immunological effects.[152] For instance, tramadol and buprenorphine do not appear to share the immunosuppressive effects demonstrated by morphine and fentanyl. Tramadol rather has been shown to have an immune-enhancing effect on several immune parameters such as NK cell activity, lymphoproliferation, and cytokine production when administered to healthy animals.[153] When tramadol was compared to morphine in experimental models of neuropathic pain[154] and surgical-induced suppression of NK activity,[155] tramadol preserve NK cell activity, while morphine suppressed it. In rat experiments, morphine but not buprenorphine has been shown to suppress NK cell activity, and T-cell and macrophage function.[156,157] In a model of surgery stress, buprenorphine was able to prevent all the biochemical and immune alterations usually associated with pain.[158] In another experiment, fentanyl, but not buprenorphine, was shown to suppress NK activity, lymphoproliferation, and cytokine production.[159]

Several studies conducted in tumor experimental models suggest opioids such as morphine and fentanyl influence tumor spread by their effects on immune function, while these have not been shown with tramadol and buprenorphine.[152] Fentanyl, for instance, at doses shown to suppress NK cell activity, was shown to increase metastatic disease in MADB106 mammary adenocarcinoma tumor model.[160] These effects were more pronounced when surgery was also performed, suggesting an additive effect on immunosuppression.[158,160] In contrast, tramadol and buprenorphine were not associated with these effects. The relevance of these findings in the palliative care population is unclear, and further research is warranted in this area.

Physiological and psychological responses to opioid use

Tolerance and physical dependence are expected physiological responses to chronic opioid use. *Tolerance* is characterized by decreasing opioid analgesic effects, requiring increased opioid doses to achieve the same degree of pain relief. In terminally ill patients, it may not be possible to know whether development of tolerance, disease progression, or both is contributing to higher opioid requirement. Tolerance also develops to several opioid side effects including nausea and respiratory depression, but not to constipation. *Physical dependence* manifests as development of withdrawal symptoms on abrupt opioid cessation, such as increased pain, agitation, insomnia, diarrhea, sweating, and palpitations. Physical dependence is frequently and incorrectly thought of as addiction. Withdrawal symptoms can be prevented by gradually tapering opioids.

In contrast to the aforementioned physiological responses, addiction and pseudo-addiction are psychological and behavioral responses toward opioids that patients may or may not develop. *Addiction* is compulsive use of drugs for nonmedical reasons, characterized by a craving for mood-altering drug effects, not pain relief. Suggestive aberrant behaviors include forgery of prescriptions, denial of drug use, stealing opioids from others, selling/buying opioids on the street, and using prescribed drugs to get "high." Addiction is uncommon in the chronic pain, and postoperative and cancer pain settings,[161-163] and opioids should not be withheld for fear that a patient will become addicted. If terminally ill patients request a strong analgesic, it is likely they have inadequate pain control. *Pseudo-addiction* is an "iatrogenic" phenomena resulting from inadequate pain management by clinicians. Patient's behavior is geared toward obtaining pain relief, such as requesting stronger pain medications, asking several providers for opioids, and frequently visiting the emergency center for pain relief. The clinician's response should always be to reassess the pain, reassure the patient, and treat pain adequately.

Opioids are potential drugs of addiction. Psychological dependence is a key feature of addiction and involves compulsive behavior to obtain and take a drug for its psychological effects. Hence, psychological dependence involves substance misuse or abuse. Fear of addiction is common in patients and physicians and can lead to underuse of opioids in palliative care populations. Opiophobia should not prevent opioids being prescribed where they are needed. In clinical practice, psychological dependence and opioid abuse are rare in patients who do not have a preexisting history of drug or alcohol abuse.[162,164] Physical dependence is often confused with psychological dependence. However, physical dependence (the appearance of withdrawal symptoms and signs when a drug is abruptly discontinued) is common when patients have been taking opioids for a period of time; this does not mean that a patient is addicted to an opioid. Abrupt discontinuation or dramatic reductions in opioid doses should be avoided. If a major dose reduction or discontinuation is desired, doses should be gradually reduced over several days. The management of pain in patients with drug and alcohol dependence is discussed in detail in Chapter 55.

REFERENCES

1   Cherny N, Ripamonti C, Pereira J et al. Strategies to manage the adverse effects of oral morphine: An evidence-based report. *J Clin Oncol* 19:2542–2554, 2001.
2   Manara L, Bianchi G, Ferretti P et al. Inhibition of gastrointestinal transit by morphine in rats results primarily from direct drug action on gut opioid sites. *J Pharmacol Exp Ther* 237:945–949, 1986.
3   Kurz A, Sessler DI. Opioid-induced bowel dysfunction: Pathophysiology and potential new therapies. *Drugs* 63:649–671, 2003.
4   De Schepper HU, Cremonini F, Park MI et al. Opioids and the gut: Pharmacology and current clinical experience. *Neurogastroenterol Motil* 16:383–394, 2004.
5   Bagnol D, Mansour A, Akil H et al. Cellular localization and distribution of the cloned mu and kappa opioid receptors in rat gastrointestinal tract. *Neuroscience* 81:579–591, 1997.
6   McKay JS, Linaker BD, Turnberg LA. Influence of opiates on ion transport across rabbit ileal mucosa. *Gastroenterology* 80:279–284, 1981.
7   De Luca A, Coupar IM. Insights into opioid action in the intestinal tract. *Pharmacol Ther* 69:103–115, 1996.
8   Pappagallo M. Incidence, prevalence, and management of opioid bowel dysfunction. *Am J Surg* 182:11S–18S, 2001.
9   Mancini I, Bruera E. Constipation in advanced cancer patients. *Support Care Cancer* 6:356–364, 1998.
10 Sykes NP. The relationship between opioid use and laxative use in terminally ill cancer patients. *Palliat Med* 12:375–382, 1998.
11 Bruera E, Suarez-Almazor M, Velasco A et al. The assessment of constipation in terminal cancer patients admitted to a palliative care unit: A retrospective review. *J Pain Symptom Manage* 9:515–519, 1994.
12 Starreveld JS, Pols MA, Van Wijk HJ et al. The plain abdominal radiograph in the assessment of constipation. *Z Gastroenterol* 28:335–338, 1990.
13 Slappendel R, Simpson K, Dubois D et al. Validation of the PAC-SYM questionnaire for opioid-induced constipation in patients with chronic low back pain. *Eur J Pain* 10:209–217, 2006.
14 Marquis P, De La Loge C, Dubois D et al. Development and validation of the Patient Assessment of Constipation Quality of Life questionnaire. *Scand J Gastroenterol* 40:540–551, 2005.
15 Bennett M, Cresswell H. Factors influencing constipation in advanced cancer patients: A prospective study of opioid dose, dantron dose and physical functioning. *Palliat Med* 17:418–422, 2003.

16 Staats PS, Markowitz J, Schein J. Incidence of constipation associated with long-acting opioid therapy: A comparative study. *South Med J* 97:129–134, 2004.

17 Allan L, Hays H, Jensen NH et al. Randomised crossover trial of transdermal fentanyl and sustained release oral morphine for treating chronic non-cancer pain. *BMJ* 322:1154–1158, 2001.

18 Mancini IL, Hanson J, Neumann CM et al. Opioid type and other clinical predictors of laxative dose in advanced cancer patients: A retrospective study. *J Palliat Med* 3:49–56, 2000.

19 Candiotti KA, Gitlin MC. Review of the effect of opioid-related side effects on the undertreatment of moderate to severe chronic non-cancer pain: Tapentadol, a step toward a solution? *Curr Med Res Opin* 26:1677–1684, 2010.

20 Afilalo M, Etropolski MS, Kuperwasser B et al. Efficacy and safety of Tapentadol extended release compared with oxycodone controlled release for the management of moderate to severe chronic pain related to osteoarthritis of the knee: A randomized, double-blind, placebo- and active-controlled phase III study. *Clin Drug Investig* 30:489–505, 2010.

21 Buynak R, Shapiro DY, Okamoto A et al. Efficacy and safety of tapentadol extended release for the management of chronic low back pain: Results of a prospective, randomized, double-blind, placebo- and active-controlled Phase III study. *Expert Opin Pharmacother* 11:1787–1804, 2010.

22 Yuan CS, Israel RJ. Methylnaltrexone, a novel peripheral opioid receptor antagonist for the treatment of opioid side effects. *Expert Opin Investig Drugs* 15:541–552, 2006.

23 Reichle FM, Conzen PF. Methylnaltrexone, a new peripheral mu-receptor antagonist for the prevention and treatment of opioid-induced extracerebral side effects. *Curr Opin Investig Drugs* 9:90–100, 2008.

24 Thomas J, Karver S, Cooney GA et al. Methylnaltrexone for opioid-induced constipation in advanced illness. *N Engl J Med* 358:2332–2343, 2008.

25 Slatkin N, Thomas J, Lipman AG, et al. Methylnaltrexone for treatment of opioid-induced constipation in advanced illness patients. *J Support Oncol* 7:39–46, 2009.

26 Lang L. The Food and Drug Administration approves methylnaltrexone bromide for opioid-induced constipation. *Gastroenterology* 135:6, 2008.

27 Paulson DM, Kennedy DT, Donovick RA et al. Alvimopan: An oral, peripherally acting, mu-opioid receptor antagonist for the treatment of opioid-induced bowel dysfunction—A 21-day treatment-randomized clinical trial. *J Pain* 6:184–192, 2005.

28 Webster L, Jansen JP, Peppin J et al. Alvimopan, a peripherally acting mu-opioid receptor (PAM-OR) antagonist for the treatment of opioid-induced bowel dysfunction: Results from a randomized, double-blind, placebo-controlled, dose-finding study in subjects taking opioids for chronic non-cancer pain. *Pain* 137:428–440, 2008.

29 Irving G, Penzes J, Ramjattan B et al. A randomized, placebo-controlled phase 3 trial (Study SB-767905/013) of alvimopan for opioid-induced bowel dysfunction in patients with non-cancer pain. *J Pain* 12:175–184, 2011.

30 Vondrackova D, Leyendecker P, Meissner W et al. Analgesic efficacy and safety of oxycodone in combination with naloxone as prolonged release tablets in patients with moderate to severe chronic pain. *J Pain* 9:1144–1154, 2008.

31 Simpson K, Leyendecker P, Hopp M et al. Fixed-ratio combination oxycodone/naloxone compared with oxycodone alone for the relief of opioid-induced constipation in moderate-to-severe noncancer pain. *Curr Med Res Opin* 24:3503–3512, 2008.

32 Lowenstein O, Leyendecker P, Hopp M et al. Combined prolonged-release oxycodone and naloxone improves bowel function in patients receiving opioids for moderate-to-severe non-malignant chronic pain: A randomised controlled trial. *Expert Opin Pharmacother* 10:531–543, 2009.

33 Lowenstein O, Leyendecker P, Lux EA et al. Efficacy and safety of combined prolonged-release oxycodone and naloxone in the management of moderate/severe chronic non-malignant pain: Results of a prospectively designed pooled analysis of two randomised, double-blind clinical trials. *BMC Clin Pharmacol* 10:12, 2010.

34 Sandner-Kiesling A, Leyendecker P, Hopp M et al. Long-term efficacy and safety of combined prolonged-release oxycodone and naloxone in the management of non-cancer chronic pain. *Int J Clin Pract* 64:763–774, 2010.

35 Schutter U, Grunert S, Meyer C et al. Innovative pain therapy with a fixed combination of prolonged-release oxycodone/naloxone: A large observational study under conditions of daily practice. *Curr Med Res Opin* 26:1377–1387, 2010.

36 Ahmedzai SH, Nauck F, Bar-Sela G et al. A randomized, double-blind, active-controlled, double-dummy, parallel-group study to determine the safety and efficacy of oxycodone/naloxone prolonged-release tablets in patients with moderate/severe, chronic cancer pain. *Palliat Med* 26:50–60, 2012.

37 McNicol E, Horowicz-Mehler N, Fisk RA et al. Management of opioid side effects in cancer-related and chronic noncancer pain: A systematic review. *J Pain* 4:231–256, 2003.

38 Clarke RS. Nausea and vomiting. *Br J Anaesth* 56:19–27, 1984.

39 Carpenter DO, Briggs DB, Strominger N. Peptide-induced emesis in dogs. *Behav Brain Res* 11:277–281, 1984.

40 Hagen NA, Foley KM, Cerbone DJ et al. Chronic nausea and morphine-6-glucuronide. *J Pain Symptom Manage* 6:125–128, 1991.

41 Bruera E, Seifert L, Watanabe S et al. Chronic nausea in advanced cancer patients: A retrospective assessment of a metoclopramide-based antiemetic regimen. *J Pain Symptom Manage* 11:147–153, 1996.

42 Bruera E, Belzile M, Neumann C et al. A double-blind, crossover study of controlled-release metoclopramide and placebo for the chronic nausea and dyspepsia of advanced cancer. *J Pain Symptom Manage* 19:427–435, 2000.

43 Vella-Brincat J, Macleod AD. Haloperidol in palliative care. *Palliat Med* 18:195–201, 2004.

44 Laugsand EA, Kaasa S, Klepstad P. Management of opioid-induced nausea and vomiting in cancer patients: Systematic review and evidence-based recommendations. *Palliat Med* 25:442–453, 2011.

45 Bruera E, Chadwick S, Brenneis C et al. Methylphenidate associated with narcotics for the treatment of cancer pain. *Cancer Treat Rep* 71:67–70, 1987.

46 Vigano A, Watanabe S, Bruera E. Methylphenidate for the management of somatization in terminal cancer patients. *J Pain Symptom Manage* 10:167–170, 1995.

47 Rozans M, Dreisbach A, Lertora JJ et al. Palliative uses of methylphenidate in patients with cancer: A review. *J Clin Oncol* 20:335–339, 2002.

48 Bruera E, Miller MJ, Macmillan K et al. Neuropsychological effects of methylphenidate in patients receiving a continuous infusion of narcotics for cancer pain. *Pain* 48:163–166, 1992.

49 Bruera E, Strasser F, Shen L et al. The effect of donepezil on sedation and other symptoms in patients receiving opioids for cancer pain: A pilot study. *J Pain Symptom Manage* 26:1049–1054, 2003.

50 Slatkin NE, Rhiner M. Treatment of opiate-related sedation: Utility of the cholinesterase inhibitors. *J Support Oncol* 1:53–63, 2003.

51 Fishbain DA, Cutler RB, Rosomoff HL et al. Are opioid-dependent/tolerant patients impaired in driving-related skills? A structured evidence-based review. *J Pain Symptom Manage* 25:559–577, 2003.

52 Clemons M, Regnard C, Appleton T. Alertness, cognition and morphine in patients with advanced cancer. *Cancer Treat Rev* 22:451–468, 1996.

53 Vainio A, Ollila J, Matikainen E et al. Driving ability in cancer patients receiving long-term morphine analgesia. *Lancet* 346:667–670, 1995.

54 Sjogren P, Banning A. Pain, sedation and reaction time during long-term treatment of cancer patients with oral and epidural opioids. *Pain* 39:5–11, 1989.

55 Sjogren P, Olsen AK, Thomsen AB et al. Neuropsychological performance in cancer patients: The role of oral opioids, pain and performance status. *Pain* 86:237–245, 2000.

56 Banning A, Sjogren P. Cerebral effects of long-term oral opioids in cancer patients measured by continuous reaction time. *Clin J Pain* 6:91–95, 1990.

57 Bruera E, Neumann CM. Management of specific symptom complexes in patients receiving palliative care. *CMAJ* 158:1717–1726, 1998.

58 Mercadante S. Opioid rotation for cancer pain: Rationale and clinical aspects. *Cancer* 86:1856–1866, 1999.

59 Walsh D, Donnelly S, Rybicki L. The symptoms of advanced cancer: Relationship to age, gender, and performance status in 1,000 patients. *Support Care Cancer* 8:175–179, 2000.

60 Lawlor PG, Gagnon B, Mancini IL et al. Occurrence, causes, and outcome of delirium in patients with advanced cancer: A prospective study. *Arch Intern Med* 160:786–794, 2000.

61 Breitbart W, Gibson C, Tremblay A. The delirium experience: Delirium recall and delirium-related distress in hospitalized patients with cancer, their spouses/caregivers, and their nurses. *Psychosomatics* 43:183–194, 2002.

62 Namba M, Morita T, Imura C et al. Terminal delirium: Families' experience. *Palliat Med* 21:587–594, 2007.

63 Morita T, Hirai K, Sakaguchi Y et al. Family-perceived distress from delirium-related symptoms of terminally ill cancer patients. *Psychosomatics* 45:107–113, 2004.

64 Bruera E, Bush SH, Willey J et al. Impact of delirium and recall on the level of distress in patients with advanced cancer and their family caregivers. *Cancer* 115:2004–2012, 2009.

65 Morita T, Tei Y, Tsunoda J et al. Increased plasma morphine metabolites in terminally ill cancer patients with delirium: An intra-individual comparison. *J Pain Symptom Manage* 23:107–113, 2002.

66 Lawlor PG. The panorama of opioid-related cognitive dysfunction in patients with cancer: A critical literature appraisal. *Cancer* 94:1836–1853, 2002.

67 Leipzig RM, Goodman H, Gray G et al. Reversible, narcotic-associated mental status impairment in patients with metastatic cancer. *Pharmacology* 35:47–54, 1987.

68 Bruera E, Miller L, McCallion J et al. Cognitive failure in patients with terminal cancer: A prospective study. *J Pain Symptom Manage* 7:192–195, 1992.

69 Farrell KR, Ganzini L. Misdiagnosing delirium as depression in medically ill elderly patients. *Arch Intern Med* 155:2459–2464, 1995.

70 Regnard CL, Tempest S. *Managing Opioid Adverse Effects. A Guide to Symptom Relief in Advanced Disease*, 4th Edn. Hochland & Hochland, Hale; p. 21, 1998.

71 Fountain A. Visual hallucinations: A prevalence study among hospice inpatients. *Palliat Med* 15:19–25, 2001.

72 Bruera E, Schoeller T, Montejo G. Organic hallucinosis in patients receiving high doses of opiates for cancer pain. *Pain* 48:397–399, 1992.

73 Pereira J, E. B. Emerging neuropsychiatric toxicities of opioids. *J Pharm Care Pain Symptom Control* 5:3–29, 1997.

74 Marsden CD, Hallet M, S. F. The nosology and patho-physiology of myoclonus. *Movement Disorders*: pp. 196–248, 1982.

75 Marsden CD, Hallet M, S. Fahn. The nosology and pathophysiology of myoclonus. In Movement Disorders, ed. C.D Marsden, and S. Fahn; London: Butterworths: pp. 196–248, 1982.

76 Sjogren P, Dragsted L, Christensen CB. Myoclonic spasms during treatment with high doses of intravenous morphine in renal failure. *Acta Anaesthesiol Scand* 37:780–782, 1993.

77 MacDonald N, Der L, Allan S et al. Opioid hyperexcitability: The application of alternate opioid therapy. *Pain* 53:353–355, 1993.

78 Babul N, Darke AC. Putative role of hydromorphone metabolites in myoclonus. *Pain* 51:260–261, 1992.

79 Kaiko RF, Foley KM, Grabinski PY et al. Central nervous system excitatory effects of meperidine in cancer patients. *Ann Neurol* 13:180–185, 1983.

80 Danziger LH, Martin SJ, Blum RA. Central nervous system toxicity associated with meperidine use in hepatic disease. *Pharmacotherapy* 14:235–238, 1994.

81 Mercadante S, Ferrera P, Villari P et al. Hyperalgesia: An emerging iatrogenic syndrome. *J Pain Symptom Manage* 26:769–775, 2003.

82 Stillman MJ, Mouline DE, Foley K. Paradoxical pain following high-dose spinal morphine. *Pain* 4(Suppl):S389, 1987.

83 Bowsher D. Paradoxical pain. *BMJ* 306:473–474, 1993.

84 Yaksh TL, Harty GJ. Pharmacology of the allodynia in rats evoked by high dose intrathecal morphine. *J Pharmacol Exp Ther* 244:501–507, 1988.

85 Mao J, Price DD, Mayer DJ. Thermal hyperalgesia in association with the development of morphine tolerance in rats: Roles of excitatory amino acid receptors and protein kinase C. *J Neurosci* 14:2301–2312, 1994.

86 Shohami E, Evron S. Intrathecal morphine induces myoclonic seizures in the rat. *Acta Pharmacol Toxicol (Copenh)* 56:50–54, 1985.

87 Hanna MH, Peat SJ, Woodham M et al. Analgesic efficacy and CSF pharmacokinetics of intrathecal morphine-6-glucuronide: Comparison with morphine. *Br J Anaesth* 64:547–550, 1990.

88 Smith MT. Neuroexcitatory effects of morphine and hydromorphone: Evidence implicating the 3-glucuronide metabolites. *Clin Exp Pharmacol Physiol* 27:524–528, 2000.

89 Gong QL, Hedner J, Bjorkman R et al. Morphine-3-glucuronide may functionally antagonize morphine-6-glucuronide induced antinociception and ventilatory depression in the rat. *Pain* 48:249–255, 1992.

90 Penson RT, Joel SP, Bakhshi K et al. Randomized placebo-controlled trial of the activity of the morphine glucuronides. *Clin Pharmacol Ther* 68:667–676, 2000.

91 Bruera E, Pereira J, Watanabe S et al. Opioid rotation in patients with cancer pain. A retrospective comparison of dose ratios between methadone, hydromorphone, and morphine. *Cancer* 78:852–857, 1996.

92 Mercadante S, Casuccio A, Fulfaro F et al. Switching from morphine to methadone to improve analgesia and tolerability in cancer patients: A prospective study. *J Clin Oncol* 19:2898–2904, 2001.

93 Quigley C. Opioid switching to improve pain relief and drug tolerability. *Cochrane Database Syst Rev* CD004847, 2004.

94 Gagnon P, Allard P, Masse B et al. Delirium in terminal cancer: A prospective study using daily screening, early diagnosis, and continuous monitoring. *J Pain Symptom Manage* 19:412–426, 2000.

95 Maddocks I, Somogyi A, Abbott F et al. Attenuation of morphine-induced delirium in palliative care by substitution with infusion of oxycodone. *J Pain Symptom Manage* 12:182–189, 1996.

96 Tuma R, DeAngelis LM. Altered mental status in patients with cancer. *Arch Neurol* 57:1727–1731, 2000.

97 Hanna MH, Elliott KM, Fung M. Randomized, double-blind study of the analgesic efficacy of morphine-6-glucuronide versus morphine sulfate for postoperative pain in major surgery. *Anesthesiology* 102:815–821, 2005.

98 Cashman JN, Dolin SJ. Respiratory and haemodynamic effects of acute postoperative pain management: Evidence from published data. *Br J Anaesth* 93:212–223, 2004.

99 Shapiro A, Zohar E, Zaslansky R et al. The frequency and timing of respiratory depression in 1524 postoperative patients treated with systemic or neuraxial morphine. *J Clin Anesth* 17:537–542, 2005.

100 Dahan A, Aarts L, Smith TW. Incidence, reversal, and prevention of opioid-induced respiratory depression. *Anesthesiology* 112:226–238, 2010.

101 Hanks GW, Twycross RG, Lloyd JW. Unexpected complication of successful nerve block. Morphine induced respiratory depression precipitated by removal of severe pain. *Anaesthesia* 36:37–39, 1981.

102 Hunt G, Bruera E. Respiratory depression in a patient receiving oral methadone for cancer pain. *J Pain Symptom Manage* 10:401–404, 1995.

103 Osborne R, Joel S, Slevin M. Morphine intoxication in renal failure; the role of morphine-6-glucuronide. *Br Med J (Clin Res Ed)* 293:1101, 1986.

104 Kaufman RD, Gabathuler ML, Bellville JW. Potency, duration of action and pA2 in man of intravenous naloxone measured by reversal of morphine-depressed respiration. *J Pharmacol Exp Ther* 219:156–162, 1981.

105 Manfredi PL, Ribeiro S, Chandler SW et al. Inappropriate use of naloxone in cancer patients with pain. *J Pain Symptom Manage* 11:131–134, 1996.

106 Tammela T, Kontturi M, Lukkarinen O. Postoperative urinary retention. I. Incidence and predisposing factors. *Scand J Urol Nephrol* 20:197–201, 1986.

107 O'Riordan JA, Hopkins PM, Ravenscroft A et al. Patient-controlled analgesia and urinary retention following lower limb joint replacement: Prospective audit and logistic regression analysis. *Eur J Anaesthesiol* 17:431–435, 2000.

108 Sillen U, Rubenson A. Central and peripheral motor effects of morphine on the rat urinary bladder. *Acta Physiol Scand* 126:181–187, 1986.

109 Dray A, Metsch R. Morphine and the centrally-mediated inhibition of urinary bladder motility in the rat. *Brain Res* 297:191–195, 1984.

110 Drenger B, Caine M, Sosnovsky M et al. Physostigmine and naloxone reverse the effect of intrathecal morphine on the canine urinary bladder. *Eur J Anaesthesiol* 4:375–382, 1987.

111 Rawal N, Mollefors K, Axelsson K et al. An experimental study of urodynamic effects of epidural morphine and of naloxone reversal. *Anesth Analg* 62:641–647, 1983.

112 Rosow CE, Gomery P, Chen TY et al. Reversal of opioid-induced bladder dysfunction by intravenous naloxone and methylnaltrexone. *Clin Pharmacol Ther* 82:48–53, 2007.

113 Herman NL, Choi KC, Affleck PJ et al. Analgesia, pruritus, and ventilation exhibit a dose-response relationship in parturients receiving intrathecal fentanyl during labor. *Anesth Analg* 89:378–383, 1999.

114 Daut RL, Cleeland CS, Flanery RC. Development of the Wisconsin Brief Pain Questionnaire to assess pain in cancer and other diseases. *Pain* 17:197–210, 1983.

115 Ballantyne JC, Loach AB, Carr DB. Itching after epidural and spinal opiates. *Pain* 33:149–160, 1988.

116 Kjellberg F, Tramer MR. Pharmacological control of opioid-induced pruritus: A quantitative systematic review of randomized trials. *Eur J Anaesthesiol* 18:346–357, 2001.

117 Katcher J, Walsh D. Opioid-induced itching: Morphine sulfate and hydromorphone hydrochloride. *J Pain Symptom Manage* 17:70–72, 1999.

118 Ko MC, Song MS, Edwards T et al. The role of central mu opioid receptors in opioid-induced itch in primates. *J Pharmacol Exp Ther* 310:169–176, 2004.

119 Waxler B, Dadabhoy ZP, Stojiljkovic L et al. Primer of postoperative pruritus for anesthesiologists. *Anesthesiology* 103:168–178, 2005.

120 Okutomi T, Saito M, Mochizuki J et al. Prophylactic epidural naloxone reduces the incidence and severity of neuraxial fentanyl-induced pruritus during labour analgesia in primiparous parturients. *Can J Anaesth* 50:961–962, 2003.

121 Lockington PF, Fa'aea P. Subcutaneous naloxone for the prevention of intrathecal morphine induced pruritus in elective Caesarean delivery. *Anaesthesia* 62:672–676, 2007.

122 Charuluxananan S, Kyokong O, Somboonviboon W et al. Nalbuphine versus propofol for treatment of intrathecal morphine-induced pruritus after cesarean delivery. *Anesth Analg* 93:162–165, 2001.

123 Charuluxananan S, Kyokong O, Somboonviboon W et al. Nalbuphine versus ondansetron for prevention of intrathecal morphine-induced pruritus after cesarean delivery. *Anesth Analg* 96:1789–1793, table of contents, 2003.

124 Kendrick WD, Woods AM, Daly MY et al. Naloxone versus nalbuphine infusion for prophylaxis of epidural morphine-induced pruritus. *Anesth Analg* 82:641–647, 1996.

125 Yeh HM, Chen LK, Lin CJ et al. Prophylactic intravenous ondansetron reduces the incidence of intrathecal morphine-induced pruritus in patients undergoing cesarean delivery. *Anesth Analg* 91:172–175, 2000.

126 Borgeat A, Stirnemann HR. Ondansetron is effective to treat spinal or epidural morphine-induced pruritus. *Anesthesiology* 90:432–436, 1999.

127 Iatrou CA, Dragoumanis CK, Vogiatzaki TD et al. Prophylactic intravenous ondansetron and dolasetron in intrathecal morphine-induced pruritus: A randomized, double-blinded, placebo-controlled study. *Anesth Analg* 101:1516–1520, 2005.

128 Charuluxananan S, Somboonviboon W, Kyokong O et al. Ondansetron for treatment of intrathecal morphine-induced pruritus after cesarean delivery. *Reg Anesth Pain Med* 25:535–539, 2000.

129 Korhonen AM, Valanne JV, Jokela RM et al. Ondansetron does not prevent pruritus induced by low-dose intrathecal fentanyl. *Acta Anaesthesiol Scand* 47:1292–1297, 2003.

130 Wells J, Paech MJ, Evans SF. Intrathecal fentanyl-induced pruritus during labour: The effect of prophylactic ondansetron. *Int J Obstet Anesth* 13:35–39, 2004.

131 Yazigi A, Chalhoub V, Madi-Jebara S et al. Prophylactic ondansetron is effective in the treatment of nausea and vomiting but not on pruritus after cesarean delivery with intrathecal sufentanil-morphine. *J Clin Anesth* 14:183–186, 2002.

132 Horta ML, Ramos L, Goncalves ZR. The inhibition of epidural morphine-induced pruritus by epidural droperidol. *Anesth Analg* 90:638–641, 2000.

133 Naji P, Farschtschian M, Wilder-Smith OH et al. Epidural droperidol and morphine for postoperative pain. *Anesth Analg* 70:583–588, 1990.

134 Facchinetti F, Volpe A, Farci G et al. Hypothalamus-pituitary-adrenal axis of heroin addicts. *Drug Alcohol Depend* 15:361–366, 1985.

135 Khan C, Malik SA, Iqbal MA. Testosterone suppression by heroin. *J Pak Med Assoc* 40:172–173, 1990.

136 Malik SA, Khan C, Jabbar A et al. Heroin addiction and sex hormones in males. *J Pak Med Assoc* 42:210–212, 1992.

137 Mendelson JH, Mendelson JE, Patch VD. Plasma testosterone levels in heroin addiction and during methadone maintenance. *J Pharmacol Exp Ther* 192:211–217, 1975.

138 Daniell HW. Narcotic-induced hypogonadism during therapy for heroin addiction. *J Addict Dis* 21:47–53, 2002.

139 Mendelson JH, Mello NK. Plasma testosterone levels during chronic heroin use and protracted astinence. A study of Hong Kong addicts. *Clin Pharmacol Ther* 17:529–533, 1975.

140 Pelosi MA, Sama JC, Caterini H et al. Galactorrhea-amenorrhea syndrome associated with heroin addiction. *Am J Obstet Gynecol* 118:966–970, 1974.

141 Abs R, Verhelst J, Maeyaert J et al. Endocrine consequences of long-term intrathecal administration of opioids. *J Clin Endocrinol Metab* 85:2215–2222, 2000.

142 Doleys D, Dinoff BL, Page L et al. Sexual dysfunction and other side effects of intraspinal opiate use in the management of chronic non-cancer pain. *Am J Pain Manage* 8:5–11, 1998.

143 Finch PM, Roberts LJ, Price L et al. Hypogonadism in patients treated with intrathecal morphine. *Clin J Pain* 16:251–254, 2000.

144 Paice JA, Penn RD, Ryan WG. Altered sexual function and decreased testosterone in patients receiving intraspinal opioids. *J Pain Symptom Manage* 9:126–131, 1994.

145 Daniell HW. Hypogonadism in men consuming sustained-action oral opioids. *J Pain* 3:377–384, 2002.

146 Daniell HW. Opioid endocrinopathy in women consuming prescribed sustained-action opioids for control of nonmalignant pain. *J Pain* 9:28–36, 2008.

147 Wong D, Gray DP, Simmonds M et al. Opioid analgesics suppress male gonadal function but opioid use in males and females does not correlate with symptoms of sexual dysfunction. *Pain Res Manage* 16:311–316, 2011.

148 Rajagopal A, Vassilopoulou-Sellin R, Palmer JL et al. Hypogonadism and sexual dysfunction in male cancer survivors receiving chronic opioid therapy. *J Pain Symptom Manage* 26:1055–1061, 2003.

149 Rajagopal A, Vassilopoulou-Sellin R, Palmer JL et al. Symptomatic hypogonadism in male survivors of cancer with chronic exposure to opioids. *Cancer* 100:851–858, 2004.

150 Dev R, Hui D, Dalal S et al. Association between serum cortisol and testosterone levels, opioid therapy, and symptom distress in patients with advanced cancer. *J Pain Symptom Manage* 41:788–795, 2011.

151 Risdahl JM, Khanna KV, Peterson PK et al. Opiates and infection. *J Neuroimmunol* 83:4–18, 1998.

152 Sacerdote P, Franchi S, Panerai AE. Non-analgesic effects of opioids: Mechanisms and potential clinical relevance of opioid-induced immunodepression. *Curr Pharm Des* 18:6034–6042, 2012.

153 Sacerdote P, Bianchi M, Manfredi B et al. Effects of tramadol on immune responses and nociceptive thresholds in mice. *Pain* 72:325–330, 1997.

154 Tsai YC, Won SJ. Effects of tramadol on T lymphocyte proliferation and natural killer cell activity in rats with sciatic constriction injury. *Pain* 92:63–69, 2001.

155 Gaspani L, Bianchi M, Limiroli E et al. The analgesic drug tramadol prevents the effect of surgery on natural killer cell activity and metastatic colonization in rats. *J Neuroimmunol* 129:18–24, 2002.

156 Ben-Eliyahu S, Page GG, Yirmiya R et al. Evidence that stress and surgical interventions promote tumor development by suppressing natural killer cell activity. *Int J Cancer* 80:880–888, 1999.

157 Gomez-Flores R, Weber RJ. Differential effects of buprenorphine and morphine on immune and neuroendocrine functions following acute administration in the rat mesencephalon periaqueductal gray. *Immunopharmacology* 48:145–156, 2000.

158 Franchi S, Panerai AE, Sacerdote P. Buprenorphine ameliorates the effect of surgery on hypothalamus-pituitary-adrenal axis, natural killer cell activity and metastatic colonization in rats in comparison with morphine or fentanyl treatment. *Brain Behav Immun* 21:767–774, 2007.

159 Martucci C, Panerai AE, Sacerdote P. Chronic fentanyl or buprenorphine infusion in the mouse: Similar analgesic profile but different effects on immune responses. *Pain* 110:385–392, 2004.

160 Shavit Y, Ben-Eliyahu S, Zeidel A et al. Effects of fentanyl on natural killer cell activity and on resistance to tumor metastasis in rats. Dose and timing study. *Neuroimmunomodulation* 11:255–260, 2004.

161 Fishbain DA, Rosomoff HL, Rosomoff RS. Drug abuse, dependence, and addiction in chronic pain patients. *Clin J Pain* 8:77–85, 1992.

162 Porter J, Jick H. Addiction rare in patients treated with narcotics. *N Engl J Med* 302:123, 1980.

163 McQuay HJ. Opioid use in chronic pain. *Acta Anaesthesiol Scand* 41:175–183, 1997.

164 Passik SD, Kirsh KL, McDonald MV et al. A pilot survey of aberrant drug-taking attitudes and behaviors in samples of cancer and AIDS patients. *J Pain Symptom Manage* 19:274–286, 2000.

45

Adjuvant analgesic drugs

RUSSELL K. PORTENOY, EVGENIA KROTOVA, DAVID LUSSIER

INTRODUCTION

The term *adjuvant analgesic* has been applied to drugs that do not have a primary indication for pain but are useful as analgesics in specific circumstances. Although several of these drugs recently have been approved for specific painful disorders, and others also are used off-label as primary analgesic treatments, the label "adjuvant" continues to be used and is particularly apt when these drugs are coadministered with opioids in populations with serious or life-threatening illness. As coanalgesics in these populations, they usually are added to an opioid regimen to improve the balance between analgesia and side effects and, in some cases, provide analgesia when opioid therapy cannot.[1,2]

In most cases, an adjuvant analgesic is added after opioid titration has resulted in a poor response (Table 45.1). If this approach is adopted, adjuvant analgesic therapy may be considered one strategy among many that may be useful to address poor opioid responsiveness.[2]

The adjuvant analgesics comprise numerous drug classes and individual agents, and the decision to try one or another may be guided by a broad categorization based on customary use. The categories include multipurpose analgesics, drugs for the treatment of neuropathic pain, drugs used specifically for bone pain, and drugs used for pain and other symptoms caused by bowel obstruction (Table 45.2).[1] Guidelines for the selection and administration of the adjuvant analgesics in populations with serious illness derive mainly from clinical experience and data extrapolated from studies in patients with noncancer pain syndromes.

MULTIPURPOSE ANALGESICS

Drugs that have been studied in diverse types of chronic pain may have sufficient evidence of broad analgesic efficacy to justify their designation as multipurpose analgesics. The classes that may be characterized in this way include the glucocorticoids, antidepressants, alpha-2 adrenergic agonists, cannabinoids, and topical therapies.

Corticosteroids

In populations with advanced illness, glucocorticoids are conventionally considered for diverse symptoms, including pain, nausea, fatigue, and anorexia. Although evidence from clinical trials is limited, clinical experience suggests that glucocorticoids may be beneficial for a variety of pain syndromes, including bone pain, neuropathic pain, pain due to bowel obstruction or to organ capsule distension, pain caused by lymphedema, and headache caused by increased intracranial pressure.[3] The mechanism of analgesia probably relates to some combination of anti-inflammatory effects and direct effects on nociceptive neural systems.

In the United States, dexamethasone is the preferred glucocorticoid for pain in serious medical illness, presumably because of its long half-life and low mineralocorticoid effects. Prednisone and methylprednisolone are acceptable alternatives. When used in the long-term management of pain or other symptoms, the typical low-dose regimen is 1–2 mg of dexamethasone orally or parenterally once or twice daily; this may be preceded by a loading dose of 10–20 mg.

A transitory (usually days to weeks) high-dose dexamethasone regimen occasionally is considered when pain is very severe and poorly responsive to an opioid; it well-accepted in the acute management of metastatic spinal cord compression.[4] The high-dose regimen begins with a loading dose of 50–100 mg of dexamethasone, which is followed by a divided daily dose that is between 50% and 100% of the loading dose. This is tapered quickly over a period of several weeks.

Acutely, the most worrisome glucocorticoid toxicity is delirium or adverse mood effects. Hyperglycemia and hypertension can occur. Long-term use is associated with the potential for many adverse effects, including myopathy,

Table 45.1 *Using adjuvant analgesics for pain management in the palliative care setting*

1. Consider optimizing the opioid regimen before introducing an adjuvant analgesic.

2. Consider the use of other strategies for pain that is poorly responsive to an opioid, including opioid rotation, aggressive management of treatment-limiting opioid side effects, neuraxial drug infusion, or trials of nonpharmacological approaches.

3. Select the most appropriate adjuvant analgesic based on a comprehensive assessment of the patient (symptoms, comorbidities, and goals of care) and the inference about the predominating type of pain.

4. When selecting an adjuvant analgesic, consider its pharmacological characteristics, actions, approved indications, unapproved indications accepted in medical practice, adverse effects, potential adverse effects, and interactions with other drugs.

5. Administer the adjuvant analgesics with the best risk:benefit ratios as first-line treatment.

6. Avoid initiating several adjuvant analgesics concurrently.

7. Initiate treatment with low doses and titrate gradually according to analgesic response and adverse effects.

8. Reassess the efficacy and tolerability of the therapeutic regimen regularly, and taper or discontinue medications that do not provide additional pain relief.

9. Consider combination therapy with multiple adjuvant analgesics in selected patients.

Source: Lussier, D. and Portenoy, R.K., Adjuvant analgesics in pain management, in, Hanks, G. Cherny, N.I., Christakis, N., Fallon, M., Kaasa, S., and Portenoy, R.K., eds., *Textbook of Palliative Medicine*, 4th edn., pp. 706–734, 2010 by permission of Oxford University Press.

Cushing's habitus, diabetes, osteoporosis, and prolonged adrenal suppression. In the context of advanced illness, these risks usually are balanced by the compelling need to provide symptomatic relief.

Antidepressant drugs

Many antidepressants, particularly the tricyclic compounds and the serotonin-norepinephrine reuptake inhibitors (SNRIs),[5,6] have analgesic efficacy. The analgesic mode of action is thought to be related to enhanced availability of monoamines within pain-modulating neural pathways in the central nervous system.

TRICYCLIC ANTIDEPRESSANTS

There is substantial evidence for the analgesic efficacy of the tricyclic antidepressant (TCAs) in a variety of pain syndromes.[7] This class includes tertiary amine compounds, such as amitriptyline, imipramine, and doxepin, and secondary amine compounds, such as nortriptyline and desipramine. The secondary amine drugs have a better side-effect profile, causing less sedation and anticholinergic side effects than the tertiary amine drugs, and are generally preferred for use in elderly or medically ill populations.

The analgesic effect of the TCAs may positively interact with their mood effects, but pain relief is not dependent on antidepressant activity. The usually effective analgesic dose is often lower than that required to treat depression, and the onset of analgesia typically occurs sooner than changes in mood.

SEROTONIN–NOREPINEPHRINE REUPTAKE INHIBITORS

SNRIs include duloxetine, milnacipran, venlafaxine, and desvenlafaxine. Evidence of analgesic efficacy is best documented for duloxetine, and this drug is an appropriate first-line agent for chemotherapy-induced neuropathy.[8,9] Venlafaxine has been shown to provide pain relief in nonmalignant painful polyneuropathy, and pain following mastectomy for breast cancer.[10,11] There have been no trials in populations with advanced medical illness, and comparative trials are lacking.

The side-effect profile of the SNRIs, which includes nausea, sexual dysfunction, and somnolence, is favorable, relative to the tertiary amine TCAs. The extent to which adverse effects occur relative to the secondary amine tricyclics is not known. In seriously ill populations with chronic pain, the first-line analgesic antidepressants typically are either a secondary amine TCA, such as desipramine or nortriptyline, or the SNRI duloxetine.

SELECTIVE SEROTONIN REUPTAKE INHIBITORS AND OTHER ANTIDEPRESSANTS

There is relatively little evidence that other classes of antidepressants are analgesic, and there have been no studies in medically ill populations. There is limited evidence for two of the SSRIs—paroxetine and citalopram[6]—and for the dual noradrenergic and dopaminergic compound bupropion.[12] The latter drug is more activating than the others and is less likely to cause sexual dysfunction; these effects may justify a trial for a patient with a serious illness and chronic pain.

Alpha₂-adrenergic agonists

The analgesic effects produced by alpha₂-adrenergic drugs presumably relate to increased activity in monoamine-dependent, endogenous pain-modulating pathways in the spinal cord and brain. Clonidine has analgesic properties in various pain syndromes, and epidural clonidine has been shown to reduce pain in patients with severe cancer pain.[13] Tizanidine is approved as an antispasticity agent, and it has been shown to have analgesic efficacy in myofascial pain syndrome and chronic headache.[14] These data support the conclusion that these drugs are multipurpose.

Table 45.2   *Classification and dose ranges of commonly used adjuvant analgesics*

Category	Drug class	Subclass	Drugs	Common starting dose	Usual effective dose
Multipurpose analgesics	Glucocorticoids		Dexamethasone	Varies	1–2 mg BID
			Prednisone	Varies	5–10 mg BID
	Antidepressants	Tricyclic antidepressants	Nortriptyline	10–25 mg qHS	50–150 mg qHS
			Desipramine	10–25 mg qHS	50–150 mg qHS
		SSRIs	Citalopram	10–20 mg qD	20–40 mg qD
		SNRIs	Venlafaxine ER	75 mg qD	150–225 mg qD
			Duloxetine	20–30 mg qD	60–120 mg qD
		Others	Bupropion	50–75 mg BID	300–450 qD
	Alpha-2 adrenergic agonists		Tizanidine	1–2 mg qHS	2–8 mg BID
	Cannabinoids		Dronabinol	2.5 mg BID	5–10 mg BID
	Topical analgesics		Lidocaine 5% patch	1–3 patches 12 h/24	
Adjuvant analgesics for neuropathic pain	All multipurpose analgesics		See earlier text	See earlier text	See earlier text
	Anticonvulsants		Gabapentin	100–300 mg BID	300–1200 mg TID
			Pregabalin	25–75 mg BID	150–300 mg BID
	Sodium channel blockers		Lidocaine IV	1–2 mg/kg over 30–60 min	2–4 mg/kg
	NMDA receptor antagonists		Ketamine	0.05–1.5 mg/kg/h	Varies
	GABA agonists		Clonazepam	0.5 mg qHS	0.5–3.0 mg qD
			Baclofen	5 mg TID	10–20 mg TID
Adjuvant analgesics for bone pain	Glucocorticoids		See earlier text	See earlier text	See earlier text
	Osteoclast inhibitors	Bisphosphonates	Pamidronate	—	60–90 mg IV monthly
	Targeted RANKL agent		Denosumab	—	120 mg SC monthly
Adjuvant analgesics for bowel obstruction	Glucocorticoids		See earlier text	See earlier text	See earlier text
	Anticholinergic drugs		Glycopyrrolate	0.1 mg qD	0.1–0.2 mg TID
	Somatostatin analogues		Octreotide	Varies	0.1–0.3 mg BID

Source: Adapted from Lussier, D. and Portenoy, R.K., Adjuvant analgesics in pain management, in , Hanks, G. Cherny, N.I., Christakis, N., Fallon, M., Kaasa, S., and Portenoy, R.K., eds., *Textbook of Palliative Medicine*, 4th edn., pp. 706–734, 2010 by permission of Oxford University Press.

The use of the alpha$_2$-adrenergic agonists as adjuvant analgesics is limited by their adverse effects, most often somnolence and hypotension. Tizanidine causes less hypotension and, for this reason, may be preferred over clonidine for a trial in medically frail patients with opioid-refractory pain who have not responded to one or more trials of analgesic antidepressants.

Cannabinoids

The available data suggest that cannabinoids may be useful as multipurpose analgesics.[15] These drugs presumably interact with an endogenous system that includes endogenous ligands, the endocannabinoids, and at least two types of receptors (known as CB1 and CB2). The endogenous system is broadly represented in both the periphery and central nervous systems, and is involved in nociception, inflammation, and other physiologic functions.

In the United States, the two commercially available cannabinoids, dronabinol (tetrahydrocannabinol [THC]) and nabilone, are marketed for indications other than pain and have modest evidence of analgesic efficacy.[15] An oromucosal spray containing THC plus cannabidiol, known as nabiximols, is undergoing development and has already been approved in several countries for the treatment of neuropathic pain due to multiple sclerosis and opioid-refractory pain due to cancer.[16]

The role of cannabinoids for pain and other indications is evolving. At present, a trial of one of the commercially available drugs usually is considered only in those patients who are poorly responsive to an opioid and have not responded to other adjuvant analgesics. The most common side effects are dizziness, somnolence, and dry mouth.

Topical analgesics

The safety associated with the limited systemic absorption of topical therapies is particularly useful in the context of medical frailty and complex medication regimens. A topical analgesic should be considered whenever the location and extent of pain makes it feasible.

The most widely used topical formulations are local anesthetics, which can be provided through a patch, or a cream or gel. Lidocaine 5% patch has been approved for the treatment of postherpetic neuralgia, and now is used for focal or regional pains of all types. Studies indicate minimal systemic absorption and a high level of safety with up to three patches worn for periods up to 24 hours.[17]

Capsaicin, the naturally occurring constituent of the chili pepper, depletes substance P from nociceptive nerve terminals, leading to decreased pain perception if used regularly. Topical application of a low-dose (0.075%–0.1%) capsaicin cream has demonstrated analgesic effects in neuropathic and joint pain.[18] Many patients experience local burning pain when initiating treatment, which is often transient. A high-concentration (8%) capsaicin patch has become available for the treatment of postherpetic neuralgia, and analgesia can persist for several months after a single application. There is yet no published experience in the use of the high-concentration patch for other focal pain conditions.

Topical NSAIDs are available as creams, and a diclofenac patch has been approved. These formulations have established efficacy in musculoskeletal pain.[19]

Numerous other drugs may be compounded into topical formulations. These include TCAs, gabapentin, ketamine, and others. Data supporting the analgesic efficacy of these agents is very limited.

ADJUVANT ANALGESICS USED FOR NEUROPATHIC PAIN

The term "neuropathic pain" is applied to those pain syndromes for which the sustaining mechanisms are presumed to be related to injury to the peripheral nervous system, central nervous system, or both. Adjuvant analgesics play an important role in the management of neuropathic pain. Although an opioid regimen usually is tried first in populations with serious or life-threatening disease and pain that is moderate or severe, adjuvant analgesics are commonly considered when a favorable balance between analgesia and side effects cannot be promptly attained.

All of the multipurpose analgesics may be used in patients with opioid-refractory neuropathic pain, and the glucocorticoids, analgesic antidepressants, and topical drugs are considered first-line therapies for these conditions.[20] Indeed, if an adjuvant analgesic is indicated for neuropathic pain, and the patient is noted to have comorbid depressed mood, a glucocorticoid or an antidepressant usually is the preferred first-line therapy. The glucocorticoid usually is selected in the setting of advanced illness and multiple other symptoms; the antidepressant typically is chosen when the disease is less advanced, or when a diagnosis of major depression is appropriate. When depressed mood is not prominent, the usual first-line drug for neuropathic pain is either a glucocorticoid—again in the proper context—or one of the gabapentinoids, specifically gabapentin or pregabalin.

Patients may require sequential drug trials if therapy is unsatisfactory, and these initial trials conventionally are selected first from among several antidepressant analgesics, both gabapentinoids, and the glucocorticoid, if appropriate. As noted, topical drugs are considered whenever pain is focal.

If these trials are not effective, and treatment with an adjuvant analgesic is still appropriate, subsequent trials are selected empirically from drugs in other categories of multipurpose analgesics or analgesics used for neuropathic pain. Many patients with severe neuropathic pain syndromes gain benefit from combinations of adjuvant analgesics.[21]

Analgesic anticonvulsants

There is good evidence that anticonvulsant drugs are useful in the management of neuropathic pain of diverse etiologies.[21,22] Analgesic effects are best established for gabapentin and pregabalin; these drugs have demonstrated efficacy in many types of neuropathic pain, including neuropathic cancer pain that is refractory to opioid analgesics, and patients may respond to one, after not responding to the other.[23–26] The gabapentinoids bind to the alpha-2 delta protein modulator of the N-type, voltage-gated calcium channel. Binding reduces calcium flux into the cell and lessens the likelihood of depolarization. Gabapentin and pregabalin both have a good safety profile, and neither has known drug–drug interactions. Both are renally excreted and dose reduction is required in the setting of renal failure. Their common side effects are dizziness, somnolence, and peripheral edema.

In the medically ill patient, gabapentin should be initiated at a daily dose of 100–300 mg at bedtime; the lower dose should be used in the setting of significant frailty or renal insufficiency. The starting dose of pregabalin usually is 50–75 mg/day, and 25 mg/day may be appropriate in those with severe frailty or renal impairment. The dose can be increased every few days. In the absence of a demonstrable analgesic ceiling dose or the development of treatment-limiting adverse effects, upward dose titration should continue until the gabapentin dose is 2700–3600 mg/day in two–three divided doses and the pregabalin dose is 300–600 mg/day in two divided doses. The drug should be stopped if there are no demonstrable benefits.

Other anticonvulsants have been studied as adjuvant analgesics. Among the older anticonvulsants, evidence of efficacy is best for carbamazepine, which remains a preferred drug for trigeminal neuralgia.[27] Although there is limited evidence supporting the use of oxcarbazepine, lamotrigine, and topiramate in neuropathic pain syndromes,[28] these drugs may be considered for trials in patients with refractory pain.

Sodium channel blockers

Systemic administration of sodium channel blockers may be analgesic.[29] Intravenous lidocaine at a dose between 1 and 4 mg/kg infused over 30 min to 1 hour has been used to treat severe neuropathic pains for many decades; this therapy is used by many pain specialists as a rapid-onset approach to address very severe neuropathic pain. The data supporting oral therapy with older sodium channel blockers, such as the antiarrhythmic mexiletine, are limited, and given their side effect profiles, a trial is considered only when sequential trials of other adjuvant analgesics have been ineffective.

A new agent, lacosamide, has a unique mechanism involving sodium channel modulation. Although there are no data in populations with severe medically illness, its side-effect profile usually is acceptable and early experience suggests that it may be considered for a trial in refractory neuropathic pain.[30]

N-methyl-d-aspartate receptor antagonists

The N-Methyl-D-aspartate (NMDA) receptor is involved in both the sensitization of central neurons and the functioning of the opioid receptor. Although studies of ketamine as an adjuvant to opioid therapy have yielded mixed results,[31–35] this drug has been widely used at subanesthetic doses to manage refractory pain in the setting of advanced illness. Ketamine treatment for pain may be delivered via brief or long-term subcutaneous or intravenous infusion, or as oral therapy. The potential for side effects, including hypertension, tachycardia, and serious psychotomimetic effects (such as a dissociative reaction), must be recognized. Treatment must be carefully monitored, and coadministration of a benzodiazepine or a neuroleptic commonly is used to reduce the risk of psychotomimetic side effects.

Other NMDA receptor antagonists, such as memantine, amantadine, and dextromethorphan, have been studied in neuropathic pain states, with mixed results.[34] They are rarely considered for trials in cancer-related neuropathic pain that has not responded to other agents.

Gamma-aminobutyric acid receptor agonists

Gamma-aminobutyric acid (GABA) receptors may be involved in pain processing. Among the GABA receptor inhibitors are the benzodiazepines, which affect the $GABA^A$ receptor subtype, and baclofen, which affects the $GABA^B$ subtype. The only $GABA^A$ inhibitor used for neuropathic pain is clonazepam, although the evidence supporting its use as an analgesic is limited. A trial in the setting of pain associated with significant anxiety is most reasonable.[35]

Baclofen is an antispasticity drug with established efficacy in trigeminal neuralgia. It is rarely used for neuropathic pain of other types, but may be considered for a trial in refractory pain.[36]

ADJUVANT ANALGESICS FOR BONE PAIN

Bone pain is the most common type of cancer pain. Focal pain can be managed with radiation therapy, and radiation is strongly indicated if pain is associated with a high risk of fracture. Interventions such as vertebroplasty or kyphoplasty, or surgical resection or stabilization or bone, also may be considered in specific circumstances. Patients with multifocal pain are usually managed with opioid therapy and other systemic analgesics, including nonsteroidal anti-inflammatory drugs and adjuvant analgesics. In addition to glucocorticoids, the adjuvant analgesics that are potentially useful in this setting include osteoclast inhibitors, specifically bisphosphonates and calcitonin; drugs that target and neutralize the ligand for receptor activator of nuclear factor-kappa B (RANKL); and radiopharmaceuticals.

Osteoclast inhibitors

Bisphosphonates, which are analogs of inorganic pyrophosphate, inhibit osteoclast activity and reduce bone resorption. For patients with metastatic bone disease, bisphosphonates reduce the risk of skeletal-related events, including pain. Analgesic efficacy has been established for many of these agents, including intravenous pamidronate, zoledronic acid, ibandronate, and clodronate, as well as oral ibandronate and clodronate.[37,38] Comparative data are very limited, and the selection of a specific drug is usually based on experience, cost, and convenience.

Although generally well tolerated, bisphosphonate administration may be associated with development of flu-like syndrome, symptomatic hypocalcemia, and impairment of renal function, which is typically transitory. Renal function should be evaluated prior to treatment, and if impaired, the starting dose should be lowered. Repeated administration of a bisphosphonate also is associated with more serious complications, specifically osteonecrosis of the jaw or femoral fracture. Patients who may be predisposed to osteonecrosis of the jaw because of poor dentition, local infection, or recent substantial dental procedures should be considered for an alternative strategy for bone pain.

The evidence that calcitonin reduces bone pain is conflicting.[39] Accordingly, this drug typically is considered only when other treatments are not available or effective.

Targeted RANKL therapies

Denosumab is a monoclonal antibody that targets RANKL, a key component in the pathway for osteoclast formation and activation. This agent has been compared to zoledronic acid in patients with metastatic bone disease from a variety of solid tumors and has been shown to have comparable benefits in preventing skeletal-related events.[40] There is no evidence that denosumab has greater analgesic efficacy than the bisphoshonates, and osteonecrosis of the jaw also is a rare complication.

Radiopharmaceuticals

Bone-seeking radionuclides, such as strontium-89 and samarium-153, may be considered for multifocal bone pain due to metastatic disease, and may be effective as monotherapy or as an adjunct to conventional radiation therapy.[1] Given the potential for bone marrow suppression, these drugs usually are considered when pain is refractory to other modalities and chemotherapy associated with bone marrow suppression is not planned.

ADJUVANT ANALGESICS USED FOR PAIN DUE TO BOWEL OBSTRUCTION

Bowel obstruction is a relatively common complication in patients with advanced intra-abdominal or pelvic tumors. If surgical decompression or palliative stent placement is not feasible, the need to control pain and other obstructive symptoms, including distension, nausea, and vomiting, becomes paramount. In some cases, decompression is best accomplished using nasogastric suctioning or venting gastrostomy. In other situations, medical management is preferred. Medical treatment usually involves hydration and symptom control using opioids and adjuvant analgesics, specifically a glucocorticoid, an anticholinergic drug, and a somatostatin analogue.[41,42]

Anticholinergic drugs

Anticholinergic drugs reduce propulsive and nonpropulsive gut motility and decrease intraluminal secretions. Hyoscine (scopolamine) can relieve pain and other symptoms from inoperable malignant bowel obstruction.[41] This agent can be administered by transdermal patch or as a continuous subcutaneous infusion. In many countries, scopolamine is available only as the hydrobromide salt, which crosses the blood–brain barrier and may produce central nervous system side effects, such as somnolence and confusion. Hyoscine butylbromide is available in some countries and is a quaternary ammonium compound with little risk of side effects related to the central nervous system, because it does not pass the blood–brain barrier. Glycopyrrolate has a pharmacological profile similar to that of hyoscine butylbromide, and also may produce fewer adverse effects because of a relatively low penetration through the blood–brain barrier. Although this drug has not been evaluated as a treatment for the symptoms of bowel obstruction, it may be preferred in patients predisposed to somnolence and confusion.

Somatostatin analogues

The somatostatin analogue, octreotide, inhibits gastric, pancreatic, and intestinal secretions, and reduces motility. These actions probably underlie the potential for analgesia and other favorable outcomes in patients with bowel obstruction. Comparative studies suggest that octreotide is superior to an anticholinergic agent alone for the symptomatic management of malignant bowel obstruction.[41,43] The cost of octreotide is substantially higher, however, and this may influence availability.

Octreotide has a good safety profile, and it may be administered as repeated subcutaneous boluses or as a continuous infusion. The starting dose of 100 mcg twice daily may be titrated upward based on efficacy. There is a long-acting formulation.

CONCLUSIONS

Scientific evidence pertaining to the utility of adjuvant analgesics has slowly but steadily evolved during the past few decades, and options for treatment have become much more numerous. Still, specific evidence of safety, efficacy, comparative efficacy and effectiveness in populations with serious or life-threatening illness remains very limited. Instead of a strong evidence base for these treatments, clinicians must rely on studies conducted in populations with chronic pain unrelated to medical illness and clinical experience.

Nonetheless, single-drug therapy or combination therapy with multiple adjuvant analgesics should be considered a potentially useful strategy to address pain that is poorly responsive to an opioid. Clinical trials in populations with well-defined pain syndromes are needed, but the limited data should not preclude empirical therapy for patients with refractory pain.

REFERENCES

1 Lussier D, Portenoy RK. Adjuvant analgesics in pain management. In: Hanks G, Cherny NI, Christakis N, Fallon M, Kaasa S, Portenoy RK, eds. *Oxford Textbook of Palliative Medicine.* 4th edn. Oxford, U.K.: Oxford University Press, 2010; pp. 706–734.

2 Mercadante S, Portenoy RK. Opioid poorly responsive cancer pain. Part 3: Clinical strategies to improve opioid responsiveness. *J Pain Symptom Manage* 2001;21:338–354.

3 Paulsen O, Aass N, Kaasa S, Dale O. Do corticosteroids provide analgesic effects in cancer patients? A systematic literature review. *J Pain Symptom Manage* November 10, 2012.

4 George R, Jeba J, Ramkumar G et al. Interventions for the treatment of metastatic extradural spinal cord compression in adults. *Cochrane Database Syst Rev* 2008:CD006716.

5 Collins SL, Moore RA, McQuay HJ, Wiffen P. Anti depressants and anticonvulsants for diabetic neuropathy and postherpetic neuralgia: A quantitative systematic review. *J Pain Symptom Manage* December 2000;20(6):449–458.

6 Saarto T, Wiffen PJ. Anti depressants for neuropathic pain. *Cochrane Database Syst Rev* 2007:CD005454.

7 Max MB, Lynch SA, Muir J et al. Effects of desipramine, amitriptyline, and fluoxetine on pain in diabetic neuropathy. *N Engl J Med* May 7, 1992;326(19):1250–1256.

8 Lunn MP, Hughes RA, Wiffen PJ. Duloxetine for treating painful neuropathy or chronic pain. *Cochrane Database Syst Rev* October 7, 2009(4):CD007115.

9 Smith EM, Pang H, Cirrincione C et al. Effect of duloxetine on pain, function, and quality of life among patients with chemotherapy-induced painful peripheral neuropathy: A randomized clinical trial. *J Am Med Assoc* April 3, 2013;309(13):1359–1367.

10 Rowbotham MC, Goli V, Kunz NR, Lei D. Venlafaxine extended release in the treatment of painful diabetic neuropathy: A double-blind, placebo-controlled study. *Pain* August 2004;110(3):697–706.

11 Reuben SS, Makari-Judson G, Lurie SD. Evaluation of efficacy of the perioperative administration of venlafaxine XR in the prevention of postmastectomy pain syndrome. *J Pain Symptom Manage* February 2004;27(2):133–139.

12   Semenchuk MR, Sherman S, Davis B. Double-blind, randomized trial of bupropion SR for the treatment of neuropathic pain. *Neurology* November 13, 2001;57(9):1583–1588.

13   Eisenach JC, DuPen S, Dubois M, Miguel R, Allin D. Epidural clonidine analgesia for intractable cancer pain. The Epidural Clonidine Study Group. *Pain* June 1995;61(3):391–399.

14   Malanga GA, Gwynn MW, Smith R, Miller D. Tizanidine is effective in the treatment of myofascial pain syndrome. *Pain Physician* October 2002;5(4):422–432.

15   Lynch ME, Campbell F. Cannabinoids for treatment of chronic non-cancer pain; a systematic review of randomized trials. *Br J Clin Pharmacol* 2011;72(5):735–744.

16   Portenoy RK, Ganae-Motan ED, Allende S et al., Nabiximols for opioid-treated cancer patients with poorly-controlled chronic pain: A randomized, placebo-controlled, graded-dose trial. *J Pain* May 2012;13(5):438–449.

17   Gammaitoni AR, Alvarez NA, Galer BS. Safety and tolerability of the lidocaine patch 5%, a targeted peripheral analgesic: A review of the literature. *J Clin Pharmacol* February 2003;43(2):111–117.

18   Derry S, Lloyd R, Moore RA, McQuay HJ. Topical capsaicin for chronic neuropathic pain in adults. *Cochrane Database Syst Rev* October 7, 2009(4) CD007393.

19   Mason L, Moore RA, Edwards JE, Derry S, McQuay HJ. Topical NSAIDs for chronic musculoskeletal pain: Systematic review and meta-analysis. *BMC Musculoskelet Disord* August 19, 2004;5:28.

20   Dworkin RH, O'Connor AB, Audette J et al. Recommendations for the pharmacological management of neuropathic pain: An overview and literature update. *Mayo Clin Proc* March 2010;85(Suppl 3):S3–S14.

21   Chaparro LE, Wiffen PJ, Moore RA, Gilron I. Combination pharmacotherapy for the treatment of neuropathic pain in adults. *Cochrane Database Syst Rev* July 11, 2012;7:CD008943.

22   Bennett MI. Effectiveness of anti epileptic or antidepressant drugs when added to opioids for cancer pain: Systematic review. *Palliat Med* July 2011;25(5):553–559.

23   Wiffen PJ, McQuay HJ, Edwards JE, Moore RA. Gabapentin for acute and chronic pain. *Cochrane Database Syst Rev* March 16, 2011(3):CD005452.

24   Moore RA, Straube S, Wiffen PJ, Derry S, McQuay HJ. Pregabalin for acute and chronic pain in adults. *Cochrane Database Syst Rev* July 8, 2009(3):CD007076.

25   Mishra S, Bhatnagar S, Goyal GN et al. A comparative efficacy of amitriptyline, gabapentin, and pregabalin in neuropathic cancer pain: A prospective randomized double-blind placebo-controlled study. *Am J Hosp Palliat Care* May 2012;29(3):177–182.

26   Toth C. Substitution of gabapentin therapy with pregabalin therapy in neuropathic pain due to peripheral neuropathy. *Pain Med* March 2010;11(3):456–465.

27   Wiffen PJ, Derry S, Moore RA, McQuay HJ. Carbamazepine for acute and chronic pain in adults. *Cochrane Database Syst Rev* January 19, 2011;(1):CD005451.

28   Eisenberg E, River Y, Shifrin A, Krivoy N. Antiepileptic drugs in the treatment of neuropathic pain. *Drugs* 2007;67(9):1265–1289.

29   Tremont-Lukas IW, Challapalli V et al. Systemic administration of local anesthetics to relieve neuropathic pain: A systematic review and meta-analysis. *Anesth Analg* December 2005;101(6):1738–1749.

30   Wymer JP, Simpson J, Sen D, Bongardt S. Efficacy and safety of lacosamide in diabetic neuropathic pain: An 18-week double-blind placebo-controlled trial of fixed-dose regimens. *Clin J Pain* June 2009;25(5):376–385.

31   Salas S, Frasca M, Planchet-Barraud B. Ketamine analgesic effect by continuous intravenous infusion in refractory cancer pain: Considerations about the clinical research in palliative care. *J Palliat Med* March 2012;15(3):287–293.

32   Hardy J, Quinn S, Fazekas B et al. Randomized, double-blind, placebo-controlled study to assess the efficacy and toxicity of subcutaneous ketamine in the management of cancer pain. *J Clin Oncol* 2012;30:3611.

33   Bell R, Eccleston C, Kalso E. Ketamine as an adjuvant to opioids for cancer pain. *Cochrane Database Syst Rev* November 14, 2012;11:CD003351.

34   Chizh BA, Headley PM. NMDA antagonists and neuropathic pain-multiple drug targets and multiple uses. *Curr Pharm Des* 2005;11(23):2977–2994.

35   Hugel H, Ellershaw JE, Dickman A. Clonazepam as an adjuvant analgesic in patients with cancer-related neuropathic pain. *J Pain Symptom Manage* 2003;26:1073–1074.

36   Yomiya K, Matsuo N, Tomiyasu S et al. Baclofen as an adjuvant analgesic for cancer pain. *Am J Hosp Palliat Care* April–May, 2009;26(2):112–118.

37   Body JJ. Bisphosphonates for malignancy-related bone disease: Current status, future developments. *Support Care Cancer* 2006;14(5):408–418.

38   Lopez-Olivo MA, Shah NA, Pratt G et al. Bisphosphonates in the treatment of patients with lung cancer and meta static bone disease: A systematic review and meta-analysis. *Support Care Cancer* November 2012;20(11):2985–2998.

39   Martinez-Zapata MJ, Roque M, Alonso-Coello P. Calcitonin for metastatic bone pain. *Cochrane Rev* 2006(3):CD003223.

40   Lipton A, Fizazi K, Stopeck AT et al. Superiority of denosumabtozoledronic acid for prevention of skeletal-related events: A combined analysis of 3 pivotal, randomised, phase 3 trials. *Eur J Cancer* November 2012;48(16):3082–3092.

41   Ripamonti C, Mercadante S, Groff L et al. Role of octreotide, scopolamine butylbromide, and hydration in symptom control of patients with inoperable bowel obstruction and nasogastric tubes: A prospective randomized trial. *J Pain Symptom Manage* 2000;19:23–34.

42   Feuer DJ, Broadley KE. Systematic review and meta-analysis of corticosteroids for the resolution of malignant bowel obstruction in advanced gynaecological and gastrointestinal cancers. Systematic Review Steering Committee. *Ann Oncol* 1999; 10:1035.

43   Mercadante S, Porzio G. Octreotide for malignant bowel obstruction: Twenty years after. *Crit Rev Oncol Hematol* September 2012;83(3):388–392.

46

Alternative routes for systemic opioid delivery

CARLA IDA RIPAMONTI, MONICA BOSCO

INTRODUCTION

It is well recognized that the oral administration of the opioid drugs is the mainstay of analgesic therapy in cancer patients. Indeed, it is safe, effective, and convenient. Moreover, the oral route for drugs makes home management simpler.

However, in some clinical situations, such as severe vomiting, bowel obstruction, severe dysphagia, or severe confusion, and in situations where rapid dose escalation is necessary, oral administration of opioids is impossible and an alternative route has to be implemented.

Recent data suggest that 53%–70% of patients with cancer-related pain require an alternative route for opioid administration hours and months before death [1,2*]. In the last few years, a number of modes for opioid administration have been explored [3]. This chapter deals with the characteristics, the main aspects of pharmacokinetics, the clinical efficacy, and indications of the following routes: rectal, sublingual, buccal (gingival, transmucosal), subcutaneous (SC), intravenous, intranasal, transdermal, and topical.

Table 46.1 shows the potential clinical applications of the most frequently used routes of opioid administration.

Table 46.2 reports the European Association for Palliative Care (EAPC) recommendations regarding the different routes of opioid administration [4].

RECTAL ROUTE

The surface area of the human rectum is small (200–400 cm^2) because of the absence of villi. Its fluid contents have a pH of 7–8. The main mechanism of absorption from the rectum is passive diffusion and is probably no different from that in the upper part of the gastrointestinal (GI) tract despite the fact that pH, surface area, and fluid content differ substantially [5]. The rectum is drained by the superior rectal vein into the portal system and by the middle and inferior rectal veins into the inferior cava vein. It is impossible to predict the quantity of drug that will bypass the hepatic filter, because there are several extensive anastomoses between the superior rectal vein that drains to the portal system and the median and inferior rectal veins that drain toward the systemic circulation [5,6]. Rectal drug vehicles may be liquid or solid [5–7]. The absorption of aqueous and alcoholic solutions may occur very rapidly, but the absorption of suppositories is generally slower and very much dependent on the nature of the suppository base, the use of surfactants, and other factors such as the presence/absence/quantity of fecal mass and the total volume content inside the rectum. Although an almost complete absence of presystemic metabolism has been found for intrarectal lidocaine in humans, several other drugs have been found to metabolize equal to or more than orally when administered intrarectally [5]. Davis et al. [7] reviewed the clinical pharmacology and therapeutic role of suppositories and rectal suspension of opioids and other analgesics.

Bioavailability studies have shown considerable interindividual variation [5–7]. Johnson et al. [8] found that after 24 hours of rectal and intravenous (IV) administration of 10 mg of morphine chloride in eight patients, the bioavailability of morphine after rectal administration was 53% ± 18% of the values obtained after IV administration. The authors conclude that probably, first-passage elimination of morphine was partially avoided by the rectal administration, since a previous study suggested that the bioavailability of oral morphine is 37% [9]. The bioavailability of free morphine and morphine-6-glucuronide was found to be comparable after oral, sublabial, and rectal administration of morphine in cancer patients [10–12].

In a comparative study [13] between 10 mg of morphine sulfate in oral solution and rectal suppository carried out in 10 patients with cancer pain, a significantly higher mean concentration of free morphine was found after rectal administration at all evaluation times throughout a period of 4.5 hours,, whereas there were no differences between the routes in mean morphine-3-glucuronide concentrations. These data suggest the presence of some avoidance of first-pass metabolism. Moolenar et al. [14] studied the rectal absorption of morphine hydrochloride from different aqueous solutions with different pH values in seven volunteers. The rectal absorption of morphine appeared to be dependent on the pH of the solution: A significant improvement in the absorption was found with a rectal solution adjusted to pH 7–8. Kaiko et al. [15] carried out a randomized cross-over multiple-dose study in 14 healthy

Table 46.1 *Potential applications of alternative routes for systemic opioid administration*

Symptoms	Sublingual	Rectal	CSI[a]	IV	Transdermal fentanyl buprenorphine	Transmucosal
Vomiting	++	++	++	++	++	____
Bowel obstruction	++	++	++	++	++	____
Dysphagia	++	++	++	++	++	____
Cognitive failure	–	+	++	++	++	____
Diarrhea	++	–	++	++	++	
Hemorrhoids anal fissures	++	–	++	++	++	____
Coagulation disorders	++	++	–	++	++	____
Severe immunosuppression	++	++	–	+	++	____
Generalized edema	++	++	–	++	–	____
Frequent dose changes	++	–	++[b]	++[b]	–	____
Titration	++	+	++[b]	++ +/–[b]	–	____
BTP	++	++	++[b]	++[b]	–	++

+, may be indicated; ++, indicated; –, contraindicated; ____, not indicated.

[a] Continuous subcutaneous infusion.

[b] Patient-controlled analgesia, PCA.

Table 46.2 *Opioid administration according to the EAPC recommendations*

A small proportion of patients develop intolerable adverse effects with oral morphine (in conjunction with a nonopioid and adjuvant analgesic as appropriate) before achieving adequate pain relief. In such patients a change to an alternative opioid or a change in the route of administration should be considered.

If patients are unable to take morphine orally, the preferred alternative route is SC. There is generally no indication for giving morphine intramuscularly for chronic cancer pain, because SC administration is simpler and less painful.

The average relative potency ratio of oral morphine to SC morphine is between 1:2 and 1:3 (i.e., 20–30 mg of morphine by mouth is equianalgesic to 10 mg by SC injection).

In patients requiring continuous parenteral morphine, the preferred method of administration is by SC infusion.

Intravenous infusion of morphine may be preferred in patients:
a. Who already have an indwelling intravenous line
b. With generalized edema
c. Who develop erythema, soreness, or sterile abscesses with SC administration
d. With coagulation disorders
e. With poor peripheral circulation

The average relative potency ratio of oral to intravenous morphine is between 1:2 and 1:3.

Rectal administration may be preferred by some patients. The equianalgesic dose by oral and rectal routes is about 1:1.

The buccal, sublingual. and nebulized routes of administration of morphine are not recommended, because at the present time, there is no evidence of clinical advantage over the conventional routes.

Oral transmucosal fentanyl citrate (OTFC) is an effective treatment for BTP in patients stabilized on regular oral morphine or an alternative step 3 opioid.

Transdermal fentanyl is an effective alternative to oral morphine but is best reserved for patients whose opioid requirements are stable. It may have particular advantages for such patients if they are unable to take oral morphine, as an alternative to SC infusion.

Spinal (epidural or intrathecal) administration of opioid analgesics in combination with local anesthetics or clonidine should be considered in patients who derive inadequate analgesia or suffer intolerable adverse effects despite the optimal use of systemic opioids and nonopioids.

Source: Data from Hanks, G.W. et al., *Br. J. Cancer*, 84/5, 587, 2001.
EAPC, European Association for Palliative Care.

men to compare the bioavailability of 30 mg of morphine sulfate tablets (MS Contin) administered orally and rectally. The results suggest that there is a slower rate of absorption for MS Contin administered rectally than when given orally.

Rectal administration of drugs can be used to produce local or systemic effects. In some countries, preparations of opioids in the form of suppositories are not commercially available. To overcome this situation, microenemas made up of liquid opioid (the same used for parenteral administration) are prepared and then given rectally as a bolus using a needleless insulin-type syringe with the advantage of a rapid absorption.

Pannuti et al. [12] found similar efficacy with oral, rectal, and sublingual application of morphine in a controlled study with 102 patients who received treatment for at least 10 days. Maloney [16] reviewed the experience with 39 terminally ill patients who received slow-release morphine as a rectal suppository. All patients had terminal cancer, and 38 patients were receiving oral slow-release morphine before starting the rectal administration. Good pain control was reported in all cases. In two patients, the slow-release morphine tablets were administered into a colostomy and in one case, a female patient with diarrhea received the tablets intravaginally. No local side effects using the standard commercial preparation of 30 mg tablets were reported. Patients were treated for an average of 11.5 days (range 1–30 days).

Long-term rectal administration of high-dose sustained-release morphine tablets is reported by Walsh and Tropiano [17]. Based on this case, the correct mg relative potency conversion ratio for rectal to IV morphine during repeated dosing appears to be 3:1, which is similar to that for the conversion from oral to IV. For rectal to oral morphine dosing, the conversion ratio seems to be 1.1.

Table 46.3 reports the randomized controlled trials (RCTs) on rectal morphine compared to oral or SC morphine [18–21 **].

Few data are available on the analgesia and tolerability of rectally administered methadone. A study [22] was carried out to assess the pharmacokinetics and pharmacodynamics of 10 mg of methadone hydrochloride administered rectally (in the form of microenema) in six opioid-naive cancer patients whose pain no longer responded to treatment with nonsteroidal anti-inflammatory drugs (NSAIDs) given at fixed times. The pharmacokinetics of rectal methadone showed rapid and extensive distribution phases followed by a slow elimination phase. The plasmatic concentrations presented a great intraindividual variability, with no correlation between analgesia and plasmatic

methadone concentration. Pain relief was statistically significant already after 30 min and continued more than 8 hours after administration. In five patients, pain control lasted between 24 and 48 hours. Only one patient reported vomiting, confusion, and vertigo after the administration of rectal methadone.

In a prospective, open study, Bruera et al. [23] demonstrated that custom-made capsules and suppositories of methadone are safe, effective, and low cost in 37 advanced cancer patients with poor pain control receiving high doses of SC hydromorphone. These patients had significant improvement in pain control with minimal toxicity, using doses higher than those reported in the literature. This study also demonstrated a large interindividual variation between methadone dosage and plasma level. Rectal methadone can be considered an effective, safe, and low-cost therapy for patients with cancer pain where oral and/or parenteral opioids are not indicated or available.

Oxycodone pectinate suppositories are available in countries such as the United Kingdom and need to be given every 8 hours. The single-dose pharmacokinetics and pharmacodynamics of oxycodone administered by IV and rectal routes were determined in 12 cancer patients. IV oxycodone was associated with a rapid onset of analgesia (5–8 min) in respect to rectal route (0.5–1 hour) but with a shorter analgesic effect (4 hours via IV route compared to 8–12 hours via rectal route) [24].

Mercadante et al. [25**] in a randomized double-blind clinical trial compared oral tramadol versus rectal tramadol. The aim of this study was to compare the analgesic activity and tolerability of tramadol by oral and rectal administration in a double-blind double dummy cross-over trial. The study included 60 cancer patients with cancer pain. Each patient initially received

Table 46.3 *RCTs on rectal morphine compared to oral or SC morphine*

Authors (Ref.)	Study design	No. of patients	Route 1	Route 2	Results
Bruera et al. [18]	Double blind cross-over	23	CR morphine sulfate, suppository every 12 hours	SC morphine, rectal / parenteral ratio 2.5:1	Comparable analgesia and side effects
Babul et al. [19]	Double blind cross-over	27	CR morphine, suppository every 12 hours	CR morphine tablets every 12 hours, conversion rate 1:1	No difference in pain and sedation; small but significant difference in nausea in favor of rectal administration
De Conno et al. [20]	Double blind, double dummy, cross-over single-dose study	34 opioid naives	Rectal morphine prepared as microenema	Oral morphine conversion rate 1:1	Rectal morphine had a faster onset of action and longer duration of analgesia than an acute dose of oral morphine. No significant difference in intensity of sedation, nausea, or number of vomiting episodes between the two routes.
Bruera et al. [21]	Randomized double blind cross-over	12, 6 evaluable	CR morphine sulfate, suppository every 12 hours	CR morphine sulfate, suppository every 24 hours	There was no significant difference between the q12h and q24h treatment groups in symptom (pain, nausea, sedation) intensity, adverse effects, and patient choice.

SC, subcutaneous; CSI continuous subcutaneous infusion; CR, controlled release; IV intravenous.

oral tramadol 50 mg drops, followed by tramadol sustained release 100 mg orally, and placebo rectally, or tramadol 100 mg rectally and placebo orally, twice a day, in a randomized sequence on each of 3 days. No differences in pain intensity (PI) and relief scores, or in other symptoms between the two treatment efficacy as judged by the clinician in patient compliance, or in patient satisfaction regarding treatment were found.

Ritschel et al. [26] have determined the absolute bioavailability of rectal administration of hydromorphone suppository in humans. They reported a maximum concentration of 3.53 ± 1.36 ng/mL, with the time taken to reach maximum concentration as 1.41 ± 0.79 hour, a bioavailability of 36% ± 0.29%, and a half-life of 3.8 hours. The low bioavailability and large interindividual variation observed when hydromorphone is administered rectally is due to various factors, namely, the type of preparation, the pH of the solutions used, the presence of feces in the ampulla, the condition of the mucosa, the placement of the agent, and the concurrent use of lubricants.

The colostomy administration route of opioids is not recommended. The results of the study of Hojsted et al. [27] comparing the pharmacokinetics of hydrochloride morphine administered via rectal and colostomic routes demonstrated that the bioavailability via colostomy showed a very wide variation, but the mean value as compared to rectal administration was 43% (range 0%–127%). The authors suspect that the main reason for lower bioavailability may be poor vascularization of the colostomy, adsorption of morphine to feces, and the presence of first-passage elimination.

There are anecdotal reports of rectal administration of controlled-release morphine, suggesting that these routes may be used for patients unable to take oral medications.

Although the studies on the rectal route reported similar efficacy and tolerability with SC or IV route [3], the rectal route of drug administration may present some disadvantages: (1) presence of feces or diarrhea when used chronically and when feces or diarrhea is present; (2) difficulty in titration and individualization of the doses; (3) interruption of absorption because of defecation; (4) presence of painful anal conditions.

This alternative route could be administered successfully in patients with breakthrough pain (BTP) and in some clinical situations how reported in Table 46.1.

With respect to SC and IV routes, the rectal route has the advantage of not requiring needles to be inserted or pumps to be carried. On the negative side, chronic and frequent rectal administration can lead to discomfort, and the presence of feces in the rectum, diarrhea, or normal peristalsis can reduce absorption.

There are some barriers to the development of rectally administered drugs. Sometimes physicians, caregivers, and patients find this route unappealing.

SUBLINGUAL AND BUCCAL ROUTES

The mouth has many areas with a potential for transmucous administration: sublingual (beneath the tongue), buccal (between the gingival edge of the upper molars and the cheek),

and gingival (between the gingival edge of the incisors and the lip). The permeability is greatest in the sublingual area and lowest at the gingival level.

The surface of the buccal and sublingual area is small (200 cm²), with a pH of 6.2–7.4. However, this region is rich in blood and lymphatic vessels and the possibility exists for rapid absorption with direct passage into the systemic circulation avoiding the hepatic first-pass metabolism [5]. The sublingual mucosa comprises a small fraction of the 200 cm² of oral mucosa, but it is the most permeable region in the oral cavity. In contrast to the buccal mucosa, which is comprised of 40–50 cell layers and is 500–800 m thick, the sublingual mucosa comprises fewer cell layers and is only 100–200 m thick. And unlike the gingival mucosa, the sublingual mucosa is nonkeratinized, thus eliminating an important barrier to drug absorption. In nonkeratinized mucosa, the outermost epithelial layers pose the major barrier to drug absorption.

The conditions for the penetration of the drug improve with the smallness of molecules, a high concentration of nonionized drug, and a high degree of lipophilicity. Thus, the amount of drug absorbed will depend on several factors including the pKa, rate of partition of the nonionized form of the drug, the lipid/water partition coefficient, molecular weight of the drug, passive diffusion, and the pH of the solution in the mouth.

Lipophilic drugs such as buprenorphine, fentanyl, and methadone are better absorbed that polar ones [28]. Salivary pH also plays a role in drug absorption.

Normal pH of saliva is 6.5 – 3 but is influenced by a number of factors including mouth-breathing, nutritional status, age, recent beverage consumption, vomiting, chemotherapy, stomatitis, and decreased salivary flow rate [9,12,13]. Even within an individual oral cavity, there is significant pH variation among the sublingual, buccal, and gingival microenvironments.

The studies on the buccal absorption of morphine report different results [5,6].

The preferred preparations are tablet form rather than liquids and pastes, which can spread all over the mouth and consequently increase the possibility of swallowing the drug. Saliva affects the absorption of the drug by dilution and by increasing the likelihood of the drug being swallowed before absorption.

Buprenorphine is one commercial opioid formulated in a sublingual preparation. Single-dose, cross-over studies have shown it to be 15 times as potent as morphine in terms of total analgesic effect [29]. The absorption half-life of sublingual buprenorphine is about 76 min, and peak plasma concentrations range from 20 to 360 min (mean 180 min) after administration, although there is a large intersubject variability [30]. A dose of 0.4 mg sublingually gives similar analgesia to 0.2–0.3 mg intramuscular (IM), with an onset of analgesia within 30–60 min of administration and a duration of 6–9 hours [31]. The long duration of analgesia with buprenorphine may be related to its affinity for the mu-opioid receptor and an unusually slow dissociation constant for the drug–receptor complex.

Robbie [32] treated 141 cancer patients with sublingual buprenorphine in doses of 0.15–0.8 mg for an average of 12 weeks. This treatment was effective in most of the patients, particularly those with pain from head and neck cancer. Drowsiness was the most common side effect, followed by dry mouth and nausea.

De Conno et al. [33] found that patients previously treated with sublingual or IM buprenorphine required a dose of morphine significantly higher than those treated with other opioids (codeine, oxycodone, dextropropoxyphene, and pentazocine) to obtain the same pain relief. Like the mixed agonist-antagonists, buprenorphine may precipitate withdrawal in patients who have received repeated doses of a morphine-like agonist and developed physical dependence. Naloxone is relatively ineffective in reversing serious respiratory depression caused by buprenorphine [34].

There are still some controversies on the efficacy of sublingual morphine [35] because of the lack of controlled clinical studies. The very few reports on the clinical effects of sublingual and buccal morphine are related to one-time dosage or anecdotal experience. Whitman [36] report that 70%–80% of 150 patients with cancer pain who were treated with sublingual morphine obtained "adequate to good pain control." Patients were treated with morphine sulfate tablets in a dose of 10–30 mg q3-4h around the clock. The main side effects reported were intolerance to the taste of the drug and occasional confusion or unpleasant dreams. Pannuti et al. [12] treated 28 patients with cancer pain with sublingual drops of morphine hydrochloride q4h. Patients were treated for an average of 5 weeks. Although the authors reported more rapid and significant pain remission for the sublingual route as compared to the rectal and oral route, no significant difference in the incidence or severity of side effects was reported. No patient required discontinuation of sublingual treatment because of toxicity. Kokki et al. [37] compared the pharmacokinetics of buccal (n = 5) and sublingual (n = 15) oxycodone (0.2 mg/kg–10 mg/mL parenteral liquid) in a randomized, open-label study of healthy, awake preoperative children (ages 6 months to 7 years) Neither the mucosal contact times nor the fates of the oxycodone-containing saliva were specified. Blood was drawn serially and serum oxycodone measured by gas chromatography/mass spectroscopy (GC/MS). Twelve of 15 (80%) in each group achieved therapeutic plasma levels that were sustained for comparable periods (sublingual: median = 175 min; range 32–62 min; buccal: median = 160 min; range 43–209 min). It seems to us that given the young ages of these study participants, the swallowing of significant amounts of the opioid was inevitable. Weinberg et al. [28] administered sublingual methadone, 5 mg (0.8 or 5 mg/mL) to healthy volunteers, and measured the quantity of drug in the saliva expectorate after 10 min. Methadone absorption was 35% at pH 3.5 and 75% at pH 8.5, a statistically significant difference. The absorption of methadone at even the lower pH was significantly greater than it was for morphine, oxycodone, hydromorphone, levorphanol and heroin. Bioavailability was not influenced by the concentration of the methadone solution.

Hagen et al. [38] found difficult to reach the adequate number for an RCT on sublingual methadone for BTP. However, on a small number of patients treated with sublingual methadone at escalating doses ranging from 2 to 18 mg, they found

a significant relief of pain, with a median onset on 5 min and no serious adverse events. Further studies are warranted [39].

Fentanyl's potency, lipophilicity, and clinical efficacy have made it the object of intense interest for a variety of transmucosal applications.

The effects of sublingual fentanyl citrate (SLFC) were assessed in 11 hospice inpatients with cancer-related BTP [40]. SLFC was started at 25 mcg (using parenteral formulation of 50 mcg/mL), and the dose was progressively increased by 25 mcg till the pain was controlled. The maximum dose used was 150 mcg as volumes greater than 3 mL were difficult to retain sublingually. Fifty-five percent of patients reported pain reduction after 10 min and 82% after 15 min. Ratings for SLFC were very good (18%), good (36%), moderate (28%), and bad (18%). Compared to the usual breakthrough medication (mostly normal-release morphine), SLFC was better (46%), the same (36%), or worse (18%). No systemic adverse effects were reported. SLFC may be an option for patients unable to tolerate oral morphine in treating BTP.

Sublingual Fentanyl at a dose of 25 μcg after 3, 6, and 9 min produced pain relief, with a minimal sedation in one patient previously treated with oral morphine and with sublingual fentanyl [41]. Sufentanyl 25 mcg is approximately equianalgesic to 70–100 mg sublingual morphine, whereas 50 mcg sublingual fentanyl is about 7–10 mg sublingual morphine [42].

Oral transmucosal fentanyl citrate (OTFC) is a synthetic opioid agonist manufactured in a matrix of sucrose and liquid glucose base and fitted onto a radiopaque plastic handle. It is a drug-delivery formulation used for management of BTP cancer pain. Doses are available in six different strengths (200, 400, 600, 800, 1200, and 1600 μcg). Absorption is via the oral mucosa. Administration of a drug through this route avoids the first-pass effect, and allows easy and rapid dose titration. From the pharmacokinetic point of view, OTFC is similar to intramuscular and IV fentanyl, whereas the plasmatic concentrations are double in respect to oral fentanyl and are reached 86 min before [43,44]. Peak effect occurs in about 20 min. Approximately 25% of the dose of fentanyl goes directly into the bloodstream through mucosal absorption and accounts for 50% of the dose that reaches the plasma. Total bioavailability is approximately 50% as duration of action ranges from 2.5 to 5 hours. The onset of analgesic effect is obtained within 5–15 min [45] when compared to the 30–60 min with normal-release oral opioids. Seventy-six percent of patients with incidental pain, predictable pain and BTP have experienced favorable results [46].

In a multicenter, randomized, double-blind, placebo-controlled trial of OTFC for cancer-related BTP carried out by Farrar et al. [47**], OTFC produced significantly larger changes in PI and better pain relief than placebo. In another controlled dose titration study [48**] in cancer patients treated with OTFC, 74% of them were successfully titrated. Moreover, OTFC provided significantly greater analgesic effect at 15, 30, and 60 min, and a more rapid onset of effect, than the usual rescue drug. There was no relationship between the total daily dose of the fixed schedule opioid regimen and the dose of OTFC required to manage BTP. As the optimal dose cannot be predicted, treatment should begin with a dose of 200 μcg and increased at 15 min intervals.

It emerged from controlled and uncontrolled studies that the adverse effects of the OTFC were similar to other opioids and very few adverse events were severe or serious.

In a double-blind, double dummy, randomized, multiple cross-over study, Coluzzi et al. [49**] compared OTFC and immediate-release morphine sulfate for management of BTP in 134 outpatients receiving a fixed scheduled opioid regimen equivalent to 60–1000 mg/day oral morphine or 50–300 mcg/hour transdermal fentanyl. Sixty-nine percent of patients (93/134) found a dose of OTFC successful, and it proved to be more effective than the immediate-release oral morphine in treating BTP.

In an open-label study [50], OTFC also showed safety and effectiveness during the long-term treatment of BTP in cancer patients cared for at home.

Mucosites, and local infection, and dry mouth may limit the use or reduce the absorption of the drug. Serum fentanyl levels achieved with OTFC are proportional to the dose administered [51]. Absolute availability is about 50%; however, the percentage absorbed by mouth and available for treating BTP is about 25%, because 75% of the drug is swallowed [51].

OTFC is approved by Food and Drug Administration (FDA) solely for the management of BTP in opioid-tolerant cancer patients [52]. It is not recommended for treating acute and or postoperative pain. Future studies are required to establish that the OTFC dose can be used as a rescue dose in patients with BP in respect to type and dose of opioid taken by the patient.

Fentanyl is also available as a rapidly disintegrating sublingual tablet that is quickly absorbed and produces a fast onset of analgesia, as documented in two randomized double-blind clinical trials compared with placebo [53].

In a prospective, multicenter phase IV study [54], sublingual fentanyl orally disintegrating tablet (sublingual fentanyl ODT) was studied in 181 patients. During the study, 3163 episodes of BTP were treated with a mean dose of 401.4 mcg per episode. In respect to baseline, a significant improvement of maximum BTP intensity appeared with sublingual fentanyl ODT (p < 0.0001) within 5 min of administration in 67.7% of episodes and maximum effect within 30 min in 63% of episodes. Quality of life assessed by means of the modified pain disability index and emotional distress assessed by HADS significantly improved during observational period of 28 days. The drug was well tolerated.

FBT is a formulation of transmucosal fentanyl designed to provide a rapid penetration of fentanyl through the buccal mucosa by using effervescence to cause PH shifts that enhance the rate and extent of fentanyl absorption. A reasonable level of salivation is needed to allow dissolution. The tablet is placed between the upper gum and cheek, above a rear molar tooth, and patients are instructed to gently rub outside of the cheek until all material is dissolved. Fentanyl is rapidly absorbed from FBT, with a mean peak plasma concentration reached in 35–90 min. The absolute bioavailability of fentanyl from FBT was greater than from OTFC. FBT is absorbed in approximately equal proportions through the buccal mucosa and the GI tract, whereas, with OTFC, the proportion absorbed through the buccal mucosa was lower (22%) than that absorbed

gastrointestinally (78%). Thus, the drug immediately available to treat BTP is double that of OTFC (48% versus 22%). Sublingual placement of FBT resulted in similar values of pharmacokinetic parameters. Patients with cancer, particularly those undergoing chemotherapy or radiotherapy, may develop oral mucositis. In patients with mild mucositis, the absorption of fentanyl with FBT was not different from that of patients without mucositis. Controlled studies have reported the efficacy and safety of FBT in opioid-tolerant cancer patients with BTP even after 10 min, after performing a titration phase to determine the effective dose. There seemed to be no relationship between effective FBT dose and the dose of baseline opioid regimen [55]. Compared with OTFC, FBT has greater bioavailability (65% FBT versus 47% OTFC) and more is absorbed transmucosally (48% FBT versus 22% OTFC) [56].

The clinical efficacy of FBT in treating BTP associated with cancer pain has been well established in two randomized, placebo-controlled trials in opioid-tolerant cancer patients. The two studies, one with 123 patients and the other with 125 patients, received FBT in a double-blind fashion. Both documented clinically significant improvement in pain scores versus placebo. The significant greater reduction (p < 0.05 and p < 0.0001, respectively) in PI was achieved after FBT administration compared with placebo as early as 15 and 10 min, respectively.

Interestingly, patients with moderate or severe pain at baseline generally experienced greater improvements in pain than those with mild pain.

In these studies, for 35% of FBT-treated episodes, the efficacy at 60 min was rated as "very good" or "excellent." Also, use of supplemental medication for pain relief occurred more frequently during episodes of BTP when patients received placebo (50%) than with FBT (23%). In these studies, the beneficial effect of an effervescent fentanyl delivery system to a clinical endpoint of pain relief was compared only with placebo. Thus, there is the need to demonstrate its effect in further studies, comparing the clinical benefits with other compounds. In the studies with FBT as well as in other studies where BTP was treated with an orally fast-acting morphine tablet, an effervescent solution [13], or with OTFC, there was no simple linear relationship between the effective dose and the dose of the background opioid regimen. Not only does such an approach lack a solid base of evidence, but also accumulating data suggest that the optimal dose of BTP medication may bear little relationship to the around-the-clock dose [31]. Such results underline the need to titrate individually to effectiveness rather than calculate the percentage of an existing opioid regimen as previously suggested [57]. Fentanyl buccal soluble film (FBSF) is a new delivery technology. This delivery system contains an inactive outer layer, which separates the underlying fentanyl layer from saliva and thus reduces the amount of swallowed fentanyl. Each film is composed of a water-soluble polymer that dissolves completely, leaving no residual product. The buccal film contains citrate, which facilitates fentanyl absorption. The film is constructed in such a way that there is a direct relationship between the surface area of the membrane and the fentanyl dose [56]. Absolute bioavailability of FBSF was

71%, with 51% absorbed through the oral mucosal and the rest through the GI tract. This result is better than those reported with OTFC. The drug is available only in few countries.

INTRANASAL ADMINISTRATION

The nasal mucosa is the only location in the body that provides a direct connection between the central nervous system and the atmosphere. Anatomically, human nasal cavity fills the space between the base of the skull and the roof of the mouth; above, it is supported by the ethmoid bones and, laterally, by the ethmoid, maxillary, and inferior conchae bones. The human nasal cavity has a total volume of 15–20 mL, and a total surface area of approximately 150 cm^2. It is divided by middle (or nasal) septum into two symmetrical halves, each one opening at the face through nostrils and extending posterior to the nasopharynx. Both symmetrical halves consist of four areas (nasal vestibule, atrium, respiratory region, and olfactory region) that are distinguished according to their anatomic and histological characteristics. Nasal vestibule is the most anterior part of the nasal cavity, just inside the nostrils, and presents an area about 0.6 cm^2. Here, there are nasal hairs, also called vibrissae, which filter the inhaled particles. Histologically, this nasal portion is covered by a stratified squamous and keratinized epithelium with sebaceous glands. These nasal vestibular characteristics are desirable to afford high resistance against toxic environmental substances, but, at the same time, the absorption of substances including drugs becomes very difficult in this region [58,59].

Drugs administered to the nasal mucosa rapidly traverse through the cribriform plate into the central nervous system by three routes: (1) directly by the olfactory neurons, (2) through supporting cells and the surrounding capillary bed, and (3) directly into the cerebrospinal fluid (CSF) [60].

Drugs sprayed onto the olfactory mucosa are rapidly absorbed by three routes: by the olfactory neurons, by the supporting cells and the surrounding capillary bed, and into the CSF. Transneuronal absorption is generally slow, whereas absorption by the supporting cells and the capillary bed is rapid. A rapid rise in systemic blood levels has been demonstrated following the nasal administration of corticosteroids. For some drugs, administration by nasal spray results in a greater ratio of CSF to plasma concentration than does IV or duodenal administration, giving evidence for diffusion of these compounds through the perineural space around the olfactory nerves, a compartment known to be continuous with the subarachnoid space.

Pharmacokinetic data in volunteers are reported for fentanyl, alfentanil, sufentanil, butorphanol, oxycodone, morphine, diamorphine, hydromorphone, methadone, heroin, and buprenorphine [61–66]. From a clinical point of view, patient-controlled intranasal (PCIN) fentanyl has been compared with oral morphine for procedural wound care in burns patients [67**]. It has been observed that PCIN fentanyl is similar in efficacy and safety to oral morphine.

A rapid onset of analgesia and potential clinical utility for the treatment of postoperative pain have been suggested for a formulation of nasal fentanyl spray [68].

Jackson et al. [69] reported the experience on the first seven applications of intranasal sufentanil via PCIN for breakthrough and incident pain in four cancer patients. The initial dose of 4.5 mcg could be repeated at 10 and 20 min till a maximum of three doses of 36 mcg/daily. Very good pain relief was achieved within 30 min and lasted for around 2 hours. No serious adverse effects were reported.

The open-label, uncontrolled study evaluated the pharmacokinetics, safety, and efficacy of a single 40 mg dose of nasal morphine gluconate administered to 11 cancer patients in response to an episode of BTP [69]. This treatment was associated with effective plasma morphine concentrations, rapid onset of pain relief, and minor side effects (nasal irritation). Patient satisfaction ratings were high.

As morphine administered nasally shows a bioavailability of the order of 10% compared with IV administration, a novel chitosan-morphine nasal formulation has been produced and tested in both healthy volunteers and in 14 cancer patients with BTP [70,71]. Morphine was rapidly absorbed (Tmax of 15 min or less), with a bioavailability of nearly 60%.

In clinical settings, encouraging results have been obtained in patients receiving 5–80 mg of nasal morphine-chitosan, with an onset of pain relief 5 min after dosing.

Finally, it is interesting to note that transnasal butorphanol has proved to be effective in the treatment of opioid-induced pruritus unresponsive to 50 mg of i.v. dyphenhydramine [72]. The efficacy of intranasal fentanyl spray (INFS) was compared with that of OTFC for the relief of cancer-related BTP in an open-label, cross-over trial. INFS constitutes a promising new treatment option for BTP, having demonstrated a rapid onset of action (median 7 min) for the relief of dental postoperative pain [73], and a clinically important reduction in pain at 10 min postadministration in cancer patients with BTP.

The primary outcome of the study—time to onset of "meaningful" pain relief—demonstrated that a statistically significant number of patients experienced faster pain relief with INFS than with OTFC. Secondary and additional efficacy outcome measures also favored INFS over OTFC, with comparisons already being both statistically significant and clinically important at 5 min. INFS offers unique advantages over existing treatment options in cancer pain management. The pharmacodynamic profile of INFS fits very closely with the temporal characteristics of BTP, and the present study has shown that "meaningful" pain relief was obtained faster in patients treated with INFS than with OTFC. PI difference was significantly greater for INFS than OTFC from 5 min postdosing, and clinically important pain relief (≥33% reduction in PI) was seen 5 min after INFS treatment in a quarter of BTP episodes. Furthermore, INFS was easy to use, with the majority of patients preferring INFS over OTFC. It was well tolerated with a safety profile that is typical for this group of opioids.

INFS represents a considerable improvement in the clinicians' armamentarium for the treatment of BTP [73].

Recently, a fentanyl pectin nasal spray (FPNS) was developed to optimize the absorption profile of fentanyl across the nasal mucosa: An RCT trial showed that FPNS provides superior pain relief compared with placebo [74]. Davies et al. [75] studied the consistency of efficacy, tolerability, and patient acceptability of FPNS versus IRMS in 110 patients experiencing one to four BTP episodes/day during a background pain treatment with oral morphine or equivalent opioids ≥60 mg/day. At baseline and during an open dose titration phase (maximum 2 weeks) followed by a double-blind, double dummy treatment phase (from 3 to 21 days) and an end-of-treatment phase (1–14 days after the last dose) the PI was evaluated by means of an 11-point numeric scale (0 = no pain; 10 = worst possible pain) and pain relief was measured on a 5-point numeric scale (0 = none, 4 = complete) and recorded on e-diary at 5, 10, 15, 30, 45, and 60 min after dosing. Moreover, the patients rated the overall satisfaction and satisfaction with speed of relief (30 and 60 min), and reliability 60 min after the nasal spray using a 4-point scale (1 = not satisfied; 4 = very satisfied). After the last treated BTP episode, patients rated the ease of use and convenience of the nasal spray.

The per-episode analysis showed that a statistical significant difference in PI scores and in pain relief was in favor of FPNS versus IRMS by 10 min after the administration (p < 0.05). Overall acceptability scores were significantly greater for FPNS than for IRMS at 30 (p < 0.01) and 60 (p < 0.05). Most of the

patients were "satisfied/very satisfied" with the convenience (79.8%) and easy to use (77.2%) of FPNS. Nobody reported significant nasal effects.

SUBCUTANEOUS ROUTE

The rate of absorption of a drug strongly depends on the blood flow to the site of absorption. In normal conditions, the perfusion of SC tissue is similar to that of muscles. However, the rate of absorption is slower. The main factors determining the SC absorption are the solubility of the drug, the site of the injection, the surface exposed, the blood pressure, the presence of cutaneous vasoconstriction, edema, or inflammatory processes in cachectic patients and those with disturbed peripheral circulation. Greater volumes are infused for SC supplementation of liquids in the dehydrated patients.

Figure 46.1 shows the plasmatic concentration of morphine when administered via continuous SC infusion or as oral slow-release tablets.

SC opioid administration can be performed both intermittently (ISCI) and continuously (CSCI). In a randomized, double-blind cross-over trial, Watanabe et al. [76] compared CSCI and ISCI of opioid for treatment of cancer pain. Eligibility criteria included stable cancer pain requiring opioid therapy, need for parenteral route, and normal cognition. Patients were randomly assigned to receive opioid by CSCI by portable pump or ISCI by Edmonton injector for 48 hours, followed by cross-over to the alternative modality for 48 hours. During each

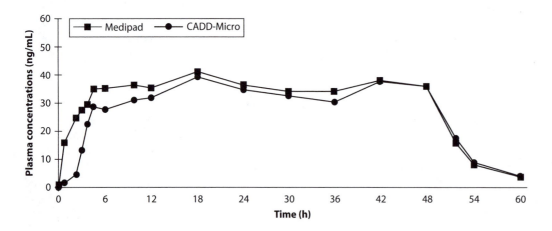

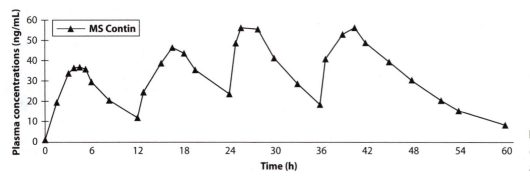

Figure 46.1 *Pharmacokinetics of oral and SC morphine: Continuous subcutaneous infusion.*

phase, placebo was administered by the alternative modality. The study was closed after 12 patients were enlisted, due to slow accrual. Eleven patients completed the study. There were no differences between CSCI and ISCI in mean visual analogue score (VAS) for pain, nausea, or drowsiness; categorical rating score of pain; number of breakthrough opioid doses per day; global rating of treatment effectiveness; or adverse effects. In all cases, patients and investigators expressed no preference for one modality over another. Further research is required to confirm that opioid administration by CSCI and ISCI provides similar analgesic and adverse effects [76]. A recent review demonstrated that CSI is effective and save for use in terminal illness [77]. Consistently with this evidence, it is gradually becoming a standard practice in palliative medicine. The SC route can also be used for patient-controlled analgesia (PCA) using portable pumps [78]. Patient-controlled analgesia (PCA) is a relatively new technique for managing pain in which patients are able to self-administer small doses of opioid analgesic when needed. This technique offers an alternative to traditional regimens and was developed in response to the undertreatment of pain in hospitalized patients. A number of uncontrolled and controlled trials have confirmed the safety and efficacy of PCA for postoperative pain in adults [79] as well as in children ranging from 5 to 15 years [78]. PCA is a very specific way of prescribing "as-needed" analgesics, because all parameters such as route, drug concentration, dose, frequency, and maximum daily or hourly dose are actually prescribed by the physician. The patient decides whether or not they should take a dose; the decision is not subject to external judgment and the administration is not slowed down by the intervention of the nurse or the doctor. A large variety of pumps are available for PCA. Most of them consist of a drug reservoir and an injection or infusion system, either manually or electronically operated. PCA devices permit the patient to choose an intermittent (demand) bolus, continuous infusion, or both intermittent and continuous modes of administration. A continuous infusion plus an intermittent bolus dose allow patients to maintain a baseline level of opioid administration plus additional doses for BTP. The device can be used to deliver the drug through continuous IV, epidural, SC infusions. Whenever the patient feels that pain relief is necessary, he/she can activate the system by pressing a button. The unit dispenses an amount of analgesic that has been programmed by the physician. In some devices, unauthorized alteration of dose parameters is excluded by a number of safety factors. A lock-out time is available in order to prevent overdosage. Other simpler and less expensive devices contain no "lock-out" system. While a "lock-out" system may be desirable for patients with confusion and/or a history of addiction, it is important to consider that oral prescriptions contain no "lock-out" mechanisms. This is a well-known therapeutic strategy in analgesia. Many different portable pumps or nonportable devices are available for CSI, including a syringe pump, disposable plastic cylinder, and battery-operated computer-driven pumps. It is important to select the most suitable solution for each patient. The disadvantages of these devices are their cost and complexity. Simpler and less expensive devices should be developed in

order to decrease the cost and increase the comfort of patients, families, and nurses. SC PCA has resulted particularly suitable also for the treatment of several types of postoperative pain [79,80]. This method is contraindicated in patients with coagulation disorders, cognitive failure, or with a history of substance abuse. Most studies of SC opioid administration have used morphine or hydromorphone. These drugs have short half-lives and hence reach the steady-state rapidly. Waldamann et al [81] reported that the blood levels of morphine during CSI are similar to those reached during continuous IV infusion. Another study in healthy volunteers provided different results, indicating that the bioavailabilities of morphine and of its main metabolites (M6G and M3G) are significantly lower after SC than after IV administration. Despite this observation, the authors concluded that the SC route is an effective method for the systemic administration of morphine [82]. No clear differences seem to exist between SC morphine and hydromorphone from both the pharmacokinetics and pharmacodynamic point of view [83**,84**]. Drugs with longer half-lives, such as methadone, have also been evaluated. In most patients, CSI of methadone produced signs of local toxicity (specifically erythema and induration). Such a toxicity is manageable by changing the position of the needle and infusing dexamethasone concurrently with the methadone [85,86]. In general, it is recommended the infusion be performed by using a 25 or 27 ga butterfly needle inserted in the anterior chest or abdomen. The SC route, with special reference to SCI, should be considered as the standard alternative route for systemic opioid delivery.

INTRAVENOUS ROUTE

IV administration of opioids permits complete systemic absorption, and produces rapid analgesia that is correlated to lipidic solubility (10–15 min for morphine, 2–5 min for methadone) but of short duration. This makes it necessary to repeat infusions at least every 4 hours.

Thus, this route of administration is painful for the patient, time-consuming for the nursing staff, and difficult to carry out in the home-setting.

Bolus administration can be substituted by continuous intravenous infusion (CIVI) using a pump. This type of administration very frequent in the cancer population during hospitalization above all in those with central venous catheters. CIVI of opioids has been reported to be effective and safe in managing cancer pain in patients who are less responsive to analgesics administered at the maximum tolerated dose by other routes [87,88]. PCA is also possible by IV route [78].

The most frequently used drugs are short-acting opioid agonists such as morphine, hydromorphone, and fentanyl [88,89**]. Because these drugs have a short half-life, the risk of delayed toxicity due to gradually increasing their plasmatic levels will be less likely than with drugs having longer half-lives such as methadone or levorphanol [141]. In the largest series reported to date, 117 consecutive cancer patients were treated with morphine (93%) or hydromorphone (7%) administered subcutaneously (87%) or intravenously (13%) with a PCA bolus set at 25% of the hourly infusion rate for BTP [90]. The mean duration of treatment was 23 days; 69% of patients were cared for at home, and the remaining patients were treated in an inpatient hospice. Most of the patients remained on PCA until death. After the initiation of PCA, 95% of patients achieved pain relief. Significant variability in opioid consumption was reported; the dose of morphine used ranged from 1 to 33 mg/hour in the SC group and from 2 to 180 mg/hour in the IV group. Complications developed in two patients (infection at the SC site in one patient and respiratory arrest within 24 hours of starting PCA in the other). The authors report that patients using the SC route who then required more than 40–50 mg/hour were switched to the IV route. PCA has been successfully used in patients presenting severe oral pain due to mucositis who required systemically administered opioid medication [78].

Over a certain period of time, some patients develop analgesic tolerance to this type of regimen, requiring frequent dose escalation. As noted earlier, if lower doses of opioid reduce psychological distress, one might rely on PCA alone during the day and a combination of PCA and continuous infusion during the night. Thus, these two modes of delivering PCA can be used together. PCA should be monitored by assessing the patient's respiratory rate and mental status and adequately modifying the opioid dosages if there is a decrease in the respiratory rate or if hypoxemia or somnolence occurs.

Although morphine is the drug of choice, clinical experience has shown that other drugs, such as methadone, hydromorphone, and fentanyl, can also be used successfully [88,91,92].

The choice of a drug for CIVI depends on the previous antalgic treatment and on the pharmacokinetic profile of the drug employed. If the patient refers a good analgesia with a particular opioid but presents adverse effects to a bolus administration (plasmatic peak toxicity or pain during the reduction of the plasmatic concentration), this is a suitable candidate for CIVI with the same drug. On the other hand, if the patient presents adverse effects at plasmatic peak and also refers poor or the absence of analgesia, the CIVI must be initiated with a different opioid. In choosing an analgesic drug, its half-life is by far the most important pharmacokinetic factor. For this reason, morphine and hydromorphone, both having short half-lives, are the preferred infusion drugs. With the use of long half-life medication such as methadone, the delay to steady-state may result in the slow onset of analgesia when CIVI is increased or in the late appearance of toxicity after analgesia appears. However, on increasing the CIVI, toxicity may develop some time after analgesic occurs.

The opioid dosage at the beginning of treatment depends on the patient's pharmacological intake. Patients treated with repeated parenteral doses can switch to CIVI with the same drug using the same daily dosage, whereas the administration of a different opioid would require a dosage reduction of between 1/2 and 2/3.

Portenoy et al. [88] reviewed the clinical experience of 36 patients who received CIVI. Mean doses during CIVI were equivalent to maximum morphine initial doses of 17 mg/hour (range 0.7–100), with maximum doses reaching 69 mg/hour (range 4–480) and 52 mg/hour (range 1–480) at the end of the treatment. Pain relief was acceptable in 28 CIVIs, unacceptable in 17, and unknown in one. The most important side effects, beginning or progressing during the CIVIs, were sedation, confusion, constipation, and myoclonus. This review suggests that CIVI is safe, that analgesia may require rapid dose escalation, and that while not all the patients had an acceptable analgesia, failure of CIVI with one medication because of incomplete cross-tolerance could be followed by effective analgesia obtained with a different opioid.

In a case report [93], hydromorphone administered via CIVI and then orally was able to prevent itching present during IV morphine administration.

Oral and IV oxycodone were compared in a single-dose study [94]. Although IV oxycodone produced a faster onset of pain relief, the duration of analgesia was about 4 hours with both routes of oxycodone administration; IV oxycodone produced significantly more adverse effects.

The pharmacokinetic of IV methadone showed rapid and extensive distribution phases followed by a slow elimination phase [95]. Manfredi et al. [96] described the dramatic beneficial effects of IV methadone in four patients in whom IV morphine and hydromorphone failed to produce adequate pain relief despite titration to dose-limiting side effects. All the patients had long-lasting pain relief without significant side effects at a methadone dose equal to 20% of the hydromorphone dose. Fitzgibbon et al. [97] described the successful use of large doses of IV methadone administered by PCA and continuous infusion for pain refractory to large doses of IV morphine. Morphine was stopped, and treatment with methadone via PCA was initiated (incremental dose 10 mg every 6 min) with a continuous infusion of methadone at a rate of 40 mg/hour. On day 3, methadone was decreased to 200 mg, with a good pain management and no adverse effects. The patient was discharged after 5 days with a dose of 220 mg/day (average daily methadone was approximately 1/10 that of morphine). After 6 weeks, the dose was increased up to 400 mg/day, with good pain control and no adverse effects.

IV methadone administered by PCA was safe and effective in controlling cancer pain, sedation, and confusion in 18 patients previously treated with IV fentanyl. A conversion ratio of 25 mcg/hour of fentanyl to 0.1 mg/hour of methadone was used to estimate the initial dose of methadone in all patients (0.25 ratio between fentanyl and methadone) [92].

Self-administered bolus doses of IV methadone equal to 50%–100% of the hourly infusion rate were allowed every 20 min and additional boluses of 100%–200% of the hourly infusion rate every 60 min. To control pain, there was a 10% increase in the median hourly infusion dose of methadone from day 1 (64.45 mg) to day 2; after day 2, the median hourly infusion dose of methadone was the same and decreased to 54 mg on day 4.

Numerous medications prolong the rate-corrected QT (QTc) interval and induce arrhythmias by blocking ionic current through cardiac potassium channels composed of subunits expressed by the human ether-a-go-go-related gene (HERG). Recent reports suggest that high doses of methadone cause torsades de pointes [98]. Kornick et al. [99] found that methadone in combination with chlorobutanol (the preservative present in the formulation of parenteral methadone) is associated with QTc interval prolongation.

Even if the titration with strong opioids is commonly performed using immediate-release oral morphine every 4 hours, there are some clinical situations such as severe pain where pain relief has to be achieved as quickly as possible. Tables 46.4 [100–102**] and 46.5 [103,104] show the studies reporting "fast

titration" resulting in rapid pain relief of moderate to severe pain in cancer patients treated with bolus doses of IV morphine or fentanyl and then switched to oral morphine or transdermal fentanyl. These authors show that "fast titration" with IV opioids is effective and safe.

At the Memorial Sloan-Kettering Cancer Center in New York, the patients on transdermal fentanyl presenting severe episodes of pain are switched (TTS removed) to CIVI of fentanyl using a transdermal:IV conversion of 1:1 [105]. PCA IV

Table 46.4   *Intravenous titration (dose finding) with morphine for severe cancer pain*

Authors (Ref.)	Study design and patient population	Initial morphine dosage and route	Following dosage and route	Results
Radbruch et al. [100]	Prospective study. 26 inpatients with uncontrolled pain, on step II opioids.	IV PCA pump programmed for 24 hours: 1 mg bolus, lock-out interval of 5 min. Max. dose of 12 mg/h.	Oral SR morphine q12h; dose on the basis of the previous IV requirements. IV-PO conversion 1:2. BTP treated with IV PCA until stable analgesia was reached.	Mean PI (NRS 0–100): At entry: 67 After 5 hours: 22 At day 7: 17 At day 14: 12 Mean morphine dosage (IV PCA) in the first 24 hours: 32 mg (range 4–78) Mean daily morphine dosage (PO + IV PCA for BTP) at PCA termination (range 2–6 days): 139 mg (range 20–376) Mean morphine dosage (PO) at day 14: 154 mg (range 20–344) No significant adverse events
Mercadante et al. [101]	Prospective study. 45 inpatients with severe (NRS ≥ 7) and prolonged pain. At entry, 30 patients. were on step II opioids, 15 were on step III opioids.	IV bolus (2 mg every 2 min), repeated until analgesia or adverse effects were reported.	Oral SR morphine; dose on the basis of the previous IV requirements. IV-PO conversion: 1:3 for lower IV dosages, 1:2 for higher IV dosages. The same IV dose was maintained for BTP in the first 24 hours	Mean PI (NRS 0–10): At entry: 8.1 After 9.7 min: 3.0 with a mean IV morphine dosage of 8.5 mg Mean daily oral morphine dosage at time to discharge: 131 mg (107–156) + 10.8 mg (IV extra doses). No significant adverse events
Harris et al. [102]	RCT. 62 strong opioid naïve in patients PI NRS ≥ 5. Patients were randomized to receive IV morphine (n = 31) or oral IR morphine (n = 31).	*IV group:* 1.5 mg bolus every 10 min until pain relief (or adverse effects). *Oral group:* IR morphine 5 mg every 4 hours in opioids naive pts. 10 mg in patients on weak opioids. Rescue dose: the same dose every 1 hour max.	*IV group:* Oral IR morphine q4h, on the basis of the previous IV requirements. IV:PO conversion 1:1. Rescue dose: the same dose every 1 hour max. *Oral group:* Follow the same scheme.	% of patients achieving satisfactory pain relief: After 1 hour: IV group, 84%; oral group, 25% (p < 0.001) After 12 hours: IV group 97%; oral group 76% (p < 0.001) After 24 hours: IV group and oral group similar *IV group:* Median morphine dosage (IV) to achieve pain relief: 4.5 mg (range 1.5–34.5). In the same group, mean morphine dosage (PO) after stabilization,: 8.3 (range 2.5–30)mg *Oral group:* Median morphine dosage to achieve pain relief: 7.2 (2.5–15) mg. No significant adverse events

IV, intravenous; PCA, patient-controlled analgesia; NRS, numerical rating scale; step II of the W.H.O. analgesic ladder; BTP, breakthrough pain.

Table 46.5 *Intravenous titration (dose finding) with fentanyl for severe cancer pain*

Authors (Ref.)	Study design and patients population	Initial morphinefentanyl dosage and route	Following dosage and route	Results
Soares et al. [103]	Prospective study. 18 outpatients' PI NRS ≥7, on oral morphine therapy for at least 2 weeks. Excluded patients with BTP and neuropathic pain.	Repeated IV bolus in four steps, with 5 min intervals. Evaluation of pain and side effects after each step. Dosage: Oral morphine converted to IV morphine (dose ratio 1:3) and then to IV fentanyl (dose ratio 1:100). Step 1 and 2: 10% of the total IV morphine taken in the previous 24 hours. Step 3 and 4: step 1 and 2 dosage increased by 50%.	The protocol was not performed to find future doses of opioids. The management of pain after the fast titration with fentanyl was 9 patients increased the previous morphine dose. 3 patients switched to the opioid. 5 patients switched to the route. 5 patients received ketamine infusion.	100% of patients achieving satisfactory pain relief. Mean time to achieve pain relief: 11 min (range 5–25 min) PI less than 4 Mean previous oral morphine dosage 276 mg (range 180–600). Mean IV fentanyl required to achieve pain relief: 214 µg (range 60–525). No significant adverse events.
Grond et al. [104]	Prospective study. 50 GI or head and neck cancer patients with severe pain. Excluded patients with BTP and opioid unresponsive pain.	Previous opioids were discontinued and PCA IV fentanyl started: demand dose 50 µg, lock-out time 5 min, hourly max dose 250 µg	On the second day TTS applied with a rate delivery calculated from the PCA dose[a] of the first 24 hours + IV fentanyl for rescue doses during first and second day, thereafter oral or SC morphine for rescue doses. If PI increased at the end of the 72 hours period and an increase of the TTS dose was ineffective, the systems were changed every 48 hours.	The patients were treated for 66 ± 101 days (3–535). The mean delivery rate was 5.9 ± 4.1 mg/day. The mean PI decreased from initially 45 ± 21 to 19 ± 15 in the titration phase and 15 ± 11 during long-term treatment. 3 patients had moderate respiratory depression moderate or severe constipation in 40% of the patients prior to study, in 18% during titration period and in 10% during long-term treatment.

IV, intravenous; NRS, numerical rating scale; BTP, breakthrough pain; GI, gastrointestinal; TTS, transdermal therapeutic system; SC, subcutaneous.

[a] PCA IV fentanyl (mg/day)   TTS fentanyl (mg/day)

PCA IV fentanyl (mg/day)	TTS fentanyl (mg/day)
0.2–0.6	0.6
0.6–1.0	1.2
1.0–1.4	1.8
1.4–1.8	2.4

fentanyl is used to administered rescue on demand doses (50%–100% of the CIVI rate). Relief of pain without serious adverse effects is reported [105].

Continuous parenteral (SC or IV) opioids improved analgesia and tolerability in 71% of cancer patients previously treated with oral opioids (codeine, tramadol, morphine, methadone) or with transdermal fentanyl. On the basis of this study, parenteral opioids may be considered a good alternative to spinal opioids [106].

CIVI of opioids used in cancer-related pain are specifically indicated in cases of generalized edema, coagulation disorders, increased frequency of SC local site infections, reduced peripheric circulation, when frequent IM or IV injections are required to maintain pain control, in the presence of prominent "bolus effects" on repetitive injection and when rapid titration of drug doses is required to produce rapid pain relief.

Opioid administration through CIVI can be carried out via central venous catheters; however, these catheters are expensive and need to be surgically implanted and require considerable nursing expertise and/or teaching the patient's family. For these reasons, CIVI should be considered only for patients with an implanted catheter and for patients who present bleeding diathesis or diminished muscle mass who develop intractable vomiting, bowel obstruction, or malabsorption.

Date of literature [107–108] show that EV and SC routes are equianalgesic for most patients when administered as a continuous infusion. Pain control and side effects are quite and acceptable. SC morphine is an excellent alternative to IV morphine in both inpatients and outpatients requiring parenteral morphine for pain. Moreover SC morphine is easier to administer.

TRANSDERMAL ROUTE

Substances with high lipid solubility and molecular weight below 800–1000 daltons (kDa) can pass through the skin. The absorption rate varies according to different factors such as the type of the vehicle, the skin characteristics (the thickness of stratum corneum) and conditions, the body surface. In general drugs that are successfully administered transdermally are those in which the daily dose is very low (no more than a few milligrams). Patient compliance with this route of administration is excellent, and skin reactions are rarely observed.

Among opioids, the potent synthetic drug "fentanyl citrate" is particularly suitable for transdermal administration, and its utility in pain therapy has been extensively evaluated. Transdermal fentanyl systems (TTS) are available in four release programs of 25, 50, 75, and 100 µg/hour, depending on the patch size, and the drug is released continuously for 3 days. A substantial amount of fentanyl remains in used systems even after 3 days of application [109]. When a TTS is removed, fentanyl continues to be absorbed into the systemic circulation from the cutaneous depot. However, opioid withdrawal symptoms may occur after discontinuation of TTS administration, as well as after conversion from other opioids to TTS [110,111]. Moreover, withdrawal symptoms were reported during chronic TTS administration and were managed with oral methadone [112].

Pharmacokinetic studies demonstrated that the rate of absorption of fentanyl from the transdermal delivery is constant, beginning 4–8 hours after placement of the patches. Steady-state is reached on the third day. However, a wide individual variability exists [113]. There is a lag period after patch application before plasma concentrations approach therapeutic levels. This lag period is highly variable, with a mean value of about 13 hours [114]. The TTS should be changed every third day. However, published data show that application intervals have to be shortened in about 25% of patients [115] at 48–60 hours because on the third day of each patch period, the need of rescue doses of short release oral morphine was major of first and second day [114,115]. In 11%–43% of patients during long-term treatment, the patch had to be changed every 48 hours [113].

The effectiveness of TTS fentanyl was first demonstrated in postoperative pain. Especially for the high incidence of respiratory depression, this use is now contraindicated. Conversely, in stable, chronic, cancer pain, this formulation offers an interesting alternative to oral morphine [114,116–118]. In comparison with oral morphine, TTS fentanyl seems to cause fewer GI side effects, with special reference to constipation [119,120]. Its usefulness in chronic, nonmalignant pain is also strongly suggested by recently published papers [121,122]. Of course, this formulation is contraindicated during the titration phase, or to control BTP.

The permeability coefficient for fentanyl is affected by temperature. A rise in body temperature to 40°C may increase the absorption rate by about one-third [119]. Acute toxicity related to increased absorption secondary to high temperature has

been reported [123]. A recent study in volunteers demonstrated that the application of local heat to the transdermal patch significantly increased systemic delivery of fentanyl [124].

Four cases of death due to the IV injection of fentanyl extracted from transdermal patches have been recently reported [125]. To minimize the problem of the "dose-dumping" due to membrane damage, and the risk of illegal diversion, a transdermal matrix patch formulation of fentanyl has been developed. Furthermore, a new system, called the electrotransport transdermal system, has been developed, which allows the drug-delivery rate to be varied electrophoretically. Further studies are necessary to verify the utility of this new formulation.

The partial agonist *buprenorphine* is another ideal candidate for delivery via a transdermal patch [126]. In the currently available formulation (buprenorphine transdermal delivery system, TDS), this drug is incorporated in a polymer adhesive matrix, from which it is released through the skin. Transdermal buprenorphine has a bioavailability of about 50%, which is comparable to that observed after sublingual administration [127]. Buprenorphine patches are available in three dosage strengths. The patches are loaded with 20, 30, or 40 mg of buprenorphine and are designed to release the opioid at a controlled rate of 35, 52.5, and 70 µg/hour, corresponding to a daily dose of 0.8, 1.2, and 1.6 mg, respectively. All the patches are designed for a 72 hours application period. They should be applied to a flat and hairless area of noninflamed skin, preferably on the upper back, subclavicular region, or chest. Following their removal, buprenorphine plasma levels slowly decrease. The manufacturers suggest that additional opioids should not be administered within 24 hours of patch removal. *Buprenorphine* TDS has been used and investigated less extensively than fentanyl TTS. The available data suggest that it may represent an effective analgesic against chronic pain [128**].

Although comparative analysis between the analgesia and the tolerability of TD and oral opioids shows that transdermal opioids are at least equivalent to the oral opioids [129], it is well known that transdermal fentanyl and transdermal buprenorphine are best reserved for patients whose opioids requirements are stable [130]. They are usually the treatment of choice for patients who are unable to swallow, patients with poor tolerance of morphine, and patients with poor compliance.

An important characteristic of the pharmacokinetics of TD buprenorphine is its safe use in patients with renal impairment. Also hemodialysis does not affect buprenorphine plasma levels, and this result leads to a stable analgesic effect [131,132].

TOPICAL OPIOIDS

The use of topical opioids in the treatment of pain in malignant and nonmalignant oropharyngeal mucositis and ulcers is based on the discovery of peripheral opioids receptors that may be enhanced by the presence of inflammation [133,134]. Moreover, morphine and its metabolites are largely undetectable systemically when applied topically to skin ulcers [135]. Kalso et al. [136] have found the efficacy of peripheral opioids injections for local analgesia, such as intra-articular morphine after knee surgery.

In a pilot randomized study, Cerchietti et al. [137] evaluated the role of morphine oral rinses administered with 15 mL of either 1 per 1000 or 2 per 1000 morphine solution in patients with painful chemoradiotherapy-induced stomatitis. Rinses with 2 per 1000 morphine solution showed better pain relief (median 80%) than those with 1 per 1000 (median 60%, p = 0.0238). No morphine was detectable in the blood through GC-MS analysis. The most important side effect due to oral morphine rinses was burning sensation.

In a next study, Cerchietti et al. [138] randomized 22 patients with painful mucositis due to chemoradiotherapy for head and neck cancer to receive morphine mouthwash (MO; 1/4 patients) or magic mouthwash (MG) composed by equal parts of lidocaine, diphenhydramine, and magnesium aluminum hydroxide (12 patients). Patients on morphine mouthwashes compared with MG group (1) had a lesser number of days (3.5) with pain (p = 0.032); (2) had a significantly lower intensity of pain (p = 0.038); (3) did not require strong opioids to relieve pain; (4) showed significant difference in the duration of severe functional impairment (p = 0.017); (5) had less local side effects (p = 0.007).

Topical morphine administered as mouthwashes during chemoradiotherapy may be considered effective in reducing painful mucositis in head and neck cancer patients.

Sublingual methadone is considered a promising therapeutic option in treating painful mucositis [139]; however, further research is necessary.

Opioids such as morphine [140] and diamorphine [141] have also been used to reduce pain in patients with ulcers as gel applications by means of Intransite Gel®, which is an aqueous gel that in contact with a wound absorbs excess exudates and produces a moist environment at the surface.

Zeppetella and Ribeiro [140] randomized 21 hospice inpatients with painful ulcers to receive topically either morphine (morphine sulfate injection 10 mg/mL in 8 g Intrasite gel) or placebo (water for injection 1 mL in 8 g Intrasite gel). After 2 days of treatment and 2 days of washout period, a cross-over was performed. Topical morphine produced significantly lower pain, as assessed by numerical rating scale (NRS) score, compared with pretreatment period and placebo group (p < 0.001) and showed no difference in rescue doses requirement. Patients reported some local effects such as itching and burning sensation. About 70% of patients under investigation preferred morphine to placebo.

In a randomized double-blind, placebo-controlled study, diamorphine gel was used in 13 patients with painful grade II or III pressure ulcers. Only seven patients completed the study. Pain score significantly improved after diamorphine gel application compared with placebo (p < 0.05). No side effects were found.

In agreement with LeBon et al. [142], we believe that despite the positive results of topical opioids on pain conditions, further research on larger sample of patients is necessary.

Key learning points

- An alternative route for opioid administration should be considered when oral administration is not possible or in the presence of poor pain control and/or adverse effects.

- The oral route is not suitable in clinical situations such as severe vomiting, bowel obstruction, dysphagia, severe confusion, and where rapid dose escalation is necessary.

- Each alternative route has indications or contraindications depending on the clinical history of the patient.

- Pharmacokinetic and pharmacodynamic characteristics of the different opioid analgesics should be carefully considered to individualize the therapy.

- The rectal route has the advantage of being simpler than the SC or IV routes; however, chronic rectal administration can lead to patient discomfort.

- Sublingual and buccal routes may deserve special attention for the administration of highly lipophilic opioids such as methadone, fentanyl, and buprenorphine.

- Continuous SCI ± extra boluses (PCA) represents the standard alternative route for systemic opioid delivery.

- IV administration is particularly indicated for "fast titration" and dose finding in patients with severe pain and in those with an implanted central venous catheter.

- The intranasal route may offer some advantages in treating BTP; however, further studies are needed.

- The transdermal route is a widely used and a comfortable way for opioid delivery. However, it should be reserved for patients whose opioid requirements are stable after the end of the "titration phase."

REFERENCES

1 Bruera E, MacMillan K, Hanson J. Palliative care in a cancer center: Results in 1984 versus 1987. *J Pain Symptom Manage* 1990; 5: 1–5.

2 Cherny NJ, Chang V, Frager G, Ingham JM, Tiseo PJ, Popp B, Portenoy R, Foley KM. Opioid pharmacotherapy in the management of cancer pain: A survey of strategies used by pain physicians for the selection of analgesic drugs and routes of administration. *Cancer* 1995; 76: 1283–1293.

3 Radbruch L, Trottemberg P, Elsner F, Kaasa S, Caraceni A. Systematic review of the role of alternative application routes for opioid treatment for moderate to severe cancer pain: An EPCRC opioid guidelines project. *Palliat Med* 2010; 25–5: 578–596.

4 Hanks GW, De Conno F, Cherny N et al. Expert Working Group of the Research Network of the European Association for Palliative Care. Morphine and alternative opioids in cancer pain: The EAPC recommendations. *Br J Cancer* 2001; 84/5: 587–593.

5 Ripamonti C, Bruera E. Rectal, buccal, and sublingual narcotics for the management of cancer pain. *J Palliat Care* 1991; 7/1: 30–35.

◆ 6 Cole L, Hanning CD. Review of the rectal use of opioids. *J Pain Symptom Manage* 1990; 5: 118–126.
◆ 7 Davis MP, Walsh D, LeGrand SB, Naughton M. Symptom control in cancer patients: The clinical pharmacology and therapeutic role of suppositories and rectal suspension. *Support Care Cancer* 2002; 10: 117–138.
● 8 Johnson T, Christensen CB, Jordening H et al. The bioavailability of rectally administered morphine. *Pharmacol Toxicol* 1988; 62: 203–205.
● 9 Sawe J, Dahlstrom B, Paalzow L et al. Morphine kinetics in cancer patients. *Clin Pharmacol Ther* 1981; 30: 629–635.
10 Breda M, Bianchi M, Ripamonti C, Zecca E, Ventafridda V, Panerai AE. Plasma morphine and morphine 6-glucuronide patterns in cancer patients after oral, subcutaneous, sublabial and rectal short-term administration. *J Clin Pharm Res* 1991; XI (2): 93–97.
11 Osborne R, Joel S, Trew D. Morphine and metabolite behaviour after different route of morphine administration: Demonstration of the importance of the active metabolite morphine 6-glucuronide. *Clin Pharmacol Ther* 1999; 47: 12–19.
12 Pannuti F, Rossi AP, Iafelice G et al. Control of chronic pain in very advanced cancer patients with morphine hydrochloride administered by oral, rectal, and sublingual route. *Pharmacol Res Commun* 1982; 14: 369–381.
13 Ellison NM, Lewis GO. Plasma concentrations following single doses of morphine sulphate in oral solution and rectal suppository. *Clin Pharmacy* 1984; 3: 614–617.
14 Moolenar F, Yska JP, Visser J et al. Drastic improvement in the rectal absorption profile of morphine in man. *Eur J Clin Pharmacol* 1985; 29: 119–121.
15 Kaiko RF, Healy N, Pav J et al. The comparative bioavailability of MS Contin tablets (controlled-release oral morphine) following rectal and oral administration. *The Edinburgh Symposium on Pain Control and Medical Education*, D. Doyle (ed.). 1989. Royal Soc of Med Serv Int'l Congresses and Symposium N° 149. Royal Soc of Med Services Ltd. Edinburgh, October 1988.
16 Maloney CM, Kesner RK, Klein G et al. The rectal administration of MS Contin: Clinical implications of use in end-stage cancer. *Am J Hospice Care*, July/Aug 1989; 6/4: 34–35.
17 Walsh D, Tropiano PS. Long-term rectal administration of high-dose sustained-release morphine tablets. *Support Care Cancer* 2002; 10: 653–655.
● 18 Bruera E, Faisinger R, Spachinsky K, Suarez-Almazor M, Inturrisi C. Clinical efficacy and safety of a novel controlled-release morphine suppository and subcutaneous morphine in cancer pain: A randomized evaluation. *J Clin Oncol* 1995; 13: 1520–1527.
● 19 Babul N, Provencher L, Laberge F, Harsanyi Z, Moulin D. Comparative efficacy and safety of controlled-release morphine suppositories and tablets in cancer pain. *J Clin Pharmacol* 1998; 38: 74–81.
● 20 De Conno F, Ripamonti C, Saita L, MacEachern T, Hanson J, Bruera E. Role of rectal route in treating cancer pain: A randomized crossover clinical trial of oral vs rectal morphine administration in opioid-naive cancer patients with pain. *JCO* 1995; 13: 1004–1008.
● 21 Bruera E, Belzile M, Neumann CM, Ford I, Harsanyi Z, Darke A. Twice-daily versus once-daily morphine sulphate controlled-release suppositories for the treatment of cancer pain. A randomized controlled trial. *Support Care Cancer* 1999; 7: 280–283.
22 Ripamonti C, Zecca E, Brunelli C, Rizzio E, Saita L, Lodi F, De Conno F. Rectal methadone in cancer patients with pain. A preliminary clinical and pharmacokinetic study. *Ann Oncol* 1995; 6: 841–843.
23 Bruera E, Watanabe S, Faisinger R, Spachynski K, Suarez-Almazor M, Inturrisi C. Custom-made capsules and suppositories of methadone for patients on high-dose opioids of cancer pain. *Pain* 1995; 62: 141–146.

24 Leow KP, Cramond T, Smith MT. Pharmacokinetics and pharmacodynamics of oxycodone when given intravenously and rectally to adults patients with cancer pain. *Anesth Analg* 1995; 80: 296–302.
25 Mercadante S, Arcuri E, Fusco F, Tirelli W, Villari P, Bussolino C et al. Randomized double-blind, double-dummy crossover clinical trial of oral vs rectal tramadol administration in opioid-naive cancer patients with pain. *Support Care Cancer* 2005; 13: 702–707.
● 26 Ritschel WA, Parab PV, Denson DD, Coyle DE, Gregg RV. Absolute bioavailability of hydromorphone after peroral and rectal administration in humans: Saliva/plasma ratio and clinical effects. *J Clin Pharmacol* 1987; 27: 647–653.
27 Hojsted J, Rubeck K, Peterson H. Comparative bioavailability of a morphine suppository given rectally and in a colostomy. *Eur J Clin Pharmacol* 1999; 39: 49–50.
● 28 Weinberg DS, Inturrisi CE, Reidewberg B et al. Sublingual absorption of selected opioid analgesics. *Clin Pharmacol Ther* 1988; 44: 335–342.
29 Wallenstein SL, Kaiko RF, Rogers AG et al. Clinical analgesic assay of sublingual buprenorphine and intramuscular morphine. In: Cooper JR, Altman F, Brown BS et al. eds. *NIDA Research Monography*. Vol. 41. Problems of drug dependence. Rockville, MD: USDHHS 1981; pp. 288–293.
30 Bullingham RES, McQuay HJ, Dwyer D et al. Sublingual buprenorphine used post-operatively: Clinical observations and preliminary pharmacokinetic analysis. *Br J Clin Pharmac* 1981; 12: 117–122.
31 Bullingham RES, McQuay HJ, Moore RA. Clinical pharmacokinetics of narcotic agonist-antagonist drug. *Clin Pharmacol* 1983; 8: 332–343.
32 Robbie DS. A trial of sublingual buprenorphine in cancer pain. *Br J Clin Pharmacol* 1979; 7: 315–317. S
33 De Conno F, Ripamonti C, Sbanotto A, Barletta L. A clinical note ob sublingual buprenorphine. *J Palliat Care* 1993; 9/3: 44–46.
34 Gal T. Naloxone reversal of buprenorphine-induced respiratory depression. *Clin Pharmacol Ther* 1989; 45: 66–71.
◆ 35 Coluzzi PH. Sublingual morphine: Efficacy reviewed. *J Pain Symptom Manage* 1998; 16: 184–192.
36 Whitman HH, Sublingual morphine: A novel route of narcotic administration. *Am J Nurs* 1984; 84: 939–940.
37 Kokki H, Rasanen I, Lasalmi M, Lethola S, Ranta VP, Vanamo K, Ojanpera I. Comparison of oxycodone pharmacokinetics after buccal and sublingual administration in children. *Clin Pharmacokinet* 2006; 45/7: 745–754.
38 Hagen NA, Moulin DE, Brascer PM, Brando PD et al. A formal feasibility study of sublingual methadone for breakthrough cancer pain. *Palliat Med* 2010; 24/7: 696–706.
39 Hagen NA, Fisher K, Stiles C. Sublingual methadone for the management of cancer related pain. *J Palliat Med* 2007; 10/2: 331–337.
40 Zeppetella G. Sublingual fentanyl citrate for cancer-related breakthrough pain: A pilot study. *Palliat Med* 2001; 15: 323–328.
41 Kunz KM, Theisen JA, Schroeder ME. Severe episodic pain: Management with sublingual sufentanyl. *J Pain Symptom Manage* 1993; 8/4: 189–190.
42 American Hospital Formulary Service. *Drug Information 1992*. Bethesda, MD: American Hospital Formulary Service, 1992: pp. 1134, 1155.
43 Streisand JB, Varvel JR, Stanki DR et al. Absorption and bioavailability of oral transmucosal fentanyl citrate. *Anesthesiology* 1991; 75: 223–229.
44 Fine PG, Marcus M, De Boer AJ et al. An open label study of oral transmucosal fentanyl citrate (OTFC) for the treatment of breakthrough cancer pain. *Pain* 1991; 45: 149.
● 45 Streisand JB, Busch MA, Egan TD et al. Dose proportionality and pharmacokinetics of oral transmucosal fentanyl citrate. *Anesthesiology* 1998; 88: 305–309.

46 Christie JM, Simmonds M, Patt R, Coluzzi P, Busch MA, Nordbrock E, Portenoy RK. Dose titration: A multicenter study of oral transmucosal fentanyl citrate for the treatment of breakthrough pain in cancer patients using transdermal fentanyl for persistent pain. *J Clin Oncol*, 1998; 16: 3238–3245.

47 Farrar JT, Clearly J, Rauck R, Busch M, Nordbrock E. Oral transmucosal fentanyl citrate: Randomized, double-blinded, placebo-controlled trial for treatment of breakthrough pain in cancer patients. *J Natl Cancer Inst* 1998; 90/8: 611–616.

● 48 Portenoy RK, Payne R, Coluzzi P, Raschko W, Lyss A, Busch MA et al. Oral transmucosal fentanyl citrate (OTFC) for the treatment of breakthrough pain in cancer patients: A controlled dose titration study. *Pain*, 1999; 79: 303–312.

● 49 Coluzzi PH, Schwartzberg L, Conroy JD, Charapata S, Gay M, Busch MA et al. Breakthrough cancer pain: A randomized trial comparing oral transmucosal fen tanyl citrate (OTFC) and morphine sulphate immediate release (MSIR). *Pain* 2001; 91: 123–130.

50 Payne R, Coluzzi P, Hart L, Simmonds M, Lyss A, Rauck R et al. Long-term safety of oral transmucosal fentanyl citrate for breakthrough cancer pain. *J Pain Symptom Manage* 2001; 22: 575–583.

51 Haronoff G, Brennan M, Pritchard D, Ginsberg B. Evidence-based oral trasmucosal fentanyl citrate (OTFC) dosing guidelines. *Pain Med* 2005; 6: 305–314.

52 Lipman AG. New and alternative noninvasive opioid dosage forms and routes of administration. *Support Oncol*, Updates 2000; 3(1): 1–8.

53 Chwieduk CM, Mc Keage K. Fentanyl syblingual in breakthrough pain in opioid-tolerant adults with cancer. *Drugs* 2010 70/17: 2281–2288.

54 Uberall MA, Muller-Schwefe Gerhard HH. Sublingual fentanyl orally disintegrating tablet in daily practice: Efficacy, safety and tolerability in patients with breakthrough cancer pain. *Curr Med Res Opin* 2011; 27/7: 1385–1394.

55 Mercadante S. The use of rapid onset opioids for breakthrough cancer pain: The challenge of its dosing. *Crit Rev Oncol/Hematol* 2011; 80: 460–465.

56 Mellar DP. Fentanyl for breakthrough pain: A systematic review. *Expert Rev Neurother*. 2011; 11/8: 1197–1216.

57 Freye E. A new transmucosal drug delivery system for patients with breakthrough cancer pain: The fentanyl effervescent buccal tablet. *J Pain Res* 2009; 2: 13–20.

58 Pires A, Fortuna A, Alves G, Falcao A. Intranasal drug delivery: How, why, and what for? *J Pharm Pharmaceut Sci* 2009; 12/13: 288–311.

59 Gopinath PG, Gopinath G, Kumar TCA. Target Site of intranasally sprayed substances and their transport across the nasal mucosa: A new insight into the intranasal route of drug-delivery. *Curr Ther Res* 1978; 23: 596–607.

60 Hilger PA. *Fundamentals of Otolaryngology, A Textbook of Ear, Nose and Throat Diseases*. 6th edn. Philadelphia, PA: WB Saunders Co; 1989; p. 184.

61 Turker S, Onur E, Ozer Y. Nasal route and drug delivery systems. *Pharm World Sci* 2004; 26: 137–142.

◆ 62 Dale O, Hjortkjaer R, Kharasch ED. Nasal administration of opioids for pain management in adults. *Acta Anaesth Scand* 2002; 46: 759–770.

63 Takala A, Kaasalainen TA, Seppala T, Kalso E, Olkkola KT. Pharmacokinetic comparison of intravenous and intranasal administration of oxycodone. *Acta Anaesth Scand* 1997; 41: 309–312.

● 64 Kendall JM, Latter VS. Intranasal diamorphine as an alternative to intramuscular morphine: Pharmacokinetic and pharmacodynamic aspects. *Clin Pharmacokinet* 2003; 42: 501–513.

65 Dale O, Hoffer C, Sheffels P, Kharasch ED. Disposition of nasal, intravenous, and oral methadone in healthy volunteers. *Clin Pharmacol Ther* 2002; 72: 536–545.

66 Coda BA, Rudy AC, Archer SM, Wermeling DP. Pharmacokinetics and bioavailability of single-dose intranasal hydromorphone hydrochloride in healthy volunteers. *Anesth Analg* 2003; 97: 117–123.

67 Finn J, Wright J, Fong J, Mackenzie E, Wood F, Leslie G, Gelavis A. A randomised crossover trial of patient controlled intranasal fentanyl and oral morphine for procedural wound care in adult patients with burns. *Burns* 2004; 30: 262–268.

68 Paech MJ, Lim CB, Banks SL, Rucklidge MW, Doherty DA. A new formulation of nasal fentanyl spray for postoperative analgesia: A pilot study. *Anaesthesia* 2003; 58: 740–744.

69 Jackson K, Ashby M, Keech J. Pilot dose finding study of intranasal sufentanil for breakthrough and incident cancer-associated pain. *J Pain Symptom Manage* 2002; 23/6: 450–452.

70 Fitzgibbon D, Morgan D, Dockter D, Barry C, Karasch. Initial pharmacokinetic, safety and efficacy evaluation of nasal morphine gluconate for breakthrough pain in cancer patients. *Pain* 2003; 106; 309–315.

● 71 Illum L, Watts P, Fisher AN, Hinchcliffe M, Norbury H, Jabbal-Gill I, Nankervis R, Davis SS. Intranasal delivery of morphine. *J Pharmacol Exp Ther* 2002; 301: 391–400.

72 Pavis H, Wilcock A, Edgecombe J, Carr D, Manderson C, Church A, Fisher A. Pilot study of nasal morphine-chitosan for the relief of breakthrough pain in patients with cancer. *J Pain Symptom Manage* 2002; 24: 598–602.

73 Mercadante S, Radbrook L, Davies A et al. A comparison of intranasal fentanyl spray with oral transmucosal fentanyl citrate for the treatment of breakthrough cancer pain: An open-label randomized crossover trial. *Curr Med Res Opin* 2009; 25: 2805–2815.

74 Portenoy RK, Burton AW, Gabrail N, Taylor D, The Fentanyl Pectin Nasal Spray 043 Study Group. A multicenter, placebo-controlled, double-blind, multiple-crossover study of fentanyl pectin nasal spray (FPNS) in the treatment of breakthrough cancer pain. *Pain* 2010; 151: 617–624.

75 Davies A, Sitte T, Elsner F, Reale Carlo, Espinosa J, Brooks D, Fallon M. Consistency of efficacy, patient acceptability and nasal tolerability of fentanyl pectin nasal spray compared with immediate-release morphine sulphate in breakthrough cancer pain. *J Pain Symptom Manage* 2011; 41: 358–366.

76 Watanabe S, Pereira J, Tarunny Y, Anson J, Bruera E. A randomized double blind crossover comparison of continuous and intermittent subcutaneous administration of opioid for cancer pain. *J Palliat Med* 2008; 11/4: 570–574.

◆ 77 Anderson SL, Shreve ST. Continuous subcutaneous infusion of opiates at the end-life. *Ann Pharmacother* 2004; 38: 1015–1123.

◆ 78 Ripamonti C, Bruera E. Current status of patient-controlled analgesia in cancer patients. *Oncology* 1997; 11: 373–384.

79 Dawson L, Brockbank K, Carr EC, Barrett RF. Improving patients' postoperative sleep: A randomised control study comparing subcutaneous with intravenous patient-controlled analgesia. *J Adv Nurs* 1999; 30: 875–881.

80 Keita H, Geachan N, Dahmani S, Couderc E, Armand C, Quazza M, Mantz J, Desmonts JM. Comparison between patient-controlled analgesia and subcutaneous morphine in elderly patients after total hip replacement. *Br J Anaesth* 2003; 90: 53–57.

81 Waldmann C, Eason J, Ramboul E. Serum morphine levels: A comparison between continuous subcutaneous and intravenous infusion in postoperative patients. *Anaesth Analg* 1984; 39: 768–773.

● 82 Stuart-Harris R, Joel SP, McDonald P, Currow P, Slevin ML. The pharmacokinetics of morphine and morphine glucuronide metabolites after subcutaneous bolus injection and subcutaneous infusion of morphine. *Br J Clin Pharmacol* 2000; 49: 207–214.

83   Moulin DE, Kreeft JH, Murray PN, Bouquillon AI. Comparison of continuous subcutaneous and intravenous hydromorphone infusions for management of cancer pain. *Lancet* 1991; 337: 465–468.

84   Miller MG, McCarthy N, O'Boyle CA, Kearney M. Continuous subcutaneous infusion of morphine vs hydromorphone: A controlled trial. *J Pain Symptom Manage* 1999; 18: 9–15.

85   Bruera E, Faisinger R, Moore M, Thibault R, Spoldi E, Ventafridda V. Local toxicity with subcutaneous methadone. Experience of two centers. *Pain* 1991; 45: 141–143.

86   Mathew P, Storey P. Subcutaneous methadone in terminally ill patients: Manageable local toxicity. *J Pain Symptom Manage* 1999; 18: 49–52.

87   Citron ML, Johnson-Early A, Fassieck BE. Safety and efficacy of continuous intravenous morphine for severe cancer pain. *Am J Med* 1984; 17: 199–204.

✱ 88   Portenoy RK, Moulin DE, Rogers A, Inturrisi CE, Foley KM. IV infusion of opioids for cancer pain: Clinical review and guidelines for use. *Cancer Treat* Report, 1986; 70: 575–581.

89   Bruera E, Brenneis C, Michaud M, MacMillan K, Hanson J, Neil MacDonald R. Patient-controlled subcutaneous hydromorphone vs continuous subcutaneous infusion for the treatment of cancer pain. *J Natl Cancer Inst* 1988; 80 (14): 1152–1154.

90   Swanson G, Smith J, Bulich R, New P, Shiffman R. Patient-controlled analgesia for chronic cancer pain in the ambulatory setting: A report of 117 patients. *J Clin Oncol* 1989; 7: 1903–1908.

✱ 91   Cherny N, Ripamonti C, Pereira J, Davis C, Fallon M, McQuay H, Mercadante S, Pasternak G, Ventafridda V for the Expert Working Group of the EAPC network. Strategies to manage the adverse effects of oral morphine: An evidence-based report. *J Clin Oncol* 2001; 19: 2542–2554.

● 92   Santiago-Palma J, Khojainova N, Kornick C et al. Intravenous methadone in the management of chronic cancer pain. Safe and effective starting doses when substituting methadone for fentanyl. *Cancer* 2001; 92: 1919–1925.

93   Catcher J, Walsh D. Opioid-induced itching: Morphine sulphate and hydromorphone hydrochloride. *J Pain Symptom Manage* 1999; 17: 70–72.

94   Leow K, Smith M, Williams B, Cramond T. Single-dose and steady-state pharmacokinetics and pharmacodynamics of oxycodone in patients with cancer. *Clin Pharmacol Ther* 1992; 52: 487–495.

◆ 95   Ripamonti C, Bianchi M. The use of methadone for cancer pain. *Hematol Oncol Clin N Am* 2002; 16: 543–555.

96   Manfredi PL, Borsook D, Chandler SW, Payne R. Intravenous methadone for cancer pain unrelieved by morphine and hydromorphone: Clinical observations. *Pain* 1997; 70: 99–101.

● 97   Fitzgibbon DR, Ready LB. Intravenous high-dose methadone administered by patient controlled analgesia and continuous infusion for the treatment of cancer pain refractory to high-dose morphine. *Pain* 1997; 73: 259–261.

98   Walker PW, Klein D, Kasza L. High dose methadone and ventricular arrhythmias: A report of three cases. *Pain* 2003; 103: 321–324.

99   Kornick CA, Kilborn MJ, Santiago-Palma J et al. QTc interval prolongation associated with intravenous methadone. *Pain* 2003; 105/3: 499–506.

● 100 Radbruch L, Loick G, Schulzeck S, Beyer A, Lynch J, Stemmler M, Lindena G, Lehmann K. Intravenous titration with morphine for severe cancer pain: Report of 28 cases. *Clin J Pain* 1999; 15/3: 173–178.

● 101 Mercadante S, Villari P, Ferrera P, Casuccio A, Fulfaro F. Rapid titration with intravenous morphine for severe cancer pain and immediate oral conversion. *Cancer* 2002; 95: 203–208.

● 102 Harris JT, Suresh Kumar K, Rajagopal MR. Intravenous morphine for rapid control of severe cancer pain. *Palliat Med* 2003; 17: 248–256.

● 103 Soares LGL, Martins M, Uchoa R. Intravenous fentanyl for cancer pain: A "fast titration" protocol for the emergency room. *J Pain Symptom Manage* 2003; 26: 876–881.

104 Grond S, Zech D, Lehmann KA, Radbruch L, Breitenbach H, Hertel D. Transdermal fentanyl in the long-term treatment of cancer pain: A prospective study of 50 patients with advanced cancer of the gastrointestinal tract or the head and neck region. *Pain* 1997; 69: 191–198.

105 Kornick CA, Santiago-Palma J, Schulman G, O'Brien PC, Weigand S, Payne R, Manfredi PL. A safe and effective method for converting patients from transdermal to intravenous fentanyl for the treatment of acute cancer-related pain. *Cancer* 2003; 97/12: 3121–3124.

106 Enting RH, Oldenmenger WH, van der Rijt C, Wilms EB, Elfrink EJ, Elswijk I, Sillevis Smitt PAE. A prospective study evaluating the response of patients with unrelieved cancer pain to parenteral opioids. *Cancer* 2002; 94: 3049–3056.

◆ 107 Mercadante S. Intravenous morphine for management of cancer pain. *Lancet Oncol* 2010; 11: 484–489.

● 108 Nelson KA, Glare PA, Walsh D, Groh ES. A prospective, within patients crossover study of continuous intravenous and subcutaneous morphine for cancer pain. *J Pain Symptom Manage* 1997; 13: 262–267.

109 Marquard KA, Tharratt RS, Musallam NA. Fentanyl remaining in a transdermal system following three days of continuous use. *Ann Pharmacother* 1995; 29: 969–971.

110 Han PKJ, Arnold R, Bond G, Janson D, Abu-Elmagd P and K. Myoclonus secondary to withdrawal from transdermal fentanyl: A case report and literature review. *J Pain Symptom Manage* 2002; 23: 66–72.

111 Hunt R. Transdermal fentanyl and the opioid withdrawal syndrome. *Palliat Med* 1996; 10: 347–348.

112 Ripamonti C, Campa T, De Conno F. Withdrawal symptoms during chronic transdermal fentanyl administration managed with oral methadone. *J Pain Symptom Manage* 2004; 27/3: 191–194.

◆ 113 Grond S, Radbruch L, Lehmann KA. Clinical pharmacokinetics of transdermal opioids: Focus on transdermal fentanyl. *Clin Pharmacokinet* 2000; 38: 59–89.

◆ 114 Gourlay GK. Treatment of cancer pain with transdermal fentanyl. *Lancet Oncology* 2001; 2: 165–172.

115 Portenoy RK, Southam MA, Gupta SK, Lapin J, Layman M, Inturrisi CE, Foley KM. Transdermal fentanyl for cancer pain. Repeated dose pharmacokinetics. *Anesthesiology* 1993; 78/1: 36–43.

● 116 Mystakidou K, Parpa E, Tsilika E, Katsouda E, Kouloulias V, Kouvaris J, Georgaki S, Vlahos L. Pain management of cancer patients with transdermal fentanyl: A study of 1828 step I, II, & III transfers. *J Pain* 2004; 5: 119–132.

117 Menten, J, Desmedt M, Lossignol D, Mullie A. Longitudinal follow-up of TTS-fentanyl use in patients with cancer-related pain: Results of compassionate-use study with special focus on elderly patients. *Curr Med Res Opin* 2002; 18: 488–498.

● 118 Radbruch L, Elsner F. Clinical experience with transdermal fentanyl for the treatment of cancer pain in Germany. *Keio J Med* 2004; 53: 23–29.

◆ 119 Muijsers RBR, Wagstaff AJ. Transdermal fentanyl. An updated review of its pharmacological properties and therapeutic efficacy in chronic cancer pain control. *Drugs* 2001; 61: 2289–2307.

120 Mystakidou K, Parpa E, Tsilika E, Mavromati A, Smyrniotis V, Georgaki S, Vlahos L. Long-term management of noncancer patients with transdermal therapeutic system fentanyl. *J Pain* 2003; 4: 298–306.

◆ 121 Kornick CA, Santiago-Palma J, Moryl N, Payne R, Obbens EA. Benefit-risk assessment of transdermal fentanyl for the treatment of chronic pain. *Drug Saf* 2003; 26: 951–973.

122 Menefee LA, Frank ED, Crerand C, Jalali S, Park J, Sanschagrin K, Besser M. The effects of transdermal fentanyl on driving, cognitive performance, and balance in patients with chronic non-malignant pain conditions. *Pain Med* 2004; 5: 42–49.

●123 Rose PG, Macfee MS, Boswell MV. Fentanyl transdermal system overdose secondary to cutaneous hyperthermia. *Anesth Analg* 1993; 77: 390–391.

124 Ashburn MA, Ogden LL, Zhang J, Love G, Basta SV. The pharmacokinetics of transdermal fentanyl delivered with and without controlled heat. *J Pain* 2003; 4: 291–297.

125 Tharp AM, Winecker RE, Winston DC. Fatal intravenous fentanyl abuse: Four cases involving extraction of fentanyl from transdermal patches. *Am J Forensic Med Pathol* 2004; 25: 178–181.

126 Böhme K. Buprenorphine in a transdermal therapeutic system—A new option. *Clin Rheumatol* 2002; Suppl 1: S13–S16.

◆127 Evans HC, Easthope SE. Transdermal buprenorphine. *Drugs* 2003; 63: 1999–2010.

●128 Sittl R, Griessinger N, Likar R. Analgesic efficacy, and tolerability of transdermal buprenorphine in patients with inadequately controlled chronic pain related to cancer and other disorders: A multicenter, randomised, double-blind, placebo-controlled trial. *Clin Ther* 2003; 25: 150–168.

●129 Apolone G., Deandrea S, Montanari M, Corli O, Greco MT, Cavuto S. Evaluation of the comparative analgesic effectiveness of transdermal and oral opioids in cancer patients: A propensity score analysis. *Eur J Pain* (accepted for publication) September 12, 2011. doi: 10.1200/J.1532-2149.2011.00020.x

*130 Ripamonti C, Bandieri E, Roila F. On behalf of the ESMO Guidelines Working Group. Management of the cancer pain: ESMO clinical practice guidelines. *Ann Oncol* 2011; Suppl6: vi69–vi77.

131 Cachia E, Ahmedzai SH. Trasdermal opioids for cancer pain. *Curr Opin Support Palliat Care* 2011; 5: 15–16.

132 Filitz J, Griessinger N, Sitti R et al. Effects of intermittent hemodialysis on buprenorphine and norbuprenorphine plasma concentrations in chronic pain patients treated wiyh TD buprenorphine. *Eur J Pain* 2006; 10: 743–748.

133 Stein C. Peripheral mechanisms of opioid analgesia. *Anesth Analg* 1993; 76: 182–191.

134 Stein C. The control of pain in peripheral tissue by opioids. *N Engl J Med* 1995; 332: 1685–1690.

135 Ribeiro MDC, Joel SP, Zeppetella G. The bioavailability of morphine applied topically to cutaneous ulcers. *J Pain Symptom Manage* 2004;27: 434–439.

136 Kalso E, Tramer MR, Carroll D et al. Pain relief from intra-articular morphine after Knee surgery: A qualitative systematic review. *Pain* 1997; 71: 127–134.

137 Cerchietti L CA, Navigante AH, Korte WM, Cohen MA et al. Potential utility of the peripheral analgesic properties of morphine in stomatitis-related pain: A pilot study. *Pain* 2003; 105: 265–273.

138 Cerchietti LCA, Navigante AH, Bonomi RL Zaderajko MA et al. Effect of topical morphine for mucositis-associated pain following concomitant chemoradiotherapy for head and neck carcinoma. *Am Cancer Soc* 2002; 95: 2230–2236.

139 Gupta A, Duckles B, Giordano J. Use of sublingual methadone for treating pain of chemotherapy-induced oral mucositis. *J Opioid Manag* 2010; 6/1: 67–69.

140 Zeppetella G, Ribeiro M. Morphine in intrasite gel applied topically to painful ulcers. *J Pain Symptom Manage* 2005; 29/2: 118–119.

141 Flock P. Pilot study to determine the effectiveness of diamorphine gel to control pressure ulcer pain. *J Pain Symptom Manage* 2003; 25: 547–554.

142 LeBon B, Zeppetella G, Higginson IJ. Effectiveness of topical administration of opioids in palliative care: A systematic review. *J Pain Symptom Manage* 2009; 37: 913–917.

47

Spinal analgesia and neurolysis

SEIJI HATTORI

INTRODUCTION

In cancer patients, "pain" is the most common symptom and will be experienced at some point in their course of illness.[1] A range of epidemiological studies in several countries suggest that pain from a wide variety of cancers is present in about 30% of patients receiving cancer treatment, and in 60%–90% with advanced illness.[2,3] Pain occurs not only at the primary site but also at the areas of metastases and multiple areas[4] affected by chemotherapy, surgery, and radiation therapy; pain also occurs due to immovability and many other conditions.[5]

Cancer pain often appears as a complex pain. It can present as somatic, visceral, and neuropathic pain that is not distinct and static but combined and progressive. Previous reports show that 80%–90% of pain in cancer patients can be effectively relieved using analgesics in accordance with a three-step analgesic ladder approach of the World Health Organization (WHO).[6,7] However, in the remaining 10%–20% of patients, this order fails to achieve adequate pain relief and high-dose opioids may be required. These patients may benefit from interventional procedures for pain treatment, when indicated as appropriate, sometimes expressed as "the fourth step in the WHO analgesic ladder."[8] The WHO analgesic ladder is a drill on how to use pharmacological therapies for cancer pain and is aimed at any medical care giver involved in managing cancer pain. It is not intended as a comprehensive guide for severe pain refractory to conventional therapies or for those patients who cannot tolerate side effects of high-dose opioids. It is well known that the patient's responses to different opioids vary greatly, and it is important to define which medication or procedure yields the most favorable balance between analgesia and side effects.[5] Interventional strategies may range from simple nerve blocks to invasive techniques such as regional or neurolytic blocks, spinal analgesia, and neurosurgical procedures. The risk/benefit of these interventions differs for each patient, and careful decision should be taken by either a pain specialist or an experienced physician.

PAIN ASSESSMENT AND SELECTION

Patient selection is the key to the effective interventional management of cancer pain. A survey among outpatients with metastatic tumors shows that 42% of patients who had pain were undermedicated and 65% of these patients were due to an underestimation of pain and discrepancy between patient and physician.[9] A comprehensive reassessment of pain is very important prior to the interventional pain treatment. In addition to physical examination of the patient and review of the disease, a thorough history of pain should be evaluated, including the onset, duration, intensity, localization, course of the pain, and neurological evaluation.[10]

Our understanding of the basic mechanisms of pain has improved considerably over the past decade. We now understand that physical injury, pain pathways, and our emotional processing of various information (i.e., anxiety, fear, anger, depression, and insomnia)[11] are interlinked in the nervous system. Therefore, failure to assess emotional, social, and psychological status prior to the intervention may lead to a poor outcome.[12]

The expectation of the result of treatment differs among patients and must be ascertained. Some patients anticipate complete pain relief, and are likely to be dissatisfied with the effectiveness of the procedure. Because cancer is progressive in nature and a patient's health is already often deteriorating at the time of an interventional pain treatment, the procedure is sometimes blamed as the trigger of their worsening. If a patient appears to maintain unrealistic expectations, the physician should attempt to understand the degree of such patient's expectation prior to interventional procedure.[13]

Selection of techniques

Selecting appropriate interventional treatment modalities is also critical. Interventional techniques can be highly effective but also have a potential to produce significant adverse effects. Therefore, a risk/benefit profile, potential complications, and/or adverse effects should be considered and carefully be explained to both the patient and his/her family members. If there are multiple choices, the procedure with least serious adverse effects is in general recommended.[14]

Another important factor is life expectancy of a patient. The options on offer can be analgesia for several days to few weeks: For example, neurolytic blocks may provide analgesia for a few months, while other techniques, such as implantable drug delivery devices, may provide good pain relief for several years. An implantable pump is appropriate in patients with a life expectancy of 1–2 years. Implantable subcutaneous ports cost less than an implantable pump and therefore are appropriate for patients with a life expectancy of less than 1 year.

Neurosurgical ablative techniques or neurolysis that have a narrow risk/benefit ratio are likely to be performed in the final phase of patients' lives.[15] However, some procedures, such as celiac plexus block for pancreatic cancer patients, may have favorable risk/benefit profile that warrant early application of neurolysis.[16]

A diagnostic nerve block using a local anesthetic agent should be used to assess the efficacy of the intended neurolytic procedure prior to conducting this irreversible procedure. Performing a nerve block is also useful to evaluate the scope of possible neurological deficit that occurs after the neurolysis. The advantages of neurolytic techniques include a reduced frequency of follow-up visits compared to regional analgesic techniques using the continuous neuraxial drug delivery system and better cost-effectiveness for patients with short life expectancy. However, neurolytic techniques may result in complications such as permanent motor loss, paresthesia, and dysesthesia.[10]

Interventional treatment may not necessarily alleviate all types of pain, and it is quite often used in combination with a systemic administration of analgesics. Moreover, due to the nature of the outcome of interventional pain treatment, doctors who practice palliative care but have never performed these procedures have a difficult time when deciding its application. Accordingly, in order to help those doctors take the decision to implement interventional techniques as treatment for pain, we have provided guidance how to apply an interventional pain modality based on the site of cancer pain.

As a basic principle for interventional cancer pain management, it is important to select from and combine following three modalities based on the status of pain: systemic administration of analgesics, neurolysis, and spinal analgesia. For cancer pain, an interventional approach mainly consists of spinal analgesia and neurolysis. Spinal analgesia can be divided into epidural analgesia and intrathecal analgesia and is best applied to treat pain in broad areas dominated by the spinal nervous system. Neurolysis is best applied when pain is localized and is restricted to the area of nervous system that is designated for neurolysis.

SPINAL ANALGESIA

Introduction

Spinal analgesia is applied when cancer pain exists at the areas innervated by the spinal nervous system. Its application should be considered when cancer pain is present at the areas from the neck to the lower extremities and mostly when systemic administration of analgesic agents is less effective. It is also applicable when there is an urgent need to alleviate pain. The site of cancer pain should be verified on the dermatome, and a catheter should be placed at the epidural space or the spinal subarachnoid space near the responsible nerve.

The following drugs are used: opioids, local analgesics, alpha (2)-adrenergic agonists clonidine, baclofen, and prialt. Local analgesics should be used at a low concentration and be adjusted to a concentration which does not induce motor and sensory block or sympathetic block. While postsurgical epidural analgesia is intended to provide temporary analgesia until wound healing is achieved, controllable analgesia and maintenance of activity of daily living (ADL) are the primary objectives in cancer pain management. Unless this is fully understood, epidural analgesia in cancer pain management may be misunderstood to induce motor impairment of the lower extremity and hypotension due to sympathetic block. Because of this misunderstanding, inappropriate decision such as hesitation to induce epidural analgesia may be made.

The commonly used conversion factors by different routes of administration are as follows: 1 mg intrathecal = 10 mg epidural = 100 mg IV = 300 mg PO morphine. However, this is relative potency estimate and physicians should adjust the dose through careful monitoring by viewing the intensity of pain.

Cancer patients may be associated with coagulopathy and impaired immunity. If epidural and intrathecal analgesia are only implemented according to using the strict indication of surgical anesthetic purposes, the majority of patients will be excluded. When palliative medicine is to be provided, benefits expected from analgesia versus procedural risk should carefully be assessed. In addition, potential complications should be explained to a patient and his/her family members in order to obtain consent before conducting the procedure.

Interventional pain procedures should be considered before making a decision to provide palliative sedation, which is an option reserved for a patient refractory to the standard management of cancer pain. In providing palliative medicine, a doctor not only should focus on risks but also should consider the potential benefit to the patient in the context of their overall health and the patient's assessment of benefit. Pain procedures may be done in patients with far advanced disease that might not be done in patients earlier in the course of illness, because the risk–benefit assessment may be different in far-advanced disease.

Epidural analgesia

ANATOMY AND PREPARATION

The epidural space is a cavity inside the spinal canal, surrounded by the yellow ligament or spinal periosteum for the external wall and dura mater for the inner wall. There are spinal nerves, fatty tissue, and venous plexus inside the cavity. The epidural space starts from foramen magnum to sacral hiatus. Spinal subarachnoid space is filled with cerebrospinal fluid, but epidural space an open space. When administering drug solution, 3–5 mL of drug solution is needed. Since immune functions of cancer patients may be suppressed, it is recommended that the procedure shall be conducted at clean procedure room or surgical theater room. Compared to placing an epidural catheter for surgery, cancer patient often cannot stay in one position for a long time and are also not able to give you favorable posture to insert epidural catheter. Therefore, trained anesthesiologists or board-certified pain clinic doctors who are familiar with the technique are preferred to conduct the procedure.

PREPARATION

Opioids to be used include morphine, fentanyl, and hydromorphone. As a local analgesic, either bupivacaine or levobupivacaine is used. Opioid administered into the epidural space is quickly absorbed and transferred to the systemic circulation. Accordingly, it reaches the brain at a relatively early phase and exerts analgesic effects. It is known that not only water-soluble opioids such as morphine but lipid-soluble drugs such as fentanyl penetrate into the epidural space, and diffuse into CSF and the brain. These can be responsible for vomiting, nausea, sedation, and delayed respiratory depression.

INDICATION

Since opioids are injected to the proximity to the CNS, water-soluble opioids such as morphine can give a 30-fold potency compared to systemic administration; therefore, superior analgesic effects can be anticipated.[17,18] However, since epidural infusion needs 90–120 mL of solution a day, the frequency of drug exchange is not suitable for home-care setting where sporadic severe pain needs to be alleviated. When systemic administration of opioids is not sufficient for pain relief, or when the dosage of opioids needs to be reduced due to intolerable side effects, epidural analgesia should be considered.[19]

When considering patient's ADL and quality of life (QoL), particularly in palliative care, intrathecal drug delivery is recommended over the epidural drug delivery.

Intrathecal analgesia

ANATOMY AND PREPARATION

Spinal subarachnoid space is a cavity surrounded by spinal dura mater and is filled with cerebrospinal fluid. Because of the presence of cerebrospinal fluid, once administered, a drug solution diffuses rapidly across the spinal subarachnoid space. Therefore, the dose adjustment should be made based on the concentration and there is no need to maintain a certain volume of drug solution as in epidural infusion.

Contraindications of intrathecal analgesia are limited; however, caution is advised with patients suffering irreversible coagulation abnormalities, severe infections, septicemia, and skin disorders at the injection or incision sites. Many cancer patients experience thrombocytopenia and/or leukopenia, and this should not be considered an absolute contraindication; when considering intrathecal analgesia, benefits and risks to a patient should be evaluated, for example, if thrombocytopenia is present, a platelet transfusion may be necessary prior to the procedure. Overall, the procedure should be investigated if leukopenia is transient or if pain relief is a priority for a patient, and the decision made by taking into account the patient's life expectancy and quality of life (QoL).

For the management of cancer pain, the administration of analgesic drugs into the intrathecal space is superior to the epidural space in many aspects. By directly administering opioids into the cerebrospinal fluid filling the spinal subarachnoid space, we can achieve direct effect on the spinal dorsal horn. On the other hand, if medication is administered into the epidural space, it must pass through the dura to reach the cerebrospinal fluid. Accordingly, the dose needs to be increased by approximately 10 times compared to the administration to the spinal subarachnoid space. In other words, the dosage required to achieve analgesic efficacy can be smaller if it is administered to the intrathecal space compared to the epidural space, and therefore, the replacement frequency of a drug filling pump will be required less often, reducing the risk of infection. Moreover, use of a subcutaneously implanted pump allows medication administration for a longer period of time before refilling is required. In addition, the dose of pain medication administered intrathecally is lower than other routes.

Additionally, when administration into the epidural space is continued for a long period of time, it may result in epidural adhesion or fibrosis, which impairs diffusion of drug solution or results in occlusion-related troubles. It is reported that such events occur more frequently than in the administration into the spinal subarachnoid space.[20,21] Finally for patients treated on an out-patient basis, home health-care, or at the end of life care, the less frequent replacement of the drug solution as administered to the intrathecal space is more desirable compared to administration into the epidural space, which requires replacement of the drug solution every 2–3 days.

Although many novel narcotics and analgesics have recently been approved, there are only two agents used for spinal analgesia: clonidine, approved in 1990, and ziconotide, approved in 2004.[22] Morphine is the primary choice for cancer pain while fentanyl is used for the management of acute pain and hydromorphone and sufentanil are used for chronic pain. In addition to these agents, it is common that clonidine, ziconotide, or diluted bupivacaine is coadministered.[23] Investigations are ongoing concerning efficacy and safety of adenosine, ketorolac, ropivacaine, meperidine, gabapentin, buprenorphine, and

Table 47.1 *Concentrations and doses of chronic intrathecal agents recommended by 2007 Polyanalgesic Consensus Conference panelists*

Drug	Maximum concentration (mg/mL)	Maximum dose/day
Morphine	20	15 mg
Hydromorphone	10	4 mg
Fentanyl	2	–
Sufentanil	0.05	–
Bupivacaine	40	30 mg
Clonidine	2	1.0 mg
Ziconotide	0.1	0.0192 mg (manufacturer recommendation)

Sources: Staats, P. et al., *Neuromodulation*, 10, 300, 2007; From Cousins, M.J., Carr, D.B., Horlocker, T.T., Bridenbaugh, P.O., eds., *Cousins and Bridenbaugh's Neural Blockade in Clinical Anesthesia and Pain Medicine*, 4th edn., Lippincott Williams & Wilkins, Philadelphia, PA, Table 40.7. With permission.

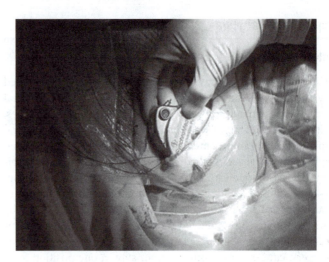

Figure 47.1 *Medtronic SynchroMed programmable intrathecal drug delivery pump. (Courtesy of Allen W. Burton.)*

octreotide.[24] The list of agents and their concentration for spinal subarachnoid administration recommended by 2007 Polyanalgesic Consensus Conference are shown in Table 47.1.

IMPLANTABLE PORT AND PUMP

In order to continue intrathecal analgesia, an indwelling catheter or infusion pump needs to be subcutaneously implanted. It is recommended for use when intraspinal analgesia is effective in achieving analgesia, when conservative pain treatment is not sufficient to achieve pain relief. When the life expectancy of a patient is at least 1–3 months, and when social backup system such as in-home care is available, it is strongly recommended. Although implantable devices approved varies between countries, their contraindication is the same: (1) hemorrhagic conditions, (2) septicemia, (3) insulin-dependent diabetes, (4) immunosuppression, (5) epidural metastases and invasion, and (6) cognitive impairment.

If a patient has bleeding tendency, there is a risk of epidural hematoma. Accordingly, careful attention and preparation is needed.[25] If skin infection is present, an indwelling catheter or an infusion pump should be placed away from the site of infection in order to avoid implanted port or pump infection and also contamination when penetrating the skin. However, if a patient is suffering from septicemia, an epidural abscess may occur and, accordingly, septicemia is strictly contraindicated. For patients with diabetes who are being treated by insulin, the probability of local infection at the site of the port or infusion pump is higher than usual, careful risk/benefit should be considered upon life expectancy and severity of pain[26] and hence, insulin is contraindicated. Patients with severely impaired immune function are also contraindicated. If the tumor has infiltrated into or metastasized to the epidural space, the point of the insertion should be away from the tumor site in order to avoid tumor penetration as if a puncture or bleeding from the tumor occurs, it may result in severe complications such as paralysis of the lower extremity. Therefore, it is better not to place epidural catheters in patients

with epidural invasion or metastasis in the epidural space.[27] Catheter insertion is often difficult in patients with cognitive dysfunction or delirium status. But when pain is the main cause of this status, by switching opioid to the intraspinal route, the dosage of opioid may be reduced and may improve these symptoms.

Due to these restrictions, many cancer patients may be contraindicated. However, if this approach appears warranted in order to achieve pain relief, its risk and benefit shall carefully be discussed between patient, family, and primary physician.

Since the capacity volume of the implantable pump (Figure 47.1)[28,29] is at best about 40 mL, it is designed and manufactured for continuous infusion into the intrathecal space. A subcutaneous implant type port (Figure 47.2) is often used when required daily volume is high and frequent refill is needed, when implantable pump is not approved by the government, or when there is financial constraint.

The pump is usually implanted into the anterior abdominal wall and a catheter tunneled to the back and into the intrathecal space. The pump has a 20–40 mL reservoir that is refilled percutaneously via the center plastic orifice every 3–4 weeks, depending on the solution and speed of administration.

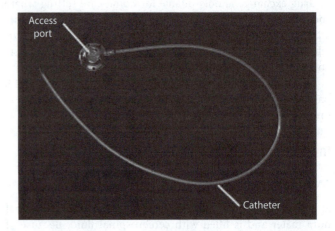

Figure 47.2 *Subcutaneous access port similar to Central Venous port and spinal subarachnoid catheter are implanted.*

An important advantage of implantable devices such as pumps and ports is their low risk of infection. The majority of infections, such as meningitis, appear to occur at the time of refilling the drug solution. Therefore, when compared to epidural analgesia that requires larger amount of analgesic agents, spinal subarachnoid analgesia with lower volume requirement may less likely to be associated with infection due to reduced frequency of refilling.

SELECTION OF THE TREATMENT BY SITE OF PAIN

Head, face, and neck pain

Sensory innervation at face and head region is achieved via the central nervous system. Accordingly, for pain manifested at these sites, neurolysis of the cranial nerve should be considered. The majority of branches from the central nervous system route through the cranial base and extend toward the facial region, and often a tumor may present adjacent to this region. If this region is destroyed anatomically, it is difficult to insert a nerve block needle and systemic administration of opioids or analgesic drugs and adjuvant drugs are likely to be recommended to achieve pain control. Among the interventional procedures commonly used, the nerve blocks appear to be trigeminal nerve block and occipital nerve block. For pain in the head and mandible regions, continuous epidural opioids to the neck region may be effective.

TRIGEMINAL NERVE BLOCK

Trigeminal nerve is the sensory nerve at facial and head region and consists of three types of nerves: ophthalmic nerve (V1), maxillary nerve (V2), and mandibular nerve (V3). A nerve block of the trigeminal nerve ganglion (gasserian ganglion) or its branches alleviates nociceptive pain and neuropathic pain relative to their nerve control region and is an established treatment for trigeminal nerve pain. A neurolytic agent or radiofrequency thermoregulation is used when destroying the nerve. This procedure is applied when pain is present at the upper portion of the face or when nerve invasion occurs. Specifically when cancer pain is present at eye-pit, maxillary antrum, or mandible, blocking of the branches by neurolysis or gasserian ganglion blocking may alleviate intolerable cancer pain.[30] If the tumor invasion and the painful area are limited, neurolysis at distal portion of branches is recommended. However, in case of cancer, it is very rare that the pathologic lesion is restricted to the area controlled by trigeminal nerve and accordingly, a trigeminal nerve block alone cannot, in general, provide adequate pain relief. In addition, if the base of the skull is destroyed by cancer infiltration or surrounding tissues are displaced by pressure or are shifted ectopically, it is often difficult to guide the tip of the needle precisely to the target site, and therefore, it is desirable that such a procedure should be performed by an experienced doctor.

If tumor is present on the needle route, bleeding may occur from tumor sites. Potential risks from bleeding include facial hematoma or intraorbital bleeding, resulting in vascular damages, and neurotoxicity induced by incorrect intravascular administration of local analgesics or neurolytic agents. In some cases, a fatal convulsive episode may occur. Neuritis after nerve block may lead to abnormal facial sensation (dysesthesia). In case of facial tumors, the size of tumor may be already quite large at the site of pain and systemic administration of opioids may be preferred to a nerve block when considering the risk/benefit profile. Siegfried and Broggi[31] reported that trigeminal nerve block was conducted in 20 patients with cancer pain and pain was alleviated in 10 patients.

With the advancement of diagnostic imaging technology, it is expected that nerve blocks will become applicable in sites where the application is currently considered difficult due to anatomical reasons.

OCCIPITAL NERVE BLOCK

The majority of the occipital region is innervated by the greater occipital nerve, a branch from the dorsal rami of C2 nerve root.

This procedure is applied for tumor or skin metastases at the occipital region or the top of the head. Originally, this nerve block was applied for postoperative wound pain after craniotomy or for the management of occipital nerve pain for the purpose of differential diagnosis of tension headache.[32] In cancer pain, it is conducted for the management of pain due to brain tumor or brain skin metastases. In general, neurolytic agents are not used and instead, local analgesics are used for palliative analgesia of the occipital region.

A greater occipital nerve block is frequently performed. The greater occipital nerve is present at 1/3 along the foramen magnum on the line that connects greater occipital protuberance and mastoid process, while lesser occipital nerve is present at the distance of 2/3 of the line. The needle is inserted at the position of lesser occipital nerve. The needle tip is directed toward the foramen magnum, and local analgesics are infiltrated from the site of greater occipital nerve. Alternatively, local analgesics are infiltrated at each site.

Since the greater occipital nerve is close to the occipital artery, by manually confirming the position of the occipital artery, we can approximate its position. Using 27-gauge needle, 2–3 mL of 0.5% bupivacaine is injected following confirmation that there is no reverse blood flow. After administration, local areas should be carefully massaged so that local analgesics become well infiltrated to ensure efficacy. Other than intravascular injection, there is almost no other complication.

Pain in upper extremities

Most common tumor type that accompanies pain at the upper extremity is the Pancoast tumor of lung cancer. Once the tumor travels from the apical portion of the lung and the thorax, it invades, compresses, and destroys the brachial plexus, which results in very severe pain and sensory and motor disorders. When cancer pain occurs in the upper extremity, analgesic agents are systemically administered and spinal analgesia should be considered. For cancer pain in the upper extremity, it is relatively rare that neurolytic procedures are appropriate. Instead, epidural analgesia is applied more frequently.

When pain is present in the upper extremity in patients with sarcoma or bone metastasis, for temporary analgesic purpose, a brachial plexus block using local analgesics may be applied. Neurolytic agents are less frequently used, but if the motor paralysis of the upper extremity is well established, neurolytic agents may be used. Many patients with motor paralysis are associated with neoplasm infiltration into the spinal nerve system or the spinal cord, making the application of nerve block difficult. This is the reason why the spinal root block or the brachial plexus block that are used for noncancer chronic pain is less often applied.

If adequate pain control cannot be achieved by systemic administration and if there is no invasion into the epidural space or the spinal subarachnoid space, a cervical epidural catheter may give certain amount of effect by infusing mixed solution of opioids and local analgesic using PCA pump.

BRACHIAL PLEXUS BLOCK

Brachial plexus consists of C5–C8 cervical spinal nerves and T1 thoracic spinal nerve. In order to reduce pain at the upper extremity, a brachial plexus block is occasionally conducted. However, since the brachial plexus is the nerve plexus responsible for sensory and motor functions of the upper extremity, the nerve block should be conducted by local anesthetics. Since use of a neurolytic agent results in motor dysfunction at the upper extremity, it is rarely employed. If cancer pain of the upper extremity exacerbates to an intolerable level, rather than using the nerve block method, continuous analgesia with systemic administration of opioids or cervical epidural infusion is more appropriate.

CERVICAL SUBARACHNOID NEUROLYSIS

This is a method in which a nerve block needle is inserted into the spinal subarachnoid space and a neurolytic agent is injected. If a patient lies on their side, 0.1–0.2 mL of 7% or 10% phenol in glycerin is gradually injected. In contrast, if a patient is turned face up, 99.5% ethanol is used for neurolysis in a similar manner. But ethanol spreads rapidly and may block other spinal nerves, so phenol is recommended. This procedure is not frequently conducted at the cervical region because needle insertion is difficult, and it is challenging to inject a neurolytic agent only at the surrounding area of the dorsal root due to the narrow diameter of the spinal cord, and any motor nerve block leads to motor disturbances of the upper extremity.

CERVICAL EPIDURAL ANALGESIA

Cancer pain may frequently appear at the upper extremity due to compression and infiltration of tumor into the brachial plexus, infiltration into the spinal cord, and brachial bone fractures due to bone metastases. In addition, it is not rare to observe progressive disturbances of sensory and/or motor functions while pain intensifies.

If adequate pain control cannot be achieved by systemic administration of opioids and analgesic adjuvants, an indwelling catheter should be placed into the cervical epidural space and epidural analgesia should be instituted early in the course of pain management. In general, morphine and low-dose bupivacaine or levobupivacaine are used.

After pain is brought under control, the future deterioration of the disease condition should be predicted more reliably based on the current status. One should consider whether a permanent catheter insertion should be placed or retry systemic administration.

Since the cervical epidural space is a narrow area and is different from the chest and lumber regions, a small amount of a drug is sufficient to achieve diffusion to an extended area. In short, the dosage is adjusted in a range of 2–4 mL/hour.

Thoracic pain

The most common cause of cancer pain in the chest area is lung cancer. Fatality rate of lung cancer is one of the highest in both male and female cancer patients, and it represents about 15% of all deaths related to malignant tumors. The causes of thoracic cancer pain are often due to thoracic wall invasion, postsurgical pain syndrome,[33] and metastases to the rib bone from other cancers. Furthermore, when breast cancer is advanced and infiltrates into the thoracic wall, the ribs and costal nerves are directly damaged, which leads to the manifestation of pain.[34] Pain is more likely to be localized to the areas of infiltration or metastasis rather than the entire chest, and neurolysis procedure is suitable. When pain is spread over deep in the chest or the entire back, thoracic metastasis, mediastinal lymph node metastasis, and psychogenic pain should be suspected.

INTERCOSTAL NERVE BLOCK

An intercostal nerve block is suitable for localized pain such as infiltration of cancer into the thoracic wall, thoracic skin metastasis, and costal metastasis. If cancer stays within the thoracic lining, patients may make complaints of visceral pain at widespread areas. In such a case, an intercostal nerve block that is expected to be effective for somatic pain may not be appropriate.[35]

The intercostal nerve runs from the spinal cord to the abdomen in parallel with the artery and vein running inside of the ribs. It has four branches and controls posterior chest, lateral chest, axillary region, and anterior chest (Figure 47.3).

At the periphery, sensory regions of the upper and lower intercostal nerves are interrelated. Accordingly, even when the target area is just a single intercostal metastatic site, it is frequently found that both upper and lower intercostal nerves need to be blocked.[36] As with thoracic infiltration, when pain is present at areas controlled by multiple intercostal nerves, spinal subarachnoid neurolysis, which will be discussed later, is appropriate. In this case, an intercostal nerve block is performed as a test block in order to evaluate temporary analgesic effect of local analgesics. After verification of analgesic effects, spinal subarachnoid neurolysis of the chest should be planned.

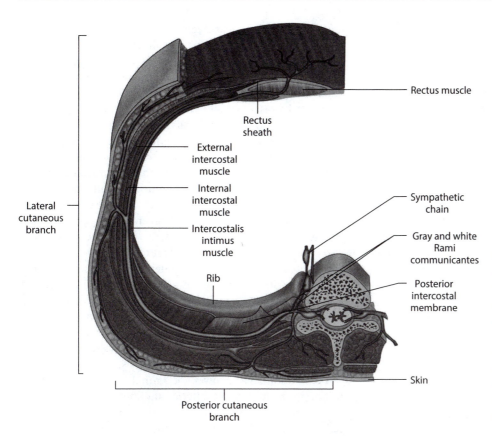

Figure 47.3 *Distribution of intercostal nerves to the rib cage. The lateral cutaneous branch runs in the skin on the side of the chest wall and is separated into the anterior and posterior branches at the middle of intercostalis intimus muscle. (From Cousins, M.J., Carr, D.B., Horlocker, T.T., Bridenbaugh, P.O., eds., Cousins and Bridenbaugh's Neural Blockade in Clinical Anesthesia and Pain Medicine, 4th edn., Lippincott Williams & Wilkins, Philadelphia, PA. With permission.)*

Neurolysis is conducted under ultrasound guidance or fluoroscopic guidance. In general, it is performed at the branch proximal to the posterior lateral cutaneous branch (Figure 47.3).

Normally, the needle size should be larger than 23 gauge. After confirmation that the contrast medium diffuses along the ribs in the groove, 3–5 mL of 10% phenol is injected per one rib. Other than chemical neurolysis, ablation may be conducted using radiofrequency thermocoagulation at the thoracic spinal nerve root. A trained pain clinic physician at clinical site should choose the best option.

This nerve block procedure can be employed relatively easily and is associated with minimum risk. Complications include pneumothorax due to pneumocentesis and acute systemic toxicity due to incorrect administration into intercostal arterial or venous vessels; therefore, after the procedure, it is recommended to perform a chest x-ray at patient follow-up. However, even when acute toxicity manifests, it is unlikely to result in a severe condition, because the injection amount is small. After neurolysis, neuropathic pain, which is often verbally described as squeezing or wearing metal jacket-like discomfort, may appear. Therefore, it is important to carefully explain potential complications to a patient and his/her family member.

THORACIC SPINAL NERVE ROOT BLOCK

For the management of thoracic pain, thoracic ganglion neurolysis may be conducted. Although it is technically similar to nerve root block, radiofrequency thermocoagulation is frequently used.

Its advantage over chemical neurolysis, in which drug solution may spread to other areas, is that radiofrequency thermocoagulation is less likely to result in such complications.

THORACIC SUBARACHNOID NEUROLYSIS

If radiofrequency thermocoagulation is not available, neurolysis agents such as phenol or alcohol are instilled into the spinal subarachnoid space to destroy the spinal nerve. While there is a report in which neurolysis agent was instilled into the epidural space, its efficacy may not be satisfactory.[37] In order to selectively destroy the dorsal root nerve in subarachnoid space, the body posture should be adjusted so that the nerve root of the target area is positioned superiorly for alcohol, while for phenol-glycerin, the target nerve root should be positioned inferiorly. In addition, in order to avoid unnecessary spreading of the drug solution to upper or lower nerve roots, the patient is better positioned laterally inflected. In case of alcohol, the affected side is positioned upward and by using the side chest pillow, the spine is slightly inflected sideways and the target nerve is uppermost. The instillation is then conducted while the abdominal side is inclined 45°. In case of phenol, the bed is folded so that the target root is positioned at the lowest point in order that phenol can drop down and stay there. After confirming the spread of contrast medium, 0.1–0.2 mL of neurolysis agent is gradually instilled. Verifying if the target pain is alleviated, an additional dose can be given if needed.

After the completion of instillation, the body position is maintained for about an hour.

Other than dysesthesia,[38] there is almost no complication. Insertion into the spinal subarachnoid space may be associated with headache and nausea, and if the procedure is performed at cervical cord or lumber cord areas, it may result in impaired mobility of extremities or bladder-rectal disorders. Accordingly, thoracic subarachnoid neurolysis is rarely used and recently is used only for patients with intractable pain and a shorter life expectancy.[39,40]

THORACIC EPIDURAL AND INTRATHECAL ANALGESIA

As discussed earlier, neurolysis is certainly recommended for localized pain; however, in case that pain is present in expanded areas, or progressive, epidural analgesia should be considered. A mixed solution of morphine, fentanyl or hydromorphone with levobupivacaine or bupivacaine (adjusted to 0.05%–0.1%) is continuously infused at the speed of 3–5 mL/hour and is titrated according to the severity of pain.

Once pain relief is achieved, it should be considered whether it is better to switch to intrathecal infusion or to maintain epidural infusion. Either implantable port or pump should be considered.

Visceral pain

ANATOMY AND INDICATION

Visceral pain originates from the organs affected by cancer and is commonly expressed as vague, dull, aching, or pressure-like. Pain from internal organs mainly comes from the celiac plexus, the superior mesenteric plexus, the inferior mesenteric plexus, and the superior hypogastric plexus via the postganglionic neuron of the autonomic nerve system (Figure 47.4).

In order to inhibit the transmission of pain stimuli to the CNS, a nerve block (neurolysis) of various nerve plexus is conducted.

The following explanations shall be provided to the patient and his/her family members, and informed consent should be obtained. The patient and family should understand that procedures related to pain management are not intended to cure or to improve the pathological condition and are only provided to alleviate pain and its efficacy is not permanent, but pain may relapse after a certain period.[41] When neurolysis is required by a cancer patient, the systemic condition of a patient tends to be already worsening and if a patient does not understand the procedure before receiving neurolysis, he or she may think that neurolysis exacerbated the disease condition.

CELIAC PLEXUS BLOCK

The celiac plexus block by a neurolytic drug is most effective for visceral pain of the upper abdomen and is a representative nerve block procedure for cancer patients. The celiac plexus receives afferent nerve fibers from upper abdominal organs such as stomach—transverse colon, pancreas, intestines, liver, and gallbladder. This block is most suitable for pancreatic cancer and gallbladder cancer and other upper abdominal cancers.[42] It is important to make a clear diagnosis if pain at the upper abdomen is a visceral pain or somatic pain as this block would be ineffective for pain related to the spinal nerve system, even if it is felt in the upper abdomen. With the advancement of diagnostic imaging technology such as Computer Assisted Tomography or CAT scan and Ultrasonography (USG), many different approaches are now reported. There is no statistically significant difference in clinical efficacy among conventional posterior approaches or between retrocrural technique, transaortic approach, and splanchnic neurolysis. A celiac plexus block can achieve analgesic effects in 70%–80% of patients immediately after nerve block. It is reported that until death, 60%–75% of patients maintained analgesic effects.[43] A recent development in the approach is to puncture the celiac plexus directly via the posterior stomach wall under ultrasound guidance (Figure 47.5).[44]

The procedure is conducted under a fluoroscope or motion-CAT scan with the patient in a prone or lateral position. A 20–21 gauge block needle is often used. The physician confirms under fluoroscope and contrast medium that the needle tip is placed in the retrocrural space and no leakage is found. Approximately 20 min after injection of local anesthetic, 99.5% alcohol 10–20 mL is injected for neurolysis.

For abdominal and lower abdominal pain, using a similar technique, a superior mesenteric ganglion block or an inferior mesenteric ganglion block can be used. However, unlike the celiac plexus block, its efficacy is not extensively reported. For pelvic pain associated with gynecological, colorectal, or genitourinary cancer, a superior hypogastric plexus block can be conducted at the level of L5, S1. Plancarte et al. reported a 43% reduction of opioid use was observed in 72% of patients who received a superior hypogastric plexus block (neurolysis).[45]

Anal pain

PHENOL SADDLE BLOCK/LUMBOSACRAL SUBARACHNOID PHENOL INJECTION

Lumbosacral spinal neurolysis is effective to treat pain in the pelvis, retroperitoneum, rectum, and pubic region. In practice, 0.2–0.3 mL of phenol is used. Since phenol is instilled along the dorsal dura mater, a patient is placed at the sitting position and is tilted toward dorsally by 15° (Figure 47.6). Vesicorectal disorder may frequently appear as a complication. The procedure is easier to perform for patients following Mile's operation or those with vesical fistula or artificial anus. Potential complications should carefully be explained to a patient when obtaining informed consent and before performing the procedure.

Pain in the lower extremity

When cancer pain is present at the lower extremity, it is due to bone metastasis to the lower extremity, lymphedema, invasion or metastasis of tumor into lumbar spine, metastatic infiltration into the lumbar epidural space, metastasis or infiltration to sacral spine, and blood flow disturbance due to megatumor within the pelvis. The majority of pain is

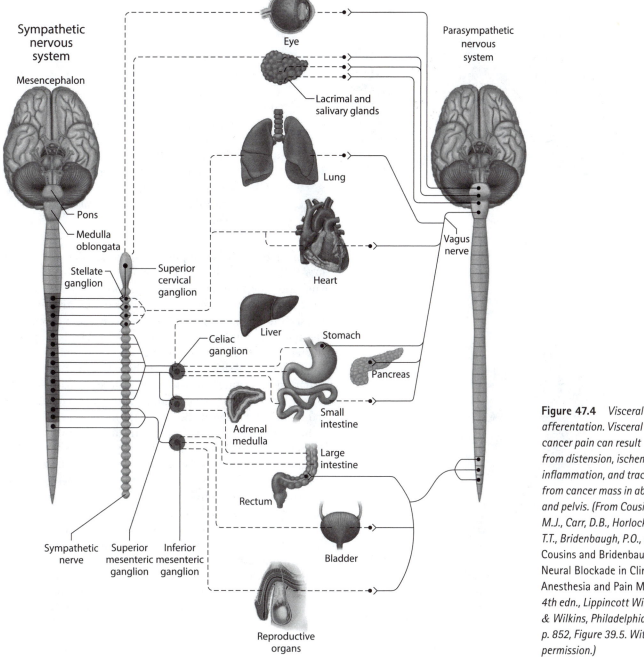

Sympathetic nervous system

Mesencephalon

Pons

Medulla oblongata

Stellate ganglion

Superior cervical ganglion

Celiac ganglion

Adrenal medulla

Sympathetic nerve

Superior mesenteric ganglion

Inferior mesenteric ganglion

Eye

Lacrimal and salivary glands

Lung

Heart

Liver

Stomach

Pancreas

Small intestine

Large intestine

Rectum

Bladder

Reproductive organs

Parasympathetic nervous system

Vagus nerve

Figure 47.4 *Visceral afferentation. Visceral cancer pain can result from distension, ischemia, inflammation, and traction from cancer mass in abdominal and pelvis. (From Cousins, M.J., Carr, D.B., Horlocker, T.T., Bridenbaugh, P.O., eds., Cousins and Bridenbaugh's Neural Blockade in Clinical Anesthesia and Pain Medicine, 4th edn., Lippincott Williams & Wilkins, Philadelphia, PA, p. 852, Figure 39.5. With permission.)*

progressive and remains less responsive even when the dosage of opioid is increased.

When attempting to alleviate cancer pain in the lower extremity, the physician must be aware that neurolysis of the lumbar spinal nerve may be associated with impaired mobility that may significantly affects ADL such as walking disturbance. Since this pain is frequently progressive, if conservative pain treatment is not sufficient to control pain, spinal analgesia is selected and the dosage should be adjusted depending on the progress of pain.

EPIDURAL ANALGESIA

For the nerve controlling the area in the lower extremity where pain is present, an indwelling catheter should be inserted into the lumbar epidural space at the height near the responsible nerve. Analgesic agents to be used include morphine, hydromorphone, or fentanyl, mixed with local anesthetic agent (levobupivacaine, bupivacaine) at the concentration of 0.05%–0.1%. Continuous infusion speed is 4–6 mL/hour. In order to manage breakthrough pain, PCA pump should be used. Once titration is achieved with an external catheter, an implantable port is implanted to prevent infection and accidental catheter withdrawal/damage.

Bone pain

There are many cancer patients who make complaint of pain due to not only bone-originated tumor such as multiple myeloma or osteosarcoma but metastasis in bone. Breast

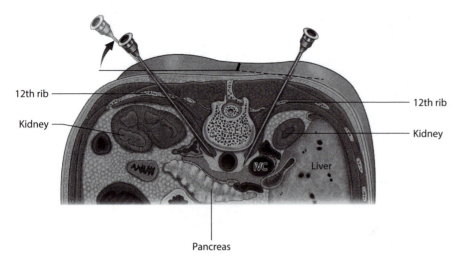

12th rib

Kidney

Pancreas

12th rib

Kidney

Liver

Figure 47.5 *A posterior approach to the splanchnic nerves and celiac plexus. (From Cousins, M.J., Carr, D.B., Horlocker, T.T., Bridenbaugh, P.O., eds., Cousins and Bridenbaugh's Neural Blockade in Clinical Anesthesia and Pain Medicine, 4th edn., Lippincott Williams & Wilkins, Philadelphia, PA. With permission.)*

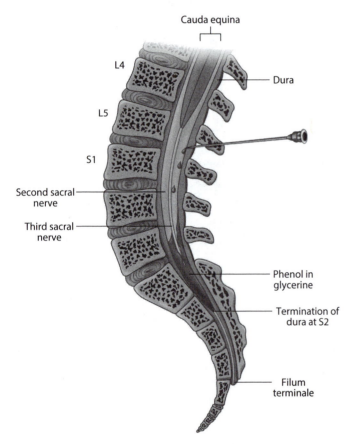

Cauda equina

L4

L5

S1

Dura

Second sacral nerve

Third sacral nerve

Phenol in glycerine

Termination of dura at S2

Filum terminale

Figure 47.6 *Saddle block with hyperbaric solution. (From Cousins, M.J., Carr, D.B., Horlocker, T.T., Bridenbaugh, P.O., eds., Cousins and Bridenbaugh's Neural Blockade in Clinical Anesthesia and Pain Medicine, 4th edn., Lippincott Williams & Wilkins, Philadelphia, PA. With permission.)*

cancer, prostate cancer, and lung cancer are frequently associated with metastasis in bone. Other cancers include stomach cancer, thyroid cancer, and lymphoma.[46] Among patients who die of breast cancer, metastasis in bone is said to be present in 80% of patients. As treatment for cancer has evolved and life expectancy prolonged, the incidence of metastasis in bone has increased accordingly. Therefore, the incidence of bone metastasis will increase in other types of cancer as well.

Among bone metastases, metastases to vertebra account for 30%–70% of cases.[47] Such patients experience lumber pain, back pain, and movement pain. Metastases to vertebra are likely to cause pathological compression fractures irrespective of a triggers such as a fall that often characterizes conventional compression fractures. The site of metastatic involvement is frequently different from sites seen in osteoporosis and steroid treatment (lower thoracic vertebra, upper lumbar vertebra).[48] Vertebrate compression fractures are associated with severe pain and lead to deterioration of systemic conditions such as reduced activity and embolic risk, thereby shortening the life prognosis.[49]

Bone pain due to metastasis and fractures due to weakening bones are treated by other anticancer therapies such as radiotherapy and chemotherapy, as well as fracture surgery, and should be given priority to manage the pathogenesis. For the management of pain, bisphosphonate therapy, opioids, analgesic adjuvant, and steroids are used.

The use of nerve blocks and spinal analgesia is limited in these cases; however, if pain is localized such as metastasis in ribs, an intercostal nerve block, a thoracic spinal nerve root block, and a thoracic spinal subarachnoid block can be applicable. It has also been reported that an intercostal nerve block by steroid injection achieved analgesic effects in metastasis in ribs.[50]

CONCLUSION

Because of increased awareness of the WHO cancer pain treatment guidelines and the introduction of a new generation of opioids, we have witnessed significant advancement in the management of patients with cancer pain. However, too much emphasis on pharmacological tools has resulted in reduced utilization of interventional procedures. Given the variability in malpractice laws between countries, it is conceivable that exclusive use of conservative pain treatments will result in order to avoid performing procedures with certain risks. If we do not conduct analgesic procedures because of such legal concerns when we are aware of its effectiveness, we may be violating the principle of medicine to do the best for our patients.

Knowledge in this area should be disseminated so that the most appropriate therapy can be offered to the patient.

There are not many interventional pain treatment options available for palliative care, and they differ from treatment for nonmalignant pain in which nerve blocks can be conducted repeatedly based on patient's condition, as the physician is under significant time pressure. For many patients with cancer pain, we have only a few opportunities to conduct pain management and accordingly, an experienced doctor should be in charge when performing interventional procedures.

Overall, when systemic administration of opioids is not sufficient to control pain, we should consider the feasibility of conducting neurolysis based on the site of pain. If it is judged that neurolysis is not suitable, the next step is to evaluate if spinal analgesia may confer sufficient pain control. Much cancer pain related to the spinal nerve system, or abdominal pain, can temporarily be managed by epidural morphine and local anesthetic. Once a conservative method is judged as no longer effective, epidural analgesia should actively be provided. Depending on the severity of pain, the dosage of epidural analgesic agents can be increased, while the dose of the systemic administration of opioid should be reduced. In parallel, we should evaluate the appropriateness of neurolysis in future treatment strategy. As time left for a patient under palliative care is limited, we should not deliberately leave uncontrollable pain as it is.

Physicians dealing with cancer pain should always be aware of what will happen next to your patient. The primary differences between patients with nonmalignant chronic pain and cancer pain are its progressive nature and the deterioration of their general condition. Therefore, selection of interventional procedures should be decided in a timely and accurate manner. Slow decision will not satisfy the patient needs and will miss the timing of interventions. Since time is of the essence in treating cancer pain, the physician should ask what benefit interventional techniques can offer to end of life care.

REFERENCES

1   World Health Organization. *World Cancer Report-International Agency for Research on Cancer*. Geneva, Switzerland: World Health Organization; 2003.

2   Caraceni A, Portenyo RK. An international survey of cancer pain characteristics and syndromes. *Pain* 1999;82:23–74.

3   Foley KM. Management of cancer pain. In: Devita VT Hellman S, Rosenberg SA, eds., *Cancer: Principles and Practice of Oncology*, 7th edn. New York: Lippincott Williams and Wilkins; 2005, pp. 2615–2649.

4   Grond S, Zech D, Schug SA et al. Validation of World Health Organization guidelines for cancer pain relied during the last days and hours of life. *J Pain Symptom Manage* 1991;6:411–422.

5   Portenoy RK, Lesage P. Management of cancer pain. *Lancet* 1999;353:1695–1700.

6   Walker VA, Hoskin PJ, Hanks GW et al. Evaluation of WHO analgesic guidelines for cancer pain in a hospital-based palliative care unit. *J Pain Symptom Manage* 1988;3:145–149.

7   Zech DF, Grond S, Lynch J et al. Validation of World Health Organization Guidelines for cancer pain relief: A 10-year prospective study. *Pain* 1995;63:645–676.

8   Miguel R. Interventional treatment of cancer pain: The fourth step in the WHO analgesic ladder? *Cancer Control* 2000;7:149–156.

9   Cleeland CS, Gonin R, Hatfield AK et al. Pain and its treatment in outpatients with metastatic cancer. *N Engl J Med* 1994;330:592–596.

10 Erdine S. Interventional treatment of cancer pain. *Eur J Cancer Suppl* 2005;3:97–106.

11 Fallon M, Hanks G, Cherny N. Principles of control of cancer pain. *BMJ* 2006;332:1022–1024.

12 Manchikanti L, Fellows B, Singh V. Understanding psychological aspects of chronic pain in interventional pain management. *Pain Phys* 2002;5:57–82.

13 Tay W, Ho K. The role of interventional therapies in cancer pain management: Review. *Ann Acad Med Singapore* 2009;38:989–997.

14 Plancarte R, Alvares J, Arrieta MC. Interventional treatment of cancer pain. *Semin Pain Med* 2003;1:34–42.

15 Mercadante S. Celiac plexus block versus analgesics in pancreatic cancer pain. *Pain* 1993;52:187–192.

16 Eisenberg E, Carr DB, Chalmers TC. Neurolytic celiac plexus block for treatment of cancer pain: A meta-analysis. *Anesth Analg* 1995;80:290–295.

17 Burton AW, Rajagopal A, Shah HN et al. Epidural and intrathecal analgesia is effective in treating refractory cancer pain. *Pain Med* 2004;5(3):239–247.

18 Baker L, Lee M, Regnard C et al. Evolving spinal analgesia practice in palliative a care. *Palliat Med* 2004;18(6):507–515.

19 Lema MJ. Invasive analgesia techniques for advanced cancer pain. *Surg Oncol Clin N Am* 2001;10(1):127–136.

20 Bahar M, Rosen M, Vickers MD. Chronic cannulation of the intradural or estradural space in the rat. *Br J Anaesth* 1984;56(4):405–410.

21 Crul BJ, Delhaas EM. Technical complications during long-term subarachnoid or epidural administration of morphine in terminally ill cancer patients: A review of 140 cases. *Reg Anesth* 1991;16(4):209–213.

22 Carr DB. Economics of patient-controlled analgesia: An annotated bibliography. In: Campbell JN, ed., *Pain 1996—An Updated Review*. Seattle, WA: IASP Press; 1996, pp. 437–439.

23 Staats P, Withworth M, Barakat M et al. The use of implanted programmable infusion pumps in the management of nonmalignant, chronic low-back pain. *Neuromodulation* 2007;10:376–380.

24 Deer T, Krames ES, Hassenbusch SJ et al. Polyanalgesic Consensus Conference 2007: Recommendations for the management of pain by intrathecal (intraspinal) drug delivery: Report of an interdisciplinary expert panel. *Neuromodulation* 2007;10:300–328.

25 Horlocker TT, Wedel DJ, Benzon H et al. Regional anesthesia in the anticoagulated patient: Defining the risks (the second ASRA Consensus Conference on Neuraxial Anesthesia and Anticoagulation). *Reg Anesth Pain Med* 2003;28:172–197.

26 Kamie J, Kasuya Y. The effects of diabetes on opioid-induced antinociception. In: Tseng LF, ed., *The Pharmacology of Opioid Peptides*. Langhorn, PA: Harwood Academic Press; 1995, p. 271.

27 Cherry DA, Gourlay GK, Cousins MJ. Extradural mass associated with lack of efficacy of epidural morphine, and undetectable CSF morphine concentrations. *Pain* 1986;25:69.

28 Laffer U, Bachmann-Mettler I, Metzger U, eds. *Implantable Drug Delivery Systems*. Basel, Switzerland: S Karger AG; 1991.

29 Penn RD, Paice JA, Gottschalk W et al. Cancer pain relief using chronic morphine infusion. Early experience with a programmable implanted drug pump. *J Neurosurg* 1984;61:302–306.

30 Waldman SD. Blockade of Gasserian ganglion. In: Waldman SD, ed., *Interventional Pain Management*. New York: WB Saunders; 2001, pp. 316–320.

31 Siegfried I, Broggi G. Percutaneous thermocoagulation of the gasserian ganglion in the treatment of pain in advanced cancer. In: Bonica JJ, Ventafridda V, eds., *Advances in Pan Research and Therapy*, Vol. 2. New York: Raven Press; 1979, pp. 463–469.

32 Ward JB. Greater occipital nerve block. *Semin Neurol* 2003;23:59–62.

33 Rogers ML, Duffy JP. Surgical aspects of chronic post-thoracotomy pain. *Eur J Cardiothorac Surg* 2000;18:711–716.

34 Wallace MS, Wallace AM, Lee J. Pain after breast surgery: A survey of 282 women. *Pain* 1996;66:195–205.

35 Moore DC. Intercostal nerve block in 4333 patients: Indications, techniques, and complications. *Anesth Analg* 1962;41:1–10.

36 Conacher ID. Percutaneous cryotherapy for post-thoracotomy neuralgia. *Pain* 1986;25:227–230.

37 Swedlow M. Subarachnoid and extradural blocks. *Adv Pain Res Ther* 1979;2:325.

38 Cousins M. In: Cousins MJ, Bridenbaugh PO, eds., *Neural Blockade in Clinical Anesthesia and Management of Pain*, 3rd edn. Philadelphia, PA: Lippincott Williams & Wilkins; 1998, pp. 1022–1033.

39 Ferrer-Brechner T. Epidural and intrachecal phenol neurolysis for cancer pain. *Anesthesiol Rev* 1982;8:14–32.

40 Candido K, Stevens RA. Intrathecal neurolytic blocks for the relief of cancer pain. *Best Pract Res Clin Anaesthesiol* 2003;17(3):407–428.

41 Tasker RR. The recurrence of pain after neurosurgical procedures. *Qual Life Res* 1994;3:S43–S49.

42 De Oliveira R, dos Reis MP, Prado WA. The effects of early or late neurolytic sympathetic plexus block on the management of abdominal or pelvic cancer pain. *Pain* 2004;110:400–408.

43 Ischia S, Ishia A, Polati E et al. Three posterior percutaneous celiac plexus block techniques. A prospective, randomized study in 61 patients with pancreatic cancer pain. *Anesthesiology* 1992;76(4):534–540.

44 Levy MJ, Topazian MD, Wiersema MJ et al. Initial evaluation of the efficacy and safety of endoscopic ultrasound-guided direct ganglia neurolysis and block. *Am J Gastroenterol* 2008;103(1):98–103.

45 Plancarte R, de Leon-Casasola OA, El-Helaly M et al. Neurolytic superior hypogastric plexus block for chronic pelvic pain associated with cancer. *Reg Anesth* 1997;22(6):562–568.

46 Buijs JT, van der Pluijm G. Osteotropic cancers: From primary tumor to bone. *Cancer Lett* 2009;273:177–193.

47 Jajan N. Palliative radiation therapy techniques. In: Fish M, Burton A, eds., *Cancer Pain Management*. New York: McGraw-Hill; 2007.

48 Alberico R et al. Neuroradiologic evaluation of the patient with cancer pain. In: de Leon Casseola O, ed., *Cancer Pain Management: Pharmacologic, Interventional and Palliative Approaches*. Philadelphia, PA: Elsevier; 2006.

49 Kado D, Browner WS, Palermo L et al. Vertebral fractures and mortality in older women: A prospective study. Study of Osteoporotic Fractures Research Group. *Arch Intern Med* 1999;159(11):1215–1220.

50 Rowell NP. Intralesional methylprednisolone for rib metastases: An alternative to radiotherapy? *Palliat Med* 1988;2(2):153–155.

51 Cousins MJ, Carr DB, Horlocker TT, Bridenbaugh PO, eds. *Cousins and Bridenbaugh's Neural Blockade in Clinical Anesthesia and Pain Medicine*, 4th edn. Philadelphia, PA: Lippincott Williams & Wilkins.

48

Anesthesiological procedures in palliative care

SARAH GEBAUER

INTRODUCTION

Most patients with cancer pain can be treated using the World Health Organization (WHO) analgesic stepladder (Zech et al. 1995). Approximately 10%–25% will need an interventional technique for pain management, which is considered the fourth step of the WHO stepladder (Miguel 2000). An interventional technique may be considered due to intolerance of opioids or pain despite optimal medical management (Miguel 2000). In general, the goals of these procedures are a decrease in pain and an improvement in quality of life and their use in children and adults (Rork et al. 2013).

NERVE BLOCKS

Definitions

Broadly speaking, regional anesthesia is the administration of medication to produce a sensory block in a specific area of the body (Rork et al. 2013). Regional analgesia provides pain relief, though not necessarily complete numbness. Colloquially, these terms are often used interchangeably. In this chapter, regional anesthesia refers to techniques that provide either anesthesia or analgesia. Neuraxial anesthesia is one aspect of regional anesthesia and is covered in the chapter on neurosurgical techniques.

Moreover, most regional anesthesia procedures, regardless of the type of nerve they affect (autonomic or peripheral) or their effect on the nerve (neurolytic or transient), are referred to as nerve blocks. Autonomic nerve blocks almost always block transmission of the sympathetic system. Most palliative sympathetic blocks are performed with neurolytic agents such as alcohol or phenol, and most peripheral nerve blocks are performed with local anesthetics.

Duration of effect

Single-shot (one-injection) regional anesthesia techniques can last from less than an hour to most of the day depending on the local anesthetic used. Peripheral nerve catheters can

provide relief for days, weeks, or even months. Neurolysis lasts 2–3 months, possibly slightly longer with alcohol (Jackson and Gaeta 2008).

Effect of blocks on components of pain

Cancer pain can be somatic, neuropathic, visceral pain, or a combination (Portenoy 2011). Noncancer patients have a variety of pain etiologies, such as ischemia, immobility, or wounds (Klinkenberg et al. 2004). Peripheral nerve blocks are often used for somatic pain and autonomic nerve blocks for visceral pain. The etiology of visceral pain is complex, and the visceral afferent fibers often travel with autonomic fibers (Cervero and Laird 1999). Decisions about which nerve(s) to block are based on the likely pathophysiology of the pain.

Contraindications, risks, and practical considerations

There is little evidence for a maximum safe international normalized ratio (INR) or minimum platelet count for neurolytic blocks (Raj et al. 2004). The American Society of Regional Anesthesia suggests an INR of 1.4 or less for deep plexus or peripheral blocks (Horlocker et al. 2010). However, less restrictive guidelines are proposed for injection sites in areas amenable to compression (Horlocker et al. 2010). The use of anticoagulants like warfarin, as well as local infection or tumor invasion, is generally considered to be a contraindication (Chambers 2008; Horlocker et al. 2010). Most risks of nerve blocks are related to the possible puncture of major vessels and organs near the nerve or failure of the block. Nerve damage and infection are also possible, though rare (Ilfeld 2011b). Blocks near major vessels are performed in the hospital due to the risk of hemodynamic collapse with intravascular injection, bleeding, or other serious complication. In the palliative care population, the need for prone positioning or transport to a radiology or gastroenterology suite may be significant barriers to care (Bhatnagar and Gupta 2011). Patients may require sedation to tolerate the procedure that may involve increased risk in some patients (Bahn and Erdek 2013).

How a neurolytic block is performed

Traditionally, fluoroscopy has been used to advance a small-bore needle to the target nerve, though CT and ultrasound guidance, including endoscopic ultrasound, are increasingly used (Bhatnagar et al. 2012). Local anesthetic may be injected first to assess for efficacy (Yuen et al. 2002), and the neurolysis with alcohol or phenol may proceed at the time of the diagnostic block or within a few weeks (Jackson and Gaeta 2008). Current data do not suggest that one method of nerve localization is markedly safer or more effective than another for most patients (Arcidiacono et al. 2011). Neurolytic blocks require no indwelling equipment, which benefits ambulatory patients (Table 48.1).

Autonomic blocks

CELIAC PLEXUS BLOCKS

Celiac plexus neurolytic blocks are among the most well-studied nerve blocks for cancer pain and affect tumors of the pancreas, stomach, gallbladder, and liver (De Leon-Casasola 2000; Mauck and Rho 2010). The plexus is located anterior to the aorta at the level of the L1 vertebrae, inferior to the origin of the celiac artery (Mauck and Rho 2010). The celiac plexus contains autonomic and visceral fibers that innervate the viscera of the upper abdomen and often travel together (Erdek et al. 2010). This block can be performed in the prone or supine position depending on technique used (De Leon-Casasola 2000). A meta-analysis of 21 studies showed that approximately 90% of patients receive partial or complete short-term pain relief, and the majority have longer-term relief (Eisenberg et al. 1995). A landmark randomized, double-blind, placebo-controlled trial of 100 patients compared neurolytic celiac plexus blocks to systemic opioid therapy. The study showed a sustained improvement in pain scores but no difference in quality of life or survival in the neurolytic celiac plexus group (Wong et al. 2004). Most studies have found that patients require opioids in addition to the neurolytic celiac plexus block, though the amount of opioids required decreases after a neurolytic celiac plexus block (Arcidiacono et al. 2011; Mercadante et al. 2003). There is debate regarding whether this technique should be used early in the course of illness or when medical therapy fails (De Oliveira et al. 2004; Tempero et al. 2010). Diarrhea, hypotension, and transient localized pain are the most common complications, and major complications occur less than 2% of the time (Eisenberg et al. 1995).

SUPERIOR HYPOGASTRIC BLOCKS

Patients with pelvic pain from with gynecologic, colorectal, and bladder pelvic tumors may respond to superior hypogastric blocks (Kroll et al. 2013). The largest study to date included 227 patients with mostly gynecological cancer, 159 of whom had a reduction in pain with a diagnostic block and therefore received a neurolytic hypogastric block (Plancarte et al. 1997). Seventy-two percent of patients had adequate pain relief for at least 3 weeks, though 38% required a second neurolytic superior hypogastric block (Plancarte et al. 1997). Mean opioid use also decreased (Plancarte et al. 1997). Major complications seem to be uncommon (Bosscher 2001).

OTHER SYMPATHETIC BLOCKS

Lumbar plexus sympathectomies have shown mixed results for painful limb ischemia (Sanni et al. 2005). Ganglion impar blocks are used for perineal pain in prostate, colorectal, and vulvar cancers (Agarwal-Kozlowski et al. 2009; Eker et al. 2008; Ho et al. 2006). Stellate ganglion blocks are typically used for sympathetically mediated pain of the head and neck, though there are also case reports and series in palliative care patients for refractory angina (Chester et al. 2000; Moore et al. 2005), postmastectomy pain (Nabil Abbas et al. 2011), and hot flashes in breast cancer survivors (Haest et al. 2012).

Peripheral nerve blocks

HOW PERIPHERAL NERVE BLOCKS ARE PERFORMED

Peripheral nerve blocks are performed with landmark guidance, nerve stimulators, and increasingly with ultrasound guidance, allowing practitioners to visualize structures and possibly decreasing the risk of unintentional venous puncture (Ilfeld 2011a). Regardless of technique, the patient is positioned for easy access to the target nerve, and the needle is guided toward the nerve. Local anesthetic is then deposited surrounding the nerve. Single-shot peripheral nerve blocks may be beneficial for patients undergoing procedures and dressing changes or with a very limited life expectancy. Catheter-based peripheral nerve blocks can be used in patients with ongoing analgesic needs.

Local anesthetics work by blocking sodium channels and vary in duration of action (French and Sharp 2012). Shorter-acting agents like lidocaine may be appropriate for scenarios such as dressing changes, while longer-acting agents like ropivacaine may be appropriate for postoperative pain management or catheter-based infusion. The concentration of the drug helps determine the density of the block. Additionally, some practitioners include adjuvants to the medication injected near the nerve. Opioids and dexamethasone are sometimes added to the local anesthetic but data to support this practice are mixed, especially when compared to systemic opioids (Desmet et al. 2013; Murphy et al. 2000).

Peripheral nerve blocks have been reported to provide pain relief for much longer than the expected duration of action of the local anesthetic (Blumenthal et al. 2011; Okell and Brooks 2009). The mechanism for this prolonged analgesia is not clear.

CATHETERS FOR PERIPHERAL NERVE ANALGESIA

In catheter-based regional anesthesia, a small catheter is threaded near the nerve. These catheters may infuse continuously, have a bolus function, or a combination of the two.

Table 48.1 *Nerve blocks*

Location of pain	Treatment options	Example of amenable pathophysiology	Effect of treatment	Selected side effects and complications	Duration of EFFECT	Setting
Upper abdomen	Celiac plexus block	Pancreatic cancer	Sympatholysis, decreased visceral pain	Diarrhea, orthostasis	Months (neurolytic)	Interventional pain, radiology, or endoscopy suites
	Neuraxial anesthesia (thoracic or upper lumbar)	Abdominal wall tumor	Analgesia of several abdominal dermatomes	Equipment failure	Months (catheter)	Bedside (external), interventional pain suite (implanted)
Pelvis	Superior hypogastric plexus	Ovarian cancer	Sympatholysis, decreased visceral pain	Need for repeat block	Months (neurolytic)	Interventional pain or radiology suites
	Neuraxial anesthesia (lumbar)	Abdominal wall tumor	Analgesia of several dermatomes	Possible loss of ambulation depending on location of catheter	Months (catheter)	Bedside (external), interventional pain suite (implanted)
Shoulder	Interscalene block (single shot or catheter)	Tumor of the humerus	Analgesia of shoulder	Diaphragmatic hemiparesis	Hours (single shot; weeks (catheter)	At bedside in hospital
Elbow	Supraclavicular, infraclavicular	Cutaneous lesions of the elbow and forearm	Analgesia below the shoulder	Risk of pneumothorax and diaphragmatic hemiparesis; likely loss of arm movement	Hours (single shot; weeks (catheter)	At bedside in hospital
Wrist and forearm	Axillary	Trauma	Analgesia below the mid-humerus	Loss of arm movement	Hours (single shot; weeks (catheter)	At bedside in hospital
	Bier block	Trauma	Analgesia below the tourniquet	Loss of forearm movement	Hours	At bedside in hospital, possibly at home
Hand	Wrist block	Trauma	Analgesia of hand	Loss of hand movement	Hours (single shot only)	At bedside, at home or in hospital
Fingers	Digital block	Trauma	Analgesia of finger	Loss of movement in that finger	Hours (single shot only)	At bedside, at home or in hospital
Leg and knee	Femoral nerve block	Femoral neck fracture	Analgesia of anterior thigh and knee, very little analgesia below the knee	Difficulty with ambulation	Hours (single shot); weeks (catheter)	At bedside in hospital
Lower leg	Popliteal sciatic (with or without saphenous block)	Tumor of the lower leg	Analgesia below the knee	Difficulty with ambulation	Hours (single shot; weeks (catheter)	At bedside in hospital
Foot	Ankle block	Diabetic foot wounds, dressing changes	Analgesia of the foot	Difficulty with ambulation	Hours (single shot only)	At bedside, at home or in hospital

Studies in postoperative patients of catheters attached to an electronic or spring-powered pump with prefilled medication show that their catheters can be easily managed at home, though the reservoir may require repeated refills for longer infusions (Ilfeld 2011a). Case reports exist of catheters being left in place for several weeks or even months (Esch et al. 2010; Pacenta et al. 2010). Some practitioners tunnel the catheter to decrease the risk of catheter migration or dislodgement (Boezaart et al. 1999).

SIDE EFFECTS OF PERIPHERAL NERVE BLOCKS

The main side effect of regional anesthesia is the loss of motor function that accompanies the loss of sensation. This may be mitigated by the choice of a lower concentration anesthetic, but full motor function is unlikely. For some patients, this may limit mobility, such as with a femoral nerve block, and for others, it may limit the ability to perform personal care, such as with a brachial plexus block.

UPPER-EXTREMITY PERIPHERAL NERVE BLOCKS

The brachial plexus, in which nerve roots from C5 to T1 form trunks, divisions, cords, and then peripheral nerves, innervates the upper extremity (Gorlin and Warren 2012). Brachial plexus infusions have been reported for pain of tumor growth in the bone, skin, and soft tissues of the arm and for Pancoast tumors (Buchanan et al. 2009; Pelaez et al. 2010; Turnbull et al. 2011; Vranken et al. 2000, 2001).

Interscalene blocks provide analgesia to the shoulder but often not to the hand (Gorlin and Warren 2012). A successful block always results in a hemiparesis of the diaphragm, with an associated decrease in pulmonary function and subjective dyspnea (Fujimura et al. 1995).

Supraclavicular blocks are performed just above the clavicle and provide analgesia below the shoulder with an associated risk of Horner's syndrome, phrenic nerve dysfunction, and pneumothorax (Bhatia et al. 2010; Maga et al. 2012).

Axillary blocks are performed at the medial aspect of the upper arm and provide reliable anesthesia to the wrist and hand with a low complication rate (Maga et al. 2012).

Wrist blocks can be performed with good success without ultrasound or nerve stimulation guidance with infiltration of local anesthetic near the radial, median, and ulnar nerves (Delaunay and Chelly 2001).

Digital blocks are safe and easy to perform, with a single subcutaneous injection of 2–3 mL of local anesthetic at the volar aspect of the base of the finger being effective (Cannon et al. 2010).

Intravenous blocks (Bier blocks) of the upper extremity are also easy to perform, reliable, and safe (Guay 2009). The arm is wrapped tightly to exsanguinate it or simply elevated; then a tourniquet is applied and a short-acting local anesthetic like lidocaine is injected into a vein in the extremity. The local anesthetic diffuses into the surrounding tissues and provides analgesia to the area below the tourniquet (Mohr 2006).

PARAVERTEBRAL BLOCKS

Paravertebral blocks are often used to decrease postoperative pain after mastectomies (Schnabel et al. 2010) and appear effective in preventing chronic mastectomy-related pain (Andreae and Andreae 2013).

LOWER-EXTREMITY BLOCKS

The femoral nerve branches from L2 to L4 nerve roots, and blocks are performed at the inguinal crease to provide analgesia for the anterior thigh, femur, and knee (Murray et al. 2010). Femoral nerve blocks and catheters have been reported for pathologic fractures and bone and muscle tumors (Koshy et al. 2010; Pacenta et al. 2010).

The sciatic nerve is most commonly blocked proximal to the crease of the knee and provides analgesia below the knee, except for the medial aspect of the lower leg in the saphenous nerve distribution (Creech and Meyr 2013).

Ankle blocks are easy to perform without ultrasound or nerve stimulator guidance by injecting local anesthetic posterior to the medial malleolus, near the dorsalis pedis artery, and posterior to the lateral malleolus and infiltrating the anterior joint line between the malleoli (Rudkin et al. 2005). This usually successful block provides anesthesia to the entire foot with few complications (Rudkin et al. 2005).

BOTULINUM TOXIN FOR PAIN MANAGEMENT

Mechanism of action

Botulinum toxin binds to the cholinergic nerve terminal and causes flaccid paralysis that lasts up to 3–6 months due to inhibition of neurotransmitter release (Chen 2012; Dressler 2012). How botulinum toxin affects pain is not well characterized, but possibilities include a decrease in neurotransmitter release relaxation of musculature surrounding a nerve (Stubblefield et al. 2008) or modulation of afferent sensory nerve firing (Yuan et al. 2009).

Studies of botulinum toxin

Botulinum toxin was first approved for spasticity and similar muscle disorders, and in recent years, interest has grown surrounding additional uses of the medication (Chen 2012). A retrospective review of cancer patients with spasticity suggested that the majority received benefit from botulinum (Fu et al. 2013). It seems to improve disabilities in patients with post-stroke spasticity, but data on pain relief are mixed (Lim et al. 2008; Marciniak et al. 2012). One prospective study of 48 patients who received botulinum injection prior to mastectomy showed a decrease in postoperative pain (Layeeque et al. 2004). There are reports of botulinum toxin being used successfully in painful radiation fibrosis syndrome (Stubblefield et al. 2008) and radiation proctitis (Vuong et al. 2011). A double-blind, crossover study of diabetic patients with painful neuropathy of the feet showed encouraging, though not definitive, results (Yuan et al. 2009).

How botulinum toxin injections are performed

Botulinum toxin injections have been performed on a wide variety of muscles throughout the body including skeletal and smooth muscle such as the bladder (Seth et al. 2013). In the case of spasticity or myofascial pain, the medication is injected into the hypertonic or painful muscle, and the amount used may vary depending on the size of the muscle (Argoff 2002). Accurate placement may be aided by electromyography or ultrasound (Lim et al. 2011).

Side effects and risks of botulinum toxin injections

Botulinum toxin is generally safe with a wide therapeutic window. Complications include local weakness and the exacerbation of preexisting weakness such as the Lambert–Eaton syndrome (Lu and Lippitz 2009). Autonomic side effects have been reported (Dressler and Benecke 2003), as well as flu-like symptoms (Baizabal-Carvallo et al. 2011) and uncommon autoimmune conditions (Dressler 2012).

CONCLUSION

Regional anesthesia and botulinum toxin can provide pain relief for ongoing or episodic pain in many parts of the body. These procedures are generally safe and should be considered for selected patients.

REFERENCES

Agarwal-Kozlowski K, Lorke DE, Habermann CR et al. CT-guided blocks and neuroablation of the ganglion impar (Walther) in perineal pain: Anatomy, technique, safety, and efficacy. *Clinical Journal of Pain.* 2009; **25**: 570–576.

Andreae MH, Andreae DA. Regional anaesthesia to prevent chronic pain after surgery: A Cochrane systematic review and meta-analysis. *British Journal of Anaesthesia.* 2013.

Arcidiacono PG, Calori G, Carrara S et al. Celiac plexus block for pancreatic cancer pain in adults. *Cochrane Database of Systematic Reviews.* 2011; **3**: CD007519.

Argoff CE. A focused review on the use of botulinum toxins for neuropathic pain. *Clinical Journal of Pain.* 2002; **18**: S177–S181.

Bahn BM, Erdek MA. Celiac plexus block and neurolysis for pancreatic cancer. *Current Pain and Headache Reports.* 2013; **17**: 310.

Baizabal-Carvallo JF, Jankovic J, Pappert E. Flu-like symptoms following botulinum toxin therapy. *Toxicon.* 2011; **58**: 1–7.

Bhatia A, Lai J, Chan VW, Brull R. Case report: Pneumothorax as a complication of the ultrasound-guided supraclavicular approach for brachial plexus block. *Anesthesia and Analgesia.* 2010; **111**: 817–819.

Bhatnagar S, Gupta R. Bedside ultrasound: A radiologic boon for placement of complex nerve blocks for abdominal malignancies. *Journal of Palliative Medicine.* 2011; **14**: 1198–1199.

Bhatnagar S, Khanna S, Roshni S et al. Early ultrasound-guided neurolysis for pain management in gastrointestinal and pelvic malignancies: An observational study in a tertiary care center of urban India. *Pain Practice.* 2012; **12**: 23–32.

Blumenthal S, Borgeat A, Neudorfer C et al. Additional femoral catheter in combination with popliteal catheter for analgesia after major ankle surgery. *British Journal of Anaesthesia.* 2011; **106**: 387–393.

Boezaart AP, De Beer JF, Du Toit C, Van Rooyen K. A new technique of continuous interscalene nerve block. *Canadian Journal of Anaesthesia.* 1999; **46**: 275–281.

Bosscher H. Blockade of the superior hypogastric plexus block for visceral pelvic pain. *Pain Practice.* 2001; **1**: 162–170.

Buchanan D, Brown E, Millar F et al. Outpatient continuous interscalene brachial plexus block in cancer-related pain. *Journal of Pain and Symptom Management.* 2009; **38**: 629–634.

Cannon B, Chan L, Rowlinson JS et al. Digital anaesthesia: One injection or two? *Emergency Medicine Journal.* 2010; **27**: 533–536.

Cervero F, Laird JM. Visceral pain. *Lancet.* 1999; **353**: 2145–2148.

Chambers WA. Nerve blocks in palliative care. *British Journal of Anaesthesia.* 2008; **101**: 95–100.

Chen S. Clinical uses of botulinum neurotoxins: Current indications, limitations and future developments. *Toxins (Basel).* 2012; **4**: 913–939.

Chester M, Hammond C, Leach A. Long-term benefits of stellate ganglion block in severe chronic refractory angina. *Pain.* 2000; **87**: 103–105.

Creech C, Meyr AJ. Techniques of Popliteal Nerve Regional Anesthesia. *Journal of Foot and Ankle Surgery.* 2013.

De Leon-Casasola OA. Critical evaluation of chemical neurolysis of the sympathetic axis for cancer pain. *Cancer Control.* 2000; **7**: 142–148.

De Oliveira R, Dos Reis MP, Prado WA. The effects of early or late neurolytic sympathetic plexus block on the management of abdominal or pelvic cancer pain. *Pain.* 2004; **110**: 400–408.

Delaunay L, Chelly JE. Blocks at the wrist provide effective anesthesia for carpal tunnel release. *Canadian Journal of Anaesthesia.* 2001; **48**: 656–660.

Desmet M, Braems H, Reynvoet M et al. I.V. and perineural dexamethasone are equivalent in increasing the analgesic duration of a single-shot interscalene block with ropivacaine for shoulder surgery: A prospective, randomized, placebo-controlled study. *British Journal of Anaesthesia.* 2013.

Dressler D. Clinical applications of botulinum toxin. *Current Opinion in Microbiology.* 2012; **15**: 325–336.

Dressler D, Benecke R. Autonomic side effects of botulinum toxin type B treatment of cervical dystonia and hyperhidrosis. *European Neurology.* 2003; **49**: 34–38.

Eisenberg E, Carr DB, Chalmers TC. Neurolytic celiac plexus block for treatment of cancer pain: A meta-analysis. *Anesthesia and Analgesia.* 1995; **80**: 290–295.

Eker HE, Cok OY, Kocum A et al. Transsacrococcygeal approach to ganglion impar for pelvic cancer pain: A report of 3 cases. *Regional Anesthesia and Pain Medicine.* 2008; **33**: 381–382.

Erdek MA, Halpert DE, Gonzalez Fernandez M, Cohen SP. Assessment of celiac plexus block and neurolysis outcomes and technique in the management of refractory visceral cancer pain. *Pain Medicine.* 2010; **11**: 92–100.

Esch AT, Esch A, Knorr JL, Boezaart AP. Long-term ambulatory continuous nerve blocks for terminally ill patients: A case series. *Pain Medicine.* 2010; **11**: 1299–1302.

French J, Sharp LM. Local anaesthetics. *Annals of the Royal College of Surgeons of England.* 2012; **94**: 76–80.

Fu J, Gutierrez C, Bruera E et al. Use of injectable spasticity management agents in a cancer center. *Supportive Care in Cancer.* 2013; **21**: 1227–1232.

Fujimura N, Namba H, Tsunoda K et al. Effect of hemidiaphragmatic pare- sis caused by interscalene brachial plexus block on breathing pat- tern, chest wall mechanics, and arterial blood gases. *Anesthesia and Analgesia.* 1995; **81**: 962–966.

Gorlin A, Warren L. Ultrasound-guided interscalene blocks. *Journal of Ultrasound in Medicine.* 2012; **31**: 979–983.

Guay J. Adverse events associated with intravenous regional anesthesia (Bier block): A systematic review of complications. *Journal of Clinical Anesthesia.* 2009; **21**: 585–594.

Haest K, Kumar A, Van Calster B et al. Stellate ganglion block for the man- agement of hot flashes and sleep disturbances in breast cancer survi- vors: An uncontrolled experimental study with 24 weeks of follow-up. *Annals of Oncology.* 2012; **23**: 1449–1454.

Ho KY, Nagi PA, Gray L, Huh BK. An alternative approach to ganglion impar neurolysis under computed tomography guidance for recurrent vulva cancer. *Anesthesiology.* 2006; **105**: 861–862.

Horlocker TT, Wedel DJ, Rowlingson JC et al. Regional anesthesia in the patient receiving antithrombotic or thrombolytic therapy: American Society of Regional Anesthesia and Pain Medicine Evidence-Based Guidelines (Third Edition). *Regional Anesthesia and Pain Medicine.* 2010; **35**: 64–101.

Ilfeld BM. Continuous peripheral nerve blocks in the hospital and at home. *Anesthesiology Clinics.* 2011a; **29**: 193–211.

Ilfeld BM. Continuous peripheral nerve blocks: A review of the published evidence. *Anesthesia and Analgesia.* 2011b; **113**: 904–925.

Jackson TP, Gaeta R. Neurolytic blocks revisited. *Current Pain and Headache Reports.* 2008; **12**: 7–13.

Klinkenberg M, Willems DL, Van Der Wal G, Deeg DJ. Symptom burden in the last week of life. *Journal of Pain and Symptom Management.* 2004; **27**: 5–13.

Koshy RC, Padmakumar G, Rajasree O. Low cost continuous femoral nerve block for relief of acute severe cancer related pain due to pathological fracture femur. *Indian Journal of Palliative Care.* 2010; **16**: 180–182.

Kroll CE, Schartz B, Gonzalez-Fernandez M et al. Factors Associated With Outcome after Superior Hypogastric Plexus Neurolysis in Cancer Patients. *Clinical Journal of Pain.* 2013.

Layeeque R, Hochberg J, Siegel E et al. Botulinum toxin infiltration for pain control after mastectomy and expander reconstruction. *Annals of Surgery.* 2004; **240**: 608–613; discussion 613–614.

Lim EC, Quek AM, Seet RC. Accurate targeting of botulinum toxin injec- tions: How to and why. *Parkinsonism & Related Disorders.* 2011; **17 (Suppl. 1)**: S34–S39.

Lim JY, Koh JH, Paik NJ. Intramuscular botulinum toxin-A reduces hemiplegic shoulder pain: A randomized, double-blind, comparative study versus intraarticular triamcinolone acetonide. *Stroke.* 2008; **39**: 126–131.

Lu DW, Lippitz J. Complications of botulinum neurotoxin. *Disease-a-Month.* 2009; **55**: 198–211.

Maga JM, Cooper L, Gebhard RE. Outpatient regional anesthesia for upper extremity surgery update (2005 to present) distal to shoulder. *International Anesthesiology Clinics.* 2012; **50**: 47–55.

Marciniak CM, Harvey RL, Gagnon CM et al. Does botulinum toxin type A decrease pain and lessen disability in hemiplegic survivors of stroke with shoulder pain and spasticity?: A randomized, double-blind, placebo-controlled trial. *American Journal of Physical Medicine and Rehabilitation.* 2012; **91**: 1007–1019.

Mauck W, Rho R. The role of neurolytic sympathetic blocks in cancer pain. *Techniques in Regional Anesthesia and Pain Management.* 2010; **14**: 32–39.

Mercadante S, Catala E, Arcuri E, Casuccio A. Celiac plexus block for pan- creatic cancer pain: Factors influencing pain, symptoms and quality of life. *Journal of Pain and Symptom Management.* 2003; **26**: 1140–1147.

Miguel R. Interventional treatment of cancer pain: The fourth step in the World Health Organization analgesic ladder? *Cancer Control.* 2000; **7**: 149–156.

Mohr B. Safety and effectiveness of intravenous regional anesthesia (Bier block) for outpatient management of forearm trauma. *CJEM.* 2006; **8**: 247–250.

Moore R, Groves D, Hammond C et al. Temporary sympathectomy in the treatment of chronic refractory angina. *Journal of Pain and Symptom Management.* 2005; **30**: 183–191.

Murphy DB, Mccartney CJ, Chan VW. Novel analgesic adjuncts for brachial plexus block: A systematic review. *Anesthesia and Analgesia.* 2000; **90**: 1122–1128.

Murray JM, Derbyshire S, Shields MO. Lower limb blocks. *Anaesthesia.* 2010; **65 (Suppl. 1)**: 57–66.

Nabil Abbas D, Abd El Ghafar EM, Ibrahim WA, Omran AF. Fluoroscopic stel- late ganglion block for postmastectomy pain: A comparison of the clas- sic anterior approach and the oblique approach. *Clinical Journal of Pain.* 2011; **27**: 207–213.

Okell RW, Brooks NC. Persistent pain relief following interscalene analgesia for cancer pain. *Anaesthesia.* 2009; **64**: 225–226.

Pacenta HL, Kaddoum RN, Pereiras LA et al. Continuous tunnelled femoral nerve block for palliative care of a patient with metastatic osteosar- coma. *Anaesthesia and Intensive Care.* 2010; **38**: 563–565.

Pelaez R, Pascual G, Aguilar JL, Atanassoff PG. Paravertebral cervical nerve block in a patient suffering from a Pancoast tumor. *Pain Medicine.* 2010; **11**: 1799–1802.

Plancarte R, De Leon-Casasola OA, El-Helaly M et al. Neurolytic superior hypogastric plexus block for chronic pelvic pain associated with cancer. *Regional Anesthesia.* 1997; **22**: 562–568.

Portenoy RK. Treatment of cancer pain. *Lancet.* 2011; **377**: 2236–2247.

Raj PP, Shah RV, Kaye AD et al. Bleeding risk in interventional pain practice: Assessment, management, and review of the literature. *Pain Physician.* 2004; **7**: 3–51.

Rork JF, Berde CB, Goldstein RD. Regional anesthesia approaches to pain management in pediatric palliative care: A review of current knowl- edge. *Journal of Pain and Symptom Management.* 2013.

Rudkin GE, Rudkin AK, Dracopoulos GC. Ankle block success rate: A prospec- tive analysis of 1,000 patients. *Canadian Journal of Anaesthesia.* 2005; **52**: 209–210.

Sanni A, Hamid A, Dunning J. Is sympathectomy of benefit in critical leg isch- aemia not amenable to revascularisation? *Interactive Cardiovascular and Thoracic Surgery.* 2005; **4**: 478–483.

Schnabel A, Reichl SU, Kranke P et al. Efficacy and safety of paravertebral blocks in breast surgery: A meta-analysis of randomized controlled tri- als. *British Journal of Anaesthesia.* 2010; **105**: 842–852.

Seth J, Khan MS, Dasgupta P, Sahai A. Botulinum toxin-what urologic uses does the data support? *Current Urology Reports.* 2013; **14**: 227–234.

Stubblefield MD, Levine A, Custodio CM, Fitzpatrick T. The role of botulinum toxin type A in the radiation fibrosis syndrome: A preliminary report. *Archives of Physical Medicine and Rehabilitation.* 2008; **89**: 417–421.

Tempero MA, Arnoletti JP, Behrman S et al. Pancreatic adenocarcinoma. *Journal of the National Comprehensive Cancer Network.* 2010; **8**: 972–1017.

Turnbull JH, Gebauer SL, Miller BL et al. Cutaneous nerve transection for the management of intractable upper extremity pain caused by invasive squamous cell carcinoma. *Journal of Pain and Symptom Management.* 2011; **42**: 126–133.

Vranken JH, Van Der Vegt MH, Zuurmond WW et al. Continuous brachial plexus block at the cervical level using a posterior approach in the management of neuropathic cancer pain. *Regional Anesthesia and Pain Medicine.* 2001; **26**: 572–575.

Vranken JH, Zuurmond WW, De Lange JJ. Continuous brachial plexus block as treatment for the Pancoast syndrome. *Clinical Journal of Pain*. 2000; **16**: 327–333.

Vuong T, Waschke K, Niazi T et al. The value of Botox-A in acute radiation proctitis: Results from a phase I/II study using a three-dimensional scoring system. *International Journal of Radiation Oncology, Biology, Physics*. 2011; **80**: 1505–1511.

Wong GY, Schroeder DR, Carns PE et al. Effect of neurolytic celiac plexus block on pain relief, quality of life, and survival in patients with unresectable pancreatic cancer: A randomized controlled trial. *JAMA*. 2004; **291**: 1092–1099.

Yuan RY, Sheu JJ, Yu JM et al. Botulinum toxin for diabetic neuropathic pain: A randomized double-blind crossover trial. *Neurology*. 2009; **72**: 1473–1478.

Yuen TS, Ng KF, Tsui SL. Neurolytic celiac plexus block for visceral abdominal malignancy: Is prior diagnostic block warranted? *Anaesthesia and Intensive Care*. 2002; **30**: 442–448.

Zech DF, Grond S, Lynch J et al. Validation of World Health Organization Guidelines for cancer pain relief: A 10-year prospective study. *Pain*. 1995; **63**: 65–76.

49

Pain management in pediatrics

REGINA OKHUYSEN-CAWLEY

INTRODUCTION

Appropriate pain management in the acutely or chronically ill child is a moral imperative. Although significant progress has been made in the last 50 years, misinformation and limited access remain widespread: It is estimated that only a small fraction of the seven million children worldwide who qualify for palliative care have integrated management utilizing pharmacologic and nonpharmacologic measures.

Perioperative and acute pain management in children are also deficient even in developed countries. Fortunately, this is changing: the seminal studies of Anand and Hickley at the end of the twentieth century underscore the importance of adequate analgesia in children subjected to deeply painful procedures and recognize that inadequate analgesia may have permanent negative repercussions in the developing brain. It is now understood that sensitivity to pain is present early in fetal life, and that pain may be safely managed with opioids even in the sickest premature infant. Myths and misconceptions limiting the use of effective medications are being replaced by rational approaches: what is painful to an adult is just as painful to any child, who may not be able to express his or her discomfort. Properly administered opioids carry very little risk of complications.

Regional and international initiatives have made dissemination of simple principles and guidelines a priority and have proposed clinically relevant research, as outlined in the comprehensively referenced *World Health Organization guidelines on the pharmacological treatment of persisting pain in children with medical illnesses*. The American Academy of Pediatrics emphasizes the importance of quality over quantity: "Add life to the child's years, rather than years to the child's life." Discernment is of particular importance in situations where symptoms become progressively more difficult to control in the face of increasing dependence on technology. A most remarkable young boy, Mattie Stepanek, beautifully articulated these concepts a few years before succumbing to a rare form of muscular dystrophy: palliative care is not about helping people die; it is about helping them live as well as possible for as long as possible, and then, when the time is certain, helping them die

gently. Recent literature suggests that significant progress has been achieved in the control of pain and distressing symptoms in dying children.

MEASURING PAIN IN CHILDREN

Neonates are babies up to 28 days after delivery; infancy encompasses the first 12 months of postnatal life. The definition of "child" from the pediatric standpoint varies regionally: Some preadolescent children are managed as adults, although they are far from mature developmentally. Thorough, systematic assessment and reassessment after intervention are crucial, ideally recording pain as a fifth vital sign in all clinical encounters. It is recognized that pain is more challenging to evaluate in infants, cognitively impaired, critically ill, and severely neglected or malnourished children. Clues to the presence of pain in pre- or nonverbal children include apathy, irritability, reluctance to move or be moved, changes in appetite or activity, sleep disturbances. Facial grimacing, moaning, and crying may occur. Neonates may become minimally responsive and even bradycardic as an energy-conserving mechanism during stressful procedures.

A number of age-appropriate pain measurement tools have emerged over the years. Commonly used scales include the Faces Pain Scale-Revised, useful for children above the age of 4, the Visual Analog Scale, for children older than 8 years. Other tools, such as the Oucher Photographic, also allow self-report in school-aged children. Neonates can be evaluated with specialized tools. Hypoactive and agitated delirium impact pain expression in the presence of advanced illness and should be recognized and treated appropriately.

The two-step strategy for pain control

The traditional three-step ladder introduced in 1986 for cancer pain relief has been revised. A simplified approach distinguishes mild from moderate to severe pain. Mild pain is appropriately managed with analgesics such as paracetamol (acetaminophen) or ibuprofen. Moderate to severe pain should

Table 49.1 *Drug considerations and dosage guidelines*

Drug	Benefits	Disadvantages	Usual starting dose	Maximum dose	Special considerations
Paracetamol (acetaminophen)	Analgesic and antipyretic; used for mild pain	Hepatotoxicity if recommended doses exceeded	10–15 mg/kg orally every 4–6 h	Not to exceed 60 mg/kg/ day; decrease dose and interval in neonates	Can be useful as an adjunct (not a substitute) in patients with severe pain
Ibuprofen	Analgesic, antipyretic; used for mild pain	Nephrotoxicity, gastric irritant, may promote bleeding	10 mg/kg orally every 6 hours	Avoid in young infants	Has anti-inflammatory effect
Morphine	Opioid Analgesic	Histamine release Dysphoria	0.05–0.1 mg/kg IV	Use appropriate precautions in young, acutely ill or debilitated children	First line; inexpensive and readily available; oral and parenteral forms
Hydromorphone	Opioid Analgesic		0.015 mg/kg IV	Longer half-life than morphine	Oral and parenteral forms
Oxycodone	Opioid Analgesic		Individualize		Oral immediate and extended release; frequently diverted
Fentanyl	Analgesia	Opioid of choice in hemodynamic instability	0.5–1 µg/kg IV	Short half-life	Parenteral, transmucosal, transdermal delivery systems
Methadone	Analgesia	Use by specialist	Individualize	Long, variable half-life	Many drug interactions; useful for neuropathic pain

be managed from its onset with opioids. The use of "weak" or intermediate-potency opioids is discouraged (Table 49.1).

The other basic principles involve treating pain at regular intervals rather than a "pro re nata" (PRN), which may translate, for practical purposes, into "patient receives nothing," as aptly described by Friedrichsdorf. Regularly scheduled, appropriately dosed opioids should be supplemented with "rescue" doses for intermittent or "breakthrough" pain. An extended-release formulation, or a drug with a long half-life methadone, is recommended for maintenance, with an immediate-release appropriate formulation for incident (pain associated with movement or activity) or breakthrough episodes, defined as those occurring unpredictably on a background of good control.

A multimodal approach inclusive of nonpharmacologic measures is recommended for all patients. Nonpharmacologic measures include those appropriate to the neonate and young infant such as environmental control, swaddling, and sucrose to more complex interventions such as hypnosis, guided imagery, and distraction in the older child.

NONOPIOID ANALGESICS

Paracetamol and ibuprofen are the mainstays of nonopioid analgesia. While they are primarily utilized worldwide for the management of mild pain and fever, paracetamol should not be overlooked in patients already receiving opioids for severe pain. Reduced doses and increased intervals are recommended for neonates and young infants, malnourished or debilitated patients. Intravenous paracetamol can be considered if enteral administration is impractical.

There are no definite advantages to using nonsteroidal analgesics other than ibuprofen, which is suitable for children older than 3 months of age. Parenteral ketorolac may be useful in selected patients, but should be used sparingly due to the risk of gastrointestinal bleeding. Meloxicam and celecoxib may be considered. Dipyrone (metamizole) is a strong analgesic and antipyretic but unfortunately carries a small but documented risk of aplastic anemia. It has been banned from many countries for this reason.

OPIOID ANALGESICS

Morphine

Morphine remains the gold standard against which all other opioids are compared. It is also the most readily available opioid worldwide, forming the basis of the essential analgesic medication formularies. It is available in several immediate- and extended-release forms. It is also the opioid that has been most extensively studied in children. The drug undergoes extensive first-pass metabolism after ingestion. It is apparent from pharmacodynamic studies that neonates and infants express enzymes required for glucuronidation in lower amounts, which contributes to a longer half-life in these babies. Babies may preferentially produce morphine-3-glucuronide, an active metabolite, which is potentially neurotoxic and devoid of analgesic activity. Morphine-6-glucuronide, the beneficial active metabolite, appears to undergo active transport across the blood–brain barrier to exert its analgesic effects on mu receptors. Morphine pharmacokinetics approximates adult profiles in the latter part of infancy as glomerular function matures. Toxicity may be observed in patients with renal failure.

ALTERNATIVE MAJOR OPIOIDS IN CHILDREN

Opioid selection depends on several factors, including the child's circumstances, prescriber preferences, and local availability. The oral route should be used as much as possible, but other approaches including intravenous, subcutaneous, rectal, and intranasal routes may be appropriate. Rotation to a different strong opioid, with reduction by 50%–75% of the calculated dose to account for cross-tolerance, may be indicated for loss of efficacy in the face of increasing side effects during titration, but there is no advantage to periodic rotation. Myoclonus, suggestive of opioid-associated neurotoxicity, must be addressed with reduction to prevent progression to seizures. There are several tables and internet resources available to assist in opioid rotation.

Fentanyl

Fentanyl is a synthetic opioid estimated to be 100 times more potent than morphine. It has the distinct advantage of producing minimal, if any, histamine release, making it very useful in the management of acutely ill children. Adequate analgesia may be achieved in the opioid-naive child with 1–2 µg/kg of ideal body weight given parenterally. The drug has a much shorter half-life than morphine or hydromorphone, making it suitable for rapid titration in the critically ill. It is suitable for continuous infusions, with the caveat that this and other synthetic opioids may rapidly induce tolerance in some patients. Chest wall rigidity has been associated with rapid infusion of large boluses. Fentanyl can be used safely in patients with renal failure, but the dose may need to be adjusted for hepatic failure. The drug is highly lipophilic, allowing for delivery as a nasal mist for children with traumatic injuries seen in emergency centers, and patients of all ages for breakthrough pain.

Fentanyl is dispensed in a variety of forms intended for chronic pain management. Transdermal patches varying from 12.5 to 100 µg/hour are available for opioid-tolerant patients, defined as those taking 30 mg or more of oral morphine equivalent per day. The patches should not be cut or modified, and should be changed every 72 hours. There is wide variability in the clinical response: onset of analgesia may occur in a matter of a few hours for some patients, and may take longer than 2 days for others, underscoring the importance of a short-acting opioid for pain until a steady-state is achieved. Toxicity may occur in patients who develop fever; absorption may be poor in the presence of severe cachexia or poor skin perfusion. Some children experience end-of-dose failure requiring a change in the patch every 48 hours. Oral bioavailability is poor, prompting the development of a variety of transmucosal preparations, including lozenges designed to dissolve within 15 min, buccal effervescent tablets, and a dissolvable film that have been marketed. These approaches may be quite costly.

Hydromorphone

Hydromorphone is approximately five times more potent than morphine. It has a longer half-life when administered intravenously. Rapid intravenous infusion may result in a euphoric feeling which some adolescents may subsequently pursue; therefore, it should be administered slowly when used intravenously. The drug has active metabolites that may accumulate in the presence of renal insufficiency. Commonly available oral formulations include solution and immediate-release tablets.

Methadone

Experience with the use of methadone is increasing, particularly in patients with cancer and neuropathic pain, given its actions as a mu-receptor agonist and NMDA-receptor antagonist. The drug has been used successfully in neonates with antenatal opioid exposure, and in neonates, infants, and children who have become habituated to opioids in the intensive care unit. The tablets and oral solution are relatively inexpensive. Methadone is widely available, an effective analgesic that is best prescribed by trained clinicians for patients with serious conditions such as cancer, given its extremely variable prolonged half-life. The recommendation to "start low and go slow" especially applies to methadone. Dosage increases are usually made no more frequently than every 72 hours, with instructions to hold one or more doses and increase the interval if excessive sedation is noted. Significant drug interactions may occur, particularly with drugs such as haloperidol, quinolones, macrolides, ondansetron, etc. Many physicians recommend monitoring the QT interval. Methadone may be extremely useful in children with chronic pain due to advancing malignancies.

Buprenorphine

The role of buprenorphine in pediatric practice is unclear at this time. Limited experience suggests that it is effective and well tolerated in children. Buprenorphine may be advantageous in patients with neuropathic pain as it affects kappa receptors in addition to mu receptor. Oral bioavailability is low due to first-pass metabolism. The drug is available as droplets for sublingual administration in many parts of the world. Although the potential for nausea exists, there is also some experience to suggest that it is less constipating than other opioids. Transdermal buprenorphine may have a role in the management of chronically ill children with limited vascular and enteral access. The transdermal patches are available in a variety of strengths, varying from 5 to 50 µg/hour, and depending on the brand, may be left in place from 96 hours to 1 week. Division of the patch is not recommended. Buprenorphine/naloxone tablets intended to treat addiction disorders in adults are extremely dangerous to children.

Oxycodone

Oxycodone is an effective strong opioid. There is some concern that it is more likely to cause respiratory depression than what is observed with morphine, but this is not common. Oxycodone is available both as an oral solution and as immediate-release and extended-release tablets. Onset of action is in about 30 min for the immediate-release form. The extended-release tablet is usually administered twice per day, although some children may require three doses to prevent end-of-dose failure.

DRUGS TO BE AVOIDED IN PEDIATRICS

Pethidine (meperidine) is no longer recommended for use in children. It is less potent than morphine, is not well absorbed enterally, and it has an active metabolite, normeperidine, which has been associated with seizures in the presence of renal insufficiency. The metabolism of codeine to morphine, essential for analgesia, depends on variable expression of the enzyme CYP2D6. Young children and even some adults are unable to metabolize it at all, while fatalities have occurred in ultrafast metabolizers. Codeine is usually marketed with paracetamol (acetaminophen), and thus carries the risk of potential ceiling effect associated with fixed drug combinations. The use of codeine as an analgesic or antitussive is discouraged in modern practice. Tramadol is a weak opioid, typically used perioperatively when morphine is unavailable. It frequently causes nausea and unfortunately has significant potential drug interactions resulting in serotonin syndrome and seizure activity. Decreased clearance may be observed in patients with hepatic dysfunction.

Other medications used in acute and chronic pain management

The extensive literature review and expert consultation that form the basis of the World Health Organization's most recent guidelines on pediatric pain management demonstrate that there is a limited role for many of the medications traditionally utilized as adjuncts for chronic pain management. A streamlined, cost-effective, individualized approach is recommended for all patients. Steroids such as dexamethasone have an important but discrete role in the management of cerebral edema, spinal cord compression, metastatic bone pain, and visceral involvement.

Patient–controlled analgesia

Patient-controlled analgesia (PCA) is available in some countries. There are several different options available depending on the child's age, intellectual development, and the expected clinical course. Children who can independently operate video games are generally able to utilize a PCA, particularly when the concept is explained to them ahead of time. There are several significant potential problems: surgical patients who are not receiving a basal infusion of the opioid may fall asleep only to awaken in severe pain; conversely, patients or their parents may push the button inappropriately to mask other symptoms or simply because they have misunderstood instructions and press the button every time it lights up. Patient and caregiver education is thus essential for proper use. Most children managed with PCAs are monitored with pulse oximetry and, in some cases, end-tidal CO_2 monitoring. Clinicians may also administer additional bolus doses as required by the child's condition, after appropriate evaluation.

Surgical patients with epidural analgesia require vigilance; epidural medications may be a combination of local anesthetics with an alfa-2 agonist, such as clonidine, and opioids. It is not unusual for epidural catheters to work erratically in children, and the function and content of the epidural catheter and the prescription should be revised if pain is present. Opioids should be used by a single route in most instances.

Continuous intravenous and subcutaneous infusions

Children with chronic conditions such as cancer frequently have implanted devices such as tunneled central venous lines, ports, or peripherally inserted central venous catheters, which may be extremely useful for palliative purposes. Peripheral intravenous catheters are impractical for long-term use; subcutaneous catheters, on the other hand, can be placed and maintained in the hospital, hospice, or home in children of all ages. They can be changed weekly, if no irritation develops. Single drugs or combinations may be delivered via small syringe drivers. Any opioid can be delivered in this fashion, although there is some concern that methadone may cause more irritation.

Rectal medications

All currently available opioids may be administered rectally in situations if necessary, but this route should be avoided in the presence of thrombocytopenia, neutropenia, or in situations where it could cause emotional distress. Medications commonly administered using this route include paracetamol (acetaminophen) and various nonsteroidal analgesics. Benzodiazepines may be administered rectally, particularly in the event of status epilepticus.

Management of opioid side effects

Transient sedation is common, and usually resolves in a few days. Excessive sedation several days into treatment with methadone, however, should be addressed with dose adjustment. Nausea is less common in children than in adults, but should be anticipated and treated, usually with agents such as ondansetron or metoclopramide. The use of promethazine and other phenothiazines is discouraged as they are central nervous depressants. Pruritus may respond to antihistamines; some patients may be managed with small subcutaneous or intravenous doses of nalbuphine. Constipation should be expected in most children requiring opioid therapy and is best managed with an agent that will stimulate the bowel and soften the stool such as a senna associated with docusate, which is ineffective when used alone. Lactulose can be used in ambulatory patients but may produce significant bowel distention and discomfort in patients who are bedridden. Milk of magnesia may be tried in some patients. Suppositories or enemas may be necessary in some cases. Subcutaneous methylnaltrexone is devoid of systemic effects but may cause severe cramping and should never be used if structural obstruction is a possibility. Urinary retention is less common than it is in adults but may respond to rotation.

Pain in the context of terminal illness

Adequate analgesia may become challenging as the underlying disease advances. Close communication with families with timely, frank discussion of prognosis and goals of care facilitates symptom management throughout the disease trajectory.

Most children with cancer respond to opioid titration or rotation to a different class. Some children require very high amounts of opioid, which is appropriate as long as intolerable side effects or neurotoxicity are not observed. An adjunct such as dexamethasone or a gabapentenoid may be useful; subanesthetic ketamine or lidocaine may be tried in refractory pain. Selected patients may benefit from image-guided interventional procedures such as nerve blocks, myelotomy, or cordotomy. Tunneled epidural catheters or refillable devices can be considered in some cases but may be associated with complications, are expensive, and may require referral to tertiary centers.

Careful interrogation of the child and caregivers and physical examination may produce clues to associated distressing symptoms such as nausea, gastroesophageal reflux, cough, constipation, bowel obstruction, urinary retention. Relief of such problems may mitigate the need for rapid opioid titration. New paresthesias or symptoms may require investigation to exclude preventable morbidity such as spinal cord compression. Sleep disorders are extremely common and should be addressed with good sleep hygiene strategies. Fatigue is extremely common and notoriously difficult to manage, but simple strategies aimed to conserve the child's energy can notably improve the quality of life.

It is important to recognize that even very young children may experience existential distress. Compassionate, culturally sensitive, and developmentally appropriate discussion with the child may be extremely beneficial. Children and families who do so may have some opportunities for special moments and closure prior to death, with fewer regrets afterward than when difficult but necessary words go unsaid.

Key learning points

- The World Health Organization emphasizes simple principles to be observed when prescribing analgesics to children:

  - Two-step approach
  - By the clock
  - By the appropriate route
  - With the child

- The range of causes for pain in pediatric palliative medicine is wide, reflecting a great variety of life-limiting conditions. The etiology of distressing symptoms and the intensity of pain are most difficult to elucidate in young and nonverbal infants.

- Children differ from adults in the pathophysiology and the pharmacology of pain management. Neonatal pharmacokinetics is very different from other periods in childhood, primarily due to immature glomerular filtration. Higher doses relative to size are commonly required in toddlers and older children when compared to adults

- Paracetamol or ibuprofen (in infants greater than 3 months of age) is indicated for mild pain. Moderate to severe pain should be managed with opioids. Risks commonly associated with opioids are minimal when they are used correctly.

- Opioids should be ordered on a scheduled basis for surgical and other types of severe pain; pain expected to persist beyond a few days should be managed with a drug with a prolonged half-life such as methadone, an extended-release preparation, or with a transdermal opioid delivery system. Immediate-release preparations should be available at all times, usually at one-sixth to one-tenth of the daily dose of the basal extended-release preparation available at short intervals, but hourly if needed. Requirement for more than two or three doses per day for 2 days signifies the need to increase the dose of the basal analgesic.

- Adjuvants should be individualized.

- All interventions should be carefully considered in terms of benefit, risk, and cost to the family. The simplest effective approach should be selected, taking into account that invasive procedures may sometimes play a part in a sound palliative care plan.

- The oral route should be preferred whenever possible. Other routes should be considered if necessary. Intramuscular injections should not be prescribed.

- Stimulant laxatives are almost always necessary and should be prescribed from the beginning of opioid therapy

- Codeine, meperidine, and medications combining opioids with paracetamol or ibuprofen should not be used.

- Nonpharmacologic measures are an integral part of pain management in patients of any age

ACKNOWLEDGMENTS

This chapter is an updated version of Chapter 50.

REFERENCES

1 World Health Organization: *WHO Guidelines on the Pharmacological Treatment of Persisting Pain in Children with Medical Illnesses.* Geneva, Switzerland: World Health Organization, 2012.
2 C Knapp, V Madden, and S Fowler-Kennedy Eds.: *Pediatric Palliative Care: Global Perspectives.* Dordrecht, the Netherlands: Springer, 2012.
3 M Silbermann et al: MECC regional initiative in pediatric palliative care: Middle Eastern course on pain management. *J Pediatr Hematol Oncol* 2012;34:S1–S11.
4 KJS Anand and PR Hickey: Pain and its effects in the human neonate and fetus. *N Engl J Med* 1987;317:1321–1329.
5 PJ Davis: Pharmacology for infants and children. *International Anesthesia Research Society 2005 Review Course Lectures,* pp. 13–15.
6 EW Boyer, EF McCance-Katz, and S Marcus: Methadone and buprenorphine toxicity in children. *Am J Addict* 2009;19:89–95.
7 LE Kelly et al: More codeine fatalities after tonsillectomy in North American children. *Pediatrics* May 2012;125(5):e1343–e1347.
8 B Zernikow, E Michel, and B Anderson: Transdermal fentanyl in childhood and adolescence: A comprehensive literature review. *J Pain* March 2007;8(3):187–207.
9 SF Friedrichsdorf et al.: Pediatric Pain Master Class Lectures, 2011.
10 SJ Friedrichsdorf: Pain management in children with advanced cancer and during end-of-life care. *Pediatr Hematol Oncol* 2010;27:257–251.
11 KPT Nguyen and NL Glass: Advances in pediatric pain management. *Adv Anesth* 2007;25:143–187.
12 E Michel, BJ Anderson, and B Zernikow: Buprenorphine TTS for children—A review of the drug's clinical pharmacology. *Pediatr Anesth* 2011;21:280–290.

50

Pain in the older adult

LINH MY THI NGUYEN, JEN-YU WEI

INTRODUCTION

Older persons are generally defined as aged 65 and older. By age 75, many people exhibit frailty and multiple chronic illnesses, and in those people older than 75, rapidly increasing morbidity, morality, and social problems result in strains on the healthcare system.[1,2] Pain assessment and management in this older frail population is more complex and necessitates individualized treatment due to both physiologic and pathologic changes such as sensory and cognitive impairment and disability. Despite these challenges, pain is usually effectively controlled in this population.

Pain can be acute or persistent in the older adult, and both types of pain warrant the proper investigation in order to diagnose and treat the underlying causes. Often, the terms "persistent pain" and "chronic pain" are synonymous. Because of the negative connotations of "chronic pain," the term "persistent pain" is preferred.[3] Commonly, the etiology of pain is multifactorial. Classifying the pain mechanism directs therapy and prognostication (Table 50.1).[4]

The most common pain management strategy is pharmacological therapy. However, evidence is lacking, because older patients have been excluded from clinical trials. Older patients appear to be more sensitive to analgesics and especially opioids.[5] Studies suggest elderly patients with postoperative and cancer pain experience higher pain relief and longer duration of action of opioids.[6,7]

Opioid treatment of persistent non-cancer-related pain is controversial. However, in the palliative population, the benefits frequently outweigh the risks. Furthermore, professional organizations endorse opioids in these appropriate situations. Fear of illicit drug use has produced reluctance of opioids in healthcare providers, patients, and families. The risk of drug abuse is low in patients taking opioids for medical treatment,[8,9] and intensive monitoring by a trained healthcare team mitigates the potential for abuse.

ASSESSMENT OF PAIN

General principles

The approach to pain management in the elderly is somewhat more complex and multifactorial, as compared to younger patients. Older patients may underreport pain or not report it at all. They also are at higher risk of side effects from drugs and complications from diagnostic and invasive procedures. Patients with cognitive impairment are at risk of undertreatment of pain due to their inability to provide an accurate pain history.

The patient's own pain report and its intensity are most accurate and reliable.[10] A verbally administered numeric rating scale 0–10 is a good first choice. However, many patients with and without cognitive impairment may have difficulty with the numeric rating scale. Alternatives for self-reporting of pain include other verbal descriptor scales, thermometers, and faces scales. It is important to personalize the scale, which is appropriate to the individual, and document the same tool at subsequent assessments.[11] Patients may deny pain; however, they may endorse "discomfort," "hurting," or "aching."[12–14]

Many patients with mild-to-moderate cognitive impairment can self-report with simple assessment tools.[15–22] Patients with sensory or cognitive impairment should be assessed with techniques adapted to the patient's handicaps.[17,23] History should also be taken from the family and other caregivers (Table 50.2).

Table 50.1   *Classification and common etiologies of pain*

Pain classification	Examples	Treatment and prognosis
Nociceptive	• Low back pain from facet joint arthritis, spondylosis • Osteoarthritis • Osteoporosis and bone fractures • Paget's disease • Rheumatoid arthritis, polymyalgia rheumatica • Gout • Degenerative disk disease • Chronic tendonitis • Ischemic disorders (e.g., claudication. peripheral vascular disease, coronary artery disease) • Myofascial pain syndromes	Usually responds well to traditional approaches including common analgesic medications and nonpharmacologic strategies
Neuropathic	• Peripheral neuropathy (e.g., diabetes, HIV, chemotherapy, nutritional, etc.) • Trigeminal neuralgia • Herpes zoster • Postherpetic neuralgia • Poststroke central/thalamic pain • Postamputation phantom limb pain • Radicular pain • Trauma	Does not respond as predictably to conventional analgesics but may respond to anticonvulsants or antiarrhythmics
Mixed or unspecified	• Recurrent headaches • Some vasculitic pain syndromes • Myofascial pain • Fibromyalgia • Chronic low back pain episodic pain	More unpredictable and may require trials of different medications or combined approaches
Other	• Rare conditions (e.g., conversion reaction)	May need psychiatric treatment but traditional analgesic interventions are not indicated

Selected 2002 AGS–guideline recommendations for the assessment of persistent pain[24]

PHARMACOLOGIC TREATMENT

General principles

Generally, older patients are at higher risk of adverse drug reactions. Age-related changes in older adults result in differences in drug effectiveness, sensitivity, and toxicity. Therefore, pharmacokinetics and pharmacodynamics properties are unique in this population (Table 50.3).[25–28]

Older adults have greater analgesic sensitivity; however, because of the heterogeneity of this population, it is difficult to predict the therapeutic dose and common side effects. Most analgesics do not recommend age-adjusted doses; however, it is generally recommend in the elderly population to initiate low doses followed by slow upward titration.

Some analgesics and adjuvants do have "geriatric dosing" and "Beers Criteria medication" recommendations, and these guidelines suggest the lowest starting doses. The American Geriatrics Society developed the 2012 Updated Beers Criteria for Potentially

Inappropriate Medication Use in Older Adults (AGS 2012 Beers Criteria) to improved medication safety.[29] These medications are known to cause adverse drug events due to their pharmacologic properties and the physiologic changes of aging. Not all criteria are applicable in patients receiving palliative and hospice. Clinicians should use this guide to identify the risks and benefits of each medication and to serve as a reminder for close monitoring so that an adverse event can be prevented or detected early.

The least invasive drug route should be used. General principles of both around the clock and as needed medications are the same in the older adult. However, for patients with cognitive impairment, the as-needed approach is not a good choice, because they are not able to request the medication appropriately. Patients should be premedicated prior to incident pain when possible, and continuous pain requires around the clock administration.

Combing pharmacological and nonpharmacological treatments including complementary and alternative medicine can enhance the analgesic control of persistent pain. Some nonpharmacological strategies have been shown to reduce pain, but these benefits are enhanced when combined with drug therapies. Physical therapy and patient and caregiver education are important interventions.[24]

Table 50.2   *Selected recommendations*

History

Cognitively intact or mild to moderate dementia
- Directly query the patient always.
- When screening, use pain synonyms (e.g., burning, discomfort, aching, soreness, heaviness, tightness).
- Standard pain scale sensitive to the patient's cognitive, language, and sensory impairments (e.g., adapted for visual, hearing, foreign language, other common handicaps in the elderly).
- Multidimensional pain scales (e.g., pain disability index, brief pain inventory).
- Patients with limited attention span and cognitive impairment should receive repeated instructions and adequate time.
- Ask about their worst pain experience over the last week.
- In mild to moderate cognitive impairment, frame the question in present tense due to impaired recall.

Moderate to severe dementia or nonverbal
- Assess pain via direct observation or history from caregivers
  - In patients with advanced dementia, unusual behaviors may indicate pain
  - Direct observation scales (e.g., PAINAD)

Physical exam
- Look for deformity, posture, leg length discrepancy.
- Look for pain behaviors (e.g., facial expressions, verbalizations/vocalizations, body movements, changes in interpersonal interactions, changes in activity patterns or routines, mental status changes).
- Physical function (e.g., measure ADL's, performance measure such as range of motion and get-up-and-go tests, etc.).
- Cognitive function for new or worsening confusion
  - Delirium assessment (e.g., MDAS, CAM)
  - Dementia assessment (e.g., SLUMS, MoCA, MMSE)

ADL, activities of daily living; BPI, brief pain inventory; CAM, confusion assessment method; MDAS, memorial delirium assessment score; MMSE, mini mental status exam; MoCA, Montreal cognitive assessment; PAINAD, pain assessment in advanced dementia; PDI, pain disability index; SLUMS, St. Louis University mental status.

Table 50.3   *Key pharmacologic changes in the older adult*

Pharmacologic concern	Normal aging
GI absorption/function	• Slowing of GI transit time may prolong effects of continuous release drugs. • Opioid-related bowel dysmotility may be enhanced.
Distribution	• Increased volume of distribution for fat-soluble drugs due to increased fat to lean body weight ratio. Results in longer effective drug half-life.
Liver metabolism	• Oxidation is variable and may decrease. May result in longer half-life.
Renal excretion	• Glomerular filtration rate decreases with age. Results in decreased excretion and prolonged effects of active metabolites.
Anticholinergic side effects	• Increased confusion, constipation, incontinence, movement disorders.

Monotherapy may not attain adequate analgesia, and therefore, combination of two or more drugs with complementary mechanisms of action may work synergistically to achieve a better outcome with less toxicity as compared to a single drug. This is known as "rational polypharmacy."

Nonopioid analgesics

Acetaminophen is effective for osteoarthritis and low back pain.[30,31] Because of its greater safety than nonsteroidal anti-inflammatory drugs (NSAIDs), acetaminophen is recommended as first-line therapy.[32] A dose titration upwards of 1000 mg of acetaminophen may control pain, and stronger medications may not be needed. The maximum safe dose is <4 g/24 hours. For patients with hepatic insufficiency or history of alcohol abuse, the maximum dose should be reduced by 50%–75%. Transient elevations of alanine aminotransferase observed in long-term users do not progress to liver dysfunction or failure when maximum doses are avoided.[33,34]

For chronic inflammatory pain (e.g., rheumatoid arthritis), NSAIDs are more effective than acetaminophen.[35] Other potential advantages of NSAIDs are that they may be better for short-term (e.g., 6 weeks) relief of osteoarthritis pain and short-term low back pain.[36–39] Although some NSAIDs at over-the-counter dosing may have a good safety profile in the general population,[40] older adults are at higher risk of NSAID side effects including gastrointestinal (GI) toxicity,[41] which increases in frequency and severity with age.[42] The GI toxicity may also be dose related and time dependent.[43,44] One study implicated NSAIDs as the cause of hospitalization for adverse drug reactions in 23.5% of cases in older adults.[45]

NSAIDs should be used cautiously in high-risk patients including those with kidney disease, which is common in the older adult due to age-related decreases in glomerular filtration rate, gastropathy, cardiovascular disease, and intravascularly depleted states such as congestive heart failure. NSAIDs were previously recommended on a trial basis; however, newer evidence suggests this is risky in the older adult. Older patients are at particular risk for NSAID-related serious or life-threatening GI bleeding and cardiovascular events,[46] and, therefore, opioids may be a safer alternative.

Opioid analgesics

Opioids are potentially effective for many patients and part of a multimodal treatment strategy for both persistent cancer and noncancer pain.[47–51] Opioids are effective in musculoskeletal disease (e.g., osteoarthritis[52] and low back pain[53,54]) and neuropathic pain syndromes (e.g., diabetic peripheral neuropathy, postherpetic neuralgia[55]).

The American Academy of Hospice and Palliative Medicine (AAHPM) recommends the starting dose for patients who are elderly, suffering from severe renal or liver disease, should be half that of the usual dose for opioid-naïve patients.[56] Again, older patients appear to be more sensitive to analgesics and especially opioids,[5] and studies suggest elderly patients with postoperative and cancer pain experience higher pain relief and longer duration of action of opioids.[6,7] "Rational polypharmacy" with agents with complementary mechanisms of action may be beneficial particularly if they experience dose-limiting side effects from a single agent.

The potential for opioid misuse and abuse should always be evaluated in every patient. However, older age is significantly associated with lower risk for opioid misuse and abuse.[57–60] Underuse of opioids may be a greater problem than misuse and abuse due to various patient-related barriers such as fear of addition, cost, side effects including constipation, and social stigma.[61]

Adjuvant drugs

Tricyclic antidepressants (e.g., amitriptyline, desipramine, and nortriptyline) were the first agents found to be effective for postherpetic neuralgia and diabetic neuropathy. Unfortunately, because of the adverse side effects in the elderly, it is often contraindicated. mixed serotonin- and norepinephrine-uptake inhibitors (SNRIs, e.g. duloxetine, venlafaxine) are effective in neuropathic pain syndromes and fibromyalgia, with a better side-effect profile as compared to tricyclic antidepressants. In contrast, SSRIs (e.g., sertraline, fluvoxamine, fluoxetine, citalopram) have not proved to be an adjuvant pain treatment.

Other drugs for pain

The evidence for the use of these drugs remains limited. As a group, they are less reliable than opioids and traditional analgesics for persistent pain. The use of these nonopioid, nontraditional drugs is a matter of clinical judgment.[62]

Muscle relaxants include cyclobenzaprine, carisoprodol, chloroxazone, methocarbamol, and others. It should be noted that cyclobenzaprine is essentially identical to amitriptyline with similar adverse effects of amitriptyline. These drugs may relieve skeletal muscle pain; however, the effects are nonspecific. These medications do not relieve muscle spasm. If muscle spasms are the etiology of pain, then benzodiazepines or baclofen should be considered, because these agents have known effects on muscle spasm. These drugs are associated with increased risk for falls in the older adults. Baclofen has been used as a second-line drug treatment for paroxysmal neuropathic pain and severe spasticity due to central nervous system and neuromuscular disorders.[63] Baclofen should be started at a low dose and slowly increased to minimize common side effects of dizziness, somnolence, and GI symptoms. Baclofen should not be abruptly discontinued due to potential for delirium and seizure and requires a slow taper.

Benzodiazepines do not have evidence to support any analgesic effect in persistent pain.[64] The high-risk profile usually outweighs any potential benefits for pain relief, although they may be justified for anxiety at the end of life, a trial for muscle spasm, and if pain coexists with these symptoms.

The use of corticosteroids, calcitonin, bisphosphonates, and topical analgesics is similar to that of younger patients. Cannabinoids have limited evidence, and in the older adult, the therapeutic window appears to be narrow because of the dysphoria and patients that use higher doses (Table 50.4).

Table 50.4 *Selected 2009 AGS guideline recommendations for persistent pain*

Nonopioids
- Acetaminophen should be considered as initial and ongoing drug therapy especially for musculoskeletal pain.
- NSAIDs may be considered rarely:
- Add either a proton pump inhibitor or misoprostol for GI protection if taking nonselective NSAID or COX-2 selective with aspirin.
- Do not use more than one NSAID.
- Patients taking aspirin should not use ibuprofen.

Opioids
- Treatment is similar to younger patients; however, the elderly may be more sensitive.

Adjuvants
- Tertiary tricyclic antidepressants (amitriptyline, imipramine, doxepin) should be avoided due to high risk of adverse effects.
- Start with lowest possible dose and titrate slowly. Some medications have delayed onset of action and therapeutic benefits (e.g., gabapentin may require 2–3 weeks).

Other drugs
- Systemic corticosteroids should be reserved for inflammatory disorders or metastatic bone pain. Osteoarthritis is not considered an inflammatory disorder.
- Consider topical agents in localized pain (e.g., lidocaine, NSAIDs, capsaicin).

REFERENCES

1   Ferrel BA. Overview of aging and pain. In: Ferrell BR, Ferrell BA eds. *Pain in the Elderly*. Seattle, WA: IASP Press, 1996, pp. 1–10.

2   He W, Sengupta M, Velkoff VA et al. *65+ in the United States: 2005*. Washington, DC: U.S. Census Bureau, Current Population Reports, U.S. Government Printing Office, 2005, pp. 23–209.

3   Weiner D, Herr K. Comprehensive interdisciplinary assessment and treatment planning: An integrative overview. In: Weiner D, Herr K, Rudy T eds. *Persistent Pain in Older Adults: An Interdisciplinary Guide for Treatment*. New York: Springer Publishing Company, 2002, pp. 18–27.

4   AGS Panel on Chronic Pain in Older Persons. The management of chronic pain in older persons. American Geriatrics Society. *J Am Geriatr Soc* 1998;46:635–651.

5   Kaiko RF, Wallenstein SL, Rogers AG et al. Narcotics in the elderly. *Med Clin North Am* 1982;66:1079–1089.

6   Kaiko RF. Age and morphine analgesia in cancer patients with postoperative pain. *Clin Pharmacol Ther* 1980;28:823–826.

7   Bellville JW, Forrest WH Jr, Miller E et al. Influence of age on pain relief from analgesics. A study of postoperative patients. *JAMA* 1971;217:1835–1841.

8   Portenoy RK. Chronic opioid therapy for persistent non-cancer pain: Can we get past the bias? *Am Pain Soc Bull* 1991;1:1,4–5.

9   Harden RN. Chronic opioid therapy: Another reappraisal. *Am Pain Soc Bull* 2002;12:1, 8–12.

10 Max MB, Payne R, Edwards WT et al. *Principles of Analgesic Drug Use in the Treatment of Acute Pain and Cancer Pain*, 4th edn. Glenville, IL: American Pain Society, 1999.

11 Ferrel BA. Pain. In: Osterweil D, Brummel-Smith K, Beck JC eds. *Comprehensive Geriatric Assessment*. New York: McGraw-Hill, 2000, pp. 381–397.

12 Parmelee PA. Assessment of pain in the elderly. In: Lawton MP, Teresi J eds. *Annual Review of Gerontology and Geriatrics*. New York: Springer Publishing Company, 1994, pp. 281–301.

13 Duggleby W, Lander J. Cognitive status and postoperative pain: Older adults. *J Pain Symptom Manage* 1994;9:19–27.

14 Miller J, Neelon V, Dalton J et al. The assessment of discomfort in elderly confused patients: A preliminary study. *J Neurosci Nurs* 1996;28:175–182.

15 Ferrell BA, Ferrell BR, Rivera L. Pain in cognitively impaired nursing home patients. *J Pain Symptom Manage* 1995:10:591–598.

16 Parmelee PA. Pain in cognitively impaired older persons. *Clin Geriatr Med* 1996;12:473–487.

17 Herr KA, Mobily PR, Kohout FJ et al. Evaluation of the faces pain scale for use with the elderly. *Clin J Pain* 1998;14:29–38.

18 Feldt KS, Warne MA, Ryden MB. Examining pain in aggressive cognitively impaired older adults. *J Gerontol Nurs* 1998;14:29–38.

19 Weiner D, Peterson B, Keffe F. Evaluating persistent pain in long term care residents: What role for pain maps? *Pain* 1998;76:249–257.

20 Wynne CF, Ling SM, Remsburg R. Comparison of pain assessment instruments in cognitively intact and cognitively impaired nursing home residents. *Geriatr Nurs* 2000;21:20–23.

21 Briggs M, Closs JS. A descriptive study of the use of visual analogue scales and verbal rating scales for the assessment of postoperative pain in orthopedic patients. *J Pain Symptom Manage* 1999;18:438–446.

22 Gloth FM III, Scheve AA, Stober BS et al. The functional pain scale: Reliability, validity and responsiveness in an elderly population. *J Am Med Dir Assoc* 2001;2:1110–1114.

23 Gagliese L, Melzack R. Age differences in the quality of chronic pain: A preliminary study. *Pain Res Manage* 1997;2:157–162.

24 AGS Panel on Persistent Pain in Older Persons. The management of persistent pain in older persons. *J Am Geriatr Society* 2002;50:S205–S224.

25 Delgado-Guay MO, Bruera E. Management of pain in the older persons with cancer. Part 2: Treatment options. *Oncology* (Williston Park) 2008;22:148–152, Discussion 152, 155, 160 passim.

26 Fine PG. Opioid analgesic drugs in older people. *Clin Geriatr Med* 2001;17:479–487.

27 Fine PG. Pharmacologic management of persistent pain in older patients. *Clin J Pain* 2004;20:220–226.

28 Pergolizzi J, Boger RH, Budd K et al. Opioids and the management of chronic severe pain in the elderly: Consensus statement of an International Expert Panel with focus on the six clinically most often used World Health Organization Step III opioids (buprenorphine, fentanyl, hydromorphone, methadone, morphine, oxycodone). *Pain Pract* 2008;8:287–313.

29 The American Geriatrics Society 2012 Beers Criteria Update Expert Panel. American geriatrics society updated beers criteria for potentially inappropriate medication use in older adults. *J Am Geriatr Soc* 2012:60:616–631.

30 Chou R, Huffman LH. Medications for acute and chronic low back pain: A review of the evidence for an American Pain Society/American College of Physicians clinical practice guidelines. *Ann Intern Med* 2007;147:505–514.

31 Zhang W, Jones A, Doherty M. Does paracetamol (acetaminophen) reduce the pain of osteoarthritis? A meta-analysis of randomized controlled trials. *Ann Rheum Dis* 2004;63:901–907.

32 Wegman A, van der Windt D, van Tulder M et al. Nonsteroidal anti-inflammatory drugs or acetaminophen for osteoarthritis of the hip or knee? A systematic review of evidence and guidelines. *J Rheumatol* 2004;31:344–354.

33 Kuffner EK, Temple AR, Cooper KM et al. Retrospective analysis of transient elevations in alanine aminotransferase during long-term treatment with acetaminophen in osteoarthritis clinical trials. *Curr Med Res Opin* 2006;22:2137–2148.

34 Watkins PB, Kaplowitz N, Slattery JT et al. Aminotransferase elevations in healthy adults receiving 4 grams of acetaminophen daily: A randomized controlled trial. *JAMA* 2006;296:87–93.

35 Weinecke T, Gotzsche PC. Paracetamol versus nonsteroidal anti-inflammatory drugs for rheumatoid arthritis. *Cochrane Database Syst Rev* 2004:CD003789.

36 Lee C, Straus WL, Balshaw R et al. A comparison of the efficacy and safety of nonsteroidal anti-inflammatory agents versus acetaminophen in the treatment of osteoarthritis: A meta-analysis. *Arthritis Rheum* 2004;51:746–754.

37 Towheed TE, Maxwell L, Judd MG et al. Acetaminophen for osteoarthritis. *Cochrane Database Syst Rev* 2006: CD004257.

38 Bjordal JM, Ljunggren AE, Klovning A et al. Non-steroidal anti-inflammatory drugs, including cyclo-oxygenase-2 inhibitors, in osteoarthritic knee pain: Meta-analysis of randomized placebo controlled trials. *BMJ* 2004;329:1317.

39 Roelof PD, Deyo RA, Koes BW et al. Non-steroidal anti-inflammatory drugs for low back pain. *Cochran Database Syst Rev* 2008: CD000396.

40 Bansal V, Dex T, Proskin H et al. A look at the safety profile of over-the-counter naproxen sodium: A meta-analysis. *J Clin Pharmacol* 2001;41:127–138.

41 Ofman JJ, MacLean CH, Straus WL et al. Metaanalysis of severe upper gastrointestinal complications of nonsteroidal anti-inflammatory drugs. *J Rheumatol* 2002;29:804–812.

42 Boers M, Tandelder MJ, van Ingen H et al. The rate of NSAID-induced endoscopic ulcers increases linearly but not exponentially with age: A pooled analysis of 12 randomised trials. *Ann Rheum Dis* 2007;66:417–418.

43 Ofman JJ, Maclean CH, Straus WL et al. Meta-analysis of dyspepsia and nonsteroidal anti-inflammatory drugs. *Arthritis Rheum* 2003;49:508–518.

44 Richy F, Bruyere O, Ethgen O et al. Time dependent risk of gastrointestinal complications induced by non-steroidal anti-inflammatory drug use: A consensus statement using a meta-analytic approach. *Ann Rheum Dis* 2004;63:759–766.

45 Franceschi M, Scarcelli C, Niro V et al. Pravalence, clinical features and avoidability of adverse drug reactions as cause of admission to a geriatric unit: A prospective study of 1756 patients. *Drug Saf* 2008;31:545–556.

46 Singh G, Wu O, Langhorne P et al. Risk of acute myocardial infarction with nonselective non-steroidal anti-inflammatory drugs: A meta-analysis. *Arthritis Res Ther* 2006;8:R153.

47 Avouac J, Gossec L, Dougados M. Efficacy and safety of opioids for osteoarthritis: A meta-analysis of randomized controlled trials. *Osteoarthritis Cartilage* 2007;15:957–965.

48 Chou R, Qaseem A, Snow V et al. Diagnosis and treatment of low back pain: A joint clinical practice guideline from the American College of Physicians and the American Pain Society. *Ann Intern Med* 2007;147:478–491.

49 Eisenberg E, McNicol ED, Carr DB. Efficacy and safety of opioid agonists in the treatment of neuropathic pain of nonmalignant origin: Systematic review and meta-analysis of randomized controlled trials. *JAMA* 2005;293:3043–3052.

50 Nicholson B, Passik SD. Management of chronic noncancer pain in the primary care setting. *South Med J* 2007;12:13–21.

51 Trescot AM, Helm S, Hansen H et al. Opioids in the management of chronic non-cancer pain: An update of American Society of the Interventional Pain Physicians' (AISPP) Guidelines. *Pain Physician* 2008;11:S5–S62.

52 Caldwell JR, Hale ME, Boyd RE at al. Treatment of osteoarthritis pain with controlled release oxycodone or fixed combination oxycodone plus acetaminophen added to nonsteroidal anti-inflammatory drugs: A double blind, randomized, multicenter, placebo controlled trail. *J Rheumatol* 1999;26:862–869.

53 Hale ME, Fleischmann R, Salzman R et al. Efficacy and safety of controlled-release versus immediate-release oxycodone: Randomized, double-blind evaluation in patients with chronic back pain. *Clin J Pain* 1999;15:179–183.

54 Rauck RL, Bookbinder SA, Bunker TR et al. The ACTION study: A randomized, open-label, multicenter trial comparing once-a-day extended-release morphine sulfate capsules (AVINZA) to twice-a-day extended-release oxycodone hydrochloride tablets (OxyContin) for the treatment of chronic, moderate to severe low back pain. *J Opioid Manage* 2006;2:155–166.

55 Dworkin RH, O'Connor AB, Backonja M et al. Pharmacologic management of neuropathic pain: Evidence-based recommendations. *Pain* 2007;132:237–251.

56 Guide to Alleviating Physical and Psychological Pain in Patients with Serious or Life-Threatening Conditions. Pocket card published by American Academy of Hospice and Palliative Medicine (AAHPM). Glenview, IL.

57 Ives TJ, Chelminski PR, Hammett-Stabler CA et al. Predictors of opioid misuse in patients with chronic pain: A prospective cohort study. *BMC Health Serv Res* 2006;6:46.

58 Reid MC, Engles-Horton LL, Weber MB et al. Use of opioid medications for chronic noncancer pain syndromes in primary care. *J Gen Intern Med* 2002;17:173–179.

59 Edlund MJ, Steffick D, Hudson T et al. Risk factors for clinically recognized opioid abuse and dependence among veterans using opioids for chronic noncancer pain. *Pain* 2007;129:355–362.

60 Ytterberg SR, Mahowald ML, Woods SR. Codeine and oxycodone use in patients with chronic rheumatic disease pain. *Arthritis Rheum* 1998;41:1603–1612.

61 Auret K, Schug SA. Underutilisation of opioids in elderly patients with chronic pain: Approaches to correcting the problem. *Drugs Aging* 2005;22:641–654.

62 Lussier D, Portenoy RK. Adjuvant analgesics in pain management. In: Douyle D, Hangs G, Cerhny N et al. eds. *Oxford Textbook of Palliative Medicine*, 3rd edn. New York: Oxford University Press, 2004, pp. 349–378.

63 Fromm GH. Baclofen as an adjuvant analgesic. *J Pain Symptom Manage* 1994;9:500–509.

64 Reddy S, Patt RB. The benzodiazepines as adjuvant analgesics. *J Pain Symptom Manage* 1994;9:510–514.

51

Neuropathic pain

PAOLO MARCHETTINI, FABIO FORMAGLIO, MARCO LACERENZA

INTRODUCTION

Diagnosing and treating neuropathic pain remains a major challenge for neurologists, oncologists, and pain specialists. Major advances in clinical, experimental, and molecular research in the past decade(s) have shed light on the multiple pathophysiological mechanisms that can generate and maintain neuropathic pain.[1] In 2011, the International Association for the Study of Pain and its Taxonomy Committee modified the definition of neuropathic pain as "pain caused by a lesion or disease of the somatosensory nervous system."[2] The 1994 definition "pain initiated or caused by a primary lesion or dysfunction in the nervous system" was changed in two aspects: The first change was made because the term "dysfunction" was raising confusion, since it allows improper labeling of nociceptive and psychogenic conditions as neurogenic/neuropathic. The second is related to the location of the damage of the nervous system that has been specified in the somatosensory system. This modification should avoid, for example, that pain associated with rigidity or spasticity, due to natural excitation of muscle nociceptors, could be considered as neuropathic pain.

The origin of these changes dates back many years[3] and encouraged a vibrant discussion among the specialists of different disciplines that converged in a consensus paper[4] published on neurology in 2008 from which the actual definition is derived, almost unmodified. Neuropathic pain originates from diseases or trauma to the peripheral or central somatosensory system and exhibits an acute or chronic temporal profile, the latter being by far more common and disabling. Pain and related neuropathic symptoms and signs may fluctuate according to the temporal evolution of the painful disease, mood and anxiety of the patient, and even weather conditions (trigeminal neuralgia).

Neuropathic pain can be spontaneous (stimulus-independent pain) with an episodic or continuous temporal profile. Episodic paroxysms are typical of trigeminal and glossopharyngeal neuralgias, but other pains in neuropathy may appear as isolated attacks or attacks of increasing intensity superimposed on continuous pain. Spontaneous symptoms are described as uncommon tactile and thermal sensations associated with numbness, tingling, pins and needles, burning, shooting, or electric-shock-like sensation. In addition, the common aching pain, attributable to the nociceptive component, may be part of the clinical picture of painful peripheral neuropathies and a frequent complaint in patients with central pain due to multiple sclerosis[5] and syringomyelia.[6]

Neuropathic pain may also be evoked. The evoking stimulus may cause massive activation of ectopic sensory discharges by acting on mechanosensitive neural pathways. The maneuvers evoking the latter are improperly called clinical signs and classically referred to by their eponyms (Lhermitte, Lasègue, and Spurling are widely known). Pain may also be evoked by direct stimulation of cutaneous nerve endings (stimulus-dependent pain) unchaining a sequence of spontaneous attacks, such as trigger point activation of tic douloureux, or remaining time locked within the original stimulus, however, with exaggeratedly intense or distorted quality. Dysesthesia, hyperalgesia, and allodynia are the terms applied to define aberrant evoked sensory phenomena. Such aberrant sensations appear following a lesion in the peripheral or central somatosensory system; obviously, similar symptoms originating from anatomically different sites and causes are likely to have different pathophysiology. Sensitization of nociceptors, ectopic activity, and multiplication of impulses are probable peripheral mechanisms of dysesthesia and hyperalgesia.[7] Dysinhibition of the spinothalamic pathway and, again, ectopic activity, are likely central mechanisms, although the evidence in humans is still weak. It is at least recognized that central pain and pain evoked by central stimuli require abnormal spinothalamic function.[8*,9*] Allodynia is a more complex condition. By definition, the term implies a painful perception evoked by stimuli (mechanical or thermal) of intensity below nociceptor threshold. Therefore, allodynia is widely viewed as the clinical "sign" of central sensitization. However, nociceptor threshold is remarkably lower than pain threshold, the pain perception requiring temporal and spatial summation of nociceptive impulses to overcome the endogenous inhibitory state. Thus, what common experience would reasonably define as stimulus of painless intensity might be sufficient to activate nociceptors.[10] Hyperactivity and multiplication of discharges in peripheral nociceptive afferents may well give rise to allodynia. Novel recordings from nociceptors in patients with allodynia due to painful neuropathies provide objective evidence for this peripheral explanation.[11]

When considering the somatotopical organization of the peripheral and central nervous systems, all neuropathic pains are perceived to occur within the innervation territory of the damaged structure. A thorough exploration of the neuroanatomical distribution of pain and sensory alteration using a pain drawing completed by the patient aids the diagnosis[3] that otherwise relies on the medical history and bedside examination. The evaluation aims at correlating sensory, motor, and autonomic signs with the anatomical localization of the lesion based on a careful history.

Autonomic signs may be a direct consequence of the nerve injury or a consequence of spinal/supraspinal reflex to nociceptive input, and care should be taken to distinguish between these phenomena.[12] Clinical neurophysiological tests such as electromyography, nerve conduction studies, evoked potentials, infrared telethermography, and quantitative mechanical and thermal threshold tests supplement the clinical diagnosis, allowing definition of nerve fibers or central sensory pathways involved.

NEUROPATHIC PAIN SYNDROMES IN PATIENTS WITH CANCER

Most of the cancer patients complain of pain in the course of their disease, in a large prevalence as a consequence of the nervous system involvement.[13] Direct activity of the growing tumors cause nerve trunk, nerve plexus, or radiculo-spinal external compression and/or infiltration.[14] In the early clinical phase, tumor compression or invasion of the peripheral or central nervous system stimulates nociceptors embedded in perinevrium and meningeal sheaths. This nociceptive nerve trunk pain[15] or meningeal pain usually responds well to analgesic drugs of nonsteroidal anti-inflammatory (NSAIDs) and opioid types. In the following phase, when the axonal membranes get damaged, typical neuropathic symptoms enter the clinical picture, and specific treatments for neuropathic pain are warranted. Cancers may damage nerves through indirect mechanisms as well: favoring nerve ischemia and infections, as herpes zoster, and in toxic, metabolic, and autoimmune (paraneoplastic) polineuropathy.

An investigation of neuropathic pain symptoms in cancer patients is useful not only to target the therapy. A neurological complication of neoplasm is frequently heralded by pain,[14,16*] and a careful neurological examination in cancer pain patients may disclose cancer recurrence, cancer progression, or other diseases such as infections.[17,18]

Cancer patients often complain of neuropathic pain. In a recent review of 22 prevalence studies on cancer pain, including 133,683 patients, neuropathic pain prevalence varied from a conservative estimate of 19% to a wide estimate of 39.1%, when mixed pain is also included. Neuropathic pain as a consequence of cancer treatments has a prevalence of 20.3%, much higher than in nonneuropathic cancer pain. Neuropathic pain nonrelated to cancer or its treatments has a prevalence of 10.2%.[19]

Neuropathic pain syndromes due to direct or indirect activity of the tumor

Classic trigeminal neuralgia is among the presenting symptoms of malignancies of middle and posterior cranial fossae.[20*] Most commonly, bone or meningeal invasion causes constant deep aching pain overlapping with paroxysmal electric-shock-like trigeminal pain. With the progression of the illness, neuropathic pain becomes continuous. Spontaneous deep burning sensation combined with sensory loss and other focal neurological signs appear following axonal loss.

Tumor invasion of mandibular canal and inferior alveolar nerve infiltration generates pain and chin dysesthesia (numb chin syndrome). This occurs more often with breast metastases and lymphoma and is a negative prognostic sign (mean life expectancy between 3 and 7 months).[21,22]

The intercostal nerve syndrome, caused by metastatic spread into a rib or by cancer thoracic wall infiltration, is a common painful syndrome caused by peripheral nerve lesion.[23] A period of deep aching pain in the chest precedes the appearance of a continuous burning pain with superimposed episodes of shooting pain with a belt distribution, culminating in the fracture of the rib. Positive and negative sensory signs may not be seen in neurological examination, for the wide overlapping of the dorsal dermatomes.

Plexopathies

Nerve plexus lesions in cancer frequently lead to pain with a neuropathic component. The nerve injury can be caused by direct invasion by the primary tumor, dissemination via adjacent lymph nodes, radiotherapy, or surgery.

Cervical plexus involvement is witnessed in primary or metastatic head or neck tumors, resulting from invasion or compression from the growing mass or from surgical and/or radiation treatment. The neuropathic pain syndrome reflects the anatomical distribution of the damaged nerve fibers. Pain and sensory symptoms can arise from the lesser and greater occipital nerve territories in the occipital region, the preauricular area supplied by the greater auricular nerve, and the anterior part of the neck and shoulder innervated by the transverse cutaneous and supraclavicular nerves and may also project to the jaw.[21*] A combination of nociceptive and neuropathic pains with positive and negative sensory symptoms in multiple nerve territories is the rule in these patients.[21,24]

Brachial plexopathy is a frequent neurological complication in patients with cancer and occurs often in lymphoma and breast and lung carcinoma. Pain usually precedes focal neurological signs, even up to 9 months; it is the most common symptom in 85% of patients.[25*] Lower plexus invasion is by far the most common, as in Pancoast syndrome, due to apical lung cancer. An aching pain in the shoulder, subscapular area, and upper back may appear some months before a burning pain in the armpit. Clinical examination usually reveals sensory loss in the intercostobrachial nerve territory, of which patients are frequently unaware.[26] The advanced clinical picture includes Horner syndrome (Figure 51.1) and focal

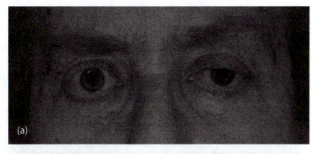

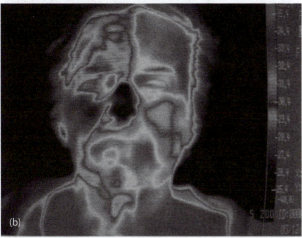

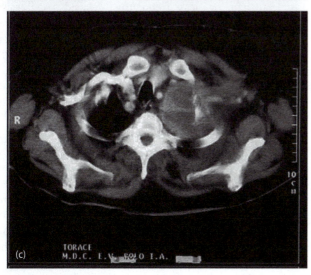

Figure 51.1 *(a) This 72-year-old woman developed aching pain in the left shoulder followed by projected burning pain in the left upper limb 4 months prior to examination. The neurological evaluation revealed Horner syndrome and signs of left lower brachial plexus involvement. (b) Telethermography revealed straightforward thermal asymmetry of the face, the left side being warmer than the right due to sympathetic denervation. (c) Computed tomography (CT) of the pulmonary apex disclosed a Pancoast tumor on the left side.*

weakness, atrophy, sensory loss in the hand. Involvement of the upper plexus (C4, C5, C6 roots) by metastatic breast carcinoma and lymphoma is less frequent. Pain is localized in the shoulder girdle, worsened by neck movement, and projected to the radial side of the hand with tingling, sensory loss, burning, and shooting sensations.[27] The combination of Lhermitte sign, Horner syndrome, and pan-plexopathy strongly suggests epidural extension, which can occur even in the absence of bony erosion.[28*]

Painful lumbosacral plexopathy, and its complications, is the most disabling condition in cancer. Pelvic tumors and metastatic malignancies almost always cause pain in the buttocks and/or legs following lumbosacral plexus invasion. The insidious onset of an aching and cramping nociceptive pain typically precedes and later merges with more specific neuropathic pain symptoms, and causalgic pain could be difficult to be seen.[28*] The anatomical distribution of weakness and sensory symptoms and signs, usually appearing after the pain, does not always correlate with CT imaging—the examination usually reveals wider invasion.[28*] Pain is projected to the thigh in the upper plexopathy (L1–L4) involvement in about a third of the cases. Pain in the leg, foot, and buttocks is associated to a lower plexopathy (L5–sacral dermatomes) and is described in half the cases. Panplexopathy is rarer and is seen in less than a fifth of patients with lumbosacral plexopathy. The presence of pain and neurological signs of lumbosacral plexopathy with normal findings on the CT of the abdomen and pelvis calls for a differential diagnosis of meningeal carcinomatosis, epidural cord compression, and cauda equina compression.

Radiculopathies and myelopathies

Painful radiculopathy in patients with cancer is usually related to direct compression or invasion of nerve roots by vertebral and paraspinal cancers or leptomeningeal metastases. There can be nociceptive focal and neuropathic pain projected along the distribution of the damaged root.[29]

Pain is the most frequent symptom in leptomeningeal carcinomatosis and often precedes other symptoms and signs by weeks. The prevalent picture is a lumbosacral polyradiculopathy, since tumor cells often seed in the lumbar sac.[24]

The clinical picture of myelopathy is often preceded by local nociceptive pain due to invasion of vertebral body or epidural space and then neuropathic pain of radicular origin. When the compression extends to the dorsal column of the spinal cord, generating focal demyelination, the presence of Lhermitte sign confirms the onset of clinical myelopathy. Pure central neuropathic pain is infrequent; it prevails a neuropathic pain originated from compression/invasion of spinothalamic pathways.[27] The pain is usually unilateral, a few myelomers below the affected level—extended down to the foot or with a patchy distribution, associated with tingling and allodynias, peculiarly due to cold and spontaneous thermal sensations.

POSTHERPETIC NEURALGIA

Postherpetic neuralgia is a painful radiculopathy following herpes zoster infection usually in the mid-thoracic dermatomes and in the ophthalmic branch of the trigeminal nerve. It is more common in altered immune states, for example, in older people and in patients with cancer (mainly leukemia and lymphomas), and it has been shown that the site of the primary tumor correlates with the site of subsequent herpes zoster infection.[29*] Neuropathic pain can be spontaneous with deep aching, burning, and shooting components or stimulus dependent with allodynia and/or hyperalgesia.[30]

Polyneuropathies

Peripheral paraneoplastic neuropathies, due to either indirect cancer activity or the immune reaction against cancer, may be painful. Altogether, these are a rare complication of cancer. An accurate diagnosis is crucial, and sometimes, it may uncover the tumor. Paraneoplastic sensory neuronopathy is a disabling condition presenting with neuropathic pain and progressive sensory loss in the limbs, trunk, and face. Burning pain and shooting sensations are present and associated with asymmetrically distributed numbness and tingling. Symptoms usually appear before, by weeks or months, the diagnosis of tumor, which most frequently is a small-cell lung cancer or less frequently a breast carcinoma. Given the high specificity (99.8%) and sensitivity (82%) of anti-Hu antibodies,[31] in patients with no evidence of cancer, a CT study of the chest should be done. Moreover, if CT scan is negative, then FDG-PET should be conducted.[32] In some patients, painful neuronopathy may be associated to mixed axonal and demyelinating sensorimotor neuropathy. In those cases, the combination of anti-Hu antibodies and anti-CV2/CRMP-5 antibodies are present.[33] Early symptomatic management of neuropathic pain is mandatory. Appropriate and successful treatment of the underlying cancer is the starting point of the therapy of paraneoplastic neuronopathy. However, immunomodulatory therapy before or together with antineoplastic treatment can be useful in patients with this condition and has been used even when the underlying tumor cannot be detected.[34]

Among other painful paraneoplastic disorders affecting the peripheral nervous system is the Guillain–Barré syndrome, which sometimes can be heralded by radicular pains and a nonsystemic vasculitic neuropathy. This subacute and progressive condition can be associated with small-cell lung cancer and lymphomas and involves sensory and motor fibers in a symmetric or asymmetric fashion. Early diagnosis of paraneoplastic vasculitis encourages combined treatment with steroids and cyclophosphamide, which yields better results than the treatment with steroids alone.[35] Severe local pain can be related to the inflammatory biochemical cascade that leads to activation/sensitization of nervi nervorum, followed by ischemia and consequent axonal damage and neuropathic pain along the anatomical distribution of the damaged nerve.

Table 51.1 summarizes the neuropathic pain syndromes in the patient with cancer along with their etiology.

IATROGENIC NEUROPATHIC PAIN IN CANCER

Bleuler, in 1924, introduced the term "iatrogenic" to define any disorder "generated or caused by medicine or medical doctors." Longer survival times and more aggressive surgical and medical treatment of cancer have led to an increase in iatrogenic painful conditions. Iatrogenic neuropathic pain in cancer patients may arise as a consequence of radiotherapy, chemotherapy, or surgical nerve lesions.[36] Pain in malignancies is often associated with cancer recurrence. The appearance of a novel painful condition deserves extensive examination aimed at early diagnosis of the cause of the pain. Informing the patient that the pain is iatrogenic and not a direct consequence of the tumor reduces their anxiety and results in a favorable response to specific treatment.

Neuropathic pain as a consequence of radiotherapy

Radiation may provoke painful myelopathy or peripheral nerve lesions. High-dose radiotherapy close to the spine causes transient or, less frequently, delayed progressive myelopathy that occasionally has the features of a central pain syndrome.[37*,38*] Sometimes, the presenting complaint of a post–radiation myeloradiculopathy is the Lhermitte sign.[39*] Painful brachial plexopathy is the most common postradiotherapy syndrome. The nerve injury may be direct or indirect, that is, infarction of the brachial plexus due to thrombosis of the subclavian artery and its branches.[40*] High-voltage radiation may cause acute painful but reversible brachial plexopathy.[41*] A delayed, but usually not painful, brachial plexopathy due to radiation fibrosis may develop several months after radiotherapy, with tingling and large fiber sensory loss within the upper plexus distribution.[42] In contrast, recurrent cancer with invasion of the peripheral nerves is often severely painful with neuropathic and nociceptive pains. Electromyographic studies help in differentiating the two conditions, with radiation being associated with myokymias more often than tumor invasion.[43]

Nearly half the data reporting on radiation-induced brachial plexus injury are from breast cancer patients who might show neurological complication in up to 39% (at 5 years follow-up) or even 50% of the cases (at 30 years follow-up).[44] The critical dose for inducing brachial plexopathy after breast radiation is 54 Gy.[45] Recent evidence shows that high-dose radiation therapy for head and neck cancer also causes

Table 51.1 *Summary of neuropathic pain syndromes in the patient with cancer and their etiologies*

Category		Clinical syndrome	Etiology
Direct activity of cancer	Nerve compression/invasion	Trigeminal neuralgia	Middle and posterior cranial fossa tumors, base of skull metastases
		Glossofaringeal neuralgia	Jugular foramen invasion, leptomeningeal metastases
		Intercostal neuralgia	Primary or metastatic lung, pleural, rib cancer
	Cervical (Compression/invasion plexopathies)	Postauricular neuralgia	Primary head and neck cancer and cervical lymph nodes metastases
		Preauricular neuralgia	Lymphoma and cervical lymph nodes metastases from breast and lung cancer
		Anterior part of the neck neuralgia	Breast metastases and lung cancer
	Brachial	Upper brachial plexus neuralgia	Primary cancer: colorectal, genito-urinary and sarcoma, lymphoma.
		Pancoast syndrome	Metastatic cancer: colorectal, breast, lymphoma, genito-urinary, melanoma, lung, gastric
	Lumbo-sacral	Upper lumbar (L1–L4) neuralgia	
		Lower lumbar (L5–S1) neuralgia	
		Sacrococcygeal neuralgia	
	Compression/invasion of nerve root	Unilateral pain in the cervical and lumbosacral radicular territories	Vertebral cancer
		Frequently, bilateral distribution in the thoracic dermatomes	Paraspinal invasion / Epidural invasion / Leptomeningeal dissemination
	Compression/invasion of spinal cord	Rarely, central pain with Brown–Séquard syndrome	Primary and metastatic cancer
	Compression/invasion of thalamo-cortical projections	Rarely, central pain with thalamic syndrome	Primary and metastatic cancer
Indirect activity of cancer	Paraneoplastic neuropathies	Sensory ganglionopathy	Small-cell lung, ovary, colon, and breast carcinomas
		Guillain–Barré syndrome	Small-cell lung cancer, lymphoma
		Nonsystemic vasculitis	
		Brachial plexopathy	
	Acute herpes zoster		Leukemia, lymphomas, postirradiation
	Postherpethic neuralgia	Frequently in the thoracic dermatomes, ophthalmic branch of the trigeminal nerve and in previously irradiated dermatomes	
	Nerve entrapment due to lymphedema	Brachial plexopathy	Postmastectomy
	Ischemic neuropathy/ies	Painful mono/multipleneuropathy	Trombosis, compression/invasion of small arteries
	Cerebral hemorrhage	Central pain with thalamic syndrome	Primary and metastatic cancer
Iatrogenic neuropathic pain in cancer	Postsurgical nerve lesion	Postneck surgery syndrome	Neck dissection
		Intercostobrachial neuralgia	Mastectomy
		Intercostal neuralgia	Thoracotomy
		Postthoracotomy pain	Thoracotomy
		Phantom pain	Limb, breast, rectal amputation
		Stump pain	
	Postradiation neuropathies	Painful brachial plexopathy acute and delayed, rarely painful lumbo-sacral plexopathy	Radiotherapy
	Postradiation myelopathy	Central pain with Brown–Séquard syndrome	
	Painful polyneuropathy associated to chemotherapy	Distal ascending pain and sensory + symptoms	Platinum compounds, vincristine, bortezomib, taxanes, and combination of them
	Inferior alveolar nerve neuropathy: numb chin syndrome	Progressive sensory loss and pain in the nerve territory	Bisphosphonates treatment

plexus injury in 8%–9% of the cases, the incidence increasing to 12% overall if patients undergoing, in addition, surgical neck dissection or chemotherapy, or both are included.[46]

Lumbosacral plexopathy, which is rarely painful, may also follow radiotherapy as a late delayed complication.[47]

Neuropathic pain as a consequence of chemotherapy

Peripheral polineuropathy is a common complication of chemotherapy. Neuropathic pain and sensory symptoms are often the limiting factor in chemotherapy with cisplatin, vincristine, bortezomib, and the taxanes. The severity of nerve damage is directly proportional to drug dosage.[48–50] Patients with pre-existing neuropathy due to diabetes mellitus, alcohol, hereditary neuropathies, paraneoplastic neuropathy, or earlier treatment with neurotoxic chemotherapy are thought to be more vulnerable to developing chemotherapy-induced peripheral neuropathy.[51] Ascending distal paresthesia and dysesthesia together with burning pain and allodynia to cold or mechanical stimuli in a glove and stocking distribution often appear after chemotherapy. The mechanisms producing the nerve injury, and in particular neuropathic pain and sensory symptoms, are not clear.

A common mechanism has been proposed for the toxicity of cisplatinum, vincristine, and taxol.[52] Vincristine therapy provokes a predominantly sensory, sometimes autonomic, subacute neuropathy in almost all patients. Cisplatinum neuropathy becomes clinically evident with cumulative dosages of the drug, nerve deterioration continuing months after drug withdrawal.[53*] The widely used paclitaxel is known to provoke neuropathic pain and sensory dysfunctions that mostly affect the hands and feet and is related to a myelinated fiber neuropathy preferentially affecting the largest fibers (with sparing of C fibers).[52]

Bortezomib is a proteasome inhibitor active against recurrent or newly diagnosed multiple myeloma,[54] and it is responsible for a primarily length-dependent sensory neuropathy affecting small fibers, often causing severe neuropathic pain. The mechanisms of bortezomib generating pain and neural toxicity are not completely understood, and in up to 30% of patients, dose modification or cessation of therapy may be necessary.[55]

Brachial and lumbosacral plexopathy may also be related to chemotherapy. Chemotherapy administration through the subclavian or iliac artery may cause an acute painful brachial or lumbosacral plexopathy, which is sometimes irreversible. This is probably due to direct damage to small vessels and thrombosis, which leads to infarction of the nerve plexus.[56*]

Postsurgical neuropathies

Postinjury neuralgia is a relatively rare event compared with the large number of nerve injuries provoked by surgical trauma, perioperative ischemia, compression, and delayed scar entrapment. Although reliable clinical data are lacking, the incidence of painful neuralgia following peripheral nerve injury seems to be about 2.5%–5% of the injuries.[57]

Post–neck surgery syndrome

Neck and nuchal pain may arise as a consequence of cutaneous nerve lesions provoked by surgical interventions for primary or metastatic head or neck tumor. Pain affects almost 50% of patients, sometimes weeks after neck dissection.[58*] According to the aggressiveness of tumor and the timing and location of the surgery, the pain may have nociceptive and neuropathic components. In half of the patients, the pain subsides in a few months, whereas in the other half, it lasts for years.[58*] In studies reporting on pain following neck surgery, 8% of patients complained of shoulder and arm pain, increasing to around 30% after a 1-year period.[58*,59,60] Shoulder pain and disability were shown to be proportional to the surgical extension; they seem to be reduced in modified radical neck dissection and selective neck dissection compared with standard radical neck dissection.[61*] Therefore, it is likely that the surgical technique influences the pain occurrence.

In recent years, the occurrence of inferior alveolar painful neuropathy is dramatically increased as a consequence of biphosphonates treatment.[62]

Pain following breast cancer surgery

More than 50% of patients have chronic pain syndromes after breast cancer surgery.[63] Acute postoperative pain has both nociceptive and neuropathic components, whereas persistent pain has predominantly a neuropathic origin. A recent, validated classification of neuropathic pain following breast cancer surgery has identified four classes: phantom breast pain, intercostobrachial neuralgia, neuroma pain, and other nerve injury pain.[63] In another study, pain occurrence correlated significantly with the surgical extension is infrequent in lumpectomy but is found in up to 72% of patients who underwent axillary lymph node dissection.[64*] In these cases, pain appearance was positively associated with the number of lymph nodes removed.[64*] Pain seems to be less frequent when careful surgical techniques are used, or when surgeons perform more interventions, as in hospitals experienced in breast surgery.[65*]

Post-thoracotomy pain

One year after thoracic surgery, up to 61% of the patients report post-thoracotomy pain. Chronic pain development is directly related to the degree of postoperative pain severity.[66*] This pain may be due to intercostal nerve lesions or to brachial plexus traction. Trans-axillary rib resection is one of the causes of brachial plexopathy.[67] Persistent chest pain may also be due to complete intercostal nerve transection, sometimes followed by painful neuroma. Seventy percent of patients undergoing thoracotomy report severe pain (usually subsiding after 2 months' time) with a neuropathic component. Progressive pain, worsening over weeks or months, and recurrence of chest pain following a pain-free period are significant negative prognostic symptoms, suspicious for cancer recurrence.[68*]

THERAPY

Pain in cancer patients may have a poor response to analgesic treatments. An explanation is the high prevalence of neuropathic pain, which is often misdiagnosed and not appropriately cured with a specific neuropathic pain treatment strategy. However, the management of chronic nonmalignant neuropathic pain, based on consecutive trials of different drugs, slowly titrated until efficacy or dose limiting side effects, is not applicable in the short survival times of a palliative care context.

Moreover, in palliative care, relief of pain is the priority, while the preservation of functionality becomes a secondary issue. Therefore, the overall side effects, and in particular the sedative effects of opioids and adjuvant drugs, may become acceptable, providing the drugs offer adequate pain control.

Neuropathic pain management is among the priorities in the palliative care research. The current recommendation of care in cancer patients is to follow the World Health Organization (WHO) ladder, choosing an analgesic regimen on the basis of pain intensity and adding complementary adjuvant drugs for neuropathic pain syndromes.[69*,70*,71]

Nerve trunk pain, that is, the nociceptive component of neuropathic pain syndromes caused by compression, invasion, or acute nerve ischemia, is treatable with NSAIDs, steroids, and eventually opioids.[13] Conversely, in the experience of most clinicians, neuropathic pain of the deafferentation type responds poorly to NSAIDs.

For a long time, opioids were considered barely effective in neuropathic pain. However, in the past decades, several retrospective reports on long-term therapy for neuropathic pain related to nonmalignant diseases and cancer have supported opioid efficacy and low risk of addiction and tolerance.[72*,73*] Since then, several clinical studies have supported the use of opioids in the treatment of peripheral neuropathic pain.[73–76,77**,79**] However, the evidence for their efficacy with regard to central pain is weak.[80,81]

Some opioids are potentially more effective than others in neuropathic pain due to their pharmacological properties: methadone[78**,79] have weak N-methyl-D-aspartate (NMDA) receptor antagonism and may be a first choice in the neuropathic pain treatment of cancer patients.

Tramadol[82**] has noradrenergic/serotonergic activity and has some evidence of efficacy in different types of neuropathic pain. Tapentadol is a novel, centrally acting analgesic that acts both as a mu-opioid receptor agonist (MOR) and as a noradrenaline reuptake inhibitor (NRI).[83,84] In clinical trials, tapentadol has proved to be efficacious in chronic pain of different origin,[85] and considering the mechanisms of action, it promises a role in mixed pain syndromes (neuropathic and nociceptive) in cancer patients.

Anticonvulsants and antidepressants, commonly referred to as adjuvant drugs, are considered effective drugs for neuropathic pain.[86***,87***,88***,89***] Gabapentin is an anticonvulsant that binds the alpha 2delta subunits of voltage-gated calcium channels and inhibits calcium cellular influx. Gabapentin has a well-documented efficacy in peripheral neuropathic pain[90**,91**,92**] and is recommended as a first choice for these syndromes.[89] In one study, Gabapentin added to opioids reduced pain in cancer patients with neuropathic pain,[93*] but it had a limited effect in a larger patient population investigated by the same group.[94**] Pregabalin shares many of the analgesic properties of Gabapentin and has better kinetics properties. Its efficacy in neuropathic pain of both peripheral[95**,96*] and central types[95*,96**] is well documented.

Carbamazepine is an old anticonvulsant that unselectively blocks sodium channels. It is still considered the gold standard treatment for trigeminal neuralgia.[97*,98**] Its analogue oxcarbazepine is also effective in trigeminal neuralgia[99*] and in painful diabetic polineuropathy, with a better tolerability profile.[100**] Lamotrigine is an antiepileptic agent that stabilizes the neural membrane, blocking voltage-sensitive sodium channels and inhibiting presynaptic release of glutamate. Its analgesic efficacy has been shown in trigeminal neuralgia,[101**] poststroke central pain,[102**] and human immunodeficiency virus (HIV)–related polyneuropathy.[103**]

Tricyclic antidepressants (TCAs) were the mainstay of neuropathic pain therapy before the introduction of the new anticonvulsants.[104***] Among these drugs, amitriptyline is the most commonly prescribed TCAs in neuropathic pain.[105] Amitriptyline reduces pain in diabetic neuropathy,[106**] central poststroke pain,[107**] while in neuropathic cancer pain patients, there is no evidence of efficacy.[108] Randomized trials of selective serotonin reuptake inhibitors have shown inconstant efficacy in neuropathic pain.[109***] The noradrenergic/serotonergic reuptake inhibitor venlafaxine has shown analgesic efficacy in diabetic polineuropathy[110] and neuropathic pain after breast cancer surgery.[111**] Duloxetine, a more balanced noradrenergic/serotonergic reuptake inhibitor, has a well-documented activity on diabetic neuropathic pain,[112] and its use in palliative medicine is rising. Cannabinoids have been proven to be effective in MS-associated pain[113] and, as smoked cannabis, in HIV neuropathy.[114] A lidocaine patch decreases pain and allodynia in postherpetic neuralgia.[115**] Intravenous lidocaine[116**] and parenteral ketamine[117**] quickly, although only transiently, reduce pain and may help control episodic neuropathic pain unresponsive to conventional analgesics.

Neuromodulation with spinal drug delivery is a recognized treatment for patients with severe refractory pain and life expectancy of at least 6 months.[118,119*] The most commonly used drugs in neuraxial analgesia are morphine, bupivacaine, clonidine, and ketamine. Recently, intrathecal ziconotide, an N-type calcium-channel blocker derived from a sea snail peptide, has shown statistically significant analgesic efficacy in advanced cancer and acquired immune deficiency syndrome (AIDS) patients with intractable pain.[120**] On the other hand, a lack of cost–benefit efficacy and concomitant poor long-term prognosis precludes electrical spinal cord stimulation.[121]

As a general rule, for treating the neuropathic component of a pain in a palliative care context, the initial approach could be based on gabapentin (particularly for peripheral pain), or pregabalin, given "round the clock" in a regular fashion with an appropriate titration dose, added to a base therapy with NSAIDS and/or opioids. Oxycodone, tramadol, tapentadol,

and, in a second line, methadone are preferred opioids. In selected cases, nonrespondents to gabapentinoids, an alternative with amitriptyline or duloxetine or other antidepressants and anticonvulsants must be considered. Opioids, and sometimes NSAIDs, may be used as rescue medication for treating breakthrough pain episodes.

Combination therapy with different class analgesics is the rule in palliative medicine. The use of different pain drugs with synergistic activity allows gaining a consistent pain relief, with lower single drug dosages and fewer side effects[122] in shorter time.

Figure 51.2 summarizes our standard approach to treating neuropathic pain in palliative care patients.

In conclusion, we emphasize the need to identify the cause of the pain, unravel its neuropathic nature, and possibly hypothesize or search for the mechanisms. A thorough investigation might lead to a more specific treatment, which even in the palliative stages could be relevant for improving the patient's autonomy, cognition, and dignity.

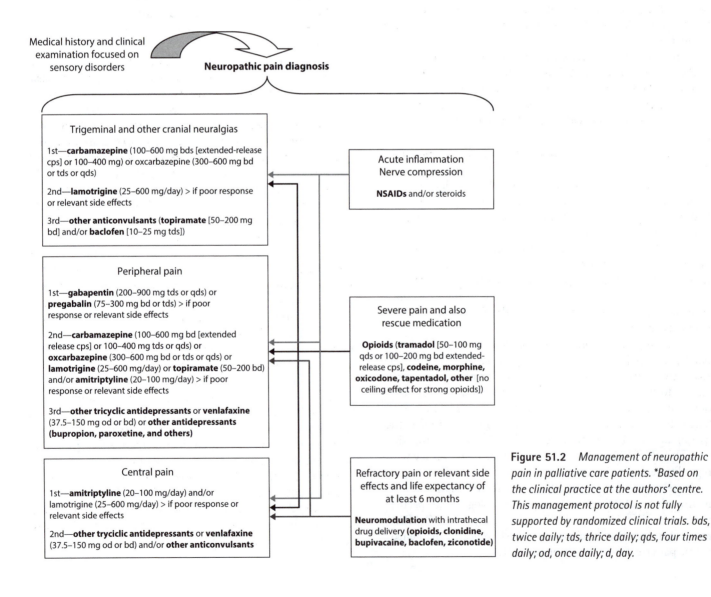

Figure 51.2 *Management of neuropathic pain in palliative care patients. *Based on the clinical practice at the authors' centre. This management protocol is not fully supported by randomized clinical trials. bds, twice daily; tds, thrice daily; qds, four times daily; od, once daily; d, day.*

Key learning points

- Neuropathic pain is not a single entity but encompasses a variety of different, complex clinical pictures with diverse pathophysiological mechanisms.

- Neuropathic pain is frequently present in cancer patients either in isolation or combined with nociceptive pain (mixed pain).

- Direct and indirect activity of cancer causes different neuropathic pain syndromes depending on the anatomy and the pathophysiology of the injured part of the nervous system.

- The number of cancer patients with neuropathic pain of iatrogenic origin is increasing due to longer survival times and the more aggressive surgical and medical treatment.

- Radiotherapy, chemotherapy, and surgery may cause multiple painful neuropathic syndromes.

- A thorough evaluation of the patient's pain points out the most appropriate treatment and enhances the patient's ability to cope.

- Treatment of neuropathic pain is moving from the empirical era to an evidence-based scientific approach. Novel adjuvant compounds have become available for neuropathic pain, supported by clinical studies on their efficacy and tolerability.

- Improved understanding of neuropathic pain pathophysiology is steering clinical research and patient management.

REFERENCES

* 1 von Hehn CA, Baron R, Woolf CJ. Deconstructing the neuropathic pain phenotype to reveal neural mechanisms. *Neuron* 2012;73:638–652.

2 Jensen TS, Baron R, Haanpää M, Kalso E, Loeser JD, Rice AS, Treede RD. A new definition of neuropathic pain. *Pain* 2011;152:2204–2205.

◆ 3 Hansson PT, Lacerenza M, Marchettini P. Aspects of clinical and experimental neuropathic pain: The clinical perspective. In: Hansson PT, Fields HL, Hill RG, Marchettini P, eds., *Neuropathic Pain: Pathophysiology and Treatment*, vol. 21. Progress in Pain Research and Management. Seattle, WA: IASP Press, 2001, pp. 1–18.

4 Treede RD, Jensen TS, Campbell JN et al. Neuropathic pain: Redefinition and a grading system for clinical and research purposes. *Neurology* 2008;70:1630–1635.

5 Osterberg A, Boivie J, Holmgren H et al. The clinical characteristics and sensory abnormalities of patients with central pain caused by multiple sclerosis. In: Gebhart GF, Hammond DL, Jensen TS, eds., *Proceedings of the 7th World Congress on Pain*, vol. 2. Progress in Pain Research and Management. Seattle, WA: IASP Press, 1994, pp. 789–796.

◆ 6 Boivie J. Central pain. In: Wall PD, Melzack R, eds., *Textbook of Pain*. Edinburgh, U.K.: Churchill Livingstone, 1999, pp. 879–914.

7 Ochoa JL, Serra J, Campero M. Pathophysiology of human nociceptor function. In: Belmonte C, Cervero F, eds., *Neurobiology of Nociceptors*. Oxford, U.K.: Oxford University Press, 1996, pp. 489–516.

● ◆ 8 Beric A. Central pain: 'New' syndromes and their evaluation. *Muscle Nerve* 1993;16:1017–1024.

● 9 Leijon G, Boivie J, Johansson I. Central post-stroke pain—Neurological symptoms and pain characteristics. *Pain* 1989;36:13–25.

● 10 Marchettini P, Simone D, Caputi G, Ochoa J. Pain from excitation of identified muscle nociceptors in humans. *Brain Res* 1996;740:109–116.

● 11 Ochoa J, Campero M, Serra J, Bostock H. Hyperexcitable polymodal and insensitive nociceptors in painful human neuropathy. *Muscle Nerve* 2005;32:459–472.

12 Bennett GJ, Ochoa JL. Thermographic observations on rats with experimental neuropathic pain. *Pain* 1991;45:61–67.

◆ 13 Vecht CJ. Cancer pain: A neurological perspective. *Curr Opin Neurol* 2000;13:649–653.

14 Gilbert MR, Grossman SA. Incidence and nature of neurologic problems in patients with solid tumors. *Am J Med* 1986;81:951–954.

● 15 Asbury AK, Fields HL. Pain due to peripheral nerve damage: An hypothesis. *Neurology* 1984;34:1587–1590.

● 16 Caraceni A, Portenoy RK. An international survey of cancer pain characteristics and syndromes. IASP Task Force on Cancer Pain. International Association for the Study of Pain. *Pain* 1999;82:263–274.

17 Gonzales GR, Elliott KJ, Portenoy RK, Foley KM. The impact of a comprehensive evaluation in the management of cancer pain. *Pain* 1991;47:141–144.

18 Manfredi PL, Gonzales GR, Sady R et al. Neuropathic pain in patients with cancer. *J Palliat Care* 2003;19:115–118.

19 Bennett MI, Rayment C, Hjermstad M et al. Prevalence and aetiology of neuropathic pain in cancer patients: A systematic review. *Pain* 2012;153:359–365.

20 Cheng TM, Cascino TL, Onofrio BM. Comprehensive study of diagnosis and treatment of trigeminal neuralgia secondary to tumors. *Neurology* 1993;43:2298–2302.

● ◆ 21 Vecht CJ, Hoff AM, Kansen PJ et al. Types and causes of pain in cancer of the head and neck. *Cancer* 1992;70:178–184.

22 Chaplin JM, Morton RP. A prospective, longitudinal study of pain in head and neck cancer patients. *Head Neck* 1999;21:531–537.

23 Abrahm JL. Palliative care for the patient with mesothelioma. *Semin Thorac Cardiovasc Surg* 2009;21:164–171.

24 Kim HH, Kim YC, Park YH et al. Cervicogenic headache arising from hidden metastasis to cervical lymph node adjacent to the superficial cervical plexus—A case report. *Korean J Anesthesiol* 2011;60:134–137.

● 25 Kori SH, Foley KM, Posner JB. Brachial plexus lesions in patients with cancer: 100 cases. *Neurology* 1981;31:45–50.

26 Marangoni C, Lacerenza M, Formaglio F et al. Sensory disorder of the chest as presenting symptom of lung cancer. *J Neurol Neurosurg Psychiatry* 1993;56:1033–1034.

27 Jaeckle KA. Neurologic manifestations of neoplastic and radiation-induced plexopathies. *Semin Neurol* 2010;30:254–262.

● 28 Jaeckle KA, Young DF, Foley KM. The natural history of lumbosacral plexopathy in cancer. *Neurology* 1985;35:8–15.

29 Rusthoven JJ, Ahlgren P, Elhakim T et al. Varicella-zoster infection in adult cancer patients. A population study. *Arch Intern Med* 1988;148:1561–1566.

● 30 Fields HL, Rowbotham M, Baron R. Postherpetic neuralgia: Irritable nociceptors and deafferentation. *Neurobiol Dis* 1998;5:209–227.

31 Molinuevo JL, Graus F, Serrano C et al. Utility of anti-Hu antibodies in the diagnosis of paraneoplastic sensory neuropathy. *Ann Neurol* 1998;44:976–980.

32 Titulaer MJ, Soffietti R, Dalmau J et al. Screening for tumours in paraneoplastic syndromes: Report of an EFNS Task Force. *Eur J Neurol* 2011;18:19–27.

33 Koike H, Tanaka F, Sobue G. Paraneoplastic neuropathy: Wide-ranging clinicopathological manifestations. *Curr Opin Neurol* 2011;24:504–510.

34 Sadeghian H, Vernino S. Progress in the management of para-neoplastic neurological disorders. *Ther Adv Neurol Disord* 2010;3:43–52.

35 Oh SJ. Paraneoplastic vasculitis of the peripheral nervous system. *Neurol Clin* 1997;15:849–863.

36 Marchettini P, Formaglio F, Lacerenza M. Iatrogenic painful neuropathic complications of surgery in cancer. *Acta Anaesthesiol Scand* 2001;45:1090–1094.

37 Marcus RB Jr., Million RR. The incidence of myelitis after irradiation of the cervical spinal cord. *Int J Radiat Oncol Biol Phys* 1990;19:3–8.

38 Jellinger K, Sturm KW. Delayed radiation myelopathy in man. *J Neurol Sci* 1971;14:389–408.

39 Lewanski CR, Sinclair JA, Stewart JS. Lhermitte's sign following head and neck radiotherapy. *Clin Oncol* 2000;12:98–103.

40 Gerard JM, Franck N, Moussa Z, Hildebrand J. Acute ischemic brachial plexus neuropathy following radiation therapy. *Neurology* 1989;39:450–451.

41 Malow BA, Dawson DM. Neuralgic amyotrophy in association with radiation therapy for Hodgkin's disease. *Neurology* 1991;41:440–441.

◆   42 Foley KM. Pain syndromes in patients with cancer. In: Bonica JJ, Ventafridda V, eds., *Advances in Pain Research and Therapy*. New York: Raven Press, 1979, pp. 59–78.

43 Lederman RJ, Wilbourn AJ. Brachial plexopathy: Recurrent cancer or radiation? *Neurology* 1984;34:1331–1335.

44 Johansson S, Svensson H, Denekamp J. Timescale evolution of late radiation injury after postoperative radiotherapy of breast cancer patients. *Int J Radiat Oncol Biol Phys* 2000;48:745–750.

45 Powell S, Cooke J, Parsons C. Radiation-induced brachial plexus injury: Follow up of two different fractionation schedules. *Radiother Oncol* 1990;18:213–220.

46 Chen AM, Hall WH, Li J, Beckett L, Farwell G, Lau DH, Purdy JA. Brachial plexus-associated neuropathy after high dose radiation therapy for head and neck cancer. *Int J Radiat Oncol Biol Phys* 2012;84(1):165–169.

●   47 Thomas JE, Cascino TL, Earle JD. Differential diagnosis between radiation and tumor plexopathy of the pelvis. *Neurology* 1985;35:1–7.

48 Alberts DS, Noel JK. Cisplatin-associated neurotoxicity: Can it be prevented? *Anticancer Drugs* 1995;6:369–383.

●   49 Casey EB, Jellife AM, Le Quesne PM, Millett YL. Vincristine neuropathy. Clinical and electrophysiological observations. *Brain* 1973;96:69–86.

50 Kaplan JG, Einzig AI, Schaumburg HH. Taxol causes permanent large fiber peripheral nerve dysfunction: A lesson for preventative strategies. *J Neurooncol* 1993;16:105–107.

◆   51 Verstappen CC, Heimans JJ, Hoekman K, Postma TJ. Neurotoxic complications of chemotherapy in patients with cancer: Clinical signs and optimal management. *Drugs* 2003;63:1549–1563.

52 Dougherty PM, Cata JP, Cordella JV et al. Taxol-induced sensory disturbance is characterized by preferential impairment of myelinated fiber function in cancer patients. *Pain* 2004;109:132–142.

53 Siegal T, Haim N. Cisplatin-induced peripheral neuropathy: Frequent off-therapy deterioration, demyelinating syndromes and muscle cramps. *Cancer* 1990;66:1117–1123.

54 Argyriou AA, Iconomou G, Kalofonos HP. Bortezomib-induced peripheral neuropathy in multiple myeloma: A comprehensive review of the literature. *Blood* 2008;112(5):1593–1599. Epub 2008 June 23.

55 Manji H. Toxic neuropathy. *Curr Opin Neurol* 2011;24(5):484–490. Review.

56 Castellanos AM, Glass JP, Young KWA et al. Regional nerve injury after intra-arterial chemotherapy. *Neurology* 1987;37:834–837.

57 Kline DG, Hudson AR, eds. *Nerve Injuries*. Philadelphia, PA: WB Saunders Company, 1995.

58 Chaplin JM, Morton RP. A prospective, longitudinal study of pain in head and neck cancer patients. *Head Neck* 1999;21:531–537.

59 Krause HR. Shoulder-arm-syndrome after radical neck dissection: Its relation with the innervation of trapezius muscle. *Int J Oral Maxillofac Surg* 1992;21:276–279.

60 Shone GR, Yardley MP. An audit into the incidence of handicap after unilateral radical neck dissection. *J Laryngol Otol* 1991;105:760–762.

61 Kuntz AL, Weymuller EA Jr. Impact of neck dissection on quality of life. *Laryngoscope* 1999;109:1334–1338.

62 Young P, Finn BC, Bruetman JE. Numb chin syndrome by biphosphonates. *Eur J Intern Med* 2008;19:557.

●◆ 63 Jung BF, Ahrendt GM, Oaklander AL, Dworkin RH. Neuropathic pain following breast cancer surgery: Proposed classification and research update. *Pain* 2003;104:1–13.

64 Hack TF, Cohen L, Katz J et al. Physical and psychological morbidity after axillary lymph nodes dissection for breast cancer. *J Clin Oncol* 1999;1:143–149.

●   65 Tasmuth T, Blomqvist C, Kalso E. Chronic post-treatment symptoms in patients with breast cancer operated in different surgical units. *Eur J Surg Oncol* 1999;25:38–43.

66 Perttunen K, Tasmuth T, Kalso E. Chronic pain after thoracic surgery: A follow up study. *Acta Anaesthesiol Scand* 1999;43:563–567.

67 Horowitz SH. Brachial plexus injury with causalgia resulting from transaxillary rib resection. *Arch Surg* 1985;120:1189–1191.

68 Kanner RM, Martini N, Foley KM. Nature and incidence of post-thoracotomy pain. *Proc Am Soc Clin Oncol* 1982;1:152.

✳   69 Grond S, Radbruch L, Meuser T et al. Assessment and treatment of neuropathic cancer pain following WHO guidelines. *Pain* 1999;79:15–20.

●   70 Stute P, Soukup J, Menzel M et al. Analysis and treatment of different types of neuropathic cancer pain. *J Pain Symptom Manage* 2003;26:1123–1131.

✳   71 Jacox A, Carr DB, Payne R. Management of Cancer Pain. AHCPR Clinical Practice Guidelines, No.9. Rockville (MD). Agency for Health Care Policy and Research (AHCPR), 1994.

●   72 Cherny NI, Thaler HT, Friedlander-Klar H et al. Opioid responsiveness of cancer pain syndromes caused by neuropathic or nociceptive mechanisms: A combined analysis of controlled, single-dose studies. *Neurology* 1994;44:857–861.

●   73 Portenoy RK, Foley KM, Inturrisi CE. The nature of opioid responsiveness and its implications for neuropathic pain: New hypotheses derived from studies of opioid infusions. *Pain* 1990;43:273–286.

74 Gimbel JS, Richards P, Portenoy RK. Controlled-release oxycodone for pain in diabetic neuropathy: A randomized controlled trial. *Neurology* 2003;60(6):927–934.

75   Rowbotham MC, Twilling L, Davies PS, Reisner L, Taylor K, Mohr D. Oral opioid therapy for chronic peripheral and central neuropathic pain. *N Engl J Med* 2003;348(13):1223–1232.

76   Bruera E, Sweeney C. Methadone use in cancer patients with pain: A review. *J Palliat Med* 2002;5(1):127–138.

✶   77   Watson CP, Babul N. Efficacy of oxycodone in neuropathic pain: A randomized trial in postherpetic neuralgia. *Neurology* 1998;50:1837–1841.

78   Morley JS, Bridson J, Nash TP et al. Low-dose methadone has an analgesic effect in neuropathic pain: A double-blind randomized controlled crossover trial. *Palliat Med* 2003;17:576–587.

79   Foley KM. Opioids and chronic neuropathic pain. *N Engl J Med* 2003;348:1279–1281.

●   80   Rowbotham MC, Twilling L, Davies PS et al. Oral opioid therapy for chronic peripheral and central neuropathic pain. *N Engl J Med* 2003;348:1223–1232.

81   Attal N, Guirimand F, Brasseur L et al. Effects of IV morphine in central pain: A randomized placebo-controlled study. *Neurology* 2002;58:554–563.

82   Sindrup SH, Andersen G, Madsen C et al. Tramadol relieves pain and allodynia in polyneuropathy: A randomised, double-blind, controlled trial. *Pain* 1999;83:85–90.

83   Tzschentke TM, Christoph T, Kögel B et al. (−)-(1R,2R)-3-(3-dimethylamino-1-ethyl-2-methyl-propyl)-phenolhydrochloride (tapentadol HCl): A novel 1-opioid receptor agonist/norepinephrine reuptake inhibitor with broad-spectrum analgesic properties. *J Pharmacol Exp Ther* 2007;323:265–276.

84   Schwartz S, Etropolski M, Shapiro DY, Okamoto A, Lange R, Haeussler J, Rauschkolb C. Safety and efficacy of tapentadol ER in patients with painful diabetic peripheral neuropathy: Results of a randomized-withdrawal, placebo-controlled trial. *Curr Med Res Opin* 2011;27(1):151–162.

85   Hoy SM. Tapentadol extended release: In adults with chronic pain. *Drugs* 2012;72(3):375–393.

● ◆   86   McQuay H, Carrol D, Jadad AR et al. Anticonvulsant drugs for management of pain: A systematic review. *BMJ* 1995;311:1047–1052.

● ◆   87   McQuay H, Tramer MR, Nye BA et al. A systematic review of antidepressants in neuropathic pain. *Pain* 1996;68:217–227.

88   Attal N, Cruccu G, Baron R, Haanpää M, Hansson P, Jensen TS, Nurmikko T. EFNS guidelines on the pharmacological treatment of neuropathic pain: 2009 revision. *Eur J Neurol* 2010;17:1113–1123.

89   Finnerup NB, Sindrup SH, Jensen TS. The evidence for pharmacological treatment of neuropathic pain. *Pain* 2010;150(3):573–581.

●   90   Backonja M, Beydoun A, Edwards KR et al. Gabapentin for the symptomatic treatment of painful neuropathy in patients with diabetes mellitus. *JAMA* 1998;280:1831–1836.

●   91   Rowbotham M, Harden N, Stacey B et al. Gabapentin for the treatment of postherpetic neuralgia. *JAMA* 1998;280:1837–1842.

92   Serpell MG, Neuropathic Pain Study Group. Gabapentin in neuropathic pain syndromes: A randomized, double-blind, placebo-controlled trial. *Pain* 2002;99:557–566.

●   93   Caraceni A, Zecca E, Martini C, De Conno F. Gabapentin as an adjuvant to opioid analgesia for neuropathic cancer pain. *J Pain Symptom Manage* 1999;17:441–445.

94   Caraceni A, Zecca E, Bonezzi C et al. Gabapentin for neuropathic cancer pain: A randomized controlled trial from the Gabapentin Cancer Pain Study Group. *J Clin Oncol* 2004;22:2909–2917.

95   Sabatowski R, Gálvez R, Cherry DA et al. Pregabalin reduces pain and improves sleep and mood disturbances in patients with post-herpetic neuralgia: Results of a randomised, placebo-controlled clinical trial. *Pain* 2004;109:26–35.

96   Richter RW, Portenoy R, Sharma U et al. Relief of painful diabetic peripheral neuropathy with pregabalin: A randomized, placebo-controlled trial. *J Pain* 2005;6:253–260.

●   97   Campbell FG, Graham JG, Zilkha KJ. Clinical trial of carbazepine (Tegretol) in trigeminal neuralgia. *J Neurol Neurosurg Psychiatry* 1966;29:265–267.

●   98   Rull JA, Quibrera R, Gonzalez-Millan H et al. Symptomatic treatment of peripheral diabetic neuropathy with carbamazepine (Tegretol): Double blind crossover trial. *Diabetologia* 1969;5:215–218.

99   Zakrzewska JM, Patsalos PN. Long-term cohort study comparing medical (oxcarbazepine) and surgical management of intractable trigeminal neuralgia. *Pain* 2002;95:259–266.

100   Dogra S, Beydoun S, Mazzola J et al. Oxcarbazepine in painful diabetic neuropathy: A randomized, placebo-controlled study. *Eur J Pain* 2005;9:543–554.

101   Zakrzewska JM, Chaudhry Z, Nurmikko TJ et al. Lamotrigine (Lamictal) in refractory trigeminal neuralgia: Results for a double blind placebo controlled crossover trial. *Pain* 1997;73:223–230.

102   Vestergaard K, Andersen G, Gottrup H et al. Lamotrigine for central poststroke pain; a randomized controlled trial. *Neurology* 2001;56:184–190.

103   Simpson DM, McArthur JC, Olney R et al. Lamotrigine for HIV-associated painful sensory neuropathies. *Neurology* 2003;60:1508–1514.

◆   104   Collins SL, Moore RA, McQuay HJ, Wiffen P. Antidepressants and anticonvulsants for diabetic neuropathy and postherpetic neuralgia: A quantitative systematic review. *J Pain Symptom Manage* 2000;20:449–458.

105   Berger A, Dukes E, Mercadante S, Oster G. Use of antiepileptics and tricyclic antidepressants in cancer patients with neuropathic pain. *Eur J Cancer Care* 2006;15(2):138–145.

●   106   Max MB, Culnane M, Schafer S et al. Amitriptyline relieves diabetic neuropathy pain in patients with normal or depressed mood. *Neurology* 1987;37:589–596.

107   Leijon G. Boivie J. Central post-stroke pain—A controlled trial of amitriptyline and carbamazepine. *Pain* 1989;36:27–36.

108   Mercadante S, Arcuri E, Tirelli W, Villari P, Casuccio A. Amitriptyline in neuropathic cancer pain in patients on morphine therapy: A randomized placebo-controlled, double-blind crossover study. *Tumori* 2002;88(3):239–242.

● ◆   109   Sindrup SH, Jensen TS. Efficacy of pharmacological treatments of neuropathic pain: An update and effect related to mechanism of drug action. *Pain* 1999;83:389–400.

110   Tasmuth T, Hartel B, Kalso E. Venlafaxine in neuropathic pain following treatment of breast cancer. *Eur J Pain* 2002;6:17–24.

111   Semenchuk MR, Sherman S, Davis B. Double-blind, randomized trial of bupropion SR for the treatment of neuropathic pain. *Neurology* 2001;57:1583–1588.

112   Kajdasz DK, Iyengar S, Desaiah D et al. Duloxetine for the management of diabetic peripheral neuropathic pain: Evidence-based findings from post hoc analysis of three multicenter, randomized, double-blind, placebo-controlled, parallel-group studies. *Clin Ther* 2007;29(Suppl.):2536–2546.

113   Iskedjian M, Bereza B, Gordon A, Piwko C, Einarson TR. Meta-analysis of cannabis based treatments for neuropathic and multiple sclerosis-related pain. *Curr Med Res Opin* 2007;23(1):17–24.

114   Abrams DI, Jay CA, Shade SB et al. Cannabis in painful HIV-associated sensory neuropathy: A randomized placebo-controlled trial. *Neurology* 2007;68:515–521.

115   Galer BS, Rowbotham MC, Perander J, Friedman E. Topical lidocaine patch relieves postherpetic neuralgia more effectively than a vehicle topical patch: Results of an enriched enrollment. *Pain* 1999;80:533–538.

●   116   Rowbotham MC, Reisner-Keller LA, Fields HL. Both intravenous lidocaine and morphine reduce the pain of postherpetic neuralgia. *Neurology* 1991;41:1024–1028.

117   Mercadante S, Arcuri E, Tirelli W et al. Analgesic effect of intravenous ketamine in cancer patients on morphine therapy: A randomized controlled, double-blind, cross-over, double dose study. *J Pain Symptom Manage* 2000;20:246–262.

◆ ✳ 118   Hassenbusch SJ, Portenoy RK, Cousins M et al. Polyanalgesic Consensus Conference 2003: An update on the management of pain by intraspinal drug delivery-report of an expert panel. *J Pain Symptom Manage* 2004;27:540–563.

●   119   Burton AW, Rajagopal A, Shah HN et al. Epidural and intrathecal analgesia is effective in treating refractory cancer pain. *Pain Med* 2004;5:239–247.

●   120   Staats PS, Yearwood T, Charapata SG et al. Intrathecal ziconotide in the treatment of refractory pain in patients with cancer or AIDS: A randomized controlled trial. *JAMA* 2004;291:63–70.

✳   121   Gybels J, Erdine S, Maeyaert J et al. Neuromodulation of pain a consensus statement prepared in Brussels, 16–18 January 1998, by the following task force of the European Federation of IASP chapters (EFIC). *Eur J Pain* 1998;2:203–209.

122   Gilron I, Bailey JM, Tu D, Holden RR, Weaver DF, Houlden RL. Morphine, gabapentin, or their combination for neuropathic pain. *N Engl J Med* 2005;352(13):1324–1334.

52

Bone cancer pain and skeletal complications

YOKO TARUMI

INTRODUCTION

Epidemiology

The skeleton is one of the most frequent sites of metastases, particularly in patients with advanced breast, prostate, and lung cancers. Metastatic breast cancer and prostate cancer are the malignancies most often responsible for malignant bone disease [1]. Tumor registry data for 11 primary tumor sites and 15 metastatic sites in 4399 patients revealed that bone metastases were present in 90%, 48%, and 39% of patients with prostate, breast, and lung cancers, respectively [2]*. The most common site of bone metastases is the axial skeleton, such as the vertebrae, pelvis, proximal ends of long bones, and skull [3].

Most patients with bone metastases will develop skeletal complications ("skeletal-related events" [SREs]) at some point during the course of their disease. Common SREs are bone cancer pain, pathologic fractures, subsequent surgery or radiation, hypercalcemia of malignancy, and spinal cord or root nerve compression [1,4**]. A population study of 35,912 patients newly diagnosed with breast cancer in Denmark during 1999–2007 revealed that 0.5% presented with bone metastases at the time of diagnoses, of whom 43.2% developed an SRE during a median of 3.4 years of follow-up; an additional 3.6% who did not have bone metastases at initial presentation subsequently developed them, of whom 46.4% developed an SRE within a median follow-up time of 0.7 years [5]*. In the same study, 5-year survival was 75.8% for those without bone metastases, 8.3% for patients with bone metastases, and 2.5% for those with both bone metastases and SREs [6]*. In a Surveillance, Epidemiology, and End Results (SEER)-Medicare database study of 126,978 men aged 65 years or older diagnosed with prostate cancer between 1999 and 2005 and followed up for a median of 3.3 years, 7.7% had bone metastasis at diagnosis (1.7%) or during follow-up (5.9%); SREs occurred in 44%. Hazard ratios for risk of death were 6.6 (95% CI = 6.4–6.9) and 10.2 (95% CI = 9.8–10.7), for men with bone metastasis but no SRE and for men with bone metastasis plus SRE, respectively, compared with men without bone metastasis [7]. Most patients with lung cancer metastatic to bone develop at least one SRE

during their lifetimes [8***]. As survival improves with new treatment modalities, the prevalence of SREs in this group is likely to increase [8***].

Bone metastases are the most common source of pain in patients with advanced malignant disease [9*].

In a prospective evaluation of 2266 cancer patients referred to a pain service, bone pain was identified in 35% of cases [10*]. Although bone cancer pain may be found in patients with an established diagnosis of malignancy, it can be also be an initial presenting symptom, with or without constitutional signs, that requires further work-up to establish the diagnosis of primary malignant disease.

Clinical characteristics of bone cancer pain

Pain caused by bone cancer may have variable temporal patterns, intensities, and characteristics, even within the same location. At its onset, bone cancer pain can be intermittent, well-localized, and achy or sharp in quality, but can progress rapidly into continuous dull and throbbing pain without any physical activity (baseline pain). Baseline pain may be eased by positioning or around-the-clock opioid analgesics. It is often provoked or aggravated by applying pressure to the affected area. With increased bone destruction and time, the pain intensifies with episodes of spontaneous aggravation of pain or movement-induced pain. The temporal flare of pain in the presence of controlled baseline pain has been referred to as "breakthrough pain," "episodic pain," or "transitory pain" [11***]. A longitudinal multicenter study of 1801 cancer patients with pain revealed that bone metastasis was one of the factors strongly associated with the presence of breakthrough pain. The presence of breakthrough pain was associated with a higher probability of death and of requiring a switch in opioid analgesics to manage analgesic failure or side effects [12*] (see Chapter 53).

Patients experiencing bone cancer pain can develop severe pain with normally nonpainful activities such as coughing, turning in bed, gentle touching, or gentle limb movements [13]. Functional status worsens as uncontrolled incident pain interferes with activities [14*,15,16*]. Thus, bone metastases and associated pain have ominous consequences for both quality and length of life.

Robust investigations of the mechanisms of bone cancer pain through preclinical models have provided insight that bone cancer pain has unique characteristics, differing from inflammatory or typical nociceptive somatic pain. It has been found to have a spectrum of neuropathic features, such as hyperalgesia, hypersensitivity to mechanical stimuli, and spontaneous pain that may be observed clinically as breakthrough or incident pain [17]. Using a self-reported screening tool, neuropathic features were identified in 17% of 98 consecutive patients with symptomatic bone metastases requiring palliative radiotherapy [14*]. However, confirmatory evidence of neuropathic pain from focused neurological assessment and appropriate imaging was not obtained [15]. To date, there has not been any classification system that defines bone cancer pain as neuropathic.

Although the most common presenting symptom of bone metastases is pain, 30%–50% of patients with bone involvement have asymptomatic bone metastases found during staging studies for primary tumors [18]. The mechanisms underlying the observation that some metastatic bones are not painful have not yet been fully explored.

MECHANISM OF BONE CANCER PAIN (SEE FIGURE 52.1)

Loss of bone homeostasis

Bone resorption (bone loss) and formation is an ongoing process occurring in both healthy and cancerous bone, directed by the influence of endocrine hormones such as parathyroid hormone (PTH) and 1,25-dihydroxyvitamin D (1,24-(OH)2D3), paracrine hormones, and cytokines. In the

setting of metastasis, the structural integrity of bone is compromised due to disruptions in the normal balance of osteolytic and osteoblastic activity [19].

Bone cancer can be osteolytic (bone destroying, as in multiple myeloma, breast, kidney, and thyroid cancer), osteosclerotic (bone-forming, as in prostate, bladder, and lung cancer), or mixed osteolytic and osteosclerotic (as in breast and lung cancer). In vivo studies have shown that cancer-induced resorption is due to the activity of osteoclasts (the cells that break down bone), and is not a direct effect of the cancer itself. Overall, osteolytic lesions result from greater osteoclast than osteoblast cellular activity, resulting in uncoupled bone resorption. That is, there is no negative feedback mechanism to halt the process [20]. Increased numbers of osteoclasts have been shown in animal models of bone cancer; these high numbers may correlate with bone cancer pain. Limiting osteoclastic activity in bone metastases may reduce bone cancer pain [21]. Both osteolytic and osteoblastic cancers are characterized by osteoclast proliferation and hypertrophy [22].

Osteoclasts are controlled by a triad of receptors and cytokines. Osteoblast and osteoclast precursors normally express the receptor activator of nuclear factor-κB ligand (RANKL), which is a member of the tumor necrosis factor family. RANKL binds to the RANK receptor on osteoclast precursors and mature osteoclasts [23]. Excessive bone resorption is prevented by the decoy receptor osteoprotegerin (OPG), produced by osteoblasts, that binds to RANKL, thus preventing interaction between RANKL and RANK [24]. This tightly controlled system is lost when cancer cells invade the bone microenvironment, inducing excessive osteolysis via the expression of RANKL or the effects of PTH-related protein (PTHr-P) on OPG and RANKL production by osteoblasts [25].

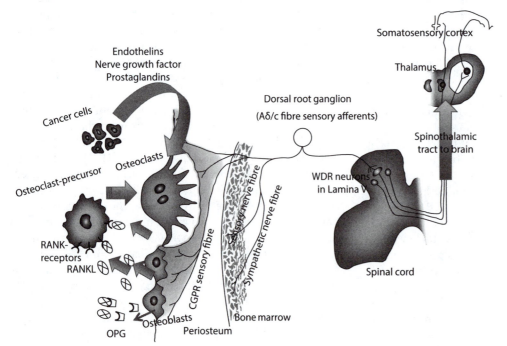

Figure 52.1 *Mechanism of bone cancer pain.*

Denosumab is a fully humanized monoclonal antibody that inhibits RANKL, and markedly reduces tumor-induced bone resorption and SREs [26]. Bisphosphonates are a class of antiresorptive compounds that are pyrophosphate analogues with a high affinity for calcium ions, causing them to rapidly and avidly bind to the mineralized matrix of bone. Bisphosphonates, once taken up by the osteoclasts, induce the loss of function and ultimately apoptosis of the osteoclasts (i.e., cell death) by impairing either the synthesis of adenosine triphosphate or cholesterol, both of which are necessary for osteoclast function and survival [27].

Neurochemicals that modulate pain

In addition to tumor-driven resorption of bone through loss of bone homeostasis, tumor cells release pronociceptive compounds including prostaglandins, nerve growth factor (NGF), and endothelins [28,29]. Nonsteroidal anti-inflammatory drugs (NSAIDs) that specifically inhibit cyclooxygenase-2 (COX-2 inhibitors) have been shown to reduce bone cancer pain, tumor burden, and bone destruction in laboratory models, while anti-NGF therapy attenuates tumor-induced nerve sprouting, neuroma formation, and bone cancer pain in a mouse model of prostate cancer-induced bone pain [30].

The cannabinoid receptor 2 (CB2 receptor) is found in the peripheral nervous system; in contrast, the cannabinoid receptor 1 (CB1 receptor) is found in central nervous system and can induce psychotropic effects. CB2 is normally expressed in osteoblasts, osteoclasts, and their precursors, and is also found in the system associated with immune responses, such as the spleen, tonsils, monocytes, B-cells, and T-cell [31]. CB2 agonists have been shown to not only produce antinociceptive and anti-inflammatory effects, but also increase bone density by increasing the number of osteoblasts and inhibiting the production of osteoclasts [32]. In a murine bone cancer model, the systemic administration of a selective CB2 agonist significantly attenuated spontaneous and evoked pain, while reducing bone loss and decreasing the incidence of cancer-induced bone fractures [31].

Innervation of bone and remodeling of dorsal horn neurons

A complex nerve supply in bone has been demonstrated in recent animal model studies. Mineralized bone and bone marrow periosteum (the thin fibrous and cellular sheath that covers the outer surface of the mineralized bone) are innervated by a combination of primary afferent sensory neurons and postganglionic sympathetic neurons [33]. The periosteum is innervated by a dense net-like mesh network of calcitonin-gene-related peptide-positive (CGRP) and 200 kDa neurofilament-positive sensory fibers that detect mechanical distortion of periosteum and bone [34].

The peripheral sensory neurons synapse with secondary ascending neurons in the spinal cord. Normally, most lamina I neurons are nociceptive-specific (NS) neurons that only respond to noxious stimuli, whereas the vast majority of lamina V cells consist of wide dynamic range (WDR) neurons, which code nonnoxious stimuli throughout the temperature and mechanical range as noxious intensities. In a rat model of bone cancer pain, the proportion of WDR neurons was increased [35]. This results in a hyperexcitable state where normally nonnoxious stimuli produce pain (hyperalgesia/allodynia).

At the spinal level, extensive neurochemical reorganization occurs, including expression of the pronociceptive opioid dynorphin, and activation of pronociceptive neuropeptide substance P and the excitatory neurotransmitter glutamate. The proliferation of astrocytes in the spinal dorsal horn of animal models bearing bone cancer supports the hypothesis that malignant bone pain is enhanced by a state of spinal sensitization [36]. These neurochemical findings have been correlated with the degree of bone destruction, and shown that malignant bone pain differs clearly from inflammatory pain or neuropathic pain [37]. The animal model has further revealed that bone cancer pain requires higher doses of morphine to control pain behaviors compared with inflammatory pain [38]. Drugs that have a role in attenuating hyperalgesia, such as gabapentin, have been demonstrated to normalize the bone cancer pain–induced dorsal horn neuronal hyperexcitability and attenuate pain behaviors in the animal model [39]. In summary, the pathophysiology of bone pain is complex and due to tissue destruction and pathological activation of the peripheral and central nervous system.

DIAGNOSTIC APPROACH

Besides the general physical examination, a musculoskeletal and neurological examination should be completed, focusing on palpable tenderness in the skeletal system and neurological deficits/alterations. Patients who have back pain with or without weakness of the limbs, paresthesias, sensory change, or bladder or bowel impairment should be carefully assessed for potential spinal cord compression or cauda equina syndrome (see Chapter XX). In all cases, it is important to emphasize that the imaging tests should be interpreted in conjunction with the clinical picture. Tables 52.1 and 52.2 provide summaries of the differential diagnoses of bone pain and diagnostic modalities.

Bone consists of 85% dense cortical bone composed of minerals and 15% porous and spongy trabecular bone composed of collagen and mineral content, which encompasses the marrow component. Most of the red marrow (made up of hematopoietic tissue) is located in the axial skeleton (e.g., vertebrae, pelvis, proximal femora), while yellow marrow (made up of fat cells) is located in appendicular bones. On plain radiographs, bone metastases may appear as areas of absent density or absent trabecular structure, which represent osteolytic lesions. Osteoblastic lesions may appear as increased density

Table 52.1 *Common presentation of bone pain and differential diagnoses*

Presentation of bone pain	Differential diagnosis to be considered		
	Cancer related	Cancer therapy related	Nonmalignant
Back pain	Spinal metastasis Pancoast syndrome Spinal cord/thecal sac/cauda equina compression Pelvic metastasis or direct invasion of tumor into pelvic structure Scapular, posterior rib metastasis may present back pain Retroperitoneal metastases	Vertebral compression fracture secondary to glucocorticoids, anti-androgen/estrogen therapy Insufficiency fracture related radiotherapy (e.g., sacrum)	Osteoporosis Immobility Paget's disease Other inflammatory conditions Infectious conditions (e.g., septic arthritis)
Hip/femur/humeral pain	Impending pathological fracture	Avascular necrosis of the femoral or humeral head related to steroid use	Avascular necrosis of the femoral or humeral head Stress fracture
Rib pain	Rib metastasis, direct invasion Intrathoracic tumor	Radiation pneumonitis Postthoracotomy neuropathy	Stress fracture New onset of herpes zoster Pleuritic chest pain related to multiple etiologies
Headache	Skull and base of skull metastasis	Chemotherapy, hormone therapy, or others	Temporal arteritis or other vasculitides

and sclerotic lesions or rims. Plain radiographs can confirm symptomatic lesions or suspicious lesions identified on bone scintigraphy (i.e., bone scan). They are also useful for assessing patients at high risk for pathological fractures. However, because 30%–75% of normal bone mineral content must be lost before osteolytic lesions in the vertebrae become apparent on plain radiographs, metastatic lesions may not be apparent on an x-ray for several months [40]. The diagnostic sensitivity of this modality for detecting bone metastases is probably in the range of 44%–50%, which is substantially less than bone scintigraphy [41]. However, plain radiographs are useful as a primary investigation and for pure lytic disease, such a multiple myeloma, in which bone scintigraphy is commonly falsely negative.

Diagnostic sensitivity of bone scintigraphy is in the range of 62%–100% and specificity is in the range of 78%–100% [41]. However, unlike plain radiographs, bone scintigraphy lacks specificity, as it may show uptake in conditions such as osteoarthritis, infection, trauma, or Paget's disease. Bone scintigraphy commonly shows an abnormality where there is osteoblastic activity, whereas it may be negative with purely lytic lesions or rapidly progressive disease, which allows little chance for new bone formation (i.e., cold spots). Diffuse accumulation of tracer throughout the skeleton may occasionally occur in disseminated skeletal disease (superscan), commonly seen in prostate cancer, leading to the false impression of a normal scan. Computed tomography (CT) with bone windows or magnetic resonance imaging (MRI) can provide detailed information on the bone and bone marrow. MRI has better contrast resolution than CT for visualizing soft tissue and the spinal cord, and CT is disadvantaged by the beam hardening artifact that obscures the adjacent soft tissues and bones. The diagnostic sensitivity and specificity of CT and MRI for the detection of bone metastases is in the range of 71%–100% and 85%–100%, respectively, with specificity of 73%–100% for MRI [41].

Table 52.2 *Comparison of diagnostic specificity/sensitivity*

	Sensitivity	Specificity	Cost	Remarks
Radiograph	Low (40%–50%)	High	Low	Useful in the • Evaluation of risk for pathological fracture • Skeletal survey for lytic lesions
Bone scintigraphy	High (62%–100%)	High (80%–100%)	Moderate	• Able to screen entire skeleton • Suffers lack of sensitivity in lytic lesions, and specificity in degenerative change, inflammatory process, and mechanical stress
CT scan	High (71%–100%)	High (85%–100%)	Moderate	
MRI	High (71%–100%)	High (73%–100%)	High	
PET scan	High	High	Very high	Detects increased metabolic activities of cancer even in early stage or bone marrow involvement only

Whole-body MRI is a new alternative to the stepwise multimodality diagnostic process for bone metastasis. The introduction of a rolling platform mounted on top of a conventional MRI examination table facilitates whole-body MR imaging within 1 hour. A recent systematic review and meta-analysis revealed a pooled sensitivity of 90.0% and pooled specificity of 91.8% for the detection of bone metastases [42***]. Positron emission tomography (PET) may have a role in early detection of soft tissue or bone metastases. A recent meta-analysis to evaluate the diagnostic properties of PET or PET/CT and bone scintigraphy in detecting bone metastases in patients with lung cancer revealed that the pooled patient-based and lesion-based sensitivity and specificity were 93% and 95% for PET, respectively, and 93% and 57% for bone scintigraphy, respectively [43***]. Although high in sensitivity and specificity that has a role in initial cancer staging to detect nodal involvement or distant metastases for consideration of surgical resection, the significance of PET in palliative care settings can be limited due to its high cost and relatively limited availability.

THERAPEUTIC APPROACH

The use of chemotherapeutic and hormonal agents has significantly improved the survival of patients with metastatic bone disease [44*,45*]. At the same time, patients with metastatic bone disease may live longer with bone cancer pain or risk of SREs. The goals of therapy are to achieve local tumor control and structural stability of bone while managing pain. This may lead to the maintenance or restoration of functional independence and improvement in quality of life, while enhancing opportunities for further life-extending therapies in some patients. Although it is important to provide immediate and effective analgesic management, clinicians should pay careful attention to possible long-term adverse effects of pharmacotherapy in patients with potential long-term survival. At the same time, nonpharmacological approaches may be considered, based on anticipated life expectancy, in order to provide maximum benefit and avoid serious harm.

Pharmacological approach

Although the provision of analgesics is the very first step to relieve suffering from bone cancer pain, and preclinical models have provided a rationale for clinical trials of drugs that target identified pain mechanisms, there is still a long way to go before mechanism-based therapy is established. Bisphosphonates and denosumab are now considered as bone-modifying agents for metastatic tumors such as breast, prostate, and multiple myeloma.

Figure 52.2 shows the flowchart for the management for bone cancer pain.

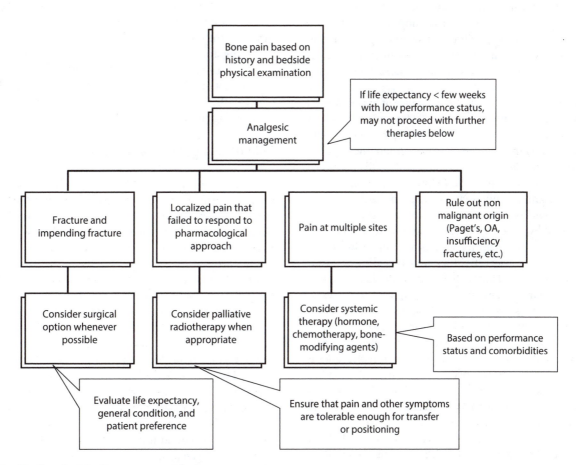

Figure 52.2   *The flowchart for the management for bone cancer pain.*

Role of bisphosphonates in SREs

The use of bisphosphonates to reduce skeletal morbidity in patients with bone metastases should be considered [46]. Randomized controlled trials of pamidronate and clodronate in patients with bony metastatic disease have shown decreased skeletal morbidity [47**,48**,49**]. Zoledronic acid has been shown to be at least as effective as pamidronate. Zoledronic acid is the most potent bisphosphonate currently available, 500–1000 times more potent than pamidronate, and the first drug in this class approved for use in all solid tumor patients with bone metastases as well as in multiple myeloma. Its use has been studied most extensively in breast cancer, prostate cancer, multiple myeloma, and lung cancer [50**,51**,52**,53**,54**,55**].

There have been three international Phase III randomized, double-blind, double-dummy, active controlled studies comparing denosumab with zoledronic acid with respect to time to first on-study SREs, and time to first and subsequent SREs (fracture, radiotherapy or surgery, and spinal cord compression) in over 5700 patients with bone metastases secondary to breast cancer, prostate cancer, and other solid tumors (non-small-cell lung cancer 40%; multiple myeloma 10% and others) [56**,57**,58**]. In this combined analysis, denosumab significantly prevented or delayed the time to first on-study SREs or hypercalcemia of malignancy. The median time to first on-study SRE was 27.7 months with denosumab versus 19.4 months with zoledronic acid (delay of 8.2 months in favor of denosumab therapy). A significant decrease in hypercalcemia of malignancy in those treated with denosumab was found, though disease progression and overall survival were similar between treatment groups, as was the incidence of all adverse events and serious adverse events.

However, there was an increased incidence of hypocalcemia in the denosumab group (9.6% versus 5.0%) and acute-phase reactions such as flu-like symptoms and acute renal toxicity (20.2% versus 8.7%) in the zoledronic acid group. Incidence of osteonecrosis of the jaw was infrequent and similar between the treatment groups, with a cumulative incidence of 1.3% in zoledronic acid group compared with 1.8% in the denosumab group. Further analysis of osteonecrosis of the jaw events suggested poor oral hygiene, dental extractions, and dental appliances accounted for the majority of cases, with up to 40% of the cases resolving with conservative therapies, including oral and/or topical antibiotics and surgical debridement after a median of 8 months. Four percent of patients required bone resection for refractory disease [59]. It is recommended that serum creatinine level be monitored prior to each dose of pamidronate and zoledronic acid, while the dosing for zoledronic acid should be adjusted when baseline serum creatinine clearance is ≥30 and ≤60 mL/min. The role of denosumab has not evaluated in patients with a creatinine clearance <30 mL/min or receiving dialysis. Monitoring for hypocalcaemia in patients with impaired creatinine clearance is recommended [60].

Thirty to fifty percentage of cancer patients with bone metastases still develop SREs while on bisphosphonate

therapy [51**]. These trials suggest a role for switching to denosumab in patients who are currently receiving oral or intravenous bisphosphonates and experience SREs or who continue to have elevated markers of bone turnover, including urinary collagen type I cross-linked N-telopeptide (Ntx) [59]. Denosumab's subcutaneous route of administration offers potential advantage in certain settings.

A trial in breast cancer patients revealed that in those with no or mild pain at baseline, median time to development of moderate or severe pain with denosumab was 296 days, compared with 176 days in those treated with zoledronic acid. Time to pain improvement was similar between treatment arms, with a median of 82 days for denosumab and a median of 85 days for zoledronic acid. A greater proportion of denosumab-treated patients reported improvements in emotional and physical well-being [59]. This result confirmed that bone-modifying agents are an adjunctive therapy for cancer-related bone pain control. However, they are not recommended as first-line treatment for cancer-related pain [60].

An economic evaluation revealed that the cost of denosumab in a 1-year period was potentially higher than zoledronic acid in hormone-refractory prostate cancer patients with bone metastases, even considering indirect drug costs [61*]. The burden of skeletal morbidity and the diagnosis and treatment of bone metastases in patients with non-small-cell lung cancer were reviewed, and found that direct costs of SREs and their subsequent supportive care are approximately $28,000 per patient. Although bone metastases often are not diagnosed until after the onset of symptoms, early treatment can delay the onset of potentially debilitating SREs. In patients with lung and other solid tumors (n = 773), zoledronic acid (4 mg via 15 min infusion every 3 weeks) delayed the median time to first on-study SREs by over 80 days compared with placebo (p = 0.009). Moreover, zoledronic acid significantly reduced the ongoing risk of SREs by 32% versus placebo (p = 0.016) [8].

Role of analgesic pharmacotherapy

Analgesic pharmacotherapy should follow the standard of cancer pain management, in view of the current lack of mechanism-specific analgesics. This includes the use of nonopioid analgesics including NSAIDs, opioid analgesics, corticosteroids, and adjuvant agents. In advanced bone cancer pain, opioids provide the mainstay for analgesia, based on clinical empirical evidence and preclinical studies. However, high doses may be required due to associated neuropathic and incident characteristics, leading to significant adverse effects [62]. Preclinical models have also shown that prolonged exposures to morphine is associated with increased osteoclast activity and upregulated interleukins (IL-1 beta), accelerated sarcoma-induced bone destruction and double the incidence of spontaneous fracture, in a dose- and naloxone-sensitive manner [63]. Furthermore, clinical studies in chronic nonmalignant pain have provided evidence for opioid-induced androgen deficiency in men and profound inhibition of ovarian sex hormone and adrenal androgen production in women (i.e., opioid-associated hypogonadotrophic hypogonadism) who chronically consume opioids, which may affect bone health [64*,65,66*]. Bone mineral density (BMD) was found to be lower in patients on methadone maintenance therapy than in normal control subjects [66*]. Although no clinical data have been published in the bone cancer pain population, further examination of the clinical impact of this phenomenon needs to be explored, considering the improving survival times for metastatic breast and prostate cancer patients.

NSAIDs inhibit the enzyme cyclooxygenase (COX). The COX-1 isoform is found in platelets, the gastrointestinal tract, kidneys, and most other human tissues. The COX-2 isoform is found predominantly in the kidneys and central nervous system, and is induced in peripheral tissues by noxious stimuli that cause inflammation and pain. In addition to peripheral effects, NSAIDs exert a central action at the brain or spinal cord level. NSAIDS are undoubtedly effective in cancer pain [67***], although there is no evidence they are uniquely more effective in bone pain compared to other pain syndromes. Adverse effects of NSAIDs include gastrointestinal ulceration and renal failure. The risk of gastrointestinal toxicity is higher with increased age, previous peptic ulcer disease, comorbid medical illnesses, use of multiple NSAIDs (including ASA) simultaneously, and use in combination with a corticosteroid. If an NSAID is prescribed for a palliative care patient, some clinicians prescribe a gastroprotective agent, although there is no strong evidence to promote this as routine practice. Effective gastroprotective agents include proton pump inhibitors, double-dose H2 receptor antagonists, and misoprostol. Misoprostol can cause diarrhea and abdominal pain, but these side effects may be less of a concern for patients who are also on opioids [68***,69***]. Renal function should be monitored on a regular basis, and adequate hydration should be ensured.

Corticosteroids are frequently prescribed in palliative care for the management of multiple symptoms. They are believed to be particularly effective for metastatic bone pain, though there has been little formal evaluation of this broad experience. Potentially life-threatening side effects occur particularly with prolonged use (e.g., osteoporosis, proximal myopathy). Therefore, it is preferable to use corticosteroids on a short-term basis, such as a couple of weeks duration, until other analgesic interventions have an opportunity to take effect. Corticosteroids can be particularly useful in the setting of short life expectancy, such as days to weeks. Preliminary evidence suggests that corticosteroids may prevent pain flare following radiotherapy [70]. Corticosteroids act directly on osteoblasts and osteocytes to induce their apoptosis and reduce bone formation and strength, and also stimulate bone resorption, increase urinary excretion of calcium, and inhibit intestinal absorption of calcium [71]. The effects are dose dependent and cumulative, with rapid onset of bone loss in the first 3–6 months of use. Even low doses, such as prednisolone 2.5 mg/day, are associated with an increased fracture risk [72].

Calcitonin is a hormone that inhibits osteoclastic bone resorption. It is used in the treatment of hypercalcemia of malignancy and for management of pain from osteoporotic compression fractures. A systematic review found only two small clinical trials evaluating calcitonin in the treatment of metastatic bone pain, concluding that available evidence does not yet support its use for this indication [73***].

One of the challenges in management of bone cancer pain is breakthrough pain or incident pain, characterized by a relatively short duration with high intensity despite successful management of baseline pain with around-the-clock opioid analgesics. Breakthrough pain is often treated with oral immediate-release opioids. A conventional, though not evidence-based, dose of breakthrough analgesic is 5%–20% of the total daily opioid dose. More recently, several formulations for oral or nasal transmucosal administration of fentanyl, specifically developed for the management of breakthrough pain, have become available. A limited number of trials of these agents in patients with breakthrough cancer pain have suggested more rapid onset of analgesia, compared to oral opioids. Studies have also shown a lack of correlation between the effective breakthrough opioid dose and the baseline opioid dose, suggesting a need to titrate the former [74***]. Further evidence is awaited on the benefits, risks, and cost of these new drugs, relative to conventional opioids.

Nonpharmacological approaches

Simple nonpharmacological methods of pain management should always be considered. Non-weight-bearing techniques, heat, ice, and sometimes gentle massage can help reduce pain. An assessment by both an occupational and physical therapist will yield information to help reduce or prevent pain. Modification of the home or workplace with equipment such as walkers, wheelchairs, and grip bars can help. Patients will have better pain relief when a combination of medications and supportive therapies is employed.

External beam radiotherapy is a standard approach to the management of painful bone metastases that cannot be adequately controlled with analgesics. It has been recognized that approximately 50% of patients will experience relief from pain within 2 weeks after completing palliative external beam radiation for bone metastases, and more than 75% will have pain relief 4 weeks after completing treatment [75**]. Radiotherapy may not be beneficial in patients whose anticipated survival time is less than 4 weeks. Radiotherapy can be administered in single or multiple fractions. A systematic review of randomized trials comparing single fractions versus multiple fractions revealed no significant difference for overall and the complete response rates; a significantly higher re-treatment rate with single fractions was evident [76***]. However, single fraction radiotherapy is less burdensome for patients and less costly for the health care system. Multiple fraction radiotherapy is preferred for previously irradiated areas, to treat or prevent pathologic fractures, and for spinal cord or cauda equina involvement [77]. A systematic review provided further insight into re-irradiation of painful bone metastases in nonresponders or recurrent pain after initial response. Overall, a pain response was achieved in 58%, although there was substantial between-study heterogeneity due to methodological differences [78***].

Radiopharmaceuticals are radioactive agents, administered intravenously, that localize specifically to metastatic bone sites and deliver radiation in a highly focal manner due to the nature of the radioactivity emitted (typically beta/electron emission). Strontium-89 and samarium-153 are the radiopharmaceuticals that have been most extensively examined in clinical trials. A systematic review has shown that radiopharmaceutical administration is associated with improved pain control (number needed to treat to achieve complete relief = 5) without conclusive evidence of effect on analgesic use [79***]. The main adverse effects are leucocytopenia and thrombocytopenia (number needed to harm = 13). Use of radiopharmaceuticals may best be considered for patients with multiple painful bone metastases where pain control with conventional analgesic regimens is unsatisfactory and local field radiotherapy is not appropriate. The selection of patients for radiopharmaceutical therapy should consider the patient's bone marrow function, performance status, recent use of other marrow suppression agents (chemotherapy or external beam radiotherapy), and suitability for alternate palliative interventions. Life expectancy should also be taken into account, since radiopharmaceuticals have an onset of analgesia typically measured in months [80***].

The goal of orthopedic surgery is to provide structural stability and promote immediate functional recovery, weight-bearing, and rehabilitation, with the least possible morbidity. The indications for operative treatment of long bone and pelvic girdle metastases include impending and pathological fractures and intractable pain [81*,82]. The operative treatment of spinal metastases is indicated for patients with spinal instability or spinal cord compression [83*,84*,85*]. Elective fixation prevents the intense pain and the loss of function associated with a pathological fracture, and requires less complex procedures than fixation of an existing pathological fracture. It is associated with shorter hospitalization and discharged home rather than facility settings [86].

Several methods have been suggested to assess the risk of pathological fractures in metastatic bone lesions. Mirel's scoring system is based on four parameters (site, radiographic appearance, size, and related pain) for predicting the risk of fracture and for recommending appropriate treatment. A total score of ≥9 reflects high risk of impending fracture and prophylactic fixation is recommended, while a total score of ≤7 reflects no risk of impending fracture and nonsurgical treatment is recommended. A higher score reflecting higher risk of fracture is given for osteolytic lesions than osteoblastic lesions, involvement of the peritrochanteric area of the femur than non-weight-bearing bones, involvement of more than half of the circumference of a bone, and association with functional pain [87]. Although Mirel's scoring system, which combines clinical and radiographic factors into one score, is the most commonly used, it has been criticized due to potential for either overuse or underuse of surgery [88*]. Spinal stability is presumed if there is transitional deformity, vertebral body collapse of >50%, tumor involvement of two of three columns, or involvement of the same column at two or more adjacent levels [89].

A prospective pilot study to evaluate orthopedic intervention in patients with painful bone metastases without fracture did not find a clear benefit to quality of life. The median survival of this group was 22 weeks, although the attrition rate was high due to deaths. A trend toward improvement in patient-rated health status scores 6 weeks after surgery was associated with an increase in the length of survival following surgery [90*]. A life expectancy of longer than 6 months is the most positive factor predicting fracture reunion postsurgery, although patients with shorter prognosis can also benefit from surgery [91*]. Decreased functional status and comorbidity can prolong recovery and increase postoperative complications such as delirium, infections, thromboembolism, and pressure ulcers. Postoperative external beam radiotherapy is necessary in most cases to obliterate residual microscopic disease and thus prevent disease progression and further osteolysis [92].

Patients with very short life expectancy would not benefit from a surgery because of the rapid general deterioration of their functional and physiological status due to the cancer and because of their inability to execute a minimal rehabilitation protocol. Consideration of the expected survival, overall medical status, quality of life, magnitude of the operation, and rehabilitation potential, all contribute to the decision-making process. Six to twelve weeks of expected survival is generally the minimum required for relatively simple procedures such as intramedullary nailing, and a minimum of 6 months is necessary for more complex procedures such as acetabular or endoprosthetic reconstruction [90].

LONG-TERM EFFECTS ON BONE HEALTH AND CANCER THERAPY

Recent improvements in cancer survival are largely due to earlier diagnosis and advancements in cancer treatments. Despite having favorable effects on cancer survival, radiotherapy, hormone treatment, and combination chemotherapy can cause long-term organ damage and functional disabilities. These effects are largely unrecognized, as they are often absent or subclinical during the active cancer treatment [93*]. Aromatase inhibitors (anastrozole, exemestane, and letrozole) massively deplete circulating estrogens by inhibiting the aromatization of androgens and their conversion to estrogens in peripheral tissues by blocking the P450 cytochrome enzyme aromatase in postmenopausal women. The substantial reduction in estrogen concentrations can lead to bone loss, and aromatase inhibitor therapy has been associated with decreased in BMD and increased fracture risk [94**,95**,96**,97**,98**]. In a clinical trial of 9366 postmenopausal women with localized breast cancer randomized to anastrozole or tamoxifen, fractures were significantly more frequent in the anastrozole group than in the tamoxifen group (11.0% versus 7.7%, respectively) after a median follow-up of 68 months, with a particularly increased risk of vertebral fractures [99**]. Similarly, in study randomizing 4895 postmenopausal women with localized breast cancer to letrozole and tamoxifen, the fracture incidence was significantly higher in the letrozole group compared with the tamoxifen group (9.3% versus 6.5%) after a median follow-up of 60.3 months [97**]. A recent prospective cohort study also revealed a high prevalence of fracture risk (low baseline BMD, elevated bone turnover markers, and low vitamin D concentrations) in postmenopausal women with early breast cancer who were to start aromatase inhibitors [100**]. Another prospective cohort study found vitamin D insufficiency and high prevalence of vertebral fractures in 497 postmenopausal women with nonmetastatic breast cancer who were to start the aromatase inhibitor therapy [101**].

In a long-term cohort study, 26,213 breast, colorectal, and prostate cancer patients who had survived over 5 years were matched with noncancer controls, using a primary care database; results revealed an elevated incidence of osteoporosis in all survivor groups, which was highest in the prostate cancer survivors [93]. Pelvic radiotherapy has been also found to contribute to insufficient fractures in uterine and cervical cancer patients [102*,103*,104*].

Based on this knowledge, the American Society of Clinical Oncology recommends screening for cancer-induced bone loss with dual energy x-ray absorptiometry (DXA) scans for all women aged ≥65 years and any postmenopausal women receiving aromatase inhibitors [46]. Guidelines from the UK further reflect the importance of global risk factors other than BMD in the selection of patients for intervention, such as low body mass index, alcohol consumption, history of fracture, premature menopause, rheumatoid arthritis or other inflammatory disease, long-term oral corticosteroid use, and family history [105]. For prostate cancer patients, all men beginning androgen deprivation therapy should have baseline DXA scans, with continued monitoring every 1–2 years for osteoporotic or osteopenic individuals [106].

Diagnosis of osteopenia and osteoporosis is based on the assessment of BMD by DXA scan, using the T-score system, which was developed to assess the risk for fracture in a 60-year-old female. Bone density is classified as normal (T-score greater than −1 SD), osteopenic (T-score −1 to −2.5 SD), or osteoporotic (T-score less than −2.5 SD) [107]. According to the UK guidelines, high-risk patients (T-score less than −2) should receive bisphosphonate therapy at osteoporosis treatment doses, in addition to lifestyle advice and calcium and vitamin D supplementation. Medium-risk patients (T-score between −2 and −1) should be given lifestyle advice plus calcium and vitamin D supplementation. Low-risk patients (T-score greater than −1) need lifestyle advice only (diet, weight-bearing exercise, reduced alcohol consumption, and cessation of smoking). The National Osteoporosis Foundation recommends that adults aged ≥50 years need 1200 mg of calcium from all sources and 800–1000 IU of vitamin daily [108].

CONCLUSION

As improvements in cancer therapy result in longer survival for patients with bone metastases, the needs for supporting individuals with bone metastases and SREs are expected to rise. At the same time, clinicians need to be aware of the long-term consequences of cancer therapies and bone cancer pain treatments on bone health. When approaching the bone cancer pain,

consideration should be given to disease trajectory, survival estimation, general health status, and patients' wishes and goals of care so that the most effective and safest treatment modalities may be provided.

Key learning points

- SREs occur in nearly half of patients with breast or prostate cancer metastatic to bone during the course of disease, and at least once in the lifetime of most patients with lung cancer with bone metastases. Bone metastases are one of the most common etiologies of cancer pain.

- Clinical characteristics of bone cancer pain include pain at rest (baseline pain) and intermittent occurrences of breakthrough pain (spontaneous or incident hyperalgesia and hypersensitivity to mechanical stimuli).

- Malignant tumor cells trigger the loss of bone homeostasis for bone resorption and formation regulated by osteoclasts and osteoblasts activities. Tumor cells release cytokines that interact with osteoclast and osteoblast activities.

- The bone marrow and periosteum are innervated by a combination of different types of afferent sensory neurons. In the spinal cord, an increased proportion of WDR neurons compared with NS neurons transmit nonnoxious stimuli as noxious stimuli, which is thought to contribute to the unique feature of hyperalgesia in bone cancer pain.

- The diagnostic sensitivity of plain radiographs for detecting bone metastases is substantially less than bone scintigraphy, although they are useful as a primary investigation and for pure lytic disease. MRI may be considered for examination of the spinal cord, rather than to screen painful bone metastases. PET scan may be useful for cancer staging for initial treatment planning but is of limited in utility in palliative care settings.

- When bone cancer pain is identified, analgesic relief is the first step in order to ensure that patients' function and quality of life are optimized. Timely surgical intervention may be necessary.

- As survival improves with new cancer treatment modalities, the prevalence of SREs in this group is likely to increase. Despite their favorable effects on cancer survival, radiotherapy, hormone treatment, and combination chemotherapy can adversely affect bone health and cause functional impairment.

REFERENCES

● 1 Coleman CN. Skeletal complications of malignancy. *Cancer* 1997;80(8 Suppl.):1588–1594.

2 Hess KR, Varadhachary GR, Wei W et al. Metastatic patterns in adenocarcinoma. *Cancer* 2006;106:1623–1633.

● 3 Rove KO, Crawfrod ED. Metastatic cancer in solid tumors and clinical outcome: Skeletal-related events. *Oncology* 2010;23:1–9. Available from: http://www.cancernetwork.com/bone-metastases/content/article/10165/1507447. (Accessed May 31, 2012).

4   Theriault RL, Lipton A, Hotobagyi GN et al. Pamidronate reduces skeletal morbidity in women with advanced breast cancer and lytic bone lesions: A randomized, placebo-controlled trial. *J Clin Oncol* 1999;17(3):846–854.

5   Jensen AØ, Jacobsen JB, NØrgaad M et al. Incidence of bone metastases and skeletal-related events in breast cancer patients: A population-based cohort study in Demark. *BMC Cancer* 2011;11:29. Available from: http://www.biomedcentral.com/1471-2407/11/29. (Accessed May 31, 2012).

6   Yong M, Jensen AØ, Jacobsen JB et al. Surbival in breast cancer patients with bone metastases and skeletal-related events: A population-based cohort study in Demark (1999–2007) *Breast Cancer Res Treat* 2011;129:495–503.

7   Sathiakumar N, Delzell E, Morrisey MA et al. Mortality following bone metastasis and skeletal-related events among men with prostate cancer: A population-based analysis of U.S. Medicare beneficiaries, 1999–2006. *Prostate Cancer Prostatic Dis* 2011;14:177–183.

8   Langer C, Hirsh V. Skeletal morbidity in lung cancer patients with bone metastases: Demonstrating the need for early diagnosis and treatment with bisphosphonates. *Lung Cancer* 2010;67:4–11.

9   Caraceni A, Portenoy RK. A working group of the IASP Task Force on Cancer Pain. An international survey of cancer pain characteristics and syndrome. *Pain* 1999;82(3):263–274.

10 Grond S, Zech D, Diefenbach C et al. Assessment of cancer pain: A prospective evaluation in 2266 cancer patients referred to a pain service. *Pain* 1996;64:107–114.

11 Haugen DF, Hjermstad MJ, Hagen N et al. Assessment and classification of cancer breakthrough pain: A systematic literature review. *Pain* 2010;149:476–482.

12 Greco MT, Corli O, Montanari M et al. Epidemiology and pattern of care of breakthrough cancer pain in a longitudinal sample of cancer patients. Results from the cancer pain outcome research study group. *Clin J Pain* 2011;27:9–18.

● 13 Clohisy DR, Mantyh PW. Bone cancer pain. *Cancer* 2003;97(3 Suppl.):866–873.

14 Kebra M, Wu JSY, Duan Q et al. Neuropathic pain features in patients with bone metastases referred for palliative radiotherapy. *J Clin Oncol* 2010;28:4892–4897.

✱ 15 Haanpaa M, Attal N, Backonja M et al. NeuPSIG guidelines on neuropathic pain assessment. *Pain* 2011;152:14–27.

16 Norgaard M, Jensen AO, Jacobsen JB, Cetin JK, Fryzek JP, Sorensen HT. Skeletal related events, bone metastasis and survival in Denmark (1999 to 2007). *J Urol* 2010;184(1):162–167.

17 Mouedden ME, Meert TF. Pharmacological evaluation of opioid and non-opioid analgesics in a murine bone cancer model of pain. *Pharmacol Biochem Behav* 2007;86:458–467.

◆ 18 Galasko CS. Diagnosis of skeletal metastases and assessment of response to treatment. *Clin Orthop* 1995;12:64–75.

◆ 19 Roodman GD. Mechanisms of bone metastasis. *N Engl J Med* 2004;350:1655–1664.

● 20 Kozlow W, Guise TA. Breast cancer metastasis to bone: Mechanisms of osteolysis and implications for therapy. *J Mammary Gland Biol Neoplasia* 2005;10:169–180.

21 Schwei MJ, Honore P, Rogers SD et al. Neurochemical and cellular recognition of the spinal cord in a murine model of bone cancer pain. *J Neurosci* 1999;19:10886–10897.

22 Honore P, Luger NM, Sabino MA et al. Osteoprotegerin blocks bone cancer-induced skeletal destruction, skeletal pain and pain-related neurochemical reorganization of the spinal cord. *Nat Med* 2000;6:521–528.

23 Lacey DL, Timms E, Tan HL et al. Osteoprotegerin ligand is a cytokine that regulates osteoclast differentiation and activation. *Cell* 1998;93(2):165–176.

24 Hofbauer LG, Khosla S, Dunstan CR et al. The roles of osteoprotegerin and osteoprotegerin ligand in the paracrine regulation of bone resorption. *J Bone Miner Res* 2000;15(1):2–12.

25 Thomas RJ, Guise TA, Yin JJ et al. Breast cancer cells interact with osteoblasts to support osteoclast formation. *Endocrinology* 1999;140(10):4451–4458.

26 Body JJ, Facon T, Coleman RE et al. A study of the biological receptor activator of nuclear factor-kappaB ligand inhibitor, denosumab, in patients with multiple myeloma or bone metastases from breast cancer. *Clin Cancer Res* 2006;12:1221–1228.

27 Drake MT, Clarke BL, Khosla S. Bisphosphonates: Mechanism of action and role in clinical practice. *Mayo Clin Proc* 2008;83:1032–1045.

28 Sabimo MA, Ghilardi JR, Jongen JL et al. Simultaneous reduction in cancer pain, bone destruction, and tumor growth by selective inhibition of cyclooxygenase-2. *Cancer Res* 2002;62:7343–7349.

29 Sevcik MA, Ghilardi JR, Peters CM et al. Anti-NGF therapy profoundly reduces bone cancer pain and the accompanying increase in markers of peripheral and central sensitization. *Pain* 2005;115:128–141.

30 Jumenez-Andrade JM, Ghilardi JR, Castaneda-Corral G et al. Preventive or late administration of antiNGF therapy attenuates tumour-induced nerve sprouting, neuroma formation, and cancer pain. *Pain* 2011;152:2564–2574.

31 Lozano-Ondoua AN, Wright C, Vardanyan A et al. A cannabinoid 2 receptor agonist attenuates bone cancer-induced pain and bone loss. *Life Sci* 2010;86:646–653.

32 Ofek O, Karsak M, Leclerc N et al. Peripheral cannabinoid receptor, CB2, regulates bone mass. *Proc Natl Acad Sci U S A* 2006;103:696–701.

33 Mach DB, Rogers SD, Sabino MC et al. Origins of skeletal pain: Sensory and sympathetic innervation of the mouse femur. *Nueroscience* 2002;113:155–166.

34 Martin CD, Jiminez-Andrade JM, Ghilardi JR, Mantyh PW. Organization of unique net-like meshwork of CGRP + sensory fibres in the mouse periosteum: Implications for the generation and maintenance of bone fracture pain. *Neurosci Lett* 2007;437:148–152.

35 Urch CE, Donovan-Rodriguez T, Dickenson AH. Alterations in dorsal horn neurons in a rat model of cancer-induced bone pain. *Pain* 2003;106:347–356.

36 Peters CM, Ghilardi JR, Keyser CP et al. Tumor-induced injury of primary afferent sensory nerve fibers in bone cancer pain. *Exp Neurol* 2005;193(1):85–100.

37 Honore P, Rogers SD, Schwei MJ et al. Murine models of inflammatory, neuropathic, and cancer pain each generates a unique set of neurochemical changes in the spinal cord and sensory neurons. *Neuroscience* 2000;98(3):585–598.

38 Lugar NM, Sabino MC, Schwei MJ et al. Efficacy of systemic morphine suggests a fundamental difference in the mechanisms that generate bone cancer vs. inflammatory pain. *Pain* 2002;99(3):397–406.

39 Donovan-Rodriguez T, Dickerson AH, Irch CE. Gabapentin normalizes spinal neuronal responses that correlate with behaviour in a rat model of cancer-induced bone pain. *Anesthesiology* 2005;102:132–140.

40 Vinholes J, Coleman R, Eastell R. Effects of bone metastases on bone metabolism: Implications for diagnosis, imaging and assessment of response to cancer treatment. *Cancer Treat Res* 1996;22(4):289–331.

◆ 41 Hamaoka T, Madewell JE, Podoloff DA, Hortobagyi GN, Ueno NT. Bone imaging in metastatic breast cancer. *J Clin Oncol* 2004;22(14):2942–2953.

42 Wu LM, Gu HY, Zheng J et al. Diagnostic value of whole-body magnetic resonance imaging for bone metastases: A systematic review and meta-analysis. *J Magn Reson Imaging* 2011;34:128–135.

43 Chang MC, CHen JH, Liang JA et al. Meta-analysis: Comparison of F-18 fluorodeoxyglucose-positron emission tomography and bone scintigraphy in the detection of bone metastasis in patients with lung cancer. *Acad Radiol* 2012;19:349–357.

44 Chia SK, Speers CH, D'yachkova Y et al. The impact of new chemotherapeutic and hormone agents on survival in a population-based cohort of women with metastatic breast cancer. *Cancer* 2007;110:973–979.

45 Ryan CJ, Elkin EP, Cowan J, Carroll PR. Initial treatment patterns and outcome of contemporary prostate cancer patients with bone metastases at initial presentation. *Cancer* 2007;110:81–86.

✳ 46 Hillner BE, Ingle JN, Chlebowski RT et al. American Society of Clinical Oncology 2003 update on the role of bisphosphonates and bone health issues in women with breast cancer. *J Clin Oncol* 2003;21(21):4042–4057.

47 Paterson AH, Powles TJ, Kanis JA et al. Double-blind controlled trial of oral clodronate in patients with bone metastases from breast cancer. *J Clin Oncol* 1993;11:59–65.

48 Hortobagyi GN, Theriault RL, Lipton A et al. Long-term prevention of skeletal complications of metastatic breast cancer with pamidronate. Protocol 19 Aredia Breast Cancer Study Group. *J Clin Oncol* 1998;16:2038–2044.

49 Powles T, Paterson A, McCloskey E et al. Reduction in bone relapse and improved survival with oral clodronate for adjuvant treatment of operable breast cancer [ISRCTN83688026]. *Breast Cancer Res* 2006;8(2):R13.

50 Lipton A, Theriault RL, Hortobagyi GN et al. Pamidronate prevents skeletal complications and is effective palliative treatment in women with breast carcinoma and osteolytic bone metastases: Long term follow up of randomized, placebo = controlled trials. *Cancer* 2000;88(5):1082–1090.

51 Rosen LS, Gordon D, Tchekmedyian NS et al. Long-term efficacy and safety of zoledronic acid in the treatment of skeletal metastases in patients with nonsmall cell lung carcinoma and other solid tumors: A randomized, Phase III, double-blind, placebo-controlled trial. *Cancer* 2004;100(12):2613–2621.

52 Rosen LS, Gordon DH, Dugan W Jr et al. Zoledronic acid is superior to pamidronate for the treatment of bone metastases in breast carcinoma patients with at least on osteolytic lesion. *Cancer* 2004;100(1):36–43.

53 Kohno N, Aogi K, Minami H et al. Zoledronic acid significantly reduces skeletal complications compared with placebo in Japanese women with bone metastases from breast cancer: A randomized, placebo-controlled trial. *J Clin Oncol* 2005;23(15):3314–3321.

54 Saad F, Gleason DM, Murray R et al. A randomized, placebo-controlled trial of zoledronic acid in patients with hormone-refractory metastatic prostate carcinoma. *J Natl Cancer Inst* 2002;94(19):1458–1468.

55 Rosen LS, Gordon D, Kaminski M et al. Long-term efficacy and safety of zoledronic acid compared with pamidronate disodium in the treatment of skeletal complications in patients with advanced multiple myeloma or breast carcinoma: A randomized, double-blind, multicenter, comparative trial. *Cancer* 2003;98(8):1735–1744.

56 Stopeck AT, Lipton A, Body JJ et al. Denosumab compared with zoledronic acid for the treatment of bone metastases in patients with advanced breast cancer: A randomized, double-blinded study. *J Clin Oncol* 2010;28(35):5132–5239.

57 Fizazi K, Carducci M, Smith M et al. Denosumab versus zoledronic acid for the treatment of bone metastases in men with castration-resistant prostate cancer: A randomized, double-blind study. *Lancet* 2011;377(9768):813–822.

58 Henry DH, Costa L, Goldwasser F et al. Randomized, double-blind study of denosumab versus zoledronic acid in the treatment of bone metastases in patients with advanced cancer (excluding breast and prostate cancer) or multiple myeloma. *J Clin Oncol* 2011;29(9):1125–1132.

◆ 59 Brown-Glaberman U, Stopeck AT. Role of denosumab in the management of skeletal complications in patients with bone metastases from solid tumors. *Biologics* 2012;6:89–99.

✳ 60 Van Poznak CH, Temin S, Yee GC et al. American Society of Clinical Oncology Executive Summary of the clinical practice guideline update on the role of bone-modifying agents in metastatic breast cancer. *J Clin Oncol* 2011;29:1221–1227.

61 Xie J, Namjoshi M, Wu EQ et al. Economic evaluation of denosumab compared with zoledronic acid in hormone-refractory prostate cancer patients with bone metastases. *J Manag Care Pharm* 2011;17:621–634.

● 62 Luger NM, Mach DB, Sevcik MA, Mantyh PM. Bone cancer pain: From model to mechanism to therapy. *J Pain Symptom Manage* 2005;29:S32–S46.

63 Kind T, Vardanyan A, Majuta L et al. Morphine treatment accelerates sarcoma-induced bone pain, bone loss, and spontaneous fracture in a murine model of bone cancer. *Pain* 2007;132:154–168.

64 Daniell HW. Opioid endocrinopathy in women consuming prescribed sustained-action opioids for control of nonmalignant pain. *J Pain* 2008;9:28–36.

● 65 Katz N, Mazer NA. The impact of opioids on the endocrine system. *Clin J Pain* 2009;25:170–175.

66 Grey A, Karla RT, Horne A et al. Decreased bone density on men on methadone maintenance therapy. *Addiction* 2010;106:349–354.

67 McNicol ED, Strassels S, Goudas L, Lau J, Carr DB. NSAIDS or paracetamol, alone or combined with opioids, for cancer pain. *Cochrane Database of Systematic Reviews* 2005, Issue 2. Art. No.: CD005180. DOI: 10.1002/14651858.CD005180.

68 Rostom A, Dube C, Wells GA, Tugwell P, Welch V, Jolicoeur E, McGowan J, Lanas A. Prevention of NSAID-induced gastroduodenal ulcers. *Cochrane Database of Systematic Reviews* 2002, Issue 4. Art. No.: CD002296. DOI: 10.1002/14651858.CD002296.

69 Rostom A, Muir K, Dube C et al. Prevention of NSAID-related upper gastrointestinal toxicity: A meta-analysis of traditional NSAIDs with gastroprotection and COX-2 inhibitors. *Drug Healthc Patient Saf* 2009;1:47–71.

70 Hird A, Zhang L, Holt T et al. Dexamethasone for the prophylaxis of radiation-induced pain flare after palliative radiotherapy for symptomatic bone metastases: A Phase II study. *Clin Oncol* 2009;21(4):329–335.

71 O'Brien CA, Jia D, Plotkin LO et al. Glucocorticoids act directly on osteoblasts and osteocytes to induce their apoptosis and reduce bone formation and strength. *Endocrinology* 2004;145:1835–1841.

◆ 72 van Staa TP. The pathogenesis, epidemiology and management of glucocorticoid-induced osteoporosis. *Calcif Tissue Int* 2006;79:129–137.

73 Martinez-Zapata MJ, Roqué i Figuls M, Alonso-Coello P, Roman Y, Català E. Calcitonin for metastatic bone pain. *Cochrane Database of Systematic Reviews* 2006, Issue 3. Art. No.: CD003223. DOI: 10.1002/14651858.CD003223.pub2.

74 Zeppetella G. Opioids for the management of breakthrough cancer pain in adults: A systematic review undertaken as part of an EPCRC opioid guidelines project. *Palliat Med* 2011;25(5):516–524.

75 Hartsell WF, Scott CB, Bruener DW et al. Randomized trial of short-versus long-course radiotherapy for palliation of painful bone metastases. *J Natl Cancer Inst* 2005;97:789–804.

76 Chow E, Harris K, Fan G et al. Palliative radiotherapy trials for bone metastases: A systemic review. *J Clin Oncol* 2007;25:1423–1436.

● 77 Dy SM, Asch SM, Naiem A, Sanati H, Walling A, Lorenz KA. Evidence-based standards for cancer pain management. *J Clin Oncol* 2008;26(23):3879–3885.

78 Huisman M, van den Bosch MA, Wijlemans JW, van Vulpen M, van der Linden YM, Verkooijen HM. Effectiveness of reirradiation for painful bone metastases: A systematic review and meta-analysis. *International Journal of Radiation Oncology, Biology, Physics* 2012; 84(1):8–14.

79 Roqué i Figuls M, Martinez-Zapata MJ, Scott-Brown M, Alonso-Coello P. Radioisotopes for metastatic bone pain. *Cochrane Database of Systematic Reviews* 2011, Issue 7. Art. No.: CD003347. DOI: 10.1002/14651858.CD003347.pub2.

80 Bauman G, Charette M, Reid R, Sathya J. Radiopharmaceuticals for the palliation of painful bone metastases—A systematic review. *Radiother Oncol* 2005;75(3):258–270.

81 Bickels J, Kollender Y, Wittig JC et al. Function after resection of humeral metastases: Analysis of 59 consecutive patients. *Clin Orthop Relat Res* 2005;437:201–208.

82 Kollender Y, Bickels J, Price WM et al. Metastatic renal cell carcinoma of bone: Indications and technique of surgical intervention. *J Urol* 2000;164:1505–1508.

83 Bauer HC. Posterior decompression with stabilization for spinal metastases. Analysis of sixty-seven consecutive patients. *J Bone Jt Surg Am* 1997;79:514–522.

84 Tomita K, Kawahara N, Kobayashi T et al. Surgical strategy for spinal metastases. *Spine* 2001;26:298–306.

85 Weigel B, Maghsudi M, Neuman C et al. Surgical management of symptomatic spinal metastases. Postoperative outcome and quality of life. *Spine* 1999;24:2240–2246.

86 Ward WG, Holsenbeck S, Dorey FJ et al. Metastatic disease of the femur: Surgical treatment. *Clin Orthop Relat Res* 2003; Issue: Volume 415 Supplement, October 2003, pp S230–S244.

◆ 87 Mirels H. Metastatic disease in long bones. A proposed scoring system for diagnosing impending pathologic fractures. *Clin Orthop Relat Res* 2003; Issue: Volume 415 Supplement, October 2003, pp S4–S13.

88 Van der Linden YM, Dijkstra PD, Kroon HM et al. Comparative analysis of risk factors for pathological fracture with femoral metastases. *J Bone Jt Surg Br* 2004;86(4):566–573.

◆ 89 Bickels J, Dadia S, Lidar Z. Current concept review: Surgical management of metastatic bone disease. *J Bone Jt Surg Am* 2009;91:1503–1516.

90 Clohisy DR, Le CT, Cheng EY, Dykes DC, Thompson RC Jr. Evaluation of the feasibility of and results of measuring health-status changes in patients undergoing surgical treatment for skeletal metastases. *J Orthop Res* 2000;18(1):1–9.

91 Nathan SS, Healey JH, Mellano D et al. Survival in patients operated on for pathologic fracture: Implications for end-of-life orthopedic care. *J Clin Oncol* 2005;23(25):6072–6082.

● 92 Frassica DA. General principles of external beam radiation therapy for skeletal metastases. *Clin Orthop Relat Res* 2003;415(Suppl.):S158–S164.

93 Khan NF, Mant C, Carpenter L et al. Long-term health outcomes in a British cohort of breast, colorectal and prostate cancer survivors: A database study. *Br J Cancer* 2011;105:S29–S37.

94 Eastell R, Adams JE, Coleman RE et al. Effect of anastrozole on bone mineral density: 5-Year results from the anastrozole, tamoxifen, alone or in combination trial 18233230. *J Clin Oncol* 2008;26:1051–1057.

95 Perez EA, Josse RG, Pritchard KI et al. Effect of letrozole versus placebo on bone mineral density in women with primary breast cancer completing 5 or more years of adjuvant tamoxifen: A companion study to NCIC CTG MA.17. *J Clin Oncol* 2006;24:3629–3635.

96 Coleman RE, Banks LM, Girgis SI et al. Skeletal effects of exemestane on bone-mineral density, bone biomarkers, and fracture incidence in postmenopausal women with early breast cancer participating in the Intergroup Exemestane Study (IES): A randomized controlled study. *Lancet Oncol* 2007;8:119–127.

97 Rabaglio M, Sun Z, Price KN et al. Bone fractures among postmenopausal patients with endocrine-responsive early breast cancer treated with 5 years of letrozole or tamoxifen in the BIG 1-98 trial. *Ann Oncol* 2009;20:1489–1498.

98 Baum M, Budzar AU, Cuzick J et al. Anastrozole alone or in combination with tamoxifen versus tamoxifen alone for adjuvant treatment of postmenopausal women with early breast cancer: First results of the ATAC randomized trial. *Lancet* 2002;359:2131–2139.

99 ATAC Trialists' Group. Results of the ATAC (Arimidex, Tamoxifen, Alone or in Combination) trial after completion of 5 years' adjuvant treatment for breast cancer. *Lancet* 2005;365:60–62.

100 Servitja S, Nogues X, Prieto-Alhambra D et al. Bone health in a prospective cohort of postmenopausal women receiving aromatase inhibitors for early breast cancer. *The Breast* 2012;21:95–101.

101 Bouvard B, Hoppe E, Soulie P et al. High prevalence of vertebral fractures in women with breast cancer starting aromatase inhibitor therapy. *Ann Oncol* 2011;23:1151–1156.

102 Oh D, Huh SJ, Yoon TC et al. Pelvic insufficiency fracture after pelvic radiotherapy for cervical cancer: Analysis of risk factors. *Int J Radiat Oncol Biol Phys* 2008;70:1183–1188.

103 Baxter NN, Habermann EB, Tepper JE et al. Risk of pelvic fractures in older women following pelvic irradiation. *JAMA* 2005;294:2587–2593.

104 Tokumaru S, Toita T, Oguchi M et al. Insufficiency fractures after pelvic radiation therapy for uterine cervical caner: An analysis of subjects in a prospective multi-institutional trial, and cooperative study of the Japan radiation oncology group and Japanese radiation oncology study group. *International Journal of Radiation Oncology Biology Physics* 2012;84(2):e195–e200. (accepted for publication March 17, 2012).

✶105 Reid DM, Doughty J, Eastell R et al. Guidance for the management of breast cancer treatment-induced bone loss: A consensus position statement from a UK expert group. *Cancer Treat Rev* 2008;34:S3–S18. Available from: http://ncrndev.org.uk/downloads/csg/Bone%20 Health%20Guidelines%20-%20FINAL.pdf. (Accessed May 31, 2012).

◆106 Ross RW, Small EJ. Osteoporosis in men treated with androgen deprivation therapy for prostate cancer. *J Urol* 2002;167:1952–1956.

●107 Licata A. Bone density vs bone quality: What's a clinician to do? *Cleve Clin J Med* 2009;79:129–137.

✶108 Institute of Medicine (U.S.) Committee to Review Dietary Reference Intakes for Vitamin D and Calcium (Summary pp1-14); Ross AC, Taylor CL, Yaktine AL, et al., editors. Dietary Reference Intakes for Calcium and Vitamin D. Washington (DC): National Academies Press (U.S.); 2011. Available from: http://www.ncbi.nlm.nih.gov/books/ NBK56070/. (Accessed June 9, 2014).

53

Breakthrough (episodic) pain in cancer patients

SHIRLEY H. BUSH

INTRODUCTION

The intensity of cancer pain commonly fluctuates over time and challenges usual cancer pain management using the World Health Organization (WHO) analgesic "ladder." It is an important clinical problem, often significantly impacting on a patient's quality of life, and can be difficult to assess and predict. A bewildering array of terminology and definitions has been used to describe this heterogeneous phenomenon, but the lack of a standardized worldwide definition has led to difficulty in comparisons of reported prevalence and management.

Background to terminology and definitions

In 1989, the Edmonton staging system for cancer pain defined "incidental pain" as "pain aggravated suddenly as a result of movements, swallowing, defecation or urination."[1] The term was later changed to "incident pain" in the subsequent Edmonton Classification System for Cancer Pain (ECS-CP).[2] In a seminal paper in 1990, Portenoy and Hagen developed a working definition for "breakthrough pain" (BTP) for a prospective survey of cancer pain patients.[3] BTP was defined as "a transitory increase in pain to greater than moderate intensity, which occurred on a baseline pain of moderate intensity or less." Opioid use was not included in the working definition, but evaluated patients had been on relatively stable doses of opioids for two consecutive days. Portenoy and Hagen's definition of BTP required controlled baseline pain.[4] A task group of the Association for Palliative Medicine of Great Britain and Ireland defined BTP as "a transient exacerbation of pain that occurs either spontaneously, or in relation to a specific predictable or unpredictable trigger, despite relatively stable and adequately controlled background pain."[5] Hagen et al. commented in their definition of BTP that "it is difficult to characterize BTP when baseline pain is not controlled"[6]; however, some authors consider BTP, irrespective of whether baseline pain is controlled.[7***] BTP has also been defined as pain that "breaks through" the regular doses of an analgesic schedule.[8]

This includes "end-of-dose failure," where pain worsens before the next scheduled dose of opioid. Conversely, not all authors think "end-of-dose failure" should be included as a subtype of BTP as it signifies that the baseline pain is not controlled.[5,7***]

The term "incident pain" is frequently used to describe pain induced by movement.[9] The definition is often broadened to describe a precipitated, stimulus-dependent, or triggered pain.[7***] McQuay and Jadad classified "incident pain" into two subtypes. The first was pain on movement that included walking, turning, lifting, coughing, and deep breathing. The other subtype was intermittent pain not related to activity or movement.[10] "Incident pain" has also been used to represent pain with a volitional precipitant, that is, induced by the patient's voluntary actions, which should be predictable.[3]

Other terms that have been used include "pain in motion"[11*] and "transitory pain."[12] In an international survey of 58 clinicians from 24 countries, where BTP was defined as an episode of "pain flare," there was a large variation in the rates of BTP identification, suggesting that the concept of BTP varies geographically.[13]

"Episodic pain" was the term agreed on by an expert working group of the European Association for Palliative Care (EAPC) in December 2000, as it translated better into different languages.[14] "Episodic pain" was defined as a transitory exacerbation of pain that changes with time, which could occur with controlled or uncontrolled baseline pain (Figure 53.1), with the term incident pain reserved for movement-related "episodic pain," usually due to bone metastases. The EAPC working group also recognized pains that are volitional and not induced by a specific movement, for example, swallowing in the presence of mucositis or touch if hyperesthesia, and non-volitional pains, for example, sneezing, coughing, laughing, or myoclonus.[14]

From these assorted terms and definitions, BTP is the commonest term that has been used in the published literature.[7***] BTP can be more usefully classified into three subtypes: incident pain, spontaneous, and "end-of-dose failure." In a recent systematic literature review, incident pain was further characterized into volitional and nonvolitional

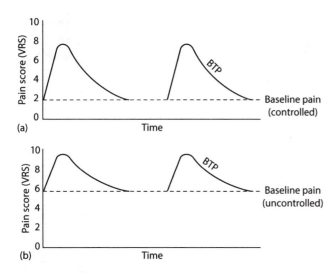

Figure 53.1 *Breakthrough pain (BTP) crescendos with (a) controlled baseline pain and (b) uncontrolled baseline pain. VRS, verbal rating scale.*

categories.[7***] Volitional (movement related) pain is usually predictable. In contrast, nonvolitional pain (nonmovement related) is usually unpredictable in nature. Spontaneous pains are independent of movement or volition, for example, neuropathic pain.[14]

ETIOLOGY OF BREAKTHROUGH PAIN

As with cancer pain etiology, BTP may be caused by the cancer or by the cancer treatment. BTP may also be due to a concurrent disorder.

BREAKTHROUGH PAIN MECHANISMS

BTP, like cancer pain, is categorized according to different anatomical and pathophysiological pain mechanisms.[15] The mechanistic categories are: nociceptive, comprising superficial somatic, deep somatic and visceral pains, and neuropathic pains. The BTP may have a different pathophysiology to the baseline pain.

PREVALENCE AND CHARACTERISTICS OF BREAKTHROUGH PAIN

The prevalence of BTP differs enormously depending on the definition and survey instrument used and the population sampled. Reported prevalence has been as low as 19%[16*] to around 90%.[17–19] Many studies report prevalence in the range of 40%–70%.[3,4,12,20,21*,22] Internationally, prevalence has been found to vary according to region with a reported prevalence of 80.1% from English-speaking countries, 69.4% from North and Western Europe, 54.8% from South America, and only 45.9% from Asia.[23]

Box 53.1 Features of typical cancer breakthrough pain

- Prevalence—40%–70%
- Frequency—3–4 times/day
- Onset—Often unpredictable
- Intensity—Moderate to severe
- Mean time to peak—3 min
- Mean duration—15–30 min

BTP is heterogeneous and commonly occurs—3–4 times/day,[3,19,24,25] although the range can markedly vary, as in the reported case of a patient with a rib fracture and cough experiencing BTP every minute.[3] Box 53.1 gives the mean time for pain to peak and the mean duration, although the upper limit of the range can be as long as 2 or even 4 hours. Most cases of BTP are exacerbations of the baseline pain, but they can be a worsening of a different pain. A minority of patients experience more than one type of BTP. The intensity of BTP is usually moderate to severe.[25]

The onset of BTP is often unpredictable, despite 20%–40% being movement related and 13%–30% classified as "end-of-dose failure."[4,18,21*] Neuropathic BTP is significantly briefer and more frequent than nociceptive BTP.[12,18]

IMPACT OF BREAKTHROUGH PAIN

Patients with BTP tend to have higher pain scores and more intense baseline pain than patients without BTP. Movement-related BTP, which is commonly due to metastatic bone disease, is relatively resistant to treatment with analgesics.[21*,26*] Only 6% of patients with pain secondary to bone metastases, who were attending a multidisciplinary pain clinic in Denmark, became pain-free "in motion" after pain treatment.[11*] In a recent international multicentre validation study of the ECS-CP, patients with incident pain required more adjuvants and higher final opioid doses.[27] Incident pain was also independently associated with a longer time to achieve stable pain control.

The presence of BTP significantly impacts on walking and causes functional interference on the Brief Pain Inventory, manifesting as increased levels of depression and anxiety.[4,21*,23] BTP often interferes with sleep and impairs quality of life by restricting social and general activities.[17] Uncontrolled BTP reminds patients of their cancer and imparts a sense of loss of control.[28] It may necessitate a change in lifestyle or even the discontinuation of work life with accompanying significant psychological distress. Cancer patients with BTP are more likely to have endured increased medical costs, due to pain-related hospitalization and physician visits.[29]

MANAGEMENT OF BREAKTHROUGH PAIN

BTP is under-recognized, and its treatment remains suboptimal.[20,22,30,31] There is a pressing need for further health care provider and patient education.[30,32] For the appropriate management of BTP, a multimodal patient-centered approach is needed while maintaining a holistic framework. The multidisciplinary and interprofessional management plan should take account of the stage of disease, illness trajectory, performance status, and the patient's goals of care. Patients' and families' fears and expectations should be explored and ongoing explanation and support provided.

Assessment of breakthrough pain

Assessment of the patient and the BTP(s) experienced should comprise a detailed history including the characteristics and mechanisms of the BTP and also the baseline pain, a thorough clinical examination, and a psychosocial evaluation. BTP assessment should include an evaluation of its interference with activities of daily living and quality of life.[7***]

The Breakthrough Pain Questionnaire was designed to characterize BTP.[3] However, the assessment algorithm used in the 1999 survey has only been partially validated.[4,7***] The Alberta Breakthrough Pain Assessment Tool (ABPAT-R) is a detailed tool for use in cancer patients.[6] It was designed to use in research as opposed to day-to-day clinical use and needs further validation. Patients often find the use of pain scales difficult and find it easier to describe their BTP in terms of severity, emotions, or impact, rather than the traditional pain descriptors (e.g., burning, stinging) used by health care professionals.[28]

Primary therapies to treat the underlying cause

Oncological interventions may be appropriate, depending on the patient's condition and anticipated prognosis. Radiotherapy is effective at reducing pain from painful bone metastases (see Chapter 88). Single and multiple fractionation schedules have been used with similar efficacy.[33***] For extensive bone metastatic disease causing pain, hemibody irradiation has been used. There is some evidence that radioisotopes, for example, strontium-89 and samarium, relieve pain over 1–6 months, but with a risk of leucocytopenia and thrombocytopenia.[34***] Bisphosphonates have been shown to be effective in reducing pain due to bone metastases[35***,36] (see Chapter 52).

There may be a role for chemotherapy or hormone therapy in responsive disease. Surgery may also be used palliatively after an assessment of benefits and attendant risks, for example, stabilization of a pathological fracture, or prophylactically for a femur at risk of fracture. Percutaneous vertebroplasty has been shown to reduce pain and improve mobility in patients with fractured spinal metastases, who have failed radiation.[37*] Some cases of bowel obstruction may be remediable with surgery, thus eliminating BTP due to colic.

Optimizing the analgesic regimen

Implementation of the principles of the WHO "ladder" should optimize the treatment of baseline pain. Opioid titration is usually required, and at times, a change in route of opioid administration is needed. BTP then regularly improves as often baseline pain has been poorly controlled. However, it is important not to oversedate the patient by increasing baseline opioid analgesia levels excessively in pursuit of around-the-clock (ATC) control of BTP crescendos, as the pain signal will often diminish with rest or time (Figure 53.2a). If opioid side effects are excessive, then opioid substitution or "switching" should be considered (see Chapters 44). Another strategy to decrease sedation from opioids is the addition of methylphenidate.[16*] Increasing the opioid dose or reducing the interval between opioid doses can manage "end-of-dose failure." For example, a few patients require 12-hourly modified release morphine to be given every 8 hours or transdermal fentanyl patches changed every 48 hours, rather than the usual 72 hours.

Depending on the pain mechanism, the use of nonopioid analgesic regimens will also improve baseline analgesia. Anti-inflammatory agents, such as nonsteroidal anti-inflammatory drugs (NSAIDs) and short-term use of steroids like dexamethasone, are indicated for pain due to bone metastases and mucosal or skin lesions. They also provide relief for pain originating from organ capsules, such as liver capsule inflammation, and from mesothelial membranes (pleura and peritoneum). Steroids also have an analgesic effect on neuropathic pain by reducing edema around peripheral nerves. The regular use of adjuvants for neuropathic pain, including tricyclic antidepressants, anticonvulsants, and antiarrhythmics, should diminish BTP from this mechanism. Patients with either multiple bone metastases and severe movement-related BTP, mucositis, or neuropathic pain have responded to ketamine, an N-methyl-D-aspartate (NMDA) receptor antagonist, given as a "burst" subcutaneous infusion for 3–5 days.[38*]

Other drugs used for BTP include antispasmodics, for example, hyoscine butylbromide for bowel spasm, oxybutynin for bladder spasm, and diazepam or baclofen for muscle spasm.

Using "rescue" analgesia for breakthrough pain

A "rescue" dose of analgesia should be administered when needed to "top up" baseline analgesia, either 20–30 min before a predictable BTP or at the onset of a BTP episode.[39] However, most patients do not take their "rescue" medication for each episode.[40] Frequently, a patient would have concluded that their prescribed "rescue" opioid medication is pointless, as their BTP episode would have resolved long before the onset of the extra pain relief. Usually an immediate release (IR) formulation of opioid is used as "rescue" medication, but sometimes, an NSAID is prescribed. If a patient is experiencing more than four BTP episodes per day, then an increase in the total daily opioid dose for baseline pain should be considered.

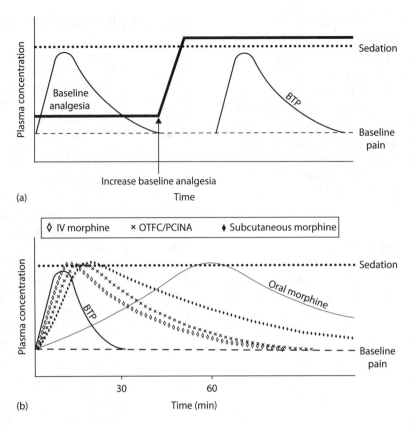

Figure 53.2   *Drug management of cancer breakthrough pain (BTP). (a) Increasing the baseline analgesia to meet the peaks of BTP, leading to overwsedation. (b) Rescue doses of analgesia—schematic representation.*

Properties of an ideal "rescue" analgesic include the following:

- Quick absorption with rapid onset of analgesia and early peak effect
- A short duration of action, but long enough to treat the BTP episode
- Minimal side effects
- A good safety profile

The drug should target the implicated pain mechanism. The ideal "rescue" analgesic would be responsive to the peaks and troughs of BTP episodes with a rapid on/off effect to counter a fluctuating pain trajectory over a short period of time, analogous to the current "gold standard" of intravenous (IV) patient-controlled analgesia (PCA). It should also be easy to self-administer, available for both inpatients and those in the community and should not be expensive. The choice of drug for the "rescue" dose and the route used will also be influenced by the accessibility of opioids and their formulations in different countries.

Routes of administration of opioid "rescue" analgesia for breakthrough pain

See Table 53.1 and Figure 53.2b.

ORAL ROUTE

For patients on an oral regularly scheduled morphine regimen for baseline pain, it has been recommended that the "rescue"

Table 53.1   *Comparing the efficacy of different routes of administration of opioids*

Route	Average time for onset of analgesia (min)	Average duration of analgesic effect (h)
IV, e.g., morphine	5	1–2
Oral transmucosal/intranasal, e.g., fentanyl series	5–15	1–2
Subcutaneous, e.g., morphine	10–15	3–4
Oral, as IR (normal) , e.g., morphine	30	4

dose be equivalent to the 4-hourly dose of morphine, that is, 16% of the 24 hours dose.[41] Other clinicians suggest 5%–10%. More recent studies suggest that an individual's "rescue" dose should be found by titration.[42*] The average time to meaningful pain relief is around 30 min with the usual IR (normal) formulation of morphine[24] contrasting with under 15 min for an effervescent IR morphine preparation.[43*] IR morphine has a mean T_{max} (time at which maximum concentration is reached) of 1 hour.[44***] Analgesia then lasts about 4 hours, indicating that the time taken for onset of analgesia and its duration are usually too prolonged for the majority of BTP episodes.

SUBCUTANEOUS ROUTE

Following a subcutaneous injection of opioid, analgesia begins within 10–15 min and lasts for 3–4 hours.[45] Mean time to pain relief with subcutaneous morphine for BTP is 17 min.[20] The majority of patients who self-administered subcutaneous rescue opioids using a "pain pen" rated its efficacy as good.[46*]

INTRAVENOUS ROUTE

Pain relief should begin within 5 min of IV administration and last for 1–2 hours.[45] On using a fixed ratio of IV morphine to oral morphine daily dose, given by bolus injection, BTP intensity was reported to be reduced by more than 50% within a mean of 16.6 min.[47*] IV administration of "rescue" doses of opioids has been found to be superior to the transmucosal route at 15 min, with both routes being equally effective at 30 min.[48***] Patients with uncontrolled bone pain have been successfully and safely managed at home by skilled and accessible staff, using a PCA pump and either the IV or subcutaneous route.[49*]

ORAL AND NASAL TRANSMUCOSAL ROUTES

These routes have the advantage of bypassing the first-pass effect of the liver. The nasal and oral mucosae are highly vascular areas, enabling rapid absorption and superior bioavailability for those drugs with suitable physicochemical properties.[50–52] Drugs meeting these requirements are lipophilic, with a high permeability coefficient, and potent. The properties of the fentanyl series of drugs make them highly suitable for transmucosal administration. The onset of action for buccal and intranasal fentanyl can occur within 10 min of administration.[48***] Fentanyl is metabolized by cytochrome P450 (CYP) 3A4. Its use should be avoided in patients who have received a mono-amine oxidase inhibitor (MAOI) within the previous 2 weeks due to an increased risk of serotonin toxicity.[53] Sufficient saliva is needed for the administration of sublingual and buccal preparations. Common adverse effects of transmucosal fentanyl are somnolence, nausea, and dizziness. Methadone also has a favorable pharmacodynamic profile. Sublingual methadone has a rapid onset of analgesic effect, occurring with a median onset of 5 min.[54*] (Methadone should only be initiated by expert physicians who are experienced in its use). Buprenorphine can be given sublingually, but sublingual absorption of morphine is poor due to low lipid solubility and over 90% ionization.[55]

Off-label sublingual administration of injectable formulations of fentanyl citrate,[56] sufentanil,[57] and alfentanil[58] has been reported. Volumes of fluid greater than 1–2 mL have been found to be problematic, due to reflex swallowing. Similarly, off-label administration of the fentanyl series by intranasal spray has been reported.[58,59*,60*] The T_{max} for their intranasal single dose administration in healthy volunteers is 5–10 min, with bioavailabilities of 65%–78%.[50] The maximum volume for one nostril in a single administration is 150–200 µL. The use of a patient-controlled intranasal analgesia (PCINA) device mimics the efficacy of IV PCA. Morphine has been administered intranasally using chitosan to enhance penetration.[61*] Adverse effects of nasal administration are mainly systemic opioid-related side effects, as opposed to nasal toxicity.

FAST-ACTING PROPRIETARY TRANSMUCOSAL FENTANYL PREPARATIONS

There has been a recent proliferation in studies of newly available products.[39,48***,62] See Table 53.2 for characteristics of these preparations. These have a role in those patients where traditional rescue analgesia has failed, causes excessive side effects, or is not sufficiently responsive to the intensity or temporal profile of their BTP. All the new formulations are comparatively expensive and availability will vary according to country. Publication bias needs to be considered in reviewing the current evidence as the majority of data on these products is from pharmaceutical industry–sponsored randomized controlled trials (RCTs).[39]

The first available proprietary transmucosal fentanyl preparation was oral transmucosal fentanyl citrate (OTFC). Double-blind RCTs showed significantly better pain relief compared to placebo or IR oral morphine.[42*,63**] The T_{max} of a 15 µg/kg dose is 22 min, with the duration of effect lasting 1–2 hours.

As studies found no fixed relationship between the total daily dose of scheduled opioid and dose of OTFC required for the BTP episode,[64*,65**] individual dose titration of all of the transmucosal fentanyl formulations is recommended,[5,48***,53] but this has been challenged.[66*,67*]

All of the transmucosal fentanyl products should only be used in adult patients on a regular strong opioid (morphine 60 mg/24 hour PO or equivalent) for chronic cancer pain for at least 1 week.[53] The optimal dose found from successful titration can be used to treat up to a maximum of four BTP episodes/24 hour. These products are not interchangeable, and retitration from the lowest available dose is essential if switching products. Safe storage and disposal is also needed.

Cases of local ulcer and dental caries have been reported with transmucosal preparations.[39] Intranasal opioids should not be used in patients with recurrent epistaxis, and concurrent use with vasoconstrictive nasal decongestants should be avoided.[53] Data from the long-term use of these products is limited.

There is a potential risk for misuse, abuse, addiction, and diversion of these medications, especially in high-risk patients. Prescriptions and aberrant behaviors need to be closely monitored.[68] In December 2011, the U.S. Food and Drug Administration (FDA) approved a single shared Risk Evaluation Mitigation Strategy (REMS) for transmucosal IR fentanyl (TIRF) dosage forms.[69]

Health care professionals may lack confidence in the appropriate prescribing and use of these newer pharmacological agents.[32] There remains a need for further education and training in this area and the development of user-friendly BTP management algorithms for day-to-day clinical practice. Patient education and counseling on the use of these products is also required.

OTHER ROUTES

The use of nebulized fentanyl has been reported in a small case series.[70] Intrapulmonary fentanyl administered with an inhaler is under development.[62]

Table 53.2   *Characteristics of currently available fast-acting transmucosal fentanyl proprietary preparations*[53,62,82,83]**

Formulation	Onset of action (min)	Duration of action (h)	Bioavailability	Notes
	(Earliest statistically significant onset from fentanyl products and placebo studies. Clinically meaningful onset usually takes longer)			
Oral transmucosal				
Oral transmucosal fentanyl citrate—OTFC (Actiq®, generic preparations are also now available)	15	1–2	Overall bioavailability: 50% (25% from rapid oromucosal absorption + 25% from slower gastrointestinal absorption, after swallowing remaining dose)	Consumed slowly over 15 min by rubbing compressed sweetened lozenge (which is attached to a plastic applicator) across the oral, particularly buccal, mucosa
Buccal				
Fentanyl buccal tablet—FBT (Fentora® [United States], Effentora® [United Kingdom])	10	≥2	65%	Enhanced buccal delivery of fentanyl: Drug delivery system utilizes effervescence to cause pH shifts
Fentanyl buccal soluble film—FBSF (Onsolis® [United States], Breakyl® [United Kingdom])	15	≥1	70%	Small bioerodible polymer film with the fentanyl-containing layer, which adheres to patient's cheek, separated from saliva by an outer layer
Sublingual				
Sublingual fentanyl tablet—SLF (Abstral®)	10	≥1	75% (estimated)	Tablet rapidly breaks down with a bioadhesive component enabling carrier particles to adhere to the sublingual mucosa
Fentanyl sublingual spray (Subsys®)	5–10	≥1	75%	Oral spray device containing a liquid formulation of nonionic fentanyl
Intranasal				
Intranasal fentanyl spray—INFS (Instanyl® [Not United States])	5	≥1	90%	Multidose device nasal spray
Fentanyl pectin nasal spray—FPNS (Lazanda® [United States] PecFent® [United Kingdom])	10	≥1	No data currently available	Aqueous nasal spray that forms a gel on contact with nasal mucosa

(For further details, see individual product monographs)

Other drugs used for breakthrough pain

Intermittent subcutaneous midazolam has been used for the temporary sedation of patients with pathological hip fractures and severe BTP.[71] Subanesthetic ketamine, in a subcutaneous bolus dose of 20–40 mg, is often used before predictable movement-related BTP, such as difficult dressing changes or repositioning of a patient with a fractured long bone. It may be combined with a bolus injection of midazolam.[72] The sublingual and intranasal routes of ketamine have also been utilized in the management of BTP, as has nitrous oxide.[73*,74**,75*]

Nonpharmacological approaches

Psychosocial interventions are a fundamental component of a multimodal approach to the management of cancer pain.[76***] Patients frequently use nonpharmacological strategies to relieve BTP including repositioning, rest and sleep, movement and exercise, heat or cold, rubbing and massage, relaxation, visualization, and distraction.[12,19,25] Transcutaneous electrical nerve stimulation (TENS) has been utilized.[77*] Referral to physiotherapy and occupational therapy is beneficial for patients with movement-related BTP. Orthotic devices, bracing, or aids may be necessary, in addition to lifestyle modification. Acupuncture may have a potential adjunctive role in the management of BTP, but more research is needed.[78]

Interventional approaches

For patients with resistant BTP, anesthetic or neurosurgical intervention may be required. Techniques used include: peripheral nerve or neurolytic blocks, spinal (intrathecal or epidural) analgesia, and percutaneous or open cordotomy.[79,80]

FUTURE DIRECTIONS

For cancer-related BTP, an internationally agreed upon definition and simple classification system are still needed for consistency in characterization. BTP has been identified as a key variable to be included in a future standardized classification system for cancer pain.[81] A validated screening tool is needed along with a well-validated and practical BTP assessment instrument for use in daily clinical practice to measure pain intensity over short periods of time. These are vital in order to standardize and further high-quality research and evidence-based clinical practice. Double-blind RCTs comparing different transmucosal products are needed. Future studies should investigate the appropriate dosing and titration techniques for "rescue" analgesia and examine the most appropriate management of different BTP mechanisms.

Key learning points

- BTP is common and challenges the WHO "ladder" for pain management.

- Current terminology and definitions are confusing.

- BTP is typically characterized by both rapid onset and brief duration.

- Thorough assessment of both breakthrough and baseline pains are vital.

- ATC analgesia for baseline pain must first be optimized.

- The parenteral and transmucosal routes are the most efficacious for "rescue" analgesia, for drugs with appropriate pharmacodynamic properties.

- BTP management should be individualized and requires both pharmacological and nonpharmacological therapeutic strategies, as well as a comprehensive multidisciplinary and interprofessional approach.

REFERENCES

1   Bruera E, MacMillan K, Hanson J, MacDonald RN. The Edmonton staging system for cancer pain: Preliminary report. *Pain*. 1989;**37**:203–209.

2   Nekolaichuk CL, Fainsinger RL, Lawlor PG. A validation study of a pain classification system for advanced cancer patients using content experts: The Edmonton Classification System for Cancer Pain. *Palliative Medicine*. 2005;**19**:466–476.

● 3   Portenoy RK, Hagen NA. Breakthrough pain: Definition, prevalence and characteristics. *Pain*. 1990;**41**:273–281.

● 4   Portenoy RK, Payne D, Jacobsen P. Breakthrough pain: Characteristics and impact in patients with cancer pain. *Pain*. 1999;**81**:129–134.

✱ 5   Davies AN, Dickman A, Reid C et al. The management of cancer-related breakthrough pain: Recommendations of a task group of the Science Committee of the Association for Palliative Medicine of Great Britain and Ireland. *European Journal of Pain*. 2009;**13**:331–338.

6   Hagen NA, Stiles C, Nekolaichuk C et al. The Alberta Breakthrough Pain Assessment Tool for cancer patients: A validation study using a Delphi process and patient think-aloud interviews. *Journal of Pain and Symptom Management*. 2008;**35**:136–152.

◆ 7   Haugen DF, Hjermstad MJ, Hagen N et al. Assessment and classification of cancer breakthrough pain: A systematic literature review. *Pain*. 2010;**149**:476–482.

◆ 8   Caraceni A, Weinstein SM. Classification of cancer pain syndromes. *Oncology*. 2001;**15**:1627–1640.

9   Portenoy RK. Treatment of temporal variations in chronic cancer pain. *Seminars in Oncology*. 1997;**24**:S16-7-12.

● 10 McQuay HJ, Jadad AR. Incident pain. *Cancer Surveys*. 1994;**21**:17–24.

11 Banning A, Sjogren P, Henriksen H. Treatment outcome in a multidisciplinary cancer pain clinic. *Pain*. 1991;**47**:129–134.

12 Petzke F, Radbruch L, Zech D et al. Temporal presentation of chronic cancer pain: Transitory pains on admission to a multidisciplinary pain clinic. *Journal of Pain and Symptom Management*. 1999;**17**:391–401.

13 Caraceni A, Portenoy RK. An international survey of cancer pain characteristics and syndromes. IASP Task Force on Cancer Pain. International Association for the Study of Pain. *Pain*. 1999;**82**:263–274.

● 14 Mercadante S, Radbruch L, Caraceni A et al. Episodic (breakthrough) pain: Consensus conference of an expert working group of the European Association for Palliative Care. *Cancer*. 2002;**94**:832–839.

● 15 Ashby MA, Fleming BG, Brooksbank M et al. Description of a mechanistic approach to pain management in advanced cancer. Preliminary report. *Pain*. 1992;**51**:153–161.

16 Bruera E, Fainsinger R, MacEachern T, Hanson J. The use of methylphenidate in patients with incident cancer pain receiving regular opiates. A preliminary report. *Pain*. 1992;**50**:75–77.

17 Fine PG, Busch MA. Characterization of breakthrough pain by hospice patients and their caregivers. *Journal of Pain and Symptom Management*. 1998;**16**:179–183.

18 Zeppetella G, O'Doherty CA, Collins S. Prevalence and characteristics of breakthrough pain in cancer patients admitted to a hospice. *Journal of Pain and Symptom Management*. 2000;**20**:87–92.

19 Swanwick M, Haworth M, Lennard RF. The prevalence of episodic pain in cancer: A survey of hospice patients on admission. *Palliative Medicine*. 2001;**15**:9–18.

20 Gómez-Batiste X, Madrid F, Moreno F et al. Breakthrough cancer pain: Prevalence and characteristics in patients in Catalonia, Spain. *Journal of Pain and Symptom Management*. 2002;**24**:45–52.

21 Hwang SS, Chang VT, Kasimis B. Cancer breakthrough pain characteristics and responses to treatment at a VA medical center. *Pain*. 2003;**101**:55–64.

22 Greco MT, Corli O, Montanari M et al. Epidemiology and pattern of care of breakthrough cancer pain in a longitudinal sample of cancer patients: Results from the Cancer Pain Outcome Research Study Group. *The Clinical Journal of Pain*. 2011;**27**:9–18.

23 Caraceni A, Martini C, Zecca E et al. Breakthrough pain characteristics and syndromes in patients with cancer pain. An international survey. *Palliative Medicine*. 2004;**18**:177–183.

24 Zeppetella G. Opioids for cancer breakthrough pain: A pilot study reporting patient assessment of time to meaningful pain relief. *Journal of Pain and Symptom Management*. 2008;**35**:563–567.

25   Davies A, Zeppetella G, Andersen S et al. Multi-centre European study of breakthrough cancer pain: Pain characteristics and patient perceptions of current and potential management strategies. *European Journal of Pain.* 2011;**15**:756–763.

26   Mercadante S, Maddaloni S, Roccella S, Salvaggio L. Predictive factors in advanced cancer pain treated only by analgesics. *Pain.* 1992;**50**:151–155.

27   Fainsinger RL, Nekolaichuk C, Lawlor P et al. An international multicentre validation study of a pain classification system for cancer patients. *European Journal of Cancer.* 2010;**46**:2896–2904.

28   Webber K, Davies AN, Cowie MR. Breakthrough pain: A qualitative study involving patients with advanced cancer. *Supportive Care in Cancer.* 2011;**19**:2041–2046.

29   Fortner BV, Okon TA, Portenoy RK. A survey of pain-related hospitalizations, emergency department visits, and physician office visits reported by cancer patients with and without history of breakthrough pain. *The Journal of Pain.* 2002;**3**:38–44.

30   Breivik H, Cherny N, Collett B et al. Cancer-related pain: A pan-European survey of prevalence, treatment, and patient attitudes. *Annals of Oncology.* 2009;**20**:1420–1433.

31   Rustøen T, Geerling JI, Pappa T et al. A European survey of oncology nurse breakthrough cancer pain practices. *European Journal of Oncology Nursing.* 2013;**17**:95–100.

32   Soden K, Ali S, Alloway L et al. How do nurses assess and manage breakthrough pain in specialist palliative care inpatient units? A multicentre study. *Palliative Medicine.* 2010;**24**:294–298.

33   Sze WM, Shelley M, Held I, Mason M. Palliation of metastatic bone pain: Single fraction versus multifraction radiotherapy. *Cochrane Database of Systematic Reviews* 2002;(1):CD004721. doi:10.1002/14651858.CD004721.

34   Roqué i Figuls M, Martinez-Zapata MJ, Scott-Brown M, Alonso-Coello P. Radioisotopes for metastatic bone pain. *Cochrane Database of Systematic Reviews* 2011;(7):CD003347. doi:10.1002/14651858. CD003347.pub2.

35   Wong RKS, Wiffen PJ. Bisphosphonates for the relief of pain secondary to bone metastases. *Cochrane Database of Systematic Reviews* 2002;(2):CD002068. doi:10.1002/14651858.CD002068.

36   Body JJ. Bisphosphonates for malignancy-related bone disease: Current status, future developments. *Supportive Care in Cancer.* 2006;**14**:408–418.

37   Cheung G, Chow E, Holden L et al. Percutaneous vertebroplasty in patients with intractable pain from osteoporotic or metastatic fractures: A prospective study using quality-of-life assessment. *Canadian Association of Radiologists Journal.* 2006;**57**:13–21.

38   Jackson K, Ashby M, Martin P et al. "Burst" ketamine for refractory cancer pain: An open-label audit of 39 patients. *Journal of Pain and Symptom Management.* 2001;**22**:834–842.

⋆ 39   Caraceni A, Hanks G, Kaasa S et al. Use of opioid analgesics in the treatment of cancer pain: Evidence-based recommendations from the EAPC. *The Lancet Oncology.* 2012;**13**:e58–e68.

40   Davies AN, Vriens J, Kennett A, McTaggart M. An observational study of oncology patients' utilization of breakthrough pain medication. *Journal of Pain and Symptom Management.* 2008;**35**:406–411.

⋆ 41   Hanks GW, Conno F, Cherny N et al. Morphine and alternative opioids in cancer pain: The EAPC recommendations. *British Journal of Cancer.* 2001;**84**:587–593.

42   Coluzzi PH, Schwartzberg L, Conroy JD et al. Breakthrough cancer pain: A randomized trial comparing oral transmucosal fentanyl citrate (OTFC) and morphine sulfate immediate release (MSIR). *Pain.* 2001;**91**:123–130.

43   Freye E, Levy JV, Braun D. Effervescent morphine results in faster relief of breakthrough pain in patients compared to immediate release morphine sulfate tablet. *Pain Practice.* 2007;**7**:324–331.

44   Collins SL, Faura CC, Moore RA, McQuay HJ. Peak plasma concentrations after oral morphine: A systematic review. *Journal of Pain and Symptom Management.* 1998;**16**:388–402.

◆ 45   Levy MH. Pharmacologic treatment of cancer pain. *New England Journal of Medicine.* 1996;**335**:1124–1132.

46   Enting RH, Mucchiano C, Oldenmenger WH et al. The "pain pen" for breakthrough cancer pain: A promising treatment. *Journal of Pain and Symptom Management.* 2005;**29**:213–217.

47   Mercadante S, Villari P, Ferrera P et al. Safety and effectiveness of intravenous morphine for episodic (breakthrough) pain using a fixed ratio with the oral daily morphine dose. *Journal of Pain and Symptom Management.* 2004;**27**:352–359.

◆ 48   Zeppetella G. Opioids for the management of breakthrough cancer pain in adults: A systematic review undertaken as part of an EPCRC opioid guidelines project. *Palliative Medicine.* 2011;**25**:516–524.

49   Swanson G, Smith J, Bulich R et al. Patient-controlled analgesia for chronic cancer pain in the ambulatory setting: A report of 117 patients. *Journal of Clinical Oncology.* 1989;**7**:1903–1908.

◆ 50   Dale O, Hjortkjaer R, Kharasch ED. Nasal administration of opioids for pain management in adults. *Acta Anaesthesiologica Scandinavica.* 2002;**46**:759–770.

◆ 51   Zhang H, Zhang J, Streisand JB. Oral mucosal drug delivery: Clinical pharmacokinetics and therapeutic applications. *Clinical Pharmacokinetics.* 2002;**41**:661–680.

52   Grassin-Delyle S, Buenestado A, Naline E et al. Intranasal drug delivery: An efficient and non-invasive route for systemic administration: Focus on opioids. *Pharmacology and Therapeutics.* 2012;**134**:366–379.

◆ 53   Twycross R, Prommer EE, Mihalyo M, Wilcock A. Fentanyl (transmucosal). *Journal of Pain and Symptom Management.* 2012;**44**:131–149.

54   Hagen NA, Fisher K, Stiles C. Sublingual methadone for the management of cancer-related breakthrough pain: A pilot study. *Journal of Palliative Medicine.* 2007;**10**:331–337.

55   Coluzzi PH. Sublingual morphine: Efficacy reviewed. *Journal of Pain and Symptom Management.* 1998;**16**:184–192.

56   Zeppetella G. Sublingual fentanyl citrate for cancer-related breakthrough pain: A pilot study. *Palliative Medicine.* 2001;**15**:323–328.

57   Gardner-Nix J. Oral transmucosal fentanyl and sufentanil for incident pain. *Journal of Pain and Symptom Management.* 2001;**22**:627–630.

58   Duncan A. The use of fentanyl and alfentanil sprays for episodic pain. *Palliative Medicine.* 2002;**16**:550.

59   Zeppetella G. An assessment of the safety, efficacy, and acceptability of intranasal fentanyl citrate in the management of cancer-related breakthrough pain: A pilot study. *Journal of Pain and Symptom Management.* 2000;**20**:253–258.

60   Good P, Jackson K, Brumley D, Ashby M. Intranasal sufentanil for cancer-associated breakthrough pain. *Palliative Medicine.* 2009;**23**:54–58.

61   Pavis H, Wilcock A, Edgecombe J et al. Pilot study of nasal morphine-chitosan for the relief of breakthrough pain in patients with cancer. *Journal of Pain and Symptom Management.* 2002;**24**:598–602.

◆ 62   Smith H. A comprehensive review of rapid-onset opioids for breakthrough pain. *CNS Drugs.* 2012;**26**:509–535.

63   Farrar JT, Cleary J, Rauck R, Busch M et al. Oral transmucosal fentanyl citrate: Randomized, double-blinded, placebo-controlled trial for treatment of breakthrough pain in cancer patients. *Journal of the National Cancer Institute.* 1998;**15**:611–616.

64 Portenoy RK, Payne R, Coluzzi P et al. Oral transmucosal fentanyl citrate (OTFC) for the treatment of breakthrough pain in cancer patients: A controlled dose titration study. *Pain.* 1999;**79**:303–312.

65 Hagen NA, Fisher K, Victorino C, Farrar JT. A titration strategy is needed to manage breakthrough cancer pain effectively: Observations from data pooled from three clinical trials. *Journal of Palliative Medicine.* 2007;**10**:47–55.

66 Mercadante S, Villari P, Ferrera P et al. Transmucosal fentanyl vs intravenous morphine in doses proportional to basal opioid regimen for episodic-breakthrough pain. *British Journal of Cancer.* 2007;**96**:1828–1833.

67 Mercadante S, Gatti A, Porzio G et al. Dosing fentanyl buccal tablet for breakthrough cancer pain: Dose titration versus proportional doses. *Current Medical Research and Opinion.* 2012;**28**:963–968.

68 Passik SD, Messina J, Golsorkhi A, Xie F. Aberrant drug-related behavior observed during clinical studies involving patients taking chronic opioid therapy for persistent pain and fentanyl buccal tablet for breakthrough pain. *Journal of Pain and Symptom Management.* 2011;**41**:116–125.

69 U.S. Food and Drug Administration. FDA approves shared system REMS for TIRF products. Available at: http://www.fda.gov/, (last accessed October 6, 2012).

70 Zeppetella G. Nebulized and intranasal fentanyl in the management of cancer-related breakthrough pain. *Palliative Medicine.* 2000;**14**:57–58.

71 del Rosario MA, Martín AS, Ortega JJ, Feria M. Temporary sedation with midazolam for control of severe incident pain. *Journal of Pain and Symptom Management.* 2001;**21**:439–442.

72 Kotlińska-Lemieszek A, Luczak J. Subanesthetic ketamine: An essential adjuvant for intractable cancer pain. *Journal of Pain and Symptom Management.* 2004;**28**:100–102.

73 Mercadante S, Arcuri E, Ferrera P et al. Alternative treatments of breakthrough pain in patients receiving spinal analgesics for cancer pain. *Journal of Pain and Symptom Management.* 2005;**30**:485–491.

74 Carr DB, Goudas LC, Denman WT et al. Safety and efficacy of intranasal ketamine for the treatment of breakthrough pain in patients with chronic pain: A randomized, double-blind, placebo-controlled, crossover study. *Pain.* 2004;**108**:17–27.

75 Parlow JL, Milne B, Tod DA et al. Self-administered nitrous oxide for the management of incident pain in terminally ill patients: A blinded case series. *Palliative Medicine.* 2005;**19**:3–8.

76 Sheinfeld Gorin S, Krebs P, Badr H et al. Meta-analysis of psychosocial interventions to reduce pain in patients with cancer. *Journal of Clinical Oncology.* 2012;**30**:539–547.

77 Bennett MI, Johnson MI, Brown SR et al. Feasibility study of Transcutaneous Electrical Nerve Stimulation (TENS) for cancer bone pain. *Journal of Pain.* 2010;**11**:351–359.

78 Paley CA, Johnson MI, Bennett MI. Acupuncture: A treatment for breakthrough pain in cancer? *BMJ Supportive & Palliative Care.* 2011;**1**:335–338.

79 Brogan SE, Winter NB. Patient-controlled intrathecal analgesia for the management of breakthrough cancer pain: A retrospective review and commentary. *Pain Medicine.* 2011;**12**:1758–1768.

80 Bhaskar AK. Interventional management of cancer pain. *Current Opinion in Supportive and Palliative Care.* 2012;**6**:1–9.

81 Knudsen AK, Brunelli C, Kaasa S et al. Which variables are associated with pain intensity and treatment response in advanced cancer patients? Implications for a future classification system for cancer pain. *European Journal of Pain.* 2011;**15**:320–327.

82 Zeppetella G. Breakthrough pain in cancer patients. *Clinical Oncology.* 2011;**23**:393–398.

83 Rauck R, Reynolds L, Geach J et al. Efficacy and safety of fentanyl sublingual spray for the treatment of breakthrough cancer pain: A randomized, double-blind, placebo-controlled study. *Current Medical Research and Opinion.* 2012;**28**:859–870.

54

Symptom burden, pain, and the problems with "somatization" diagnosis

CARRIE J. AIGNER, DIANE M. NOVY

INTRODUCTION

Symptoms such as unexplained pain, fatigue, nausea, headache, dizziness, and insomnia are common complaints among people seen in palliative care settings.[1***,2*] Although symptoms such as these are often described as "somatic" in nature, this characterization might not be appropriate, especially in palliative care settings. Most patients in medical settings, including pain centers, do not meet the criteria of somatization as defined by the DSM-IV. Among palliative care patients in particular, these symptoms may be part of the overall symptom burden, which includes aspects of the illness, side effects of medical treatment, or psychological suffering. Given the complex symptom profile and high symptom burden among patients in palliative care, caution must be used when assigning a somatic disorder diagnosis in this population.

SYMPTOM BURDEN

Patients receiving palliative care typically have a high symptom burden.[3**] Fatigue is one of the most commonly reported symptoms in palliative care patients.[4*] One study of patients in palliative care found that fatigue was reported by 80% of cancer patients and 99% of patients following chemotherapy.[4*] The authors proposed that many factors influenced fatigue in cancer patients including aspects of the disease, the cancer treatment, and a psychological component of suffering.[5*] This study highlights the problems with classifying symptoms such as fatigue as "somatic" in medical populations, where patients often have complex symptom profiles and a high symptom burden.

It is estimated that about one in four patients with advanced cancer receiving palliative care experience depression.[2,6*] Empirical evidence supports a relation among symptoms such as pain, nausea, and fatigue, and negative mood states such as depression and anxiety in many medical settings.[1***] In palliative care settings, depression and anxiety have consistently been found to relate to greater reporting of medical symptoms.[2,6*] For example, among advanced cancer patients in palliative care, greater depression and anxiety symptoms are associated with greater symptoms of fatigue, drowsiness, and pain and lower quality of life.[2,7*] Patients with chronic cancer pain show similar symptom profiles, with those in greater pain reporting more negative affect such as depression, anxiety, and anger.[8,9*,10*]

The relation between pain and negative mood states is also found in patients with chronic noncancer pain. Patients with chronic noncancer pain typically report more symptoms of depression and anxiety and experience more somatic symptoms such as fatigue, headache, and nausea, compared to patients without pain.[1,8,9,11***] This relation between pain and negative mood states holds even when taking into account the severity of the medical illness. As an illustration, patients with chronic medical illness and comorbid depression have been found to report a significantly higher number of somatic symptoms than those with a chronic medical illness but no depression, even when controlling for the severity of the medical illness.[12*]

Thus, the relation between negative mood and physical symptoms is supported by research findings with a wide variety of patients across various treatment settings. The commonly observed associations between mood, pain, and other somatic symptoms highlight the difficulty, if not futility, in attempting to separate these symptoms into "real" body symptoms and psychological symptoms. Moreover, this research highlights the problematic nature of the "somatic" label, as symptoms such as headache, nausea, and fatigue have multiple and complex causes and may not fit a traditional definition of somatization, especially in palliative care populations.

TRADITIONAL VIEWS OF SOMATIZATION

Current diagnostic criteria for somatization disorders reflect a focus on medically unexplained or unaccounted for symptoms, but proposed changes to the Diagnostic and Statistical Manual of Mental Disorders (DSM)-IV suggest a possible shift away from this conceptualization. The Diagnostic and Statistical Manual of Mental Disorders (DSM)-IV[13] defines somatoform disorders as a group of specific disorders or problems characterized by persistent bodily symptoms or concerns that cannot be fully accounted for by a diagnosable disease. Somatization disorder is one of a group of disorders known as somatoform disorders. Hypochondriasis, for example, is the persistent, unfounded worry or conviction, despite adequate medical assurance to the contrary, that one has a serious medical illness. Somatization is a chronic condition consisting of multiple and specific categories of medically unexplained physical complaints that occur over a prolonged period of time. Pain disorder involves the persistence of medically unexplained pain symptoms. In the medical literature, the term "functional somatic syndrome" refers to several syndromes in which the symptoms and subsequent suffering and disability are not fully explained by demonstrable tissue abnormality.[14*] These patients may express symptoms such as gastrointestinal symptoms and fatigue in addition to pain. Individuals who meet diagnostic criteria for functional somatic syndromes, as defined in the medical literature, have higher rates of somatoform disorders, as defined in the DSM-IV, and higher rates of anxiety and depression.[14*]

CURRENT VIEWS OF SOMATIZATION

In actuality, most patients in medical settings, including pain clinics, do not meet the strict criteria of somatization as defined by the current version of the DSM (DSM-IV). As previously noted, the distinction between medically explained and unexplained symptoms can be problematic. Prevalence rates for medically unexplained symptoms in pain populations vary widely, with estimates ranging from 0% to 80%.[15*,16*,8,9*] When making diagnoses of somatization disorders, physicians have acknowledged that many patient-reported somatic symptoms cannot easily be classified as either medically explainable or unexplainable.[8,9*]

The more traditional conceptualizations of somatization disorders seen in the DSM-IV and medical literature focus on "medically unexplained symptoms" as a defining feature of somatization. Recent shifts in the conceptualization of somatization can be seen in plans for the upcoming edition of the DSM (DSM-5).[17] In the DSM-5, "medically unexplained symptoms" will likely no longer be a core feature of the diagnosis for somatoform disorders. Instead, for the newly proposed "somatic symptom disorders," for example, it has been suggested that diagnosis be dependent on the presence of both somatic symptoms and psychological symptoms (e.g., dysfunctional cognition related to illness), regardless of whether medical symptoms are unexplained. These proposed changes reflect an appreciation for the close relation between psychological and physical symptoms and the difficulty inherent in classifying symptoms as "medically unexplained." If adopted, these changes would support a conceptualization of physical and psychological symptoms as interacting processes best treated with a multidisciplinary team approach, rather than separate, distinct symptom clusters treated in isolation. This conceptualization is consistent with a more comprehensive perspective of pain, such as that proposed by the International Association for the Study of Pain (ISAP), which takes into account both physiological and psychological factors when describing a person's overall experience of pain.[18,19***]

THEORIES OF PAIN

All patients experience pain and illness differently. The overall suffering and discomfort experienced by each patient will depend on multiple factors including aspects of the disease and treatment, how the patient interprets and experiences illness and pain, social support available to the patient, ability to cope with stressors, psychological distress, depression, and anxiety. Thus, multiple and complex factors are involved in the experience of pain.

Theories of pain provide some insight into the potential mechanisms involved in pain perception. One such theory proposes that a sensitizing effect to physiological events in some patients may heighten bodily awareness and increase pain.[14*] Support for this theory can be found in research on patients with chronic pain conditions such as fibromyalgia, which has found that these patients have increased responsiveness and sensitivity to various sensory stimulation, including pain, auditory tones, and tactile stimuli.[20*] A similar perspective, supported by work from Geisser and colleagues,[21*] presents a neurobiological model of pain in which a patient's tendency to focus on bodily symptoms activates pain facilitation neurons. The activation of these neurons is believed to sharpen the perception of the painful stimulus. Consistent with this theory, some people attend to and focus on pain and pain-related stimuli to a greater degree, a practice that has been found to be related to greater pain reporting.[22***]

A third perspective draws from cognitive-behavioral theories of pain. Cognitive-behavioral perspectives propose that pain can be examined on three dimensions: (1) an affective dimension, which describes pain-related affect (depression, anxiety, anger), (2) a behavioral dimension, which includes maladaptive behaviors related to pain (inactivity, avoiding others), and (3) a cognitive dimension, including maladaptive beliefs and thoughts about pain (e.g., belief that one cannot function when in pain). These various dimensions all influence a person's overall experience of pain. Moreover, this model supports bidirectional relations between dimensions.

As an illustration, negative mood can lead to changes in pain behaviors, such as inactivity, thus leading to deconditioning in some patients and increasing the body's vulnerability to illness and injury. Negative mood state may also affect the interpretation of physical changes, such that the body's cues and signals (e.g., heart palpitations, shortness of breath) are inaccurately interpreted as more enduring symptoms or conditions.[23*] Additionally, pain can also influence mood states. For example, the way in which a person interprets their chronic pain condition (e.g., the degree to which they believe the pain will interfere with daily living) can influence the later development of depression symptoms.[24**]

Lastly, cultural, social, and institutional factors that emphasize physical symptoms rather than psychological factors may also contribute to a heightened focus on physical symptoms.[25*] Research has found that some patients with chronic pain report certain experiences, such as affective distress, as pain.[25*] Additionally, qualitative examination of patient and provider beliefs suggests that cultural factors can influence how physicians respond to patients' problems, the relationship between health care providers and patients, and how patients respond to illness, including the reporting of pain and psychological symptoms.[26*]

TREATMENT RECOMMENDATIONS

The discussion presented in this chapter highlights the multifaceted and interactive nature of pain, physical complaints, and psychological symptoms. It is important to recognize that in palliative care, symptoms such as pain, nausea, and fatigue will likely reflect aspects of the chronic medical condition or its treatment. Additionally, each patient will experience pain differently. The overall suffering and discomfort experienced by each patient will depend on multiple factors such as how the patient interprets and experiences illness and pain, social support available to the patient, psychological distress, depression, and anxiety. Given the high concordance of psychological symptoms with physical complaints and research findings presenting evidence for the interactive nature of these symptoms, the use of a multidisciplinary treatment approach is recommended. In the treatment of pain, multidisciplinary teams often include professionals from pain medicine, palliative care, psychology, social work, and nursing. Treatment models in which these disciplines are integrated fully into the treatment team are ideal, but utilizing these services on a consulting basis may be necessary in some settings due to financial, geographic, or institutional constraints. Multidisciplinary approaches to pain management have consistently been found to be more effective than other forms of treatment for chronic pain.[27*] Additionally, research demonstrates that incorporating routine screening for psychological distress in cancer pain patients leads to improved detection of psychological symptoms and more appropriate referrals to specialized services.[8,28*]

> ## Box 54.1 Management guidelines for somatization
>
> - Utilize a multidisciplinary team approach.
> - Rule out diagnosable medical disease.
> - Assess for psychological distress.
> - Consider the cultural and social context.
> - Build a collaborative relationship with the patient.
> - Provide a caring physician attitude.
> - Make appropriate referrals to specialized services.

A multidisciplinary approach to pain management may help to address potential difficulties that can occur when treating some patients presenting with somatic complaints. When appropriate, involve other services including psychology and social work in the patient's treatment. We also recommend using caution in assigning a somatoform disorder or other psychiatric diagnosis, as these labels may invalidate patients' physical symptoms or unfairly alter the perception of the patient held by other providers. Moreover, as demonstrated in this article, diagnosis of somatization disorders is unreliable and can be complicated in patients with chronic medical conditions. Pain management guidelines, based in part on suggestions presented by Barsky and Borus[29*] and Purcell[30*], are presented in Box 54.1.

SUMMARY

In summary, symptoms such as unexplained pain, fatigue, nausea, headache, dizziness, and insomnia are common complaints among people with medical conditions. Among palliative care patients, these symptoms may be related to aspects of the illness, side effects of medical treatment, or psychological suffering. Given the complex symptom profile and high symptom burden among patients in palliative care, we recommend using caution when assigning a somatic disorder diagnosis. The upcoming version of the DSM (DSM 5) may include changes to the diagnosis of somatization disorder in which "medically unexplainable symptoms" would no longer be a required diagnostic criterion. These proposed changes reflect an appreciation for the close relation between psychological and physical symptoms and the difficulty inherent in classifying symptoms as "medically unexplained." Negative mood is associated with greater pain and greater symptom reporting among patients with both chronic noncancer and cancer pain. Theories of pain perception offer insights into the relation among mood, somatic symptoms, and pain, which suggest that these symptoms are interactive, rather than distinct, independent symptoms. This conceptualization of pain supports a multidisciplinary treatment approach where psychological treatment and other specialized services are integrated at all stages of care.

Key learning points

- Patients in palliative care consistently report more symptoms such as pain, fatigue, sleep difficulties, and headache.

- Negative mood is associated with greater pain and physical complaints among patients with both chronic noncancer and cancer pain.

- The labeling of medical symptoms as "somatic" may be problematic in palliative care settings as these symptoms may be related to aspects of the illness, side effects of medical treatment, or psychological suffering.

- In the DSM-5, "medically unexplained symptoms" will likely no longer be a core feature of the diagnosis for somatoform disorders.

- The changes in the DSM support a conceptualization of physical and psychological symptoms as interacting processes best treated with a multidisciplinary approach, rather than separate, distinct symptoms clusters treated in isolation.

- This conceptualization is consistent with a more comprehensive perspective of pain, such as that proposed by the ISAP), which takes into account both physiological and psychological factors of pain.

- Multidisciplinary approaches to pain management, which include professionals from pain medicine, palliative care, psychology, social work, and nursing, have been found to be more effective than other forms of treatment for chronic pain.

REFERENCES

1 Fishbain D, Lewis J, Gao J et al. Is chronic pain associated with somatization/hypochondriasis? An evidence-based structured review. *Pain Practice* 2009; **9**: 449–467.

2 Delgado-Guay M, Parson H, Li Z et al. Symptom distress in advanced cancer patients with anxiety and depression in the palliative care setting. *Supportive Care Cancer* 2009; **17**: 573–579.

◆ 3 Temel J, Greer J, Muzikansky A et al. Early palliative care for patients with metastatic non-small-cell lung cancer. *The New England Journal of Medicine* 2010; **363**: 733–742.

4 Radbruch L, Strasser F, Elsner F et al. Fatigue in palliative care patients-an EAPC approach. *Palliative Medicine* 2008; **22**: 13–32.

5 Strasser F, Walker P, Bruera E. Palliative pain management: When both pain and suffering hurt. *Journal of Palliative Care* 2005; **21**: 69–79.

6 Rayner L, Lee W, Price A et al. The clinical epidemiology in palliative care and the predictive value of somatic symptoms: Cross-sectional survey with four-week follow-up. *Palliative Medicine* 2010; **25**: 229–241.

7 Lloyd-Williams M, Dennis M, Taylor F. A prospective study to determine the association between physical symptoms and depression in patients with advance cancer. *Palliative Medicine* 2004; **18**: 558–563.

8 Berry M, Palmer J, Bruera E, Novy D. Predictors of unexplained somatic symptoms in cancer and noncancer pain. Paper presented at *American Psychological Association Annual Meeting*, July 2004.

9 Novy D, Berry M, Palmer J et al. Somatic symptoms in patients with chronic noncancer and cancer pain. *Journal of Pain and Symptom Management* 2005; **29**: 603–612.

10 Zimmerman L, Story K, Gaston-Johansson F, Rowles J. Psychological variables and cancer pain. *Cancer Nursing* 1996; **19**: 44–53.

◆ 11 Romano J, Turner J. Chronic pain and depression: Does the evidence support a relationship. *Psychological Bulletin* 1985; **97**: 18–34.

12 Katon W, Lin E, Roenke K. The association of depression and anxiety with medical symptom burden in patients with chronic medical illness. *General Hospital Psychiatry* 2007; **29**: 147–155.

✳ 13 American Psychiatric Association. *Diagnostic and Statistical Manual of Mental Disorders*. 4th edn. Washington, DC: American Psychiatric Association; 1994.

14 Barsky A, Goodson D, Lane R. The amplification of somatic symptoms. *Psychosomatic Medicine* 1988; **50**: 510–519.

15 Kroenke D, Spitzer R, Williams J et al. Physical symptoms in primary care: Predicators of psychiatric disorders and functional impairment. *Archives of Family Medicine* 1994; **3**: 774–779.

16 Sikorski J, Stampfer H, Cole R. Psychological aspects of chronic low back pain. *Australiian and New Zealand Journal of Surgery* 1996; **66**: 297–297.

17 Somatic Symptom Disorders. American Psychiatric Association: DSM-5 Development, 2012; www.dsm5.org/proposedrevision.

✳ 18 International Association for the Study of Pain Subcommittee on Taxonomy. *Classification of Chronic Pain: Descriptions of Chronic Pain Syndromes and Definitions of Pain Terms*. Amsterdam, the Netherlands: Elsevier; 1986.

◆ 19 Novy D, Nelson D, Francis D, Turk D. Perspectives of chronic pain: An evaluative comparison of restrictive and comprehensive models. *Psychological Bulletin* 1995; **118**: 238–247.

20 Geisser M, Strader Donnell C, Petzke F et al. Comorbid somatic symptoms and functional status in patients with fibromyalgia and chronic fatigue syndrome: Sensory amplification as a common mechanism. *Psychosomatics* 2008; **49**: 235–242.

21 Geisser M, Gaskin M, Robinson M. The relationship of depression and somatic focus to experimental and clinical pain in chronic pain patients. *Psychology and Health* 1993; **8**: 415–420.

22 VanDamme S, Legrain V, Vogt J, Crombez G. Keeping pain in mind: A motivational account of attention to pain. *Neuroscience and Biobehavioral Reviews* 2010; **34**: 204–213.

23 Mechanic D. The experience and reporting of common physical complaints. *Journal of Health and Social Behavior* 1980; **21**: 146–155.

24 Rudy T, Kerns R, Turk D. Chronic pain and depression: Toward a cognitive-behavioral mediation model. *Pain* 1988; **35**: 129–140.

25 Dworkin S, Wilson L, Masson D. Somatizing as a risk factor for chronic pain. In: Grzesiak R, Ciccone D eds. *Psychological Vulnerability to Chronic Pain*. New York: Springer; 1994, pp. 28–54.

26 Bates M, Rankin-Hill L, Sanchez-Ayendez M. The effects of the cultural context of health care on treatment of and response to chronic pain and illness. *Social Science and Medicine* 1997; **45**: 1433–1447.

27 Loeser J. Multidisciplinary pain management. In: Merskey H, Loeser J, Dubner R eds. *The Paths of Pain 1975–2005*. Seattle, WA: IASP Press, 2005, pp. 1433–1447.

28 Ford S, Fallowfield L, Lewis S. Can oncologists detect distress in their out-patients and how satisfied are they with their performance during bad news consultations? *British Journal of Cancer* 1994; **70**: 767–770.

29 Barsky A, Borus J. Functional somatic syndromes. *Annals of Internal Medicine* 1999; **130**: 910–921.

30 Purcell T. The somatic patient. *Emergency Medicine Clinics of North America* 1991; **9**: 137–159.

55

Pain in patients with alcohol and drug dependence

JULIE R. PRICE, STEVEN D. PASSIK, KENNETH L. KIRSH

INTRODUCTION

Substance abuse and dependence are difficult problems, both theoretically and clinically, in the arena of pain management and palliative care.[1***] Physicians and other medical staff need to be continually mindful of the potential for substance abuse and diversion. The severity of substance-related problems varies significantly: patients with pain and advanced disease unilaterally escalating drug doses, using medications to treat other symptoms, or prescriptions that are being mishandled. The clinician is therefore challenged to understand such happenings and plan interventions accordingly. Once these aberrant behaviors are identified, the clinician must decide on a course of action that is fair and in the best interests of the patient as well as his or her own career. The problem of alcoholism, drug abuse, and chemical dependency spans a continuum from formal psychiatric disorders to problematic behaviors in the absence of these disorders; thus, proper identification, assessment, and clinical management of the entire spectrum of substance-related problems are critically important for the optimal treatment of patients in palliative care settings.

PREVALENCE

Nearly half of the U.S. population aged 15–54 has used illicit drugs, and an estimated 6%–15% has a substance use disorder of some type.[2–4*] In 2011, the Substance Abuse and Mental Health Services Administration's (SAMHSA) National Survey on Drug Use and Health reported that an estimated 20.6 million persons (8% aged 12 or older) had been classified with substance abuse or dependence based on the Diagnostic and Statistical Manual of Mental Disorders, 4th edition (DSM-IV), which is a decrease from the prior year (22.2 million).[5*] As a result of this high prevalence, and the association between drug abuse and life-threatening diseases, problems with substance abuse-related issues are commonly encountered in palliative care settings.[6*] In diverse patient populations with progressive life-threatening diseases, a remote or current history of drug abuse presents a constellation of physical and psychosocial issues that carry a stigma that can both complicate the management of the underlying disease and undermine palliative therapies. Clearly, the interface between the therapeutic use of potentially abusable drugs and the abuse of these drugs is complex and must be understood to optimize palliative care.

Substance abuse appears to be less frequent among palliative care patients as compared to the prevalence of substance use disorders in society at large, in general medical populations, and in emergency medical departments.[2–4*,7] This relatively low prevalence was also reported in the Psychiatric Collaborative Oncology Group study that assessed psychiatric diagnoses in ambulatory cancer patients from several tertiary care hospitals.[8*] Following structured clinical interviews, less than 5% of 215 cancer patients met the Diagnostic and Statistical Manual for Mental Disorders (DSM-III) criteria for a substance use disorder.[9*] Thus, the problem reflects a minority of patients, but one that can only be adequately and successfully treated when their substance problems are noted by staff and their needs addressed.[10,11*]

CURRENT DEFINITIONS OF ABUSE AND DEPENDENCE

The pharmacological phenomena of tolerance and physical dependence are commonly confused with abuse and true substance dependence as defined by the DSM-IV. All the definitions applied to medical patients have been developed from substance-abusing populations without medical illness, as well as sociocultural considerations, which may lead to mixed messages in the clinical setting. The clarification of this terminology is an essential step in improving the diagnosis and management of substance abuse in the palliative care setting.

Tolerance, a pharmacological property defined by the need for increasing doses to maintain effects, has been of particular concern during opioid therapy.[12,13] Clinicians and patients both commonly express concerns that tolerance to analgesic effects may compromise the benefits of therapy and lead to the requirement for progressively higher, and ultimately unsustainable, doses.

Notwithstanding these concerns, extensive clinical experience with opioid analgesic in the medical context has not confirmed that tolerance causes substantial problems.[14-16] Although tolerance to a variety of opioid effects can be reliably observed in animal models,[17**] and tolerance to nonanalgesic effects, such as respiratory depression and cognitive impairment,[10*] occurs routinely in the clinical setting, analgesic tolerance does not appear to routinely interfere with the clinical efficacy of opioid analgesic. Most patients can attain stable doses associated with a favorable balance between analgesia and side effects for prolonged periods. Dose escalation, when it is required, usually heralds the appearance of a progressive painful lesion.[18-24*] Unlike tolerance to the side effects of the opioids, clinically meaningful analgesic tolerance appears to be a rare phenomenon, and is rarely the cause for dose escalation.

Physical dependence is defined solely by the occurrence of a withdrawal syndrome following abrupt dose reduction or administration of an antagonist.[12,13,25*] Neither the dose nor the duration of administration required to produce clinically significant physical dependence in humans is known. Most practitioners assume that the potential for withdrawal exists after opioids have been administered repeatedly for only a few days.

There is great confusion among clinicians about the differences between physical dependence and true substance dependence. Physical dependence, like tolerance, has been suggested to be a component of substance dependence, and the avoidance of withdrawal has been postulated to create behavioral contingencies that reinforce drug-seeking behavior.[26-29] These speculations, however, are not supported by the experience acquired during opioid therapy for chronic pain. Physical dependence does not preclude the uncomplicated discontinuation of opioids during multidisciplinary pain management of nonmalignant pain, and opioid therapy is routinely stopped without difficulty in the cancer patients whose pain disappears following effective antineoplastic therapy.[30] Indirect evidence for a fundamental distinction between physical dependence and substance dependence is even provided by animal models of opioid self-administration, which have demonstrated that persistent drug-taking behavior can be maintained in the absence of physical dependence.[31**]

CONCERNS OVER CURRENT DEFINITIONS

These definitions of tolerance and physical dependence highlight deficiencies in the nomenclature applied to substance abuse. The terms "addiction" and "addict" are particularly troublesome and are often inappropriately applied to describe both aberrant drug use and phenomena related to tolerance or physical dependence. Clinicians and patients may use the word "addicted" to describe compulsive drug-taking in one patient and nothing more than the possibility for withdrawal in another. Thus, it is not surprising that patients, families, and staff become very concerned about the outcome of opioid treatment when this term is applied, which often leads to misperceptions about this mode of therapy for all involved.[32]

The accurate assessment of drug-related behaviors in patients with advanced medical disease usually requires detailed information about the role of the drug in the patient's life. The existence of mild mental clouding or the time spent out of bed may be less meaningful than other outcomes, such as nonadherence to drug-related therapy, or behaviors that jeopardize relationships with physicians, other healthcare providers or family members.

ALTERNATIVE APPROACH FOR DEFINING ABUSE AND DEPENDENCE IN THE MEDICALLY ILL

Previous definitions that include phenomena related to physical dependence or tolerance cannot be the model terminology for medically ill populations who receive potentially abusable drugs for legitimate medical purposes. A more appropriate definition of substance dependence notes that it is a chronic disorder characterized by "the compulsive use of a substance resulting in physical, psychological or social harm to the user and continued use despite that harm."[33] This definition appropriately emphasizes that substance dependence is, fundamentally, a psychological and behavioral syndrome. Any appropriate definition of substance abuse or dependence must include the concepts of loss of control over drug use, compulsive drug use, and continued use despite harm.

Spectrum of aberrant drug–taking behavior

If drug-taking behavior in a medical patient can be characterized as aberrant, a differential diagnosis for this behavior can be explored. A true substance dependence disorder is only one of several possible explanations. Of the behaviors likely to represent true substance dependence, some recent research suggests that multiple unsanctioned dose escalations and obtaining opioids from multiple prescribers may have some specific relevance.[34] If the problem is not substance dependence, the challenging diagnosis of pseudoaddiction must be considered if the patient is reporting distress associated with unrelieved symptoms. Behaviors such as aggressively complaining about the need for higher doses, or occasional unilateral drug escalations, may be signs that the patient's pain is undermedicated. Also, impulsive drug and alcohol use may indicate the existence of another psychiatric disorder, which may have therapeutic implications. For example, patients with borderline personality disorder can express fear and rage through aberrant drug-taking and behave impulsively and self-destructively during pain therapy.[35] Similarly, patients who self-medicate psychiatric conditions such as anxiety, panic, depression or even periodic dysphoria, and loneliness can present as aberrant drug takers. In such instances, careful diagnosis and treatment of these additional problems can at times obviate the need for such self-medication.[36] Other rule-outs for substance dependence include mild encephalopathy and criminal intent through diversion or sale of medications.

In assessing the differential diagnosis for drug-related behavior, it is useful to consider the degree of aberrancy. The less aberrant behaviors (such as aggressively complaining about the need for medications) are more likely to reflect untreated distress of some type, rather than substance dependence-related concerns. Conversely, the more aberrant behaviors (such as injection of an oral formulation) are more likely to reflect true substance dependence. Although empirical studies are needed to validate this conceptualization, it may be a useful model when evaluating aberrant behaviors.

Empirical validation of the aberrant drug-taking concept

The spectrum of aberrant drug-taking has been used as a heuristic to guide the assessment of problematic drug-taking in several recent studies. The studies performed to date all involve small samples, though they have shown the utility of the spectrum concept as an assessment tool yielding important implications for clinicians.

The first study examined the relationship between aberrant drug-taking behaviors and adherence in patients with a history of substance abuse receiving chronic opioid therapy for nonmalignant pain. Dunbar and Katz examined outcomes and drug-taking in a sample of 20 patients with diverse histories of drug abuse during a year of chronic opioid therapy.[37] During the study, 11 patients followed the drug regimen and 9 did not. The authors examined patient characteristics and aberrant drug-taking behaviors that differentiated the two groups. The patients who did not abuse the therapy were current alcohol abusers only (or had remote histories of polysubstance abuse), were in a solid drug-free recovery as evidenced by participation in 12-step programs, and had good social support. The patients who abused the therapy were polysubstance abusers, were not participating in 12-step programs, and had poor social support. The specific behaviors that were recorded more frequently by those who abused the therapy were unscheduled visits and multiple phone calls to the clinic, unsanctioned dose escalations, and obtaining opioids from more than one source.

A second study examined the relationship between aberrant drug-taking and the presence or absence of a psychiatric diagnosis of substance use disorder in pain patients. Compton and colleagues studied 56 patients seeking pain treatment in a multidisciplinary pain program who were referred for "problematic drug-taking."[38*] The patients underwent structured psychiatric interviews, and the sample was divided between those qualifying and not qualifying for the psychiatric diagnoses of substance use disorders. The authors then examined the subjects' reports of aberrant drug-taking behaviors on a structured interview assessment. Those with a substance use disorder were more likely to have engaged in unsanctioned dose escalations, received opioids from multiple sources, and a subjective impression of loss of control of their prescribed medications.

Passik and researchers examined the self-reports of aberrant drug-taking attitudes and behaviors in samples of cancer (n = 52) and acquired immune deficiency syndrome (AIDS) (n = 111) patients with a questionnaire designed for the purposes of the study.[32*] Reports of past drug use and abuse were more frequent than present reports in both groups. Current aberrant drug-related behaviors were seldom reported. Attitude items, however, revealed that patients would consider engaging in aberrant behaviors, or would possibly excuse them in others, if pain or symptom management were inadequate. Overall, patients greatly overestimated the risk of substance dependence in pain treatment. Experience with this questionnaire suggests that patients with both cancer and AIDS respond in a forthcoming fashion to drug-taking behavior questions and describe attitudes and behaviors which may be highly relevant to the diagnosis and management of substance use disorders.

Such studies will help us to better understand the particular diagnostic meanings of the various behaviors so that clinicians may recognize which are the true "red flags" in a given population. Far too often, anecdotal accounts shape the way clinicians view these behaviors. Some behaviors are regarded almost universally as aberrant despite limited systematic data to suggest that this is the case. Consider, for example, the patient who requests a specific pain medication, or a specific route or dose. Such behavior often reflects a patient who is knowledgeable about what works for him or her, but is almost always greeted with suspicion on the part of practitioners. Other behaviors may be found to be common in medically ill non-substance-abusing populations, and although they seem aberrant based upon their face value, they may have little predictive value for true substance dependence.

RISK OF ABUSE AND DEPENDENCE IN THE MEDICALLY ILL

Risk in patients without prior drug abuse

An extensive worldwide experience in the long-term management of cancer pain with opioid drugs has demonstrated that opioid administration in cancer patients with no prior history of substance abuse is only rarely associated with the development of significant abuse or dependence.[27,39–50*] Indeed, concerns about abuse in this population are now characterized by an interesting paradox: Although the lay public and inexperienced clinicians still fear the development of substance abuse or dependence when opioids are used to treat cancer pain, specialists in cancer pain and palliative care widely believe that the major problem related to potential abuse is not the phenomenon itself, but rather the persistent undertreatment of pain driven by inappropriate fear that it will occur.

The traditional view of long-term opioid therapy is negative, and early surveys of substance abusers, which noted that a relatively large proportion began their abuse as medical patients while utilizing opioid analgesics for pain, provided some indirect support for this perspective.[51–53*] The most influential of these surveys recorded a history of medical opioid use for pain in 27% of white male abusers and 1.2% of black male abusers.[53*]

Surveys of substance-abusing populations, however, do not provide a valid measure of the liability associated with chronic opioid therapy in populations without known abuse. Prospective patient surveys are needed to define this risk accurately. One project evaluated 11,882 inpatients who had no prior history of substance abuse and were administered an opioid while hospitalized; only four cases of substance abuse or dependence could be identified subsequently.[54*] A national survey of burn centers could find no cases of abuse in a sample of more than 10,000 patients without prior drug abuse history who were administered opioids for pain, and a survey of a large headache clinic identified opioid abuse in only three of 2369 patients admitted for treatment, most of whom had access to opioids.[55,56*]

Other data suggest that the medically ill patient with chronic pain is sufficiently different from the patient with substance abuse/dependence issues without painful disease, and that the risk of abuse or dependence during opioid therapy is likely to be low. For example, surveys of cancer patients and postoperative patients indicate that euphoria, a phenomenon believed to be common during the abuse of opioids, is extremely uncommon following administration of an opioid for pain; dysphoria is observed more typically, especially in those who receive meperidine.[57*] Although the psychiatric comorbidity identified in substance abuse populations could be an effect, rather than a cause, of aberrant drug-taking, the association suggests the existence of psychological risk factors for substance dependence.

The inaccurate perception that opioid therapy inherently yields a relatively high likelihood of substance abuse or dependence has encouraged assumptions that are not supportable in populations without a prior history of substance abuse. Perhaps the most important, the relevance of genetic predisposition to substance abuse, which was suggested in a twin study that demonstrated a significant concordance rate for aberrant drug-related behaviors.[58*] A more critical evaluation of the extant literature actually yields little substantive support for the view that large numbers of individuals with no personal or family history of substance abuse or dependence, no affiliation with a substance-abusing subculture, and no significant premorbid psychopathology will develop abuse or dependence de novo when administered potentially abusable drugs for appropriate medical indications.[24*,58*,59*,60–63*]

Risk in patients with current or remote drug abuse

There is very little information about the risk of substance abuse or dependence during, or after, the therapeutic administration of a potentially abusable drug to patients with a current or remote history of substance abuse or dependence. Anecdotal reports suggest that successful long-term opioid therapy in patients with cancer pain or chronic nonmalignant pain is possible, particularly if the history of substance abuse or dependence is remote.[37*,64*,65*] Indeed, one study showed that patients with AIDS-related pain were able to be successfully treated with morphine whether or not they were substance users or nonusers. In fact, the major difference found was that substance users required considerably more morphine to reach

stable pain control.[66*] However, a modicum of caution should be employed. For example, although there is no empirical evidence that the use of short-acting drugs or the parenteral route is more likely to lead to problematic drug-related behaviors than other therapeutic approaches, it may be prudent to avoid such therapies in patients with histories of substance abuse.

CLINICAL MANAGEMENT

Aberrant drug-taking among palliative care patients (with or without a prior history of substance abuse) represents a serious and complex clinical occurrence. Perhaps the more difficult situations involve the patient who is actively abusing illicit or prescription drugs or alcohol concomitantly with medical therapies. The following guidelines can be useful whether the patient is an active drug abuser, has a history of substance abuse, or is not adhering with the therapeutic regimen.

Multidisciplinary approach

A multidisciplinary team approach is recommended for the management of substance abuse in the palliative care setting. Mental health professionals with specialization in substance abuse can be instrumental in adherence. Providing care to these patients can lead to feelings of anger and frustration among staff. Such feelings can unintentionally compromise the level of patient care surrounding the patient's pain management and contribute to feelings of isolation and alienation by the patient. A structured multidisciplinary approach can be effective in helping the staff better understand the patient's needs and develop effective strategies for controlling pain and aberrant drug use simultaneously. Staff meetings can be helpful in establishing treatment goals, facilitating adherence, and coordinating the multidisciplinary team.

Assessment

The first member of the medical team to suspect problematic drug-taking or a history of drug abuse should alert the patient's palliative care team, thus beginning the multidisciplinary assessment and management process.[67***] A physician should assess the potential of withdrawal or other pressing concerns and begin involving other staff (i.e., social work, psychology, and/or psychiatry) to initiate the planning of management strategies. Obtaining as detailed as possible the information about a history of duration, frequency, and desired effect of drug use is crucial. Frequently, clinicians avoid asking patients about substance abuse out of fear that they will anger the patient or that they are incorrect in their suspicion of abuse. However, such approaches will likely contribute to continued problems with treatment adherence and frustration among staff. Empathic and truthful communication is always the best approach.

The use of a careful, graduated interview approach can be instrumental in slowly introducing the assessment of drug use. This approach entails starting the assessment interview with broad questions about the role of drugs (e.g., nicotine, caffeine) in the patient's life and gradually becoming more specific in focus to include illicit drugs. This interviewing style also assists in the detection of coexisting psychiatric disorders that may be present. Comorbid psychiatric disorders can significantly contribute to aberrant drug-taking behavior. Anxiety, mood, and personality disorders are the most commonly encountered.[68,69] The assessment and treatment of comorbid psychiatric disorders can greatly enhance management strategies and reduce the risk of relapse. The patient's desired effects from illicit drugs can often be a clue to comorbid psychiatric disorders (i.e., drinking to quell panic symptoms).

In addition, we must always keep in mind that a spectrum of nonadherence exists and that this spectrum is distinct for pain patients versus those who use these medications for nonmedical purposes (Figure 55.1).[70] Nonmedical users can be seen as self-treating personal issues, purely as recreational users, or as having a more severe and consistent substance use disorder or "addiction." On the other hand, pain patients are more complex and their behaviors might range from strict adherence to chemically coping to a frank substance use disorder or "addiction." Thus, it is important to be careful when assessing patients who are thought to have problematic drug-taking, or at increased risk for substance abuse, that you might be uncovering some of the gray areas of nonadherence.

Development of a multidisciplinary treatment plan

Drug abuse is often a chronic, progressive disorder. Therefore, the development of clear treatment goals is essential for the management of drug abuse/dependence. Team members should not expect a complete remission of the patient's substance use problems. The distress of coping with a life-threatening illness and the availability of prescription drugs for symptom control can make complete abstinence an unrealistic goal.[71] Rather, a harm reduction approach should be employed that aims to enhance social support, maximize treatment adherence, and contain harm done through episodic relapse. The following guidelines are recommended for the management of patients with a substance disorder.

1. The clinician should first establish a relationship based on empathic listening and accept the patient's report of distress.
2. It is important to utilize nonopioid and behavioral interventions when possible, but not as substitutes for appropriate pain management.
3. The team should consider tolerance, route of administration, and duration of action when prescribing medications for pain and symptom management. Preexisting tolerance should be taken into account for patients who are actively abusing drugs or are being maintained on methadone maintenance programs. Failure to realize any existing tolerance can result in undermedication and contribute to the patient's attempts to self-medicate.
4. The team should consider using longer-acting drugs (e.g., fentanyl patch and sustained-release opioids). The longer duration and slow onset may help to reduce aberrant drug-taking behaviors when compared to the rapid onset and increased frequency of dosage associated with short-acting drugs.[72*]
5. The team should make plans to frequently reassess the adequacy of pain and symptom control, as well as adherence via use of urine drug screens and any other forms of monitoring.[72*]

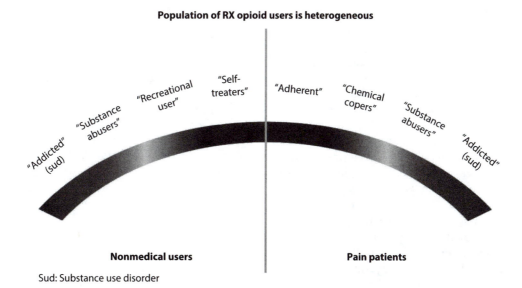

Population of RX opioid users is heterogeneous

"Addicted" (sud)   "Substance abusers"   "Recreational user"   "Self-treaters"   "Adherent"   "Chemical copers"   "Substance abusers"   "Addicted" (sud)

Nonmedical users   **Pain patients**

Sud: Substance use disorder

Figure 55.1 *The spectrum of adherence for pain patients versus the spectrum of illicit use by nonmedical users. (From Kirsh, K.L. and Passik, S.D., Exp. Clin. Psychopharmacol., 16(5), 400, 2008.)*

Patients in recovery

Pain management with patients in recovery presents a unique challenge. Depending on the structure of the recovery program (e.g., Alcoholics Anonymous, methadone maintenance programs), a patient may fear ostracism from the program's members or may have an increased fear regarding susceptibility to re-addiction. The first choice should be to explore nonopioid therapies with these patients, which may require referral to a pain center.[73] Alternative therapies may include the use of nonsteroidal anti-inflammatory drugs, anticonvulsants (for neuropathic components), bio-feedback, electrical stimulation, neuroablative techniques, acupuncture, or cognitive behavioral management. If the pain condition is so severe that opioids are required, care must be taken to structure their use with opioid management contracts, random urine toxicology screens, and occasional pill counts. If possible, attempts should be made to include the patient's recovery program sponsor to garner their cooperation and aid in successful monitoring of the condition.

Patients with advanced disease

Managing substance abuse or dependence problems in patients with advanced cancer is labor-intensive and can be extremely time-consuming. In fact, many clinicians might opt to overlook a patient's use of alcohol or illicit drugs, viewing these behaviors as a last source of pleasure for the patient. However, substance abuse or dependence issues have deleterious impact on palliative care efforts. Proper management plays an important part in the success of palliative efforts to reduce suffering and increase quality of life. Complete abstinence may not be a realistic outcome, but reduction in use can certainly have positive effects for the patient.[74]

CONCLUSION

Although the most prudent actions on the part of clinicians cannot obviate the risk of all aberrant drug-related behaviors, clinicians must recognize that virtually, any drug that acts on the central nervous system can be abused. The effective management of patients with pain who engage in aberrant drug-related behavior necessitates a comprehensive approach that recognizes the biologic, chemical, social, and psychiatric aspects of substance abuse, and provides practical means to manage risk, treat pain effectively, and assure patient safety. An accepted nomenclature for abuse and dependence and an operational approach to the assessment of patients with medical illness are prerequisites to an accurate definition of risk in populations with and without histories of substance abuse.

Key learning points

- Substance abuse and dependence are difficult challenges in practice and theory when addressing pain management issues in palliative care patients.

- Traditional definitions for defining substance abuse (i.e., those focusing on tolerance and physical dependence) are subpar for application in the medically ill population. Rather, a focus on use despite harm is a better approach for identifying patients at risk.

- It is important to embrace an understanding of aberrant drug-taking as a spectrum of behaviors that can be viewed as potentially problematic by prescribers.

- The use of opioid analgesics in patients without a history of abuse is very unlikely to create a problem unless the patient has genetic, social, and familial vulnerabilities, and a predisposition toward abuse. In essence, we do not "create addicts" simply by prescribing opioids.

- Managing patients with known alcohol or other drug abuse/dependence creates a complex clinical management challenge that is best addressed through a multidisciplinary team approach.

REFERENCES

1   Kirsh KL, Whitcomb LA, Donaghy K, Passik SD. Abuse and addiction issues in medically ill patients with pain: Attempts at clarification of terms and empirical study. *Clin J Pain* 2002; 4(Suppl.): S52–S60.
2   Colliver JD, Kopstein AN. Trends in cocaine abuse reflected in emergency room episodes reported to DAWN. *Publ Health Rep* 1991; 106: 59–68.
3   Groerer J, Brodsky M. The incidence of illicit drug use in the United States, 1962–1989. *Br J Addict* 1992; 87: 1345–1351.
4   Regier DA, Meyers JK, Dramer M et al. The NIMH epidemiologic catchment area program. *Arch Gen Psychiatry* 1984; 41: 934–937.
5   Substance Abuse and Mental Health Services Administration, Results from the 2011 National Survey on Drug Use and Health: Summary of National Findings, NSDUH Series H-44, HHS Publication No. (SMA) 12-4713. Rockville, MD: Substance Abuse and Mental Health Services Administration; 2012.
6   Wells KB, Golding JM, Burnam MA. Chronic medical conditions in a sample of the general population with anxiety, affective, and substance use disorders. *Am J Psychiatry* 1989; 146: 1440–1445.
7   Burton RW, Lyons JS, Devens M, Larson DB. Psychiatric consults for psychoactive substance disorders in the general hospital. *Gen Hosp Psychiatry* 1991; 13: 83–87.
8   Derogatis LR, Morrow GR, Fetting J et al. The prevalence of psychiatric disorders among cancer patients. *JAMA* 1983; 249: 751–758.
9   American Psychiatric Association. *Diagnostic and Statistical Manual for Mental Disorders-III*. Washington, DC: American Psychiatric Association, 1983.
10 Bruera E, Macmillan K, Hanson JA, MacDonald RN. The cognitive effects of the administration of narcotic analgesics in patients with cancer pain. *Pain* 1989; 39: 13–17.

11 Bruera E, Moyano J, Seifert L et al. The frequency of alcoholism among patients with pain due to terminal cancer. *J Pain Symptom Manage* 1995; 10: 599–606.

12 Dole VP. Narcotic addiction, physical dependence and relapse. *N Engl J Med* 1972; 286: 988–994.

13 Martin WR, Jasinski DR. Physiological parameters of morphine dependence in man—Tolerance, early abstinence, protracted abstinence. *J Psychiatr Res* 1969; 7: 9–13.

14 Portenoy RK. Opioid therapy for chronic nonmalignant pain: Current status. In: Fields HL, Liebeskind JC, eds. Progress in pain research and management, Vol. 1. *Pharmacological Approaches to the Treatment of Chronic Pain: New Concepts and Critical Issues.* Seattle, WA: IASP Publications, 1994, pp. 247–249.

15 Portenoy RK. Opioid tolerance and efficacy: Basic research and clinical observations. In: Gebhardt G, Hammond D, Jensen T, eds. *Proceedings of the Seventh World Congress on Pain.* Progress in Pain Research and Management, Vol. 2. Seattle, WA: IASP Press, 1994, pp. 595–597.

16 Foley KM. Clinical tolerance to opioids. In: Basbaum AI, Besson J-M, eds. *Towards a New Pharmacotherapy of Pain.* Chichester, U.K.: John Wiley & Sons, 1991, pp. 181–186.

17 Ling GSF, Paul D, Simantov R, Pasternak GW. Differential development of acute tolerance to analgesia, respiratory depression, gastrointestinal transit and hormone release in a morphine infusion model. *Life Sci* 1989; 45: 1627–1633.

18 Twycross RG. Clinical experience with diamorphine in advanced malignant disease. *Int J Clin Pharmacol Ther Toxicol* 1974; 9: 184–188.

19 Kanner RM, Foley KM. Patterns of narcotic drug use in a cancer pain clinic. *Ann N Y Acad Sci* 1981; 362: 161–167.

20 Chapman CR, Hill HF. Prolonged morphine self-administration and addiction liability: Evaluation of two theories in a bone marrow transplant unit. *Cancer* 1989; 63: 1636–1639.

21 France RD, Urban BJ, Keefe FJ. Longterm use of narcotic analgesics in chronic pain. *Soc Sci Med* 1984; 19: 1379–1385.

22 Portenoy RK, Foley KM. Chronic use of opioid analgesics in nonmalignant pain: Report of 38 cases. *Pain* 1986; 25: 171–175.

23 Urban BJ, France RD, Steinberger DL et al. Longterm use of narcotic antidepressant medication in the management of phantom limb pain. *Pain* 1986; 24: 191–196.

24 Zenz M, Strumpf M, Tryba M. Long-term opioid therapy in patients with chronic nonmalignant pain. *J Pain Symptom Manage* 1992; 7: 69–75.

25 Redmond DE, Krystal JH. Multiple mechanisms of withdrawal from opioid drugs. *Annu Rev Neurosci* 1984; 7: 443–478.

26 Wikler A. *Opioid Dependence: Mechanisms and Treatment.* New York: Plenum Press, 1980.

27 World Health Organization. *Cancer Pain Relief and Palliative Care.* Geneva, Switzerland: World Health Organization, 1990.

28 World Health Organization. *Technical Report No. 516, Youth And Drugs.* Geneva, Switzerland: World Health Organization, 1973.

29 American Psychiatric Association. *Diagnostic and Statistical Manual for Mental Disorders-IV.* Washington, DC: American Psychiatric Association, 1994.

30 Halpern LM, Robinson J. Prescribing practices for pain in drug dependence: A lesson in ignorance. *Adv Alcohol Subst Abuse* 1985; 5: 184–187.

31 Dai S, Corrigal WA, Coen KM, Kalant H. Heroin self-administration by rats: Influence of dose and physical dependence. *Pharmacol Biochem Behav* 1989; 32: 1009–1012.

32 Passik S, Kirsh, KL, McDonald M et al. A pilot survey of aberrant drug-taking attitudes and behaviors in samples of cancer and AIDS patients. *J Pain Symptom Manage* 2000; 19: 274–286.

33 Rinaldi RC, Steindler EM, Wilford BB, Goodwin D. Clarification and standardization of substance abuse terminology. *JAMA* 1988; 259: 555.

34 Passik SD, Kirsh KL, Whitcomb LA et al. A new tool to assess and document pain outcomes in chronic pain patients receiving opioid therapy. *Clin Ther* 2004; 26: 552–561.

35 Hay JL, Passik SD. The cancer patient with borderline personality disorder: Suggestions for symptom-focused management in the medical setting. *Psychooncology* 2000; 9: 91–100.

36 Khantzian EJ, Treece C. DSM-III psychiatric diagnosis of narcotic addicts. *Arch Gen Psychiatry* 1985; 42: 1067–1071.

37 Dunbar SA, Katz NP. Chronic opioid therapy for nonmalignant pain in patients with a history of substance abuse: Report of 20 cases. *J Pain Symptom Manage* 1996; 11: 163–170.

38 Compton P, Darakjian J, Miotto K. Screening for addiction in patients with chronic pain with 'problematic' substance use: Evaluation of a pilot assessment tool. *J Pain Symptom Manage* 1998: 16: 355–363.

39 Jorgensen L, Mortensen M-J, Jensen N-H, Eriksen J. Treatment of cancer pain patients in a multidisciplinary pain clinic. *Pain Clin* 1990; 3: 83–87.

40 Moulin DE, Foley KM. Review of a hospital-based pain service. In: Foley KM, Bonica JJ, Ventafridda V, eds. *Advances in Pain Research and Therapy*, Vol. 16. Second International Congress on Cancer Pain. New York: Raven Press, 1990, pp. 413–420.

41 Schug SA, Zech D, Dorr U. Cancer pain management according to WHO analgesic guidelines. *J Pain Symptom Manage* 1990; 5: 27–33.

42 Schug SA, Zech D, Grond S et al. A long-term survey of morphine in cancer pain patients. *J Pain Symptom Manage* 1992; 7: 259–265.

43 Ventafridda V, Tamburini M, DeConno F. Comprehensive treatment in cancer pain. In: Fields HL, Dubner R, Cervero F, eds. *Advances in Pain Research and Therapy*, Vol. 9. Proceedings of the Fourth World Congress on Pain. New York: Raven Press, 1985, pp. 617–621.

44 Ventafridda V, Tamburini M, Caraceni A et al. A validation study of the WHO method for cancer pain relief. *Cancer* 1990; 59: 850–854.

45 Walker VA, Hoskin PJ, Hanks GW, White ID. Evaluation of WHO analgesic guidelines for cancer pain in a hospital-based palliative care unit. *J Pain Symptom Manage* 1988; 3: 145–153.

46 Health and Public Policy Committee, American College of Physicians. Drug therapy for severe chronic pain in terminal illness. *Ann Intern Med* 1983; 99: 870–876.

47 Ad Hoc Committee on Cancer Pain, American Society of Clinical Oncology. Cancer pain assessment and treatment curriculum guidelines. *J Clin Oncol* 1992; 10: 1976–1984.

48 Agency for Health Care Policy and Research, U.S. Department of Health and Human Services. *Clinical Practice Guideline Number 9: Management of Cancer Pain.* Washington, DC: U.S. Department of Health and Human Services, 1994.

49 American Pain Society. *Principles of Analgesic Use in the Treatment of Acute Pain and Cancer Pain.* Skokie, IL: American Pain Society, 1992.

50 Zech DFJ, Grond S, Lynch J et al. Validation of the World Health Organization Guidelines for cancer pain relief: A 10 year prospective study. *Pain* 1995; 63: 65–68.

51 Kolb L. Types and characteristics of drug addicts. *Ment Hyg* 1925; 9: 300–306.

52 Pescor MJ. *The Kolb Classification of Drug Addicts.* Washington, DC: Public Health Reports Suppl 155, 1939–1942.

53 Rayport M. Experience in the management of patients medically addicted to narcotics. *JAMA* 1954; 156: 684–691.

54 Porter J, Jick H. Addiction rare in patients treated with narcotics. *N Engl J Med* 1980; 302: 123–124.

55 Perry S, Heidrich G. Management of pain during debridement: A survey of U.S. burn units. *Pain* 1982; 13: 267–272.

56 Medina JL, Diamond S. Drug dependency in patients with chronic headache. *Headache* 1977; 17: 12–16.

57 Kaiko RF, Foley KM, Grabinski PY et al. Central nervous system excit-atory effects of meperidine in cancer patients. *Ann Neurol* 1983; 13: 180–187.

58 Grove WM, Eckert ED, Heston L et al. Heritability of substance abuse and antisocial behavior: A study of monozygotic twins reared apart. *Biol Psychiatry* 1990; 27: 1293–1297.

59 Gardner-Nix JS. Oral methadone for managing chronic nonmalignant pain. *J Pain Symptom Manage* 1996; 11: 321–328.

60 Potter JS, Hennessy G, Borrow JA et al. Substance use histories in patients seeking treatment for controlled-release oxycodone depen-dence. *Drug Alcohol Depend* 2004; 76: 213–215.

61 Meuser T, Pietruck C, Radruch L et al. Symptoms during cancer pain treatment following WHO guidelines: A longitudinal follow-up study of symptom prevalence, severity, and etiology. *Pain* 2001; 93: 247–257.

62 McCarberg BH, Barkin RC. Long-acting opioids for chronic pain: Pharmacotherapeutic opportunities to enhance compliance, quality of life, and analgesia. *Am J Ther* 2001; 8: 181–186.

63 Aronoff GM. Opioids in chronic pain management: Is there a significant risk of addiction? *Curr Rev Pain* 2000; 4: 112–121.

64 Macaluso C, Weinberg D, Foley KM. Opioid abuse and misuse in a cancer pain population [abstract]. *J Pain Symptom Manage* 1988; 3: S24–S25.

65 Gonzales GR, Coyle N. Treatment of cancer pain in a former opioid abuser: Fears of the patient and staff and their influence on care. *J Pain Symptom Manage* 1992; 7: 246–249.

66 Kaplan R, Slywka J, Slagle S et al. A titrated analgesic regimen com-paring substance users and non-users with AIDS-related pain. *J Pain Symptom Manage* 2000; 19: 265–271.

67 Lundberg JC, Passik SD. Alcohol and cancer: A review for psycho-oncol-ogists. *Psychooncology* 1997; 6: 253–266.

68 Regier DA, Farmer ME, Rae, DS et al. Comorbidity of mental disorders with alcohol and other drug abuse. *JAMA* 1985; 264: 2511–2518.

69 Penick E, Powell B, Nickel E et al. Comorbidity of lifetime psychiat-ric disorders among male alcoholics. *Alcohol Clin Exp Res* 1994; 18: 1289–1293.

70 Kirsh KL, Passik SD. The interface between pain and drug abuse the evolution of strategies to optimize pain management while minimizing drug abuse. *Exp Clin Psychopharmacol* 2008; 16(5): 400–404.

71 Passik SD, Portenoy RK. Substance abuse issues in palliative care. In: Berger A, Portenoy R, Weissman D, eds. *Principles and Practice of Supportive Oncology*. Philadephia, PA: Lippincott Raven Publishers, 1998.

72 Passik S, Schreiber J, Kirsh KL et al. A chart review of the ordering and documentation of urine toxicology screens in a cancer center: Do they influence patient management? *J Pain Symptom Manage* 2000; 19: 40–44.

73 Parrino M. State methadone treatment guidelines. TIPS 1 DHHS Publication No. (SMA) 93-1991. Washington, DC.

74 Passik S, Theobald D. Managing addiction in advanced cancer patients: Why bother? *J Pain Symptom Manage* 2000; 19: 229–234.

PART 9

Gastrointestinal systems

56

Pathophysiology of cachexia–anorexia syndrome

EGIDIO DEL FABBRO

INTRODUCTION

The cachexia–anorexia syndrome (CAS) is a multifactorial syndrome characterized by involuntary loss of skeletal muscle and fat, reduced quality of life, and decreased survival. Unlike starvation, the loss of weight in the CAS cannot be fully reversed by nutritional support (Table 56.1.). This chapter describes the complex interactions between disease and host that leads to variable combinations of increased resting energy expenditure (REE), inhibition of protein synthesis, proteolysis, lipolysis, and dysregulation of neurohormonal mechanisms to enhance appetite.

The CAS is a marker for poor prognosis and is psychologically distressing[1] for both patients and their families.[2] The syndrome impairs physical function, body image, and sense of self.[3] Although typically associated with cancer, cachexia is also common to many seemingly disparate chronic illnesses such as AIDS, COPD HIV, tuberculosis and malaria, rheumatoid arthritis, COPD,[4] congestive heart failure,[5] kidney failure,[6] and liver failure. There are very few studies in the scientific literature investigating large population samples, but an estimated 5 million people in the United States alone may be coping with cachexia.[7]

The considerable variation in the prevalence of cachexia depends on the disease type and the clinical definition of the CAS, for example, more inclusive definitions of cancer cachexia suggest a prevalence of 85% in patients with advanced cancer, which decreases to 12% when using alternate diagnostic criteria.[8] Cachexia is reported to range from about 10% in conditions such as CHF[9] to about 80% in patients with specific tumor types such as pancreatic and gastric cancers.[10] However, despite the high prevalence, patients with pancreatic cancer do not universally experience cachexia; this may be due to variations in the genotype of the host or the phenotype of the tumor.[11] In a large study of more than 3000 patients, one third of patients with pancreatic or gastric cancer experienced weight loss >10%, although it is noteworthy that any weight loss was associated with poorer prognosis.[5] Despite heterogeneity in the prevalence of cachexia and its effect on morbidity and mortality among the different disease states, there is substantial evidence for similar mechanisms causing the CAS.

These common mechanisms are important therapeutic targets since a successful intervention for the syndrome could be applicable to patients with different chronic illnesses.

PRIMARY CACHEXIA AND SECONDARY CAUSES OF WEIGHT LOSS

The cause of weight loss and poor appetite is likely to be multifactorial within each individual patient. The concepts of primary cachexia and secondary causes of weight loss are useful clinically but may also be relevant for distinguishing the mechanisms of the CAS. Primary cachexia refers to the direct effects of the disease (e.g., by tumor and tumor products) as well as the host response to the disease, for example, chronic inflammation. Secondary causes are additional factors that decrease appetite and food intake or exacerbate fat and muscle loss. These include treatable contributors to the weight loss of primary cachexia such as nutritional impact symptoms (NIS) and comorbid metabolic abnormalities (e.g., adrenal insufficiency, thyroid dysfunction, and vitamin B12 deficiency). Other causes of weight loss that have a predominant starvation component such as gastrointestinal obstruction are also included in the category of secondary causes and may be amenable to endoscopic (e.g., stent placement or dilatation) or surgical treatment. Table 56.1 shows some of the key differences between primary cachexia and pure starvation.

Weight loss in patients with cachexia will occur despite caloric supplementation and can be differentiated from starvation by hormonal abnormalities such as insulin and ghrelin resistance and frequently also by increased REE. Unfortunately, patients with cancer and weight loss often have a combination of primary cachexia and additional secondary causes that exacerbate decreased caloric intake, such as uncontrolled symptoms. Nutrition impact symptoms in these patients may include nausea, vomiting, constipation, diarrhea, defecation after meal (dumping syndrome), severe pain, dyspnea, anxiety or depression, stomatitis, dysgeusia, difficulty chewing, xerostomia, and dysphagia. A retrospective study from a cachexia clinic at a comprehensive cancer center found that most patients with involuntary weight loss had three or more uncontrolled NIS.[12] Finally, even though the

Table 56.1 *Starvation versus cachexia*

	Starvation	Cachexia
Caloric intake	↓↓	↓
REE	↓	↓↑ or ↔
Body fat	↓↓	↓
Lean body mass	↓	↓
Acute phase reactants	↔	↑ or ↔
Insulin	↓	↑

↔ Unchanged
↓ Reduce
↓↓ Markedly reduced
↓↑ Increased or reduced
↑ Increased

categories of primary cachexia and secondary causes of weight loss are a useful clinical framework, a symptom such as early satiety may be more difficult to categorize as either primary or secondary since the etiology of this particular symptom may be quite varied and could include the anorexigenic neuropeptidergic effects of cytokines, autonomic dysfunction (AD) producing gastroparesis, organomegaly due to tumor burden, and severe constipation.

MECHANISMS OF THE CACHEXIA–ANOREXIA SYNDROME (FIGURE 56.1)

The mechanisms causing weight loss, poor appetite, and wasting of muscle and fat in patients with chronic illness are multifactorial. However, none of the mechanisms that contribute to this syndrome should be viewed in isolation since they are all interrelated. They include inflammation, endocrine abnormalities, autonomic nervous system (ANS) dysfunction, NIS, and disease-specific factors as illustrated in Figure 56.1.

Although there are multiple mechanisms causing the CAS, an aberrant proinflammatory response to chronic disease has been proposed as the unifying, dominant mechanism since inflammation has extensive, detrimental effects on cell metabolism, protein synthesis, endocrine homeostasis, and the ANS.

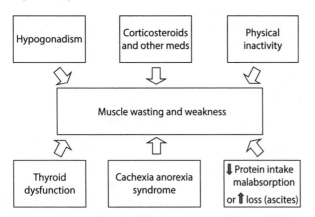

Figure 56.1 *Contributors to muscle wasting in patients with chronic illness. CRP, C-reactive protein; PIF, proteolysis-inducing factor; ROS, reactive oxygen species; TNF, tumor necrosis factor; ZAG, zinc α-2 glycoprotein.*

Inflammation

CYTOKINES

Chronic inflammation and cytokines are associated with sickness behavior and a variety of symptoms including fatigue, depression, and anorexia. Chronic inflammation also has effects peripherally on skeletal muscle and adipose tissue causing catabolism and decreased anabolism. Cytokines are small proteins produced by a variety of cells including lymphocytes and macrophages that act as intercellular messengers, influencing the brain, peripheral muscle, and fat. These humoral messengers are important modulators of the immune system along with cellular mechanisms and neural circuits.[13]

Peripheral effects

Although skeletal muscle wasting in patients with chronic disease is multifactorial (Figure 56.2), specific cytokines such as interleukin (IL)-6, tumor necrosis factor (TNF), and Interferon (INF)-λ are implicated in the pathogenesis. Proinflammatory cytokines can induce wasting by targeting particular skeletal muscle gene products. Skeletal muscle is composed of core myofibrillar proteins, including myosin heavy chain (MyHC), actin, troponin, and tropomyosin. Transcription of the MyHC gene and many other muscle genes is regulated in part by the nuclear transcription factor MyoD. Myogenic cell cultures and animal models of tumor-induced cachexia show MyHC to be a selective target for procachectic inflammatory cytokines by inhibiting MyoD (via TNF-α and IFN-γ) and activating the ligase-dependent ubiquitin–proteasome pathway (via IL-6).[14] The ubiquitin ligase-dependent proteasome pathway is a major cellular mechanism that degrades proteins and regulates skeletal muscle wasting in cancer and other disease states. The preferential loss of the MyHC relative to troponin, tropomyosin, and actin may alter the ratio between thick and thin filaments, possibly inducing further atrophy in order to restore balance to the functional contractile lattice.[15] These preclinical studies suggest that at least a dual combination of inflammatory cytokines is necessary for muscle wasting. This premise is supported by recent clinical trials using single-agent etanercept[16] or infliximab[17] that produced no improvement in cachexia-related clinical outcomes.

More recent studies have also revealed that lipolysis plays an important role in the pathogenesis of muscle wasting associated with cancer cachexia. Animal models show that muscle wasting induced by circulating cytokines may be modulated by genetic ablation of adipose triglyceride lipase (ATL).[18] Animals with and without ATL activity were injected with tumor cells, resulting in high circulating levels of inflammatory cytokines such as IL-6, TNF-α, and lipid-mobilizing factor (ZAG) in both groups. However, only the animals with ATL activity experienced adipose tissue wasting and subsequent muscle loss accompanied by an increased expression of the ubiquitin–proteasome pathway (Figure 56.3).

Cytokines have other actions that promote catabolism and decrease anabolism including insulin resistance, the production of reactive oxygen species (ROS), acute phase proteins, and increased REE.

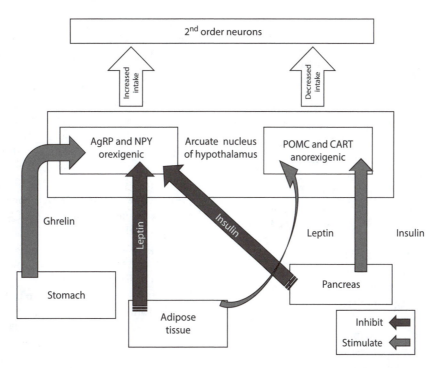

Figure 56.2   *Hormones regulating appetite. AgRP, agouti-related protein; CART, cocaine- and amphetamine-regulated transcript; NPY, neuropeptide Y.*

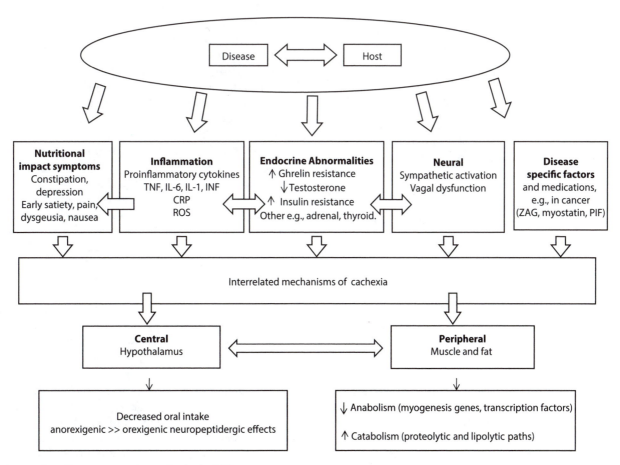

Figure 56.3   *Contributors to muscle wasting in the CAS.*

Central effects

Systemic proinflammatory cytokines stimulate the expression of cytokines within the hypothalamus and can also influence the brain through second messengers such as nitric oxide, prostanoids, or neural pathways.[19] Reciprocal circadian rhythms of two peripheral hormones, anorexigenic leptin from adipocytes and orexigenic ghrelin from the stomach, are major afferent signals for the appetite-regulating network in the hypothalamus[20] (see Figure 56.2). Cytokines produce effects that mimic the anorexigenic signals of leptin and suppress orexigenic signals from neuropeptides such as ghrelin and agouti-related peptide (AgRP). Proinflammatory cytokines are also implicated in causing anorexia by stimulating neural pathways within the arcuate nucleus of the hypothalamus to secrete anorexigenic peptides such as α-melanocyte-stimulating hormone (α-MSH).[21] α-MSH inhibits feeding and increases energy expenditure by activating melanocortin receptors, primarily the type 4 melanocortin receptor (MC4-R). Agouti-related peptide (AgRP) is an endogenous antagonist that binds to MC4-R, thereby inhibiting the effect of anorexigenic melanocortin peptides. The expression of AgRP is stimulated by fasting, by gastric ghrelin crossing the blood brain barrier, and by locally produced hypothalamic ghrelin and is inhibited by leptin. In mice with renal cachexia, central administration of AgRP increases weight and lean body mass and decreases the proinflammatory cytokines within the muscle.[22] In healthy animals, orally administered selective MC4-R antagonists that penetrate the blood–brain barrier increase food intake, and in mice with C26 adenocarcinoma, selective MC4-R antagonists prevent tumor-induced loss of body weight, fat mass, and lean body mass.[23] One possible mechanism whereby central nervous system signaling alone can induce a catabolic process in muscle is via interleukin 1β (IL-1β). The process is dependent on hypothalamic-pituitary-adrenal (HPA) axis activation, since CNS IL-1β-induced atrophy is abolished by adrenalectomy.[24] Activation of the HPA axis appears to be an integral part of the catabolic response to inflammation in that glucocorticoids probably act in concert with cytokines to promote muscle atrophy. There is also prior experimental evidence that leukemia inhibitory factor[25] and IL-6[26] can stimulate pituitary corticotrophs directly, leading to the release of ACTH independent of hypothalamic signaling. In addition, cytokines also have other central effects that decrease oral intake indirectly by generating symptoms such as early satiety (via IL-1)[27] and depression (IL-6).[28]

Clinical studies and proinflammatory cytokines

Although cytokines are important in the pathogenesis of cachexia and could prove to be useful therapeutic targets, the relationship between serum cytokines and clinical outcomes is inconsistent.

Several clinical studies have demonstrated an association between cancer cachexia and elevated serum cytokines. Compared to noncachectic lung cancer patients, those with >5% weight loss within 6 months displayed elevated TNF-α serum levels and increased TNF-α gene expression in peripheral blood mononuclear cells.[29] Another prospective study in newly diagnosed Non Small Cell Lung Cancer (NSCLC) patients[30] found IL-6 was increased and correlated with poor nutritional status, impaired performance status, and shorter survival. A study of pancreatic cancer patients at MD Anderson similarly found[31] that high IL-6, IL-10, and IL-8 serum levels were associated with poor performance status and/or weight loss, compared to healthy volunteers. Also in patients with advanced prostate cancer, the serum[32] levels of TNF α, IL-6, and IL-8 were elevated in those with cachexia, compared to those without cachexia. Finally, there are preliminary studies showing inhibition of specific proinflammatory cytokines improves clinical outcomes. A review[33] of small, early-phase clinical trials that used monoclonal antibodies (mAb) to IL-6 in patients with multiple myeloma, renal cell carcinoma, and B-lymphoproliferative disorders concluded that anti-IL-6 mAb treatment decreased C-reactive protein (CRP) levels and the incidence of cachexia.

Other investigators have not found significant correlations between proinflammatory serum cytokines and weight loss.[34] A recent study of NSCLC[35] patients with weight loss ≥10% compared to those with <10% showed TNF-α and IL-6 levels did not differ between groups. A Japanese study in cachectic gastric and colorectal patients found production of IL-12 was lowest in the patients with distant metastasis and cachexia, but levels of IL4, IL-6, and IL-10 did not differ significantly.[36] Lastly, a multi-institutional cachexia trial found little clinical utility in measuring serum cytokines.[37] Baseline serum IL-6 predicted a diminished survival only after adjustment for age and cancer site, while no correlations were observed between serum cytokine concentrations (IL-6, TNF α, IL-1) and changes in weight or appetite.

Local rather than systemic cytokine production may be important for muscle atrophy. In precachectic lung cancer patients, CRP levels were elevated and associated with reduced exercise capacity despite maintenance of muscle mass and unaltered Ubiquitin Proteasome System (UPS) or nuclear factor κB (NF-κB)-dependent activation on muscle biopsy. The investigators hypothesize that transition of systemic to local inflammation is required to initiate the UPS-dependent muscle wasting of cachexia.[38] A study comparing cancer patients with and without cachexia to noncancer patients found plasma levels of TNF-α were not significantly elevated in cachectic patients, and no correlation was found between TNF-α and weight loss or appetite scores. Again, the authors suggested that TNF-α may act in a paracrine rather than an endocrine fashion and that serum levels may not accurately reflect tissue concentrations.[39] Similarly, the relationship between serum cytokines and cachexia in patients with COPD is unclear, since recent studies have shown no association between clinical outcomes and elevated levels of IL-6 or TNF-α.[40]

Other reasons for the inconsistent relationship between cachexia and serum cytokine levels include differences in tumor phenotype, tumor stage, type of cytokine assays, or a genetic variation in the immune response.[41] In future, a genetic predisposition to systemic inflammation and cachexia could be identified through gene polymorphisms, allowing treatment to be initiated earlier, thereby improving the chances of a therapeutic response. Candidates include single-nucleotide polymorphisms (SNPs) of IL-6, TNF, and IL-10.[42] However, a large exploratory study of 1853 patients found no associations with loss of appetite and 93 SNP candidates that had potential for a genetic predisposition.[43]

C-REACTIVE PROTEIN

CRP is a useful prognostic marker in a variety of cancers and appears to be a good surrogate marker for IL-6.[44] An elevated preoperative serum level of CRP is an independent prognostic factor for patients with colorectal cancer[45] and hepatocellular cancer,[46] and a CRP-based prognostic score predicts survival in patients with metastatic renal cancer[47] and in metastatic breast cancer.[48] There are recent studies that suggest CRP is more than a marker and that it may play an active role in the development of inflammation[49] and fibrosis associated with chronic disease.[50] In a study of 226 patients with upper gastrointestinal malignancy, dietary intake serum CRP concentrations and stage of disease were identified as independent variables in determining degree of weight loss.[51] Similarly, in patients with inoperable non-small cell lung cancer, an increase in CRP was associated with increased weight loss and reduced albumin, performance status, and survival.[52]

NF-κB

NF-κB is a transcriptional factor that regulates the expression of many genes involved in inflammation including cyclooxygenase inhibitors (COX-2), nitric oxide synthase, TNFα, and IL-6. NF-κB is also involved in many aspects of oncogenesis and apoptosis and is considered a potential antitumor target, even though NF-κB inhibition carries a theoretical risk of immunosuppression, given its critical role in innate and adaptive immune responses.[53] As regards muscle atrophy, TNF-α inhibits myogenesis in vitro by activating NF-κB, which leads to degradation of MyoD transcripts.[54] More recently in a mouse model of cancer cachexia, two novel drugs were tested that specifically inhibited NF-κB by targeting the IκB kinase (IKK) complex. The drugs prevented the development of tumor-induced systolic dysfunction and atrophy.[55] NF-κB also appears to be essential in the proteolysis-inducing factor (PIF)-induced expression of the ubiquitin–proteasome pathway.[56]

Muscle atrophy

Muscle wasting associated with cachexia is caused by a decrease in protein synthesis and an increase in protein degradation or a combination of both.[57] In addition to the UPS discussed earlier that degrades the MyHC, there are at least three other proteolytic pathways that degrade muscle including lysosomal, calcium-dependent, and caspase-dependent paths.[58] Positive regulators of muscle growth such as insulin-like growth factor 1 (IGF-1) are downregulated in cachexia while negative regulators such as myostatin are upregulated. Growth hormone (GH) regulates liver IGF-1 expression with downstream anabolic effects on skeletal muscle. In a

hepatoma animal model, IGF-1 administration attenuated the development of cachexia and improved quality of life and survival.[59] Other factors such as angiotensin II have also been shown to downregulate anabolism produced by IGF-1.[60] The regulating factors for muscle catabolism and anabolism are influenced by various factors derived from both tumor/disease and host, including inflammation, cations such as Ca^{2+} and Mg^{2+}, cytokines, exercise, and hormones.

MYOSTATIN

In addition to proinflammatory cytokines (discussed earlier), the extracellular cytokine myostatin plays an important role in negatively regulating muscle mass. Myostatin mutations in animals and humans[61] result in dramatic hypertrophy of muscle and improved strength. Myostatin upregulation has been observed in the pathogenesis of muscle wasting associated with different diseases (i.e., cancer, heart failure, HIV).[62] Active myostatin binds to the activin type IIB (ActRIIB) cell membrane receptor leading to the inhibition of transcription factors such as myoD. There are at least four other extracellular inhibitors that can prevent binding of myostatin to the ActRIIB receptor, including follistatin and growth and differentiation factor-associated serum protein 1 (GASP-1). Recently, myostatin was shown to be secreted experimentally by C26 colon cancer cells. Exposure to C26 medium resulted in myotubular atrophy due to the upregulation of muscle-specific E3 ligases, atrogin-1 and MuRF1 (muscle RING-finger protein 1), and enhanced activity of the ubiquitin–proteasome pathway. The C26 conditioned medium (CM) also activated ActRIIB/Smad and NF-κB signaling and reduced the activity of the IGF-1/phosphoinositide 3-kinase (PI3K)/Akt pathway. Antagonists to myostatin prevented C26 CM-induced wasting in muscle cell cultures.[63] Future therapeutic targets for muscle wasting associated with cachexia could include either myostatin or the ActRIIB receptor.[64]

Fat atrophy

Body fat is lost more rapidly than lean tissue in progressive cancer cachexia.[65] Similar to muscle atrophy, the loss of adipose tissue results partly from reduced food intake as well as from tumor factors and systemic inflammatory cytokines that either inhibit lipogenesis or promote lipolysis. Samples of white adipose tissue in patients with cancer cachexia showed fat cell size was decreased but adipocyte numbers were normal, suggesting that there was no major fat cell death.[66] Preliminary studies show the expression and secretion of an adipokine zinc-α2-glycoprotein (ZAG) is increased in cachectic cancer patients and correlates with weight loss. Recombinant ZAG was also found to stimulate lipolysis in human adipocytes.[67]

Anabolic hormones

A relative deficiency or resistance to anabolic hormones such as testosterone, insulin, and ghrelin contributes to the muscle wasting and poor appetite associated with cachexia.

GHRELIN

Ghrelin is a 28-amino acid peptide produced by gastric endocrine cells[68] that increases appetite and gastrointestinal motility and reduces inflammation. Besides its GH-secretagogue activity, ghrelin is the only orexigenic circulating hormone that has been identified in humans,[69] and fasting plasma ghrelin levels are inversely related to body mass index.[70] Ghrelin also appears to inhibit muscle atrophy by another mechanism that is independent of GH[71] and is able to counteract angiotensin-induced muscle catabolism in a mouse model.[72] Individuals with caloric restriction or anorexia nervosa have markedly elevated fasting levels of ghrelin that return to normal when body weight increases.[73] Similarly, patients with cancer cachexia have increased active ghrelin levels, likely as a compensatory response to weight loss.[74] In spite of the elevated levels, there appears to be a resistance to ghrelin's orexigenic effects in patients with cachexia. In animals with cancer-induced cachexia, ghrelin has been shown to reduce fat oxidation and increase adiposity, caloric intake, and body weight.[75] Ghrelin may modulate other mechanisms that contribute to cachexia, including inflammation[76] and gastroparesis[77] by stimulating gastric emptying, small intestinal transit, and fecal output, while decreasing IL-6, TNF-α, and the anorectic effect of IL-1.

ANDROGENS

Androgens exert both direct and indirect anabolic effects on muscle. Testosterone and other androgens directly increase muscle mass and strength by augmenting the synthesis of myosin[78] and perhaps by also upregulating the expression of the androgen receptor. Other indirect mechanisms include antiglucocorticoid effects and interactions with the GH/IGF-1 axis since testosterone treatment increases muscle IGF-1 levels.[79] Newly diagnosed male patients with cancer that have low testosterone and low luteinizing hormone levels (suggestive of secondary hypogonadism) have significantly greater weight loss than those with normal testosterone. Low testosterone levels are associated with a poor prognosis in male patients with cancer cachexia,[80] and cross-sectional studies have also shown associations with poor appetite,[81] decreased quality of life, and fatigue. Various medications that are used for the control of symptoms in palliative care can cause hypogonadism including glucocorticoids, megestrol acetate,[82] and opioids.

INSULIN

Although insulin decreases appetite centrally, it has peripheral anabolic effects on muscle and adipose tissue. Insulin has a major role in controlling muscle proteolysis, and increases in endogenous insulin result in a decrease in muscle protein degradation[83] by the ubiquitin–proteasome pathway. Cachexia is typically associated with insulin resistance in animal models[84] and in humans,[85] and exogenous administration improves clinical outcomes such as survival and quality of life in cancer cachexia.[86]

Catabolic hormones

Disruption of endocrine homeostasis plays a key role in skeletal muscle atrophy and the disequilibrium between anabolic and catabolic signaling pathways in cancer, COPD, and CHF. Neurohormonal activation is implicated in the development of cardiac cachexia, since patients have been shown to have markedly increased norepinephrine levels compared with noncachectic CHF patients.[87] Additional features suggesting the presence of a catabolic/anabolic imbalance was a twofold increase in cortisol levels and decreased levels of the anabolic steroid dehydroepiandrosterone. Preclinical experiments with cardiac cachexia animal models have identified aldosterone as an important mediator of muscle wasting. Aldosterone/salt treatment (ALDOST) is known to produce a chronic immunostimulatory stressor state.[88] Rats given ALDOST, in order to mimic the elevated plasma ALDOST levels found in human CHF, experienced muscle wasting over 4 weeks.[89] Muscle atrophy in these animal models was associated with a downregulation of IGF-1, increased intracellular Ca^{2+} and ROS, and upregulation of the UPS. Weight gain and muscle recovery was seen after the withdrawal of ALDOST. Epinephrine and norepinephrine are known to play key roles in lipolysis, but more recently, B-type natriuretic peptide (BNP) has also been shown to induce lipolysis in patients with CHF. Lipolysis by BNP_{1-32} is increased in CHF patients compared with control subjects, which suggests that BNP might play an important role in excessive free fatty acids (FFA) mobilization and related metabolic abnormalities that include cardiac cachexia.[90] In patients with cardiac cachexia, ZAG levels correlate with circulating levels of FFA and norepinephrine, suggesting the downstream involvement of ZAG in sympathetic-mediated lipolysis.[91]

Increased resting energy expenditure

Increased REE may represent an increase in futile metabolic cycles such as the Cori cycle (which converts the large amount of lactate produced by the tumor back to glucose in the liver) or may be due to an increased expression and activity of mitochondrial uncoupling proteins, which are involved in the control of energy metabolism and cause increased thermogenesis. Increased REE is more likely to be associated with particular tumor types[92] and is also found in some patients without evidence of metastatic disease.[93] Similar abnormalities have been reported in patients with CHF,[94] rheumatoid arthritis,[95] and kidney failure. Underweight COPD patients had increased REE, reduced serum and adipose tissue leptin, and increased serum adiponectin, suggesting adipokines play a role in the energy imbalance of COPD-related cachexia.[96]

Reactive oxygen species

Although ROS are present in the body as normal products of O_2 energy metabolism, they are potentially toxic, and, therefore, the human body has a complex system of endogenous antioxidants to protect against the oxidative damage mediated by ROS. Endogenous antioxidants include enzymes such as glutathione peroxidase, catalase, and superoxide dismutase as well as non-enzymatic defenses, such as glutathione, histidine peptides, the iron-binding proteins transferrin and ferritin, lipoic acid, reduced coenzyme Q10 (CoQ10), melatonin, urate, and plasma proteinthiols.[97] ROS are activated by a number of cachexia mechanisms and are potent activators of the NF-κB signaling cascade. There is experimental and clinical evidence for the role of ROS in cachexia. ROS oxidize proteins and modulate the proteasomal system in rat models of cancer cachexia.[98] Animals inoculated with tumor cells had increased muscle wasting, lipid hydroperoxide, and superoxide dismutase and decreased antioxidant glutathione levels and total radical antioxidant capacity, with increased mRNA atrogin-1 expression. Other experiments in cachectic mouse models[99] have shown decreased activity of antioxidant enzymes are responsible for elevated superoxide levels in skeletal muscle. Another link, between ROS and purine metabolism may play a role in cancer cachexia, since xanthine oxidase inhibition reduces inflammatory signals, ROS, proteolytic activity, and tissue degradation in an animal model of cachexia.[100]

In humans, some clinical trials have incorporated antioxidants as part of multimodality therapy, showing improved lean body mass and spontaneous physical activity in patients with cancer cachexia.[101] Potent antioxidants such as melatonin demonstrated promise in open-label trials[102] but were not effective in a recent double-blind placebo-controlled study.[103]

Autonomic nervous system dysfunction

Clinical manifestations of AD are well described in patients with advanced cancer,[104] rheumatoid arthritis, HIV, CHF,[105,106] and COPD.[107] Whether the gastrointestinal (chronic nausea and early satiety) and cardiovascular (postural hypotension, fixed heart rate) manifestation represent the same underlying mechanism is unknown. Vagal nerve dysfunction can contribute to the CAS through gastroparesis, disruption of neurohormonal feeding signals, and proinflammatory effects.[108] Compared to normal volunteers, patients with cancer cachexia have a global reduction in heart rate variability parameters[109] affecting parasympathetic and sympathetic components. However, despite the high prevalence of AD, a cross-sectional study in patients with advanced cancer found no associations between AD and weight loss, history of diabetes, history of chronic heart failure, and previous neurotoxic chemotherapy.[110]

CONCLUSION

The pathophysiology of the CAS is characterized by a complex cascade of multiple interrelated mechanisms that include the secretion of tumor products and cytokines, an aberrant proinflammatory response, neuroendocrine dysregulation, ANS failure, diminished appetite, and increased muscle proteolysis and lipolysis. Future interventions for this syndrome are likely to require a multimodal therapeutic approach that targets the mechanisms simultaneously.

REFERENCES

1   Hopkinson JB. The emotional aspects of cancer anorexia. *Curr Opin Support Palliat Care* December 2010;4(4):254–258.

2   McClement S. Cancer anorexia-cachexia syndrome: Psychological effect on the patient and family. *J Wound Ostomy Continence Nurs* July–August 2005;32(4):264–268.

3   Chochinov HM, Hack T, Hassard T, Kristjanson LJ, McClement S, Harlos M. Dignity in the terminally ill: A cross-sectional, cohort study. *Lancet* December 2002;360(9350):2026–2030.

4   Schols AM, Broekhuizen R, Weling-Scheepers CA, Wouters EF. Body composition and mortality in chronic obstructive pulmonary disease. *Am J Clin Nutr* July 2005;82(1):53–59.

5   von Haehling S, Lainscak M, Springer J, Anker SD. Cardiac cachexia: A systematic overview. *Pharmacol Ther* March 2009;121(3):227–252.

6   Cheung WW, Paik KH, Mak RH. Inflammation and cachexia in chronic kidney disease. *Pediatr Nephrol* 2010;25:711–724.

7   Morley JE, Thomas DR, Wilson MM. Cachexia: Pathophysiology and clinical relevance. *Am J Clin Nutr* 2006;83(4):735–743.

8   Wallengren O, Lundholm K, Bosaeus I. Diagnostic criteria of cancer cachexia: Relation to quality of life, exercise capacity and survival in unselected palliative care patients *Support Care Cancer* January 13, 2013;21:1569–1577.

9   Christensen HM, Kistorp C, Schou M, Keller N, Zerahn B, Frystyk J, Schwarz P, Faber J. Prevalence of cachexia in chronic heart failure and characteristics of body composition and metabolic status. *Endocrine* June 2013;43(3):626–634.

10 Dewys WD, Begg C, Lavin PT et al. Prognostic effect of weight loss prior to chemotherapy in cancer patients. Eastern Cooperative Oncology Group. *Am J Med* October 1980;69(4):491–497.

11 Monitto CL, Berkowitz D, Lee KM, Pin S, Li D, Breslow M, O'Malley B, Schiller M. Differential gene expression in a murine model of cancer cachexia. *Am J Physiol Endocrinol Metab* August 2001;281(2):E289–E297.

12 Del Fabbro E, Hui D, Dalal S, Dev R, Nooruddin ZI, Bruera E. Clinical outcomes and contributors to weight loss in a cancer cachexia clinic. *J Palliat Med* September 2011;14(9):1004–1008.

13 Andersson U, Tracey KJ. Neural reflexes in inflammation and immunity. *J Exp Med* 2012;209:1057–1068.

14 Acharyya S, Ladner KJ, Nelsen LL et al. Cancer cachexia is regulated by selective targeting of skeletal muscle gene products. *J Clin Invest* August 2004;114(3):370–378.

15 Chamberlain JS. Cachexia in cancer—Zeroing in on myosin. *N Engl J Med* November 2004;351(20):2124–2125.

16 Jatoi A, Dakhil SR, Nguyen PL et al. A placebo-controlled double-blind trial of etanercept for the cancer anorexia/weight loss syndrome: Results from N00C1 from the North Central Cancer Treatment Group. *Cancer* September 2007;110(6):1396–1403.

17 Wiedenmann B, Malfertheiner P, Friess H et al. A multicenter, phase II study of infliximab plus gemcitabine in pancreatic cancer cachexia. *J Support Oncol* January 2008;6(1):18–25.

18 Das SK, Eder S, Schauer S et al. Adipose triglyceride lipase contributes to cancer-associated cachexia. *Science* 2011;333:233–238.

19 Inui A. Cancer anorexia-cachexia syndrome: Are neuropeptides the key? *Cancer Res* September 15, 1999;59(18):4493–4501.

20 Kalra SP, Ueno N, Kalra PS. Stimulation of appetite by ghrelin is regulated by leptin restraint: Peripheral and central sites of action. *J Nutr* May 2005;135(5):1331–1335.

21 Grossberg AJ, Scarlett JM, Marks DL. Hypothalamic mechanisms in cachexia. *Physiol Behav* July 14, 2010;100(5):478–489.

22 Cheung WW, Mak RH. Melanocortin antagonism ameliorates muscle wasting and inflammation in chronic kidney disease. *Am J Physiol Renal Physiol* November 1, 2012;303(9):F1315–F1324.

23 Weyermann P, Dallmann R, Magyar J et al. Orally available selective melanocortin-4 receptor antagonists stimulate food intake and reduce cancer-induced cachexia in mice. *PLoS One* 2009;4(3):e4774.

24 Braun TP, Zhu X, Szumowski M et al. Central nervous system inflammation induces muscle atrophy via activation of the hypothalamic-pituitary-adrenal axis. *J Exp Med* November 21, 2011;208(12):2449–2463.

25 Akita S, Webster J, Ren SG et al. Human and murine pituitary expression of leukemia inhibitory factor. Novel intrapituitary regulation of adrenocorticotropin hormone synthesis and secretion. *J Clin Invest* 1995;95:1288–1298.

26 Bethin KE, Vogt SK, Muglia LJ. Interleukin-6 is an essential, corticotropin-releasing hormone-independent stimulator of the adrenal axis during immune system activation. *Proc Natl Acad Sci USA* August 1, 2000;97(16):9317–9322.

27 McCarthy DO, Daun JM. The role of prostaglandins in interleukin-1 induced gastroparesis. *Physiol Behav* 1992;52(2):351–353.

28 Lutgendorf SK, Weinrib AZ, Penedo F et al. Interleukin-6,cortisol, and depressive symptoms in ovarian cancer patients. *J Clin Oncol* 2008;26(29):4820–4827.

29 Fortunati N, Manti R, Birocco N et al. Pro-inflammatory cytokines and oxidative stress/antioxidant parameters characterize the biohumoral profile of early cachexia in lung cancer patients. *Oncol Rep* 2007;18(6):1521–1527.

30 Martin F, Santolaria F, Batista N et al. Cytokine levels (IL-6 and IFN-gamma), acute phase response and nutritional status as prognostic factors in lung cancer. *Cytokine* 1999;11(1):80–86.

31 Ebrahimi B, Tucker SL, Li D, Abbruzzese JL, Kurzrock R. Cytokines in pancreatic carcinoma: Correlation with phenotypic characteristics and prognosis. *Cancer* 2004;101(12):2727–2736.

32 Pfitzenmaier J, Vessella R, Higano CS, Noteboom JL, Wallace D Jr, Corey E. Elevation of cytokine levels in cachectic patients with prostate carcinoma. *Cancer* 2003;97(5):1211–1216.

33 Trikha M, Corringham R, Klein B, Rossi JF. Targeted anti-interleukin-6 monoclonal antibody therapy for cancer: A review of the rationale and clinical evidence. *Clin Cancer Res* 2003;9(13):4653–4665.

34 Maltoni M, Fabbri L, Nanni O et al. Serum levels of tumour necrosis factor alpha and other cytokines do not correlate with weight loss and anorexia in cancer patients. *Support Care Cancer* 1997;5(2):130–135.

35 Kayacan O, Karnak D, Beder S et al. Impact of TNF-alpha and IL-6 levels on development of cachexia in newly diagnosed NSCLC patients. *Am J Clin Oncol* 2006;29(4):328–335.

36 Shibata M, Nezu T, Kanou H, Abe H, Takekawa M, Fukuzawa M. Decreased production of interleukin-12 and type 2 immune responses are marked in cachectic patients with colorectal and gastric cancer. *J Clin Gastroenterol* April 2002;34(4):416–420.

37 Jatoi A, Egner J, Loprinzi CL et al. Investigating the utility of serum cytokine measurements in a multi-institutional cancer anorexia/weight loss trial. *Support Care Cancer* 2004;12(9):640–644.

38 Op den Kamp CM, Langen RC, Minnaard R et al. Pre-cachexia in patients with stages I–III non-small cell lung cancer: Systemic inflammation and functional impairment without activation of skeletal muscle ubiquitin proteasome system. *Lung Cancer* April 2012;76(1):112.

39 Garcia JM, Garcia-Touza M, Hijazi RA et al. Active ghrelin levels and active to total ghrelin ratio in cancer-induced cachexia. *J Clin Endocrinol Metab* 2005;90(5):2920–2926.

40 Wagner PD. Possible mechanisms underlying the development of cachexia in COPD. *Eur Respir J* 2008;31(3):492–501.

41 Tan BH, Deans DA, Skipworth RJ, Ross JA, Fearon KC. Biomarkers for cancer cachexia: Is there also a genetic component to cachexia? *Support Care Cancer* 2008;16(3):229–234.

42 Deans DA, Tan BH, Ross JA, Rose-Zerilli M, Wigmore SJ, Howell WM, Grimble RF, Fearon KC. Cancer cachexia is associated with the IL10 -1082 gene promoter polymorphism in patients with gastroesophageal malignancy. *Am J Clin Nutr* April 2009;89(4):1164–1172.

43 Solheim TS, Fayers PM, Fladvad T et al. Is there a genetic cause of appetite loss?-an explorative study in 1,853 cancer patients. *J Cachexia Sarcopenia Muscle* 2012;3(3):191–198.

44 Guthrie GJ, Roxburgh CS, Horgan PG, McMillan DC. Does interleukin-6 link explain the link between tumour necrosis, local and systemic inflammatory responses and outcome in patients with colorectal cancer. *Cancer Treat Rev* February 2013;39(1):89–96.

45 Groblewska M, Mroczko B, Wereszczyńska-Siemiatkowska U et al. Serum interleukin 6 (IL-6) and C-reactive protein (CRP) levels in colorectal adenoma and cancer patients. *Clin Chem Lab Med* 2008;46:1423–1428.

46 Hashimoto K, Ikeda Y, Korenaga D et al. The impact of preoperative serum C-reactive protein on the prognosis of patients with hepatocellular carcinoma. *Cancer* 2005;103:1856–1864.

47 Ramsey S, Lamb GW, Aitchison M, Graham J, McMillan DC. Evaluation of an inflammation-based prognostic score in patients with metastatic renal cancer. *Cancer* 2007;109:205–212.

48 Al Murri AM, Bartlett JM, Canney PA et al. Evaluation of an inflammation-based prognostic score (GPS) in patients with metastatic breast cancer. *Br J Cancer* 2006;94:227–230.

49 Meng S, Zhang L, Zhao L et al. Effects of C-reactive protein on CC chemokine receptor 2-mediated chemotaxis of monocytes. *DNA Cell Biol* January 2012;31(1):30–35.

50 Zhang R, Zhang YY, Huang XR et al. C-reactive protein promotes cardiac fibrosis and inflammation in angiotensin II-induced hypertensive cardiac disease. *Hypertension* 2010;55(4):953–960.

51 Deans DA, Tan BH, Wigmore SJ et al. The influence of systemic inflammation, dietary intake and stage of disease on rate of weight loss in patients with gastro-oesophageal cancer. *Br J Cancer* 2009;100:63–69.

52 Scott HR, McMillan DC, Forrest LM et al. The systemic inflammatory response, weight loss, performance status and survival in patients with inoperable non-small cell lung cancer. *Br J Cancer* 2002;87:264–267.

53 Carbone C, Melisi D. NF-κB as a target for pancreatic cancer therapy. *Expert Opin Ther Targets* April 2012;16 Suppl 2:S1–S10.

54 Guttridge DC, Mayo MW, Madrid LV, Wang CY, Baldwin AS. NF-B induced loss of MyoD messenger RNA: Possible role in muscle decay and cachexia. *Science* 2000;289:2363–2366.

55 Wysong A, Couch M, Shadfar S et al. NF-κB inhibition protects against tumor-induced cardiac atrophy in vivo. *Am J Pathol* 2011;178(3):1059–1068.

56 Smith HJ, Wyke SM, Tisdale MJ. Role of protein kinase C and NF-B in proteolysis-inducing factor-induced proteasome expression in C2C12 myotubes. *Br J Cancer* 2004;90:1850–1857.

57 Tisdale MJ. Mechanisms of cancer cachexia. *Physiol Rev* April 2009;89(2):381–410.

58 Lenk K, Schuler G, Adams V. Skeletal muscle wasting in cachexia and sarcopenia: Molecular pathophysiology and impact of exercise training. *J Cachexia Sarcopenia Muscle* September 2010;1(1):9–21.

59 Schmidt K, von Haehling S, Doehner W, Palus S, Anker SD, Springer J. IGF-1 treatment reduces weight loss and improves outcome in a rat model of cancer cachexia. *J Cachexia Sarcopenia Muscle* 2011;2(2):105–109.

60 Brink M, Wellen J, Delafontaine P. Angiotensin II causes weight loss and decreases circulating insulin-like growth factor I in rats through a pressor-independent mechanism. *J Clin Invest* 1996;97:2509–2516.

61 Schuelke M, Wagner KR, Stolz LE, Hübner C, Riebel T, Kömen W, Braun T, Tobin JF, Lee SJ. Myostatin mutation associated with gross muscle hypertrophy in a child. *N Engl J Med* June 24, 2004;350(26):2682–2688.

62 Elkina Y, von Haehling S, Anker SD, Springer J. The role of myostatin in muscle wasting: An overview. *J Cachexia Sarcopenia Muscle* September 2011;2(3):143–151.

63 Lokireddy S, Wijesoma IW, Bonala S et al. Myostatin is a novel tumoral factor that induces cancer cachexia. *Biochem J* August 15, 2012;446(1):23–36.

64 Fearon KC, Glass DJ, Guttridge DC. Cancer cachexia: Mediators, signaling, and metabolic pathways. *Cell Metab* August 8, 2012;16(2):153–166.

65 Fouladiun M, Körner U, Bosaeus I et al. Body composition and time course changes in regional distribution of fat and lean tissue in unselected cancer patients on palliative care-correlations with food intake, metabolism, exercise capacity, and hormones. *Cancer* May 15, 2005;103(10):2189–2198.

66 Rydén M, Agustsson T, Laurencikiene J, Britton T, Sjölin E, Isaksson B, Permert J, Arner P. Lipolysis--not inflammation, cell death, or lipogenesis--is involved in adipose tissue loss in cancer cachexia. *Cancer* October 1, 2008;113(7):1695–1704.

67 Mracek T, Stephens NA, Gao D, Bao Y, Ross JA, Rydén M, Arner P, Trayhurn P, Fearon KC, Bing C. Enhanced ZAG production by subcutaneous adipose tissue is linked to weight loss in gastrointestinal cancer patients. *Br J Cancer* February 1, 2011;104(3):441–447.

68 Kojima M, Hosoda H, Date Y, Nakazato M, Matsuo H, Kangawa K. Ghrelin is a growth-hormone-releasing acylated peptide from stomach. *Nature* 1999;402:656–660.

69 Wren AM, Seal LJ, Cohen MA et al. Ghrelin enhances appetite and increases food intake in humans. *J Clin Endocrinol Metab* 2001;86:5992.

70 Cummings DE, Weigle DS, Frayo RS et al. Plasma ghrelin levels after diet-induced weight loss or gastric bypass surgery. *N Engl J Med* 2002;346:1623–1630.

71 Porporato PE, Filigheddu N, Reano S et al. Acylated and unacylated ghrelin impair skeletal muscle atrophy in mice. *J Clin Invest* February 1, 2013;123(2):611–622.

72 Sugiyama M, Yamaki A, Furuya M et al. Ghrelin improves body weight loss and skeletal muscle catabolism associated with angiotensin II–induced cachexia in mice. *Regul Pept* October 10, 2012;178(1–3):21–28.

73 Soriano-Guillen L, Barrios V, Campos-Barros A, Argente J. Ghrelin levels in obesity and anorexia nervosa: Effect of weight reduction or recuperation. *J Pediatr* 2004;144:36–42.

74 Garcia JM, Garcia-Touza M, Hijazi RA, Taffet G, Epner D, Mann D, Smith RG, Cunningham GR, Marcelli M. Active ghrelin levels and active to total ghrelin ratio in cancer-induced cachexia. *J Clin Endocrinol Metab* 2005;90:2920–2926.

75 Tschop M, Smiley DL, Heiman ML. Ghrelin induces adiposity in rodents. *Nature* 2000;407:908–913.

76 Dixit VD, Schaffer EM, Pyle RS et al. Ghrelin inhibits leptin- and activation-induced proinflammatory cytokine expression by human monocytes and T cells. *J Clin Invest* July 2004;114:57–66.

77 Greenwood-Van Meerveld B, Kriegsman M, Nelson R. Ghrelin as a target for gastrointestinal motility disorders. *Peptides* 2011;32:2352–2356.

78 Brodsky IG, Balagopal P, Nair KS. Effects of testosterone replacement on muscle mass and muscle protein synthesis in hypogonadal men--a clinical research center study. *J Clin Endocrinol Metab* 1996;81:3469–3475.

79 Muniyappa R, Sorkin JD, Veldhuis JD et al. Long-term testosterone supplementation augments overnight growth hormone secretion in healthy older men. *Am J Physiol Endocrinol Metab* 2007;293(3):E769–E775.

80 Del Fabbro E, Hui D, Nooruddin ZI et al. Associations among hypogonadism, C-reactive protein, symptom burden, and survival in male cancer patients with cachexia: A preliminary report. *J Pain Symptom Manage* June 2010;39(6):1016–1024.

81 Garcia JM, Li H, Mann D et al. Hypogonadism in male patients with cancer. *Cancer* June 15, 2006;106(12):2583–2591.

82 Dev R, Del Fabbro E, Bruera E. Association between megestrol acetate treatment and symptomatic adrenal insufficiency with hypogonadism in male patients with cancer. *Cancer* September 15, 2007;110(6):1173–1177.

83 Honors MA, Kinzig KP. The role of insulin resistance in the development of muscle wasting during cancer cachexia. *J Cachexia Sarcopenia Muscle* March 2012;3(1):5–11.

84 Asp ML, Tian M, Wendel AA, Belury MA. Evidence for the contribution of insulin resistance to the development of cachexia in tumor-bearing mice. *Int J Cancer* 2010:126:756–763.

85 Winter A, MacAdams J, Chevalier S. Normal protein anabolic response to hyperaminoacidemia in insulin-resistant patients with lung cancer cachexia. *Clin Nutr* October 2012;31(5):765–773.

86 Lundholm K, Körner U, Gunnebo L et al. Insulin treatment in cancer cachexia: Effects on survival, metabolism, and physical functioning. *Clin Cancer Res* May 1, 2007;13:2699.

87 Anker SD, Chua TP, Swan JW et al. Hormonal changes and catabolic/anabolic imbalance in chronic heart failure: The importance for cardiac cachexia. *Circulation* 1997;96:526–534.

88 Gerling IC, Sun Y, Ahokas RA et al. Aldosteronism: An immunostimulatory state precedes the proinflammatory/fibrogenic cardiac phenotype. *Am J Physiol Heart Circ Physiol* 2003;285:H813–H821.

89 Cheema Y, Zhao W, Zhao T et al. Reverse remodeling and recovery from cachexia in rats with aldosteronism. *Am J Physiol Heart Circ Physiol* August 15, 2012;303(4):H486–H495.

90 Polak J, Kotrc M, Wedellova Z et al. Lipolytic effects of B-type natriuretic peptide 1–32 in adipose tissue of heart failure patients compared with healthy controls. *J Am Coll Cardiol* September 6, 2011;58(11):1119–1125.

91 Tedeschi S, Pilotti E, Parenti E. Serum adipokine zinc α2-glycoprotein and lipolysis in cachectic and noncachectic heart failure patients: Relationship with neurohormonal and inflammatory biomarkers. *Metabolism* January 2012;61(1):37–42.

92 Fredrix EW, Soeters PB, Wouters EF, Deerenberg IM, von Meyenfeldt MF, Saris WH. Effect of different tumor types on resting energy expenditure. *Cancer Res* November 15, 1991;51(22):6138–6141.

93 Jatoi A, Daly BD, Hughes VA et al. Do patients with nonmetastatic non-small cell lung cancer demonstrate altered resting energy expenditure? *Ann Thorac Surg* August 2001;72(2):348–351.

94 Wang AY, Sea MM, Tang N et al. Energy intake and expenditure profile in chronic peritoneal dialysis patients complicated with circulatory congestion. *Am J Clin Nutr* November 2009;90(5):1179–1184.

95 Binymin K, Herrick A, Carlson G, Hopkins S. The effect of disease activity on body composition and resting energy expenditure in patients with rheumatoid arthritis. *J Inflamm Res* 2011;4:61–66.

96 Brúsik M, Ukropec J, Joppa P et al. Circulatory and adipose tissue leptin and adiponectin in relationship to resting energy expenditure in patients with chronic obstructive pulmonary disease. *Physiol Res* December 14, 2012;61(5):469–480.

97 Mantovani G, Madeddu C, Macciò A. Cachexia and oxidative stress in cancer: An innovative therapeutic management. *Curr Pharm Des* 2012;18(31):4813–4818.

98 Guarnier FA, Cecchini AL, Suzukawa AA, Maragno AL, Simão AN, Gomes MD, Cecchini R. Time course of skeletal muscle loss and oxidative stress in rats with Walker 256 solid tumor. *Muscle Nerve* December 2010;42(6):950–958.

99   Sullivan-Gunn MJ, Campbell-O'Sullivan SP, Tisdale MJ, Lewandowski PA. Decreased NADPH oxidase expression and antioxidant activity in cachectic skeletal muscle. *J Cachexia Sarcopenia Muscle* September 2011;2(3):181–188.

100   Springer J, Tschirner A, Hartman K et al. Inhibition of xanthine oxidase reduces wasting and improves outcome in a rat model of cancer cachexia. *Int J Cancer* November 1, 2012;131(9):2187–2196.

101   Mantovani G, Macciò A, Madeddu C et al. Randomized phase III clinical trial of five different arms of treatment in 332 patients with cancer cachexia. *Oncologist* 2010;15(2):200–211.

102   Lissoni P. Is there a role for melatonin in supportive care? *Support Care Cancer* 2002;10:110–116.

103   Del Fabbro E, Dev R, Hui D, Palmer L, Bruera E. Effects of melatonin on appetite and other symptoms in patients with advanced cancer and cachexia: A double-blind placebo-controlled trial. *J Clin Oncol* 2013;31:1271–1276.

104   Bruera E, Chadwick S, Fox R, Hanson J, MacDonald N. Study of cardiovascular autonomic insufficiency in advanced cancer patients. *Cancer Treat Rep* 1986;70:1383–1387.

105   Martins CDD, Chianca DA, Fernandes LG. Cardiac autonomic balance in rats submitted to protein restriction after weaning. *Clin Exp Pharmacol Physiol* 2011;38:89–93.

106   Scott EM, Greenwood JP, Pernicova I, Law GR, Gilbey SG, Kearney MT, Mary DA. Sympathetic activation and vasoregulation in response to carbohydrate ingestion in patients with congestive heart failure. *Can J Cardiol* February 2013;29(2):236–242.

107   Andreas S, Anker SD, Scanlon PD, Somers VK. Neurohumoral activation as a link to systemic manifestations of chronic lung disease. *Chest* 2005;128:3618–3624.

108   Matteoli G, Boeckxstaens GE. The vagal innervation of the gut and immune homeostasis. *Gut* August 2013;62(8):1214–1222.

109   Chauhan A, Sequeria A, Manderson C et al. Exploring autonomic nervous system dysfunction in patients with cancer cachexia: A pilot study. *Auton Neurosci* 2012;166(1–2):93–95.

110   Strasser F, Palmer JL, Schover LR et al. The impact of hypogonadism and autonomic dysfunction on fatigue, emotional function, and sexual desire in male patients with advanced cancer: A pilot study. *Cancer* December 15, 2006;107(12):2949–2957.

57

Overview of the management of the anorexia/weight loss syndrome

CARA BONDLY, AMINAH JATOI

OVERVIEW AND DEFINITIONS

The anorexia/weight loss syndrome occurs in patients with a variety of illnesses, including cancer, acquired immune deficiency syndrome (AIDS), and congestive heart failure. The cancer anorexia/weight loss syndrome is particularly devastating and is characterized by loss of appetite and weight, and functional decline, which occurs as a result of tissue wasting, in particular, muscle wasting. This syndrome affects approximately two-thirds of patients who die from advanced cancer.[1]

Weight loss of 10% is a well-accepted diagnostic criterion for severe malnutrition. However, among patients with cancer, previous studies have clearly shown that the anorexia/weight loss syndrome can be invoked if an involuntary weight loss of even 6% has occurred. This degree of weight loss has been observed in conjunction with incurable cancer, progressive debility, and a decline in performance status.[2]

From a clinical standpoint, the assessment of nutritional status is often viewed as multifaceted, if not cumbersome. A variety of approaches are utilized, and these span anything from a quick hands-off assessment shortly after entering a patient's room to a detailed modeling of nutritional parameters into a single risk assessment to an elaborate assessment of body composition that includes measurement of total body potassium, ingestion and sampling of tritiated water, and dual x-ray absorptiometry. All these approaches have their merits. However, we believe that the most clinically useful, practical, and validated measurement is patient-reported weight loss. As discussed earlier, weight loss of 6% or greater over the preceding 6 months predicts a poor prognosis among cancer patients, and everyone will agree that it is relatively simple to acquire.

The anorexia/weight loss syndrome is distressing to patients and their families; in their eyes, the patient is "starving." Walsh et al. interviewed 1000 patients with advanced cancer referred to a palliative care program. Anorexia was tied for third, superseded only by pain and fatigue, as the most prevalent and bothersome symptom experienced by these patients.[3] Some of the distress associated with this symptom may be derived specifically from loss of appetite, but, at the same time, this decline in oral intake brings with it tremendous turmoil for the patient and family. This fear of "starvation," as noted earlier, provides an extra emotional burden in the setting of an incurable, refractory malignancy.

Although these patients are not starving (Table 57.1), the anorexia/weight loss syndrome does portend an unfavorable prognosis in patients with cancer as well as in patients with human immunodeficiency virus (HIV) infection and congestive heart failure. In the cancer setting, Dewys et al. formally analyzed the impact of weight loss on prognosis. They retrospectively evaluated 3047 patients from 12 different Eastern Cooperative Oncology Group clinical trials. Patient-reported weight loss of more than 5% over the preceding 6 months predicted early mortality independently of tumor stage, histology, and patient performance status. This weight loss was also associated with a trend toward lower chemotherapy response rates.[4] Similarly, Quinten examined appetite scores among over 1800 cancer patients who were followed prospectively. Again, loss of appetite was a strong and statistically significant predictor of survival, and gradations in loss of appetite also demonstrated a prognostic effect.[4b] Along these same lines, Anker et al. demonstrated a much worse prognosis among congestive heart failure patients who had lost weight compared with those who had maintained their weight. Both groups of patients had similar degrees of left ventricular dysfunction.[5] Finally, in HIV-infected patients, weight loss has been associated with increased mortality,[6–12] accelerated disease progression,[12] and impairment of strength and functional status.[13] Thus, in several disease states, involuntary weight loss clearly predicts a shortened survival (Figure 57.1).

There are multiple readily observable clinical factors that contribute to involuntary weight loss in patients with chronic diseases such as cancer, HIV, or congestive heart failure. In cancer patients, the systemic and local effects of the tumor and side effects from anticancer treatments all contribute, whereas fatigue, anxiety, depression, and pain appear also to contribute, to the weight loss. These patients face many challenges

Table 57.1   *Cancer anorexia/weight loss versus starvation*

Cancer anorexia/weight loss	Starvation
Loss of fat and lean tissue	Loss of fat
No hunger	Hunger
Resting energy expenditure sometimes increased	Drop in resting energy expenditure
Specific mediators have been implicated	Specific mediators not as well implicated

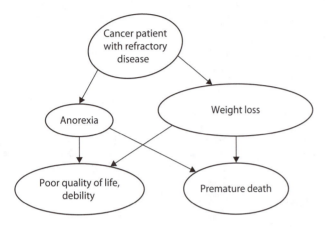

Figure 57.1   *The anorexia/weight loss syndrome is associated with diminished survival and quality of life.*

in maintaining adequate caloric intake, including difficulty swallowing due to obstructing tumors or nerve compromise, mucositis, dry mouth, odor sensitivity, taste changes, diarrhea, constipation, and nausea and vomiting. Changes in the capacity to recognize and taste sweetness in foods occur in over a third of cancer patients. Bitterness, sourness, and saltiness are less frequently affected.[14,15] Multiple theories have been proposed regarding this change in taste, including zinc deficiency, alterations in brain neuropeptides, and opioid peptides.[16–18] Alterations have also been described in the gastrointestinal tract of weight-losing patients, and these almost certainly play a role in the weight loss of these patients. Early satiety is seen in weight-losing cancer patients even without direct tumor involvement of the gastrointestinal tract. Proinflammatory cytokines such as interleukin (IL)-1β and central corticotropin-releasing factor have been implicated in early satiety.[19,20] Central corticotropin-releasing factor may also induce delayed gastric emptying and gastric stasis, ultimately resulting in early satiety.[18,21,22]

PATHOPHYSIOLOGY

The anorexia/weight loss syndrome is a complex metabolic derangement that includes anorexia, early satiety, weakness, and anemia, as well as weight loss. Patients experience inadequate energy intake, possibly increased resting energy expenditure, and abnormalities induced by proinflammatory cytokines.[23] Bruera et al. demonstrated that weight-losing cancer patients consumed 3200 kJ (800 Cal) per day less than patients without

weight loss.[24] This observation is important, because it shows that weight loss occurs not only as a result of inappropriately spent energy sources but also as a result of diminished energy intake. At the same time, however, multiple studies have shown that provision of increased energy through increased oral nutritional support does not result in weight gain.[25,26] In the anorexia/weight loss syndrome, unlike starvation, loss of skeletal muscle in relation to adipose tissue is accelerated. In contrast, starvation results in preferential consumption of fat rather than glucose as the primary fuel, perhaps in an effort to spare lean body mass.[27]

The exact pathophysiology of the cancer anorexia/weight loss syndrome has not yet been clearly defined, but the development of this syndrome is associated with multiple hormonal and metabolic alterations. Leptin is a hormone secreted by adipose tissue in response to changes in weight. Levels of circulating leptin decline as weight loss occurs and, through complex feedback mechanisms, stimulates food intake in healthy people.[2] In weight-losing cancer patients, however, the leptin system appears to be dysregulated; studies are inconsistent on whether weight loss is truly associated with a drop in serum leptin.[28] In addition to leptin, several cytokines have also been implicated as mediators of weight loss and anorexia. These include tumor necrosis factor α (TNFα), IL-1, IL-6, and interferon γ (IFNγ). High levels of serum TNFα, IL-1β, and IL-6 have been found in some patients with cancer. When elevated levels of these cytokines are present, they seem to correlate with the progression of the tumor.[29–31] However, a recent North Central Cancer Group study has questioned the role of serum cytokines and hypothesized instead that cytokines in the peripheral blood mononuclear cells may be more reflective of what occurs at the tissue level.[32] Several studies have also shown that administration of these cytokines to healthy patients reduces food intake and reproduces the features of anorexia/weight loss syndrome.[17,27–33] Hypermetabolism, which is defined as an elevation in the resting energy expenditure, is sometimes a feature of this syndrome. Some studies suggest that this occasional phenomenon may be caused by induction of the mitochondrial uncoupling protein in muscle and adipose tissue. The induction of this protein may be due to cytokine activation. Ultimately, these mechanisms lead to increased heat production and muscle wasting.[17,34]

A variety of changes in nutrient metabolism have also been described in weight-losing patients (Box 57.1). Glucose metabolism is altered in weight-losing cancer patients. Lactate is

---

Box 57.1   Mediators of the cancer anorexia/weight loss syndrome

- TNFα
- IL-1β
- IL-6
- Lipid-mobilizing factor
- Leptin (possibly)
- IFNγ

produced in excess quantities by many solid tumors and is converted back to glucose via the Cori cycle in the liver.[35,36] This cycle of producing glucose from lactate uses ATP in a highly inefficient manner. Possibly, this process contributes to the increased resting energy expenditure mentioned earlier. In one study, a 40% increase in hepatic glucose production was observed in weight-losing cancer patients.[35–37] Changes in lipid metabolism have also been described in patients with the cancer anorexia/weight loss syndrome. These include increased lipid mobilization, decreased lipogenesis, and decreased activity of lipoprotein lipase, which is responsible for clearance of triglyceride from plasma.[18,35,36] A lipid-mobilizing factor has also been isolated.[27,36,38,39] Studies in animal models have suggested that lipid-mobilizing factor may contribute to loss of body fat and increased resting energy expenditure.[39]

Along with the changes in glucose and lipid metabolism, changes in protein metabolism have also been documented in weight-losing cancer patients. During starvation, glucose utilization by the brain is replaced by the use of ketone bodies derived from fat. This process decreases the amino acid–driven gluconeogenesis by the liver. In weight-losing cancer patients, however, amino acids are not spared and lean body mass is depleted.[2] Skeletal muscle biopsies from patients with cancer have demonstrated both increased rates of protein synthesis and increased rates of protein degradation.[40,41] The cancer cachectic factor is a 24 kDa proteoglycan that has recently been implicated as a mediator in cancer-associated weight loss. Utilizing a rodent model, Todorov et al.[42] found that direct injection of this "cancer cachectic factor" into the body results in weight loss. In contrast, if an antibody to the "cancer cachectic factor" is administered 24 hours before the injection, this same wasting effect is not observed. Providing provocative clinical data, these investigators found that this proteoglycan is highly specific for weight loss in patients with cancer as opposed to weight loss from trauma or sepsis or the mere presence of cancer with no weight loss. Recent clinical findings raise questions of the relevance of this cancer cachectic factor in cancer patients, but nonetheless, these data merit mention as an illustration of the complexity of this whole process of cancer-related weight loss[42b,42c].

In general, the pathophysiology of the cancer anorexia/weight loss syndrome continues to be studied, and much of what is described earlier still requires further investigation. Nonetheless, the available data clearly point to pathophysiological mechanisms that are markedly different from those observed in classic starvation. Thus, the most important point of the preceding discussion is that caloric repletion is not the answer to managing this syndrome and that other approaches, such as counseling patients on prognosis and, on occasion, pharmacological manipulation of the appetite, should be considered.

THERAPEUTIC OPTIONS

Treatment of the anorexia/weight loss syndrome has led to only modest improvements in clinical outcome. In the cancer anorexia/weight loss syndrome, treating the underlying

malignancy appears to reverse at least some aspects of the syndrome. Geels et al. examined 300 patients who were receiving chemotherapy for breast cancer, a relatively chemotherapy-sensitive solid tumor. Patients completed questionnaires that included an assessment of appetite, and a direct relation between tumor response and improvement in appetite was observed. Specifically, 82% of patients with a complete or partial response to chemotherapy also reported an improvement in appetite.[43] To our knowledge, no major studies have examined weight or body composition in cancer survivors or in patients whose cancer responds dramatically to cancer therapy to assess what sort of changes in weight or eating patterns occur in these settings. However, the aforementioned data suggest that at least some aspects of the cancer anorexia/weight loss syndrome can be reversed with chemotherapy.

CALORIC SUPPLEMENTATION

Intuitively, and at a first glance, caloric supplementation seems to be the ideal approach for managing weight loss in patients with the cancer anorexia/weight loss syndrome. This strategy, however, has been shown to be beneficial in only a few, specific situations, particularly in the cancer setting. Indeed, it is our contention that, by definition, patients who benefit from nutritional supplementation do not truly have the cancer anorexia/weight loss syndrome. Cancer patients who do sometimes benefit from nutritional support include those with perioperative cancer, those who have undergone stem cell or bone marrow transplantation, and those who are receiving radiation for head and neck cancer. The unifying theme behind all these situations is that these patients all appear to have potentially curable malignancies or a high likelihood of long-term tumor response.

In contrast, in patients with advanced, incurable, metastatic disease, no benefit has been derived from parenteral or enteral nutritional support. McGeer et al. published a meta-analysis showing no benefit with parenteral nutrition in cancer patients receiving chemotherapy. In fact in this meta-analysis, patients receiving parenteral nutrition experienced higher rates of infectious complications compared with patients receiving no parenteral nutrition.[44] Similarly, Ovesen et al. found that among cancer patients receiving chemotherapy, dietary counseling did lead to increased caloric intake, but this increased caloric intake did not result in improved survival, tumor response rates, or quality of life.[26] More recently, Baldwin and others conducted a meta-analysis that included 13 randomized studies that evaluated oral nutritional supplementation.[26b] These investigators observed that dietary supplementation resulted in increased nutritional intake and weight but had no effect on survival. Importantly, this study also observed tremendous heterogeneity among studies and large differences in quality, findings that suggest that perhaps further research in this field is indicated. For now, however, caloric supplementation does not appear to have strong justification in patients with advanced cancer. With regard to patients with congestive heart failure, there have been no large controlled studies of nutritional strategies in the management of cardiac-associated anorexia/weight loss. However, in patients with clinically stable congestive heart failure and no evidence of severe malnutrition, nutritional support alone has not been shown to carry a significant effect on clinical status.[45]

Unlike studies in cancer and congestive heart failure patients, studies of total parenteral nutrition in HIV-infected patients with severe wasting have shown significant improvement in weight. The patients receiving total parenteral nutrition experienced an 8 kg weight increase compared with a 3 kg weight loss in patients receiving no parenteral nutrition.[46] The effects of total parenteral nutrition on lean body mass were greatest in HIV-infected patients with documented malabsorption compared with patients with active secondary infections.[47]

Is there ever a situation among patients with incurable, metastatic cancer where nutritional support, such as total parenteral nutrition, appears to benefit patients? As emphasized earlier, we believe that this approach is outside the standard of care for most patients with cancer. However, case reports and small series suggest that occasionally, these patients may benefit from total parenteral nutrition. Certainly, selection bias may result in the publication of the most favorable outcomes. The Mayo Clinic published a report on a 20-year retrospective experience with total parenteral nutrition in this group of patients.[48] Overall, the use of total parenteral nutrition at this institution was quite conservative; only 52 patients with incurable cancer, or 15% of all patients treated at home, received this intervention. Although most patients did poorly, 16 did live for 1 year or longer, presumably as a result of the total parenteral nutrition. In an attempt to tease out predictive factors in order to provide guidance on who might benefit from total parenteral nutrition from a practice perspective, no such predictive factor emerged. Thus, the conclusion of this study was that clinical discretion—in the setting of a multidisciplinary approach and after in-depth discussions with the patient and family members—should guide management when this nonstandard approach is considered.

In cancer, the limited role of increased caloric intake emphasizes the need to discuss goals and realistic expectations of any intervention for patients suffering from the anorexia/weight loss syndrome. First, the healthcare provider should determine who actually is most bothered by the decreased oral intake and weight loss. Is it the patient or the family? Often, family members, and not the patient, are more distressed by these signs and symptoms. Family members often feel tremendous guilt over their inability to convince their loved ones to increase their oral intake and thereby presumably stop ongoing weight loss. Their attempts to encourage oral intake can become a source of frustrating disagreement between patients and their families. Second, frank discussions with patients and their family members regarding the fact that a simple increased oral intake of food is unlikely to prolong life or improve quality of life in terminally ill cancer patients often relieve this source of anxiety.

Studies of patients near the end of life indicate that they usually do not feel hunger and dehydration even in the absence of nutritional or fluid supplementation.[49] These findings should be explicitly conveyed to family members. Therefore, patients should base the use of pharmacological measures to improve appetite, as discussed later, on their own wishes for appetite improvement rather than on the guilt and frustration of family members. Third, it is important to point out to patients and family members that symptoms such as loss of appetite and weight often occur at the end of life. The major role of dietary counseling in this setting is to provide education that the cancer anorexia/weight loss syndrome is common, out of the patient's control, and not representative of lack of volition on the part of the patient.

Emerging qualitative data point to the importance of all the points previously discussed.[49b] In a recent qualitative study from Hopkinson and others, a patient was quoted as saying, "I'm forced to eat. I don't eat." The unsettling nature of this comment points to the importance of potentially utilizing this symptom of loss of appetite as a point of departure for discussing end-of-life issues.

PHARMACOLOGICAL INTERVENTIONS

When the decision is made to initiate pharmacological treatment for the cancer anorexia/weight loss syndrome, progestational agents or glucocorticoids are reasonable options. These two classes of agents are the only ones that have been shown in multiple, placebo controlled, randomized trials to stimulate appetite.

PROGESTATIONAL AGENTS

Progestational agents used in the management of this syndrome include megestrol acetate and medroxyprogesterone acetate. Megestrol acetate is a synthetic, orally active derivative of naturally occurring progesterone. Medroxyprogesterone acetate is also available as an injectable, depot formulation, although, to our knowledge, the depot formulation has not been used extensively for appetite stimulation. Multiple studies suggest that progestational agents improve appetite in patients with advanced cancer and anorexia. Some have speculated that this effect is exerted partially by the downregulation of IL-6, although some studies refute this mechanism of action. Approximately 15 published, placebo-controlled trials in cancer patients have evaluated the appetite-stimulating effects of megestrol acetate. Thirteen of these studies demonstrated that megestrol acetate improved appetite.[50] For example, in a North Central Cancer Treatment Group trial, Loprinzi et al. examined 133 cancer patients in a placebo-controlled trial and found that those who received megestrol acetate at 800 mg/day manifested both an increase in appetite and an increase in nonfluid weight.[51]

A recent meta-analysis by Pascual Lopez et al. included 26 studies published between 1990 and 1999 investigating the effectiveness of megestrol acetate in the treatment of anorexia/weight loss syndrome in comparison with placebo and other drugs used in the treatment of cachexia. All together, 3368 patients were included in the meta-analysis. Eighty-six percent of patients had cancer, 11% had HIV, and 2% had other illnesses (failure to round up apparently precluded summing to 100%), including cystic fibrosis in 12 children and a wide range of other diseases in the geriatric population. In general, the study revealed an increase in appetite and weight gain with megestrol acetate. Results regarding quality of life were somewhat less clear cut. However, when the Karnofsky performance index was used as surrogate marker for quality of life, the overall results were in favor of megestrol.[52]

Megestrol acetate has been shown to have a dose-related benefit starting at doses of 160 mg. The optimal dosage is generally considered 800 mg/day, and increasing the dose beyond this level provides no further benefit.[53] It is generally recommended that patients start at 160 mg/day and titrate upward according to clinical response.[2] However, the clinician may choose to start at 800 mg/day if a rapid clinical decline is anticipated, and the option of gradual titration is thought to be unavailable.

Progestational agents are reasonably well tolerated for the most part. However, adverse effects of both megestrol acetate and medroxyprogesterone include thromboembolic phenomena, breakthrough uterine bleeding, peripheral edema, hyperglycemia, hypertension, adrenal suppression, and adrenal insufficiency.[2] The risk of thromboembolic events with the use of megestrol acetate is minimal. In Pascual Lopez et al.'s meta-analysis, the only statistically significant adverse effect observed in patients receiving megestrol acetate versus placebo was edema with a relative risk of 1.67.[52] However, a history of thromboembolism remains a definite contraindication to initiating megestrol acetate for the anorexia/weight loss syndrome, as the risk: benefit ratio is too great. Whereas use of progestational agents for the anorexia/weight loss syndrome in cancer or HIV patients may provide benefit, their use in weight-losing congestive heart failure has not been extensively studied. Progestational agents promote fluid retention and may therefore lead to deleterious side effects in this particular patient group. In general, their use in congestive heart failure patients is not routinely recommended.

GLUCOCORTICOIDS

In addition to progestational agents, corticosteroids have been extensively studied as a treatment approach for the anorexia/weight loss syndrome. These agents are thought to exert their effects through the suppression of inflammatory mediators and possibly through a direct effect on appetite centers in the hypothalamus.[54] Moertel et al. published the first placebo-controlled trial investigating the effectiveness of corticosteroids in the cancer anorexia/weight loss syndrome. This study included 116 patients with advanced gastrointestinal malignancies. At 4 weeks, 55% of patients in the corticosteroid group reported an improvement in appetite compared with 26% in the placebo group.[55] Multiple subsequent studies have demonstrated similar results with corticosteroids in the treatment of cancer-associated anorexia.

Which are better: corticosteroids or progestational agents? In a North Central Cancer Treatment Group study, Loprinzi et al. answered this question by a randomized controlled trial in 475 weight-losing and/or anorexic cancer patients. Patients were randomly assigned to receive megestrol acetate 800 mg daily versus dexamethasone 0.75 mg four times daily versus the androgen fluoxymesterone. Fluoxymesterone did not provide favorable results. However, the key point of this trial was that, at the doses studied, megestrol acetate and dexamethasone provided equivalent orexigenic effects. Toxicity was different in these two effective arms. Myopathy was more frequent in the dexamethasone group: 6% and 18% in the megestrol acetate and dexamethasone groups, respectively. Other adverse effects that were seen more commonly in the dexamethasone group included cushingoid changes (1% vs. 6%) and peptic ulcer disease (0% vs. 3%). Twenty-five percent of megestrol acetate–treated patients and 36% of dexamethasone-treated patients discontinued therapy because of either their wishes and/or toxicity.[56]

Based on these findings, corticosteroids are generally reserved for patients in whom megestrol acetate is contraindicated, such as in those with thromboembolism. Patients with a limited life expectancy, and therefore likely to receive only short-term benefits, may prefer corticosteroids.[54] For other patients who do not fall into these categories, progestational agents may be viewed as a more favorable choice.

INEFFECTIVE OR RELATIVELY INEFFECTIVE AGENTS

Other pharmacological agents have been proposed as possible treatments for the cancer anorexia/weight loss syndrome. The list of agents that have not proved as effective in large randomized, comparative trials is extensive (see Box 57.2) and includes fluoxymesterone (as discussed earlier).

Box 57.2 What does not work?

- Dronabinol
- Cyproheptadine
- Pentoxifylline
- Hydrazine sulfate
- Dietary counseling as a single intervention
- Eicosapentaenoic acid

OTHER PROMISING AGENTS

Other agents appear more promising and merit further study (Box 57.3). First, in cancer patients, melatonin appears promising. This is a pineal gland hormone that has been demonstrated to decrease the level of circulating TNFα. In one study, the addition of melatonin to chemotherapy for lung cancer resulted in improved response and survival rates and a reduced incidence of myelosuppression, neuropathy, and weight loss in the group treated with melatonin compared with the control group.[57] Although promising, this finding needs to be confirmed in larger trials. Second, thalidomide is another promising agent that may work in the treatment of cancer anorexia/weight loss syndrome by means of TNFα inhibition. Bruera et al. observed in their study that the majority of cancer patients who were at the end of life reported an overall improved sense of well-being with this agent.[58] Finally, phase III testing of the androgen oxandrolone has been recently completed following promising pilot data.

In AIDS patients, modest doses of thalidomide have been associated with a significant improvement in well-being and weight gain.[59] There is now accumulating evidence that the combination of aggressive nutritional counseling, appetite stimulants, progressive strength training, and anabolic hormones can reverse weight loss and increase lean body mass. This approach requires further study, but at this point appears promising. The first goals of therapy for these patients should be treatment of any secondary infections and optimization of antiretroviral therapy.[60] Nutritional strategies employed in these patients with some success include total parenteral nutrition, β-hydroxy-β-methylbutyrate, and high-quality oral proteins including whey protein supplements. Improvement in weight has been shown with the use of megestrol acetate. Physiological testosterone administration in hypogonadal men with AIDS wasting has been shown to result in sustained improvement in lean body mass. Another agent associated with improvement in lean body mass in HIV patients is growth hormone.[61] Again, further study of all these approaches appears to be indicated.

Multiple drugs have been investigated as potential treatments for the anorexia/weight loss syndrome in the setting of congestive heart failure. Freeman et al. suggested that fish oil supplementation reduces circulating levels of IL-1 and improves cachexia in dogs.[61] Specific anticytokine therapies have been tested in this patient population. Etanercept, an anti-TNFα antibody, was studied in a large-scale trial. Unfortunately, the trial was stopped early based on unfavorable preliminary results.[62] There are preliminary data that the angiotensin inhibitor enalapril can prevent the development of weight loss in congestive heart failure patients although definitive evidence is lacking.[63] Hryniewicz et al. reported promising results with the use of β blocker therapy in patients with anorexia/weight loss and congestive heart failure. In this study, 27 patients with baseline anorexia/weight loss were treated with carvedilol or long-acting metoprolol. Compared with a similar control group, the patients treated with β blocker therapy demonstrated a significantly greater weight gain.[64] Anecdotal evidence has been reported supporting the use of short-term, high-dose growth hormone therapy in cardiac anorexia/weight loss patients. Two case reports of three "cachectic" patients stated that there were profound increases in muscle mass and strength without significant side effects.[65,66] The use of anabolic steroids has also been proposed as a treatment option for patients with cardiac anorexia/weight loss, but the side effects of these medications often limit their usefulness in this patient population. Interestingly, treatment with left ventricular assist devices provides little benefit with regard to weight gain in this patient population.[67]

Finally, earlier research on muscle physiology has prompted the initiation of a handful of ongoing clinical trials that examine some agents with what appear to be truly novel mechanisms of action. First, myostatin is a protein that, under normal circumstances, plays an important role in checking muscle growth and reducing extreme muscle hypertrophy. Clinical case reports had shown that patients who harbored gene mutations did in fact demonstrate extreme muscle hypertrophy. Recent preclinical data from Zhou and others show that myostatin inhibition leads to improvements in body weight and survival in tumor-bearing animals. Such data have given rise to early clinical trials in cancer patients.[67b] Second, anamorelin is an oral ghrelin mimetic that has recently undergone preliminary testing in cancer patients. Garcia described a placebo-controlled, double-blind crossover study that included 16 patients.[67c] Anamorelin resulted in weight gain and improvement in appetite and was also well tolerated. Based on such results, further evaluation in a larger trial is ongoing. Finally, JAK (Janus kinase family of enzymes) is a group of proteins involved in the signaling of inflammatory cytokines, which have also been invoked to explain the etiology of cancer cachexia.[67d] Mutations of these proteins are associated with several hematologic malignancies, including myelofibrosis, and inhibition of these JAK proteins has demonstrated improvements in spleen size, weight gain, and general well-being in some patients with these malignancies. Such findings suggest that perhaps cancer patients who are suffering from cancer-associated weight loss might gain an improvement in symptoms and potentially even a survival advantage. Thus, clinical trials are underway to test JAK inhibition in cancer patients in an effort to treat cancer-associated

---

Box 57.3 Some of the agents that merit further study

- Ghrelin
- Neuropeptide Y
- TNF inhibitors
- Oxandrolone
- Thalidomide
- Adenosine triphosphate
- Melatonin
- anti-myostatin therapy
- anamorelin

weight loss. On a long-term basis, it is hoped that the identification of agents that show real efficacy in treating this syndrome will lead to multiagent trials that in turn will lead to great strides in the control of all aspects of cancer-associated loss of weight and appetite.

Key learning points

- Anorexia and weight loss are devastating aspects of a syndrome that complicates several chronic diseases.

- When present, the anorexia/weight loss syndrome is not only psychologically difficult for patients and their families but portends a worse outcome.

- The goals of nutritional/pharmacological management of this syndrome vary for individual patients depending on their underlying disease, but the approach is primarily palliative in nature.

- Aggressive nutritional support, particularly with total parenteral nutrition, is beneficial in only a few well-defined circumstances.

- Pharmacological interventions that are considered reasonable, particularly in patients with advanced cancer or HIV, include progestational agents or corticosteroids.

- Management of the cancer anorexia/weight loss syndrome is challenging, because this syndrome represents a set of complex metabolic aberrations, but the exact pathophysiology remains unclear.

- Certainly, the most pressing issues surrounding this syndrome center around its etiology and finding effective means to palliate associated symptoms, improve quality of life, and prolong survival.

- Future research should focus on gaining a better grasp on pathophysiology for purposes of eventually developing better therapies.

REFERENCES

1 Splinter TA. Cachexia and cancer: A clinicians view. *Ann Oncol* 1992; 3: 25–27.

2 Inui A. Cancer anorexia-cachexia syndrome: Current issues in research and management. *Cancer J Clin* 2002; 52: 72–91.

3 Walsh D, Donnelly S, Rybicki L. The symptoms of advanced cancer: Relationship to age, gender and performance status in 1000 patients. *Support Care Cancer* 2000; 8: 175–179.

4 Dewys WD, Begg C, Lavin PT et al. Prognostic effect of weight loss prior to chemotherapy in cancer patients. Eastern Cooperative Oncology Group. *Am J Med* 1980; 69: 491–497.

4b Quinten C, Coens C, Mauer M et al. Baseline quality of life as a prognostic indicator of survival: A meta-analysis of individual patient data from EORTC clinical trials. *Lancet Oncol* 2009; 10: 865–871.

5 Anker S, Ponikowski P, Varney S et al. Wasting as an independent risk factor for mortality in chronic heart failure. *Lancet* 1997; 349: 1050–1053.

6 Kotler D, Tierney AR, Wang J, Pierson RN Jr. Magnitude of body-cell-mass depletion and the timing of death from wasting in AIDS. *Am J Clin Nutr* 1989; 50: 444–447.

7 Chlebowski R, Grosvenor MB, Bernhard NH et al. Nutritional status, gastrointestinal dysfunction and survival in patients with AIDS. *Am J Gastroenterol* 1989; 84: 1288–1293.

8 Guenter P, Muurahainen N, Simons G et al. Relationships among nutritional status, disease progression, and survival in HIV infection. *J Acquir Immune Defic Syndr* 1993; 6: 1130–1138.

9 Palenicek J, Graham NM, He YD et al. Weight loss prior to clinical AIDS as a predictor of survival. *J Acquir Immune Defic Syndr* 1995; 10: 366–373.

10 Semba R, Caiaffa WT, Graham NM et al. Vitamin A deficiency and wasting as predictors of mortality in human immunodeficiency virus-infected injection drug users. *J Acquir Immune Defic Syndr* 1995; 171: 1196–1202.

11 Suttmann U, Ockenga J, Selberg O et al. Incidence and prognostic value of malnutrition and wasting in human immunodeficiency virus-infected outpatients. *J Acquir Immune Defic Syndr* 1995; 8: 239–246.

12 Wheeler D, Gibert CL, Launer CA et al. Weight loss as a predictor of survival and disease progression in HIV infection. *J Acquir Immune Defic Syndr* 1998; 18: 80–85.

13 Grinspoon S, Corcoran C, Rosenthal D et al. Quantitative assessment of cross-sectional muscle area, functional status and muscle strength in men with AIDS wasting syndrome. *J Clin Endocrinol Metab* 1999; 84: 201–206.

14 Dewys WD. Anorexia as a general effect of cancer. *Cancer* 1979; 41: 2013–2019.

15 Dewys WD, Walters K. Abnormalities of taste sensation in cancer patients. *Cancer* 1975; 36: 1888–1896.

16 Glass MJ, Billington CJ, Levine AS. Opioids and food intake: Distributed functional neural pathways? *Neuropeptides* 1999; 33: 360–368.

17 Inui A. Cancer anorexia-cachexia syndrome: Are neuropeptides the key? *Cancer Res* 1999; 59: 4493–4501.

18 Nelson KA, Walsh D, Sheehan FA. The cancer anorexia-cachexia syndrome. *J Clin Oncol* 1994; 12: 213–225.

19 Fujimiya M, Inui A. Peptidergic regulation of gastrointestinal motility in rodents. *Peptides* 2000; 21: 1565–1582.

20 Tache Y, Garrick T, Raybould H. Central nervous system action of peptides to influence gastrointestinal motor function. *Gastroenterology* 1990; 98: 517–528.

21 Inui A, Okano H, Miyamoto M et al. Delayed gastric emptying in bulimic patients. *Lancet* 1995; 346: 1240.

22 Okano H, Inui A, Ueno N et al. EM523L, a nonpeptide motilin agonist, stimulates gastric emptying and pancreatic polypeptide secretion. *Peptides* 1996; 17: 895–900.

23 Capra S, Ferguson M, Ried K. Cancer: Impact of nutrition intervention outcome–Nutrition issues for patients. *Nutrition* 2001; 17: 769–772.

24 Bruera E, Carraro S, Roca E et al. Association between malnutrition and caloric intake, emesis, psychological depression, glucose taste and tumour mass. *Cancer Treat Rep* 1984; 68: 873.

25 Evans WK, Nixon DW, Daly JM et al. A randomized study of oral nutritional support versus ad lib nutritional intake during chemotherapy for advanced colorectal and non-small cell lung cancer. *J Clin Oncol* 1987; 5: 113.

26 Ovesen L, Allingstrup L, Hannibal J et al. Effect of dietary counseling on food intake, body weight, response rate, survival and quality of life in cancer patients undergoing chemotherapy: A prospective, randomized study. *J Clin Oncol* 1993; 11: 2043.

26b Baldwin C, Spiro A, Ahern R. Emery PW. Oral nutritional interventions in malnourished patients with cancer: A systematic review and meta-analysis. *J Natl Cancer Inst* 2012; 104: 371–385.

27 Tisdale MJ. Biology of cachexia—A review. *J Natl Cancer Inst* 1997; 89: 1763.

28   Jatoi A, Loprinzi CL, Sloan JA et al. Neuropeptide y, leptin, and chole-cystokinin 8 in patients with advanced cancer and anorexia. A North Central Cancer Treatment Group exploratory investigation. *Cancer* 2001; 92: 629–633.

29   Moldawer LL, Rogy MA, Lowry SF. The role of cytokines in cancer cachexia. *J Parenter Enteral Nutr* 1992; 16: 43–49.

30   Noguchi Y, Yoshikawa T, Matsumoto A et al. Are cytokines possible mediators of cancer cachexia? *Surg Today* 1996; 26: 467–475.

31   Matthys P, Billiau A. Cytokines and cachexia. *Nutrition* 1997; 13: 763–770.

32   Jatoi A, Egner J, Loprinzi CL et al. Investigating the utility of serum cytokine measurements in a multi-institutional cancer anorexia/weight loss study. *Support Care Cancer* 2004; 12: 640–644.

33   Gelin J, Moldawer LL, Lonnroth C et al. Role of endogenous tumor necro-sis factor alpha and interleukin 1 for experimental tumor growth and the development of cancer cachexia. *Cancer Res* 1991; 51: 415–421.

34   Bessesen DH, Faggioni R. Recently identified peptides involved in the regulation of body weight. *Semin Oncol* 1998; 25: 28–32.

35   Barber MD, Ross JA, Fearon KC. Cancer cachexia. *Surg Oncol* 1999; 8: 133–141.

36   Tisdale MJ. Metabolic abnormalities in cachexia and anorexia. *Nutrition* 2000; 16: 1013–1014.

37   Tayek JA. A review of cancer cachexia and abnormal glucose metabo-lism in humans with cancer. *J Am Coll Nutr* 1992; 11: 445–456.

38   Hirai K, Hussey HJ, Barber MD et al. Biological evaluation of a lipid-mobilizing factor isolated from the urine of cancer patients. *Cancer Res* 1998; 58: 2359–2365.

39   Tisdale MJ. Cancer anorexia and cachexia. *Nutrition* 2001; 17: 438–442.

40   Baracos VE. Regulation of skeletal muscle protein turnover in cancer associated cachexia. *Nutrition* 2000; 16: 1015–1018.

41   Lundholm K, Bylund AC, Holm J, Schersten T. Skeletal muscle metabo-lism in patients with malignant tumor. *Eur J Cancer* 1976; 12: 465–473.

42   Todorov P, Variuk P, McDevitt T et al. Characterization of a cancer cachectic factor. *Nature* 1996; 379: 739–742.

42b Wieland BM, Stewart GD, Skipworth RJ et al. Is there a human homo-logue to the murine proteolysis-inducing factor? *Clin Cancer Res* 2007; 13: 4984–4992.

42c Jatoi A, Foster N, Wieland B et al. The proteolysis inducing factor: In search of its clinical relevance in patients with metastatic gastric/esophageal cancer. *Dis Esoph* 2006; 19: 241–247.

43   Geels P, Eisenhauer E, Bezjak A et al. Palliative effect of chemotherapy: Objective tumor response is associated with symptom improvement in patients with metastatic breast cancer. *J Clin Oncol* 2000; 18: 2395–2405.

44   McGeer AJ, Detsky AS, O'Rourke K. Parenteral nutrition in cancer patients undergoing chemotherapy: A meta-analysis. *Nutrition* 1990; 6: 233.

45   Broqvist M, Arnqvist H, Dahlstrom U et al. Nutritional assessment and mus-cle energy metabolism in severe chronic congestive heart failure—Effects of long-term dietary supplementation. *Eur Heart J* 1994; 15: 1641–1650.

46   Kotler D, Tierney AR, Ferraro R et al. Enteral alimentation and repletion of body cell mass in malnourished patients with acquired immunodefi-ciency syndrome. *Am J Clin Nutr* 1991; 53: 149–154.

47   Kotler D, Tierney AR, Culpepper-Morgan JA et al. Effect of home total par-enteral nutrition on body composition in patients with acquired immuno-deficiency syndrome. *J Parenter Enteral Nutr* 1990; 14: 454–458.

48   Hoda D, Jatoi A, Burnes J et al. Should patients with advanced, incur-able cancers ever be sent home with total parenteral nutrition? *Cancer* 2005; 103: 863–868.

49   Vullo-Navich K, Smith S, Andrews M et al. Comfort and incidence of abnormal serum sodium, bun, creatinine, and osmolality in dehydration of terminal Illness. *Am J Hosp Palliat Care* 1993; 15: 77–84.

49b Hopkinson JB, Wright DNM, Foster C. Management of weight loss and anorexia. *Ann Oncol* (supplement) 2008; 19: 289–293.

50   Jatoi A, Kumar S, Sloan JA, Nguyen PL. On appetite and its loss. *J Clin Oncol* 2000; 59: 166.

51   Loprinzi CL, Ellison NM, Schaid DJ et al. Controlled trial of megestrol acetate for the treatment of cancer anorexia and cachexia. *J Natl Cancer Inst* 1990; 82: 1127–1132.

52   Pascual Lopez A, Roque i Figuls M, Urrutia Cuchi G et al. Systematic review of megestrol acetate in the treatment of anorexia-cachexia syn-drome. *J Pain Symptom Manage* 2004; 27: 360–369.

53   Loprinzi CL, Michalak JC, Schaid DJ et al. Phase III evaluation of four doses of megestrol acetate as therapy for patients with cancer anorexia and/or cachexia. *J Clin Oncol* 1993; 11: 762–767.

54   Jatoi A, Loprinzi CL. Drug therapy for cancer-associated anorexia. In: Ripamonti C, Bruera E (eds). *Gastrointestinal Symptoms in Advanced Cancer Patients.* New York: Oxford University Press, 2002: pp. 361–372.

55   Moertel CG, Schutt AJ, Reitemeier RJ, Hahn RG. Corticosteroid therapy of preterminal gastrointestinal cancer. *Cancer* 1974; 33: 1607.

56   Loprinzi CL, Kugler JW, Sloan JA et al. Randomized comparison of megestrol acetate versus dexamethasone versus fluoxymesterone for the treatment of cancer anorexia/cachexia. *J Clin Oncol* 1999; 17: 3299.

57   Lissoni P, Paolorossi F, Ardizzoia A et al. A randomized study of chemo-therapy with cisplatin plus etoposide versus chemoendocrine therapy with cisplatin, etoposide and the pineal hormone melatonin as a first-line treatment of advanced non-small cell lung cancer patients in poor clinical state. *J Pineal Res* 1997; 23: 15–19.

58   Bruera E, Neumann CM, Pituskin E et al. Thalidomide in patients with cachexia due to terminal cancer: Preliminary report. *Ann Oncol* 1999; 10: 857–859.

59   Klausner JD, Makonkawkeyoon S, Akarasewi P et al. The effect of thalido-mide on the pathogenesis of human immunodeficiency virus type 1 and M. tuberculosis infection. *J Acquir Immune Defic Syndr* 1996; 11: 247–257.

60   Grinspoon S, Mulligan K, Department of Health and Human Services Working Group on the Prevention and Treatment of Wasting and Weight Loss. Weight loss and wasting in patients infected with human immunodeficiency virus. *Clin Infect Dis* 2003; 36: S69–S78.

61   Freeman L, Rush JE, Kehayias JJ et al. Nutritional alterations and the effect of fish oil supplementation in dogs with heart failure. *J Vet Intern Med* 1998; 12: 440–448.

62   Johnston C. IHFS: Etanercept no benefit in treating heart failure—International study stopped prematurely. July 2001. Available at: www.pslgroup.com/dg/2001D6.htm, (accessed October 17, 2005).

63   Anker S. Weight loss in chronic heart failure and the impact of treat-ment with ACE inhibitors—Results from the SOLVD treatment trial. *Circulation* 1999; 100: 1–78.

64   Hryniewicz K, Androne AS, Hudaihed A, Katz SD. Partial reversal of cachexia by beta adrenergic receptor blocker therapy in patients with chronic heart failure. *J Card Fail* 2003; 9: 464–468.

65   Cuneo RC, Wilmshurst P, Lowy C et al. Cardiac failure responding to growth hormone. *Lancet* 1989; 1: 838–839.

66   O'Driscoll JG, Green DJ, Ireland M et al. Treatment of end-stage cardiac failure with growth hormone. *Lancet* 1997; 34: 1068.

67   Clark AL, Loebe M, Potapov EV et al. Ventricular assist device in severe heart failure: Effects on cytokines, complement and body weight. *Eur Heart J* 2001; 22: 2275–2283.

67b Zhou X, Wang JL, Lu J et al. Reversal of cancer cachexia and muscle wasting in ActRIIB antagonism leads to prolonged survival. *Cell* 2010; 142: 531–543.

67c Garcia JM, Friend J, Allen S. Therapeutic potential of anamorelin, a novel, oral ghrelin mimetic, in patients with cancer-related cachexia: A multicentre, randomized, double-blind, crossover, pilot study. *Support Care Cancer* 21: 129–137, 2013.

67d Verstovsek S, Kantarjian H, Mesa RA et al. Safety and efficacy INCB018424, a JAK1 and JAK2 inhibitor, in myelofibrosis. *N Engl J Med* 2010; 363: 1117–1127.

58

Nausea/vomiting

SEBASTIANO MERCADANTE

INTRODUCTION

Nausea and vomiting have long been presented as common and distressing symptoms affecting the majority of patients. In fact, these gastrointestinal symptoms are demeaning, reduce patients' quality of life, and affect compliance with therapy. Nausea occurs both at an early stage and in the advanced stage of cancer disease and has been associated with a shortened survival [1]. The frequency reported in literature varies according to the setting: primary tumor, concurrent treatment, stage and life expectancy, different evaluation tools or study design, and sex. For example, nausea and vomiting occur more frequently in women, probably due to cancer type and increased sensitivity to drugs [2]. It has been reported as affecting up to 70% of patients in the last months of life [3**].

It is reasonable to principally distinguish two forms of nausea and vomiting: that associated with chemotherapy and other oncological treatments, and the chronic multifactorial nausea and vomiting, commonly observed in advanced cancer or associated with progressive diseases. Other than in cancer patients, patients with progressive neurological diseases such as central nervous diseases, peripheral nervous diseases, dysfunction of neuromuscular junction, and muscle diseases may also develop nausea and vomiting with different mechanisms [4].

DEFINITIONS

Accurate use of terminology and an understanding of the symptom experience are essential for reliable, valid assessment and measurement. Three components of vomiting are recognized: nausea, retching, and emesis. Nausea is an unpleasant sensation of the need to vomit and is associated with autonomic symptoms, including pallor, cold sweats, tachycardia, and diarrhea. It may occur without retching or vomiting. It is not clear if nausea and vomiting represent different points along the spectrum of outputs from the vomiting center, or if they are related, but independent, phenomena. Nausea, differently from vomiting and retching, which are objective and definitive signs, arises from subjective components and dimensions unique to the individual.

While nausea is an expression of autonomic stimulation, characterized by a decrease in gastric tone and peristalsis and associated with an increase in the tone of duodenum, retching and vomiting are mediated by somatic nerves. Retching is an attempt to vomit without bringing anything up. It is characterized by a spasmodic movement of the diaphragm and abdominal musculature with the glottis closed, and denotes the labored rhythmic respiratory activity that frequently precedes emesis. The vomiting act involves forceful contraction of the abdominal muscles, contraction of pylorus and antrum, a raised gastric cardias, diminished lower esophageal sphincter pressure, and esophageal dilatation. Intestinal contents are commonly present in vomited material, implying a possible reverse peristalsis [5]. Hypersalivation and cardiac rhythm disturbances are frequently associated phenomena. Although the neural pathways that mediate nausea are not known, evidence suggests that they are the same pathways that mediate vomiting.[4] It may be that mild activation leads to nausea, whereas more intense activation leads to retching or vomiting.

PATHOPHYSIOLOGY AND CAUSES OF NAUSEA AND VOMITING

The distress resulting from these symptoms may escalate over time with the continuing symptom experience, regardless of the frequency, duration, and severity. Although people may experience seemingly identical symptoms, the cause of the symptoms and each person's response to the symptoms may vary, so that an accurate assessment of the individual's symptoms and recognition of the possible causes forms the basis for customized treatments.

Vomiting involves a complex set of activities that suggests a central neurological control by a vomiting center. Stimulation of the dorsal portion of the lateral reticular formation in the vicinity of the fasciculus solitarius produces vomiting. This vomiting center is anatomically adjacent to the medullary centers that control respiration and salivation. The emetic pattern generator is in the third ventricle, close to the area postrema, but lying fully within the blood–brain barrier. It contains D_2-receptors, histaminic (H_1) receptors, muscarinic-cholinergic receptors, serotonin (5-hydroxytryptamine [5-HT] 2 and 3) receptors, which are emetogenic, and m_2-opioid receptors, which are antiemetic at this location. Intracranial lesions are an important cause of nausea and vomiting. The increased intracranial pressure compresses and stimulates the emetic center on the floor of the fourth ventricle. Circumscribed lesions—vascular lesions, neoplasm, or local inflammatory lesions of the brain—may directly affect the emetic center or its afferent pathways. The emetic center may also be stimulated through ventricular dilatation without increased intracranial pressure, as in low-pressure hydrocephalus. Infectious diseases of the central nervous system may also produce vomiting [3**,6,7].

Psychological or emotional factors may also contribute to the generation of nausea at this level, where there is a group of motor nuclei, including the nucleus ambiguous, ventral and dorsal respiratory groups, and the dorsal motor nucleus of the vagus.

An additional important area, the chemoreceptor trigger zone (CTZ), is sensitive to chemical stimuli, and lies in the floor of the fourth ventricle in the brain stem and is able to stimulate the vomiting center. This area is outside the blood–brain barrier and is bathed in the systemic circulation. The CTZ contains emetic receptors for dopamine (D_2), serotonin (5-HT$_3$), acetylcholine (ACHr), and opioids (mu$_2$), which when stimulated provide input for the vomiting center sited in the third ventricle. High plasma concentrations of emetogenic substances, such as calcium ions, urea, morphine, and digoxin, may stimulate dopamine receptors in this area. Anorexia, dehydration, weight loss, abnormal metabolites, and toxins produced by associated infections may also contribute. Moreover, it also receives input from the vestibular apparatus and the vagus (see Box 58.1). The deeper layers of the area postrema are partly formed of the nucleus tractus solitarius, which predominantly contains 5-HT receptors and is considered the main central connection of the vagus. Visceral afferent impulses arising from the gastrointestinal tract may reach the medullary vomiting center by way of the vagus, without traversing the CTZ [3**,6–8].

Box 58.1 Factors stimulating the CTZ

- Glycosides
- Opioids
- Ergot derivatives
- Chemotherapeutic agents, enterotoxins, salicylates
- Metabolic abnormalities: Uremia, hypercalcemia, hyponatremia, diabetic ketoacidosis
- Hypoxia
- Radiation sickness

Vomiting is an integrated somatovisceral process. The central emetic pattern generator coordinates emetic processes, receiving and integrating input from various sources. The efferent pathways are mainly somatic, involving the vagus nerve, the phrenic nerves, and the spinal nerves. Changes in tone and mobility of the stomach during vomiting are likely mediated by visceral efferent neurons. Once the vomiting center has been sufficiently stimulated, the vomiting reflex is initiated. The person takes a deep breath which is held, the glottis closes to avoid aspiration of vomitus, the soft palate elevates to close off the nasal passage, and finally the diaphragm and abdominal muscles contract. As a consequence, intra-abdominal pressure squeezes the stomach between the two sets of muscles, and the gastrointestinal sphincter relaxes, allowing the expulsion of gastric contents [5].

RECEPTORS AND NEUROTRANSMITTERS

Different neuromediators are implicated in the genesis of gastrointestinal symptoms, including dopamine, serotonin (via 5-HT$_3$ receptors), histamine, norepinephrine, gamma-aminobutyric acid (GABA), acetylcholine, and enkephalin.[6] The CTZ is also implicated in delaying the reflex of gastric emptying, and production of taste aversion, which could contribute to vomiting. Acoustic neuroma, bone metastases at the base of the skull, brain tumors, or metastases affecting the vestibular apparatus are possible other causes of vestibular stimulation of H_1 receptors and muscarinic cholinergic receptors. In addition to the direct afferent pathways from the gastrointestinal tract to the vomiting center, the anatomical region of the area postrema receives emetic impulses from the pharynx, heart, peritoneum, mesenteric vasculature, and bile ducts. Impulses from these peripheral receptors are also transmitted directly to the vomiting center.

Drugs, particularly aspirin and opioids, directly stimulate the vestibular apparatus, which in turn provides input to the vomiting center. Receptors in the gastrointestinal tract play an equally important part in the pathogenesis and treatment of nausea and vomiting, particularly 5-HT$_3$, 5-HT$_4$, and D_2 receptors. Activation of D_2 receptors produces gastroparesis. Vagus receptors include 5-HT$_3$ receptors, which are emetogenic, and 5-HT$_4$ receptors, which enhance the propulsion, resulting in a prokinetic effect. This effect is mediated by the cholinergic myenteric plexus, so that it could be inhibited by anticholinergics. Various stimuli, notably bowel distension and inflammation, may produce massive release of 5-HT from enterochromaffin cells contained in the bowel wall. Slowed gastric emptying and constipation, frequently observed in patients progressively immobilized and anorectic, may activate the same process. The activation of these peripheral receptors leads to the stimulation of the vomiting center via vagal and sympathetic afferents. There are also corticobulbar afferents to the vomiting center that mediate vomiting in response to some smells, sights, and tastes, and may play a role in psychogenic vomiting. Stress, anxiety, and nausea from any cause induce delayed gastric emptying via peripheral dopaminergic receptors on the

Table 58.1 *Receptor site affinities of principal antiemetics*

	Dopamine D$_2$ antagonist	Histamine H$_1$ antagonist	Acetylcholine antagonist	5-HT$_2$ antagonist	5-HT$_3$ antagonist	5-HT$_4$ agonist
Metoclopramide	++				+	++
Domperidone	++					
Ondansetron					+++	
Cyclizine		++	++			
Hyoscine			+++			
Haloperidol	+++					
Prochlorperazine	++	+				
Chlorpromazine	++	++	+			
Levomepromazine	++	+++	++	+++		

5-HT, 5-hydroxytryptamine

myenteric plexus interneurons. Therefore, nausea and vomiting are influenced by a complex network of central and peripheral factors that interact with each other. The receptor site affinities of principal antiemetics are listed in Table 58.1.

SPECIFIC CONDITIONS ASSOCIATED WITH VOMITING

Chemotherapy-induced nausea and vomiting

Although chemotherapy and radiation may no longer be indicated for curative reasons in patients with advanced disease, they may provide symptom palliation. Chemotherapy-induced nausea and vomiting is one the most feared effects of cancer treatment and is associated with a significant deterioration in quality of life. These symptoms also may result in nonadherence to or dose reductions in chemotherapy [6].

There are different levels of emetic potential of chemotherapeutic agents. The emetogenic potential is high, in nearly all patients, with cisplatin, decarbazine, melphalan in high doses, and nitrogen mustard [9]. A preemptive treatment with antiemetics is mandatory for the highest levels. Neurotransmitters, such as dopamine, acetylcholine, histamine, and serotonin, are involved in the emetogenic pathways stimulated by chemotherapy and radiation. It has been suggested that chemotherapy causes release of serotonin from enterochromaffin cells of the gastrointestinal tract, which then stimulate emesis via both the vagus and greater splanchnic nerve as well as stimulating the area postrema of the brain, which is rich in serotonin receptors. Thus, serotonin receptors, both central and peripheral, are particularly important in the pathophysiology of acute emesis, and drugs that inhibit this group of receptors are the cornerstone of the prevention and treatment of chemotherapy-related nausea and vomiting. Contributing factors include emetogenic potential of the chemotherapy drug combination, dosages, route, time of day, and length of administration, other therapies, anxiety, previous episodes, sex, and age [10]. Five categories are used to classify this phenomenon: acute, delayed, anticipatory, breakthrough, and refractory. The incidence of acute emesis, occurring in the first 24 hours after chemotherapy, reflects several treatment-related factors, including

the environment in which chemotherapy is administered, the emetogenicity of and doses of drugs administered, and patient-related factors. Delayed emesis develops more than 24 hours after chemotherapy administration. Delayed emesis is more common in patients who experienced acute emesis and typically occurs after carboplatin, doxorubicin, or cyclophosphamide. For cisplatin, emesis reaches peak intensity in 2–3 days and can last up to a week. Vomiting that occurs within 5 days after prophylactic use of antiemetic agents or requires a rescue medication is called breakthrough emesis. If vomiting occurs in subsequent chemotherapy cycles when antiemetic prophylaxis and rescue have failed in earlier cycles, it is known as refractory emesis. Finally, anticipatory nausea and vomiting occurs on the day or some hours before the expected chemotherapy, and often symptoms present in particular conditions, such as talking or thinking about the treatment. It affects a third of patients attending for chemotherapy. A psychological mechanism of association is probable, and is strongly related to the intensity of adverse effects associated with the previous chemotherapy, and the number of treatments received. Younger age, expectation, and motion sickness are well-recognized risk factors for developing anticipatory nausea and vomiting, probably due to the higher doses used and anxiety [6].

Disorders affecting the central nervous system

Different neurological diseases may produce a disturbance in central control of gut motility, resulting in gastrointestinal syndromes, such as vomiting or intestinal pseudo-obstruction with or without gastric stasis (Table 58.2).

Lesions of various origin of the spinal cord, above T$_5$, may isolate the spinal sympathetic control from the influence of high centers. This results in a delayed gastric emptying and delay in duodenal progression. In the early period, severe gastric stasis and dilatation, and ileus are commonly present. In cases of long-term loss of function, patients who develop quadriplegia are more likely to have gut complications than those with paraplegia. The incidence of gastroesophageal reflux is increased and gastric emptying impaired. Chronic constipation may worsen the clinical picture, possibly facilitating the development of nausea and vomiting. Neuropathies are frequently encountered in patients with cancer [4].

Table 58.2   *Nervous system diseases associated with nausea and vomiting*

Disease group	Mechanisms
Central nervous system	
Cerebral and brainstem disorders	
Multiple sclerosis	Gastroparesis
Parkinson disease	Gastrointestinal dysmotility
Cerebral masses	Compression of vomiting center
Spinal cord disorders	
Amyotrophic lateral sclerosis	Gastric atony, ileus
Poliomyelitis	Gastric atony, ileus
Autonomic dysfunction, gastric atony	Esophageal dysfunction
Peripheral nervous system	
Alcohol-related gastroparesis	Gastritis (acute), neuropathy—impaired esophageal peristalsis
Myenteric plexus dysfunction	Pseudo-obstruction
(Chagas disease, Hirschsprung disease, achalasia, ganglioneuromatosis)	
Neuromuscular junction	
Myasthenia gravis	Oropharyngeal incoordination
Muscle disease	
Myotonic dystrophy	Dysphagia, gastric atony, pseudo-obstruction
Dermatomyositis-polymyositis	Dysphagia, gastric atony, pseudo-obstruction
Oculopharyngeal muscular dystrophy	Dysphagia
Duchenne muscular dystrophy	Dysphagia, pseudo-obstruction
Familiar visceral neuropathy	Dysphagia, pseudo-obstruction

Source: Twycross, R. and Back, I., *Eur. J. Palliat. Care*, 5, 39, 1998.

Autonomic failure

Autonomic failure is more common in patients with poor performance status often associated with anorexia-cachexia syndrome. The mechanisms remain unclear and appear to be multifactorial—tumor invasion of nervous tissue, malnutrition, damage from chemotherapy or radiotherapy, drugs, preexisting disease—and could be considered a sort of paraneoplastic syndrome, producing gastroparesis [11].

Other disorders may affect the extrinsic gastrointestinal innervation. There is evidence that vagal autonomic neuropathy may be responsible for gastric motor disturbances in diabetic patients with gastroparesis. It is well known that the motility disorder involves not only the stomach, but also the upper small bowel. This has been commonly attributed to gastric motor dysfunction with delayed gastric emptying. Peripheral neuropathy, manifestations of autonomic neuropathy, with bladder dysfunction, sweat disorder, orthostatic hypotension, impotence, nephropathy, and retinopathy are frequently found, as gastroparesis is commonly reported in patients with longstanding, insulin-dependent poorly controlled diabetes.[11] Neurological diseases, such as dystrophia myotonica and progressive muscular dystrophy, amyloidosis, collagen vascular diseases, and autoimmune neurological diseases, may affect parietal structures of the gastrointestinal tract, inducing motility dysfunction, which can precipitate nausea and vomiting.[2] Radiation injury is another important cause of gastrointestinal dysmotility. Early vomiting is probably due to direct mucosal injury, whereas late vomiting and gastrointestinal stasis may be related to radiation-induced inflammation or strictures [5,12].

Metabolic disorders

Significant gastrointestinal disturbances may be associated with thyroid and parathyroid disorders. Intestinal pseudo-obstruction may develop both in hyperthyroidism and hypothyroidism. The role of gastrointestinal hormones in disorders of upper intestinal motility remains unclear [8].

Drug-induced nausea and vomiting

Many drugs commonly cause nausea and vomiting. Adrenergic agents, such as β-agonists, generally delay gastric emptying, whereas β blockers enhance gastric emptying. Clonidine, an α_2 agonist, may induce nausea and vomiting. Anticholinergic agents, such as some tricyclic antidepressants, inhibit contractile activity and delay gastric emptying.

Dopamine agonists, opioids, digitalis, and chemotherapeutic agents such as cisplatin remain the major offenders. Opioids have central and peripheral actions. Centrally, they may stimulate the emetic center via D_2 receptors of the CTZ, richly distributed in the area postrema. In addition, they induce a relevant delay in gastric emptying and a delay in intestinal transit. Nausea occurs when there is relaxation of the esophageal sphincter tone, delayed gastric emptying, and poor duodenum motility. The narcotic bowel syndrome is characterized by a picture similar to pseudo-obstruction. Nonsteroidal anti-inflammatory drugs (NSAIDs) may induce nausea and vomiting by damaging gastric mucosa and activating peripheral ascending impulses. A central effect of alcohol on the CTZ has been recognized, other than the well-known consequence of damage to the gastric mucosa [13].

ASSESSMENT AND DIAGNOSIS

Like pain, nausea is a subjective experience and presents all of the problems inherent in measuring pain. Nausea is usually assessed by visual analogue or numerical scales. Vomiting can be objectively recorded as events in a manner reminiscent of the methodology used to study antiemesis related to chemotherapy.

Many factors should be considered when choosing antiemetic treatment. History, examination, and review of the ongoing drug regimen are generally helpful in finding the cause of gastrointestinal symptoms in the neurological population. A multitude of medications, including opioids, digoxin, antibiotics, imidazoles, and cytotoxics, can cause nausea and vomiting by acting on the CTZ, whereas NSAIDs, iron supplements, antibiotics, and tranexamic acid may damage gastric mucosa. Opioids, tricyclics, phenothiazines, and anticholinergics induce gastric stasis. Finally, selective serotonin reuptake inhibitors and cytotoxic drugs may induce 5-HT$_3$ receptor stimulation. Uncontrolled pain *per se* may be a cause of nausea and vomiting.

In patients with neurological diseases such as diabetic neuropathy, or with advanced cancer, autonomic failure occurs with gastroparesis, nausea, vomiting, and constipation. Movement-related nausea with vomiting suggests either vestibular dysfunction or mesenteric traction. Nausea increasing with head motion, with tinnitus, decreased hearing, or skull tenderness is suggestive of vestibular involvement due to drug toxicity and local lesions. Presence of vertigo may be helpful in distinguishing the two conditions. Candidal infection may produce pharyngeal irritation, activating the afferent arm of the vomiting circuit via the vagus nerve and should be suspected in patients taking steroids.

Emesis produced with cough occurs at the end or during a coughing paroxysm and is associated with chronic pulmonary disease, esophageal fistulas, and brain metastases. Morning vomiting, sometimes projectile, associated with cognitive changes or neurological deficits may be due to brain tumors or secondaries. Papilledema may be a possible associated sign. Neck stiffness and headache may be signs of underlying meningitis. Computed tomography (CT) or magnetic resonance imaging (MRI) can confirm the diagnosis. Nausea produced by hyperglycemia or hypercalcemia is associated with polyuria and polydipsia. Patients treated for prolonged periods with steroids for chronic neurological disease may develop Addison disease after abrupt suspension of medication.

Vomiting that occurs in relation to meals is frequently of diagnostic importance. Patients with gastric outlet obstruction or gastric atony often will complain of vomiting several hours after eating. In contrast, patients who vomit as a result of viral gastroenteritis or psychogenic causes are usually symptomatic in the immediate postprandial period. Appropriate screening tests include a biochemistry profile consisting of electrolytes, blood urea nitrogen, creatinine, glucose, albumin, and calcium. In patients taking digoxin or anticonvulsants, the plasma drug levels should be considered. A pattern of infrequent large-volume vomitus which relieves nausea suggests a partial bowel obstruction. Abdominal examination and an abdominal x-ray are helpful to screen for situations involving subobstruction. Abdominal CT and ultrasound may be required to complete the investigation. Emotional experience may trigger psychogenic vomiting.

TREATMENT

Long periods or repeated episodes of vomiting can lead to dehydration. To avoid this, it is important to replace fluids lost through vomiting. In some circumstances, it is necessary to administer fluids and drugs by the parenteral route, either subcutaneously or intravenously. Treating any identifiable cause of nausea and vomiting is the first step. Reversible causes include hypercalcemia, hyperglycemia, hypocortisolism, hyponatremia, uremia, obstipation, and increased intracranial pressure. Bisphosphonates for hypercalcemia and dexamethasone for intracranial tumors are the first-line treatments in these specific conditions. Identifiable offending drugs should be stopped. A range of environmental and psychological factors contribute to the experience of nausea. A calm and reassuring environment may be useful, avoiding exposure to foods precipitating nausea. Control of malodor from decubitus ulcers is mandatory. Behavioral techniques, relaxation exercises, and benzodiazepines may be helpful for anticipatory nausea.

Generally, widely accepted management guidelines are not available, except for the treatment of nausea and vomiting associated with chemotherapy. The use of the modern antiemetic regimens based on combinations of drugs has dramatically reduced the incidence, which was reported to be about 80% in the past decades [6].

The pharmacological treatment of nausea and vomiting in the palliative care setting does not have solid data to provide specific information. The fact that different agents cause nausea and vomiting by different mechanisms prompted researchers to develop regimens with multiple drug with different mechanisms of action [14***]. Although the mechanism considered to play the predominant role in the induction of nausea and vomiting is the activation of the CTZ; gastrointestinal stimulation or damage, vestibular and cortical mechanisms, or alterations of taste and smell, all may equally contribute in different ways in producing these symptoms.

Many classes of medication have been used as antiemetics. If vomiting prevents drug absorption, a nonoral route should be used at first. Patients should be re-evaluated at regular intervals to optimize the dose or to switch drugs. The choice of medication depends upon drug receptor selectivity and drug interactions, as patients are frequently receiving several medications that potentially interact with or antagonize the antiemetics. The afferent pathway involved and the group of antiemetics that antagonize the involved neuroreceptors are key factors that influence the choice of the first drug, that is, a mechanistic approach should be the basis for choosing first-line antiemetic drugs. The sites and possible receptor mechanisms of the principal antiemetic drugs are listed in Table 58.1.

An important principle is to use combinations of antiemetics with different modes of action [15,16], primarily based on starting with a metoclopramide regimen. On the other hand, antiemetics may have specific adverse effects in patients with neurological diseases. Moreover, anticholinergic medications may antagonize the prokinetic effects of drugs acting via the cholinergic system in the myenteric plexus [3**].

In a systematic review of the efficacy of antiemetics in the treatment of nausea in patients with terminal cancer, uncontrolled studies had high response rates (75%–93%) to standard regimens, whereas randomized controlled trials reported much lower response rates (23%–36% percent for nausea, 18%–52% for vomiting), regardless of an empirical or a more selective clinical approach [17***].

Antiemetic drugs are commonly grouped into five categories, including prokinetic agents, dopamine antagonists, antihistamines, anticholinergics, and serotonin antagonists. However, most of them are broad agents working at multiple receptor sites. Moreover, there are novel and old drugs not included in these groups, such as corticosteroids, cannabinoids, benzodiazepines, and neurokinin-1 receptor antagonists. The use of octreotide will be described in the chapter regarding bowel obstruction.

Prokinetic agents

The prokinetic antiemetics activate 5-HT_4 receptors and antagonize 5-HT_3 receptors and D_2 receptors, favoring acetylcholine release from myenteric plexus neurons in the upper gastrointestinal tract. Metoclopramide, in addition to its recognized dopamine antagonist action, also acts as a weak serotonin antagonist and can stimulate gastrointestinal motility by increasing acetylcholine release, which explains the potential for central adverse effects, such as extrapyramidal reactions. Metoclopramide, usually combined with steroids, appears to be as effective as the "setrons" (see below) in preventing delayed emesis, and is cheaper than specific antiserotonin agents. Metoclopramide enhances the transit of the contents of the gastrointestinal tract as far as the jejunum, speeding gastric emptying, and decreasing small intestinal transit time, probably by increasing cholinergic activity through the activation of 5-HT_4 receptors. In high doses, metoclopramide also has 5-HT_3 receptor antagonist activity. Although in same studies

the efficacy was similar to that observed with placebo [18**], metoclopramide in doses of 60 mg daily was quite effective in a cancer population with chronic nausea. Three percent of patients required other antiemetics because of extrapyramidal side effects [19*]. Controlled-release metoclopramide 40 mg every 12 hours, significantly reduced nausea, without producing the pertinent adverse effects in patients with a history of cancer-associated dyspepsia syndrome [20**]. Metoclopramide use confers an increased risk for the initiation of treatment generally reserved for the management of Parkinson disease in patients with drug-induced parkinsonian symptoms [22*].

Domperidone, a D_2 antagonist analogous of metoclopramide that poorly crosses the blood–brain barrier, acts primarily on gastric D_2 receptors and D_2 receptors in the CTZ, which are outside the blood–brain barrier, facilitating gastric motor activity and emptying. Extrapyramidal adverse effects are less likely, because it does not cross the blood–brain barrier [2,3**].

Dopamine antagonists

Phenothiazines and butyrophenones belong to the class of D_2 antagonists. Haloperidol has a relatively narrow spectrum and is a potent D_2 antagonist with negligible anticholinergic activity, so it produces less sedation than phenothiazines but greater extrapyramidal reactions [3**]. Haloperidol has been widely used in the management of nausea and vomiting due to chemical or toxic causes, nonrelated to cancer treatment. Despite the lack of evidence and the need for objective evaluation, about half of patients are expected to have a benefit [21]. Antiemetic doses are lower than antipsychotic doses. It is less likely than phenothiazines to cause sedation, but causes more extrapyramidal side effects [3**].

Phenothiazines possess a broader spectrum of activity with dopaminergic, cholinergic, and histamine receptor antagonism. Hypotension, sedation, and decreased salivary flow are the main adverse effects. Central and hemodynamic adverse effects are more likely with major tranquilizers like chlorpromazine. Levomepromazine is a phenothiazine closely related chemically to chlorpromazine. Its proven analgesic properties make it unique among the phenothiazines. It is efficacious and generally nonsedative in doses of 5–12.5 mg/day. It is a potent antagonist at 5-HT_2, H_1, D_2, and a_1-receptors [3**]. Methotrimeprazine is a phenothiazine antipsychotic used in palliative care for the management of terminal agitation and nausea/vomiting. The administration of low-dose methotrimeprazine proved to be useful in patients with advanced malignancy [22].

Olanzapine, an atypical antipsychotic, possesses a unique neurotransmitter binding profile that is similar to methotrimeprazine. It blocks multiple neurotransmitters, particularly at the D_2 and 5-HT_3 receptors. It has been shown to relieve nausea in some patients with advanced cancer who fail to respond to the usual antiemetics [23–25]. Olanzapine has been also used to reduce the incidence of delayed emesis in patients receiving moderate to highly emetogenic chemotherapy and is well tolerated [6].

ANTIHISTAMINES

There are many drugs in this class, including promethazine and cyclizine, all of which have potential as antiemetics because they exert a H_1 receptor antagonism in the vomiting center of medulla, the vestibular nucleus, and the CTZ, although they belong to phenothiazine family. They also have an antimuscarinic effect, blocking the cholinergic receptors on intestinal smooth muscles. Promethazine has been largely used for motion sickness and vestibular disorders, but may also help with nausea related to raised intracranial pressure. The antiemetic dose of promethazine is 25 mg orally or intravenously every 4–6 hours. Cyclizine has more antimuscarinic activity, making it useful for bowel obstruction as well as movement-related nausea [3**]. Cyclizine is effective in nausea associated with motion sickness, pharyngeal stimulation, bowel obstruction, and increased intracranial pressure. Drowsiness and antimuscarinic effects are the main adverse effects [2,8].

Anticholinergics

Hyoscine is a naturally occurring compound, which competitively inhibits the action of acetylcholine and other muscarinic agonists. The primary indication of hyoscine is motor sickness and labyrinthic disturbances. Because it relaxes smooth muscle and reduces gastrointestinal secretions via blockade of muscarinic receptors, it is also used for the management of gastrointestinal symptoms in patients with inoperable bowel obstruction. Unlike the other antimuscarinic agents, hyoscine produces central nervous system depression in therapeutic doses—manifesting as drowsiness, euphoria, amnesia, disorientation, restlessness, and hallucinations [2]. The anticholinergic effects of hyoscine are a potential problem in the elderly. The butylbromide salt does not cross the blood–brain barrier and is less sedating [3**].

Setron family

As mentioned above, serotonin receptors, both central and peripheral, are particularly important in the pathophysiology of acute emesis and drugs that target this group of receptors underpin the prevention and treatment of chemotherapy-related nausea and vomiting. The role of the $5\text{-}HT_3$ receptor was recognized during the evaluation of the mechanism of high-dose metoclopramide, which, unlike other D_2 receptor antagonists, has a good capacity to reduce the emesis induced by cisplatin administration.

Several $5\text{-}HT_3$ antagonists are commercially available, including ondansetron, granisetron, tropisetron, dolasetron, and palonosetron. Many randomized controlled trials have demonstrated that these agents have equivalent antiemetic activity and safety at the recommended doses, despite differences in structure and pharmacokinetic profiles [26**], both orally and intravenously, due to their good bioavailability following oral administration. These drugs are well tolerated,

and central adverse effects are not commonly observed with serotonin antagonists, unless for constipation which may be of concern in advanced cancer patients. Palonosetron, compared with older $5\text{-}HT_3$ receptor antagonists, has a higher potency and a significantly longer half-life. It is used in a single dose of 0.25 mg for the prevention of acute and delayed nausea and vomiting associated with initial and repeat courses of moderately and highly emetogenic cancer chemotherapy [6].

The effect of the setrons on the serotonin-mediated emetic pathways may lend itself to the management of chronic nausea. Ondansetron, a selective $5\text{-}HT_3$ antagonist, has been used in palliative care setting in patients not responding to conventional treatments. In 9 of 16 patients with advanced human immunodeficiency disease, the treatment was effective and well tolerated [27]. However, in a controlled study, the efficacy of ondansetron at relatively large doses was similar to that reported with placebo [18]. Tropisetron-containing combinations or tropisetron as a single agent are much more effective in the control of emesis in patients with advanced cancer than the conventional antiemetic combination of chlorpromazine plus dexamethasone [28*]. Not being antidopaminergic, setrons are potentially useful when the risk of extrapyramidal reactions is high, such as in children or elderly people who have neurological diseases with an extrapyramidal component. They appear to have no effect on motion sickness [2].

Neurokinin-1 receptor antagonists

These substances inhibit the effects of substance P on the nucleus tractus solitarius. In early clinical trials, the neurokinin-1 receptor antagonist aprepitant was effective in the prevention of acute and delayed chemotherapy-induced nausea and vomiting associated with single or multiple cycles of highly emetogenic chemotherapy, when combined with best available therapy, including a $5\text{-}HT_3$ receptor antagonist and dexamethasone. Aprepitant is used in doses of 125 mg on day one and then 80 mg once daily on days 2 and 3 and is generally well tolerated [29]. Fosaprepitant and casopitant represent the new generation of neurokinin-1 receptor antagonists [6].

Benzodiazepines

The sedative properties of benzodiazepines may enhance the effectiveness of other antiemetic regimen. Benzodiazepines in combination with dopamine antagonists were found more appropriate for use in breakthrough and anticipatory symptoms or in preventing the delayed phase of chemotherapy-induced nausea and vomiting [7].

Steroids

Dexamethasone has synergistic or additive antiemetic effects combined with setrons, metoclopramide, or phenothiazines. The mechanism remains unknown. The antiemetic actions of dexamethasone are not well characterized, except for use in the treatment of nausea and vomiting due to increased intracranial pressure. Adverse effects include glucose intolerance, myopathy, osteopenia, and infections [2,8].

Dronabinol

Cannabinoids appear to be of low antiemetic efficacy, and adverse effects may occur. The mechanism of the antiemetic effect of cannabinoids is unknown. It has been hypothesized that an indirect inhibition of the vomiting center in the medulla occurs as a result of binding to opioid receptors in the forebrain. Dronabinol has been used in diffuse metastatic disease in the gastrointestinal tract mucosa for intractable nausea and vomiting unresponsive to conventional antiemetics [30].

Key learning points

- Nausea and vomiting are frequent symptoms reported by cancer patients. Several causes are recognized, including curative and symptomatic treatments, as well as disease itself.

- Different and complex systems are involved in the mechanisms producing these symptoms.

- Except for chemotherapy-induced vomiting, no clear guidelines have been produced for the remaining conditions, particularly in advanced-stage disease, when multiple factors may play a role in producing or exacerbating nausea and vomiting.

- Different classes of antiemetics or their combinations are usually chosen according to the supposed mechanism with variable efficacy.

- The need for controlled studies is justified by the finding that uncontrolled studies show high response rates, whereas randomized controlled studies have shown lower response rates.

REFERENCES

1 Chang VT, Hwang SS, Kasimis B et al. Shorter symptom assessment instruments: The Condensed memorial Symptom Assessment Scale (CMSAS). *Cancer Invest* 2004;22:526–536.

2 Twycross R, Back I. Nausea and vomiting in advanced cancer. *Eur J Palliat Care* 1998;5:39–45.

3 Glare PA, Dunwoodie D, Clark K et al. Treatment of nausea and vomiting in terminally ill patients. *Drugs* 2008;68:2575–2590.

4 Mercadante S. Nausea and vomiting. In: Voltz R, Bernat JL, Borasio GD eds. *Palliative Care in Neurology*. Oxford, U.K.: Oxford University Press, 2004.

5 Nailor R, Rudd JA. Emesis and anti-emesis. In: Hanks GW ed. *Cancer Surveys, Vol. 21. Palliative Medicine: Problem Areas in Pain and Symptom Management*. New York: Cold Spring Harbor Laboratory Press, 1994: pp. 117–135.

6 Navari RM. Pharmacological management of chemotherapy-induced nausea and vomiting. *Drugs* 2009;69:515–533.

7 Perwitasari DA, Geldrblom H, Atthobari J et al. Anti-emetic drugs in oncology: Pharmacology and individualization by pharmacogenetics. *Int J Clin Pharm* 2011;33:33–43.

8 Fallon B. Nausea and vomiting unrelated to cancer treatment. In: Berger AM, Portenoy RK, Weissman DE eds. *Principles and Practice of Supportive Oncology*. Philadelphia, PA: Lippincott Williams & Wilkins, 1998: pp. 179–190.

9 Grunberg SM, Osoba D, Hesketh PJ et al. Evaluation of new antiemetic agents and definition of antineoplastic agent emetogenivity—An update. *Support Care Cancer* 2005;13:80–84.

10 Rhodes V, McDaniel R. Nausea, vomiting, and retching: Complex problems in palliative care. *CA Cancer J Clin* 2001;51:232–248.

11 Bruera E, Sweeney C. Chronic nausea and vomiting. In: Berger AM, Portenoy RK, Weissman DE eds. *Principles and Practice of Supportive Oncology*, 2nd edn. Philadelphia, PA: Lippincott Williams & Wilkins, 2002: pp. 222–232.

12 Lee M, Feldman M. Nausea and vomiting. In: Slesinger MH, Fordtran JS eds. *Gastrointestinal Disease*. Philadelphia, PA: WB Saunders Co, 1993: pp. 509–523.

13 Mercadante S. Diarrhea, malabsorption, constipation. In: Berger A, Von Roenn J, Shuster J. *Principles and Practice of Palliative Care and Supportive Oncology*, 3rd edn. Philadelphia, PA: Lippincott Williams & Wilkins, 2007: pp. 163–176.

14 Kris MG, Hesketh PJ, Somerfield MR et al. American Society of Clinical Oncology guideline for antiemetics in oncology: An update 2006. *J Clin Oncol* 2006;24:2932–2947.

15 Bentley A, Boyd K. Use of clinical pictures in the management of nausea and vomiting: A prospective audit. *Palliat Med* 2001;15:247–253.

16 Herndon CM, Jackson KC, Hallin PA. Management of opioid-induced gastrointestinal effects in patients receiving palliative care. *Pharmacotherapy* 2002;22:240–250.

17 Glare P, Pereira G, Kristjanson LJ et al. Systematic review of the efficacy of antiemetic in the treatment of nausea in patients with far-advanced cancer. *Support Care Cancer* 2004;12:432–440.

18 Hardy J, Daly S, McQuade B et al. A double-blind, randomised parallel group, multi-national, multi-centre study comparing ondansetron 24 mg p.o. with placebo and metoclopramide 10 mg tds p.o. in the treatment of opioid induced nausea and emesis in cancer patients. *Support Care Cancer* 2002;10:231–236.

19 Bruera E, Seifert L, Watanabe S et al. Chronic nausea in advanced cancer patients: A retrospective assessment of a metoclopramide-based antiemetic regimen. *J Pain Symptom Manage* 1996;11:147–153.

20 Bruera E, Balzile M, Neumann C et al. A double-blind, crossover study of controlled-release metoclopramide and placebo for the chronic nausea and dyspepsia of advanced cancer. *J Pain Symptom Manage* 2000;19:427–435.

21 Hardy JR, O'Shea A, White C, Gilshenan K, Welch L, Douglas C. The efficacy of haloperidol in the management of nausea and vomiting in patients with cancer. *J Pain Symptom Manage* 2010;40:111–116.

22 Kennett A, Hardy J, Shah S, A'Hern R. An open study of methotrimeprazine in the management of nausea and vomiting in patients with advanced cancer. *Support Care Cancer* 2005;13:715–721.

23 Passik SD, Kirsh KL, Theobald DE et al. A retrospective chart review of the use of olanzapine for the prevention of delayed emesis in cancer patients. *J Pain Symptom Manage* 2003;25:485–488.

24 Srivastava M, Brito-Dellan N, Davis MP et al. Olanzapine as an antiemetic in refractory nausea and vomiting in advanced cancer. *J
Palliat Med* 2003;6:251–255.

25 Brown J. A retrospective chart review of the use of olanzapine for
the prevention of delayed emesis in cancer patients. *J Pain Symptom
Manage* 2003;25:485–488.

● 26 Hesketh PJ. Chemotherapy-induced nausea and vomiting. *N Engl J
Med* 2008;358:2482–2494.

27 Currow DC, Coughlan M, Fardell B, Cooney NJ. Use of ondansetron in
palliative medicine. *J Pain Symptom Manage* 1997;13:302–307.

28 Mystakidou K, Befon S, Liossi C, Vlachos L. Comparison of tropisetron and chlorpromazine combinations in the control of nausea and
vomiting in patients with advanced cancer. *J Pain Symptom Manage*
1998;15:176–184.

29 Curran MP, Robinson DM. Aprepitant. A review of its use in the prevention of nausea and vomiting. *Drugs* 2009;69:1853–1878.

30 Walsh D, Nelson KA, Mahomoud FA. Established and potential therapeutic application of cannabinoids in oncology. *Support Care Cancer*
2003;11:137–143.

59

Constipation and diarrhea

JAY R. THOMAS

INTRODUCTION/NORMAL GASTROINTESTINAL PHYSIOLOGY

The gastrointestinal (GI) tract is a complex organ system that in disease conditions can cause significant distress, including constipation and diarrhea. To understand the pathophysiology and treatment of these conditions requires an understanding of normal GI physiology.

Normal GI function includes secretion, absorption, transport, and storage [1,2]. The details of these processes vary throughout the GI tract, but there are common themes. In terms of intestinal motility, there are two basic forms of contraction: segmental and peristaltic. Segmental contraction serves to mix luminal contents in place and expose different surfaces to the mucosa to be acted upon by secretion or absorption. Peristalsis involves increased muscular tone proximally coordinated with decreased muscular tone distally so that contraction leads to forward movement of luminal contents. In the small intestine, during fasting states, "migrating motor complexes" occur about every 90 min to sweep luminal contents from the duodenum to the ileum. About 90 min is needed to traverse this distance. In the colon, "mass movements" occur on average from one to three times per day; these movements propel luminal contents over large distances.

A local GI event also must be coordinated with other GI processes and systemic events. For example, under "fight or flight conditions," GI perfusion and motility are decreased. After a meal, the gastrocolonic reflex leads to increased colonic motility. Finally, when the rectum is full, the rectosphincteric reflex leads to relaxation of the internal anal sphincter.

These events are regulated via neurocrine, endocrine, paracrine, autocrine, and immune mechanisms. Under the serosa, the smooth muscle system of the GI tract consists of an outer longitudinal layer and an inner circular layer, whereas the lumen is lined with the mucosal layer. In general, the smooth muscle cells are in electrical contact via gap junctions, allowing synchronous contraction after stimulation by the neurotransmitter acetylcholine.

Nervous system control is mediated by both intrinsic and extrinsic systems. The intrinsic enteric nervous system consists of the myenteric plexus that resides between the layers of smooth muscle and the submucosal plexus that resides just beneath the mucosa. This enteric "brain" consists of 400–600 million neurons, including afferent neurons, efferent neurons, and interneurons utilizing neurotransmitters, such as acetylcholine, serotonin, vasoactive intestinal peptide (VIP), somatostatin, endogenous opioids, and nitric oxide. Projections from enteric neurons to the spinal cord and brain have been identified [3]. Ninety-five percent of the body's serotonin resides in the GI tract, and many of the subtypes of serotonin receptors have been identified there. The 5HT1p and 5HT4 serotonin receptor subtypes seem particularly important in mediating contractility [4].

The extrinsic system consists of the autonomic nervous system. Parasympathetic input is derived from the vagus and pelvic nerves, whereas sympathetic input arises from the thoracolumbar spine.

The interstitial cells of Cajal (ICC) commingle with the neurons and smooth muscle cells of the GI tract [5]. The ICC are electrically coupled via gap junctions and generate oscillating "slow wave" activity that is conveyed to the smooth muscle via gap junctions also. These slow waves set the periodicity of smooth muscle action potentials that occur at the peak of slow wave electrical activity. Finally, enterochromaffin cells line the mucosa. They contain serotonin that can be released by perturbation of their luminal surface by luminal contents.

Integration of input from all these systems determines the patterns of secretion, absorption, and motility that are established. For example, a meal triggers cholecystokinin release that, through a series of secondary messengers, ultimately leads to increased colonic motility. Under stressful conditions, sympathetic input to the GI tract is increased, which leads to decreased blood flow, decreased secretion, and decreased motility. When luminal contents physically distort the mucosal enterochromaffin cells, they release their serotonin stores, leading to a wave of communication, ultimately ending in smooth muscle contraction.

About 9 L of fluid passes through the GI tract each day. About 2 L is ingested orally, and secretion from the salivary glands, stomach, liver, pancreas, and small intestine accounts for about 7 L of fluid. After absorption in the small intestine, about 1–2 L enters the colon. The colon has an absorptive capacity of 3–4 L/day [6], and about 0.2 L is excreted each day.

Disruption of this complex orchestration of communication at the level of pacemaker cells, nerves, muscle, or transmitters can lead to bowel dysfunction, triggering either constipation or diarrhea.

CONSTIPATION

Definition/epidemiology

The Rome III criteria are a research definition for functional constipation (Table 59.1) [7]. This definition highlights the physical characteristics of stool, frequency of bowel movements, and subjective perceptions of distress as important to constipation. It is a common and distressing symptom in palliative care despite not formally meeting this research definition. In North America, functional constipation ranges from 2% to 27% in the general population [8]. In patients with advanced illness such as cancer, Sykes found that the prevalence of constipation before onset of severe disease was similar to this prevalence of the population at large. After diagnosis, 54% of patients reported constipation half of the time [9]. In another study of advanced cancer patients, constipation was present in 64% of patients not on opioids and approached 90% when they were on strong opioids [10]. Constipation is associated with other symptoms (Table 59.2) that augment its distress, which can be experienced as greater than pain in this population [11].

Table 59.1 Rome III criteria for functional constipation

1. Must include *two or more* of the following:
   a. Straining during at least 25% of defecations
   b. Lumpy or hard stools in at least 25% of defecations
   c. Sensation of incomplete evacuation for at least 25% of defecations
   d. Sensation of anorectal obstruction/blockage for at least 25% of defecations
   e. Manual maneuvers to facilitate at least 25% of defecations (e.g., digital evacuation, support of the pelvic floor)
   f. Fewer than three defecations per week
2. Loose stools are rarely present without the use of laxatives.
3. Insufficient criteria for irritable bowel syndrome.

* Criteria fulfilled for the last 3 months with symptom onset at least 6 months prior to diagnosis.

Table 59.2 Symptoms associated with constipation

- Anorexia
- Abdominal distension
- Abdominal pain
- Nausea and/or vomiting
- Flatulence
- Pseudodiarrhea (see section on diarrhea)
- Fecal impaction/GI obstruction
- Dyspnea (from limiting diaphragmatic excursion)
- Urinary retention
- Delirium

Causes

Common causes of constipation are listed in Table 59.3. There may also be general factors correlated with increased age often present in advanced illness that contribute to constipation. These include altered diet with decreased fiber content, decreased exercise, and age itself, which has been correlated with loss of enteric neurons [12]. Given the prevalence of 2%–27% in the general population, functional constipation is likely to be comorbid in a subset of palliative care patients. However, secondary causes of constipation are much more common, and in serious illness, there may be multiple coexisting etiologies. Endocrine/metabolic causes include diabetes, hypothyroidism, and hypercalcemia. Nerve function can be perturbed by diseases like Parkinson's, direct invasion by tumor, or paraneoplastic syndromes. Intrinsic or extrinsic luminal compression from masses can mechanically lead to constipation. Psychologic conditions such as depression have been linked to an increased incidence of constipation [13]. Medications, such as calcium channel blockers, anticholinergic agents, antiserotonergic agents, and opioids, are prime mediators of constipation.

Because of mu receptor agonists' (e.g., morphine) prominence in constipation in palliative care, the existence of targeted therapies for opioid-induced constipation, and the therapeutic

Table 59.3 Causes of constipation

- Primary/idiopathic
  - Slow transit constipation
  - Normal transit constipation
  - Pelvic floor dyssynergia
- Secondary
  - Endocrine/metabolic
    - Hypothyroidism
    - Hypercalcemia
    - Hypokalemia
    - Dehydration
  - Nervous system
    - Peripheral nervous system
      - Autonomic neuropathy (including diabetic neuropathy)
      - Neuropathy (tumor invasion, paraneoplastic syndrome)
      - Hirschsprung disease
      - Chagas disease
    - Central nervous system
      - Brain or spinal cord lesion
      - Multiple sclerosis
      - Parkinson's disease
      - Depression
  - Mechanical
    - Intrinsic and extrinsic luminal compression
  - Myopathy/Collagen vascular
    - Myotonic dystrophy
    - Dermatomyositis
    - Amyloidosis
    - Systemic sclerosis
  - Medications (see Table 59.4)

Table 59.4 *Medications commonly associated with constipation*

- Opioids
- 5-Hydroxytryptamine (5-HT$_3$) blockers
- Anticholinergic (antispasmodics, antidepressants, and phenothiazines)
- Haloperidol
- Anticonvulsants
- Iron
- Calcium-channel blockers
- Vinca alkaloids
- Aluminum (antacids)
- Calcium
- Barium sulfate
- Ganglionic blockers
- Diuretics
- Antihypertensives

role of opioids in diarrhea, we will further explore their action. Mu receptors are present in the central and peripheral nervous systems, as well as the GI tract. In humans, mu receptors are consistently distributed between the myenteric and submucosal plexi, and between the small and large intestines. There is no evidence of mu receptors on the mucosal cells, the ICC, or the smooth muscle cells [14].

The role of endogenous opioids in GI tract normal function remains largely unknown. It is believed that they play a role in normal physiologic control of motility based on experiments with systemic antagonists. When normal opioid-naive volunteers are treated with systemic opioid antagonists, such as naloxone, measurable decreases in GI transit time are observed [15].

Exogenous mu agonists are known to affect the GI tract in several ways. It is known that there are central nervous system–mediated GI effects. If opioids are introduced intrathecally (either intraspinally or supraspinally), slowing of GI motility and decreased intestinal secretion are observed [16–18]. However, it is also clear that opioids can work peripherally at the level of the GI tract itself. Opioids, such as loperamide, that do not cross the blood–brain barrier can induce GI slowing [19], isolated denervated segments of bowel show opioid-mediated slowing [20], and peripherally acting opioid antagonists that do not cross the blood–brain barrier (alvimopan and methylnaltrexone) can prevent opioid-mediated slowing. In response to exogenous opioids, decreased motility occurs at multiple levels in the GI tract, including the stomach, small intestine, and large intestine [21].

Opioid receptors, including the mu receptor, are members of the seven-transmembrane-spanning G-protein-coupled receptor superfamily. Mu receptors predominantly interact with G$_i$/G$_o$ proteins, leading to (1) decreased levels of intracellular cAMP, (2) increased potassium conductance, making neurons less likely to fire, and (3) decreased calcium conductance, leading to decreased neurotransmitter release. In the central nervous system, these mu receptor modulatory effects

decrease neurotransmission. Direct recording from enteric neurons supports a similar inhibition of neuronal firing occurring in the GI tract also [22,23].

Studies in various animals have demonstrated that under the influence of opioids, the outer longitudinal smooth muscle relaxes, but the inner circular smooth muscle has increased tone [21]. It is believed that excitatory neurons that innervate the longitudinal smooth muscle are inhibited in their release of acetylcholine, leading to a decrease in tone. However, it is believed that the circular smooth muscle is tonically active and is under the constant control of inhibitory neurons containing inhibitory neurotransmitters VIP and nitric oxide. Opioids inhibit this tonic inhibition, leading to increased tone in the circular muscle layer. In vitro, peristalsis is blocked when trying to traverse an area under opioid effect. The net effect is increased segmental contraction but a decrease in productive forward peristalsis. A byproduct of this disruption of peristalsis, and resulting stasis of luminal contents is that there is increased passive absorption of fluids, leading to dryer and harder stools.

It is also clear that opioids play a direct role in decreasing GI secretions [24]. Opioids are known to be able to inhibit secretions induced by cholera toxin, VIP, prostaglandin E1 (PGE1), and dibutyryl cyclic AMP(adenosine monophosphate). This opioid-mediated secretory inhibition can itself be inhibited by serotonin and adrenergic receptor antagonists. This fact implicates serotonin and norepinephrine as downstream mediators of the opioid effect.

Overall, opioid inhibition of peristalsis and secretion causes constipation. Unfortunately, tolerance to this effect develops slowly or not at all.

Assessment

A history should include past medical history, medications (both prescription and non-prescription), and a complete review of systems, as important clues to secondary causes of constipation may be identified. Furthermore, the review of systems may identify symptoms indicative of important complications of constipation such as nausea/vomiting with fecal obstruction and urinary retention with fecal impaction.

Because of individual variability in bowel movement patterns, constipation in a patient should be assessed in the context of that patient's experience. It is important to know the patient's prior stool pattern and frequency to determine if chronic constipation was present at baseline before significant illness and, if not, to establish a baseline for comparison. It is also important to determine not only the only overall pattern of bowel movements and the last occurrence but also their characteristics. This characterization includes volume, consistency, straining, sensation of incomplete emptying, and whether any intervention was needed such as a medication, suppository, or manual manipulation. It is not unusual for a patient to complain of diarrhea, after passing a small volume of loose stool that in reality is due to leakage of liquid stool around an impaction.

A general physical exam is indicated with particular attention to the rectal exam. Abdominal examination may reveal distension, tenderness, firmness, or the presence of fecal mass, particularly in the descending colon. Several features can help distinguish between a fecal mass and a tumor. Fecal masses usually indent with deep palpation and can have a crepitus-like feeling because of the presence of entrapped gas. Over time the fecal mass will move [25]. Auscultation can detect high-pitched, hyperactive sounds, characteristic of intestinal obstruction or loss of bowel sounds, signifying ileus.

The rectal exam may identify decreased sphincter tone indicative of neurologic issues, the presence of hemorrhoids or fissures that may explain stool retention to avoid pain, strictures, tissue masses, prolapse, and the presence of stool and its consistency in the rectal vault. An empty rectal vault may indicate proximal impaction or obstruction. Firm stool may indicate an impaction, and the rectal exam may be therapeutic with disimpaction. Finally, having the patient bear down as if to have a bowel movement may identify sphincter contraction instead of relaxation and the failure of the perineum to descend consistent with anal dyssynergia.

In the general population, diagnostic laboratory tests are not recommended [26], but in a palliative care population with multiple potential secondary causes for constipation, tests for complete blood count, complete metabolic panel, and thyroid stimulating hormone are warranted.

Because the diagnosis of constipation by history and physical examination alone has been shown to be unreliable and inaccurate [27], a plain abdominal radiograph can assess stool burden throughout the colon. It is not uncommon for a patient to have fairly frequent bowel movements, but for plain films to show extensive fecal burden throughout the colon. Sykes has proposed a radiographic scoring system [28].

In a subset of patients with worrisome signs and symptoms of mucosal lesion, a colonoscopy may be indicated. In some cases of high impaction, endoscopic procedures may be therapeutic to resolve an obstruction.

For patients without a clear diagnosis or who have not responded to symptomatic therapy, more advanced diagnostic procedures such as colonic transit studies, defecography, and manometry may be indicated but are beyond the scope of this chapter.

Treatment

If secondary causes of constipation are identified, attempts can be made to reverse them within the context of goals of care. For anal dyssynergia, biofeedback relaxation training [29,30] and botulinum toxin [31,32] injection into muscles with increased tone such as the puborectalis may be effective. For other forms of functional constipation and constipation that persists despite reversing known causes, there are general measures and specific pharmacologic interventions that can be used. In treatment resistant cases, if consistent with goals of care, partial or total colectomy is sometimes pursued.

GENERAL MEASURES

It is useful to synergize pharmacologic interventions with normal physiologic processes. For example, timing interventions with a patient's normal toileting schedule and taking advantage of the gastrocolonic response to meals may improve outcomes. In general, greater volume of stool causes luminal stretch that triggers peristalsis. Therefore, hydration and high dietary fiber content are usually advantageous. The best evidence exists for psyllium [8,33]. Psyllium husk is a fibrous hydrophilic substance whose volume increases 10-fold with hydration. In a double-blind, randomized study comparing the stool softener docusate 100 mg bid to psyllium 5.1 g bid, psyllium was superior in softening stool and increasing water content [34]. However, colonic bacterial digestion of fiber can cause increased gas bloating and discomfort. Furthermore, in patients with advanced medical illness, when hydration is often suboptimal, added dietary bulk fiber such as psyllium may actually worsen constipation and should be avoided. Finally, activity may correlate with an improvement in constipation [35].

STOOL SOFTENERS

Stool softeners, such as docusate sodium, are detergents that are thought to break up the fat content of stool, allowing water to penetrate more effectively. They may also increase luminal fluid secretion [36]. As mentioned earlier, psyllium may be superior. Moreover, several studies including a randomized, double-blind study comparing sennosides with placebo to sennosides with docusate showed no improvement with the addition of the stool softener [37–41] and do not support docusate's efficacy. Thus, given cost, pill burden, and the possibility of side effects, it is not recommended.

OSMOTIC AGENTS

Osmotic agents such as magnesium salts, lactulose, sorbitol, and polyethylene glycol (PEG) pull water along with luminal contents to keep the stool softer and more voluminous. Magnesium salts tend to cause urgent liquid stools, making them less convenient for many patients. Extensive use of magnesium containing osmotics can lead to magnesium toxicity, especially in patients with preexisting renal insufficiency. Some patients find the disaccharide osmotics such as lactulose and sorbitol to be unpalatable. Moreover, when they reach the colon, bacteria can metabolize them, leading to gas production and bloating. Studies have shown lactulose and sorbitol to be equally efficacious; however, sorbitol is cheaper [42]. PEG 3350 exists with electrolytes and without. The number refers to the average molecular weight of the compound. PEG 3350 with electrolytes (e.g., Golytely) is reconstituted in a large volume of water and is designed not to affect the net flux of electrolytes or water across the GI mucosa. PEG 3350 also exists without electrolytes (Miralax). As a tasteless, odorless powder, it can be mixed with foods or liquids, increasing palatability. PEG 3350 is not metabolized by colonic flora, and therefore, there may be less gas bloating. In a randomized, double-blind, placebo-controlled trial, PEG was found to be efficacious for chronic constipation [43]. Interestingly, PEG was found to decrease colonic transit time, implying increased motility [44]. A comparison of PEG with and without electrolytes in a geriatric population showed both preparations to be equally effective. Although PEG without electrolytes led to a statistically significant lowering of plasma sodium levels, this change was not clinically significant [45]. Compared to lactulose, studies have shown PEG to be more effective and better tolerated [46,47]; however, it is more expensive.

STIMULANT LAXATIVES

Stimulant laxatives such as senna, bisacodyl, and sodium picosulfate appear to increase intestinal propulsive activity and secretion through unclear mechanisms [48,49]. They are all prodrugs that must be activated by intestinal activity. Senna becomes active only upon reaching the colon where bacteria metabolize it. Bisacodyl and sodium picosulfate are both converted to a common active metabolite. Whereas bisacodyl is activated in the small intestine and increases contractility in both the small and large intestines, sodium picosulfate is activated only in the colon. Because of its earlier activation in the small intestine, there may be more cramping with bisacodyl. Sodium picosulfate is available in many countries, but in the United States, it is only available in combination with other agents as a colonoscopy preparation. Bisacodyl can also be given as a rectal suppository.

Although senna has been used extensively, there are no good clinical trials. Recently, both bisacodyl and sodium picosulfate have undergone randomized, double-blind, placebo-controlled trials, establishing their efficacy in chronic constipation [50,51]. Chronic use of senna and bisacodyl has also been questioned due to concerns of colonic neurotoxicity and increased risk for colon cancer. Several studies in animals and humans have lessened these concerns [52–54].

LUBIPROSTONE

Lubiprostone is a selective chloride channel (ClC-2) activator that induces chloride-rich intestinal secretion and also increases motility without altering serum electrolytes. Randomized, double-blind, placebo-controlled trials have led to Food and Drug Administration (FDA) approval for chronic constipation [55–57], irritable bowel syndrome with constipation in women greater than 18 years old [58], and opioid-induced constipation in patients with noncancer pain (data not published at the time of writing). In the chronic constipation phase 3 trials, patients received lubiprostone 24 mcg bid or placebo for 3 weeks after establishing a baseline frequency of spontaneous bowel movements (SBMs) per week. In the first of the studies, at the 1-week primary outcome timepoint, lubiprostone had significantly increased SBMs to 5.69 per week compared to 3.46 for placebo. Baseline frequency was 1.37 and

1.47 SBMs per week for lubiprostone versus placebo, respectively. Compared to placebo, stool consistency, straining, and constipation severity were all significantly better with lubiprostone. The most common side effect was nausea experienced by about 30% of patients.

LINACLOTIDE

Linaclotide is a synthetic peptide agonist at the guanylate cyclase C receptor on the luminal surface of the intestinal epithelium that the FDA has approved for the treatment of chronic constipation. Receptor binding leads to increased intracellular and extracellular cyclic guanosine monophosphate levels that through second messengers lead to activation of the cystic fibrosis transmembrane conductance regulator. The net effect is increased secretion of bicarbonate- and chloride-rich fluid into the lumen and increased motility [59]. In two randomized, double-blind, placebo-controlled trials, 1276 patients with chronic constipation were treated with oral linaclotide 145 mcg, 290 mcg, or placebo daily for 12 weeks [60]. The primary outcome was ≥3 complete spontaneous bowel movements (CSBMs) per week and an increase of ≥1 CSBMs over baseline during at least 9 out of the 12 weeks. Both linaclotide doses were significantly better than placebo for the primary outcome. Overall, in both studies, about 20% of patients achieved the primary outcome versus 5% with placebo. There was also significant improvement of linaclotide versus placebo in secondary outcomes, including weekly CSBMs, weekly SBMs, stool consistency, straining severity, abdominal symptoms, and constipation severity. The most common side effect was diarrhea that caused linaclotide discontinuation in about 4%.

OPIOID ANTAGONISTS

Methylnaltrexone has been FDA approved for the treatment of opioid-induced constipation in patients with advanced illness receiving palliative care. As stated previously, opioids are thought to cause constipation by binding to mu receptors in the GI tract, leading to decreased secretion, decreased productive forward peristalsis, and increased passive fluid absorption. Methylnaltrexone, by virtue of its positive charge, is restricted from crossing the blood–brain barrier, and therefore does not reverse central nervous system–mediated analgesia. In two randomized, double-blind, placebo-controlled, phase 3 trials, patients with advanced illness and opioid-induced constipation received methylnaltrexone or placebo subcutaneously either as a one-time dose or every other day over 2 weeks [61,62]. Primary endpoints included having a bowel movement within 4 hours of receiving drug in both studies and, in the longer study, having a bowel movement within 4 hours after dosing in ≥2 of the first 4 doses. Overall, methylnaltrexone 0.15 mg/kg caused bowel movements in 50%–60% of patients within 4 hours versus about 15% with placebo. The most common side effect was abdominal pain in about 20%. Methylnaltrexone has also proved effective for opioid-induced constipation in patients with chronic nonmalignant pain [63].

Alvimopan is another peripherally restricted opioid receptor antagonist, but it is only FDA approved for restricted short-term hospital use for postoperative ileus and not for constipation.

LUBRICANTS

There are also lubricating suppositories as well as enemas that can work mechanically to soften the leading edge of hard, dry stool. Examples include glycerol suppositories, oil enemas, and tap water small volume enemas. Large volume enemas, in addition to being lubricating, can cause luminal distention and thus trigger peristalsis. Many different types of enemas are used clinically, but there are no studies to guide practice. A systematic review of sodium phosphate enemas has raised concerns [64]. The authors advise caution in elderly patients with comorbid chronic kidney disease and altered intestinal motility who may be most susceptible to water and electrolyte disturbances. In their review, this seemed most common with sodium phosphate enemas that were multiply dosed or retained for long periods. However, the authors point out that given the widespread use, the number of patients with side effects reported in the literature is minimal.

OTHER POTENTIAL AGENTS

Given acetylcholine's key role in smooth muscle contraction, neostigmine, an acetylcholinesterase inhibitor, has been used in acute colonic pseudo-obstruction (Ogilvie's syndrome) [65]. Results were impressive, but systemic side effects of bradycardia and increased respiratory secretions are a concern, and therefore, neostigmine is not recommended for chronic use.

Given serotonin's role in GI tract modulation and our increasing understanding of the multiple subtypes of serotonin receptors, several serotonergic agents have been studied. The 5-HT4 agonist tegaserod has been FDA approved for constipation-predominant irritable bowel syndrome [66] The 5-HT4 agonist, prucalopride, has been approved for chronic constipation in Canada and Europe [67,68], but not in the United States; another 5-HT4 agonist, velusetrag, gave encouraging results in a phase 2 trial.

Studies have also demonstrated potential roles for additional agents such as colchicine [69,70], misoprostol [71,72], neurotrophin-3 [73], and the bile acid transporter inhibitor, A3309 [74]. The role that any of these classes of agents may play in palliative care remains to be seen.

RECOMMENDATIONS FOR MANAGEMENT

It is often necessary to synergize medications that work through different mechanisms to achieve optimal results. Once a patient is constipated, before a baseline regimen will be successful, a combination of oral and rectal interventions is often required. There is frequently a leading, hard, dry edge to the stool that must be mobilized. If impaction is present,

manual rectal excavation is often needed. An enema, such as a tapwater enema, and a stimulant suppository, such as bisacodyl, can be used to soften and mobilize the stool, respectively. Oral osmotic agents, such as PEG 3350, can also be used in larger doses to aid in this mobilization [75].

Once mobilized, there is no clear order in which to enlist medications for a routine bowel regimen. There are few comparative clinical trials to guide therapy. Based on the evidence, docusate, the stool softener, is not recommended. Many clinicians would opt to start with a stimulant laxative or an osmotic. Osmotic agents such as PEG not only increase stool water content and volume, but also increase motility. The initial agent is titrated in general to achieve a soft, easy-to-pass bowel movement at least every other day. If this goal is not achieved, especially in a palliative care population, aggressive measures to restore bowel movements are indicated to avoid impaction, including the use of suppositories or enemas. If rectal interventions continue to be required to promote bowel movements, the baseline oral bowel regimen should be titrated up to maximal doses, and then continue with the addition of a mechanistically different agent. For opioid-induced constipation, specific opioid antagonists, such as methylnaltrexone, can be considered.

Given that osmotics like PEG, lubiprostone, and linaclotide all seem to increase luminal fluid and motility, further comparative studies will be needed to elucidate the role of the newer agents in palliative care.

Table 59.5 provides typical dosing regimens for some of the most commonly used medications.

DIARRHEA

Definition/physiology/pathophysiology

Some define diarrhea as the passage of ≥3 loose or watery bowel movements per day. Another definition depends on passing ≥200 g of stool per day based on a typical diet. Half of the mass of a normal bowel movement is bacteria, and fiber and water account for most of the rest of the weight. The net water content is the result of the balance between secretion and absorption, with absorption also affected by transit time, which controls contact time between luminal contents and the intestinal epithelium. As stated previously, these events are regulated via neurocrine, endocrine, paracrine, autocrine, and immune mechanisms. About 9 L of fluid passes through the GI tract each day. About 2 L is ingested orally, and secretion from the salivary glands, stomach, liver, pancreas, and small intestine accounts for about 7 L of fluid. After absorption in the small intestine, about 1–2 L enters the colon. The colon has an absorptive capacity of 3–4 L/day [6], and about 0.2 L is excreted each day.

The balance between absorption and secretion determines the net amount of luminal fluid. In the small intestine, it is thought villus cells mediate absorption and crypt cells mediate secretion. Some absorption is passive following electrochemical gradients. When energy is needed for absorption, active

Table 59.5 *Classification, dosages, and pharmacological properties of laxatives*

Laxative	Onset of action (h)	Mechanism	Usual adult dose	Comments
Bulk forming agents	12–24	Hold water in stool and cause distension		Patients should be able to increase fluid intake; otherwise, fluid impaction might occur
Natural (psyllium)			7 g/day	
Synthetic (methylcellulose)			4–6 g/day	
Saline laxatives	0.5–3	Draw fluid into the intestine		Avoid in patients with renal or heart failure
Magnesium hydroxide			30 mL	
Magnesium citrate			200 mL	
Hyperosmolar agents	Variable, generally 24–48	Increase stool osmolarity, leading to accumulation of fluid in the colon		Might cause flatulence and distension
PEG			8–25 g/day	
Lactulose			15–30 mL	
Sorbitol			15–30 mL	
Contact cathartics	6–10	Stimulate peristalsis by direct action on the myenteric plexus. Reduce net absorption of water and electrolytes		Additive risk of hepatotoxicity when docusate is used in combination with other contact cathartics
Anthraquinones			Variable	
Diphenylmethane			65–130 mg	
Castor oil	2–6		15–60 mL	
Docusate	24–72		100–800 mg	
Emollient laxatives	6–8	Lubricant and stool softener		
Mineral oil			15–45 mL/day	Might lead to serious lipoid pneumonia if aspiration occurs
Prokinetic agents	Variable	Decrease transit time through intestine		For refractory constipation. Might be useful in colonic inertia secondary to spinal cord injury
Metoclopramide			40–120 mg/day	
Domperidone			30–80 mg/day	

transport of sodium via Na,K-ATPases creates a gradient with a high concentration of sodium in the lumen. Absorption uses the energy from this gradient to cotransport sugar or amino acids in conjunction with sodium. Water passively follows solute.

Crypt cells possess a cyclic-AMP-dependent chloride channel on their luminal surface, named, the cystic fibrosis transmembrane conductance regulator (CFTR). When adenyl cyclase is activated, levels of cyclic-AMP rise and activate the CFTR, leading to secretion of chloride into the lumen. The negatively charged chloride attracts the positively charged sodium, leading to the net secretion of sodium chloride and the passive following of water.

Pathologic processes can disrupt this normally tight regulation between absorption and secretion. Cholera toxin can aberrantly activate adenyl cyclase, leading to increased chloride secretion and profuse watery diarrhea. With inflammation due to a variety of sources, the mucosal lining of the intestine is damaged, leading to passive loss of protein-rich fluid, disruption of absorption, and under the influence of prostaglandins and cytokines, increased secretion, creating diarrhea.

Types of diarrhea can also be categorized by duration. Acute diarrhea is defined as ≤14 days, persistent diarrhea is defined as >14 days but <30 days, and chronic diarrhea is defined as >30 days. These categories can also have mechanistic value. Most, but not all, acute diarrhea is infectious. Most chronic diarrhea is noninfectious, but there are also exceptions.

In this section, we will present the causes, assessment, specific treatments for diarrhea, and symptomatic relief of the diarrhea while waiting for specific treatments to work, when diarrhea persists despite underlying treatment, or when there is no treatment.

Causes

Tables 59.6 and 59.7 list many causes of acute and chronic diarrhea. In general, diarrhea can be categorized as related to disordered motility, secretion, inflammation, or osmosis/

Table 59.6 *Causes of diarrhea*

- Disordered motility
  - Hyperthyroidism
  - Diabetic autonomic neuropathy
  - Irritable bowel syndrome
  - Postvagotomy diarrhea
- Secretory
  - Acute
    - Infection
      - Viral (e.g., rotavirus)
      - Noninvasive bacteria (e.g., enterotoxigenic *E. coli*)
      - Protozoa
  - Chronic
    - Infection (e.g., HIV)
    - Inflammatory bowel disease
      - Ulcerative colitis
      - Crohn's disease
      - Microscopic colitis
    - Neuroendocrine tumors
      - Carcinoid syndrome
      - VIPoma
      - Gastrinoma
    - Bile salts postcholecystectomy
    - Medications (see Table 59.7)
- Inflammatory
  - Acute
    - Infection
      - Invasive bacteria (e.g., *Shigella*)
    - Toxin (e.g., *C. difficile* toxin)
  - Chronic
    - Infection (e.g., invasive parasitic ambiasis)
    - Inflammatory bowel disease
      - Ulcerative colitis
      - Crohn's disease
    - Chemotherapy
    - Radiation therapy
    - Graft-versus-host disease
- Osmotic/malabsorption
  - Pancreatic insufficiency
  - Celiac disease
  - Lactase deficiency
  - Small intestinal bacterial overgrowth
  - Ingested osmotic
    - Nonabsorbable sugars (e.g., lactulose, sorbitol, mannitol)
    - Phosphate- or magnesium-containing products

Table 59.7 *Drugs commonly associated with diarrhea in palliative care*

- Laxatives
- Antibiotics
- Antiretrovirals
- Antacid (containing magnesium)
- Olestra, orlistat (lipase inhibitor)
- Colchicine
- Neomycin
- Theophylline
- Thyroxine
- Metformin
- Cholinergic drugs (glaucoma eye drops)
- Cholinesterase inhibitors
- Metoclopramide
- Chemotherapy
- Misoprostol
- Nonsteroidal anti-inflammatory drugs (NSAIDs)

bowel disease disrupt the mucosa, leading to increased secretion and decreased absorption as detailed earlier. Lactase deficiency leads to the inability to break down lactose to monosaccharides that are absorbable. Lactose therefore is nonabsorbable, carries osmotic weight, pulls water into the intestinal lumen, and causes diarrhea. Interesting, lactase activity can be lost temporarily after intestinal mucosal damage. Thus, lactose-containing products should be avoided in many forms of diarrhea.

Assessment

History should completely characterize the diarrhea, including duration, frequency, volume, consistency, presence of greasy stools that float, malodor, diarrhea during the night, and presence of blood or mucous [76–78]. Large, watery diarrhea is often due to small intestinal derangement, while smaller more frequent stools are likely colonic in origin. Greasy, floating, malodorous stools could signify fat malabsorption. Diarrhea during times of fasting, such as overnight when osmotic sources would be minimized, could indicate a secretory diarrhea. The presence of bloody stool is consistent with severe inflammation. The rest of a complete history should also be done including past medical history, family history, medications including nonprescription ones and recent antibiotic use, travel history, and sexual history. Antibiotic use can predispose to *C. difficile* colitis, recent travel may identify sources for possible infectious agents, and sexual history could identify risk factors for HIV that can itself cause diarrhea or increase risk for infectious diarrheas.

A complete physical exam should be done with particular emphasis on fever and signs of dehydration, abdominal exam for masses and pain, and digital rectal exam monitoring for structural abnormalities and the presence of gross or microscopic blood.

malabsorption. Some causes of diarrhea may involve several of these categories. Diabetic autonomic neuropathy may increase motility, decreasing time for absorption, resulting in diarrhea. Noninvasive infectious agents, such as cholera and its toxin, trigger increased secretion without disrupting the intestinal mucosa, as detailed earlier. Invasive infectious agents, such as *Shigella*, and diseases like inflammatory

Diagnostic tests may not be needed in acute diarrhea that is short-lived and without signs of severe illness. Stool cultures are positive only 1%–5% of the time in acute diarrhea, implying that many are viral and therefore self-limited [78]. However, in 87% of patients with severe diarrheal illness, bacteria were cultured [79]. Guidelines suggest further diagnostic workup if severe illness is present as indicated by the presence of one or more of the following: fever, dehydration, stool with blood and/or mucus, severe abdominal pain, hospitalization, recent antibiotic use, and being an elderly or immunocompromised patient. Diagnostic workup could entail complete blood count with differential, thyroid function, complete metabolic panel, stool cultures, fecal occult blood, fecal leukocytes, stool fat quantitation, stool osmotic gap, ova and parasites, and endoscopy. An elevated white count could indicate a systemic infection, and eosinophilia could indicate a parasitic infection. Fecal leukocytes could indicate an inflammatory diarrhea, but the test although reasonably sensitive is not specific; however, lactoferrin and calprotectin are more sensitive and specific for leucocytes [77]. Increased stool fat content is consistent with malabsorption, and an increased stool osmotic gap supports osmotic diarrhea. Guidelines indicate ova and parasite tests are not cost effective unless diarrhea is persistent (>14 days), travel history is supportive, there is exposure to daycare infants, immunocompromise is present or suspected, or bloody diarrhea is present without fecal leucocytes as this is associated with amebiasis [80]. Endoscopy may be useful to obtain tissue to establish a diagnosis. Flexible sigmoidoscopy is sufficient most of the time, but colonoscopy has some advantages, being able to reach the terminal ileum to examine the small intestine [80].

Treatment

If the etiology for diarrhea is identified, treatment can be directed at the underlying cause if consistent with goals of care. Supportive and symptomatic therapy can be instituted while waiting for specific treatments to work, when diarrhea persists despite underlying treatment, or when there is no underlying treatment. One general measure is to ensure adequate hydration.

For acute diarrhea, guidelines recommend empiric antibiotic therapy be reserved for those suspected with moderate to severe travel-related diarrhea, those with probable invasive bacterial diarrhea as evidenced by fever and stool with blood, mucus, or pus, the immunocompromised, and the elderly. Of note, if enterotoxigenic *E. coli* is suspected, antibiotics are not recommended. They have been found to be ineffective and may increase the risk of hemolytic uremic syndrome. A potential clue to this condition is bloody stool accompanied by abdominal pain but without significant fever.

For less severe acute diarrhea, without fever or bloody stools, antidiarrheals can be used to empirically to reduce the diarrhea volume and frequency as described later.

For identified acute or chronic diarrhea etiologies, appropriate treatments can be instituted. Appropriate antibiotics for infections, immunosuppressants for inflammatory bowel disease, pancreatic supplements for pancreatic insufficiency, bile sequestrants for bile salt–related diarrhea, and discontinuation of offending medications are a few examples.

For symptomatic relief of diarrhea independent of cause, loperamide is first-line therapy. It is a potent mu receptor agonist [81] that is excluded from the central nervous system by active transport of the P-glycoprotein of the blood–brain barrier [82]. Therefore, it is restricted peripherally and has no centrally mediated analgesic effects. As described previously in the constipation section, mu receptor agonists in the GI tract decrease secretion, disrupt productive forward peristalsis, and promote increased passive fluid absorption. Opioids have been shown in vitro to completely block the secretory effect of cholera toxin [24]. Loperamide has additionally been shown to increase anal sphincter tone [83]. It has a half-life of 11 hours and is typically dosed orally at 4 mg initially with another 2 mg after each episode of diarrhea to a maximum of 16 mg/day. For chemotherapy-induced diarrhea, it is used at up to 24 mg/day [84]. For chronic diarrhea, given its half-life, it can be dosed bid with good effect, and has been observed to be used for years without tolerance [85].

Diphenoxylate, another mu receptor agonist, is available in a 2.5 mg tablet together with 25 mcg of atropine. Diphenoxylate does cross the blood–brain barrier and the subtherapeutic atropine component is added as a deterrent to abuse, which limits how high it can be titrated for clinical effects. Clinically, loperamide is preferred.

For loperamide-resistant diarrhea, octreotide, a longer acting synthetic analog of somatostatin, has been used. Somatostatin is found in the enteric nervous system, both the submucosal and myenteric plexi, and in the endocrine-like D cells of the stomach, pancreas, and gut. Octretotide in the GI tract reduces splanchnic and portal blood flow, decreases GI motility, reduces gastric, biliary, pancreatic, and small intestine secretion, and increases electrolyte and water absorption by inhibiting secretion of insulin, glucagon, gastrin, peptide YY, neurotensin, VIP, and substance P [86]. It also can inhibit serotonin release in carcinoid, glucagon in glucagonoma, and VIP in VIPoma. Octreotide is typically started at 100 mcg tid, but has been titrated to 2500 mcg tid. It has been found useful in both chemotherapy and radiation-induced diarrhea [84], graft-versus-host disease–related diarrhea [87], and HIV-related diarrhea [88,89].

With a careful assessment, treatment of identified causes of diarrhea, and symptomatic treatment, we are successful in controlling most diarrhea, but unfortunately, there is still a subset of treatment-resistant diarrhea that causes significant suffering in palliative care. While waiting for research to bring new options, the palliative care interdisciplinary team's psychosocial and spiritual support for the patient and family remains paramount.

Key learning points

Constipation

The prevalence of chronic functional constipation ranges from 2% to 27% in the general population and means that a subset of palliative care patients with constipation may have it as a component of their presentation.

A careful bowel history is needed to determine baseline and current patterns, including frequency, volume, consistency, straining, and sensation of incomplete evacuation.

A patient may complain of "diarrhea" that may be leakage of loose stool around an impaction.

A rectal exam is an essential component of the evaluation of constipation.

There is a dearth of evidence to guide the pharmacologic treatment of constipation, especially comparative studies.

The use of docusate, stool softener, is not supported by current evidence.

There is no clear evidence that chronic use of stimulant laxatives is detrimental.

Osmotics such as PEG not only increase stool water and volume, but also increase motility.

The role of lubiprostone and linaclotide in palliative care, which increase luminal fluid and GI motility similarly to osmotics, requires more research.

Methylnaltrexone is a peripherally acting mu receptor antagonist, which does not reverse centrally mediated analgesia that may be effective for opioid-induced constipation.

Rectal interventions, including suppositories and enemas, may be important to soften and mobilize the hard, dry leading edge of stool before baseline oral regimens can be effective.

Diarrhea

A careful history can give insight into the likely cause of diarrhea: disordered motility, secretory, inflammatory, or osmotic/malabsorptive.

Many causes of diarrhea lead to temporary secondary lactase deficiency, and therefore, lactose-containing products should be avoided until function returns.

Loperamide is a peripherally restricted mu receptor agonist that is the first line therapy for the symptomatic relief of diarrhea.

For loperamide-resistant diarrhea, octreotide, with its vasoactive, antisecretory, antimotility, and proabsorptive properties, is our best therapy for severe chemotherapy-induced diarrhea, graft-versus-host disease–associated diarrhea, and HIV-related diarrhea.

REFERENCES

1   Johnson LR (ed.). *Gastrointestinal Physiology*, 6th edn. Philadelphia, PA: Mosby Elsevier; 2001.
2   Feldman M, Friedman LS, Sleisenger MH (eds.). *Feldman: Sleisenger & Fordtran's Gastrointestinal and Liver Disease*, 7th edn. Philadelphia, PA: Saunders; 2002.
3   Furness J. *The Enteric Nervous System.* Oxford, U.K.: Blackwell; 2006.
4   Gershon MD. Review article: Serotonin receptors and transporters—Roles in normal and abnormal gastrointestinal motility. *Aliment Pharmacol Ther.* 2004;20 Suppl 7:3–14. PubMed PMID: 15521849. eng.
5   Cook IJ, Brookes SJ. Motility of large intestine. In: Feldman M, Friedman LS, Sleisenger MH (eds.) *Feldman: Sleisenger & Fordtran's Gastrointestinal and Liver Disease*, 7th edn. Philadelphia, PA: Saunders; 2002.
6   Debongnie JC, Phillips SF. Capacity of the human colon to absorb fluid. *Gastroenterology.* 1978;74(4):698–703. PubMed PMID: 631507.
7   Longstreth GF, Thompson WG, Chey WD, Houghton LA, Mearin F, Spiller RC. Functional bowel disorders. *Gastroenterology.* 2006;130(5):1480–1491. PubMed PMID: 16678561.eng.
8   Brandt LJ, Prather CM, Quigley EM, Schiller LR, Schoenfeld P, Talley NJ. Systematic review on the management of chronic constipation in North America. *Am J Gastroenterol.* 2005;100 Suppl 1:S5–S21. PubMed PMID: 16008641.
9   Sykes NP. The pathogenesis of constipation. *J Support Oncol.* 2006;4(5):213–218. PubMed PMID: 16724641.eng.
10 Sykes NP. The relationship between opioid use and laxative use in terminally ill cancer patients. *Palliat Med.* 1998;12(5):375–382. PubMed PMID: 9924600.
11 Holmes S. Use of a modified symptom distress scale in assessment of the cancer patient. *Int J Nurs Stud.* 1989;26(1):69–79. PubMed PMID: 2707983.
12 Gomes OA, de Souza RR, Liberti EA. A preliminary investigation of the effects of aging on the nerve cell number in the myenteric ganglia of the human colon. *Gerontology.* 1997;43(4):210–217. PubMed PMID: 9222749.eng.
13 Garvey M, Noyes R, Jr., Yates W. Frequency of constipation in major depression: Relationship to other clinical variables. *Psychosomatics.* 1990;31(2):204–206. PubMed PMID: 2330403.
14 Sternini C, Patierno S, Selmer IS, Kirchgessner A. The opioid system in the gastrointestinal tract. *Neurogastroenterol Motil.* 2004;16 Suppl 2:3–16. PubMed PMID: 15357847.
15 Kaufman PN, Krevsky B, Malmud LS, Maurer AH, Somers MB, Siegel JA et al. Role of opiate receptors in the regulation of colonic transit. *Gastroenterology.* 1988;94(6):1351–1356. PubMed PMID: 2834257.eng.
16 Galligan JJ, Burks TF. Centrally mediated inhibition of small intestinal transit and motility by morphine in the rat. *J Pharmacol Exp Ther.* 1983;226(2):356–361. PubMed PMID: 6875849.eng.
17 Porreca F, Heyman JS, Mosberg HI, Omnaas JR, Vaught JL. Role of mu and delta receptors in the supraspinal and spinal analgesic effects of [D-Pen2, D-Pen5]enkephalin in the mouse. *J Pharmacol Exp Ther.* 1987;241(2):393–400. PubMed PMID: 3033214.eng.
18 Jiang Q, Sheldon RJ, Porreca F. Opioid modulation of basal intestinal fluid transport in the mouse: Actions at central, but not intestinal, sites. *J Pharmacol Exp Ther.* 1990;253(2):784–790. PubMed PMID: 2160010.eng.
19 Basilisco G, Camboni G, Bozzani A, Paravicini M, Bianchi PA. Oral naloxone antagonizes loperamide-induced delay of orocecal transit. *Dig Dis Sci.* 1987;32(8):829–832. PubMed PMID: 3608730.eng.
20 Van Nueten JM, Van Ree JM, Vanhoutte PM. Inhibition by met-enkephalin of peristaltic activity in the guinea pig ileum, and its reversal by naloxone. *Eur J Pharmacol.* 1977;41(3):341–342. PubMed PMID: 837977.eng.

21 Wood JD, Galligan JJ. Function of opioids in the enteric nervous system. *Neurogastroenterol Motil.* 2004;16 Suppl 2:17–28. PubMed PMID: 15357848.eng.

22 North RA, Henderson G. Action of morphine on guinea-pig myenteric plexus and mouse vas deferens studied by intracellular recording. *Life Sci.* 1975;17(1):63–66. PubMed PMID: 167255.

23 Morita K, North RA. Opiates and enkephalin reduce the excitability of neuronal processes. *Neuroscience.* 1981;6(10):1943–1951. PubMed PMID: 7301113.

24 De Luca A, Coupar IM. Insights into opioid action in the intestinal tract. *Pharmacol Ther.* 1996;69(2):103–115. PubMed PMID: 8984506.

25 Wald A. *Textbook of Gastroenterology.* Philadelphia, PA: Lippincott Williams & Wilkins; 2003: pp. 895–907.

26 American College of Gastroenterology Chronic Constipation Task F. An evidence-based approach to the management of chronic constipation in North America. *Am J Gastroenterol.* 2005;100 Suppl 1:S1–S4. PubMed PMID: 16008640.

27 Starreveld JS, Pols MA, Van Wijk HJ, Bogaard JW, Poen H, Smout AJ. The plain abdominal radiograph in the assessment of constipation. *Zeitschrift fur Gastroenterologie.* 1990;28(7):335–338. PubMed PMID: 2238762.

28 Sykes N. In: Doyle D HG, MacDonald N (eds.) *Palliative Medicine.* Oxford, U.K.: Oxford University Press; 1993: pp. 299–310.

29 Rao SS, Seaton K, Miller M, Brown K, Nygaard I, Stumbo P et al. Randomized controlled trial of biofeedback, sham feedback, and standard therapy for dyssynergic defecation. *Clin Gastroenterol Hepatol.* 2007;5(3):331–338. PubMed PMID: 17368232.

30 Heymen S, Scarlett Y, Jones K, Ringel Y, Drossman D, Whitehead WE. Randomized, controlled trial shows biofeedback to be superior to alternative treatments for patients with pelvic floor dyssynergia-type constipation. *Dis Colon Rectum.* 2007;50(4):428–441. PubMed PMID: 17294322.

31 Farid M, Youssef T, Mahdy T, Omar W, Moneim HA, El Nakeeb A et al. Comparative study between botulinum toxin injection and partial division of puborectalis for treating anismus. *Int J Colorectal Dis.* 2009;24(3):327–334. PubMed PMID: 19039596.

32 Farid M, El Monem HA, Omar W, El Nakeeb A, Fikry A, Youssef T et al. Comparative study between biofeedback retraining and botulinum neurotoxin in the treatment of anismus patients. *Int J Colorectal Dis.* 2009;24(1):115–120. PubMed PMID: 18719924.

33 Ramkumar D, Rao SS. Efficacy and safety of traditional medical therapies for chronic constipation: Systematic review. *Am J Gastroenterol.* 2005;100(4):936–971. PubMed PMID: 15784043.

34 McRorie JW, Daggy BP, Morel JG, Diersing PS, Miner PB, Robinson M. Psyllium is superior to docusate sodium for treatment of chronic constipation. *Aliment Pharmacol Ther.* 1998;12(5):491–497. PubMed PMID: 9663731.

35 Holdstock DJ, Misiewicz JJ, Smith T, Rowlands EN. Propulsion (mass movements) in the human colon and its relationship to meals and somatic activity. *Gut.* 1970;11(2):91–99. PubMed PMID: 5441889.

36 Moriarty KJ, Kelly MJ, Beetham R, Clark ML. Studies on the mechanism of action of dioctyl sodium sulphosuccinate in the human jejunum. *Gut.* 1985;26(10):1008–1013. PubMed PMID: 2414161.

37 Goodman J, Pang J, Bessman AN. Dioctyl sodium sulfosuccinate—An ineffective prophylactic laxative. *J Chronic Dis.* 1976;29(1):59–63. PubMed PMID: 1254685.

38 Chapman RW, Sillery J, Fontana DD, Matthys C, Saunders DR. Effect of oral dioctyl sodium sulfosuccinate on intake-output studies of human small and large intestine. *Gastroenterology.* 1985;89(3):489–493. PubMed PMID: 2410320.

39 Fain AM, Susat R, Herring M, Dorton K. Treatment of constipation in geriatric and chronically ill patients: A comparison. *South Med J.* 1978;71(6):677–680. PubMed PMID: 78527.

40 Castle SC, Cantrell M, Israel DS, Samuelson MJ. Constipation prevention: Empiric use of stool softeners questioned. *Geriatrics.* 1991;46(11):84–86. PubMed PMID: 1718823.

41 Tarumi Y, Wilson MP, Szafran O, Spooner GR. Randomized, double-blind, placebo-controlled trial of oral docusate in the management of constipation in hospice patients. *J Pain Symptom Manage.* 2013;45(1):2–13. PubMed PMID: 22889861.

42 Lederle FA, Busch DL, Mattox KM, West MJ, Aske DM. Cost-effective treatment of constipation in the elderly: A randomized double-blind comparison of sorbitol and lactulose. *Am J Med.* 1990;89(5):597–601. PubMed PMID: 2122724.

43 Dipalma JA, Cleveland MV, McGowan J, Herrera JL. A randomized, multicenter, placebo-controlled trial of polyethylene glycol laxative for chronic treatment of chronic constipation. *Am J Gastroenterol.* 2007;102(7):1436–1441. PubMed PMID: 17403074.

44 Klauser AG, Muhldorfer BE, Voderholzer WA, Wenzel G, Muller-Lissner SA. Polyethylene glycol 4000 for slow transit constipation. *Zeitschrift fur Gastroenterologie.* 1995;33(1):5–8. PubMed PMID: 7886986.

45 Seinela L, Sairanen U, Laine T, Kurl S, Pettersson T, Happonen P. Comparison of polyethylene glycol with and without electrolytes in the treatment of constipation in elderly institutionalized patients: A randomized, double-blind, parallel-group study. *Drugs Aging.* 2009;26(8):703–713. PubMed PMID: 19685935.

46 Attar A, Lemann M, Ferguson A, Halphen M, Boutron MC, Flourie B et al. Comparison of a low dose polyethylene glycol electrolyte solution with lactulose for treatment of chronic constipation. *Gut.* 1999;44(2):226–230. PubMed PMID: 9895382.

47 Freedman MD, Schwartz HJ, Roby R, Fleisher S. Tolerance and efficacy of polyethylene glycol 3350/electrolyte solution versus lactulose in relieving opiate induced constipation: A double-blinded placebo-controlled trial. *J Clin Pharmacol.* 1997;37(10):904–907. PubMed PMID: 9505981.

48 Manabe N, Cremonini F, Camilleri M, Sandborn WJ, Burton DD. Effects of bisacodyl on ascending colon emptying and overall colonic transit in healthy volunteers. *Aliment Pharmacol Ther.* 2009;30(9):930–936. PubMed PMID: 19678812. Pubmed Central PMCID: 2862903.

49 Hardcastle JD, Wilkins JL. The action of sennosides and related compounds on human colon and rectum. *Gut.* 1970;11(12):1038–1042. PubMed PMID: 4929273. Pubmed Central PMCID: 1553168.

50 Kamm MA, Mueller-Lissner S, Wald A, Richter E, Swallow R, Gessner U. Oral bisacodyl is effective and well-tolerated in patients with chronic constipation. *Clin Gastroenterol Hepatol.* 2011;9(7):577–583. PubMed PMID: 21440672.

51 Mueller-Lissner S, Kamm MA, Wald A, Hinkel U, Koehler U, Richter E et al. Multicenter, 4-week, double-blind, randomized, placebo-controlled trial of sodium picosulfate in patients with chronic constipation. *Am J Gastroenterol.* 2010;105(4):897–903. PubMed PMID: 20179697.

52 Heinicke EA, Kiernan JA. Resistance of myenteric neurons in the rat's colon to depletion by 1,8-dihydroxyanthraquinone. *J Pharm Pharmacol.* 1990;42(2):123–125. PubMed PMID: 1972397.

53 Nascimbeni R, Donato F, Ghirardi M, Mariani P, Villanacci V, Salerni B. Constipation, anthranoid laxatives, melanosis coli, and colon cancer: A risk assessment using aberrant crypt foci. *Cancer Epidemiol Biomarkers Prev.* 2002;11(8):753–757. PubMed PMID: 12163329.

54 Nusko G, Schneider B, Schneider I, Wittekind C, Hahn EG. Anthranoid laxative use is not a risk factor for colorectal neoplasia: Results of a prospective case control study. *Gut.* 2000;46(5):651–655. PubMed PMID: 10764708.

55 Johanson JF, Ueno R. Lubiprostone, a locally acting chloride channel activator, in adult patients with chronic constipation: A double-blind, placebo-controlled, dose-ranging study to evaluate efficacy and safety. *Aliment Pharmacol Ther.* 2007;25(11):1351–1361. PubMed PMID: 17509103. eng.

56 Johanson JF, Morton D, Geenen J, Ueno R. Multicenter, 4-week, double-blind, randomized, placebo-controlled trial of lubiprostone, a locally-acting type-2 chloride channel activator, in patients with chronic constipation. *Am J Gastroenterol*. 2008;103(1):170–177. PubMed PMID: 17916109.

57 Barish CF, Drossman D, Johanson JF, Ueno R. Efficacy and safety of lubiprostone in patients with chronic constipation. *Dig Dis Sci*. 2010;55(4):1090–1097. PubMed PMID: 20012484.

58 Drossman DA, Chey WD, Johanson JF, Fass R, Scott C, Panas R et al. Clinical trial: Lubiprostone in patients with constipation-associated irritable bowel syndrome—Results of two randomized, placebo-controlled studies. *Aliment Pharmacol Ther*. 2009;29(3):329–341. PubMed PMID: 19006537.

59 Andresen V, Camilleri M, Busciglio IA, Grudell A, Burton D, McKinzie S et al. Effect of 5 days linaclotide on transit and bowel function in females with constipation-predominant irritable bowel syndrome. *Gastroenterology*. 2007;133(3):761–768. PubMed PMID: 17854590.

60 Lembo AJ, Schneier HA, Shiff SJ, Kurtz CB, MacDougall JE, Jia XD et al. Two randomized trials of linaclotide for chronic constipation. *N Engl J Med*. 2011;365(6):527–536. PubMed PMID: 21830967.

61 Thomas J, Karver S, Cooney GA, Chamberlain BH, Watt CK, Slatkin NE et al. Methylnaltrexone for opioid-induced constipation in advanced illness. *N Engl J Med*. 2008;358(22):2332–2343. PubMed PMID: 18509120. Epub 2008/05/30. eng.

62 Slatkin N, Thomas J, Lipman AG, Wilson G, Boatwright ML, Wellman C et al. Methylnaltrexone for treatment of opioid-induced constipation in advanced illness patients. *J Support Oncol*. 2009;7(1):39–46. PubMed PMID: 19278178. Epub 2009/03/13. eng.

63 Michna E, Blonsky ER, Schulman S, Tzanis E, Manley A, Zhang H et al. Subcutaneous methylnaltrexone for treatment of opioid-induced constipation in patients with chronic, nonmalignant pain: A randomized controlled study. *J Pain*. 2011;12(5):554–562. PubMed PMID: 21429809.

64 Mendoza J, Legido J, Rubio S, Gisbert JP. Systematic review: The adverse effects of sodium phosphate enema. *Aliment Pharmacol Ther*. 2007;26(1):9–20. PubMed PMID: 17555417.

65 Ponec RJ, Saunders MD, Kimmey MB. Neostigmine for the treatment of acute colonic pseudo-obstruction. *N Engl J Med*. 1999;341(3):137–141. PubMed PMID: 10403850.

66 Novick J, Miner P, Krause R, Glebas K, Bliesath H, Ligozio G et al. A randomized, double-blind, placebo-controlled trial of tegaserod in female patients suffering from irritable bowel syndrome with constipation. *Aliment Pharmacol Ther*. 2002;16(11):1877–88. PubMed PMID: 12390096.

67 Quigley EM, Vandeplassche L, Kerstens R, Ausma J. Clinical trial: The efficacy, impact on quality of life, and safety and tolerability of prucalopride in severe chronic constipation—A 12-week, randomized, double-blind, placebo-controlled study. *Aliment Pharmacol Ther*. 2009;29(3):315–328. PubMed PMID: 19035970.

68 Muller-Lissner S, Rykx A, Kerstens R, Vandeplassche L. A double-blind, placebo-controlled study of prucalopride in elderly patients with chronic constipation. *Neurogastroenterol Motil*. 2010;22(9):991–998, e255. PubMed PMID: 20529205.

69 Verne GN, Davis RH, Robinson ME, Gordon JM, Eaker EY, Sninsky CA. Treatment of chronic constipation with colchicine: Randomized, double-blind, placebo-controlled, crossover trial. *Am J Gastroenterol*. 2003;98(5):1112–1116. PubMed PMID: 12809836.

70 Taghavi SA, Shabani S, Mehramiri A, Eshraghian A, Kazemi SM, Moeini M et al. Colchicine is effective for short-term treatment of slow transit constipation: A double-blind placebo-controlled clinical trial. *Int J Colorectal Dis* 2010;25(3):389–394. PubMed PMID: 19705134.

71 Roarty TP, Weber F, Soykan I, McCallum RW. Misoprostol in the treatment of chronic refractory constipation: Results of a long-term open label trial. *Aliment Pharmacol Ther*. 1997;11(6):1059–1066. PubMed PMID: 9663830.

72 Soffer EE, Metcalf A, Launspach J. Misoprostol is effective treatment for patients with severe chronic constipation. *Dig Dis Sci*. 1994;39(5):929–933. PubMed PMID: 8174433.

73 Parkman HP, Rao SS, Reynolds JC, Schiller LR, Wald A, Miner PB et al. Neurotrophin-3 improves functional constipation. *Am J Gastroenterol*. 2003 Jun;98(6):1338–1347. PubMed PMID: 12818279.

74 Chey WD, Camilleri M, Chang L, Rikner L, Graffner H. A randomized placebo-controlled phase IIb trial of a3309, a bile acid transporter inhibitor, for chronic idiopathic constipation. *Am J Gastroenterol*. 2011;106(10):1803–1812. PubMed PMID: 21606974. Pubmed Central PMCID: 3188811.

75 Youssef NN, Peters JM, Henderson W, Shultz-Peters S, Lockhart DK, Di Lorenzo C. Dose response of PEG 3350 for the treatment of childhood fecal impaction. *J Pediatr*. 2002;141(3):410–414. PubMed PMID: 12219064.

76 Thielman NM, Guerrant RL. Clinical practice. Acute infectious diarrhea. *N Engl J Med*. 2004 1;350(1):38–47. PubMed PMID: 14702426.

77 Fine KD, Schiller LR. AGA technical review on the evaluation and management of chronic diarrhea. *Gastroenterology*. 1999;116(6):1464–1486. PubMed PMID: 10348832.

78 Guerrant RL, Van Gilder T, Steiner TS, Thielman NM, Slutsker L, Tauxe RV et al. Practice guidelines for the management of infectious diarrhea. *Clin Infect Dis*. 2001;32(3):331–351. PubMed PMID: 11170940.

79 Dryden MS, Gabb RJ, Wright SK. Empirical treatment of severe acute community-acquired gastroenteritis with ciprofloxacin. *Clin Infect Dis*. 1996;22(6):1019–1025. PubMed PMID: 8783703.

80 DuPont HL. Guidelines on acute infectious diarrhea in adults. The Practice Parameters Committee of the American College of Gastroenterology. *Am J Gastroenterol*. 1997;92(11):1962–1975. PubMed PMID: 9362174.

81 Shannon HE, Lutz EA. Comparison of the peripheral and central effects of the opioid agonists loperamide and morphine in the formalin test in rats. *Neuropharmacology*. 2002;42(2):253–261. PubMed PMID: 11804622.

82 Sadeque AJ, Wandel C, He H, Shah S, Wood AJ. Increased drug delivery to the brain by P-glycoprotein inhibition. *Clin Pharmacol Ther*. 2000;68(3):231–237. PubMed PMID: 11014404.

83 Hallgren T, Fasth S, Delbro DS, Nordgren S, Oresland T, Hulten L. Loperamide improves anal sphincter function and continence after restorative proctocolectomy. *Dig Dis Sci*. 1994;39(12):2612–2618. PubMed PMID: 7995187.

84 Benson AB, 3rd, Ajani JA, Catalano RB, Engelking C, Kornblau SM, Martenson JA, Jr. et al. Recommended guidelines for the treatment of cancer treatment-induced diarrhea. *J Clin Oncol*. 2004;22(14):2918–2926. PubMed PMID: 15254061.

85 Heel RC, Brogden RN, Speight TM, Avery GS. Loperamide: A review of its pharmacological properties and therapeutic efficacy in diarrhoea. *Drugs*. 1978;15(1):33–52. PubMed PMID: 342229.

86 Gyr KE, Meier R. Pharmacodynamic effects of Sandostatin in the gastrointestinal tract. *Digestion*. 1993;54 Suppl 1:14–19. PubMed PMID: 8103010.

87 Ippoliti C, Champlin R, Bugazia N, Przepiorka D, Neumann J, Giralt S et al. Use of octreotide in the symptomatic management of diarrhea induced by graft-versus-host disease in patients with hematologic malignancies. *J Clin Oncol*. 1997;15(11):3350–3354. PubMed PMID: 9363865.

88 Cello JP, Grendell JH, Basuk P, Simon D, Weiss L, Wittner M et al. Effect of octreotide on refractory AIDS-associated diarrhea. A prospective, multicenter clinical trial. *Ann Intern Med*. 1991 1;115(9):705–710. PubMed PMID: 1929038.

89 Romeu J, Miro JM, Sirera G, Mallolas J, Arnal J, Valls ME et al. Efficacy of octreotide in the management of chronic diarrhoea in AIDS. *Aids*. 1991 Dec;5(12):1495–1499. PubMed PMID: 1814331.

60

Malignant ascites

JEREMY KEEN

MALIGNANT ASCITES

A survey of Canadian physicians and their management of malignant ascites produced comments such as "generally impossible to manage," "it is a frustrating clinical situation," and "a practical and effective solution is needed."[1]

This chapter will aim to review briefly the pathophysiology of ascites formation in malignant disease and then to examine the prevalence, associated symptoms, and, in more detail, the reported methods of clinical management.

The primary concerns in the management of ascites are questions related to the role of diuretic therapy, imaging, and the method of paracentesis, each of which remains poorly tested in formal trials. However, new work in the pathophysiology of ascites formation may lead to more individualized and novel methods of management.

INCIDENCE/PREVALENCE

Problems related to the presence of malignant ascites have been reported to be present in 3.6%–6% of patients admitted to palliative care units.[2,3] The development of ascites is most frequently associated with a primary diagnosis of ovarian carcinoma, developing in 37.7% of cases in one retrospective review.[4] Pancreaticobilary and gastric carcinomas were the other significant underlying primary malignant diagnoses (ascites developing in 21% and 18.3% of cases respectively) while oesophageal, colorectal, and breast carcinomas were each found to be responsible for 3%–4% of cases. The presence of ascites is usually an indicator of advanced disease and, unfortunately, is detectable at the time of initial diagnosis in over half of the patients in whom it develops.[5] Patients with ovarian cancer, however, do have a significantly longer median survival from the time of development of ascites compared with those with other malignancies.[6] In one review, the median survival of those with ascites and ovarian cancer was just under 2 years compared with a median of less than 6 months for all cancer types with ascites.[4] This may relate to ascites being a complication of relatively early stage ovarian cancer and its relative

sensitivity to cytotoxic chemotherapy. However, in one study of patients with stage III and IV disease receiving chemotherapy, the presence of ascites at the start of treatment reduced 5-year survival from 46% to 5%.[7] In another study of debulking surgery for patients with stage IV disease, the presence of ascites was the only independent predictive factor for early tumor progression.[8] Control of ascites often requires repeated inpatient episodes that, in one series of patients with ovarian cancer, showed a rapid increase in frequency over the last year of life to a median of seven admissions in the last 3 months.[9]

SYMPTOMS

Symptoms requiring palliation relate to increased intra-abdominal pressure and include; discomfort in abdominal wall, dyspnea, anorexia, early satiety, nausea and vomiting, esophageal reflux, poor mobility, insomnia related to general discomfort, pain in the groins and subcostal regions, and lower limb edema (Table 60.1). Abdominal compartment syndrome with resultant multisystem failure has also been recently reported.[10] Easily overlooked can be the significant negative effect of abdominal distension on body image.

PATHOPHYSIOLOGY

The accumulation of ascites is a result of an imbalance in the normal state of influx and efflux of fluid from the peritoneal cavity. The absorption of radiolabeled serum albumin after intraperitoneal injection has been measured in humans to be 4–5 mL/hour.[11] Drainage of peritoneal fluid occurs via the lymphatic system with the open-ended diaphragmatic lymphatics probably providing the major pathway.

A decreased rate of fluid efflux may occur as a result of blockage of the lymphatic system by tumor, and this has been shown histologically in association with malignant ascites in animal models.[12] In human subjects, one study demonstrated that 32 of 38 patients with malignant ascites showed no lymphatic absorption of radiolabeled sulfur colloid that had been

Table 60.1 *Malignant ascites in 1000 consecutive admissions to St. Columba's Hospice (January 1, 1997–October 16, 1999—personal communication)*

Number of admissions with ascites	36 (3.6% of all admissions)
With visceral pain	15 (42% of those with ascites)
With nausea	13 (36%)
With dyspnea	9 (25%)
With pain, nausea, and dyspnea	3 (8%)

injected into the peritoneum.[13] Conversely, 13 of 14 control subjects with either no ascites or nonmalignant ascites did demonstrate lymphatic uptake of the colloid.

It is unlikely that a reduced rate of fluid efflux alone is sufficient to cause the accumulation of massive amounts of ascitic fluid. Indeed, the rate of efflux has been shown to increase as ascites accumulates and intra-abdominal pressure increases, possibly up to rates approaching 80 mL/hour.[14]

The rate of fluid influx into the peritoneal space may be increased in malignancy as a result of two distinct mechanisms. Each mechanism will result in ascitic fluid of different biochemical properties and may respond to different modes of treatment.

1. Increased hepatic venous pressure, as an anatomical consequence of multiple hepatic metastases, or single large (sometimes benign) tumors causing a Budd-Chiari syndrome.[15] An increase in venous pressure results both in fluid leakage into the peritoneum from the sinusoids and, via an increase in plasma renin concentration, in the retention of salt and water in the kidneys. The ascitic fluid resulting from this mechanism is similar to that seen as a result of cirrhosis and has the properties of a transudate.

2. An exudate, of relatively high protein concentration, may be produced as a result of increased vascular permeability. Tumor neovasculature is thought to be intrinsically leaky, allowing extravasation of fluid and, from peritoneal tumor deposits, would contribute to ascites formation. However, it has long been recognized that ascitic fluid also arises from the areas of peritoneum unaffected by tumor.[14] Beecham and colleagues observed a marked neovascularization of the parietal peritoneum in patients with malignant ascites and ovarian carcinoma.[16]

In rats, there appears to be an increase in the permeability of peritoneal capillaries after cell-free malignant ascitic fluid is infused intraperitoneally.[5] The permeability of normal microvessels, such as those that line the peritoneal cavity, can be increased by a variety of cytokines, including transforming growth factors α and β, epidermal growth factor, and vascular endothelial growth factor (VEGF).[17] Cytokines may be secreted by tumor cells and/or inflammatory monocytes and macrophages.

VEGF is expressed by the normal ovary during the phases of follicular development and copora lutea formation,[18] and in one series, the degree of tumor expression was related to patient survival.[19] VEGF not only increases capillary permeability but also stimulates angiogenesis, facilitating tumor growth and also, potentially, the observed neovascularization of normal peritoneum. Animal experiments have demonstrated a significant relationship between the degree of tumor cell expression of VEGF and the observed levels of angiogenesis and ascites production.[20,21] VEGF has been detected in high concentrations in malignant as opposed to nonmalignant ascites and associated with metastases from a variety of primary sites.[22–24] The exception has been the observation of high levels of VEGF in ovarian hyperstimulation syndrome, also associated with ascites formation.[25] The potential for therapeutic interventions that target the production or actions of VEGF will be discussed later.

In an individual patient, the relative contribution of these two principal mechanisms of ascitic fluid production can be estimated from the calculation of the serum-ascites albumin gradient. The serum-ascites gradient is calculated by subtracting the albumin concentration of the ascitic fluid from that within a serum specimen obtained on the same day. The gradient correlates with the portal venous pressure, and a value of ≥11 g/L is indicative of a transudate and the presence of portal hypertension.[26] This may be of importance in assessing the likelihood of response to diuretic therapy with an aldosterone antagonist.

The formation of chylous ascites is a complication of retroperitoneal tumor spread or its treatment and arises either from damage to lymphatic vessels or through the obstruction of lymphatic flow through lymph nodes or the pancreas.

DIAGNOSIS

The diagnosis of the presence of ascites in an individual is usually straightforward, relying on relevant clinical history and examination.[27] Where there is doubt, usually with typical symptoms present in a patient with an obese abdomen or with potential bowel obstruction, ultrasound examination can detect as little as 100 mL of free fluid in the peritoneum.[28] Computerized tomography is equally as accurate but not always as easily available as ultrasound. Plain abdominal x-rays may be helpful in excluding not only signs suggestive of bowel obstruction but also positive signs of ascites such as a *ground glass* appearance, loss of psoas shadows and organ definition, and increased spacing of intestinal loops.

Clearly, the presence of ascites in a patient with known malignancy cannot always be assumed to be secondary to the presence of intra-abdominal tumor, and other causes, such as cirrhosis, congestive heart failure, nephrotic syndrome, tuberculosis, and pancreatitis, which necessitate specific modalities of treatment, must be excluded.

Several tests have been proposed to differentiate malignant ascites from other forms of ascites such as fluid levels of sialic acid,[29] telomerase,[30] ß-HCG,[31] fibronectin,[32] or, in one study, a combination of total protein, lactate dehydrogenase, tumor necrosis factor-α, C4, and haptoglobin.[33] Such diagnostic tests may, of course, be helpful in terms of prognosis and possibly decisions regarding antitumor therapy but not as an aid to decisions about other forms of palliative treatment.

MANAGEMENT

The palliation of all symptoms related to malignant disease follows the same broad principles of totally individualized care based on the best evidence available from larger populations. Guidelines and treatment algorithms for the management of problems such as ascites have been developed and are helpful,[17,34,35] but the temptation is to manipulate every patient into particular protocols or guidelines and lose sight of the individual risk–benefit analyses for certain management plans.

Antitumor therapy

For the relief of symptoms resulting from complications, such as ascites, which reflect tumor activity, specific antitumor therapy should always be considered, particularly for patients with ovarian or breast carcinoma. The development of ascites often complicates ovarian carcinoma relatively early in the course of the disease and is, in fact, a presenting feature in a third of all cases.[36] Malik et al.[37*] demonstrated a complete clearance or significant reduction of ascites in 46% of patients with ovarian cancer treated with systemic cytotoxic chemotherapy. Significant response in ovarian cancer can be observed with second- and even third-line chemotherapy, an approach which should, therefore, always be considered.

Cytotoxic agents have been given intraperitoneally from as early as the 1950s.[38] There has been a resurgence of interest with the development of a hyperthermic intraperitoneal chemotherapy (HIPEC) that appears to allow greater tissue penetration and reduce the levels of drug resistance.[39] More recently, the use of laparoscopy and HIPEC has been proposed to allow the division of adhesions to optimize the access of infused cytotoxic to the peritoneal surface as well as to facilitate the positioning of inflow tube and outflow drains to form a closed-loop irrigation system.[40] Of 14 individuals with malignant ascites treated with this technique, all had ascites controlled with no reported morbidity or mortality connected with the procedure. A multi-institutional analysis of the outcome of 52 individuals treated with laparoscopic HIPEC demonstrated a complete resolution of ascites in 94% with a mean hospital stay of 2.3 days and complicated by only two minor wound infections and a deep venous thrombosis.[41]

HIPEC has been used in combination with aggressive cytoreductive surgery, which in some series has been associated with high rates of morbidity, but, if individuals are selected carefully, this approach may result in good control of ascites and a prolonged survival with a variety of primary tumor types.[42*,43*,44]

Chylous ascites, when associated with retroperitoneal lymphoma and a consequent disruption of normal lymphatic drainage pathways, may be expected to show some response to chemotherapy if it is the first- or second-line treatment. Radiotherapy may also have a role in the relief of symptoms of lymphoma.

The success of the intracavitary instillation of a variety of agents in the control of malignant pleural effusions has encouraged a similar approach to the treatment of malignant

Table 60.2 *Agents that have been employed for intraperitoneal instillation in the management of peritoneal malignancy and ascites*

[198]Au
[32]CrPO$_4$
Thiotepa
Fluorouracil
Mustine
Bleomycin
Cisplatinum
Carboplatin
Etoposide
Mitomycin C
Adriamycin
Docetaxel
Mitoxantrone
Interferon-γ
Interferon-α
Interferon-β
Tumor necrosis factor
Interleukin-2
Radiolabeled monoclonal antibodies
Metalloproteinase inhibitors
Corticosteroids
Bevacizumab
Catumaxomab
Rituximab
Corynebacterium parvum
OK-432 (extract from *S. pyogenes*)

ascites. There have been numerous small trials and case series reporting the use of radioisotopes, cytotoxics, and, more recently, biological agents and response modifiers to reduce ascitic fluid formation (Table 60.2). One phase II study found that intraperitoneal instillation of the corticosteroid triamcinolone hexacetonide resulted in a significant slowing of ascites accumulation.[45*] The effect was noted particularly in patients with an albumin serum-ascites gradient of <11 g/L. The authors postulated the effect to have been mediated through a steroid-induced reduction of the secretion of VEGF.

Other approaches

Initial preclinical trials with anti-VEGF antibodies, anti-VEGF receptor antibodies, and an inhibitor of VEGF receptor tyrosine kinase activity[46] have been reported to show a reduction in ascites formation in animal models. Transfection of a mutated gene controlling the production of VEGF has decreased ascites production in mice.[47] Clinical trials of the humanized VEGF antibody, bevacizumab, given both systemically and intraperitoneally have been promising.[48*,49] More recently, aflibercept, a decoy VEGF receptor that binds and neutralizes VEGF, has shown good inhibitory effects on ascites production, but parenteral therapy in phase II trials was associated with a relatively high level of side effects, principally intestinal perforation.[50*,51**] Tumor necrosis factor has been found to block the reaccumulation of ascites in an animal model by inhibiting the expression of VEGF mRNA,[52] and an early clinical study suggested the benefit from the administration of recombinant TNFα.[53*] Interestingly, a recent report of the use of the anti-TNF agent infliximab showed a reduction in the levels of VEGF and angiogenesis in the synovia of patients with psoriatic arthritis.[54*] VEGF expression and associated angiogenesis have also been shown to be reduced by ketoprofen,[55] green tea,[56] and angiotensin-converting enzyme inhibitors.[57]

Epithelial cell adhesion molecule (EpCAM) is a cell surface glycoprotein that mediates epithelial cell to cell adhesion. It is found to be expressed in the majority of epithelial carcinomas, including those responsible for most incidences of malignant ascites, and is a tempting target for immunotherapy. The normal peritoneal cavity is lined by mesothelial cells that do not express EpCAM. Catumaxomab is a trifunctional monoclonal antibody that binds to EpCAM, and the T-lymphocyte surface antigen, CD3 and is designed to recruit not only T cells but also cytokine-producing accessory cells.[58] A phase II/III clinical trial of intraperitoneal infusions of catumaxomab in individuals with malignant ascites and EpCAM positive tumors resulted in an increase in *puncture-free survival* and a delayed deterioration in the quality of life when compared with a standard approach of serial paracenteses alone.[59**,60**] However, side effects were common, and the protocol called for four repeat intraperitoneal infusions over a 10-day period.

Matrix metalloproteinases are a group of enzymes that, after the loss of normal inhibitory control during tumor development, potentiate tumor invasion and metastases. In early clinical trials, metalloproteinase inhibitors have been reported to be of benefit.[61*]

Octreotide, a somatostatin analog, has been suggested to have therapeutic potential for a myriad of different disorders, and indeed, there has been a small case series demonstrating a reduction in malignant ascites in two of three patients treated.[62*] The physiological mechanism remains unclear although one other report does suggest a benefit to patients with hepatic cirrhosis and ascites.[63]

Diuretic therapy

Diuretic therapy remains the mainstay of the treatment of patients with ascites of nonmalignant origin, but the role of diuretics in the management of malignant ascites remains controversial. A recent Canadian survey of the management of malignant ascites reported that while 98% of physicians used paracentesis, only 61% prescribed diuretics, and of these, one quarter felt them to be ineffective.[1] The rates of response to diuretics in reported studies range from 38%[64*] to 86%.[65*] Theoretically, it would be expected that those patients who demonstrate raised plasma renin activity and hence increased sodium and water retention would have a greater likelihood of response to diuretics. These patients are those who tend to demonstrate a serum-ascites albumin gradient of ≥11 g/L, where ascites is formed exclusively or principally as a result of intrahepatic metastases. A small study of the use of diuretics in patients with ascites and either massive hepatic metastases, *peritoneal carcinomatosis*, or chylous ascites only demonstrated a reduction in the estimated ascitic volume in the group with hepatic metastases.[66*] Each of the three patients in the group with hepatic metastases had raised plasma renin levels and a high serum-ascites albumin gradient and responded to the aldosterone antagonist spironolactone. In another small series, 13 of 15 patients with malignant ascites responded to spironolactone therapy.[65*] Plasma renin levels were measured in only five patients but were found to have risen in each case. There is a significant body of evidence relating to the optimum use of diuretics in ascites secondary to cirrhosis, where 90% of patients would be expected to respond to the treatment.[26] The majority of trials report the use of spironolactone, but given the long half-life of the parent drug and its active metabolites, there is often a delay of up to 2 weeks before the onset of a significant diuresis. Amiloride, an alternative potassium-sparing diuretic, has a much faster onset of action. Although amiloride is not a classical mineralocorticoid receptor antagonist, it appears to interfere with aldosterone effects in model systems.[67] Interestingly, both amiloride and spironolactone interfere with the effect of aldosterone on endothelial cells. Amiloride with a faster onset of action may be a more appropriate choice for patients with relatively short prognoses or in whom the early prevention of reaccumulation of ascites after paracentesis is desired. The use of a loading dose of spironolactone has not been reported, and the usual regime comprises a starting dose of 100 mg as a single daily dose, increasing at 2- to 3-day intervals to 400 mg if needed and tolerated. Regular girth measurement may be a more appropriate method of monitoring the response to treatment than daily weights and accurate fluid balance recordings. The response to diuretics is thought to occur, in part, as a result of a redistribution of fluid within body compartments rather than being wholly dependent on a diuresis.[68] The addition of a loop diuretic may improve the speed of response with one study reporting a rapid initial response to the use of an intravenous infusion of frusemide during the accumulation period of spironolactone therapy.[69]

The initiation of spironolactone therapy is not infrequently associated with nausea unrelated to electrolyte imbalance. The most debilitating side effects, however, relate to intravascular volume depletion and include postural hypotension, uremia, and, in some cases, renal failure. A proportion of patients will have a concurrent paraneoplastic autonomic neuropathy and resultant postural hypotension[70] that will be augmented by an aggressive diuretic therapy. Hepatic encephalopathy is an additional potential complication of aggressive diuresis in patients with limited residual hepatic function. It is important to monitor the response to diuretics and titrate the dose to a maintenance level to lessen the chance of side effects.

Paracentesis

Abdominal paracentesis remains the most commonly employed modality of treatment for malignant ascites.[1] It affords quick symptomatic relief in a population that often has a relatively short prognosis and for whom diuretic therapy, if effective, may include a significant lag period and be associated with postural hypotension.

The reported techniques and equipment used for the procedure are numerous and particularly among palliative care physicians appear to allow a full expression of their creativity. The most significant differences in approach relate to the cannula or catheter used for puncturing the peritoneum, the rate of ascitic fluid drainage, and the necessity or not of maintenance of intravascular volume with albumin, colloid, or crystalloid infusions. A Cochrane Review published in 2010 could find no evidence to support particular methods of paracentesis with no answers to questions relating to the length of time that a drain should remain in place, the use of intravenous replacement of fluid, the clamping of drains, and the recording of vital observations during drainage.[71***]

The large experience of the potential problems associated with paracentesis in patients with hepatic cirrhosis, particularly hypotension and renal impairment, has colored the approach of many to the procedure in malignant ascites. It is likely that, in the absence of a serum-ascites gradient of ≥11 g/L, these complications of paracentesis are rare in patients with malignant ascites, and fluid maybe drained off relatively rapidly with no need to routinely administer intravenous colloid or albumin.[35] Indeed, the use of vacuum bottles allowing several liters to be removed in a matter of minutes, with apparently few complications, has been reported to be particularly useful in the outpatient clinic or even the patient's home.[72]

A study of 35 patients with ascites and ovarian cancer demonstrated a direct correlation between the measured value of intraperitoneal pressure and the severity of symptoms reported.[73*] Another recent study helps to confirm that raised intra-abdominal pressure and related symptoms can be significantly relieved after the drainage of just a *few liters* over 2 hours.[74*] The group of patients reported had a mean of 5.3 L drained over 24 hours but no significant improvement in symptom relief (of those assessed) after 24 hours than that noted after only 2 hours of drainage. Indeed ,only dyspnea (and not discomfort, nausea, or vomiting) was improved significantly more at 72 hours than at 2 hours of ascitic drainage. It would be of interest if the perception of body image had been factored into these studies.

Since symptoms can often be relieved by the removal of relatively small volumes of ascites over a short period, this is to be recommended particularly in the very frail with a limited prognosis. One to two liters of fluid can be removed simply over 30 min via a plastic intravenous cannula. The insertion of the cannula is simple and, if used in conjunction with a local infiltration of local anesthetic, is a relatively comfortable procedure. The removal of such a modest volume is unlikely to cause symptomatic hypovolemia, and the use of a small cannula for a short time is highly unlikely to cause local complications.

Clearly, however, ascites is likely to reaccumulate, and should a prognosis be more than a few days, then frequent recurrent small-volume paracenteses will be required. There has been increasing recent evidence of the effectiveness, safety, tolerability, and potential financial savings afforded by the use of the PleurX system of indwelling peritoneal catheters and vacuum drainage bottles. Indeed, in England and Wales, the National Institute for Health and Clinical Excellence (NICE) issued a report in 2012 recommending the use of this system in the National Health Service (NHS) for individuals with malignant ascites likely to require repeated large-volume paracenteses for palliation of symptoms.[75] The NICE committee acknowledged the paucity of robust evidence directly comparing the use of indwelling catheters with other approaches to ascitic drainage. The system would result in savings to the NHS if regular large-volume paracenteses involved an overnight stay in the hospital but not if performed on a day-case or outpatient basis. Until this technology becomes more widely available and each budget-holding health authority is convinced of the advantages of a PleurX, or similar system, over regular low-tech drainage, it is likely that most clinicians will continue to give consideration to the less frequent drainage of larger volumes of ascites through some form of temporary catheter. Peritoneal dialysis, suprapubic urinary bladder, and self-retaining nephrostomy catheters have all been described as useful drainage devices.

Stephenson and Gilbert reported the successful introduction of guidelines for paracentesis into an oncology unit that resulted in reductions in the use of ultrasound to mark sites for drainage, the mean duration of drainage, and length of inpatient stay.[35] Catheters were left in for no more than 6 hours with up to 5 L being drained and intravenous fluids only considered if patients were hypotensive, dehydrated, or known to have severe renal impairment. Patients without peripheral edema may be particularly prone to hypovolemia. It is prudent to monitor blood pressure during the procedure with intravascular volume replenished by intravenous infusion of either colloid or plasma protein solution should hypotension develop. A low threshold for the administration of intravenous fluid should be present for patients with high serum-ascitic albumin gradient who do not respond to diuretics and are treated by paracentesis.

After the withdrawal of the drain, there is a likelihood of a continued leakage of fluid from the drain site. This can be lessened by the use of a *Z-technique* when introducing the catheter through the skin and then the peritoneal wall. Some operators tie a purse string suture around the site, some place a stoma bag over the site until the leakage stops, and others have suggested the application of enbucrilate adhesive to seal the skin.[76]

Complications of paracentesis relate mainly to the potential for a relatively rapid shift of fluid between body compartments. One study reported two deaths from hypotension in a series of 109 consecutive paracenteses performed on 43 patients.[77*] More likely in malignant ascites are procedural complications including bowel perforation, peritonitis, and localized cellulitis surrounding the drain site. One study reported 2 deaths from peritonitis in a series of 127 paracenteses in 100 patients.[12*] Infection was a particular problem in a reported case series of patients with permanent implanted drains.[78*] A reported series of 10 patients treated with tunneled PleurX catheters recorded no catheter-related infections with a mean catheter survival of 70 days.[79*] In this series, serial serum albumin measurements demonstrated a progressive decline. However, one case report of the use of an implanted peritoneal dialysis catheter reported only one superficial infection in 17 months during which time the patient drained 1000–1500 mL of ascites twice a week.[80] Interestingly, this same patient maintained serum albumin levels despite such prolonged and frequent drainage. However, anecdotal experience would suggest that many patients feel extremely tired for several days following paracentesis, and both hyponatremia and a progressive fall in plasma albumin concentration with repeated paracenteses have been recorded in some series. Patients with severely compromised hepatic function are at particular risk of hepatic failure and encephalopathy over the first 24 hours after ascitic drainage.

Peritoneovenous shunting

Potential problems of repeated paracentesis such as intravascular hypovolemia, hypoalbuminemia, infection and visceral damage, and the expense, discomfort, and the inconvenience of repeated hospital admissions have prompted the development of alternative drainage procedures. Peritoneovenous shunting was established in the mid-1970s[81] and remains the most common procedure performed. Shunting of ascitic fluid into the stomach[82] and urinary bladder[83] has also been reported but has presented too many technical difficulties to be useful at present. There have, however, been no randomized controlled trials to date comparing peritoneovenous shunting with repeated abdominal paracentesis.

Two forms of shunt have been commonly used, the original Le Veen (production now discontinued) and the Denver shunt. Both are designed to allow the drainage of ascites into the central venous system, usually via the internal jugular or femoral veins. They may be placed surgically, laparoscopically, or percutaneously with a comparative study reporting no difference in performance or complication rate of each of these techniques.[84*] The most common reason for shunt failure is lumen occlusion, which appears to occur more frequently during the drainage of malignant ascites than cirrhotic ascites (for the control of which these shunts were first described). The Denver shunt has the theoretical advantage of a manual pumping mechanism to facilitate ascitic flow and clearance of debris. However, no statistical difference in the performance of the two shunts could be found in one comparative study.[85*]

Successful resolution of ascites and symptom relief with the use of peritoneovenous shunts has been reported in between 62% and 87% of patients.[64,86–89] One noncontrolled study showed, in addition, a maintenance of serum albumin levels in comparison to a progressive decrease in patients treated with repeated paracentesis.[64*] This same study measured *quality of life* by a single question and VAS scale and found a nonsignificant trend to an improvement with either paracenteses or shunts and no difference between the two methods of drainage. In the previously quoted survey of physicians' practice, only 12 of 44 respondents had used peritoneovenous shunts, and 7 found them to be useful.[1] The apparent reluctance to use this method is probably a result of the significant complication rate of both the operative procedure and the ongoing operation of the shunt. There is a significant operative mortality in

patients with malignant ascites quoted as 13% in one of the larger studies,[86] although this is less than that associated with the procedure for ascites associated with cirrhosis. While this high mortality rate is in part to be expected in a frail population undergoing a general anesthetic or even local anesthetic and sedation, specific procedure-related mortality is more commonly a result of pulmonary edema. This complication of a sudden increase in fluid volume within the central venous system can be avoided, in part, by removing a proportion of the ascites (50%–70% quoted in one study[90]) at operation to reduce pressure and hence flow through the shunt. Many centers would still advocate *intensive* monitoring with central venous pressure lines for the first 24 hours after surgery.

Overall, complication rates of peritoneovenous shunts of between 25% and 50% are reported.[64,86,87] The most common complication is shunt occlusion, either, more commonly, from thrombosis of the venous terminal or alternatively from debris in the peritoneal end. Two studies reported alterations in the laboratory measurements of coagulation parameters (increased concentration of fibrinogen degradation products) consistent with subclinical disseminated intervascular coagulation (DIC) in all patients with patent shunts.[85*,91*] Indeed, while such findings may be used as surrogate evidence of shunt patency, frank DIC remains a rare complication. One recent review of 341 individuals undergoing the placement of a shunt found DIC to be a complication in 9.3% but with no associated mortality.[92] The incidence of DIC is greater in patients with shunts and cirrhotic ascites possibly as a result of a higher concentration of plasminogen activator inhibitor in malignant ascites with consequently less potential for fibrinolytic activity.[93] The incidence of postoperative DIC can be reduced by the removal of a significant proportion of the ascitic volume intraoperatively.[91] Other complications include thromboembolism, vena caval thrombosis, hepatic encephalopathy, peritonitis, and tumor seeding to the subcutaneous tissues of the anterior abdominal wall.

The potential effects of the introduction of tumor cells from the peritoneal cavity into the circulation via the shunt have been examined in a small series of postmortem examinations.[94] The study reported a variety of observations but concluded that metastases, although occurring in some patients as a direct result of shunt placement, are not clinically significant and do not alter a prognosis. This is likely to be related to the short prognosis of the majority of patients who develop malignant ascites.

Peritoneovenous shunts are clearly unsuitable for patients with loculated ascites and are not advised if the ascites is hemorrhagic or chylous or the patient has poor cardiac or renal function or a tendency to hepatic encephalopathy. Patients with elevated bilirubin levels have an increased risk of intravascular coagulation with shunting.[95*] Portal hypertension, massive pleural effusion, and coagulation disorders are relative contraindications.[96,97] The presence of malignant cells in ascitic fluid, if no antitumor treatment is to be given, correlates with a poor prognosis (median survival of 26 days compared with 140 days if cytology is negative) and is thus also a relative contraindication.[98] A recently reported series of patients with ascites and nongynecological primary tumors showed the best outcomes of peritoneovenous shunts to occur in patients with normal renal function and tumors of nongastrointestinal primary origin.[99] The relatively long survival of patients with ascites and gynecological malignancies and the potential savings in terms of repeated hospitalizations for paracentesis make peritoneovenous shunting an option to be considered in all cases.

SUMMARY

The burden of ascites as a complication of malignancy remains highly significant, particularly for the individual patient but also in terms of the health care resources consumed in clinical management. Despite numerous small studies of the intraperitoneal administration of various radioisotopes, immune/biological response modifiers, and cytotoxic agents, including recent interest in hyperthermic chemotherapy, management continues to rely upon the use of diuretics, abdominal paracentesis, and peritoneovenous shunts.

However, it is from recent studies into the pathophysiology of ascites production in intra-abdominal malignancy that new and specific ways to slow or halt ascitic fluid production are likely to emerge. In particular, the present interest in the role of VEGF in tumor angiogenesis along with the realization of the role of peritoneal neovascularization in ascites production has highlighted a possible new, specific, target for therapy. One would hope, given the high frequency of occurrence of this complication of malignancy, that there would be good levels of recruitment to large multicentre trials. However, surprisingly, such trials have not been a feature of research into ascites management to date.

DIURETICS

- Most effective if serum-ascites albumin gradient is <11 g/L.
- Spironolactone requires high doses and does have a significant lag time. Amiloride, a faster acting diuretic that interferes with the effects of aldosterone, is potentially useful but has not been assessed in formal trials.

PARACENTESIS

- Most widely used method of managing malignant ascites.
- Symptomatic relief is often afforded with the removal of a relatively small volume of ascites. For patients with a prognosis measured in days. consider using an intravenous cannula to drain ascitic fluid for minimal discomfort.
- For patients with a longer prognosis, larger volumes of ascites may be drained relatively quickly without the necessity of intravenous fluid replacement in all individuals.
- Consider the use of implanted/tunneled catheters with regular drainage performed by the patient at home.

PERITONEOVENOUS SHUNTS

- Associated with significant morbidity but potentially useful if ascites is rapidly recurrent after paracentesis and is diuretic-resistant.
- Most useful for patients with gynecological (principally ovarian) and nongastrointestinal primary tumors and normal renal function.
- Complications can be significantly reduced if the sufficiently large volume of the ascitic fluid is removed at the time of shunt insertion.

REFERENCES

1   Lee CW, Bociek G, Faught W. A survey of practice in management of malignant ascites. J. Pain Symptom. Manage. 1998;16:96–101.
2   Keen J, Fallon M. Malignant ascites. In Ripamonti C, Bruera E eds. Gastrointestinal Symptoms in Advanced Cancer Patients. Oxford, U.K.: Oxford University Press, 2002; pp. 279–290.
3   Preston N. New strategies for the management of malignant ascites. Eur. J. Cancer Care (Engl.) 1995;4;178–183.
4   Ayantunde AA, Parsons SL. Pattern and prognostic factors in patients with malignant ascites: A retrospective study. Ann. Oncol. 2007;18:945–949
5   Garrison RN, Kaelin LD, Galloway RH, Heuser LS. Malignant ascites. Clinical and experimental observations. Ann. Surg. 1986;203:644–651.
6   Parsons SL, Lang MW, Steele RJ. Malignant ascites: A 2-year review from a teaching hospital. Eur. J. Surg. Oncol 1996;22:237–239.
7   Puls LE, Duniho T, Hunter JE, Kryscio R, Blackhurst D, Gallion H. The prognostic implication of ascites in advanced-stage ovarian cancer. Gynecol. Oncol. 1996;61:109–112.
8   Zang RY, Zhang ZY, Cai SM et al. Cytoreductive surgery for stage IV epithelial ovarian cancer. J. Exp. Clin. Cancer Res. 1999;18:449–454. www.nice.org.uk/guidance/MTG9
9   von Gruenigen VE, Frasure HE, Reidy AM, Gil KM. Clinical disease course during the last year in ovarian cancer. Gynecol. Oncol. 2003;90:619–624.
10 Etzion Y, Barski L, Almog Y. Malignant ascites presenting as abdominal compartment syndrome. Am. J. Emerg. Med. 2004;22;430–431.
♦ 11 Parsons SL, Watson SA, Steele RJ. Malignant ascites. Br. J. Surg. 1996;83:6–14.
12 Feldman GB, Knapp RC, Order SE, Hellman S. The role of lymphatic obstruction in the formation of ascites in a murine ovarian carcinoma. Cancer Res. 1972;32:1663–1666.
13 Coates G, Bush RS, Aspin N. A study of ascites using lymphoscintigraphy with 99m Tc-sulphur colloid. Radiology 1973;107:577–583.
14 Hirabayashi KI, Graham J. Genesis of ascites in ovarian cancer. Am. J. Obstet. Gynecol. 1970;106:492–497.
15 Sebastian S, Tuite D, Crotty P, Torreggiani W, Buckley MJ. Painful ascites. Gut 2004;53:1344, 1355.
16 Beecham JB, Kucera P, Helmkamp BF, Bonfiglio TA. Peritoneal angiogenesis in patients with ascites. Gynecol. Oncol. 1983;15:142.
17 De Simone GG. Treatment of malignant ascites. Prog. Palliat. Care 1999;7:10–16.
18 Yamamoto S, Konishi I, Tsuruta Y et al. Expression of vascular endothelial growth factor (VEGF) during folliculogenesis and corpus luteum formation in the human ovary. Gynecol. Endocrinol. 1997;11:371–381.

19   Yamamoto S, Konishi I, Mandai M et al. Expression of vascular endothelial growth factor (VEGF) in epithelial ovarian neoplasms: Correlation with clinicopathology and patient survival, and analysis of serum VEGF levels. *Br. J. Cancer* 1997;76:1221–1227.

20   Yoneda J, Kuniyasu H, Crispens MA, Price JE, Bucana CD, Fidler IJ. Expression of angiogenesis-related genes and progression of human ovarian carcinomas in nude mice. *J. Natl. Cancer Inst.* 1998;90:447–454.

21   Huang S, Robinson JB, Deguzman A, Bucana CD, Fidler IJ. Blockade of nuclear factor-kappaB signaling inhibits angiogenesis and tumorigenicity of human ovarian cancer cells by suppressing expression of vascular endothelial growth factor and interleukin 8. *Cancer Res.* 2000;60:5334–5339.

22   Zebrowski BK, Liu W, Ramirez K, Akagi Y, Mills GB, Ellis LM. Markedly elevated levels of vascular endothelial growth factor in malignant ascites. *Ann. Surg. Oncol.* 1999;6:373–378.

23   Verheul HM, Hoekman K, Jorna AS, Smit EF, Pinedo HM. Targeting vascular endothelial growth factor blockade: Ascites and pleural effusion formation. *Oncologist* 2000;5 (Suppl 1):45–50.

24   Kraft A, Weindel K, Ochs A et al. Vascular endothelial growth factor in the sera and effusions of patients with malignant and nonmalignant disease. *Cancer* 1999;85:178–187.

25   Gomez R, Simon C, Remohi J, Pellicer A. Administration of moderate and high doses of gonadotropins to female rats increases ovarian vascular endothelial growth factor (VEGF) and VEGF receptor-2 expression that is associated to vascular hyperpermeability. *Biol. Reprod.* 2003;68:2164–2171.

26   Runyon BA. Care of patients with ascites. *N. Engl. J. Med.* 1994;330: 337–342.

27   Williams JW, Jr., Simel DL. The rational clinical examination. Does this patient have ascites? How to divine fluid in the abdomen. *JAMA* 1992;267:2645–2648.

28   Goldberg BB, Goodman GA, Clearfield HR. Evaluation of ascites by ultrasound. *Radiology* 1970;96:15–22.

29   Colli A, Buccino G, Cocciolo M, Parravicini R, Mariani F, Scaltrini G. Diagnostic accuracy of sialic acid in the diagnosis of malignant ascites. *Cancer* 1989;63:912–916.

30   Tangkijvanich P, Tresukosol D, Sampatanukul P et al. Telomerase assay for differentiating between malignancy-related and nonmalignant ascites. *Clin. Cancer Res.* 1999;5:2470–2475.

31   Gerbes AL, Hoermann R, Mann K, Jungst D. Human chorionic gonadotropin-beta in the differentiation of malignancy-related and nonmalignant ascites. *Digestion* 1996;57:113–117.

32   Colli A, Buccino G, Cocciolo M, Parravicini R, Mariani F, Scaltrini G. Diagnostic accuracy of fibronectin in the differential diagnosis of ascites. *Cancer* 1986;58:2489–2493.

33   Alexandrakis MG, Moschandrea J, Kyriakou DS, Alexandraki R, Kouroumalis E. Use of a variety of biological parameters in distinguishing cirrhotic from malignant ascites. *Int. J. Biol. Markers* 2001;16:45–49.

✱ 34   Regnard C, Mannix K. Management of ascites in advanced cancer—A flow diagram. *Palliat. Med.* 1989;4:45–47.

35   Stephenson J, Gilbert J. The development of clinical guidelines on paracentesis for ascites related to malignancy. *Palliat. Med.* 2002;16:213–218.

36   Lifshitz S. Ascites, pathophysiology and control measures. *Int. J. Radiat. Oncol Biol. Phys.* 1982;8:1423–1426.

37   Malik I, Abubakar S, Rizwana I, Alam F, Rizvi J, Khan A. Clinical features and management of malignant ascites. *J. Pak. Med. Assoc.* 1991;41:38–40.

38   Weisberger AS, Levine B, Storaasli JP. Use of nitrogen mustard in treatment of serous effusions of neoplastic origin. *JAMA* 1955;159:1704–1707.

◆ 39   Witkamp AJ, de Bree E, Van Goethem R, Zoetmulder FA. Rationale and techniques of intra-operative hyperthermic intraperitoneal chemotherapy. *Cancer Treat. Rev.* 2001;27:365–374.

40   Garofalo A, Valle M, Garcia J, Sugarbaker PH. Laparoscopic intraperitoneal hyperthermic chemotherapy for palliation of debilitating malignant ascites. *Eur. J. Surg. Oncol.* 2006;32:682–685.

◆ 41   Valle M, Van der Speeten K, Garafalo A. Laparoscopic hyperthermic intraperitoneal peroperative chemotherapy (HIPEC) in the management of refractory malignant ascites: A multi-institutional retrospective analysis in 52 patients. *J Surg. Oncol.* 2009;100:331–334.

42   de Bree E, Romanos J, Michalakis J et al. Intraoperative hyperthermic intraperitoneal chemotherapy with docetaxel as second-line treatment for peritoneal carcinomatosis of gynaecological origin. *Anticancer Res.* 2003;23:3019–3027.

43   Loggie BW, Perini M, Fleming RA, Russell GB, Geisinger K. Treatment and prevention of malignant ascites associated with disseminated intraperitoneal malignancies by aggressive combined-modality therapy. *Am. Surg.* 1997;63:137–143.

◆ 44   Sangisetty SL, Miner TJ. Malignant ascites: A review of prognostic factors, pathophysiology and therapeutic measures. *World J. Gastrointest. Surg.* 2012; 4: 87–95.

45   Mackey JR, Wood L, Nabholtz J, Jensen J, Venner P. A phase II trial of triamcinolone hexacetanide for symptomatic recurrent malignant ascites. *J. Pain Symptom Manage.* 2000;19:193–199.

46   Xu L, Yoneda J, Herrera C, Wood J, Killion JJ, Fidler IJ. Inhibition of malignant ascites and growth of human ovarian carcinoma by oral administration of a potent inhibitor of the vascular endothelial growth factor receptor tyrosine kinases. *Int. J. Oncol.* 2000;16:445–454.

47   Huang S, Robinson JB, Deguzman A, Bucana CD, Fidler IJ. Blockade of nuclear factor-kappaB signaling inhibits angiogenesis and tumorigenicity of human ovarian cancer cells by suppressing expression of vascular endothelial growth factor and interleukin 8. *Cancer Res.* 2000;60:5334–5339.

48   Numnum TM, Rocconi RP, Whitworth J, Barnes MN. The use of bevacizumab to palliate symptomatic ascites in patients with refractory ovarian carcinoma. *Gynecol. Oncol.* 2006;102:425–428.

◆ 49   Kobold S, Hegewisch-Becker, Oechsle K, Jordan K et al. Intraperitoneal VEGF inhibition using bevacizumab: A potential approach for the symptomatic treatment of malignant ascites? *Oncologist* 2009;14:1242–1251.

50   ColomboN, MangiliG, MammolitiS, KallingM et al. A phase II study of aflibercept in patients with advanced epithelial ovarian cancer and symptomatic malignant ascites. *Gynecol. Oncol.* 2012;125:42–47.

51   GotliebWH, Amant F, Advani S, Goswami C et al. Intravenous aflibercept for treatment of recurrent symptomatic malignant ascites in patients with advanced ovarian cancer: A phase 2, randomised, double-blind, placebo-controlled study. *Lancet Oncol.* 2012;13:154–162.

52   Stoelcker B, Echtenacher B, Weich HA, Sztajer H, Hicklin DJ, Mannel DN. VEGF/Flk-1 interaction, a requirement for malignant ascites recurrence. *J. Interferon Cytokine Res.* 2000;20:511–517.

53   Rath U, Kaufmann M, Schmid H et al. Effect of intraperitoneal recombinant human tumour necrosis factor alpha on malignant ascites. *Eur. J. Cancer* 1991;27:121–125.

54   Canete JD, Pablos JL, Sanmarti R et al. Antiangiogenic effects of anti-tumor necrosis factor alpha therapy with infliximab in psoriatic arthritis. *Arthritis Rheum.* 2004;50:1636–1641.

55   Sakayama K, Kidani T, Miyazaki T et al. Effect of ketoprofen in topical formulation on vascular endothelial growth factor expression and tumor growth in nude mice with osteosarcoma. *J. Orthop. Res.* 2004;22:1168–1174.

56   Kojima-Yuasa A, Hua JJ, Kennedy DO, Matsui-Yuasa I. Green tea extract inhibits angiogenesis of human umbilical vein endothelial cells through reduction of expression of VEGF receptors. *Life Sci.* 2003;73:1299–1313.

57 Yoshiji H, Kuriyama S, Noguchi R, Fukui H. Angiotensin-I converting enzyme inhibitors as potential anti-angiogenic agents for cancer therapy. *Curr. Cancer Drug Targets.* 2004;4:555–567.

58 Ammouri L, Prommer EE. Palliative treatment of malignant ascites: Profile of catumaxomab. *Biologics.* 2010;4:103–110.

59 Heiss MM, Murawa P, Koralewski P, Kutarska E et al. The trifunctional antibody catumaxomab for the treatment of malignant ascites due to epithelial cancer: Results of a prospective randomized phase II/III trial. *Int. J. Cancer.* 2010;127:2209–2221.

60 Wimberger P, Gilet H, Gonschior A-K, Heiss MM et al. Deterioration in quality of life (QoL) in patients with malignant ascites: Results from a phase II/III study comparing paracentesis plus catumaxomab with paracentesis alone. *Ann. Oncol.* 2012;23:1979–1985.

61 Beattie GJ, Smyth JF. Phase I study of intraperitoneal metalloproteinase inhibitor BB94 in patients with malignant ascites. *Clin. Cancer Res.* 1998;4:1899–1902.

62 Cairns W, Malone R. Octreotide as an agent for the relief of malignant ascites in palliative care patients. *Palliat. Med.* 1999;13:429–430.

63 McCormick PA, Chin J, Greenslade L, Karatapanis S. Cardiovascular effects of octreotide in patients with hepatic cirrhosis. *Hepatology.* 1995;21:1255–1260.

◆ 64 Gough IR, Balderson GA. Malignant ascites. A comparison of peritoneovenous shunting and nonoperative management. *Cancer* 1993;71;2377–2382.

65 Greenway B, Johnson PJ, Williams R. Control of malignant ascites with spironolactone. *Br. J. Surg.* 1982;69:441–442.

66 Pockros PJ, Esrason KT, Nguyen C, Duque J, Woods S. Mobilization of malignant ascites with diuretics is dependent on ascitic fluid characteristics. *Gastroenterology* 1992;103:1302–1306.

67 Oberleithner H, Ludwig T, Riethmuller C et al. Human endothelium: Target for aldosterone. *Hypertension* 2004;43:952–956.

68 Twycross RG, Lack SA. *Ascites. Control of Alimentary Symptoms in Far Advanced Cancer.* Edinburgh, U.K.: Churchill Livingstone, 1986: pp. 282–299.

69 Amiel SA, Blackburn AM, Rubens RD. Intravenous infusion of frusemide as treatment for ascites in malignant disease. *Br. Med. J.* 1984;288:1041.

70 Bruera E, Chadwick S, Fox R, Hanson J, MacDonald N. Study of cardiovascular autonomic insufficiency in advanced cancer patients. *Cancer Treat. Rep.* 1986;70:1383–1387.

◆ 71 Keen A, FitzgeraldD, BryantA, DickinsonHO. Management of drainage for malignant ascites in gynaecological cancer. *Cochrane Database Syst. Rev.* 2010;1:CD007794.

∗ 72 Moorsom D. Paracentesis in a home care setting. *Palliat. Med.* 2001;15:169–170.

73 Gotleib WH, Feldman B, Feldman-Moran O et al. Intraperitoneal pressures and clinical parameters of total paracentesis for palliation of symptomatic ascites in ovarian cancer. *Gynecol. Oncol.* 1998;71:381–385.

74 McNamara P. Paracentesis—An effective method of symptom control in the palliative care setting? *Palliat. Med.* 2000;14:62–64.

◆ 75 National Institute for Health and Clinical Excellence. The PleurX peritoneal catheter drainage system for vacuum-assisted drainage of treatment-resistant, recurrent malignant ascites. NICE Medical Technology Guidance 9. 2012

76 Blackwell N, Burrows M. A sticky tip. *Palliat. Med.* 1994;8:256–257.

77 Ross GJ, Kessler HB, Clair MR, Gatenby RA, Hartz WH, Ross LV. Sonographically guided paracentesis for palliation of symptomatic malignant ascites. *AJR Am. J. Roentgenol.* 1989;153:1309–1311.

78 Belfort MA, Stevens PJ, DeHaek K, Soeters R, Krige JE. A new approach to the management of malignant ascites; a permanently implanted abdominal drain. *Eur. J. Surg. Oncol.* 1990;16:47–53

79 Richard HM, III, Coldwell DM, Boyd-Kranis RL, Murthy R, Van Echo DA. Pleurx tunnelled catheter in the management of malignant ascites. *J. Vasc. Interv. Radiol.* 2001;12:373–375.

80 Bui CDH, Martin CJ, Currow DC. Effective community palliation of intractable malignant ascites with a permanently implanted abdominal drain. *J. Palliat. Med.* 1999;2:319–321

81 Le Veen HH, Christoudias G, Moon IP, Luft R, Falk G, Grosberg S. Peritoneovenous shunting for ascites. *Ann. Surg.* 1974;180:580–590.

82 Lorentzen T, Sengelov L, Nolsoe CP, Khattar SC, Karstrup S, von der MH. Ultrasonically guided insertion of a peritoneo-gastric shunt in patients with malignant ascites. *Acta Radiol.* 1995;36:481–484.

83 Stehman FB, Ehrlich CE. Peritoneo-cystic shunt for malignant ascites. *Gynecol. Oncol.* 1984;18:402–407.

84 Clara R, Righi D, Bortolini M, Cornaglia S, Ruffino MA, Zanon C. Role of different techniques for the placement of Denver peritoneovenous shunt (PVS) in malignant ascites. *Surg. Laparosc. Endosc. Percutan. Tech.* 2004;14:222–225.

85 Edney JA, Hill A, Armstrong D. Peritoneovenous shunts palliate malignant ascites. *Am. J. Surg.* 1989;158:598–601.

86 Schumacher DL, Saclarides TJ, Staren ED. Peritoneovenous shunts for palliation of the patient with malignant ascites. *Ann. Surg. Oncol.* 1994;1:378–381.

87 Helzberg JH, Greenberger NJ. Peritoneovenous shunts in malignant ascites. *Dig. Dis. Sci.* 1985;30:1104–1107.

◆ 88 Adam RA, Adam YG. Malignant ascites: Past, present, and future. *J. Am. Coll. Surg.* 2004;198:999–1011.

◆ 89 Zanon C, Grosso M, Apra F et al. Palliative treatment of malignant refractory ascites by positioning of Denver peritoneovenous shunt. *Tumori* 2002;88:123–127.

90 Holm A, Halpern NB, Aldrete JS. Peritoneovenous shunt for intractable ascites of hepatic, nephrogenic, and malignant causes. *Am. J. Surg.* 1989;158:162–166.

91 Reinhold RB, Lokich JJ, Tomashefski J, Costello P. Management of malignant ascites with peritoneovenous shunting. *Am. J. Surg.* 1983;145:455–457.

◆ 92 White MA, Agle SC, Padia RK, Zervos EE. Denver peritoneovenous shunts for the management of malignant ascites: A review of the literature in the post LeVeen Era. *Am. Surg.* 2011;77:1070–1075.

93 Scott-Coombes DM, Whawell SA, Vipond MN, Crnojevic L, Thompson JN. Fibrinolytic activity of ascites caused by alcoholic cirrhosis and peritoneal malignancy. *Gut* 1993;34:1120–1122.

94 Tarin D, Price JE, Kettlewell MG, Souter RG, Vass AC, Crossley B. Mechanisms of human tumor metastasis studied in patients with peritoneovenous shunts. *Cancer Res.* 1984;44:3584–3592.

95 Schwartz ML, Swaim WR, Vogel SB. Coagulopathy following peritoneovenous shunting. *Surgery* 1979;85:671–676.

96 Markey W, Payne JA, Straus A. Hemorrhage from esophageal varices after placement of the LeVeen shunt. *Gastroenterology* 1979;77:341–343.

97 Qazi R, Savlov ED. Peritoneovenous shunt for palliation of malignant ascites. *Cancer* 1982;49:600–602.

98 Cheung DK, Raaf JH. Selection of patients with malignant ascites for a peritoneovenous shunt. *Cancer* 1982;50:1204–1209.

99 Bieligk SC, Calvo BF, Coit DG. Peritoneovenous shunting for nongynecologic malignant ascites. *Cancer* 2001;91:1247–1255.

61

Jaundice

NATHAN I. CHERNY, BATSHEVA WERMAN

In developed countries, jaundice in patients with terminal illness is most commonly encountered in advanced malignancy. In this setting, it is generally caused by obstruction of biliary drainage, extensive hepatocellular failure due to liver infiltration by metastases, or a combination of both. Indeed, cancer-related jaundice is one of the most common causes of severe jaundice; in a recent series from Sweden, it accounted for 58 of 173 sequential cases [1]. Less commonly in developed countries, but more commonly in developing countries, it may be due to end-stage chronic liver disease.

GENERALIZED HEPATIC DYSFUNCTION

Jaundice is a common feature of generalized hepatic dysfunction. Intrahepatic cholestasis involves either diffuse injury to small bile ducts or metabolic derangements in the bile secretory apparatus at the level of the hepatocyte and canaliculus. Intrahepatic cholestasis is typically not associated with ductal dilatation and is not amenable to mechanical interventions.

End-stage chronic liver disease or fulminant acute liver disease

Jaundice is a common feature in both of these scenarios. In chronic liver disease, there are often other associated clinical features including palmar erythema, spider nevi, gynecomastia, and signs of portal hypertension [2].

Cancer infiltration

Jaundice caused by extensive tumor infiltration of the liver by primary liver cancer or intrahepatic metastases is a sign of very extensive dysfunction, and it is usually accompanied by other features of liver failure. Gastrointestinal malignancies are especially prone to spread to the liver because of its portal venous drainage. Extra-abdominal tumors such as bronchogenic carcinoma, breast cancer, and malignant melanoma often spread hematogenously to the liver. Irrespective of the site of origin of the tumor, jaundice associated with extensive tumor infiltration of the liver is a sign of far-advanced disease and is an adverse prognostic factor associated with a relatively short anticipated survival [3–8].

Patients commonly display signs of incipient encephalopathy and ascites and have evidence of hypoalbuminemia and laboratory findings of coagulopathy. Ultrasonic or CT imaging of the liver usually demonstrates extensive involvement of the liver by metastases.

The role of antitumor therapies in this setting depends on the likelihood of anticipated response, the performance status of the patient, and the goals of care. Among patients with tumors that are sensitive to systemic therapies (chemotherapy, hormonal therapy, tyrosine kinase inhibitors, or immunotherapy), occasional patients will achieve a remission with adequate restoration of liver function to facilitate resolution of jaundice. In patients with unresponsive disease, liver failure ensues with progression until death. Administration of antitumor therapies in this situation requires great caution since many agents require dose modification in the setting of liver failure and some are contraindicated [9].

BILIARY OBSTRUCTION

Cancer-related cholestasis

Tumors may obstruct biliary flow within the liver parenchyma, at the porta hepatis or at any point along the common bile duct until the ampulla of Vater.

Proximal obstruction at the ductal confluence may be caused by cholangiocarcinoma, gallbladder carcinoma, intrabiliary metastases, or adenopathy in the porta hepatis secondary to a variety of metastases [10,11]. Rarely sarcoid reaction in hilar lymph nodes has been associated with obstructive jaundice in cases of cholangiocarcinoma [12].

Obstruction of the common bile duct is most commonly caused by cancer of the head of pancreas, ampullary carcinoma, or less commonly cholangiocarcinoma or gallbladder carcinoma [13–15]. Among patients with hepatocellular carcinoma, bile duct thrombosis is one of the main causes for obstructive jaundice, and the reported incidence is 1.2%–9% [16].

Thrombi can be benign (clots, pus, or sludge), malignant, or a combination of both. Rarely, rupture of hepatocellular carcinoma into the common bile duct may cause a fluctuating obstruction by floating tumor debris [17].

Extensive tumor metastases within the liver may produce intrahepatic cholestasis by obstructing smaller intrahepatic ducts. Diffuse infiltration of malignant cells along hepatic sinusoids with consequent cholestasis also may occur, especially in small cell carcinoma of the lung and in lymphoma.

Chronic cholestatic liver disease

Primary biliary cirrhosis and primary sclerosing cholangitis are both chronic progressive liver diseases with predominant cholestatic features.

AIDS cholangiopathy

AIDS may be associated with a number of biliary tract abnormalities [18]. Patients with advanced immunodeficiency may develop acalculous cholecystitis, focal distal biliary stenosis at the ampulla of Vater, or multifocal stenoses of the biliary tree that resembles primary biliary cirrhosis. AIDS cholangiopathy is strongly associated with colonization of bile with cryptosporidia, cytomegalovirus, or microsporidia. Patients typically describe right upper quadrant abdominal pain and diarrhea and often have abnormal liver test results, particularly elevated alkaline phosphatase. The diagnosis may be suggested when an ultrasound (U.S.) examination of the gallbladder reveals edema of the wall; endoscopic retrograde cholangiopancreatography (ERCP) demonstrates strictures and delayed emptying and may permit direct sampling of bile for pathogens. These syndromes are late complications of AIDS that, although rarely fatal of itself, indicate a poor prognosis.

Chronic graft–versus–host disease

After bone marrow transplantation, chronic graft-versus-host disease may be associated with an intrahepatic cholestasis syndrome [19]. Liver involvement is characterized by mononuclear infiltration of portal tracts with obliteration of small bile ductules, similar to that seen in primary billiary cirrhosis (PBC). Intensive immunosuppression may control the graft-versus-host reaction, and if this fails, ursodeoxycholic acid may improve cholestasis; however, the cholestasis often progresses to biliary cirrhosis.

CLINICAL PRESENTATION

Patients with advanced jaundice experience generalized malaise, weakness, easy fatigability, nausea, anorexia, and pruritus. Itch is common but it does not occur in all cases.

Introduction of bacteria into bile above an obstructing lesion can cause ascending cholangitis, a purulent infection of the biliary tree and liver. Contributing factors include high biliary pressure and stasis. In the absence of infection, however, cholestasis

may be well tolerated for very long periods of time. Common presenting features of cholangitis include fever, right upper quadrant pain, confusion, or hypotension. Chronic biliary obstruction, regardless of cause, eventually leads to cirrhosis with all its complications. The mechanism by which an increased bile secretory pressure leads to cirrhosis has not as yet been established, but it can occur with either extrahepatic or intrahepatic obstruction.

INVESTIGATION

Clinical evaluation often yields substantial information in the assessment of the cancer patient who presents with jaundice. It is important to ascertain the tumor type and history to date, if known. The presence of pale stools is strongly suggestive of cholestasis. The abdomen is examined for evidence of hepatomegaly, ascites, and features of portal hypertension. Patients should undergo a brief mental status examination and neurological examination for evidence of asterixis and features of Parkinson's like psychomotor retardation [20].

DIAGNOSTIC EVALUATION

Blood tests

The diagnosis of jaundice is confirmed by the finding of hyperbilirubinemia. Serum bilirubin concentration in normal adults is less than 1–1.5 mg/dL and varies directly with bilirubin production and inversely with hepatic bilirubin clearance. A serum bilirubin value of 3 mg/dL is usually required for jaundice or scleral icterus to be clinically evident.

Other initial studies should include a complete blood cell count as well as liver function tests including activities of alkaline phosphatase (ALP) and alanine and aspartate aminotransferases (ALT and AST), albumin, and prothrombin time. Both gamma-glutamyl transpeptidase (GGT) and ALP are typically elevated in patients with cholestasis; the combination of an elevated ALP and normal GGT suggests that the ALP elevation is due to release of ALP from bone. Conversely, an isolated elevation of GGT may result from certain drugs (e.g., phenytoin) or alcohol even in the absence of liver disease.

Imaging studies

Imaging studies help identify the presence or absence of intrahepatic metastases, the presence of intrahepatic or extrahepatic cholestasis, and the site of obstruction if present.

Ultrasound

Transabdominal U.S. is a noninvasive test that can identify the presence or absence of metastases and determine whether the intrahepatic and/or extrahepatic biliary system is dilated. The sensitivity of abdominal ultrasonography for the detection of biliary obstruction in jaundiced patients ranges from 55% to 91%, and the specificity ranges from 82% to 95% [21,22]. Given the sensitivity limitations of this approach, a negative U.S. should not preclude further imaging when there is a compelling clinical suspicion of obstruction.

Computerized tomography

Computerized tomography (CT) may be preferred when precise definition of anatomic structure and information about the level of obstruction are desired [22]. It provides a more comprehensive analysis of the liver and extrahepatic abdomen and pelvis than U.S. Both CT and U.S. may occasionally fail to identify dilated ducts in obstructed patients with cirrhosis and poorly compliant hepatic parenchyma or in patients with primary sclerosing cholangitis. Conversely, the presence of dilated ducts in a patient who has previously undergone cholecystectomy does not necessarily signify obstruction.

Endoscopic retrograde cholangiopancreatography

ERCP is highly accurate in the diagnosis of biliary obstruction, with a sensitivity of 89%–98% and specificity of 89%–100% [21,22]. If dilated ducts are identified, it is generally appropriate to visualize the biliary tree directly by ERCP. ERCP involves passing an endoscope into the duodenum, introducing a catheter into the ampulla of Vater, and injecting contrast medium into the distal common bile duct and or pancreatic duct. Choledochoscopy and bile duct brushing cytology are potentially useful techniques to distinguish between obstructions due to intraluminal mass, infiltrating ductal lesions, or extrinsic mass compression. Furthermore, if a focal cause for biliary obstruction is identified (e.g., choledocholithiasis, biliary stricture), therapeutic maneuvers to relieve obstruction (e.g., sphincterotomy, stone extraction, dilation, stent placement) can be performed during the procedure. ERCP is not a benign procedure and significant adverse events occur in 0.5%–2% of patients. Risks include respiratory depression, aspiration, bleeding, perforation, cholangitis, and pancreatitis.

Percutaneous transhepatic cholangiography

Percutaneous transhepatic cholangiography (PTC) involves percutaneous passage of a needle through the hepatic parenchyma and injection of contrast medium into the proximal biliary tree through a peripheral bile duct. PTC is often preferred when the level of biliary obstruction is proximal to the common hepatic duct or in which altered anatomy precludes ERCP. When, however, bile ducts are not dilated, this approach may be technically difficult and it may be unsuccessful in up to 25% of attempts. As with ERCP, interventional procedures, such as balloon dilation and stent placement, can be performed at the time of PTC.

Magnetic resonance cholangiopancreatography

Magnetic resonance cholangiopancreatography (MRCP) is a technical refinement of standard magnetic resonance imaging

that permits rapid clear-cut delineation of the biliary tree without the requirement of intravenous contrast agents. This approach is superior to ERCP in interpreting the cause and depicting the anatomical extent of the perihilar obstructive jaundice and is particularly distinctive in cases associated with tight biliary stenosis and along segmental biliary stricture [23–25]. It is particularly useful when patients are at high risk for complications from ERCP or PTC. In patients with hilar tumors and bilateral biliary tree obstruction, MRCP can determine the dominant ductal drainage for the liver segments for subsequent stent placement [26]. Limitations of this approach include image artifacts (caused by fluid within the adjacent duodenum, duodenal diverticula, and ascites).

Endoscopic ultrasonography

Endoscopic U.S. is a valuable imaging test for diagnosing and staging pancreatic cancer. In skilled hands, it is more accurate than spiral CT scanning [27,28] or MRCP [29]. This approach is particularly useful when no visible mass is observed on routine imaging studies. In this setting, it has both high positive and negative predictive values [27]. Endoscopic ultrasonography (EUS) is particularly useful in the diagnosis of cancer of papilla of Vater [28].

MANAGEMENT OF BILIARY OBSTRUCTION

Symptomatic management

Biliary obstruction that is asymptomatic in a patient who has a short life expectancy does not require intervention. In many cases, however, jaundice is associated with symptoms of itch, anorexia, and fatigue. Indeed, studies that have evaluated the quality of life of patients before and after relief of biliary obstruction highlight improvements in itch, anorexia, fatigue, and global well-being [30,31].

Surgical management

Historically, the approach to obstructive jaundice has been biliary bypass surgery. However, randomized trials and a meta-analysis [32] have demonstrated that endoscopically placed stents are as successful as surgical bypass but with lower morbidity and procedure-related mortality rates and that most can be successfully managed using stents or percutaneous drains.

Endoscopic biliary stent

Endoscopic placement of biliary endoprostheses can provide effective drainage without the burden and stigma of an external drain [33]. It is successful in more than 90% of attempts; it is associated with procedure-related mortality of about 1%. Transient complication of cholangitis, fever, or hemorrhage is common and occurs in about 20% of patient attempts [34]. Median survival for stented patients was 4.9 months [34].

Combined percutaneous-endoscopic procedures have been described for patients in whom endoscopic insertion is unsuccessful [35–37]. In this approach, a guidewire and fine-bore catheter is introduced percutaneously, and the biliary tree is decompressed. The guidewire is advanced through the obstruction and into the duodenum. An endoscopist then introduces a stent over the guidewire. Once adequate internal drainage has been achieved, the percutaneously placed guidewire and catheter may be withdrawn.

Stent blockage is a major problem with Teflon catheters. Obstruction has been attributed to adherence of bacteria to the wall of the stent, resulting in the production of a biofilm that traps debris and ultimately occludes the lumen [38]. Occlusion of Teflon or plastic endoprostheses generally is managed with repeat endoscopy and stent replacement. Exchange of endoprostheses may be done as long as duodenal intubation with an adequate endoscope remains possible, but does require a second endoscopy. Early prophylactic stent exchange at 3–6 months has been advocated, but an optimal time has not been defined. In patients whose stents have occluded but who are not candidates for endoscopic replacement, percutaneous stenting may be palliative.

Self-expanding metal prostheses were introduced to overcome the problem of occlusion. The most commonly used device, the Wallstent®, consists of a stainless steel mesh that is mounted on a 9 Fr delivery catheter. Metal stents have a larger diameter (8–10 mm), most are not removable, and they are much more expensive than plastic. They are introduced into the bile duct enclosed in a sheath that is then retracted enabling the stent to expand against the wall of the bile duct. However, metal stents also are permanent and much more expensive than plastic. Meta-analysis of 7 prospective trials in which patients with biliary obstruction were randomized to stenting with either polyethylene or metal stents found that placement is seen in at least 95% of patients and is independent of stent material. There is no impact of type of stent on survival, but the duration of patency is greater for metal stents, resulting in fewer episodes of cholangitis and fewer total days in the hospital [39].

Covered metal stents have lower rates of tumor ingrowth and a potential advantage of removability [40]. These advantages must be balanced against higher rates of stent migration due to the limited ability of the stents to embed surrounding tissues because of the overlying covering.

Percutaneous transhepatic cholangiographic drainage

Percutaneous drainage can be achieved with an internal–external catheter that can drain externally or, if the obstruction can be passed, internally [41–43]. Even when biliary obstructions are complete, in many instances, an interventional radiologist can negotiate through a stricture with a combination of guidewires and catheters under fluoroscopic guidance. Transhepatic catheters are designed with side holes both above and below the level of obstruction in the biliary tree; the tip of the catheter resides within the bowel, so that bile drains through the catheter across the obstruction and out of the side holes into the duodenum.

Transhepatic catheters are associated with complications of obstruction, leakage, and infection [44]. Usually, transhepatic biliary catheters are routinely changed every 2 months to avoid any chance of obstruction.

The percutaneous approach to biliary cannulation (PTC) can also be used to inset expandable metallic stents. Experience comparing direct stent insertion with an approach of delayed stenting after initial drainage and dilatation demonstrated substantially less morbidity with the more direct approach [45]. In a series of 224 patients, there were no procedure-related deaths, and the clinical success rate within the first 30 days was 88% [46].

Endoscopic ultrasound–guided biliary drainage

Traditionally, patients who had failed ERCP have been offered PTC or surgical biliary decompression, both of which are associated with higher morbidity. Endoscopic-U.S.-guided biliary drainage has been developed as a less invasive alternative for biliary drainage [47]. In a single-step procedure, it aims to establish biliary drainage using transgastric puncture of the intrahepatic duct or the common bile duct. This approach is feasible in patients with inaccessible papillae due to duodenal obstruction, surgically altered anatomy or hilar block due to cholangiocarcinoma or gallbladder cancer. This approach may also be safer than PTC since the bile duct is accessed using Doppler to avoid blood vessels in the needle path [47]. The most common complications are biliary leakage and pneumoperitoneum that is usually self-limited. Biliary leakage may occur predominantly with extrahepatic duct puncture, transluminal drainage, and larger hole. The procedure is technically complex, and it is only performed by specialist endoscopists who are skilled at both ERCP and EUS. It requires surgical backup and is not yet widely available.

Special case: Obstruction at the bifurcation of the hepatic ducts

Patients with biliary obstruction at the bifurcation of the hepatic ducts present a difficult challenge, and there is much controversy as to the importance of establishing drainage of both liver lobes in malignant hilar obstruction. MRCP can be used to determine the dominant ductal drainage for the liver segments thus directing stent placement. In a series of 35 patients who underwent MRCP, with subsequent unilateral stent deployment at ERCP, jaundice resolved in 86% [26].

SYMPTOMATIC MANAGEMENT OF CHOLESTATIC PRURITUS

Pruritus is the major symptom of obstructive jaundice [48,49]. Pruritus may occur with any type of liver disease but is primarily associated with acute or chronic cholestasis. It has been estimated to occur in 20%–50% of jaundiced patients. The intensity of the pruritus varies from mild to severe. It can be persistent or intermittent, and it may be generalized or localized to specific parts of the body, commonly the soles of the feet and palms of the hands.

The pathogenesis of cholestatic pruritus is complex and multifactorial [50]. Indirect evidence suggests that it may be caused at least in part by dermal itch receptor stimulation by a bile acid, a bile acid derivative, or some other substance that undergoes enterohepatic circulation. Recent studies have implicated lysophosphatidic acid (LPA). Not all jaundiced patients suffer from pruritus, but those with pruritus have highly elevated levels of serum autotaxin (ATX), the enzyme that converts lysophosphatidylcholine into LPA [51,52]. A central mechanism, associated with altered neurotransmission in the brain, has also been imputed based on observations that opioid and serotonin antagonists reduce scratching activity in cholestatic patients.

The management of pruritus in this setting is often difficult, and it should involve specific antipruritic therapies along with general supportive measures.

Anion exchange resins

Anion exchange resins, which are given by mouth, bind bile acids and other anionic compounds in the intestine, resulting in increased fecal excretion of bound substances. Thus, they decrease the enterohepatic circulation of bile acids. The most widely administered treatment for the pruritus of cholestasis has been the basic anion exchange resin cholestyramine, but other resins, colestipol and colesevelam, are also available [50]. The maximum recommended dose of cholestyramine is 16 g/24 hour. The resins should be taken at least 2 hours apart from other medications so as not to interfere in their absorption. Cholestyramine is not very palatable, and it should be diluted in water or juice. The most common side effects of resin treatment are bloating and constipation. It is prudent to monitor the prothrombin time during prolonged administration of these agents, because treatment may result in malabsorption of fat-soluble vitamins. The American Association for the Study of Liver Diseases (AASLD) recommends this as an initial approach for cholestatic itch in the setting of primary biliary cirrhosis [53].

Rifampicin

Rifampicin (like phenobarbital, discussed later) is a pregnane X receptor agonist that strongly induces hepatic microsomal oxidizing enzymes and biotransformation transporters (i.e., CYP3A4, UGT1A1, and MRP2) that may promote the metabolism and/or the secretion of the potential endogenous pruritogens. Additionally, it competes with bile acid uptake by hepatocytes and modifies secondary bile acid synthesis in the gut lumen (through its antimicrobial effects). Substantial effectiveness in the relief of cholestatic itch is supported by multiple small trials and 2 meta-analyses [54,55]. When effective, the

onset of effect is relatively rapid. The usual dose is 300–600 mg/day in divided oral doses [54,55]. The long-term administration of rifampicin for pruritus is associated with occasional hepatotoxicity, and patients require regular monitoring of serum ALT levels [56].

Opioid antagonists

The observation that intravenous naloxone can reduce cholestatic pruritus [57,58] prompted trials of therapy with orally administered antagonists nalmefene and naltrexone. In an open-label study of nalmefene, it was associated with a significant subjective amelioration of pruritus, as measured by a visual analogue scale of pruritus and a significant decrease in scratching activity. Most patients required up to 30–80 mg/day but with substantial variability [59]. Naltrexone at doses of 50 mg/day has been studied in 2 placebo-controlled studies of cholestatic prurits without apparent toxicity and with subjective relief [60,61]; these findings are supported by several case reports [62–65]. In a small study, some patients achieved relief with buprenorphine [66].

Medications with limited evidence of benefit

Despite common application in this setting, antihistamines are rarely effective in this setting [50]. Phenobarbital may relieve pruritus in individual patients, but its utility has not been supported in controlled trials [67]. The barbiturate phenobarbital has sedative effects as well as effects on the liver. This drug nonspecifically increases the activity of the hepatic microsomal enzyme system by enzyme induction, and it is hypothesized that it may act by enhancing the excretion of pruritogens. A recent systematic review concluded that the 5-HT3 antagonist ondansetron had negligible effect on cholestatic or uremic pruritus on the basis of a limited number of studies [68]. Finally, propofol, at subhypnotic doses of 15 mg, was reported to ameliorate the cholestatic pruritus in a small placebo-controlled trial [69,70].

Other measures

In addition to these specific therapies, simple measures have been recommended. Such measures include the use of emollients and mild fragrance-free soaps (e.g., fragrance-free Dove, Basis, Aveeno), less frequent bathing, wearing light clothing, and frequent cutting of fingernails.

REFERENCES

1   Bjornsson E, Ismael S, Nejdet S, Kilander A. Severe jaundice in Sweden in the new millennium: Causes, investigations, treatment and prognosis. *Scand J Gastroenterol.* 2003;38(1):86–94.

2   Heidelbaugh JJ, Bruderly M. Cirrhosis and chronic liver failure: Part I. Diagnosis and evaluation. *Am Fam Physician.* 2006;74(5):756–762.

3   Fischerman K, Petersen CF, Jensen SL, Christensen KC, Efsen F. Survival among patients with liver metastases from cancer of the colon and rectum. *Scand J Gastroenterol Suppl.* 1976;37:111–115.

4   Bengmark S, Domellof L, Hafstrom L. The natural history of primary and secondary malignant tumours of the liver. 3. The prognosis for patients with hepatic metastases from pancreatic carcinoma verified by laparotomy. *Digestion.* 1970;3(1):56–61.

5   O'Reilly SM, Richards MA, Rubens RD. Liver metastases from breast cancer: The relationship between clinical, biochemical and pathological features and survival. *Eur J Cancer.* 1990;26(5):574–577.

6   Hoe AL, Royle GT, Taylor I. Breast liver metastases—Incidence, diagnosis and outcome [see comments]. *J R Soc Med.* 1991;84(12):714–716.

7   Hogan BA, Thornton FJ, Brannigan M, Browne TJ, Pender S, O'Kelly P et al. Hepatic metastases from an unknown primary neoplasm (UPN): Survival, prognostic indicators and value of extensive investigations. *Clin Radiol.* 2002;57(12):1073–1077.

8   Polee MB, Hop WC, Kok TC, Eskens FA, van der Burg ME, Splinter TA et al. Prognostic factors for survival in patients with advanced oesophageal cancer treated with cisplatin-based combination chemotherapy. *Br J Cancer.* 2003;89(11):2045–2050.

9   Superfin D, Iannucci AA, Davies AM. Commentary: Oncologic drugs in patients with organ dysfunction: A summary. *Oncologist.* 2007;12(9):1070–1083.

10 Koea J, Holden A, Chau K, McCall J. Differential diagnosis of stenosing lesions at the hepatic hilum. *World J Surg.* 2004;28(5):466–470.

11 Takamatsu S, Teramoto K, Kawamura T, Kudo A, Noguchi N, Irie T et al. Liver metastasis from rectal cancer with prominent intrabile duct growth. *Pathol Int.* 2004;54(6):440–445.

12 Onitsuka A, Katagiri Y, Kiyama S, Mimoto H, Nakamura T, Toda K et al. Hilar cholangiocarcinoma associated with sarcoid reaction in the regional lymph nodes. *J Hepatobiliary Pancreat Surg.* 2003;10(4):316–320.

13 Holzinger F, Schilling M, Z'Graggen K, Stain S, Baer HU. Carcinoma of the cystic duct leading to obstructive jaundice. A case report and review of the literature [see comments]. *Dig Surg.* 1998;15(3):273–278.

14 Hu J, Pi Z, Yu MY, Li Y, Xiong S. Obstructive jaundice caused by tumor emboli from hepatocellular carcinoma. *Am Surg.* 1999;65(5):406–410.

15 NIH state-of-the-science statement on endoscopic retrograde cholangiopancreatography (ERCP) for diagnosis and therapy. *NIH Consens State Sci Statements.* 2002;19(1):1–26.

16 Qin LX, Tang ZY. Hepatocellular carcinoma with obstructive jaundice: Diagnosis, treatment and prognosis. *World J Gastroenterol.* 2003;9(3):385–391.

17 Chen MF, Jan YY, Jeng LB, Hwang TL, Wang CS, Chen SC. Obstructive jaundice secondary to ruptured hepatocellular carcinoma into the common bile duct. Surgical experiences of 20 cases. *Cancer.* 1994;73(5):1335–1340.

18 Yusuf TE, Baron TH. AIDS cholangiopathy. *Curr Treat Options Gastroenterol.* 2004;7(2):111–117.

19 Arai S, Lee LA, Vogelsang GB. A systematic approach to hepatic complications in hematopoietic stem cell transplantation. *J Hematother Stem Cell Res.* 2002;11(2):215–229.

20 Lewis M, Howdle PD. The neurology of liver failure. *QJM.* 2003;96(9):623–633.

21 Pasanen PA, Partanen KP, Pikkarainen PH, Alhava EM, Janatuinen EK, Pirinen AE. A comparison of ultrasound, computed tomography and endoscopic retrograde cholangiopancreatography in the differential diagnosis of benign and malignant jaundice and cholestasis. *Eur J Surg.* 1993;159(1):23–29.

22 Saini S. Imaging of the hepatobiliary tract. *N Engl J Med.* 1997;336(26):1889–1894.

23 Kaltenthaler E, Vergel YB, Chilcott J, Thomas S, Blakeborough T, Walters SJ et al. A systematic review and economic evaluation of magnetic resonance cholangiopancreatography compared with diagnostic endoscopic retrograde cholangiopancreatography. *Health Technol Assess.* 2004;8(10):iii, 1–89.

24 Romagnuolo J, Bardou M, Rahme E, Joseph L, Reinhold C, Barkun AN. Magnetic resonance cholangiopancreatography: A meta-analysis of test performance in suspected biliary disease. *Ann Intern Med.* 2003;139(7):547–557.

25 Liang C, Mao H, Wang Q, Han D, Li Yuxia L, Yue J et al. Diagnostic performance of magnetic resonance cholangiopancreatography in malignant obstructive jaundice. *Cell Biochem Biophys.* 2011;61(2):383–388.

26 Hintze RE, Abou-Rebyeh H, Adler A, Veltzke-Schlieker W, Felix R, Wiedenmann B. Magnetic resonance cholangiopancreatography-guided unilateral endoscopic stent placement for Klatskin tumors. *Gastrointest Endosc.* 2001;53(1):40–46.

27 Agarwal B, Abu-Hamda E, Molke KL, Correa AM, Ho L. Endoscopic ultrasound-guided fine needle aspiration and multidetector spiral CT in the diagnosis of pancreatic cancer. *Am J Gastroenterol.* 2004;99(5):844–850.

28 Maluf-Filho F, Sakai P, Cunha JE, Garrido T, Rocha M, Machado MC et al. Radial endoscopic ultrasound and spiral computed tomography in the diagnosis and staging of periampullary tumors. *Pancreatology.* 2004;4(2):122–128.

29 Ainsworth AP, Rafaelsen SR, Wamberg PA, Durup J, Pless TK, Mortensen MB. Is there a difference in diagnostic accuracy and clinical impact between endoscopic ultrasonography and magnetic resonance cholangiopancreatography? *Endoscopy.* 2003;35(12):1029–1032.

30 Luman W, Cull A, Palmer KR. Quality of life in patients stented for malignant biliary obstructions. *Eur J Gastroenterol Hepatol.* 1997;9(5):481–484.

31 Abraham NS, Barkun JS, Barkun AN. Palliation of malignant biliary obstruction: A prospective trial examining impact on quality of life. *Gastrointest Endosc.* 2002;56(6):835–841.

32 Moss AC, Morris E, Leyden J, MacMathuna P. Malignant distal biliary obstruction: A systematic review and meta-analysis of endoscopic and surgical bypass results. *Cancer Treat Rev.* 2007;33(2):213–221.

33 Cipolletta L, Rotondano G, Marmo R, Bianco MA. Endoscopic palliation of malignant obstructive jaundice: An evidence-based review. *Dig Liver Dis.* 2007;39(4):375–388.

34 Naggar E, Krag E, Matzen P. Endoscopically inserted biliary endoprosthesis in malignant obstructive jaundice. A survey of the literature. *Liver.* 1990;10(6):321–324 [the above reports in MacintoshPCUNIX TextHTML format].

35 Hall RI, Denyer ME, Chapman AH. Percutaneous-endoscopic placement of endoprostheses for relief of jaundice caused by inoperable bile duct strictures. *Surgery.* 1990;107(2):224–227.

36 Tsang TK, Crampton AR, Bernstein JR, Ramos SR, Wieland JM. Percutaneous-endoscopic biliary stent placement. A preliminary report. *Ann Intern Med.* 1987;106(3):389–392.

37 Wayman J, Mansfield JC, Matthewson K, Richardson DL, Griffin SM. Combined percutaneous and endoscopic procedures for bile duct obstruction: Simultaneous and delayed techniques compared. *Hepatogastroenterology.* 2003;50(52):915–918.

38 Huibregtse K, Carr-Locke DL, Cremer M, Domschke W, Fockens P, Foerster E et al. Biliary stent occlusion—A problem solved with self-expanding metal stents? European Wallstent Study Group. *Endoscopy.* 1992;24(5):391–394.

39 Moss AC, Morris E, Leyden J, MacMathuna P. Do the benefits of metal stents justify the costs? A systematic review and meta-analysis of trials comparing endoscopic stents for malignant biliary obstruction. *Eur J Gastroenterol Hepatol.* 2007;19(12):1119–1124.

40 Saleem A, Leggett CL, Murad MH, Baron TH. Meta-analysis of randomized trials comparing the patency of covered and uncovered self-expandable metal stents for palliation of distal malignant bile duct obstruction. *Gastrointest Endosc.* 2011;74(2):321–327.e1–e3.

41 Born P, Rosch T, Triptrap A, Frimberger E, Allescher HD, Ott R et al. Long-term results of percutaneous transhepatic biliary drainage for benign and malignant bile duct strictures. *Scand J Gastroenterol.* 1998;33(5):544–549.

42 Tipaldi L. A simplified percutaneous hepatogastric drainage technique for malignant biliary obstruction. *Cardiovasc Intervent Radiol.* 1995;18(5):333–336.

43 Gunther RW, Schild H, Thelen M. Percutaneous transhepatic biliary drainage: Experience with 311 procedures. *Cardiovasc Intervent Radiol.* 1988;11(2):65–71.

44 Nomura T, Shirai Y, Hatakeyama K. Bacteribilia and cholangitis after percutaneous transhepatic biliary drainage for malignant biliary obstruction. *Dig Dis Sci.* 1999;44(3):542–546.

45 Inal M, Aksungur E, Akgul E, Oguz M, Seydaoglu G. Percutaneous placement of metallic stents in malignant biliary obstruction: One-stage or two-stage procedure? Pre-dilate or not? *Cardiovasc Intervent Radiol.* 2003;26(1):40–45.

46 Inal M, Akgul E, Aksungur E, Demiryurek H, Yagmur O. Percutaneous self-expandable uncovered metallic stents in malignant biliary obstruction. Complications, follow-up and reintervention in 154 patients. *Acta Radiol.* 2003;44(2):139–146.

47 Chavalitdhamrong D, Draganov PV. Endoscopic ultrasound-guided biliary drainage. *World J Gastroenterol.* 2012;18(6):491–497.

48 Mela M, Mancuso A, Burroughs AK. Review article: Pruritus in cholestatic and other liver diseases. *Aliment Pharmacol Ther.* 2003;17(7):857–870.

49 Bosonnet L. Pruritus: Scratching the surface. *Eur J Cancer Care (Engl).* 2003;12(2):162–165.

50 Bergasa NV. Pruritus in chronic liver disease: Mechanisms and treatment. *Curr Gastroenterol Rep.* 2004;6(1):10–16.

51 Elferink RPJO, Kremer AE, Beuers U. Mediators of pruritus during cholestasis. *Curr Opin Gastroenterol.* 2011;27(3):289–293.

52 Elferink RPJO, Kremer AE, Martens JJWW, Beuers UH. The molecular mechanism of cholestatic pruritus. *Dig Dis.* 2011;29(1):66–71.

53 Lindor KD, Gershwin ME, Poupon R, Kaplan M, Bergasa NV, Heathcote EJ. Primary biliary cirrhosis. *Hepatology.* 2009;50(1):291–308.

54 Tandon P, Rowe BH, Vandermeer B, Bain VG. The efficacy and safety of bile Acid binding agents, opioid antagonists, or rifampin in the treatment of cholestasis-associated pruritus. *Am J Gastroenterol.* 2007;102(7):1528–1536.

55 Khurana S, Singh P. Rifampin is safe for treatment of pruritus due to chronic cholestasis: A meta-analysis of prospective randomized-controlled trials. *Liver Int.* 2006;26(8):943–948.

56 Talwalkar JA, Souto E, Jorgensen RA, Lindor KD. Natural history of pruritus in primary biliary cirrhosis. *Clin Gastroenterol Hepatol.* 2003;1(4):297–302.

57 Terra SG, Tsunoda SM. Opioid antagonists in the treatment of pruritus from cholestatic liver disease. *Ann Pharmacother.* 1998;32(11):1228–1230.

58 Bergasa NV, Talbot TL, Alling DW, Schmitt JM, Walker EC, Baker BL et al. A controlled trial of naloxone infusions for the pruritus of chronic cholestasis. *Gastroenterology.* 1992;102(2):544–549.

59 Bergasa NV, Schmitt JM, Talbot TL, Alling DW, Swain MG, Turner ML et al. Open-label trial of oral nalmefene therapy for the pruritus of cholestasis. *Hepatology.* 1998;27(3):679–684.

60 Wolfhagen FH, Sternieri E, Hop WC, Vitale G, Bertolotti M, Van Buuren HR. Oral naltrexone treatment for cholestatic pruritus: A double-blind, placebo-controlled study. *Gastroenterology.* 1997;113(4):1264–1269.

61 Mansour-Ghanaei F, Taheri A, Froutan H, Ghofrani H, Nasiri-Toosi M, Bagherzadeh AH et al. Effect of oral naltrexone on pruritus in cholestatic patients. *World J Gastroenterol.* 2006;12(7):1125–1128.

62 Zellos A, Roy A, Schwarz KB. Use of oral naltrexone for severe pruritus due to cholestatic liver disease in children. *J Pediatr Gastroenterol Nutr.* 2010;51(6):787–789.

63 Malekzad F, Arbabi M, Mohtasham N, Toosi P, Jaberian M, Mohajer M et al. Efficacy of oral naltrexone on pruritus in atopic eczema: A double-blind, placebo-controlled study. *J Eur Acad Dermatol Venereol.* 2009;23(8):948–950.

64 LaSalle L, Rachelska G, Nedelec B. Naltrexone for the management of post-burn pruritus: A preliminary report. *Burns.* 2008;34(6):797–802.

65 Chang Y, Golkar L. The use of naltrexone in the management of severe generalized pruritus in biliary atresia: Report of a case. *Pediatr Dermatol.* 2008;25(3):403–404.

66 Juby LD, Wong VS, Losowsky MS. Buprenorphine and hepatic pruritus. *Br J Clin Pract.* 1994;48(6):331.

67 Laatikainen T. Effect of cholestyramine and phenobarbital on pruritus and serum bile acid levels in cholestasis of pregnancy. *Am J Obstet Gynecol.* 1978;132(5):501–506.

68 To TH, Clark K, Lam L, Shelby-James T, Currow DC. The role of ondansetron in the management of cholestatic or uremic pruritus—A systematic review. *J Pain Symptom Manage.* 2012;44(5):725–730.

69 Borgeat A, Wilder-Smith OH, Mentha G. Subhypnotic doses of propofol relieve pruritus associated with liver disease. *Gastroenterology.* 1993;104(1):244–247.

70 Borgeat A, Wilder-Smith O, Mentha G, Huber O. Propofol and cholestatic pruritus. *Am J Gastroenterol.* 1992;87(5):672–674.

62

Malignant bowel obstruction

CARLA IDA RIPAMONTI, ALEXANDRA M. EASSON, HANS GERDES

DEFINITION AND EPIDEMIOLOGY

Bowel obstruction is defined as any process preventing the movement of bowel contents. MBO was defined using the following criteria: clinical evidence of bowel obstruction (history/physical/radiological examination) and bowel obstruction beyond the ligament of Treitz, in the setting of a diagnosis of intra-abdominal cancer with incurable disease *or* a diagnosis of non-intra-abdominal primary cancer with clear intraperitoneal disease [1,2].

Bowel obstruction may be a mode of presentation of intra-abdominal and pelvic malignancy or a feature of recurrent disease following anticancer therapy. MBO is well recognized in gynecologic patients with advanced cancer. Retrospective and autopsy studies found the frequency at approximately 5.5%–51% of patients with gynecological malignancy [3–8]. MBO is particularly frequent in patients with ovarian cancer where it is the most frequent cause of death [5,6,8]. Patients with stage III and IV ovarian cancer and those with high-grade lesions are at higher risk for MBO as compared to patients with lower-stage or low-grade tumors [9,10].

The reported frequency of bowel obstruction ranges from 10% to 28% in colorectal cancer [2,11].

Bowel obstruction can be partial or complete, single or multiple. Benign causes are reported in nearly half the patients with colorectal cancer and in approximately 6% of patients with gynecological cancer [2,11]. The small bowel is more commonly involved than the large bowel (61% vs. 33%) and both are involved in over 20% of the patients [3–7].

Several pathophysiological mechanisms may be involved in the onset of bowel obstruction, and there is variability in both presentation and etiology (Table 62.1). Any mechanism limiting or preventing the propulsion of the intestinal content from passing distally induces a cascade of events producing definitive bowel obstruction (Figure 62.1).

At least three factors occur in bowel obstruction: (1) accumulation of gastric, pancreatic, and biliary secretions that are a potent stimulus for further intestinal secretions; (2) decreased absorption of water and sodium from the intestinal lumen; and (3) increased secretion of water and sodium into the lumen as distension increases [12,13] (Figure 62.1). As a result of the breakdown of the sequence and reabsorption in the gastrointestinal (GI) tract, there is a loss of fluids and electrolytes. The pancreatic, biliary, and GI secretions accumulate in the bowel above the obstruction, and the volume of secretions tends to increase following intestinal distension and the consequent increase in the surface area, thus producing a vicious circle of secretion–distension–secretion [12,13]. Depletion of water and salt in the lumen is considered the most important "toxic factor" in bowel obstruction.

Signs and symptoms: Assessment and differential diagnosis

In cancer patients, compression of the bowel lumen develops slowly and often remains partial. The initial symptoms are frequently abdominal cramps, nausea, vomiting, and abdominal distension that usually present periodically and resolve spontaneously. These episodes are frequently followed by passage of gas or loose stools. GI symptoms caused by the sequence of distension–secretion–motor activity of the obstructed bowel (Figure 62.1) occur in different combinations and intensity depending on the site of obstruction and tend to worsen (Table 62.2). Vomiting can be assessed in terms of numbers, volume, and overall duration. Other symptoms such as nausea, pain (both colicky and/or continuous), xerostomia, somnolence, dyspnea, and even sensation of hunger can be present and can be evaluated with visual analog, numerical, or verbal scales. The assessment of patients with suspected MBO should consider (1) other causes of nausea, vomiting, and constipation; (2) metabolic abnormalities; (3) type and dosages of drugs; (4) nutritional and hydration status; (5) bowel movements and the presence of overflow diarrhea; (6) presence of abdominal fecal masses, distension

Table 62.1 *Pathophysiological mechanisms of MBO*

Mechanical obstruction is caused by
1. Extrinsic occlusion of the lumen due to an enlargement of the primary tumor or recurrence, mesenteric and omental masses, abdominal or pelvic adhesions (caused by either the tumor or secondary to surgery), postirradiation fibrosis
2. Intraluminal occlusion of the lumen due to neoplastic mass or annular tumoral dissemination
3. Intramural occlusion of the lumen due to intestinal linitis plastica
Functional obstruction (or adynamic ileus) is caused by intestinal motility disorders consequently to the following:
   a. Tumor infiltration of the mesentery or bowel muscle and nerves (carcinomatosis), malignant involvement of the celiac plexus.
   b. Paraneoplastic neuropathy in patients with lung cancer.
   c. Chronic intestinal pseudo-obstruction (CIP) mainly due to diabetes mellitus, previous gastric surgery, and other neurological disorders. These factors may affect extrinsic neural control to viscera. Vagal dysfunction is confirmed in a majority of patients with CIP associated with diabetes or neurologic disorders.
   d. Paraneoplastic pseudo-obstruction.

Other causes such as inflammatory edema, fecal impaction, constipating drugs (such as opioids, anticholinergics), and dehydration are likely to contribute to the development of bowel obstruction or to worsen the clinical picture.

to all the abdomen or above the obstacle, ascites, as well as painful sites; and (7) presence of feces in the rectal ampulla (rectal exploration).

From the metabolic point of view, dehydration, electrolyte losses, and disorders of acid–base balance are frequently associated with bowel obstruction. The hypovolemic state may induce a functional renal failure due to a decrease of the renal flow and, as a consequence, of the glomerular filtration. Different respiratory patterns may be observed, depending on the level of obstruction. Whereas the level is high, metabolic alkaloses, hypochloremy and hypokalemy, due to a prevalent loss of gastric secretions, determine hypoventilation; if the level of obstruction is distal, the secondary deficit is global including chlorum, sodium, potassium, and bicarbonates owing to intestinal stasis of biliary, pancreatic, intestinal, as well as gastric secretions. The dehydration reflects the accumulation of fluids and electrolytes in the third space. With a low level of obstruction, including ileum or colon, acidosis prevails due to ischemic tessual lesions or septic complications.

The diagnosis of intestinal obstruction is established or suspected on clinical grounds and usually confirmed with abdominal radiographs demonstrating air–fluid levels. However, there is no point in proceeding with any of these if the patient is too ill or has declined surgery.

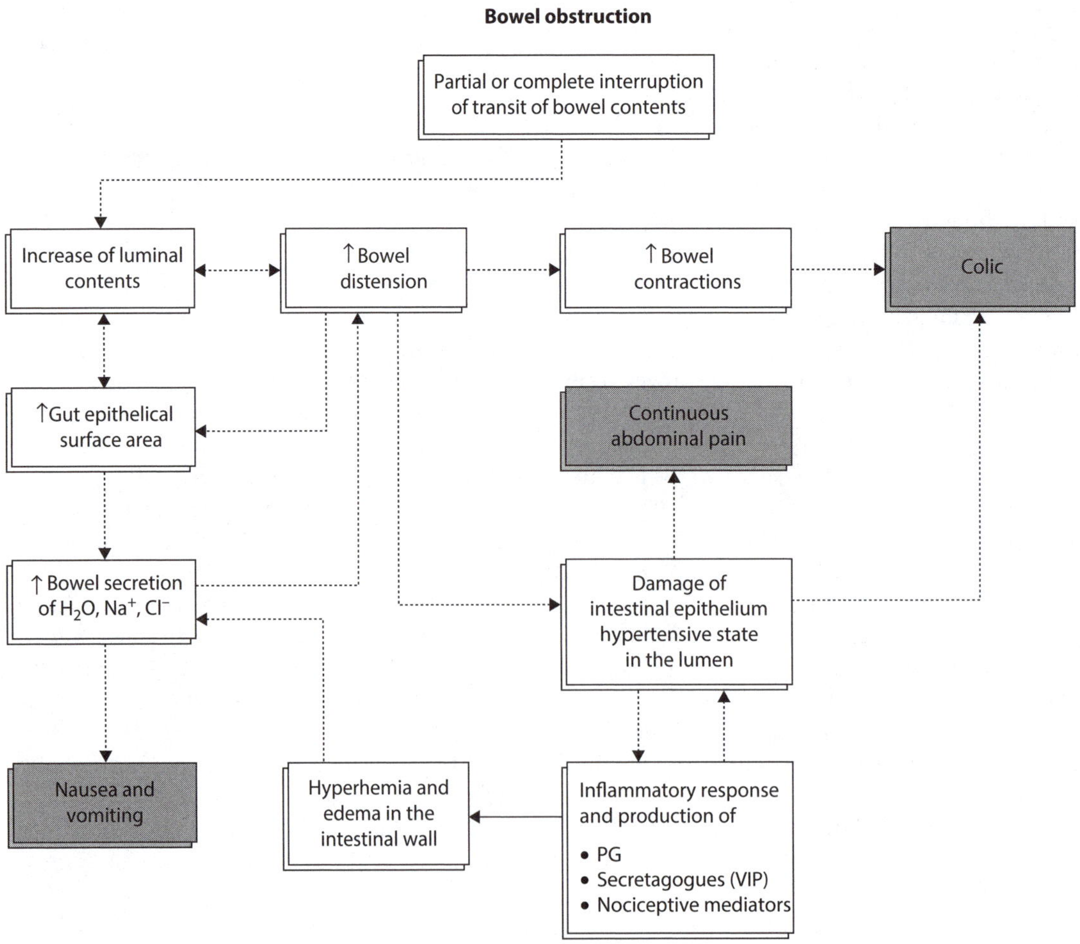

Figure 62.1 *Definitive bowel obstruction.*

Table 62.2   *Common symptoms in cancer patients with MBO*

Vomiting	Intermittent or continuous	It develops early and in large amounts in gastric, duodenum, and small-bowel obstruction and develops later in large-bowel obstruction.	Biliary vomiting is almost odorless and indicates an obstruction in the upper part of the abdomen. The presence of bad smelling and fecaloid vomiting can be the first sign of an ileal or colic obstruction.
Nausea	Intermittent or continuous		
Colicky pain	Variable intensity and localization due to distension proximal to the obstruction; secondary to gas and fluid accumulation, most of which are produced by the gut.	If it is intense, periumbilical, and occurring at brief intervals, it may be an indication of an obstruction at the jejunal–ileal level. In large-bowel obstruction, the pain is less intense, deeper, and occurring at longer intervals and spreads toward the colon wall.	An overall acute pain that begins intensely and becomes stronger, or a pain that is specifically localized, may be a symptom of a perforation or an ileal or colic strangulation. A pain that increases with palpation may be due to peritoneal irritation or the beginning of a perforation.
Continuous pain	Variable intensity and localization	It is due to abdominal distension, tumor mass, tumor mass growth compressing the intestine, intestinal distension, and/or hepatomegaly.	
Dry mouth		It is due to severe dehydration, metabolic alterations, but above all, it is due to the use of drugs with anticholinergic properties.	
Constipation	Intermittent or complete	In case of complete obstruction, there is no evacuation of feces and no flatus.	In case of partial obstruction, the symptom is intermittent.
Overflow (paradoxical) diarrhea		It is the result of bacterial liquefaction of the fecal material blocked in the sigma or rectum.	

MANAGEMENT OF BOWEL OBSTRUCTION: THERAPEUTIC APPROACHES

The management of patients with MBO is one of the greatest challenges for physicians who care for cancer patients. This management has to be highly personalized according to the stage of the illness, the prognosis, the possibility of further antineoplastic therapies, and the general status and choices of the patients. Figure 62.2 shows an algorithm for a decision-making process in patients with MBO.

In the face of a clearly incurable situation, significant patient discomfort and suffering must be balanced with the need to simplify the care of those patients with a short time to live.

A multidisciplinary working group of the EAPC reviewed issues regarding bowel obstruction and published clinical practice recommendations for the management of MBO in patients with end-stage cancer [7].

Surgical procedures

Palliative interventions, either open, laparoscopic, endoscopic, or fluoroscopic, may benefit patients with MBO and are generally considered when bowel obstruction symptoms do not resolve after 24–48 hours of NGT decompression. Each patient must be assessed individually to decide whether an invasive intervention is feasible and appropriate (Table 62.3). Although the diagnosis and location of obstruction can be suggested by the history, physical exam, and plain or contrast radiography, cross-sectional imaging by computed tomography (CT) scanning or magnetic resonance imaging (MRI) is essential in decision making. CT will diagnose the site and cause of obstruction in 70%–95% of cases [14], compared to 23% for ultrasound and 7% for plain film radiography [15]. CT will also rule out closed-loop obstruction and intestinal ischemia, which requires emergency management. Newer technology in CT scanning such as spiral and multidetector scanners, combined with the intravenous and oral ± rectal contrast, provides a better global assessment of the abdomen and pelvis and, when coupled with multiplanar reconstruction, can help identify the transition point(s) in bowel obstruction, thereby determining the site, cause, and severity of obstruction [16,17]. MRI may provide similar information, but is not as widely available as CT scanning, and local expertise in its use in the assessment of bowel obstruction may be limited. The expected results with MRI should be similar to CT scanning, but the data on the sensitivity, specificity, and accuracy are lacking. Once the site and cause of obstruction are known, a decision can be made about management. The procedure that is the most likely to successfully relieve symptoms for the greatest length of time with reasonable morbidity is chosen [18].

Complete surgical resection of a tumor is most desirable. However, it is only worthwhile if the entire tumor in that area can be resected with negative margins. The exception can be ovarian or some GI cancers where intraperitoneal chemotherapy can treat the residual disease after a "debulking" operation

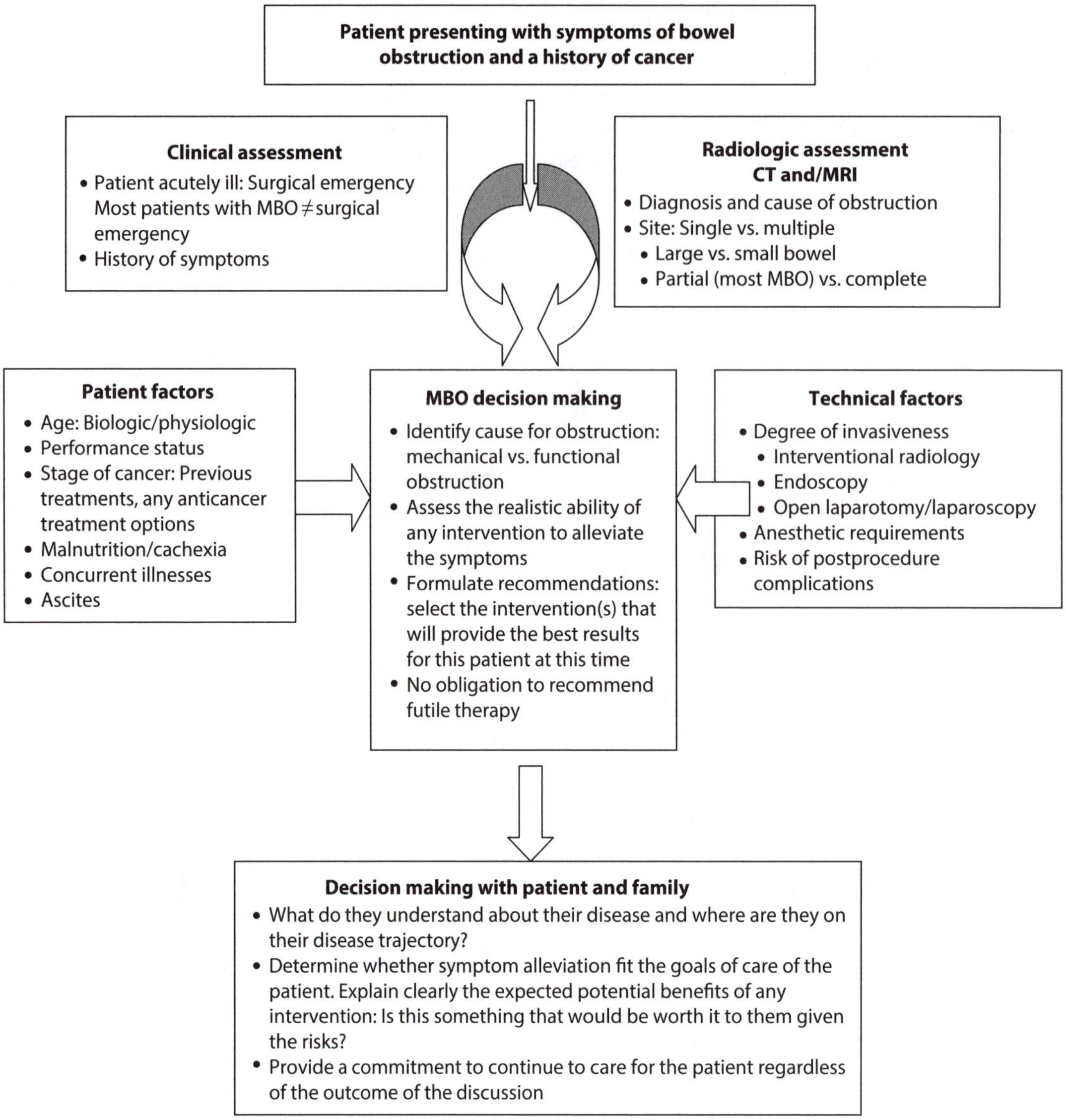

Figure 62.2 *Algorithm for assessing and managing a patient with MBO.*

Table 62.3 *Radiological investigations*

Plain radiography	Abdominal radiography taken in supine and standing position to document the dilated loops of bowel, air–fluid interfaces, or both.
Contrast radiography	Help to evaluate dysmotility and partial obstruction and to define the site and extent of obstruction.
	Barium can interfere with subsequent endoscopic studies or cause severe impaction or aspiration pneumonia.
	Gastrografin (diatrizoate meglumine) is useful in such cases; moreover, it often provides excellent visualization of proximal obstructions and can reduce luminal edema and help resolve partial obstructions. Contrast studies of the stomach, gastric outlet, and small bowel can distinguish obstructions from metastases, radiation injury, or adhesions.
	The diagnosis of a motility disorder is revealed by the slow passage of barium through undilated bowel with no demonstrable point of obstruction.
	Retrograde, transrectal contrast studies (barium or water-soluble medium enema) can rule out and diagnose isolated or concomitant obstruction of the large bowel.
CT	Abdominal CT is useful to evaluate the global extent of disease, to perform staging, and to assist in the choice of surgical, endoscopic, or simple pharmacological palliative intervention for the management of the obstruction.
Endoscopy	Once a site of obstruction is identified in either the gastric outlet or colon, endoscopic studies may be helpful to evaluate the exact cause of the obstruction. This is particularly important when endoscopic treatment approaches, such as stent placement, are considered.

Table 62.4 *Prognostic indicators of low likelihood of clinical benefit from surgery of MBO*

1. Obstruction secondary to cancer
2. *Intestinal motility problems due to diffuse intraperitoneal carcinomatosis
3. +Widespread tumor
4. +Patients over 65 in association with cachexia
5. *Ascites requiring frequent paracentesis
6. +Low serum albumin level and low serum prealbumin level
7. +Previous radiotherapy of the abdomen or pelvis
8. +Poor nutritional status
9. *Diffuse palpable intra-abdominal masses
10. +Liver metastases, distant metastases, pleural effusion, or pulmonary metastases producing dyspnea
11. *Multiple partial bowel obstructions with prolonged passage time on radiograph examination
12. +Elevated blood urea nitrogen levels, elevated alkaline phosphatase levels, advanced tumor stage, short diagnosis to obstruction interval
13. +Poor performance status
14. *A recent laparotomy, which demonstrated that further corrective surgery was not possible
15. *Previous abdominal surgery, which showed diffuse metastatic cancer
16. *Involvement of proximal stomach
16. +Extra-abdominal metastases producing symptoms difficult to control (e.g., dyspnea)

Source: Modified from Ripamonti, C. et al., *Support. Care Cancer*, 19, 23, 2001.
    Data from retrospective studies.
Absolute* and relative+ contraindications to surgery.

of all obvious diseases. Otherwise, debulking of a tumor is not generally beneficial, as the tumor will only grow back in the absence of anticancer therapy (Table 62.4).

If the tumor cannot be resected, but there is healthy nonobstructed bowel before and after the site of obstruction, a side-to-side bypass can be performed. This will restore bowel continuity and allow the patient to eat and maintain their nutritional status. In the case of distal obstruction, a stoma can be created out of the most distal unaffected bowel segment. In order to maintain one's nutrition orally, it is necessary to have a minimum of 100 cm of proximal bowel before a stoma, so the length of proximal bowel should be measured prior to creating a proximal stoma. Proximal stomas also have high outputs and may cause significant fluid balance problems. Finally, in the absence of any other options, a gastrostomy tube may be placed to avoid the need for an NGT.

The likelihood of long-term relief of obstruction after surgery depends on the location of the bowel obstruction, with large-bowel obstruction successfully relieved in 80% of cases versus 25% if both large and small bowels are involved [19]. The number of obstructed sites also affects the likelihood of success; a single site of obstruction has a high likelihood of success as compared to multiple sites of obstruction. It is worth emphasizing that MBO from generalized carcinomatosis is a distinct entity that responds poorly, or not at all, to surgical intervention and these patients are not surgical candidates [7,13,20,21].

Surgical decision making

In addition to the aforementioned technical factors, surgical decision making must take into account the individual patient and their disease. Performance status remains one of the best predictors of lower complication rates and improved survival [22]. Patient factors associated with poor surgical outcomes include advanced age (both physiological and chronological); poor nutritional status, psychological health, and social support; ascites; and/or concurrent illness and comorbidities [23,24]. Disease factors such as tumor type, grade and extent, time from primary presentation, and history of response to and availability of anticancer treatments also affect decision making. Slow-growing, well-differentiated tumors are more likely to be associated with better outcomes and longer survival. The best predictor of the future is the place of the disease in the past and its response to treatment, due to the biology and inherent growth characteristics of the tumor. Patients with bulky liver or lung metastatic disease will generally die sooner than those with localized pelvic or intraperitoneal disease and are therefore less likely to benefit from surgery.

The selection of patients who will benefit from these procedures is an ongoing challenge. Because the management of MBO is rarely an emergency, time can and should be taken to develop an appropriate individualized treatment plan with the patient and family. In the face of an incurable, progressive illness, the balance between honesty and maintaining hope and optimism can be difficult to achieve but is necessary to avoid futile treatments and harm to the patient [25]. It may be easier to offer a treatment just to do something; the more difficult decision may be not to do something when it is not going to help. However, there is little guidance on what should be considered a futile treatment as the definition will vary depending on the patient's goals and values and the clinician's experience [7,26].

A decision-making approach can be outlined as follows (Figure 62.2). The clinician first decides which, if any, treatments are appropriate or feasible. This can only be done after a thorough evaluation, including imaging, to assess the current state of the illness, avoiding intraoperative surprises or emergencies. The patient is asked about their understanding of where they are on their disease trajectory and about their expectations, goals, and values. Their current medical condition and expected prognosis are discussed. All treatment options including surgery, endoscopy, interventional radiology, and aggressive medical management should be discussed, along with the complication rates and the expected success of each intervention. Reasonable treatment goals are set, and a plan is developed with the patient, whether this is continued anticancer therapy, withdrawal of inappropriate therapies, or vigorous palliative care. These goals should address the relief of suffering and improving quality of life (QOL). This may take time as the patient comes to terms with their disease.

With careful preoperative planning, it is possible to determine before the operation in most cases which operation is most likely to succeed; however, the final decision will be made in the operating room. The possibility that no surgical procedure may be possible must also be discussed, and the patient and family must be prepared for that option. Finally, there must be a commitment to ongoing care with a clear care plan whatever the outcome of the surgery. Several recent papers from large cancer centers have followed patients prospectively with MBO. Significant symptom relief can be obtained by selecting appropriate patients either for surgery or stenting with minimal procedural mortality [22,24,27,28].

Nutritional considerations

Any malignancy may influence a patients' nutritional status, whether due to the disease itself or to anticancer treatments such as chemotherapy or radiation. Nutritional status is further impaired by the inability to eat with MBO. The European Society for Clinical Nutrition and Metabolism (ESPEN) defined severe malnutrition as existing when patients have at least one of the following risk factors: weight loss ≥10%–15% within 6 months, body mass index (BMI) ≤18 kg/m², and serum albumin ≤30 g/L (without evidence of renal and/or liver dysfunction) [29]. Cachexia is a catabolic–metabolic state common in advanced cancer, where the patient is metabolically breaking down intrinsic muscle, protein, and fat [30]. Cachexia is associated with inflammation, hypercatabolism, hormonal changes, and the production of tumor factors. There is no consensus in the literature how to best diagnose cachexia. Cachexia is not reversible by increasing nutritional intake and represents end-stage disease, and therefore, interventions to improve oral intake will not be helpful. Unfortunately, in advanced cancer patients, cachexia, MBO, and poor nutritional status are often seen together, and it can be difficult to identify if the weight loss can be reversed if the obstruction is relieved.

The use of parenteral nutrition (PN) in unrelieved MBO from advanced cancer is generally not recommended. Recent guidelines by ESPEN were published for the use of PN in patients who will undergo a surgical procedure [29] and for cancer patients who will not undergo a surgical intervention [31]. For those patients who meet the ESPEN definition for severe malnutrition (BMI under 18.5–22 kg/m² depending on age) in whom a surgery is planned and who cannot be enterally fed, ESPEN recommends starting PN 7–10 days preoperatively to decrease the rate of postoperative infections, length of stay in hospital, and postoperative mortality. Short-term postoperative PN is indicated for malnourished patients who required emergency surgery and therefore could not receive PN preoperatively [29]. For those patients with advanced cancer and poor nutritional status who will not have surgery, PN is considered ineffective if the reason for the poor nutritional status is not located in the GI tract. Also, PN does not have a role as a supplement while patients are on either chemotherapy, radiation treatment, or both therapies simultaneously and also are able to receive oral or enteral nutrition adequately [31].

Once the obstruction is relieved, the value of an oral nutritional support programs for advanced cancer patients is unclear. Several early reports suggest a benefit for active nutritional intervention in advanced cancer patients [32,33]. However, in advanced head and neck cancer patients undergoing radiation, the group randomized to the nutritional support program lost less weight but had an overall poorer outcome [34], and a review of nutritional support program in lung cancer patients also demonstrated no survival benefit [35].

Stenting and venting procedures

Over the past two decades, there has been increasing experience in the use of self-expanding metallic stents (SEMS) in the management of MBO of the gastric outlet, proximal small bowel, and colon. SEMS may be used in the treatment of acute small-bowel or colonic obstruction, associated with the initial presentation of potentially resectable disease, where the goal of stenting is to convert an emergent operation to a safer, elective one that can be curative or provide an opportunity to deliver neoadjuvant therapy prior to a curative operation [36]. For patients presenting with bowel obstruction from recurrent or metastatic disease, curative treatment is unlikely, so stenting provides a quick and safe procedure palliating the patient's symptoms with a very brief hospital stay or, in some cases, a 1-day visit to the ambulatory surgery center. This approach now provides an important alternative to palliative surgery.

Endoscopic management of gastroduodenal and proximal jejunal obstruction

Patients presenting with malignant gastric outlet obstruction (GOO) or small-bowel obstruction often present with severe abdominal pain with distension, nausea, vomiting, and dehydration, severely reducing their QOL. Although it sometimes occurs early in the course of disease, obstruction most often represents a late consequence of pancreatic cancer, gastric cancer, gall bladder cancer, and cholangiocarcinoma. This can also result from metastases of a variety of extra-abdominal malignancies, such as breast and lung cancer.

Advances in endoscopy and interventional radiology now permit the insertion of SEMS, resulting in rapid relief of obstruction, and it is now performed in many centers, including community hospitals, with technical success rates for stent placement reported to be >90% and clinical success for resolution of nausea and vomiting and improved oral consumption reported over 75% [37–42]. The major limiting factor is the ability to reach and traverse the point of obstruction with an endoscope or guidewire especially when the obstructing tumor is located beyond the ligament of Treitz.

Durable palliation of obstructive symptoms is variable as a result of multiple factors affecting the patency of the stents, such as effects of anticancer therapy (chemotherapy and radiation) on continued tumor growth, the long-term survival of the patient, and the location and characteristics of the original tumor stricture. In one multicenter prospective trial, 56% of patients experienced an improvement in solid food intake by 1 week, and 80% by 1 month, and this effect lasted till death or last follow-up in 48%, and 66% of patients did not require any reintervention, demonstrating the excellent durability of palliative stenting [43]. In the limited comparative studies published, endoscopic stent placement has been associated with shorter hospital stay with lower periprocedural mortality in patients with GOO secondary to pancreatic cancer [44,45] and with more rapid food intake compared to surgical bypass [44–46]. Stent placement has even been shown to be effective in palliating symptoms from obstruction in the setting of limited degrees of peritoneal carcinomatosis [47].

Delayed stent failure can occur, however, from food impaction or reobstruction caused by tumor ingrowth, but there is some evidence that additional cancer chemotherapy or radiation therapy can slow the development of tumor ingrowth and prolong the patency of the stents [48]. Stent migration also can occur, sometimes in association with cancer treatment, if there is reduction in the size of the tumor [48]. In most cases, reobstruction due to tumor ingrowth can be managed with placement of a second stent or tumor ablation by Nd:YAG laser or argon plasma coagulator [50–51]. In comparative studies, those managed with SEMS in the initial palliative management of malignant obstruction did just as well initially as patients managed with surgical bypass but had a greater need for reintervention because of delayed stent occlusion [46,52].

The overall safety of procedures to insert SEMS has been considered very acceptable with bleeding and perforation occurring in about 3%–4% in published reports [37–41]. Delayed erosion and perforation also occur but are inconsistently reported [53].

The effect of palliative treatments on the patient's QOL in malignant GOO has not been widely studied, and those that have been published show very modest results [54,55]. In one prospective, nonrandomized study, Schmidt et al. showed that stent placement in the treatment of malignant gastric and/or duodenal obstruction was associated with a shorter hospital stay than surgical bypass, but both procedures were associated with improvements in nausea, vomiting, ability to eat, and several measures of QOL [55]. In another prospective study examining QOL in patients with malignant GOO, Mehta and coauthors randomized 27 patients to receive laparoscopic gastrojejunostomy or endoscopic stent placement. Stent placement was associated with less pain and shorter hospital stay, with a greater improvement in physical health following stent placement relative to those managed surgically [54].

When faced with decisions on the best treatment for patients with malignant gastric or duodenal obstructions, clinicians need to consider multiple factors including the nature and extent of the malignancy, prior treatment, medical comorbidities and performance status, the overall prognosis, and the available technical expertise. Surgical bypass should be the preferred option for patients with a good performance status, a slowly progressive disease, and a relatively long life expectancy (>60 days). If the site of obstruction is distal in the jejunum or ileum or if there are multiple sites of obstruction, endoscopic stenting is not likely to succeed, so surgical intervention or drainage gastrostomy should be considered. Patients who are best suited for endoscopic stenting are those with a short proximal tumor, at a single site, or those with an intermediate to high performance status and an intermediate life expectancy of greater than 30 days. Patients with rapidly progressive disease, evidence of advanced carcinomatosis with moderate to severe ascites, multiple levels of obstruction on cross-sectional imaging, a poor performance status, or a very short life expectancy of less than 30 days are best served by medical palliation of symptoms or the insertion of a drainage percutaneous endoscopic gastrostomy (PEG).

Endoscopic management of malignant small-bowel obstruction

Much of the experience with endoscopic management of small-bowel obstruction comes from that which has just been reviewed in the setting of gastroduodenal obstruction previously. Most gastroscopes are unable to reach beyond the ligament of Treitz, and colonoscopes are unable to reach very far retrograde into the terminal ileum, so most cases of small-bowel obstruction are not amenable to endoscopic stenting.

The recent development of long enteroscopes that can be advanced far into the small intestine through an overtube with pleating of the small bowel has permitted some investigators to report success in stenting areas of the small intestine not previously accessible to standard endoscopes. Most of these reports are anecdotal, but with time, increasing interventional endoscopist experience and further development of the enteroscopes, the stents, and manipulating tools, the ability to treat midjejunal and ileal points of malignant obstruction may become more available, and such patients will have another option for treatment [56–58]. The selection of patients appropriate for such interventions will, however, remain challenging.

Endoscopic management of malignant colorectal obstruction

The endoscopic management of malignant large-bowel obstruction has paralleled the experience reported with the treatment of malignant esophageal and gastroduodenal obstruction. The procedure can be performed by sigmoidoscopy, colonoscopy, or transnasal wire-guided approaches under fluoroscopy alone. Published series have shown technical success rates for insertion of metallic stents ranging from 80% to 100%, with clinical improvement in symptoms reported in more than 75% of patients [36,59,60]. Many patients treated with stents have a durable relief of symptoms until death from progression of disease, but as has been seen with the use of stents in other parts of the body, restenosis occurs, usually caused by tumor ingrowth through the interstices of the stent or stent migration. This can usually be managed with insertion of another stent, endoscopic dilation, or laser ablation [59–62].

Two analyses of pooled data from the multiple reported case series have been published [63,64]. Both report clinical success rates of 88% and 91%, defined as resolution of obstructive symptoms following the insertion of stents. The limitations to success are a very proximal location of obstruction in the proximal colon and the ability to traverse a tortuous or tightly obstructing tumor with the endoscope or a guide-wire. A greater success with stenting primary colorectal cancer has been noted, with lesser success for obstruction caused by extrinsic compression from metastatic or locally invasive pelvic tumors [62,65,66].

Limited data on cost-effectiveness of colorectal stenting are available in published reports, with some calculations suggesting a potential reduction in the estimated cost of palliation for such patients of approximately 50% compared to surgery [63]. This is predominantly attributed to a reduced hospital stay with stenting.

A recent multicenter study was completed demonstrating similar results with a newer generation of nitinol SEMS, called the Wallflex [67]. This study, like most others, demonstrates the ease of use, high technical and short-term clinical efficacy, and low overall and serious complication rate. As in stenting in other parts of the GI tract, these procedures have acceptable published safety rates, with bleeding and perforation occurring in less than 5% of cases [63,64,68]. One limitation of stent use in malignant colorectal obstruction is the location of obstruction involving the lower rectum. Although not widely published, stent placement for tumors that obstruct the mid- or lower rectum may result in relief of obstruction but an insufficient remaining rectal reservoir, resulting in the development of intractable tenesmus and incontinence, which severely impairs QOL [69]. It is best to recognize such patients as inappropriate for treatment with a stent and consider performing surgical diversion or other palliative approaches.

The proper evaluation of the efficacy of palliative treatments requires a careful assessment of the effect of each treatment on symptoms and the QOL and less attention on survival. In one prospective, nonrandomized study evaluating the effect of endoscopic stenting and surgical diversion in palliating malignant colorectal obstruction, symptoms improved significantly after either treatment but were more durable after stenting than after surgery. Although there was a trend, neither stenting nor surgery had a significant effect on overall QOL [67]. This and other studies demonstrate how difficult it is to actually quantify the benefits of therapeutic interventions in the dying patient.

Drainage percutaneous endoscopic gastrostomy in bowel obstruction

Often efforts to reconstitute the patency of the GI tract fail or are considered inappropriate due to the extent of intraperitoneal disease or the realization of the medical futility of such attempts. Such patients experience intractable nausea and vomiting, which may benefit from the insertion of an NGT, but this may be associated with severe nasopharyngeal discomfort, pain with swallowing, speaking, and coughing, or be cosmetically unacceptable, and confine the patient at home.

In such patients, gastric venting with PEG tube placement has become a widely acceptable alternative for palliating nausea and vomiting [69,70]. Endoscopic or radiographically guided placement of drainage PEG tubes is a rapid and safe method of

achieving symptomatic relief without the risks of a traditional surgical procedure. Original clinical guidelines following the early experience with PEG tubes for nutritional support suggested that patients with advanced abdominal malignancies or prior surgery were contraindicated for PEG placement due to the presence of ascites, adhesions, or tumor infiltration of the stomach, but published studies have shown that endoscopic PEG placement can be safely performed and can provide meaningful palliation of the severe nausea and vomiting occurring with such irreversible forms of bowel obstruction [69–71].

In an early series, Campagnutta et al. [69] reported on 34 patients with bowel obstruction from gynecological malignancies that were palliated with drainage PEG. Using 15 and 20 Fr. tubes, 94% had PEGs successfully placed, and 84.4% had resolution of symptoms, with return of the ability to consume liquids or soft food for a median of 74 days.

In a retrospective study, 28 Fr. PEG tube placement was feasible in 98% of patients with advanced recurrent ovarian cancer, even in patients with tumor encasing the stomach, diffuse carcinomatosis, and ascites [70]. This approach has also been used to temporarily palliate symptoms in patients still undergoing systemic anticancer therapy. However, for most patients with MBO from advanced peritoneal carcinomatosis, drainage PEG tubes only help reduce some of the symptoms associated with MBO such as nausea and vomiting and often require additional efforts at controlling pain from the distension associated with ascites or direct tumor effect in the abdomen and elsewhere.

In some cases where the stomach has been partially or completely removed, the insertion of a venting PEG becomes impossible, so a drainage PEJ (percutaneous endoscopic jejunostomy) tube may have to be attempted, to serve the same purpose of decompressing the fluid-distended GI tract [72]. The selection of the appropriate procedure, if any, for patients with advanced abdominal malignancy and obstruction is difficult. The application of these procedures should be considered in a favorable manner as when available, they do help transition patients with incurable disease out of the hospital to the home or terminal care facilities in greater comfort.

PHARMACOLOGICAL MANAGEMENT OF SYMPTOMS

The pharmacological management of bowel obstruction due to advanced cancer focuses on the treatment of nausea, vomiting, pain, and other symptoms without the use of an NGT. If a central venous catheter has been previously inserted, this can be used to administer drugs for symptom control. Continuous subcutaneous infusion of drugs using a portable syringe driver allows the parenteral administration of different drug combinations, produces minimal discomfort for the patient, and is easy to use in a home setting.

Drug therapy comprising analgesics, antisecretory drugs, and antiemetics, without using an NGT, was first described by Baines et al. [73]. Several authors have confirmed the efficacy of this approach [3–7]. Medications should be tailored to each patient regarding the drugs to be administered, the dosages, the drug associations, and the route of their administration [7]. In most bowel-obstructed patients, oral administration is not suitable, and alternative routes have to be considered. Most of the recommended drugs can be administered in association via parenteral continuous infusion.

To relieve continuous abdominal pain, opioid analgesics via continuous subcutaneous or intravenous infusion are necessary in most of the patients. The dosage has to be titrated for each patient until pain relief is achieved. Anticholinergics may be administered in association to opioids to control colicky pain [7] (Figure 62.3).

Vomiting can be managed using two different pharmacological approaches and reduced to an acceptable level for the patient (e.g., 1–2 times/day): (1) drugs such as anticholinergics (scopolamine butylbromide [SB], glycopyrrolate) and/or octreotide, which reduce GI secretions, and (2) antiemetics acting on the central nervous system, alone or in association with drugs to reduce GI secretions (Figure 62.3).

Recently, a meta-analysis compared the effectiveness of histamine-2 receptor antagonists and proton-pump inhibitors (PPIs) in reducing gastric secretions in patients with MBO. It was done based on seven randomized controlled trials (RCTs). In total, 445 patients were included, 223 received ranitidine and 222 different PPIs (omeprazole, lansoprazole, pantoprazole, and rabeprazole). Both drugs were able to reduce the gastric secretions, and between them, ranitidine was the most potent [74]. Based on this report, we cannot make final conclusions, but these findings represent another tool available in the management of this condition and something that needs further investigation.

Several authors recommend the use of *corticosteroids* for the symptoms due to bowel obstruction because it can reduce peritumoral inflammatory edema, thus improving intestinal motility. No robust trials have been carried out and administration routes and dosing of these drugs have not been standardized as yet. A systematic review showed a tendency but not significant reduction in symptoms in the steroids group compared to the placebo. In terms of mortality, there are no differences between both groups. The role of corticosteroids in treating bowel obstruction is still controversial [75]. However, the coadministration of octreotide, corticosteroids, and metoclopramide produced a prompt resolution of GI symptoms and recovery of bowel movements within 5 days [76].

SB is a frequently used drug for both vomiting and colicky pain by some palliative care centers [73,77–79]. This drug differs from both atropine and scopolamine hydrobromide in having a low lipid solubility. It does not penetrate the blood–brain barrier as well as these other drugs and, consequently, may produce fewer side effects, such as somnolence and hallucinations, when administered in combination with opioids. The anticholinergic activity of SB decreases the tonus and peristalsis in smooth muscle and decreases the secretions in the GI tract. The antiemetic, antisecretory, as well the analgesic role of SB administered subcutaneously by a syringe driver has been well documented by different authors. Dry mouth is reported to be the most significant side effect, but the patients tolerated it by sucking ice cubes and drinking small sips of water. Also anticholinergic agents such as scopolamine hydrobromide or butylbromide and glycopyrrolate reduce colicky pain and the volume of intestinal secretions. *Glycopyrrolate*, which is used as an antisecretory drug in the United States, is more potent than scopolamine hydrobromide and may be effective in some patients who fail to respond to scopolamine [80]. It has little central nervous system penetration and is unlikely to cause the delirium that has been associated with tertiary amine anticholinergics.

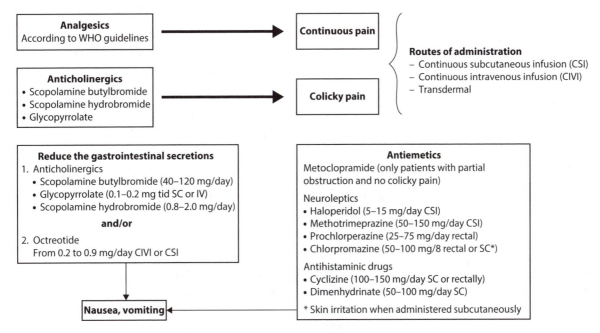

Figure 62.3 *Symptomatic pharmacological approach.*

Octreotide, a synthetic analog of somatostatin that has a more potent biological activity and a longer half-life, has also been used to manage the symptoms of bowel obstruction. Somatostatin and its analogs have been shown to inhibit the release and activity of GI hormones, modulate GI function by reducing gastric acid secretion, slow intestinal motility, decrease bile flow, increase mucous production, and reduce splanchnic blood flow. It reduces GI contents and increases absorption of water and electrolytes at intracellular level, via cAMP and calcium regulation. Submucosal somatostatin-containing neurons, activated by octreotide, inhibit excitatory nerves, mainly by an inhibition of acetylcholine output. As a result, muscle relaxation can occur, ameliorating the spastic activity responsible for colicky pain. These effects may be due to the VIP inhibition, which is increased in experimental bowel obstruction and is known to have adverse effects on intestinal secretions, splanchnic flow, and peristalsis [81].

The inhibitory effect of octreotide on both peristalsis and GI secretions reduces bowel distension and the secretion of water and sodium by the intestinal epithelium, thereby reducing vomiting and pain. The drug may therefore break the vicious circle represented by secretion, distension, and contractile hyperactivity. Octreotide has been shown to have a potent anti-VIP effect resulting in the inhibition of intestinal secretions [82,83]. Also in the in vitro experiments on rabbit ileum, somatostatin was able to stimulate water and NaCl absorption and inhibit HCO_3 secretion and to inhibit water secretion in the jejunum [13,84].

Experimental studies suggest that the principal mechanism of fluid secretion in bowel obstruction depends on VIP-induced inflammatory events [13,81,85]. Another inhibitory mechanism of hormonal release occurs through the activation of a G protein, which, on stimulating the potassium channels, determines the hyperpolarization of the cell, with the consequent blockage of the flux of calcium to the cell [86]. Octreotide may be administered by subcutaneous bolus or continuous subcutaneous or intravenous infusion. Its half-life is about 1.5 hours after intravenous or subcutaneous administration, and its kinetics are linear. The recommended starting dose is 0.3 mg/day subcutaneously. The dose can be titrated upward until symptom control is achieved in general 0.6–0.9 mg/day. Octreotide is an expensive drug, and its cost–benefit ratio should be carefully considered, especially for prolonged treatment. However, the cost of the drug should be interpreted in the widest possible sense, that is, if the use of a drug results in a more rapid improvement of GI symptoms that potentially limits the bed stay or the admission to an inpatient unit in addition to a better QOL of the patient [87].

Many experimental studies evaluated the efficacy of somatostatin and octreotide in respect to placebo on intestinal distension, electrolyte losses, and ischemia [13].

Efficacy of octreotide before surgery for bowel obstruction

Surgical GI complications are common, and postoperative outcome is poor in advanced cancer patients. As luminal contents accumulate proximal to the obstruction, the bowel becomes distended, and the increase in intraluminal pressure stimulates intestinal fluid secretion, which further stretches the bowel wall. The consequent pathological findings are an accumulation of fluids and gases above the obstruction with altered motility producing distension, wall edema, vessel congestion, necrosis, and perforation of the bowel above the obstruction and the presence of peritoneal fluids. Obstructed patients are hypovolemic, tachycardic, and frequently hypotensive as a result of fluids and electrolytes sequestered in the gut wall and in its lumen. Successful surgery may be compromised by these alterations and higher morbidity and mortality are expected [88].

Octreotide at a daily dose of 0.3 mcg has been preoperatively administered in patients undergoing surgery for bowel obstruction due to cancer. The patients were managed by an intravenous replacement of fluids and electrolytes, NGT, and antibiotics. The diameter of the bowel above the obstruction was normal, and no local gross pathological findings due to the accumulation of fluids in the lumen, such as edema, vessel congestion, or necrosis of the bowel above the obstruction, commonly observed in this situation, were observed. Samples of intestine above and below the obstruction revealed a normal anatomic and biochemical pattern. Intestinal anastomosis after resection was successful [89]. These preliminary results were confirmed in a randomized, double-blind, clinical trial carried out on 54 consecutive patients with mechanical bowel obstruction. Patients who received octreotide preoperatively required surgery less often than patients who did not receive the drug. Moreover, severe dilatation and necrosis of the bowel proximal to the area of obstruction were significantly less frequent as compared with those patients who did not receive the drug preoperatively [90].

Efficacy of octreotide in patients with GI symptoms due to inoperable malignant bowel obstruction

Many studies, although uncontrolled, strongly support the use of octreotide in reducing GI secretions, nausea, and vomiting in patients with MBO [3,5,7,12,88–101]. In many cases, the NGT can be removed. Reported effective doses range from 100 to 600 mcg/day either as a continuous infusion or as intermittent subcutaneous boluses. Octreotide has been coadministered with numerous other agents including morphine, haloperidol, and SB.

Table 62.5 shows the efficacy of octreotide administration in the control of GI symptoms due to bowel obstruction [12,91–95] reported in some studies. All the authors were able to show the efficacy on emesis in cancer patients with intractable continual vomiting due to small-/large-bowel obstruction that was unresponsive to conventional therapy (prochlorperazine, metoclopramide, cyclizine, and dexamethasone). Octreotide was administered subcutaneously in association or not with opioid analgesics and with antiemetics.

Symptom control was maintained until death. No adverse effects were attributable to the drugs. The NGT was removed in most patients.

Table 62.5   *Role of octreotide in MBO*

Author(s)	No of PTS	Site of cancers Site of obstruction	Symptom(s)	OCT dose/route ±Other drugs	Results
Khoo et al. [91]*	5	Various intra-abdominal Small bowel	Intractable vomiting unresponsive to conventional therapy	0.1–0.5 mg/day Scb at start than CSI	Vomiting stopped within 1 hour from start of treatment. The only patient with an NGT presented a reduction in aspirate from 2000 mL/day to under 300 mL/day. No important toxicity was reported.
Mercadante et al. [92]*	2	Intra-abdominal Small and/or large bowel ± carcinomatosis	Abdominal pain and vomiting (1°) Colic pain and vomiting despite the use of NGT and haloperidol (2°)	0.3–0.2 mg/day +0.9 mg buprenorphine CSI 0.9 mg/day +3 mg haloperidol	Pain and vomiting disappeared within 24 hours. NGT was removed. No adverse effects were reported. Within 24 hours, NGT secretions decreased from 2600 to 350 mL/day and vomiting disappeared. NGT was removed. No further need for analgesics or IV fluids. No adverse effects were reported.
Mercadante et al. [93]	14	Various intra-abdominal Small and/or large bowel	Nausea, vomiting Unresponsive to haloperidol or chlorpromazine	0.3–0.6 mg/day Scb or CSI + haloperidol + analgesics	Vomiting was controlled in 12 patients and reduced in 2. In two out of three patients, NGT was removed and the symptoms controlled. No important toxicity was reported.
Riley et al. [12]	24	Various intra-abdominal Small and/or large bowel	Intractable vomiting not responsive to a combination of antiemetics, steroids, and/or NGT drainage for 24 hours	0.1–1.2 mg/day Scb or CSI	Fourteen patients had no further vomiting, and four patients showed some improvements with a dose from 0.1–0.6 mg/day. There was a reduction of aspirate in all five patients with NGT. Six patients did not respond despite dosages of 0.6–1.2 mg/day. No adverse effects were reported also at higher dosages.
Mangili et al. [94]	13	Ovary Small and/or large bowel	Vomiting not responsive to metoclopramide and haloperidol	0.3–0.6 mg/day Scb or CSI ± analgesics	Vomiting was controlled in all cases within 3 days (range 1–6). In eight patients with an NGT, there was a reduction of secretions, and NGT was removed. No adverse effects were reported.
Steadman et al. [95]*	1	Pancreas Small bowel	Vomiting and drowsiness with diamorphine, cyclizine, hyoscine	0.2 mg/day + diamorphine	Good symptom relief without causing unwanted uncomfortable drowsiness

In the presence of marked and diffuse bowel distension, the administration of octreotide may reduce GI secretions and thus allow an appropriate site for PEG placement to be obtained [96].

These studies, although uncontrolled, support the use of octreotide in the management of GI symptoms due to inoperable MBO. Reported effective doses range from 0.1 to 0.6 mg/day either as a continuous parenteral infusion or as intermittent subcutaneous or intravenous boluses. Octreotide, administered in association, respectively, with morphine or hyoscine butylbromide (HB) or haloperidol (0.5–1.2 mg/mL), does not show visual precipitation when mixed in the syringe [7].

Comparative studies between octreotide and scopolamine butylbromide

Three randomized trials have compared octreotide with HB [102–104]. In all of these trials, octreotide was superior in the control of symptoms compared to HB.

Two randomized prospective studies were carried out to compare the antisecretory effects of octreotide (0.3 mg/day) and SB (60 mg/day) administered by continuous subcutaneous infusion for 3 days in 17 patients with inoperable bowel obstruction having an NGT [102] and in 15 patients without NGT [103]. In both studies, 50% of the patients were cared for at home, and the other half were hospitalized in surgical wards. In both studies, the hospitalized patients received significantly more parenteral hydration (2000 vs. 500 mL daily) in respect to the patients cared for at home.

In the study of Ripamonti et al. [102], octreotide was shown to significantly reduce the amount of GI secretions already at T_2 ($p = 0.016$) and T_3 ($p = 0.020$). The NGT could be removed in all 10 home care patients and in 3 hospitalized patients without changing the dosage of the drug. In three patients, it was possible to remove the NGT when the octreotide was added to SB (one patient) or when the SB dose was doubled and parenteral hydration was reduced (one patient). Also in these patients, octreotide showed a trend toward better efficacy than SB.

It can be hypothesized that in the hospitalized patients, the major difficulty in removing the NGT was associated with the higher amount of parenteral hydration.

In the second study [103], octreotide treatment induced a significantly rapid reduction in the number of daily episodes of vomiting and intensity of nausea when compared to SB-treated patients, examined at the different time intervals.

In the third RCT, Mystakidou et al. [104] evaluated the efficacy of octreotide in the management of nausea, vomiting, and abdominal pain, secondary to MBO in inoperable cancer patients. Sixty-eight terminally ill patients were enrolled, and the patients were randomly assigned into two equal groups. One group received SB 60–80 mg/day and chlorpromazine 15–25 mg/day, and the comparative group received octreotide 0.6–0.8 mg/day and chlorpromazine 15–25 mg/day. The drugs were administered via continuous subcutaneous infusion. Patients on octreotide presented significant less intensity of nausea and quantity of vomiting episodes. The survival time ranged from 7 to 61 days [104].

The association of the two drugs (octreotide and SB) may reduce GI secretions and vomiting whenever one drug alone is ineffective [101,102].

Partial or reversible bowel obstruction

Other than reducing the GI symptoms in definitive bowel obstruction, octreotide may be useful in reversing clinical conditions of subobstruction, as it can reduce the hypertensive state in the lumen, producing the sequence distension–secretion, which is propedeutic to definitive obstruction if not treated [89,97]. The most important mechanism in these circumstances is functional and can be reversible, if an aggressive treatment is initiated early before fecal impaction and edema render MBO irreversible. An early and intensive pharmacological treatment may not only reduce GI symptoms but also reverse MBO, in clinical conditions commonly considered definitive [97].

Mercadante et al. [105] studied 15 consecutive advanced cancer patients with inoperable MBO receiving octreotide in combination with metoclopramide, corticosteroids, and an initial bolus of amidotrizoate (a mixture of sodium diatrizoate, meglumine diatrizoate, and a wetting agent [polysorbate 80]). Recovery of bowel transit appeared in 1–5 days in 14 of 15 patients till death.

Few studies have addressed the use of long-acting octreotide in patients with advanced malignancies who developed MBO at some point during the course of the disease [106,107]. The efficacy and safety of octreotide long-acting release (LAR) at the dose of 30 mg on day 1 and octreotide for 2 weeks were evaluated in a pilot study of 15 patients with advanced ovarian cancer. Of 13 evaluable patients, 3 patients had a major efficacy to LAR treatment with reduction in GI symptoms, 2 had minor response, 4 patients had no response, and 4 had progressive symptoms. No significant toxicities were due to LAR [106].

We do think this is an interesting finding, but based on only small numbers of patients, we are unable to make further conclusions at the present time. It will be interesting to see more research in this area because this drug might be used potentially in the ambulatory setting. Recognizing that octreotide is an expensive therapy and considering the fact that the goal of the treatment is the improvement in the QOL of the patient and based on the strong evidence available in the literature that supports a real benefit with the use of this medication, the authors of this chapter consider that octreotide should be part of the treatment once the patient is diagnosed despite the cost.

Key learning points

1. Malignant bowel obstruction (MBO) is a distressing outcome above all in patients with abdominal and pelvic cancer in the advanced and terminal stage of disease.

2. Surgery should not routinely be undertaken in patients with poor prognostic criteria such as intra-abdominal carcinomatosis, poor performance status, and massive ascites.

3. Medical measures such as analgesics, antisecretory drugs, and antiemetics administered alone or in combination should be used to relieve symptoms.

4. Endoscopic management of MBO should always be considered.

5. A nasogastric tube (NGT) should be used only as a temporary measure, and a venting gastrostomy should be considered if drugs fail in reducing vomiting to an acceptable level.

6. Total parenteral nutrition (TPN) should be considered only for patients who may die for starvation rather than from tumor spread.

7. Parenteral hydration is sometimes indicated to correct nausea, and regular mouth care is the treatment of choice for dry mouth.

8. A collaborative approach by surgeons and physicians can offer patients an individualized and appropriate symptom management plan.

REFERENCES

1   Anthony T, Baron T, and Mercadante S et al. Report of the clinical protocol committee: Development of randomized trials for malignant bowel obstruction. *J Pain Symptom Manage* 2007; 34: S49–S59.

2   Krouse RS. The international conference on malignant bowel obstruction: A meeting of the minds to advance palliative care research. *J Pain Symptom Manage* 2007; 34: S1–S6.

◆ 3   Baines M. The pathophysiology and management of malignant intestinal obstruction. In: Doyle D, Hanks GWC, and MacDonald N, eds., *Oxford Test Book of Palliative Medicine*, 2nd ed. Oxford University Press, Oxford, U.K.; New York, 1998: p. 526.

◆ 4   Ripamonti C. Malignant bowel obstruction. In: Ripamonti C and Bruera E, eds., *Gastrointestinal Symptoms in Advanced Cancer Patients*. Oxford University Press, Oxford, U.K.; New York, 2002: Vol. 12, p. 235.

◆ 5   Ripamonti C and Mercadante S. Pathophysiology and management of Malignant Bowel obstruction. In: Doyle D, Hanks G et al., eds., *Oxford Textbook of Palliative Medicine*, 3rd ed. Oxford University Press, Oxford, U.K.; New York, 2004: Vol. 8, pp. 496–506.

● 6   Krebs HB and Goplerud DR. Mechanical intestinal obstruction in patients with gynecologic disease: A review of 368 patients. *Am J Obstet Gynecol* 1987; 157: 577–579.

✱ 7   Ripamonti C, Twycross R, Baines M, Bozzetti F, Capri S, De Conno F, Gemlo B et al. Clinical-practice recommendations for the management of bowel obstruction in patients with end-stage cancer. *Support Care Cancer* 2001; 19: 23–34.

◆ 8   Feuer DJ, Broadley KE, Shepherd JH, and Barton DPJ. Systematic review of surgery in malignant bowel obstruction in advanced gynecological and gastrointestinal cancer. *Gynecol Oncol* 1999; 75: 313–322.

● 9   Tunca JC, Buchler DA, Mack EA, Ruzicka FF, Crowley JJ, and Carr WF. The management of ovarian-cancer-caused bowel obstruction. *Gynecol Oncol* 1981; 12: 186–192.

● 10 Krebs HB and Goplerud DR. Surgical management of bowel obstruction in advanced ovarian carcinoma. *Obstet Gynecol* 1983; 61: 327–330.

11 Correa R, Ripamonti CI, Dodge JE, and Easson AM. Malignant bowel obstruction. In: Davis M et al. eds., *Supportive Oncology*. Elsevier/Saunders, Philadelphia, PA, 2011; Vol. 30, pp. 326–341.

12 Riley J and Fallon MT. Octreotide in terminal malignant obstruction of the gastrointestinal tract. *Eur J Palliat Care* 1994; 1: 23–28.

◆ 13 Ripamonti C, Panzeri C, Groff L et al. The role of somatostatin and octreotide in bowel obstruction: Pre-clinical and clinical results. *Tumori* 2001; 87: 1–9.

14 Furukawa A, Yamasaki M, Takahashi M, Nitta N, Tanaka T, Kanasaki S, Yokoyama K, Murata K, and Sakamoto T. CT diagnosis of small bowel obstruction: Scanning technique, interpretation and role in the diagnosis. *Semin Ultrasound CT MR* 2003; 24(5): 336–352.

15 Suri S, Gupta S, Sudhakar P J, Venkataramu N K, Sood B, and Wig JD. Comparative evaluation of plain films, ultrasound and CT in the diagnosis of intestinal obstruction. *Acta Radiol* 1999; 40(4): 422–428.

16 Angelelli G, Moschetta M, Binetti F, Cosmo T, and Stabile Ianora AA. Prognostic value of MDCT in malignant large-bowel obstructions. *Radiol Med* 2010; 115(5): 747–757.

17 Angelelli G, Moschetta M, Sabato L, Morella M, Scardapane A, and Stabile Ianora AA. Value of "protruding lips" sign in malignant bowel obstructions. *Eur J Radiol* 2011; 80(3): 681–685.

18 Krouse RS. Surgical palliation of bowel obstruction. *Gastroenterol Clin North Am* 2006; 35(1): 143–151.

19 Bryan D, Radbod R, and Berek J. An analysis of surgical versus chemotherapeutic intervention for the management of intestinal obstruction in advanced ovarian cancer. *Int J Gynecol Cancer* 2004; 16: 125–134.

20 Helyer LK, Law CH, Butler M, Last LD, Smith AJ, and Wright FC. Surgery as a bridge to palliative chemotherapy in patients with malignant bowel obstruction from colorectal cancer. *Ann Surg Oncol* 2007; 14(4): 1264–1271.

21 Abbas SM and Merrie AE. Resection of peritoneal metastases causing malignant small bowel obstruction. *World J Surg Oncol* 2007; 5(1): 122.

22 Wright FC, Chakraborty A, Helyer L, Moravan V, and Selby D. Predictors of survival in patients with non-curative stage IV cancer and malignant bowel obstruction. *J Surg Oncol* 2010; 101(5): 425–429.

23 Medina-Franco H, Garcia-Alvarez MN, Ortiz-Lopez LJ, Cuairan JZ. Predictors of adverse surgical outcome in the management of malignant bowel obstruction. *Rev Invest Clin* 2008; 60(3): 212–216.

24 Imai K, Yasuda H, Koda K, Suzuki M, Yamazaki M, Tezuka T, Kosugi C et al. An analysis of palliative surgery for the patients with malignant bowel obstruction. *Gan To Kagaku Ryoho* 2010; 37(Suppl 2): 264–267.

25 Hancock K, Clayton JM, Parker SM, Wal der S, Butow PN, Carrick S, Currow D et al. Truth-telling in discussing prognosis in advanced life-limiting illnesses: A systematic review. *Palliat Med* 2007; 21(6): 507–517.

26 Hofmann B, Haheim LL, and Soreide JA. Ethics of palliative surgery in patients with cancer. *Br J Surg* 2005; 92(7): 802–809.

27 Dalal KM, Gollub MJ, Miner TJ, Wong WD, Gerdes H, Schattner MA, Jaques DP, and Temple LK. Management of patients with malignant bowel obstruction and stage IV colorectal cancer. *J Palliat Med* 2011; 14(7): 822–828.

28 Chakraborty A, Selby D, Gardiner K, Myers J, Moravan V, and Wright F. Malignant bowel obstruction: Natural history of a heterogeneous patient population followed prospectively over two years. *J Pain Symptom Manage* 2011; 41(2): 412–420.

29 Braga M, Ljungqvist O, Soeters P, Fearon K, Weimann A, and Bozzetti F. ESPEN guidelines on parenteral nutrition: Surgery. *Clin Nutr* 2009; 28(4): 378–386.

30 MacDonald N, Easson AM, Mazurak VC, Dunn GP, and Baracos VE. Understanding and managing cancer cachexia. *J Am Coll Surg* 2003; 197(1): 143–161.

31 Bozzetti F, Arends J, Lundholm K, Micklewright A, Zurcher G, and Muscaritoli M. ESPEN guidelines on parenteral nutrition: Non-surgical oncology. *Clin Nutr* 2009; 28(4): 445–454.

32 Varker KA, Ansel A, Aukerman G, and Carson WE, III. Review of complementary and alternative medicine and selected nutraceuticals: Background for a pilot study on nutrigenomic intervention in patients with advanced cancer. *Altern Ther Health Med* 2012; 18(2): 26–34.

33 Paccagnella A, Morassutti I, and Rosti G. Nutritional intervention for improving treatment tolerance in cancer patients. *Curr Opin Oncol* 2011; 23(4): 322–330.

34 Rabinovitch R, Grant B, Berkey BA, Raben D, Ang KK, Fu KK, and Cooper JS. Impact of nutrition support on treatment outcome in patients with locally advanced head and neck squamous cell cancer treated with definitive radiotherapy: A secondary analysis of RTOG trial 90-03. *Head Neck* 2006; 28(4): 287–296.

35 Rueda JR, Sola I, Pascual A, and Subirana CM. Non-invasive interventions for improving well-being and quality of life in patients with lung cancer. *Cochrane Database Syst Rev* 2011; 2011(9): CD004282.

36   Mainar A, De Gregorio MA, Tejero E et al. Acute colorectal obstruction: Treatment with self-expandable metallic stents before scheduled surgery: Results of a multicenter study. *Radiology* 1999; 210: 65–69.

37   Lowe AS, Beckett CG, Jowett S et al. Self-expandable metal stent placement for the palliation of malignant gastroduodenal obstruction: Experience in a large, single, UK centre. *Clin Radiol* 2007; 62: 738–744.

38   Telford JJ, Carr-Locke DL, Baron TH et al. Palliation of patients with malignant gastric outlet obstruction with the enteral Wallstent: Outcomes from a multicenter study. *Gastrointest Endosc* 2004; 60: 916–920.

39   Dormann A, Meisner S, Verin N et al. Self-expanding metal stents for gastroduodenal malignancies: Systematic review of their clinical effectiveness. *Endoscopy* 2004; 36: 543–550.

40   Nassif T, Prat F, Meduri B et al. Endoscopic palliation of malignant gastric outlet obstruction using self-expandable metallic stents: Results of a multicenter study. *Endoscopy* 2003; 35: 483–489.

41   Costamagna G, Tringali A, Spicak J et al. Treatment of malignant gastroduodenal obstruction with a nitinol self-expanding metal stent: An international prospective multicentre registry. *Dig Liv Dis,* 2012; 44(1): 37–43.

42   Arya N, Bair D, Arya P, and Pham J. Community experience of colonic stenting in patients with acute large bowel obstructions. *Can J Surg* 2011; 54(4): 283–285.

43   Piesman M, Kozarek RA, Brandbur JJ et al. Improved oral intake after palliative duodenal stenting for malignant obstruction: A prospective multicenter clinical trial. *Am J Gastro* 2009; 104: 2403–2411.

44   Espinel J, Sanz O, Vivas S et al. Malignant gastrointestinal obstruction: Endoscopic stenting versus surgical palliation. *Surg Endosc* 2006; 20: 1083–1087.

45   Lillemoe KD, Cameron JL, Hardacre JM et al. Is prophylactic gastrojejunostomy indicated for unresectable periampullary cancer? A prospective randomized trial. *Ann Surg* 1999; 230: 322–328. Discussion 328–330.

46   Jeurnink SM, Steyerberg EW, Hof GV et al. Gastrojejunostomy versus stent placement in patients with malignant gastric outlet obstruction: A comparison in 95 patients. *J Surg Oncol* 2007; 96: 389–396.

47   Mendelsohn RB, Gerdes H, Markowitz AJ et al. Carcinomatosis is not a contraindication to enteral stenting in selected patients with malignant gastric outlet obstruction. *Gastrointest Endosc* June 2011; 73(6): 1135–1140. Epub April 5, 2011.

48   Kim JH, Son HY, Shin JH et al. Metallic stent placement in the palliative treatment of malignant gastroduodenal obstructions: Prospective evaluation of results and factors influencing outcome in 213 patients. *Gastrointest Endosc* 2007; 66: 256–264.

49   Holt AP, Patel M, Ahmed MM. Palliation of patients with malignant gastroduodenal obstruction with self-expanding metallic stents: The treatment of choice? *Gastrointest Endosc* 2004; 60: 1010–1017.

50   Jang JK, Song HY, Kim JH et al. Tumor overgrowth after expandable metallic stent placement: Experience in 583 patients with malignant gastroduodenal obstruction. *Am J Roentgenol* June 2011; 196(6): W831–W836.

51   Dafnis G._Repeated coaxial colonic stenting in the palliative management of benign colonic obstruction. *Eur J Gastroenterol Hepatol* January 2007; 19(1): 83–86.

52   Wong YT, Brams DM, Munson L et al. Gastric outlet obstruction secondary to pancreatic cancer: Surgical vs endoscopic palliation. *Surg Endosc* 2002; 16: 310–312.

53   Phillips MS, Gosain S, Bonatti H et al. Enteral stents for malignancy: A report of 46 consecutive cases over 10 years, with critical review of complications. *J Gastrointest Surg* November 2008; 12(11): 2045–2050. Epub July 22, 2008.

54   Mehta S, Hindmarsh A, Cheong E et al. Prospective randomized trial of laparoscopic gastrojejunostomy versus duodenal stenting for malignant gastric outflow obstruction. *Surg Endosc* 2006; 20: 239–242.

55   Schmidt C, Gerdes H, Hawkins W et al. A prospective observational study examining quality of life in patients with malignant gastric outlet obstruction. *Am J Surg* 2009; 198: 92–99.

56   Lennon AM, Chandrasekhara V, Shin EJ et al. Spiral-enteroscopy-assisted enteral stent placement for palliation of malignant small-bowel obstruction. *GIE* 2010; 71(2): 422–425.

57   Ross AS, Semrad C, Waxman I et al. Enteral stent placement by double balloon enteroscopy for palliation of malignant small bowel obstruction. *GIE* 2006; 65(5): 835–837.

58   Lee H, Park JC, Shin SK et al. Preliminary study of enteroscopy-guided, self-expandable metal stent placement for malignant small bowel obstruction. *J Gastroenterol Hepatol* 2012; 27(7): 1181–1186.

59   Camunez F, Echenagusia A, Simo G et al. Malignant colorectal obstruction treated by means of self-expanding metallic stents: Effectiveness before surgery and in palliation. *Radiology* 2000; 216: 492–497.

60   Law WL, Chu KW, Ho JW et al. Self-expanding metallic stent in the treatment of colonic obstruction caused by advanced malignancies. *Dis Colon Rectum* 2000; 43: 1522–1527.

61   Nash CL, Markowitz AJ, Schattner M et al. Colorectal stents for the management of malignant large bowel obstruction. *Gastrointest Endo* 2002; 55: AB216.

62   Pothuri B, Guiguis A, Gerdes H et al. The use of colorectal stents for palliation of large bowel obstruction due to recurrent gynecologic cancer. *Gynecol Oncol* 2004; 95: 513–517.

63   Khot UP, Wenk Lang A, Murali K et al. Systematic review of the efficacy and safety of colorectal stents. *Br J Surg* 2002; 89: 1096–1102.

64   Sebastian S, Johnston S, Geoghegan T et al. Pooled analysis of the efficacy and safety of self-expanding metal stenting in malignant colorectal obstruction. *Am J Gastro* 2004; 99: 2051–2057.

65   Caceres A, Zhou Q, Iasonos A et al. Colorectal stents for palliation of large-bowel obstructions in recurrent gynecologic cancer: An updated series. *Gynecol Oncol.* March 2008; 108(3): 482–485.

66   Nagula S, Ishil N, Nash C et al. Quality of life and symptom control after stent placement or surgical palliation of malignant colorectal obstruction. *J Am Coll Surg* 2010; 210: 45–53.

67   Meisner S, Gonzalez-Huix F, Vandervoort JG et al. Self-expandable metal stents for relieving malignant colorectal obstruction: Short-term safety and efficacy within 30 days of stent procedure in 447 patients. *Gastro Endo* 2011; 74(4): 876–884.

68   Dohmoto M, Hunerbein M, and Schlag PM. Application of rectal stents for palliation of obstructing rectosigmoid cancer. *Surg Endosc* 1997; 11: 758–761.

69   Campagnutta E, Cannizzaro R, Gallo A et al. Palliative treatment of upper intestinal obstruction by gynecological malignancy: The usefulness of percutaneous endoscopic gastrostomy. *Gynecol Oncol* 1996; 62: 103–105.

70   Pothuri B, Montemarano M, Gerardi M et al. Percutaneous endoscopic gastrostomy tube placement in patients with malignant bowel obstruction due to ovarian carcinoma. *Gynecol Oncol* 2005; 96: 330–334.

71   Vashi PG, Dahlk S, Vashi RP et al. Percutaneous endoscopic gastrostomy tube occlusion in malignant peritoneal carcinomatosis-induced bowel obstruction. *Eur J Gastroenterol Hepatol.* November 2011; 23(11): 1069–1073.

72   Piccinni G, Angrisano A, Testini M et al. Venting direct percutaneous jejunostomy (DPEJ) for drainage of malignant bowel obstruction in patients operated on for gastric cancer. *Support Care Cancer* 2005; 13: 535–539.

● 73   Baines M, Oliver DJ, and Carter RL. Medical management of intestinal obstruction in patients with advanced malignant disease: A clinical and pathological study. *Lancet* 1985; 2: 990–993.

74   Clark K, Lam L, and Currow D. Reducing gastric secretions—A role for histamine 2 antagonists or proton pump inhibitors in malignant bowel obstruction? *Support Care Cancer* 2009; 17(12): 1463–1468.

◆ 75   Feuer DJ and Broadley KE, members of the systematic review steering committee. Systematic review and meta-analysis of corticosteroids for the resolution of malignant bowel obstruction in advanced gynaecological and gastrointestinal cancers. *Ann Oncol* 1999; 10: 1035–1041.

76   Porzio G, Aielli F, Verna L, Galletti B, Shoja E, Razavi G, and Ficorella C. Can malignant bowel obstruction in advanced cancer patients be treated at home? *Support Care Cancer* 2011; 19: 431–433.

77   Ventafridda V, Ripamonti C, Caraceni A et al. The management of inoperable gastrointestinal obstruction in terminal cancer patients. *Tumori* 1990; 76: 389–393

78   Fainsinger RL, Spachynski K, Hanson J et al. Symptom control in terminally ill patients with malignant bowel obstruction. *J Pain Symptom Manage* 1994; 9: 12–18.

79   De Conno F, Caraceni A, Zecca E et al. Continuous subcutaneous infusion of hyoscine butylbromide reduces secretions in patients with gastrointestinal obstruction. *J Pain Sympt Manage* 1991; 6: 484–486.

80   Davis MP, Furste A. Glycopyrrolate: A useful drug in the palliation of mechanical bowel obstruction. *J Pain Symptom Manage* 1999; 18: 153–154.

81   Basson MD, Fielding LP, Bilchik AJ, Zucker KA, Ballantyne GH, Sussman J, Adrian TE, Modlin IM. Does vasoactive intestinal polypeptide mediate the pathophysiology of bowel obstruction? *Am J Surg* 1989; 157: 109–115.

82   Nellgard P, Bojo L, and Cassuto J. Importance of vasoactive intestinal peptide and somatostatin for fluid losses in small-bowel obstruction. *Scan J Gastroenterol* 1995; 30: 464–469.

83   Neville R, Fielding P, Cambria RP, and Modlin I. Vascular responsiveness in obstructed gut. *Dis Col Rect* 1991; 34: 229–235.

84   Dharmsathaphorn K, Binder HJ, and Dobbins WJ. Somatostatin stimulates sodium and chloride absorption in the rabbit ileum. *Gastroenterology* 1980; 78: 1559–1565.

85   Nellgard P and Cassuto J. Inflammation as a major cause of fluid losses in small-bowel obstruction. *Scand J Gastroenterol* 1993; 28: 1035–1041.

86   Yatani A, Birnbaumer L, and Brown AM. Direct coupling of the somatostatin receptor to potassium channels by a G protein. *Metabolism* 1990; 39(9 Suppl): 91–95.

87   Ripamonti C and Mercadante S. How to use octreotide for malignant bowel obstruction. *J Support Oncol* 2004; 2/4: 357–364.

88   Yamaner S, Bugra D, Muslumanoglu M, Bulut T, Cubukcu O, and Ademoglu E. Effects of octreotide on healing of intestinal anastomosis following small bowel obstruction in rats. *Dis Colon Rectum* 1995; 38/3: 308–312.

● 89   Mercadante S, Avola G, Maddaloni S, Salamone G, Aragona F, and Rodolico V. Octreotide prevents the pathological alterations of bowel obstruction in cancer patients. *Support Care Cancer* 1996; 4: 393–394.

90   Sun X, Li X, and Li H. Management of intestinal obstruction in advanced ovarian cancer: An analysis of 57 cases. *Chung Hua Chung Liu Tsa Chih* 1995; 17: 39–42.

91   Khoo D, Riley J, and Waxman J. Control of emesis in bowel obstruction in terminally ill patients. *Lancet* 1992; 339: 375–376.

● 92   Mercadante S and Maddaloni S. Octreotide in the management of inoperable gastrointestinal obstruction in terminal cancer patients. *J Pain Symptom Manage* 1992; 7(8): 496–498.

93   Mercadante S, Spoldi E, Caraceni A, Maddaloni S, and Simonetti MT. Octreotide in relieving gastrointestinal symptoms due to bowel obstruction. *Palliat Med* 1993; 7: 295–299.

94   Mangili G, Franchi M, Mariani A, Zanaboni F, Rabaiotti E, Frigerio L, Bolis PF, and Ferrari A. Octreotide in the management of bowel obstruction in terminal Ovarian cancer. *Gynecol Oncol* 1996; 61: 345–348.

95   Steadman K and Franks A. A woman with malignant bowel obstruction who did not want to die with tubes. *Lancet* 1996; 347: 944.

96   Sartori S, Trevisani L, Nielsen I, Tassinari D, and Righini E. Identification of a safe site for percutaneous endoscopic gastrostomy placement in patients with marked bowel distension: May octreotide have a role? *Endoscopy* 1994; 26: 710–711.

● 97   Mercadante S, Kargar J, and Nicolosi G. Octreotide may prevent definitive intestinal obstruction. *J Pain Symptom Manage* 1997; 13: 352–355.

98   Fainsinger RL, MacEachern T, Miller MJ et al. The use of hypodermoclysis for rehydration in terminally ill cancer patients. *J Pain Sympt Manage* 1994; 9: 298–302.

99   Shima Y, Ohtsu A, Shirao K and Sasaki Y. Clinical efficacy and safety of octreotide (SMS201–995) in terminally ill Japanese cancer patients with malignant bowel obstruction. *Jpn J Clin Oncol* 2008; 38: 354–359.

100   Hisanaga T, Shinjo T, Morita T, Nakajima N, Ikenaga M, Tanimizu M, Kizawa Y, Maeno T, Shima Y, and Hyodo I. Multicenter prospective study on efficacy and safety of Octreotide for inoperable malignant bowel obstruction. *Jpn J Clin Oncol* 2010; 40: 739–745.

101   Mercadante S. Scopolamine butylbromide plus octreotide in unresponsive bowel obstruction. *J Pain Symptom Manage* 1998; 16(5): 278–279.

102   Ripamonti C, Mercadante S, Groff L, Zecca E, De Conno F, and Casuccio A. Role of octreotide, scopolamine butylbromide and hydration in symptom control of patients with inoperable bowel obstruction having a nasogastric tube. A prospective, randomized clinical trial. *J Pain Symptom Manage* 2000; 19(1): 23–34.

103   Mercadante S, Ripamonti C, Casuccio A, Zecca E, and Groff L. Comparison of octreotide and hyoscine butylbromide in controlling gastrointestinal symptoms due to malignant inoperable bowel obstruction. *Support Care Cancer* 2000; 8: 188–191.

104   Mystakidou K, Tsilika E, Kalaidopoulou O, Chondros K, Georgaki S, and Papadimitriou L. Comparison of octreotide administration vs conservative treatment in the management of inoperable bowel obstruction in patients with far advanced cancer: A randomized, double- blind, controlled clinical trial. *Anticancer Res* 2002; 22: 1187–1192.

105   Mercadante S, Ferrera P, Villari P, and Maeeazzo A. Aggressive pharmacological treatment for reversing bowel obstruction. *J Pain Symptom Manage* 2004; 28: 412–416.

106   Matulonis UA, Seiden MV, Roche M, Krasner C, Fuller AF, Atkinson T, Kornblith A, and Person R. Long-acting octreotide for the treatment and symptomatic relief of bowel obstruction in advanced ovarian cancer. *J Pain Symptom Manage* 2005; 30: 563–569.

107   Massacesi C and Galeazzi G. Sustained release octreotide may have a role in the treatment of malignant bowel obstruction. *Palliat Med* 2006; 20: 715–716.

63

Endoscopic treatment of gastrointestinal symptoms

PASQUALE SPINELLI

INTRODUCTION

Most tumors, and 99% of the digestive ones, are *endo*cavitary, and thus, *endo*scopy is the most suitable approach for them, for diagnostic as well as therapeutic purposes. Endocavitary treatment of cancer may lead to the cure of superficial, locally extending, nonmetastatic lesions or palliation of noncurable tumors. Digestive cancers form about 20% of all diagnosed cancers; when these are advanced, most of them are poorly responsive to curative treatments; consequently, patients not responding to curative treatment will need symptomatic, palliative treatment.

Palliative care has appropriately been receiving increased attention in recent years. Palliation, by itself, can be defined as the treatment of the symptoms of a disease. Palliative treatment is planned when it is impossible to treat a disease for cure. Palliation would be better defined by dividing it into the following:

- Palliative care—which includes the treatments required during the course of patients with advanced tumors from a stage of specific disease status to the stage of terminal events
- Control of symptoms—which concerns an earlier stage in the natural history of the disease, when there is an acceptable disease-related quality of life[1]

In view of these distinctions, palliative treatments to control symptoms should start as soon as the disease is classified as incurable.[2] It could happen at the time of the diagnosis if conditions preventing curative treatments already exist. Palliation must be undertaken if anticancer treatments are not considered advisable because of general or local reasons, such as in cases where anticancer treatments would waste the time and resources that could be used for a more tolerable and profitable symptomatic approach.

Diagnosis of a solid cancer must be followed by the staging, as therapeutic options and prognosis are strictly related to the stage. Staging procedures are based on sophisticated and precise diagnostic tools so that the oncologist should be able to separate localized from diffused and curable from noncurable diseases in the majority of cases. In fact, all suitable diagnostic possibilities must be considered to identify patients with noncurable disease as early as possible and, thus, avoid giving them inefficacious, sometime toxic, and always costly anticancer treatments, instead managing their symptoms appropriately.[3] Before deciding on palliative care to treat only the symptoms and waiving the possibility of directly treating the disease, the following points should be considered:

- The different curative potentials of surgery, radiotherapy, chemotherapy, immunotherapy, and any other kind of certified treatments
- Risk factors in a particular patient
- Side effects of a treatment
- Quality of the remaining life of the patient
- Weighing up the real impact of the therapeutic procedures with regard to the expected benefits[4*]

With the availability of a variety of new prognostic indicators in the form of molecular, clinical, and pathological testing, the possibility that they could also be used for distinguishing potentially curable from noncurable patients has emerged. Analysis of gene expression patterns may be useful in the future for predicting the response to an anticancer treatment.[4,5*]

PALLIATIVE TREATMENTS: GENERAL CONCEPTS

Surgery

Surgery can be indicated in various contexts and is generally the first option to be considered.[6**] From the surgeon's standpoint, therapy is considered palliative when resection of all known tumor sites is no longer possible or advisable. Since a cure, as it is commonly defined, is not possible, the success of the therapy is determined by the alleviation of the suffering. A part of the gastrointestinal tract may be resected in the presence of painful obstructive symptoms with the aim of relieving pain, restoring the lumen, and reducing bleeding by removing a tumor. Bypass operations, indicated in cases of nonresectable tumor masses, may be performed through traditional laparotomy and also through laparoscopic access, achieving the double goal of minimum trauma and quick recovery. The appropriate use of surgery in these settings can improve the quality of life of patients with cancer.

Radiotherapy

In the presence of unresectable tumors, radiotherapy reduces the tumor volume. It does seem to be of benefit in selected cases with large cancers because it may reduce the mass and make it resectable. Under specific circumstances, it can be given together with endoscopic treatments, thus combining endoluminal with the extraluminal benefits of mass reduction. In some cancers causing local symptoms, reduction of the size of the tumor and of the extravisceral extension of the tumor with radiation therapy results in partial control of pain. This treatment can be used alone or in combination with other anti-cancer treatments.[7]

Among the different radiotherapeutic options, brachyther-apy can better localize radiation dose with limited side effects; this is important when treating previously irradiated areas.[8]

Chemotherapy

Chemotherapy using multiagent regimens has an advantage for palliation of unresectable or metastatic cancer in cases of medium survival, but there is no confirmed advantage in cases of long-term survival. Chemotherapy is used to reduce the size of masses and to alleviate symptoms. Furthermore, in patients who have locally advanced, unresectable disease and in patients in whom tumors are resected with positive margins, the dura-tion of survival can be increased with palliative chemotherapy and irradiation.[9] Along with chemotherapy, endoscopic treat-ments aimed at immediately relieving the obstruction of an occluded cavity may be strongly advisable in selected cases, allowing for functional recovery.[10]

PALLIATIVE CARE FOR GASTROINTESTINAL SYMPTOMS

From the endoscopic point of view, both primary digestive cancers and their metastases can compromise esophageal, tracheobronchial, biliary, and urinary functions, depending on their location. In consideration of these concepts, pallia-tive care should not be limited to the patients with pretermi-nal disease, but greatly expanded, starting with the control of symptoms as soon as the disease is classified as incurable and avoiding unnecessary anticancer treatments. As stated earlier in this chapter, when a solid cancer is diagnosed, the disease must be staged, as therapeutic options and prognosis are related to the stage. Since the disease is staged through precise diagnostic procedures, one should be able to separate localized from diffused and curable from noncurable cancers in most cases.

The continuing increase of the lifespan that has happened in recent years entails a constant increase in the incidence of age-related malignant neoplasms; advanced age, together with related risk factors, reduces the possibility of performing radi-cal treatments and opens the doors to palliative treatments. In current clinical practice, however, most patients are treated with curative intent, even when palliation of symptoms would have been the right choice. Furthermore, the majority of clini-cal trials currently in progress are evaluating the response to treatments in terms of decrease in the volume of the tumor mass and global survival but neglecting the evaluation of the impact of the treatment toxicity and of the general side effects on the quality of life and on the relationships of the patients with the people around them.

Although the primary purpose of a palliative procedure is not to increase survival, the treatment of severe symptoms (nutritional, respiratory, or metabolic) as in tumors resulting in stenosis of the esophagus, trachea, or intestinal, biliary, or urinary tracts very often results in an effective extension of the survival time. Consequently, palliation becomes, in many cases, not just the simple treatment of symptoms, but it offers to the patient a wide range of therapeutic opportunities during the entire course of the disease.

Endoscopic palliative treatments aim to obtain the best pos-sible quality of life with immediate and durable benefits with negligible trauma, side effects, and incidence of complications related to the proposed advantages. Although these objectives seem to be obvious, it often happens that these simple prin-ciples—essential to the correct approach to the oncological patient—are not adopted and patients are submitted to treat-ments that are not suited to their requirements and their health status. In everyday practice, it frequently happens that patients who only need control of symptoms related to the size and site of the tumor masses and to their relations with the surround-ing anatomical structures are overtreated.

Palliative treatment of an oncological patient under these conditions must be tailored so that the quality of life offered by the treatment is more consistent with their lifestyle, and, when possible, it should be planned in agreement with the patient. This is because there are different ways to achieve relief from one symptom. The physician must be able to inform the patient about the different methods available so that they can choose the one that fits better with their preferred lifestyle. For exam-ple, esophageal stenosis can be relieved by a nasogastric tube, by a laser treatment, by a gastrostomy, or by a palliative radio-chemotherapy: patients must be informed about these options so that they can decide which one is the most suitable for their way of life.

In the field of clinical research, human resources are insuffi-cient, and dedicated researchers are spread out among numer-ous—and partly curative—projects and not focused on specific palliation research. This is of concern also to endoscopic pallia-tive treatments, as these are less widely known and used than they should be, considering the palliative opportunities they offer to oncological patients. Methodologically appropriate research is needed to bring into focus the indications of these methods and disseminate awareness about them.

Gastrointestinal symptoms may be produced by digestive or extradigestive tumors. Most of these tumors affect the digestive cavities and grow into them, occupying the spaces required for the digestive functions. The gastrointestinal tract has cavities that function as "containers" or as "canals" (stomach, esophagus, intestine, biliary, and pancreatic tract). Tumors reduce the space available and impair the functions of containing and flowing; moreover, tumors that infiltrate and ulcerate the walls of these cavities generate symptoms; in particular, they cause hemorrhage, obstruction, perforation, and fistula formation. The most important symptoms of digestive tumors are dysphagia, salivation, vomiting, jaundice, pain, and hemorrhage. All these symptoms can be treated by endoscopic modalities.

Dysphagia

Dysphagia is the most severe symptom of pharyngo-esophageal tumors. Malignant dysphagia can be in relation to the presence of a primary or secondary esophageal tumor, or it can be consequent to a surgical treatment or to a radiotherapy or chemotherapy. Dysphagia can be defined as an abnormal swallowing, characterized by difficulty in transferring solid or liquid food from the mouth to the stomach; it is the initial symptom of an esophageal cancer in 90% of cases, but it may also be caused by compression or infiltration by thyroid or lung tumors, mediastinal lymphomas, or metastatic involvement of the mediastinum, mainly by breast cancer. Dysphagia can be associated with pain (odynophagia) and aspiration of food and saliva into the trachea and bronchi and with chronic cough, asthma, laryngitis, and, eventually, pneumonia.

Beyond the most common causes, in oncological patients, dysphagia may occur due to the following:

- Neurological reasons, for example, cricopharyngeal dysphagia because of recurrent nerve palsy due to perineural and neural infiltration by tumor tissue; neurological dysphagia may also occur due to vagal or sympathetic tumoral infiltration, with the involvement of the skull base or due to brain metastases.
- Mucositis related to candidosis, bacterial infection, herpes, radiotherapy, chemotherapy.
- Asthenia/cachexia.

From the mechanical viewpoint, a patient becomes dysphagic when the diameter of the esophageal lumen is less than 14 mm, but an uncertain feeling of trouble in swallowing is generally complained of some weeks or months before the diagnosis of esophageal cancer.

Esophagoscopy is indicated when a patient complains of dysphagia; its performance can be indicated in the various phases of diagnosis, staging, and treatment. It allows the surgeon to characterize and exactly locate a tumor, to measure its length and appreciate the circular extent and the size of the residual esophageal lumen, and to obtain histological confirmation of the clinical diagnosis. Echoendoscopy is extremely useful for determining the level of infiltration of the lesion across the esophageal wall, the involvement of neighboring anatomical structures, and the eventual presence of metastatic

lymph nodes. Infiltration of the wall interrupts the progression of peristaltic contraction and stops, temporarily or definitively, the progression of food; this interruption is related to the extent of the obstruction, and it causes a variety of symptoms, depending on whether it is partial or total. Partial obstruction can stop solid food but allows passage of liquids; total obstruction, which stops the flow of liquids too, causes liquids to collect above the site of the obstruction and between the obstruction and the upper esophageal sphincter.

Regurgitation, salivation, odynophagia

Long-standing stenoses can cause incompetence—permanent or episodic—of the upper esophageal sphincter and the regurgitation of undigested material together with the possibility of inhalation; the amount of this collection is related to the level of the obstruction, being much larger when the lesion is close to the cardia; moreover, total obstruction stops the passage of saliva and causes the onset of another invalidating symptom, that is, salivation.

The patient complaining of salivation is obliged to spit or dribble continuously and walks around with a bag full of handkerchiefs—deprived of a social life. Dysphagia can be associated with odynophagia, generally caused by inflammation of the esophageal wall or by candidiasis or herpes-virus; odynophagia too may cause salivation. Salivation and regurgitation often cause coughing as patients attempt to swallow and may simulate an esophago-respiratory fistula. This false diagnosis can be confirmed by a bronchogram due to the regurgitation of contrast medium when performing an esophagogram; it may be further confirmed by the fact that, after insertion of a stent into a stenotic esophagus, cough on swallowing disappears not because the inexistent fistula has been closed, but because, after the opening of the esophageal transit, there is no more esophago-respiratory regurgitation. Consequently, the diagnosis of esophago-respiratory fistula must be confirmed by a tracheo-bronchoscopy, although nasal regurgitation is suggestive of the presence of a tracheo-esophageal or broncho-esophageal fistula. When dealing with an oncological patient for palliative purposes, one should learn to give the patient the opportunity to fully explain the symptoms of the disease. A combination of an accurate clinical history and the results of the investigations often allows planning of treatment with a reduced number and frequency of traumatic and time-consuming examinations in these patients with a limited survival time.

Palliative endoscopic options for dysphagia

NASOGASTRIC TUBE

The objective of esophagoscopic treatment of dysphagia and its sequelae is based on crossing the obstacle that prevents the passage of food: this can be achieved by a nasogastric tube, by restoring the esophageal lumen by dilation, laser treatment, photodynamic treatment, or prostheses insertion or performing a gastrostomy. These different options have specific indications.[10] The purpose of inserting a nasogastric tube is feeding liquid food, and it is an alternative to a gastrostomy. The indication is restricted to cases in which the stenotic obstacle cannot be dilated more than 4–5 mm; this mainly happens when there is postoperative or postradiotherapy fibrotic stenosis that makes forced dilation dangerous as there is a possibility of perforation.

There are several different disadvantages of the nasogastric tube:

- Esthetic—the patient is obliged to live with the tube coming out of his or her nose
- Functional—the external surface of the tube adheres strictly to the inner surface of the stenotic tract, and this prevents saliva from being swallowed, leading to salivation
- Sensuous—with food introduced through the tube, the patient is unable to enjoy its taste, one of the few pleasant sensations remaining at this stage of the life.

These disadvantages have also to be considered when planning to perform a gastrostomy, because, except for the presence of the nasal tube, patients complain of these symptoms after the creation of a gastrostomy.

DILATION

Dilation can be performed by pneumatic balloon dilators or by plastic bougies: both can slide along a guidewire and enlarge the esophageal lumen up to 20 mm. There are also balloons that can be introduced through the operative channel of the endoscope and guided into the stenotic tract under direct vision; the drawback of the dilation is that the stenosis will recur in 1–3 weeks, and dilations must be frequently repeated.

LASER TREATMENT

This aims to reopen the esophageal lumen through the thermal coagulation–destruction of the cancer tissue: power laser radiation increases the local temperature of the irradiated tissues and causes the tissue water to evaporate. The neodymium:yttrium aluminum garnet (Nd:YAG) laser is the most frequently used due to the depth of the penetration of its radiation into the cancer tissue. The treatment is precise and safe in appropriate hands, and the esophageal lumen can be fully restored so as to obtain a satisfactory eating function; the mean duration of the patency of the lumen is estimated to be 4–8 weeks.[11]

Laser treatments were more popular before the end of last century. Most centers abandoned laser techniques in favor of stents, easier to be inserted, safer, and maintaining a more durable palliation.[12]

PHOTODYNAMIC THERAPY

Photodynamic therapy (PDT) uses photosensitizing drugs from the group of porphyrins that are selectively fixed by the tumor. The photosensitizer, activated by light, produces singlet oxygen that is toxic for biological tissues and causes a necrotic effect; unlike the procedures, discussed earlier, which are performed to allow the passage of food, the necrotic effect of PDT needs 4–8 days to become apparent, and the relief from obstruction lasts for 5–10 weeks.[13] However, patients submitted to PDT have to avoid direct sunlight for 4–6 weeks because of the skin photosensitization.[14]

PROSTHESES

The fate of all these procedures is the recurrence of the obstruction due to the regrowth of the tumor, unless a prosthesis is inserted after dilation of the stenotic tract.[15] Both disposal plastic and metallic prostheses are available. The plastic ones require full dilation of the lumen (17 mm to insert a 15 mm prosthesis), unlike the metallic ones, that, being expandable, can be introduced through a narrow (7–9 mm) passage, to reach, at the end of the expansion, an internal diameter of 20–22 mm, allowing an optimal and immediate transit for any kind of food.[16] The insertion of an expandable prosthesis is no more traumatic than a flexible esophagoscopy.

A new horizon is open by the drug-eluting stents. Gemcitabine-eluting metal stents were prepared for potential application as drug delivery systems for localized treatment of malignant tumors in the digestive tract. The controlled release of gemcitabine from covered drug-eluting stents may increase the patency of these stents as well as cancer-related stenosis.[17]

The differences between plastic and expandable prostheses are as follows: the plastic ones have a narrower lumen and give rise to a larger number of complications (migration, perforation, obstruction by solid food) whereas the expandable ones are much more expensive, cannot be removed, and, being woven as meshes, cannot be used to close fistulas. Recently, covered stents to be used in cases with fistulas have been manufactured, but the possibility of migration is higher than with noncovered stents, particularly when inserted through the cardia. Prostheses can be obstructed by large morsels or by regrowth of the tumor. The best results are obtained when the prosthesis does not interfere with the mechanism of a sphincter (the pharyngo-esophageal or the cardiac sphincter).[18] When the cardiac sphincter is infiltrated by the tumor, and the prosthesis keeps it open, the valvular antireflux mechanism is impaired, and the gastric content flows back into the esophagus. The acid gastric secretion can be responsible for supra-prosthetic esophagitis, and this condition causes dysphagia even though the esophagus is patent. However, in patients submitted to gastrectomy or operated on with techniques including vagotomy, in which the gastric environment is alkaline, the reflux through the prosthesis may give rise to an alkaline esophagitis. While in the first group of patients, drugs that increase the pH, such as proton pump inhibitors, are indicated, in the second group, with alkaline esophagitis, these drugs worsen the dysphagic symptoms. Therefore, special attention must be paid to the medical treatment of patients with patent prosthesis complaining of resistant dysphagia. Special prostheses with antireflux mechanisms have been recently manufactured, but definite results of their use are not yet available.[19] The use of biodegradable stents in malignant esophageal strictures for the treatment of dysphagia can be considered as a new frontier.[20] When the pharyngo-esophageal sphincter is involved and the insertion of the prosthesis keeps it open, the patient must adapt the swallowing mechanism to this new condition, and that may need some days or weeks to be perfected.

In patients predicted to have a long survival, the evolution of the cancer through the esophageal wall can be in the form of the development of a fistula, connecting the esophageal lumen with the skin of the neck, the trachea, a bronchus, the mediastinum, or the pleural space. Prostheses are equally used in these patients to bypass the fistula, allowing immediate passage of the oral intake. Fistulas can be consequent to tumor infiltration or previous surgery or radiotherapy.[21] Insertion of a prosthesis to bypass a fistula allows immediate restoration of oral feeding and curing of concomitant dermatitis (in cervical fistulas), bronchopneumonia (in tracheo- and broncho-esophageal fistulas), mediastinitis (in mediastinal fistulas), and pleural effusions (in esophago-pleural fistulas). Obviously, only plastic stents or covered mesh stents can be used in the indication of closing a fistulous passage, because a simple mesh stent would allow the filtration of liquids through the mesh.[20] Covered stents have a tendency to migrate, and their application must be carefully evaluated, because an eventual removal may be extremely difficult. The new self-expanding plastic stents have been used in the treatment of thoracic leaks after esophagectomy for cancer; these stents can be easily removed after the fistula repair, and their application reduces leak-related morbidity and mortality and can be considered as a cost-effective alternative to surgery and other endoscopic treatments.[20]

If an esophago-tracheal or an esophago-bronchial fistula cannot be treated by inserting a stent into the esophagus (no concomitant stenosis to avoid migration of the stent), the prosthesis can be inserted into the respiratory tract to close the tracheal or the bronchial opening to avoid aspiration pneumonia, a frequent cause of death in these patients. Generally, plastic stents are used. The most widely marketed are the Dumon stents, introduced with a rigid tracheo-bronchoscope under general anesthesia. These stents have the advantage that they can be easily repositioned in case of migration or removed if the fistula closes, as it can happen in postsurgical cases.

PERCUTANEOUS GASTROSTOMY

Percutaneous gastrostomy is considered only when there is no possibility to carry out one of the previously described procedures. Percutaneous endoscopic gastrostomy (PEG) consists of the insertion of a feeding/venting tube into the stomach, through the abdominal wall under direct endoscopic control, to choose the best position to access the gastric cavity. Such a tube can be advanced to reach the jejunum, thus becoming a jejunostomy, and it can also be used for decompressing an obstructed intestine.

Bleeding and vomiting

Endoscopic treatment can be beneficial for bleeding and vomiting, when these symptoms result mainly from intragastric or pancreatic tumors infiltrating the gastric wall. Polypoid or ulcerated, they may be endoscopically treated because they produce symptoms linked to the bleeding or to the food progression. This second group of symptoms is generally linked to the compression of the gastric antrum. Malignant ulcerations

bleed and produce anemic conditions, speeding up the progression toward cachexia. Decisions concerning the management of a bleeding gastrointestinal cancer need to consider the general clinical condition of the patient and the burden and the extent of the disease.

PALLIATIVE ENDOSCOPIC OPTIONS FOR BLEEDING AND VOMITING

To stop bleeding, endoscopic laser photocoagulation, unipolar or multipolar electrocoagulation, cryotherapy, and injection of sclerosing drugs can be used for cytoreductive as well as hemostatic purposes. These treatments are effective, but the duration of the effect is limited and the recurrence of the bleeding is a rule. The progression of the infiltration of the gastric wall and the presence of polypoid intragastric masses, mainly in the antrum, obstructs the gastric passage and causes gastric distension, nausea, and, finally, vomiting. Because all these symptoms are produced by gastric obstruction, they disappear when the obstruction is relieved after an endoscopic treatment performed through the administration of thermal energy (electrocoagulation and laser [argon beam] coagulation) or positioning a stent. Duodenal obstructions, as well as the gastric ones, can also be treated by performing a translaparoscopic bypass between the gastric body and the first jejunal loop, although expandable prostheses are also used to bypass duodenal and gastric compressive and stenosing lesions. Duodenum and gastric antrum can be obstructed by primary or metastatic tumors. Malignant lymph nodes and pancreatic and ampullary cancers are the most frequent causes of duodenal obstruction. Together with biliary tumors, these conditions are responsible for biliary obstruction and cause malignant jaundice.

Malignant jaundice

After the first cannulation of the papilla of Vater performed by Classen and Demling[23,25] and the consequent operative procedures, jaundice became one of the most important fields of application of the endoscopic techniques.

Biliary obstruction causes malignant jaundice. The obstruction can be caused by biliary, pancreatic, or metastatic cancer or by lymphomas, obstructing the common bile duct or the hepatic ducts. It is generally concomitant with whitish stools, brown urine, and diffuse itching. Pancreatic cancer is the most common cause of malignant biliary obstruction, followed by cholangiocarcinoma, carcinoma of the papilla of Vater, and metastatic tumors. When biliary obstruction and the consequent jaundice occur, the patient has advanced stage disease and palliation of the jaundice is the real purpose of the treatment.

PALLIATIVE ENDOSCOPIC OPTIONS FOR MALIGNANT JAUNDICE

An endoscopic approach[22,24] by inserting biliary endoprostheses through the transpapillary route has become the palliative treatment of choice, particularly for distal stenoses located at the choledochal level. When the obstruction is located into the hepatic hilum, the endoscopic approach is more difficult. However, palliative treatments that are alternatives to the endoscopic ones (surgical and percutaneous) have higher costs and complications and a lower success rate. They are indicated in case of failure of the endoscopic procedure.[26] Moreover, the endoscopic approach allows a careful inspection of the alimentary tract and particularly of the antro-pyloric and duodenal area: this inspection is useful because of the frequent association of biliary and duodenal obstruction.

Insertion of gastroduodenal prostheses can relieve a concomitant obstruction of the gastric outlet and of the gastro-duodenal passage. To obtain endoscopic biliary drainage, the obstructed biliary tract must be crossed with a guidewire introduced through the papilla under endoscopic guidance; a guide catheter is then passed over it, and, lastly, a plastic prosthesis is pushed through the stenotic tract and allows bile to flow. These plastic stents present a main late complication consisting of the occlusion with biliary sludge; in this case, they must be removed and replaced with new ones; it generally happens within 6 months after the stent is introduced. Metallic expandable prostheses, similar to those used in the coronary vessels, in the urethra and in the tracheo-bronchial tree, have been proposed for the biliary tract. They have a low occlusion and complication rate, are easy to place, and can be considered as a permanent procedure in the malignant jaundice.

The main advantages of the endoscopic approach are the low rate of trauma and the immediate effect.

In fact, whitish stools become well-stained in the 24–48 hours after the procedure, the urine loses progressively its intensive brown color, and itchiness disappears. When endoscopic drainage is impossible, percutaneous, video-laparoscopic, or open surgical routes can be used: the first one allows the insertion of a transhepatic tube, whereas the second and third allow a wide exploration of the peritoneal cavity and the performance of a bilio-digestive bypass.[22,24]

Constipation

Constipation is a very frequent symptom; more than 50% of advanced cancer patients need to be treated for the infrequent passage of hard stool. The cause should be clarified. When caused by anticancer chemotherapeutic drugs (mainly vincristine), opioids, metabolic problems like hypokalemia, or global electrolyte imbalances, it is mostly of the type of a dynamic ileus and is frequently accompanied by generalized abdominal pain. Intestinal obstruction by endoluminal masses or by extraintestinal compressions is more frequently accompanied by colicky pain.

PALLIATIVE ENDOSCOPIC OPTIONS FOR CONSTIPATION

Long-standing constipation resistant to common treatments must be managed in an effective way, but the safety of the treatment is compulsory. Endoscopy can help in the purpose of perfecting the diagnosis as well as treating the distension. These

patients are generally submitted to nasogastric intubation or other venting procedures for gastroduodenal decompression. A transanal approach can be necessary so that after cleaning enemas have been performed at low pressure, colonoscopy with large channel endoscopes allows gas and liquid aspiration and distension of the bowel wall. It must be performed carefully, injecting small quantities of warm water to clean the lumen, considering that the bowel wall is often very fragile because of concomitant ischemic lesions.

PALLIATIVE OPTIONS FOR OBSTRUCTION

A cancer growing into the intestinal lumen will obstruct the progression of intestinal content. Obstruction can also occur due to metastatic involvement of the mesenteric lymph nodes or diffuse peritoneal nodular metastases, for example, in papillary carcinomas, mainly, ovarian and pancreatic. About 10% of intestinal obstructions are caused by malignancies; up to 30% of obstructions result in resolution. More than 60% of malignant obstructions are caused by recurrent cancers.[30,31]

The plan of investigations and the treatment in each case is tailored to the individual patient. If a patient, already treated for an intestinal tumor, presents with abdominal distension, vomiting, constipation, and crampy pain, and plain X-ray of the abdomen shows air–fluid levels and bowel distension, the first choice is endoscopy. This is to locate precisely the cause of the obstruction and to perform, when possible, the first palliative treatment by dilation, laser, or stenting.

Surgery

Surgery is indicated consequent to endoscopic examination and to restaging examinations. Surgical procedures can be classified as bowel resections, preparing ostomy or bypass operations; the kind of procedure is related to the position of the stenosing lesion and to the type of previous surgery. Providing optimal palliative care for the patient with advanced colorectal cancer is a complex and challenging process and may be a departure from the traditional surgical satisfaction derived from the complete excision of a malignancy. However, surgeons aspiring excellence in palliative care will likely find this a rewarding endeavor.[23,25]

Considering the pros and the cons of the different surgical procedures, on the one hand, bypass operations and diverting stomas do not remove the tumor and consequently do not interfere with symptoms related to its presence, such as bleeding and pain due to infiltration of anatomical structures (peritoneum in intraabdominal cancers or periosteum in the pelvic localizations) although they alleviate symptoms due to obstruction, and, on the other hand, surgical removal, when possible, alleviates all the tumor-related symptoms, but morbidity and mortality rates are higher in patients who undergo palliative versus curative surgery.

When only palliation of symptoms is possible, the purpose of surgery is to bypass the stenotic tract, removing the malignancy. Before surgery, some points must be noted, such as the location of the lesion, whether it is single or multiple, the degree of the stenosis, the viability of the bowel wall, the real and ultimate cause of symptoms (malignancy, adherences, bands), and the likelihood of spontaneous resolution.

Persistence of bowel obstruction has a strong influence on prognostic outcome, and in a multivariate analysis, it was the only symptom that had an independent effect. Consequently, it must be managed and possibly interrupted as soon as possible. Conventional medical treatment has to be established with nasogastric or nasojejunal intubation and supply of intravenous fluids and electrolytes. The patient must be monitored with serial physical examinations performed by the same physician, enemas should be performed to clean the colon, and a colonoscopy should be done with the purpose of localizing and possibly treating the obstructing lesion. This type of examination must be performed carefully by an experienced endoscopist because of the fragility of the patient and of the intestinal wall, the hypersensitivity to pain, and the risk of perforation.

Endoscopic options

Endoscopic procedures to be considered in case of obstruction are dilation, electrocoagulation, laser coagulation, cryotherapy, and, lastly, endoprostheses, all of them with low mortality and morbidity.[26] Any treatment has to be performed only in patients presenting symptoms (obstruction, pain, bleeding) clearly attributable to the tumor and must be directed to bypass the symptom. In asymptomatic patients, any palliative treatment must be deferred. Patients to be submitted to palliation are those with very advanced and nonremovable cancers. They generally present with cachexia and weight loss, and surgical operations carry a high mortality, about 10%, and a survival rate of around 5% at 5 years.

There are different endoscopic possibilities of treatment, related to the kind of the obstructing lesion and in particular to its shape and to the tumor bulk, growing into the lumen or infiltrating the bowel wall. In the first case—the presence of an obstructing mass—the mass has to be removed to reopen the intestinal lumen; this can be done through an endoscopic laser treatment. In the second case—lesion infiltrating the bowel wall—a trans-stenotic guidewire has to be introduced under endoscopic visual guidance and a dilator slid on it; once dilation has been achieved, the fecal transit can been reestablished, the emergency problem overcome, and the bowel cleaned. If the tumor is operable, the lesion can be resected or a bypass operation performed through a surgical laparotomy or a laparoscopic procedure, which is planned for the following days; if the patient is inoperable because of high risk conditions or because the lesion is not removable, the endoscopic alternative is the only feasible option. To keep open the intestinal lumen and maintain the bowel functions, an expandable prosthesis must be inserted in these cases to obtain a durable effect.[28] The results of the endoscopic treatments can be summarized as follows:

- Dilation with inflatable balloons has a high rate of success (~90%), but stenosis recurs in 1–2 weeks.
- Similar rate of success is obtained with Nd:YAG laser, but the duration of the dilation is longer.

- Insertion of a prosthesis with a correct technique and indication allows the patency of the large bowel to be maintained in more than 80% of treated patients. We started to insert stents in primary rectal tumors and in recurrences in rectal anastomoses with a success rate of more than 90%. In most of our cases, patency of the stent lasts until death.[29]

CONCLUSION

The features of endoscopic palliation are as follows: (1) achievement of an immediate result in the control of symptoms and in the restoration of a normal function, whereas other options of palliation, like radiotherapy and chemotherapy and surgery, are generally more risky and need incomparably longer times to become effective; (2) absence of contraindications and side effects; and (3) the possible combination of endoscopic treatments with any other form of treatment.

Palliative treatments, in each case, should be tailored to the individual patient, and some clinical benefit, subject to the patient's capacity to undergo the treatments, consisting of a decrease or disappearance of symptoms and of improvement of performance status, should be the primary endpoint.[30]

Key learning points

- Palliative treatments should start to control the symptoms as soon as the disease is classified as incurable.

- Digestive cancers form about 20% of all diagnosed cancers, and most of them, when advanced, are poorly responsive to curative treatments; consequently, patients not responding to curative treatment will need symptomatic, palliative treatments.

- Before deciding to treat only symptoms, we should consider the different curative options offered by surgery, radiotherapy, chemotherapy, and immunotherapy, through a multidisciplinary approach.

- Gastrointestinal symptoms may be produced by digestive or extradigestive tumors. Most of them affect the digestive cavities and grow into them, occupying spaces required for digestive functions.

- Tumors reduce the spaces and impair the functions of containing and flowing, and they infiltrate and ulcerate the walls of these cavities, thus producing symptoms; in particular, they cause hemorrhages, obstructions, perforations, and fistulas.

- More than 95% of the digestive tumors are endocavitary, and endoscopy is the most suitable approach for precise and selective treatment.

REFERENCES

◆ 1 Nelson KA. The cancer anorexia–cachexia syndrome. *Semin Oncol* 2000;27:64.

◆ 2 Baines MJ. Symptom control in advanced gastrointestinal cancer. *Eur J Gastroenterol Hepatol* 2000;12:375–379.

◆ 3 Ikeda M. Significant host and tumor-related factors for predicting prognosis in patients with esophageal carcinoma. *Ann Surg* 2003;238:197–202.

◆ 4 Brown JM, Wouters BG. Apoptosis, p53, and tumor cell sensitivity to anticancer agents. *Cancer Res* 1999;59:1391–1399.

5 Jernvall P, Makinen MJ, Karttunen TJ et al. Loss of heterozygosity at 18q21 is indicative of recurrence and therefore poor prognosis in a subset of colorectal cancers. *Br J Cancer* 1999;79:903–908.

● 6 Silberman AW. Surgical debulking of tumors. *Surg Gynecol Obstet* 1982;155:577–585.

✶ 7 Morris DE. Clinical experience with retreatment for palliation. *Semin Radiat Oncol* 2000;10:210–221.

● 8 De Vita VT, Schein PS. The use of drugs in combination for the treatment of cancer. *N Engl J Med* 1973;288:998.

9 Lipsky MH, Chu MY, Yee LK et al. Predictive sensitivity of human cancer cells to anticancer agents in vivo. *Proc Am Assoc Cancer Res* 1994;35:371.

◆ 10 Goodwin WJ, Byers PM. Nutritional management of the head and neck cancer patients. *Med Clin North Am* 1993;77:597–610.

11 Spinelli P, Dal Fante M, Mancini A. Endoscopic palliation of malignancies of the upper gastrointestinal tract using Nd:YAG laser: Results and survival in 308 treated patients. *Lasers Surg Med* 1991;11:550–555.

12 Lightdale CJ, Heier SK, Marcon NE et al. Photodynamic therapy with porfimer sodium versus thermal ablation therapy with Nd:YAG laser for palliation of esophageal cancer: A multicenter randomized trial. *Gastrointest Endosc* 1995;42:507–512.

◆ 13 Lightdale CJ. Role of photodynamic therapy in the management of advanced esophageal cancer. *Gastrointest Endosc Clin North Am* 2000;10:397–408.

✶ 14 Spinelli P, Cerrai FG, Meroni E. Pharingo-esophageal prostheses in malignancies of the cervical esophagus. *Endoscopy* 1991;23:213–214.

◆ 15 Boyce HW Jr. Stents for palliation of dysphagia due to esophageal cancer [editorial]. *N Engl J Med* 1993;329:1345–1346.

✶ 16 Decker P, Lippler J, Decker D, Hirner A. Use of the Polyflex stent in the palliative therapy of esophageal carcinoma: Results in 14 cases and review of the literature. *Surg Endosc* 2001;15:1444–1447.

17 Moon S, Yang S, Na K. An acetylated polysaccharide-PTFE membrane-covered stent for the delivery of gemcitabine for treatment of gastrointestinal cancer and related stenosis. *Biomaterials* 2011;32:3603–3610.

18 Dormann AJ, Eisendrath P, Wigginghaus B et al. Palliation of esophageal carcinoma with a new self-expanding plastic stent. *Endoscopy* 2003;35:207–211.

19 O'Donnell CA, Fullarton GM, Murray GD et al. A comparison of the effectiveness of metallic stents and plastic endoprostheses in the palliation of oesophageal cancer: A pilot randomised controlled trial. *Br J Surg* 2002;89:985.

◆ 20 Boyce HW Jr. Palliation of dysphagia of esophageal cancer by endoscopic lumen restoration techniques. *Cancer Control* 1999;6:73–83.

21 Krokidis M, Burke C, Spiliopoulos S et al. The use of biodegradable stents in malignant esophageal strictures for the treatment of dysphagia before neoadjuvant treatment of radical radiotherapy: A feasibility study. *Cardiovasc Interv Radiol* 2013;36:1047–1054.

✶ 22 Hünerbein M, Stroszczynski C, Moesta KT, Schlag PM. Treatment of thoracic anastomotic leaks after esophagectomy with self-expanding plastic stents. *Ann Surg* 2004;240:801.

● 23 Classen M, Koch H, Demling L. Diagnostische Bedeutung des endoscopischen Kontrastdarstellung des Pankreas-gang-systems. *Leber Magen Darm* 1972;2:79–81.

◆ 24 Costamagna G. Therapeutic biliary endoscopy. *Endoscopy* 2000;32:209.

● 25 Bismuth H, Casting D, Traynor O. Resection or palliation: Priority of surgery in the treatment of hilar cancer. *World J Surg* 1988;12:39–47.

✶ 26 Matthew R, Dixon A, Michael J, Stamos B. Strategies for palliative care in advanced colorectal cancer. *Dig Surg* 2004;21:344–351.

◆ 27 Spinelli P, Mancini A, Dal Fante M. Endoscopic treatment of gastrointestinal tumors: Indications and results of laser photocoagulation and photodynamic therapy. *Semin Surg Oncol* 1995;11:307–318.

28 Spinelli P, Mancini A. Use of self-expanding metal stents for palliation of rectosigmoid cancer. *Gastrointest Endosc* 2001;53:203–206.

29 Baron Th, Rey JF, Spinelli P. Expandable metal stent placement for malignant colorectal obstruction. *Endoscopy* 2002;34:823–830.

30 Emmert M, Pohl-Dernick K, Wein A et al. Palliative treatment of colorectal cancer in Germany: Cost of care and quality of life. *Eur J Health Econ* 2013;4:629–638.

31 Ronnekleiv-Kelly SM, Kennedy GD. Management of stage IV rectal cancer: Palliative options. *World J Gastroenterol* 2011;17:835–847.

32 Suh JP, Kim SW, Cho YK et al. Effectiveness of stent placement for palliative treatment in malignant colorectal obstruction and predictive factors for stent occlusion. *Surg Endosc* 2010;24:400–406.

PART 10

Fatigue

64

Pathophysiology of fatigue

CLAUDIA GAMONDI, HANS NEUENSCHWANDER

INTRODUCTION

Fatigue is one of the most frequent symptoms in palliative care patients, still remaining one of the less understood in its genesis.[1,2]

Fatigue is reported as a symptom that heavily interferes with daily life. The prevalence is estimated to be between 32% and 90% among advanced cancer patients, 54% and 85% in AIDS, 69% and 82% in heart disease, 68% and 80% in COPD, and 73% and 87% in renal disease.[3–8**]

Fatigue becomes a leading, nonspecific symptom that accompanies patients from diagnosis to death. Fatigue can be one of the symptoms that lead to a diagnosis; it may occur during etiologic or palliative treatments such as in oncology, with antiretroviral therapy in AIDS, or dialysis and may represent a major difficulty during rehabilitation and remain one of the major complaints in the end of life.

Fatigue commonly has a major impact on function, regardless of the underlying illness. Descriptive studies show an inverse relation between fatigue and various indicators of quality of life.[9–15*] Some studies have explored the gender difference in fatigue: data suggest that there is no gender difference, even if there are some indications, that women generally report higher rates of symptoms than men.[16–21] Fatigue may easily interfere with social and physical activities, may influence the patient's decision making, and may lead a patient to refuse a potentially curative treatment. During the past few years, in palliative care, there has been an increasing awareness of the importance of this symptom not only in oncology but also in other chronic degenerative disease such as in multiple sclerosis (MS) and chronic organ failure.

The basic mechanisms by which fatigue is caused are not well understood. Occasionally, one predominant abnormality is present and appears to be the main contributor to the symptom, but in most cases, several abnormalities and many symptoms coexist, all differently contributing to the genesis and severity of fatigue.

Some of the pathways leading to fatigue in chronic degenerative illnesses are partially understood, but the interactions within these "generating fatigue pathways" in a specific disease or in a given patient remain unclear. In oncology, for example, the clinical picture is very often determined not only by the presence of multiple cofactors but more likely by the synergistic effect of having multiple problems leading to fatigue.[22]

In the following section, we will describe different pathways that can lead to fatigue. These pathways can be disease specific or not.

CYTOKINES, TUMOR-INDUCED PRODUCTS, AND INFLAMMATION IN CANCER AND OTHER DISEASES

Cancer by itself is able to release a number of substances, termed "asthenins," able to interfere with host metabolism. Cancer can also mediate the production of cytokines, such as tumor necrosis factor-alpha (TNF-α), interleukin (IL)-1, IL-6, and IL-2, which are active in the muscle tissue and in the central nervous system (Figure 64.1).

Inflammation is a predominant pathway leading to fatigue. In chronic heart failure, chronic beta-adrenergic stimulation and enhanced angiotensin II activity as well as the effects of inflammatory cytokines (e.g., TNF-α and IL-6) and reactive oxygen species are mediating the skeletal muscle dysfunction, playing a role in the multifactorial genesis of fatigue.[23]

Some encouraging results on breast cancer survivors showed improvement in physical aspects of fatigue with a higher dietary intake of omega-3 and omega-6 fatty acids, with the hypothesis that by decreasing inflammation, fatigue could be influenced.[24]

Fatigue, cachexia, and muscle

Cachexia is observed in cancer and in many other chronic degenerative diseases. Malnutrition, muscle mass loss, and progressive cachexia are valid reasons for fatigue, and they are strongly related to each other. The relationship between fatigue, cachexia, and muscle loss is complex. Cancer patients

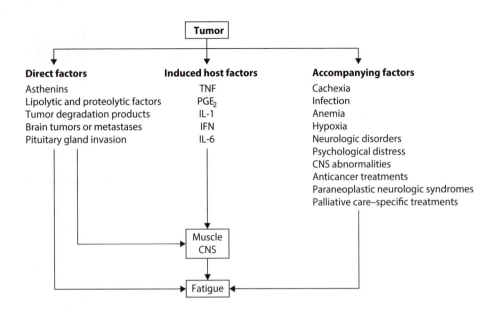

Figure 64.1 *Fatigue-generating mechanisms. TNF, tumor necrosis factor; IFN, interferon; IL, interleukin; PGE, prostaglandin E; CNS, central nervous system.*

present a catabolic metabolism: they show increased rate of metabolism and energy expenditure compared with control groups with similar weight loss; in addition, they show an increased need for amino acids, which leads to protein breakdown.[25–27]

Cachexia in cancer is characterized by severe muscle abnormalities leading to muscle loss: reactive oxygen and nitrogen species have been proposed as underlying mechanisms. The inefficiency of the antioxidant enzymes may be responsible for the development of both oxidative and nitrosative stress in cancer-induced cachexia.[28]

In cancer, there is an atrophy of type II muscle fibers, responsible for anaerobic performance.[1]

Muscles of cancer-bearing animals show alterations in the activity of various enzymes, distribution of isoenzymes, and synthesis and breakdown of myofibrillar and sarcoplastic proteins.[27,29] In humans, there is an evidence of excessive lactate production in tumor-free muscle tissue: this represents an expression of both weakness and pathophysiological mechanism.[30,31]

In patients with chronic heart failure, cardiac cachexia is common: tissue and enzymatic changes influence skeletal muscle metabolism and autonomic function. All muscles are involved, including those with ventilatory function, contributing to impaired exercise capacity and muscle fatigue.[32,33]

However, fatigue does not necessarily relate to the degree of myocardial dysfunction, indicating that potential peripheral hypoperfusion is not the single cause of fatigue in these patients.[34]

A significant correlation between muscular fatigability and reduced electromyographic activity was found in patients with chronic heart failure.[35] A reduction in skeletal muscle protein stores may result from endogenous TNF or from TNF administered as antineoplastic therapy.[36] Thorud et al., in a study conducted on rats with congestive heart failure, observed that elevated circulatory concentrations of TNF-α and monocyte chemoattractant protein-1 are a frequent finding. These molecules are supposed to stimulate matrix metalloproteinase activity and thereby contribute to distort the normal contractile muscle function, increasing skeletal muscle fatigue.[37] Prolonged bed rest and immobility lead to loss of muscle mass and reduced cardiac output. This deconditioning results in reduced endurance for exercise and activities of daily living and may be compounded by other muscle abnormalities in patients with cancer.[38,39]

Franssen et al. pointed out the contribution of starvation, deconditioning, and aging to alterations of peripheral skeletal muscle in chronic organ diseases, such as chronic obstructive pulmonary disease and chronic heart and renal failure.[40] Studies have demonstrated that endurance training can reduce fatigue and improve physical performance in cancer patients while they are receiving chemotherapy and bone marrow or autologous stem cell transplantation.[41–46]

Aerobic training and combination of exercise modalities in patients with heart failure are shown to be effective in decreasing global rating of symptoms, including fatigue.[47]

Physical inactivity due to the neurological impairment can be a cause of fatigue in poststroke, reported between 30% and 68% of stroke survivors. The hypothesis is that physical deconditioning plays a crucial role, by building up a vicious, self-perpetuating cycle.[48] Data supporting this hypothesis show that limb muscle strength on both sides is significantly lower in patients after stroke compared with controls.[49]

As contributors to fatigue, neurohormonal and immune abnormalities may play a crucial role.[50] However, in a number of conditions, this relationship is not as close as expected: patients with breast cancer or lymphomas might complain of profound fatigue, but they have low incidence of cachexia.[51] Furthermore, patients with chronic fatigue syndrome or major depression show no malnutrition but high incidence of fatigue. On the other hand, in diseases such as anorexia nervosa, there is severe malnutrition without fatigue.[1]

Anemia and hypoxia

Anemia is a common finding in patients with malignant disease. It can be caused by the cancer itself, or it can be cancer induced or due to correlated factors such as bleeding, hemolysis, nutritional deficiencies, iron deficiency, and antineoplastic treatment such as chemotherapy or radiotherapy or by cancer-independent factors. Hemoglobin levels below 8 g/dL are associated with profound fatigue.[1]

In some circumstances, anemia may be a major factor in cancer-related fatigue and impairment of quality of life in cancer patients.[5,52,53] For individual patients, it is difficult to discern the real impact of anemia from that of other competing contributing factors to fatigue. The impact of anemia varies depending on factors such as the rapidity of onset, patient's age, plasma volume status, and the number and severity of comorbidities.[54]

In patients with mean levels of hemoglobin between 9 and 11 g/dL receiving chemotherapy, the correction of anemia has been shown to be effective in ameliorating quality of life, activity levels, and energy levels.[52] The difficulty in conducting research in this field is correlating hemoglobin levels with degree of fatigue and its potential alterability.

In a study conducted among women undergoing pelvic radiotherapy for uterine cancer, Ahlberg et al. observed an increase in fatigue during treatment and no significant correlation between general fatigue and hemoglobin levels after 3 weeks of therapy.[55] Combined data from three randomized, placebo-controlled trials on erythropoietin alfa, the recombinant form of human erythropoietin, revealed an association between increased hematocrit and an improvement in overall quality of life.[56] Patients with an increase in hematocrit of 6% had significant improvement in energy level and daily activities. Three large, prospective, nonrandomized, multicenter, community trials similarly observed that epo alfa-treated patients who experienced a rise in hemoglobin reported significant improvements in energy level, activity level, functional status, and overall quality of life.[52,53,57,58]

Since none of these studies had fatigue as a primary endpoint, caution in interpreting these findings remains mandatory. Many of these studies refer to fatigue under chemotherapy, and many are supported by industries. Mercadante et al. in a consecutive sample of patients with hemoglobin levels of 8 ± 0.5 g/dL measured fatigue before, after 1 day, and 15 days after a single blood transfusion. Significant changes in fatigue and dyspnea were found immediately after transfusion, although the effect was partially lost 15 days after transfusion.[59] These results upon transfusions and fatigue are confirmed by a Cochrane review: Preston et al. concluded that around one-third of patients may not benefit of blood transfusions and that duration of response is short in those who do. Authors driven the attention on the risk of harm from blood transfusion in frail, ill patients at the end of life, potentially related to fluid overload or higher plasma viscosity.[60]

In COPD, hypoxia and hypoxemia are cofactors associated with fatigue. Data show that also impaired fat-free mass and loss of fatigue-resistant muscle fibers are associated with fatigue in these patients.[61,62]

Low oxygen levels may be associated with changes in cognitive function and stimulate affective areas of the brain, mainly in the frontal lobe, which is associated with motivational process, leading to low motivation and depression.[61]

In sickle-cell disease, fatigue is emerging as a leading symptom, together with pain. Hypoxemia can cause muscle weakness and produce oxidative stress, and sickled erythrocytes disrupt the vascular endothelium and stimulate the production of proinflammatory cytokines, particularly IL-1, IL-6, and TNF-α.[63]

Infection

Correlation between fatigue and infection is well documented. Fatigue can be a prodromal symptom and it can outlast the infection for weeks and months.[64,65] In cancer patients, because of the immunodepression, acute and chronic infections are very common, and one of the underlying mechanisms of pathophysiology is the production of some mediators of inflammatory response, such as TNF-α.[66] The production of some cytokines (TNF-α, IL-1, IL-2, IL-6, interferon [IFN]) and the consequent activation of the inflammatory reaction can, in some cases, be considered the main mechanism leading to the cachexia–anorexia syndrome.[29,67,68] It can be assumed that there is a similar underlying mechanism in the genesis of infection-induced fatigue.

Metabolic and endocrine disorders

In chronic advanced illness, many metabolic and endocrine disorders, such as diabetes mellitus and Addison disease, or electrolytic disorders are common as comorbidities and characterized by fatigue as a leading symptom. Dysfunction of the hypothalamic–pituitary–adrenal (HPA) axis is a field of research. Abnormalities of the HPA axis have been postulated as possible additional factors in the chronic fatigue syndrome.[1]

There is also evidence suggesting that IFN-α initiates a cytokine cascade that affects the HPA and hypothalamic–pituitary–gonadal axis, thus affecting regulation of glucocorticoid and sex steroid hormone secretion. However, the clinical significance of these observations has not yet been established.[69] There is clear evidence that hormonal deficiency syndromes, such as hypothyroidism, occur in a relatively large portion of patients receiving systemic IFN-α therapy.

Some authors, after acknowledging the limitations of current clinical data, have concluded that adrenal and gonadal axis dysfunction also must be considered in patients with IFN-α-induced fatigue.[70] The possibility of hypothyroidism must be considered. However, diagnosis of hypothyroidism in cancer patients might be complicated by the occurrence of the "sick euthyroid syndrome" (SES). This syndrome is defined as the decrease of serum-free triiodothyronine with normal free L-thyroxin and thyrotropin.[71] Recent reports have shown that IL-6 plays a key role in the pathogenesis of SES: some authors have demonstrated that IL-6 can suppress the thyroid function.[72–74]

Kumar et al. conducted a prospective observational study on 198 consecutive breast cancer patients receiving adjuvant chemotherapy.[75] Changes in anthropometric data, fatigue, nutritional intake, physical activity, and thyroid and steroid hormones were monitored from start to end of the chemotherapy and 6 months after therapy. They concluded that cytotoxic agents may influence thyroid function in this population, contributing to and progressively worsening symptoms such as weight gain, amenorrhea, fatigue, and lowered physical activity. They suggested screening breast cancer patients for thyroid function at diagnosis or at the beginning of the adjuvant treatment.[75]

The role of testosterone has also been studied: the findings from Burnes and colleagues suggest that testosterone works in conjunction with a specific acid-sensing ion channel (ASIC3) involved in muscle pain to protect against muscle fatigue.

There can be a biological link in female and male mice between testosterone and the pathways leading to pain and fatigue. This could explain why more women than men are diagnosed with chronic pain and fatigue conditions like fibromyalgia and chronic fatigue syndrome.[76]

In humans, age-associated hypogonadism occurs in 30% of men after the age of 55. It is associated with decreased muscle mass, bone mineral density, and libido, hemoglobin levels and with anorexia, fatigue, and irritability.[77] Even if some of these symptoms overlap with those of depression, the association between the two disorders is unclear. There is some evidence that there is an increased incidence of depressive illness and a shorter time to diagnosis of depression in hypogonadal men.[78] In male patients with cancer, hypogonadism is correlated with fatigue, and androgen insufficiency can be caused by anorexia–cachexia syndrome.

Profound hypogonadism with low levels of serum testosterone or estrogen coupled with low levels of pituitary gonadotropins has been noted in male and female patients receiving intrathecal opioids.[79,80] Hormone levels are related to the opioid consumed, dosage and dosage form, nonopioid medication use, and several personal characteristics.[81] A recent study demonstrated that cancer survivors who were chronic opioid consumers experienced symptomatic hypogonadism with significantly higher levels of depression, fatigue, and sexual dysfunction.[82] The reduction in opioid consumption can dramatically increase libido and sexual function with a possible mechanism involving opioid-related effects on the HPA axis.[83*]

A high prevalence of decreased testosterone levels in HIV-infected patients has also been demonstrated, together with some other common endocrine abnormalities.[84]

Low levels of testosterone are also demonstrated in chronic heart failure.[34]

Hormonal ablative therapy in prostate cancer patients can double the incidence of fatigue, and the replacement therapy in hypogonadic and testosterone-depleted HIV patients results in an improvement of energy, libido, and hemoglobin levels.[1]

Psychological distress

The prevalence of depression in cancer patients varies: major depression has a prevalence of 0%–38% and depression spectrum syndromes from 0% to 58%. In palliative care, the reported prevalence of depression varies from 17% to 42%.[85] In psychiatric patients, fatigue is a common somatic symptom of clinical depression, and it is included in the diagnostic criteria for major depressive disorders, bipolar disorders, and dysthymic disorders. Anderson et al. conclude that patients with cancer report significantly more severe fatigue and fatigue-related interference in their daily life activities than the community-dwelling subjects. Furthermore, patients with depressive disorders reported more severe fatigue and more interference with their daily lives due to fatigue than either cancer or community individuals.[86]

Several investigators have suggested that depression and fatigue may have overlapping but not equivalent physiopathological mechanisms: this could explain why patients with clinical depression who respond to antidepressant medication may continue to experience residual fatigue.[87] In a large representative sample of cancer patients where the most frequently reported problem was fatigue, 37.8% met criteria for general distress in the clinical range.[88] This finding supports the view of the chronic stress condition mentioned earlier. In addition, a recent study supports the evidence that in treating depression with sustained released (SR) bupropion, there can be a reduction of the symptom fatigue experienced by cancer patients.[89]

HIV-related fatigue is strongly associated with psychological factors such as depression and anxiety, together with sleep disturbances and comorbidities.[90,91]

In general, psychological distress seems to play a role in HIV-related fatigue, and there is some evidence showing that in HIV-infected patients, those reporting fatigue can be significantly more disabled than those not reporting it, and in high levels of psychological distress, the fatigued HIV-positive population can have much poorer quality of life compared with HIV patients without fatigue.[92,93]

Central nervous system abnormalities

Abnormalities of the CNS can themselves be a cause of fatigue, and, at the same time, the brain is also the area where fatigue is perceived.[1]

Mental fatigue, with decreased concentration capacity, is common in neuroinflammatory and neurodegenerative diseases.

Some authors postulated that the proinflammatory cytokines such as TNF-α, IL-1β, and IL-6 can be involved in the pathophysiology of mental fatigue through their ability to interfere with glial activity in the brain, altering metabolic supply for the neurons.[94]

In MS, neuronal factors such as dysfunction of premotor, limbic, basal ganglia, or hypothalamic areas, the disruption of the neuroendocrine axis, alterations in serotoninergic pathways, changes in neurotransmitter levels, and altered CNS functioning caused by a disruption of the immune response are identified in the genesis of fatigue.[95]

Reports indicate also that fatigue can be related to hypometabolism in certain brain areas and correlates with the gravity of axonal damage, brain atrophy, and impairment of inhibitory circuits in their primary motor cortex.[96–99]

In Parkinson's disease, dopamine deficiency is supposed to play a role in contributing to central fatigue.[100]

Some of the abovementioned mechanism of fatigue can be implicated in primary or secondary CNS tumors, which by causing endocrine abnormalities or producing hormones and neurotransmitters can lead to fatigue. Chronic pain creates a persistent activation of the reticular activating system, which seems to be responsible for the experience of fatigue.

Etiological treatments

Symptoms in patients with HIV under antiretroviral regimens have been associated with decreased compliance and quality of life.[101,102]

In patients with HIV and AIDS, muscle aches, numbness in the extremities, and fatigue are reported in literature as concomitant symptoms, regardless of the antiretroviral drug therapy,[103] but remains very controversial to what extent the antiretroviral therapy plays a role in generating or aggravating fatigue in these patients.

Anticancer treatments have a high impact on energy levels: most of the patients complain of fatigue while receiving chemotherapeutic agents.[104–107] Several studies have shown a correlation between fatigue and different types of oncological treatment: it has been observed that 65%–100% of patients undergoing radiotherapy and up to 82%–96% of those receiving chemotherapy suffer from fatigue during treatment.[108] In supportive care, drugs used to control nausea and vomiting are themselves contributors to fatigue. However, it may be difficult, in the individual patient, to demonstrate if fatigue is more related to treatment or to the underlying disease.

In a multivariate analysis, 43% of the variance in fatigue was ascribed to disease-related symptoms and 35% to toxicity of treatment.[108] Radiotherapy and chemotherapy can result in anemia, diarrhea, anorexia, and weight loss, all contributors to fatigue. For example, treatment with dexamethasone may be beneficial to reduce postchemotherapy symptoms induced by irinotecan, specifically anorexia and fatigue.[109**] In patients treated with biological response modifiers such as IFN-α, fatigue is an important dose-limiting side effect.

Autoimmune thyroid disease, another contributor to fatigue, is a well-recognized consequence of IFN-α therapy and may be mediated by the induction of IFN-γ production by lymphocytes.[70] Recent data suggest that IFN-α depression may be composed of two overlapping syndromes: a depression-specific syndrome characterized by mood, anxiety, and cognitive complaints and a neurovegetative syndrome characterized by fatigue, anorexia, and psychomotor slowing.[110]

Patients with acute lymphoblastic leukemia receiving cranial radiotherapy experience fatigue, depression, and sleepiness.[111]

Fann et al. in a study conducted on delirium episodes in patients undergoing hematopoietic stem cell transplantation observed that affective distress and fatigue were common and appeared to be associated most with psychosis-behavioral

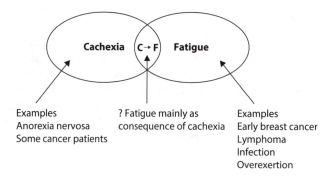

Figure 64.2 *Possible relation between cachexia and fatigue.*

delirium symptoms.[112] The new emerging feature called "chemo brain" should stimulate further research in the possible relation between delirium and fatigue (Figure 64.2).[113]

Paraneoplastic neurological syndromes

Even though quite rare, these neurological complications of cancer are probably underestimated. Sometimes, these symptoms can precede the outbreak of the malignant disease by months or even more or may lead to the diagnosis of cancer. Box 64.1 shows some of the syndromes associated with fatigue. Lung cancer has the highest incidence of paraneoplastic syndrome.[114]

Symptom control–oriented treatments

OPIOIDS

Nearly 90% of patients with advanced cancer receive opioids[1]; these drugs are known to act on the reticular system and cause sedation and drowsiness, which can be perceived by patients as a dimension of fatigue. Opioids may interfere with concentration and can contribute to mental fatigue. On the other hand, their effect in relieving pain may contribute to a less sleep deprivation and possibly to less fatigue.

> ## Box 64.1 Paraneoplastic neurological syndromes associated with fatigue
>
> - Progressive multifocal leukoencephalopathy
> - Peripheral paraneoplastic neurological syndrome
> - Paraneoplastic encephalomyelitis
> - Ascending acute polyneuropathy
> - Amyotrophic lateral sclerosis
> - Neuromuscular paraneoplastic syndromes: Dermatomyositis, polymyositis, Eaton–Lambert syndrome, myasthenia gravis
> - Subacute motor neuropathy
> - Subacute necrotic myelopathy

ANTIDEPRESSANTS

Common side effects of antidepressants are weight gain, sexual dysfunction, sleep disturbances, fatigue, apathy, and cognitive impairment. Selective serotonin reuptake inhibitors and atypical antidepressants (e.g., venlafaxine, bupropion, and nefazodone) show relatively favorable short-term as well as long-term tolerability compared with older drugs (e.g., tricyclics and monoamine oxidase inhibitors).[115]

ANXIOLYTICS

All central actions of the benzodiazepines are based on a common molecular mechanism. Reactions that are CNS depressant, such as sedation, fatigue, ataxia, impairment of motor coordination, and intellectual functions including memory are most frequent, especially in the elderly.[116]

ANTIEMETICS

There is clear evidence that almost all antiemetics might cause fatigue. In an anecdotal report, however, five female patients with chronic fatigue syndrome were eligible to receive oral granisetron for 1 month: the treatment with granisetron resulted in significant improvement in fatigue and functional impairment. Activity level showed no significant increase.[117] The significance of this finding has still to be assessed.

STEROIDS

On the one hand, steroids can be a cause of weakness by inducing myopathy, and on the other hand, they can be part of the treatment of asthenia and their withdrawal can contribute to worsening of the symptom.

Other symptoms as contributors to fatigue

Uncontrolled pain or dyspnea exacerbates fatigue. Poorly controlled symptoms may lead to insomnia, depression, and anxiety, all contributors to fatigue.[1] Autonomic dysfunction, a common finding in patients with advanced cancer, characterized in others by postural hypotension, fixed heart rate, and gastroparesis, is in many cases an important contributor to fatigue.

Sleep disturbance, defined as insomnia or hypersomnia occurring nearly every day, may appear as a self-standing symptom or as an epiphenomenon of depression. Among cancer patients, it has received limited attention in clinical studies: it is estimated to range from 23% to over 50%.[86] There is a correlation between sleep patterns and fatigue: most patients with chronic fatigue syndrome complain of unrefreshing sleep. It can be supposed that the perceived sleep quality is of greater importance than the sleep characteristics. There is some evidence that sleep disturbance is associated with patient's fatigue level: a recent study, conducted in patients undergoing radiotherapy, found a correlation between improvement in sleep patterns and decrease in fatigue.[118] The relation between sleep disturbance and fatigue in cancer patients may be related to disease and treatment-induced abnormalities in cytokine levels. Many cytokines involved in cancer and cancer treatments have been associated with fatigue and sleep disorders. For example, injection of TNF-α or IL-1 induces non-REM sleep, and IFN-α reduces the amount of both slow-wave and REM sleep.[119] Anderson et al. indicate that symptoms of sleep disturbance are highly prevalent among cancer patients and that sleep disturbance is a significant predictor of severe fatigue in these patients.[86]

Key learning points

- Fatigue is a leading symptom in patients with malignant and nonmalignant disease. In the mean time, it is the most underestimated condition that impairs function and quality of life. It has unfortunately still to be considered a mostly silent symptom, because it is underreported by the patient and underestimated and therefore undertreated by the caring teams.

- Even though quite often fatigue, or at least a part of it, might be attributed to other findings (symptoms, therapy side effects) therefore considered as an epiphenomenon, there is now enough evidence that fatigue is a self-standing symptom complex. In this sense, it deserves to be considered as a syndrome.

- Fatigue is almost always a multifactorial symptom. However, in several cases, one of the contributing factors may be apparently predominant. For this reason, it is worth investigating the different possible causes, with respect to important therapeutic consequences.

- Research in the field of fatigue is needed. Research should be focused in recognizing common pathways leading to fatigue, independently from specific underlying diseases. Clinical researchers should also have an interest in the study of sleep disturbances, endocrine dysfunction, psychiatric conditions, and the therapeutic balance between utility and futility of physical training and rest. A proper classification of this symptom is still missing.

REFERENCES

1 Sweeney C, Neuenschwander H, Bruera E. Fatigue and asthenia. In: Doyle D, Hanks G, Cherny NI, Calman K, eds. *Oxford Textbook of Palliative Medicine*, 3rd edn. Oxford, U.K.: Oxford University Press, 2004: 560–568.

2 Radbruch L, Strasser F, Elsner F, Ferraz Gonçalves J, Løge J, Kaasa S, Nauck F, Stone P and the Research Steering Committee of the European Association for Palliative Care. Fatigue in palliative care patients—An EAPC approach. *Palliat Med* 2008; 22: 13–32.

3 Bruera E. Research into symptoms other than pain. In: Doyle D, Hanks G, MacDonald N, eds. *Oxford Textbook of Palliative Medicine*, 2nd edn. Oxford, U.K.: Oxford University Press, 1998: 179–185.

4   Coyle N, Adelhardt J, Foley KM et al. Character of terminal illness in the advanced cancer patient: Pain and other symptoms during the last 4 weeks of life. *J Pain Symptom Manage* 1990; 5: 83–93.

5   Cella DF, Tulsky DS, Gray G et al. The functional assessment of cancer therapy scale: Development and validation and of the general measure. *J Clin Oncol* 1993; 11: 570–579.

6   Vogelzang NJ, Breitbart W, Cella D et al. Patient, caregiver and oncologist perception of cancer related–Fatigue: Result of a tripart assessment survey. The Fatigue Coalition. *Semin Hematol* 1997; 34: 4–12.

7   Portenoy RK, Thaler HT, Kornblith AB et al. Symptom prevalence, characteristics and distress in a cancer population. *Qual Life Res* 1994; 3: 183–189.

◆ 8   Solano JP, Gomes B, Higginson IJ. A comparison of symptom prevalence in far advanced cancer, AIDS, heart disease, chronic obstructive pulmonary disease and renal disease. *JPSM* 2006, January; 31: 58–69.

9   Dodd MJ, Miaskowski C, Paul SM. Symptom cluster and their effect on the functional status of patients with cancer. *Oncol Nurs Forum* 2001; 28: 465–470.

10   Schwartz AL. Fatigue mediates the effects of exercise on quality of life. *Qual Life Res* 1999; 8: 529–538.

11   Ferrell BR, Grant M, Dean GE et al. 'Bone tired': The experience of fatigue and its impact on quality of life. *Oncol Nurs Forum* 1996; 23: 1539–1547.

12   Servaes P, van der Werf S, Prins J et al. Fatigue in disease-free cancer patients compared with fatigue in patients with chronic fatigue syndrome. *Support Care Cancer* 2001; 9: 11–17.

13   Hickok JT, Morrow GR, McDonald S et al. Frequency and correlates of fatigue in lung cancer patients receiving radiation therapy: Implications for management. *J Pain Symptom Manage* 1996; 11: 370–377.

14   Akechi T, Kugaya A, Okamura H et al. Fatigue and its associated factors in ambulatory cancer patients: A preliminary study. *J Pain Symptom Manage* 1999; 17: 42–48.

15   Stone P, Hardy J, Broadley K et al. Fatigue in advanced cancer: A prospective controlled cross-sectional study. *Br J Cancer* 1999; 79: 1479–1486.

16   Heinonen H, Volin L, Uutela A et al. Gender associated differences in the quality of life after allogenic BMT. *Bone Marrow Transplant* 2001; 28: 503–509.

17   Pater JL, Zee B, Palmer M et al. Fatigue in patients with cancer: Results with the National Cancer Institute of Canada Clinical Trials Group studies employing the EORT QLQ-C30. *Support Care Cancer* 1997; 5: 410–413.

18   Walsh D, Donnelly S, Rybicki L. The symptoms of advanced cancer: Relationship to age, gender and performance status in 1000 patients. *Support Care Cancer* 2000; 8: 175–179.

19   Kronke K, Wood Rd, Mangelsdrorff AD et al. Chronic fatigue in primary care. Prevalence, patient characteristics, and outcome. *JAMA* 1998; 260: 929–934.

20   Van Wijk CM, Kolk AM. Sex differences in physical symptoms: The contribution of symptom perception theory. *Soc Sci Med* 1997; 45: 231–246.

21   Verbrugge LM. Gender and health: An update on hypotheses and evidence. *J Health Soc Behav* 1985; 26: 156–182.

22   Bruera E. Cancer-related fatigue: A multidimensional syndrome. *J Support Oncol* 2010; 8: 175–176.

◆ 23   Haehling S, Doehner W, Anker SD. Nutrition, metabolism, and the complex pathophysiology of cachexia in chronic heart failure. *Cardiovasc Res* 2007; 73: 298–309.

24   Alfano CM, Imayama I, Neuhouser ML, Kiecolt-Glaser JK, Smith AW, Meeske K, McTiernan A, Bernstein L, Baumgartner KB, Ulrich CM, Ballard-Barbash R. Fatigue, inflammation, and ω-3 and ω-6 fatty acid intake among breast cancer survivors. *J Clin Oncol* 2012; 30(12): 1280–1287.

25   Argiles JM, Moore-Carrasco R, Busquets S et al. Catabolic mediators as targets for cancer cachexia. *Drug Discov Today* 2003; 15: 838–844.

26   Legaspi A, Jeevanadam M, Stanes HF et al. Whole body lipid and energy metabolism in the cancer patient. *Metabolism* 1987; 10: 958–963.

27   Nelson KA, Walsh D, Shehan FA. The cancer anorexia–cachexia syndrome. *J Clin Oncol* 1994; 12: 213–225.

28   Barreiro E, de la Puente B, Busquets S et al. Both oxidative and nitrosative stress are associated with muscle wasting in tumour-bearing rats. *FEBS Lett* 2005; 579: 1646–1652.

29   Theologides A. Anorexins, asthenins, and cachectins in cancer. *Am J Med* 1986; 81: 696–698.

30   Bruera E, Brenneis C, Michaud M et al. Association between involuntary muscle function and asthenia, nutritional status, lean body mass, psychometrical assessment and tumour mass in patient with advanced breast cancer. *Proc Am Soc Clin Oncol* 1987; 6: 261.

31   Holroyde CP, Axelrod RS, Skutches CL et al. Lactate metabolism in patient with metastatic colorectal cancer. *Cancer Res* 1979; 39: 4900–4904.

◆ 32   Mangner N, Matsuo Y, Schuler G, Adams V. Cachexia in chronic heart failure: Endocrine determinants and treatment perspectives. *Endocrine* 2012, August. 19.

33   Bellinger AM, Mongillo M, Marks AR. Stressed out: The skeletal muscle ryanodine receptor as a target of stress. *J Clin Invest* 2008; 118: 445–453.

34   Aukrust P, Ueland T, Gullestad L, Yndestad A. Testosterone: A novel therapeutic approach in chronic heart failure? *J Am Coll Cardiol* 2009; 54(10): 928–929.

35   Schulze PC, Linke A, Schoene N et al. Functional and morphological skeletal muscle abnormalities correlate with reduced electromyographic activity in chronic heart failure. *Eur J Cardiovasc Prev Rehabil* 2004; 11: 155–161.

36   St Pierre BA, Kasper CE, Lindsey AM. Fatigue mechanisms in patients with cancer: Effects of tumour necrosis factor and exercise on skeletal muscle. *Oncol Nurs Forum* 1992; 19: 419–425.

37   Thorud HM, Stranda A, Birkeland JA et al. Enhanced matrix metalloproteinase activity in skeletal muscles of rats with congestive heart failure. *Am J Physiol Regul Integr Comp Physiol* 2005; 289: R389–R394.

38   Germain P, Guell A, Marini JF. Muscles strength during bed-rest with and without muscle exercise as a countermeasure. *Eur J Appl Physiol Occup Physiol* 1995; 71: 342–348.

39   Levine BD, Zuckerman JH, Pawelczyk JA. Cardiac atrophy after bedrest deconditioning: A nonneural mechanism for orthostatic intolerance. *Circulation* 1997; 96: 517–525.

◆ 40   Franssen FM, Wouters EF, Schols AM. The contribution of starvation, deconditioning and ageing to the observed alterations in peripheral skeletal muscle in chronic organ diseases. *Clin Nutr* 2002; 21: 1–14.

41   Dimeo FC, Stieglitz RD, Novelli-Fischer U et al. Effects of physical activity on the fatigue and psychologic status of cancer patients during chemotherapy. *Cancer* 1999; 85: 2273–2277.

42   Dimeo F, Fetscher S, Lange W et al. Effects of aerobic exercise on the physical performance and incidence of treatment related complications after high dose chemotherapy. *Blood* 1997; 90: 3390–3394.

43   Dimeo F, Bertz H, Finke J et al. An aerobic exercise program for patients with haematological malignancies after Bone Marrow Transplantation. *Bone Marrow Transplant* 1996; 18: 1157–1160.

44   Dimeo FC. Effects of exercise on cancer-related fatigue. *Cancer* 2001; 92(6 Suppl.): 1689–1693.

45   Dimeo F, Schwartz S, Fietz T et al. Effects of endurance training on the physical performance of patients with hematological malignancies during chemotherapy. *Support Care Cancer* 2003; 11: 623–628.

46   Crevenna R, Zielinski C, Keilani MY et al. Aerobic endurance training for cancer patients. *Wien Med Wochenschr* 2003; 153: 212–216.

47   Corvera-Tindel T, Doering LV, Woo MA et al. Effects of a home walking exercise program on functional status and symptoms in heart failure. *Am Heart J* 2004; 147: 339–346.

♦ 48   Duncan F, Kutlubaev MA, Dennis MS, Greig C, Mead GE. Fatigue after stroke: A systematic review of associations with impaired physical fitness. *Int J Stroke* 2012; 7(2): 157–162.

49   Carin-Levy G, Greig C, Young A, Lewis S, Hannan J, Mead G. Longitudinal changes in muscle strength and mass after acute stroke. *Cerebrovasc Dis* 2006; 21: 201–207.

50   Anker SD, Sharma R. The syndrome of cardiac cachexia. *Int J Cardiol* 2002; 85: 51–66.

♦ 51   Bruera E, Brenneis C, Michaud M et al. Association between asthenia and nutritional status, lean body mass, anaemia, psychological status, and tumour mass in patients in advanced breast cancer. *J Pain Symptom Manage* 1989; 4: 59–63.

52   Glaspy J, Bukowski R, Steinberg D et al. Impact of therapy with epoetin alfa on clinical outcomes in patients with nonmyeloid malignancies during cancer chemotherapy in community oncology practice. Procrit Study Group. *J Clin Oncol* 1997; 15: 1218–1234.

53   Demetri GD, Kris M, Wade J et al. Quality-of-life benefit in chemotherapy patients treated with epoetin alfa is independent of disease response or tumour type: Results from a prospective oncology study. Procrit Study Group. *J Clin Oncol* 1998; 16: 3412–3425.

54   Johnston E, Crawford J. The haematological support of the cancer patient. In: Berger A, Portenoy RK, Weissman DE, eds. *Principles and Practice of Supportive Oncology*. Philadelphia, PA: Lippincott-Raven Publishers, 1998, pp. 549–569.

55   Ahlberg K, Ekman T, Gaston-Johansson F. Levels of fatigue compared to levels of cytokines and haemoglobin during pelvic radiotherapy: A pilot study. *Biol Res Nurs* 2004; 5: 203–210.

56   Abels RI. Recombinant human erythropoietin in the treatment of the anaemia of cancer. *Acta Haematol* 1992; 1(87 Suppl.): 4–11.

57   Glaspy J. The impact of epoetin alfa on quality of life during cancer chemotherapy: A fresh look at an old problem. *Semin Hematol* 1997; 34(3 Suppl. 2): 20–26.

58   Gabrilove J. Overview: Erythropoiesis, anaemia, and the impact of erythropoietin. *Semin Hematol* 2000; 37(4 Suppl. 6): 1–3.

59   Mercadante S, Ferrera P, Villari P, David F, Giarratano A, Riina S. Effects of red blood cell transfusion on anemia-related symptoms in patients with cancer. *J Palliat Med* 2009; 12(1): 60–63.

♦ 60   Preston NJ, Hurlow A, Brine J, Bennett MI. Blood transfusions for anaemia in patients with advanced cancer. *Cochrane Database Syst Rev* 2012; 2: CD009007.

61   Lewko A, Bidgood PL, Garrod R. Evaluation of psychological and physiological predictors of fatigue in patients with COPD. *BMC Pulm Med* 2009; 9: 47.

62   Evans WJ, Lambert CP. Physiological basis of fatigue. *Am J Phys Med Rehabil* 2007; 86: 29–46.

63   Ameringer S, Smith WR. Emerging biobehavioral factors of fatigue in sickle cell disease. *Nurs Scholarsh* 2011; 43(1): 22–29.

64   Jones JF, Ray CG, Minnich LL et al. Evidence for active Epstein-Barr virus infection in patients with persistent, unexplained illnesses: Elevated anti-early antigen antibodies. *Ann Intern Med* 1985; 102: 1–7.

65   Straus SE, Tosato G, Armstrong G et al. Persisting illness and fatigue in adults with evidence of Epstein-Barr virus infection. *Ann Intern Med* 1985; 102: 7–16.

66   Neuenschwander H, Bruera E. Pathophysiology of cancer asthenia. In: Portenoy RK, Bruera E, eds. *Topics in Palliative Care*, Vol. 2. Oxford, U.K.: Oxford University Press, 1998.

67   Beutler B, Cerami A. Cachectin: More than a tumour necrosis factor. *N Engl J Med* 1987; 316: 379–385.

68   Tisdale MJ. New cachexie factors. *Curr Opin Clin Nutr Metab Care* 1998; 1: 253–256.

69   Gisslinger H, Svoboda T, Clodi M et al. Interferon-alpha stimulates the hypothalamic-pituitary-adrenal axis in vivo and in vitro. *Neuroendocrinology* 1993; 57: 489–495.

70   Jones TH, Wadler S, Hupart KH. Endocrine-mediated mechanism of fatigue during treatment with interferon-alpha. *Semin Oncol* 1998; 25(1 Suppl. 1): 54–63.

71   Vexiau P, Perez-Castiglioni P, Socie G et al. The 'euthyroid sick syndrome': Incidence, risk factors and prognostic value soon after allogeneic Bone Marrow Transplantation. *Br J Haematol* 1993; 85: 778–782.

72   Kimura T, Kanda T, Kotajima N et al. Involvement of circulating interleukin-6 and its receptor in the development of euthyroid sick syndrome in patients with acute myocardial infarction. *Eur J Endocrinol* 2000; 143: 179–184.

73   Kotajima N, Kanda T, Kimura T et al. Studies on circulating interleukin-6 and thyroid functions in acute myocardial infarction. *Rinsho Byori* 2000; 48: 276–281.

74   Davies PH, Black EG, Sheppard MC et al. Relation between serum interleukin-6 and thyroid hormone concentrations in 270 hospital in-patients with non-thyroidal illness. *Clin Endocrinol* (Oxford) 1996; 44: 199–205.

75   Kumar N, Allen KA, Riccardi D et al. Fatigue, weight gain, lethargy and amenorrhea in breast cancer patients on chemotherapy: Is subclinical hypothyroidism the culprit? *Breast Cancer Res Treat* 2004; 83: 149–159.

76   Burnes LA, Kolker SJ, Danielson JF, Walder RY, Sluka KA. Enhanced muscle fatigue occurs in male but not female ASIC3 mice. *Am J Physiol Regul Integr Comp Physiol* 2008; 294(4): R1347–R1355.

77   Cavallini G, Caracciolo S, Vitali G et al. Carnitine versus androgen administration in the treatment of sexual dysfunction, depressed mood, and fatigue associated with male aging. *Urology* 2004; 63: 641–646.

78   Shores MM, Sloan KL, Matsumoto AM et al. Increased incidence of diagnosed depressive illness in hypogonadal older men. *Arch Gen Psychiatry* 2004; 61: 162–167.

79   Finch PM, Roberts LJ, Price L et al. Hypogonadism in patients treated with intrathecal morphine. *Clin J Pain* 2000; 16: 251–254.

80   Roberts LJ, Finch PM, Pullan PT et al. Sex hormone suppression by intrathecal opioids: A prospective study. *Clin J Pain* 2002; 18: 144–148.

81   Daniell HW. Hypogonadism in men consuming sustained-action oral opioids. *J Pain* 2002; 3: 377–384.

♦ 82   Rajagopal A, Vassilopoulou-Sellin R, Palmer JL et al. Symptomatic hypogonadism in male survivors of cancer with chronic exposure to opioids. *Cancer* 2004; 100: 851–858.

83   Rajagopal A, Bruera E. Improvement in sexual function after reduction of chronic high-dose opioid medication in a cancer survivor. *Pain Med* 2003; 4: 379–383.

84   Rabkin JG, Wagner GJ, Rabkin R. A double-blind, placebo-controlled trial of testosterone therapy for HIV-positive men with hypogonadal symptoms. *Arch Gen Psychiatry* 2000; 57(2): 141–147.

85 Massie MJ. Prevalence of depression in patients with cancer. *J Natl Cancer Inst Monogr* 2004: 57–57.

86 Anderson KO, Getto CJ, Mendoza TR et al. Fatigue and sleep disturbance in patients with cancer, patients with clinical depression, and community-dwelling adults. *J Pain Symptom Manage* 2003; 25: 307–318.

87 Menza MA, Kaufmann KR, Castellanos A. Modafinil augmentation of antidepressant treatment in depression. *J Clin Psychiatry* 2000; 61: 378–381.

88 Carlson LE, Angen M, Cullum J et al. High levels of untreated distress and fatigue in cancer patients. *Br J Cancer* 2004; 90: 2297–2304.

89 Cullum JL, Wojciechowski AE, Pelletier G et al. Bupropion sustained release treatment reduces fatigue in cancer patients. *Can J Psychiatry* 2004; 49: 139–144.

90 Voss JG. Predictors and correlates of fatigue in HIV/AIDS. *J Pain Symptom Manage* 2005; 29: 173–184.

91 Jong E, Oudhoff LA, Epskamp C, Wagener MN, van Duijn M, Fischer S, van Gorp EC. Predictors and treatment strategies of HIV-related fatigue in the combined antiretroviral therapy era. *AIDS* 2010; 24(10): 1387–1405.

92 Henderson M, Safa F, Easterbrook P, Hotopf M. Fatigue among HIV-infected patients in the era of highly active antiretroviral therapy. *HIV Med* 2005; 6: 347–352.

93 Phillips K, Sowell R, Rojas M, Tavakoli A, Fulk L, Hand G. Physiological and psychological correlates of fatigue in HIV disease. *Biol Res Nurs* 2004; 6: 59–74.

94 Rönnbäck L, Hansson E. On the potential role of glutamate transport in mental fatigue. *J Neuroinflamm* 2004; 1(1): 22.

◆ 95 Krupp LB. Fatigue in multiple sclerosis: Definition, pathophysiology and treatment. *CNS Drugs* 2003; 17(4): 225–234.

96 Roelcke U, Kappos L, Lechner-Scott J et al. Reduced glucose metabolism in the frontal cortex and basal ganglia of multiple sclerosis patients with fatigue: A 18F-fluorodeoxyglucose positron emission tomography study. *Neurology* 1997; 48(6): 1566–1571.

97 Marrie RA, Fisher E, Miller DM, Lee JC, Rudick RA. Association of fatigue and brain atrophy in multiple sclerosis. *J Neurol Sci* 2005; 228: 161–166.

98 Tartaglia MC, Narayanan S, Francis SJ et al. The relationship between diffuse axonal damage and fatigue in multiple sclerosis. *Arch Neurol* 2004; 61: 201–207.

99 Liepert J, Mingers D, Heesen C, Baumer T, Weiller C. Motor cortex excitability and fatigue in multiple sclerosis: A transcranial magnetic stimulation study. *Mult Scler* 2005; 11: 316–321.

100 Lou JS, Kearns G, Benice T, Oken B, Sexton G, Nutt J. Levodopa improves physical fatigue in Parkinson's disease: A double-blind, placebo-controlled, crossover study. *Mov Disord* 2003; 18: 1108–1114.

101 Ammassari A, Antinori A, Aloisi MS et al. Depressive symptoms, neurocognitive impairment, and adherence to highly active antiretroviral therapy among HIV-infected persons. *Psychosomatics* 2004; 45(5): 394–402.

102 Burgoyne RW, Rourke SB, Behrens DM, Salit IE. Long-term quality-of-life outcomes among adults living with HIV in the HAART era: The interplay of changes in clinical factors and symptom profile. *AIDS Behav* 2004; 8(2): 151–163.

103 Wantland DJ, Mullan JP, Holzemer WL, Portillo CJ, Bakken S, McGhee EM. Additive effects of numbness and muscle aches on fatigue occurrence in individuals with HIV/AIDS who are taking antiretroviral therapy. *J Pain Symptom Manage* 2011; 41(2): 469–477.

104 Greene D, Nail LM, Fieler VK et al. A comparison of patient reported side effects among three chemotherapy regimens for breast cancer. *Cancer Pract* 1994; 2: 57–62.

105 Stone P, Richards M, A'Hern R et al. Fatigue in patients with cancers of the breast or prostate undergoing radical radiotherapy. *J Pain Symptom Manage* 2001; 22: 1007–1015.

106 Irvine D, Vincent L, Graydon JE et al. The prevalence and correlates of fatigue in patients receiving treatment with chemotherapy and radiotherapy. A comparison with fatigue experience by healthy individuals. *Cancer Nurs* 1994; 17: 367–378.

107 Blesch KS, Paice JA, Wickham R et al. Correlates of fatigue in people with breast or lung cancer. *Oncol Nurs Forum* 1991; 18: 81–87.

108 Lawrence DP, Kupelnick B, Miller K et al. Report on the occurrence, assessment, and treatment of fatigue in cancer patients. *J Natl Cancer Inst Monographs* 2004: 40–50.

109 Inoue A, Yamada Y, Matsumura Y et al. Randomized study of dexamethasone treatment for delayed emesis, anorexia and fatigue induced by irinotecan. *Support Care Cancer* 2003; 11: 528–532.

110 Raison CL, Demetrashvili M, Capuron L et al. Neuropsychiatric adverse effects of interferon-alpha: Recognition and management. *CNS Drugs* 2005; 19: 105–123.

111 Proctor SJ, Kernaham J, Taylor P. Depression as component of postcranial irradiation somnolence syndrome. *Lancet* 1981; 1: 1215–1216.

112 Fann JR, Alfano CM, Burington BE et al. Clinical presentation of delirium in patients undergoing hematopoietic stem cell transplantation. *Cancer* 2005; 15: 810–820.

113 Wefel JS, Lenzi R, Theriault R et al. 'Chemobrain' in breast carcinoma?: A prologue. *Cancer* 2004; 101: 466–475.

114 Jurado Gamez B, Garcia de Lucas MD, Gudin Rodriguez M. Lung cancer and paraneoplastic syndromes. *An Med Interna* 2001; 18: 440–446.

115 Cassano P, Fava M. Tolerability issues during long-term treatment with antidepressants. *Ann Clin Psychiatry* 2004; 16: 15–25.

116 Klotz U. Effects and side effects of benzodiazepines. *Anasth Intensivster Notfallmed* 1988; 23: 122–126.

117 Prins J, Bleijenberg G, van der Meer JW. The effect of granisetron, a 5-HT3 receptor antagonist, in the treatment of chronic fatigue syndrome patients—A pilot study. *Neth J Med* 2003; 61: 285–289.

118 Sharpley A, Clements A, Hawton K et al. Do patients with 'pure' chronic fatigue syndrome (neurasthenia) have abnormal sleep? *Psychosom Med* 1997; 59: 592–596.

119 Kubota T, Majde JA, Brown RA et al. Tumour necrosis factor receptor fragment attenuates interferon-gamma-induced non-REM sleep in rabbits. *J Neuroimmunol* 2001; 119: 192–198.

65

Physical activity in palliative and supportive care

SONYA S. LOWE, KERRY S. COURNEYA

INTRODUCTION

Quality of life (QoL) is the primary goal of palliative care, which the World Health Organization defines as the interdisciplinary and holistic management of progressive, advanced disease wherein prognosis is limited.[1] Palliative care is unique in that "it lacks a specific disease, bodily organ, or life stage to call its own."[2] Recently, there is increasing recognition that the benefits of palliative care can extend to earlier stages in the cancer trajectory[3] and can encompass noncancer populations.[4] Hence, the contemporary scope of palliative care has broadened such that there is little consensus regarding the definition of the palliative patient in clinical trials.[5] Despite these challenges, it is recognized that the closer the patient is toward death, the greater the disease and symptom burden becomes, thus making palliation the sole goal of care.[6]

Physical activity (PA) can be defined as any bodily movement produced by the skeletal muscles that results in a substantial increase in energy expenditure over resting levels; exercise can be defined as any form of PA undertaken by an individual during leisure time and performed repeatedly over an extended period with the goal of improving fitness or health.[7] Self-reported physical functioning (PF) can be defined as self-perception of individual capacity or performance[8]; objective PF can be defined as the sensoriomotor performance of an individual that includes fundamental and complex activities of daily living.[9] Multiple meta-analyses have demonstrated that exercise can positively affect cardiorespiratory fitness, mood, cancer-related fatigue (CRF), PF, mood, and overall QoL in cancer patients.[10,11] The 2010 American College of Sports Medicine Roundtable on Exercise Guidelines for Cancer Survivors concluded that exercise training is safe during and after cancer treatments, and results in improvements in PF, QoL, and CRF in several cancer survivor groups.[12] The American Cancer Society's updated guidelines recommend regular PA to cancer patients both during and after treatment for improved QoL.[13]

Although there is substantial evidence to support the efficacy of PA interventions in improving QoL outcomes in cancer survivors, there are no current PA recommendations or guidelines specific to palliative cancer care.[14] Since this chapter's predecessor was published in 2006,[15] there have been two systematic reviews pertaining to this area of interest. In January 2009, Lowe et al. published a systematic review of PA as a supportive care intervention in palliative cancer patients; the authors defined palliative cancer as progressive, incurable, and locally recurrent or metastatic cancer, with a clinician-estimated life expectancy of 12 months or less.[16] Five observational studies and one randomized controlled trial were included, with significant heterogeneity in terms of study design, participants, and interventions administered. Overall, there was preliminary evidence that at least some palliative cancer patients were able to tolerate PA interventions, with some demonstrating improvement in QoL outcomes postintervention.

In July 2009, Beaton et al. published a systematic review of the effects of exercise interventions for patients with metastatic cancer.[17] The authors did acknowledge that "not all patients with metastatic or advanced cancer are in the palliative or end-of-life phase," and quoted the example of average survival for breast cancer patients after metastasis being "18 to 24 months, and many patients exceed this period."[17] These statements are in keeping with the 2010 American College of Sports Medicine Roundtable on Exercise Guidelines for Cancer Survivors, in which the survivorship category of the cancer control continuum includes patients with advanced cancer that are stable and whose survival may be years in duration.[12] Five observational studies and three randomized controlled trials were included, with significant heterogeneity in interventions, participants, and outcomes measured. Overall, there was insufficient evidence to support efficacy of exercise as an intervention in patients with metastatic cancer, and further research was warranted.[17] Despite the paucity of evidence, the 2010 American College of Sports Medicine Roundtable on Exercise Guidelines for Cancer Survivors recommended that "the advice to 'avoid inactivity', even in cancer patients with existing disease or undergoing difficult treatments, is likely helpful."[12]

CANCER–RELATED FATIGUE, PHYSICAL FUNCTIONING, AND QUALITY OF LIFE IN PALLIATIVE CANCER PATIENTS

Fatigue (69%), weakness (66%,) and lack of energy (61%) were among the five most prevalent symptoms in a retrospective study of 1000 patients in an American palliative medicine program.[18] Between 60% and 90% of advanced cancer patients report experiencing CRF, and rate CRF as the symptom with the most negative impact on overall QoL.[19] Pathophysiologically, CRF is postulated to be related to the tumor itself, through peripheral energy depletion or central hypothalamic-pituitary-adrenal axis or serotonin dysfunction, as well as interactions between tumor load and subsequent proinflammatory cytokine production, including interleukin-1, interleukin-6, and tumor necrosis factor-α.[20] In combination with neurohormonal and metabolic abnormalities, autonomic failure, and anorexia-cachexia affecting loss of lean body mass tissues at the end stages of cancer, the most devastating repercussion of CRF is loss of PF.

Decline in PF is among the most common symptoms of advanced cancer patients, with potential contributors being disease progression, deconditioning, pain, direct tumor and paraneoplastic effects, cancer treatments, and subsequent complications.[21] Not only does loss of PF result in deconditioning and impaired mobility, it is likewise linked to loss of independence in activities of daily living and increasing dependency on caregivers. "Loss of the ability to do what one wants" has been identified as one of the highest-rated end-of-life concerns from the perspective of both patients and caregivers.[22] In the hospice setting, Wallston et al. (1988) report that 22% of terminal cancer patients wish to be physically able to do what they choose to do, even in the last 3 days of life[23]; Yoshioka (1994) reports that 88% of terminal cancer patients in hospice had a strong desire for mobility.[24] The fear of functional decline and increasing caregiver dependency may have marked psychosocial ramifications; loss of autonomy and becoming a burden to others has been identified as among the top reasons for requests for euthanasia.[25]

Progressive cancer is inevitably accompanied by a decline in PF,[26,27] which has been identified as an important determinant of QoL in advanced cancer patients in palliative care.[6] Progressive anorexia-cachexia and low lean body mass, all contribute to declining PF in advanced cancer patients,[28] particularly in the last 6 months of life.[29] Deconditioning, pain, poor balance, and focal weakness were among the most prevalent functional disabilities identified in palliative care inpatients.[30] Given the heterogeneity inherent within the palliative cancer population, the assessment of PF poses challenges with respect to sensitivity at either end of the PF spectrum.

Following their systematic literature review of PF assessment instruments, Helbostad et al. (2009) employed the International Classification of Functioning and Health and a palliative cancer care expert panel to identify two major PF domains: mobility and self-care.[31] The authors' hypothesis is that self-care activities are basic prerequisites for mobility at higher levels, with self-care items increasing sensitivity of the instrument at the lower end of the PF spectrum.[31] Based on that work, Helbostad et al. (2011) subsequently conducted a cross-sectional study of 604 responses from palliative cancer patients and 186 responses from chronic pain patients, which determined good psychometric properties of a computer-administered PF mobility (PF-M) scale.[32]

PA is one potential intervention that may address both CRF and loss of PF in palliative cancer care. Multiple recent reviews have demonstrated the efficacy of exercise interventions in improvement of fatigue,[33,34] PF, and QoL outcomes in cancer survivors.[10,11] Two recent systematic reviews have highlighted the paucity of evidence examining PA interventions in palliative cancer patients[16] and patients with metastatic cancer,[17] respectively. The past 5 years have seen a rapid increase in the quantity and quality of studies examining PA and PF in this patient population. This present chapter is an updated summary of the available evidence related to exercise and physical function in palliative cancer care. For the purposes of this chapter, palliative cancer is defined as progressive, incurable, and locally recurrent or metastatic disease.

A literature review of all studies examining PA and PF in palliative cancer patients was conducted on the following electronic databases in May 2012: The Cochrane Central Register of Controlled Trials, MEDLINE, EMBASE, CINAHL, and PubMED. Study participants had to be 18 years of age or older, and also have a diagnosis of progressive, incurable, and locally recurrent or metastatic cancer, regardless of tumor type or type of cancer treatment. Key words that related to cancer (i.e., neoplasm, carcinoma, tumor), palliative (i.e., terminally ill, hospice, end of life, end stage), and PA (i.e., exercise, exercise therapy, PF) were combined and searched. Reference lists of included studies were hand-searched for additional studies. To be included in the review, a study had to be written in the English language and published in a peer-reviewed journal. Abstracts without the corresponding full paper were not included. A decision was made a priori to exclude studies that involved a mixed population of different disease stages or treatment (i.e., curative versus palliative intent), if they did not report data or analyze data separately for palliative patients. We found 6 qualitative studies, 17 observational studies, and 16 interventional studies that examined PA and PF in palliative cancer patients. Details of the studies are reported in Tables 65.1 through 65.5, and we briefly summarize them here.

QUALITATIVE STUDIES OF PHYSICAL ACTIVITY IN PALLIATIVE CANCER PATIENTS

Mackey et al. (2000) conducted a qualitative single-case study with replication exploring the experience of three older women with cancer receiving hospice care, with the aim of informing physical therapy assessment and care in this setting.[35] Social relationships, spirituality, outlook on mortality, and meaningful PA were identified as key themes; in particular, the participants mourned the loss of familiar physical activities, which

Table 65.1 *Summary of qualitative studies examining PA in palliative cancer patients*

Authors	Sample	Design	Aim	Key themes
Mackey et al. (2000)	3 older women with cancer receiving hospice care	Qualitative single-case study with replication using grounded theory analysis	Explore the hospice patient experience in order to inform physical therapy and assessment	1. Social relationships 2. Spirituality 3. Outlook on mortality 4. Meaningful PA
Paltiel et al. (2009)	5 participants from Oldervoll et al.'s (2006) phase II pilot study	Semistructured interviews using phenomenological-hermeneutical analysis	Explore the meaning of the exercise intervention for the individual participant	1. Perception of the group 2. Sense of belonging and commitment 3. Secure and caring setting for group 4. Emphasis on enhancing coping 5. Underlying qualifications of professional guidance during intervention 6. Poor suitability of public gym for intervention type
Selman and Higginson (2010)	New Delhi: 8 carers, 3 patients, and 2 teachers London: 6 patients, 1 teacher, 1 assistant	Semistructured interviews using thematic analysis	Explore and compare the yoga classes offered by palliative care services in New Delhi and London, and the experience of participants and teachers at those services	1. Content of the classes 2. Participants' symptoms and problems 3. Preconceptions and meaning of yoga 4. Effects of yoga 5. Challenges 6. Recommendations for services
Gulde et al. (2011)	11 palliative home care cancer patients enrolled in some form of PA under guidance of physiotherapist	Semistructured interviews using qualitative content analysis	Explore how palliative cancer patients with poor performance status experience their participation in PA with the guidance of a professional physiotherapist	1. Routines of everyday life: Something to do and being together with others in similar situation 2. Less fatigue 3. Professional guidance: Physiotherapist as tutor and motivator 4. Hope
Adamsen et al. (2011)	15 formerly sedentary advanced lung cancer patients undergoing chemotherapy and participating in a hospital-based, supervised group intervention	Individual semistructured interviews (n = 15) and one semistructured focus group interview (n = 8) using thematic analysis	Explore the feasibility and experienced health benefits and barriers of participation in the intervention from the patients' perspective	Individual interviews: 1. Diagnosis, shock, and participating in team sports despite no previous interest 2. Motivation to participate: Experienced physical weakness, fatigue, pain, and unspoken desire to combat illness through own actions 3. Benefits: Strength training helps weak body achieve well-being, despite fatigue, soreness, and pain 4. Fitness training: Tough challenge 5. Relaxation training: Much needed break 6. Paradox: So tired but more energetic Focus group interview: 1. Diagnosis, shock, and participating in team sports despite no previous interest 2. Exercise program's volume, content, and duration 3. Importance of exercising in group with those in similar circumstance 4. Exercising at home: Great instructions but lack of discipline to perform solo

(Continued)

Table 65.1 (*Continued*)   *Summary of qualitative studies examining PA in palliative cancer patients*

Authors	Sample	Design	Aim	Key themes
Selman et al. (2012)	18 cancer patients in hospice day care	Mixed methods study	1. Measure yourself concerns and well-being questionnaire 2. Content analysis of qualitative data relating to patient concerns, well-being, other things affecting health and most important aspects of service	1. Significant improvement in concern/problem score 2. Mobility/fitness and breathing problems were the top categories of concerns or problems with which patients reported they required help 3. Social benefits of attending classes, enjoyment and relaxing nature, improvements in mobility and breathing ability

held special meaning in their lives before cancer diagnosis.[35] The authors concluded that the "to further maximize meaning for patients who are dying, while maximizing endurance and conserving energy, physical therapists may foster continuity of those physical activities that have held particular meaning in the patients' lives."[35]

Seven months postintervention, Paltiel et al. (2009) randomly selected five participants from Oldervoll et al.'s (2006) phase II pilot study for semistructured interviews exploring the meaning of the exercise intervention for the individual participant.[36] Participants identified themes of perception of the group, with emphasis on sense of belonging and commitment, and a secure and caring setting for the group with emphasis on enhancing coping, underlying qualifications of professional guidance during the intervention, and poor suitability of public gym for this type of intervention.[36]

Selman and Higginson (2010) conducted semistructured interviews with yoga teachers, patients, and carers from yoga classes offered by palliative care services in New Delhi and London.[37] The intervention consisted of 90 min yoga classes offered once weekly at both respective sites, with the New Delhi yoga teachers being based in the Bihar philosophy and the London yoga teacher being based in the Sivananda tradition; the exact content of the classes was not reported. Six major themes emerged including class content, participants' symptoms and difficulties, preconceptions and the meaning of yoga, challenges and recommendations for services. In particular, psychological benefits were a shared theme between both sites, with participants describing "improved well-being, emotional balance, and ability to cope."[37] Symptom burden posed physical limitations for some patients to participate in yoga; however, participants did describe a sense of achievement and inspiration from others when overcoming these challenges.[37]

Gulde et al. (2011) conducted semistructured interviews in 11 cancer patients from palliative home care units in Sweden and who were enrolled in some form of PA under the guidance of a physiotherapist.[38] Three of the study participants passed away within 3 months of interview. The patients identified themes of routines of everyday life, less fatigue, professional guidance, and hope as being significant in their experience of PA. The authors concluded that these themes should be incorporated into physiotherapist recommendations for individualized PA programs in this population.[38]

Adamsen et al. (2011) conducted individual semistructured interviews and a focus group interview of 15 formerly sedentary patients with advanced lung cancer undergoing a hospital-based, supervised group intervention involving resistance, cardiovascular, and relaxation training for 4 hours/week and a concurrent unsupervised home-based exercise program, over a 6-week period.[39] Fifteen percent of participants had stage IV non–small cell lung cancer and 13% had small cell lung cancer, although survival was not reported; all participants were undergoing chemotherapy, and 67% of participants were also undergoing radiotherapy. The average attendance rate for the hospital-based group intervention was 76%, whereas the participants failed to comply with the home-based exercise program. The participants identified key themes of the desire to combat the illness through their own actions, increasing body well-being despite fatigue and pain, and the challenge of fitness training concomitant with the desirable break of relaxation training; the participants reported benefits of the hospital-based group intervention including social support, motivation, and supervision by trained professional.[39]

Selman et al. (2012) conducted a mixed-methods study evaluating 6-week group classes of yoga and Lebed Method dance therapy on 18 cancer patients in hospice day care.[40] Seventy-eight percent of participants had a cancer diagnosis, with 83% of participants designated as "palliative" treatment status; "mobility/fitness" was identified as participant's most prevalent concerns. The yoga classes included postures, breathing techniques, relaxation through visualizations, and positions in a 90 min format, whereas the Lebed method classes included slow, smooth, and minimal resistance movements done seated or standing, with no more than four repetitions on each side of the body, in a 60 min format. The authors reported the greatest improvement in mean change scores for patient concerns for both yoga and Lebed method therapies, with improvement in well-being being clinically significant for participants in the yoga group; participants reported psycho-spiritual benefit as being among the most important aspects of both programs.[40]

Table 65.2 *Summary of observational studies examining self-reported PA in palliative cancer patients*

Authors	Sample	Design	Physical activity measure	Other measures	Outcomes
Clark et al. (2007)	128 advanced cancer patients receiving outpatient chemotherapy Breast (n = 21) Digestive (n = 17) Lung (n = 13) Gynecologic (n = 12) Genitourinary (n = 9) Neurologic (n = 5) Head and neck (n = 4) Other (n = 21)	Cross-sectional survey	1. Self-efficacy for PA via Likert scale 2. Exercise frequency via Godin Lesiure-time exercise questionnaire 3. Outcome expectations, perceived barriers and benefits. interest in and plans for PA via closed and open-ended items	1. Mood via positive affect negative affect scales (PA-NAS) 2. QoL via (FACT-G)	FACT-G Physical well-being subscale (t = 0.63, p = 0.53) Overall QoL rating mean 7.1 (1.9) PA-NAS Positive affect (t = 2.18, p < 0.05) Negative affect (t = 0.59, p = 0.58)
Lowe et al. (2009, 2010, 2012)	50 advanced cancer patients from palliative home care and outpatient clinics Lung (n = 15) Genitourinary (n = 11) Breast (n = 8) Gastrointestinal (n = 8) Hematological (n = 4) Head and neck (n = 2) Other (n = 2)	Cross-sectional survey	1. PA via modified items from PA scale for the elderly	1. QoL via McGill Quality of Life Questionnaire (MQoL) 2. Symptoms via Edmonton Symptom Assessment System (ESAS) 3. PF via abbreviated version of the late-life function and disability instrument (LLFDI)	MQOL Total score Walking ≥ 30 min/day (d = 0.59, p = 0.046) LLFDI Total function score Walking ≥ 30 min/day (d = −0.32, p = 0.261) Edmonton Symptom Assessment System (ESAS) fatigue subscale Walking ≥ 30 min/day (d = −0.31, p = 0.273) Majority of participants were interested in and felt able to participate in a PA intervention with walking being the preferred modality, and home-based preference
Oechsle et al. (2011)	53 patients with incurable cancer undergoing outpatient palliative chemotherapy Gastrointestinal (n = 11) Hematological (n = 11) Pancreas, liver, gallbladder (n = 9) Lung (n = 9) Other solid tumors (n = 7) Breast (n = 6)	Cross-sectional survey	1. Questionnaire for measurement of habitual PA 2. International Physical Activity Questionnaire 3. New questionnaire soliciting Physical habits, demographics, and interest in PA	European Organization for Research and Treatment of Cancer Quality of Life Questionnaire (EORTC QLQ-C13)	Significantly positive correlations between "work index" and QoL (p = 0.004), physical function (p = 0.02), and "hours of PA per week" and QoL (p < 0.05) QoL scores significantly higher in patients with sportive activities ≥ 9MET h/week 60% of participants were willing to participate in an individually adapted activity training program

(Continued)

Table 65.2 (Continued)   *Summary of observational studies examining self-reported PA in palliative cancer patients*

Authors	Sample	Design	Physical activity measure	Other measures	Outcomes
Maddocks et al. (2011)	200 incurable cancer patients from outpatient oncology clinics or day-case chemotherapy suite	Cross-sectional survey	1. Exercise behavior via Godin leisure time exercise questionnaire	1. Six different therapeutic exercise programs illustrated by looping short video clip with accompanying text 2. 19-item questionnaire developed specifically for study examining preference for type of exercise program and program delivery preferences	More than 80% of participants felt physically capable of undertaking exercise programs involving resistance training, whole body vibration, or neuromuscular electrical stimulation Neuromuscular electrical stimulation most preferred type of exercise among participants who felt able to undertake exercise currently. Majority of participants preferred to undertake exercise at home, alone, and unsupervised.

OBSERVATIONAL STUDIES OF SELF-REPORTED PHYSICAL ACTIVITY IN PALLIATIVE CANCER PATIENTS

Clark et al. (2007) conducted a cross-sectional survey on 128 advanced cancer patients receiving chemotherapy, with an estimated life expectancy of greater than 6 months but less than 5 years.[41] Breast cancer was the most common diagnosis amongst participants; however, the presence or location of metastatic disease and actual survival were not reported. Positive outcome expectations for PA, positive mood, and higher current exercise level were related to self-efficacy, and fatigue was identified as the most significant barrier to PA. Overall, 89% of participants intended to maintain or increase their current PA level, and 47% of participants were probably to definitely interested in receiving professional support for PA.[41]

Lowe et al. (2009) conducted a pilot survey of 50 advanced cancer patients recruited from outpatient palliative care clinic and palliative home care, with a median survival of 104 days from time of survey to time of death.[42] Walking was the most common reported PA. There was a positive association between patient-reported PA and QoL, with those who reported walking more than 30 min/day associated with higher total QoL scores on the McGill Quality of Life Questionnaire.[42] The majority of participants indicated that they would be interested in and felt able to participate in a PA program, with walking being the preferred mode of PA, and a strong preference for home-based programs.[43] Affective attitude, self-efficacy, and intention were the strongest correlates of total PA levels.[44]

Oechsle et al. (2011) conducted a cross-sectional study of 53 incurable cancer patients undergoing outpatient palliative

chemotherapy in Germany.[45] Gastrointestinal, hematological, and lung were the most prevalent malignant diagnoses, with lung, retroperitoneal, and liver being the most prevalent sites of metastases. Median time from diagnosis was 30 months; however, median survival from time of questionnaire to time of death was not reported. The authors reported positive associations between hours of PA per week and QoL, with QoL scores being significantly higher in patients engaged in sportive activities requiring greater than 9 metabolic equivalent hours per week. Sixty percent of participants indicated interest in participating in an individually prescribed PA intervention.[45]

Maddocks et al. (2011) conducted a questionnaire study exploring the acceptability of six different exercise programs in 200 incurable cancer patients and Eastern Cooperative Oncology Group (ECOG) Performance Status of 0–2 recruited from outpatient oncology clinics or day-case chemotherapy suite in the United Kingdom.[46] Greater than 80% of participants felt physically capable of engaging in exercise programs using resistance training, whole body vibration, or neuromuscular electrical stimulation, whereas approximately 50% of participants felt capable of engaging in walking, treadmill walking, or cycling programs. Among the most common reasons for not feeling capable were dyspnea, fatigue, pain, and leg weakness. Two-thirds of participants reported feeling prepared to engage in one or more exercise programs at the time of questionnaire, with the most preferred type of exercise being neuromuscular electrical stimulation based on perceived practicality and convenience; walking and resistance training were among the most preferred activities, with a clear preference for home exercise without supervision.

Table 65.3   *Summary of observational studies examining objective PA in palliative cancer patients*

Authors	Sample	Design	PA measure	Other measures	Outcomes
Dahele et al. (2007)	20 ambulatory outpatients with advanced upper gastrointestinal cancer receiving palliative chemotherapy (esophagus: n = 8, gastric: n = 6, gastroesophageal junction: n = 2, pancreatic: n = 2, other: n = 2) and 13 age-matched healthy controls	Prospective	activPAL™ ambulatory PA meter	1. Functional assessment of anorexia and cachexia therapy (FAACT) 2. functional assessment of chronic illness therapy–fatigue (FACIT-F) 3. European Organization for Research and Treatment of Cancer (EORTC) QLQ-C30	EORTC QLQ-C30 Global health/QoL subscale Correlation between estimated total energy expenditure (r = −0.029, p = 0.905) and average steps per day (r = 0.047, p = 0.848) EORTC QLQ-C30 Physical functioning subscale Correlation between estimated total energy expenditure (r = 0.352, p = 0.139) and average steps per day (r = 0.370, p = 0.113) FACIT-F Trial outcome index Correlation between estimated total energy expenditure (r = 0.59, **p = 0.009**) and average steps per day (r = 0.59, **p = 0.008**) EORTC QLQ-C30 Fatigue subscale Correlation between estimated total energy expenditure (r = −0.281, p = 0.244) and average steps per day (r = −0.398, p = 0.091) FAACT (anorexia/cachexia) Trial outcome index Correlation between estimated total energy expenditure (r = 0.40, p = 0.089) and average steps per day (r = 0.41, p = 0.080) Cancer patients undergoing palliative chemotherapy spent more time lying/sitting (p = 0.0005) and less time in stepping (p = 0.003) than controls. Median number of total steps taken during week by cancer patients approximately 43% fewer than healthy controls (p = 0.002).
Fouladiun et al. (2007)	53 weight-losing outpatients with systemic cancer (pancreas: n = 18, esophagus/ventriculum: n = 13, colorectal: n = 4, unknown: n = 3, other: n = 4) and 8 age-matched controls	Prospective	ActiGraph™ accelerometer	Exercise testing on treadmill SenseWear PRO2 armband sensor body monitoring system QoL via SF-36 Resting energy expenditure via indirect calorimetry Body weight and composition via dual-energy x-ray absorptiometry	QoL was globally reduced in cancer patients (p < 0.01) with significantly reduced spontaneous PA, which continued to decline over follow-up period Patient survival was not predicted by spontaneous PA

(Continued)

Table 65.3 (Continued)   Summary of observational studies examining objective PA in palliative cancer patients

Authors	Sample	Design	PA measure	Other measures	Outcomes
Skipworth et al. (2011)	49 advanced cancer patients (aerodigestive: n = 56%, urogenital: 18%, breast: n = 13%) and healthy controls	Prospective	activPAL™ ambulatory PA meter	Karnofsky performance status Step count, number of transitions, and time spent upright against video study Energy expenditure against doubly labeled water and indirect calorimetry	Step count error was significantly higher in patients with non-self-caring Karnofsky Performance Status (KPS) 40–60 compared to self-caring KPS 70–100 (p = 0.006). Absolute errors for mean time spent in different body positions, number of transfers, mean energy expenditure, and total energy expenditure were low Inaccuracy of step count, particularly in non-self-caring patients
Ferriolli et al. (2012)	162 cancer patients (advanced palliative care undergoing palliative radiotherapy: n = 59 (main tumor sites of breast, prostate, and lung), advanced palliative care undergoing palliative chemotherapy: n = 37 (main tumor sites of upper gastrointestinal) and 20 healthy volunteers	Prospective	activPAL™ ambulatory PA meter	Performance status via World Health Organization (WHO)/ ECOG and Karnofsky scales QoL via European Organization for Research and Treatment of Cancer QoL Questionnaire–C30	Patients with advanced cancer took 45% few steps and spent an extra 2.8 h/day lying/sitting (p = 0.001). Significant correlations between PA and physical and role domains and fatigue subscale of EORTC QLQ-C30
Maddocks and Wilcock (2012)	43 patients with locally advanced (stage IIIb) and 41 patients with metastatic (stage IV) lung cancer (non–small cell lung cancer: n = 84, small cell lung cancer: n = 8, mesothelioma: n = 5)	Prospective	activPAL™ ambulatory PA meter	Performance status via ECOG	Patients with ECOG 0–2 took average 4200 steps/day and spent just over 4 hours upright Mean decline in both step count and time spent upright (standing or stepping) between ECOG categories was relatively large (>30%)

The authors concluded "success is more likely the sooner the programme commences after diagnosis rather than waiting until significant loss in function has occurred."[46]

OBSERVATIONAL STUDIES OF OBJECTIVE PHYSICAL ACTIVITY IN PALLIATIVE CANCER PATIENTS

In their pilot study of objective PA monitoring using the activ-PAL™ accelerometer in 20 patients with advanced upper gastrointestinal cancer receiving palliative chemotherapy versus 13 age-matched healthy controls, Dahele et al. (2007) reported significant reductions in estimated total energy expenditure, medium time spent upright, and median steps taken per day in the patient group.[47] Data on median survival of participants was not reported. There was no association between objective PA and the European Organization for Research and Treatment

of Cancer Quality of Life Questionnaire (EORTC QLQ-C30) global health score, although how much value patients place upon PA as a component of overall QoL is yet to be determined. Dahele et al. (2007) conclude that further research is required to explore whether PA can be used as a simple, objective, functional endpoint in advanced cancer patients.[47]

Fouladiun et al. (2007) evaluated Actigraph-measured spontaneous physical and rest activities in relation to nutritional state, energy metabolism, exercise capacity, and health-related QoL in 53 unselected weight-losing cancer patients versus age-matched noncancer patients.[48] The cancer patients exhibited significantly reduced spontaneous PA, which declined over time along with progression in their disease, and which correlated only weakly with maximum exercise capacity. Weight loss, self-reported PF, and bodily pain were all predictive of variations in overall daily PA. Only weight loss and serum albumin levels predicted patient survival, suggesting that daily physical and rest activity is a measure reflective of complex mental, physiologic, and metabolic interactions.[48]

Table 65.4 *Summary of observational studies of exercise capacity and PF in palliative cancer patients*

Authors	Sample	Design	Exercise capacity/PF	Other measures	Outcomes
Fouladiun et al. (2005)	311 unselected weight-losing cancer patients who were receiving palliative care (colorectal: n = 84, pancreas: n = 74, upper gastrointestinal: n = 73, liver-biliary: n = 51, breast: n = 3, melanoma: n = 5, other: n = 21)	Longitudinal	Treadmill walking to maximal exercise power	Blood serology (albumin, Erythrocyte Sedimentation Rate (ESR), C-Reactive Protein (CRP), Liver Function Tests (LFTs)) Radioimmunoassay of serum insulin, IGF-1, leptin, ghrelin Body composition via dual energy x-ray absorptiometry (DEXA) and body weight Energy expenditure via indirect calorimetry Dietary records	Resting energy expenditure and maximum exercise capacity remained unchanged in patients with decreased body weight and decreased lean tissue mass over time consistent with progressive cancer cachexia
Montoya et al. (2006)	99 stage III or stage IV non-small cell lung cancer patients recruited from outpatient thoracic centre	Prospective	SFA	Karnofsky performan ce status Edmonton symptom assessment system Brief fatigue inventory functional assessment of cancer therapy-lung (FACT-L)	Good adherence to SFA Low to moderate correlation between SFA changes on SFA and subjective fatigue assessments
Lundholm et al. (2007)	138 unselected advanced gastrointestinal cancer patients recruited from surgical department (esophageal/gastric: n = 53, liver/bile duct: n = 12, pancreas: n = 44, colorectal: n = 15, primary unknown: n = 5, miscellaneous: n = 9)	Randomized controlled trial of best supportive palliative care ± insulin treatment	Maximum physical capacity via MediGraph exercise testing Actigraph system monitoring daily PA	Body composition via dual energy x-ray absorptiometry Blood serology Resting energy expenditure via indirect calorimetry QoL via SF-36 and EORTC QL40	Insulin treatment increased metabolic efficiency during exercise (derived as oxygen consumed per watt produced at maximum work load), which may imply facilitated PF Insulin treatment did not increase maximum exercise capacity and spontaneous PA, which may be more dependent on cardiovascular and mental functioning than integrative metabolism Self-reported QoL indicated that positive objective metabolic effects of insulin treatment may not be translated into improved self-scored PF
Kasymjanova et al. (2009)	45 newly diagnosed non-small cell lung cancer patients recruited from outpatient oncology clinic	Prospective	6 min walk test for exercise capacity once on initial assessment, once prechemotherapy, and once after two cycles of chemotherapy	Blood serology: CRP and Hb levels ECOG performance status Survival	Patients with initial 6 MW 400 m ≤ had significantly greater survival time than those with initial 6 MW < 400 m (hazard ratio 0.44; 95% CI; 0.23–0.83 (p = 0.001)
Machado et al. (2010)	50 stage IIIB (n = 35) and stage IV (n = 15) non-small cell lung cancer patients undergoing paclitaxel and platinum derivative chemotherapy recruited from lung cancer outpatient clinic	Nonrandomized longitudinal trial	6 min walk distance prechemotherapy, postchemotherapy and 6 months after start of chemotherapy	ECOG performance status level Body mass index	Increased number of asymptomatic participants after 6-month follow-up accounted for improved performance status over course of chemotherapy, no significant changes in body mass index or 6 min walk distance

(Continued)

Table 65.4 (*Continued*)   *Summary of observational studies of exercise capacity and PF in palliative cancer patients*

Authors	Sample	Design	Exercise capacity/PF	Other measures	Outcomes
England et al. (2012)	41 incurable lung cancer patients recruited from outpatient clinic (non–small cell lung cancer: n = 26, mesothelioma: n = 11, small cell lung cancer: n = 4)	Prospective	exercise performance via incremental shuttle walking test Peripheral muscle power via leg extensor power	Inspiratory muscle strength via sniff nasal inspiratory pressure Lung function via simple spirometry Mastery over breathlessness via mastery domain of the chronic respiratory disease questionnaire	Only inspiratory muscle strength and peripheral muscle power were significantly related to and predictive of exercise performance
Jones et al. (2012)	118 consecutive metastatic non–small cell lung cancer patients recruited from university health system	Prospective	Functional capacity via 6 min walk distance	Exercise behavior via Godin leisure-time exercise questionnaire ECOG performance status level Survival	Functional capacity via 6 min walk distance was a strong independent predictor of survival in advanced non–small cell lung cancer
Low et al. (2012)	101 consecutive patients recruited from specialist palliative day care therapy unit for rehabilitation (noncancer: n = 14, first remission: n = 29, first recurrence: n = 16, metastatic disease: n = 42)	Cross-sectional	Physical function via 1 min timed sit-to-stand test and timed 2 min walking test	Acceptance measured using Acceptance and Action Questionnaire-II Psychological status using Kessler-10 Mortality within 6 months entry into study	Positive correlation between acceptance and sit to stand (r = 0.27) and distance walked (r = 0.21), suggesting it may be possible to improve physical mobility by increasing patient's acceptance via an acceptance and commitment therapy–based intervention

Skipworth et al. (2011) tested the criterion-based validity of activPAL™ step count, number of transitions and time spent upright against video observations, and activPAL energy expenditure against doubly labeled water and indirect calorimetry in 49 advanced cancer patients versus healthy controls.[49] The majority of participants had advanced gastrointestinal and lung cancer, although location of metastatic disease and survival were not reported. Although absolute errors for activPAL mean time spent in different body positions, number of transfers, and mean energy expenditure were low, the authors reported that activPAL step count was significantly higher in non-self-caring participants (Karnofsky performance status 40–60) versus self-caring participants (Karnofsky performance status 70–100). The authors concluded that the variability in results due to step count inaccuracy warranted further research.[49]

Ferriolli et al. (2012) examined objective PA using the activPAL monitor in 162 cancer patients, including 59 patients receiving palliative radiotherapy for bone metastases and 37 patients receiving palliative chemotherapy for advanced upper gastrointestinal cancer which were designated "advanced palliative care stage."[50] Data on median survival of participants was not reported. Advanced palliative care patients demonstrated 45% fewer steps and increased time in the lying/sitting position compared to patients with early-stage disease, and there were moderate correlations between objective PA and the physical, role, and fatigue domains of the EORTC QLQ-C30 scale. The authors concluded that objective monitoring of daily PA may have the potential as an objective endpoint in clinical management and research trials of this population.[50]

Maddocks and Wilcock (2012) measured objective PA levels using the activPAL monitor in 43 patients with locally advanced (stage IIIb) and 41 patients with metastatic (stage IV) lung cancer.[51] Data on median survival of participants were not reported. The authors determined that patients with an ECOG PS 0–2 took an average of 4200 steps/day and spent approximately 4 hours/day in the upright position, which is significantly less than that reported for healthy older adults and those with nonmalignant disease. There was significant variation in PA across ECOG PS categories, with the authors concluding that further research was needed to improve scale sensitivity.[51]

OBSERVATIONAL STUDIES OF EXERCISE CAPACITY AND PHYSICAL FUNCTIONING IN PALLIATIVE CANCER PATIENTS

Fouladiun et al. (2005) conducted a longitudinal study examining correlations between time course changes in body composition, food intake, metabolism, exercise capacity, and hormones in 311 unselected cancer patients receiving palliative

Table 65.5 *Summary of interventional studies of PA in palliative cancer patients*

Authors	Sample	Design	Exercise intervention	Measures	Outcomes
Yoshioka (1994)	301 terminal cancer patients who received physical therapy in a hospice facility (Stomach (55) Lung (43) Breast (38) Rectum (28) Uterus (23) Liver (21) Colon (18) Ovary (11) Pancreas (10) Other (55)	Retrospective study of patients Cross-sectional questionnaire study of families of deceased patients	Techniques used singly or in combination: 1. Positioning for cancer pain 2. Therapeutic exercise aimed at muscle strength, range of motion, and balance 3. Activities of daily living exercises aimed at enabling function 4. Endurance training aimed at physical fitness 5. Chest physiotherapy 6. Swallowing exercises 7. Intermittent pneumatic compression for edema 8. Thermotherapy 9. Acupuncture 10. Brace/sling/splint	Barthel mobility index	Barthel mobility index (maximum 47 points) Average score increased from 12.4 to 19.9 after rehabilitation program Questionnaire to 169 families of deceased patients: 78% were satisfied with rehabilitation program, 63% considered program to be effective
Porock et al. (2000)	9 home hospice care patients Bowel (n = 4) Pancreas (n = 2) Melanoma (n = 1) Breast (n = 1) Oral (n = 1) Metastases (n = 7) Active RT (n = 1) Active chemo (n = 2)	Single group pre- to postintervention study	Unsupervised home-based exercise program based on individualized "Duke energizing exercise plan" with range of physical activities throughout the day, with frequency and duration set according to Winningham's half rule of thumb for 28 days	QoL via Graham and Longman's QoL scale Fatigue via MFI Anxiety and Depression via Hospital Anxiety and Depression Scale (HADS) Symptom Distress via McCorkle and Young's SDS	Graham & Longman's Scale Mean QoL rating: 5.3 (Day 0) 6.1 (Day 7) 6.6 (Day 14) Incomplete data for HADS, adherence, and withdrawals.
Crevenna et al. (2003b)	55-year-old male with advanced hepatocellular cancer with lung and brain metastases undergoing palliative thalidomide therapy	Case report	Supervised aerobic exercise program Bicycle ergometer cycling with workload systematic increase to maintain training HR at 60% of maximum workload of first symptom-limited exercise test. 60 min per session, 2 sessions per week for 6 weeks.	Symptom-limited ergometric bicycle exercise test: 1. Peak work capacity, endurance capacity, and HR 2. 6 min walk 3. Grimsby's self-reported physical performance questionnaire 4. QoL via SF-36 5. Self-reported benefit in physical performance, mental state, satisfaction and QoL	No adverse events reported. 100% compliance with training sessions. Participant commented on "being persistently and positively motivated by the physicians" SF-36 General health perception subscale: Pre: 65, Post: 62 SF-36 PF subscale: Pre:65, Post:85 SF-36 Vitality/fatigue subscale: Pre:25, Post:50 SF-36 Pain subscale: Pre: 22, Post: 41

(Continued)

Table 65.5 (Continued)   *Summary of interventional studies of PA in palliative cancer patients*

Authors	Sample	Design	Exercise intervention	Measures	Outcomes
Crevenna et al. (2003a)	48-year-old female with advanced breast cancer with lung, liver, and bone metastases undergoing palliative chemotherapy and radiotherapy	Case report	Supervised aerobic exercise program Bicycle ergometer cycling with workload increased to maintain training HR at 60% of maximum workload of first symptom-limited exercise test. 60 min per session, 3 sessions per week for 52 weeks.	Symptom-limited ergometric bicycle exercise test: 1. VO_2max, peak work capacity, and HR 2. Lung function via respiratory quotient 3. QoL via SF-36 4. Self-reported physical performance, mental state, fatigue, sleep, satisfaction, and QoL	No adverse events reported Participant attributed benefit to persistent and positive motivation by the physicians Incomplete data reporting from SF-36
Kelm et al. (2003)	58-year-old male with rectal adenocarcinoma (pT3N0M1) with liver metastases undergoing postop intrahepatic chemotherapy	Case report	Supervised whole body strength and endurance training: 1. Strength training machines at 40%–60% of 1-repetition maximum up to 5 series of 20 repetitions. 2. Treadmill/bicycle/upper body ergometer 10 min each with resistance and speed controlled to HR between 130–150 bpm. 6-week postop and every 2 weeks between chemotherapy cycles for total of 13 weeks	Upper extremity and lower extremity strength: 1. RM 2. Endurance by reduction in HR and lactate concentration 3. Lung function by Forced Expiratory Volume in 1 Second (FEV1), Forced Vital Capacity (FVC), and Vital Capacity (VC) 4. QoL by GIQLI score 5. Immune function by NK cell count	GIQLI Pre: 106, Post: 129 +21.6% difference
Headley et al. (2004)	38 women with stage IV breast cancer patients receiving chemotherapy	Randomized controlled longitudinal trial	Unsupervised home-based seated exercise program using armchair fitness: gentle exercise video, 30 min per session, 3 sessions per week for 12 weeks	1. Fatigue and QoL via the FACIT-F 2. Perceived intensity via the Borg rating of perceived exertion scale	FACIT-F Total scores: t[49] = 2.31; **p = 0.0254** Experimental group's decline in total well-being occurred at a slower rate than in control group FACIT-F Functional well-being subscale: no significant difference between groups at any time point FACIT-F Fatigue subscale: t[49] = 2.78; **p = 0.0078** Experimental group's decline in fatigue occurred at a slower rate than in control group
Crevenna et al. (2006)	47-year-old female with advanced lung cancer with brain and bone metastases	Case report	Neuromuscular electrical stimulation on bilateral gluteal and thigh muscles in 60 min sessions, five sessions per week for a total of four weeks	6 min walk distance Timed-up-and-go QoL via SF-36	6 min walk distance improved by 44% Improvement in timed-up-and-go, demonstrating improvement in mobility Improvements in PF, vitality, bodily pain, and general health subscales of SF-36

Study	Sample	Design	Intervention	Outcome measures	Results	Comments
						Useful palliative treatment in patients with brain and bone metastases wherein risk of seizures and pathological fractures may preclude volitional training
McDonald et al. (2006)	Six patients with advanced progressive illnesses and recruited from palliative day care	Single group pre- to postintervention trial	Once-weekly 40 min Dru Yoga sessions over a 12-week period. Each session included activation, energy block release, posture and sequences, and relaxation phases	Questionnaire regarding patient feedback and perceived benefits and challenges	5 patients completed all 12 sessions, over 57% reported a positive response to the program, greater than 60% of participants reported interest in attending more sessions	
Oldervoll et al. (2005, 2006)	34 palliative cancer patients from outpatient clinic and hospice. Gastrointestinal (n = 16), Breast (n = 5), Genitourinary (n = 5), Lung (n = 1), Miscellaneous (n = 7), Metastases (n = 27), Active chemo (n = 9), Active hormone therapy (n = 3)	Single group pre- to post intervention trial	Supervised group exercise program (3–8 patients per group) with personalized circuit training stations focused on UE/LE muscle strength, standing balance, and aerobic endurance with 50 min per session, 2 sessions per week for 6 weeks	1. Physical performance via 6 min walk, timed sit-to-stand, functional reach 2. Fatigue via FQ 3. QoL via EORTC QLQ-C30	Adherence rate to exercise sessions 10.6/12. 46% attrition rate. EORTC QLQ-C30 Global QoL subscale: Pre:61(21) Post:64(20) $p = 0.26$ EORTC QLQ-C30 PF subscale: Pre:65(20), Post:67(22) $p = 0.62$ Fatigue Questionnaire Total fatigue subscale: Pre:17.5(4.7), Post:15.5(5.8) $p = 0.06$ Mental fatigue subscale: Pre:5.3(1.7), Post:5.1(2.0) $p = 0.42$ Physical fatigue subscale: Pre:12.2(3.6), Post:10.4(4.1) $p = 0.04$ EORTC QLQ-C30 Nausea/vomiting: Pre:18(25), Post:14(19) $p = 0.26$ Pain: Pre:41(35), Post:37(34) $p = 0.36$ Dyspnea: Pre:42(33), Post:30(31) $p = 0.006$ Appetite loss: Pre:37(38), Post:28(35) $p = 0.07$	

(Continued)

Table 65.5 (continued) *Summary of interventional studies of PA in palliative cancer patients*

Authors	Sample	Design	Exercise intervention	Measures	Outcomes
Hui et al. (2008)	21 terminal cancer patients from hospital palliative day care unit	Single group pre- to post intervention trial	Group Tai Chi classes, with three classes per week for total of 18 consecutive weeks Each class included 30 min of general mobilizing exercises based on 18-form Tai Chi training	Functional status via modified version of functional ambulation classification (MFAC) Mobility via timed up and go test (TUG) Flexibility via functional reach test (FRT) Balance via Berg's Balance Scale (BBS) Overall handicap via Chinese version London handicap scale (LHS)	Significant improvements in mean MFAC (p = 0.034), TUG (p = 0.017), FRT (p = 0.000), and BBS (p = 0.001) scores postintervention Improvements in independence (p = 0.012), mobility (p = 0.001) domains of LHS
Maddocks et al. (2009)	16 non–small cell lung cancer patients recruited from thoracic oncology clinics	Randomized controlled pilot study	Daily neuromuscular electrical stimulation of quadricep muscles for 4 weeks	Quadricep muscle strength via Cybex NORM dynamometer Exercise endurance via endurance shuttle walk test Free-living PA via activPAL™ accelerometer	Median (range) adherence to program was 80% No significant differences in outcomes between groups
Temel et al. (2009)	25 newly diagnosed advanced stage non–small cell lung cancer patients (stage IIIB with pleural or pericardial effusions: n = 4, stage IV: n = 21)	Single group pre- to post intervention trial	Twice weekly group exercise sessions for 12 week period Groups of 8–10 patients, each session lasting approximately 90–120 min in duration. Sessions included 10 min warm-up period, 30 min aerobic exercise (15 min on treadmill, 15 min on upright bicycle) to achieve 70–85% maximum HR or perceived exertion of 13, 30–40 min strength training component (3 sets of 10 repetitions of 6 different exercises, 3 upper extremity, and 3 lower extremity movements, starting at 60% of 1RM and increasing to 80% of 1RM over course of 16 sessions	Symptom-limited submaximal modified Bruce treadmill test, progressing to 85% of participant's age-predicted maximal HR Functional exercise capacity via 6 min walk test Muscle strength via maximal amount of weight that each muscle group can move through available ROM FACT-G, FACT-L, HADS	44% of patients completed all 16 planned sessions. Study completers experienced significant reduction in lung cancer symptoms and no deterioration in 6 min walk test or muscle strength
Buss et al. (2010)	49 home and stationary hospice advanced cancer patients with life expectancy of 1–3 months	Nonrandomized controlled trial	Individually supervised kinesitherapy exercises 3 times/week, for 20–30 min in duration, for period of 3–4 weeks	Rotterdam symptom checklist Brief fatigue inventory Visual analogue fatigue scale	Fatigue intensity decreased significantly after 3 weeks in intervention group, whereas fatigue intensity increased after 2 weeks of observation QoL in intervention group remained stable throughout the study, whereas tendency toward deterioration of QoL with time passing in control group

Author (year)	Study design	Population	Intervention	Outcomes measured	Results
Tatematsu et al. (2011)	Retrospective study	48 hospitalized cancer patients referred to palliative care team	Walking and/or range of motion exercise (at least one of these), others (Activities of Daily Living (ADL) training, resistance training, stretching, etc), daily frequency (except weekends) for 20 min/day. Participants enrolled in exercise therapy at the time of onset of delirium symptoms	Administered antipsychotic drug doses; Survival time	Administered doses of antipsychotic medications significantly lower in exercise group compared to nonexercise group
Oldervoll et al. (2011)	Multicenter randomized controlled trial	231 advanced cancer patients with life expectancy ≤2 years recruited from day care palliative care units and outpatient oncological units (exercise vs. usual care) Gastrointestinal (34% vs. 29%) Breast (19% vs. 26%) Lung (17% vs. 16%) Urological (13% vs. 13%) Gynecological (7% vs. 4%) Hematological (2% vs. 5%) Other (8% vs. 9%)	60 min group exercise session supervised by physiotherapist given twice weekly over 8-week period Program includes warm-up, circuit training with 6 stations (lower limb strengthening, balance, upper limb strengthening, general functioning, lower limb strengthening, aerobic endurance)	Fatigue questionnaire: primary endpoint of fatigue Physical performance tests: 1. Sit to stand 2. Grip strength 3. Maximal step length 4. Shuttle walk test	36% of exercise group lost to follow-up compared to 23% usual care group, primarily due to disease progression Adherence rate was 69% for participants in exercise group who completed pre- and posttesting 6 min walk test (EMD 60 m, $p = 0.008$), grip strength test (EMD 2.0, $p = 0.01$) Fatigue questionnaire No significant between-group effects in physical fatigue (Estimated Mean Difference (EMD) −0.3, $p = 0.62$) total fatigue (EMD −0.3, $p = 0.53$) or mental fatigue (EMD −0.3, $p = 0.53$)
Lopez-Sendin et al. (2012)	Randomized controlled pilot study	24 terminal cancer patients admitted to hospital oncology department (lung: n = 12, melanoma: n = 3, sarcoma: n = 2, pancreas: n = 3, breast: n = 2, other: n = 3)	Physiotherapy intervention included several different therapeutic massage techniques, passive mobilization, active-assisted or active-resisted exercises, and local- and global-resisted exercises, proprioceptive neuromuscular facilitation Choice, duration, and strength of each session determined by the therapist based on patient response to intervention Control group received simple hand contact placed on areas of pain and maintained for same period as intervention group	Primary outcome: Brief pain inventory (BPI) Memorial pain assessment card Memorial Symptom Assessment Scale	Significant improvements in intervention group for Brief Pain Inventory (BPI) worst pain, BPI pain right now, BPI index, Memorial Symptom Assessment Scale (MSAS) psychological subscales

care during 4–62 months of follow-up.[52] The authors reported that although there was loss of body fat and lean tissue mass concurrent with decrease in serum albumin and increased biomarkers of systemic inflammation, "resting energy expenditure and maximum exercise capacity remained unchanged in the same patients."[52] The authors postulated that nutrient uptake may be preferential toward lean tissue mass, hence maintaining the same level in maximum exercise capacity.[52]

Montoya et al. (2006) conducted a prospective study of 100 ambulatory patients with stage III or IV non–small cell lung cancer to determine PF using the SFA test, and to explore the association between objective physical function and patient-reported QoL.[53] The SFA test was comprised of eight items (including putting on a sock, tying a belt, putting coins in a cup, reaching above the head, standing up and sitting down, reaching forward, walking for 50 ft, and 6 min walk). Montoya et al. (2006) reported only low to moderate correlations between the SFA test and self-reported fatigue scores, suggesting that objective and subjective assessment of PF offers differing yet complementary information in this sample of advanced lung cancer patients.[53]

Lundholm et al. (2007) conducted a randomized controlled trial of insulin treatment plus best available palliative support in 138 unselected patients with mainly advanced gastrointestinal malignancy, with a median survival of 128 days.[54] Although there was a positive association between insulin treatment and increased metabolic efficiency, this did not affect maximum exercise capacity or spontaneous PA levels as measured by Actigraph system. The authors concluded that cardiovascular and mental functioning may have more impact on maximum exercise testing and spontaneous PA levels, than integrative metabolism, in this patient population.[54]

Kasymjanova et al. (2009) examined the 6 min walk test as a prognostic tool in 45 advanced non–small cell lung cancer patients both before and after two cycles of chemotherapy.[55] All participants had stage IIIA or higher disease, with an overall median survival of 11.1 months. There was a statistically significant decline in 6 min walk distance after two cycles of chemotherapy, with a distance of greater than or equal to 400 m on baseline testing being predictive of survival after adjusting for covariates.[55]

Machado et al. (2010) conducted a nonrandomized longitudinal trial examining performance status, body mass index, and 6 min walk distance in 50 non–small cell lung cancer patients undergoing chemotherapy.[56] Thirty percent of the participants presented with stage IV disease, and 46% of the participants showed worsening of performance status or passed away before or after the 6-month follow-up period. Although the increased number of asymptomatic participants after 6-month follow-up accounted for improved performance status over the course of chemotherapy, there were no significant changes in body mass index or 6 min walk distance, suggesting maintenance of physical condition during the chemotherapy period.[56]

England et al. (2012) examined factors related to exercise performance using the incremental shuttle walking test in 41 incurable lung cancer patients with a median survival of 47 weeks.[57] England et al. (2012) determined that inspiratory muscle strength using sniff nasal inspiratory pressure, and peripheral muscle power using leg extensor power, was positively associated with and predictive of exercise performance. The authors concluded that rehabilitation efforts focusing on inspiratory and peripheral muscle training should be explored in this patient group.[57]

Jones et al. (2012) examined functional capacity using the 6 min walk test and self-reported exercise behavior in 118 consecutive metastatic non–small lung cancer patients.[58] Participants reporting lower PA levels likewise had lower median survival (12.89 versus 25.63 months), suggesting that functional capacity using the 6 min walk test is an independent predictor of survival in advanced non–small cell lung cancer.[58]

Low et al. (2012) conducted a cross-sectional study of 101 consecutive specialist palliative care day therapy patients examining the association between experiential acceptance, as measured by the Acceptance and Action Questionnaire-II, and psychological well-being and functional status, as measured by a timed 2 min walking test and 1 min sit-to-stand test.[59] Participants' cancer diagnosis and location of metastatic disease were not reported; however, the authors noted that 15% of participants died within 6 months from study recruitment. The authors reported a positive association between experiential acceptance and sit-to-stand and 2 min walking test, suggesting that improvements in physical mobility may be possible via increasing acceptance using an acceptance and commitment therapy intervention.[59]

INTERVENTIONAL STUDIES OF PHYSICAL ACTIVITY IN PALLIATIVE CANCER PATIENTS

Yoshioka (1994) conducted a retrospective study of 301 consecutive terminal cancer patients receiving a rehabilitation program under the supervision of a trained physical therapist in a hospice, from 1987 to 1993.[24] The rehabilitation program consisted of the following components, which were used singly or in combination: positioning for relief of cancer pain, therapeutic exercise aimed at muscular strength, range of motion and balance, activities of daily living exercises aimed at enabling function, endurance training aimed at physical fitness, chest physiotherapy, swallowing exercises, intermittent pneumatic compression for edema, thermotherapy, acupuncture, and use of brace, sling, or splint for pain relief. No data regarding exercise type, duration, intensity, or frequency was given. Median time from start of rehabilitation until death was 35 days, and median time from end of rehabilitation program until death was 12 days. The average score of the Barthel mobility index improved from 12.4 to 19.9 postintervention, with 63% of deceased patients' families indicating that the rehabilitation program had been effective. Yoshioka (1994) concluded that "the rehabilitative care can continue to the day of death, depending, of course, on the assessment of the condition of the patient by physical therapists, nurses and/or families."[24]

Porock et al. (2000) conducted a single group post intervention study of unsupervised home-based PA program in nine home hospice care patients.[60] No staging or survival information was reported. The intervention consisted of an individualized "Duke Energizing Exercise Plan" with range of physical activities throughout the day, with frequency and duration set according to Winningham's half rule of thumb for 28 days.[60] Mean QoL ratings measured via Graham and Longman's QOL scale increased over the duration of the intervention, although physical function, fatigue, symptoms, and physical fitness outcomes were not reported.[60]

Crevenna et al. (2003) reported two case studies of supervised aerobic exercise in a 55-year-old male with advanced hepatocellular cancer with lung and brain metastases,[61] and a 48-year-old female with advanced breast cancer with lung, liver, and bone metastases.[62] The intervention consisted of bicycle ergometer cycling for 60 min/session, with two sessions per week for 6 weeks for the former case study and three sessions per week for 52 weeks for the latter. There was improvement in general health perception, PF, and vitality/fatigue as measured by Short Form-36 (SF-36), and an increased in peak oxygen uptake and peak work capacity postintervention.[61,62]

Kelm et al. (2003) reported a case study of supervised whole-body strength and endurance training in a 58-year-old male with rectal adenocarcinoma with liver metastases during postoperative intrahepatic chemotherapy.[63] The intervention consisted of strength training component using machines at 40%–60% of one repetition maximum, up to five series of 20 repetitions, and treadmill/bicycle/upper-body ergometer for 10 min each with resistance and speed controlled to maintain heart rate between 130 and 150 beats/min.[63] The training commenced 6 weeks postoperatively, and every 2 weeks between chemotherapy cycles, for a total of 13 weeks. There was improvement in the gastrointestinal QoL index postintervention, and improvements in forced expiratory volume in 1 s, forced vital capacity and inspiratory vital capacity postintervention.[63]

Headley et al. (2004) conducted a randomized, controlled longitudinal trial of an unsupervised home-based seated exercise program in 38 stage IV breast cancer patients receiving chemotherapy.[64] Life expectancy or median survival time was not reported. The intervention consisted of 30 min sessions of seated exercise using armchair fitness: gentle exercise video, for a total of three sessions per week for 12 weeks. Data for adherence and intensity of activity were incomplete. There was a statistically significant slowing of decline in fatigue and total well-being, as measured by the functional assessment of chronic illness therapy—fatigue version IV, in the experimental versus control group.[64] Symptoms, self-reported PF, and objective physical fitness outcomes were not reported.

Crevenna et al. (2006) reported a case study of neuromuscular electrical stimulation in a 47-year-old female with advanced lung cancer with brain and bone metastases.[65] The neuromuscular electrical stimulation protocol used biphasic, symmetric pulses was administered on the bilateral gluteal and thigh muscles in 60 min sessions, five sessions per week for a total of 4 weeks. There was improvement in the 6 min walk and the timed-up-and-go tests postintervention, as well as improvement in the SF-36 QoL scales; adherence was 100%, and no adverse events were encountered during the training period.

The authors concluded that neuromuscular electrical stimulation may be a useful palliative treatment in patients with brain and bone metastases, wherein the risk of seizures and pathological fractures would prohibit volitional exercise training.[65]

McDonald et al. (2006) conducted a pilot study of a once-weekly 40 min Dru Yoga session over a 12-week period with a sample of six patients in a palliative day care setting.[66] Dru yoga "involves gentle flowing physical movements, performed slowly with awareness and often with many repetitions of each movement/posture"; each session was comprised of activation, energy block release, posture, sequences, and relaxation phases. All patients had advanced progressive illnesses; however, information regarding cancer diagnosis, metastatic disease burden, and survival was not reported. Five patients completed all 12 sessions, and over 57% reported a positive response to the program; greater than 60% of participants reported interest in attending more sessions. Participants' comments highlighted the positive aspects of gentle exercises, mind–body connection, and relaxation.[66]

Oldervoll et al. (2006) conducted a phase II pilot study of a twice-weekly supervised group exercise program on QoL, fatigue, and objective physical performance in 34 incurable cancer patients with clinician-estimated life expectancy between 3 months and 1 year.[67] Sixty-three percent of patients were willing to participate in the exercise intervention, and 54% of the participants completed the entire 6-week intervention, with the most frequent reason for withdrawal being disease progression and pain.[68] After the 6-week-long program, the distance walked in 6 min was increased and timed sit-to-stand was reduced; there were improvements in emotional functioning and physical fatigue postintervention.[67]

Hui et al. (2008) conducted a pilot study of group Tai Chi classes in 21 terminal cancer patients from a hospital palliative day care unit.[69] Group classes included 30 min of general mobilizing exercise based on the 18-form tai chi training, with three courses per week for a total of 18 consecutive weeks. No data regarding cancer diagnosis, survival, or adherence was reported. The authors reported significant improvements in functional ambulation classification, timed up and go test, functional reach test and Berg's balance scale postintervention, with improvements in mean scores of independence and mobility domains of the Chinese version London handicap scale, postintervention.[69]

Maddocks et al. (2009) conducted a randomized controlled pilot study of a 4-week program of daily neuromuscular electrical stimulation of the quadriceps muscle in 16 patients with non–small cell lung cancer and ECOG performance status of 0 or 1 recruited from thoracic oncology clinics in the United Kingdom.[70] Median adherence was 80%; however, there were no statistically significant differences between treatment and usual groups in dynamometer-assessed quadriceps muscle strength, exercise endurance as assessed by the shuttle walk test, or free-living PA levels as assessed by activPAL accelerometer.[70]

Temel et al. (2009) conducted a pilot study of twice-weekly aerobic exercise and weight training sessions facilitated by a physical therapist over an 8-week period in 25 newly diagnosed advanced stage non–small cell lung cancer patients.[71] Eighty-four percent of participants had stage IV non–small cell lung cancer, and seventy-two percent of participants were undergoing initial chemotherapy. With their primary endpoint being adherence to the exercise program, the authors reported that 44% of participants were able to complete all 16 planned sessions, and 24% of participants attended at least 6 sessions prior to withdrawing from the study due to health status deterioration. Of the 11 participants who completed the intervention program, there was a statistically significant improvement in the functional assessment of cancer therapy–lung (FACT-L) lung cancer subscale score and in elbow extension postintervention, with no deterioration in 6 min walk test or other measures of muscle strength capacity.[71]

Buss et al. (2010) conducted a nonrandomized controlled trial of kinesitherapy in 49 home and stationary hospice patients in Poland.[72] The intervention group performed exercises 3 times/week, for 20–30 min in length, over a period of 3–4 weeks; although the authors stated that "exercises were individually supervised by a physiotherapist, following a carefully worked out pattern," neither a definition of kinesitherapy nor a description of the specific exercises was reported. The sample was described as "far advanced cancer patients under hospice care, with the life expectancy of 1–3 months"; however, participant characteristics, including cancer diagnosis and location of metastatic disease, were not reported. The authors demonstrated that in the intervention group, the intensity of fatigue decreased significantly after 3 weeks of kinesitherapy; the intensity of fatigue in the control group, however, increased after 2 weeks of observation. The overall QoL in the intervention group, as measured by the Rotterdam symptom checklist, remained stable over the course of 4 weeks, whereas that of the control group deteriorated.[72]

Tatematsu et al. (2011) conducted a retrospective study examining the effects of exercise therapy on antipsychotic drugs used to treat delirium symptoms in 48 hospitalized cancer patients who were referred to the palliative care team.[73] Participants were divided into exercise and nonexercise therapy groups depending on whether exercise therapy was being used for early ambulation at the time of onset of delirium; although there were no significant baseline differences between groups, 35% of the exercise group and 42% of the nonexercise group participants had a survival of less than 6 months. The authors reported that despite the fact that doses of opioid medication did not differ significantly between groups, the administered dose of antipsychotic medications was significantly lower in the exercise group compared to the nonexercise group, suggesting that delirium symptoms may have been attenuated in patients who received exercise therapy.[73]

Oldervoll et al. (2011) conducted a multicenter randomized controlled trial of 231 cancer patients recruited from day care palliative care units and outpatient oncology departments in Norway.[74] Among the patients who successfully completed the intervention, the median survival times were 16.3 months in the physical exercise versus 17.1 months in the usual care group. The PA intervention consisted of twice-weekly physiotherapist-supervised group exercise sessions for an 8-week period, which included circuit training focused on lower and upper limb muscle strength, standing balance, and aerobic endurance. The average adherence rate was 69%, and 36% of participants in the intervention group were lost to follow-up, primarily due to disease progression. There were no significant between-group effects in physical fatigue as measured by the fatigue questionnaire; however, significant improvement in physical performance tests, including shuttle walk test, sit to stand, handgrip strength, and maximal step length, was found in the physical exercise versus usual care groups. The authors concluded that their specific exercise intervention was less feasible for patients with a life expectancy of less than 6 months.[74]

Lopez-Sendin et al. (2012) conducted a randomized controlled pilot study examining the effects of physical therapy, including massage and exercise, on pain and mood in 24 terminal cancer patients admitted to a hospital oncology department.[75] The majority of participants had a diagnosis of lung cancer, with the majority of tumor metastases being osseous in location; although there were no significant between-group baseline differences, the authors reported a 25.8 month time of diagnosis in the intervention group, versus 17.5 months in the control group. The intervention consisted of therapeutic massage techniques in combination with passive mobilization, active-assisted or active-resisted exercises, and local- and global-resisted exercises, with the choice, intensity, and duration of each session being tailored to the individual participant by the physical therapist; the control group received simple hand contact to areas of pain and maintained for the same period as the intervention group. Each session was 30–35 min in duration over a 2-week period. The authors reported significant improvements in pain and psychological outcomes in the intervention group, although the control group also demonstrated improvements in the Brief Pain Inventory least pain, and Memorial Symptom Assessment Scale physical scores.[75]

FUTURE RESEARCH DIRECTIONS

Although there has been an increase in the evidence examining PA interventions in advanced cancer patients, there are significant gaps in the literature that remain to be addressed. First and foremost, there is an urgent need for consensus regarding the definition of the palliative patient.[5] The 2010 American College of Sports Medicine Roundtable on Exercise Guidelines for Cancer Survivors characterizes patients in the palliation phase of the cancer control continuum as those with progressive disease and who are at the end of life.[12] The adjective "palliative," however, has been attributed to a wide range of patient characteristics: having incurable disease, undergoing noncurative chemotherapy or radiotherapy, having pain or other symptoms related to cancer and its treatment and which require interdisciplinary management, receiving palliative care services via specialist consultation or at palliative care hospice, clinician-estimated life expectancy, or being at the end of life. In their survey of Dutch general practitioners, Borgsteede et al. (2006) demonstrated significant differences in the elicited patient populations based on the different inclusive criteria of "noncurative treatment," "palliative care," and "death was expected"; the authors recommended that future research should include a combination of different criteria, including the intent of the palliative care provided as well as an assessment of the participant's life expectancy as an indicator of their chronological status along the cancer trajectory.[76] In lieu of clinician estimates, use of a validated prognostic tool may aid in defining the patient population more precisely.

An alternative categorization would be to use palliative performance status (PPS) level. The PPS scale has been widely used, validated, and shown to be predictive of prognosis in palliative cancer populations.[7] The PPS also incorporates aspects of both self-care and mobility, which have been identified as key components of PF in palliative care populations.[31] Determining the optimal type of PA intervention at each PPS level would be a priority so as to include as many patients of varying functional abilities for as long as possible during their disease course. Along with more thorough characterization of the functional trajectory of disease, future research should aim toward encouraging mobility in as many palliative cancer patients as possible, in view of decreasing symptom burden and maintaining overall QoL.

The traditional purview of palliative care being limited to the end of life has been challenged by more recent studies confirming the QoL and survival benefits of palliative care earlier in the cancer trajectory, even from time of initial diagnosis.[78] This shift in the scope of palliative care may redirect research on PA interventions toward tumor-specific TNM stage and metastatic site-specific populations, rather than by clinician-estimated life expectancy alone. This does not, however, preclude the need to investigate whether PA interventions are beneficial throughout the cancer trajectory, up to and including the end of life. There is a critical gap in the evidence with respect to what PA interventions are feasible in patients who have extremely limited mobility or who are bed-bound. What type of PA is most beneficial at which point of the disease trajectory has yet to be determined.

Given the loss of functioning and progressive debility that accompanies advanced cancer, there have been emerging preliminary studies on assessment tools and outcome measures for PF and PA in this population. There is significant heterogeneity in terms of assessment instruments and outcome measures used for PF and PA, which makes it challenging to compare intervention effects across studies.[79] Further research is needed to validate and compare assessment tools for self-reported PF and self-reported PA, as well as outcome measures for objective PF and objective PA levels.

Although fatigue has been identified as a primary outcome in many of the studies involving PA interventions in advanced cancer patients, there are emerging studies examining the effect of these interventions on other symptoms that are relevant to palliative care, including delirium and pain. Although there are a few qualitative studies exploring the meaning of PA to advanced cancer patients, there are none examining the primary psychological outcomes of PA interventions in advanced cancer patients. Given the high symptom burden faced by advanced cancer patients with progressive disease, and the

correlation between loss of PF and request for euthanasia, this would be an area deserving of critical attention.

The growing research interest in this field has provided stimulus for future studies. Rief et al. (2011) recently published a prospective, randomized controlled trial protocol in parallel-group design to examine the effect of isometric muscle training of the spine musculature in patients with spinal bony metastases under radiation therapy.[80] Galvao et al. (2012) recently published a randomized clinical trial protocol investigating the efficacy and safety of a multimodal (resistance, aerobic, and flexibility) exercise program in prostate cancer patients with bone metastases.[81] Given the interest in sedentary behavior, together with the 2010 American College of Sports Medicine Roundtable on Exercise Guidelines for Cancer Survivors recommendation to "avoid inactivity,"[12] future studies examining the effects of reducing sedentary behavior on QoL in palliative cancer patients would be warranted.

CLINICAL IMPLICATIONS

Despite the emerging nature of the evidence base of PA and PF in palliative cancer care, there are a number of noteworthy implications for clinicians. First, for those advanced cancer patients who express interest in PA, it is incumbent on the clinician to conduct a thorough clinical history and pertinent physical examination related to the patient's current level of functioning, including level of mobility and self-care, and current level of PA, including type, intensity, duration, and frequency. Second, the clinician should conduct a detailed symptom assessment, including pain and fatigue, as poorly managed symptoms may impact the patient's ability to tolerate, as well as gain any potential benefit from, PA. The etiologies underlying symptoms should be elucidated, and both nonpharmacological and pharmacological therapies should be considered to target the underlying etiologies and ameliorate the resulting symptoms. Third, multidisciplinary team involvement, including physical therapy and rehabilitation services, would be important for expertise and ongoing supervision of the patient's activity and function goals. Comprehensive, holistic assessment and multidisciplinary collaboration is critical in tailoring PA prescription based on the advanced cancer patient's abilities and functional status.

Based on the current evidence, palliative cancer patients are encouraged to consider PA under the specific direction and guidance of the multidisciplinary team. Walking can be performed to tolerance in most individuals, and is reported to be among the most preferred activities in this population.[43] Repetition of specific functional tasks may assist in preserving basic activities of daily living, and assisted range of motion exercises may be encouraged to minimize muscle contractures and to slow muscle deconditioning. Although there is emerging evidence that PA interventions can improve physical performance outcomes in this population,[74] the overall goal should be that of energy conservation, maintaining or even slowing the decline of PF for as long as possible.

SUMMARY AND CONCLUSIONS

Since this chapter's predecessor was published in 2006,[15] there has been a marked rise in observational studies and limited trials examining PA interventions and PF in advanced cancer populations. The observational studies demonstrate that some advanced cancer patients express interest in PA, and that for some advanced cancer patients, PA is positively associated with QoL. The limited trials suggest that advanced cancer patients are able to tolerate some PA, which may improve select PF and QoL outcomes. Further development and validation of self-report instruments and objective tools to assess PF and PA levels are warranted, as standardization of instruments and tools is critical in comparing outcomes between studies. The nature and degree of benefit in PF and QoL may be dependent on tumor type, TNM stage, and site of metastases. The window of patient ability to participate in PA interventions, however, and the potential benefit in QoL outcomes are limited by disease progression and proximity to end of life. Overall, there is preliminary evidence of benefit from PA interventions for palliative cancer patients; although the current evidence base does not support general recommendations for this population, tailored PA recommendations based on individual abilities may be appropriate.

ACKNOWLEDGMENT

SSL is supported by the full-time Roche Fellowship in Translational Cancer Research Award from the Alberta Cancer Foundation. KSC is supported by the Canada Research Chairs Program.

REFERENCES

1   Ventrafridda V. According to the 2002 WHO definition of palliative care... *Palliative Medicine*. 2006;20:159.
2   Clark, D. Between hope and acceptance: The medicalisation of dying. *British Medical Journal*. 2002;324:905–907.
3   Von Roenn JH, Temel J. The integration of palliative care and oncology: The evidence. *Oncology (Williston Park)*. 2011;25(13):1258–1260, 1262, 1264–1265.
4   Fitzsimons D, Mullan D, Wilson JS et al. The challenge of patients' unmet palliative care needs in the final stages of chronic illness. *Palliative Medicine*. 2007;21(4):313–322.
5   Van Mechelen W, Aertgeerts B, De Ceulaer K, Thoonsen B, Vermandere M, Warmenhoven F, van Rijswijk E, De Lepeleire J. Defining the palliative care patient: A systematic review. *Palliative Medicine*. 2013;27(3):197–208.
6   Cohen SR, Leis A. What determines the quality of life of terminally ill cancer patients from their own perspective? *Journal of Palliative Care*. 2002;8:48–58.
7   Bouchard C, Shephard RJ. Physical activity, fitness and health: The model and key concepts. In: Bouchard C, Shephard RJ, Stephens T (eds.), *Physical Activity, Fitness, and Health. International Proceedings and Consensus Statement*. Champaign, IL: Human Kinetics Publishers, 1994, pp. 77–88.
8   U.S. Department of Health and Human Services. *Physical Activity and Health: A Report of the Surgeon General*. McLean, VA: International Medical Publisher, 1996.
9   Jette AM. State of the art in functional status assessment. In: Rothstein JM, Rothstein JMS (eds.), *Measurement in Physical Therapy*. New York: Churchill Livingstone, 1985, pp. 137–168.
10 Ferrer RA, Huedo-Medina TB, Johnson BT, Ryan S, Pescatello LS. Exercise interventions for cancer survivors: A meta-analysis of quality of life outcomes. *Annals of Behavioral Medicine*. 2011;41(1):32–47.
11 Fong DY, Ho JW, Hui BP et al. Physical activity for cancer survivors: Meta-analysis of randomized controlled trials. *British Medical Journal*. 2012;344:e70. doi:10.1136/bmj.e70.
12 Schmitz KH, Courneya KS, Matthews C et al. American College of Sports Medicine roundtable on exercise guidelines for cancer survivors. *Medicine and Science in Sports and Exercise*. 2010;42(7):1409–1426.
13 Rock CL, Doyle C, Demark-Wahnfried W et al. Nutrition and physical activity guidelines for cancer survivors. *CA: A Cancer Journal for Clinicians*. 2012;62(4):243–274.
14 Eyigor S. Physical activity and rehabilitation programs should be recommended on palliative care for patients with cancer. *Journal of Palliative Medicine*. 2010;13(10):1183–1184.
15 Courneya KS, Vallance JKH, McNeely ML, Peddle CJ. Exercise, physical function, and fatigue in palliative care. In: Bruera E, Higginson IJ, Ripamonti C, von Gunten C (eds.), *Textbook of Palliative Medicine*. London, U.K.: Edward Arnold (Publishers) Ltd, 2006, pp. 629–639.
16 Lowe SS, Watanabe SM, Courneya KS. Physical activity as a supportive care intervention in palliative cancer patients: A systematic review. *Journal of Supportive Oncology*. 2009;7(1):27–34.
17 Beaton R, Pagdin-Friesen W, Robertson C, Vigar C, Watson H, Harris SR. Effects of exercise intervention on persons with metastatic cancer: A systematic review. *Physiotherapy Canada*. 2009;61(3):141–153.
18 Walsh D, Donnelly S, Rybicki L. The symptoms of advanced cancer: Relationship to age, gender and performance status in 1,000 patients. *Supportive Care in Cancer*. 2000;8(3):175–179.
19 Munch TN, Stromgren AS, Pedersen L, Petersen MA, Hoermann L, Groenvold M. Multidimensional measurement of fatigue in advanced cancer patients in palliative care: An application of the multidimensional fatigue inventory. *Journal of Pain and Symptom Management*. 2006;31(6):533–541.
20 Barnes EA, Bruera E. Fatigue in patients with advanced cancer: A review. *International Journal of Gynecological Cancer*. 2002;12(5):424–428.
21 Cheville A. Rehabilitation of patients with advanced cancer. *Cancer*. 2001;92:1039–1048.
22 Axelsson B, Sjoden PO. Quality of life of cancer patients and their spouses in palliative home care. *Palliative Medicine*. 1998;12:29–39.
23 Wallston KA, Burger C, Smith RA, Baugher RJ. Comparing the quality of death for hospice and non-hospice cancer patients. *Medical Care*. 1988;26:177–182.
24 Yoshioka H. Rehabilitation for the terminal cancer patient. *American Journal of Physical Medicine & Rehabilitation*. 1994;73:199–206.
25 Van der Maas PJ, van der Val G, Haverkate I, de Graaff CL, Kester JG, Onwuteaka-Philipsen BD, van der Heide A, Bosma JM, Willems DL. Euthanasia, physician-assisted suicide, and other medical practices involving the end of life in the Netherlands, 1990–1995. *New England Journal of Medicine*. 1996;335(22):1699–1705.
26 Jordhoy MS, Fayers P, Loge JH, Ahlner-Elmqvist M, Kaasa S. Quality of life in palliative cancer care: Results from a cluster randomized trial. *Journal of Clinical Oncology*. 2001;19:3884–3894.
27 Elmqvist MA, Jordhoy MS, Bjordal K, Kaasa S, Jannert M. Health-related quality of life during the last three months of life in patients with advanced cancer. *Supportive Care in Cancer*. 2009;17(2):191–198.

28   Fearon KC. Cancer cachexia: Developing multimodal therapy for a multidimensional problem. *European Journal of Cancer.* 2008;44(8):1124–1132.

29   McCarthy EP, Phillips RS, Zhong Z, Drews RE, Lynn J. Dying with cancer: Patients' function, symptoms, and care preferences as death approaches. *Journal of the American Geriatrics Society.* 2000;48:S110–S121.

30   Montagnini M, Lodhi M, Born W. The utilization of physical therapy in a palliative care unit. *Journal of Palliative Medicine.* 2003;6(1):11–17.

31   Helbostad JL, Holen JC, Jordhoy MS, Ringdal GI, Oldervoll L, Kaasa S. A first step in the development of an international self-report instrument for physical functioning in palliative cancer care: A systematic literature review and an expert opinion evaluation study. *Journal of Pain and Symptom Management.* 2009;37(2):196–205.

32   Helbostad JL, Oldervoll LM, Fayers PM, Jordhoy MS, Fearon KCH, Strasser F, Kaasa S. Development of a computer-administered mobility questionnaire. *Supportive Care in Cancer.* 2011;19:745–755.

33   Brown JC, Huedo-Medina TB, Pescatello LS, Pescatello SM, Ferrer RA, Johnson BT. Efficacy of exercise interventions in modulating cancer-related fatigue among adult cancer survivors: A meta-analysis. *Cancer Epidemiology, Biomarkers & Prevention.* 2011;20(1):123–133.

34   McMillan EM, Newhouse IJ. Exercise is an effective treatment modality for reducing cancer-related fatigue and improving physical capacity in cancer patients and survivors: A meta-analysis. *Applied Physiology, Nutrition, and Metabolism.* 2011;36:892–903.

35   Mackey KM, Sparling JW. Experiences of older women with cancer receiving hospice care: Significance for physical therapy. *Physical Therapy.* 2000;80:459–468.

36   Paltiel H, Solvoll E, Loge JH, Kaasa S, Oldervoll L. "The healthy me appears": Palliative cancer patients' experiences of participation in a physical group exercise program. *Palliative and Supportive Care.* 2009;7:459–467.

37   Selman L, Higginson IJ. 'A softening of edges': A comparison of yoga classes at palliative care services in New Delhi and London. *International Journal of Palliative Nursing.* 2010;16(11):548–554.

38   Gulde I, Oldervoll LM, Martin C. Palliative cancer patients' experience of physical activity. *Journal of Palliative Care.* 2011;27(4):296–302.

39   Adamsen L, Stage M, Laursen J, Rorth M, Quist M. Exercise and relaxation intervention for patients with advanced lung cancer: A qualitative feasibility study. *Scandinavian Journal of Medicine and Science in Sports.* 2012;22(6):804–815.

40   Selman LE, Williams J, Simms V. A mixed-methods evaluation of complementary therapy services in palliative care: Yoga and dance therapy. *European Journal of Cancer Care.* 2012;21:87–97.

41   Clark MM, Vickers KS, Hathaway JC, Smith M, Looker SA, Petersen LR, Pinto BM, Rummans TA, Loprinzi CL. Physical activity in patients with advanced-stage cancer actively receiving chemotherapy. *Journal of Supportive Oncology.* 2007;5(10):487–493.

42   Lowe SS, Watanabe SM, Baracos VE, Courneya KS. Associations between physical activity and quality of life in cancer patients receiving palliative care: A pilot survey. *Journal of Pain and Symptom Management.* 2009;38(5):785–796.

43   Lowe SS, Watanabe SM, Baracos VE, Courneya KS. Physical activity interests and preferences in palliative cancer patients. *Supportive Care in Cancer.* 2010;18:1469–1475.

44   Lowe SS, Watanabe SM, Baracos VE, Courneya KS. Determinants of physical activity in palliative cancer patients: An application of the Theory of Planned Behavior. *Journal of Supportive Oncology.* 2012;10(1):30–36.

45   Oechsle K, Jensen W, Schmidt T, Reer R, Braumann KM, de Wit M, Bokemeyer C. Physical activity, quality of life, and the interest in physical exercise programs in patients undergoing palliative chemotherapy. *Supportive Care in Cancer.* 2011;19:613–619.

46   Maddocks M, Armstrong S, Wilcock A. Exercise as a supportive therapy in incurable cancer: Exploring patient preferences. *Psychooncology.* 2011;20:173–178.

47   Dahele M, Skipworth RJE, Wall L, Voss A, Preston T, Fearon KCH. Objective physical activity and self-reported quality of life in patients receiving palliative chemotherapy. *Journal of Pain and Symptom Management.* 2007;33(6):676–685.

48   Fouladiun M, Korner U, Gunnebo L, Sixt-Ammilon P, Bosaeus I, Lundholm K. Daily physical-rest activities in relation to nutritional state, metabolism, and quality of life in cancer patients with progressive cachexia. *Clinical Cancer Research.* 2007;13(21):6379–6385.

49   Skipworth RJE, Stene GB, Dahele M et al. Patient-focused endpoints in advanced cancer: Criterion-based validation of accelerometer-based activity monitoring. *Clinical Nutrition.* 2011;30:812–821.

50   Ferriolli E, Skipworth RJE, Hendry P et al. Physical activity monitoring: A responsive and meaningful patient-centered outcome for surgery, chemotherapy, or radiotherapy? *Journal of Pain and Symptom Management.* 2012;43(6):1025–1035.

51   Maddocks M, Wilcock A. Exploring physical activity level in patients with thoracic cancer: Implications for use as an outcome measure. *Supportive Care in Cancer.* 2012;20:1113–1116.

52   Fouladiun M, Korner U, Bosaeus I, Daneryd P, Hyltander A, Lundholm KG. Body composition and time course changes in regional distribution of fat and lean tissue in unselected cancer patients on palliative care—Correlations with food intake, metabolism, exercise capacity, and hormones. *Cancer.* 2005;103:189–198.

53   Montoya M, Fossella F, Palmer JL, Kaur G, Pace EA, Yadav R, Simmonds M, Gillis T, Bruera E. Objective evaluation of physical function in patients with advanced lung cancer: A preliminary report. *Journal of Palliative Medicine.* 2006;9(2):309–316.

54   Lundholm K, Korner U, Gunnebo L, Sixt-Ammilon P, Fouladiun M, Daneryd P, Bosaeus I. Insulin treatment in cancer cachexia: Effects on survival, metabolism and physical functioning. *Clinical Cancer Research.* 2007;13(9):2699–2706.

55   Kasymjanova G, Correa JA, Kreisman H, Dajczman E, Pepe C, Dobson S, Lajeunesse L, Sharma R, Small D. Prognostic value of the six-minute walk in advanced non-small cell lung cancer. *Journal of Thoracic Oncology.* 2009;4(5):602–607.

56   Machado L, Bredda Saad IV, Honma HN, Morcillo AM, Zambon L. Evolution of performance status, body mass index, and six-minute walk distance in advanced lung cancer patients undergoing chemotherapy. *The Jornal Brasileiro de Pneumologia.* 2010;36(5):588–594.

57   England R, Maddocks M, Manderson C, Wilcock A. Factors influencing exercise performance in thoracic cancer. *Respiratory Medicine.* 2012;106:294–299.

58   Jones LW, Hornsby WE, Goetzinger A et al. Prognostic significance of functional capacity and exercise behavior in patients with metastatic non-small cell lung cancer. *Lung Cancer.* 2012;76(2):248–252.

59   Low J, Davis S, Drake R, King M, Tookman A, Turner K, Serfaty M, Leurent B, Jones L. The role of acceptance in rehabilitation in life-threatening illness. *Journal of Pain and Symptom Management.* 2012;43(1):20–28.

60   Porock D, Kristjanson LJ, Tinnelly K, Duke T, Blight J. An exercise intervention for advanced cancer patients experiencing fatigue: A pilot study. *Journal of Palliative Care.* 2000;16(3):30–36.

61   Crevenna R, Schmidinger M, Keilani M, Nuhr M, Nur H, Zoch C, Zielinski C, Fialka-Moser V, Quittan M. Aerobic exercise as additive palliative treatment for a patient with advanced hepatocellular cancer. *Wiener Medizinische Wochenschrift.* 2003;153:237–240.

62   Crevenna R, Schmidinger M, Keilani M, Nuhr M, Fialka-Moser V, Zettinig G, Quittan M. Aerobic exercise for a patient suffering from metastatic bone disease. *Supportive Care in Cancer.* 2003;11(2):120–122.

63 Kelm J, Ahlhelm R, Weissenbach P, Schliesing P, Regitz T, Deubel G, Engel C. Physical training during intrahepatic chemotherapy. *Archives of Physical Medicine and Rehabilitation.* 2003;84:687–690.

64 Headley JA, Ownby KK, John LD. The effect of seated exercise on fatigue and quality of life in women with advanced breast cancer. *Oncology Nursing Forum.* 2004;31(5):977–983.

65 Crevenna R, Marosi C, Schmidinger M, Fialka-Moser V. Neuromuscular electrical stimulation for a patient with metastatic lung cancer—A case report. *Supportive Care in Cancer.* 2006;14:970–973.

66 McDonald A, Burjan E, Martin S. Yoga for patients and carers in a palliative day care setting. *International Journal of Palliative Nursing.* 2006;12(11):519–523.

67 Oldervoll LM, Loge JH, Paltiel H, Asp MB, Vidvei U, Wiken AN, Hjermstad MJ, Kaasa S. The effect of a physical exercise program in palliative care: A phase II study. *Journal of Pain and Symptom Management.* 2006;31(5):421–430.

68 Oldervoll LM, Loge JH, Paltiel H, Asp MB, Vidvei U, Hjermstad MJ, Kaasa S. Are palliative cancer patients willing and able to participate in a physical activity program? *Palliative and Supportive Care.* 2005;3:281–287.

69 Hui ES, Cheng JO, Cheng HK. Benefits of Tai Chi in palliative care for advanced cancer patients. *Palliative Medicine.* 2008;22(1):93–94.

70 Maddocks M, Lewis M, Chauhan A, Manderson C, Hocknell J, Wilcock A. Randomized controlled pilot study of neuromuscular electrical stimulation of the quadriceps in patients with non-small cell lung cancer. *Journal of Pain and Symptom Management.* 2009;38(6):950–956.

71 Temel JS, Greer JA, Goldberg S, Vogel PD, Sullivan M, Pirl WF, Lynch TJ, Christiani DC, Smith MR. A structured exercise program for patients with advanced non-small cell lung cancer. *Journal of Thoracic Oncology.* 2009;4(5):595–601.

72 Buss T, de Walden-Galuszko K, Modlinska A, Osowicka M, Lichodziejewska-Niemierko M, Janiszewska J. Kinesitherapy alleviates fatigue in terminal hospice cancer patients—An experimental, controlled study. *Supportive Care in Cancer.* 2010;18:743–749.

73 Tatematsu N, Hayashi A, Narita K, Tamaki A, Tsuboyama T. The effects of exercise therapy on delirium in cancer patients: A retrospective study. *Supportive Care in Cancer.* 2011;19:765–770.

74 Oldervoll LM, Loge JH, Lydersen S et al. Physical exercise for cancer patients with advanced disease: A randomized controlled trial. *The Oncologist.* 2011;16:1649–1657.

75 Lopez-Sendin N, Alburquerque-Sendin F, Cleland JA, Fernandez-de-las-Penas C. Effects of physical therapy on pain and mood in patients with terminal cancer: A pilot randomized clinical trial. *The Journal of Alternative and Complementary Medicine.* 2012;18(5):480–486.

76 Borgsteede SD, Deliens L, Francke AL, Stalman WA, Willems DL, van Eijk JT, van der Wal G. Defining the patient population: One of the problems for palliative care research. *Palliative Medicine.* 2006;20(2):63–68.

77 Lau F, Cloutier-Fisher D, Kuziemsky C, Black F, Downing M, Borycki E, Ho F. A systematic review of prognostic tools for estimating survival time in palliative care. *Journal of Palliative Care.* 2007;23(2):93–112.

78 Temel JS, Greer JA, Muzikansky A et al. Early palliative care for patients with metastatic non-small cell lung cancer. *New England Journal of Medicine.* 2010;363(8):733–742.

79 Jordhoy MS, Ringdal GI, Helbostad JL, Oldervoll L, Loge JH, Kaasa S. Assessing physical functioning: A systematic review of quality of life measures developed for use in palliative care. *Palliative Medicine.* 2007;21:673–682.

80 Rief H, Jensen AD, Bruckner T, Herfarth K, Debus J. Isometric muscle training of the spine musculature in patients with spinal bony metastases under radiation therapy. *BMC Cancer.* 2011;11:482.

81 Galvao DA, Taaffe DR, Cormie P et al. Efficacy and safety of a multi-modal exercise program in prostate cancer patients with bone metastases: A randomized controlled trial. *BMC Cancer.* 2011;11:517.

66

Assessment and management of fatigue

SRIRAM YENNURAJALINGAM, EDUARDO BRUERA

INTRODUCTION

Fatigue is subjective sensation of weakness, lack of energy, or becoming easily tired.[1-4] It is one of the most common and chronic symptom experienced by advanced cancer.[5] Fatigue is debilitating and profoundly impacts the quality of life (QOL) of the patients and their families.[6] With the availability of effective treatments for pain and nausea, screening and treatment of fatigue have become a major focus of symptom management in advanced cancer.[5]

Definition

Cancer-related fatigue (CRF) is defined as a "distressing persistent, subjective sense of physical, emotional and/or cognitive tiredness or exhaustion related to cancer or cancer treatment that is not proportional to recent activity and interferes with usual functioning"[2] (NCCN guidelines 2010). In contrast to muscle fatigue, clinical fatigue is a multidimensional phenomenon and includes three major components: (1) generalized weakness, resulting in inability to initiate certain activities; (2) easy fatigability and reduced capacity to maintain performance; and (3) mental fatigue resulting in impaired concentration, loss of memory, and emotional lability. Despite the distinction to the three major dimensions (physical, affective, and cognitive), it is unresolved whether these dimensions are stable and reproduced in more general settings.[7] Due to the limitation in distinction and reproducibility of various dimensions, there is also an emerging thought among fatigue researchers of more having a "case definition" for CRF that may best capture and describe what constitutes clinically significant fatigue in subgroups of patients with advanced cancer.[1]

Frequency

Fatigue is reported to be prevalent in most studied population including patients with cancer and palliative care patients. The frequency of fatigue has been reported to be approximately 60%–90% in patients with advanced cancer.[8-12] The wide range of these estimates likely reflects variable diagnostic criteria used to define CRF. For example, using an International Classification of Diseases, 10th revision (ICD-10 definition criteria), the frequency of fatigue was reported to be 49.8%, far less than that reported in previous studies using a numeric rating scale (NRS) of 0–10.[13]

Moderate-to-severe persistent fatigue affects the patient's QOL and ability to perform activities that add meaning to their life. Fatigue has been associated with other symptoms as symptom cluster including pain, anxiety, depression, cachexia, and insomnia. Assessment and treatment of this common symptom, however, is difficult as it is a complex, subjective symptom and often underreported. Most commonly assessment of severity can be used to guide the management (Figure 66.1).

The pathophysiology of fatigue has already been discussed in the previous chapters, and it is clear that fatigue is usually multifactorial in patients receiving palliative care.[3] Physiological, psychological, and situational factors can contribute to fatigue. The most frequent contributing factors in patients with advanced cancer include weight loss, depression, dyspnea, deconditioning, isolation, and polypharmacy.[2,10,14] Chronic diseases can produce factors such as circulating cytokines, inflammation, and autonomic failure that may mediate fatigue.[15,16]

Although few published studies have correlated fatigue and cytokines near or at the end of life, several lines of evidence implicate cytokines in the pathophysiology of fatigue.[17] First, cytokine levels are increased in nononcologic conditions characterized by fatigue, such as chronic fatigue syndrome. Second, fatigue is a major adverse effect of cytokines administered for therapeutic purposes including interleukins (IL), tumor necrosis factor-α (TNF-α), and interferon (IFN).[18] Finally, upregulation of proinflammatory cytokines is correlated with fatigue in several malignancies.[9,15]

In this chapter, we will discuss the assessment and management of fatigue in advanced cancer.

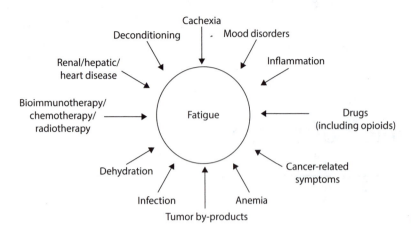

Figure 66.1   *Contributors to fatigue.*

ASSESSMENT OF FATIGUE

Fatigue is a complex, subjective, chronic, multifactorial, and multidimensional symptom.[4,19,20] Therefore, a systematic evaluation is essential. Fatigue assessment involves characterizing its severity and temporal features (onset, course, duration, and daily pattern); exacerbating and relieving factors, associated distress, and impact on daily life; and identifying treatable causes.[3,4] Several scales have been developed to quantify fatigue (Table 66.1). These instruments measure the severity and assess various dimensions of fatigue.

These include the Edmonton Symptom Assessment Scale (ESAS) fatigue item,[21] which evaluates the average severity of fatigue in the last 24 hours (in 0–10 scale wherein "0" is no fatigue and "10" is the worst fatigue imaginable).[4] In addition to the ESAS fatigue item, various other scales are commonly used: these include EORTC fatigue items,[22] Brief Fatigue Inventory (BFI),[23] Functional Assessment of Chronic Illness Therapy–Fatigue (FACIT-F) subscale,[24] and most recently PROMIS fatigue item bank short form.[25] CRFs have been classified into various subtypes based on severity or cutoff scores. The National Comprehensive Cancer Network (NCCN) guidelines on CRF recommend that a simple 0–10 NRS be used to assess CRF intensity during the past week (0 = no fatigue; 10 = worst fatigue you can imagine).[1] Patients can be grouped by their severity responses into subtypes such as 0 = none; 1–3 = mild; 4–6 = moderate; and 7–10 = severe. A CRF severity score of 4 or more can be used to indicate that further work-up, referrals, and treatment may be needed.[1,2] Cutoff scores are sometimes used to identify the optimal level for detecting cases of clinically significant fatigue defined by exceeding the established threshold of "caseness." The cutoff scores, however, vary according to how they are used to define a subgroup and by the CRF measure used. For example, FACIT-F score of 43 or less indicates clinically significant fatigue, and on a 0–10 NRS scale, a cutoff score of 4 or greater has been used as an eligibility criteria for entry into clinical trials.[10,26] Several multidimensional instruments are more frequently used in research rather than routine clinical settings.

These include Multidimensional Fatigue Symptom Inventory–Short Form (MFSI-SF), Fatigue Symptom Inventory (FSI), and Multidimensional Fatigue Inventory.

Assessment of fatigue in clinical practice

Assessment of fatigue in palliative practice might be a challenge, and fatigue is probably often neglected or overlooked.[27] Physicians' neglect of fatigue might have historical reasons, but it is probably related to the nonspecificity of fatigue as a symptom and also due to the fact that there are limited effective treatments available. By asking, the physician might fear ending up in a long consultation, taking several tests, not finding any treatment options, and ending up with presenting general advice. For these reasons, physicians probably omit to address fatigue, and the lack of documentation on treatment alternatives might further support such a nihilistic or avoidant approach. The physicians' beliefs about fatigue are therefore of relevance.[28] However, the prevalence of fatigue, the overall aim of palliative care to prioritize the patients' QOL, and the burden fatigue imposed on the patients and their families both psychologically and functionally do not support an avoidant approach. In fact, many patients are relieved just by being asked, they feel assured by adequate information tailored to their level of knowledge, and many are well aware of the limited possibilities for documented treatment alternatives. The clinical assessment of fatigue as a symptom follows general guidelines for symptom assessment in palliative care.[3,4] Fatigue assessment involves characterizing its severity, temporal features (onset, course, duration, and daily pattern), exacerbating and relieving factors, associated distress, and impact on daily life. To measure fatigue severity, routine use of a simple NRS such as the fatigue item in the ESAS might be useful for both the physician and patient. Fatigue is for most the complex, subjective experience, and hence, in patients who are deemed to have clinically significant fatigue, it is essential to further assess the predominant dimension, physical, psychosocial, or cognitive domain that is interfering with optimal function. However, evaluation should include a detailed history

Table 66.1 *Fatigue-specific instruments in cancer patients*

Instruments	Reliability, cronbach coefficient	Population base	No. of items	Comments
Unidimensional instruments				
FACIT-F	0.93–0.95, test–retest reliability r = 0.87 over 3–7 days	Patients with cancer and receiving treatment	41 items, self-administered or interview, 10 min.	Multidimensional fatigue subscales of FACT assess global fatigue severity and QOL.
ESAS	0.79, test–retest reliability 0.65	Elderly patients receiving palliative care	Patients rate the severity of 9 symptoms including fatigue on 11-point (0–10) visual analog scales, self-administered or interview, 5 min.	Global fatigue severity.
Profile of mood states (vigor and fatigue)	0.89, test–retest reliability r = 0.65	Patients with cancer and many chronic conditions	8 items for vigor, 7 items for fatigue.	Global fatigue severity.
Short form-36-version 1 vitality (energy/fatigue) subscale[35]	0.87	Adults with cancer and other populations	1–2 min for 4-item subscale.	Vitality, energy level, and fatigue.
PROMIS fatigue short form	0.994	Adults with cancer and other populations	Each question has five response options ranging in value from one to five. It assesses fatigue over the past 7 days.	Fatigue frequency, duration, and intensity and impact of fatigue on physical, mental, and social activities.[a]
BFI	0.82–0.97	Patients with cancer and receiving treatment	9 items, self-administered, 5 min.	Severity and effect of fatigue on daily functioning in the past 24 hours.
FSI[31]	0.90	Patients with cancer and receiving treatment	13 items, self-administered.	Fatigue intensity and duration and interference in QOL in the past week.
EORTC QLQ (FS)	0.80–0.85	Patients with cancer and receiving treatment	3 items, self-administered.	It has been noted to have a ceiling effect in advanced cancer patients and is not recommended as a single measure in this group.
Multidimensional instruments				
Multidimensional fatigue inventory	0.80 validity (r ≤ 0.78)	Cancer patients receiving radiotherapy, patients with chronic fatigue syndrome, psychology students, medical students, army recruits, and junior physicians	20-item self-report instrument.	Multidimensional scale including general fatigue, physical fatigue, mental fatigue, reduced motivation, and reduced activity.
Multidimensional assessment of fatigue	0.93	Adults with rheumatoid arthritis, HIV-positive adults, multiple sclerosis, coronary heart disease, or cancer	16 items, self-administered, 5 min.	Subjective aspects of fatigue including quantity, degree, distress, impact, and timing are assessed.
MFSI-SF	0.87–0.96	Patients with different types of cancer	30-item instrument.	Global, somatic, affective, cognitive, and behavioral symptoms of fatigue.

(Continued)

Table 66.1 (Continued)   *Fatigue-specific instruments in cancer patients*

Instruments	Reliability, cronbach coefficient	Population base	No. of items	Comments
Revised piper fatigue scale	0.85–0.97	Patients with CRF or chronic hepatitis C infections	22-item measure.	Multidimensional, assesses global fatigue severity to evaluate the efficacy of intervention strategies.
Fatigue questionnaire	0.79–0.89	Adults with cancer and other populations	11-item instrument.	One of the few multidimensional instruments that is brief and easy to use but also has robust psychometric properties.

Sources: Table in part was adapted from an article Yennurajalingam, S. and Bruera, E., *J. Am. Med. Assoc.*, 297(3), 295, 2007; Minton, O. and Stone, P., *Ann. Oncol.*, 20(1), 17, 2009.
a http://www.assessmentcenter.net/documents/PROMIS%20Scoring%20SF%20Fatigue%207a.pdf

and focused physical examination and laboratory investigations based on clinical suspicion so as to identify treatable causes (Table 66.2).[4]

Management of fatigue

To be able to manage fatigue adequately, the contributing factors, often multiple, need to be determined (Figure 66.1), some of which may be irreversible. Once appropriate assessment is completed, the therapeutic approach to fatigue can be divided into treating underlying causes and symptomatic treatment (Figure 66.1).

Routine assessment and management of fatigue is essential for optimal management. The NCCN guidelines for CRF recommend screening all patients at regular intervals. For mild fatigue, educating the patient and their caregivers along with close monitoring at regular intervals is advised. When patients report moderate or severe CRF, which is significant

enough to affect their QOL, a focused history evaluation helps to delineate contributing factors (medications/side effects, cancer-related symptoms such as pain, nausea, drowsiness, lack of appetite, shortness of breath, emotional distress, sleep disturbance, anemia, nutritional deficit/imbalance, decreased functional status, and comorbidities). Treating the reversible factors with the use of evidence-based interventions tailored based on individual needs is important (Figure 66.2).

Cancer

The complex association between cancer and fatigue has not been completely defined. There is little doubt, however, that most patients with cancer at some time in their illness develop fatigue, and especially in the terminal phase, this is thought to be as a direct result of the cancer.[29–31] In a cross-sectional follow-up study of 459 Hodgkin disease patients, fatigue was

Table 66.2   *Assessment modalities for the causes of unexplained fatigue at the end of life*

Medical condition	Assessment modality
Anemia	Complete blood cell count, serum vitamin B_{12}, folate, iron, transferrin saturation, ferritin levels, fecal occult blood tests, and, if abnormal test results, further evaluation for blood loss
Medication adverse effects and polypharmacy	Anticholinergics, antihistamines, anticonvulsants, neuroleptics, opioids, central α-antagonists, β-blockers, diuretics, selective serotonin reuptake inhibitors and tricyclic antidepressants, muscle relaxants, and benzodiazepines
Cognitive or functional impairment	Assessments such as ADL, IADL, MMSE, and "get up and go" test
Mood disorders	Assessment of depression and anxiety following the *DSM-IV* criteria
Adverse effects of primary disease treatment	Recent radiation therapy, chemotherapy, surgery
Malnutrition	Serum albumin, prealbumin, cholesterol
Infections	Blood cultures, urine culture, chest radiography, HIV antibody, RPR, PPD skin test
Other contributing medical conditions	Directed based on clinical finding

Sources: Evaluations of fatigue are based on the article Yennurajalingam, S. and Bruera E., *J. Am. Med. Assoc.*, 297(3), 295, 2007; Hickok, J.T. et al., *J. Pain Symptom Manage.*, 30(5), 433, 2005.
Abbreviations: ADL, activities of daily living; *DSM-IV, Diagnostic and Statistical Manual of Mental Disorders, Fourth Edition*; HIV, human immunodeficiency virus; IADL, instrumental activities of daily living; MMSE, mini-mental state examination; PPD, purified protein derivative; RPR, rapid plasma reagin.

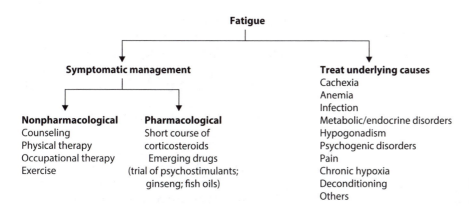

Figure 66.2 *Therapeutic approaches to the management of fatigue.*

significantly higher than in controls from the general population.[32] In patients with cancer, there is a complex interaction occurring between tumor and host, which is not well understood but is thought to result in fatigue in several ways. Tumors produce proteolytic and lipolytic factors, which can interfere with host metabolism. These factors are thought to play a role in the development of cancer cachexia with which there is complex overlap and interplay with fatigue[33] as discussed in other chapters in this book and also in the following. Moreover, there may be other substances induced or released directly by the tumor, which can also lead to fatigue.[16,34] Tumors can also act by direct invasion of brain tissue, particularly the pituitary gland, and cause fatigue by both direct (disturbance in cognition) or indirect (endocrine disturbances via the pituitary axis) mechanisms.[16] Management in this case is essentially treating the cancer. The successful treatment of the malignancy can result in significant and sustained improvement in fatigue.[35] Fatigue is generally perceived as a sign of progression of disease by the patient and family members, which adds to anxiety and unnecessary interventions. The patient and caregivers must be educated about how common fatigue is as a complication of cancer and its treatment. They must also be counseled and educated about what to anticipate during and after therapy is completed with regard to fatigue and mechanisms by which this common symptom can be managed.

Many of the cancer therapies and symptomatic treatment of other effects of the cancer such as pain can themselves result in transient and/or prolonged fatigue, and management of this is discussed in the following.

Therapies and medications

CHEMOTHERAPY AND RADIOTHERAPY

These treatment modalities in patients with cancer cause a specific fatigue syndrome.[36–38] In isolation, they both can cause fatigue, but this is augmented further when both modalities are given concurrently. Bower et al. in a longitudinal study in 763 breast carcinoma survivors found that the patients with both radiation and chemotherapy were more likely to be fatigued than radiation alone.[39] Fatigue associated with chemotherapy tends to have a cyclical pattern. It occurs within the first few days of starting therapy, gets to

a peak at about the time the white blood cell count is at its lowest level, and then improves in the week or so thereafter. The cycle is repeated with each cycle of chemotherapy and worsens with subsequent cycles, suggestive of a cumulative dose-related toxic effect.[37,40] Multiple chemotherapeutic agents have been studied in fatigue either in isolation or in combination with most generating some degree of fatigue. Different types of cancer have also been studied with specific chemotherapeutic regimens with varying degrees of fatigue noted depending on the cancer and the regimen.[37,41–43] A longitudinal, prospective, controlled study assessed 104 women with breast cancer receiving adjuvant chemotherapy and 102 controls. Tools used included the Functional Assessment of Cancer Treatment-General Quality of Life questionnaire, with subscales for fatigue and endocrine symptoms, and the High Sensitivity Cognitive Screen. 83 patients and 81 controls were assessable at the end of 1 and 2 years, respectively. Differences between patients and controls were significant for both scales. It showed that fatigue, menopausal symptoms, and cognitive dysfunction were important adverse effects of chemotherapy that improved in most patients with time.[43] Radiotherapy causes a different pattern of fatigue when given alone.[38] It tends to start more abruptly soon after treatment and diminishes soon thereafter but may get progressively worse as therapy continues.[44,45] Fatigue has been noted to diminish but not completely resolve when short breaks in therapy occur, for example, at weekends.[44]

BIOLOGICAL THERAPY

Biological response-modifying agents such as IFN-α cause fatigue in 70% of patients who receive this therapy.[31] Fatigue is one of the most important dose-limiting side effects of this type of therapy. The mechanism here is unknown though some investigators have postulated diffuse encephalopathy may occur.[32*,33*]

Management of fatigue in these situations is essentially symptomatic and nonpharmacological. Patients and their caregivers need to be counseled and educated prior to commencing therapy about the anticipated fatigue associated with the different treatment modalities, and that treatment-related fatigue does not necessarily correlate to disease progression. Exercise, without overexertion, as well as physical and occupational therapy during treatment can help minimize the sometimes overwhelming fatigue and prevent deconditioning. One common side effect of chemotherapy, which may impact fatigue and has been associated with symptom improvement if treated early, is anemia. This will be discussed later in this chapter.

OPIOIDS

A large proportion of cancer patients experiencing pain are on opioids. This group of medications has significant effects on the reticular system and can cause sedation, cognitive changes, and fatigue in some but not all patients. The central acting effects would explain the mental fatigue, but it is more likely that the drowsiness or somnolence is what is perceived as fatigue by some patients.[46] A trial of dose reduction if pain is well controlled and fatigue is becoming the predominant symptom can be effective. Psychostimulants such as methylphenidate (MP) and donepezil have been used to improve opioid-induced fatigue.[47,48] Chronic opioid use has been implicated in causing male hypogonadism and contributing to symptoms of fatigue.[49] If treatment of hypogonadism by hormone replacement or decreasing dose of opioid is the best approach is yet to be identified.

Cytokine modulation

Circulating cytokines and inflammatory proteins are thought to be associated with many of the symptoms exhibited in patients with advanced cancer such as fatigue, pain, depression, cachexia, and sleep disorders.[16,33,50] These products have also been associated with infections, the effects of cancer treatments including chemotherapy and radiation therapy, and with the presence of the cancer itself. One of the mechanisms shown in laboratory studies by which cytokines mediate symptoms is via a number of signals through the hypothalamic–pituitary–adrenal (HPA) axis.[16,51] Since fatigue is one of the most common symptoms in advanced cancer, researchers have proposed that one possible explanation for fatigue in this patient population is the increased secretion of proinflammatory cytokines, such as IL-2, IL-6, IFN-α, and TNF-α, in response to both the disease and its treatment.[41,42] Several lines of evidence support cytokines in the pathophysiology of fatigue. These include

- The occurrence of fatigue as a major side effect of cytokines used in the treatment of cancer patients[36,52]
- The elevation of cytokine levels seen in chemotherapy treatments for cancer[53]
- The upregulation of proinflammatory cytokines seen in several malignancies and their correlation with fatigue[42,48,49]

Treatment in this case can be challenging and depends to some extent on the mechanism. Evidence to date strongly supports a role for cytokine modulation with agents such as corticosteroids, cyclooxygenase (COX) 1 and 2 inhibitors (nonsteroidal anti-inflammatory drugs, nabumetone), thalidomide, monoclonal antibodies (anti-TNF, infliximab), and specific soluble receptor antagonists, some of which are currently being studied to modulate the effects of cytokines on the brain and other sites.[54,55]

Treatment of cachexia

Cachexia has been covered in detail elsewhere in this book, but there are a number of important points to note with cachexia in association with fatigue.[33] There is a complex overlap between cachexia and fatigue especially in advanced cancer. Cachexia can be reversible when due to malnutrition or starvation or in catabolic states such as acute or chronic infections. However, when due to underlying illness usually in the terminal phase such as cancer, AIDS, end-stage cardiac disease, or chronic obstructive airway disease, it is often more difficult to reverse.[33,56] The significant loss of muscle mass in cachexia could explain the profound weakness and fatigue with which it is associated.[57] Of note though is that fatigue can be present in the absence of significant weight loss and vice versa where profound cachexia and malnutrition may exist without fatigue.

Treatment for cachexia secondary to malnutrition or starvation involves nutritional support. Though there is no evidence that aggressive nutritional therapy improves the QOL in advanced cancer patients or that parenteral feeding has much impact on fatigue,[56] in patients where cachexia is deemed to be secondary to malnutrition, these are exactly the measures that should be employed. In such patients, aggressive nutritional support can result in reversing the cachexia and associated fatigue. The majority of cachexia in palliative care patients is unfortunately irreversible and treatment is often symptomatic. In addition to established agents in use including progestins (megestrol acetate), corticosteroids, and prokinetics (metoclopramide), many newer agents are being studied such as thalidomide, cannabinoids, and omega-3 fatty acids found in fish oils.[58] Treatment of secondary cachexia by treating symptoms like constipation, nausea, dysgeusia, dysphagia, and early satiety with simple pharmacologic measures also helps with treatment of cachexia/anorexia and consequent weight gain.[59]

Management of autonomic failure

Autonomic failure is a common outcome of advanced cancer[60,61] but can also occur in other noncancer diseases encountered in palliative care such as Parkinson's disease. Symptoms associated with autonomic failure include postural hypotension with or without intermittent episodes of syncope, gastrointestinal symptoms such as nausea, vomiting, diarrhea or constipation, and anorexia.[61] Some of these symptoms may contribute directly or indirectly to fatigue such as postural hypotension, anorexia, and persistent diarrhea. A subset of chronic fatigue syndrome has been associated with autonomic dysfunction, but this association has not been studied much in advanced diseases encountered in palliative care. Low heart rate variability (HRV) and increased norepinephrine levels have been associated with fatigue in advanced cancer population. Exercise is known to increase HRV and hence might benefit with management of fatigue in advanced cancer population with autonomic failure.[62]

Autonomic failure is usually irreversible and can be difficult to treat in the setting of fatigue. Midodrine, a specific a_1 sympathomimetic agent, has been used to manage autonomic failure in other conditions such as diabetes and might have a therapeutic role in autonomic failure in the palliative care population. In a double-blind, randomized, crossover study with midodrine and ephedrine, eight patients with refractory orthostatic hypotension secondary to autonomic failure were assessed. Midodrine produced a significant increase in both systolic and diastolic blood pressure with associated improved ability to stand as compared with ephedrine and placebo.[63] Another double-blind, placebo-controlled, four-way, crossover trial looked at 25 patients with neurogenic orthostatic hypotension. Patients were randomized to receive either placebo or three different doses of midodrine (2.5, 10, or 20 mg) on successive days. Supine and standing blood pressures were measured sequentially, and midodrine was shown to significantly increase standing systolic blood pressure (peaking at 1 hour after dosing) with mean score of global improvement of symptoms being significantly higher for midodrine at doses of 10 and 20 mg compared with placebo.[64] Other measures, including discontinuing all possible contributing medications, plasma volume expansion with increased salt intake and use of fludrocortisone, wearing pressure stockings, and rising up in stages and slowly for patients with postural hypotension used in other causes of autonomic failure, might also be applicable in this patient population.[65]

Neurological disorders

A number of neurological disorders are associated with fatigue, some of which may be the primary disease such as amyotrophic lateral sclerosis (ALS), myasthenia gravis, Parkinson's disease, multiple sclerosis, and other demyelinating diseases.[2] On the other hand, some neurological disorders occur as a result of the terminal disease and may sometimes precede the disease by quite a long time, such as the paraneoplastic syndromes including Eaton–Lambert syndrome and dermatomyositis/polymyositis (Table 66.3).[66] Treatment here is disease specific, though

Table 66.3 *Paraneoplastic neurological syndromes associated with fatigue*

Syndrome	Association
Progressive multifocal leukoencephalopathy	Lymphoma, leukemia
Paraneoplastic encephalomyelitis	70% lung, 30% other malignancies
Subacute motor neuropathy	For example, after irradiation in lymphoma
Subacute necrotic myelopathy	Lung cancer
Peripheral paraneoplastic neuropathy	Often precedes the primary
Ascending acute polyneuropathy (GBS)	Lymphoma
Dermatomyositis/polymyositis	Associated with malignancy in 50%
Eaton–Lambert syndrome	Small cell lung cancer
Myasthenia gravis	Lymphoma, thymoma (30%)
ALS	Primary disorder with fatigue

GBS, Guillain–Barré syndrome.

most of these diseases are progressive despite treatment and both the disease and associated fatigue become irreversible, at which point symptomatic therapies, both pharmacological and nonpharmacological, are introduced (see Figure 66.2).

Treating anemia

Anemia is a common entity seen in cancer patients, either as a complication of chemotherapy or as a disease presentation in itself, more so with hematological malignancies. Low Hb and duration of anemia have been found to correlate with negative symptoms in patients with cancer including fatigue, QOL, depression, and vertigo. However, in the setting of advanced cancer, the etiology of fatigue is multidimensional and the contribution of anemia is yet to be defined.[14,67] In the patient group in which mild to moderate levels of anemia may exacerbate fatigue, there is evidence that treating less severe anemia improves energy levels and QOL includes those receiving chemotherapy. In patients with advanced disease and in the palliative care patient population, anemia is probably overdiagnosed as a cause for fatigue. Fatigue measured on a scale of 0–10 in a retrospective study of 147 patients seen in palliative care consultation with a median hemoglobin level of 11.6 g/dL did not show significant correlation between fatigue and hemoglobin level though there was a trend (P = 0.09).[68] There is little doubt that anemia is prevalent in such disease states, especially advanced cancer, but it is unclear at what hemoglobin level the treatment of anemia either with blood transfusions or epoetin impacts fatigue. Unfortunately, treatment of anemia in advanced cancer in palliative settings has not been studied with randomized, controlled trial (RCT). The two mainstays of treatment of anemia are blood transfusions and synthetic erythropoietin (EPO).

1. *Synthetic EPO*: EPO and darbepoetin are synthetic drugs administered subcutaneously either weekly or every 3 weeks. Several trials in the past have shown benefit of EPO with respect to decrease in need for RBC transfusions and improved QOL and Hb levels. In an open-label study, 2342 patients from community-based hospitals, with malignancies undergoing chemotherapy, were treated with epoetin alfa. A total of 1047 patients completed the full 4 months of epoetin therapy and showed significant increase in mean self-rated scores of energy level, activity level, and overall QOL. These improvements correlated with the magnitude of the hemoglobin increase.[69] Another prospective community-based study with 2289 patients with nonmyeloid malignancies receiving chemotherapy received epoetin for 16 weeks. Patients reported improvement in QOL parameters, which correlated with significant increases in hemoglobin levels independent of tumor response.[70] Some authors, however, believe that the improvement noted in treating this level of anemia may be secondary to improvement in exertional dyspnea rather than fatigue per se.

   Osterborg et al. conducted a placebo-controlled, randomized trial of epoetin alpha in severely anemic transfusion-dependent patients with advanced hematologic malignancy. They concluded an improvement of QOL and anemia with most benefit seen ≥2 g/dL Hb. In 2008, FDA revisited the safety data and has black box warning on EPO as several studies in breast, head, and neck malignancies reported decreased survival, Venous Thromboembolism (VTE), and cardiac risks. The recommendation for use of EPO in cancer patients is to limit its use for chemotherapy-related anemia at the lowest dose possible to keep Hb around 12 g/dL and dose reduction for Hb >12.[71,72]

2. *Blood transfusion*: In a Cochrane review by Preston et al., the effect of blood transfusion for treating anemia in patients with advanced cancer was analyzed.[73] Twelve studies with 653 participants were identified, and the primary outcome in 5 studies was improvement of fatigue for 2–7 days with the effect waning after 14 days. The studies used different measures for assessment and quantification of fatigue. Few patients in some studies died at or after 14 days of transfusion, which could be attributed to transfusion or simply the patients being sicker. The result of this review demonstrated the short-term response with concerns about risk and safety of blood transfusion in advanced disease. In managing fatigue thought to be associated with anemia, assessment of the underlying cause as well as the acuity of anemia becomes important as this may influence the choice of treatment. The goals of care need to be determined on an individual basis as well as overall prognosis since transfusions would give almost immediate results and EPO could take up to 4 weeks to show response.[74]

Pain

Some authors have found a strong correlation between pain intensity/severity and fatigue in patients with cancer.[75] It is more likely that there is an indirect correlation with chronic uncontrolled pain causing psychological distress and insomnia, thus impacting fatigue. Moreover, as mentioned earlier, some of the treatment modalities of pain can cause fatigue, for example, opioids. As such, detailed assessment and targeting treatment toward the associated factors and symptoms, as well as achieving good pain control, would be the most appropriate management here.

Other comorbidities

INFECTION

Patients with advanced cancer and other advanced disease states seen in palliative care are at increased risk of infection due to relative and sometimes profound immunosuppression. Fatigue is often associated with infections, especially when the course is protracted or when infections are recurrent. Prolonged viral infections are especially notorious for producing long-lasting episodes of fatigue.[76–78] Fatigue may occur as a prodromal symptom and persist sometimes long

after the infection has resolved. Chronic infection and cancer induce the same cytokine mediators for cachexia such as IL-6 and TNF-α,[78,79] so it is possible that they share similar mediators for fatigue as well due to the overlap between cachexia and fatigue described earlier. Vigilance in avoiding recurrent infections is important here, and having a low threshold for using appropriate antimicrobial therapy can minimize some of these infections.

PSYCHOLOGICAL DISTRESS

Depression and anxiety are discussed in more detail elsewhere in this book, but a few key points are worth mentioning here due to the strong correlation between these disorders and fatigue. Symptoms of psychological distress and adjustment disorders with depressive or anxious moods are much more common in this patient population than major psychiatric disorders.[80] The incidence of depression in this group tends to be overestimated. Self-reported scales suggest a prevalence as high as 25%, but in fact, only 6% of cancer patients are estimated to have major depression and 2% have anxiety disorders.[81] Fatigue can be the prevalent symptom in any of these disorders. It is sometimes difficult to tease out cause and effect as depression, for instance, may be the cause of or occur as a result of fatigue. Some groups have found significant association between fatigue and psychological distress, but again, this is by no means the only variable causing fatigue, reiterating the multifactorial contributors to fatigue. Furthermore, treatment of depression using antidepressant may not improve fatigue.[82]

Treatment here is by large symptomatic with good, expressive, supportive counseling, though antidepressants may sometimes be indicated especially when depressive mood makes up a large component of the adjustment disorder.[83]

INSOMNIA

Lack of sleep occurs for multiple reasons, which themselves may be indirectly causing fatigue. Sleep may be disturbed because of uncontrolled symptoms such as pain, depression or anxiety, mild delirium with sleep cycle inversion, drugs, and suboptimal conditions causing poor sleep hygiene. Insomnia is less likely therefore to be an independent variable in the etiology of fatigue, and though it can cause fatigue, it does not cause physical weakness.[53]

Appropriately assessing the patient and treating the underlying contributing factors such as pain and psychogenic disorders, as well as teaching good sleep hygiene, can improve the insomnia and may sometimes be more effective in the long run than using hypnotics and sedatives, which sometimes may be indicated for short-term use.[83]

METABOLIC AND ENDOCRINE ABNORMALITIES

These are often very reversible causes of fatigue, which can be easy to treat.[4] It is therefore important when a patient presents with fatigue to run a simple chemistry panel as part of the work-up. Abnormalities such as hyponatremia, hypokalemia,

hypomagnesemia, hypercalcemia, and hyper- or hypoglycemia can be readily diagnosed and corrected with simple
measures such as hydration and replacement therapy. A lot of
these electrolyte disturbances cause physical/muscle weakness,
which can cause significant fatigue. Endocrine disorders are
easily missed but can also often be readily reversible or treatable causes of fatigue. Addison disease, for instance, causes
significant fatigue, and although this is now uncommon in
Western society, hypoadrenalism per se is still fairly common.
Many drugs can cause secondary hypoadrenalism, which has
identical symptoms to the primary disorder, for example, steroids (when discontinued abruptly). Other common endocrine
disorders such as diabetes and hypothyroidism should also be
excluded and, if diagnosed, treated promptly with appropriate
replacement therapies.

HYPOGONADISM

This condition deserves a separate mention from the other
endocrine disorders due to recent research interest in this as
a cause of fatigue with associated loss of muscle mass. Low
testosterone results in loss of muscle mass, fatigue, reduced
libido, and reduced hemoglobin.[84,85] Two large patient groups
encountered in palliative care, namely, cancer patients and
patients with AIDS, have been found to have testosterone deficiency, which in males can often be easily reversible by replacement therapy with testosterone. Some antineoplastic therapies
as well as both systemic and intrathecal opioids have been
shown to cause hypogonadotropic hypogonadism,[85–87] and a
low threshold for measuring testosterone levels and offering
replacement therapy is key in managing fatigue in this patient
population. Hormonal ablative therapy has been shown to
double the incidence of fatigue in men with prostate cancer,
but of note is that this is one patient population in which testosterone replacement therapy is contraindicated.

CHRONIC HYPOXIA

The association here with fatigue is probably best studied in
chronic airway disease where oxygen therapy has been shown to
improve QOL in patients with fatigue as one of the symptoms.
In a prospective, longitudinal study of 43 consecutive chronic
obstructive pulmonary disease (COPD) patients fulfilling criteria for long-term oxygen therapy and 25 patients not fulfilling
criteria, there was significant improvement noted in health-
related QOL in patients on long-term oxygen therapy. This
improvement in symptoms included fatigue, emotional, and
mental function and was sustained over a 6-month period.[88]

The use of supplemental oxygen in decreasing dyspnea and
fatigue or improving exercise tolerance has not been shown to
be beneficial in cancer patients with mild hypoxemia. A double-blind, randomized, controlled, crossover trial with 31 lung
cancer patients without severe hypoxemia (O_2 saturation level
>90%) assessed whether or not oxygen is more effective than
air in decreasing dyspnea and fatigue and increasing physical performance. There was no significant difference observed
between treatment and control groups in dyspnea, fatigue, or

physical performance.[89] Earlier studies showed that patients
with cancer who had hypoxemia and dyspnea at rest benefit
from oxygen therapy, but further studies are required to determine whether oxygen therapy could improve fatigue or exercise tolerance in hypoxia patients with advanced disease.[90]

SYMPTOMATIC MANAGEMENT OF FATIGUE

This can be divided into pharmacological and nonpharmacological management.

Pharmacological management

Pharmacological management can be further divided into
established and emerging agents (Box 68.1).

ESTABLISHED AGENTS

Unfortunately, there is no single agent that can be used to
treat fatigue in advanced diseases effectively. This is probably
because of the multifactorial etiologies contributing to fatigue.
However, a number of agents have been studied and shown to
be effective in treating fatigue, often in combination targeting
the multifactorial and multidimensional etiology of fatigue.

CORTICOSTEROIDS

Corticosteroids are commonly used in palliative care for the
management of symptoms. The mechanism of action of corticosteroids on fatigue is not well understood. Corticosteroids
are presumed to decrease fatigue by their effect on (a) inflammatory cytokines like IL-1, IL-6, and TNF-α, which have
been implicated in pathogenesis of CRF, and (b) effect on the
HPA axis as dysregulation of the HPA axis has been associated with chronic fatigue syndrome. Some smaller studies have
also implicated the altered cortisol response to stress in cancer
patients related to persistent fatigue and symptom clusters.

Studies have been done on steroids, dexamethasone, and
methylprednisolone and have shown improvement in fatigue.
In a double-blind, controlled study by Moertel et al., 116
patients with advanced gastrointestinal cancer, with dexamethasone given at a dose of 0.75 and 1.5 mg four times daily, showed
improvement in appetite and sense of well-being.[91] There was,
however, no associated weight gain or improvement in performance status. There was also initial symptomatic improvement
in the placebo group, but after 4 weeks, this disappeared, and
at this point, dexamethasone showed a statistically significant
advantage over placebo. Other groups found methylprednisolone caused improvement in activity level quite rapidly, but this
was not sustained over a 3-week period. Forty terminally ill
cancer patients were studied in a 14-day randomized, double-
blind, crossover trial comparing methylprednisolone with placebo. The daily dose was 32 mg, and end points studied were
pain, appetite, nutritional status, psychiatric status, daily activity, and performance. Appetite and daily activity increased in

77% and 21% of patients, respectively, with 71% and 57% reduction in depression and analgesic use, respectively.[92] In a recent randomized, placebo-controlled study by Yennurajalingam et al. (2013) with 84 advanced cancer patients, oral dexamethasone 8 mg/day for 14 days was found to be effective in relieving CRF as compared to placebo. The mean (standard deviation) improvement in the FACIT-F subscale at day 15 was significantly higher in the dexamethasone group than in the placebo (9 [10.3] vs. 3.1 [9.59], P = 0.008). The numbers of grade ≥3 adverse effects did not differ between groups (17/62 vs. 11/58, P = 0.27). Corticosteroids to treat fatigue are probably best used on a short-term basis, as long-term use is associated with increased incidence of side effects including myopathy, which could potentially make fatigue worse. Moreover, studies have shown that the beneficial effects generally last between 2 and 4 weeks. Other beneficial effects of steroids that may impact fatigue include the effect on nausea, appetite, and pain.[55]

Progestational steroids

Cancer cachexia is known to contribute to fatigue in cancer patients and weight loss has been associated with increased mortality. A number of studies in terminally ill patients given megestrol acetate have shown a rapid improvement within 1 week to 10 days, in a number of symptoms including fatigue, appetite, calorie intake, and nutritional status. Doses used range from 160 to 480 mg/day. In a randomized, double-blind, crossover study with 53 evaluable patients with advanced solid tumors not responsive to hormone therapy, megestrol acetate given at a dose of 160 mg three times daily for 10 days reported a significant improvement in appetite, activity, and well-being. There was also significant improvement in overall fatigue score. There was no significant change in nausea, nutrition, or energy intake. The mechanism of action of megestrol acetate is unclear and may be due to the glucocorticoid or anabolic activity or due to effects on cytokine release or a combination. In a Cochrane review by Minton et al. involving three studies on progestational steroids, no benefit of these for treatment of fatigue was found. Known side effects of these agents include thromboembolic events, adrenal suppression with insufficiency upon abrupt discontinuation, hypertension, hyperglycemia, breakthrough uterine bleeding, and skin photosensitivity.[93]

Psychostimulants

MP is a known drug therapy for ADD, used mainly in children. Prior studies found that MP blocks the reuptake of norepinephrine and dopamine into the presynaptic neuron by its action on the dopamine transporter, and this results in the increased release of these monoamines into the extraneuronal space.[94] There is also evidence that MP results in significant improvement in activity level in patients on large doses of opioids. In a randomized, double-blind, crossover study, 28 patients with chronic pain due to advanced cancer (on opioids) were treated with MP (10 mg with breakfast and 5 mg with lunch) for 3 days. Activity improved and drowsiness decreased

on MP. The intensity of pain and the number of extra doses of analgesics also decreased.[95] The effect of MP in this patient population may therefore be an indirect effect by improving opioid-induced sedation as well as improving pain. Also of note are the rapid-onset antidepressant effects of psychostimulants such as MP, which may indirectly impact fatigue.

Multiple studies have been conducted to study the efficacy and safety of MP in the management of fatigue in cancer patients.[96] The studies have been heterogeneous with mixed results, different sample size, dose, and duration of therapy. In a most recent study by Bruera et al. of 141 evaluable advanced cancer patients, neither MP nor its combination with nurse counseling intervention improved fatigue compared to placebo or control.[97] In another phase III, double-blind, placebo-controlled study by Moraska et al., 148 cancer patients were assigned to receive MP (up to 54 mg/day) versus placebo for 4 weeks with primary end point to measure efficacy of MP in improvement of CRF.[98] There was no evidence that MP, as compared with placebo, improved CRF (P = 0.35). However, patients with stage III and IV disease had fatigue improvement with MP (19.7 with MP vs. 2.1 with placebo; P = 0.02). Also those with severe fatigue (score of 8–10) at baseline, the mean change in usual fatigue on MP was higher than placebo (26 vs. 16), which was not statistically significant. Similar findings were seen in a retrospective study by Yennurajalingam (2010) with higher baseline fatigue scores, and response on day 1 of the treatment was associated with overall response of fatigue to MP.[99]

The effect of modafinil on fatigue in cancer patient was studied by Jean-Pierre et al. in a phase III, double-blind, placebo-controlled, randomized trial with 631 patients on chemotherapy.[100] Modafinil 200 mg once a day dose was used, and BFI-3 was utilized as a measure of fatigue in this study. The results showed statistically significant response for those with severe fatigue (BFI score ≥ 7) with average BFI-3 scores of 7.2 in the modafinil group as compared to placebo with an average score of 7.6 (P -0.033), although there were no significant differences in BFI-3 in the patients with mild to moderate fatigue. Therefore, modafinil can be used in cancer patients with severe fatigue, but more studies are needed for optimal utilization of the drug.

Other psychostimulants studied in noncancer palliative groups include modafinil and amantadine in multiple sclerosis[101] and armodafinil in human immunodeficiency virus (HIV)[102] and ALS.[103] Modafinil, a psychostimulant, is effective and well tolerated for the treatment of excessive daytime sleepiness (EDS) in patients with narcolepsy and conditions such as Parkinson's disease and obstructive sleep apnea. It was studied in HIV-positive and ALS patients and was found to improve symptoms of fatigue, depression, and sleepiness.[104]

Currently, there is insufficient evidence to use psychostimulants for the management of fatigue in cancer patients without opioid-related sedation.[96]

Testosterone

Low testosterone is common in men with advanced cancer. Low testosterone has been associated with high inflammatory markers and high symptom burden in patients with advanced cancer.[105] Treatment with testosterone replacement has been beneficial in the management of symptoms in non-cancer patients. The use of testosterone and its derivatives and other androgenic anabolic steroids has been shown, predominantly in patients with hypogonadism due to HIV disease, to increase muscle mass, improve energy and libido, and increase hemoglobin levels. In a prospective longitudinal study over a 3-year period, 18 hypogonadal men who had never been treated were given transdermal testosterone. The mean testosterone level reached the normal range by 3 months of treatment and remained normal for the duration of treatment. Outcomes measured were bone mineral density, fat-free mass, prostate volume, erythropoiesis, energy, and sexual function. The full effect on bone mineral density took 24 months, but the full effects on the other tissues and energy levels took 3–6 months.[106] A randomized, double-blind, placebo-controlled study in a group of hypogonadal men with AIDS wasting looked at the effects of testosterone administration on the depression score. Fifty-two hypogonadal males with AIDS demonstrated significantly higher scores on the BECK DEPRESSION INVENTORY (BDI) than matched eugonadal men also with AIDS. The hypogonadal men were then treated with testosterone, and there was a significant decrease noted in the BDI score for the 39 patients who completed the study.[107*] The correlation between depression and fatigue has been made earlier, and hence by improving depression in this way, fatigue could potentially improve. Testosterone deficiency has also been shown to occur as a result of cancer therapy including radiation and chemotherapy as well as in the hormonal treatment of certain cancers such as prostate cancer (where testosterone replacement is not possible). A preliminary randomized, controlled study was recently conducted by Del Fabbro et al. to evaluate the efficacy of testosterone replacement for fatigue in male hypogonadic patients with advanced cancer.[108] A total of 26 patients were evaluated with 12 on replacement and 14 on placebo for the primary outcome at day 29. The intervention group had improvement in fatigue scores (mean [SD] −5.5 ± 19 for placebo and 3.9 ± 14 for testosterone, $P = 0.09$). Adverse events were similar between groups.

EMERGING PHARMACOLOGICAL AGENTS

Fatigue, as stated earlier in this chapter, is the most common symptom in palliative patients and yet is probably one of the most difficult symptoms to treat. Multiple agents have been studied and found not to be effective in the treatment of fatigue, such as mazindol, donepezil,[109] and L-carnitine.[110] With regard to the established agents, results are often short term or they are associated with unacceptable side effects, for example, corticosteroids with myopathy in long-term use or megestrol acetate with associated thrombotic risk. This often makes them unsuitable for many in this patient population. Moreover, because of the multifactorial complex etiology of fatigue, it has been challenging to find a single effective pharmacological agent to treat fatigue. Currently, a number of agents are under investigation for the treatment of fatigue, some of which are discussed in the following.

Ginseng is a Chinese herbal medicine, which comes in three forms—the Asian (*Panax* ginseng), the American (*Panax quinquefolius*), and the Siberian (*Eleutherococcus senticosus*) variety. It is presumed to help fatigue by reducing the impact on environmental stress (adaptogen). However, there are limited studies conducted in cancer patients. In a recent randomized, double-blind, dose evaluation pilot study by Barton et al. with 282 cancer patients, Wisconsin ginseng (*Panax quinquefolius*) was tried in a dose of 750, 1000, and 2000 mg/day in twice-daily dosing versus placebo.[111] There was no difference in symptom improvement in patients on 750 mg versus placebo, although 40% of patients who completed 8 weeks of treatment with the 1000 and 2000 mg doses noted moderate benefit as compared to 17% of the patients on the placebo arm. No significant toxicities were noted despite patients being on cytotoxic therapy. In a recently completed study, Wisconsin ginseng at a dose of 2000 mg daily for 2 months was found to be effective compared to placebo in reducing fatigue in cancer patients. In a subset of patients receiving chemotherapy, it was found to be effective in 4 weeks.[112] There were no significant side effects between the treatment and placebo arm.

Other emerging and proposed agents for targeting the treatment of fatigue in palliative care include a melanocyte-stimulating hormone and monoclonal antibodies against TNF-α such as infliximab and COX-1 and COX-2 inhibitors, to name a few. Herbal remedies are often used by patients with CRF. *Ginkgo biloba*, for example, has some activity against TNF, and the potential benefits of natural products in fatigue should also be explored with good clinical studies.[113]

Nonpharmacological management

EDUCATION

Educating the patient and caregivers about the possible causes of fatigue and informing them of how frequent a symptom is at this stage in their disease may help them have more realistic expectations. Also providing them with information about the different modalities of treatment, some of which can be self-implemented, such as education about sleep hygiene and progressive limitation in physical activity can help empower the patient.[83,114]

Counseling

Counseling a patient about what symptoms to expect, including fatigue, with disease progression or with cancer treatment helps to better prepare them for the symptom when it occurs. Counseling for coping with other symptoms, such as adjustment disorder with depressed mood and anxiety, which may impact fatigue, could also help with improving fatigue. Cognitive behavioral therapy (CBT) has shown benefit in chronic fatigue syndrome, neurological disorders, and primary insomnia. The benefits of this therapy in cancer population have been studied as well. Gielissen et al. conducted a study with 112 cancer survivors with unexplained fatigue, who were randomly allocated to intervention (CBT) versus no intervention (waiting list) and assessed at baseline and 6 months.[115] There was significant improvement in fatigue severity (−13.3; 95% CI, 8.6–18.1) and in functional impairment (−38.2; 95% CI, 197.1–569.2) in CBT versus no intervention group. Fifty-four percent of CBT group had clinically significant improvement in fatigue severity as compared to 4% of waiting list group. Similar results were seen with regard to improvement in functional impairment (50% vs. 18% in CBT vs. waiting list, respectively). In another RCT by Espie et al., with 150 cancer patients, CBT was used as an intervention to study the effect on sleep quality with fatigue, QOL as secondary measures.[116] Patients with CBT intervention had statistically significant improvement in physical fatigue measured by the Functional Assessment of Cancer Therapy (FACT) scale as well as FSI at posttreatment and at 6-month follow-up.

Exercise (overexertion/deconditioning) has been discussed in detail in other chapters of this book. It is important, however, to mention this again briefly here as it does impact the management of fatigue. Impaired muscle function may be one of the underlying mechanisms in fatigue (at least the physical component to fatigue). There are a number of studies showing muscle alterations in cancer patients and the association between reduced muscle mass in cachexia and fatigue.[117,118] Prolonged bed rest or immobility has been shown to cause deconditioning with associated loss of muscle mass and decreased cardiac output. This state results in reduced endurance both for normal activities of daily living and exercise. Normal exercise has been shown to have a beneficial effect on muscle and cardiovascular fitness; however, overexertion is a frequent cause of fatigue in noncancer patients. This is an important problem to recognize in younger cancer patients who are trying to maintain their social and professional lives while receiving aggressive antineoplastic therapies such as chemotherapy and radiotherapy.[119]

Several meta-analyses now support the benefits of exercise for treatment of fatigue in patients receiving cancer treatment and in cancer survivors. In a Cochrane analysis by Cramp et al. in 2008,[120] involving 28 RCTs, similar results were compiled. Most of these studies show that a clear benefit of exercise on fatigue is in cancer survivors, patients with breast cancer, and patients with less advanced disease. In an RCT by Oldervoll et al. in 2011, 231 patients with advanced cancer and life expectancy ≤2 years were randomized to a physical exercise under supervision versus usual care.[121] The exercise included warm-up, circuit training, stretching, and relaxation for 60 min twice a week for 8 weeks. The primary outcome was physical fatigue measured by the Fatigue Questionnaire, and physical performance was a secondary outcome measured by the shuttle walk test (SWT) and handgrip strength (HSG) test. Analyses showed that fatigue was not significantly reduced (P-0.2), but physical performance (SWT and HGS test) was significantly improved (P-0.001 for both) after 8 weeks of exercise. In a smaller study by Buss et al. with 49 hospice patients with 30 patients receiving kinesitherapy and 19 without kinesitherapy, the results were different. In this study, patients exercised under physiotherapist's supervision three times a week, for 20–30 min, for 3–4 weeks.[122] The patients in the exercise group had significant

improvement in fatigue after 3 weeks (P < 0.0001) as compared to the control group in which the fatigue deteriorated. Hence, based on the prior studies, exercise improves fatigue and physical functioning in patients with less advanced disease and cancer survivors, although with advanced illness, the type and amount of exercise need to be defined.

Therefore, exercise is recommended as part of the therapy for fatigue in cancer patients,[2] and physiotherapists and occupational therapists should suggest suitable exercises and help achieve increased activity.

CONCLUSION

Fatigue is a multifactorial symptom, which is extremely common in advanced cancer. Approach to the management of this complex symptom must therefore be multidimensional to be effective. Detailed assessment is key to appropriate management, and as noted here, there is still a lot of research to be done to offer adequate therapy to this patient population for such a common symptom.

Key learning points

- Fatigue is a common yet complex multifactorial symptom in palliative care.

- To offer appropriate treatment, a detailed assessment is important.

- Treat reversible causes and then add in symptomatic treatment if indicated—pharmacological as well as nonpharmacological.

- Multiple agents are emerging with constant research, but it will be difficult to find a single agent to manage this complex symptom.

REFERENCES

1. Piper BF, Cella D. Cancer-related fatigue: Definitions and clinical subtypes. *Journal of the National Comprehensive Cancer Network*. August 1, 2010;8(8):958–966.
2. Berger AM, Abernethy AP, Atkinson A et al. Cancer-related fatigue. *Journal of the National Comprehensive Cancer Network*. August 1, 2010;8(8):904–931.
3. Radbruch L, Strasser F, Elsner F et al. Fatigue in palliative care patients—An EAPC approach. *Palliative Medicine*. January 1, 2008;22(1):13–32.
4. Yennurajalingam S, Bruera E. Palliative management of fatigue at the close of life. *JAMA*. January 17, 2007;297(3):295–304.
5. Butt Z, Rosenbloom SK, Abernethy AP et al. Fatigue is the most important symptom for advanced cancer patients who have had chemotherapy. *Journal of the National Comprehensive Cancer Network*. May 1, 2008;6(5):448–455.
6. Hofman M, Ryan JL, Figueroa-Moseley CD, Jean-Pierre P, Morrow GR. Cancer-related fatigue: The scale of the problem. *The Oncologist*. May 1, 2007;12(Suppl. 1):4–10.

7 Lundh Hagelin C, Wengström Y, Åhsberg E, Fürst C. Fatigue dimensions in patients with advanced cancer in relation to time of survival and quality of life. *Palliative Medicine.* March 1, 2009;23(2):171–178.

8 Cella D, Lai J-s, Chang C-H, Peterman A, Slavin M. Fatigue in cancer patients compared with fatigue in the general United States population. *Cancer.* 2002;94(2):528–538.

9 Okuyama T, Tanaka K, Akechi T et al. Fatigue in ambulatory patients with advanced lung cancer: Prevalence, correlated factors, and screening. *Journal of Pain and Symptom Management.* 2001;22(1):554–564.

10 Spichiger E, Müller-Fröhlich C, Denhaerynck K, Stoll H, Hantikainen V, Dodd M. Prevalence and contributors to fatigue in individuals hospitalized with advanced cancer: A prospective, observational study. *International Journal of Nursing Studies.* 2012;49(9):1146–1154.

11 Su W-H, Yeh E-T, Chen H-W, Wu M-H, Lai Y-L. Fatigue among older advanced cancer patients. *International Journal of Gerontology.* 2011;5(2):84–88.

12 Cella D, Davis K, Breitbart W, Curt G. Fatigue coalition. Cancer-related fatigue: Prevalence of proposed diagnostic criteria in a United States sample of cancer survivors. *Journal of Clinical Oncology.* July 15, 2001;19(14):3385–3391.

13 Yeh ET, Lau SC, Su WJ, Tsai DJ, Tu YY, Lai YL. An examination of cancer-related fatigue through proposed diagnostic criteria in a sample of cancer patients in Taiwan. *BMC Cancer.* 2011;11:387.

14 Yennu S, Urbauer D, Bruera E. Factors associated with the severity and improvement of fatigue in patients with advanced cancer presenting to an outpatient palliative care clinic. *BMC Palliative Care.* 2012;11(1):16.

15 Bower JE, Ganz PA, Irwin MR, Kwan L, Breen EC, Cole SW. Inflammation and behavioral symptoms after breast cancer treatment: Do fatigue, depression, and sleep disturbance share a common underlying mechanism? *Journal of Clinical Oncology.* September 10, 2011;29(26):3517–3522.

16 Miller AH, Ancoli-Israel S, Bower JE, Capuron L, Irwin MR. Neuroendocrine-immune mechanisms of behavioral comorbidities in patients with cancer. *Journal of Clinical Oncology.* 2008;26(6):971–982.

17 Inagaki M, Isono M, Okuyama T et al. Plasma interleukin-6 and fatigue in terminally Ill cancer patients. *Journal of Pain and Symptom Management.* 2008;35(2):153–161.

18 Haroon E, Anand R, Chen X et al. 178. Interferon-alpha-induced fatigue is associated with alterations in CNS glutamate metabolism as measured by magnetic resonance spectroscopy. *Brain, Behavior, and Immunity.* 2012;26(Suppl. 1):S49–S50.

19 Barnes EA, Bruera E. Fatigue in patients with advanced cancer: A review. *International Journal of Gynecological Cancer.* 2002;12(5):424–428.

20 Minton O, Stone P. A systematic review of the scales used for the measurement of cancer-related fatigue (CRF). *Annals of Oncology.* January 1, 2009;20(1):17–25.

21 Bruera E, Kuehn N, Miller MJ, Selmser P, Macmillan K. The Edmonton Symptom Assessment System (ESAS): A simple method for the assessment of palliative care patients. *Journal of Palliative Care.* 1991;7(2):6.

22 Knobel H, Loge JH, Brenne E, Fayers P, Hjermstad MJ, Kaasa S. The validity of EORTC QLQ-C30 fatigue scale in advanced cancer patients and cancer survivors. *Palliative Medicine.* December 1, 2003;17(8):664–672.

23 Mendoza TR, Wang XS, Cleeland CS et al. The rapid assessment of fatigue severity in cancer patients. *Cancer.* 1999;85(5):1186–1196.

24 Cella DF, Tulsky DS, Gray G et al. The functional assessment of cancer therapy scale: Development and validation of the general measure. *Journal of Clinical Oncology.* March 1, 1993;11(3):570–579.

25 Yost KJ, Eton DT, Garcia SF, Cella D. Minimally important differences were estimated for six patient-reported outcomes measurement information system-cancer scales in advanced-stage cancer patients. *Journal of Clinical Epidemiology.* 2011;64(5):507–516.

26 Butt Z, Wagner L, Beaumont J et al. Use of a single-item screening tool to detect clinically significant fatigue, pain, distress, and anorexia in ambulatory cancer practice. *Journal of Pain and Symptom Management.* 2008;35:20–30.

27 Passik SD. Abstract: Impediments and solutions to improving the management of cancer-related fatigue. *JNCI Monographs.* July 1, 2004;2004(32):136.

28 Portenoy RK. Cancer-related fatigue: An immense problem. *The Oncologist.* October 1, 2000;5(5):350–352.

29 Stone P, Hardy J, Broadley K, Tookman AJ, Kurowska A, A'Hern R. Fatigue in advanced cancer: A prospective controlled cross-sectional study. *British Journal of Cancer.* 1999;79(9–10):1479–1486.

30 Coyle N, Adelhardt J, Foley KM, Portenoy RK. Character of terminal illness in the advanced cancer patient: Pain and other symptoms during the last four weeks of life. *Journal of Pain and Symptom Management.* 1990;5:83–93.

31 Donnelly S, Walsh D. The symptoms of advanced cancer. *Seminars in Oncology.* 1995;22:67–72.

32 Loge JH, Abrahamsen AF, Ekeberg Ø, Kaasa S. Hodgkin's disease survivors more fatigued than the general population. *Journal of Clinical Oncology.* January 1, 1999;17(1):253.

33 Fearon Kenneth CH, Glass David J, Guttridge Denis C. Cancer cachexia: Mediators, signaling, and metabolic pathways. *Cell Metabolism.* 2012;16(2):153–166.

34 Barsevick A, Frost M, Zwinderman A, Hall P, Halyard M. I'm so tired: Biological and genetic mechanisms of cancer-related fatigue. *Quality of Life Research.* 2010;19(10):1419–1427.

35 Goldstein D, Bennett BK, Webber K et al. Cancer-related fatigue in women with breast cancer: Outcomes of a 5-year prospective cohort study. *Journal of Clinical Oncology.* May 20, 2012;30(15):1805–1812.

36 Wang XS, Shi Q, Williams LA et al. Inflammatory cytokines are associated with the development of symptom burden in patients with NSCLC undergoing concurrent chemoradiation therapy. *Brain, Behavior, and Immunity.* 2010;24(6):968–974.

37 Wang XS, Fairclough DL, Liao Z et al. Longitudinal study of the relationship between chemoradiation therapy for non–small-cell lung cancer and patient symptoms. *Journal of Clinical Oncology.* September 20, 2006;24(27):4485–4491.

38 Hickok JT, Morrow GR, Roscoe JA, Mustian K, Okunieff P. Occurrence, severity, and longitudinal course of twelve common symptoms in 1129 consecutive patients during radiotherapy for cancer. *Journal of Pain and Symptom Management.* 2005;30(5):433–442.

39 Bower JE, Ganz PA, Desmond KA et al. Fatigue in long-term breast carcinoma survivors. *Cancer.* 2006;106(4):751–758.

40 Wang XS, Shi Q, Williams LA et al. Serum interleukin-6 predicts the development of multiple symptoms at nadir of allogeneic hematopoietic stem cell transplantation. *Cancer.* 2008;113(8):2102–2109.

41 Jacobsen PB, Hann DM, Azzarello LM, Horton J, Balducci L, Lyman GH. Fatigue in women receiving adjuvant chemotherapy for breast cancer: Characteristics, course, and correlates. *Journal of Pain and Symptom Management.* 1999;18(4):233–242.

42 Brant JM, Beck SL, Dudley WN, Cobb P, Pepper G, Miaskowski C. Symptom trajectories during chemotherapy in outpatients with lung cancer colorectal cancer, or lymphoma. *European Journal of Oncology Nursing.* 2011;15(5):470–477.

43 Fan HGM, Houédé-Tchen N, Yi Q-L et al. Fatigue, menopausal symptoms, and cognitive function in women after adjuvant chemotherapy for breast cancer: 1- and 2-year follow-up of a prospective controlled study. *Journal of Clinical Oncology.* November 1, 2005;23(31):8025–8032.

44 Miaskowski C, Paul SM, Cooper BA et al. Trajectories of fatigue in men with prostate cancer before, during, and after radiation therapy. *Journal of Pain and Symptom Management.* 2008;35(6):632–643.

45 Dirksen SR, Kirschner KF, Belyea MJ. Association of symptoms and cytokines in prostate cancer patients receiving radiation treatment. *Biological Research for Nursing.* May 30, 2013;16:250–257.

46 Yennurajalingam S, Palmer JL, Zhang T, Poulter V, Bruera E. Association between fatigue and other cancer-related symptoms in patients with advanced cancer. *Support Care Cancer.* October 1, 2008;16(10):1125–1130.

47 Bruera E, Fainsinger R, MacEachern T, Hanson J. The use of methylphenidate in patients with incident cancer pain receiving regular opiates. A preliminary report. *Pain.* 1992;50(1):75–77.

48 Bruera E, Strasser F, Shen L et al. The effect of donepezil on sedation and other symptoms in patients receiving opioids for cancer pain: A pilot study. *Journal of Pain and Symptom Management.* 2003;26(5):1049–1054.

49 Rajagopal A, Vassilopoulou-Sellin R, Palmer JL, Kaur G, Bruera E. Symptomatic hypogonadism in male survivors of cancer with chronic exposure to opioids. *Cancer.* 2004;100(4):851–858.

50 Bower JE, Lamkin DM. Inflammation and cancer-related fatigue: Mechanisms, contributing factors, and treatment implications. *Brain, Behavior, and Immunity.* 2013;30(Suppl.):S48–S57.

51 Chrousos GP. The hypothalamic–pituitary–adrenal axis and immune-mediated inflammation. *New England Journal of Medicine.* 1995;332(20):1351–1363.

52 Bower JE, Ganz PA, Tao ML et al. Inflammatory biomarkers and fatigue during radiation therapy for breast and prostate cancer. *Clinical Cancer Research.* September 1, 2009;15(17):5534–5540.

53 Liu L, Mills PJ, Rissling M et al. Fatigue and sleep quality are associated with changes in inflammatory markers in breast cancer patients undergoing chemotherapy. *Brain, Behavior, and Immunity.* 2012;26(5):706–713.

54 Lee BN, Dantzer R, Langley KE et al. A cytokine-based neuroimmunologic mechanism of cancer-related symptoms. *Neuroimmunomodulation.* 2004;11(5):279–292.

55 Yennurajalingam S, Frisbee-Hume S, Palmer JL et al. Reduction of cancer-related fatigue with dexamethasone: A double-blind, randomized, placebo-controlled trial in patients with advanced cancer. *Journal of Clinical Oncology.* September 1, 2013;31(25):3076–3082.

56 Stewart GD, Skipworth RJ, Fearon KC. Cancer cachexia and fatigue. *Clinical Medicine.* March 1, 2006;6(2):140–143.

57 Blum D, Omlin A, Baracos VE et al. Cancer cachexia: A systematic literature review of items and domains associated with involuntary weight loss in cancer. *Critical Reviews in Oncology/Hematology.* 2011;80(1):114–144.

58 Mantovani G, Madeddu C. Cancer cachexia: Medical management. *Supportive Care in Cancer.* January 1, 2010;18(1):1–9.

59 Del Fabbro E, Hui D, Dalal S, Dev R, Nooruddin ZI, Bruera E. Clinical outcomes and contributors to weight loss in a cancer cachexia clinic. *Journal of Palliative Medicine.* 2011;14(9):1004–1008.

60 Fadul N, Strasser F, Palmer JL et al. The association between autonomic dysfunction and survival in male patients with advanced cancer: A preliminary report. *Journal of Pain and Symptom Management.* 2010;39(2):283–290.

61 Walsh D, Nelson K. Autonomic nervous system dysfunction in advanced cancer. *Supportive Care in Cancer.* October 1, 2002;10(7):523–528.

62 Fagundes CP, Murray DM, Hwang BS et al. Sympathetic and parasympathetic activity in cancer-related fatigue: More evidence for a physiological substrate in cancer survivors. *Psychoneuroendocrinology.* 2011;36(8):1137–1147.

63 Fouad-Tarazi FM, Okabe M, Goren H. Alpha sympathomimetic treatment of autonomic insufficiency with orthostatic hypotension. *The American Journal of Medicine.* 1995;99(6):604–610.

64 Low PA, Gilden JL, Freeman R, Sheng K, McElligott M. Efficacy of midodrine vs. placebo in neurogenic orthostatic hypotension: A randomized, double-blind multicenter study. *The Journal of the American Medical Association.* 1997;277(13):1046–1051.

65 Shibao C, Okamoto L, Biaggioni I. Pharmacotherapy of autonomic failure. *Pharmacology and Therapeutics.* 2012;134(3):279–286.

66 Wokke JHJ. Fatigue is part of the burden of neuromuscular diseases. *Journal of Neurology.* July 1, 2007;254(7):948–949.

67 Hwang SS, Chang VT, Rue M, Kasimis B. Multidimensional independent predictors of cancer-related fatigue. *Journal of Pain and Symptom Management.* 2003;26(1):604–614.

68 Munch T, Zhang T, Willey J, Palmer J, Bruera E. The association between anemia and fatigue in patients with advanced cancer receiving palliative care. *Journal of Palliative Medicine.* 2005;8:1144–1149.

69 Glaspy J, Bukowski R, Steinberg D, Taylor C, Tchekmedyian S, Vadhan-Raj S. Impact of therapy with epoetin alfa on clinical outcomes in patients with nonmyeloid malignancies during cancer chemotherapy in community oncology practice. Procrit Study Group. *Journal of Clinical Oncology.* March 1, 1997;15(3):1218–1234.

70 Demetri GD, Kris M, Wade J, Degos L, Cella D. Quality-of-life benefit in chemotherapy patients treated with epoetin alfa is independent of disease response or tumor type: Results from a prospective community oncology study. Procrit Study Group. *Journal of Clinical Oncology.* October 1, 1998;16(10):3412–3425.

71 Fishbane S, Jhaveri KD. The new label for erythropoiesis stimulating agents: The FDA'S sentence. *Seminars in Dialysis.* 2012;25(3):263–266.

72 Smith RE, Aapro MS, Ludwig H et al. Darbepoetin alfa for the treatment of anemia in patients with active cancer not receiving chemotherapy or radiotherapy: Results of a phase III, multicenter, randomized, double-blind, placebo-controlled study. *Journal of Clinical Oncology.* March 1, 2008;26(7):1040–1050.

73 Preston NJ, Hurlow A, Brine J, Bennett MI. Blood transfusions for anaemia in patients with advanced cancer. *Cochrane Database of Systematic Reviews.* 2012;2:CD009007.

74 Mercadante S, Ferrera P, Villari P, David F, Giarratano A, Riina S. Effects of red blood cell transfusion on anemia-related symptoms in patients with cancer. *Journal of Palliative Medicine.* 2009;12(1):60–63.

75 Fishbain DA, Cole B, Cutler RB, Lewis J, Rosomoff HL, Fosomoff RS. Is pain fatiguing? A structured evidence-based review. *Pain Medicine.* 2003;4(1):51–62.

76 Kenyon JC, Lever AML. XMRV, prostate cancer and chronic fatigue syndrome. *British Medical Bulletin.* June 1, 2011;98(1):61–74.

77 Piraino B, Vollmer-Conna U, Lloyd AR. Genetic associations of fatigue and other symptom domains of the acute sickness response to infection. *Brain, Behavior, and Immunity.* 2012;26(4):552–558.

78 Harden LM, du Plessis I, Poole S, Laburn HP. Interleukin-6 and leptin mediate lipopolysaccharide-induced fever and sickness behavior. *Physiology & Behavior.* 2006;89(2):146–155.

79 Dantzer R. Cytokine-induced sickness behaviour: A neuroimmune response to activation of innate immunity. *European Journal of Pharmacology.* 2004;500(1–3):399–411.

80 Wilson KG, Chochinov HM, Graham Skirko M et al. Depression and anxiety disorders in palliative cancer care. *Journal of Pain and Symptom Management.* 2007;33(2):118–129.

81 Brenne E, Loge JH, Kaasa S, Heitzer E, Knudsen AK, Wasteson E. Depressed patients with incurable cancer: Which depressive symptoms do they experience? *Palliative & Supportive Care.* 2013;11(6):491–501.

82 Morrow GR, Hickok JT, Roscoe JA et al. Differential effects of paroxetine on fatigue and depression: A randomized, double-blind trial from the University of Rochester Cancer Center community clinical oncology program. *Journal of Clinical Oncology.* December 15, 2003;21(24):4635–4641.

83   de Raaf PJ, de Klerk C, Timman R, Busschbach JJV, Oldenmenger WH, van der Rijt CCD. Systematic monitoring and treatment of physical symptoms to alleviate fatigue in patients with advanced cancer: A randomized controlled trial. *Journal of Clinical Oncology*. February 20, 2013;31(6):716–723.

84   Garcia JM, Li H, Mann D et al. Hypogonadism in male patients with cancer. *Cancer*. 2006;106(12):2583–2591.

85   Strasser F, Palmer JL, Schover LR et al. The impact of hypogonadism and autonomic dysfunction on fatigue, emotional function, and sexual desire in male patients with advanced cancer. *Cancer*. 2006;107(12):2949–2957.

86   Burney BO, Hayes TG, Smiechowska J et al. Low testosterone levels and increased inflammatory markers in patients with cancer and relationship with cachexia. *Journal of Clinical Endocrinology and Metabolism*. May 1, 2012;97(5):E700–E709.

87   Blick G, Khera M, Bhattacharya RK, Nguyen D, Kushner H, Miner MM. Testosterone replacement therapy outcomes among opioid users: The Testim Registry in the United States (TRiUS). *Pain Medicine*. 2012;13(5):688–698.

88   Eaton T, Lewis C, Young P, Kennedy Y, Garrett JE, Kolbe J. Long-term oxygen therapy improves health-related quality of life. *Respiratory Medicine*. 2004;98(4):285–293.

89   Bruera E, Sweeney C, Willey J, Palmer JL, Strasser F, Morice RC, Pisters K. A randomized controlled trial of supplemental oxygen versus air in cancer patients with dyspnea. *Palliative Medicine*. 2003;17(8):659–663.

90   Bruera E, de Stoutz N, Velasco-Leiva A, Schoeller T, Hanson J. Effects of oxygen on dyspnoea in hypoxaemic terminal-cancer patients. *The Lancet*. 1993;342(8862):13–14.

91   Moertel CG, Schutt AJ, Reitemeier RJ, Hahn RG. Corticosteroid therapy of preterminal gastrointestinal cancer. *Cancer*. 1974;33(6):1607–1609.

92   Bruera E, Roca E, Cedaro L, Carraro S, Chacon R. Action of oral methylprednisolone in terminal cancer patients: A prospective randomized double-blind study. *Cancer Treatment Reports*. 1985;69(7–8):751–754.

93   Minton O, Richardson A, Sharpe M, Hotopf M, Stone P. Drug therapy for the management of cancer-related fatigue. *The Cochrane Database of Systematic Review*. 2010;(7):CD006704.

94   Volkow ND, Wang G-J, Fowler JS et al. Relationship between blockade of dopamine transporters by oral methylphenidate and the increases in extracellular dopamine: Therapeutic implications. *Synapse*. 2002;43(3):181–187.

95   Bruera E, Chadwick S, Brenneis C, Hanson J, MacDonald RN. Methylphenidate associated with narcotics for the treatment of cancer pain. *Cancer Treatment Reports*. 1987;7(1):67–70.

96   Minton O, Richardson A, Sharpe M, Hotopf M, Stone PC. Psychostimulants for the management of cancer-related fatigue: A systematic review and meta-analysis. *Journal of Pain and Symptom Management*. 2011;41(4):761–767.

97   Bruera E, Yennurajalingam S, Palmer JL et al. Methylphenidate and/or a nursing telephone intervention for fatigue in patients with advanced cancer: A randomized, placebo-controlled, phase II trial. *Journal of Clinical Oncology*. July 1, 2013;31(19):2421–2427.

98   Moraska AR, Sood A, Dakhil SR et al. Phase III, randomized, double-blind, placebo-controlled study of long-acting methylphenidate for cancer-related fatigue: North Central Cancer Treatment Group NCCTG-N05C7 trial. *Journal of Clinical Oncology*. August 10, 2010;28(23):3673–3679.

99   Yennurajalingam S, Palmer JL, Chacko R, Bruera E. Factors associated with response to methylphenidate in advanced cancer patients. *The Oncologist*. February 1, 2011;16(2):246–253.

100   Jean-Pierre P, Morrow GR, Roscoe JA et al. A phase 3 randomized, placebo-controlled, double-blind, clinical trial of the effect of modafinil on cancer-related fatigue among 631 patients receiving chemotherapy. *Cancer*. 2010;116(14):3513–3520.

101   Vucic S, Burke D, Kiernan MC. Fatigue in multiple sclerosis: Mechanisms and management. *Clinical Neurophysiology*. 2010;121(6):809–817.

102   Rabkin JG, McElhiney MC, Rabkin R. Treatment of HIV-related fatigue with armodafinil: A placebo-controlled randomized trial. *Psychosomatics*. 2011;52(4):328–336.

103   Rabkin JG, Gordon PH, McElhiney M, Rabkin R, Chew S, Mitsumoto H. Modafinil treatment of fatigue in patients with ALS: A placebo-controlled study. *Muscle & Nerve*. 2009;39(3):297–303.

104   Tyne H, Taylor J, Baker G, Steiger M. Modafinil for Parkinson's disease fatigue. *Journal of Neurology*. March 1, 2010;257(3):452–456.

105   Dev R, Hui D, Dalal S et al. Association between serum cortisol and testosterone levels, opioid therapy, and symptom distress in patients with advanced cancer. *Journal of Pain and Symptom Management*. 2011;41(4):788–795.

106   Snyder PJ, Peachey H, Berlin JA et al. Effects of testosterone replacement in hypogonadal men. *Journal of Clinical Endocrinology and Metabolism*. August 1, 2000;85(8):2670–2677.

107   Grinspoon S, Corcoran C, Askari H et al. Effects of androgen administration in men with the AIDS wasting syndrome a randomized, double-blind, placebo-controlled trial. *Annals of Internal Medicine*. 1998;129(1):18–26.

108   Fabbro E, Garcia JM, Dev R et al. Testosterone replacement for fatigue in hypogonadal ambulatory males with advanced cancer: A preliminary double-blind placebo-controlled trial. *Supportive Care in Cancer*. September 1, 2013;21(9):2599–2607.

109   Bruera E, El Osta B, Valero V et al. Donepezil for cancer fatigue: A double-blind, randomized, placebo-controlled trial. *Journal of Clinical Oncology*. August 10, 2007;25(23):3475–3481.

110   Cruciani RA, Zhang JJ, Manola J, Cella D, Ansari B, Fisch MJ. L-Carnitine supplementation for the management of fatigue in patients with cancer: An eastern cooperative oncology group phase III, randomized, double-blind, placebo-controlled trial. *Journal of Clinical Oncology*. November 1, 2012;30(31):3864–3869.

111   Barton D, Soori G, Bauer B et al. Pilot study of *Panax quinquefolius* (American ginseng) to improve cancer-related fatigue: A randomized, double-blind, dose-finding evaluation: NCCTG trial N03CA. *Supportive Care in Cancer*. February 1, 2010;18(2):179–187.

112   Barton DL, Liu H, Dakhil SR et al. Wisconsin Ginseng (*Panax quinquefolius*) to improve cancer-related fatigue: A randomized, double-blind trial, N07C2. *Journal of the National Cancer Institute*. August 21, 2013;105(16):1230–1238.

113   Finnegan-John J, Molassiotis A, Richardson A, Ream E. A systematic review of complementary and alternative medicine interventions for the management of cancer-related fatigue. *Integrative Cancer Therapies*. July 1, 2013;12(4):276–290.

114   Reif K, de Vries U, Petermann F, Görres S. A patient education program is effective in reducing cancer-related fatigue: A multi-centre randomised two-group waiting-list controlled intervention trial. *European Journal of Oncology Nursing*. 2013;17(2):204–213.

115   Gielissen MFM, Verhagen S, Witjes F, Bleijenberg G. Effects of cognitive behavior therapy in severely fatigued disease-free cancer patients compared with patients waiting for cognitive behavior therapy: A randomized controlled trial. *Journal of Clinical Oncology*. October 20, 2006;24(30):4882–4887.

116   Espie CA, Fleming L, Cassidy J et al. Randomized controlled clinical effectiveness trial of cognitive behavior therapy compared with treatment as usual for persistent insomnia in patients with cancer. *Journal of Clinical Oncology*. October 1, 2008;26(28):4651–4658.

117 Roberts BM, Frye GS, Ahn B, Ferreira LF, Judge AR. Cancer cachexia decreases specific force and accelerates fatigue in limb muscle. *Biochemical and Biophysical Research Communications.* 2013;435(3):488–492.

118 Stene GB, Helbostad JL, Balstad TR, Riphagen II, Kaasa S, Oldervoll LM. Effect of physical exercise on muscle mass and strength in cancer patients during treatment—A systematic review. *Critical Reviews in Oncology/Hematology.* 2013;88(3):573–593.

119 Segal RJ, Reid RD, Courneya KS et al. Randomized controlled trial of resistance or aerobic exercise in men receiving radiation therapy for prostate cancer. *Journal of Clinical Oncology.* January 20, 2009;27(3):344–351.

120 Cramp F, Daniel J. Exercise for the management of cancer-related fatigue in adults. *The Cochrane Database of Systematic Review.* 2008;14(11):CD006145.

121 Oldervoll LM, Loge JH, Lydersen S et al. Physical exercise for cancer patients with advanced disease: A randomized controlled trial. *The Oncologist.* November 1, 2011;16(11):1649–1657.

122 Buss T, Walden-Gałuszko K, Modlińska A, Osowicka M, Lichodziejewska-Niemierko M, Janiszewska J. Kinesitherapy alleviates fatigue in terminal hospice cancer patients—An experimental, controlled study. *Supportive Care in Cancer.* June 1, 2010;18(6):743–749.

PART 11

Respiratory systems

67

Dyspnea

JAY R. THOMAS

DEFINITION/SCOPE

Dyspnea is a prevalent source of suffering for palliative care patients. Many use the synonymous term breathlessness to refer to dyspnea, which is most simply defined as an uncomfortable sensation or awareness of breathing. The American Thoracic Society defines dyspnea as "a subjective experience of breathing discomfort that consists of qualitatively distinct sensations that vary in intensity" [1].

These definitions highlight dyspnea's subjective nature. Furthermore, they support the concept that psychological, social, and spiritual/existential issues can amplify the dyspnea-related suffering. This concept is similar to total pain or total suffering. As discussed below in the section "Pathophysiology of Dyspnea", functional brain imaging is leading to an understanding of dyspnea's perception that supports this tenet.

Dyspnea in palliative medicine must be approached within the context of a patient's goals of care. Dependent on these goals, investigations to identify and interventions to reverse sources of dyspnea may be warranted. While waiting for underlying etiologies to be reversed, clinicians should still pursue palliation of dyspnea. Sometimes, sources of dyspnea are irreversible or their reversal is incapable of restoring a patient to a subjectively defined state of quality of life. In these cases, symptomatic relief of dyspnea may be the goal.

The epidemiology and pathophysiology of dyspnea will be presented first. Next, the identification and treatment of reversible causes of dyspnea will be briefly presented. Other sources for more in-depth coverage of treatment for specific etiologies are indicated. The management of congestive heart failure (CHF) and chronic obstructive pulmonary disease (COPD) will be presented in Chapters 94 and 97, respectively. The primary focus of this chapter will be to present the evidence base for the symptomatic relief of dyspnea.

EPIDEMIOLOGY

Dyspnea is a common complaint in both cancer and noncancer diagnoses. In a representative population sample of 988 Americans living at home identified by their physicians as being terminally ill with a prognosis of less than 6 months, 71% had shortness of breath [2]. Depending on the stage of cancer, dyspnea prevalence ranges from 21% to 90% [3–5]. When there is primary or metastatic lung involvement, dyspnea is understandable; however, it is also a common complaint of patients with no direct lung involvement. In one study, 24% of cancer patients had dyspnea with no known cardiopulmonary pathology [5]. Moreover, cancer is often diagnosed in patients who have significant underlying cardiopulmonary problems, such as COPD and CHF, the two most common noncancer causes of chronic progressive dyspnea.

Worldwide, there are no good estimates of the incidence and prevalence of noncancer conditions causing dyspnea. The World Health Organization (WHO) estimates deaths in 2008 from noncancer conditions that are likely to be associated with dyspnea as follows: cardiovascular disease, ~8 million; lower respiratory infections, ~3.5 million; COPD, ~3.3 million; asthma, ~0.24 million; and iron deficiency anemia, ~0.14 million [6].

Dyspnea, due to its prevalence and associated suffering, is a significant burden to patients, caregivers, and society. For both cancer and noncancer patients, studies have significantly correlated increasing dyspnea intensity with lower quality of life [7,8].

PATHOPHYSIOLOGY OF DYSPNEA

Functional brain imaging (positron-emission tomography and functional magnetic resonance imaging) may be identifying areas involved in the perception and modulation of dyspnea [9–16]. There are many similarities in brain structures involved in the perception of both pain and dyspnea, although there are also likely to be differences. Like pain, it is hypothesized that in addition to a perception of dyspnea intensity, there are also affective components consisting of unpleasantness and an emotional response, such as anxiety or fear [17]. These studies used normal volunteers with differing sources of experimental dyspnea, for example, increased work of breathing or hypercapnia. How well these results translate to patients with dyspnea remains to be seen.

One area implicated in all dyspnea studies to date is the anterior insula, part of the limbic system. Other areas potentially involved include the anterior cingulate and the amygdala. Interestingly, the anterior insula has also been implicated in the perception not only of pain but also hunger and thirst [18–24]. Thus, it is intriguing to speculate that there may be some commonality to the perception of unpleasant sensations and an emotional response.

To assess the impact of emotions and attention on the perception of dyspnea, von Leupoldt et al. tested healthy volunteers made dyspneic using inspiratory resistive load [25,26]. While exposed to a constant resistive load, the subjects were exposed to standardized pictures from the International Affective Picture System with positive, neutral, and negative emotional content in one experiment or had their attention distracted by reading texts in another. Although subjects rated dyspnea intensity similarly under the varying experimental conditions, the perceived unpleasantness of the dyspnea improved as the images changed from negative to positive or as attention was distracted. This impact of emotions or attention on the degree of suffering felt from a specific physiologic stimulus is similar in pain perception and may support the palliative medicine tenet that the optimal treatment of physical suffering requires addressing patient psychosocial/spiritual/existential issues.

What signals are transmitted to the brain for processing that trigger dyspnea? Although incompletely understood, most studies indicate two types of signals: (1) the work of breathing and (2) chemoreception of oxygen and carbon dioxide levels [27,28]. The respiratory center in the medulla and pons coordinates the activity of the diaphragm, the intercostal muscles, and accessory muscles of respiration (see Figure 67.1). In addition,

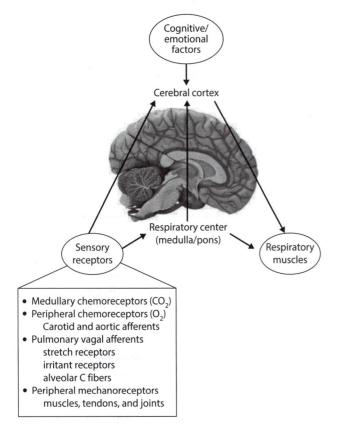

Figure 67.1 *The respiratory center in the medulla and pons coordinates the activity of the diaphragm.*

animal studies have identified neural connections between the medullary respiratory center and the cortex, including the anterior insula [29]. These connections support the hypothesis that the respiratory center may send signals concomitantly to activate respiratory muscles as well as to the cortex leading to conscious perception of breathing.

The respiratory center receives sensory information from multiple sources. Peripheral mechanoreceptors in muscles, tendons, and joints send information regarding lung expansion and contractile force. The increased effort required for breathing against increased resistance (e.g., COPD), or breathing with weakened muscles (e.g., neuromuscular disease or cachexia), may be sensed as dyspnea. This sense of effort probably comes not only from the increased work of ventilation relayed by mechanoreceptors but also from the increased strength of central nervous system efferent signals required to activate the muscles of breathing. As mentioned previously, these efferent signals appear to be sent concomitantly to the cortex where they may contribute to dyspnea.

There are also pulmonary vagal afferents including (1) pulmonary stretch receptors activated by lung inflation; (2) pulmonary irritant receptors triggered by certain chemicals, airflow, and smooth muscle tone; and (3) alveolar C fibers responding to pulmonary interstitial and capillary pressure. These afferents may also send information directly to the cerebral cortex. An example of the role vagal afferents may play is elucidated by an experiment comparing dyspnea induced by bronchoconstriction to that induced by an external increase in breathing load [30]. The work of breathing was similar in both cases, but bronchoconstriction induced more dyspnea. Moreover, inhaled lidocaine, a nonselective sodium channel blocker, prevented dyspnea from bronchoconstriction, whereas dyspnea from external resistance was unchanged. This result implies pulmonary afferents are involved in some causes of dyspnea.

There are central and peripheral chemoreceptors that sense oxygen and carbon dioxide levels. Medullary chemoreceptors predominantly sense hypercapnia. Carotid and aortic body chemoreceptors predominantly sense hypoxemia. These sensations can lead to dyspnea independent of increased respiratory effort [31,32]. Despite common belief, hypoxemia appears to be less significant in dyspnea. First, it requires moderately severe levels of hypoxemia to trigger peripheral chemoreceptors [33]. Secondly, the compensatory increase in ventilation triggered by hypoxemia drives down the CO_2 level, which then partially negates hypoxemia's dyspneic effect.

The concept of neuromechanical dissociation proposes that when there is a mismatch between what the brain desires for respiration and the sensory feedback it receives, dyspnea is enhanced [34]. For example, when researchers limit the inspiratory flow rate at which a subject is allowed to breathe, dyspnea results despite there being no change in respiratory work or chemical status [35].

Therefore, multiple independent and potentially additive mechanisms can trigger dyspnea, but individual mechanisms may trigger qualitatively different perceptions. Questionnaires have identified different words used by patients to describe dyspnea that may have mechanistic implications. For example, the bronchospasm of asthma is often characterized as "tightness," whereas hypercapnia is often described as "air hunger" [31,36,37]. Experimental hypercapnia with limited ventilatory response led to descriptions of "air hunger" and was experienced as more unpleasant than experimental hyperpnea against increased external resistance that led to descriptions of "rapid deep breathing" and "work/effort," despite similar dyspnea intensity [17]. Further study will determine whether treatment can be reliably based on this "language of dyspnea." Although these experimental dyspnea models used normal volunteers, they may help elucidate the pathophysiology of dyspnea and serve as models to test potential clinical interventions.

ASSESSMENT AND IDENTIFICATION OF CAUSES OF DYSPNEA

Table 67.1 lists the important elements of a thorough assessment. The degree of assessment is determined by the burdens and benefits of interventions in the context of patient goals of care.

Patient self-report is the only accurate measure of dyspnea. Although objective measures such as respiratory rate or arterial blood gas determinations may imply dyspnea and possibly help identify etiologies, they do not directly measure dyspnea. For example, patients may be hypoxic and tachypneic and

Table 67.1   *Dyspnea Assessment*

History
Characterization of dyspnea (onset, description, quantification, associated symptoms, exacerbators, and relievers)
Past medical history (including smoking history, occupational history, prior radiation or chemotherapy)
Psychosocial/spiritual history

Physical
Observation (cachexia, cyanosis, clubbing, breathing pattern)
Vital signs
Cardiac exam (rhythm, adventitious sounds, murmurs, jugular venous distention, paradoxical pulse)
Pulmonary exam (hyperinflation, stridor, adventitious sounds)
Ascites
Peripheral edema

Additional studies
Laboratory studies (complete blood count, arterial blood gas, B-type natriuretic peptide)
Pulse oximetry
Pulmonary function tests
Electrocardiogram
Echocardiogram
Angiography
Imaging studies (chest x-ray, computed tomography, magnetic resonance imaging, positron-emission tomography, ventilation–perfusion scan)

Table 67.2   *Causes of dyspnea*

Infection
Anemia
Deconditioning
Hypoxia
Hypercapnia
Metabolic acidosis
Bronchospasm
Pulmonary edema
Pleural effusion
Restrictive processes (chest wall restriction, decreased lung compliance)
Pneumothorax
Pulmonary embolus
Muscle weakness (neuromuscular diseases, cachexia, steroid myopathy, phrenic nerve paralysis)
Airway mechanical obstruction
Lymphangitic carcinomatosis
Pulmonary hypertension
Pericardial effusion
Ascites
Psychosocial/spiritual issues

"look dyspneic" but, when well palliated, report they have no sense of dyspnea. Validated scales such as the one-dimensional visual analog scale [38] or the Borg scale [39] are clinically useful to quantify the intensity of dyspnea. The multidimensional dyspnea profile (MDP) is a validated 12-item tool that, in addition to immediate intensity, also quantifies the immediate unpleasantness, sensory qualities, and emotional response to dyspnea [40]. On a 0–10 rating scale, subjects/patients rate breathing sensations from none to maximum sensation, unpleasantness from neutral to unbearable, sensory qualities (muscle work or effort, hunger for air, mental effort, tight, breathing a lot), and emotional response (depression, anxiety, frustration, anger, and fear). Subjects/patients are instructed to rate the intensity of breathing sensations "like the loudness of sound, regardless of whether the sensation is pleasant or unpleasant; for example, a sensation could be intense without being unpleasant."

After thorough assessment, it may be possible to identify and treat underlying causes of dyspnea. Table 67.2 lists common causes for dyspnea associated with malignant and nonmalignant processes.

SYMPTOMATIC MANAGEMENT OF DYSPNEA

Opioids

Opioids are first-line therapy for the symptomatic relief of dyspnea. Unfortunately, the mechanism is not well understood.

Endogenous opioids are implicated in the control of dyspnea in both normal volunteers and patients with COPD [41,42]. COPD patients, whose mean forced expiratory volume in 1 s (FEV_1) was 50% of predicted, were noted to have a significant increase in circulating beta-endorphin after exercise. Importantly, when given intravenous naloxone, a systemically acting opioid antagonist, versus saline placebo, dyspnea on exertion was enhanced. This result implies antagonism of endogenous opioids that were working to dampen dyspnea.

Opioid receptors are located throughout the peripheral and central nervous system. They are also located throughout the lung with the highest concentration in the alveoli [43]. As previously noted, functional brain imaging has identified loci in the brain believed to be involved in dyspnea such as the anterior insula that also seem to be involved in perceiving other types of suffering such as pain. Indeed, functional brain imaging of mu opioid receptor activity is consistent with colocalization at these structures [44], and opioids decreased insular activation after breath holding [45]. Thus, it is possible that opioids modulate the perception of dyspnea in a manner similar to that of pain.

There is evidence that opioids can be safe and effective in treating dyspnea in experimental and several clinical populations.

Banzett et al. demonstrated that one type of experimental dyspnea was opioid responsive [46]. Opioid-naïve volunteers made dyspneic by hypercapnia with restricted ventilation completed the multidimensional dyspnea profile and predominantly endorsed significant air hunger. After intravenous morphine administration (0.07 mg/kg; ~5 mg for a 70 kg person) versus placebo, dyspnea discomfort was reduced 65%. There was also a significant reduction in dyspnea-related anxiety. Although ventilation was reduced 28%, this did not correlate with the reduction in dyspnea nor was it a clinically significant respiratory depression in this opioid-naïve population.

In clinical trials, opioids' efficacy has been seen in cancer-related dyspnea [47–49], CHF [50–52], idiopathic pulmonary fibrosis [53], amyotrophic lateral sclerosis [54], and COPD [55,56]. Moreover, a systematic meta-analysis [57]*** identified double-blind, randomized, placebo-controlled studies that assessed opioids' efficacy in treating dyspnea from any cause. Nine studies tested oral or parenteral opioids (7 for COPD, 1 for cancer, and 1 for CHF), demonstrating a statistically significant overall subjective improvement in dyspnea. A COPD subgroup analysis also demonstrated opioids' effectiveness. Importantly, no deaths were attributed to opioids. Patients did experience opioid side effects such as nausea, lethargy, and constipation, highlighting the need to treat these predictable side effects proactively with chronic use. Despite known opioid lung receptors and anecdotal reports that nebulized opioids improve dyspnea, a subgroup analysis of nine studies using nebulized opioids (seven for COPD, one for cancer, and one for interstitial lung disease) in this meta-analysis failed to show any benefit.

What guidance does the literature give in terms of prescribing opioids for dyspnea? In opioid-naïve cancer patients, as little as 5 mg of subcutaneous morphine was effective in controlling dyspnea without causing harm [49]**. The effect lasted for 4 hours, which is consistent with morphine's known half-life and effect for pain relief. Interestingly, this morphine dose is roughly equivalent to that used in opioid-naïve volunteers for experimentally induced dyspnea [46]. Allard et al. showed that a 25% increase in the baseline opioid dose

Table 67.3 *Opioid dosing recommendations for opioid-naïve patients*

1. Start with oral morphine or equivalent 2.5–5 mg.
2. Based on response at the time of maximum serum concentration (~1 hour po, ~ 30′ SQ/IM, ~6′ IV), the dose may be repeated or titrated up (for continued mild to moderate dyspnea, the dose can be titrated up 25%–50%; for moderate to severe dyspnea, the dose can be titrated up 50%–100%).
3. Calculate 24-hours opioid requirements and provide equivalent as long-acting opioid.
4. Allow 5%–15% of the 24-hours opioid dose for breakthrough dyspnea every hour as needed.

for cancer pain provided relief of dyspnea for up to 4 hours [48]*. Long-acting opioids have also shown to be effective for dyspnea [56,58]. In Currow et al.'s observational study, opioid-naïve COPD patients were treated with once-a-day long-acting morphine titrating from 10 to 30 mg/day to achieve at least a 10% improvement over baseline dyspnea. Sixty-two percent of patients achieved this benefit with the majority responding to the 10 mg dose. A subset of these responders continued to benefit for the 3-month duration of the trial.

Extrapolating from these results and by analogy with pain treatment, a reasonable regimen to control chronic dyspnea would include both a sustained release opioid for baseline control and an immediate-release opioid for breakthrough dyspnea (Table 67.3). A conservative trial of low-dose opioid such as 2.5–5 mg of oral morphine or equivalent for an opioid-naïve patient is warranted. Oral opioid peak serum levels are reached in about 1 hour. If patients remain symptomatic, an appropriate opioid dose can be safely given again. Once daily basal opioid requirements have been identified using short-acting opioids, an appropriate dose of a long-acting opioid can be prescribed with an immediate-release opioid dose for breakthrough dyspnea calculated at up to 25% of the daily dose. At appropriate opioid dosing, based on experimental and clinical studies, there is no significant risk of respiratory depression. Patients can be monitored for any adverse events. The half-life of short-acting opioids ensures that any adverse events are equally short-lived. In the rare event of a severe opioid adverse event, specific antagonists are effective.

Oxygen

Many clinicians use oxygen for dyspnea independent of etiology or presence of hypoxemia. There is evidence of oxygen's benefit in COPD patients who are hypoxic at baseline or who become significantly hypoxic with exertion. Often, however, patients report improved dyspnea with oxygen when they are not hypoxemic or when they remain hypoxemic despite oxygen.

Two randomized, double-blind, trials have addressed this issue. Philip et al. found no significant difference between oxygen and air for dyspnea relief in advanced cancer patients [59]. In a small subset of hypoxic patients, they found no significant difference in dyspnea between oxygen and air despite improvement in oxygen saturation and correction of hypoxia in most patients treated with oxygen. In a larger trial, Abernethy et al. also found no significant difference in the relief of dyspnea between oxygen and air in patients with $PaO_2 > 55$ mm Hg who were dyspneic at rest or with minimal exertion [60]. The majority of patients had COPD, but there were also patients with dyspnea due to cancer and a few with other etiologies including CHF.

A partial explanation for these results may be that oxygen has a placebo effect, potentially due to the medical symbolism inherent in its use. However, another explanation comes from studies on normal volunteers and patients that demonstrate stimulation of the trigeminal nerve (V2 branch) dampens dyspnea [61–64] (all **). Galbraith et al. demonstrated in a randomized, controlled, crossover trial that an inexpensive handheld fan could improve dyspnea when directed at the face but not the leg in patients with baseline dyspnea due to multiple etiologies including COPD, cancer, and heart disease.

Thus, if patients are hypoxemic and symptomatic, it is rational to attempt to reverse hypoxemia and dyspnea with oxygen. If dyspnea palliation is unsuccessful, oxygen need not be continued simply because of the hypoxemia. The use of oxygen must be individualized. In hypoxemic COPD patients, oxygen may decrease mortality without significantly affecting quality of life. However, oxygen also has burdens that must be included in decisions about its use. Oxygen is costly and explosive, restricts mobility, affects self-image, and may cause CO_2 retention in some patients. If these burdens outweigh its benefits, it should not be used. However, independent of dyspnea etiology, one can consider a fan that provides cool, moving air across the trigeminal nerve distribution.

Anxiolytics

Benzodiazepines are frequently prescribed for anxiety that coexists with dyspnea. Moreover, benzodiazepines are thought to be active at brain structures implicated in the perception of dyspnea [65]. Overall, however, the data on benzodiazepine efficacy for dyspnea is mixed.

One placebo-controlled single-blind study of four COPD patients demonstrated that moderate diazepam doses improved dyspnea [66]. Navigante et al. performed single-blind, non–placebo-controlled studies using midazolam on advanced cancer patients with significant dyspnea at rest but excluded patients with decompensated COPD, CHF, or severe renal or hepatic failure [67,68]. In their first study, they accrued patients with a life expectancy of <1 week. Patients were randomized to receive round-the-clock parenteral morphine, midazolam, or the combination. At 24 and 48 hours, the combination was significantly better than either individual arm. In the investigators' judgment, there was no severe sedation or respiratory depression attributable to the treatments. In their second study, ambulatory patients with moderate to severe dyspnea at rest were randomized to a rapid outpatient titration of oral morphine or midazolam to achieve at least a 50% reduction in dyspnea and then followed for 4 days receiving their identified dose round-the-clock. Interestingly, all patients achieved at least 50% dyspnea

reduction during the titration phase. Both groups maintained a significant dyspnea reduction versus baseline during the rest of the study, but midazolam was significantly better.

However, double-blind studies on healthy subjects or COPD patients with diazepam or alprazolam and a systematic review/meta-analysis failed to show any benefit over placebo [69–72] (all **). Larger, well-controlled trials will be required to further elucidate the role of benzodiazepines in dyspnea.

In experimental dyspnea, opioids have been shown to decrease anxiety [46]. In addition, pulmonary rehabilitation [73] and psychoeducational interventions [74] have been shown to reduce dyspnea-related anxiety. Potentially, these effects may be mediated by the brain structures implicated in dyspnea perception.

Nevertheless, some patients may continue to have anxiety despite appropriate opioid dosing or other interventions, or they may have an underlying anxiety disorder. In these cases, it is rational and safe to prescribe benzodiazepines in conjunction with opioids. As long as dosing guidelines are followed, there is no fear of respiratory depression.

Other psychoactive agents have also been studied. Buspirone, a non-benzodiazepine anxiolytic, has yielded conflicting results in two studies [75,76]. The major tranquilizer, chlorpromazine, was tested in a small randomized, double-blind trial in healthy volunteers [77].** Chlorpromazine 25 mg orally was able to significantly reduce dyspnea compared to placebo without increasing sedation. Larger studies will be needed to clarify its role in dyspnea. However, for dyspneic patients with a component of delirium or agitation, it may be a reasonable choice.

Lidocaine

As previously cited, inhaled lidocaine decreased dyspnea experimentally induced by bronchoconstriction [30]. Similarly, inhaled lidocaine compared to placebo was able to decrease adenosine-induced dyspnea while not affecting adenosine-induced tachycardia [78]. Presumably, these results are due to inhibition of pulmonary vagal afferents. However, small studies of patients with interstitial lung disease [79] and cancer [80] failed to show any difference between inhaled lidocaine and saline. Larger studies are needed to determine whether any subset of dyspnea is responsive to inhaled lidocaine.

FUROSEMIDE

In controlled experimental settings with volunteers, inhaled furosemide decreased dyspnea generated by breath holding, hypercapnia, and hypercapnia together with increased work of breathing [81–83]. Uncontrolled studies have raised the possibility that furosemide may be beneficial for cancer dyspnea [84,85]; however, a small randomized, placebo-controlled trial in cancer patients did not support this effect [86]. In two randomized double-blind placebo-controlled, crossover studies, 40 mg of inhaled furosemide versus placebo decreased exercise-related dyspnea in COPD [87,88]. FEV_1 and forced vital capacity (FVC) did improve after furosemide treatment indicating bronchodilation. No changes were observed in blood gas parameters, heart rate, and respiratory rate.

The effect of inhaled furosemide on dyspnea is not completely understood. Although at least in some studies it can affect diuresis, this seems unlikely to explain the effect given the absence of heart failure and pulmonary edema. In the COPD studies, inhaled furosemide did induce bronchodilation, so in patients with bronchoconstriction, this effect may partially explain its efficacy. However, research also indicates inhaled furosemide can sensitize slowly adapting stretch receptors that send messages via the vagus nerve to the brain [89]. Lung expansion is known to reduce the sensation of air hunger; thus, it is hypothesized that activation of these stretch receptors may mimic lung inflation giving sensory feedback to the brain reducing neuromechanical dissociation.

Given the mixed results in clinical trials, clear guidance for furosemide's role in treating dyspnea awaits further study.

NONPHARMACOLOGIC THERAPIES

Pulmonary rehabilitation

In addition to exercise training, pulmonary rehabilitation typically uses an interdisciplinary team to teach breathing control, activity pacing, and relaxation techniques and provide psychosocial support. In both COPD and cancer dyspnea, this approach can improve dyspnea, exercise tolerance, emotional states such as anxiety, and quality of life [90–92].** Table 67.4 lists common nonpharmacologic techniques. A systematic review of nonpharmacologic interventions found moderate strength of evidence to support walking aids and breathing techniques used in these programs and high strength of

Table 67.4 *Nonpharmacologic interventions*

Pursed lip breathing to increase end-expiratory pressure that in turn prevents alveolar collapse and thus improves oxygenation.
Diaphragmatic breathing.
Use of walking aids such as a wheelchair to reduce metabolic demands.
Use of a fan blowing on the face in the trigeminal V2 distribution.
Leaning forward while sitting or standing and supporting the thorax by bracing the arms against a chair or a patient's knees has been shown to increase ventilatory capacity.
Simple repositioning to improve ventilation and perfusion matching when a disease process affects the lungs asymmetrically.
Keeping a room well ventilated while maintaining a line of sight to the outside.
Educating patients and their caregivers about the underlying causes of dyspnea and proactive techniques to treat dyspnea in order to reestablish some sense of control of their lives.
Education on the optimal preemptive use of medications such as opioids or bronchodilators before known exertional triggers to improve exercise tolerance.

evidence to support chest wall vibration and neuromuscular electrical stimulation [93]. As presented earlier, a simple hand-held fan may help relieve dyspnea from multiple etiologies.

Integrative therapies

In a randomized, placebo-controlled, single-blind trial, acupuncture was tested in COPD [94]. Sixty-eight patients were randomized to receive either real or placebo acupuncture at 11 sites weekly for 12 weeks. After a 6-min walk test, modified Borg 10-point dyspnea scores fell significantly from baseline (5.5–1.9) for real acupuncture with no change seen with sham treatment. Interestingly, secondary outcomes showed real acupuncture led to significant improvement in 6-min walk distance, oxygen saturation during the walk, and quality of life. Additionally, measures of pulmonary function, including FVC, FEV_1 percent predicted, and diffusing capacity of carbon monoxide (D_{LCO}), improved with real acupuncture. Although the mechanism of these objective physiologic changes is unclear, the study was single-blind, and multiple secondary outcomes were tested potentially leading to spurious statistical results, the primary outcome appears very promising and warrants further study.

Other integrative therapies such as mindfulness, relaxation therapy, and music therapy have not been shown to improve dyspnea to date [93,95].

Noninvasive positive pressure ventilation

Noninvasive positive pressure ventilation (NIPPV) has been used in respiratory failure, including neuromuscular disease, COPD, and cancer. Both lung failure (primarily hypoxia) and respiratory pump failure (primarily hypercapnia) have been treated. For COPD, NIPPV has been shown to decrease dyspnea and increase exercise tolerance [96]. Opioids have been shown to produce similar effects. It would be interesting to compare them and test for additive effects to improve functional status and quality of life.

NIPPV has been also been used in lieu of endotracheal intubation. Its use has been deemed palliative when it is used in patients who have elected "do not intubate" (DNI) but in whom there is a possible survival benefit outweighing its burdens and in patients without expected survival whose main goal is comfort. As opposed to endotracheal intubation, NIPPV often allows a patient to continue verbal communication. Azoulay et al. performed a multisite intensive care unit prospective observational study of patients who received NIPPV [97]. About 20% (134 patients) of those who received NIPPV were DNI. Most of these patients had COPD but about 25% had cancer. About 56% of this group survived to discharge and about 40% survived to 90 days postdischarge. Of those who responded at 90 days, there was no significant decrease in quality of life from baseline prior to admission as recalled by patients at admission. Thus, NIPPV may restore some quality of life to DNI patients or enable some to achieve short-term goals. This benefit must be carefully weighed against the burdens of the intervention for each individual and potentially the family and society. The efficacy of NIPPV for symptomatic relief of dyspnea compared to other interventions or its role in dyspnea refractory to other interventions remains unclear. Further studies are needed to elucidate the optimal role of NIPPV in palliative care.

REFRACTORY DYSPNEA

Rarely, some patients may have severe dyspnea that is refractory to interventions. In such cases where the patient has a short life expectancy, palliative sedation is an ethical and legal option with patient or surrogate informed consent.

Key learning points

1. The physiologic basis of dyspnea is still being elucidated but is likely related to afferent signals sent to the brain reporting chemical signals (O_2, CO_2) and the work of breathing, with subsequent cerebral processing likely giving an affective component.

2. Dyspnea is a subjective phenomenon that can only be quantified by asking a patient.

3. When consistent with a patient's goals of care, an attempt to identify and reverse the underlying causes of dyspnea is reasonable. While waiting for an etiology to be reversed, effective palliation is still indicated.

4. When interventions to reverse the causes of dyspnea are not possible or when these interventions are not consistent with a patient's goals of care, opioids are the best therapy for the symptomatic relief of dyspnea.

5. Benzodiazepines are not a first-line therapy for dyspnea but can safely be used adjunctively with opioids.

6. For symptomatic relief, oxygen can rationally be tried if hypoxia is present but does not need to be continued if symptoms remain unabated. Stimulation of the trigeminal nerve distribution with cool, moving air is reasonable for symptomatic relief of dyspnea independent of cause.

7. Dyspnea must also be understood in the context of a whole person, and all sources of suffering must be addressed for optimal symptom control.

REFERENCES

1 Parshall MB, Schwartzstein RM, Adams L, Banzett RB, Manning HL, Bourbeau J et al. An official American Thoracic Society statement: Update on the mechanisms, assessment, and management of dyspnea. *Am J Respir Crit Care Med.* February 15, 2012;185(4):435–452. PubMed PMID: 22336677.

2 Emanuel EJ, Fairclough DL, Slutsman J, Emanuel LL. Understanding economic and other burdens of terminal illness: The experience of patients and their caregivers. *Ann Intern Med.* March 21, 2000;132(6):451–459. PubMed PMID: 10733444.

3 Muers MF, Round CE. Palliation of symptoms in non-small cell lung cancer: A study by the Yorkshire Regional Cancer Organisation Thoracic Group. *Thorax.* April 1993;48(4):339–343. PubMed PMID: 7685550.

4 Higginson I, McCarthy M. Measuring symptoms in terminal cancer: Are pain and dyspnoea controlled? *J R Soc Med.* May 1989;82(5):264–267. PubMed PMID: 2474072.

5 Reuben DB, Mor V. Dyspnea in terminally ill cancer patients. *Chest.* February 1986;89(2):234–236. PubMed PMID: 3943383.

6 World Health Organization, Beaglehole R, Irwin A, Prentice T. *The World Health Report 2004: Changing History.* Geneva, Switzerland: World Health Organization, 2004, p. xvii, 169pp.

7 Gupta D, Lis CG, Grutsch JF. The relationship between dyspnea and patient satisfaction with quality of life in advanced cancer. *Support Care Cancer.* May 2007;15(5):533–538. PubMed PMID: 17120067.

8 Moy ML, Reilly JJ, Ries AL, Mosenifar Z, Kaplan RM, Lew R et al. Multivariate models of determinants of health-related quality of life in severe chronic obstructive pulmonary disease. *J Rehabil Res Dev.* 2009;46(5):643–654. PubMed PMID: 19882497. Pubmed Central PMCID: 2774920.

9 Evans KC, Banzett RB, Adams L, McKay L, Frackowiak RS, Corfield DR. BOLD fMRI identifies limbic, paralimbic, and cerebellar activation during air hunger. *J Neurophysiol.* September 2002;88(3):1500–1511. PubMed PMID: 12205170.

10 Banzett RB, Mulnier HE, Murphy K, Rosen SD, Wise RJ, Adams L. Breathlessness in humans activates insular cortex. *Neuroreport.* July 14, 2000;11(10):2117–2120. PubMed PMID: 10923655.

11 Brannan S, Liotti M, Egan G, Shade R, Madden L, Robillard R et al. Neuroimaging of cerebral activations and deactivations associated with hypercapnia and hunger for air. *Proc Natl Acad Sci USA.* February 13, 2001;98(4):2029–2034. PubMed PMID: 11172070.

12 Liotti M, Brannan S, Egan G, Shade R, Madden L, Abplanalp B et al. Brain responses associated with consciousness of breathlessness (air hunger). *Proc Natl Acad Sci USA.* February 13, 2001;98(4):2035–2040. PubMed PMID: 11172071.

13 Parsons LM, Egan G, Liotti M, Brannan S, Denton D, Shade R et al. Neuroimaging evidence implicating cerebellum in the experience of hypercapnia and hunger for air. *Proc Natl Acad Sci USA.* February 13, 2001;98(4):2041–2046. PubMed PMID: 11172072.

14 Peiffer C, Poline JB, Thivard L, Aubier M, Samson Y. Neural substrates for the perception of acutely induced dyspnea. *Am J Respir Crit Care Med.* March 2001;163(4):951–957. PubMed PMID: 11282772.

15 Peiffer C, Costes N, Herve P, Garcia-Larrea L. Relief of dyspnea involves a characteristic brain activation and a specific quality of sensation. *Am J Respir Crit Care Med.* February 15, 2008;177(4):440–449. PubMed PMID: 18048808.

16 von Leupoldt A, Sommer T, Kegat S, Baumann HJ, Klose H, Dahme B et al. The unpleasantness of perceived dyspnea is processed in the anterior insula and amygdala. *Am J Respir Crit Care Med.* February 8, 2008;177(9):1026–1032. PubMed PMID: 18263796.

17 Banzett RB, Pedersen SH, Schwartzstein RM, Lansing RW. The affective dimension of laboratory dyspnea: Air hunger is more unpleasant than work/effort. *Am J Respir Crit Care Med.* June 15, 2008;177(12):1384–1390. PubMed PMID: 18369200. Pubmed Central PMCID: 2427058.

18 Baciu MV, Bonaz BL, Papillon E, Bost RA, Le Bas JF, Fournet J et al. Central processing of rectal pain: A functional MR imaging study. *AJNR Am J Neuroradiol.* November–December 1999;20(10):1920–1924. PubMed PMID: 10588119.

19 Binkofski F, Schnitzler A, Enck P, Frieling T, Posse S, Seitz RJ et al. Somatic and limbic cortex activation in esophageal distention: A functional magnetic resonance imaging study. *Ann Neurol.* November 1998;44(5):811–815. PubMed PMID: 9818938.

20 Derbyshire SW, Jones AK, Gyulai F, Clark S, Townsend D, Firestone LL. Pain processing during three levels of noxious stimulation produces differential patterns of central activity. *Pain.* December 1997;73(3):431–445. PubMed PMID: 9469535.

21 Iadarola MJ, Berman KF, Zeffiro TA, Byas-Smith MG, Gracely RH, Max MB et al. Neural activation during acute capsaicin-evoked pain and allodynia assessed with PET. *Brain.* May 1998;121(Part 5):931–947. PubMed PMID: 9619195.

22 Peyron R, Garcia-Larrea L, Gregoire MC, Costes N, Convers P, Lavenne F et al. Haemodynamic brain responses to acute pain in humans: Sensory and attentional networks. *Brain.* September 1999;122(Part 9):1765–1780. PubMed PMID: 10468515.

23 Denton D, Shade R, Zamarippa F, Egan G, Blair-West J, McKinley M et al. Correlation of regional cerebral blood flow and change of plasma sodium concentration during genesis and satiation of thirst. *Proc Natl Acad Sci USA.* March 2, 1999;96(5):2532–2537. PubMed PMID: 10051677.

24 Tataranni PA, Gautier JF, Chen K, Uecker A, Bandy D, Salbe AD et al. Neuroanatomical correlates of hunger and satiation in humans using positron emission tomography. *Proc Natl Acad Sci USA.* April 13, 1999;96(8):4569–4574. PubMed PMID: 10200303.

25 von Leupoldt A, Mertz C, Kegat S, Burmester S, Dahme B. The impact of emotions on the sensory and affective dimension of perceived dyspnea. Psychophysiology. July 2006;43(4):382–386. PubMed PMID: 16916434.

26 von Leupoldt A, Seemann N, Gugleva T, Dahme B. Attentional distraction reduces the affective but not the sensory dimension of perceived dyspnea. *Respir Med.* April 2007;101(4):839–844. PubMed PMID: 16971103.

27 Manning HL, Schwartzstein RM. Pathophysiology of dyspnea. *N Engl J Med.* December 7, 1995;333(23):1547–1553. PubMed PMID: 7477171.

28 Dyspnea. Mechanisms, assessment, and management: A consensus statement. American Thoracic Society. *Am J Respir Crit Care Med.* January 1999;159(1):321–340. PubMed PMID: 9872857.

29 Gaytan SP, Pasaro R. Connections of the rostral ventral respiratory neuronal cell group: An anterograde and retrograde tracing study in the rat. *Brain Res Bull.* December 1998;47(6):625–642. PubMed PMID: 10078619.

30 Taguchi O, Kikuchi Y, Hida W, Iwase N, Satoh M, Chonan T et al. Effects of bronchoconstriction and external resistive loading on the sensation of dyspnea. *J Appl Physiol.* December 1991;71(6):2183–2190. PubMed PMID: 1778911.

31 Banzett RB, Lansing RW, Reid MB, Adams L, Brown R. 'Air hunger' arising from increased PCO_2 in mechanically ventilated quadriplegics. *Respir Physiol.* April 1989;76(1):53–67. PubMed PMID: 2499025.

32 Lane R, Cockcroft A, Adams L, Guz A. Arterial oxygen saturation and breathlessness in patients with chronic obstructive airways disease. *Clin Sci (Lond).* June 1987;72(6):693–698. PubMed PMID: 3595075.

33 Eyzaguirre C, Zapata P. Perspectives in carotid body research. *J Appl Physiol.* October 1984;57(4):931–957. PubMed PMID: 6150019.

34 O'Donnell DE, Webb KA. Exertional breathlessness in patients with chronic airflow limitation. The role of lung hyperinflation. *Am Rev Respir Dis.* November 1993;148(5):1351–1357. PubMed PMID: 8239175.

35 Manning HL, Molinary EJ, Leiter JC. Effect of inspiratory flow rate on respiratory sensation and pattern of breathing. *Am J Respir Crit Care Med.* March 1995;151(3 Part 1):751–757. PubMed PMID: 7881666.

36 Simon PM, Schwartzstein RM, Weiss JW, Fencl V, Teghtsoonian M, Weinberger SE. Distinguishable types of dyspnea in patients with shortness of breath. *Am Rev Respir Dis.* November 1990;142(5):1009–1014. PubMed PMID: 2240820.

37 Binks AP, Moosavi SH, Banzett RB, Schwartzstein RM. "Tightness" sensation of asthma does not arise from the work of breathing. *Am J Respir Crit Care Med.* January 1, 2002;165(1):78–82. PubMed PMID: 11779734.

38 Adams L, Chronos N, Lane R, Guz A. The measurement of breathlessness induced in normal subjects: Validity of two scaling techniques. *Clin Sci (Lond).* July 1985;69(1):7–16. PubMed PMID: 4064556.

39 Borg GA. Psychophysical bases of perceived exertion. *Med Sci Sports Exerc.* 1982;14(5):377–381. PubMed PMID: 7154893.

40 Meek PM, Banzett R, Parshall MB, Gracely RH, Schwartzstein RM, Lansing R. Reliability and validity of the multidimensional dyspnea profile. *Chest.* June 2012;141(6):1546–1553. PubMed PMID: 22267681. Pubmed Central PMCID: 3367480.

41 Akiyama Y, Nishimura M, Kobayashi S, Yoshioka A, Yamamoto M, Miyamoto K et al. Effects of naloxone on the sensation of dyspnea during acute respiratory stress in normal adults. *J Appl Physiol.* February 1993;74(2):590–595. PubMed PMID: 8458774.

42 Mahler DA, Murray JA, Waterman LA, Ward J, Kraemer WJ, Zhang X et al. Endogenous opioids modify dyspnoea during treadmill exercise in patients with COPD. *Eur Respir J.* April 2009;33(4):771–777. PubMed PMID: 19213787.

43 Zebraski SE, Kochenash SM, Raffa RB. Lung opioid receptors: Pharmacology and possible target for nebulized morphine in dyspnea. *Life Sci.* 2000;66(23):2221–2231. PubMed PMID: 10855942.

44 Henriksen G, Willoch F. Imaging of opioid receptors in the central nervous system. *Brain.* May 2008;131(Part 5):1171–1196. PubMed PMID: 18048446. Pubmed Central PMCID: 2367693.

45 Pattinson KT, Governo RJ, MacIntosh BJ, Russell EC, Corfield DR, Tracey I et al. Opioids depress cortical centers responsible for the volitional control of respiration. *J Neurosci.* June 24, 2009;29(25):8177–8186. PubMed PMID: 19553457.

46 Banzett RB, Adams L, O'Donnell CR, Gilman SA, Lansing RW, Schwartzstein RM. Using laboratory models to test treatment: Morphine reduces dyspnea and hypercapnic ventilatory response. *Am J Respir Crit Care Med.* October 15, 2011;184(8):920–927. PubMed PMID: 21778294. Pubmed Central PMCID: 3208656.

47 Bruera E, MacEachern T, Ripamonti C, Hanson J. Subcutaneous morphine for dyspnea in cancer patients. *Ann Intern Med.* November 1, 1993;119(9):906–907. PubMed PMID: 8215003.

48 Allard P, Lamontagne C, Bernard P, Tremblay C. How effective are supplementary doses of opioids for dyspnea in terminally ill cancer patients? A randomized continuous sequential clinical trial. *J Pain Symptom Manage.* April 1999;17(4):256–265. PubMed PMID: 10203878.

49 Mazzocato C, Buclin T, Rapin CH. The effects of morphine on dyspnea and ventilatory function in elderly patients with advanced cancer: A randomized double-blind controlled trial. *Ann Oncol.* December 1999;10(12):1511–1514. PubMed PMID: 10643545.

50 Chua TP, Harrington D, Ponikowski P, Webb-Peploe K, Poole-Wilson PA, Coats AJ. Effects of dihydrocodeine on chemosensitivity and exercise tolerance in patients with chronic heart failure. *J Am Coll Cardiol.* January 1997;29(1):147–152. PubMed PMID: 8996307.

51 Williams SG, Wright DJ, Marshall P, Reese A, Tzeng BH, Coats AJ et al. Safety and potential benefits of low dose diamorphine during exercise in patients with chronic heart failure. *Heart.* September 2003;89(9):1085–1086. PubMed PMID: 12923038.

52 Johnson MJ, McDonagh TA, Harkness A, McKay SE, Dargie HJ. Morphine for the relief of breathlessness in patients with chronic heart failure—A pilot study. *Eur J Heart Fail.* December 2002;4(6):753–756. PubMed PMID: 12453546.

53 Allen S, Raut S, Woollard J, Vassallo M. Low dose diamorphine reduces breathlessness without causing a fall in oxygen saturation in elderly patients with end-stage idiopathic pulmonary fibrosis. *Palliat Med.* March 2005;19(2):128–130. PubMed PMID: 15810751.

54 Clemens KE, Klaschik E. Morphine in the management of dyspnoea in ALS. A pilot study. *Eur J Neurol.* May 2008;15(5):445–450. PubMed PMID: 18355309.

55 Light RW, Muro JR, Sato RI, Stansbury DW, Fischer CE, Brown SE. Effects of oral morphine on breathlessness and exercise tolerance in patients with chronic obstructive pulmonary disease. *Am Rev Respir Dis.* January 1989;139(1):126–133. PubMed PMID: 2492170.

56 Abernethy AP, Currow DC, Frith P, Fazekas BS, McHugh A, Bui C. Randomised, double blind, placebo controlled crossover trial of sustained release morphine for the management of refractory dyspnoea. *Br Med J.* September 6, 2003;327(7414):523–528. PubMed PMID: 12958109.

57 Jennings AL, Davies AN, Higgins JP, Gibbs JS, Broadley KE. A systematic review of the use of opioids in the management of dyspnoea. *Thorax.* November 2002;57(11):939–944. PubMed PMID: 12403875.

58 Currow DC, McDonald C, Oaten S, Kenny B, Allcroft P, Frith P et al. Once-daily opioids for chronic dyspnea: A dose increment and pharmacovigilance study. *J Pain Symptom Manage.* September 2011;42(3):388–399. PubMed PMID: 21458217.

59 Philip J, Gold M, Milner A, Di Iulio J, Miller B, Spruyt O. A randomized, double-blind, crossover trial of the effect of oxygen on dyspnea in patients with advanced cancer. *J Pain Symptom Manage.* December 2006;32(6):541–550. PubMed PMID: 17157756.

60 Abernethy AP, McDonald CF, Frith PA, Clark K, Herndon JE, 2nd, Marcello J et al. Effect of palliative oxygen versus room air in relief of breathlessness in patients with refractory dyspnoea: A double-blind, randomised controlled trial. *Lancet.* September 4, 2010;376(9743):784–793. PubMed PMID: 20816546. Pubmed Central PMCID: 2962424.

61 Schwartzstein RM, Lahive K, Pope A, Weinberger SE, Weiss JW. Cold facial stimulation reduces breathlessness induced in normal subjects. *Am Rev Respir Dis.* July 1987;136(1):58–61. PubMed PMID: 3605841.

62 Liss HP, Grant BJ. The effect of nasal flow on breathlessness in patients with chronic obstructive pulmonary disease. *Am Rev Respir Dis.* June 1988;137(6):1285–1288. PubMed PMID: 3144198.

63 Burgess KR, Whitelaw WA. Effects of nasal cold receptors on pattern of breathing. *J Appl Physiol.* January 1988;64(1):371–376. PubMed PMID: 3128527.

64 Galbraith S, Fagan P, Perkins P, Lynch A, Booth S. Does the use of a handheld fan improve chronic dyspnea? A randomized, controlled, crossover trial. *J Pain Symptom Manage.* May 2010;39(5):831–838. PubMed PMID: 20471544.

65 Paulus MP, Feinstein JS, Castillo G, Simmons AN, Stein MB. Dose-dependent decrease of activation in bilateral amygdala and insula by lorazepam during emotion processing. *Arch Gen Psychiatry.* March 2005;62(3):282–288. PubMed PMID: 15753241.

66 Mitchell-Heggs P, Murphy K, Minty K, Guz A, Patterson SC, Minty PS et al. Diazepam in the treatment of dyspnoea in the 'Pink Puffer' syndrome. *Q J Med.* Winter 1980;49(193):9–20. PubMed PMID: 6776586.

67 Navigante AH, Castro MA, Cerchietti LC. Morphine versus midazolam as upfront therapy to control dyspnea perception in cancer patients while its underlying cause is sought or treated. *J Pain Symptom Manage.* May 2010;39(5):820–830. PubMed PMID: 20471543.

68 Navigante AH, Cerchietti LC, Castro MA, Lutteral MA, Cabalar ME. Midazolam as adjunct therapy to morphine in the alleviation of severe dyspnea perception in patients with advanced cancer. *J Pain Symptom Manage.* January 2006;31(1):38–47. PubMed PMID: 16442481.

69 Stark RD, Gambles SA, Lewis JA. Methods to assess breathlessness in healthy subjects: A critical evaluation and application to analyse the acute effects of diazepam and promethazine on breathlessness induced by exercise or by exposure to raised levels of carbon dioxide. *Clin Sci (Lond).* October 1981;61(4):429–439. PubMed PMID: 6793277.

70 Woodcock AA, Gross ER, Geddes DM. Drug treatment of breathlessness: Contrasting effects of diazepam and promethazine in pink puffers. *Br Med J (Clin Res Ed).* August 1, 1981;283(6287):343–346. PubMed PMID: 6788319.

71 Man GC, Hsu K, Sproule BJ. Effect of alprazolam on exercise and dyspnea in patients with chronic obstructive pulmonary disease. *Chest.* December 1986;90(6):832–836. PubMed PMID: 3780329.

72 Simon ST, Higginson IJ, Booth S, Harding R, Bausewein C. Benzodiazepines for the relief of breathlessness in advanced malignant and non-malignant diseases in adults. *Cochrane Database Syst Rev.* 2010;(1):CD007354. PubMed PMID: 20091630.

73 Carrieri-Kohlman V, Gormley JM, Eiser S, Demir-Deviren S, Nguyen H, Paul SM et al. Dyspnea and the affective response during exercise training in obstructive pulmonary disease. *Nurs Res.* May–June 2001;50(3):136–146. PubMed PMID: 11393635.

74 Chan CW, Richardson A, Richardson J. Managing symptoms in patients with advanced lung cancer during radiotherapy: Results of a psycho-educational randomized controlled trial. *J Pain Symptom Manage.* February 2011;41(2):347–357. PubMed PMID: 21131165.

75 Argyropoulou P, Patakas D, Koukou A, Vasiliadis P, Georgopoulos D. Buspirone effect on breathlessness and exercise performance in patients with chronic obstructive pulmonary disease. *Respiration.* 1993;60(4):216–220. PubMed PMID: 8265878.

76 Singh NP, Despars JA, Stansbury DW, Avalos K, Light RW. Effects of buspirone on anxiety levels and exercise tolerance in patients with chronic airflow obstruction and mild anxiety. *Chest.* March 1993;103(3):800–804. PubMed PMID: 8449072.

77 O'Neill PA, Morton PB, Stark RD. Chlorpromazine—A specific effect on breathlessness? *Br J Clin Pharmacol.* June 1985;19(6):793–797. PubMed PMID: 4027121.

78 Burki NK, Sheatt M, Lee LY. Effects of airway anesthesia on dyspnea and ventilatory response to intravenous injection of adenosine in healthy human subjects. *Pulm Pharmacol Ther.* 2008;21(1):208–213. PubMed PMID: 17442602.

79 Winning AJ, Hamilton RD, Guz A. Ventilation and breathlessness on maximal exercise in patients with interstitial lung disease after local anaesthetic aerosol inhalation. *Clin Sci (Lond).* March 1988;74(3):275–281. PubMed PMID: 3345636.

80 Wilcock A, Corcoran R, Tattersfield AE. Safety and efficacy of nebulized lignocaine in patients with cancer and breathlessness. *Palliat Med.* 1994;8(1):35–38. PubMed PMID: 7514070.

81 Nishino T, Ide T, Sudo T, Sato J. Inhaled furosemide greatly alleviates the sensation of experimentally induced dyspnea. *Am J Respir Crit Care Med.* June 2000;161(6):1963–1967. PubMed PMID: 10852774.

82 Minowa Y, Ide T, Nishino T. Effects of inhaled furosemide on CO_2 ventilatory responsiveness in humans. *Pulm Pharmacol Ther.* 2002;15(4):363–368. PubMed PMID: 12220941.

83 Moosavi SH, Binks AP, Lansing RW, Topulos GP, Banzett RB, Schwartzstein RM. Effect of inhaled furosemide on air hunger induced in healthy humans. *Respir Physiol Neurobiol.* April 16, 2007;156(1):1–8. PubMed PMID: 16935035.

84 Shimoyama N, Shimoyama M. Nebulized furosemide as a novel treatment for dyspnea in terminal cancer patients. *J Pain Symptom Manage.* January 2002;23(1):73–76. PubMed PMID: 11779672.

85 Kohara H, Ueoka H, Aoe K, Maeda T, Takeyama H, Saito R et al. Effect of nebulized furosemide in terminally ill cancer patients with dyspnea. *J Pain Symptom Manage.* October 2003;26(4):962–967. PubMed PMID: 14575057.

86 Wilcock A, Walton A, Manderson C, Feathers L, El Khoury B, Lewis M et al. Randomised, placebo controlled trial of nebulised furosemide for breathlessness in patients with cancer. *Thorax.* October 2008;63(10):872–875. PubMed PMID: 18408049.

87 Ong KC, Kor AC, Chong WF, Earnest A, Wang YT. Effects of inhaled furosemide on exertional dyspnea in chronic obstructive pulmonary disease. *Am J Respir Crit Care Med.* May 1, 2004;169(9):1028–1033. PubMed PMID: 14977622.

88 Jensen D, Amjadi K, Harris-McAllister V, Webb KA, O'Donnell DE. Mechanisms of dyspnoea relief and improved exercise endurance after furosemide inhalation in COPD. *Thorax.* July 2008;63(7):606–613. PubMed PMID: 18250181.

89   Sudo T, Hayashi F, Nishino T. Responses of tracheobronchial receptors to inhaled furosemide in anesthetized rats. *Am J Respir Crit Care Med.* September 2000;162(3 Part 1):971–975. PubMed PMID: 10988115.

90   Lacasse Y, Goldstein R, Lasserson TJ, Martin S. Pulmonary rehabilitation for chronic obstructive pulmonary disease. *Cochrane Database Syst Rev.* 2006;(4):CD003793. PubMed PMID: 17054186.

91   Paz-Diaz H, Montes de Oca M, Lopez JM, Celli BR. Pulmonary rehabilitation improves depression, anxiety, dyspnea and health status in patients with COPD. *Am J Phys Med Rehabil.* January 2007;86(1):30–36. PubMed PMID: 17304686.

92   Bredin M, Corner J, Krishnasamy M, Plant H, Bailey C, A'Hern R. Multicentre randomised controlled trial of nursing intervention for breathlessness in patients with lung cancer. *Br Med J.* April 3, 1999;318(7188):901–904. PubMed PMID: 10102851.

93   Bausewein C, Booth S, Gysels M, Higginson I. Non-pharmacological interventions for breathlessness in advanced stages of malignant and non-malignant diseases. *Cochrane Database Syst Rev.* 2008;(2):CD005623. PubMed PMID: 18425927.

94   Suzuki M, Muro S, Ando Y, Omori T, Shiota T, Endo K et al. A randomized, placebo-controlled trial of acupuncture in patients with chronic obstructive pulmonary disease (COPD): The COPD-acupuncture trial (CAT). *Arch Intern Med.* June 11, 2012;172(11):878–886. PubMed PMID: 22905352.

95   Mularski RA, Munjas BA, Lorenz KA, Sun S, Robertson SJ, Schmelzer W et al. Randomized controlled trial of mindfulness-based therapy for dyspnea in chronic obstructive lung disease. *J Altern Complement Med.* October 2009;15(10):1083–1090. PubMed PMID: 19848546.

96   van 't Hul A, Kwakkel G, Gosselink R. The acute effects of noninvasive ventilatory support during exercise on exercise endurance and dyspnea in patients with chronic obstructive pulmonary disease: A systematic review. *J Cardiopulm Rehabil.* July–August 2002;22(4):290–297. PubMed PMID: 12202851.

97   Azoulay E, Kouatchet A, Jaber S, Lambert J, Meziani F, Schmidt M et al. Noninvasive mechanical ventilation in patients having declined tracheal intubation. *Intensive Care Med.* February 2013;39(2):292–301. PubMed PMID: 23184037.

68

Other respiratory symptoms (cough, hiccup, and secretions)

SARAH MOLLART, TABITHA THOMAS, ROSEMARY WADE, SARA BOOTH

INTRODUCTION

In this chapter, we consider the difficult respiratory symptoms apart from breathlessness. We present the latest evidence on the pathophysiology and treatment of these symptoms, but in all of these, a rounded palliative care approach is needed if the best control possible is to be achieved.

All patients with advanced disease have concerns and problems that go beyond the simple pathophysiology of their illness. Some advanced diseases progress rapidly barely giving the family time to adjust to the dreadful deterioration in their loved one's condition. Others occur in young people, when culturally it seems particularly cruel and where the patients themselves are alienated from the condition of most of their contemporaries. The person with advanced disease will usually have carers, loved ones, friends, and family, who will all be affected by the illness, and in palliative care, those closest or most significant to the patient will be cared for. Some patients may have no relatives, friends, or informal carers and this poses a problem in itself.

Each symptom has its own section where the latest research evidence is presented on the current understanding of pathophysiology and management. This chapter ends with a table that complements these sections, describing and discussing a general palliative care approach to rare but unpleasant difficult respiratory symptoms, where the evidence base is slender and multiple approaches to treatment often required.

COUGH

Cough is common in the general population and is generally self-limiting or can be managed by treating the precipitating cause.[1] Intractable cough associated with advanced disease is a distressing symptom. Approximately 65% of patients with lung cancer complain of cough at presentation, and as it is generally not well controlled, its incidence and severity remain constant throughout the disease course.[2] Cough is also common in patients with any type of advanced cancer. In one survey, 37%

of such patients complained of cough, and 38% of these rated it as moderate or severe.[3]

Relentless coughing can have a profound impact on quality of life. It leads to exhaustion, breathlessness, musculoskeletal pain, vomiting, and incontinence. Disturbed sleep affects both patients and partners with consequent strain on family and social relationships.

Physiology

Under normal conditions, cough serves as a reflex defense mechanism to remove inhaled material or inflammatory products. The reflex begins with either mechanical or chemical stimulation of irritant receptors in the epithelium of the respiratory tract. Impulses are then transmitted via vagal afferents to the medulla oblongata where a cough response is coordinated. Cough involves the initial inspiration of air to a high lung volume, followed by glottis closure and the development of high intrapleural pressure. When the glottis opens, a biphasic turbulent blast of air is produced as a result of the high pressure and the dynamic compression of the central airways. At high airflow velocities, the surface of the mucus is sheared off and droplets are propelled into the airway lumen. However, in a variety of disease processes, cough may become nonproductive and excessive and damage the airway mucosa.[4]

Pathogenesis

An effective cough, resulting in mucus displacement, depends upon

- The velocity of the airstream
- The tenacity of the mucus
- A functioning mucociliary transport system

Thus, weak respiratory and abdominal muscles, for example, in paraplegic patients, reduce the ability to produce a high expiratory pressure, reducing the velocity of airflow and producing an ineffective cough. Vocal cord paralysis, associated with left upper lobe lung cancers, prevents complete glottis closure. This impairs the generation of sufficient intrathoracic pressure to produce an efficient cough. Mucus tenacity increases when the water content of mucus decreases, which leads to ineffective clearance. Finally, a functioning mucociliary apparatus is required to move mucus from the periphery to the more central airways from where it can be expelled by coughing.

On a receptor level, the upregulation of various cough receptors, primarily capsaicin receptor and transient receptor potential vanilloid-1 (TRPV1), is thought to be responsible for heightened cough sensitivity, in almost all forms of chronic cough.[5]

Causes

Any form of malignant lung disease can cause an inflammatory or mechanical stimulus to cough. It may be the direct result of the tumor itself or a consequence of consolidation associated with bronchial obstruction, aspiration, or tracheoesophageal fistulae. In addition, the combination of pain and cachexia diminishes cough effectiveness and increases susceptibility to infection. Some tumors, particularly bronchoalveolar carcinoma, actively secrete mucus and therefore continuously stimulate the cough reflex. Occasionally, cough associated with increasing breathlessness is the result of an interstitial pneumonitis associated with radiotherapy.

There are many nonmalignant causes of chronic cough, which may be relevant in palliative care patients. Smoking is a prime cause in adults and induces airway inflammation and mucus hypersecretion and causes damage to mucociliary apparatus. Lung damage due to smoke or persistent infection leads to chronic bronchitis and bronchiectasis. Management is usually directed at treating the underlying cause, that is, treating infection and increasing cough clearance, rather than cough suppression.

In nonsmoking, immunocompetent adults with a normal chest radiograph, who are not taking an angiotensin-converting enzyme (ACE) inhibitor and who do not have exposure to irritants, the three most common causes of cough are upper airway cough syndrome (formerly postnasal drip syndrome[6]) due to various rhinosinus conditions, asthma, and gastroesophageal reflux disease. In 20% of patients, cough is due to more than one of these causes[1]; some may even have all three. For each, cough may be the only symptom. Each of these diagnoses should therefore be considered if the cause of cough is not otherwise clear.[7]

Assessment

Cough may make an important contribution to symptoms such as pain, nausea, insomnia, and breathlessness, and its treatment can therefore have considerable benefits. As well as looking for an underlying cause, care should be taken to determine whether cough frequency or difficulty with expectoration is most troublesome. Once this is established, it helps make the decision as to whether therapy should be curative, protussive, or antitussive. Management is, of course, related to the patient's prognosis: if cough is severe and the prognosis short, there may

be no time to treat infection or reflux, and a powerful opioid antitussive might be more appropriate. It's important that when considering the possibility of the three common benign causes of chronic cough (upper airway cough syndrome, asthma, and gastroesophageal reflux disease), neither the history (character and timing of cough) nor the presence or absence of sputum production is of much diagnostic value.[8]

Management strategies

SUPPORTIVE

The severity of a cough may be used as a gauge of disease progression by some patients, particularly if it was the presenting symptom of their cancer. Paroxysms of coughing are distressing to experience and alarming to watch and can lead to a fear that death will occur during an attack. Discussion, reassurance, and the establishment of a management plan to use during a coughing fit are helpful for both patients and carers.

STOP ACE INHIBITORS

Among approximately 10% of users, ACE inhibitors cause a cough, which tends to be a class effect and is not dose related. Cough of any cause can be aggravated by ACE inhibitors and this effect can take up to 4 weeks to resolve once the drug is stopped.[9**]

PHARMACOLOGICAL

Pharmacological therapy can be used to treat an underlying cause or to modify the cough, in which case it is either protussive or antitussive. *Protussive* therapy makes the cough more effective and therefore less distressing and is also useful if the cough is providing a useful physiological function, for example, clearing sputum. *Antitussive* therapy involves cough suppression. There is a paucity of evidence available regarding the pharmacological treatment of cough, so little formal guidance for treatment strategies. There is some evidence for the drugs described here, but their use should be balanced against their potential side effects, and the local availability of drugs must also be taken into account. There are some drugs available that have not become widely used but their use should be considered for individual patients.

Treatment of the underlying cause

DECONGESTANTS AND ANTIHISTAMINES

"Upper airway cough syndrome" is the most common cause of chronic cough. A variety of mechanisms have been postulated. Secretions from the nose or sinuses drip into the hypopharynx and stimulate the cough reflex. Symptoms of nasal congestion or discharge or a history of a recent cold is relatively sensitive but not necessarily specific,[4] and ultimately a diagnosis of upper airway cough syndrome is made if cough shows a response to therapy. Sedative antihistamines and decongestants have been shown to be beneficial[10**,11*] but the effect is gradual and can take up to 2 weeks.

BRONCHODILATORS

Cough may be the only, or predominant, symptom of asthma: cough-variant asthma.[12] In those with asthma or airway hyperresponsiveness, cough will respond transiently to bronchodilator therapy with β_2 agonists[13*] and in the long term has been shown to respond to sodium necrodomil,[14**] antileukotriene agents,[15*] and corticosteroids.[16*] In addition, the bronchodilator ipratropium bromide has been found to be useful as an antitussive in patients with chronic obstructive pulmonary disease by decreasing both sputum production and cough.[17**]

CORTICOSTEROIDS

Inhaled (and sometimes oral) corticosteroids are important in the management of both asthma and nonasthmatic eosinophilic bronchitis (a disorder characterized by cough and eosinophilic airway inflammation).[18] A dry cough associated with increasing dyspnea in those who have recently received radiotherapy to the lung should raise the suspicion of radiation pneumonitis.[19] Interstitial pneumonitis is also a rare complication of some chemotherapeutic agents.[20,21] If appropriate, radiological imaging should be carried out to confirm the diagnosis, as both are likely to respond to steroids.

PROTON PUMP INHIBITORS/ANTACIDS

It is thought that gastroesophageal reflux may be the cause of cough even in the absence of gastrointestinal symptoms. The cough may take a number of weeks to resolve in healthy subjects treated with antacids.[22] A double-blind randomized placebo-controlled trial has shown a statistically significant improvement in cough both in patients treated with esomeprazole 20 mg twice daily and the placebo group, with no significant difference between the groups, suggesting a marked placebo effect in the treatment of cough.[23**] Greater improvement of cough was seen in those in the treatment group who were also exhibiting dyspeptic symptoms, suggesting that treatment should be restricted to these patients.

ONCOLOGICAL AND ENDOBRONCHIAL TREATMENT

Oncological treatments may be helpful in palliating cough. Radiotherapy can improve cough in non-small-cell lung cancer in about 50% of patients.[24*] Retreatment can be beneficial for those with cough who have previously received radiotherapy (palliation lasted for more than 50% of their remaining life span in one study).[25,26*] Intraluminal brachytherapy for endobronchial lesions improved cough at 6 weeks in 62% of patients,[27*] but a recent review suggests that external beam radiation alone is more effective at palliating cough than brachytherapy alone.[28***]

Chemotherapy can provide good palliation of cough. Studies have shown significant benefit from gemcitabine monotherapy, with 73% of those with moderate-to-severe cough noticing an improvement in cough, which lasted 2–5 months.[29]

A range of endobronchial treatments are available, including laser therapy, electrocautery, argon plasma coagulation, photodynamic therapy, cryotherapy, and intraluminal stent insertion. The main indication for endobronchial therapies in palliative care is for the relief of malignant central airway obstruction and, in the case of the first three, management of hemoptysis. Brachytherapy is the only endobronchial therapy for which relief of cough has been specifically mentioned as a treatment outcome. Other therapies have reported more global symptom relief.[30] If a patient with cancer who has been discharged from oncological care develops intractable cough, it is important to refer them back for assessment or at least discuss them with the oncologist, so that an important treatment option for this difficult symptom is not overlooked.

Protussive cough enhancers (mucoactive agents)

EXPECTORANTS

Expectorants improve cough effectiveness by increasing airway water or the volume of airway secretions. Simple hydration has not been shown to improve cough and may be detrimental, since overhydration has been shown to decrease airway clearance in some patients with chronic cough.[31*]

HYPERTONIC SALINE

Nebulized hypertonic saline has been shown to enhance mucociliary clearance. As well as stimulating mucociliary transport, it is postulated that hypertonic saline breaks the ionic bonds within mucus gel and therefore lowers viscosity and elasticity.[32] The effect appears to be concentration dependent: patients with cystic fibrosis were found to have better cough clearance with increasing concentrations of nebulized hypertonic saline.[33*] Therefore, more evidence exists for the use of nebulized hypertonic saline as opposed to normal saline, which tends to be administered routinely.

GUAIFENESIN

This expectorant is found in many over-the-counter preparations, but the evidence is mixed. One placebo-controlled trial showed that patients treated with guaifenesin maintained steady levels of sputum production compared with a decline in those taking placebo.[34**] Guaifenesin has recently been shown to decrease cough reflex sensitivity in patients with upper respiratory tract infection.[35] Other trials have shown guaifenesin to have no effect on cough due to chronic bronchitis.[36*,37*]

MUCOLYTIC AGENTS

Mucolytic medications increase the expectoration of sputum by depolymerizing either the mucin network (classic mucolytics) or the DNA–actin polymer network (peptide mucolytics), thereby reducing its viscosity and aiding cough clearance.[38]

CLASSIC MUCOLYTICS, E.G., CARBOCYSTEINE

These mucolytics hydrolyze the disulfide bonds that link mucin monomers within sputum. Although they have some benefit in reducing the number and length of exacerbations of chronic bronchitis,[39***] their relevance for patients with advanced cancer is unclear. Oral preparations are gastric irritants.

PEPTIDE MUCOLYTICS

Recombinant DNase is approved for use in patients with cystic fibrosis, though the American College of Chest Physicians' 2006 guidelines on treatment of chronic cough do not recommend its use for this indication.[40] It reduces the size of DNA molecules within mucus, thereby reducing sputum viscosity and aiding clearance. Though it has been shown to improve forced expiratory volume in one second (FEV_1), reduce exacerbations, and improve quality of life in cystic fibrosis patients, it has shown no benefit for patients with chronic bronchitis and is not generally used for symptom control in other conditions.[38]

CHEST PHYSIOTHERAPY

Advice from a physiotherapist on cough technique is important. "Huffing," a technique that involves forcible exhalation with the glottis open from a medium-to-low lung volume, can be helpful for weak, breathless patients with extensive disease.

Cough assist machines (mechanical insufflation–exsufflation) are effective for improving airway clearance for patients with neuromuscular disease, and the long-term home use of such devices is well tolerated.[41]

Cough suppression

HOME REMEDIES/OVER-THE-COUNTER PREPARATIONS

Any sweet thickened drink will help relieve cough, and many popular "cough medicines" and herbal remedies rely on the presence of demulcents such as sugars and gum arabic, which absorb fluid and produce a soothing covering in the throat. They are probably most useful if the cough is due to receptor irritation in the oropharynx.[42] Butamirate citrate linctus has been shown to reduce cough in lung cancer but not in other conditions.[43**]

ANTITUSSIVES

Relatively little is known about how antitussive drugs inhibit cough.[44] Some have a predominantly central mode of action, for example, opioids, whereas others are thought to work peripherally. The concept of "opioid-resistant cough" appears in the literature as a distinct entity[45*,46**,47*] and may be due to either peripheral or central sensitization of the cough reflex. A number of antitussives are discussed in the following. As discussed earlier, there is a paucity of large trials to guide treatment.

OPIOIDS AND RELATED COMPOUNDS

The antitussive activity of opioids is distinct from their analgesic effect and some opioid-related antitussives have no analgesic effect at all. In palliative care patients, it is often necessary to treat both cough and pain, in which case a strong opioid analgesic is appropriate. If cough persists while a patient is taking a strong opioid for pain relief, there is no evidence currently available to support adding a separate opioid that has greater antitussive activity for cough.

Morphine

A recent double-blind placebo-controlled study of patients with chronic cough, without significant lung disease, showed a mean 40% reduction in daily cough scores for patients taking modified-release morphine sulfate 5 mg twice daily.[48**] The patients enrolled to the study had previously failed to respond to trials of specific antitussive therapy: an open-label extension showed a benefit from modified-release morphine sulfate 10 mg twice daily for those who had not had significant benefit from 5 mg. In "responders," maximum benefit was seen within 5 days.

Codeine

Codeine's antitussive activity is much greater than its analgesic action and has been extensively studied both clinically and experimentally.[49***] There is conflicting evidence. A 4 hours dose of 30–60 mg has been seen to be effective but has all the typical opioid side effects such as nausea, drowsiness, and constipation. A significant dose-dependent relationship with "cough counts" (but not patients' evaluations of its effectiveness) has been shown by one study.[50**] A more recent crossover study in patients with stable COPD showed no difference between codeine and placebo when ambulatory cough recording, cough symptom score, and visual analogue scales were measured.[51**] The popularity of codeine as a treatment for cough may be partially due to ease of prescribing, because of its noncontrolled drug status, rather than any unique pharmacological properties.[48**]

Hydrocodone

Hydrocodone is one of the metabolites of codeine and has analgesic and antitussive activity. It was used in a phase II open-label study in cancer patients with cough as an alternative to codeine because it had been found to be better tolerated.[52*] A median dose of 10 mg a day was associated with the best response (most patients achieved greater than 50% improvement in cough frequency). Most patients were using other opioids for analgesia.

Methadone

The dextroisomer of methadone is particularly active and is a more potent antitussive than codeine or morphine.[49*] Methadone linctus can be given at a dose of 1–2 mg every 4–6 hours, reducing to twice daily with prolonged use. Because of its long half-life and potential to accumulate, it should be used with caution and under specialist supervision.

OPIOID-RELATED ANTITUSSIVES WITH NO ANALGESIC ACTIVITY

Pholcodine

This is structurally related to codeine and possibly has greater antitussive activity, but no analgesic action. It has few side effects and does not give rise to tolerance or dependence.[49**]

Dextromethorphan

Dextromethorphan is a nonnarcotic codeine analogue and is the active ingredient in many over-the-counter preparations. It is the most commonly used antitussive in the United States and compares favorably to codeine in patients with chronic cough. In one comparative study, both were effective in reducing cough frequency at a dose of 20 mg, but dextromethorphan was preferred by the majority of patients and had fewer side effects.[53**]

Dimemorfan

Dimemorfan is widely used in Japan. Although an opioid derivative, dimemorfan is thought to have a central antitussive activity, independent of the narcotic antitussive mechanism. It shows marked or moderate efficacy in about 50% of patients treated at doses of 20 mg three times daily. It does not cause dependence and has no analgesic action.[54**]

NONOPIOID ANTITUSSIVE DRUGS

Sodium Cromoglycate

Sodium cromoglycate may suppress unmyelinated C-fibers involved in the afferent pathway of the cough reflex. A small trial in patients with neoplastic, irritative cough that had been unresponsive to conventional treatment found there was a significant reduction in cough among those receiving inhaled sodium cromoglycate when compared with placebo.[46**] It typically took 36–48 hours before the effect of the drug could be observed.

Benzonatate

Benzonatate is thought to act peripherally by anesthetizing stretch receptors. It has been described in a case series as useful for opioid-resistant cough in cancer patients at a dose of 100 mg three times daily and has few side effects.[47*]

Levodropropizine

Levodropropizine has been shown to be as effective as dihydrocodeine in patients with malignant involvement of the lung at a dose of 75 mg three times daily. There was significantly less somnolence reported in the levodropropizine group.[55**] The side effect profile of levodropropizine was also significantly better when it was compared to dextromethorphan in patients with moderate nonproductive cough, although both had similar antitussive activity.[56**]

Moguisteine

Moguisteine has been shown to produce a significant reduction in cough when compared with placebo (42% vs. 14%, respectively). Patients received moguisteine syrup, 200 mg three times daily, or placebo over a period of 4 days.[57**] In a separate study, a dose of 100 mg three times daily was found to be equally as effective as codeine 15 and 30 mg.[58**]

Glaucine

This centrally acting antitussive is mainly available in eastern Europe (and should not be confused with a beta-blocker, metipranolol, which is marketed in Europe under the same name[4]). Antitussive effects and side effect profile were significantly better than codeine in one randomized controlled trial.[59**] Both drugs were taken at a dose of 30 mg three times daily.

Baclofen

Baclofen has been shown to have a cough suppressant effect in animal studies[60] and also to reduce irritant-induced cough in humans.[61,62] However, no double-blinded or placebo-controlled studies of pathological cough have been carried out, and it is not recommended unless there is no alternative.[40]

LOCAL ANESTHETICS

Experimentally, local anesthetics delivered either intravenously or by inhalation have been shown to inhibit the cough response to a variety of stimuli.[44] Nebulized bupivacaine has been used for persistent cough in the palliative care setting, on the basis of case reports only.[63*] Its use is limited by its unpleasant taste, risk of aspiration, risk of bronchospasm, and short duration of action and frequent tachyphylaxis.

SEROTONIN-SELECTIVE REUPTAKE INHIBITORS

It has been postulated that serotonin-selective reuptake inhibitors may be beneficial in opioid-resistant dry cough based on observations that increased serotonin levels depress the cough reflex in cats.[64] One case series reported paroxetine to be effective for cancer patients with cough for whom codeine had been ineffective.[45*] However, there is no controlled data available.[65]

SPEECH THERAPY

There is some evidence that speech pathology management techniques can reduce the symptom severity in chronic cough. In a single-blinded randomized placebo-controlled trial,[66**] these techniques led to a significant improvement in cough scores. Techniques included education (that there is no physiological benefit from cough, that there is capacity for voluntary cough control), strategies to reduce cough (identify warning signs for cough and replace with modified swallow technique, pursed lip breathing, or relaxed throat breath), reduction of laryngeal irritation (increased hydration, decreased exposure to irritating stimuli), and psychoeducational counseling (internalizing locus of control, acceptance that treatment is hard work, setting realistic goals).

Approach to managing cough in the palliative care population

If the patient has a *very poor prognosis*—consider cough suppression alone, or no intervention.

Consider history, examination, and appropriate investigations, which may include chest radiograph and spirometry. Manage any pathology accordingly, considering disease-directed therapies:

- Antibiotics
- Mucolytic agents
- Radiotherapy, chemotherapy, endobronchial therapies

Stop ACE inhibitors.

Consider smoking cessation counseling.

Consider benign causes of cough, remembering that presentations are commonly "atypical." The American College of Chest Physicians recommends stepwise empirical treatment, in the following order[67]:

- Upper airway cough syndrome arising from rhinosinusitis: Sedative antihistamines and/or decongestants.[10**,11*]

- Asthma: Most respond to inhaled bronchodilators and inhaled corticosteroids (some may need treatment with a leukotriene receptor antagonist and/or a short course of oral steroids).[16*,68]

- Gastroesophageal reflux disease: Prokinetics, antacids, and proton pump inhibitors/H2 antagonists.

- Nonasthmatic eosinophilic bronchitis: Difficult to differentiate clinically from asthma.[69] Most patients respond to inhaled corticosteroids.[18]

Commence other treatments—protocol from Association for Palliative Medicine task group[70] (reproduced with permission):

- Prescribe simple linctus: A demulcent cough preparation for which there is no empirical evidence, but which is simple and safe.

- Give a therapeutic trial of inhaled sodium cromoglycate: There is evidence from only one small RCT,[46**] but it is relatively safe and well tolerated. The main limitation is the need to use an inhaler device.

- Prescribe an opioid or opioid derivative:
  a. Dextromethorphan: Weak evidence[53**] but low toxicity, which can be purchased in many countries without a prescription.
  b. Morphine: The most recent evidence suggests significant benefit over placebo,[48**] but this was in patients without significant lung disease. Start with morphine sulfate modified release, 5 mg 12 hours, unless the patient is already on morphine for other reasons, then titrate upwards to effect.
  c. Codeine: Historical evidence is weak and most recent evidence shows no benefit over placebo[50**] although this was in COPD patients with stable disease. Codeine should probably not be chosen over dextromethorphan or morphine.

HICCUP

Chronic hiccup is an infrequent but distressing problem and can be a sign of serious underlying pathology. It can lead to fatigue, insomnia, depression, and weight loss and therefore has a significant effect on quality of life.

Physiology

Hiccup may exist as an exercise to coordinate respiratory muscles in the fetus but serves no known physiological purpose in the adult.[71] The reflex arc consists of

1. Afferent input via the vagus nerve and phrenic nerves and the thoracic sympathetic chain
2. A central mediator thought to be in the cervical spine and brain stem
3. An efferent limb via motor fibers of the phrenic nerve and intercostal nerves

Pathophysiology

The pathophysiology of chronic hiccup is poorly understood but often results from a persistent disturbance of one of the components of the reflex arc. Conditions associated with hiccup can be grouped into three main causes:

1. *Physical Causes along the Anatomical Distribution of the Phrenic and Vagus Nerves*
   This may include esophagogastric, subphrenic, and hepatic disease and mediastinal disease (see Box 68.1).
2. *Central Nervous System Involvement*
   A review of 71 patients with neurologically induced hiccups found the majority of causes were located in the brain stem (medulla oblongata 66% and pons 17%), with lateral medullary infarcts being the most frequent cause. However, the involvement of midbrain and cerebrum in 13% of patients with neurologically induced hiccups would suggest there is also a descending influence.[72] There also appears to be a complex association of hiccups with Parkinson's disease: one study found a higher incidence of frequent or persistent hiccups in those with Parkinson's disease compared to healthy controls,[73] and hiccups are a recognized complication of therapeutic pallidotomy.[74] It is not clear whether it is the disease or its treatment that influences the development of hiccups, as both have been implicated.[75–77]
3. *Metabolic and Drug-Induced Causes*
   Steroids in particular have been linked with the onset of hiccup and are thought to lower the threshold for synaptic transmission in the brain.[78] Corticosteroids and cisplatin together increase the likelihood of developing hiccups.[79]

Box 68.1 Conditions associated with intractable hiccup

Peripheral causes interrupting the vagus or phrenic nerve

Gastritis

Gastric distension

Bowel obstruction

Gastroesophageal reflux

Subphrenic and hepatic disease

Pleural effusion

Lateral myocardial infarction

Mediastinal disease

Thoracic aortic aneurysm

Central causes

Brain stem infarction (in particular lateral medullary infarction)

Demyelinating conditions: multiple sclerosis (MS), neuromyelitis optica (NMO)

Tumor

Hemorrhage

Meningitis

Tuberculoma

Sarcoidosis

Parkinson's disease

Metabolic/toxic causes

Corticosteroids

Hyponatremia

Uremia

Hypocalcaemia

Hypocapnia

Alcohol

Midazolam

Table 68.1 *Medications used to treat hiccup*

Drug	Evidence	Common side effects
Gabapentin and pregabalin. Starting dose 100–300 mg tds	Reported to be effective in a number of case series.[112–117]	Drowsiness, dizziness, and ataxia
Baclofen 5 mg tds orally, increasing dose by 5 mg every 3 days until effective or maximum dose reached	A number of case series and an extremely small randomized crossover trial support its use.[118–121]	Sedation—particularly in renal failure
Metoclopramide	Used with success in a case series of 14 patients with a variety of conditions.[122]	Few side effects and not sedative
Haloperidol	Licensed for use in intractable hiccup but evidence for efficacy in case reports only. Commonly used in palliative care.	Extrapyramidal side effects and sedation (usually at higher doses)
Chlorpromazine	Licensed for use in intractable hiccup but scant evidence for efficacy.	Hypotension and sedation
Nifedipine 30–60 mg/day (orally)	Four patients in a series of seven gained complete relief and a fifth felt improvement with nifedipine.[123]	Headache, vasodilatation, and peripheral edema

Management strategies

It is important to consider the probable or possible etiology (Box 68.1): treatment of the underlying cause is more likely to be successful than medication. However, in many cases, the cause is untreatable or cannot be found. As with all symptoms, an assessment of the extent and impact of the symptom on the patient and family should be documented to establish the benefit of any treatments. Rare and self-limiting symptoms like hiccup are particularly difficult to research and there are few published trials. The pharmacological treatments discussed here are those for which there is a small amount of evidence or which have found their way into general use (Table 68.1).

Nonpharmacological strategies

While there are many "traditional" remedies for acute bouts of hiccups, which often involve some form of pharyngeal stimulation or diaphragmatic splinting, for example, a cold key on the back of the neck or drinking water from the wrong side of a cup, these are unlikely to be successful for intractable hiccup. Nonpharmacological interventions that have been used with success include phrenic nerve stimulation[80] and phrenic nerve block.[81] Acupuncture at pressure points GV26 and P6 has also been successful.[82]

SECRETIONS

Respiratory secretions that block the upper airway can be particularly distressing and require palliation. Two scenarios that are specific to palliative care are discussed in this chapter: noisy secretions at the end of life (rattle) and massive bronchorrhea (usually related to bronchoalveolar carcinoma of the lung).

NOISY SECRETIONS AT THE END OF LIFE (RATTLE)

Prospective studies of terminally ill cancer patients have reported the incidence of death rattle to be between 41% and 56%.[83-86] Rates in smaller observational studies vary widely.

Pathophysiology

Noisy, rattly breathing is thought to be caused by an accumulation of secretions as the cough and swallowing reflexes deteriorate in the final days and hours of life. The noise occurs when the secretions bubble with respiration. Airway secretions are a combination of pooled saliva and mucus arising from the bronchial mucosa. The degree to which each source contributes to rattle varies and has led to suggestions that there may be two distinct types: type 1 a consequence of pooled salivary secretions when a patient has lost their swallowing reflex and type 2 caused mainly by bronchial secretions when the patient is too weak to cough effectively.[87] Both salivary glands and bronchial secretory glands are stimulated by cholinergic nerves acting at muscarinic M3 receptors. Bronchial mucus production also occurs in response to many other stimuli such as inflammation and infection, and these too play a part in the development of rattle. An alternative classification distinguishes between "real" death rattle, due to nonexpectorated, nonpathological secretions, and "pseudo death rattle" caused by bronchial or other secretions in the presence of pulmonary disease.[88] Rattle resulting from predominantly bronchial secretions is likely to be poorly responsive to antimuscarinic medication.

Among cancer patients, it seems that cerebral tumors and malignant lung involvement may predispose to death rattle.[95,98] It is possible that some cases of refractory death rattle associated with cerebral tumors are due to neurogenic pulmonary edema, which is also unresponsive to anticholinergic agents.[89]

Management strategies

Good terminal care often implies "dying peacefully." Controlling death rattle can be an important component of this but is probably only effective in a third to a half of treated patients[90,95] Although some relatives and staff find the noise very distressing, qualitative studies show that some do not mind it or may take comfort from the fact that death is imminent.[91-93] Therefore, it is vital that time is spent giving explanation and reassurance to relatives, and it is important that staff feel confident to do this.[94]

POSITIONING

Repositioning the patient to a lateral or more upright position to promote drainage of secretions is often recommended. In one study, nonpharmacological interventions such as repositioning and suction improved symptoms in 31% of patients.[96]

SUCTIONING

This can be appropriate if secretions have accumulated in the pharynx and are easily reachable but can cause significant distress to some patients.[97] Assessment should be made on an individual basis and depend upon the extent to which the excessive secretions are causing distress.

Pharmacological management

The aim of anticholinergic medication is to reduce salivary and bronchial secretions and dilate the airways to allow a more laminar flow. Such drugs have a lesser effect on bronchial secretions, for reasons outlined earlier, and have no effect on those secretions that have already accumulated.[98] They are therefore more likely to be effective in preventing rattle if used early.

Clinical guidelines have been published giving guidance for doses of anticholinergic medication in death rattle, based on one-off doses in healthy volunteers.[95]

Table 68.2 *Anticholinergic medications used for death rattle*

	Cross blood–brain barrier[a]	Stat dose (sc)	Continuous SC infusion in 24 hours (mg)	Comments
Atropine	Yes	300–600 µg	1.2–2.4	No evidence to support its use, but could be considered if no alternative is available.
Hyoscine hydrobromide	Yes	400 µg	1.2–2	Available in transdermal patches in doses 0.5–1.5 mg for use over 24–72 h. Multiple patches can be used.
Hyoscine butylbromide	No	20 mg	400–120	Poor oral absorption.
Glycopyrrolate	No	400 µg	1.2–2.4	

Note: Anticholinergic drugs for death rattle.
SC, subcutaneous.
[a] Sedation, antiemetic, confusion.

Two RCTs have compared the effects of different anticholinergic medications,[96,97]**and one study compared octreotide with hyoscine hydrobromide.[98]** No study has shown conclusive evidence of one drug being superior to another.[99]*** All can cause dry mouth and urinary retention and those that cross the blood–brain barrier are more sedative. Although this can be beneficial, they may also cause confusion and agitation, particularly in the elderly.

BRONCHORRHEA

Bronchorrhea is defined as the production of >100 mL of sputum per day. Excessive sputum production is seen in benign lung diseases such as bronchiectasis and chronic bronchitis. However, massive bronchorrhea, in which liters of clear frothy sputum are generated, is usually associated with malignancy and can lead to severe fluid and electrolyte depletion in addition to respiratory distress. It is most commonly associated with bronchioloalveolar carcinoma (BAC) but has previously been described in metastatic pancreatic, colonic, and cervical adenocarcinoma.[100-102] The major airway mucin gene, MUC5AC, is highly expressed in BAC. Epidermal growth factor (EGF) ligands also stimulate the production of mucin, and this may explain why the EGFR-TK inhibitors, gefitinib, and erlotinib have been reported to achieve rapid and complete resolution of bronchorrhea related to BAC.[103-106] In each case, sputum production completely resolved within a few days and seemed to be independent of tumor response[114] or EGF receptor mutation status.[115]

Management strategies

BRONCHORRHEA SECONDARY TO MALIGNANCY

Bronchorrhea caused by an underlying malignancy will diminish if the tumor responds to therapy. However, in BAC, the response to gefitinib was so rapid (within a matter of hours in one case) the authors suggest that its activity on mucin production is independent of tumor response. This is also borne out by the fact that although the disease progressed on gefitinib, the bronchorrhea did not recur.

Nebulized indomethacin[107] and subcutaneous octreotide[108] have also been reported to be successful in treating malignancy-associated bronchorrhea.

BRONCHORRHEA SECONDARY TO NONMALIGNANT LUNG DISEASE

There has been one randomized, controlled trial that compared nebulized indomethacin at a dose of 2 mL three times daily (1.2 µg/mL) with placebo in patients with bronchorrhea associated with chronic bronchitis, diffuse panbronchiolitis,

and bronchiectasis. Sputum production was significantly reduced and breathlessness improved.[109] Based on evidence that erythromycin inhibits bronchial hypersecretion in vivo and from epithelial cells in vitro, there are case reports of its successful use in benign and malignant causes of bronchorrhea (Table 68.3).[110,111]

Key learning points

Cough

- Intractable cough is rare but causes significant distress to patients and relatives.
- Simple, safe treatments should always be tried, for example, linctus, sugary drinks, and sipping cold water when cough begins.
- Treat any contributory causes where possible and appropriate.
- There is no one ideal antitussive agent; this is an area where research is urgently needed to give definitive guidance.
- There is a greater range of antitussive agents available than generally used, and clinicians need to consult the literature to make the best choice for patients.
- Opioids are still the most widely available antitussive therapy but may not be appropriate in early disease.

Hiccup

- Investigate and treat or remove the underlying cause if possible. Check basic parameters such as blood electrolytes and remedy abnormalities. See Box 68.1.
- Treat gastric distension and reflux with prokinetics and proton pump inhibitors. It may be necessary to administer drugs such as metoclopramide parenterally via a syringe driver if oral drug absorption is likely to be poor, for example, in malignant bowel obstruction.
- Failing the aforementioned, gabapentin is increasingly becoming the recommended second-line medication for intractable hiccups.[112]
- Consider nonpharmacological interventions if pharmacological therapy fails or is not tolerated.

Secretions

- Explanation and reassurance to family and carers is vital.
- Simple measures such as repositioning the patient can help.
- If using medication, use a stat dose followed by a subcutaneous infusion of an anticholinergic drug (see Table 68.2) at the earliest sign of rattle.
- Suction may be useful on occasion but risks causing more distress.

Table 68.3 *Palliative care approach for difficult respiratory symptoms*

Problem	Intervention	Reasons	If Management fails
Psychological issues exacerbating the symptom, e.g., depression, anxiety	Therapeutic listening. Taking a detailed history of the symptom may be therapeutic in itself. Often with intractable, rarely experienced symptoms such as hiccup, the doctors and other clinicians the patient has met thus far will have been unsure what to do and may just have taken a rushed history. Take as detailed a history as usual for pain, asking all the same sorts of questions. This will contribute to understanding etiology and may be therapeutic. Ensure you uncover the patient and carer's belief(s) about etiology and fears that possibly unnecessarily exacerbating symptom. After assessment, try a first-line treatment, preferably the one with the most evidence, but explain that a period of trial and substitution may follow before the right drug/combination of drugs or other interventions. Explain you believe that by careful adjustment of appropriate interventions, you will be able to improve the symptom, although complete control may be impossible. Assess whether psychological symptoms need specialist help. Do not forget to increase self-management strategies and support including anxiety management strategies and help from other services.	If you need to keep changing therapeutic interventions, without explaining that the patient has a rare/difficult symptom, the patient may feel everything is going wrong or that you do not know what you are doing. Explain from the outset that it may take time to achieve maximum symptom control; this will prevent anxiety.	1. Review your diagnosis of etiology, returning to diagnoses you have excluded, e.g., subphrenic abscess causing hiccups is notoriously difficult to detect. Consult with other clinicians, e.g., radiologist who may help to make a better diagnosis. Show that you are not giving up on understanding the etiology or treatment of symptom. Specialist psychological help may be necessary for intractable anxiety/depression.
Carer distress	Therapeutic listening. Many carers express surprise when attention is paid to their needs separately. Focusing on the carer's individual needs can have a disproportionately positive effect on morale. In addition, you can find out about carer's health (it is clear that carers' health suffers due to chronic stress of long-term caring). You can find out the sorts of support that an individual carer would use or those already in place to build upon. Most carers are elderly with health problems of their own. Encourage ways to make this practically possible (volunteer sitters). Help might come from referral to Carer support services at the local hospital/ community or voluntary organizations, e.g., volunteer sitters, Specialist psychological support, and Alert primary care team.	It is still uncommon for carers' needs to be addressed; even when someone has been a carer for many years, this is particularly common when the patient registered with one practice and the carer with another. The carer's GP may have no concept of seriousness of problems at home. If this is the situation, get carer's permission to contact their primary care team. Service commissioners often do not consider carer interventions to be fundable—you need to find a way around this. There is increased mortality/morbidity in carers; therefore, it is important to encourage the carers to look after themselves.	If the carer is clearly distressed and needs help but will not accept it, you are in a very difficult position. A distressed carer is unlikely to be able to offer support to an unwell patient, and they may even become very distressed when the patient suffers episodes of coughing or increased secretions and can make things worse for the patient. If the patient is at the very end of his life, carer distress or carer exhaustion may be a reason for an admission for hospice for end-of-life care, although this is best avoided as a sole reason for admission. Carer distress that cannot be relieved is also a pointer for getting specialist bereavement support.

(Continued)

Table 68.3 (*Continued*)   *Palliative care approach for difficult respiratory symptoms*

Problem	Intervention	Reasons	If Management fails
Carer exhaustion	Many of the same interventions follow for those of distress, but the main intervention and the most effective one is to anticipate carer exhaustion and prevent it. Interventions will include the following: • Early control of the patient's symptom. • Helping the carer to understand where sources of help are available for them early on. • Warning the carer about carer exhaustion and putting in a balanced plan of support so the carer has time out and time off. • Encouraging the carer to look after himself or herself from the word go, e.g., good diet, adequate exercise, and time off. • Education in relaxation or other strategies to reduce impact of stress. • Ensuring the carer has support of his or her own. • Ensuring the carer understands what is happening with patient's medical condition.	Carer exhaustion is likely to lead to carer ill health, and carer exhaustion can mean that eventually the situation at home will break down possibly leading to an emergency admissions. Admission to hospital, particularly in the last days or hours of life, is always distressing and with careful planning can often be avoided. It is your responsibility as a clinician to think about the carer and to anticipate the exhaustion that they may not believe will happen.	If the carer is exhausted but will not accept extra help, find out if there is another member of the family with whom you can discuss the situation ideally with the carer present. It may be that the carer's primary care team (contacted with their permission) can intervene. Find out if a clinician looking after the carer for their own illness can also make some helpful recommendations.
Alienation from doctors or medical system.	Therapeutic listening. Your detailed history of the difficult symptom may be a revelation to the patient. They may be used to feeling brushed off or the conversation being closed down when they try and talk about their difficult symptom. This is particularly likely for those with intractable difficult symptoms where clinicians are unsure what to do. A psychologically informed approach is particularly important in these circumstances. It is very hard when a patient or carer criticizes a fellow professional, but you can make the family feel that clinicians will always prioritize "sticking together" if you simply defend or interpret the clinicians' actions immediately. It is not helpful either to criticize colleagues even if, from what you have heard, you are uncertain that everything was done as well as it should have been. The most important thing initial response is to empathize with the patient. You may offer to liaise with that clinician or urge the patient to talk to the clinician himself or herself about his or her difficulties. The earliest intervention would be to support the patient. If you are at all concerned about what has happened, you must ensure that the patient safety has not been compromised and if there is any doubt, discuss with colleagues or your manager.	If you rush to defend the hospital, the doctor, the nurse, or other clinician, you will only make the individual feel that they are up against a bureaucratic system, which is only interested in defending itself rather than ensuring that patients get the right treatment. It is important to make the patient and carer feel heard and to suggest alternative ways in which they can navigate their way around the system. You also need to be confident about the management of the case, but this is not usually the problem.	If in spite of all your efforts, the patient and/or carer remains cynical, distressed, upset, and suspicious of the hospital, community, and medical or clinical system; all you can do is be consistently trustworthy and reliable and communicate well and make sure that you explain clearly what you are doing. You may not be able to manage the symptom completely as well as you would like. It is very difficult with those discussed in this chapter, but making a serious persistent attempt to do this and being on the patient and carer's side and clearly working to help them usually make some difference to symptom control.

(*Continued*)

Table 68.3 (*Continued*) *Palliative care approach for difficult respiratory symptoms*

Problem	Intervention	Reasons	If Management fails
Anger at lack of success of previous therapeutic interventions	Listen, listen, listen and do not try to damp down the anger. Make empathetic remarks in everyday language, e.g., "it sounds as if you're totally fed up with everything" or "it sounds as if you have had a rotten time" or "it sounds as if things have been very difficult" rather than using psychotherapeutic terminology. Try and understand who is the most angry—the patient or the carer—and therefore who needs more attention in this area. Set out a clearly written plan with what you will do if the drugs or other interventions fail on this occasion so that the patient/carer can see that several steps ahead you have an idea of what to do.	If one tries to answer anger with an explanation which the patient may feel puts them in the wrong, or dismisses their concerns, the distress and anger are only going to get worse. However much you may feel that management has been correct in every way and that the symptom is simply very difficult to control, patients and carers can feel that they have not been listened to, which may replicate their experience up to that point. Try and ensure that you are the one who does listen and comes up with consistent, clear plans. On the other hand, do not accept abuse, violence, and the threat of violence or become an emotional punch bag. Anger at the lack of success of therapeutic interventions can be anger about the illness itself.	If the patient is angry but in a controlled, articulate way, you may just have to live with listening to that every time you visit, while keeping your own management plan as consistent as possible. If the patient or carer is at all threatening or you feel uncomfortable, you must remove yourself from them and probably only visit with someone else. If they are in a hospice or an institution, it is easier to set boundaries and to ensure that no one member of staff becomes the person who gets the anger all the time. If someone is totally unable to control themselves verbally, it may be better to leave and say that you will come back when the person is feeling a bit calmer to discuss things, rather than endlessly listening to a barrage of angry complaint. It is very different if there is any hint of poor management or negligence of any sort.

REFERENCES

1 Harding SM. Chronic cough: Practical considerations. *Chest* 2003;123:659–660.

2 Muers MF and Round CE. Palliation of symptoms in non-small cell lung cancer: A study by the Yorkshire Regional Cancer Organisation Thoracic Group. *Thorax* 1993;48:339–343.

3 Donnelly S, Walsh D, and Rybicki L. The symptoms of advanced cancer: Identification of clinical and research priorities by assessment of prevalence and severity. *J Palliat Care* 1995;11:27–32.

◆ 4 Irwin SI, Boulet L-P, Cloutier MM et al. Managing cough as a defence mechanism and as a symptom: A consensus panel report of the American College of Chest Physicians. *Chest* 1998;114:S133–S181.

5 Groneberg DA, Niimi A, Dinh QT et al. Increased expression of transient receptor potential vanilloid-1 in airway nerves of chronic cough. *Am J Respir Crit Care Med* 2004;170:1276–1280.

◆ 6 Pratter MR. Chronic upper airway cough syndrome secondary to rhinosinus diseases (previously referred to as postnasal drip syndrome): ACCP evidence-based clinical practice guidelines. *Chest* January 2006;129(Suppl. 1):63S–71S.

◆ 7 Pratter MR. Overview of common causes of chronic cough: ACCP evidence-based clinical practice guidelines. *Chest* January 2006;129(Suppl. 1):59S–62S.

8 Mello CJ, Irwin RS, and Curley FJ. Predictive values of the character, timing, and complications of chronic cough in diagnosing its cause. *Arch Intern Med* 1996;156,997–1003.

9 Lacourciere Y, Brunner H, Irwin R et al. Effects of modulators of the renin-angiotensin-aldosterone system on cough. Losartan Cough Study Group. *J Hypertens* 1994;12:1387–1393.

10 Curley FJ, Irwin RS, Pratter MR et al. Cough and the common cold. *Am Rev Respir Dis* 1988;138:305–511.

11 Pratter MR, Bartter T, Akers S, and DuBois J. An algorithmic approach to chronic cough. *Ann Intern Med* 1993;119:977–983.

12 Corrao WM, Braman SS, and Irwin RS. Chronic cough as the sole presenting manifestation of bronchial asthma. *N Engl J Med* 1979;300:633–637.

13 de Benedictis FM, Canny GJ, and Levison H. Methacholine inhalational challenge in the evaluation of chronic cough in children. *J Asthma* 1986;23:303–308.

14 A double-blind multicenter group comparative study of the efficacy and safety of nedocromil sodium in the management of asthma. North American Tilade Study Group. *Chest* 1990;97:1299–1306.

15 Spector SL and Tan RA. Effectiveness of montelukast in the treatment of cough variant asthma. *Ann Allergy Asthma Immunol* 2004;93:232–236.

16 Cheriyan S, Greenberger PA, and Patterson R. Outcome of cough variant asthma treated with inhaled steroids. *Ann Allergy* 1994;73:478–480.

17 Sutton PP, Gemmell HG, Innes N et al. Use of nebulised saline and nebulised terbutaline as an adjunct to chest physiotherapy. *Thorax* 1988;43:57–60.

18 Desai D and Brightling C. Cough due to asthma, cough-variant asthma and non-asthmatic eosinophilic bronchitis. *Otolaryngol Clin North Am* February 2010;43(1):123–130.

19 Abratt RP, Morgan GW, Silvestri G, and Willcox P. Pulmonary complications of radiation therapy. *Clin Chest Med* 2004;25:167–177.

20 Kudrik FJ, Rivera MP, Molina PL et al. Hypersensitivity pneumonitis in advanced non-small-cell lung cancer patients receiving gemcitabine and paclitaxel: Report of two cases and a review of the literature. *Clin Lung Cancer* 2002;4:52–56.

21 Fassas A, Gojo I, Rapoport A et al. Pulmonary toxicity syndrome following CDEP (cyclophosphamide, dexamethasone, etoposide, cisplatin) chemotherapy. *Bone Marrow Transplant* 2001;28:399–403.

◆ 22 Harding SM and Richter JE. The role of gastroesophageal reflux in chronic cough and asthma. *Chest* 1997;111:1389–1402.

23 I Faruqi S, Molyneux ID, Fathi H, Wright C, Thompson R, and Morice AH. Chronic cough and esomeprazole: A double-blind placebo-controlled parallel study. *Respirology* October 2011;16(7):1150–1156.

24 Langendijk JA, ten Velde GP, Aaronson NK et al. Quality of life after palliative radiotherapy in non-small cell lung cancer: A prospective study. *Int J Radiat Oncol Biol Phys* 2000;47:149–155.

25 Kramer GW, Gans S, Ullmann E et al. Hypofractionated external beam radiotherapy as retreatment for symptomatic non-small-cell lung carcinoma: An effective treatment? *Int J Radiat Oncol Biol Phys* 2004;58:1388–1393.

26 Gressen EL, Werner-Wasik M, Cohn J et al. Thoracic reirradiation for symptomatic relief after prior radiotherapeutic management for lung cancer. *Am J Clin Oncol* 2000;23:160–163.

27 Gollins SW, Burt PA, Barber PV, and Stout R. High dose rate intraluminal radiotherapy for carcinoma of the bronchus: Outcome of treatment of 406 patients. *Radiother Oncol* 1994;33:31–40.

28 Ung YC, Yu E, Falkson C, Haynes AE, Stys-Norman D, and Evans WK; Lung Cancer Disease Site Group of Cancer Care Ontario's Program in Evidence-Based Care. The role of high-dose-rate brachytherapy in the palliation of symptoms in patients with non-small-cell lung cancer: A systematic review. *Brachytherapy* 2006;5:189–202.

29 Thatcher N, Jayson G, Bradley B et al Gemcitabine: Symptomatic benefit in advanced non-small cell lung cancer. *Semin Oncol* 1997;24:S8-6–S8-12.

◆ 30 Paul A, Kvale. Chronic cough due to lung tumors: ACCP evidence-based clinical practice guidelines. *Chest* 2006;129:147S–153S.

31 Shim C, King M, and Williams MH, Jr. Lack of effect of hydration on sputum production in chronic bronchitis. *Chest* 1987;92:679–682.

32 King M and Rubin BK. Pharmacological approaches to discovery and development of new mucolytic agents. *Adv Drug Deliv Rev* 2002;54:1475–1490.

33 Robinson M, Hemming AL, Regnis JA et al. Effect of increasing doses of hypertonic saline on mucociliary clearance in patients with cystic fibrosis. *Thorax* 1997;52:900–903.

34 Parvez L, Vaidya M, Sakhardande A et al. Evaluation of antitussive agents in man. *Pulm Pharmacol* 1996;9:299–308.

35 Dicpinigaitis PV and Gayle YE. Effect of guaifenesin on cough reflex sensitivity. *Chest* 2003;124:2178–2181.

36 Kuhn JJ, Hendley JO, Adams KF et al. Antitussive effect of guaifenesin in young adults with natural colds: Objective and subjective assessment. *Chest* 1982;82:713–718.

37 Thomson ML, Pavia D, and McNicol MW. A preliminary study of the effect of guaiphenesin on mucociliary clearance from the human lung. *Thorax* 1973;28:742–747.

38 Rubin BK. The pharmacologic approach to airway clearance: Mucoactive agents. *Respir Care* 2002;47:818–822.

◆ 39 Poole PJ and Black PN. Oral mucolytic drugs for exacerbations of chronic obstructive pulmonary disease: Systematic review. *Br Med J* 2001;322:1271–1274.

◆ 40 Bolser DC. Cough suppressant and pharmacologic protussive therapy: ACCP evidence-based clinical practice guidelines. *Chest* January 2006;129(Suppl. 1):238S–249S.

41 Bento J, Gonçalves M, Silva N, Pinto T, Marinho A, and Winck JC. Indications and compliance of home mechanical insufflation-exsufflation in patients with neuromuscular diseases. *Arch Bronconeumol.* August 2010;46(8):420–425.

42 Ziment I. Herbal antitussives. *Pulm Pharmacol Ther* 2002;15:327–333.

43 Charpin J and Weibel MA. Comparative evaluation of the antitussive activity of butamirate citrate linctus versus clobutinol syrup. *Respiration* 1990;57:275–279.

44 Bolser DC. Mechanisms of action of central and peripheral antitussive drugs. *Pulm Pharmacol* 1996;9:357–364.

45 Zylicz Z and Krajnik M. What has dry cough in common with pruritus? Treatment of dry cough with paroxetine. *J Pain Symptom Manage* 2004;27:180–184.

46 Moroni M, Porta C, Gualtieri G et al. Inhaled sodium cromoglycate to treat cough in advanced lung cancer patients. *Br J Cancer* 1996;74:309–311.

47 Doona M and Walsh D. Benzonatate for opioid-resistant cough in advanced cancer. *Palliat Med* 1998;12:55–58.

48 Morice AH, Menon MS, Mulrennan SA et al. Opiate therapy in chronic cough. *Am J Respir Crit Care Med* 2007;175:312–315.

49 Eddy NB, Friebel H, Hahn KJ, and Halbach H. Codeine and its alternates for pain and cough relief. 4. Potential alternates for cough relief. *Bull World Health Organ* 1969;40:639–719.

50 Sevelius H, McCoy JF, and Colmore JP. Dose response to codeine in patients with chronic cough. *Clin Pharmacol Ther* 1971;12:449–455.

51 Smith J, Owen E, Earis J, and Woodcock A. Effect of codeine on objective measurement of cough in chronic obstructive pulmonary disease. *J Allergy Clin Immunol* 2006;117:831–835.

52 Homsi J, Walsh D, Nelson KA et al. A phase II study of hydro-codone for cough in advanced cancer. *Am J Hosp Palliat Care* 2002;19:49–56.

53 Matthys H, Bleicher B, and Bleicher U. Dextromethorphan and codeine: Objective assessment of antitussive activity in patients with chronic cough. *J Int Med Res* 1983;11:92–100.

54 Ida H. The nonnarcotic antitussive drug dimemorfan: A review. *Clin Ther* 1997;19:215–231.

55 Luporini G, Barni S, Marchi E, and Daffonchio L. Efficacy and safety of levodropropizine and dihydrocodeine on nonproductive cough in primary and metastatic lung cancer. *Eur Respir J* 1998;12:97–101.

56 Catena E and Daffonchio L. Efficacy and tolerability of levo-dropropizine in adult patients with non-productive cough. Comparison with dextromethorphan. *Pulm Pharmacol Ther* 1997;10:89–96.

57 Aversa C, Cazzola M, Clini V et al. Clinical trial of the efficacy and safety of moguisteine in patients with cough associated with chronic respiratory diseases. *Drugs Exp Clin Res* 1993;19:273–279.

58 Barnabe R, Berni F, Clini V et al. The efficacy and safety of moguisteine in comparison with codeine phosphate in patients with chronic cough. *Monaldi Arch Chest Dis* 1995;50:93–97.

59 Gastpar H, Criscuolo D, and Dieterich HA. Efficacy and tolerability of glaucine as an antitussive agent. *Curr Med Res Opin* 1984;9:21–27.

60 Bolser D, DeGennaro FC, O'Reilly S et al. Peripheral and central sites of action of GABA-B agonists to inhibit the cough reflex in the cat and guinea pig. *Br J Pharmacol* 1994;113:1344–1348.

61 Dicpinigaitis P and Dobkin JB. Antitussive effect of the GABA-agonist baclofen. *Chest* 1997;111:996–999.

62 Dicpinigaitis P, Dobkin JB, Rauf K et al. Inhibition of capsaicin-induced cough by the γ-aminobutyric acid agonist baclofen. *J Clin Pharmacol* 1998;38:364–367.

63 Howard P, Cayton RM, Brennan SR, and Anderson PB. Lignocaine aerosol and persistent cough. *Br J Dis Chest* 1977;71:19–24.

64 Kamei J. Role of opioidergic and serotonergic mechanisms in cough and antitussives. *Pulm Pharmacol* 1996;9:349–356.

65 Eccles R. The powerful placebo in cough studies? *Pulm Pharmacol Ther* 2002;15:303–308.

66 Vertigan AE, Theodoros DG, Gibson PG, and Winkworth AL. Efficacy of speech pathology management for chronic cough: A randomised placebo controlled trial of treatment efficacy. *Thorax* 2006;61:1065–1069.

67 Pratter MR, Brightling CE, Boulet LP, and Irwin RS. An empiric integrative approach to the management of cough: ACCP evidence-based clinical practice guidelines. *Chest* January 2006;129(Suppl. 1):222S–231S.

◆ 68 Dicpinigaitis PV. Chronic cough due to asthma: ACCP evidence-based clinical practice guidelines. *Chest* January 2006;129(Suppl. 1):75S–79S.

69 Turcotte SE and Lougheed MD. Cough in asthma. *Curr Opin Pharmacol* June 2011;11(3):231–237.

✷ 70 Wee B, Browning J, Adams A, Benson D, Howard P, Klepping G, Molassiotis A, and Taylor D. Management of chronic cough in patients receiving palliative care: Review of evidence and recommendations by a task group of the Association for Palliative Medicine of Great Britain and Ireland. *Palliat Med* September 12, 2012;26(6):780–787.

71 Orr CF and Rowe DB. Helicobacter pylori hiccup. *Intern Med J* 2003;33:133–134.

72 Keane JR. Hiccups due to central nervous system disease: Analysis of 71 inpatients. *Can J Neurol Sci* 2010;37(6):870–872.

73 Miwa H and Kondo T. Hiccups in Parkinson's disease: An overlooked non-motor symptom? *Parkinsonism Relat Disord* 2010;16(4):249–251.

74 Hua Z, Guodong G, Quinchuan L et al. Analysis of complications of radiofrequency pallidotomy. *Neurosurgery* 2003;52:89–101.

75 Sharma P, Morgan JC, and Sethi KD. Hiccups associated with dopamine agonists in Parkinson disease. *Neurology* 2006;66(5):774.

76 Yardimci N, Benli S, and Zileli T. A diagnostic challenge of Parkinson's disease: Intractable hiccups. *Parkinsonism Relat Disord* 2008;14(5):446–447.

77 Wilcox SK, Garry A, and Johnson MJ. Novel use of amantadine: To treat hiccups. *J Pain Symptom Manage* 2009;38(3):460–465.

78 Dickerman RD and Jaikumar S. The hiccup reflex arc and persistent hiccups with high dose anabolic steroids: Is the brainstem the steroid responsive locus? *Clin Neuropharmacol* 2001;24:62–64.

79 Liaw CC, Wang CH, Chang HK et al. Cisplatin-related hiccups: Male predominance, induction by dexamethasone, and protection against nausea and vomiting. *J Pain Symptom Manage* 2005;30(4):359–366.

80 Schulz-Stubner S and Kehl F. Treatment of persistent hiccups with transcutaneous phrenic and vagal nerve stimulation. *Intensive Care Med* 2011;37(6):1048–1049.

81 Renes SH, van Geffen GJ, Rettig HC, Gielen MJ, and Scheffer GJ. Ultrasound-guided continuous phrenic nerve block for persistent hiccups. *Reg Anesth Pain Med* 2010;35(5):455–457.

82 Dietzel J, Grundling M, Pavlovic D, and Usichenko TI. Acupuncture for persistent postoperative hiccup. *Anaesthesia* 2008;63(9):1021–1022.

83 Back IN, Jenkins K, Blower A, and Beckhelling J. A study comparing hyoscine hydrobromide and glycopyrrolate in the treatment of death rattle. *Palliat Med* 2001;15:329–336.

84 Morita T, Tsunoda J, Inoue S, and Chihara S. Risk factors for death rattle in terminally ill cancer patients: A prospective exploratory study. *Palliat Med* 2000;14:19–23.

85 Lichter I and Hunt E. The last 48 hours of life. *J Palliat Care* 1990;6:7–15.

86 Morita T, Hyodo I, Yoshimi T et al. Incidence and underlying etiologies of bronchial secretion in terminally ill cancer patients: A multicentre, prospective observational study. *J Pain Symptom Manage* 2004;27:533–539.

87 Bennet MI. Death rattle: An audit of hyoscine use and review of management. *J Pain Symptom Manage* 1996;12:229–233.

88 Wildiers H, Menten J. Death rattle: Prevalence, prevention and treatment. *J Pain Symptom Manage* 2002;23(4):310–317.

89 Macleod AD. Neurogenic pulmonary edema in palliative care. *J Pain Symptom Manage* 2002;23:154–156.

90 Hughes A, Wilcock A, Corcoran R et al. Audit of three antimuscarinic drugs for managing retained secretions. *Palliat Med* 2000;14:221–222.

91 Wee B, Coleman PG, Hillier R et al. The sound of death rattle I: Are relatives distressed by hearing this sound? *Palliat Med* 2006;20:171–175.

92 Wee B, Coleman PG, Hillier R et al. The sound of death rattle II: How do relatives interpret the sound? *Palliat Med* 2006;20:177–181.

93 Wee B, Coleman PG, Hillier R et al. Death rattle: Its impact on staff and volunteers in palliative care. *Palliat Med* 2008;22:173–176.

94 Watts T and Jenkins K. Palliative care nurses' feelings about death rattle. *J Clin Nurs* 1999;8:615–616.

✷ 95 Bennet M, Lucas V, Brennan M et al. Using anti-muscarinic drugs in the management of death rattle: Evidence based guidelines for palliative care. *Palliat Med* 2002;16:369–374.

96 Likar R, Rupacher E, Kager H et al. Comparing the efficacy of glycopyrronium bromide and scopolamine-hydrobromide in patients with death rattle. A prospective randomised study [Die Wirkung von Glycopyrroniumbromid im vergleich mit scopolamine-hydrobromicum bein terminalen rasseln:eine randomisierte doppelblinde piot-studie]. *Mid Eur J Med* 2008;120:679–683.

97 Wildiers H, Dhaenekint C, Demeulenaere P et al. Atropine, hyoscine butylbromide, or scopolamine are equally effective for the treatment of death rattle in terminal care. *J Pain Symptom Manage* 2009;38:124–133.

98 Clark K, Currow DC, Agar M et al. A pilot phase II randomized, cross over, double blinded, controlled efficacy study of octreotide versus hyoscine hydrobromide for control of noisy breathing at the end of life. *J Pain Palliat Care Pharmacother* 2008;22:131–138.

99 Wee B and Hillier R. Interventions for noisy breathing in patients near to death. *Cochrane Database Syst Rev* 2008;(1):CD005177.

100 Lembo T and Donnelly TJ. A case of pancreatic carcinoma causing massive bronchial fluid production and electrolyte abnormalities. *Chest* 1995;108:1161–1163.

101 Shimura S and Takishima T. Bronchorrhea from diffuse, lymphangitic metastasis of colon carcinoma to the lung. *Chest* 1994;105:308–310.

102 Epaulard O, Moro O, Langin T et al. Bronchorrhea revealing cervix adenocarcinoma metastatic to the lung. *Lung Cancer* 2001;3131:331–334.

103 Kitazaki T, Fukuda M, Soda H et al. Novel effects of gefitinib on mucin production in bronchioloalveolar carcinoma; two case reports. *Lung Cancer* 2005;49:125–128.

104 Popat N, Raghavan N, and McIvor A. Severe bronchorrhea in a patient with bronchioloalveolar carcinoma. *Chest* 2012;141:513–514.

105 Milton D, Kris M, Gomez J et al. Prompt control of bronchorrhea in patients with bronchioloalveolar carcinoma treated with gefitinib. *Support Care Cancer* 2005;13:70–72.

106 Thotathil Z. Erlotinib effective against refractory bronchorrhea from advanced non small cell lung cancer. *J Thoracic Oncol* 2007;2:881–882.

107   Homma S, Kawabata M, Kishi K et al. Successful treatment of refractory bronchorrhea by inhaled indomethacin in two patients with bronchioloalveolar carcinoma. *Chest* 1999;115:1465–1468.

108   Hudson E, Lester J, Attanoos R et al. Successful treatment of bronchorrhea with octreotide in a patient with adenocarcinoma of the lung. *J Pain Symptom Manage* 2006;32:200–202.

109   Tamaoki J, Chiyotani A, Kobayashi K et al. Effect of indomethacin on bronchorrhea in patients with chronic bronchitis, diffuse panbronchiolitis, or bronchiectasis. *Am Rev Respir Dis* 1992;145:458–452.

110   Suga T, Sugiyama Y, Fujii T, and Kitamura S. Bronchioloalveolar carcinoma with bronchorrhea treated with erythromycin. *Eur Respir J* 1994;7:2249–2251.

111   Marom Z and Goswami S. Respiratory mucus hypersecretion (bronchorrhea): A case discussion-possible mechanism(s) and treatment. *J Allergy Clin Immunol* 1991;87:1050–1055.

112   Tegeler ML and Baumrucker SJ. Gabapentin for intractable hiccups in palliative care. *Am J Hosp Palliat Care* 2008;25(1):52–54.

113   Hernandez JL, Pajaron M, Garcia-Regata O, Jimenez V, Gonzalez-Macias J, and Ramos-Estebanez C. Gabapentin for intractable hiccup. *Am J Med* 2004;117(4):279–281.

114   Moretti R, Torre P, Antonello RM, Ukmar M, Cazzato G, and Bava A. Gabapentin as a drug therapy of intractable hiccup because of vascular lesion: A three-year follow up. *Neurologist* 2004;10(2):102–106.

115   Porzio G, Aielli F, Verna L, Aloisi P, Galletti B, and Ficorella C. Gabapentin in the treatment of hiccups in patients with advanced cancer: A 5-year experience. *Clin Neuropharmacol* 2010;33(4):179–180.

116   Petroianu G, Hein G, Stegmeier-Petroianu A, Bergler W, Rüfer R. Gabapentin 'add-on therapy' for idiopathic chronic hiccup. *J Clin Gastroenterol* 2000;30:321–324.

117   Jatzko A, Stegmeier-Petroianu A, and Petroianu GA. Alpha-2-delta ligands for singultus (hiccup) treatment: Three case reports. *J Pain Symptom Manage* 2007;33(6):756–760.

118   Walker P, Watanabe S, and Bruera E. Baclofen, a treatment for chronic hiccup. *J Pain Symptom Manage* 1998;16:125–132.

119   Petroianu G, Hein G, and Petroianu A. Idiopathic chronic hiccup: Combination therapy with cisapride, omeprazole and baclofen. *Clin Ther* 1997;19:1031–1038.

120   Guelaud C, Similowski T, Bizec JL et al. Baclofen therapy for chronic hiccup. *Eur Resp J* 1995;8:235–237.

121   Ramirez FC and Graham DY. Treatment of intractable hiccup with baclofen: Results of a double-blind randomized, controlled, crossover study. *Am J Gastroenterol* 1992;87:1789–1791.

122   Madanagopolan N. Metoclopramide in hiccup. *Curr Med Res Opin* 1975;3:371–374.

123   Lipps DC, Jabbari B, Mitchell MH, and Daigh JD. Nifedipine for intractable hiccups. *Neurology* 1990;40:531–532.

PART 12

Neuropsychiatrics

69

Depression/anxiety

TATSUO AKECHI, YOSUKE UCHITOMI

INTRODUCTION

The length and quality of life of patients with serious chronic illnesses such as cancer are influenced not only by their malignant disease but also by comorbid medical and psychological conditions, such as depression and anxiety. For example, recent study investigating the effect of cancer diagnosis demonstrates that cancer diagnosis can produce acute stress associated with higher suicide rate and cardiovascular death especially in the first weeks, and these effects prolong at least 6 months after diagnosis.[1] The complexity of care for these patients makes it particularly challenging to ascertain whether a patient is struggling with serious depression. Moreover, compared with the statistics on the overall population of general medical patients, there are fewer data to draw upon that would help clinicians determine what treatments are effective for depression in the advanced cancer or other advanced disease settings. This chapter will examine the assessment and treatment of depression in general medical patients and in patients with cancer.

PREVALENCE, EFFECT, AND ASSESSMENT OF DEPRESSION

General medical patients

To better understand how to recognize and treat depression in patients with cancer, it is useful to first review the existing paradigms for finding and treating depression in the primary care setting. Depression is estimated to affect 121 million people worldwide, and 5.8% of men and 9.5% of women will experience a depressive episode every year.[2] The prevalence of major depression in primary care setting is 5%–9%.[3] Depression is two to three times more common in patients with chronic medical illnesses.[4] Physicians recognize psychological distress in about two-thirds of the general medical

patient population and prescribe antidepressants for about half of those distressed patients.[5] Major depressive disorders can cause severe decrement in health.[6] Depressive symptoms are associated with a higher-than-normal risk of physical decline and with long-term mortality in older adults[7,8]; depression is also a risk factor for diabetes, coronary heart disease, and stroke,[4,9***] and it is associated with a greater use of healthcare services.[10] In addition, comorbid depression is associated with increased medical symptom burden, functional impairment, medical costs, poor adherence to self-care regimens, and increased risk of morbidity and mortality in patients with chronic medical disorders.[4]

The standard paradigm for identifying depression in the primary care setting is to view depression as a syndromal diagnosis made on the basis of patient history and the exclusion of competing diagnoses, using criteria from the Diagnostic and Statistical Manual of Mental Disorders (DSM)-I5.[11] Major depression is defined as depressed mood or anhedonia (loss of interest in pleasurable activities) that lasts for at least 2 weeks plus the presence of three or four other specific psychological or somatic symptoms. If two to four rather than more than five symptoms are present, then the patient may be defined as having minor depression, an other specified diagnosis in the DSM-IV-5.[12] The U.S. Preventive Services Task Force recommends depression screening in clinical practices that have systems in place to ensure accurate diagnosis and effective treatment and follow-up.[3] Unfortunately, such systems are not available in most primary care practices or oncology/hematology subspecialty practices.

The decision regarding whether to treat a patient for depression in the primary care setting is not always made on the basis of rigid diagnostic criteria; it often arises from clinical judgment about the severity and duration of symptoms and the likelihood of spontaneous recovery within a supportive environment.[13] Between 50% and 60% of cases of major depression respond to initial therapy with antidepressants, psychotherapy, or both.[13] Although previous study suggests that minor depression has similar response rates to antidepressants or psychotherapy over placebo, recent meta-analysis investigating the effect of antidepressants on minor depression reveals that there is unlikely to be a clinically important advantage for antidepressants.[14***] Depression may be treated by a patient's primary care physician, who can use either a collaborative care model that involves augmentation with one or more visits with a mental healthcare provider or a stepped-care approach in which patients whose depression does not respond to initial therapy are referred to a mental healthcare provider.[15]

Depression is the first leading cause of disability adjusted life years (DALY) lost excluding death, and the third leading cause of DALY including death in the world according to the most recent WHO estimates.[16] Moreover, this burden is expected to rise in the next 20 years. Thus, depression is now recognized as an important cause of long-term disability and dependency.[17] It produces not only serious suffering,[18] but also worsens quality of life,[19] reduces adherence to medical treatments,[20] can lead to suicide,[21] is a psychological burden on the family,[22***] and prolongs hospitalization.[23] Fortunately, depression is treatable, and thus, cost-effective interventions to improve the detection and treatment of depression are important.

Cancer: A paradigm for serious chronic illness

Mitchell et al. reported findings with regard to meta-analysis including 70 studies with 10,071 individuals across 14 countries in oncological and hematological settings, and they demonstrated that prevalence of major depression was 14.9% (95% confidence interval: 12.2–17.7), minor depression 19.2% (9.1–31.9), adjustment disorders 19.4% (14.5–24.8), and dysthymia 2.7% (1.7–4.0).[24***] In palliative care settings studies including 24 studies with 4007 individuals across seven countries, they also found that prevalence of major depression was 14.3% (11.1–17.9), minor depression 9.6% (3.6–18.1), and adjustment disorders 15.4% (10.1–21.6).[24] Thus, the best estimate is that major depression has a point prevalence of 10%–20% in cancer patients, irrespective of cancer stage. This prevalence is similar to that seen in patients with other chronic medical illnesses.

Although some comprehensive cancer centers have adequate behavioral healthcare resources, most hospitals and oncology clinics rely on general psychiatry and psychology staff and resources. Limited funding for mental healthcare resources is a serious problem, and care is often fragmented among private practitioners, for-profit and not-for-profit clinics, and community mental health centers.[25] This is a report by American psycho-oncologist: the situations, however, are similar or even much worse in other countries including Asian nations.[26] Limited resources in standard areas of care also affect the research environment.

Even though it may be ideal to use a two-stage strategy that combines an assessment of severity with an assessment of the number of depressive symptoms, it is far more common to perform only a short instrument to assess symptom

---

Box 69.1　Self-report measures used to assess depressive symptoms in cancer patients

- Hospital and Anxiety Depression Scale (HADS)
- Zung Self-Rating Depression Scale (ZSRDS)
- Brief version, Zung Self-Rating Depression Scale (BZSDRS)
- Beck Depression Inventory (BDI)
- Beck Depression Inventory, Short Form (BDI-SF)
- Center for Epidemiologic Studies Depression Scale (CES-D)
- Brief Symptom Inventory (BSI)
- Rotterdam Symptom Checklist (RSCL)
- Geriatric Depression Scale (GDS)
- Profile of Mood States (POMS)
- Profile of Mood States, Short Form (POMS-SF)
- General Health Questionnaire (GHQ)
- Edinburg Postnatal Depression Scale (EPD)

---

severity in the typical environment where time and resources are limited. Numerous symptom scales have been used to assess depression symptom severity at a specific time or over time. The most commonly reported instruments are shown in Box 69.1.

Challenges in the assessment of depression in cancer patients

Patients, family members, and healthcare providers sometimes believe that feeling down, depressed, or hopeless is perfectly natural and understandable in the context of living with cancer. Clinicians are encouraged to acknowledge the difficulty and disappointment that often confront cancer patients and their families,[27] but depression and hopelessness are not accepted by expert clinicians as an inevitable consequence of living with cancer. In addition, cancer patients often have physical symptoms of depression (so-called neurovegetative symptoms), such as sleep disturbance, psychomotor retardation, appetite disturbance, poor concentration, and low energy, as a consequence of their underlying illness or treatment, thus confounding the diagnosis of depression. Indeed, depression is just one of the many symptoms that clinicians must recognize and manage in inpatients and outpatients with cancer. For example, roughly two-thirds of outpatients with cancer experience pain, and more than a third report significant disruption in daily function associated with the pain.[28] For patients with advanced cancer, fatigue, pain, lack of energy, weakness, and appetite loss are the most frequent symptoms, occurring in more than 50% of patients.[29***] It may be that the problem of concurrent symptoms is the most relevant difference between depression in the general medical setting and in the cancer care setting. Relatively few cancer

---

Box 69.2 Common barriers to the assessment of depression in patients with cancer

Overlap of physical symptoms of depression and symptoms of cancer or its treatment

- Clinician's underrecognition of hopelessness, feelings of worthlessness, or suicidal ideation
- Clinician's uncertainty about how to interpret screening instrument cut-offs
- Lack of clinician's routine discussion with patients and family about low mood, not like pain assessment
- Limited understanding by cancer professionals regarding which patients are most at risk
- Time constraints in busy oncology settings
- Cost constraints limiting access to professionals with behavioral health training
- Few mental health programs and specialists connecting with oncology
- Poor continuity of care over the trajectory of illness
- Stigma concerning mental illness or weakness perceived by the patient/family
- Patient/family fear that revealing depression will lead to undertreatment of the cancer

---

Box 69.3 Examples of 1- or 2-question screening methods for depression

One question

- "Are you depressed?" (Chochinov et al.[30])
- "Please grade your mood during the past week by assigning it a score from 0 to 100, with a score of 100 representing your usual relaxed mood. A score of 60 is considered a passing grade." (Akizuki et al.[31])

Two questions

- "Have you often been bothered by feeling down, depressed, or hopeless?"[32]
- "Have you often been bothered by having a lack of interest or pleasure in doing things?" (Whooley et al.[32])

---

care providers have sufficient knowledge and skills to assess and treat depression in this context, and it is often difficult to decide whether the depressive symptoms should be the primary focus of treatment or whether these symptoms may improve if other problems are better managed.

The large number of instruments and techniques used to assess cancer patients for depression does not seem to translate into an overall improvement in the assessment of depression in this complex population of patients. A "Don't ask, don't tell" policy appears to be in place all too often.[25] A list of 11 of the most significant barriers to the assessment of depression is presented in Box 69.2.

With a growing appreciation for the need to simplify the starting point in assessing depression, the use of 1- or 2-item screening techniques has become popular (Box 69.3). Chochinov et al.[30] have studied a simple 1-item survey and found it to have acceptable psychometric properties in patients with advanced cancer. Akizuki et al.[31] have described a clever 1-item survey that was tested in 275 patients and was found to correlate well with both the hospital anxiety and depression scale (HADS) ($r = 0.66$) and the distress thermometer ($r = 0.71$). At optimal cut-offs, the sensitivity (80%) and specificity (61%) for diagnosing major depression and adjustment disorders for this 1-item survey were similar to those of the HADS and distress thermometer. Finally, Whooley et al.[32] have used 2-item screening in medically ill patients who did not have cancer with an

approach that targeted depressed mood and anhedonia. This 2-item screening approach has been endorsed by the U.S. Preventive Health Task Force for use in primary care settings.[3,33] Recent meta-analysis investigating the screening performance of one or two simple verbal questions in the detection of depression in cancer settings demonstrated the findings as follows: a simple 1-item "depression" survey, sensitivity of 72%, specificity of 83%; a simple 1-item "loss of interest" survey, sensitivity of 83%, specificity of 86%; two questions "depression and loss of interest" survey; sensitivity of 91%, specificity of 86%.[34***] The author concluded that simple surveys perform well at excluding depression in the nondepressed but perform poorly at confirming depression and that the "two question" method is significantly more accurate than either single question. In addition, based on this finding, the author emphasizes that clinicians should not rely on these simple questions alone and should be prepared to assess the patient more thoroughly.

The HADS[35***] has also been investigated as a screening tool for depression and anxiety in cancer patients and this instrument has been translated into more than 20 languages. A meta-analysis published in 2010 investigating the accuracy of the HADS as a screening tool in cancer patients demonstrates that the HADS had a sensitivity of 82%, a specificity of 77% for depression (no studies for anxiety).[36] The authors conclude that the HADS is recommended as a screening tool but not case-finding instrument.

In addition to brief screening approaches specific to depression, a more global approach to distress screening has been developed by Holland and endorsed by the National Comprehensive Cancer Network.[37] This approach involves a thermometer with a numerical scale ranging from 0 to 10 for the patient to indicate "How much distress you have been experiencing in the past week, including today?" This is coupled with a 34-item checklist organized into practical areas, family issues, emotional issues, spiritual/religious issues, and physical symptoms. This approach embeds depression screening in a broad context that can be less stigmatizing to some patients. The drawback of this approach is that it is not easy to use in face-to-face discussions between the physician and the patient. Rather, it is well suited to a practice setting in which other providers are available to do the screening and initiate an appropriate response to the patient on the basis of the information provided. In general, the distress screening approach works best in a resource-rich environment. Now distress thermometer approach is introduced and used in several countries.[38–40]

Non-Western, for example, Japanese, patients still had difficulty with Western biopsychiatric concepts of depression. Sadness, worry, and stress, not depression, were more commonly used terms; thus, mental health providers need more euphemisms: worry, maybe sadness, stress, anxiety. These patients are reluctant to discuss with psychological issues, especially emotional disclosure to their physicians. They would like not to view their condition as an individual issue. Focusing on community and contextual factors, such as family, work, financial, and housing issues, was seen as more acceptable. The physicians might avoid the term "depression" during these discussions.[41]

TREATMENT OF DEPRESSION

General medical patients

Antidepressant therapy and psychotherapy seem to be equally effective for treating mild-to-moderate depression in the general medical population.[15,42] For treating severe depression, antidepressant therapy combined with psychotherapy may be better than psychotherapy alone.[42] Antidepressants are also effective for treating depression in patients with concomitant life-threatening physical illnesses. In 2011, a systematic review of randomized trials comparing antidepressants with placebo to treat depression in patients with life-threatening illness was published; the review comprised 25 studies including more than 1100 patients with a variety of life-threatening illness including cancer, renal failure, chronic obstructive pulmonary disease, chronic heart failure, Parkinson's disease, multiple sclerosis, and HIV/AIDS.[43***] Depression treated with antidepressants was significantly more likely to improve than that treated with placebo (4–5 weeks odds ratio 1.93; 95% CI 1.15–3.42; 6–8 weeks odds ratio 2.25; 95% CI 1.38–3.67; 9–18 weeks odds ratio 2.71; 95% CI 1.50–4.91). However, at 4–5 weeks, the study also showed that approximately nine patients would need to be treated to produce one recovery that would not have occurred with placebo alone (number needed to treat [NNT] 9; 95% CI 4.3–81.0). The NNT decreased over time: 6–8 weeks NNT 6; 95% CI 3.9–8.8; 9–18 weeks NNT 5; 95% CI 2.9–9.9.[43]

More than 24 antidepressants that work by at least 7 distinct mechanisms of action are available.[44] However, no single drug or category of drugs has proved most effective for

relieving depressive symptoms or treating the syndrome of major depression (see Box 69.4, for a summary of antidepressant agents),[13,45**,46***] although one previous study suggests existence of differences for efficacy and acceptability among second-generation antidepressants.[47***]

Box 69.4 Commonly used antidepressants grouped by mechanism of action

Selective serotonin reuptake inhibitors (SSRIs)

- Sertraline
- Citalopram
- Escitalopram
- Fluoxetine

Comment: These agents are frequently used. They have few anticholinergic or cardiovascular side effects and, therefore, not fatal in overdose. Sexual dysfunction, insomnia, headache, or nausea may occur with any of these agents.

Noradrenergic and specific serotonergic antidepressants

- Mirtazapine

Comment: This agent is frequently used for patients with poor appetite and/or insomnia, because they cause sedation and weight gain. For this reason, it can be dosed at night to improve sleep and given to patients who have poor appetite.

Serotonin and norepinephrine reuptake inhibitor (SNRIs)

- Venlafaxine
- Duloxetine

Comment: In addition to its effect on depression, this agent has been used to decrease the frequency and intensity of hot flashes and neurotoxicity induced by chemotherapy in cancer patients. Dose-related sustained hypertension is an important possible side effect to monitor. May cause sexual dysfunction, insomnia, headache, constipation, or nausea.

Dopamine and norepinephrine reuptake inhibitor

- Bupropion

Comment: This agent is also indicated to improve rates of successful smoking cessation. Sometimes used to avoid the sexual dysfunction seen with other agents. Does not treat anxiety. Known to lower the seizure threshold. May cause insomnia, agitation, confusion, headache, or weight loss.

Psychostimulants

- Methylphenidate
- Pemoline
- Dextroamphetamine

Comment: These agents are known for the rapid onset of action in terms of antidepressant efficacy. They are activating agents also used to counteract opioid-induced sedation. Generally given in the waking hours (morning and early afternoon). Should be avoided in patients with unstable ischemia or cardiac arrhythmias. Drug tolerance, abuse, and dependence can occur. May cause nervousness, agitation, insomnia, or nausea.

Tricyclic antidepressants

- Nortriptyline
- Amitriptyline
- Doxepin
- Desipramine

Comment: These agents are generally not used because they can cause cardiac arrhythmias, and overdoses are lethal. Baseline electrocardiography is recommended. Often used as adjuvant analgesics at doses subtherapeutic for depression. May cause sexual dysfunction, weight gain, anticholinergic effects (dry mouth, sedation, or constipation), or orthostatic hypotension.

Cancer patients

CHOOSING PATIENTS FOR TREATMENT

The largest barrier to the effective treatment of depression in patients with cancer is the difficulty in recognizing patients who are depressed and need treatment.[48] The factors associated with increased risk of depression in cancer patients are shown in Box 69.5. Because of the complexity of assessing patients in modern cancer care environments, many cases of depression are missed, and the patients with more severe symptoms, ironically, are more easily overlooked. Investigators in Indiana, USA, working in the community setting[49] evaluated 1109 outpatients with cancer and found that physicians were most accurate at correctly identifying the absence of depression. However, when depression was severe, only 13% of affected patients were correctly classified by their oncologists. In general, oncologists and oncology nurses appear to be most responsive to sad, tearful patients with minor depression rather than patients with a flat affect, feelings of pervasive guilt or worthlessness, or suicidal thoughts. In a sense, sicker patients may create thicker smokescreens that impede easy recognition of the underlying problem. These patients are particularly vulnerable, and their inability to advocate for themselves may be part of the illness.[25]

Symptom research is an emerging interest within the discipline of academic general medicine.[49,50] Within this new paradigm, symptoms are conceptualized in terms of a functional disturbance of the nervous system. There is a growing appreciation for the physical changes in the nervous system associated with depression and its treatment.[51,52] Understanding depressive symptoms in the context of symptom science rather than solely within the standard psychiatric paradigm is being explored in the context of cancer care to try to overcome some of the barriers to recognition and management of depression in this population.

TREATMENT OPTIONS

Drugs used to treat depression in cancer patients are quite similar to those used in the primary care setting; these include

---

Box 69.5 Risk factors for depression in cancer

Social and environmental factors

- Recent losses (e.g., spouse, family, friends, animals)
- Financial stressors
- Poor social support
- Sexual and/or physical abuse
- Childhood trauma or parental loss

Psychiatric factors

- Family and own history of depressive disorder
- History of substance abuse

Cancer-related factors

- Advanced stage of disease
- Poor performance status
- Poor pain control

Cancer treatment factors

- Corticosteroids
- Interferon alfa
- Interleukin-2
- Amphotericin-B
- Procarbazine
- L-Asparaginase
- Paclitaxel

---

tricyclic antidepressants, Selective serotonin reuptake inhibitor (SSRIs), newer antidepressants, and psychostimulants. The essential medicines recommended by the International Association for Hospice and Palliative Care for treatment of depression in palliative care are amitriptyline, citalopram (or any other SSRIs except paroxetine and fluvoxamine), and mirtazapine (or any other generic dual action noradrenergic and specific serotonergic antidepressants or SNRIs).[53] Specific examples of commonly used antidepressants grouped by mechanism of action are presented in Box 69.4. The National Institutes of Health consensus statement regarding symptom management in cancer states that "depression related to cancer is not substantially different from depression in other medical conditions, but treatments may need to be adapted or refined for cancer patients."[54] One refinement for patients with cancer, particularly in the palliative care setting, is the growing interest in the use of psychostimulants to treat depression.[55***,56*] Especially depressive terminally ill patients with estimated prognosis of less than a couple of weeks are best treated by psychostimulants. Another refinement that is often important to cancer patients is being mindful of potentially important drug interactions that can occur with antidepressants that are metabolized using the cytochrome P450 (CYP) enzyme system of the liver.[57] In particular, agents such as fluoxetine and nefazodone that inhibit the CYP 3A4 enzyme system may increase the effects of some commonly used chemotherapeutic agents. Fluoxetine may also influence and paroxetine (CYP 2D6 inhibitors) can probably affects on the effect of tamoxifen that is the usual endocrine therapy for hormone receptor-positive breast cancer in premenopausal women.[58,59*] Moreover, because many patients with cancer are older adults with complex medical problems, other coadministered drugs may be influenced by the antidepressants. Among commonly used antidepressants for physically ill patients, sertraline and citalopram may be recommended for first-line treatment, because these drugs appear to be less potential for serious pharmacokinetic drug interaction.[60]

Psychological therapies include psychoeducational interventions, behavioral therapy including relaxation training, cognitive behavioral therapy, interpersonal therapy, supportive psychotherapy, group therapy, and supportive-expressive psychotherapy. In practice, all psychological therapies are patient-centered but very flexibly provided depending on each patient's physical condition and needs. Electroconvulsive therapy, an invasive modality known to be effective for severe depression, is rarely used and has not been studied for depression in the context of cancer care. Some recent studies have demonstrated the effectiveness of ketamine[61**] and scopolamine,[62**] commonly used drugs in palliative care setting, and light therapy[63***] on depression in physically healthy people. These therapies may be worth for testing their efficacy for the treatment of depression among cancer patients. Finally, both pharmacological and psychological therapies have been shown to be efficacious in treating depression in cancer, it is unknown that their relative and combined efficacy and their role in the treatment that is less severe and occurs in association with advanced disease.[64]

RANDOMIZED TRIALS

With all of these challenges in mind, it is not surprising that data from controlled trials regarding the efficacy of treatment of depression in cancer patients are sparse. Thirteen published controlled randomized trials have investigated the effects of an antidepressant drug for depression in cancer patients (Table 69.1). A total of 1546 patients were included; none of these studies included children, and seven of the studies[65**,66**,67**,68**,69**,70**,71**] included women only. The trend in these studies was in favor of the treatment arm than placebo, but the small sample size of the individual trials, short follow-up duration, and lack of reporting of adverse events/tolerability limit the conclusions that can be made from this body of research. In addition, no specific antidepressant has proved more effective for relieving depression in cancer patients. As the previous systematic review investigating the effectiveness of pharmacological treatment for depression in cancer patients suggested, there is some evidence that cancer patients with depression are responsive to pharmacological treatment although more data are needed regarding the safety and efficacy of antidepressants.[72***]

Psychological therapies are most often applied in addition to drug treatments for depressed patients, but this kind of therapy can also be used alone to treat moderate to severe depression.[15] In fact, there are very few studies in the medically ill in which the effect of psychotherapy has been described with sufficient methodological detail.[73] There are several published systematic reviews and meta-analyses of controlled trials of psychological interventions for decreasing psychological distress in cancer patients (Table 69.2). Although the findings of these reviews are not consistent probably due to differences in the focus of the reviews, the methods used to summarize findings across studies, and the manner in which recommendations were reached, psychoeducational interventions, behavioral therapy, cognitive behavioral therapy, supportive and supportive-expressive psychotherapy are effective for ameliorating depression for cancer patients.[74]

It is useful to note that application of unwanted (but received) intervention has been uniquely associated with poor psychosocial adjustment.[75] As such, clinicians would do well to make support available to cancer patients but to respect the boundaries that some patients set regarding such services.

A recent study, investigating the effect of provision of early palliative care by palliative care team consisting of board-certified palliative care physicians and advanced-practice nurses for advanced lung cancer patients on quality of life and psychological distress including depression, demonstrated that early palliative care itself contributes to improvement in quality of life and ameliorating depression.[76**] This study suggests the usefulness of patient-centered early palliative care itself for reducing depression in cancer patients.

UNIQUE ISSUES IN END-OF-LIFE CARE

Ambiguity surrounding the definition of end-of-life care makes this particular literature difficult to interpret and apply. The 1-item screening question "Are you depressed?" explored by Chochinov involved a cohort of 197 palliative care inpatients and had perfect sensitivity and specificity of 1.0 in this single study.[30] However, in a palliative care cohort of 74 patients in the United Kingdom receiving only palliative and supportive day care, Lloyd-Williams et al. found that 27% of patients had depression by semistructured interview criteria, and the single-item screening question had a sensitivity of 55%, a specificity of 74%, a positive predictive value of 44%, and a negative predictive value of 82%.[77] The similar findings with regard to poor screening performance of the 1-item screening question are also shown in Japanese study (a sensitivity of 47%, a specificity of 97%).[78] Nevertheless, even use of the 14-item HADS had significant limitations in another UK study in a hospice population, as the positive predictive value of this instrument using a cut-off threshold of 20 was only 48% with a sensitivity of 77% and specificity of 89%.[79] Overall, there are insufficient data in end-of-life patient populations to distinguish the assessment issues from those that have been described for cancer patients in general.[80***] It should be noted, however, that the occurrence of counter-transference of hopelessness on the part of families

Table 69.1   *Clinical trials comparing antidepressant with placebo or other antidepressants for depression in patients with cancer*

Author	Antidepressants	Subjects	Inclusion criteria for depression	Main findings
Costa (1985)[65**]	A. Mianserin (N = 36) B. Placebo (N = 37)	Women with cancer	Major depression	Depression is more improved in mianserin group.
Van Heeringen (1996)[66**]	A. Mianserin (N = 28) B. Placebo (N = 27)	Early breast cancer patients receiving radiation therapy	Major depression	Depression is more improved in mianserin group.
Razavi (1996)[99**]	A. Fluoxetine (N = 45) B. Placebo (N = 46)	Mixed cancer patients	Major depression or adjustment disorders	NS
Holland (1998)[67**]	A. Fluoxetine (N = 21) B. Desipramine (N = 17)	Adult women with advanced cancer	Major depression or adjustment disorders	NS
Pezzella (2001)[68**]	A. Paroxetine (N = 88) B. Amitriptyline (N = 87)	Adult women with breast cancer	Major depression	NS
Tasmuth (2002)[69**]	A. Venlafaxine (N = 13) B. Placebo (N = 13)	Patients with breast cancer and neuropathic pain	None	NS
Morrow (2003)[100**]	A. Paroxetine (N = 277) B. Placebo (N = 272)	Fatigued patients with cancer receiving chemotherapy	None	Depression is more improved in paroxetine group.
Fisch (2003)[101**]	A. Fluoxetine (N = 83) B. Placebo (N = 80)	Advanced cancer patients	Depressed mood and/or anhedonia revealed by 2-question survey	Depression is more improved in fluoxetine group.
Roscoe (2005)[70**]	A. Paroxetine (N = 44) B. Placebo (N = 50)	Breast cancer patients receiving chemotherapy	None	Depression is more improved in paroxetine group.
Musselman (2006)[71**]	A. Paroxetine (N = 13) B. Desipramine (N = 11) C. Placebo (N = 11)	Breast cancer patients	Major depression	NS
Stockler (2007)[102**]	A. Sertraline (N = 95) B. Placebo (N = 94)	Advanced cancer patients	Depressive but not with major depression	NS
Cankurtaran (2008)[103*]	A. Mirtazapine (N = 20) B. Imipramine (N = 13)	Cancer patients	Major depression or adjustment disorders or anxiety disorders	Depression is more improved in mirtazapine group.
Lydiatt (2008)[104**]	A. Citalopram (N = 13) B. Placebo (N = 12)	Head and neck cancer patients	Without major depression	NS

NS, not statistically significant.

and clinicians may discourage dying patients from seeking assessment and treatment for depression.[81]

Regarding the treatment of patients with depression toward the end of life, several consensus statements have been published.[18,73,81,82] These statements are limited by the paucity of evidence, but several themes emerge across these statements. First, there should be a low threshold for treating patients with suspected depression using short-term therapeutic trials of carefully selected interventions.[18,73] In addition, the rapid onset of the action of psychostimulants makes this class of drugs particularly appealing in patients toward the very end of life although one guideline does not recommend the use of psychostimulants due to three being evidence of adverse effects and inadequate evidence of efficacy.[82] At all events, because patients' survival time largely determines susceptibility to pharmacological treatment and it is hard to achieve drug response in patients whose survival time is very limited,

possible symptom management including sleep disturbance and agitation, even not focused on depression fundamentally, should be provided.[83] In addition, novel psychotherapeutic interventions focused on issues related to meaning and/or dignity[84**,85**] have shown promising results in the terminally ill.

Finally, one of the more dreaded issues in managing patients with serious illness toward the end of life is the problem of patients who express desire for death. Desire for death statements may indicate that a patient is depressed or suicidal, but may also be a way of coping or expressing suffering.[86,87] Depressive disorders and delirium are the most common underlying psychiatric disorders of suicidal ideation in patients with potentially fatal illnesses.[88,89] However, the presence of a potentially fatal illness, by itself, only carries a modest two- to fourfold increased risk for suicide.[21,90***] Challenging aspects of assessing patients with desire for death include evaluation and treatment of depression and delirium, assessing the adequacy of palliative care overall,

Table 69.2 *Systematic reviews and meta-analysis of psychotherapy for depression and anxiety in cancer patients*

Author	Psychotherapy	Included studies	Effect size or results Depression	Anxiety	Main findings
Devine[105]***	Psycho-education	R and Non-R	$d = 0.54$ (95% CI 0.43 to 0.65)	$d = 0.56$ (95% CI 0.42 to 0.70)	Psycho-education is effective for both depression and anxiety.
Sheard[106]***	Psychological intervention	R	$d = 0.36$ (95% CI 0.06 to 0.66) ($d = 0.19$ with positive outliers removed)	$d = 0.42$ (95% CI 0.08 to 0.74)	Preventative psychological interventions may have a moderate clinical effect upon anxiety but not depression.
Luebbert[107]***	Relaxation training	R	$d = 0.54$ (95% CI 0.30 to 0.78)	$d = 0.45$ (95% CI 0.23 to 0.67)	Relaxation training is effective for both depression and anxiety.
Redd[108]***	Behavioral intervention for side effects	R and Non-R	NA	Positive results reported in 17 of 19 studies	Behavioral intervention is effective for ameliorating anxiety associated with aversive side effects.
Barsevick[109]***	Psycho-education	R and Non-R	Positive results reported in 29 of 46 studies.	NA	Psycho-education is effective for depression.
Newell[110]***	Psychological intervention	R	No intervention strategy can be recommended.	Music therapy can be tentatively recommended.	Music therapy can be tentatively recommended for reducing anxiety, although no intervention strategy can be recommended for reducing depression.
Ross[111]***	Psychological intervention	R	Positive results reported in 9 of 17 studies.	Positive results reported in 10 of 24 studies.	The question of whether psychosocial intervention among cancer patients has a beneficial effect remains unresolved.
Akechi[112]***	Psychological intervention for advanced cancer	R	SMD = −0.44 (95% CI −0.08 to −0.80)	SMD = −0.68 (95% CI 0.01 to −1.37)	Psychotherapy is effective for depression in advanced cancer patients.

R, randomized studies; Non-R, nonrandomized studies; CI, confidence interval; SMD, standardized mean difference.

and dealing with broader issues such as personality, family dynamics, as well as important ethnic and cultural issues.[91,92] It is important to understand that most patients appreciate being asked about their mood in depth, including questions about desire for death or suicide.[93]

MANAGING ANXIETY

Because anxiety is a response to threat, most patients living with cancer or a serious chronic illness experience some kinds of anxiety. Thus, anxiety is an inevitable human reaction to serious medical illness. On the other hand, anxiety ranges from adaptive to pathological ones. In psychiatry, clinically pathological anxiety is diagnosed with anxiety disorders including generalized anxiety disorders (GAD), panic disorders, posttraumatic disorders, and so on[11] and a certain amount of cancer patients actually have these disorders.[94,95] However, in practice, these criteria may be difficult to apply to cancer patients (e.g., A diagnosis of a DSM-5[11] defines GAD requires excessive anxiety and worry, difficulty in controlling the worry, plus 3 or more additional symptoms of anxiety occurring more days than not for at least 6 months). Rather anxiety may be encountered as a component of an adjustment disorder, depressive disorders, delirium, or organic anxiety disorder.

Symptoms that are uniquely attributable to anxiety include physical symptoms such as tremor, sweating, tachycardia, hyperventilation, and restlessness. Psychological symptoms of anxiety include worry, rumination, and fear.[96] In the palliative care setting, it may not be easy to distinguish the somatic causes of anxiety from the psychological ones.[97] The common causes of anxiety symptoms in palliative care are outlined in Box 69.6.

For patients with pervasive worry and autonomic hyperreactivity, pharmacotherapy may be indicated. The categories of medications used to treat anxiety are listed in Box 69.7. The essential medicines recommended by the International Association for Hospice and Palliative Care for treatment of anxiety in palliative care are diazepam, lorazepam, and midazolam.[53] Unfortunately, there is an overall lack of evidence on the role of benzodiazepines and most other anxiolytics in palliative care patients.[98]*** Benzodiazepines are the most commonly prescribed agents, and they are effective first-line agents. These medications may cause significant sedation or trigger delirium in patients who are on other psychoactive medications (including opioids) or who are particularly frail. These drugs should be used cautiously and, when feasible, should be discontinued. The short-acting benzodiazepines lorazepam and alprazolam are used most frequently. For patients

Box 69.6 Common causes of anxiety symptoms in palliative care

Situational

- Recent diagnosis of serious illness
- Impending surgery or chemotherapy
- Impending diagnostic imaging
- Perceived risk for receiving bad news
- Fear of death/existential anxiety

Symptom-related

- Pain
- Dyspnea
- Palpitations
- Nausea

Metabolic disturbances

- Hypercalcemia
- Hypoglycemia
- Carcinoid syndrome
- Pulmonary embolus
- Paraneoplastic syndrome

Drug-associated

- Akathisia due to antipsychotics or antiemetics (dopamine-2 antagonists)
- Steroids
- Bronchodilators
- Psychostimulants
- Thyroid replacement
- Allergic reactions
- Substances or withdrawal from substances

Psychiatric disorders

- Delirium
- Depressive disorders
- Panic disorder
- Posttraumatic stress disorder
- Phobias
- Generalized anxiety disorder

Box 69.7 Drug therapy of anxiety

Benzodiazepines

- Alprazolam
- Diazepam
- Lorazepam
- Clonazepam
- Midazolam

Antidepressant agents

- SSRI and newer antidepressants
- Tricyclic antidepressants

Neuroleptic agents

- Haloperidol
- Atypical antipsychotics

Other drug therapies

- Buspirone
- β blockers (for autonomic symptom relief)
- Sedative hypnotics (for relief of insomnia)
- Antihistamines

Key learning points

- Depression and anxiety are common in patients with serious illness.

- Despite a body of research that spans several decades and includes hundreds of clinical trials, one can make no strong recommendations about the effectiveness of antidepressants or psychological interventions at improving depression or anxiety outcomes for patients with cancer and other serious chronic illnesses.

- Simple, direct questions to explore issues about mood, anxiety, or desire for death are important and appreciated by patients.

- An awareness of the potential for drug interactions with antidepressants and some other drugs commonly used in palliative care is important.

- Patients with serious chronic illnesses would benefit from multidisciplinary care that includes access to specialists in behavioral health when needed.

with coexisting delirium, risperidone, quetiapine, olanzapine, or other neuroleptic agents are useful for the management of symptoms. Antihistamines and other sedative hypnotic agents can also provide useful anxiolysis, particularly at night when insomnia is an issue. Finally, most psychotherapies shown as effective for reducing depression are also useful for ameliorating anxiety in cancer patients.[74]

REFERENCES

1 Fang F, Fall K, Mittleman MA et al. Suicide and cardiovascular death after a cancer diagnosis. *N Engl J Med* 2012;366:1310–1318.
2 Barley EA, Murray J, Walters P, Tylee A. Managing depression in primary care: A meta-synthesis of qualitative and quantitative research from the UK to identify barriers and facilitators. *BMC Fam Pract* 2011;12:47.

✳ 3   US Preventive Services Task Force. Screening for depression: Recommendations and rationale. *Ann Intern Med* 2002;136:760–764.

● 4   Katon WJ. Epidemiology and treatment of depression in patients with chronic medical illness. *Dialogues Clin Neurosci* 2011;13:7–23.

◆ 5   Hirschfeld RM, Keller MB, Panico S et al. The National Depressive and Manic-Depressive Association consensus statement on the under-treatment of depression. *JAMA* 1997;277:333–340.

● 6   Moussavi S, Chatterji S, Verdes E, Tandon A, Patel V, Ustun B. Depression, chronic diseases, and decrements in health: Results from the World Health Surveys. *Lancet* 2007;370:851–858.

7   Kazama M, Kondo N, Suzuki K, Minai J, Imai H, Yamagata Z. Early impact of depression symptoms on the decline in activities of daily living among older Japanese: Y-HALE cohort study. *Environ Health Prev Med* 2011;16:196–201.

8   Gallo JJ, Bogner HR, Morales KH, Post EP, Ten Have T, Bruce ML. Depression, cardiovascular disease, diabetes, and two-year mortality among older, primary-care patients. *Am J Geriatr Psychiatry* 2005;13:748–755.

● 9   Pan A, Sun Q, Okereke OI, Rexrode KM, Hu FB. Depression and risk of stroke morbidity and mortality: A meta-analysis and systematic review. *JAMA* 2011;306:1241–1249.

10   Herrman H, Patrick DL, Diehr P et al. Longitudinal investigation of depression outcomes in primary care in six countries: The LIDO study. Functional status, health service use and treatment of people with depressive symptoms. *Psychol Med* 2002;32:889–902.

11   APA. *Diagnostic and Statistical Manual of Mental Disorders*, 5th edn. text revision. Washington, DC: American Psychiatric Association; 2013.

12   Williams JW, Jr., Noel PH, Cordes JA, Ramirez G, Pignone M. Is this patient clinically depressed? *JAMA* 2002;287:1160–1170.

◆ 13   Whooley MA, Simon GE. Managing depression in medical outpatients. *N Engl J Med* 2000;343:1942–1950.

● 14   Barbui C, Cipriani A, Patel V, Ayuso-Mateos JL, van Ommeren M. Efficacy of antidepressants and benzodiazepines in minor depression: Systematic review and meta-analysis. *Br J Psychiatry* 2011;198:11–16.

15   Kroenke K. A 75-year-old man with depression. *JAMA* 2002;287:1568–1576.

● 16   WHO, The global burden of disease: 2004 update; 2008. Available at: http://www.who.int/healthinfo/global_burden_disease/2004_report_update/en/index.html.

17   Prince M, Livingston G, Katona C. Mental health care for the elderly in low-income countries: A health systems approach. *World Psychiatry* 2007;6:5–13.

◆ 18   Block SD. Assessing and managing depression in the terminally ill patient. ACP-ASIM End-of-Life Care Consensus Panel. American College of Physicians—American Society of Internal Medicine. *Ann Intern Med* 2000;132:209–218.

19   Grassi L, Indelli M, Marzola M et al. Depressive symptoms and quality of life in home-care-assisted cancer patients. *J Pain Symptom Manage* 1996;12:300–307.

20   Colleoni M, Mandala M, Peruzzotti G, Robertson C, Bredart A, Goldhirsch A. Depression and degree of acceptance of adjuvant cytotoxic drugs. *Lancet* 2000;356:1326–1327.

● 21   Henriksson MM, Isometsa ET, Hietanen PS, Aro HM, Lonnqvist JK. Mental disorders in cancer suicides. *J Affect Disord* 1995;36:11–20.

● 22   Hodges LJ, Humphris GM, Macfarlane G. A meta-analytic investigation of the relationship between the psychological distress of cancer patients and their carers. *Soc Sci Med* 2005;60:1–12.

23   Prieto JM, Blanch J, Atala J et al. Psychiatric morbidity and impact on hospital length of stay among hematologic cancer patients receiving stem-cell transplantation. *J Clin Oncol* 2002;20:1907–1917.

● 24   Mitchell AJ, Chan M, Bhatti H et al. Prevalence of depression, anxiety, and adjustment disorder in oncological, haematological, and palliative-care settings: A meta-analysis of 94 interview-based studies. *Lancet Oncol* 2011;12:160–174.

◆ 25   Greenberg DB. Barriers to the treatment of depression in cancer patients. *J Natl Cancer Inst Monogr* 2004;(32):127–135.

26   Gotay CC. Disparities in the impact of cancer. In: Holland J, Brietbart W, Jacobsen PB, Lederberg MS, Loscalzo M, eds., *Psyho-Onocology*. New York: Oxford University Press; 2010, pp. 503–508.

27   Quill TE, Arnold RM, Platt F. "I wish things were different": Expressing wishes in response to loss, futility, and unrealistic hopes. *Ann Intern Med* 2001;135:551–555.

● 28   Cleeland CS, Gonin R, Hatfield AK et al. Pain and its treatment in outpatients with metastatic cancer. *N Engl J Med* 1994;330:592–596.

● 29   Teunissen SC, Wesker W, Kruitwagen C, de Haes HC, Voest EE, de Graeff A. Symptom prevalence in patients with incurable cancer: A systematic review. *J Pain Symptom Manage* 2007;34:94–104.

● 30   Chochinov HM, Wilson KG, Enns M, Lander S. "Are you depressed?" Screening for depression in the terminally ill. *Am J Psychiatry* 1997;154:674–676.

31   Akizuki N, Akechi T, Nakanishi T et al. Development of a brief screening interview for adjustment disorders and major depression in patients with cancer. *Cancer* 2003;97:2605–2613.

32   Whooley MA, Avins AL, Miranda J, Browner WS. Case-finding instruments for depression. Two questions are as good as many. *J Gen Intern Med* 1997;12:439–445.

33   Pignone MP, Gaynes BN, Rushton JL et al. Screening for depression in adults: A summary of the evidence for the U.S. Preventive Services Task Force. *Ann Intern Med* 2002;136:765–776.

● 34   Mitchell AJ. Are one or two simple questions sufficient to detect depression in cancer and palliative care? A Bayesian meta-analysis. *Br J Cancer* 2008;98:1934–1943.

35   Zigmond AS, Snaith RP. The hospital anxiety and depression scale. *Acta Psychiatr Scand* 1983;67:361–370.

● 36   Mitchell AJ, Meader N, Symonds P. Diagnostic validity of the Hospital Anxiety and Depression Scale (HADS) in cancer and palliative settings: A meta-analysis. *J Affect Disord* 2010;126:335–348.

✳ 37   Holland JC, Bultz BD. The NCCN guideline for distress management: A case for making distress the sixth vital sign. *J Natl Compr Canc Netw* 2007;5:3–7.

38   Carlson LE, Groff SL, Maciejewski O, Bultz BD. Screening for distress in lung and breast cancer outpatients: A randomized controlled trial. *J Clin Oncol* 2010;28:4884–4891.

39   Akizuki N, Yamawaki S, Akechi T, Nakano T, Uchitomi Y. Development of an Impact Thermometer for use in combination with the Distress Thermometer as a brief screening tool for adjustment disorders and/or major depression in cancer patients. *J Pain Symptom Manage* 2005;29:91–99.

40   Grassi L, Rossi E, Caruso R et al. Educational intervention in cancer outpatient clinics on routine screening for emotional distress: An observational study. *Psychooncology* 2011;20:669–674.

41   Furler J, Kokanovic R, Dowrick C, Newton D, Gunn J, May C. Managing depression among ethnic communities: A qualitative study. *Ann Fam Med* 2010;8:231–236.

✳ 42   American Psychiatric Association. Practice guideline for the treatment of patients with major depressive disorder, third edition. *Am J Psychiatry* 2010;167(Suppl.):1–118.

● 43   Rayner L, Price A, Evans A, Valsraj K, Hotopf M, Higginson IJ. Antidepressants for the treatment of depression in palliative care: Systematic review and meta-analysis. *Palliat Med* 2011;25:36–51.

44 Stahl SM. Basic psychopharmacology of antidepressants, part 2: Estrogen as an adjunct to antidepressant treatment. *J Clin Psychiatry* 1998;59(Suppl. 4):15–24.

45 Kroenke K, West SL, Swindle R et al. Similar effectiveness of paroxetine, fluoxetine, and sertraline in primary care: A randomized trial. *JAMA* 2001;286:2947–2955.

● 46 Gartlehner G, Hansen RA, Morgan LC et al. Comparative benefits and harms of second-generation antidepressants for treating major depressive disorder: An updated meta-analysis. *Ann Intern Med* 2011;155:772–785.

● 47 Cipriani A, Furukawa TA, Salanti G et al. Comparative efficacy and acceptability of 12 new-generation antidepressants: A multiple-treatments meta-analysis. *Lancet* 2009;373:746–758.

48 Akechi T, Ietsugu T, Sukigara M et al. Symptom indicator of severity of depression in cancer patients: A comparison of the DSM-IV criteria with alternative diagnostic criteria. *Gen Hosp Psychiatry* 2009;31:225–232.

49 Aronowitz RA. When do symptoms become a disease? *Ann Intern Med* 2001;134:803–808.

50 Kroenke K, Harris L. Symptoms research: A fertile field. *Ann Intern Med* 2001;134:801–802.

51 Holden C. Neuroscience. Drugs and placebos look alike in the brain. *Science* 2002;295:947.

52 Vastag B. Decade of work shows depression is physical. *JAMA* 2002;287:1787–1788.

● 53 De Lima L. International Association for Hospice and Palliative Care list of essential medicines for palliative care. *Ann Oncol* 2007;18:395–399.

✳ 54 NIH State-of-the-Science Statement on symptom management in cancer: Pain, depression, and fatigue. *NIH Consens State Sci Statements* 2002;19:1–29.

◆ 55 Rozans M, Dreisbach A, Lertora JJ, Kahn MJ. Palliative uses of methylphenidate in patients with cancer: A review. *J Clin Oncol* 2002;20:335–339.

56 Meyers CA, Weitzner MA, Valentine AD, Levin VA. Methylphenidate therapy improves cognition, mood, and function of brain tumor patients. *J Clin Oncol* 1998;16:2522–2527.

● 57 Miguel C, Albuquerque E. Drug interaction in psycho-oncology: Antidepressants and antineoplastics. *Pharmacology* 2011;88:333–339.

● 58 Henry NL, Stearns V, Flockhart DA, Hayes DF, Riba M. Drug interactions and pharmacogenomics in the treatment of breast cancer and depression. *Am J Psychiatry* 2008;165:1251–1255.

59 Kelly CM, Juurlink DN, Gomes T et al. Selective serotonin reuptake inhibitors and breast cancer mortality in women receiving tamoxifen: A population based cohort study. *BMJ* 2010;340:c693.

✳ 60 National Institute for Health and Clinical Excellence. *Depression in Adults with a Chronic Physical Health Problem: Treatment and Management*. Leicester, U.K.: British Psychological Society; 2010.

● 61 Zarate CA, Jr., Singh JB, Carlson PJ et al. A randomized trial of an N-methyl-D-aspartate antagonist in treatment-resistant major depression. *Arch Gen Psychiatry* 2006;63:856–864.

● 62 Furey ML, Drevets WC. Antidepressant efficacy of the antimuscarinic drug scopolamine: A randomized, placebo-controlled clinical trial. *Arch Gen Psychiatry* 2006;63:1121–1129.

● 63 Golden RN, Gaynes BN, Ekstrom RD et al. The efficacy of light therapy in the treatment of mood disorders: A review and meta-analysis of the evidence. *Am J Psychiatry* 2005;162:656–662.

● 64 Li M, Fitzgerald P, Rodin G. Evidence-based treatment of depression in patients with cancer. *J Clin Oncol* 2012;30:1187–1196.

● 65 Costa D, Mogos I, Toma T. Efficacy and safety of mianserin in the treatment of depression of women with cancer. *Acta Psychiatr Scand Suppl* 1985;320:85–92.

● 66 van Heeringen K, Zivkov M. Pharmacological treatment of depression in cancer patients. A placebo-controlled study of mianserin. *Br J Psychiatry* 1996;169:440–443.

67 Holland JC, Romano SJ, Heiligenstein JH, Tepner RG, Wilson MG. A controlled trial of fluoxetine and desipramine in depressed women with advanced cancer. *Psychooncology* 1998;7:291–300.

68 Pezzella G, Moslinger-Gehmayr R, Contu A. Treatment of depression in patients with breast cancer: A comparison between paroxetine and amitriptyline. *Breast Cancer Res Treat* 2001;70:1–10.

69 Tasmuth T, Hartel B, Kalso E. Venlafaxine in neuropathic pain following treatment of breast cancer. *Eur J Pain* 2002;6:17–24.

70 Roscoe JA, Morrow GR, Hickok JT et al. Effect of paroxetine hydrochloride (Paxil) on fatigue and depression in breast cancer patients receiving chemotherapy. *Breast Cancer Res Treat* 2005;89:243–249.

71 Musselman DL, Somerset WI, Guo Y et al. A double-blind, multicenter, parallel-group study of paroxetine, desipramine, or placebo in breast cancer patients (stages I, II, III, and IV) with major depression. *J Clin Psychiatry* 2006;67:288–296.

◆ 72 Williams S, Dale J. The effectiveness of treatment for depression/depressive symptoms in adults with cancer: A systematic review. *Br J Cancer* 2006;94:372–390.

◆ 73 Stiefel R, Die Trill M, Berney A, Olarte JM, Razavi A. Depression in palliative care: A pragmatic report from the Expert Working Group of the European Association for Palliative Care. *Support Care Cancer* 2001;9:477–488.

◆ 74 Jacobsen PB, Jim HS. Psychosocial interventions for anxiety and depression in adult cancer patients: Achievements and challenges. *CA Cancer J Clin* 2008;58:214–230.

75 Reynolds JS, Perrin NA. Mismatches in social support and psychosocial adjustment to breast cancer. *Health Psychol* 2004;23:425–430.

● 76 Temel JS, Greer JA, Muzikansky A et al. Early palliative care for patients with metastatic non-small-cell lung cancer. *N Engl J Med* 2010;363:733–742.

● 77 Lloyd-Williams M, Dennis M, Taylor F, Baker I. Is asking patients in palliative care, "are you depressed?" Appropriate? Prospective study. *BMJ* 2003;327:372–373.

78 Akechi T, Okuyama T, Sugawara Y, Shima Y, Furukawa TA, Uchitomi Y. Screening for depression in terminally ill cancer patients in Japan. *J Pain Symptom Manage* 2006;31:5–12.

79 Le Fevre P, Devereux J, Smith S, Lawrie SM, Cornbleet M. Screening for psychiatric illness in the palliative care inpatient setting: A comparison between the Hospital Anxiety and Depression Scale and the General Health Questionnaire-12. *Palliat Med* 1999;13:399–407.

● 80 Wasteson E, Brenne E, Higginson IJ et al. Depression assessment and classification in palliative cancer patients: A systematic literature review. *Palliat Med* 2009;23:739–753.

81 APM's Ad Hoc Committee on End-of-Life Care. Psychiatric aspects of excellent end-of-life care: A position statement of the Academy of Psychosomatic Medicine. *J Palliat Med* 1998;1:113–115.

✳ 82 Rayner L, Price A, Hotopf M, Higginson IJ. The development of evidence-based European guidelines on the management of depression in palliative cancer care. *Eur J Cancer* 2011;47:702–712.

83 Shimizu K, Akechi T, Shimamoto M et al. Can psychiatric intervention improve major depression in very near end-of-life cancer patients? *Palliat Support Care* 2007;5:3–9.

● 84 Chochinov HM, Kristjanson LJ, Breitbart W et al. Effect of dignity therapy on distress and end-of-life experience in terminally ill patients: A randomised controlled trial. *Lancet Oncol* 2011;12:753–762.

● 85 Breitbart W, Poppito S, Rosenfeld B et al. Pilot randomized controlled trial of individual meaning-centered psychotherapy for patients with advanced cancer. *J Clin Oncol* 2012;30:1304–1309.

86 Nissim R, Gagliese L, Rodin G. The desire for hastened death in individuals with advanced cancer: A longitudinal qualitative study. *Soc Sci Med* 2009;69:165–171.

● 87 Rodin G, Lo C, Mikulincer M, Donner A, Gagliese L, Zimmermann C. Pathways to distress: The multiple determinants of depression, hopelessness, and the desire for hastened death in metastatic cancer patients. *Soc Sci Med* 2009;68:562–569.

● 88 Chochinov HM, Wilson KG, Enns M et al. Desire for death in the terminally ill. *Am J Psychiatry* 1995;152:1185–1191.

89 Akechi T, Nakano T, Akizuki N et al. Clinical factors associated with suicidality in cancer patients. *Jpn J Clin Oncol* 2002;32:506–511.

◆ 90 Harris EC, Barraclough BM. Suicide as an outcome for medical disorders. *Medicine (Baltimore)* 1994;73:281–296.

91 Cohen LM, Steinberg MD, Hails KC, Dobscha SK, Fischel SV. Psychiatric evaluation of death-hastening requests. Lessons from dialysis discontinuation. *Psychosomatics* 2000;41:195–203.

◆ 92 Mann JJ. A current perspective of suicide and attempted suicide. *Ann Intern Med* 2002;136:302–311.

93 Meyer HA, Sinnott C, Seed PT. Depressive symptoms in advanced cancer. Part 2. Depression over time; the role of the palliative care professional. *Palliat Med* 2003;17:604–607.

94 Spencer R, Nilsson M, Wright A, Pirl W, Prigerson H. Anxiety disorders in advanced cancer patients: Correlates and predictors of end-of-life outcomes. *Cancer* 2010;116:1810–1819.

◆ 95 Stark DP, House A. Anxiety in cancer patients. *Br J Cancer* 2000;83:1261–1267.

◆ 96 Stiefel F, Razavi D. Common psychiatric disorders in cancer patients. II. Anxiety and acute confusional states. *Support Care Cancer* 1994;2:233–237.

97 Roth AJ, Massie MJ. Anxiety and its management in advanced cancer. *Curr Opin Support Palliat Care* 2007;1:50–56.

● 98 Jackson KC, Lipman AG. Drug therapy for anxiety in palliative care. *Cochrane Database Syst Rev* 2004;10:CD004596.

99 Razavi D, Allilaire JF, Smith M et al. The effect of fluoxetine on anxiety and depression symptoms in cancer patients. *Acta Psychiatr Scand* 1996;94:205–210.

●100 Morrow GR, Hickok JT, Roscoe JA et al. Differential effects of paroxetine on fatigue and depression: A randomized, double-blind trial from the University of Rochester Cancer Center Community Clinical Oncology Program. *J Clin Oncol* 2003;21:4635–4641.

●101 Fisch MJ, Loehrer PJ, Kristeller J et al. Fluoxetine versus placebo in advanced cancer outpatients: A double-blinded trial of the Hoosier Oncology Group. *J Clin Oncol* 2003;21:1937–1943.

●102 Stockler MR, O'Connell R, Nowak AK et al. Effect of sertraline on symptoms and survival in patients with advanced cancer, but without major depression: A placebo-controlled double-blind randomised trial. *Lancet Oncol* 2007;8:603–612.

103 Cankurtaran ES, Ozalp E, Soygur H, Akbiyik DI, Turhan L, Alkis N. Mirtazapine improves sleep and lowers anxiety and depression in cancer patients: Superiority over imipramine. *Support Care Cancer* 2008;16:1291–1298.

104 Lydiatt WM, Denman D, McNeilly DP, Puumula SE, Burke WJ. A randomized, placebo-controlled trial of citalopram for the prevention of major depression during treatment for head and neck cancer. *Arch Otolaryngol Head Neck Surg* 2008;134:528–535.

●105 Devine EC, Westlake SK. The effects of psychoeducational care provided to adults with cancer: Meta-analysis of 116 studies. *Oncol Nurs Forum* 1995;22:1369–1381.

●106 Sheard T, Maguire P. The effect of psychological interventions on anxiety and depression in cancer patients: Results of two meta-analyses. *Br J Cancer* 1999;80:1770–1780.

●107 Luebbert K, Dahme B, Hasenbring M. The effectiveness of relaxation training in reducing treatment-related symptoms and improving emotional adjustment in acute non-surgical cancer treatment: A meta-analytical review. *Psychooncology* 2001;10:490–502.

●108 Redd WH, Montgomery GH, DuHamel KN. Behavioral intervention for cancer treatment side effects. *J Natl Cancer Inst* 2001;93:810–823.

●109 Barsevick AM, Sweeney C, Haney E, Chung E. A systematic qualitative analysis of psychoeducational interventions for depression in patients with cancer. *Oncol Nurs Forum* 2002;29:73–84; quiz 5–7.

●110 Newell SA, Sanson-Fisher RW, Savolainen NJ. Systematic review of psychological therapies for cancer patients: Overview and recommendations for future research. *J Natl Cancer Inst* 2002;94:558–584.

● 111 Ross L, Boesen EH, Dalton SO, Johansen C. Mind and cancer: Does psychosocial intervention improve survival and psychological well-being? *Eur J Cancer* 2002;38:1447–1457.

●112 Akechi T, Okuyama T, Onishi J, Morita T, Furukawa T. Psychotherapy for depression among incurable cancer patients. *Cochrane Database Syst Rev* 2008;(2):CD005537.

70

Delirium

YESNE ALICI, WILLIAM BREITBART

INTRODUCTION

A variety of mental syndromes can be seen in patients with advanced disease. These mental syndromes could fall under one of the following subcategories of the Diagnostic and Statistical Manual of Mental Disorders, Fourth Edition–Text Revision (DSM-IV-TR)[1]:

- Delirium, dementia, amnestic disorders, and other cognitive disorders
- Mental disorders due to a general medical condition (including catatonic disorder and personality change)
- Mood disorder due a general medical condition
- Anxiety disorder due a general medical condition
- Psychotic disorder due to a general medical condition
- Substance-related disorders.

While virtually all of these mental syndromes can be seen in the patient with advanced disease, the most common are delirium, dementia, and mood and anxiety disorders due to a general medical condition. Cognitive disorders are unfortunately all too common in patients with advanced illness. With mental disorders due to a general medical condition or medications where cognitive impairment is limited, or relatively intact, the more prominent symptoms tend to consist of anxiety, mood disturbance, delusions, hallucinations, or personality change. For instance, the patient with mood disturbance meeting criteria for major depression who is severely hypothyroid or on high-dose corticosteroids is most accurately diagnosed as having a mood disorder due to a general medical condition or substance-induced mood disorder, respectively (particularly if medical factors are judged to be the primary etiology related to the mood disturbance). Similarly, the patient with hyponatremia or on acyclovir for central nervous system (CNS) herpes who is experiencing visual hallucinations but has a normal level of alertness and attention span with minimal cognitive deficits is more accurately diagnosed as having a psychotic disorder due to a general medical condition or a substance-induced psychotic disorder, respectively.

Delirium is a common and often serious neuropsychiatric complication in palliative care settings that is characterized by concurrent disturbances of the level of alertness (consciousness), attention, thinking, perception, memory, psychomotor behavior, mood, and sleep–wake cycle. Disorientation, fluctuation, and waxing and waning of these symptoms, as well as an acute or abrupt onset of such disturbances, are other critical features of delirium. Delirium is a sign of significant physiological disturbance, usually involving multiple causes, including infections, organ failure, and medication adverse effects. Delirium, in contrast with dementia, is conceptualized as a *reversible* process. Reversibility of the process of delirium is often possible even in the patient with advanced illness; however, it may *not* be reversible in the last 24–48 hours of life, and this influences the outcomes of its management.[2] This is most likely due to the fact that irreversible processes such as multiple organ failure are occurring in the final hours of life. Delirium occurring in these last days of life is often referred to as terminal restlessness or terminal agitation in the palliative care literature.

Delirium is associated with significant morbidity and mortality. Increased health-care costs, prolonged hospital stays, and long-term cognitive decline are well-recognized outcomes of delirium.[3–5] Delirium is a harbinger of impending death in terminally ill patients, causing significant distress for patients, family members, and staff.[5–9] In a study of the "Delirium Experience" of terminally ill cancer patients, Breitbart and colleagues found that 54% of patients recalled their delirium experience after recovery from delirium.[6] Factors predicting delirium recall included the degree of short-term memory impairment, delirium severity, and the presence of perceptual disturbances (the more severe, the less likely recall). The most significant factor predicting distress for patients was the presence of hallucinations and delusions. Patients with hypoactive delirium were just as distressed as patients with hyperactive delirium. Predictors of spouse distress included the patients' Karnofsky Performance Status (the lower the Karnofsky, the worse the spouse distress), and predictors of nurse distress included delirium severity and perceptual disturbances. A survey of 300 bereaved Japanese families showed that two-thirds of the families found delirium in the family members to be highly distressing.[7] Symptoms that caused the most distress included agitation and cognitive impairment. In a study of 99 patients with advanced cancer who had recovered from delirium, 74% remembered their delirium episode.[8] Patients who recalled their delirium episode reported a higher level of distress than patients with no recall. Family caregivers of those patients reported higher levels of distress compared to nurses and physicians caring for patients with delirium.[8] Another study on caregivers has shown that the family members of delirious terminally ill patients were 12 times more likely to develop an anxiety disorder than caregivers of nondelirious patients.[9] These findings highlight the importance of not only treating the causes and controlling the symptoms of delirium but also informing the caregivers of the medical nature of delirium and the potential treatment options to reduce caregiver distress.

Delirium can interfere dramatically with the recognition and control of other physical and psychological symptoms such as pain in later stages of illness.[5] Uncontrolled pain can cause agitation. Patients with delirium use a significantly greater number of "breakthrough" doses of opioids at night compared with patients without delirium due to sleep–wake cycle reversal.[11] On the other hand, agitation due to delirium may be misinterpreted as uncontrolled pain, resulting in inappropriate escalation of opioids, potentially worsening delirium.[12] A recent retrospective study of 284 hospice patients sought to identify factors that contribute to impairment of communication capacity in terminally ill cancer patients.[13] The study demonstrated that communication capacity was frequently impaired in terminally ill cancer patients and the degree of impairment was significantly associated with higher doses of opioids. Patients with delirium were also found to have difficulty communicating their needs, emphasizing the importance of further investigations to explore new strategies for maintaining communication capacity in this population.[13]

Unfortunately, delirium is often underrecognized or misdiagnosed and inappropriately treated or untreated in terminally ill patients.[5] The diversity of the signs and symptoms of delirium and the fluctuating clinical course primarily lead to underrecognition and mistreatment of delirium. Practitioners caring for patients with life-threatening illnesses must be able to diagnose delirium accurately, undertake appropriate assessment of the etiologies, and be familiar with the risks and benefits of the pharmacological and nonpharmacological interventions currently available in managing delirium among the terminally ill. Improved recognition of delirium with delirium assessment tools validated in palliative care settings and the terminally ill is the first step toward better management of delirium. Implementation of delirium assessment strategies to routine care should become the standard of care to rule out this disabling condition in palliative care settings.[10]

This chapter provides an overview of the prevalence as well as the main clinical features of delirium, including its subtypes, differential diagnosis, and assessment of etiologies. Pharmacological and nonpharmacological interventions and controversies common to the management of delirium in palliative care settings are also summarized.

DELIRIUM IN PALLIATIVE CARE SETTINGS

Prevalence of delirium

Delirium is one of the most common mental disorders encountered in general hospital practice. Delirium is highly prevalent in cancer and AIDS patients with advanced disease, particularly in the terminally ill, in the last weeks of life, with prevalence rates ranging from 20% to 88%.[5,14–19] The wide range of prevalence reports in the literature is due to the diverse and complex nature of delirium and heterogeneity of sample populations, setting of care, and the assessment scale used.[5]

Prospective studies conducted in inpatient palliative care settings have found a delirium occurrence rate of 20%–42% upon admission, and an incident delirium developing during admission in 32%–45% of patients.[14,15,17–19] Massie and coworkers found delirium in 25% of 334 hospitalized cancer patients seen in psychiatric consultation and in 85% of terminal cancer patients.[14] Pereira and coworkers found the prevalence of cognitive impairment in cancer inpatients to be 44%, and just prior to death, the prevalence rose to 62.1%.[15] A prospective study of 69 patients with head and neck cancer undergoing outpatient treatment showed that six patients (8.6%) developed delirium during treatment. More importantly, the prevalence and incidence of subsyndromal delirium were 7.2% and 45.3%, respectively.[16] Among patients undergoing myeloablative hematopoietic stem cell transplantation, delirium has been found to occur in up to 50% of patients during the 4 weeks after conditioning and stem cell infusion.[20]

Pathophysiology of delirium

The study of the pathophysiology of delirium is vital to our understanding of the phenomenology, prognosis, treatment, and prevention of delirium. As reflected by its diverse phenomenology, delirium is a dysfunction of multiple regions of the brain, a global cerebral dysfunction. Despite many different etiologies, symptoms of delirium are largely stereotypical, with a set of core symptoms. It appears that this diversity of physiological disturbances translates into a common clinical expression that may relate to dysfunction of a final common neuroanatomical and/or neurochemical pathway.[21] Investigators through brain imaging and lesion studies have postulated that the final common pathway involves the prefrontal cortex, posterior parietal cortex, temporo-occipital cortex, anteromedial thalamus, and right basal ganglia with an imbalance in the neurotransmitters acetylcholine and dopamine.[21] The literature on the pathophysiology of delirium has continued to expand within the last decade. An in-depth review of pathophysiology of delirium is available elsewhere.[22]

Diagnosing delirium

The diagnostic "gold standard" is the clinician's assessment using the DSM-IV-TR criteria for delirium.[1] The essential features of delirium are as follows: disturbance of consciousness with reduced ability to focus, sustain, or shift attention; change in cognition that is not better accounted by a preexisting, established, or evolving dementia or development of a perceptual disturbance; development of the disturbance over a short period of time, usually hours to days, and fluctuation of symptoms during the course of the day; and evidence from the history, physical examination, or laboratory tests that the delirium is a direct physiologic consequence of a general medical condition, substance intoxication or withdrawal, use of a medication, or toxin exposure—or a combination of these factors.[1]

The clinical features of delirium are quite numerous and include a variety of neuropsychiatric symptoms that are also common to other psychiatric disorders such as depression, dementia, and psychosis.[5,23] Main features of delirium include prodromal symptoms (e.g., restlessness, anxiety, sleep disturbances, and irritability); rapidly fluctuating course; abrupt onset of symptoms; reduced attention span (easily distractible); altered level of alertness; increased or decreased psychomotor activity; disturbance of sleep–wake cycle; affective symptoms (emotional lability, sadness, anger, and euphoria); altered perceptions (misperceptions, illusions, delusions, and hallucinations); disorganized thinking and incoherent speech; disorientation to time, place, or person; and memory impairment (cannot register new material) or impairment in other cognitive domains (dysnomia, sensorimotor aphasia, dysgraphia, constructional apraxia, executive dysfunction) (Table 70.1). The DSM-IV-TR criteria for delirium does not address the prodromal or affective symptoms (i.e., depressed mood) of delirium, which might be more prominent in patients with delirium in palliative care settings and also associated with worse outcomes.[5] Neurological examination abnormalities may include motor abnormalities (tremor, asterixis, myoclonus, and reflex and tone changes) and/or signs of frontal release (grasp, palmomental, glabellar tap, and snout reflexes).[5]

Table 70.1 *Clinical features of delirium*

Disturbance in the level of alertness (consciousness)

Attentional disturbances

Rapidly fluctuating clinical course and abrupt onset of symptoms

Disorientation

Cognitive disturbances (i.e., memory impairment, executive dysfunction, apraxia, agnosia, visuospatial dysfunction, and language disturbances)

Increased or decreased psychomotor activity

Disturbance of sleep–wake cycle

Mood symptoms (depression, mood lability)

Perceptual disturbances (hallucinations or illusions) or delusions

Disorganized thought process

Incoherent speech

Neurological findings (may include asterixis, myoclonus, tremor, frontal release signs, changes in muscle tone)

Source: Adapted from Breitbart, W. and Alici, Y., *JAMA*, 300, 2898, 2008.

Cognitive impairment was found to be the most common symptom noted in phenomenology studies with disorientation occurring in 78%–100%, attention deficits in 62%–100%, memory deficits in 62%–90%, and diffuse cognitive deficits in 77%.[24] Disturbance of consciousness was recorded in 65%–100% of patients with delirium. In addition, disorganized thinking was found in 95%, language abnormalities in 47%–93%, and sleep–wake cycle disturbances in 49%–96%.[24] A phenomenology study by Meagher and colleagues has found the sleep–wake cycle abnormalities (97%) and inattention (97%) to be the most frequent symptoms in patients with delirium; disorientation was found to be the least common symptom.[25]

The clinical presentation of delirium may vary based on the age of the patients. A phenomenology study of different age groups has shown that childhood delirium presents more likely with severe perceptual disturbances, severe delusions, severe lability of mood, and agitation when compared with delirium in adult and geriatric patient populations.[26] More severe cognitive symptoms were observed in geriatric patients with delirium.[26]

It is important to emphasize that clinicians should assess for subsyndromal delirium (i.e., delirium that does not meet the full *DSM-IV-TR* criteria for a diagnosis of delirium) or prodromal signs of delirium to timely recognize and treat this disabling condition in palliative care settings.[27]

Delirium screening and diagnostic tools

The diagnostic gold standard for delirium is the clinician's assessment utilizing the DSM-IV-TR criteria as outlined earlier.[28-34] A number of scales or instruments have been developed that can aid the clinician in rapidly screening for cognitive impairment disorders (dementia or delirium), establishing a diagnosis of delirium, and assessing delirium severity. A detailed review of these assessment tools is available elsewhere.[28] Several examples of delirium assessment tools currently used in palliative care settings include the Memorial Delirium Assessment Scale (MDAS),[29,30] the Delirium Rating Scale-Revised 98,[31] and the Confusion Assessment Method (CAM).[32,33] Of those, the MDAS and the CAM have been validated in palliative care settings.[30,33] Each of these scales has good reliability and validity.[28-33] A systematic review of the evidence on the accuracy of bedside instruments in diagnosing delirium in adult patients identified 25 prospectively conducted studies (n = 3027 patients) describing the use of 11 instruments.[34] Considering the instrument's ease of use, test performance, and clinical importance of the heterogeneity in the confidence intervals (CIs) of the likelihood ratios (LR), the CAM was found to have the best available supportive data as a bedside delirium instrument (summary-positive LR, 9.6; 95% CI, 5.8–16.0; summary-negative LR, 0.16; 95% CI, 0.09–0.29). Of all scales, the Mini Mental Status Examination (MMSE) (score < 24) was the least useful for identifying a patient with delirium (LR, 1.6; 95% CI, 1.2–2.0). The authors concluded that the choice of instrument may be dictated by the amount of time available and the discipline of the examiner; however, the best evidence supported the use of the CAM, which took 5 min to administer.[34]

Subtypes of delirium

Three clinical subtypes of delirium, based on psychomotor behavior and the level of alertness, have been described.[35,36] These subtypes include the "hyperactive" subtype, the "hypoactive" subtype, and a "mixed" subtype with alternating features of hyperactive and hypoactive delirium.[5,18,35–41]

In the palliative care setting, hypoactive delirium is most common and is frequently misdiagnosed as depression or severe fatigue.[5] Despite the frequency of hypoactive delirium, hypoactive delirium has been found to be underdetected when compared with the detection rates of hyperactive or mixed subtypes of delirium in palliative care settings.[37]

Research suggests that the hyperactive form is most often characterized by hallucinations, delusions, hypervigilance, and psychomotor agitation, while the hypoactive form is characterized by psychomotor retardation, lethargy, sedation, and reduced awareness of surroundings.[5] Delirium phenomenology studies suggest that cognitive performance is similar across motor subtypes of delirium. A study of 100 consecutive cases of DSM-IV-TR delirium across motor subtypes (33 patients with hypoactive, 18 with hyperactive, 26 with mixed, and 23 patients with no motor alteration were included) in a palliative care unit showed that patients with mixed motoric subtype had more severe delirium, with highest scores for DRS-R-98 sleep–wake cycle disturbance, hallucinations, delusions, and language abnormalities.[38] Cognitive performance did not differ across hyperactive, mixed, and hypoactive motor groups. Authors concluded that motor variants in delirium have similar cognitive profiles, but mixed cases differ in the expression of several noncognitive features. A recent phenomenology study showed that although perceptual disturbances and delusions were more prevalent in hyperactive (70.2% and 78.7%, respectively) than in hypoactive delirium (50.9% and 43.4%, respectively), the prevalence of perceptual disturbances and delusions in hypoactive delirium was much higher than previously reported, deserving clinical attention and intervention.[39]

The mean prevalence of hypoactive delirium was reported to be 48% (ranging from 15% to 71%) in comparison to hyperactive delirium that occurred in 13%–46% of patients in the palliative care settings.[5,36,40] In a hospice setting, 29% of 100 acute admissions were found to have delirium; 86% of these had the hypoactive subtype.[18] The prototypically agitated delirious patient most familiar to clinicians may actually constitute less than half of patients with delirium in the terminally ill.

There is evidence suggesting that specific delirium subtypes may be related to specific etiologies of delirium and may have unique pathophysiologies, differential responses to treatment, and prognosis.[5,18,41–44] Hypoactive delirium has been shown to be associated with higher rates of mortality than hyperactive delirium.[18,41] Hypoactive delirium has been found to occur with hypoxia, metabolic disturbances, and anticholinergic medications. Hyperactive delirium has been correlated with alcohol and drug withdrawal, drug intoxication, or medication adverse effects.[5,18,41] A randomized controlled trial of haloperidol and chlorpromazine found that both drugs were equally effective in hypoactive and hyperactive subtypes of delirium, whereas an open label trial of olanzapine found poorer treatment response with hypoactive delirium.[42,43] A recent case-matched study comparing the efficacy of haloperidol and aripiprazole in the treatment of delirium has shown no significant differences in treatment results between the two medications for patients with hypoactive or hyperactive delirium.[44]

Differential diagnosis of delirium

Many of the clinical features and symptoms of delirium can also be associated with other psychiatric disorders such as depression, mania, psychosis, and dementia. Delirium, particularly the "hypoactive" subtype, is often initially misdiagnosed as depression. Symptoms of major depression, including altered level of psychomotor activity (hypoactivity), insomnia, reduced ability to concentrate, depressed mood, and even suicidal ideation, can overlap with symptoms of delirium, making an accurate diagnosis more difficult. In distinguishing delirium from depression, particularly in the context of advanced disease, an evaluation of the onset and temporal sequencing of depressive and cognitive symptoms is particularly helpful. Importantly, the degree of cognitive impairment in delirium is much more severe and pervasive than in depression, with a more abrupt temporal onset. Also, in delirium the characteristic disturbance in the level of alertness is present, while it is usually not a feature of depression. Similarly, a manic episode may share some features of delirium, particularly a "hyperactive" or "mixed" subtype of delirium. Again, the temporal onset and course of symptoms, the presence of a disturbance in the level of alertness as well as of cognition, and the identification of a presumed medical etiology or medications for delirium are helpful in differentiating these disorders. Past psychiatric history or family history of mood disorders is usually evident in patients with depression or a manic episode. Symptoms such as severe anxiety and autonomic hyperactivity can lead the clinician to an erroneous diagnosis of panic disorder. Delirium that is characterized by vivid hallucinations and delusions must be distinguished from a variety of psychotic disorders. In delirium, such psychotic symptoms occur in the context of a disturbance in the level of alertness and impaired attention span, as well as memory impairment and disorientation, which is not the case in other psychotic disorders. Delusions in delirium tend to be poorly organized and of abrupt onset, and hallucinations are predominantly visual or tactile rather than auditory as is typical of schizophrenia. Finally, the development of these psychotic symptoms in the context of advanced medical illness makes delirium a more likely diagnosis. It is important to note that not all patients with agitation have delirium. Patients with uncontrolled pain, medication-induced akathisia, and panic attacks may also present with agitation. The diagnosis of delirium is reserved for patients who meet the diagnostic criteria for delirium.

The most challenging differential diagnostic issue is whether the patient has delirium, or dementia, or a delirium superimposed upon a preexisting dementia. Both delirium and dementia are cognitive impairment disorders and so share such common clinical features as impaired memory, thinking, judgment, aphasia, apraxia, agnosia, executive dysfunction, and disorientation. Delusions and hallucinations can be seen in patients with dementia. The patient with dementia is alert and does not have a disturbance in the level of alertness that is characteristic of delirium. The temporal onset of symptoms in dementia is more subacute and chronically progressive. It is the abrupt onset, fluctuating course, and disturbances of consciousness that differentiate delirium from dementia. It is also important to note that delirium represents an acute change from the patient's baseline cognitive functioning, even if the patient has dementia or other cognitive disturbances at baseline. Delirium superimposed on an underlying dementia can be encountered such as in the case of an older patient, an AIDS patient, or a patient with a paraneoplastic syndrome. Reversibility of the process of delirium is often possible even in the patient with advanced illness as opposed to dementia. However, as noted previously, delirium may not be reversible in the last 24–48 hours of life. Clinically, a number of scales or instruments aid clinicians in the diagnosis of delirium, dementia, or delirium superimposed on dementia.[28,34] Boettger and colleagues reviewed the treatment and phenomenological characteristics of 100 cancer patients with delirium superimposed on dementia (DD) in contrast to patients with delirium in the absence of dementia (ND).[45,46] Patients in the DD (n = 18) group, compared to the ND group (n = 82), had significantly greater levels of disturbance of consciousness and impairments in all cognitive domains (i.e., orientation, short-term memory, and concentration). There were no significant differences between the DD and ND groups in terms of the presence or severity of hallucinations, delusions, psychomotor behavior, and sleep–wake cycle disturbances. The MDAS scores at baseline were significantly higher in DD (21.1) compared to NDD (17.6). Over the course of treatment, MDAS scores were significantly higher in DD with 11.7 compared with 7.0 in NDD. After 3 days of management, delirium resolution rates were significantly lower in DD with 18.2% compared to 53.9% in NDD, and at 7 days, delirium resolution rates were 50% and 83%, respectively. Researchers concluded that when delirium is superimposed on dementia, the delirium may present with more severe cognitive symptoms, may respond poorly to treatment, and may resolve at a lower rate when compared to nondemented patients with delirium.[45,46]

Management of delirium in palliative care settings

The standard approach to the management of delirium includes a search for underlying causes, correction of those factors, and management of the symptoms of delirium (utilizing both pharmacological and nonpharmacological interventions).[10] Treatment of the symptoms of delirium should be initiated before, or in concert with, a diagnostic assessment of the etiologies to minimize distress to patients, staff, and family members. In the terminally ill patient who develops delirium in the last days of life ("terminal" delirium), the management

of delirium is unique, presenting a number of dilemmas, and the desired clinical outcome may be significantly altered by the dying process. The desired and often achievable outcome is a patient who is awake, alert, calm, comfortable, cognitively intact, not psychotic, not in pain, and communicating coherently with family and staff.

ASSESSMENT OF ETIOLOGIES OF DELIRIUM

The underlying etiologies of delirium are multiple (Table 70.2). In the medical setting, the diagnostic workup typically includes an assessment of potentially reversible causes, for example, dehydration or medication, as well as those that are potentially irreversible, for example, sepsis or major organ failure. The clinician should obtain a detailed history from the family and staff of the patient's baseline mental status and verify the current fluctuating mental status. Predisposing delirium risk factors should be reviewed in detail, including old age, physical frailty, multiple medical comorbidities, dementia, admission to the hospital with infection or dehydration, visual impairment, deafness, polypharmacy, renal impairment, and malnutrition.[3] Physical examination should seek evidence of infection, dehydration, fecal impaction, urinary retention, or organ (e.g., liver, pulmonary, and renal) failure.[5] Medication adverse effects should be reviewed as a possible cause. It is important to inquire about alcohol or other substance use disorders to be able to recognize and treat alcohol or other substance-induced withdrawal delirium. Opioids, corticosteroids, benzodiazepines, and anticholinergics are commonly associated with delirium particularly in the elderly and the terminally ill.[5,47] In palliative care settings, medications used for symptom control (e.g., antihistamines, opioids, tricyclic antidepressants, and corticosteroids) have been shown to significantly increase the overall burden of anticholinergic adverse effects, increasing the risk for delirium.[47] Gaudreau et al. prospectively studied the association of medication use with the development of delirium in[42] patients with cancer and found that daily doses of benzodiazepines above 2 mg, corticosteroids above 15 mg, and opioids above a morphine equivalent daily dose of 90 mg were

Table 70.2   *Causes of delirium in patients with advanced disease*

Direct CNS causes
    Primary brain tumors
    Metastatic spreads to CNS
    Seizures (including nonepileptiform status epilepticus)
Indirect causes
    Metabolic encephalopathy due to organ failure
    Electrolyte imbalance
    Treatment side effects from chemotherapeutic agents, corticosteroids, radiation therapy, opioids, anticholinergics, antiemetics, antivirals, and other medications and therapeutic modalities
    Infections
    Hematological abnormalities
    Nutritional deficiencies
    Paraneoplastic syndromes

associated with the development of delirium.[48] Laboratory tests can identify metabolic abnormalities (e.g., hypercalcemia, hyponatremia, hypoglycemia), hypoxia, or disseminated intravascular coagulation. In some instances, an electroencephalogram (to rule out seizures), brain imaging studies (to rule out brain metastases, intracranial bleeding, or ischemia), and lumbar puncture (to rule out leptomeningeal carcinomatosis or meningitis) may be appropriate.[5]

When confronted with delirium in the terminally ill or dying patient, a differential diagnosis should always be formulated as to the likely etiology or etiologies including underlying medical conditions, such as infections, electrolyte disturbances, organ failure, uncontrolled pain, and medication adverse effects. However, the clinician must take an individualized and judicious approach to such testing, consistent with the goals of care. There is an ongoing debate as to the appropriate extent of diagnostic evaluation that should be pursued in a dying patient with a terminal delirium. Most palliative care clinicians would undertake diagnostic studies only when a clinically suspected etiology can be identified easily, with a minimal use of invasive procedures, and treated effectively with simple interventions that carry minimal burden or risk of causing further distress. A survey of 270 physicians from 4 disciplines (palliative care, medical oncology, geriatrics, and geriatric psychiatry) found that about 85% of specialists would order basic blood tests when confronted with delirium in patients with advanced cancer; more than 40% of specialists reported that they would not do any investigation in patients with terminal delirium.[49] Diagnostic workup in pursuit of an etiology for delirium may be limited by either practical constraints such as the setting (home, hospice) or the focus on patient comfort so that unpleasant or painful diagnostics may be avoided. Most often, however, the etiology of terminal delirium is multifactorial or may not be determined. When a distinct cause is found for delirium in the terminally ill, it is often irreversible or difficult to treat. Studies, however, in patients with earlier stages of advanced cancer have demonstrated the potential utility of a thorough diagnostic assessment. When such diagnostic information is available, specific therapy may be able to reverse delirium. In a study of patients with advanced cancer admitted to hospice, the overall delirium reversibility rate was only 20% and the 30-day mortality rate was 83%.[50] Reversibility of delirium was highly dependent on the etiology: hypercalcemia was reversible in 38%; medications in 37%; infection in 12%; and hepatic failure, hypoxia, disseminated intravascular coagulation, and dehydration each in less than 10%. Leonard and colleagues found a 27% recovery rate from delirium among patients in palliative care. Patients with irreversible delirium experienced greater disturbances of sleep and cognition. Mean (SD) time until death was 39.7 (69.8) days for 33 patients with reversible delirium vs. 16.8 (10.0) days for 88 patients with irreversible delirium.[2] In a prospective study of delirium in patients on a palliative care unit, investigators reported that the etiology of delirium was multifactorial in a great majority of cases.[51] Even though delirium occurred in 88% of dying patients in the last week of life, delirium was reversible in approximately 50% of episodes. Causes of delirium that were most associated with

reversibility included dehydration and psychoactive or opioid medications. Major organ failure and hypoxic encephalopathies were less likely to be reversed in terminal delirium.[51]

In light of the several studies on the reversibility of delirium, the prognosis of patients who develop delirium is defined by the interaction of the patients' baseline physiologic susceptibility to delirium (e.g., predisposing factors), the precipitating etiologies, and any response to treatment. If a patient's susceptibility or resilience is modifiable, then targeted interventions may reduce the risk of delirium upon exposure to a precipitant and enhance the capacity to respond to treatment. Conversely, if a patient's vulnerability is high and resistant to modification, then exposure to precipitants enhances the likelihood of developing delirium and may diminish the probability of a complete restoration of cognitive function.

NONPHARMACOLOGICAL INTERVENTIONS

In addition to seeking out and potentially correcting underlying causes of delirium, nonpharmacological and supportive therapies are important. In fact, in the dying patient, they may be the only steps taken. Fluid and electrolyte balance, nutrition, measures to help reduce anxiety and disorientation, and interactions with and education of family members may be useful. Measures to help reduce anxiety and disorientation (i.e., structure and familiarity) include a quiet, well-lit room with familiar objects, a visible clock or calendar, and the presence of family.

In nonpalliative care settings, there is evidence that nonpharmacological interventions result in faster improvement in delirium and slower deterioration in cognition. However, these interventions were not found to have any beneficial effects on mortality or health-related quality of life when compared with usual care.[52–57] Nonpharmacological interventions used in these studies include oxygen delivery, fluid and electrolyte administration, ensuring bowel and bladder function, nutrition, mobilization, pain treatment, frequent orientation, use of visual and hearing aids, and environmental modifications to enhance a sense of familiarity (Table 70.3).[52–57] Low implementation rates of all the components of the interventions were identified as the main limiting factor in the interpretation of the study results in a majority of nonpharmacological intervention trials.[58] Physical restraints should be avoided in patients who are at risk for developing delirium and for those with delirium. Physical restraints have been identified as an independent risk factor for the persistence of delirium at discharge.[59] Recent evidence suggests that restraint-free management of patients should be the standard of care for prevention and treatment of delirium.[60] One-to-one observation may be necessary while maintaining the safety of the patient without the use of any restraints.

PHARMACOLOGICAL INTERVENTIONS IN DELIRIUM

While no medications have been approved by the U.S. Food and Drug Administration (FDA) for treatment of delirium, treatment with antipsychotics or sedatives is often required

Reducing polypharmacy

Control of pain

Sleep hygiene (minimize noise and interventions at bedtime)

Monitor for dehydration and fluid-electrolyte disturbances

Monitor nutrition

Monitor for sensory deficits, provide visual and hearing aids

Encourage early mobilization (minimize the use of immobilizing catheters, IV lines, and physical restraints)

Monitor bowel and bladder functioning

Reorient the patient frequently

Place an orientation board, clock, or familiar objects in patient rooms

Encourage cognitively stimulating activities

Adapted from Breitbart, W. and Alici, Y. *JAMA*, 300, 2898, 2008.

a Nonpharmacological interventions are supported by the U.S. Preventive Services Task Force (USPSTF) Level I evidence in reducing the incidence of delirium in nonpalliative care settings.

b Nonpharmacological interventions are supported by the USPSTF Level I evidence in faster improvement of delirium and in slower deterioration in cognition following an episode of delirium in nonpalliative care settings. However, these interventions were not found to have any effects on mortality or health-related quality of life when compared with usual care.

to control the symptoms of delirium in palliative care settings.[10] There have been an increasing number of delirium prevention and treatment studies published within the last decade (Table 70.4). Antipsychotics, cholinesterase inhibitors, and alpha-2 agonists are the three groups of medications studied in randomized controlled trials in different patient populations. In palliative care settings, the evidence is supportive of short-term low-dose use of antipsychotics in the control of symptoms of delirium with close monitoring for possible side effects especially in older patients with multiple medical comorbidities (Tables 70.5 and 70.6).[10] It is also recommended that nonpharmacological interventions in the routine care of patients at risk for delirium and patients with delirium be implemented, based on the evidence from the medically ill older persons.[10] Following is a brief description of each medication class with a review of the evidence of their use in the treatment of delirium in palliative care settings.

Antipsychotics

Antipsychotics, formerly known as neuroleptics, are a group of medications primarily indicated for schizophrenia, bipolar disorder, and other mood disorders. The mechanisms by which these drugs ameliorate disturbances of thought and affect in psychotic states are not fully understood, but presumably, they act by blocking the postsynaptic mesolimbic dopamine receptors. Typical (conventional or first-generation) and atypical (second-generation) antipsychotics differ in their effects on the different dopamine and serotonin receptor subtypes. Typical antipsychotics are traditionally known to be associated with

a higher incidence of extrapyramidal side effects (EPS) due to their effects on the striatal dopamine 2 (D2) receptors. On the other hand, atypical antipsychotics (i.e., risperidone, olanzapine, quetiapine, ziprasidone, and aripiprazole) have been associated with weight gain, and metabolic syndrome, but significantly less risk for EPS. There have been case reports, case series, retrospective chart reviews, open-label trials, randomized controlled comparison trials, and, most recently, placebo-controlled trials with both typical and atypical antipsychotics in the treatment of delirium.[42–44,61–73] Study populations mostly include general medically ill patients, postoperative patients, and patients in intensive care unit settings, and only a few focus specifically on patients with delirium in palliative care settings. Table 70.4 presents a summary of all the randomized controlled antipsychotic trials for the treatment of delirium published to date. More than a dozen open-label studies with antipsychotics can be found elsewhere.[61,62]

The American Psychiatric Association (APA) practice guidelines published in 1999 recommended the use of antipsychotics as the first-line pharmacological option in the treatment of symptoms of delirium.[23] The APA guidelines recommend the use of low-dose haloperidol (i.e., 1–2 mg per oral [PO] every 4 hours PRN or 0.25–0.5 mg PO every 4 hours for the elderly) as the treatment of choice in cases where medications are necessary.[23] Haloperidol is considered to be the preferred antipsychotic in the treatment of delirium in patients with advanced disease due to its efficacy and tolerability (few anticholinergic effects, lack of active metabolites, and availability in different routes of administration).[5] In general, doses of haloperidol need not exceed 20 mg in a 24 hours period; however, some clinicians advocate higher doses (up to 250 mg/24 hour of haloperidol intravenously) in selected cases.[74] Typically 0.5–1.0 mg haloperidol (PO, intravenous [IV], intramuscular [IM], subcutaneous [SC]) is administered, with repeat doses every 45–60 min titrated against target symptoms of agitation, paranoia, and fear.[23] An IV route can facilitate rapid onset of medication effects. If IV access is unavailable, IM or SC routes of administration could be used with switch to the oral route when possible. The majority of delirious patients can be managed with oral haloperidol. Parenteral doses are approximately twice as potent as oral doses. Haloperidol is administered by the SC route by many palliative care practitioners.[5] It is important to note that the FDA has issued a warning about the risk of QTc prolongation and torsades de pointes on electrocardiogram with IV haloperidol; therefore, monitoring QTc intervals closely among medically ill patients on IV haloperidol has become the standard clinical practice.[75] A common strategy in the management of symptoms related to delirium is to add parenteral lorazepam to a regimen of haloperidol.[5] Lorazepam (0.5–1.0 mg every 1–2 hours PO or IV) along with haloperidol may be more effective in rapidly sedating the agitated delirious patient and may minimize EPS associated with haloperidol.[76] An alternative strategy is to switch from haloperidol to a more sedating antipsychotic such as chlorpromazine, especially in the intensive care unit setting where close blood pressure monitoring is feasible. It is important to monitor for anticholinergic and hypotensive adverse effects of chlorpromazine, particularly in elderly patients.[5]

Table 70.4 *Randomized control trials with antipsychotics in the treatment of delirium*

	Intervention	Dose and duration, mean (SD)	Results	Comments
Breitbart et al.[42]	Double-blind RCT of terminally ill AIDS patients: 11, haloperidol; 13, chlorpromazine; and 6, lorazepam for treatment of delirium.	1.4 (1.2) mg/day haloperidol, 36 (18.4) mg/day chlorpromazine, 4.6 (4.7) mg/day lorazepam used for up to 6 days.	DRS scores significantly improved in haloperidol and chlorpromazine groups ($p < 0.05$). No significant extrapyramidal symptoms were observed.	Lorazepam group was discontinued early due to worsening of delirium symptoms.
Hu et al.[66]	Double-blind RCT of hospitalized patients: 75, olanzapine; 72, IM haloperidol; and 29, oral placebo for the treatment of delirium	4.5 (4) mg/day olanzapine, 7 (2.3) mg/day haloperidol, and placebo, used for 7 days	The improvement in DRS scores were significantly higher in the olanzapine (72%) and haloperidol (70%) groups vs. placebo (29.7%) ($p < 0.01$). Increased rates of extrapyramidal symptoms observed in the haloperidol group.	Comparison of oral olanzapine and oral placebo with IM haloperidol hinders the quality of double-blind study design.
Kim et al.[71]	A randomized, single-blind, comparative clinical trial comparing the effectiveness of risperidone (n = 17) and olanzapine (n = 15) in the treatment of delirium among mostly oncology patients.	Study period: 7 days. The mean starting doses were 0.6(0.2) mg/day risperidone and 1.8(0.6) mg/day olanzapine. The mean doses at last observation were 0.9(0.6) mg/day risperidone and 2.4(1.7) mg/day olanzapine.	Significant within-group improvements in the DRS-R-98 scores over time were observed in both treatment groups; the response (defined as a 50% reduction in the DRS-R-98 scores) rates did not differ significantly between the two groups (risperidone group: 64.7%, olanzapine group: 73.3%).	The response to risperidone was significantly poorer in patients >or =70 years of age compared with those aged <70 years. There was no significant difference in the safety profiles, including extrapyramidal symptoms (EPSs), between the two groups.
Han and Kim[65]	Double-blind RCT of hospitalized patients: 12, haloperidol; 12, risperidone for the treatment of delirium	1.7 (0.84) mg/day haloperidol, 1 (0.4) mg/day risperidone, used for 7 days.	MDAS scores improved significantly in both groups, but no significant difference between groups was observed.	Researchers were not able to provide tablets identical in appearance, which might have hindered the double-blind study design. No significant difference in adverse effects observed.

Study	Description	Dosage	Results	Safety
Girard et al.[68]	Placebo-controlled randomized feasibility trial of intensive care unit patients: 35 haloperidol, 30 ziprasidone, 36 placebo for the treatment of delirium.	Patients in the haloperidol group received 15.0 mg/day (10.8–17.0 mg/day), and patients in the ziprasidone group received 113.3 mg/day (81.0–140.0 mg/day) for an average of 4 days.	There were no differences in the number of days alive without delirium between the three treatment groups. The study did not find any differences in other outcomes such as ventilator-free days, hospital length of stay, or mortality.	The study reported no difference in any safety concerns (i.e., akathisia, neuroleptic malignant syndrome, extrapyramidal symptoms, QT prolongation, or arrhythmias). The adverse events were similar between the three groups with no serious events.
Devlin et al.[69]	Placebo-controlled randomized pilot trial of intensive care unit patients with delirium who had an as-needed haloperidol order: 18 quetiapine or 18 placebo for the treatment of delirium	Quetiapine 110 mg (88–191 mg) for 102 hours (84–168); placebo group for 186 (108–228) p = 0.04.	Quetiapine add-on was associated with a shorter time to first resolution of delirium [1.0 (inter quartile range [IQR], 0.5–3.0) vs. 4.5 days (IQR, 2.0–7.0; p = 0.001)], and a reduced duration of delirium [36 (IQR, 12–87) vs. 120 hours (IQR, 60–195; p = 0.006)].	The incidence of EPSs was similar between groups, however, more somnolence was observed with quetiapine (22% vs. 11%; p = 0.66).
Tahir et al.[70]	Placebo-controlled randomized trial in medical and surgical patients with delirium: 21 patients with quetiapine and 20 patients with placebo.	The mean dose of quetiapine was 40 mg on day 4; 25 mg on day 1; 37.5 mg on day 10.	The quetiapine group recovered 82.7% (37.1%) faster (p = 0.026) than the placebo group in terms of DRS-R-98 severity score. However, there was no difference in the total DRS-R-98 scores at anytime.	The study reported no difference in any safety concerns between medication and placebo arms.
Grover et al.[67]	A single-blind randomized controlled trial to compare the efficacy and safety of olanzapine (n = 23) and risperidone (n = 21) vs. haloperidol (n = 20) in patients with delirium admitted to medical and surgical wards.	A flexible dose regimen (haloperidol, 0.25–10 mg; risperidone, 0.25–4 mg; olanzapine, 1.25–20 mg) was used.	There was a significant reduction in DRS-R98 severity scores over the period of 6 days, but there was no difference between the three medication groups.	Researchers concluded that risperidone and olanzapine are as efficacious as haloperidol in the treatment of delirium.

Source: Adapted from Breitbart, W. and Alici, Y., J. Clin. Oncol., 30(11), 1206, April 10, 2012.

Table 70.5 *Antipsychotic medications used in the treatment of delirium*

Medication	Dose range	Routes of administration	Side effects	Comments
Typical antipsychotics				
Haloperidol[b]	0.5–2 mg every 2–12 h	PO, IV, IM, SC	Extrapyramidal adverse effects can occur at higher doses. Monitor QT interval on electrocardiogram (EKG).	Remains the gold-standard therapy for delirium. May add lorazepam (0.5–1 mg every 2–4 h) for agitated patients. Double-blind controlled trials support efficacy in the treatment of delirium. A pilot placebo-controlled trial suggests lack of efficacy when compared to placebo.
Chlorpromazine[b]	12.5–50 mg every 4–6 h	PO, IV, IM, SC, PR	More sedating and anticholinergic compared with haloperidol. Monitor blood pressure for hypotension. More suitable for use in ICU settings for closer blood pressure monitoring.	May be preferred in agitated patients due to its sedative effect. Double-blind controlled trials support efficacy in the treatment of delirium. No placebo-controlled trials.
Atypical antipsychotics				
Olanzapine[b]	2.5–5 mg every 12–24 h	PO,[a] IM	Sedation is the main dose-limiting adverse effect in short-term use.	Older age, preexisting dementia, and hypoactive subtype of delirium have been associated with poor response. Double-blind comparison trials with haloperidol and risperidone support efficacy in the treatment of delirium. A pilot placebo-controlled prevention trial suggested worsening in delirium severity. A placebo-controlled study is supportive of efficacy in reducing delirium severity and duration.
Risperidone[b]	0.25–1 mg every 12–24 h	PO[a]	Extrapyramidal adverse effects can occur with doses >6 mg/day. Orthostatic hypotension.	Double-blind comparison trials support efficacy in the treatment of delirium. No placebo control trials.
Quetiapine[b]	12.5–100 mg every 12–24 h	PO	Sedation, orthostatic hypotension.	Sedating effects may be helpful in patients with sleep–wake cycle disturbance. Pilot placebo-controlled trials suggest efficacy in the treatment of delirium. However, studies allowed for the concomitant use of haloperidol, which makes the results difficult to interpret.
Ziprasidone	10–40 mg every 12–24 h	PO, IM	Monitor QT interval on EKG.	Placebo-controlled, double blind trial suggests lack of efficacy in the treatment of delirium.
Aripiprazole[c]	5–30 mg every 24 hours	PO,[a] IM	Monitor for akathisia.	Evidence is limited. A prospective open-label trial suggests comparable efficacy to haloperidol. No placebo-controlled trials.

Source: Adapted from Breitbart, W. and Alici, Y., *J. Clin. Oncol.*, 30(11), 1206, April 10, 2012.

[a] Risperidone, olanzapine, and aripiprazole are available in orally disintegrating tablets. There have been no intervention or prevention trials with the use of recently released antipsychotics, including paliperidone, iloperidone, asenapine, or lurasidone in the treatment or prevention of delirium.

[b] Despite shortcomings of the studies described in the text there is USPSTF Level I evidence for the use of haloperidol, risperidone, olanzapine, and quetiapine in the treatment of delirium.

[c] There is USPSTF Level II-2 evidence for the use of aripiprazole in the treatment of delirium.

A 2004 Cochrane review on drug therapy for delirium in the terminally ill concluded that haloperidol was the most suitable medication for the treatment of patients with delirium near the end of life, with chlorpromazine being an acceptable alternative based on one randomized controlled trial with haloperidol, chlorpromazine, and lorazepam.[63]

A 2007 Cochrane review, comparing the efficacy and the incidence of adverse effects between haloperidol and atypical antipsychotics, concluded that, like haloperidol, selected atypical antipsychotics (risperidone and olanzapine) were effective in managing delirium.[64] Haloperidol doses greater than 4.5 mg/day resulted in increased rates of extrapyramidal

Table 70.6 *Recommendations on monitoring patients with delirium for antipsychotic side effects in palliative care settings*[a]

EKG—Baseline, and with every dose increase [consider daily monitoring if on high doses (e.g., haloperidol > 5–10 mg daily), patients with underlying unstable cardiac disease, patients with electrolyte disturbances, patients on other QT prolonging medications,[b] medically frail, older patients; patients with unstable cardiac diseases or those on IV antipsychotics may require continuous monitoring in consultation with cardiology]

Fasting blood glucose—Baseline, and weekly

Body mass index—Baseline, and weekly

EPS (including parkinsonism, dystonia, akathisia, neuroleptic malignant syndrome)—Baseline, and daily

Blood pressure, pulse—Baseline, and at least daily (continuous monitoring may be required in medically unstable patients; orthostatic measurements should be considered with antipsychotics with alpha-1 antagonist effects such as chlorpromazine, risperidone, and quetiapine)

Source: Adapted from Breitbart, W. and Alici, Y., *J. Clin. Oncol.*, 30(11), 1206, April 10, 2012.

[a] Recommendations are based on the Consensus Development Conference on antipsychotic drugs and obesity and diabetes.

[b] The risk of QT prolongation is directly correlated with higher antipsychotic doses, with parenteral formulations (e.g., IV haloperidol) of antipsychotics, and with certain medications (e.g., ziprasidone, thioridazine). In individual patients, an absolute QTc interval of >500 ms or an increase of 60 ms (or more than 20%) from baseline is regarded as indicating an increased risk of torsades des pointes. Discontinuation of the antipsychotic and a consultation with cardiology should be considered, especially if there is continued need for the use of antipsychotics.

symptoms compared with the atypical antipsychotics, but low-dose haloperidol (i.e., less than 3.5 mg/day) was not shown to result in a greater frequency of extrapyramidal adverse effects.[64]

Recent randomized and placebo-controlled trials support the recommendations of the APA guidelines for the management of delirium in that low-dose haloperidol (i.e., 1–2 mg PO every 4 hours as needed or 0.25–0.5 mg PO every 4 hours for the elderly) continues to be the first-line agent for the treatment of symptoms of delirium.[62,64–67] Based on the current evidence, atypical antipsychotics could be considered as an effective alternative to haloperidol, particularly in patients who are sensitive or intolerant to the use of haloperidol.[65–72] None of the antipsychotics were found to be superior when compared to others in the treatment of delirium symptoms, and evidence for efficacy in the improvement of the symptoms of delirium exists for the following atypical antipsychotics: quetiapine, olanzapine, risperidone, and aripiprazole.[42,43,61–72] In light of the existing literature, risperidone may be used in the treatment of delirium, starting at doses ranging from 0.25 to 1 mg and titrated up as necessary with particular attention to the risk of EPS, orthostatic hypotension, and sedation at higher doses. Olanzapine can be started between 2.5 and 5 mg nightly and titrated up with the sedation being the major limiting factor, which may be favorable in the treatment of hyperactive delirium. The current literature on the use of quetiapine suggests a starting dose of 25–50 mg and a titration up to 100–200 mg a day (usually at twice daily divided doses). Sedation and

orthostatic hypotension are the main dose-limiting factors. A starting dose of 10–15 mg daily for aripiprazole is suggested based on open-label studies, with a maximum dose of 30 mg daily. Of the atypical antipsychotics, olanzapine, aripiprazole, and ziprasidone are available in IM formulations. The use of SC olanzapine has been recently studied with promising results.[73]

Important considerations in starting treatment with any antipsychotic for delirium should include EPS risk, sedation, anticholinergic side effects, cardiac arrhythmias, and possible drug–drug interactions (Table 70.6). Despite the growing evidence for the use of antipsychotics in the treatment of symptoms of delirium, there have been concerns regarding the safety of antipsychotics, especially in older patients with dementia.[1] The FDA has issued a black box warning of increased risk of mortality associated with the use of antipsychotics in elderly patients with dementia-related behavioral disturbances. This warning was based on a meta-analysis by Schneider et al. of 17 placebo-controlled trials involving patients with dementia.[77] The risk of death in patients treated with atypical antipsychotic agents was 1.6–1.7 times greater than in those who received placebo. Most deaths were associated with cardiovascular disease or infection. A second retrospective study of nearly 23,000 older patients found higher mortality rates associated with typical than with atypical antipsychotics—whether or not they had dementia.[78] This finding led to an extension of the FDA warning to typical antipsychotics.[79] A recent retrospective cohort study of Medicaid enrollees in Tennessee demonstrated an increased risk of serious ventricular arrhythmias and sudden cardiac death among the users of both typical and atypical antipsychotics, which expanded the diagnostic categories and the age groups at risk.[80] A retrospective, case control analysis of 326 elderly hospitalized patients with delirium at an acute care community hospital, comparing the risk of mortality among patients who received an antipsychotic versus those who did not, showed that of the 111 patients who received an antipsychotic, a total of 16 patients died during that hospitalization. The odds ratio (OR) of association between antipsychotic use and death was 1.53 (95% C.I. 0.83–2.80) in univariate and 1.61 (95% C.I. 0.88–2.96) in multivariate analysis.[81] The researchers concluded that among elderly patients with delirium, administration of antipsychotics was not associated with a statistically significant increased risk of mortality.[81] However, prospective, randomized-controlled studies with a larger sample size are needed to clarify this conclusion.

Caution is advised when using antipsychotic medications, especially in elderly patients with dementia, due to the FDA warnings described earlier. Therefore, the use of nonpharmacological interventions is critical to reduce the need to use antipsychotic medications whenever possible. It is also important to recognize that antipsychotics have complex mechanisms of action, mostly affecting multiple neurotransmitter systems that can lead to unwanted side effects. Therefore, the benefits of initiating antipsychotic treatment for delirium should be weighed against risks associated with its use. As mentioned previously, in palliative care settings, the evidence is most clearly supportive of the short-term low-dose use of antipsy-chotics for the control of the symptoms of delirium, with close monitoring for possible side effects, especially in older patients with multiple medical comorbidities.[10]

Psychostimulants

The use of psychostimulants in the treatment of hypoactive subtype of delirium has been suggested.[82–84] However, studies with psychostimulants in treating delirium are limited to case reports and one open-label study.[82–84] The risks of precipitat-ing agitation and exacerbating psychotic symptoms should be carefully evaluated when psychostimulants are considered in the treatment of delirium in palliative care settings.[10]

Cholinesterase inhibitors

Impaired cholinergic function has been implicated as one of the final common pathways in the neuropathogenesis of delirium.[22] Despite the case reports of beneficial effects of donepezil and rivastigmine, a 2008 Cochrane review[85] concluded that there is currently no evidence from controlled trials supporting the use of cholinesterase inhibitors in the treatment of delirium.

A pilot, double-blind, placebo-controlled trial with riv-astigmine in the treatment of patients with delirium in general hospital settings failed to show any differences between rivastig-mine and placebo groups in the duration of delirium.[86] A recent European multicenter study conducted in intensive care units comparing rivastigmine and placebo for the treatment of delir-ium was stopped prematurely because of increased mortality in the rivastigmine group. No common cause of mortality could be identified among patients who died while on rivastigmine.[87]

The use of cholinesterase inhibitors in delirium have not been studied in palliative care settings. On the basis of the existing evidence from general hospital and critical care set-tings, cholinesterase inhibitors cannot be recommended in the treatment of delirium.[10]

Other agents

While antipsychotics are most effective in diminishing agita-tion, clearing the sensorium and improving cognition are not always possible in delirium, which complicates the last days of life. Approximately 30% of dying patients with delirium do not have their symptoms adequately controlled with antipsychotic medications.[88–91] Processes causing delirium may be ongoing and irreversible during the active dying phase. In such cases, a reasonable choice is the use of sedative agents such as ben-zodiazepines (e.g., midazolam and lorazepam), propofol, or opioids to achieve a state of quiet sedation.[88–93] Delirium has, in fact, been identified as the main indication for the use of palliative sedation in up to 82% of cases in symptom control studies among the terminally ill.[88–97] Clinicians are often con-cerned that the use of sedating medications may hasten death via respiratory depression, hypotension, or even starvation. However, studies have shown that the use of opioids and psy-chotropic agents in hospice and palliative care settings is asso-ciated with longer rather than shorter survival.[94–97]

Dexmedetomidine, a selective α(2)-adrenergic receptor ago-nist that is indicated in the United States for the sedation of mechanically ventilated adult patients in intensive care settings and in nonintubated adult patients prior to and/or during surgical and other procedures, has been considered for the prevention and treatment of delirium in the palliative care settings and enhance-ment of analgesia.[98–100] Clinical trials with dexmedetomidine in the intensive care unit settings have shown mixed results for the prevention and treatment of delirium.[98,99] There have not been any studies with dexmedetomidine for the treatment of delirium in palliative care settings to the best of our knowledge.

Prevention of delirium

Given the increased morbidity and mortality associated with delirium, effective strategies that prevent delirium should be a high priority in palliative care settings.

Nonpharmacological interventions have been studied in the prevention of delirium among older patient populations in gen-eral hospital settings with promising results.[5,101–103] The use of nonpharmacological interventions in the prevention of delirium has been shown to reduce the incidence of delirium in general medical settings. The study effect sizes suggested statistically significant reductions in delirium incidence by about one-third with multicomponent interventions.[102,103] A simple multicom-ponent preventive intervention was found to be ineffective in reducing delirium incidence or severity among cancer patients (n = 1516) receiving end-of-life care.[104] No difference was observed between the intervention and the usual-care groups in delirium incidence (OR 0.94, p = 0.66), delirium severity (1.83 vs. 1.92; p = 0.07), total days in delirium (4.57 vs. 3.57 days; p = 0.63), or duration of first delirium episode (2.9 vs. 2.1 days; p = 0.96).[104]

A summary of nonpharmacological interventions used in the delirium treatment and prevention trials described earlier is included in Table 70.3. These preventive interventions might be adapted to the needs of patients near the end of life, allowing families to work to actively maintain patient comfort.[5,58]

A variety of pharmacological interventions have also been considered in the prevention of delirium. Antipsychotics, cho-linesterase inhibitors, melatonin, and dexmedetomidine have been studied in the prevention of delirium in randomized controlled delirium prevention studies conducted in different settings.[98–100,103,105–108]

A 2007 Cochrane review of delirium prevention studies in different patient populations concluded that the evidence on the effectiveness of interventions to prevent delirium was sparse; therefore; no recommendations could be made regarding the use of pharmacological interventions for the prevention of delirium.[102]

Studies published since 2007 have shown mixed results with cholinesterase inhibitors, antipsychotics, melatonin, and dex-medetomidine. Those studies could be summarized as follows.

A double-blind, randomized, placebo-controlled trial of rivastigmine conducted among 120 patients aged 65 or older undergoing elective cardiac surgery[107] did not show a statis-tically significant difference between placebo and rivastig-mine groups. Delirium developed in 17 out of 57 (30%) and

18 out of 56 (32%) patients in the placebo and rivastigmine groups, respectively (p = 0.8).

A 2010 study by Larsen and colleagues[109] tested the efficacy of perioperative olanzapine administration to prevent postoperative delirium in elderly patients (n = 400) after joint-replacement surgery in a randomized, double-blind, placebo-controlled trial. The incidence of postoperative delirium was lower in the olanzapine group compared to the placebo group for both knee- and hip-replacement surgery patients (14.3% [n = 28] versus 40.2% [n = 82]; 95% CI: 17.6–34.2; p < 0.0001). However, delirium lasted longer in the olanzapine group than in the placebo group (2.2 [SD = 1.3] versus 1.6 [SD = 0.7] days; p = 0.02). The severity of delirium (expressed as the maximum DRS-R-98 score on the first day of delirium) was also greater in the olanzapine-treated group than in the placebo group (16.44 [SD: 3.7] versus 14.5 [SD: 2.7]; p = 0.02).

A study published in 2012 by Wang et al. evaluated the efficacy and safety of short-term low-dose IV haloperidol (0.5 mg IV bolus injection followed by continuous infusion at a rate of 0.1 mg/h for 12 hours) for delirium prevention in critically ill older patients (n = 457) following noncardiac surgery in a prospective, randomized, double-blind, and placebo-controlled design. The incidence of delirium during the first 7 days after surgery was 15.3% (35/229) in the haloperidol group and 23.2% (53/228) in the control group (p = 0.031), supporting the efficacy of haloperidol use to prevent delirium in the studied patient population. There was no significant difference with regard to all-cause 28-day mortality between the two groups (0.9% [2/229] vs. 2.6% [6/228]; p = 0.175). No drug-related side effects were documented.[111]

A randomized, double-blinded, placebo-controlled study[112] (n = 145) conducted in the Internal Medicine service of a tertiary care centre evaluated the efficacy of low-dose exogenous melatonin (0.5 mg every night for 14 days or until discharge) in decreasing the incidence of delirium. Melatonin was associated with a lower risk of delirium (12.0% vs. 31.0%, p = 0.014), with an OR, adjusted for dementia and comorbidities of 0.19 (95% CI: 0.06–0.62). However, results were not different when patients with prevalent delirium were excluded.

As noted earlier, although more recent trials have suggested haloperidol, olanzapine, dexmedetomidine (noted in the previous section), and melatonin to be effective in the prevention of delirium, there are no pharmacological agents proven effective in the prevention of delirium in palliative care settings. Based on the current literature, no recommendations can be made regarding the use of medications in the prevention of delirium among palliative care patients.

Controversies in the management of terminal delirium

Several aspects of the use of antipsychotics and other pharmacological agents in the management of delirium in the dying patient remain controversial in some circles. A study by Agar and colleagues[49] showed that physicians from different disciplines manage terminal delirium differently. According to a survey of 270 physicians from different disciplines, medical oncologists were found to be more likely to manage terminal delirium with benzodiazepines or benzodiazepine and antipsychotic combinations. On the other hand, palliative care physicians were more likely to use antipsychotics to manage delirium symptoms, including hypoactive subtype of delirium.

Some have argued that pharmacological interventions with antipsychotics or benzodiazepines are inappropriate in the dying patient. Delirium is viewed by some as a natural part of the dying process that should not be altered. In particular, there are clinicians who care for the dying who view hallucinations and delusions, which involve dead relatives communicating with, or in fact welcoming dying patients to heaven, as an important element in the transition from life to death. Clearly, there are many patients who experience hallucinations and delusions during delirium that are pleasant and in fact comforting, and many clinicians question the appropriateness of intervening pharmacologically in such instances. Another concern that is often raised is that these patients are so close to death that aggressive treatment is unnecessary. Parenteral antipsychotics or sedatives may be mistakenly avoided because of exaggerated fears that they might hasten death through hypotension or respiratory depression. Many are unnecessarily pessimistic about the possible results of neuroleptic treatment for delirium. They argue that since the underlying pathophysiological process often continues unabated (such as hepatic or renal failure), no improvement can be expected in the patient's mental status. There is concern that antipsychotics or sedatives may worsen delirium by making the patient more confused or sedated.

Clinical experience in managing delirium in dying patients suggests that the use of antipsychotics in the management of agitation, paranoia, hallucinations, and altered sensorium is safe, effective, and often quite appropriate.[5] Management of delirium on a case-by-case basis seems wisest. The agitated delirious dying patient should probably be given antipsychotics to help restore calm. A "wait and see" approach, prior to using antipsychotics, may be appropriate with some patients who have a lethargic or somnolent presentation of delirium or those who have frankly pleasant or comforting hallucinations. Such a "wait and see" approach must, however, be tempered by the knowledge that a lethargic or "hypoactive" delirium may very quickly and unexpectedly become an agitated or "hyperactive" delirium that can threaten the serenity and safety of the patient, family and staff. Similarly, hallucinations and delusions during a delirium that are pleasant and comforting can quickly become menacing and terrifying. It is important to remember that by their nature, the symptoms of delirium are unstable and fluctuate over time.

Finally, perhaps the most challenging of clinical problems is management of the dying patient with a "terminal" delirium that is unresponsive to standard antipsychotic interventions, whose symptoms can only be controlled by sedation to the point of a significantly decreased level of consciousness. Before undertaking interventions, such as midazolam or propofol infusions, where the best achievable goal is a calm and comfortable but sedated and unresponsive patient, the clinician must first take several steps. The clinician must have a discussion with the family (and the patient if there are lucid moments when the patient appears to have capacity), eliciting their concerns and wishes for the type of care that can best honor their desire to provide comfort and symptom control during the dying process. The clinician should describe the optimal achievable goals of therapy as they currently exist. Family members should be informed that the goal of sedation is to provide comfort and symptom control, not to hasten death. They should also be told to anticipate that sedation may result in a premature sense of loss and that they may feel their loved one is in some sort of limbo state, not yet dead, but yet no longer alive in the vital sense. The distress and confusion that family members can experience during such a period can be ameliorated by including the family in the decision making and emphasizing the shared goals of care. Sedation in such patients is not always complete or irreversible; some patients have periods of wakefulness despite sedation, and many clinicians will periodically lighten sedation to reassess the patient's condition. Ultimately, the clinician must always keep in mind the goals of care and communicate these goals to the staff, patients, and family members. The ethical concerns of palliative sedation have been reviewed in an article by Lo and Rubenfeld.[93] The clinician must weigh each of the issues outlined earlier in making decisions on how to best manage the dying patient who presents with delirium that preserves and respects the dignity and values of that individual and family.

Prognostic implications of delirium in the terminally Ill

It is important to emphasize the prognostic value of delirium in terminally ill patients. Delirium is a relatively reliable predictor of approaching death in the coming days to weeks.[58] The death rates among hospitalized elderly patients with delirium over the 3-month postdischarge period range from 22% to 76%, the wide range most likely reflecting the variability in underlying general medical conditions contributing to delirium in elderly patients.[59] In the palliative care setting, several studies provide support that delirium reliably predicts impending death in patients with advanced cancer.[113] Bruera and colleagues[114] demonstrated a significant association between delirium and the likelihood of dying within 4 weeks. In Japan, Morita and colleague[115] showed that delirium predicted poor short-term prognosis in patients admitted to hospice. Caraceni and colleagues[116] evaluated the impact of delirium on patients for whom chemotherapy was no longer considered effective and had been referred to palliative care programs. The length of survival of patients with delirium differed significantly from those without delirium. Compared with an overall median survival of 39 days in their study, delirious patients died, on average, within 21 days. Mori and colleagues[117] retrospectively reviewed 166 consecutive cancer patients admitted to a palliative care unit to determine the association between changes in symptoms and inpatient mortality among advanced cancer patients. One hundred and thirty-four patients (80.7%) were discharged alive, and 32 (19.3%) died during hospitalization. Persistent delirium was significantly associated with inpatient mortality (OR 2.59, 95% CI: 0.09–6.17, p = 0.031), although presence of baseline delirium was not.

Given prognostic significance of delirium, recognizing an episode of delirium in the late phases of palliative care is critically important in treatment planning and in advising family members on what to expect.

CONCLUSION

Palliative care clinicians commonly encounter delirium as a major complication of terminal illness. Proper assessment, diagnosis, and management of delirium are essential in improving the quality of life and minimizing morbidity in palliative care settings for patients, families, and health care professionals.

Key learning points

- Delirium occurs in up to 85% of patients prior to death.
- Hypoactive subtype of delirium is as common and as distressing as the hyperactive subtype of delirium.
- There are typically three or more etiologies for delirium in the palliative care setting.
- In the terminally ill, delirium is reversible in only 50% of cases compared with more than 80% of cases in patients with earlier stage disease.
- The management of delirium involves the concurrent search for and treatment of the underlying etiology while actively controlling the symptoms of delirium.
- Delirium often is a harbinger of impending death. Issues of end-of-life care treatment preferences are ideally dealt with prior to the onset of delirium.
- Delirium is associated with high levels of distress in patients, family members, and nurses. Education of family members and nurses in the palliative care setting is important.
- Current evidence is supportive of the short-term use of antipsychotics in the treatment of symptoms of delirium (i.e., agitation, sleep–wake cycle disturbances, delusions, hallucinations) with close monitoring for possible side effects especially in elderly patients with multiple medical comorbidities. The choice of antipsychotic medication for the treatment of delirium should be based on the clinical presentation of the patient and the side effect profile of each antipsychotic drug, as none of the antipsychotics were found to be superior to others in comparison trials.
- It is strongly recommended to implement nonpharmacological interventions in the routine care of patients who are either at risk for delirium and for patients with established delirium, based on the evidence from nonpalliative care settings. There are no known risks associated with the use of nonpharmacological interventions
- Sedation may be necessary in up to 30% of patients with delirium unresponsive to antipsychotics.

REFERENCES

1 American Psychiatric Association. *Diagnostic and Statistical Manual of Mental Disorders.* 4th edn, text revision. Washington, DC: American Psychiatric Association Press; 2000.

2 Leonard M, Raju B, Conroy M et al. Reversibility of delirium in terminally ill patients and predictors of mortality. *Palliat Med* 2008;22(7):848–854.

◆ 3 Inouye SK. Delirium in older persons. *N Engl J Med* 2006;354:1157–1165.

4 Witlox J, Kalisvaart KJ, de Jonghe JF et al. Cerebrospinal fluid beta-amyloid and tau are not associated with risk of delirium: A prospective cohort study in older adults with hip fracture. *J Am Geriatr Soc* 2011;59:1260–1267.

◆ 5 Breitbart W, Alici Y. Agitation and delirium at the end of life: "We couldn't manage him." *JAMA* 2008;300:2898–2910.

6 Breitbart W, Gibson C, Tremblay A. The delirium experience: Delirium recall and delirium related distress in hospitalized patients with cancer, their spouses/caregivers, and their nurses. *Psychosomatics* 2002;43:183–194.

7 Morita T, Hirai K, Sakaguchi Y et al. Familyperceived distress from delirium-related symptoms of terminally ill cancer patients. *Psychosomatics* 2004;45:107–113.

8 Bruera E, Bush SH, Willey J et al. Impact of delirium and recall on the level of distress in patients with advanced cancer and their family caregivers. *Cancer* May 1, 2009;115(9):2004–2012.

9 Buss MK, Vanderwerker LC, Inouye SK, Zhang B, Block SD, Prigerson HG. Associations between caregiver-perceived delirium in patients with cancer and generalized anxiety in their caregivers. *J Palliat Med* 2007;10(5):1083–1092.

10 Breitbart W, Alici Y. Evidence-based treatment of delirium in patients with cancer. *J Clin Oncol* April 10, 2012;30(11):1206–1214.

11 Gagnon B, Lawlor PG, Mancini IL, Pereira JL, Hanson J, Bruera ED. The impact of delirium on the circadian distribution of breakthrough analgesia in advanced cancer patients. *J Pain Symptom Manage* 2001;22(4):826–833.

12 Coyle N, Breitbart W, Weaver S, Portenoy R. Delirium as a contributing factor to 'Crescendo' pain: Three case reports. *J Pain Symptom Manage* 1994;9:44–47.

13 Morita T, Tei Y, Inouye S. Impaired communication capacity and agitated delirium in the final week of terminally ill cancer patients: Prevalence and identification of research focus. *J Pain Symptom Manage* 2003;26:827–834.

14 Massie MJ, Holland J, Glass E. Delirium in terminally ill cancer patients. *Am J Psychiatry* 1983;140(8):1048–1050.

15 Pereira J, Hanson J, Bruera E. The frequency and clinical course of cognitive impairment in patients with terminal cancer. *Cancer* 1997;79(4):835–842.

16 Bond SM, Dietrich MS, Shuster JL Jr, Murphy BA. Delirium in patients with head and neck cancer in the outpatient treatment setting. *Support Care Cancer* May 2012;20(5):1023–1030. Epub May 5, 2011.

17 Lawlor PG, Gagnon B, Mancini IL et al. Occurrence, causes, and outcome of delirium in patients with advanced cancer: A prospective study. *Arch Intern Med* 2000;160(6):786–794.

18 Spiller JA, Keen JC. Hypoactive delirium: Assessing the extent of the problem for inpatient specialist palliative care. *Palliat Med* 2006;20(1):17–23.

19 Gagnon P, Charbonneau C, Allard P et al. Delirium in terminal cancer: A prospective study using daily screening, early diagnosis, and continuous monitoring. *J Pain Symptom Manage.* 2000;19(6):412–426.

20 Fann JR, Roth-Roemer S, Burington BE et al. Delirium in patients undergoing hematopoietic stem cell transplantation. *Cancer* 2002;95:1971–1981.

21 Trzepacz PT. Is there a final common neural pathway in delirium? Focus on acetylcholine and dopamine. *Semin Clin Neuropsychiatry* 2000;5:132–148.

◆ 22 Maldonado JR: Pathoetiological model of delirium: A comprehensive understanding of the neurobiology of delirium and an evidence-based approach to prevention and treatment. *Crit Care Clin* 2008;24:789–856.

★ 23 American Psychiatric Association. Practice guidelines for the treatment of patients with delirium. *Am J Psychiatry* 1999;156(5 suppl):1–20.

24 Meagher DJ, Trzepacz PT. Delirium phenomenology illuminates pathophysiology, management, and course. *J Geriatr Psychiatry Neurol* Fall 1998;11(3):150–156.

25 Meagher DJ, Moran M, Raju B, Gibbons D, Donnelly S, Saunders J, Trzepacz PT. Phenomenology of delirium. Assessment of 100 adult cases using standardized measures. *Br J Psychiatry* February 2007;190:135–141.

26 Leentjens AF, Schieveld JN, Leonard M, Lousberg R, Verhey FR, Meagher DJ. A comparison of the phenomenology of pediatric, adult, and geriatric delirium. *J Psychosom Res* February 2008;64(2):219–223.

27 Gagnon PR. Treatment of delirium in supportive and palliative care. *Curr Opin Support Palliat Care* March 2008;2(1):60–66.

28 Smith MJ, Breitbart WS, Platt MM. A critique of instruments and methods to detect, diagnose, and rate delirium. *J Pain Symptom Manage* 1994;10(1):35–77.

29 Breitbart W, Rosenfeld B, Roth A. The memorial delirium assessment scale. *J Pain Symptom Manage* 1997;13:128–137.

30 Lawlor P, Nekolaichuck C, Gagnon B et al. Clinical utility, factor analysis and further validation of the Memorial Delirium Assessment Scale (MDAS). *Cancer* 2000;88:2859–2867.

31 Trzepacz PT, Mittal D, Torres R, Kanary K, Norton J, Jimerson N. Validation of the delirium rating scale-revised-98: Comparison with the delirium rating scale and the cognitive test for delirium. *J Neuropsychiatry Clin Neurosci* 2001;13(2):229–242.

32 Inouye B, Vandyck C, Alessi C. Clarifying confusion: The confusion assessment method, a new method for the detection of delirium. *Ann Intern Med* 1990;113:941–948.

33 Ryan K, Leonard M, Guerin S et al. Validation of the confusion assessment method in the palliative care setting. *Palliat Med* 2009;23:40–55.

34 Wong CL, Holroyd-Leduc J, Simel DL, Straus SE. Does this patient have delirium?: Value of bedside instruments. *JAMA* August 18, 2010;304(7):779–786.

35 Meagher DJ, O'Hanlon D, O'Mahony E, Casey PR, Trzepacz PT. Relationship between symptoms and motoric subtype of delirium. *J Neuropsychiatry Clin Neurosci* 2000;12(1):51–56.

36 Stagno D, Gibson C, Breitbart W. The delirium subtypes: A review of prevalence, phenomenology, pathophysiology, and treatment response. *Palliat Support Care* 2004;2(2):171–179.

37 Fang CK, Chen HW, Liu SI, Lin CJ, Tsai LY, Lai YL. Prevalence, detection and treatment of delirium in terminal cancer inpatients: A prospective survey. *Jpn J Clin Oncol* January 2008;38(1):56–63.

38 Leonard M, Donnelly S, Conroy M, Trzepacz P, Meagher DJ. Phenomenological and neuropsychological profile across motor variants of delirium in a palliative-care unit. *J Neuropsychiatry Clin Neurosci* Spring 2011;23(2):180–188.

39 Boettger S, Breitbart W. Phenomenology of the subtypes of delirium: Phenomenological differences between hyperactive and hypoactive delirium. *Palliat Support Care* 2011;9:129–135.

40   Ross CA, Peyser CE, Shapiro I, Folstein MF. Delirium: Phenomenologic and etiologic subtypes. *Int Psychogeriatr* 1991;3(2):135–147.

41   Kiely DK, Jones RN, Bergmann MA, Marcantonio ER. Association between psychomotor activity delirium subtypes and mortality among newly admitted postacute facility patients. *J Gerontol A Biol Sci Med Sci* 2007;62(2):174–179.

42   Breitbart W, Marotta R, Platt MM, Weisman H, Derevenco M, Grau C, Corbera K, Raymond S, Lund S, Jacobson P. *Am J Psychiatry* February 1996;153(2):231–237. PMID:8561204.

43   Breitbart W, Tremblay A, Gibson C. *Psychosomatics* May–June 2002;43(3):175–182. PMID:12075032.

44   Boettger S, Friedlander M, Breitbart W et al. Aripiprazole and haloperidol in the treatment of delirium. *Aust N Z J Psychiatry* 2011;45:477–482.

45   Boettger S, Passik S, Breitbart W. Delirium super imposed on dementia versus delirium in the absence of dementia: Phenomenological differences. *Palliat Support Care* December 2009;7(4):495–500.

46   Boettger S, Passik S, Breitbart W. Treatment characteristics of delirium super imposed on dementia. *Int Psychogeriatr* December 2011;23(10):1671–1676. Epub June 28, 2011.

47   Agar M, Currow D, Plummer J et al. Changes in anticholinergic load from regular prescribed medications in palliative care as death approaches. *Palliat Med* 2009;23:257–265.

48   Gaudreau JD, Gagnon P, Harel F et al. Psychoactive medications and risk of delirium in hospitalized cancer patients. *J Clin Oncol* 2005;23:6712–6718.

49   Agar M, Draper B, Phillips PA, Phillips J, Collier A, Harlum J, Currow D. Making decisions about delirium: A qualitative comparison of decision making between nurses working in palliative care, aged care, aged care psychiatry, and oncology. *Palliat Med* October 2012;26(7):887–896.

50   Morita T, Tei Y, Tsunoda J, Inoue S, Chihara S. Underlying pathologies and their associations with clinical features in terminal delirium of cancer patients. *J Pain Symptom Manage.* 2001;22(6):997–1006.

51   Lawlor P, Gagnon B, Mancini I et al. The occurrence, causes and outcomes of delirium in advanced cancer patients: A prospective study. *Arch Intern Med* 2002;160:786–794.

52   Cole MG, Primeau FJ, Bailey RF et al. Systematic intervention for elderly inpatients with delirium: A randomized trial. *CMAJ* 1994;151(7):965–970.

53   Cole MG, McCusker J, Bellavance F et al. Systematic detection and multidisciplinary care of delirium in older medical inpatients: A randomized trial. *CMAJ* 2002;167(7):753–759.

54   Pitkälä KH, Laurila JV, Strandberg TE, Tilvis RS. Multicomponent geriatric intervention for elderly in patients with delirium: A randomized, controlled trial. *J Gerontol A Biol Sci Med Sci* 2006;61(2):176–181.

55   Pitkala KH, Laurila JV, Strandberg TE, Kautiainen H, Sintonen H, Tilvis RS. Multicomponent geriatric intervention for elderly in patients with delirium: Effects on costs and health-related quality of life. *J Gerontol A Biol Sci Med Sci* 2008;63(1):56–61.

56   Milisen K, Lemiengre J, Braes T, Foreman MD. Multicomponent intervention strategies for managing delirium in hospitalized older people: Systematic review. *J Adv Nurs* 2005;52(1):79–90.

57   Flaherty JH, Steele DK, Chibnall JT et al. An ACE unit with a delirium room may improve function and equalize length of stay among older delirious medical inpatients. *J Gerontol A Biol Sci Med Sci* 2010;65:1387–1392.

58   Casarett DJ, Inouye SK. American College of Physicians-American Society of Internal Medicine End-of-Life Care Consensus Panel. Diagnosis and management of delirium near the end of life. *Ann Intern Med* 2001;135(1):32–40.

59   Inouye SK, Zhang Y, Jones RN, Kiely DK, Yang F, Marcantonio ER. Risk factors for delirium at discharge: Development and validation of a predictive model. *Arch Intern Med.* 2007;167(13):1406–1413.

60   Flaherty JH, Little MO. Matching the environment to patients with delirium: Lessons learned from the delirium room, a restraint-free environment for older hospitalized adults with delirium. *J Am Geriatr Soc* November 2011;59(Suppl 2):S295–S300.

61   Boettger S, Breitbart W. A typical antipsychotics in the management of delirium: A review of the empirical literature. *Palliat Support Care* 2005;3(3);227–237.

62   Flaherty JH. The evaluation and management of delirium among older persons. *Med Clin North Am* 2011:95(3);555–577, xi.

♦ 63   Jackson KC, Lipman AG. Drug therapy for delirium in terminally ill patients. *Cochrane Database Syst Rev* 2004;(2):CD004770.

♦ 64   Lonergan E, Britton AM, Luxenberg J, Wyller T. Antipsychotics for delirium. *Cochrane Database Syst Rev* 2007;(2):CD005594.

65   Han CS, Kim Y. A double-blind trial of risperidone and haloperidol for the treatment of delirium. *Psychosomatics* 2004;45(4):297–301.

66   Hu H, Deng W, Yang H. A prospective random control study comparison of olanzapine and haloperidol in senile delirium. *Chongging Med J* 2004;8:1234–1237.

67   Grover S, Kumar V, Chakrabarti S. Comparative efficacy study of haloperidol, olanzapine and risperidone indelirium. *J Psychosom Res* October 2011;71(4):277–281. Epub March 2, 2011.

68   Girard TD, Pandharipande PP, Carson SS et al. Feasibility, efficacy, and safety of antipsychotics for intensive care unit delirium: The MIND randomized, placebo-controlled trial. *Crit Care Med* 2010;38(2):428–437.

69   Devlin JW, Roberts RJ, Fong JJ et al. Efficacy and safety of quetiapine in critically ill patients with delirium: A prospective, multicenter, randomized, double-blind, placebo-controlled pilot study. *Crit Care Med* 2010;38(2):419–427.

70   Tahir TA, Eeles E, Karapareddy V et al. A randomized controlled trial of quetiapine versus placebo in the treatment of delirium. *J Psychosom Res* 2010;69(5):485–490.

71   Kim SW, Yoo JA, Lee SY et al. Risperidone versus olanzapine for the treatment of delirium. *Hum Psychopharmacol* 2010;25(4):298–302.

72   Kim KY, Bader G, Kotlyar V, Gropper D. Treatment of delirium in older adults with quetiapine. *J Geriatr Psychiatry Neurol* 2003;16(1):29–31.

73   Elsayem A, Bush SH, Munsell MF, Curry E 3rd, Calderon BB, Paraskevopoulos T, Fadul N, Bruera E. Subcutaneous olanzapine for hyperactive or mixed delirium in patients with advanced cancer: A preliminary study. *J Pain Symptom Manage* November 2010;40(5):774–782. Epub August 21, 2010.

74   Fernandez F, Holmes V, Adams F, Kavanaugh J. Treatment of severe refractory agitation with a haloperidol drip. *J Clin Psychiatry* 1988;49(6):239–241.

75   U.S. Food and Drug Administration. Information for healthcare professionals: Haloperidol (marketed as Haldol, Haldol Decanoate and Haldol Lactate). 2007. http://www.fda.gov/drugs/drugsafety/postmarketdrugsafetyinformationforpatientsandproviders/drugsafetyinformationforheathcareprofessionals/ucm085203.htm. Last accessed June 3rd, 2013.

76   Menza M, Murray G, Holmes V. Controlled study of extrapyramidal reactions in the management of delirious medically ill patients: Intravenous haloperidol versus haloperidol plus benzodiazepines. *Heart Lung* 1988;17:238–241.

● 77   Schneider LS, Dagerman KS, Insel P. Risk of death with atypical antipsychotic drug treatment for dementia: Meta-analysis of randomized placebo-controlled trials. *JAMA* 2005;294(15):1934–1943.

● 78   Wang PS, Schneeweiss S, Avorn J et al. Risk of death in elderly users of conventional vs. atypical antipsychotic medications. *N Engl J Med* 2005;353(22):2335–2341.

79   U.S. Food and Drug Administration. Information for healthcare professionals: Antipsychotics. 2008 http://www.fda.gov/cder/drug/InfoSheets/HCP/antipsychotics_conventional.htm. Last accessed June 3rd 2014.

80 Ray WA, Chung CP, Murray KT, Hall K, Stein CM. A typical antipsychotic drugs and the risk of sudden cardiac death. *N Engl J Med* 2009;360(3):225–235.

81 Elie M, Boss K, Cole MG et al. A retrospective, exploratory, secondary analysis of the association between antipsychotic use and mortality in elderly patients with delirium. *Int Psychogeriatr* 2009;21(3):588–592.

82 Gagnon B, Low G, Schreier G. Methylphenidate hydrochloride improves cognitive function in patients with advanced cancer and hypoactive delirium: A prospective clinical study. *J Psychiatry Neurosci* 2005;30(2):100–107.

83 Keen JC, Brown D. Psychostimulants and delirium in patients receiving palliative care. *Palliat Support Care* 2004;2(2):199–202.

84 Morita T, Otani H, Tsunoda J, Inoue S, Chihara S. Successful palliation of hypoactive delirium due to multi-organ failure by oral methylphenidate. *Support Care Cancer* 2000;8(2):134–137.

◆ 85 Overshott R, Karim S, Burns A. Cholinesterase inhibitors for delirium. *Cochrane Database Syst Rev* 2008;(1):CD005317.

86 Overshott R, Vernon M, Morris J, Burns A. Rivastigmine in the treatment of delirium in older people: A pilotstudy. *Int Psychogeriatr* August 2010;22(5):812–818.

87 Van Eijk MM, Roes KC, Honing ML et al. Effect of rivastigmine as an adjunct to usual care with haloperidol on duration of delirium and mortality in critically ill patients: A multicentre, double-blind, placebo-controlled randomised trial. *Lancet* 2010;376:1829–1837.

88 Ventafridda V, Ripamonti C, DeConno F, Tamburini M, Cassileth BR. Symptom prevalence and control during cancer patients' last days of life. *J Palliat Care* 1990;6(3):7–11.

89 Fainsinger RL, Waller A, Bercovici M et al. A multicentre international study of sedation for uncontrolled symptoms in terminally ill patients. *Palliat Med* 2000;14(4):257–265.

90 Rietjens JA, van Zuylen L, van Veluw H, van der Wijk L, van der Heide A, van der Rijt CC. Palliative sedation in a specialized unit for acute palliative care in a cancer hospital: Comparing patients dying with and without palliative sedation. *J Pain Symptom Manage* 2008;36(3):228–234.

91 Connor SR, Pyenson B, Fitch K, Spence C, Iwasaki K. Comparing hospice and nonhospice patient survival among patients who die within a three-year window. *J Pain Symptom Manage* 2007;33(3):238–246.

92 Mercadante S, DeConno F, Ripamonti C. Propofol in terminal care. *J Pain Symptom Manage* 1995;10(8):639–642.

93 Lo B, Rubenfeld G. Palliative sedation in dying patients: "we turn to it when everything else hasn't worked." *JAMA* 2005;294(14):1810–1816.

94 Sykes N, Thorns A. Sedative use in the last week of life and the implications for end-of-life decision making. *Arch Intern Med* 2003;163(3):341–344.

95 Morita T, Chinone Y, Ikenaga M et al. Efficacy and safety of palliative sedation therapy: A multicenter, prospective, observational study conducted on specialized palliative care units in Japan. *J Pain Symptom Manage* 2005;30(4):320–328.

96 Bercovitch M, Adunsky A. Patterns of high-dose morphine use in a home-care hospice service: Should we be afraid of it? *Cancer.* 2004;101(6):1473–1477.

97 Vitetta L, Kenner D, Sali A. Sedation and analgesia-prescribing patterns in terminally ill patients at the end of life. *Am J Hosp Palliat Care* 2005;22(6):465–473.

98 Pandharipande PP, Sanders RD, Girard TD et al. Effect of dexmedetomidine versus lorazepam on outcome in patients with sepsis: An a priori-designed analysis of the MENDS randomized controlled trial. *Crit Care* 2010;14(2):R38.

99 Riker RR, Shehabi Y, Bokesch PM et al. Dexmedetomidine vs. midazolam for sedation of critically ill patients: A randomized trial. *JAMA* 2009;301(5):489–499.

100 Prommer E. Reviewarticle: Dexmedetomidine: Does it have potential in palliative medicine? *Am J Hosp Palliat Care* June 2011;28(4):276–283.

101 Inouye SK, Bogardus ST Jr, Charpentier PA et al. A multicomponent intervention to prevent delirium in hospitalized older patients. *N Engl J Med* 1999;340(9):669–766.

102 Siddiqi N, Stockdale R, Britton AM, Holmes J. Interventions for preventing delirium in hospitalised patients. *Cochrane Database Syst Rev* April 2007;18(2):CD005563.

★103 National Institute for Health and Clinical Excellence. Delirium: Diagnosis, prevention and management (clinical guideline 103). Published July 2010. Accessed at www.nice.org.uk/nicemedia/live/13060/49909/49909.pdfon14August2012.

104 Gagnon P, Allard P, Gagnon B, Mérette C, Tardif F. Delirium prevention in terminal cancer: Assessment of a multicomponent intervention. *Psychooncology* December 19, 2010;21:187–194.

105 Liptzin B, Laki A, Garb JL, Fingeroth R, Krushell R. Donepezil in the prevention and treatment of post-surgical delirium. *Am J Geriatr Psychiatry* December 2005;13(12):1100–1106.

106 Sampson EL, Raven PR, Ndhlovu PN et al. A randomized, double-blind, placebo-controlled trial of donepezil hydrochloride (Aricept) for reducing the incidence of postoperative delirium after elective total hip replacement. *Int J Geriatr Psychiatry* April 2007;22(4):343–349.

107 Gamberini M, Bolliger D, Lurati Buse GAM et al. Rivastigmine for the prevention of post operative deliriumin elderly patients undergoing elective cardiac surgery—A randomized controlled trial. *Crit Care Med* May 2009;37(5):1762–1768.

108 Kalisvaart KJ, de Jonghe JF, Bogaards MJ et al. Haloperidol prophylaxis for elderly hip-surgery patients at risk for delirium: A randomized placebo-controlled study. *J Am Geriatr Soc* 2005;53(10):1658–1666.

109 Larsen KA, Kelly SE, Stern TA et al. Administration of olanzapine to prevent post operative delirium in elderly joint-replacement patients: A randomized, controlled trial. *Psychosomatics* September–October 2010;51(5):409–418.

110 Prakanrattana U, Prapaitrakool S. Efficacy of risperidone for prevention of postoperative delirium in cardiac surgery. *Anaesth Intensive Care* October 2007;35(5):714–719.

111 Wang W, Li HL, Wang DX, Zhu X, Li SL, Yao GQ, Chen KS, Gu XE, Zhu SN. Haloperidol prophylaxis decreases delirium incidence in elderly patients after noncardiac surgery: A randomized controlled trial*. *Crit Care Med* March 2012;40(3):731–739.

112 Al-Aama T, Brymer C, Gutmanis I, Woolmore-Goodwin SM, Esbaugh J, Dasgupta M. Melatonin decreases delirium in elderly patients: A randomized, placebo-controlled trial. *Int J Geriatr Psychiatry* July 2011;26(7):687–694.

113 Dhillon N, Kopetz S, Pei BL, Fabbro ED, Zhang T, Bruera E. Clinical findings of a palliative care consultation team at a comprehensive cancer center. *J Palliat Med* March 2008;11(2):191–197.

114 Bruera E, Miller L, McCallion J, Macmillan K, Krefting L, Hanson J. Cognitive failure in patients with terminal cancer: A prospective study. *J Pain Symptom Manage* 1992;7(4):192–195.

115 Morita T, Tsunoda J, Inoue S, Chihara S. Survival prediction of terminally ill cancer patients by clinical symptoms: Development of a simple indicator. *Jpn J Clin Oncol* 1999;29(3):156–159.

116 Caraceni A, Nanni O, Maltoni M et al. Impact of delirium on the short term prognosis of advanced cancer patients. Italian Multicenter Study Group on Palliative Care. *Cancer* 2000;89(5):1145–1149.

117 Mori M, Parsons HA, DelaCruz M, Elsayem A, Palla SL, Liu J, Li Z, Palmer L, Bruera E, Fadul NA. Changes in symptoms and inpatient mortality: A study in advanced cancer patients admitted to an acute palliative care unit in a comprehensive cancer center. *J Palliat Med* September 2011;14(9):1034–1041. Epub August 11, 2011.

71

Sleep disturbances in advanced cancer patients

SANDRA L. PEDRAZA, DAVE BALACHANDRAN, SRIRAM YENNURAJALINGAM

INTRODUCTION

Sleep disturbances (SDs) can be defined as any symptom or condition that interferes with normal sleep [1]. They are very common in patients with advanced cancer [2], with a prevalence reported to be between 24% and 95% in this population [3]. However, this problem is usually neglected in treatment strategies for advanced cancer, as many studies have focused on patients with early-stage disease and on survivors [4]. SDs in the cancer population can present as a temporary symptom associated with the cancer or as part of depression or anxiety disorders, and physicians often assume that the SD will resolve when the underlying problem is treated [4–6].

The sleep disorders are a group of pathologic conditions that have been defined based on clinical presentation and diagnostic criteria [7]. There is a classification system published by the American Academy of Sleep Medicine (AASM) (see Table 71.1) that standardizes the diagnosis of sleep disorders and is especially useful in the research setting [8]. This system recognizes six major sleep disorder categories: insomnia, sleep-related breathing disorders, hypersomnia, circadian rhythm sleep disorders, parasomnias, and sleep-related movement disorders. Of those disorder categories, the most common in advanced cancer patients, compared with the general population, is insomnia, which accounts for 35% of the diagnoses in these patients [9,10].

Insomnia is a complex complaint that can be defined as a difficulty initiating sleep, trouble staying asleep, with prolonged nocturnal awakenings, early morning awakening with inability to resume sleep, or impairment of daytime functioning. Insomnia can appear as an isolated disorder or as a symptom that accompanies a different disorder. Differentiating between these two situations is very important since the approach to treatment can differ between the two. The international classification of sleep disorders [7] and the DSM-IV (Diagnostic and Statistical Manual of Mental Disorders, Fourth Edition) [11] typically used in clinical research categorize insomnia duration as transient (1 month or less), short term (between 1 and 6 months), and chronic (6 months or more).

The prevalence of sleep disorders in cancer patients is about twice that in the general population. Screening tests used for sleep disorder are heavily weighted toward diagnosing insomnia; therefore, it is not surprising that the most common SDs found by Sela et al. in palliative cancer patients were difficulty falling asleep (40%), difficulty staying asleep (63%), and not feeling rested in the morning (72%) [1]. Adjustment insomnia (acute insomnia) and insomnia due to medical conditions (comorbid insomnia) are the most common new-onset SD subtypes. The general criteria for insomnia in adults are presented in Table 71.2 [12].

The prevalence of SDs varies depending upon the type of cancer. For example, breast cancer patients have a high frequency of insomnia and fatigue, whereas lung cancer patients have the highest prevalence of SDs in general, owing to coughing, difficulty breathing, and nocturia that lead to frequent awakenings that disrupt the patient's sleep pattern. Proper diagnostic criteria and classification schemes have not been used when studying the frequency of sleep disorders in individuals with cancer, making it somewhat difficult to establish the incidence and prevalence of conditions other than insomnia [2].

In this chapter, we will describe normal sleep architecture and discuss the mechanisms of cancer-related SD. We will then turn to assessment and diagnosis of SD, through subjective self-reports and more objective medical tests such as polysomnography (PSG). We will conclude by summarizing the treatments available, ranging from nonpharmacological methods to SD medications.

PATHOPHYSIOLOGY OF SLEEP DISORDERS IN CANCER PATIENTS

Normal sleep architecture

The normal sleep physiology has been divided into two distinct physiologic types: rapid eye movement (REM) and non–rapid eye movement (NREM) sleep. The latter is subdivided in stages numbered from N1 to N3. The last stage is known as slow-wave sleep based on the electroencephalography. Perhaps the most

Table 71.1 *International classification of disorders*

1. Insomnia
   a. Adjustment insomnia (acute insomnia)
   b. Psychophysiological insomnia
   c. Paradoxical insomnia
   d. Idiopathic insomnia
   e. Insomnia due to mental disorder
   f. Inadequate sleep hygiene
   g. Behavioral insomnia of childhood
   h. Insomnia due to drug or substance
   i. Insomnia due to medical condition
   j. Insomnia not due to substance or known physiological condition, unspecified (nonorganic insomnia, not otherwise specified (NOS))
   k. Physiological (organic) insomnia, unspecified
2. Sleep-related breathing disorders
   a. Central sleep apnea syndromes
      i. Primary central sleep apnea
      ii. Central sleep apnea due to Cheyne–Stokes breathing pattern
      iii. Central sleep apnea due to high-altitude periodic breathing
      iv. Central sleep apnea due to medical condition, not Cheyne–Stokes
      v. Central sleep apnea due to drug or substance
      vi. Primary sleep apnea of infancy
   b. OSA syndromes
      i. OSA, adult
      ii. OSA, pediatric
   c. Sleep-related hypoventilation/hypoxemic syndromes
      i. Sleep-related nonobstructive alveolar hypoventilation, idiopathic
      ii. Congenital central alveolar hypoventilation syndrome
   d. Sleep-related hypoventilation/hypoxemia due to medical conditions
      i. Sleep-related hypoventilation/hypoxemia due to pulmonary parenchymal or vascular pathology
      ii. Sleep-related hypoventilation/hypoxemia due to lower airway obstruction
      iii. Sleep-related hypoventilation/hypoxemia due to neuromuscular and chest wall disorders
   e. Other sleep apnea/sleep-related breathing disorders
3. Hypersomnia of central origin not due to a circadian rhythm disorder or other cause of disturbed nocturnal sleep
   a. Narcolepsy with cataplexy
   b. Narcolepsy without cataplexy
   c. Narcolepsy due to medical conditions
   d. Narcolepsy unspecified
   e. Recurrent hypersomnia
      i. Kleine–Levin syndrome
      ii. Menstrual-related hypersomnia
   f. Idiopathic hypersomnia with long sleep time
   g. Idiopathic hypersomnia without long sleep time
   h. Behaviorally induced insufficient sleep syndrome
   i. Hypersomnia due to medical conditions
   j. Hypersomnia due to drug or substance
   k. Hypersomnia not due to substance or known physiological condition (nonorganic hypersomnia, NOS)
   l. Physiological (organic) hypersomnia, unspecified (organic hypersomnia, NOS)

4. Circadian rhythm sleep disorder
   a. Circadian rhythm disorder, delayed sleep-phase type (delayed sleep-phase disorder)
   b. Circadian rhythm disorder, advanced sleep-phase type (advanced sleep-phase disorder)
   c. Circadian rhythm disorder, irregular sleep–wake type (irregular sleep–wake rhythm)
   d. Circadian rhythm disorder, free-running type (nonentrained type)
   e. Circadian rhythm disorder, jet lag type (jet lag disorder)
   f. Circadian rhythm disorder, shift work type (shift work disorder)
   g. Circadian rhythm disorder, due to medical conditions
   h. Other circadian rhythm disorder (circadian rhythm disorder, NOS)
   i. Other circadian rhythm disorder due to drug or substance
5. Parasomnia
   a. Disorders of arousal from NREM sleep
      i. Confusional arousals
      ii. Sleepwalking
      iii. Sleep terrors
   b. Parasomnias usually associated with REM sleep
      i. REM sleep behavior disorder
      ii. Recurrent isolated sleep paralysis
      iii. Nightmare disorder
   c. Other parasomnias
      i. Sleep-related dissociative disorders
      ii. Sleep enuresis
      iii. Sleep-related groaning (catathrenia)
      iv. Exploding head syndrome
      v. Sleep-related hallucinations
      vi. Sleep-related eating disorder
      vii. Parasomnia, unspecified
      viii. Parasomnias due to drug or substance
      ix. Parasomnias due to medical conditions
6. Sleep-related movement disorder
   a. Restless legs syndrome
   b. Periodic limb movement disorder
   c. Sleep-related leg cramps
   d. Sleep-related bruxism
   e. Sleep-related rhythmic movement disorder
   f. Sleep-related movement disorder, unspecified
   g. Sleep-related movement disorder due to drug or substance
   h. Sleep-related movement disorder due to medical conditions
7. Isolated symptoms, apparently normal variants and unresolved issues
   a. Long sleepers
   b. Short sleepers
   c. Snoring
   d. Sleep talking
   e. Sleep starts (hypnic jerks)
   f. Benign sleep myoclonus of infancy
   g. Hypnagogic foot tremor and alternating leg muscle activation during sleep
   h. Propriospinal myoclonus at sleep onset
   i. Excessive fragmentary myoclonus

(Continued)

Table 71.1 (Continued) *International classification of disorders*

8. Other sleep disorders
   a. Other physiological (organic) sleep disorder
   b. Other sleep disorder not due to substance or known sleep disorder
   c. Environmental sleep disorder

Sources: Adapted from American Academy of Sleep Medicine, *International Classification of Sleep Disorders: Diagnostic and Coding Manual*, 2nd edn., American Academy of Sleep Medicine, Westchester, IL, 2005; T. Freedom, *Disease-a-Month*, 57, 323, 2011.

Table 71.2 *General criteria for insomnia in adults*

1. Difficulty initiating sleep, difficulty maintaining sleep, or waking up too early or sleep that is chronically nonrestorative or poor in quality
2. Sleep difficulty occurring despite adequate opportunities and circumstances for sleep
3. Patient reports at least 1 of the following forms of daytime impairment related to the nighttime sleep difficulty:
   - Fatigue or malaise
   - Attention, concentration, or memory impairment—social or vocational dysfunction
   - Mood disturbance or irritability
   - Daytime sleepiness
   - Motivation, energy, or initiative reduction
   - Proneness for errors or accidents at work or while driving
   - Tension, headache, or gastrointestinal symptoms in response to sleep loss
   - Concerns or worries about sleep

Source: Adapted from American Academy of Sleep Medicine, *International Classification of Sleep Disorders: Diagnostic and Coding Manual*, 2nd edn., American Academy of Sleep Medicine, Westchester, IL, 2005.

important difference between NREM and REM sleep is the presence of voluntary muscle paralysis with evidence of electroencephalographic activity in the latter. During REM sleep, people experience dreams and significant autonomic variability [13]. Sleepers experience complete paralysis of voluntary skeletal muscles, which is mediated through changes in the brain stem that causes activation of downgoing inhibitory pathways on the brain stem and spinal cord [14].

During a normal sleep night, individuals progress between different sleep stages, from light (stage 1) to deep or slow-wave sleep, returning to more light stages and to REM sleep in between. A normal night sleep consists of several of these fluctuations (between 4 and 6). The distinction between the physiological stages of sleep is important because certain pathologies present exclusively during certain stages (parasomnias) or are exacerbated during specific phases (such as sleep-disordered breathing during REM sleep) [15,16].

Mechanisms of cancer-related SD

Just as many aspects of sleep physiology are still not understood, the precise mechanism by which cancer leads to SDs also remains unknown. Several models have been developed to explain sleep–wake disorders in the context of cancer. All these models appear to coincide in the multifactorial nature of the disorder and the hypothesis that physiological, psychological, and behavioral phenomena play an important role in the development of deviations from normal sleep and pathologic changes [17]. The most commonly cited hypothesis in patients with cancer is based on the Speilman3-factor model: predisposing factors that increase the individual's vulnerability to insomnia (gender, age, and a family history of insomnia); precipitating factors that trigger the onset of insomnia (disease-specific biological factors, cancer-related emotional factors, functional loss, treatment, pain, and delirium); and perpetuating factors that maintain insomnia over time (maladaptive sleep behaviors and misconceptions about sleep). The most important contributors for each category of factors are summarized in Table 71.3 [10].

This model assumes that predisposing factors are rarely modifiable and that many cancer patients may have preestablished sleep disorders, thus making the determination of true risk factors difficult, especially since some populations have been studied preferentially (e.g., breast cancer patients). The cancer-specific-related risk factors for SDs may be subdivided into disease-specific, treatment-related, or associated phenomenon. Patients with cancer share demographic and age risk factors for SDs with the normal population. The single most important unmodifiable risk factor for sleep–wake disturbances is age, especially since cancer tends to be diagnosed in older patients. The cancer-specific factors may be subdivided into disease-specific, treatment-related, or associated phenomena [12]. These cancer-specific factors have been divided into pathophysiological changes induced by the disease, symptoms that may interfere with normal sleep initiation or maintenance, and changes in lifestyle that could contribute to disturbances in the sleep–wake cycle.

Table 71.3 *Key etiologic factors of insomnia in cancer patients*

Predisposing factors	Precipitating factors	Perpetuating factors
• Psychiatric disorders	• Pain	• Poor sleep habits (excessive time spent in bed, napping, irregular sleep schedules)
• Female sex	• Medical illness	
• Advancing age	• Mutilating surgery	
• Hyperarousability	• Hospitalization	
• Family history of insomnia	• Radiation therapy	• Dysfunctional reactions to sleep (anxiety associated with the act of sleeping)
• Personal history of insomnia	• Bone marrow transplantation	
• Misconceptions about the causes of insomnia	• Medications (antiemetic drugs, hormonal therapy, chemotherapy)	• Unrealistic sleep requirements
	• Delirium	• Misattributions of daytime impairments

Source: Adapted from Savard, J. and Morin, C.M., *J. Clin. Oncol.*, 19, 895, February 1, 2001.

Cancer can affect the patient's sleep by contributing to symptoms that are known to cause sleep–wake disruption. Changes in sleep architecture have been described with decrease in slow-wave sleep and REM sleep and corresponding increases in stages N1 and N2 sleep [18]. Symptoms such as urinary disturbances can cause patients to awaken frequently, disturbing their sleep cycles. Several agents used to treat malignancies also can lead to symptoms such as neuropathy or pain that can further disrupt the sleep–wake cycle.

Pain has been proposed as an important factor leading to insomnia, although there have been very few trials to support this widely accepted association [2,19]. Likewise, inadequate pain management can lead to significant changes in insomnia occurrence and severity. In a study of symptom assessment, Meuser et al. showed that adequate pain control may actually be associated with a decrease in the incidence of insomnia [20]. Another important aspect of pain in cancer patients is that it is frequently treated with opioids, which can cause changes in the normal sleep physiology and may lead to respiratory depression with exacerbation of other sleep disorders [21].

Mood and anxiety disorders, which appear to interfere significantly with normal sleep, are the most common psychiatric diagnoses in cancer patients and have been demonstrated to cause disruption of the sleep architecture, as in depression [22–24]. In contrast, anxiety can lead to increased arousal with patients experiencing difficulty falling asleep. Despite the extensive association between affective problems and anxiety with SDs, there is very little evidence that this association is exclusive to the cancer population, suggesting that the symptoms may precede the cancer diagnosis [25,26]. Severe emotional distress, not uncommon in this group of patients, may further alter the patient's ability to maintain sleep.

There is growing interest in the potential role of cytokines in the development of specific symptoms in cancer patients. Elevated levels of proinflammatory cytokines have been found in patients with cancer [27]. Cytokines exert their effect in the brain through different pathways including the liberation of prostaglandin E2, elevating the body temperature, and stimulating the hypothalamic–pituitary–adrenal (HPA) axis that in turn may lead to changes in the sleep–wake cycle. Because symptoms experienced by this population may resemble those suffered by individuals with infections, cytokines have been studied as potential mediators of most chemotherapy and cancer-related symptoms [28,29]. Some cancer patients receiving interleukin-2 and tumor necrosis factor alpha as treatment for their underlying malignancy develop systemic signs of inflammation and the appearance of symptoms such as fever, fatigue, anorexia, and insomnia [2].

Further experimental data from animal models suggest the important role of these cytokines in sleep. For example, interleukin-1 and tumor necrosis factor alpha increased intracellular calcium concentrations in gamma amino butyric acid (GABA) producing cultured rat hypothalamic neurons [30]. In addition, studies done in rats have shown that the administration of interleukin-1 or TNF can induce and increase slow-wave sleep when administered topically to the somatosensory cortex under the dura [31]. It also appears that the effects of the cytokines on sleep may be modulated through the serotonin system, since the dorsal raphe, the main serotoninergic system in the brain, has receptors for interleukin-1 and exposure to cytokines increases NREM sleep in rats [32]. Additionally, most of the effects of interleukin-1 on sleep are lost with disruption of the serotoninergic system in the brain [33,34]. Finally, other animal models have demonstrated that the infusion of interleukin-1 to the preoptic nucleus of the hypothalamus can change the firing rates of active neurons, further substantiating the potential role of these cytokines in sleep [35].

Interleukin-6, another cytokine that may be involved in the regulation of sleep, is important in the modulation of response to interleukin-1 among other functions. Interleukin-6 shows a normal diurnal variation in levels that mirror changes in the sleep–wake cycle [36] and can also increase slow-wave sleep and reduce REM sleep in humans [37]. Interestingly, clinical studies using the tumor necrosis factor alpha receptor antagonist etanercept have shown a decrease in plasma interleukin-6 levels as well as daytime sleepiness in sleep apnea patients [38]. There are clinical studies showing that interleukin-6 levels may correlate with the amount of sleep and that sleep deprivation may change the normal temporal pattern of circadian interleukin-6 secretion [39].

Thus, growing evidence supports the role of cytokines as sleep modulatory substances. Most of the data come from animal experiments, but some clinical data are slowly appearing. One important aspect from a therapeutic standpoint is the modulation potential of these protein levels as a treatment for SD.

ASSESSMENT OF SLEEP DISORDERS

The most important aspect during assessment of SD in cancer patients is characterizing the sleep difficulty and identifying the causes, exacerbating factors, and comorbidities that trigger the SD. Taking into consideration that cancer patients occasionally do not report SD to their physicians, a thorough history is essential to identify the factors that contribute to SD. The patients should be able to provide this information, and their partners should be asked to contribute to the sleep history to rule out other sleep disorders such as restless legs syndrome or obstructive sleep apnea (OSA) [40,41].

Several screening and evaluation tests are available for detecting and diagnosing SD. The first group of the tests relies on self-reports about sleep latency, quality, satisfaction, and awakenings. This information is usually gathered with sleep quality questionnaires, sleep history questionnaires, sleep diaries, and daytime sleepiness questionnaires [13]. The Pittsburgh sleep quality index (PSQI), the standard for self-reported sleep data, is a frequently used tool in clinical research. The PSQI measures the quality and patterns of sleep and differentiates "poor" from "good" sleep by measuring subjective sleep quality, sleep latency, sleep duration, habitual sleep efficiency, SD, use of sleeping medication, and daytime dysfunction [42]. The Edmonton symptom assessment scale (ESAS) evaluates the prevalence and severity of 10 self-reported symptoms commonly experienced by cancer patients over the previous 24 hours: pain, fatigue, nausea, depression, anxiety, drowsiness, dyspnea, loss of appetite, sense of well-being, and sleep. The severity of each symptom is rated on a numerical scale of 0–10, where 0 means that the symptom is absent, and 10 indicates the worst possible severity [43]. The cutoff point of the presence of ESAS sleep symptom is 3 out of 10 for the screening of SD. This cutoff has a sensitivity of 86% and a specificity of 53% [3].

Another way to document SDs and to monitor the effect of interventions is with sleep diaries, which are more objective than patient or partner recall. Several sleep diary models collect various kinds of data, but in general, the patient records daily information on time to initiation of sleep, total sleep time, and number of awakenings. Daytime sleepiness and sleep-related habits are recorded as well [44]. The daytime sleepiness inventories are aimed at finding the repercussions of impaired sleep on the patient's daytime functioning.

Because of the subjective nature of the self-reported instruments, it is often recommended that researchers and physicians also use objective measures of SD. The standard for detection of specific sleep and wake states is PSG [45]. PSG records several bioelectrical signals such as electroencephalogram (EEG), heart rate, respiratory rate, upper airway flow, presence of snoring, EMG, and leg movement to characterize the sleep architecture and detect SD. Another frequently used test in the diagnosis of SD is actigraphy, which uses an accelerometer to monitor activity throughout the day. With the use of computer algorithms, actigraphy calculates sleep time, latency, and awakenings. Unlike subjective measures, which can differ significantly from the polysomnogram, actigraphy correlates well with polysomnographic data [46]. Both PSG and actigraphy complement the self-reported SD. These tests help us gather more objective information about stages of sleep in hospital settings or sleep–wake patterns of patients in their own homes [47].

Laboratory investigations may be considered when associated medical conditions are causing SD. For example, ferritin measurement can help diagnose restless legs syndrome, and a physical examination of the head and neck can help identify OSA as a cause of daytime tiredness and fatigue secondary to SD. The STOP-Bang (snoring, tired, observed, blood pressure–BMI, age, neck circumference, gender) questionnaire was developed as a screening tool for OSA in surgical patients and preoperative clinics. This questionnaire is short and easy to apply and has a sensitivity between 93% and 100% for moderate-to-severe OSA [48].

TREATMENT OF SLEEP DISTURBANCES

SD has a negative effect on quality of life in patients suffering from advanced cancer and other diseases, emphasizing the need to treat this condition [49]. Management of the underlying pathology is paramount in order to lessen the somatic, psychological, and social effects of SD experienced by cancer patients.

Symptoms such as fatigue, impaired daytime functioning, and mood disturbances are commonly reported by advanced cancer patients and could be secondary to SD [10]. Therefore, the development of interventions aimed at improving SD can help alleviate these symptoms and increase patients' coping capacity [10]. A multimodal approach with pharmacological and nonpharmacological interventions has been used to treat SD in advanced cancer patients, but data on the effectiveness of these measures in this specific population are limited [50].

Nonpharmacological interventions

The AASM strongly recommends educating patients about sleep hygiene measures [51] (see Table 71.4). These interventions alone have not been demonstrated to be effective against insomnia but are easy to implement and have a high possibility of improving sleep when combined with other therapeutic interventions such as cognitive behavioral treatment (CBT). Awareness of good sleep hygiene may also help the patient identify abnormal behavior that can interfere with restful sleep.

Several nonpharmacological therapies to treat insomnia have been tried in the general population. The most commonly evaluated modalities include behavioral and CBTs. CBT is a supportive counseling intervention aimed at eliminating factors associated with chronic insomnia, reducing the severity of perpetuating factors below the insomnia threshold, and deactivating the hyperarousal [12]. Importantly, two meta-analyses revealed that some of these interventions might have efficacy against insomnia [10]. Not all measures of sleep quality have responded equally well to CBT. The largest therapeutic effects have been obtained for sleep-onset latency, sleep quality ratings, and duration of awakenings.

Table 71.4   *Commonly recommended sleep hygiene measures*

1. Maintain a regular bed and wake time schedule including weekends.
2. Establish a regular, relaxing bedtime routine such as soaking in a hot bath and then reading a book or listening to soothing music.
3. Create a sleep-conducive environment that is dark, quiet, comfortable, and cool.
4. Sleep on a comfortable mattress and pillows.
5. Use your bedroom only for sleep and sex.
6. Finish eating at least 2–3 hours before your regular bedtime.
7. Exercise regularly. It is best to complete your workout at least a few hours before bedtime.
8. Avoid caffeine (e.g., coffee, tea, soft drinks, chocolate) close to bedtime. It can keep you awake.
9. Avoid nicotine (e.g., cigarettes, tobacco products). When used close to bedtime, it can lead to poor sleep.
10. Avoid alcohol close to bedtime.

Sources: Adapted from National Sleep Foundation, *Healthy Sleep Tips*, http://www.sleepfoundation.org/article/sleep-topics/healthy-sleep-tips, Reviewed 05/23/2012; Adapted from American Academy of Sleep Medicine, *International Classification of Sleep Disorders: Diagnostic and Coding Manual*, 2nd edn., American Academy of Sleep Medicine, Westchester, IL, 2005.

The National Institutes of Health State-of-the-Science Conference on Insomnia concluded that CBT is as effective as hypnotic medications are for the short-term management of insomnia [2]. CBT's effects are also longer lasting than those of pharmacological agents, and in general, CBT may have other benefits for the patient's quality of life. The *American Academy of Sleep Medicine's Practice Parameters*, published in 2006, recommended behavioral and psychological interventions as a standard for the treatment of chronic comorbid insomnia [12]. Other techniques that have proven beneficial include stimulus control, relaxation, sleep restriction, and multicomponent therapy that are part of CBT.

Several studies have evaluated the effectiveness of CBT for the treatment of insomnia in the cancer population. A recent review reports that four randomized controlled trials and nine quasi-experimental studies have shown that in general, CBT is an effective intervention that leads to improvement of several sleep outcome measures including sleep quality using the PSQI [12]. These studies have been performed in different cancer populations, including patients undergoing active treatment and survivors. Among other interventions, supportive expressive group therapy showed an increase in the wake-latency time in breast cancer patients [52]. Objective measures, such as actigraphy, and subjective measures, such as sleep diaries and questionnaires, showed improvement with CBT in a randomized controlled crossover study done by Fiorentino et al. [53].

Complementary interventions that have been tested include progressive muscle relaxation, which decreased sleep latency in patients with multiple cancers; hypnosis interventions, which

decreased hot flashes in breast cancer patients; and bright-light therapy, which may improve SD and fatigue in breast cancer patients during chemotherapy [2,12]. Exercise interventions such as stretching, concentrating, and strengthening affect the circadian phase (evening exercise produced substantial phase advances for evening exercises). Regular exercise for a sustained period of time may help to improve sleep latency and quality [47]. Exercise may prove beneficial for cancer patients, but further studies are required before these interventions can be widely recommended [12].

Pharmacological interventions

Pharmacotherapy is the most common SD intervention in the general population and cancer patients. Table 71.5 summarizes the most commonly used hypnotic agents in the cancer population. The newer, short-acting benzodiazepines have a more selective hypnotic effect with less residual side effects than do long-acting benzodiazepines. Benzodiazepines interact with the GABA-A receptor, increasing the conductance to chloride and therefore hyperpolarizing the neurons [54]. In general, benzodiazepines cause central nervous system depression, with amnestic and hypnotic effects, and have been shown to decrease sleep latency and duration in short-term studies in the general population [55,56]. However, objective data from polysomnographic studies show that self-reported measures may overestimate the effect on sleep latency [57]. There are many different benzodiazepines with variable half-lives depending on their metabolism. This becomes important when using long

Table 71.5 *Commonly used hypnotic medications*

Activity		Initial dose (mg)	Considerations
Ultrashort acting	Zaleplon	5–10	Little to no anxiolytic effect; costly
Short-onset brief duration	Triazolam	0.125	Rapid sleep induction; limited effect on sleep maintenance
	Alprazolam	0.5–1	
Short-onset, intermediate duration of action	Zolpidem	5–10	No clear advantage over benzodiazepines; costly; minimal anxiolytic effect
	Zoplicone	5–7.5	
	Eszopiclone	3	
Intermediate onset, duration	Lorazepam	0.5–4	Adequate effect on sleep induction and maintenance; risk of daytime drowsiness
	Temazepam	7.5–15	
Longer latency to onset, prolonged activity	Clonazepam	0.5–2	Slow sleep induction with increased risk of accumulation of metabolites; high risk of daytime sedation
	Chlordiazepoxide	50–100	
	Diazepam	5–10	
Longer Latency to onset, prolonged activity (off-label for insomnia)	Amitryptiline	25–100	Increased risk of daytime sedation, confusion, constipation, and cardiac conduction abnormalities
	Imipramine	25–100	
	Doxepin	25–100	
	Trazodone	25–100	
	Mirtazapine	15–30	
Variable activity (off-label for insomnia)	Haloperidol	0.5–5	Used in sleep disturbance related to psychosis or delirium
	Risperidone	0.5–1	
	Olanzapine	5–10	
	Quetiapine	25	

Source: Adapted from Delgado-Guay, M. and Yennurajalingam, S., in *Oxford American Handbook of Hospice and Palliative Medicine*, S. Yennurajalingam, E. Bruera, eds., Oxford University Press, New York, pp. 115–126, 2011.

half-life medications, since residual effects with impairment of daytime functioning may occur, especially in the elderly, leading to an increased risk of falls and hip fractures [58]. Another important concern in elderly cancer patients is the potential of benzodiazepines to cause delirium, cognitive impairment, and respiratory depression when combined with opioids [59–62]. These adverse interactions have been described with methadone even at a low dose [63]. In addition, very little information is available on the long-term efficacy of these agents, and the well-known pharmacological effects, such as the patient's tolerance and dependence on these agents, may make them undesirable for long-term use [64].

Antidepressant medications with sedative properties, such as trazodone, amitriptyline, and doxepin, can be beneficial for depressed patients with SD [10]. Since selective serotonin reuptake inhibitors (SSRIs) have very low sedative effects, the use of SSRIs is limited to depression-related insomnia. Venlafaxine can be used to treat both hot flashes and SD in breast cancer patients; however, no beneficial effects for sleep have been reported. SSRI and serotonin norepinephrine reuptake inhibitors (SNRIs) can produce SD as well owing to their pharmacological action over the 5-HT2 and 5-HT3 receptors [65].

Side effects associated with antidepressants, such as orthostasis (mostly with trazodone), anticholinergic activity, nausea, and constipation, should be considered before prescribing these medications for cancer patients [65]. Tricyclic antidepressants can decrease sleep latency, reduce awakenings, and increase sleep quality, but they also can cause concerning side effects, such as daytime sedation, an anticholinergic effect, and cardiovascular problems, especially in older patients [65–67].

Mirtazapine is a good option for managing multiple distressing symptoms in cancer patients. A noradrenergic and specific serotonergic antidepressant with antagonistic effects on 5-HT2 and 5-HT3 receptors, mirtazapine, can improve nausea, vomiting, and insomnia. An advantageous side effect associated with mirtazapine is weight gain because this agent increases appetite and thus improves anorexia in cancer patients. Benzodiazepines should not be use with mirtazapine because of the risk of sedation [68].

Melatonin, a naturally existing hormone produced in the pineal gland, regulates circadian rhythm by regulating the suprachiasmatic nucleus of the hypothalamus through G-protein-coupled receptors (MT1–MT3). The use of melatonin in the treatment of sleep disorders is still controversial. Data from several meta-analyses suggest that melatonin's effects are limited to delayed sleep-phase syndrome [69]. One of the suggested reasons for melatonin's failure to achieve results against insomnia in clinical trials is the lack of consistency in the melatonin presentations, which has led to the development of specific melatonin (MT1–MT2) agonists that have received FDA approval for the treatment of insomnia. Because of the lack of conclusive data for melatonin use in the cancer population, the routine use of this supplement or its agonists cannot be recommended [50], even though melatonin appears to be very safe with few side effects.

CONCLUSION

SDs have a negative effect on quality of life in the advanced cancer patient. Fatigue, impaired daytime functioning, and mood disturbances are commonly reported in this population and could be secondary to SDs. Both subjective and objective screening tools are available for evaluation of SD in the cancer population. Interventions that are aimed at improving SDs help alleviate these symptoms and increase the copying capacity. Management of these symptoms usually requires a multimodality approach with the use of nonpharmacological and pharmacological measures to obtain long-lasting results.

REFERENCES

1   R. A. Sela, S. Watanabe, C. L. Nekolaichuk, Sleep disturbances in palliative cancer patients attending a pain and symptom control clinic. *Palliative & Supportive Care* 3, 23 (March 2005).

2   L. Liu, S. Ancoli-Israel, Sleep disturbances in cancer. *Psychiatric Annals* 38, 627 (September 1, 2008).

3   M. Delgado-Guay, S. Yennurajalingam, H. Parsons, J. L. Palmer, E. Bruera, Association between self-reported sleep disturbance and other symptoms in patients with advanced cancer. *Journal of Pain and Symptom Management* 41, 819 (2011).

4   T. Akechi et al., Associated and predictive factors of sleep disturbance in advanced cancer patients. *Psycho-Oncology* 16, 888 (October 2007).

5   C. M. Morin et al., Cognitive behavioral therapy, singly and combined with medication, for persistent insomnia: A randomized controlled trial. *The Journal of the American Medical Association* 301, 2005 (May 20, 2009).

6   J. Savard, S. Simard, H. Ivers, C. M. Morin, Randomized study on the efficacy of cognitive-behavioral therapy for insomnia secondary to breast cancer, part I: Sleep and psychological effects. *Journal of Clinical Oncology: Official Journal of the American Society of Clinical Oncology* 23, 6083 (September 1, 2005).

7   American Academy of Sleep Medicine, *International Classification of Sleep Disorders: Diagnostic and Coding Manual*, 2nd edn. American Academy of Sleep Medicine, Westchester, IL (2005).

8   T. Freedom, Classification of sleep disorders. *Disease-a-Month* 57, 323 (July 2011).

9   B. Hearson, J. A. Sawatzky, Sleep disturbance in patients with advanced cancer. *International Journal of Palliative Nursing* 14, 30 (January 2008).

10 J. Savard, C. M. Morin, Insomnia in the Context of Cancer: A review of a neglected problem. *Journal of Clinical Oncology* 19, 895 (February 1, 2001).

11 American Psychiatric Association, *Diagnostic and Statistical Manual of Mental Disorders*, 4th edn. American Psychiatric Association, Washington, DC (2000).

12 A. M. Berger, Update on the state of the science: Sleep–wake disturbances in adult patients with cancer. *Oncology Nursing Forum* 36, E165 (July 2009).

13 C. Vena, K. Parker, M. Cunningham, J. Clark, S. McMillan, Sleep–wake disturbances in people with cancer. Part I: An overview of sleep, sleep regulation, and effects of disease and treatment. *Oncology Nursing Forum* 31, 735 (July 2004).

14 Y. Hishikawa, T. Shimizu, Physiology of REM sleep, cataplexy, and sleep paralysis. *Advances in Neurology* 67, 245 (1995).

15   C. A. Goldstein, Parasomnias. *Disease-a-Month* **57**, 364 (2011).

16   R. Primhak, R. Kingshott, Sleep physiology and sleep-disordered breathing: The essentials. *Archives of Disease in Childhood* **97**, 54 (January 1, 2012).

17   J. L. Otte, J. S. Carpenter, Theories, models, and frameworks related to sleep–wake disturbances in the context of cancer. *Cancer Nursing* **32**, 90 (March–April 2009).

18   E. J. Stepanski, H. J. Burgess, Sleep and cancer. *Sleep Medicine Clinics* **2**, 67 (2007).

19   P. M. Silberfarb, P. J. Hauri, T. E. Oxman, P. Schnurr, Assessment of sleep in patients with lung cancer and breast cancer. *Journal of Clinical Oncology: Official Journal of the American Society of Clinical Oncology* **11**, 997 (May 1993).

20   T. Meuser et al., Symptoms during cancer pain treatment following WHO-guidelines: A longitudinal follow-up study of symptom prevalence, severity and etiology. *Pain* **93**, 247 (September 2001).

21   J. E. Dimsdale, D. Norman, D. DeJardin, M. S. Wallace, The effect of opioids on sleep architecture. *Journal of Clinical Sleep Medicine: Official Publication of the American Academy of Sleep Medicine* **3**, 33 (February 15, 2007).

22   A. Bottomley, Depression in cancer patients: A literature review. *European Journal of Cancer Care* **7**, 181 (September 1998).

23   J. Fleming, Sleep architecture changes in depression: Interesting finding or clinically useful. *Progress in Neuro-Psychopharmacology & Biological Psychiatry* **13**, 419 (1989).

24   L. R. Derogatis et al., The prevalence of psychiatric disorders among cancer patients. *The Journal of the American Medical Association* **249**, 751 (February 11, 1983).

25   N. Breslau, T. Roth, L. Rosenthal, P. Andreski, Sleep disturbance and psychiatric disorders: A longitudinal epidemiological study of young adults. *Biological Psychiatry* **39**, 411 (March 15, 1996).

26   B. Cimprich, Pretreatment symptom distress in women newly diagnosed with breast cancer. *Cancer Nursing* **22**, 185 (June 1999).

27   R. J. Dunlop, C. W. Campbell, Cytokines and advanced cancer. *Journal of Pain and Symptom Management* **20**, 214 (September 2000).

28   L. J. Wood, L. M. Nail, A. Gilster, K. A. Winters, C. R. Elsea, Cancer chemotherapy-related symptoms: Evidence to suggest a role for proinflammatory cytokines. *Oncology Nursing Forum* **33**, 535 (May 2006).

29   T. Rich et al., Elevated serum cytokines correlated with altered behavior, serum cortisol rhythm, and dampened 24-hour rest-activity patterns in patients with metastatic colorectal cancer. *Clinical Cancer Research: An Official Journal of the American Association for Cancer Research* **11**, 1757 (March 1, 2005).

30   A. De, L. Churchill, F. Obal, Jr., S. M. Simasko, J. M. Krueger, GHRH and IL1 beta increase cytoplasmic Ca(2+) levels in cultured hypothalamic GABAergic neurons. *Brain Research* **949**, 209 (September 13, 2002).

31   H. Yoshida et al., State-specific asymmetries in EEG slow wave activity induced by local application of TNFalpha. *Brain Research* **1009**, 129 (May 29, 2004).

32   A. Manfridi et al., Interleukin-1 beta enhances non-rapid eye movement sleep when microinjected into the dorsal raphe nucleus and inhibits serotonergic neurons in vitro. *The European Journal of Neuroscience* **18**, 1041 (September 2003).

33   L. Imeri, M. Mancia, M. R. Opp, Blockade of 5-hydroxytryptamine (serotonin)-2 receptors alters interleukin-1-induced changes in rat sleep. *Neuroscience* **92**, 745 (1999).

34   C. Gemma, L. Imeri, M. G. de Simoni, M. Mancia, Interleukin-1 induces changes in sleep, brain temperature, and serotonergic metabolism. *The American Journal of Physiology* **272**, R601 (February 1997).

35   M. N. Alam et al., Interleukin-1 beta modulates state-dependent discharge activity of preoptic area and basal forebrain neurons: Role in sleep regulation. *The European Journal of Neuroscience* **20**, 207 (July 2004).

36   J. Bauer et al., Interleukin-6 serum levels in healthy persons correspond to the sleep–wake cycle. *The Clinical Investigator* **72**, 315 (March 1994).

37   E. Spath-Schwalbe et al., Acute effects of recombinant human interleukin-6 on endocrine and central nervous sleep functions in healthy men. *The Journal of Clinical Endocrinology and Metabolism* **83**, 1573 (May 1998).

38   A. N. Vgontzas et al., Marked decrease in sleepiness in patients with sleep apnea by etanercept, a tumor necrosis factor-alpha antagonist. *The Journal of Clinical Endocrinology and Metabolism* **89**, 4409 (September 2004).

39   L. Redwine, R. L. Hauger, J. C. Gillin, M. Irwin, Effects of sleep and sleep deprivation on interleukin-6, growth hormone, cortisol, and melatonin levels in humans. *The Journal of Clinical Endocrinology and Metabolism* **85**, 3597 (October 2000).

40   M. J. Sateia, K. Doghramji, P. J. Hauri, C. M. Morin, Evaluation of chronic insomnia. An American Academy of Sleep Medicine review. *Sleep* **23**, 243 (March 15, 2000).

41   A. Chesson, Jr. et al., Practice parameters for the evaluation of chronic insomnia. An American Academy of Sleep Medicine report. Standards of Practice Committee of the American Academy of Sleep Medicine. *Sleep* **23**, 237 (March 15, 2000).

42   D. J. Buysse, C. F. Reynolds, 3rd, T. H. Monk, S. R. Berman, D. J. Kupfer, The Pittsburgh Sleep Quality Index: A new instrument for psychiatric practice and research. *Psychiatry Research* **28**, 193 (May 1989).

43   E. Bruera, N. Kuehn, M. J. Miller, P. Selmser, K. Macmillan, The Edmonton Symptom Assessment System (ESAS): A simple method for the assessment of palliative care patients. *Journal of Palliative Care* **7**, 6 (Summer 1991).

44   H. Babkoff, A. Weller, M. Lavidor, A comparison of prospective and retrospective assessments of sleep. *Journal of Clinical Epidemiology* **49**, 455 (April, 1996).

45   L. de Souza et al., Further validation of actigraphy for sleep studies. *Sleep* **26**, 81 (February 1, 2003).

46   R. J. Cole, D. F. Kripke, W. Gruen, D. J. Mullaney, J. C. Gillin, Automatic sleep/wake identification from wrist activity. *Sleep* **15**, 461 (October, 1992).

47   A. Berger et al., Sleep/wake disturbances in people with cancer and their caregivers: State of the science. *Oncology Nursing Forum* **32**, E98 (2005).

48   F. Chung et al., STOP questionnaire: A tool to screen patients for obstructive sleep apnea. *Anesthesiology* **108**, 812 (May 2008).

49   B. V. Fortner, E. J. Stepanski, S. C. Wang, S. Kasprowicz, H. H. Durrence, Sleep and quality of life in breast cancer patients. *Journal of Pain and Symptom Management* **24**, 471 (2002).

50   M. Delgado-Guay, S. Yennurajalingam, Symptom Assessment, In *Oxford American Handbook of Hospice and Palliative Medicine*, S. Yennurajalingam, E. Bruera, eds., Oxford University Press, New York (2011), pp. 115–126.

51   T. Morgenthaler et al., Practice parameters for the psychological and behavioral treatment of insomnia: An update. An american academy of sleep medicine report. *Sleep* **29**, 1415 (November 2006).

52   P. Fobair et al., Psychosocial intervention for lesbians with primary breast cancer. *Psycho-Oncology* **11**, 427 (September–October 2002).

53   L. Fiorentino et al., Individual cognitive behavioral therapy for insomnia in breast cancer survivors: A randomized controlled crossover pilot study. *Nature and Science of Sleep* **2010**, 1 (December 1, 2009).

54   P. Polc, Enhancement of GABAergic inhibition: A mechanism of action of benzodiazepines, phenobarbital, valproate and L-cycloserine in the cat spinal cord. *Electroencephalography and Clinical Neurophysiology. Supplement* **36**, 188 (1982).

55   P. D. Nowell et al., Benzodiazepines and zolpidem for chronic insomnia: A meta-analysis of treatment efficacy. *The Journal of the American Medical Association* **278**, 2170 (December 24–31, 1997).

56   L. Parrino, M. G. Terzano, Polysomnographic effects of hypnotic drugs. A review. *Psychopharmacology* **126**, 1 (July 1996).

57 A. M. Holbrook, R. Crowther, A. Lotter, C. Cheng, D. King, Meta-analysis of benzodiazepine use in the treatment of insomnia. *Canadian Medical Association Journal = journal de l'Association medicale canadienne* **162**, 225 (January 25, 2000).

58 A. K. Wagner et al., Benzodiazepine use and hip fractures in the elderly: Who is at greatest risk? *Archives of Internal Medicine* **164**, 1567 (July 26, 2004).

59 A. Foy et al., Benzodiazepine use as a cause of cognitive impairment in elderly hospital inpatients. *The Journals of Gerontology. Series A, Biological Sciences and Medical Sciences* **50**, M99 (March 1995).

60 J. T. Hanlon et al., Benzodiazepine use and cognitive function among community-dwelling elderly. *Clinical Pharmacology and Therapeutics* **64**, 684 (December 1998).

61 S. Paterniti, C. Dufouil, A. Alperovitch, Long-term benzodiazepine use and cognitive decline in the elderly: The Epidemiology of Vascular Aging Study. *Journal of Clinical Psychopharmacology* **22**, 285 (June 2002).

62 L. E. Tune, F. W. Bylsma, Benzodiazepine-induced and anticholinergic-induced delirium in the elderly. *International Psychogeriatrics/IPA* **3**, 397 (Winter 1991).

63 J. M. Corkery, F. Schifano, A. H. Ghodse, A. Oyefeso, The effects of methadone and its role in fatalities. *Human Psychopharmacology* **19**, 565 (December 2004). Published 2012.

64 U. Busto, E. M. Sellers, Pharmacologic aspects of benzodiazepine tolerance and dependence. *Journal of Substance Abuse Treatment* **8**, 29 (1991).

65 M. Fava et al., Acute efficacy of fluoxetine versus sertraline and paroxetine in major depressive disorder including effects of baseline insomnia. *Journal of Clinical Psychopharmacology* **22**, 137 (April 2002).

66 G. M. Saletu-Zyhlarz et al., Insomnia in depression: Differences in objective and subjective sleep and awakening quality to normal controls and acute effects of trazodone. *Progress in Neuro-Psychopharmacology & Biological Psychiatry* **26**, 249 (February 2002).

67 S. H. Sindrup, T. S. Jensen, Efficacy of pharmacological treatments of neuropathic pain: An update and effect related to mechanism of drug action. *Pain* **83**, 389 (December 1999).

68 S. W. Kim et al., Effectiveness of mirtazapine for nausea and insomnia in cancer patients with depression. *Psychiatry and Clinical Neurosciences* **62**, 75 (February 2008).

69 E. J. Sanchez-Barcelo, M. D. Mediavilla, D. X. Tan, R. J. Reiter, Clinical uses of melatonin: Evaluation of human trials. *Current Medicinal Chemistry* **17**, 2070 (2010).

70 National Sleep Foundation. *Healthy Sleep Tips.* http://www.sleepfoundation.org/article/sleep-topics/healthy-sleep-tips. Reviewed 05/23/2012.

72

Counseling in palliative care

KIMBERLEY MILLER, DAVID W. KISSANE

Psychotherapeutic interventions and support may be offered to the individual patient living with advanced cancer, but palliative care also recognizes the needs of the "second order"[1] or "hidden" patients[2] among families and caregivers. Although the incidence of distress found in studies varies, approximately 15%–40% of cancer patients will develop significant anxiety and/or depressive symptoms, and even higher rates are found at the end of life.[3–6] Among caregivers of the terminally ill, one study using structured psychiatric interviews found that 33% had psychiatric morbidity,[7] most commonly major depression, anxiety, or adjustment disorders. When self-report questionnaires are used, these frequencies become higher.[8–10] A systematic review has shown that those suffering from or at risk of psychological distress show a greater effect size in responding to psychological treatments compared to those with minimal or no distress.[11] Therefore, identifying and intervening with patients and families at high risk is an important therapeutic and cost-minimizing principle.

The approach to counseling will vary according to needs and clinical indications.[12,13] Services may be delivered individually, some will be more effective when targeting the couple, and meeting with the immediate or extended caregiving family is both helpful and cost-effective. Self-help or professionally led groups are beneficial in promoting support, while focused family therapy and multifamily groups present other options.

In this chapter, the indications for counseling, varied models of intervention, issues for therapists, and process challenges in the delivery of the counseling will be reviewed alongside the evidence for effectiveness of outcome.

WHAT ISSUES PRESENT FOR COUNSELING?

Patients present often with a concern or worry, sometimes with a symptom and rarely with a labeled disorder. The concern may be phrased as a question, buried in a bewildered maze of thoughts and feelings or projected as a problem onto another family member. Whatever the presentation—whether emotional, attitudinal, behavioral, or conative—each request

for help challenges the clinician to recognize what is relevant and organize this meaningfully. Understanding the person with their gamut of life's experiences and influences, successes and failures, accomplishments and omissions, shame and secrets, and health or illness is at the heart of being able to respond to the whole person as a unique individual within their culture, family, and social world.[14]

Clinicians respond to such complexity with organizational schemata that structure the phenomena into recognizable patterns and hierarchies. Training, skill, and experience are crucial here if order is to emerge from potential chaos and be channeled constructively towards improved coping and beneficial outcome.[15] Nevertheless, health professionals need to suspend any preconceptions and listen intently, lest the real needs of the patient are ignored with an inherent inability to heal, even if the disease is being treated. During the final weeks and days of life, matters existential, relational, and spiritual come to the fore and may be more important ultimately than physical symptom management.[16]

How do clinicians organize patients' concerns to aid comprehension and plan consequent intervention? While listening to the narrative of illness, themes are identified and clustered into groups. Common themes include (1) loss, (2) emotional response, (3) meaning, and (4) coping. Loss is myriad in its presentations during the course of illness, and unless normalized as universal yet forever challenging, grief may not be well supported. When loss corresponds with expectations consonant with the life cycle, acceptance results readily; when illness is out of step with this natural order, distress, resentment, and profound grief develop easily. Identifying relevant emotions and any meaning attributed to illness is pertinent. Concepts of the inevitability of change or transitions associated with aging prove helpful, while adaptation as a response invokes some form of coping to optimize outcome and sustain quality of life.

The biopsychosocial and existential/spiritual model is one framework for organizing common issues that present for counseling during palliative care.[17] Its value lies in its integration of the somatic with psychological, social, and spiritual concerns. Table 72.1 illustrates typical issues without seeking to be exhaustive in its coverage of potential themes.

Table 72.1 *Biopsychosocial and spiritual orientation to common issues that may arise in counseling during palliative care*

Biological	Psychological	Social	Spiritual
Specific somatic symptoms, e.g., pain, fatigue, insomnia	*Emotional responses*, e.g., sadness, grief, anger, fear, anxiety, depression	*Instrumental care*, e.g., nursing, pharmacy	*Meaning of illness*, e.g., dying, punishment, spiritual doubt
Reduced physical function, e.g., frailty, impairment, disability	*Adaptation*, e.g., courage, acceptance, rejection, suicidality	*Occupational and physical therapies*, e.g., respite, aides	*Dignity of person*, e.g., respect, valuing accomplishments
Altered bodily appearance, e.g., disfigurement	*Sense of self*, e.g., self-esteem, shame, stigma, loss of worth	*Relational*, e.g., marital, family, sexual, intimacy	*Freedom and control*, e.g., choice, mastery, being a burden
Treatment processes, e.g., radiation, chemotherapy	*Decision making*, e.g., quality of life and treatment adherence	*Financial and supportive*, e.g., burden, withdrawal	*Rituals*, e.g., prayer, connection with the sacred

WHAT DIAGNOSES POTENTIALLY UNDERPIN THESE CONCERNS?

Sometimes therapists offer counseling about specific issues or focused requests like "what do I say to my children?" In these circumstances, direct exploration of options and role play will assist readily. Generally, however, the process of making a clinical diagnosis is pivotal to considering all of the therapeutic options available to ease distress and promote healing. The beauty of diagnosis is that it should trigger a comprehensive treatment plan, one based on experience, clinical wisdom, and, indeed, evidence of effectiveness. In this sense, no counseling should occur in palliative care without a competent, thorough clinical assessment leading to a thoughtful management plan. The clinician is thus always the professional.[18]

Moreover, just as each physical symptom should lead to an assessment, examination, differential diagnosis, and continued reevaluation of response to treatment, so too should each emotional theme generate its differential and continued exploration. Thus, is the sadness an expression of grief or depression?[19] Is the fear grounded in reality or excessive because of coping style? Does a pattern of low self-esteem increase embarrassment or sense of stigma? Does the loss of meaning constitute demoralization or depression?[20,21] Is concern about being a burden driven by altruism, independence, or shame at loss of control? Before considering what the applicable model of intervention is, these golden rules are vital: always take a careful history; examine the mental state; understand what has predisposed to, precipitated, or perpetuated such distress; and formulate why this person is ill in this manner and at this time.

Table 72.2 overviews the common clinical diagnoses that are suitable for counseling. In terms of psychiatric nosological systems, these fall into grief reactions, situational or adjustment disorders, anxiety and depression, existential concerns, and relational and V-code categories. DSM-V, with more emphasis on the dimensional severity on any disorder, will not change the basic diagnoses, except for the addition of adjustment disorder related to bereavement.[22] Other common diagnoses such as delirium, dementia, psychoses, and a range of other organic states are not suitable for psychotherapy primarily, pharmacotherapy being the mainstay of treatment. For a number of conditions including anxiety and depressive disorders, combinations of psychotropic and psychotherapeutic treatment are indicated.[23]

Table 72.2 *Common psychiatric diagnoses that lead to counseling therapies*

Category	Examples
Adjustment disorder	Coping with intense grief, social withdrawal
Anxiety disorder	Panic attacks, nightmares, insomnia
Depressive disorder	Anhedonia, unhappiness, lost interest
Demoralization disorder	Loss of meaning, loss of hope, suicidality
Relational disorder	Marital and family dysfunction, personality disorders, sexual dysfunction
Existential disorder	Spiritual despair, concern about being a burden, need to be in control, profound aloneness
Organic psychiatric disorder	Delirium, medication side effects, alcohol and substance abuse, or withdrawal

INDICATIONS FOR COUNSELING

Distress, formal psychiatric disorder, concern about coping, and lack of sufficient social supports are the common indications for counseling.[24] Sometimes it can be as simple as unmet information needs, but in general, we try to distinguish those who can be supported by all members of the multidisciplinary care team from those who warrant referral for specialist counseling. The latter involves particularly clinicians trained in social work, psychology, or psychiatry.

Risk factors for poorer coping include

1. *Factors in the person*: Past history of depression or psychiatric disorder, cumulative life events, high levels of perceived stress or poor coping
2. *Factors in the illness*: Onset at a young age; delay in diagnosis; recent diagnosis with rapid disease progression;

long, intensive treatments or complications of treatment; specific cancers—pancreatic, neuroendocrine, lymphomas

3. *Factors in the environment*: Poor social supports, family dysfunction, socioeconomic deprivation, potential to leave young children behind

Whenever one or more of these factors are present, consideration of the benefits of supportive counseling proves worthwhile.[25] Once an established psychiatric disorder exists, referral should be axiomatic.

Because of the large research literature showing that psychiatric disorders are often missed (for instance[26–28]), usually through normalization of distress as what is expected, many services utilize a model of screening to assist recognition of those in greater need of psychosocial care.[29,30] A randomized controlled trial of computer-assisted screening and referral for intervention has demonstrated an ability to reduce depressive disorders in oncology patients.[31] Many services today use a triage mechanism to refer patients with milder levels of distress to social workers and those with more severe distress to psychologists or psychiatrists.

MODELS OF COUNSELING

A number of schools of psychotherapy exist, many developed originally for specific clinical circumstances, but generally these are applied eclectically by counselors so that aspects of these different models are combined to suit the clinical predicament of the patient or family. Table 72.3 summarizes the common models of psychotherapy. The following case example will illustrate how each psychotherapeutic model can be used.

> Soon after moving back to his hometown with Sue, his common law girlfriend of 9 years, George, a 29-year-old man was diagnosed with stage IV renal cell carcinoma, involving extensive retroperitoneal and para-aortic lymphadenopathy. They had both just completed their education and hoped to marry and start their family, while beginning their careers and living closer to their families. Sadly, George's cancer was found to have metastasized quickly to his lungs, bones, and liver.

> As the cancer progressed, George required regular subcutaneous injections of Dilaudid for pain control. He began to feel more helpless and worried that he was placing too large a burden on Sue, who was giving him the injections around the clock, with help from a visiting nurse service. George's underlying fear was that Sue would grow weary of this, her view of him would shift from partner to patient, and that they would drift apart, as his health deteriorated.

Psychoeducational interventions

Whether delivered individually, to groups, or to families, the provision of information about the illness and its treatment

Table 72.3 *Models of psychotherapy*

Targets of therapy	Categories of therapy
Individual	• Psychoeducational
	• Supportive expressive
	• Grief therapy
Couple	• Existential psychotherapy
	• Cognitive behavioral therapy
Group	• Interpersonal psychotherapy
	• Psychodynamic therapies
Family	• Narrative and dignity therapies
	• Spiritual and meaning-centered therapies
Community	• Systemic therapies

is foundational and a counseling component of all clinical encounters. In their meta-analysis of 116 studies, Devine and Westlake[32] proved that psychoeducational models have a large effect size, which should not be surprising, as the outcome measure in such studies is simply the acquisition of new knowledge. Studies of unmet needs have nevertheless identified information provision as a major concern of patients with cancer,[33] highlighting its importance at all stages of illness. The efficacy of psychoeducation improves when delivered by individuals with medical expertise.[34]

> In George's case, nursing education covered pain and other symptom management, the nature of his cancer and its treatment, the anticipated process of dying, and how Sue could optimize her role and coordinate care with other members of George's family.

Supportive psychotherapy

Supporting a patient and family through cancer is best done by listening to the story of illness and its treatment, exploring the meaning of the diagnosis and prognosis, allowing the therapist to convey a level of understanding, and thereby developing a trusting relationship with them. The counselor employs a range of therapeutic techniques including questions that seek clarification and invite sharing of emotions; comments that affirm, reassure, encourage, or explain; and suggestions that guide, promote acceptance, and optimize support. This approach is the most generic form of counseling and its techniques are found in all other models of psychotherapy. Although cited in group work, the following goals are also pursued in individual supportive therapy: building bonds, expressing emotions about the illness and its impact on relationships, detoxifying death and dying, redefining life priorities, mobilizing supports, and improving coping and communication.[35–37] Evidence for its effectiveness in advanced cancer is strongest for supportive-expressive group therapy (SEGT)[38] where randomized controlled trials have demonstrated its ability to reduce emotional distress, anxiety, and depression.[39]

The unfairness of George's illness occurring out of step with his expected life cycle was acknowledged, their grief at the many losses normalized, their courage affirmed and their commitment to each other understood. Helping George and Sue to share their feelings and consider how best to support one another lead to affirmation of their greater sense of closeness that this tragedy brought. Accompaniment and commitment were key principles in sustaining continuity of care for them.

Grief therapy

Loss is found universally in illness and is experienced through disease, disfigurement, disability, dependency, depression, and death.[40] Although a variant on supportive psychotherapy, the model of counseling developed for the bereaved[41,42] serves well also as a response to the cumulative experience of loss during any journey with advanced disease. Grief is the interest owed on the debt of investment.[43] The tasks involved include promoting the sharing of emotion, normalizing the sadness, educating about the pattern of distress (waves of emotionality) and time course of mourning, interpreting any displacement of anger, and encouraging adaptive coping responses. Education about the dual track model of grief work,[44] with movement from emotional preoccupation with the loss to refocusing on the living, can help avoid premature grief. Such counseling techniques should be applied by all clinicians working in palliative medicine.

Counseling the bereaved becomes an important dimension of comprehensive palliative care, those at high risk being identified through recognition of (1) personal vulnerability, such as past history of psychiatric disorder; (2) relational problems like dependence or ambivalence; (3) a death experienced as in some way shocking, unexpected, or traumatic; and (4) the presence of family dysfunction or perception of being unsupported or disenfranchised. Group work is especially helpful for the isolated.[45]

Existential psychotherapy

Bred from existentialism, "the study of the experience of living life to its fullest,"[46] concepts of self-awareness, freedom, and responsibility in making choices in one's life, ultimate aloneness and our human need for relatedness, the meaning of life, and the inevitable reality of death[47] are explored and confronted in the dying population. The common sources of existential distress are summarized in Table 72.4 with suitable models of counseling for specific challenges.[48] The counselor helps to define the particular existential challenge that each patient perceives and invites consideration of realistic ways of responding. Built upon processes of confrontation, reaction formation, and inviting choice about those aspects of life that should be most valued, and informed by the narrative story of their life, patients are helped to live authentic and purposeful lives with a particular focus on living in the present moment. Recent end-of-life models of therapy (dignity and meaning centered) have developed from existential psychotherapy.[49]

In George's case, questions were asked about the meaning of their relationship, what they valued in life and each other, what priorities they had in living life out fully, and what benefits Sue found in caring for George. Open acknowledgment of the potential for death helped identify the preciousness of each moment. Grief was checked to the extent that it risked spoiling continued living; the random nature of George's illness was contrasted with their spiritual wonder about life's mysteries.

Cognitive behavioral therapy

Cognitive behavioral therapy (CBT) involves teaching the patient to make connections between emotional events or triggers, associated automatic thoughts or beliefs, and resultant feelings or behaviors. This model, well known in the general psychiatry literature for successfully treating anxiety and depressive disorders,[50–52] can be delivered by palliative care professionals[53] and has been further developed specifically for cancer patients.[54–56] Homework is assigned between sessions, allowing the patient to practice identifying thought patterns that accompany distressing experiences associated with their illness. This is reviewed in the session, where cognitive reframing and disputing of negative automatic thoughts is taught, placing a more realistic framework in place. In working with advanced cancer patients, their concerns should not be simply dismissed, shifting to an unrealistic positive stance. Rather, validating their experience remains paramount, while helping them to understand that their pattern, for example, that of catastrophizing or overgeneralizing, likely contributes to further psychological distress. In the palliative population, existential themes may be understood through cognitive therapy,[57] exploring and examining guilt about prior lifestyle choices, feelings of burden, hopelessness, helplessness, perceived loss of control, anxiety about disfigurement, perceived rejection by friends, and fear of the dying process.

A focus on problem solving and active coping, including assertiveness training and anger management, may also be employed.[58] Additional behavioral interventions include relaxation training through progressive muscular relaxation, guided imagery,[59,60] massage,[61] and hypnosis or meditation,[62–64] together with activity scheduling, exposure, and systematic desensitization as commonly used in the general psychiatry to treat depression and anxiety.

Mind reading and negative predictions were identified as the cognitive distortions being used and alternative explanations were suggested to George. As well, he was urged to clarify this with Sue, who was devastated to learn that he was feeling this way. She explained that providing him with pain relief was a privilege and that it made her feel helpful. Sue acknowledged that she was tired, but suggested that she was no more tired than he was and that they were in this together for the long haul. She felt, more than ever before in their relationship, that they were very much partners in this and reassured him that this was only going to continue to bring them closer together.

Table 72.4 *Adaptive and maladaptive responses to existential challenges and relevant counseling*

Nature of existential challenge	Features of successful adaptation	Form of existential distress when problematic	Common symptoms experienced	Related psychiatric disorders	Suitable model of therapy
1. Death	Courageous awareness of and acceptance of dying; saying goodbye	Death anxiety	Fear of the process of dying or the state of being dead; panic at somatic symptoms; distress at uncertainty	Anxiety disorders, panic disorder, agoraphobia, generalized anxiety disorder, acute stress disorder, adjustment disorder with anxious mood	Psychoeducational, cognitive behavioral therapy, existential psychotherapy, psychodynamic therapy
2. Loss	Sad at reality of loss yet resigned to the occurrence of illness	Complicated grief	Intense tearfulness, grief, and waves of emotionality, progressing into symptoms of depression	Depressive disorders	Supportive psychotherapy, grief therapy, interpersonal psychotherapy
3. Aloneness	Accompanied and supported by family and friends	Profound loneliness	Isolated, alienated, and sense of complete aloneness in life	Dysfunctional family, absence of social support, relationship problems	Interpersonal psychotherapy, family-focused therapy, supportive group therapy
4. Freedom	Acceptance of frailty and reduced independence	Loss of control	Angst at loss of control; obsessional mastery; indecisive, nonadherent to treatments; fear of dependency	Phobic disorders, obsessive–compulsive disorders, substance abuse disorders	Supportive psychotherapy, interpersonal psychotherapy, psychodynamic therapy
5. Meaning	Sense of fulfillment	Demoralization	Pointlessness, hopelessness, futility, loss of role, desire to die	Demoralization syndrome, depressive disorders	Interpersonal psychotherapy, narrative and dignity-conserving therapies, meaning-centered therapies, existential therapy
6. Dignity	Sense of worth despite disfigurement or handicap	Worthlessness	Shame, horror, body image concerns, fear of being a burden	Adjustment disorders	Narrative and dignity-conserving therapies, supportive psychotherapy, grief therapy
7. Mystery	Reverence for the unknowable and sacred	Spiritual doubt and despair	Guilt, loss of faith, loss of connection with the transcendent	Adjustment, anxiety, and depressive disorders	Meaning-centered therapy, life narrative therapies

Psychodynamic psychotherapy

Psychodynamic therapy examines the interplay between emotional and motivational factors and how they impact psychological states and behavior. Several principles from psychodynamic psychotherapy are commonly employed in working with the medically ill population, including advanced cancer patients.[65–67] Patterns of prior coping and relationship difficulties may be revealed in the threat of loss, and recognition of such patterns in earlier life may increase understanding and aid resolution of conflicts. Identifying and exploring defenses, examining core conflicts, and working with transference and countertransference issues are useful processes in supporting the dying patient with cancer.[68] Defenses such as denial and regression may, in fact, be adaptive and promote functioning, while death awareness can also coexist with a strong will to live in those patients with advanced cancer.[69] Such defenses may serve to alleviate distress such as depression, anxiety, or helplessness, assuming they do not result in disruption of appropriate medical treatment or fulfillment of goals, including the organization of one's final affairs. Projected feelings of helplessness may develop in therapists treating patients facing the terminal phase of illness. Understanding this as a countertransference response increases the therapist's insight into what the patient is experiencing, guiding what the focus of therapeutic work might therefore be. Derived from relational theory, attachment theory, and existential therapy, a brief 3- to 6-session individual psychotherapy, *Managing Cancer and Living Meaningfully* (CALM), has been found to provide substantial benefit for patients with advanced cancer prior to end of life.[70] A large randomized controlled mixed-method trial is currently underway. Therapeutic elements of CALM include the supportive relationship, authenticity, modulation of affect, encouragement of reflective functioning, renegotiation of attachment security, joint creation of meaning, shifting frame and flexibility, and facing the limits and boundaries related to mortality, interpretation, and ultimately, termination.[71]

> In reminiscing about his childhood, George recalled how often his mother complained about the extra washing of his sporting clothes caused and how when the washing wasn't done; he had to miss his beloved events. He felt abandoned by his mother at such times, but retreated from any argument as her verbal lashings were fierce. When George asked the therapist if the sessions were too upsetting for her, she drew a comparison between his fears of being a burden to the therapist and to Sue, akin to how he felt a burden to his mother in childhood. It dawned on George that his fear of Sue retreating from his care was based on his old pattern of relating and not something coming from Sue.

Life narrative and dignity-conserving therapies

The narrative account of the person's life aims to generate an understanding of the patient's reaction to and meaning attributed to their illness from the perspective of their overall philosophy and approach to life.[72] Links are made between prior coping during early life experiences and current responses to their cancer experience. The therapist summarizes her understanding of the coherent developmental story to promote a sense of accomplishment, fostering celebration and sense of fulfillment while highlighting roles, relationships, and any apparent purpose of the patients' life. A shared consensus is sought about all that has been accomplished.[72,73]

Chochinov has developed a model of dignity-conserving care for patients approaching death.[74,75] Efforts to improve their self-worth and promote respect are at its core. Each person's illness-related concerns, independence, and spiritual and psychological concerns and how these impact on their sense of dignity are explored. A key goal is to promote hope, autonomy, and sense of control while also addressing spiritual concerns. Dignity-conserving psychotherapy invites the patient to give a narrative account on tape of important aspects of their life that they would most want remembered. This is transcribed, edited, and given to the patient, as well as being a legacy for their family. Topics that prompt this life review in the dignity-conserving model include the following: the individual's life story; how they want their families to remember them; vital roles they have played within their family, job, and community; accomplishments they are most proud of; hopes and dreams for relatives and friends; words of advice to pass along to others; things they want to say to family that have not been said before or that they want to say again; and words that might provide comfort to their family and friends. Although dignity therapy was not found to be better than client-centered care or standard palliative care in reducing overall distress, patients reported that it

was significantly more likely to be helpful, improve quality of life, increase sense of dignity, change how their family saw and appreciated them, and be helpful to their family.[76]

Meaning-centered psychotherapy

Spiritual suffering arises from doubt about earlier beliefs and religious practices and whether there is any greater meaning to life and death. For the religious, loss of connectedness with the transcendent is problematic; for the atheist, the absence of meaning in the chaos of "life-considered-random" can render existence pointless. Individual and group meaning-centered psychotherapies have been developed that promote a sense of meaning and purpose,[77-79] adopting many principles from Viktor Frankl's "logotherapy".[80] Patients are active members in their own treatment, sharing experiences that have helped promote a sense of meaning, peace, and purpose. Exercises are assigned as homework and reviewed at subsequent meetings. The model is being tested in individual and group formats. Sense of personal responsibility, attitudes, creative and experiential values, and the meaning they bring to life are explored.[81]

> George identified the joy that Sue had brought into his life as giving him a special sense of purpose through their relationship together. He lamented nonetheless that they wouldn't reproduce now and that he would not leave a child behind. He told Sue that he wanted her to find someone else after his death and that she should have children early on in this next relationship. Sue told George that she would take some of his gentleness into any future parenting she did, so that he would live on through his influence on her.

Systemic therapies

Whether focused on the marital, parental, or sibling systems, the family of origin, or current nuclear family, the mutual and reciprocal influence of one party upon another can be an important consideration therapeutically. Furthermore, insight into recurring patterns across generations helps families to vary these "scripts" and choose a new direction in their relationships.[82] While couple[83] and family therapies are classical examples of systemic therapies, the concepts can also be applied in individual counseling. Family-focused grief therapy (FFGT) is one preventive model that targets at-risk families during palliative care and continues with the bereaved post-death, aiming to optimize family functioning so that complicated grief and depression are prevented.[84] Families with poor communication, reduced cohesion, and a muted style of dealing with anger respond best to FFGT.[9,85] Care needs to be exercised with the most dysfunctional or hostile families to respect any salutary solution to family conflict through separations and distance, so that conflict is not rekindled by family meetings.[86,87] Thus, modest goals are set with these very dysfunctional families. FFGT has much to offer families at risk in palliative care, its brief and focused approach delivering cost-effectiveness alongside continuity of care into bereavement.

George and Sue were brought together with their parents and siblings, the broader family rallying to support the young couple. Open communication about the cancer and its treatment ensured their grief was shared, hope fostered, and respite organized to protect Sue from exhaustion. As teamwork grew, each family's sense of celebration of George's life became apparent, and support was sustained for Sue throughout the subsequent period of bereavement.

THERAPIST AND PROCESS ISSUES

Professionals working with palliative care patients and their families generally include medical practitioners, nurses or nurse practitioners, social workers, psychologists, psychiatrists, pastoral care workers, and other integrative medicine or allied health clinicians.[88-90] Trained volunteers and health-care aides also play a supportive role. All disciplines should have broad knowledge about palliative medicine as well as a general ability to support dying patients and their families compassionately. The whole of the multidisciplinary treatment team makes a contribution to psychosocial care.

When it comes to developing skill and expertise in the specific models of counseling described in this chapter, formal training is needed. Research confirms that patients respond better to brief interventions provided by well-trained and skilled therapists compared to longer courses of treatment given by less psychologically trained staff.[11]

The core elements of any counseling comprise the relationship that is established, the explanatory model of intervention used, the procedure for promoting change, and the healing that in turn induces further benefit. A number of therapeutic factors are common to all models of intervention. For instance, developing a strong working relationship, often termed a therapeutic alliance, with the patient and their caregivers is foundational.[91] Other key factors include engaging in active listening, allowing patients to ventilate their feelings about their experience, validating their concerns, providing support, and building trust and respect.[92] Exploration of prior losses, especially deaths in the family, and how members coped with their related grief is illuminating.

Irrespective of the model of intervention, some degree of emotional and cognitive learning occurs as each patient is invited to take responsibility for change and well-being. Jerome Frank[93,94] emphasized the restoration of hope and sense of mastery over whatever one can accomplish as being at the heart of all therapeutic improvement. As gains are achieved, consolidation grows from renewed confidence, while response prevention strategies are generally worthwhile. For much of this work, a delicate balance is needed between promoting hope and supporting grief, these two themes often evolving in parallel. Availability, particularly at a time when patients are being told that life-prolonging treatment is no longer an option, can decrease any sense of abandonment. As well, psychological intervention may help patients to adhere to supportive care measures in a way that will improve the quality of life remaining.

Winnicott's model of a facilitating environment is helpful, in which the counselor provides a secure relationship, whose structure creates an experience in which "holding" and "containment" of distress are achieved.[95,96] In palliative care, the boundaries under which this structure would be established ordinarily are modified, so that appropriate and compassionate touch is permitted, access and responsiveness are the norm, and the therapist's warmth, empathy, and unconditional regard help create the holding frame. Nevertheless, an emphasis still exists on appropriate restriction of therapist self-disclosure, here and now feelings being sensitively shared while greater caution is exercised over one's personal life. Disclosure of a gay orientation may be helpful to homosexual patients, but disclosure of personal cancer or illness experiences is generally unwise, the focus of the therapy being truly directed towards the patient.

In the setting of medical illness, most counseling needs to be brief and focused for pragmatic reasons. Given this, the skill and experience of the therapist is especially pertinent, with clinical judgments determining what is worthy of constructive focus and what is wisely left as a long-term or irremediable pattern of behavior. Personality disorders would not be addressed at the individual therapy level, and entrenched family conflict might be respected as ultimately a difference of opinion best resolved by accepting distance between relatives. Selection of a model of therapy is usually eclectic and based on clinical experience, combining elements from several models in response to the prevailing symptoms or predicaments that the patient presents.

Flexibility in number, frequency, and duration of sessions, location of appointments, and modality of treatment used are necessary parts of working with the palliative care population. Telephone support may substitute for direct patient care. Physical symptoms, side effects of treatments, and stage of illness all significantly impact on delivery of services and a change in medical status may necessitate a shift in therapeutic focus. An open flexible approach is best maintained throughout the course of treatment. The potential for psychopharmacological treatment is always considered alongside any counseling and its need monitored.

EFFECTIVENESS OF COUNSELING AND LIMITATIONS

Several meta-analyses have examined the effectiveness of psychological interventions for the treatment of anxiety and depression in patients with cancer.[11,88,97,98] Jacobsen et al. found moderate to large effect sizes in their meta-analyses of interventions for depression in cancer and positive results in 41%–63% of the systematic reviews of the topic[88]. Psychotherapy for depression among incurable cancer patients is useful in treating depressive states, but no studies were identified that focused on major depression.[99] A review of eight manualized interventions for treatment of existential distress revealed that only one SEGT met the criteria for "probably efficacious" treatment.[100] The others were felt to be promising, but requiring additional research due to methodological problems, including need for replication. Research limitations in this field were felt to include challenges related to issues of recruitment and attrition, data analyses, follow-up assessments, confounding factors, and operationalization of outcomes.

Group therapy is at least as effective as individual counseling. Length of treatment is important, with more than 8 hours of counseling generating a greater effect size for anxiety compared to when only 4–7 hours is given.[97] Similarly, length of therapy improves outcome in treating depression. More experienced therapists increase the effect size for both anxiety and depression compared with less experienced counselors.[97] These findings challenge palliative care services to hire appropriately skilled counselors.

The latter concept may have relevance when one seeks to understand the findings from systematic analyses that palliative care service interventions do not significantly improve the outcome for caregivers of the dying patient.[101,102] Community programs over the world have saved costs through engaging unskilled counselors. Another explanation for the apparent absence of proven impact on carers is the absence of targeting "at-risk" carers with preventive interventions. Unless services employ screening to identify high-risk individuals and families, many delightful folk, who will otherwise cope admirably, receive expensive therapies and hide the benefit in studies available to those with more limited coping.

Finally, a caveat is needed about the risks of counseling. Just as pharmacotherapy can induce side effects, sometimes with deleterious consequences, so also can counseling cause harm. Research suggests that about 10% of counseling interventions generate untoward effects, such as worsening anxiety, depression, or marital and family conflict. This limitation calls for skill and experience being derived from formal training in the models of intervention and in one of the basic psychosocial disciplines, so that therapists can identify any deterioration and introduce corrective strategies. When counseling is delivered by trained and experienced professionals, it has much to offer in ameliorating distress and suffering.

Key learning points

- High rates of distress exist among patients, caregivers, and family members during palliative care.

- Counseling interventions have proven efficacy in relieving distress, anxiety, and depression.

- The training and experience of the therapist strongly influences the effectiveness of interventions.

- Outcome is progressively improved by longer interventions.

- Group interventions are at least as efficacious as individual therapies; family group counseling may be more cost-effective when applicable.

- While psychoeducational, supportive, and grief therapies are the mainstay of psychotherapeutic approaches, interpersonal, narrative, and meaning-centered models offer promise in ameliorating existential distress.

REFERENCES

1 Rait D, Lederberg M. The family of the cancer patient. In: Holland JC, Rowland JH, eds. *Handbook of Psychooncology: Psychological Care of the Patient with Cancer*. New York: Oxford University Press; 1989, pp. 585–597.

2 Wiley S. Who cares for family and friends? Providing palliative care at home. Nursing monograph. Darlinghurst, New South Wales, Australia: St. Vincent's Healthcare; 1998, pp. 4–7. Available at http://www.clininfo.health.nsw.gov.au/hospolic/stvincents/stvin98/a2.html

3 Lo C, Zimmerman C, Rydall A, Walsh A, Jones JM, Moore MJ, Shepherd FA, Gagliese L, Rodin G. Longitudinal study of depressive symptoms in patients with metastatic gastrointestinal and lung cancer. *Journal of Clinical Oncology* 2010; 28: 3084–3089.

4 Lloyd-Williams M, Reeve J, Kissane DW. Distress in palliative care patients: Developing patient-centred approaches to clinical management. *European Journal of Cancer* 2008; 44: 1133–1138.

5 Mitchell AJ. Screening procedures for psychosocial distress. In: Holland JC, Breitbart WS, Jacobsen PB, Lederberg MS, Loscalzo MJ, McCorkle R, eds. *Psycho-Oncology*, 2nd edn. New York: Oxford University Press; 2010, pp. 389–396.

6 Massie MJ, Lloyd-Williams M, Irving G, and Miller K. The prevalence of depression in people with cancer. In: Kissane DW, Maj M, Sartorius N, eds. *Depression and Cancer*. Chichester, U.K.: Wiley-Blackwell; 2011, pp. 1–36.

7 Maguire P, Walsh S, Keeling F, Jeacock J, Kingston R. Physical and psychological needs of patients dying from colo-rectal cancer. *Palliative Medicine* 1999; 13: 45–50.

8 Given B, Wyatt G, Given C. Burden and depression among caregivers of patients with cancer at the end of life. *Oncology Nursing Forum* 2004; 31: 1105–1115.

9 Kissane DW, McKenzie M, Bloch S, Moskowitz C, McKenzie DP, O'Neill I. Family focused grief therapy: A randomized controlled trial in palliative care and bereavement. *American Journal of Psychiatry* 2006; 163: 1208–1218.

10 Northouse LL, Mood DW, Schafenacker A. Randomized clinical trial of a family intervention for prostate cancer patients and their spouses. *Cancer* 2007; 110: 2809–2818.

11 Sheard T, Maguire P. The effect of psychological interventions on anxiety and depression in cancer patients: Results of two meta-analyses. *British Journal of Cancer* 1999; 80 (11): 1770–1780.

12 National Breast Cancer Centre & National Cancer Control Initiative. *Clinical Practice Guidelines for the Psychosocial Care of Adults with Cancer*. Camperdown, New South Wales, Australia: National Breast Cancer Centre; 2003.

13 Holland JC, Bultz BD, National Comprehensive Cancer Network (NCCN). The NCCN guideline for distress management: A case for making distress the sixth vital sign. *Journal of the National Comprehensive Cancer Network* 2007; 1: 3–7.

14 Cassell EJ. *The Nature of Suffering and the Goals of Medicine*. New York: Oxford University Press; 1991.

15 Watson M, Kissane DW, eds. *Handbook of Psychotherapy in Cancer Care*. Chichester, U.K.: Wiley-Blackwell; 2011.

16 Sheldon F. *Psychosocial Palliative Care*. Cheltenham, U.K.: Thornes; 1997.

17 Kissane DW. Psychospiritual and existential distress. The challenge for palliative care. *Australian Family Physician* 2000; 29: 1022–1025.

18 Roth AJ, Hoge MA. Training psychiatrists and psychologists in psycho-oncology. In: Holland JC, Breitbart WS, Jacobsen PB, Lederberg MS, Loscalzo MJ, McCorkle R, eds. *Psycho-Oncology*, 2nd edn. New York: Oxford University Press; 2010, pp. 582–587.

19 Lichtenthal WG, Prigerson HG, Kissane DW. Bereavement: A special issue in oncology. In: Holland JC, Breitbart WS, Jacobsen PB, Lederberg MS, Loscalzo MJ, McCorkle R, eds. *Psycho-Oncology*, 2nd edn. New York: Oxford University Press; 2010, pp. 537–543.

20 Kissane DW, Clarke DM, Street AF. Demoralization syndrome—A relevant psychiatric diagnosis for palliative care. *Journal of Palliative Care* 2001; 17: 12–21.

21 Kissane DW, Treece C, Breitbart W, McKeen NA, Chochinov HM. Dignity, meaning and demoralization: Emerging paradigms in end-of-life care. In: Chochinov HM, Breitbart W, eds. *Handbook of Psychiatry in Palliative Medicine*, 2nd edn. Oxford, U.K.: Oxford University Press; 2009, pp. 324–340.

22 American Psychiatric Association. Diagnostic and statistical manual of disorders DSM-V. 2013. http://www.dsm5.org/Proposed Revision/Pages/proposedrevision.aspx?rid=367, accessed 3/25/2012.

23 Kissane DW, Smith GC. Consultation-liaison psychiatry in an Australian oncology unit. *Australian & New Zealand Journal of Psychiatry* 1996; 30: 397–404.

24 Burton M, Watson M. *Counselling People with Cancer*. Chichester, U.K.: Wiley; 1998.

25 Lederberg MS, Holland JC. Supportive psychotherapy in cancer care: An essential ingredient of all therapy. In: Watson M, Kissane DW, eds. *Handbook of Psychotherapy in Cancer Care*. Chichester, U.K.: Wiley-Blackwell; 2011, pp. 3–14.

26 Wasteson E, Brenne E, Higginson IJ et al. Depression assessment and classification in palliative care patients: A systematic literature review. *Palliative Medicine* 2009; 23: 739–753.

27 Thune-Boyle IC, Myers LB, Newman SP. The role of illness beliefs, treatment beliefs, and perceived severity of symptoms in explaining distress in cancer patients during chemotherapy treatment. *Behavioral Medicine* 2006; 32: 19–29.

28 Passik SD, Dugan W, McDonald MV. Oncologists' recognition of depression in their patients with cancer. *Journal of Clinical Oncology* 1998; 16: 1594–1600.

29 Zabora J, Loscalzo MJ. Comprehensive psychosocial programs: A prospective model of care. *Oncology* 1996; 11: 14–18.

30 Mitchell AJ. Pooled results from 38 analyses of the accuracy of distress thermometer and other ultra-short methods of detecting cancer-related mood disorder. *Journal of Clinical Oncology* 2007; 25: 4670–4681.

31 McLachlan SA, Allenby A, Matthews J, Wirth A, Kissane DW, Bishop M, Beresford J, Zalcberg J. Randomized trial of coordinated psychosocial interventions based on patient self-assessments versus standard care to improve the psychosocial functioning of patients with cancer. *Journal of Clinical Oncology* 2001; 19: 4117–4125.

32 Devine EC, Westlake SK. The effects of Psychoeducational care provided to adults with cancer: Meta-analysis of 166 studies. *Oncology Nursing Forum*, 1995; 22: 1369–1381.

33 Newell S, Sanson-Fisher RW, Grigis A, Ackland S. The physical and psychosocial experiences of patients attending an outpatient medical oncology department: A cross-sectional study. *European Journal of Cancer Care* 1999; 8: 73–82.

34 Zimmerman T, Heinrichs N, Baucom DH. "Does one size fit all?" Moderators in psychosocial interventions for breast cancer patients: A meta-analysis. *Annals of Behavioral Medicine* 2007; 34: 225–239.

35 Goodwin P, Leszcz M, Ennis M et al.. The effect of group psychosocial support on survival in metastatic breast cancer. *New England Journal of Medicine* 2001; 345: 1719–1726.

36 Kissane DW, Grabsch B, Clarke, DM et al. Supportive-expressive group therapy for women with metastatic breast cancer: Survival and psychosocial outcome from a randomized controlled trial. *Psycho-Oncology* 2007; 16: 277–286.

37 Spiegel D, Butler L, Giese-Davis J et al. Effects of supportive-expressive group therapy on survival of patients with metastatic breast cancer. *Cancer* 2007; 110: 1130–1138.

38 Spiegel D, Classen C. *Group Therapy for Cancer Patients*. New York: Basic Books; 2000.

39 Cunningham AJ, Edmonds CV, Jenkins GP, Pollack H, Lockwood GA, Warr D. A randomized controlled trial of the effects of group psychological therapy on survival in women with metastatic breast cancer. *Psycho-Oncology* 1998; 7: 508–517.

40 Holland JC, Lewis S. *The Human Side of Cancer*. New York: Harper; 2000.

41 Worden JW. *Grief Counseling and Grief Therapy*. 2nd edn. New York: Springer; 1991.

42 Christ GH. *Healing Children's Grief*. New York: Oxford University Press; 2000.

43 Yalom ID. *The Gift of Therapy. Reflections on Being a Therapist*. London, U.K.: Piatkus; 2001.

44 Stroebe M, Schut H. The dual process model of coping with bereavement: Rationale and description. *Death Studies* 1999; 23: 197–224.

45 Yalom ID, Vinogradov S. Bereavement groups: Techniques and themes. *International Journal Group Psychotherapy* 1988; 38: 419–446.

46 Spira JL. Existential psychotherapy. In: Chochinov HM, Breitbart W. *Handbook of Psychiatry in Palliative Medicine*. New York: Oxford University Press; 2000, pp. 197–214.

47 Fischer C. Existential therapy. In: Covey G, editor. *Theory and Practice of Counseling and Psychotherapy*. 2nd edn. San Francisco, CA: Brooks/Cole Publishing; 1982, pp. 67–75.

48 Kissane DW, Yates P. Psychological and existential distress. In: O'Connor M, Aranda S, eds. *Palliative Care Nursing: A Guide to Practice*. 2nd edn. Melbourne, Victoria, Australia: Ausmed; 2003.

49 Yalom ID. *Existential Psychotherapy*. New York: Basic Books; 1980.

50 Clum GA, Clum GA, Surls R. A meta-analysis of treatments for panic disorder. *Journal of Consultation Clinical Psychology* 1993; 61: 317–326.

51 van Balkom AJLM, van Oppen P, Vermeulen AWA, van Dyck RV, Nauta MCE, Vorst HCM. A meta-analysis on the treatment of obsessive compulsive disorder: A comparison of antidepressants, behavior and cognitive therapy. *Clinical Psychology Review* 1994; 14: 359–381.

52 Gloaquenu K, Cotraux J, Cucherat M, Blackburn IM. A meta-analysis of the effects of cognitive therapy with depressed patients. *Journal Affective Disorder* 1998; 49: 59–72.

53 Mannix KA, Blackburn IM, Garland A, Gracie J, Moorey S, Reid B, Standart S, Scott J. Effectiveness of brief training in cognitive behaviour therapy techniques for palliative care practitioners. *Palliative Medicine* 2006; 20: 579–584.

54 Moorey S, Greer S. *Cognitive Behaviour Therapy for People with Cancer*, 2nd edn. Oxford, U.K.: Oxford University Press; 2002.

55 Moorey S, Cort E, Kapari M, Monroe B, Hansford P, Mannix K, Henderson M, Fisher L, Hotopf M. A cluster randomized controlled trial of cognitive behavioural therapy for common mental disorders in patients with advanced cancer. *Psychological Medicine* 2009; 39: 713–723.

56 Kissane DW, Bloch S, Smith GC, Miach P, Clarke DM, Ikin J, Love A, Ranieri N, McKenzie DP. Cognitive-existential group psychotherapy for women with primary breast cancer: A randomized controlled trial. *Psycho-Oncology* 2003; 12: 532–546.

57 Kissane DW, Bloch S, Miach P, Smith GC, Seddon A, Keks N. Cognitive-Existential group therapy for patients with primary breast cancer—Techniques and themes. *Psycho-Oncology* 1997; 6: 25–33.

58 Horne D, Watson M. Cognitive-behavioural therapies in cancer care. In: Watson M, Kissane DW, eds. *Handbook of Psychotherapy in Cancer Care*. Chichester, U.K.: Wiley-Blackwell; 2011, pp. 15–26.

59 Baider LB, Peretz T, Hadani PE, Koch U. Psychological intervention in cancer patients: A randomized study. *General Hospital Psychiatry* 2001; 23: 272–277.

60 Walker LG, Walker MB, Ogston K, Heys SD, Ah-see AK, Miller ID, Hutcheon AW, Sarkar TK, Eremin O. Psychological, clinical and pathological effects of relaxation training and guided imagery during primary chemotherapy. *British Journal of Cancer* 1999; 80 (1/2): 262–268.

61 Soden K, Vincent K, Craske S, Lucas C, Ashley S. A randomized controlled trial of aromatherapy massage in a hospice setting. *Palliative Medicine* 2004; 18: 87–92.

62 Carlson L, Ursuliak Z, Goodey E, Angen M, Speca M. The effects of a mindfulness meditation-based stress reduction program on mood and symptoms of stress in cancer outpatients: 6-month follow-up. *Support Care Cancer* 2001; 9: 112–123.

63 Payne DK. Mindfulness interventions for cancer patient. In: Watson M, Kissane DW, eds. *Handbook of Psychotherapy in Cancer Care.* Chichester, U.K.: Wiley-Blackwell; 2011, pp. 39–47.

64 Lewis EJ, Sharp MD. Relaxation and image based therapy. In: Watson M, Kissane DW, eds. *Handbook of Psychotherapy in Cancer Care.* Chichester, U.K.: Wiley-Blackwell; 2011, pp. 49–58.

65 Kent LK, Blumenfield M. Psychodynamic psychiatry in the general medical setting. *Journal of the American Academy of Psychoanalysis and Dynamic Psychiatry* 2011; 39: 41–62.

66 Nash SS, Kent LK, Muskin PR. Psychodynamics in medically ill patients. *Harvard Review of Psychiatry* 2009; 17: 389–397.

67 Rodin G, Zimmerman C. Psychoanalytic reflections on mortality: A reconsideration. *Journal of the American Academy of Psychoanalysis and Dynamic Psychiatry* 2008; 36: 181–196.

68 Straker N. Psychodynamic psychotherapy for cancer patients. *Journal of Psychotherapy Practice and Research* 1998; 7(1): 1–9.

69 Rodin G, Zimmerman C, Rydall A, Jones J, Shepherd FA, Moore M, Fruh M, Donner A, Gagliese L. The desire for hastened death in patients with metastatic cancer. *Journal of Pain and Symptom Management* 2007; 33: 661–675.

70 Nissim R, Freeman E, Lo C, Zimmerman C, Gagliese L, Rydall A, Hales S, Rodin G. Managing Cancer and Living Meaningfully (CALM): A qualitative study of a brief individual psychotherapy for individuals with advanced cancer. *Palliat Med* 2014; 28: 234–242.

71 Lo C, Hales S, Jung J, Chiu A, Panday T, Rydall A, Nissim R, Malfitano C, Petricone-Westwood D, Zimmermann C, Rodin G. *Managing cancer and Living Meaningfully (CALM): Phase 2 trial of a brief individual psychotherapy for patients with advanced cancer. Palliative Medicine* 2012; 26: 713–721.

72 Viederman M. Psychodynamic life narrative in a psychotherapeutic intervention useful in crisis situations. *Psychiatry* 1983; 46: 236–246.

73 Snedker Boman B. Narrative therapy. In: Watson M, Kissane DW, eds. *Handbook of Psychotherapy in Cancer Care.* Chichester, U.K.: Wiley-Blackwell; 2011, pp. 69–77.

74 Chochinov HM. Dying, dignity and new horizons in palliative end-of-life care. *CA Cancer Journal for Clinicians* 2006; 56: 84–103.

75 Chochinov HM, McKeen NA. Dignity therapy. In: Watson M, Kissane DW, eds. *Handbook of Psychotherapy in Cancer Care.* Chichester, U.K.: Wiley-Blackwell; 2011, pp. 79–88.

76 Chochinov HM, Kristjanson L, Breitbart W, McClement S, Fack TF, Hassard T, Harlos M. Effect of dignity therapy on distress and end-of-life experience in terminally ill patients: A randomized controlled trial. *Lancet* 2011; 12: 753–762.

77 Breitbart W, Rosenfeld B, Gibson C. Meaning-centered group psychotherapy for patients with advanced cancer: A pilot randomized controlled trial. *Psychooncology* 2010; 19: 21–28.

78 Breitbart W, Applebaum A. Meaning-centered group psychotherapy. In: Watson M, Kissane DW, eds. *Handbook of Psychotherapy in Cancer Care.* Chichester, U.K.: Wiley-Blackwell; 2011, pp. 138–148.

79 Breitbart W, Poppito S, Rosenfeld B, Vickers AJ, Li Y, Abbey J, Olden M, Pessin H, Lichtenthal W, Sjoberg D, Cassileth BR. Pilot randomized controlled trial of individual meaning-centered psychotherapy for patients with advanced cancer. *Journal of Clinical Oncology* 2012; 30: 1304–1309.

80 Frankl VF. *Man's Search for Meaning,* 4th edn. Boston, MA: Beacon Press; 1992.

81 Breitbart W, Gibson C, Poppito S, Berg A. Psychotherapeutic interventions at the end of life: A focus on meaning and spirituality. *Cancer Journal Psychiatry* 2004; 49: 366–372.

82 Kissane DW, Zaider TI. Focused family therapy in palliative care and bereavement. In: Watson M, Kissane DW, eds. *Handbook of Psychotherapy in Cancer Care.* Chichester, U.K.: Wiley-Blackwell; 2011, pp. 185–197.

83 Zaider TI, Kissane DW. Couples therapy in advanced cancer: Using intimacy and meaning to reduce existential distress. In: Watson M, Kissane DW, eds. *Handbook of Psychotherapy in Cancer Care.* Chichester, U.K.: Wiley-Blackwell; 2011, pp. 161–173.

84 Kissane DW, Bloch S. *Family Focused Grief Therapy: A Model of Family-Centered Care during Palliative Care and Bereavement.* Buckingham, U.K.: Open University Press; 2002.

85 Chan EK, O'Neill I, McKenzie M, Love A, Kissane DW. What works for therapists conducting family meetings: Treatment integrity in Family Focused Grief Therapy during palliative care and bereavement. *Journal of Pain and Symptom Management* 2004; 27: 502–512.

86 Dumont I, Kissane DW. Techniques for framing questions in conducting family meetings in palliative care. *Palliative & Supportive Care* 2009; 7:163–170.

87 Del Gaudio F, Zaider TI, Brier M, Kissane DW. Challenges in providing family-centered support to families in palliative care. *Palliative Medicine* 2012; in press.

88 Jacobsen PB, Jim HS. Psychosocial interventions for anxiety and depression in adult cancer patients: Achievements and challenges. *CA Cancer Journal for Clinicians* 2008; 58: 214–230.

89 Strong V, Waters R, Hibberd C et al. Management of depression for people with cancer (SMaRT oncology 1): A randomized trial. *Lancet* 2008; 372: 40–48.

90 Walker J, Sharpe M. Depression care for people with cancer: A collaborative care intervention. *General Hospital Psychiatry* 2009; 31: 436–441.

91 Rodin G, Walsh A, Zimmermann C et al. The contribution of attachment security and social support to depressive symptoms in patients with metastatic cancer. *Psycho-Oncology* 2007; 16: 1080–1091.

92 Massie MJ, Popkin MK. Depression. In: Holland JC, Rowland JH, eds. *Handbook of Psycho-Oncology.* New York: Oxford University Press; 1989, pp. 518–541.

93 Frank J. The role of hope in psychotherapy. *International Journal of Psychiatry* 1968; 5: 383–395.

94 Frank J. The restoration of morale. *American Journal of Psychiatry* 1974; 131: 271–274.

95 Davis M, Wallbridge D. *Boundary and Space. An Introduction to the Work of D. W. Winnicott.* New York: Brunner/Mazel; 1981.

96 Winnicott DW. *The Maturational Processes and the Facilitating Environment.* London, U.K.: Karnac Books and The Institute of Psycho-analysis; 1990.

97 Devine EC, Westlake SK. The effects of psychoeducational care provided to adults with cancer: Meta-analysis of 116 studies. *Oncology Nursing Forum* 1995; 22: 1369–1381.

98 Osborn R, Demoncada A, Feuerstein M. Psychosocial interventions for depression, anxiety, and quality of life in cancer survivors: Meta-analyses. *International Journal of Psychiatry in Medicine* 2006; 36: 13–34.

99 Akechi T, Okuyama T, Onishi J, Morita T, Furukawa TA. Psychotherapy for depression among incurable cancer patients (Review). *Cochrane Database of Systematic Review* 2010; 16: CD005537.

100 LeMay K, Wilson K. Treatment of existential distress in life threatening illness: A review of manualized interventions. *Clinical Psychology Review* 2008; 28: 472–493.

101 Higginson IJ, Finlay IG, Goodwin DM, Hood K, Edwards AG, Cook A, Douglas HR, Normand CE. Is there evidence that palliative care teams alter end-of-life experiences of patients and their caregivers? *Journal of Pain and Symptom Management* 2003; 25: 150–168.

102 Harding R, Higginson IJ. What is the best way to help caregivers in cancer and palliative care? A systematic literature review of interventions and their effectiveness. *Palliative Medicine* 2003; 17:63–74.

73

Hope in end-of-life care

CHERYL L. NEKOLAICHUK

The biggest pain to go through in the end...
is the gradual drop-away of visitors.
I hope my friends keep their promises.
Promises about sitting with me
and being with me when that time comes
                    A palliative care patient (May 29, 2012)

INTRODUCTION

The progressive, unpredictable nature of a terminal illness—marked by debilitating symptoms, body image distortions, and multiple losses—propels patients and their families onto a pathway of uncertainty, fear, and, for some, despair. Traditional roles may be reversed or erased, as patients feel marginalized from society. External messages of "There is no cure" become internal messages of "There is no hope," as they wrestle with their own mortality. In a study involving advanced cancer patients, 48% of participants reported at least some sense of hopelessness.[1]

Despite these substantive challenges, patients at end of life strive to maintain hope within their caring circles. In interviews with 120 terminally ill cancer patients, 99% of respondents rated *having a sense of hope* as a very important existential concern.[2] Based on a review of research studies, Lin and Bauer-Wu[3] identified *living with meaning and hope* as one of six essential themes of psychosocial spiritual well-being in patients with advanced cancer. In a qualitative study focusing on information needs, patients with advanced cancer identified the *provision of hope and need for hopeful messages* as one of the two most important concerns regarding information content.[4]

Health-care professionals equally emphasize the importance of hope in the delivery of palliative care. Numerous position papers and literature reviews highlight the need for intentionally incorporating hope within end-of-life care.[5–11] Janssens et al.[12] have further embedded the concept within a philosophy of care for palliative care, consisting of three realms—medical, psychosocial, and spiritual—with hope as a central existential phenomenon within the spiritual realm.

Despite these overwhelming endorsements, the systematic integration of hope within routine clinical practice remains relatively underdeveloped. Beginning with an overview of the therapeutic value of hope, this chapter will address the following questions for intentionally integrating hope within end-of-life care:

- What is the nature of hope in palliative care?
- How can we enhance our approaches for assessing hope in people who are terminally ill?
- What types of hope-enhancing strategies and interventions would be most appropriate for this unique population?

THERAPEUTIC VALUE OF HOPE IN ILLNESS

The therapeutic value of hope in chronic and life-threatening illnesses is well documented. Hope has been positively linked to effective coping,[13–15] enhanced quality of life,[16–18] spiritual well-being,[19] and healing.[20–22] In contrast, hopelessness may be associated with low levels of perceived emotional support,[23,24] depression,[24,25] suicidal intent,[26] desire for hastened death,[27] and pain.[27,28] Studies in terminally ill patients have revealed that hopelessness is a strong predictor of poorer health-related quality of life,[29] desire for hastened death,[30,31] will to live,[32] and suicidal intent.[33]

Although these findings are significant, some caution is warranted in making cross-study comparisons. Study samples were quite diverse, including patients with human immunodeficiency virus (HIV)/acquired immune deficiency syndrome (AIDS)[19,23,24] and cancer,[13,16,30,31,33] depressed patients,[21,22,25,26] patients with long-term disabilites,[14,20] and older patients,[17] and were not entirely limited to the terminal illness phase. The use of different measures to assess hope or hopelessness across studies further limits meaningful comparisons. Future research studies, focusing on relationships between hope, symptom expression, and positive health indicators, such as quality of life, well-being, and coping, need to specifically target the terminally ill, using consistent measurement approaches appropriate for this population.

NATURE OF HOPE IN PALLIATIVE CARE

What does hope mean to you as a health-care provider?

What does hope mean to the patients for whom you provide care?

In health care, the concept of hope has been closely linked with treatments and cures.[34-36] When hope for a cure is no longer viable, health-care professionals and patients may give up hope. Although the situation may be hopeless, there is always hope for the individual.[37] A key challenge is to understand the nature of hope in palliative care.

A diversity of conceptual frameworks exists in the literature, with no consensus for a universal definition of hope. A critique of the hope literature revealed seven themes associated with these differing perspectives[38] (see Figure 73.1), accompanied by the following assumptions:

- *Universality*: Hope is both a universal and an intensely personal experience.
- *Dimensionality*: Hope is a complex concept, ranging from unidimensional to multidimensional aspects of a person's experience.
- *Intangibility*: Hope has both tangible and intangible components, some of which may never be elucidated.
- *Temporality*: Hope appears to imply some sense of temporality, although this may not necessarily be limited to a future orientation. It is also possible that some components of hope may not be bound by time.
- *Predictability*: The experience of hope may have both predictable and unpredictable components.
- *Value based*: The value of hope appears to be embedded in personal experience.
- *Reality based*: Hope appears to be connected with some sense of realism, although the viewpoints of reality remain unclear.

These seven themes provide a cohesive framework for understanding the nature of hope in palliative care.

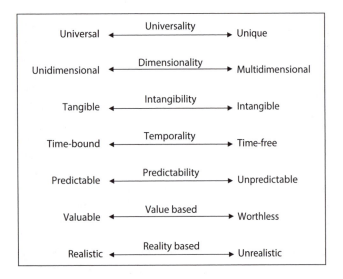

Figure 73.1 *Thematic analysis of the concept of hope.*

Universality

Although hope is a universal human experience, it is also intensely unique. A number of qualitative studies, focusing on the terminally ill patient's experience of hope, have been conducted in diverse settings, such as palliative home care,[39-43] inpatients,[44-47] outpatient clinics,[36,44,39,48-50] and nonmedical settings.[37,51-53] Samples varied, including patients with cancer,[39,40,44,45] HIV/AIDS,[37,51-53] amyotrophic lateral sclerosis (ALS),[54] and end-stage renal disease.[48] In contrast, one study involved interviewing nurses about their perceptions of hope in palliative care patients with cancer.[49]

Dimensionality

A diversity of conceptual frameworks for hope has emerged, ranging from unidimensional to multidimensional models. Of the many diverse frameworks, Dufault and Martocchio's model,[55] qualitatively derived from a sample of older cancer and terminally ill patients, provides a useful initial framework for understanding hope in the terminally ill. Dufault and Martocchio proposed a multidimensional framework for hope, consisting of six dimensions: cognitive, affective, behavioral, affiliative, contextual, and temporal. Each of these dimensions may be impacted in different ways when a person is facing a terminal illness.

Intangibility

The experience of hope may have both tangible and intangible components. Dufault and Martocchio[55] described these two types of hope as particularized and generalized hopes. Particularized hopes are hopes that are directed toward specific goals. For terminally ill patients, specific hopes may change over time,[56,57] for example, shifting from hope for a cure to hope for symptom relief, a special time with family, or a peaceful death. In contrast, generalized hopes represent an intangible inner experience of hope that is not connected to any specific goal. This invisible part of hope may be difficult to articulate and is often experienced at a deep, spiritual level.

Temporality

Although most definitions for hope include a future orientation, this may not always be appropriate for the terminally ill.[5] For some people, with strong faith beliefs, hope may be tied to a future beyond this life. For others, the experience of hope may be interwoven with past, present, and future experiences[5,55,58,59]; may be lived in the present[16]; or may transcend time.[55,60] It is important to have some understanding of how patients view hope in terms of time, potentially deemphasizing the future component.

Predictability

The uncertainty of advancing disease raises fears in most patients who are terminally ill. Although frameworks do differ, some models have included uncertainty as an inherent part of the hope experience.[58,61] Exploring a person's fears, as well as focusing on predictable aspects of a person's life, helps buffer the uncertainties of progressive illness.

Value based

Few could argue with the potential therapeutic benefits that hope offers to the dying. Not everyone, however, may value hope positively, particularly if they have been previously disappointed by hope. For example, patients who direct all their hopes toward finding a cure are often devastated when they are told that their condition is incurable. The challenge is to be able to help patients develop a broad hoping repertoire, including hopes beyond a cure.[5]

Reality based

Often, people may concurrently hold two opposing hopes, such as hope for a cure and hope for a peaceful death.[38,62] This may be troubling for some professional caregivers and family members, who might view this as unrealistic or unhealthy denial. In contrast, Jevne and Nekolaichuk[63] describe this phenomenon as a normal way for patients to prioritize their hopes:

> It is important to listen to the descriptive words that they [patients] attach to their hopes, acknowledging the range (and depth) of their hopes. One elderly patient who was forced to stop traveling due to a progression of his disease described his hope to travel as a 'forlorn' hope. Another palliative patient who expressed a hope for peace in the world described that particular hope as a 'big' hope. Yet another patient who hung onto a hope for a cure, despite being told that her cancer was incurable, suggested that it 'may not be a very realistic' hope, but that 'miracles do happen.' For a patient who believed in life after death, her hope to be united with God was her 'ultimate' hope. (p. 195)

Professional caregivers need to normalize these apparently polarizing views, balancing the provision of honest truthful information with the maintenance of hope.[62,64]

ASSESSMENT OF HOPE

> How can you tell how hopeful a person is?
>
> What do you need to know to understand a person's experience of hope?

Although a variety of hope assessment approaches have been developed in clinical practice,[61] few have been developed specifically for palliative care.[5,10,65] Given the frailty of this population, assessments need to be relatively brief, psychometrically sound in terms of quantitative measures, and closely linked with the development of hope-enhancing strategies and interventions. In some cases, the assessment itself may be a therapeutic intervention. The Herth Hope Index[66] is a well-validated measure that has been used extensively in the palliative care population. Although psychometric findings are generally favorable across different cultures, in one validation study involving Swedish palliative patients, the authors cautioned against its use in Swedish clinical palliative settings, due to linguistic, conceptual, and cultural translation difficulties.[67]

Given the complexity of the hope experience, quantitative measures need to be combined with qualitative assessments. An example of a qualitative hope assessment framework for palliative care appears in Table 73.1.[5] This framework is based on an empirically derived model of hope, consisting of three dimensions: personal spirit, risk, and authentic caring.[68] Personal spirit is a predominant personal dimension, represented by a core theme of meaning. Risk, a situational dimension, is primarily represented by an underlying theme of uncertainty. Authentic caring, a relational dimension, is characterized by the complementary themes of credibility and caring. Thus, a person's experience of hope may be associated with finding meaning in life, taking risks in spite of uncertainty, and developing caring, credible relationships.

Table 73.1 *A hope assessment framework for terminally ill patients*

Theme	Questions for the health–care professional	Questions for the patient
Personal spirit	What is meaningful in this person's life?	What gives you meaning in your life?
	What is this person's relationship with time?	How has your hope changed over time?
	How might past, present, and future experiences influence this person's experience of hope?	Tell me about a time in your past that has influenced your hope in some way.
Risk	What is this person's tolerance for uncertainty?	How have you handled times of uncertainty in the past? What are you most afraid of?
	How can I enhance this person's hope, beyond a hope for a cure?	Without taking away your hope for a cure, what else might keep you going in the event that a cure is not possible?
Authentic caring	Who authentically cares about this person?	Who in your world cares about you?
	How can I provide truthful information to this person, yet still remain hopeful?	Whom do you care about?

Source: Adapted from Nekolaichuk, C.L. and Bruera, E., *J. Palliat. Care*, 14, 36, 1998.

HOPE-ENHANCING STRATEGIES AND INTERVENTIONS

How do you enhance hope for someone who appears to have given up?

How do you serve as a model of hope for your patients?

There are many descriptions of hope-enhancing strategies and interventions for the terminally ill, based on literature reviews,[69] research studies,[8,56,70–74] theoretical perspectives,[75] and clinical experience.[76–78] In a systematic review of nursing literature, Holt[79***] identified 14 hope intervention themes, the 6 most common being positive relationships, patient self-worth, patient control, goal setting, use of distraction, and family support.

Despite the interest in this area, there are very few hope-focused intervention studies, specifically targeted for the terminally ill population. Duggleby and colleagues have developed a Living with Hope Program (LWHP), which they evaluated in senior palliative home care patients.[80**] Using a mixed-method concurrent nested experimental design, patients in the LWHP arm had significantly higher hope (p = 0.005) and quality of life (p = 0.027) than those in the standard care comparison group. They have also pilot tested a parallel program for caregivers of family members with advanced cancer.[81*] Using a quasi-experimental design, Herth[82*] demonstrated the effectiveness of an eight-session hope-enhancing nursing intervention program in a convenience sample of patients with first recurrence of cancer. Patients in the treatment arm had significantly higher levels of hope and quality of life immediately after and at 3-, 6-, and 9-month posttreatment than the comparison group. A follow-up evaluation of this intervention program was also conducted with the treatment group.[83*] In contrast, other studies involving advanced cancer patients have included hope or hopelessness as an outcome of specific therapeutic interventions, such as meaning-centered therapy,[84**] dignity therapy,[85**,86**] forgiveness therapy,[87*] or life review,[88**] with mixed results.

Others have demonstrated the effectiveness of hope-specific interventions in nonpalliative populations, such as homeless veterans[89*] and patients newly diagnosed with cancer.[90*] Based on a quasi-experimental design, Tollett and Thomas[89*] studied the effect of rational thought on levels of hope in a sample of 40 homeless veterans. Rustoen et al.[90*] conducted

a quasi-experimental study to evaluate the effect of an eight-session hope-focused nursing intervention on hope and quality of life in patients newly diagnosed with cancer. In both of these studies, hope was significantly higher after the intervention than in the comparison groups.

The use of explicit hope-enhancing interventions needs to be integrated with implicit approaches, in which hope is modeled by the professional caregiver's hopeful presence and orientation.[63] An example of an integrated hope intervention framework for cancer patients appears in Table 73.2. This framework was derived from a thematic analysis of the literature, patient interviews, and clinical experiences. It consists of seven hope-enhancing themes: caring, communication, commitment, coping, creating, community, and celebrating. Within each theme, specific strategies for enhancing hope are proposed, some of which may be explicit while others may be implicit (see Jevne and Nekolaichuk[63] for detailed descriptions of additional strategies). Although this framework was developed for cancer patients, many of these strategies could be applied to the terminally ill. Further research is needed to extend its use in this population.

SUMMARY

How might we create a space for hope in end-of-life care?

This chapter highlighted three specific challenges for intentionally integrating hope within clinical practice:

- The need to understand the nature of hope at end of life
- The need to develop brief, psychometrically sound measures and complementary qualitative assessment frameworks
- The need to develop and evaluate specific hope-enhancing interventions for the terminally ill

The lack of well-developed assessment approaches and effective hope-enhancing interventions, targeted specifically for the terminally ill, has impeded progress in this area. Through collaborative efforts involving patients, clinicians, and researchers, appropriate hope assessment frameworks and hope-focused interventions need to be developed and eventually become part of routine end-of-life care.

Table 73.2 *The seven Cs: A hope intervention framework*

Theme	Questions for the patient
Caring	Tell me about a time in your life when you experienced a moment of caring.
Communication	Tell me about what it is like to be ill. How has your hope changed since you have become ill?
Commitment	What would be one small thing that you might do on a regular basis to help strengthen your hope?
Coping	What has helped you through difficult times in the past?
Creating	If you were to create a "hope kit," what things would you put in it?
Community	How is hope experienced in your community (culture)?
Celebrating	If you were to plan a celebration of hope, what might you do?

Source: Adapted from Jevne, R.F. and Nekolaichuk, C.L., Threat and hope in coping with cancer for health care professionals. In: Jacoby, R., Keinan, G., eds. *Between Stress and Hope: From a Disease-Centered to a Health-Centered Perspective*, Praeger Publishers, Westport, CT, pp. 187–212, 2003.

Key learning points

- Patients, health-care providers, and health researchers have all acknowledged the important role of hope in terminal illness.

- Hope is an inherent part of being human. Although it is a universal human experience, it is also an intensely personal one. It is important to understand what hope means to each person with a terminal illness.

- Hope assessments and interventions are closely intertwined. Assessment is a continuous process and may be a type of intervention. Interventions are closely linked to the types of assessments that are conducted.

- Although many assessment and intervention approaches for hope have been proposed, few have been developed for and validated in the terminally ill.

- Systematic approaches for hope assessment and intervention need to be developed and integrated into routine clinical practice in end-of-life care.

REFERENCES

1 Wilson KG, Graham IG, Viola RA et al. Structured interview assessment of symptoms and concerns in palliative care. *Can J Psychiatry* 2004; **49**: 350–357.

2 Greisinger AJ, Lorimor RJ, Aday LA et al. Terminally ill cancer patients: Their most important concerns. *Cancer Pract* 1997; **5**: 147–154.

3 Lin H, Bauer-Wu SM. Psycho-spiritual well-being in patients with advanced cancer: An integrative review of the literature. *J Adv Nurs* 2003; **44**: 69–80.

4 Kirk P, Kirk I, Kristjanson LJ. What do patients receiving palliative care for cancer and their families want to be told? A Canadian and Australian qualitative study. *BMJ* 2004; **328**: 1343.

◆ 5 Nekolaichuk CL, Bruera E. On the nature of hope in palliative care. *J Palliat Care* 1998; **14**: 36–42.

6 Bustamante JJ. Understanding hope. Persons in the process of dying. *Int Forum Psychoanal* 2001; **10**: 49–55.

7 Duggleby W. Hope at the end of life. *J Hosp Palliat Nurs* 2001; **3**: 51–57, 64.

◆ 8 Herth KA, Cutcliffe JR. The concept of hope in nursing 3: Hope and palliative care nursing. *Br J Nurs* 2002; **11**: 977–983.

◆ 9 Sullivan MD. Hope and hopelessness at the end of life. *Am J Geriatr Psychiatry* 2003; **11**: 393–405.

10 Parker-Oliver D. Redefining hope for the terminally ill. *Am J Hosp Palliat Care* 2002; **19**: 115–120.

11 McClement SE, Chochinov HM. Hope in advanced cancer patients. *Eur J Cancer* 2008; **44**: 1169–1174.

12 Janssens RMJ, Zylicz Z, Ten Have HAM. Articulating the concept of palliative care: Philosophical and theological perspectives. *J Palliat Care* 1999; **15**: 38–44.

● 13 Herth KA. The relationship between level of hope and level of coping response and other variables in patients with cancer. *Oncol Nurs Forum* 1989; **16**: 67–72.

14 Elliott TR, Witty TE, Herrick S, Hoffman JT. Negotiating reality after physical loss: Hope, depression, and disability. *J Pers Soc Psychol* 1991; **61**: 608–613.

15 Van Laarhoven HWM, Schilderman J, Bleijenberg G et al. Coping, quality of life, depression, and hopelessness in cancer patients in a curative and palliative, end-of-life care setting. *Cancer Nurs* 2011; **34**: 302–314.

16 Post-White J, Ceronsky C, Kreitzer MJ et al. Hope, spirituality, sense of coherence, and quality of life in patients with cancer. *Oncol Nurs Forum* 1996; **23**: 1571–1579.

17 Staats S. Quality of life and affect in older persons: Hope, time frames, and training effects. *Curr Psychol Res Rev* 1991; **10**: 21–30.

18 Pipe TB, Kelly A, LeBrun G et al. A prospective descriptive study exploring hope, spiritual well-being, and quality of life in hospitalized patients. *Med Surg Nurs* 2008; **17**: 247–257.

19 Carson V, Soeken KL, Shanty J, Terry L. Hope and spiritual well-being: Essentials for living with AIDS. *Perspect Psychiatr Care* 1990; **26**: 28–34.

20 Udelman HD, Udelman DL. Hope as a factor in remission of illness. *Stress Med* 1985; **1**: 291–294.

21 Udelman DL, Udelman HD. A preliminary report on anti-depressant therapy and its effects on hope and immunity. *Soc Sci Med* 1985; **20**:1069–1072.

22 Udelman DL, Udelman HD. Affects, neurotransmitters, and immuno-competence. *Stress Med* 1991; **7**: 159–162.

23 Zich J, Temoshok L. Perceptions of social support in men with AIDS and ARC: Relationships with distress and hardiness. *J Appl Soc Psychol* 1987; **17**: 193–215.

24 Rabkin JG, Williams JBW, Neugebauer R et al. Maintenance of hope in HIV-spectrum homosexual men. *Am J Psychiatry* 1990; **147**: 1322–1326.

● 25 Beck AT, Weissman A, Lester D, Trexler L. The measurement of pessimism: The hopelessness scale. *J Consult Clin Psychol* 1974; **42**: 861–865.

● 26 Beck AT, Steer RA, Kovacs M, Garrison B. Hopelessness and eventual suicide: A 10-year prospective study of patients hospitalized with suicidal ideation. *Am J Psychiatry* 1985; **142**: 559–563.

27 Arnold EM. Factors that influence consideration of hastening death among people with life-threatening illnesses. *Health Soc Work* 2004; **29**: 17–26.

28 Hsu TH, Lu MS, Tsou TS, Lin CC. The relationship of pain, uncertainty and hope in Taiwanese lung cancer patients. *JPSM* 2003; **26**: 835–842.

29 Mystakidou K, Tsilika E, Parpa E et al. The relationship between quality of life and levels of hopelessness and depression in palliative care. *Depress Anxiety* 2008; **25**: 730–736.

● 30 Breitbart W, Rosenfeld B, Pessin H et al. Depression, hopelessness, and desire for hastened death in terminally ill patients with cancer. *JAMA* 2000; **284**: 2907–2911.

● 31 Rodin G, Lo C, Mikulincer M, Donner A, Gagliese L, Zimmerman C. Pathways to distress: The multiple determinants of depression, hopelessness, and the desire for hastened death in metastatic cancer patients. *Soc Sci Med* 2009; **68**: 562–569.

32 Chochinov HM, Hack T, Hassard T et al. Understanding the will to live in patients nearing death. *Psychosomatics* 2005; **46**: 7–10.

● 33 Chochinov HM, Wilson KG, Enns M, Lander S. Depression, hopelessness, and suicidal ideation in the terminally ill. *Psychosomatics* 1998; **39**: 366–370.

● 34 Perakyla A. Hope work in the care of seriously ill patients. *Qual Health Res* 1991; **1**: 407–433.

35 Nuland SB. *How We Die: Reflections on Life's Final Chapter.* New York: Alfred A Knopf, 1994.

● 36 Eilott J, Olver IN. Hope and hoping in the talk of dying cancer patients. *Soc Sci Med* 2007; **64**: 138–149.

● 37 Hall BA. The struggle of the diagnosed terminally ill person to maintain hope. *Nurs Sci Quart* 1990; **3**: 177–184.

◆ 38 Nekolaichuk CL. Diversity or divisiveness? A critical analysis on hope. In: Cutcliffe JRM, McKenna H, eds. *Essential Concepts in Nursing*. Oxford, U.K.: Elsevier, 2005, pp. 179–212.

39 Benzein E, Norberg A, Saveman BI. The meaning of the lived experience of hope in patients with cancer in palliative home care. *Palliat Med* 2001; **15**: 117–126.

40 Appelin G, Bertero C. Patients' experiences of palliative care in the home: A phenomenological study of a Swedish sample. *Cancer Nurs* 2004; **27**: 65–70.

41 Olsson L, Östlund G, Strang P, Grassman EJ, Friedrichsen M. The glimmering embers: Experiences of hope among cancer patients in palliative home care. *Palliat Support Care* 2011; **9**: 43–54.

42 Duggleby W, Wright K. Transforming hope: How elderly palliative patients live with hope. *CJNR* 2005; **37**: 70–84.

43 Duggleby W, Holtslander L, Steeves M, Duggleby-Wenzel S, Cunningham S. Discursive meaning of hope for older persons with advanced cancer and their caregivers. *Can J Aging* 2010; **29**: 361–367.

44 Flemming K. The meaning of hope to palliative care cancer patients. *Int J Palliat Nurs* 1997; **3**: 14–18.

45 Salander P, Bergenheim T, Henriksson R. The creation of protection and hope in patients with malignant brain tumors. *Soc Sci Med* 1996; **42**: 985–996.

46 Mok E, Wai ML, Chan LN, Lau KP, Ng JSC, Chan KS. The meaning of hope from the perspective of Chinese advanced cancer patients in Hong Kong. *Int J Palliat Nurs* 2010; **16**: 298–305.

47 Hong IWM, Ow R. Hope among terminally ill patients in Singapore: An exploratory study. *Soc Work Health Care* 2007; **45**: 85–105.

48 Weil CM. Exploring hope in patients with end stage renal disease on chronic hemodialysis. *Nephrol Nurs J* 2000; **27**: 219–224.

49 Benzein E, Saveman BI. Nurses' perception of hope in patients with cancer: A palliative care perspective. *Cancer Nurs* 1998; **21**: 10–16.

50 Eliott J, Olver IN. Hope, life, and death: A qualitative analysis of dying cancer patients' talk about hope. *Death Stud* 2009; **33**: 609–638.

51 Kylma J, Vehvilainen-Julkunen K, Lahdevirta J. Hope, despair and hopelessness in living with HIV/AIDS: A grounded theory study. *J Adv Nurs* 2001; **33**: 764–775.

52 Ezzy D. Illness narratives: Time, hope and HIV. *Soc Sci Med* 2000; **50**: 605–617.

53 Wong-Wylie G, Jevne RF. Patient Hope: Exploring the interactions between physicians and HIV seropositive individuals. *Qual Health Res* 1997; **7**: 32–56.

54 Fanos JH, Gelinas DF, Foster RS, Postone N, Miller RG. Hope in palliative care: From narcissism to self-transcendence in amyotrophic lateral sclerosis. *J Palliat Med* 2008; **11**: 470–475.

● 55 Dufault K, Martocchio BC. Hope: Its spheres and dimensions. *Nurs Clin North Am* 1985; **20**: 379–391.

56 Herth K. Fostering hope in terminally-ill people. *J Adv Nurs* 1990; **15**: 1250–1259.

57 Reynolds MA. Hope in adults, ages 20–59, with advanced stage cancer. *Palliat Support Care* 2008; **6**: 259–264.

58 Stephenson C. The concept of hope revisited for nursing. *J Adv Nurs* 1991; **16**: 1456–1461.

59 Jevne RF, Nekolaichuk CL, Boman J. *Experiments in Hope: Blending Art and Science with Service*. Edmonton, Alberta, Canada: Hope Foundation of Alberta, 1999.

◆ 60 Yates P. Towards a reconceptualization of hope for patients with a diagnosis of cancer. *J Adv Nurs* 1993; **18**: 701–706.

◆ 61 Farran CJ, Herth KA, Popovich JM. *Hope and Hopelessness: Critical Clinical Constructs*. Thousand Oaks, CA: Sage, 1995.

62 Clayton JM, Hancock K, Parker S et al. Sustaining hope when communicating with terminally ill patients and their families: A systematic review. *Psycho-Oncology* 2008; **17**: 641–659.

◆ 63 Jevne RF, Nekolaichuk CL. Threat and hope in coping with cancer for health care professionals. In: Jacoby R, Keinan G, eds. *Between Stress and Hope: From a Disease-Centered to a Health-Centered Perspective*. Westport, CT: Praeger Publishers, 2003, pp. 187–212.

64 Innes S, Payne S. Advanced cancer patients' prognostic information preferences: A review. *Palliat Med* 2009; **23**: 29–39.

65 Nekolaichuk CL, Bruera E. Assessing hope at end-of-life: Validation of an experience of hope scale in advanced cancer patients. *Palliat Support Care* 2004; **2**: 243–253.

● 66 Herth K. Abbreviated instrument to measure hope: Development and psychometric evaluation. *J Adv Nurs* 1992; **17**: 1251–1259.

67 Benzein E, Berg A. The Swedish version of Herth Hope Index—An instrument for palliative care. *Scand J Caring Sci* 2003; **17**: 409–415.

● 68 Nekolaichuk CL, Jevne RF, Maguire TO. Structuring the meaning of hope in health and illness. *Soc Sci Med* 1999; **48**: 591–605.

◆ 69 MacLeod R, Carter H. Health professionals' perception of hope: Understanding its significance in the care of people who are dying. *Mortality* 1999; **4**: 309–317.

70 Cutcliffe JR. How do nurses inspire and instil hope in terminally ill HIV patients? *J Adv Nurs* 1995; **22**: 888–895.

71 Herth K. Contributions of humor as perceived by the terminally ill. *Am J Hosp Care* 1990; **7**: 36–40.

72 Herth K. Engendering hope in the chronically and terminally ill: Nursing interventions. *Am J Hosp Palliat Care* 1995; **12**: 31–39.

73 Kennett CE. Participation in a creative arts project can foster hope in a hospice day centre. *Palliat Med* 2000; **14**: 419–425.

74 Duggleby W, Wright K. Elderly palliative care cancer patients' descriptions of hope-fostering strategies. *Int J Palliat Nurs* 2004; **10**: 352–359.

75 Gum A, Snyder CR. Coping with terminal illness: The role of hopeful thinking. *J Palliat Med* 2002; **5**: 883–894.

76 Centers LC. Beyond denial and despair: ALS and our heroic potential for hope. *J Palliat Care* 2001; **17**: 259–264.

77 Aldridge D. Spirituality, hope, and music therapy in palliative care. *Arts Psychother* 1995; **22**: 103–109.

78 Jevne RF. *It All Begins with Hope: Patients, Caregivers and the Bereaved Speak Out*. San Diego, CA: LuraMedia, 1991.

◆ 79 Holt J. A systematic review of the congruence between people's needs and nurses' interventions for supporting hope. *Online J Knowledge Synthesis Nurs* 2001; **8**: 10.

● 80 Duggleby WD, Degner L, Williams A et al. Living with hope: Initial evaluation of a psychosocial hope intervention for older palliative home care patients. *J Pain Symptom Manage* 2007; **33**: 247–257.

81 Duggleby W, Wright K, Williams A et al. Developing a Living with Hope program for caregivers of family members with advanced cancer. *J Palliat Care* 2007; **23**: 24–31.

● 82 Herth K. Enhancing hope in people with a first recurrence of cancer. *J Adv Nurs* 2000; **32**: 1431–1441.

83 Herth K. Development and implementation of a hope intervention program. *Oncol Nurs Forum* 2001; **28**: 1009–1017.

84 Breitbart W, Rosenfeld B, Gibson C et al. Meaning-centered group psychotherapy for patients with advanced cancer: A pilot randomized controlled trial. *Psycho-Oncology* 2010; **19**: 21–28.

85 Chochinov HM, Kristjanson L, Breitbart et al. Effect of dignity therapy on distress and end-of-life experience in terminally ill patients: A randomised controlled trial. *Lancet Oncol* 2011; **12**: 753–762.

86 Hall S, Goddard C, Opio D. A novel approach to enhancing hope in patients with advanced cancer: A randomized phase II trial of dignity therapy. *BMJ Support Palliat Care* 2011; **1**: 315–321.

87 Hansen MJ, Enright RD, Baskin TW, Klatt J. A palliative care intervention in forgiveness therapy for elderly terminally ill cancer patients. *J Palliat Care* 2009; **25**: 51–60.

88 Ando M, Morito T, Akechi T, Okamoto T. Efficacy of short-term life-review interviews on the spiritual well-being of terminally ill cancer patients. *J Pain Symptom Manage* 2010; **39**: 993–1002.

89 Tollett JH, Thomas SP. A theory-based nursing intervention to instill hope in homeless veterans. *Adv Nurs Sci* 1995; **18**: 76–90.

90 Rustoen T, Wiklund I, Hanestad BR, Moum T. Nursing intervention to increase hope and quality of life in newly diagnosed cancer patients. *Cancer Nurs* 1998; **21**: 235–245.

Assessment and management of other problems

74

Dehydration and rehydration

ROBIN L. FAINSINGER

INTRODUCTION

There are many facets to the often complicated and controversial topic of dehydration and rehydration of palliative care populations. The ongoing divergent opinion is well illustrated by the following statements:

> Research is limited but suggests that artificial hydration in imminently dying patients influences neither survival nor symptom control.[1]
> The best available evidence suggests that hydration of advanced cancer patients plays an important role in maintaining cognitive function and is therefore an important factor in the prevention and reversal of delirium in this population.[2]

Superimposed on these conflicting medical comments are other complex issues:

> Terminal dehydration is a controversial topic, weighted heavily with historic symbolism, and strong religious, societal, and cultural conflicts.[3]

Some of these issues can be illustrated with the following examples.

Scenario 1

A 70-year-old woman living in an isolated rural community in southern Africa develops increasing abdominal discomfort. She has been active and in good health, although she has lost approximately 3 kg of weight over the last 2 months. She develops severe nausea and vomiting and inability to maintain an adequate oral intake. The family's access to transportation that would enable them to travel to the nearest hospital 10 km away is limited. Her extended family nurses her at home, and after a few days, she is able to resume a reasonable oral intake, her strength improves, and she resumes her role with household maintenance and care of her grandchildren.

Scenario 2

A 70-year-old woman living in a wealthy country with universal health care develops increasing abdominal discomfort. She has been active and in good health, although she notes that she has lost approximately 3 kg of weight over the last few months. Extensive diagnostic imaging and subsequent liver biopsy confirm pancreatic cancer with liver metastases. She develops severe nausea and vomiting and presents to the emergency department of her local hospital with clinical evidence of dehydration. She is rehydrated with intravenous fluids and admitted for investigation. No evidence of bowel obstruction is found on diagnostic imaging. The patient improves, resumes a reasonable oral intake, and is discharged home.

Scenario 1

Over the course of the next few weeks, the woman develops increasing abdominal pain, poor appetite and loss of weight, and intermittent nausea and vomiting. She is fortunate that a mobile health clinic has now started to visit her isolated community on a monthly basis. The nurse practitioner doing the examination notes that the patient looks cachectic and has an enlarged, tender liver. She suspects that the patient is dying from an unknown gastrointestinal primary with extensive intra-abdominal metastatic disease. The family and patient are provided with an explanation of the suspected diagnosis and prognosis. The clinic is able to provide a free prescription of morphine liquid and an explanation of dietary supplements they could use to prevent constipation. The nurse practitioner is aware of the options for hydration supplementation including intravenous, hypodermoclysis, and rectal hydration. However, for a variety of reasons, including economic and the increased burden this would place on the family caregivers, all of these options are rejected. Instead, the family is given suggestions to assist the patient to continue to drink as long as this is comfortable for her, as well as some suggestions to provide mouth care. The nurse practitioner wishes the patient and family well and indicates that they should return for a follow-up visit when the mobile clinic is back in their community. The nonverbal communication in the room indicates that all of them understand that the nurse practitioner does not really expect to see them for a follow-up visit.

Scenario 2

Over the next few weeks, increasing abdominal pain requires escalating morphine doses to achieve good control. The patient expresses a preference to remain at home as she deteriorates. However, the patient and her husband indicate to the family physician that their religious beliefs are that everything possible should be done to maintain life for as long as possible. Intermittent nausea and vomiting result in the oral morphine being changed to the subcutaneous route, and increasing abdominal pain requires increasing the morphine to 100 mg subcutaneously per day. The family physician discusses the option of parenteral hydration. Hypodermoclysis at 1 L overnight is instituted. A daughter and son now arrive to assist and support their father in caring for their mother. The son has worked as a hospice nurse and questions the value of ongoing hydration at this point. The daughter is a nephrologist who believes that hydration is necessary to maintain normal renal function and avoid the accumulation of morphine metabolites that may cause side effects. The patient and her husband have had extensive discussions over the years with their family physician who has a good understanding of how their spirituality affects their decision making. Although respecting their children's opinions, the couple rely heavily on their family physician to provide information and direction on appropriate management.

These scenarios highlight some of the complexity that surrounds this widely debated and controversial topic. At the center of the discussion, irrespective of the setting and circumstances, is the desire to keep patients as comfortable as possible while avoiding unnecessary management or procedures. However, there is no doubt that the definition of "unnecessary" will have great international variation. Clinicians with the responsibility to make these decisions will need to sort through expressions of opinion, information on pathophysiology and biochemical changes, research looking at a variety of outcomes, differing family and cultural expectations, and consensus statements. This diverse information then has to be individually applied to the specific trajectory and circumstances of patients and their families.

WHAT IS DEHYDRATION?

As has been pointed out in past reviews, use of the term dehydration in considering this issue is often inaccurate.[2,4] Fluid deficit is the state of water loss with or without electrolytes, which includes the subtypes of volume depletion and dehydration. Dehydration should be understood as total body water deficit that is predominantly intracellular and associated with hypernatremia. Volume depletion implies a deficit in the intravascular fluid volume and can be isotonic, hyponatremic, or hypernatremic (Figure 74.1).

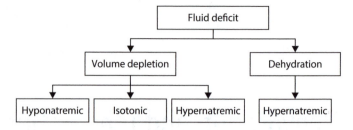

Figure 74.1 *Types of fluid deficit.*

Table 74.1 *Factors associated with fluid deficits*

Decreased intake	Increased fluid loss
Asthenia	Bowel resection
Anorexia	Diarrhea
Coma	Diuretics
Delirium	Diabetes mellitus/insipidus
Dementia	Fistulas
Depression	Fever/sweating
Dysphagia	Hypercalcemia
Nausea	Vomiting

A variety of factors can be associated with fluid deficits (Table 74.1). Any of these etiologies for fluid deficit can occur at any stage of a palliative care illness and multiple possible mechanisms can occur simultaneously.

The assessment of risk or presence of fluid deficits is based on a variety of factors that can be determined by history, physical examination, and laboratory findings. The history is of obvious value in determining the possible risk factors listed in Table 74.1. There are sometimes practical difficulties in estimating the accuracy of fluid intake estimates and potential fluid loss through urine and fecal incontinence. Symptoms of fluid deficit can include behavior and cognitive changes, fatigue, thirst, nausea, and dry mouth. The classic signs of fluid deficit include dry mouth, reduced skin turgor, postural hypotension, tachycardia, reduced jugular venous pressure, sunken eyes, and reduced sweating. However, all of these problems need to be interpreted with caution as they can be associated with other causes present in aging, cachexia, advanced cancer, and side effects due to commonly used medications.

Laboratory evaluation can provide some helpful information in evaluating fluid deficits but will obviously depend on the setting of care and whether such investigations are acceptable to the patient, family, and health-care team. The common findings present in volume-depleted patients include elevated levels of urea, creatinine, plasma proteins, hematocrit, and sodium. It is worth noting that a systematic review attempted to clarify the physical diagnosis of hypovolemia in adults.[5***] The authors concluded that in patients with vomiting, diarrhea, or decreased oral intake, few findings, with the exception of serum electrolytes, urea, and creatinine values, have proven value.

HYDRATION CONTROVERSY

There is no controversy that palliative care populations should be encouraged to maintain an adequate oral intake to prevent fluid deficit. However, there are many literature reports illustrating opposing viewpoints on the use of supplemental parenteral hydration. These have been considered from both clinical and ethical viewpoints.[6–16] Historical reviews on this topic have referenced a similar collection of clinical anecdotes and opinions. The arguments for and against hydrating palliative care populations are summarized in Box 74.1.[11,12]

It would appear that the arguments for initiating or maintaining parenteral hydration in palliative care populations originate from the standard medical approach to fluid deficits. Thus, it would be reasonable to expect that most patients dying in hospitals will have an intravenous line unless they have undergone rapid deterioration or unanticipated demise. This was originally demonstrated by a Canadian report[17] where 73 of 106 cancer patients dying in a tertiary care hospital were noted to have intravenous fluids administered. A more recent retrospective study on the use of artificial hydration in an acute care hospital in England[1] noted that of 111 patients, 65% were hydrated during the last week of life and 46% were being hydrated at the time of death. The mean rate of parenteral hydration was 2000 mL/day. The results suggest that artificial hydration is no longer necessarily considered routine hospital practice for dying patients in this setting.

In order to clarify the routine practice of physicians involved in end-of-life care in Edmonton, Canada, the routine management of parenteral hydration for patients dying in a palliative care unit and acute care hospital while receiving or not receiving consult advice from the palliative care program was reported.[18] A retrospective chart review of 50 consecutive patients dying at each of the three sites was included. The majority of patients at all sites received hydration ranging from 66% to 98% of patients during the last week of life. However, the volume of hydration was noted to be significantly lower in the palliative care unit site.

A survey questionnaire of Japanese physicians attempted to clarify attitudes towards terminal dehydration. Results revealed that physicians with more positive attitudes towards intravenous hydration were less involved in end-of-life care and more likely to regard fluid as a necessary physiological requirement, consider it a minimum standard of care, and believe that this was beneficial for palliating symptoms.[19] A Canadian study distributed a questionnaire to 18 palliative care physicians in major Canadian centers in an attempt to clarify the routine practice of physicians involved in end-of-life care.[20] Results demonstrated a wide range of practice. Physicians estimated that they ordered parenteral hydration in a median of 6%–10% of patients (range 0%–100%). The routes of parenteral hydration were intravenous hydration, with a median of 30% (range 0%–100%), and hypodermoclysis, with a median of 70% (range 0%–100%). The estimated average volume range per 24 hours was between 200 and 2400 mL. A survey of 238 palliative care physicians in Latin America reported that 60% prescribed parenteral hydration to 40%–100% of their patients in the last weeks of life. These results differ from traditional hospice philosophy, and the report concludes that clinical perceptions of benefit drive practice to prescribe or withhold parenteral hydration based on individualized treatment decisions.[21]

It is easy to imagine the problems inflicted on advanced palliative care populations by a policy of maintaining intravenous hydration with volumes in excess of 3 L/day. Under this circumstance, complications such as increased respiratory and gastrointestinal symptom distress can be anticipated. The literature reports against parenteral hydration would suggest that some health-care professionals looking after palliative care populations have reacted to overuse of intravenous fluids and concluded that no parenteral hydration is the preferred approach. This has been reinforced by anecdotal literature reports noting that many palliative care

---

Box 74.1 Hydration in palliative care

Against parenteral hydration

- Symptom distress is not experienced by comatose patients.

- Dying is prolonged by parenteral fluids.

- There is less urine and thus less problem with incontinence and catheter use.

- Decreased gastrointestinal fluid associated with dehydration results in less nausea and vomiting.

- Decreased respiratory secretions will result in less cough and pulmonary edema.

- The severity of edema and ascites is decreased.

- Dehydration can act as a natural anesthetic for the central nervous system.

- Parenteral hydration is uncomfortable and limits patient mobility.

For parenteral hydration

- Parenteral hydration assists in making dying patients more comfortable.

- There is no evidence that parenteral hydration prolongs life.

- Fluid deficits can cause restlessness, confusion, and neuromuscular irritability.

- Oral hydration is provided to dying patients complaining of thirst, and therefore, parenteral hydration should be an option.

- Emphasis on the poor quality of life of palliative care populations detracts from efforts to improve comfort and life quality.

- Parenteral hydration is considered a minimum standard of care.

- Withholding parenteral fluid from palliative care populations may result in withholding therapies to other compromised patient groups.

patients appear to die comfortably without parenteral hydration. Nevertheless, a review of the literature indicates that these reports are mostly based on unsubstantiated data.[12] There are other issues worth considering[11,12,22–25]:

- Fluid deficit as a cause of confusion and restlessness in nonterminally ill patients is well recognized. The problems of delirium and agitation have been well reported in palliative care populations.[2]
- Reduced intravascular volume and glomerular filtration rate caused by fluid deficits are well accepted as a cause of prerenal failure.[2,4] Opioid metabolite accumulation in the presence of renal failure, resulting in confusion, myoclonus, and seizures, has been well documented.

Reports with regard to agitated delirium and terminal restlessness have frequently appeared in the palliative care literature. Discussion of these problems has generally centered on the need for pharmacological management, which often includes sedation.[26–28] Ventafridda et al.[29] reported 9% of patients requiring sedation for agitated delirium in a study of unendurable symptoms experienced by patients with cancer during their last days of life. This prompted a report by our group[30] that agitated delirium was the most frequent problem requiring sedation in the last week of life in 10% of our patients. A later report noted that the severity of agitated delirium requiring sedation had decreased to 3% in our palliative care unit.[31] We speculated that this resulted from a change in our practice to include more frequent use of hypodermoclysis for hydration, switching opioids earlier when toxicity developed, and the use of less sedating treatments such as haloperidol for delirium, decreasing the prevalence and difficulty of managing agitated delirium in this setting.[32]

Reports in the palliative care literature have continued to note innovative approaches to the pharmacological management of symptoms associated with agitated delirium, including the use of intravenous propofol.[33–35] A retrospective chart review of 76 consecutive patients dying at St. Luke's Hospice in Cape Town, South Africa, found that 29% of patients required sedation for agitated delirium. Although none of these patients were treated with parenteral hydration, patients requiring sedation were noted to require significantly higher doses of opioids during a longer admission.[36]

Further reports on the use of sedation have suggested that agitated delirium appears to be less problematic in a number of different settings in Edmonton,[37] where parenteral hydration is more common practice,[18] compared with requirements for sedation in a number of other international settings.[38] As a result, it has been suggested that dehydration could be a reversible component of agitated delirium, which may be ignored by an approach that focuses on a sedative pharmacological solution to this apparently common and certainly distressing situation.[39*] Thus, it may be illogical for a patient to receive medications for agitated delirium, myoclonus, and seizures, if in some circumstances these problems could be prevented or corrected by the use of parenteral hydration.

HYDRATION RESEARCH

Research into the use of hydration in palliative care settings has focused on three dimensions[40]:

- The association between biochemical findings and hydration status
- The association between biochemical findings and clinical symptoms
- The association between hydration status and clinical symptoms

Biochemical findings and hydration status

There is no controversy that dehydration is a cause of renal failure.[41–43] However, while parenteral hydration is accepted standard management in many settings, the impact of fluid deficit and rehydration on the renal function and electrolyte balance of palliative care populations is still questioned.[10,44–47]

Ellershaw et al.[48] undertook a biochemical investigation in 82 patients with advanced cancer. The patients were taking oral sips of fluid and no longer able to tolerate oral medication. Our group[49] reported biochemical investigation of 100 consecutive patients, 69 of whom received hypodermoclysis at an average volume of 1203 ± 505 mL/day. A comparison of these two reports[50] has been published (Table 74.2). Morita et al.[51] published further results on the biochemistry of terminally ill cancer patients and concluded that relatively small amounts of parenteral hydration may result in less abnormal biochemistry, particularly with regard to renal function.

Biochemical findings/hydration status and clinical symptoms

Much of the early literature on this issue was based on anecdotal opposing viewpoints and case reports.[52,53] However, many reports have now attempted to study this issue more carefully. Burge[46] reported a cross-sectional survey studying the quantitative assessment of the dehydration experience in patients with advanced cancer. The study concluded that parenteral hydration on the basis of fluid intake and laboratory measures were not helpful if the aim was to reduce thirst. McCann et al.[54] studied 48 consecutive patients with regard to symptom prevalence and management of hunger and thirst in terminally ill patients not receiving parenteral hydration. Symptoms of hunger, thirst, and dry mouth were apparently well managed with oral sips and mouth care.

Table 74.2   *Comparison of biochemical findings in patients taking oral fluids (sips)[47] and those receiving hypodermoclysis[48]*

	Fainsinger et al.[48]		Ellershaw et al.[47]	
	Mean	Normal range	Mean	Normal range
Urea (mmol/L)	8.8	3.2–8.2	15.5	2.5–6.5
Creatinine	101	62–133	177	60–120 (μmol/L)

Ellershaw et al.[48] investigated the relationship between symptoms and dehydration in 82 patients not provided with parenteral hydration. No significant association was demonstrated between the level of hydration and respiratory tract secretions, thirst, and dry mouth. However, they did acknowledge that the effect of renal failure and possible consequences of agitation and confusion were not assessed. Musgrave et al.[55] studied the effect of intravenous fluids on a group of patients with advanced cancer dying in a hospital oncology unit. No relationship was demonstrated between level of thirst, intravenous fluids, and biochemical parameters. A subsequent study[56] also failed to demonstrate any relation between intravenous fluids, fluid balance, and the prevalence of crepitations, ascites, and leg edema. A retrospective chart review of 117 and 162 patients admitted to a palliative care unit in 1988–1989 and 1991–1992 assessed the impact of a change in practice with regard to management of dehydration and cognitive impairment.[57*] The authors concluded that the data suggested that routine cognitive assessment, opioid rotation, and hydration may reduce the frequency of agitated confusion in terminally ill cancer patients. Although hydration may have had a role, it was not possible to determine the relative contribution. A partial replication of this study considered the role of hydration and an incomplete opioid substitution on the prevalence of agitated delirium.[58] No significant decrease in the occurrence of agitated delirium was noted.

Ashby et al.[59] measured plasma concentrations of morphine and metabolites in 36 hospice patients. They concluded that morphine metabolites may be a causal aggravating factor in nausea and vomiting and cognitive impairment in palliative care patients with significant renal impairment. Lawlor et al.[60*] completed prospective serial assessments of 113 patients with advanced cancer in a delirium study. Univariate analysis demonstrated reversibility associated with psychoactive medications and dehydration. They concluded that although delirium is multifactorial, hydration using hypodermoclysis may be one of the potential useful measures to consider.

Bruera et al. published the first randomized, controlled, double-blind study of parenteral hydration in terminally ill cancer patients. This was a multicenter study where patients with clinical and biochemical evidence of dehydration and history of an oral intake of less than 1 L of fluid per day were randomly assigned to receive 1000 mL (treatment group) or 100 mL (placebo group) of normal saline over 4 hours for 2 days. The outcome measures were patient- and investigator-rated symptoms of fatigue, sedation, myoclonus, hallucinations, and a global sense of well-being. A significant improvement in sedation and myoclonus scores was noted in the hydration treatment group.[61] A follow-up study using similar methodology and 6 hospices in the Houston area included 129 patients randomly assigned to hydration or placebo and found no significant differences. The authors concluded that in this population, hydration of 1000 mL/day does not improve symptoms, quality of life, or survival compared to placebo. They did comment that further research in other patient populations such as delirium

associated with dehydration and opioid toxicity should be explored in future studies.[62**]

A review by Burge[63***] concluded that there is little clinical evidence to guide patients, families, and clinicians in treatment decisions regarding fluid intake during the terminal phase of life. A subsequent systematic review by Viola et al.[64***] summarized existing evidence regarding fluid status effects and fluid therapy. Six studies were selected for inclusion and the authors concluded that given the study limitations, it was impossible to draw firm conclusions regarding clinical care. A Cochrane review (updated in 2011) concluded that there was insufficient quality research for practice recommendations in the use of alternative hydration assistance for palliative care patients.[65***]

ETHICAL, SOCIAL, AND CULTURAL CONSIDERATIONS

There are other important issues to consider in regard to the use of parenteral hydration.[66] Patient and family attitudes, level of comfort with the situation, and education and healthcare workers' attitudes, level of education, and biases in presentation all influence the decision-making process.

Unfortunately, artificial nutrition and hydration are often considered as the same issue in ethical and clinical discussion papers. This causes unnecessary confusion, as the arguments and rationale for providing nutritional calories via artificial means as opposed to hydration should be considered independently.

Morita et al.[67] studied patients' and family members' perceptions about rehydration to identify factors contributing to decision making. The survey included 121 Japanese hospice patients with insufficient oral intake. Patient performance status, fluid retention symptoms, denial, physician recommendations, patients' and family members' beliefs with regard to hydration effect on patient distress, and family anxiety about withholding rehydration were significantly associated with decision making. The main determinants for rehydration were the patient performance status, fluid retention symptoms, denial, and care receiver's beliefs about the effects of rehydration on patient distress.

A Canadian study[68] identified issues of importance to family caregivers with regard to administering parenteral hydration to patients with advanced cancer. Factors influencing caregivers included symptom distress issues, ethical and emotional considerations, information exchanged between health professionals and families, and culture. Perceived benefits of artificial hydration were central to the ethical, emotional, and cultural considerations involved in caregivers' decision making. An article presenting the values of the Jewish faith with regard to terminal dehydration[69] illustrates the difficulty of applying cultural and ethnic research and opinion. Letters in response varied from describing this as an "excellent article"[70] to "extremely offensive in its references to Jewish people."[71]

Malia et al. noted that artificial hydration in palliative care is a controversial practice in the United Kingdom and applied

Q methodology to identify issues of most concern to patients in influencing decisions. The importance of considering the different views patients bring to their decision making and the need to involve them in making unbiased informed treatment choices are nicely demonstrated in this novel research study.[72] Cohen et al. used phenomenological interviews with patients and caregivers in home hospice care in the United States to understand how they viewed parenteral hydration. Findings differed from traditional hospice beliefs in that this was described by some participants as enhancing comfort, dignity, and quality of life.[73]

It has been proposed that terminal dehydration or voluntary cessation of drinking may provide an alternative to physician-assisted suicide. Miller and Meier[74] suggested that terminal dehydration accompanied by standard palliative care management offers patients a way to escape agonizing, incurable conditions that they consider to be worse than death, without requiring transformation of the law and medical ethics. Quill et al.[75] suggested that voluntary cessation of "eating and drinking are clinical options that may be acceptable to a patient and physician and do not require fundamental changes in the law."

Craig[76] argued passionately that a blanket policy of no hydration, as initially endorsed in a national guideline end-of-life care pathway in the United Kingdom, was ethically indefensible. Her primary concern was that the value of hydration is underestimated and could increase deaths associated with palliative sedation. Craig[77] has devoted a book to this issue, in which she stated, "My personal role in the hydration debate has been to highlight the ethical, legal and medical dangers of a regime of sedation without hydration in the dying and draw attention to the plight of dissenting relatives."

ALTERNATIVE HYDRATION TECHNIQUES

There is universal agreement that the best and most convenient route to correct fluid deficits is increasing or improving oral intake. However, where this is impossible or inadequate, there are some circumstances where parenteral hydration may be of benefit. It is often misunderstood that we are not necessarily all seeing patients in the same trajectory of illness. Clinical circumstances evolve[78] and a physically independent and cognitively intact patient at an early stage of a palliative illness is likely to be viewed very differently to the same patient a number of months later who is now cognitively impaired and physically dependent. However, if a decision is made to use parenteral hydration, there are considerations with regard to the type of fluid, volume, and route of administration. There is no doubt that intravenous hydration is the route of choice in acute care institutions. There are obvious disadvantages such as difficulty finding venous access, pain, infection, limitations to mobility, and displaced lines, particularly with confused patients. Nevertheless, it should be noted that a report from an Italian palliative care program stated that 82% of palliative care patients will have an intravenous line and receive a range of 1–1.5 L of fluid per day.[79] In addition, they stated that

although hypodermoclysis has been suggested as an alternative, experience suggests that it is not less stressful for palliative care patients and that the intravenous route is preferred.

Nasogastric tubes and gastrostomy

Nasogastric tubes are generally uncomfortable for patients and prolonged use, particularly in palliative care populations, should be avoided where possible.[80,81] Percutaneous gastrostomies are commonly used with head and neck or esophageal cancer patients with increasing dysphagia who may benefit from nutrition as well as hydration.[82] As patients deteriorate, there is a need to review the goals of care with regard to enteral nutrition. However, difficulty with discontinuing management and ease of access can result in ongoing enteral nutrition and hydration in circumstances where this might not otherwise have been instituted.

Hypodermoclysis

The safety of hypodermoclysis has been well documented and reported in noncancer patients.[83*,84*] There have also been studies in palliative care patients demonstrating the ease of administration and minimal toxicity.[49*,85*,86*]

The procedure is simple and associated with minimal pain. A butterfly needle is inserted subcutaneously and attached to a fluid line that can run via gravity or an infusion pump. It requires minimal training for insertion and surveillance, and family caregivers can be trained to supervise this management in the home. There is evidence of increasing acceptance of hypodermoclysis in the acute care setting.[18] It is generally recommended that solutions with some electrolytes are used, as nonelectrolyte solutions have been reported to draw fluid into the interstitial space.[11*,12*,87*] Initial recommendation suggested rates of infusion limited to a maximum of 100–120 mL/hour; however, patients can tolerate boluses up to 500 mL/hour.[88*]

Traditionally, the use of hypodermoclysis was assisted by adding hyaluronidase to promote absorption in a dose ranging from 150 to 750 units/L. Initially, smaller volumes of hyaluronidase were demonstrated to be just as effective.[88] However, a shortage of hyaluronidase led to clinical experience and anecdotal reports suggesting good absorption of hypodermoclysis without hyaluronidase. This resulted in a report of 24 consecutive patients receiving hypodermoclysis without hyaluronidase.[89*] Hydration was maintained for a mean 12 ± 9 days, with an infusion varying in range between 20 and 300 mL/hour. Three patients were demonstrated to tolerate twice daily boluses of 500 mL over 1 hour. The average infusion site duration was 3.3 ± 3.6 days. These results and the increasing difficulty obtaining hyaluronidase have resulted in the ongoing clinical observation that most patients tolerate hypodermoclysis without requiring the addition of hyaluronidase. This is now standard practice in our setting with rates up to 80 mL/hour well tolerated by most patients. However, recombinant human hyaluronidase has been reported in clinical studies and may have a future role in improving the absorption of subcutaneously administered fluids.[90]

Proctoclysis

As noted, intravenous hydration can be uncomfortable, expensive, and difficult to maintain in the home, while even hypodermoclysis can be expensive and too complicated in some settings. The potential advantage of the rectal administration of fluid, particularly in resource-limited developing countries, prompted a trial of rectal hydration in terminally ill cancer patients.[91*] Proctoclysis was offered to 17 adult patients with a fluid deficit where resources were inadequate for the use of hypodermoclysis. Tap water was used and the rectal infusion was increased from 100 mL to a maximum of 400 mL/hour, unless fluid leakage occurred before the maximum volume was achieved. The mean daily volume, hourly rate, and duration were reported as 1035 ± 150 mL/day, 224 ± 58 mL/hour, and 14 ± 8 days, respectively. Rectal hydration was noted to be well tolerated with minimal side effects in the majority of patients. A follow-up report[92*] included 78 advanced cancer patients receiving rectal hydration. Volumes infused, patient tolerance, and side effects were similar to the earlier report, confirming that this is a safe, effective, and low-cost technique for rehydration in terminally ill palliative care populations.

CONCLUSION

Reconsider the varying circumstances and sociocultural circumstances of the two patients described in the introduction to this chapter. Discussion of management of these two patients, the manner in which information should be presented to them, literature interpretation as reviewed earlier, and the biases of health-care providers and the circumstances in which we work will have significant implications on how we consider the issue of fluid deficit and rehydration. We can perhaps achieve consensus that dehydration is a cause of renal failure and that hypodermoclysis is a safe and effective way of providing rehydration. There may be some agreement that rehydration of palliative care populations may result in better biochemical parameters at the end of life. There is certainly much evidence to recommend that if terminally ill patients are not rehydrated, medications such as opioids should be gradually decreased to avoid accumulation and unnecessary side effects. There is likely to be consensus that the major clinical issue is to consider whether rehydration will cause benefit or harm to palliative care patients unable to sustain adequate oral intake.

The need to consider individual circumstances and predictions of life expectancy in evaluating the potential benefits of rehydration is a recurring theme.[2,11,93] Although starting from different perspectives, there is some consensus[10,39,64] that

- Available data are inadequate for final conclusions on this issue
- Careful individual assessment of the relevance of fluid deficit to each clinical situation is essential
- Further carefully designed research trials are required[61,62]

Key learning points

- Hydration in palliative care is a controversial topic with divergent opinions.
- Fluid deficits can cause confusion and renal failure.
- Hydration research is inconclusive in guiding clinical care.
- Hypodermoclysis is an excellent alternative for rehydration in palliative care populations.
- Diverse clinical and sociocultural circumstances need to be considered.
- Evidence recommends that if terminally ill patients are not rehydrated, medications should be decreased to avoid accumulation and side effects.
- Rehydration may be helpful in some individual situations.
- Patient and family preferences need to be understood and incorporated into the treatment plan.

REFERENCES

1 Soden K, Hoy A, Hoy W et al. Artificial hydration during the last week of life in patients dying in district general hospital. *Palliative Medicine* 2002; **16**:542–543.

● 2 Lawlor P. Delirium and dehydration: Some fluid for thought? *Support Care Cancer* 2002; **10**:445–454.

3 Huffman JL, Dunn GP. The paradox of hydration in advanced terminal illness. *Journal of the American College of Surgeons* 2002; **194**:835–839.

● 4 Sarhill N, Walsh D, Nelson K, Davis M. Evaluation and treatment of cancer related fluid deficits: Volume depletion and dehydration. *Support Care Cancer* 2001; **9**:408–419.

5 McGee S, Abernethy WB, Simel DI. Is this patient hypovolemic? *Journal of the American Medical Association* 1999; **281**:1022–1029.

6 Craig GM. On withholding nutrition and hydration in the terminally ill: Has palliative medicine gone too far? *Journal of Medical Ethics* 1994; **20**:139–143.

7 Ashby M, Stoffell B. Artificial hydration and alimentation at the end of life: A reply to Craig. *Journal of Medical Ethics* 1995; **21**:135–140.

8 Dicks B. Rehydration or dehydration? *Support Care Cancer* 1994; **2**:88–90.

9 Dunlop RJ, Ellershaw JE, Baines MJ et al. On withholding nutrition and hydration in the terminally ill: Has palliative medicine gone too far? A reply. *Journal of Medical Ethics* 1995; **21**:141–143.

10 Dunphy K, Finlay I, Rathbone G et al. Rehydration in palliative and terminal care: If not—Why not? *Palliative Medicine* 1995; **9**:221–228.

● 11 Fainsinger RL, Bruera E. The management of dehydration in terminally ill patients. *Journal of Palliative Care* 1994; **10**:55–59.

12 Fainsinger RL, Bruera E. Hypodermoclysis for symptom control vs the Edmonton Injector. *Journal of Palliative Care* 1991; **7**:5–8.

13 Meares CJ. Terminal dehydration. A review. *American Journal of Hospice and Palliative Care* 1994; **11**:10–14.

14 Slomka J. What do apple pie and motherhood have to do with feeding tubes and caring for the patient? *Archives Internal Medicine* 1995; **155**:1258–1263.

15   Smith SA. Patient induced dehydration—Can it ever be therapeutic? *Oncology Nursing Forum* 1995; **22**:1487–1491.

16   Wilkes E. On withholding nutrition and hydration in the terminally ill: Has palliative medicine gone too far? A commentary. *Journal of Medical Ethics* 1994; **20**:144–145.

17   Burge FI, King DB, Wilson D. Intravenous fluids and the hospitalized dying: A medical last rite? *Canadian Family Physician* 1990; **86**:883–886.

18   Lanuke K, Fainsinger RL, de Moissac D. Hydration management at the end of life. *Journal of Palliative Medicine* 2004; **7**:257–263.

19   Morita T, Shima Y, Adachi I. Attitudes of Japanese physicians towards terminal dehydration: A nationwide study. *Journal of Clinical Oncology* 2002; **20**:4699–4704.

20   Lanuke K, Fainsinger RL. Hydration management in palliative care settings—A survey of experts. *Journal of Palliative Care* 2004; **19**:278–279.

21   Torres-Vigil I, Mendoza TR, Alonso-Babarro A et al. Practice patterns and perceptions about parenteral hydration in the last weeks of life; a survey of palliative care physicians in Latin America. *Journal of Pain and Symptom Management* 2012; **43**:47–58.

22   Fainsinger RL, Bruera E, Watanabe S. Rehydration in palliative care. *Palliative Medicine* 1996; **10**:165–166.

23   Fainsinger RL. Deshydratation et soins palliatifs. In: Roy DJ, Rapin C, eds. *Les annales de soins palliatifs.* Vol. 3. Montreal, Quebec, Canada: Centre de Bioethique. Institut de Recherches Cliniques de Montreal, 1995; pp. 171–180.

24   Fainsinger RL. Nutrition and hydration for the terminally ill. *Journal of the American Medical Association* 1995; **273**:1736.

25   MacDonald SM, Fainsinger RL. Symptom control: The problem areas. *Palliative Medicine* 1994; **8**:167–168.

26   Burke AL, Diamond PL, Hulbert J. Terminal restlessness—Its management and the role of midazolam. *Medical Journal of Australia* 1999; **155**:485–487.

27   Back IN. Terminal restlessness in patients with advanced malignant disease. *Palliative Medicine* 1992; **6**:293–298.

28   Lichter I, Hunt E. The last 48 hours of life. *Journal of Palliative Care* 1990; **6**:7–15.

● 29   Ventafridda V, Ripamonti C, De Conno F et al. Symptom prevalence and control during cancer patients last days of life. *Journal of Palliative Care* 1990; **6**:7–11.

● 30   Fainsinger RL, Bruera E, Miller MJ et al. Symptom control during the last week of life on a palliative care unit. *Journal of Palliative Care* 1991; **7**:5–11.

31   Fainsinger RL, MacEacheron T, Miller MJ et al. The use of hypodermoclysis for rehydration in terminally ill cancer patients. *Journal of Palliative Care* 1992; **8**:70.

32   Fainsinger RL, Tapper M, Bruera E. A perspective on the management of delirium in the terminally ill. *Journal of Palliative Care* 1993; **9**:4–8.

33   Mercadante S, De Conno F, Ripamonti C. Propofol in terminal care. *Journal of Pain and Symptom Management* 1995; **10**:639–642.

34   Moyle J. Use of propofol in palliative medicine. *Journal of Pain and Symptom Management* 1995; **10**:643–646.

35   Morita T, Inoue S, Chihara S. Sedation for symptom control in Japan: The importance of intermittent use and communication with family members. *Journal of Pain and Symptom Management* 1996; **12**:32–38.

36   Fainsinger RL, Landman W, Hoskings M, Bruera E. Sedation for uncontrolled symptoms in a South African hospice. *Journal of Pain and Symptom Management* 1998; **16**:145–152.

37   Fainsinger RL, deMoissac D, Mancini I, Oneschuk D. Sedation for delirium and other symptoms in terminally ill patients in Edmonton. *Journal of Palliative Care* 2000; **16**:5–10.

38   Fainsinger RL, Waller A, Bercovici M et al. A multi-centre international study of sedation for uncontrolled symptoms in terminally ill patients. *Palliative Medicine* 2000; **14**:257–265.

● 39   Fainsinger RL, Bruera E. When to treat dehydration in a terminally ill patient? *Support Care Cancer* 1997; **5**:205–211.

● 40   Morita T, Ichiki T, Tsunoda J et al. Three dimensions of the rehydration—Dehydration problem in a palliative care setting. *Journal of Palliative Care* 1999; **15**:60–61.

41   Badr K, Ichikawa I. Prerenal failure: A deleterious shift from renal compensation to decompensation. *New England Journal of Medicine* 1988; **319**:623–629.

42   Brady HR, Singer GG. Acute renal failure. *Lancet* 1995; **346**:1533–1540.

43   Weinberg A, Minakar KL. Dehydration. Evaluation and management in older adults. *Journal of the American Medical Association* 1995; **274**:1552–1556.

44   Waller A. Letter to the Editor. *American Journal of Hospice and Palliative Care* 1995; **7**:5–6.

45   Oliver D. Terminal dehydration [letter]. *Lancet* 1994; **ii**:631.

46   Burge FI. Dehydration symptoms of palliative care cancer patients. *Journal of Pain and Symptom Management* 1993; **8**:454–464.

47   Waller A, Hershkowitz M, Adunsky A. The effect of intravenous fluid infusion on blood and urine parameters of hydration and on the state of consciousness in terminal cancer patients. *American Journal of Hospice and Palliative Care* 1994; **11**:22–27.

48   Ellershaw JE, Sutcliffe JM, Saunders CM. Dehydration and the dying patient. *Journal of Pain and Symptom Management* 1995; **10**:192–197.

49   Fainsinger RL, MacEacheron T, Miller MJ et al. The use of hypodermoclysis for rehydration in terminally ill cancer patients. *Journal of Pain and Symptom Management* 1994; **9**:298–302.

50   Fainsinger RL. Biochemical dehydration in terminally ill cancer patients. *Journal of Palliative Care* 1999; **15**:59–61.

51   Morita T, Ichika T, Tsunoda J et al. Biochemical dehydration and fluid retention symptoms in terminally ill cancer patients whose death is impending. *Journal of Palliative Care* 1998; **14**:60–62.

52   Andrews M, Bell ER, Smith SA et al. Dehydration in terminally ill patients. Is it appropriate palliative care? *Postgraduate Medical Journal* 1993; **93**:201–208.

53   Yan E, Bruera E. Parenteral hydration of terminally ill cancer patients. *Journal of Palliative Care* 1991; **7**:40–43.

54   McCann RM, Hall WJ, Groth-Juncker A. Comfort care for the terminally ill patients. The appropriate use nutrition and hydration. *Journal of the American Medical Association* 1994; **272**:1263–1266.

55   Musgrave CF, Bartle N, Opstad J. The sensation of thirst in dying patients receiving IV hydration. *Journal of Palliative Care* 1995; **11**:17–21.

56   Musgrave CF. Fluid retention and intravenous hydration in the dying. *Palliative Medicine* 1996; **10**:53.

● 57   Bruera E, Franco JJ, Maltoni M et al. Changing pattern of agitated impaired mental status in patients with advanced cancer: Association with cognitive monitoring, hydration, and opioid rotation. *Journal of Pain and Symptom Management* 1995; **10**:287–291.

58   Morita T, Tei U, Ionoue S. Agitated terminal delirium and association with partial opioid substitution and hydration. *Journal of Palliative Medicine* 2003; **6**:557–563.

59   Ashby M, Fleming B, Wood M et al. Plasma morphine and glucuronide (M3G & M6G), concentrations in hospice in-patients. *Journal of Pain and Symptom Management* 1997; **14**:157–167.

● 60   Lawlor PG, Gagnon B, Mancini IL et al. Occurrence, causes, and outcome of delirium in patients with advanced cancer. *Archives of Internal Medicine* 2000; **160**:786–794.

61 Bruera E, Sala R, Rico MA et al. Effects of parenteral hydration in terminally ill cancer patients: A preliminary study. *Journal of Clinical Oncology* 2005; **23(10)**:2366–2371.

62 Bruera E, Hui D, Dalal S et al. Parenteral Hydration in patients with advanced cancer: A multicenter, double blind, placebo controlled randomized trail. *Journal of Clinical Oncology* 2013; **31(1)**:111–118.

63 Burge Fl. Dehydration and provision of fluids in palliative care. What is the evidence? *Canadian Family Physician* 1996; **42**:2383–2388.

64 Viola RA, Wells GA, Peterson J. The effects of fluid status and fluid therapy on the dying: A systematic review. *Journal of Palliative Care* 1997; **13**:41–52.

65 Good P, Cavenagh J, Mather M, Ravenscroft P. Medically assisted hydration for adult palliative care patients. *Cochrane Database of Systematic Reviews* 2008; **2**:CD006273. doi:10.1002/14651858. CD006273.pub2. Review content assessed as up-to-date: 13 February 2011.

66 Baumrucker S. Science, hospice, and terminal dehydration. *American Journal of Hospice and Palliative Care* 1999; **16**:502–503.

67 Morita T, Tsunoda J, Inoue S et al. Perceptions and decision-making on rehydration of terminally ill cancer patients and family members. *American Journal of Hospice Palliative Care* 1999; **16**:509–516.

68 Parkash R, Burge F. The family's perspective on issues of hydration in terminal care. *Journal of Palliative Care* 1997; **13**:23–27.

69 Bodell J, Weng MA. The Jewish patient in terminal dehydration: A hospice ethical dilemma. *American Journal of Hospice Palliative Care* 2000; **17**:185–188.

70 Schur TG. Life and afterlife in Jewish tradition. *American Journal of Hospice and Palliative Care* 2000; **17**:296–297.

71 Rothstein JM. Out of context? *American Journal of Hospice and Palliative Care* 2000; **17**:297.

72 Malia C, Bennett MI. What influences patients' decisions on Artificial Hydration at the End of Life? A Q-methodology Study. *Journal of Pain and Symptom Management* 2011; **42(2)**:192–201.

73 Cohen MZ, Torres-Vigil I, Burbach BE et al. The meaning of parenteral hydration to family caregivers and patients with advanced cancer receiving hospice care. *Journal of Pain and Symptom Management* 2012; **43**:855–865.

74 Miller FG, Meier DE. Voluntary death: A comparison of terminal dehydration and physician-assisted suicide. *Annals of Internal Medicine* 1998; **128**:559–562.

75 Quill TE, Meier DE, Block SD et al. The debate over physician-assisted suicide: Empirical data and conversant views. *Annals of Internal Medicine* 1998; **128**:552–558.

76 Craig G. Palliative care in overdrive: Patients in danger. *American Journal of Hospice and Palliative Care* 2008; **25(2)**:155–160.

77 Craig G. *Challenging Medical Ethics 1: No Water—No Life: Hydration in the Dying.* 2004; Fairway Folio (Christian Publishing Services), Cheshire, UK.

78 Fainsinger R. Dehydration. In: MacDonald N. ed. *Palliative Medicine: A Case-Based Manual.* New York: Oxford University Press, 1998, pp. 91–99.

79 Mercadante S, Villari P, Ferrera P. A model of acute symptom control unit: Pain relief and palliative unit of La Maddalena Cancer Centre. *Support Care Cancer* 2003; **11**:114–119.

80 Fainsinger RL, Spachynski K, Hanson J et al. Symptom control in terminally ill patients with malignant bowel obstruction. *Journal of Pain and Symptom Management* 1994; **9**:12–18.

81 Ripamonti C, Mercadante S, Groff L et al. Role of octreotide, scopolamine butylbromide and hydration in symptom control of patients with inoperable bowel obstruction and nasogastric tubes: A prospective randomized trial. *Journal of Pain and Symptom Management* 2000; **19**:23–24.

82 Steiner N, Bruera E. Methods of hydration in palliative care patients. *Journal of Palliative Care* 1998; **14**:6–13.

83 Constans T, Dutertre J, Froge E. Hypodermoclysis in dehydrated elderly patients: Local effects with and without hyaluronidase. *Journal of Palliative Care* 1991; **7**:10–12.

84 Molloy DJ, Cunje A. Hypodermoclysis and the care of old adults. An old solution for new problems? *Canadian Family Physician* 1992; **38**:2038–2043.

85 Hays H. Hypodermoclysis for symptom control in terminal cancer. *Canadian Family Physician* 1985; **31**:1253–1256.

86 Bruera E, Legris M, Keuhn N, Miller MJ. Hypodermoclysis for the administration of fluids and narcotic analgesics in patients with advanced cancer. *Journal of Pain and Symptom Management* 1990; **5**:218–220.

87 Turner T, Cassano A. Subcutaneous dextrose for rehydration of elderly patients—An evidence based review. *BioMed Central Geriatrics* 2004; **4**:2.

88 Bruera E, de Stoutz ND, Fainsinger RL et al. Comparison of two different concentrations of hyaluronidase in patients receiving one hour infusions of hypodermoclysis. *Journal of Pain and Symptom Management* 1995; **10**:505–509.

89 Centeno C, Bruera E. Subcutaneous hydration with no hyaluronidase in patients with advanced cancer. *Journal of Pain and Symptom Management* 1999; **17**:305–306.

90 Pirrello R., Ting Chen C, Thomas SH. Initial experiences with subcutaneous recombinant human hyaluronidase. *Journal of Palliative Medicine* 2007; **10(4)**:861–864.

91 Bruera E, Schoeller T, Pruvost M. Proctoclysis for hydration of terminal cancer patients. *Lancet* 1994; **344**:1699.

92 Bruera E, Pruvost M, Schoeller T. Proctoclysis for hydration of terminally ill cancer patients. *Journal of Pain and Symptom Management* 1998; **15**:216–219.

93 Dalal S, Del Fabbro E, Bruera E. Is there a role for hydration at the end-of-life? *Current Opinion Supportive Palliative Care* 2009; **3**:72–78.

75

Fever, sweats, and hot flashes

AHSAN AZHAR, SHALINI DALAL

INTRODUCTION

Fever, sweats, and hot flashes are commonly encountered in the terminally ill and cancer patients. These may sometimes be associated with considerable morbidity and mortality. Although infection remains the most common etiology of fever in patients, irrespective of whether they are receiving chemotherapy or not, fever is commonly seen in patients in the absence of infection as well. Fever is also one of the most common symptoms experienced by elderly people at the end of life.[1,2] Similarly, hot flashes are reported by the majority of menopausal women and, in some women, can be a major source of distress.[3,4] Less well recognized is the impact of hot flashes on individuals with cancer, particularly women with a history of breast cancer and men with prostate cancer. In women with a history of breast cancer, approximately two-thirds experience hot flashes.[5,6] Optimal management of fevers, chills, sweats, and hot flashes is therefore of vital consideration in symptom management. As detailed in this chapter, it is contingent on meticulous patient assessment, on ascertaining the likely etiology, if possible, and on the implementation of appropriate treatment interventions befitting the patient-determined goals of care.

FEVER

Fever, as defined in *Stedman's Medical Dictionary*, is a "complex physiologic response to disease mediated by pyrogenic cytokines and characterized by a rise in core temperature, generation of acute phase reactants, and activation of immune systems."[7] More commonly, fever is defined as the elevation of core body temperature above normal. Normal average adult core body temperature is 37°C (98.6°F) and displays a circadian rhythm with body temperatures being the lowest in the predawn hours, at 36.1°C (97°F) or lower, and rising to 37.4°C (99.3°F) or higher in the afternoon. In oncology practice, a single reading of temperature of more than 38.3°C (101°F) or three readings (each taken at least an hour apart) of temperatures more than 38°C (100.4°F) is considered significant.

Pathophysiology of fever

Much like other fundamental aspects of human biology, core body temperature is closely regulated by intricate control mechanisms, involving a complex interplay of autonomic, endocrine, and behavioral responses. Integral to this process is the hypothalamus, which functions much like a thermostat, balancing heat production with heat loss. Fever is considered a hallmark of immune system activation, resulting in a regulated rise in body temperature. The regulation of this phenomenon is accomplished by the actions of two types of endogenous immunoregulatory proteins called cytokines, some functioning as pyrogens and others as antipyretics. This is described later and illustrated in Figure 75.1.

A number of exogenous substances, often referred to as exogenous pyrogens, have been found to be capable of evoking fever in animal models.[8] Of these, lipopolysaccharide (LPS), a cell wall product derived from Gram-negative bacteria, has been the most extensively studied. Exogenous pyrogens induce the production of proinflammatory cytokines, such as interleukin (IL)-1b and IL-6 (Castleman's disease, pheochromocytoma, and renal cell carcinoma), interferon α (INFα), and tumor necrosis factor (TNF), like in Hodgkin's disease, which act as humoral mediators influencing brain structures involved in resetting the hypothalamic set-point.[9] Cytokines are thought to exert their effect on the brain via direct and indirect mechanisms.[10–13]

Peripherally produced cytokines reach the central nervous system (CNS) directly by crossing at leaky areas in the blood–brain barrier via circumventricular vascular organs, which are networks of enlarged capillaries surrounding the hypothalamic regulatory centers.[14,15] In disease states such as bacterial infections, the blood–brain barrier can be compromised further, leading to an influx of cytokines from the periphery. This can account for several of the neurological manifestations associated with sickness behavior, including fever.[16,17] Cytokines are also produced locally within the CNS,[11] and may account for the hyperpyrexia of CNS hemorrhage. Among the cytokines measurable in the blood plasma during LPS-induced fever, circulating levels of IL-6 have shown the best correlation with fever.[18,19]

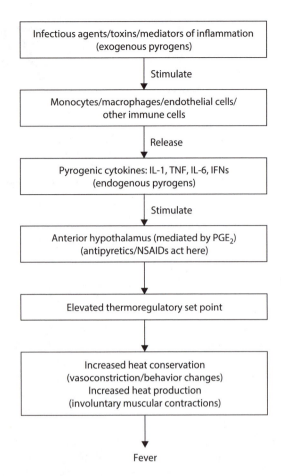

Figure 75.1 *Pathophysiology of fever. IL, interleukin; TNF, tumor necrosis factor; IFN, interferon; PGE, prostaglandin E; NSAID, nonsteroidal anti-inflammatory drug.*

Although not fully understood, it is proposed that cytokines stimulate the central production of the inducible enzyme cyclooxygenase (COX)-2, and subsequently stimulate the production of prostaglandins of the E series.[20,21] These prostaglandins activate thermoregulatory neurons of the anterior hypothalamic area to elevate body temperature.[22] Peripherally produced cytokines can also communicate with the brain indirectly in several ways, including the stimulation of terminal fibers of the autonomic nervous system.[23,24] Norepinephrine is the principal neurotransmitter, although several others such as acetylcholine, endorphins, enkephalins, substance P, somatostatin, and vasoactive intestinal polypeptide (VIP) have also been implicated.[25]

Etiology of fever (Box 75.1)

INFECTIONS

Nearly two-thirds of fever in patients with prolonged neutropenia may be attributed to infections,[26] a major cause of morbidity in patients with cancer. Fever in a cancer patient should be considered indicative of infection unless proven otherwise, with appropriate assessments being instituted in a timely fashion. Febrile neutropenic patients (absolute neutrophil count

---

Box 75.1 Etiology of fever in cancer patients

- Blood transfusion reaction
- CNS metastasis
- Drug associated (e.g., cytotoxic agents, antibiotics, IFN)
- Infections
- Radiation induced (e.g., radiation pneumonitis)
- Thrombosis
- Tumor (paraneoplastic fever)

[ANC] $\leq 500/mm^3$) represent an absolute emergency. In patients with advanced Alzheimer's disease, physical consequences of the progression of dementia predispose them to infection and fever, especially to aspiration pneumonia, urinary tract infections,[27–30] and decubiti.

PARANEOPLASTIC FEVER

Fever may be a common presentation for some malignancies and their progression may parallel the occurrence of fevers. Although Hodgkin disease has classically been associated with Pel–Epstein fevers (recurring periods of fever lasting for 3–10 days at a time), several other malignancies are also associated with paraneoplastic fevers and include acute leukemias, lymphomas, renal cell carcinoma, bone sarcomas, adrenal carcinomas, and pheochromocytomas. Solid tumors such as breast, lung, and colon cancer are less often associated with paraneoplastic fevers. However, the presence of liver metastasis from these tumors may result in fever. In addition, any solid tumor causing obstruction can result in fever.

Malignancy is often found during the workup of patients presenting with fever of unknown origin. While earlier reports found an incidence of 20%, a later study reported malignancy as the cause of fever in 15% of patients.[31] In patients with cancer presenting with fever of unknown origin, paraneoplastic fever was found to be the most common etiology.[32] Although the exact mechanism of tumor-associated fever is unclear, it is thought to involve inflammatory cytokines such as TNFα, IL-1, and IL-6, which are produced either by host macrophages in response to the tumor or by the tumor itself.[33,34]

TRANSFUSION-ASSOCIATED FEVER

Febrile and allergic nonhemolytic transfusion reactions (NHTRs) are the most common adverse effects of blood transfusions.[35,36] These reactions are generally not life threatening, but they are expensive in their management, evaluation, and associated blood product wastage. The true incidence of febrile NHTRs (FNHTRs) is not well established in patients with cancer. In a large retrospective study, the incidence of side effects following transfusion of 100,000 units of packed red blood cells to more than 25,000 cancer patients over a 4-year period was found to be at 0.3% (of these, 51.3% were FNHTRs, 36.7% were allergic urticarial reactions, and 17% were hemolytic reactions).[37] This is comparable to other studies where the incidence has ranged from 0.2% to 0.7%.[38,39]

The occurrence of fever is usually caused by the presence of antibodies to antigens on the donor's white blood cells. Its prevention by using leukodepleted blood components was demonstrated more than two decades ago.[40-42] Some studies have shown a correlation with storage time of platelets and the release of cytokines as another reason for the occurrence of FNHTRs.[43-45]

Infection may also be a source of fever in patients receiving blood transfusions.[46-48] The prevalence of bacteria is estimated to be about 0.04%–2%, depending on the type of components, the number and age of the evaluated components, and the detection methods used. It is estimated that 1 in. each 1000/2000 units of platelet concentrates (obtained from whole blood or apheresis) is contaminated with bacteria.[49-52] The incidence of bacterial contamination in red cell concentrates is much lower and almost zero for fresh frozen plasma and cryoprecipitate.

DRUG FEVER

Drug-associated fever is usually a diagnosis of exclusion, except for some drugs such as biological response modifiers, amphotericin B, and bleomycin, where the occurrence of fever may be predictable. Other drugs commonly implicated as a cause of fever include antibiotics, cardiovascular drugs, anticonvulsants, cytotoxic agents, and growth factors. In one retrospective study of 148 episodes of drug fever, antimicrobials were found to be the most common offending agent (31%).[53] Cytotoxic agents accounted for 11 episodes (7.4%).

In a retrospective chart review of 50 patients who had received at least 100 mg of amphotericin B for at least 3 days, the incidence of fever and chills was 34% and 56%, with rates of 2.6 and 3.5 mean episodes per patient per treatment course, respectively.[54] Interferon therapy is associated with acute "flu-like" syndrome consisting of fever, chills, fatigue, myalgias, arthralgia, and headaches, with some variation according to type of IFN, route of administration, schedule, dose, and age of patient.[55] The administration of growth factors is also associated with fever, being more common following granulocyte macrophage colony–stimulating factor (GM-CSF) administration than granulocyte colony–stimulating factor (G-CSF) administration. Bleomycin-associated fever occurs in 20%–50% of patients and is more common when it is administered intravenously. Fever is also associated with other cytotoxic agents such as cisplatin, streptozocin, 5-fluorouracil, and therapy with monoclonal antibodies.[56-59] In addition to antibiotics, common drugs in palliative care setting, which can mimic rise in body temperature, include antipsychotics (neuroleptic malignant syndrome [NMS]) and antidepressants (serotonin syndrome).[60] See fever versus hyperthermia in the following. Withdrawal from opioids can also present in similar manner.

Evaluation of fever

Assessment of fever requires a careful study of history, medication review, and a thorough physical examination to include all major body systems. Patients should undergo meticulous evaluation of the skin and all body orifices, including mouth, ears, nose, throat, urethra, vagina, rectum, venipuncture sites, biopsy site, skin folds (i.e., breast, axilla, abdomen, and groin), and interdigital spaces. In nearly two-thirds of neutropenic patients, the initial evaluation may not identify a focus of infection.[33] This may relate in part to the high frequency of empirical treatment with broad-spectrum antibiotics, which may make it harder to determine the site of infection. Careful physical examinations should be repeated at least daily in patients with neutropenia, even after the initiation of empirical antibiotics. It must be remembered that immunocompromised patients may be vulnerable to more than one infection and that different organisms may emerge during a single febrile episode.

Interventions for fever

GOALS OF CARE

The presence of fever may be associated with potential metabolic consequences including dehydration, increased oxygen consumption, and metabolic rate,[61,62] which may be especially pronounced in debilitated terminally ill patients. If prolonged, fevers may be associated with increased nutritional demands and debilitating fatigue. Although fever may be beneficial for enhancing host defense,[63,64] other factors such as the patient's comfort and physiological responses also deserve consideration. Suppression of fever may help alleviate uncomfortable, constitutional symptoms of fatigue, myalgias, diaphoresis, and chills. In addition to constitutional symptoms, focal findings related to the etiology of fever may also contribute to symptom burden. For example, abscess formation is often associated with pain, while uncomfortable dyspnea and cough can be related to pneumonia. The specific interventions used for fever management are determined by the underlying etiology, together with patient-determined goals of care. Workup of fever can lead to unnecessary and prolonged hospitalization as well as additional costs for patients near the end of their life, resulting in significant suffering.[65] Patients with advanced cancer may opt not to treat the underlying etiology of fever and seek only nonspecific palliative measures. For patients who can communicate, it may be beneficial to be certain that if the fever is uncomfortable, and whether curing the fever is more uncomfortable than the fever itself for the patient. Although empiric, there is no compelling reason to think that treatment of fever actually reduces suffering for dying, unresponsive patients.[66] Individuals seeking comfort-oriented care exclusively may decline parenteral antibiotic treatment of pneumonia to avoid hospitalization and remain at home. For others, treating the underlying etiology of fever with more aggressive interventions, such as surgical drainage of a painful abscess, will offer symptom palliation and potentially contribute to improvement in quality of life and even life prolongation. Aggressive treatment of infection does not improve survival rates among persons with severe dementia and has been associated with accelerated progression of the severity of dementia.[67] Antibiotics and other aggressive measures are often associated with numerous deleterious outcomes, including renal failure and ototoxicity, allergic or drug reactions, rash, diarrhea, blood dyscrasias, antibiotic resistance, use of intravenous lines and mechanical restraints, prolonged time to death, and increased costs.[68,69]

NONSPECIFIC INTERVENTIONS

During febrile episodes, increasing fluid intake, removing excess clothing and linens, tepid water bathing or sponging, and use of antipyretics may offer relief. In the very sick, administration of fluids intravenously or subcutaneously may be warranted. Other comfort measures include the application of lubricant to dried lips and keeping mucous membranes moist with ice chips. Convective cooling via increasing air circulation by fans or using an airflow blanket may be effective to reduce temperatures and improve patient comfort.[70*] Ensure that clothes and bed linens are dry and changed as needed. Again, patient preferences must always be given priority. Noisy and labor-intensive measures, which can distract family and other caregivers from more meaningful interactions at the death-bed, should be avoided. Education and reassurance is of paramount importance in such situations.[66]

Antipyretic agents such as acetaminophen, aspirin, or nonsteroidal anti-inflammatory drugs (NSAIDS) act by lowering the elevated thermal set-point by the inhibition of enzyme COX. Although these agents are commonly administered to hospitalized patients to enhance patient comfort,[71] no studies have been done in the cancer population with fever, and carefully controlled efficacy studies have not quantified the degree to which the antipyretics therapy enhances the comfort of febrile patients in other populations. Although theoretically, patients with pulmonary and cardiovascular disorders may benefit from antipyretic therapy by minimizing the impact of increased metabolic demands, the risk versus benefit of this approach has not been determined. Similarly, antipyretic therapy has not been demonstrated to prevent febrile seizures in children.[72] Several studies have confirmed that increasing the dose of acetaminophen from moderate dosage (10 mg/kg every 4 hours, maximum 5 doses/day) to relatively higher dosage (15–20 mg/kg every 4 hours, maximum 5 doses/day) in children failed to reduce the rate of recurrence of febrile seizures.[73]

Fever control may be enhanced by combining physical methods with antipyretics. In children, a randomized placebo-controlled trial of sponging with ice water, isopropyl alcohol, or tepid water (with or without acetaminophen) demonstrated that all combinations enhanced fever control, but comfort was greatest in children receiving placebo or sponging, followed by those who received acetaminophen combined with tepid water sponging.[74] Discomfort was found to be greatest when sponging with ice water or isopropyl alcohol with or without concomitant administration. Like acetaminophen, aspirin may be effective in reducing fever, but should be used with caution in patients with or at risk of thrombocytopenia due to its antiplatelet effects. In children, aspirin use is contraindicated due to the risk of Reye syndrome with fever related to certain viral etiologies, including varicella and influenza.[75] NSAIDs should also be used cautiously in the cancer population, as they inhibit platelet function and may also cause gastrointestinal hemorrhage and adversely affect renal function.

PRIMARY INTERVENTIONS DIRECTED AT THE ETIOLOGY OF FEVER

Infections

Patients should be instructed to seek medical help if a fever develops when the neutrophil count is low or declining. In febrile neutropenic patients, broad-spectrum antibiotics should be initiated immediately even before culture results are available,[76] as mortality rate is 70% for patients not receiving antibiotics within 48 hours.[77] Initial antibiotic use is guided by the knowledge of the treating institution's antimicrobial spectrum and antibiotic resistance pattern, as well as the suspected cause. Although there is general consensus that empirical therapy is appropriate, there is no consensus as to which antibiotics or combinations of antibiotics should be used. The Infectious Diseases Society of America (IDSA) Fever and Neutropenia Guidelines Panel recommends empirical antibiotics based on the patient's clinical condition and risk for complications, and determination of the need of vancomycin in the initial regimen.[78] These four protocols are depicted in Table 75.1.

Treatment regimens are further modified by the duration of fever and individual patient risk factors such as the presence of central lines or other artificial devices, history of steroid use, and history of injection drug use. After a specific pathogen is isolated, antibiotic therapy is then changed to provide optimal therapeutic response. The single most important determinant of successful discontinuation of antibiotics is the neutrophil count. If infection is not identified after 3 days of treatment, if the neutrophil count is >500 cells/mm^3 for 2 consecutive days, and if the patient is afebrile for >48 hours, antibiotic therapy may be discontinued. For neutropenic hosts with persistent or recurrent fevers after 1 week of broad-spectrum antibiotic therapy, the addition of an antifungal agent is recommended, as continued granulocytopenia is usually associated with the development of nonbacterial opportunistic infections, particularly candidiasis and aspergillosis.[79] Acyclovir is the drug of choice in the treatment of herpes simplex or varicella zoster viral infection. Ganciclovir has activity against cytomegalovirus (CMV). Both agents can be used prophylactically in the management of patients at high risk for these infections. Foscarnet is useful in the treatment of CMV and acyclovir-resistant herpes simplex virus.

Various investigators have developed models predicting risk groups of febrile neutropenia, with implications for management strategies. Therapeutic options under evaluation include

Table 75.1 *Empiric antibiotic regimens for unexplained neutropenic fever in the cancer population*

Regimen	Route	Antibiotic selection	Comments
1	Oral	Ciprofloxacin *plus* amoxicillin–clavulanate	• For use in select *adult* patients • Patients mostly in remission and at low risk for serious life threatening infections • Can be used on an outpatient basis if ready access to care, no signs of focal infection and no signs or symptoms suggestive of systemic infection other than fever
2	Intravenous	Choose one: cefepime, ceftazidime, imipenem, or meropenem	• Mono-drug choice is as effective as multiple drug combinations for uncomplicated neutropenic patients • Monitor closely for poor response, emergence of secondary infection(s) and drug resistance
3	Intravenous	Aminoglycoside plus antipseudomonal penicillin or ceftazidime or carbapenem	• Advantages include potential synergistic effects against some Gram-negative bacilli • Potential minimal emergence of drug-resistant strains during treatment
4	Intravenous	Vancomycin plus antibiotics from regimens 2 or 3 above	• Restrict to • Institutions with high prevalence of infections with penicillin-resistant Gram-positive bacteria • Suspected catheter-related cellulitis or bacteremia • Gram-positive bacteremia • Evidence of septic shock

Source: Data from Milner, L.V. and Butcher, K., *Transfusion*, 18(4), 493, July–August 1978.

early hospital discharge, home intravenous antibiotic therapy, and oral antibiotic regimens. Due to rapid changes in the field, the reader is directed to specialized sources for specific management recommendations of febrile neutropenia.

Paraneoplastic fever

The best management for paraneoplastic fevers is the treatment of the underlying neoplasm with definitive antineoplastic therapy. If not possible, NSAIDs have been considered as the mainstay of treatment,[66] with naproxen being the most extensively studied. However, indomethacin and diclofenac have also been found to be effective.[80**] Several studies suggesting that neoplastic fevers are more responsive to NSAIDs than infectious fevers, leading to advocacy of the "naproxen test" to differentiate between neoplastic and non-neoplastic fevers.[65,81,82] However, this approach has not been validated.[83] Thalidomide, an immune-modulatory agent, has been shown to have modulatory and/or suppressive effects on several cytokines such as TNFα, IL-1, and IL-6,[84,85] all involved in paraneoplastic fever and which, theoretically, may have a role in the treatment of cancer patients with fever and sweats.[86] Despite reports of its antipyretic and antidiaphoretic activity,[87,88] this agent has not been formally tested in clinical studies with cancer patients for fever or sweat control. Strategies, using the IL-1 receptor antagonist model, have been explored in paraneoplastic fever aimed at blocking IL-6 signaling pathways.[13]

Transfusion-associated fever

Many institutions have moved toward leukoreduced transfusions in an effort to decrease incidence of FNHTRs, and several countries have even restricted the manufacture and transfusion of blood products to prestorage leukodepleted blood components only. A retrospective analysis conducted at Johns Hopkins Hospital examined the frequency of transfusion reactions associated with the transfusion of red blood cells (RBCs), between July 1994 and December 2001.[89] The study directly compared two time periods before and after the initiative toward leukoreduction. In the initial period (July–December 1994) before the initiative to move toward leukoreduction, 96% of RBC inventory was non-leukoreduced. In the study period after leukoreduction (July–December 2001) 99.5% of RBC inventory was leukoreduced. When comparing these two time periods, the incidence of FNHTRs decreased from 0.37% to 0.19% ($P = 0.0008$). The trend over the entire 7.5-year study period confirmed the decrease in FNHTRs as the percentage of leukoreduced RBCs increased. The incidence of allergic NHTRs remained unchanged. The decreased incidence of FNHTRs with leukoreduction has been found in other studies as well.[90–93] Common clinical practice prior to blood product transfusions includes premedication with acetaminophen/diphenhydramine with or without steroids. The use of erythropoietin for cancer-related anemia may decrease the need of blood transfusions and may be used for cancer-related anemia. The risks versus benefits, including cost, of such prophylactic treatments to avoid or delay transfusions needs to be carefully reviewed as they are not devoid of side effects, including reduction in survival.[94–97]

Drug fever

Drug-associated fever responds to cessation of the offending agent, when possible. Response to fever and related symptoms, with biological response modifier administration, is type, route, dose, and schedule dependent. These factors may sometimes be altered for fever control without compromising with efficacy. Liposomal amphotericin B is as effective as conventional amphotericin B for empirical antifungal therapy in patients with fever and neutropenia, but is associated with decreased toxicity, including occurrence of fever and chills.[98] Caspofungin has also shown promising responses.[79] Fever may also be attenuated by the use of acetaminophen, NSAIDs, with or without steroid, premedication. It is common clinical practice to administer meperidine to attenuate severe chills associated with a febrile reaction, although empirical data confirming its efficacy are not available. Index of suspicion should be kept higher when using multiple antidepressants or antipsychotics and while rotating or suddenly stopping opioids or any drugs of abuse when patient gets admitted (withdrawal).

Fever versus hyperthermia

Although in the vast majority of patients, an elevated body temperature usually represents a fever, there are instances where elevated temperatures could be secondary to hyperthermia. These include heat stroke syndromes, certain metabolic diseases (hyperthyroidism), and drugs that interfere with thermoregulation. With fever, thermoregulatory mechanisms remain intact, but the hypothalamic thermal set-point is raised by exposure to endogenous pyrogens,[99] leading to behavioral and physiological responses to elevate body temperature. In contrast, during hyperthermia, the setting of the thermoregulatory center remains unchanged[66] at normothermic levels, while body temperature increases in an uncontrolled fashion and overrides the ability to lose heat. Hyperthermia thus results from overwhelming of the peripheral heat-dissipating mechanisms by disease, drugs, or from excessive heat, be it external or internal.[100]

Atropine may increase endogenous heat production by interfering with thermoregulation: It blocks sweating and vasodilation, thereby raising core temperature. Hyperthermia also occurs with NMS, an idiosyncratic reaction to drugs that block the dopamine receptor. Haloperidol and chlorpromazine, which are conventional antipsychotic agents, can be the common offenders.[101,102] Atypical antipsychotic medications, including clozapine, risperidone, olanzapine, and quetiapine, have also been associated with NMS.[103,104] There are also case reports of other medications causing NMS, including venlafaxine, promethazine, and metoclopramide.[105,106] NMS typically occurs within several days of the initiation of treatment, while dosages and serum concentration of these medications are usually within the therapeutic range. The probability of developing NMS is directly related to the antidopaminergic potency of the neuroleptic agent. In addition, specific polymorphisms of the dopamine D_2 receptor may predispose some patients to NMS.[107] Use of multiple antidepressants can present with serotonin syndrome.[60] Great care should be taken not to predispose a patient to withdrawal of opioids or sudden stoppage of a drug of abuse, especially immediately after the patient gets admitted.

It is important to make the distinction between fever and hyperthermia, since management approaches to these distinct syndromes differ. There is no rapid way to differentiate elevated core temperature due to fever from hyperthermia, and a diagnosis of hyperthermia is often made because of a preceding history of heat exposure or use of certain drugs that interfere with normal thermoregulation. On physical examination, the skin is hot but dry in heat stroke syndromes and in patients taking drugs that block sweating.

Antipyretic agents act by lowering the elevated thermal set-point and are used in the treatment of fever, but are ineffective in hyperthermia, where the thermal set-point is normal. In hyperthermia, drugs that interfere with vasoconstriction such as phenothiazines and those that block muscle contractions or shivering are useful. However, these are not true antipyretics as they can reduce body temperature independently of hypothalamic control. Shivering may be suppressed with intravenous benzodiazepines such as diazepam or lorazepam. Chlorpromazine intravenously (25–50 mg) may also be used for this purpose if NMS is not suspected.

In patients diagnosed with hyperthermia, physical cooling should be started immediately with techniques such as removing bedclothes, sponging the patient with tepid water, and using bed fans. More rapid reductions in body temperature can be achieved by sponging the patient with alcohol or by using hypothermic mattresses or ice packs. Immersion in ice water is the most effective means of physical cooling, but it should be reserved for true hyperthermic emergencies, such as heat stroke. In true emergencies, treatment may also include the intravenous or intraperitoneal administration of cool fluid, gastric lavage or enemas with ice water, and even extracorporeal circulation. No matter what technique is used, the body temperature must always be monitored closely to avoid hypothermia.

SWEATS

In patients with advanced disease or those receiving palliative care, the prevalence of sweating (hyperhidrosis) ranges from 14% to 28%, is frequently nocturnal (nocturnal diaphoresis or night sweats), and is moderate to severe in intensity.[108–111] Although night sweats have been defined as drenching sweats that require the patient to change bedclothes, this definition may not describe the majority of patients who complain of the symptom. Sweating is a feature unique to humans (and apes) in which skin loses heat thru evaporation and helps in regulating body temperatures when exposed to hot environment. Patients with inherited disorder of anhidrotic ectodermal hypoplasia as well as infants and frail elderly fail to sweat sufficiently to maintain cooler body temperatures.[111] In the literature, night sweats have also been associated with a variety of medical problems including malignancies (e.g., lymphomas), some infections including tuberculosis, autoimmune diseases, and drugs. Common malignancies associated with night sweats include lymphomas, leukemia, renal cell carcinoma, and Castleman's disease. The classic presentation of tuberculosis includes fever, weight loss, and night sweats. AIDS-related infections might also cause night sweats, including *Mycobacterium avium* complex (MAC) infection and CMV syndromes. The differential diagnosis for night sweats is broad, and Box 75.2 lists some of these conditions.

Box 75.2 Etiology of night sweats

Malignancy

- Castleman's disease
- Leukemia
- Lymphoma
- Renal cell carcinoma

Infections

- Endocarditis
- Fungal infections
- Human immunodeficiency virus
- Infectious mononucleosis
- Lung abscess
- Mycobacterium avium complex
- Tuberculosis

Others

- Anxiety
- Chronic fatigue syndrome
- Diabetes insipidus
- Gastroesophageal reflux disease
- Granulomatous disease
- Obstructive sleep apnea
- Rheumatologic diseases

Endocrine

- Acromegaly
- Diabetes insipidus
- Diabetes mellitus (nocturnal hypoglycemia)
- Endocrine tumors (pheochromocytoma, carcinoid tumor)
- Hyperthyroidism (thyrotoxicosis)
- Orchiectomy
- Perimenopausal and postmenopausal women

Drugs

- Antihypertensives
- Antipyretics: Salicylates, acetaminophen
- Drugs of abuse: Alcohol, heroin
- Leuprolide
- Niacin
- Opioids: Morphine, diamorphine, methadone, butorphanol
- Phenothiazines
- Selective estrogen receptor modulator drugs (SERMs): tamoxifen and raloxifene
- Selective serotonin receptor inhibitors

Patients presenting with night sweats warrant a detailed evaluation including history and physical examination aimed at revealing associated symptoms to help narrow down the broad differential diagnosis and guide further workup. Compensatory hyperhidrosis can usually occur in normal sweat-producing skin areas in response to anhidrosis in other areas of skin. The prevalence of sweats and their impact on quality of life in the cancer population is not well established and requires further description. Clinically, hot flashes are often seen in association with sweats. By far this is the most common cause of sweats encountered in clinical medicine, experienced by the majority of perimenopausal and postmenopausal women, and hence, this topic is being covered in detail later.

HOT FLASHES

Hot flashes, experienced by three-quarters of menopausal women, are described as a sudden onset of an uncomfortable sensation of intense heat, accompanied by skin flushing, warmth, and sweating, usually of the chest and face.[4] Hot flashes typically last for 2–4 min and are often accompanied by palpitations and anxiety, and may be triggered by emotional stress, anxiety, alcohol, and certain foods.[112] Factors associated with a greater risk of hot flashes are listed in Box 75.3.[113-116] Approximately two-thirds of women with history of breast cancer experience hot flashes.[5] In postmenopausal women with a history of breast cancer, predictors of hot flash severity include higher body mass index, a high school education or less, younger age at diagnosis, and tamoxifen use (selective estrogen receptor modulators, SERMs).[117,118] For patients starting tamoxifen, hot flashes typically increase in the first 2–3 months, followed by a plateau and then gradual dissipation.[119]

In men treated with androgen ablation for locally advanced or metastatic prostate cancer, 50%–88% experience hot flashes.[120,121] Patients with other cancers are also affected with hot flashes; however, data on this is limited. The rapid menopause associated with cancer treatments does not allow for a gradual adjustment of falling estrogen levels, and this may explain why hot flashes resulting from cancer treatment tend to be more profound.

Pathophysiology

The prevailing hypothesis relates the development of hot flashes to lowering of estrogen levels leading to complex neuroendocrine mechanisms, including alterations in the level of hypothalamic neurotransmitters, which resets the thermostat to a lower level with a narrower range, as compared with those who do not experience hot flashes.[122,123] A small rise in core body temperature has been found to occur 15 min prior to hot flashes in 60% of hot flash episodes.[124] This subtle elevation in core body temperature stimulates mechanisms of heat dissipation, resulting in cutaneous vasodilation and sweating, the two central components of the hot flash syndrome.

Box 75.3 Factors associated with hot flashes

Abrupt menopause

- Chemotherapy
- Drugs
- Radiation
- Surgery

Cancer type

- Breast
- Prostate

Early menopause

Ethnicity

- African women
- Western women

Lack of exercise

High body mass index

Low education

Low estrogen levels

Low socioeconomic status

Smokers

Box 75.4 Treatment interventions for hot flashes in patients with cancer

Hormonal agents

- Androgens
- Estrogens
- Progestational agents

Nonhormonal agents

- α-Adrenergic agents
- Antidepressants
- β-Blockers
- Gabapentin
- Veralipride
- Vitamin E

CAM approaches

- Herbal medications
- Acupuncture
- Behavioral interventions

Two most recognized neurotransmitters involved in hypothalamic thermoregulatory processes are norepinephrine and serotonin. Catecholestrogens (estrogenic metabolites) abundant in the hypothalamus stimulate the production of β-endorphins. Both catecholestrogens and endorphins inhibit the production of hypothalamic norepinephrine. Loss of this negative feedback in low estrogenic states results in rise of norepinephrine levels and an upregulation of certain hypothalamic serotonin receptors responsible for resetting of the thermostat.[125] Norepinephrine is believed to be responsible for the rise in core temperature prior to onset of hot flashes.[124] In men, it is uncertain if low testosterone levels or decline in estrogen levels or both are responsible for development of the hot flash syndrome.

Assessment and treatment of hot flashes

Hot flashes should be routinely assessed as a component of systematic symptom surveys, and if present, a careful assessment of hot flash frequency, intensity, duration, potential triggers, and impact on quality of life is advised in order to construct an individualized treatment plan. Patient self-report diaries with hot flash frequency, intensity, possible trigger factors, and associated distress can be helpful to clinicians to formulate treatment recommendations.[126] Hot flash score is determined by multiplying the daily frequency of hot flashes by their average severity. Box 75.4 lists the possible options for management of hot flashes.

HORMONE REPLACEMENT THERAPY

Estrogen

Estrogen replacement is effective for treatment of hot flashes in 80%–90% of patients, regardless of underlying etiology.[127**,128,129*130**] However, some women have absolute or relative contraindications to hormone replacement therapy (HRT), and others are reluctant to take hormones due to perceived risks and side effects. The Women's Health Initiative Study evaluated the risks and benefits of estrogen plus progestin therapy in healthy postmenopausal women.[131**] The estrogen plus progestin arm was stopped prematurely in women with an intact uterus at a mean follow-up of 5.2 years (61.3) due to detection of a 1.26 times increased breast cancer risk (95% CI 1.00–1.59). Observed benefits of HRT on hip fractures and colon cancer risk were far outweighed by increased risks of venous thromboembolic disease, breast cancer, stroke, and coronary artery disease. Another population-based, case–control study of 975 postmenopausal women diagnosed with breast cancer supports an increased risk of breast cancer with combined HRT.[132] In this cohort, HRT use was associated with an increased risk of breast cancer, including lobular, ductal, and estrogen and progesterone receptor positive tumors.

Progestational agents

Progestational agents have comparable efficacy to estrogens for hot flash reduction. Agents studied include megestrol acetate and transdermal progesterone, and the long-acting intramuscular preparation, depo-medroxyprogesterone acetate (DMPA).[133**134**135*]

Despite benefit of amelioration of hot flashes, there is ongoing debate about safety of progesterone in patients with breast, uterine, or prostate cancer. In men with prostate cancer, several investigators have reported a decline in prostate-specific antigen (PSA) levels after withdrawal of megestrol acetate, raising concerns that its use may be harmful in this population.[136–138] Risk associated with progestin use in women with a history of breast cancer is unknown at this time, as is its effect on the outcome of tamoxifen treatment. Some data have suggested that progestational agents may increase epithelial cell proliferation, an undesirable effect in breast cancer.[139,140] There is also some evidence of antitumor activity in breast cancer.[141]

Tibolone

Tibolone, a synthetic steroid compound with combined estrogenic, progestogenic, and androgenic properties, has been reported to reduce hot flashes.[142*143] One study of postmenopausal women receiving tamoxifen after surgery for breast cancer found a significant reduction in the severity of hot flashes with tibolone compared with placebo (0.4 vs. 0.2, respectively, $P = 0.031$) but no change in the daily number of hot flashes with either tibolone or placebo ($P = 0.219$).[144**] Tibolone is not available in the United States.

NONHORMONAL AGENTS

Nonhormonal agents are gaining popularity as therapy for hot flash reduction due to the heightened concerns about the risks of using HRT. These include pharmacotherapies as well as complementary and alternative medicinal approaches.

Antidepressants

Several large placebo-controlled, randomized trials have shown the beneficial effects of antidepressants from the selective serotonin reuptake inhibitors (SSRIs) and selective serotonin and norepinephrine reuptake inhibitors (SNRIs) class in hot flash management. In the Mayo Clinic study, breast cancer survivors and menopausal women experiencing hot flashes were assigned to receive one of three different dose levels of venlafaxine (37.5, 75, and 150 mg daily), or placebo for 4 weeks.[145**] A dose-related diminution in average hot flashes scores from baseline was noted (27% in the placebo subjects vs. 37%, 61%, and 61% for the three venlafaxine groups, respectively). Similar beneficial results have been found in studies with paroxetine and fluoxetine.[146**,147**] Preliminary studies with other newer antidepressants, including citalopram and mirtazapine, have also shown good results in standard starting doses.[148*,149*]

Of note, many of the SSRIs can inhibit the cytochrome P450 enzyme system involved in the hepatic metabolism of tamoxifen, a drug commonly used in the treatment of breast cancer. In a prospective study, coadministration of paroxetine with tamoxifen was shown to result in decreased concentrations of 4-hydroxy-N-desmethyl-tamoxifen, an active tamoxifen metabolite (also known as endoxifen).[150] Women with the wild-type CYP2D6 genotype demonstrated greater decreases in endoxifen levels than those with a variant genotype ($P = 0.03$). Given the widespread use of SSRIs for the treatment of mood disorders and hot flashes, the interactions of SSRIs with tamoxifen merit further study.

OTHER NONHORMONAL AGENTS

Several other agents have been found to be useful in hot flash management. In a placebo-controlled, randomized study of 59 postmenopausal women, gabapentin was more effective than placebo in reducing hot flash frequency (45% vs. 29%, respectively) and hot flash composite score (54% vs. 31%, respectively).[151,152] Gabapentine appears to decrease hot flashes in men to similar degree as in women.[153] Clonidine, a central acting α_2-adrenergic receptor agonist, has been shown to have modest benefits in hot flash reduction in several studies in healthy postmenopausal women, breast cancer survivors on tamoxifen, and men with prostate cancer, but with significant dose-related side effects,[154**,155**] especially dry mouth, constipation, and sleeping problems. The North Central Cancer Treatment Group (NCCTG), in a randomized, placebo-controlled crossover trial of vitamin E in women with a history of breast cancer, found a minor decrease with treatment, with a mean reduction of 1 flash/day, without adverse effects.[156**] This reduction is unlikely to be of meaningful clinical benefit. Bellergal, a combination of belladonna and phenobarbital, was widely used in the past for hot flash management. Although several reports favor its use over placebo,[157] this therapy cannot be recommended in view of the risk of phenobarbital dependence and dose-dependent anticholinergic side effects of belladonna, including dry mouth, constipation, blurry vision, and dizziness.

COMPLEMENTARY AND ALTERNATIVE MEDICINE APPROACHES

Eighty percent of women in the 45–60 age groups have reported the use of nonprescription therapies for the management of menopausal symptoms.[158] Often perceived to be safer than hormone replacement therapy, complementary and alternative medicine (CAM) may provide users with a sense of personal control over their healthcare.

Soy phytoestrogens are weak estrogens found in plant foods, and while dietary supplementation with natural soy products appears to be a benign intervention, long-term effects are not known. Two randomized, placebo-controlled studies show no clinical benefit of soy over placebo for hot flash management.[159**,160**] Breast cancer risk in the general population and risk of recurrence in breast cancer survivors has not yet been clarified, nor has its effect on hormonally mediated antitumor therapies, such as tamoxifen and the aromatase inhibitors. Black cohosh (*Cimicifuga racemosa*) is approved in Germany for the treatment of hot flashes. The anecdotal clinical and observational experience suggests black cohosh may produce 25%–30% more efficacy than placebo for menopausal symptoms, including hot flashes.[161] In a randomized, double-blind, placebo-controlled study on breast cancer survivors in the United States, however, efficacy of black cohosh was not significantly different from placebo.[162**] The high prevalence of tamoxifen use in study participants may have confounded study results. Red clover, which contains isoflavones (phytoestrogens) and dong quai (Angelica sinensis, "female ginseng"), has not been found to be beneficial in the management of hot flashes.

Acupuncture has been suggested as a remedy for hot flashes. In a randomized controlled study, Wyon et al. compared the efficacy of electro-acupuncture with oral estradiol treatment and superficial needle insertion on hot flash reduction in 45 postmenopausal women.[163**] They found that electro-acupuncture decreased the number of hot flashes significantly over time, but not to the same extent as the estrogen treatment. No significant difference in effect was found between electro-acupuncture and the superficial needle insertion. In a small pilot study of prostate cancer patients who underwent castration therapy, a substantial decrease (70% reduction) in hot flash symptoms was noted at 10 weeks, with a sustained reduction of 50% at 3 months.[164*] Further studies are warranted to determine efficacy and potential mechanisms of action of acupuncture as a modality of therapy for the treatment of hot flashes.

Behavioral methods may play a role in hot flash management. Studied methods include relaxation response training[165**] and paced respirations.[166**] These may be used as primary alternatives for patients who do not want to take medications or as an adjunct for individuals who achieve suboptimal relief with other interventions. The beneficial effects may be related to the decreased adrenergic tone mediated by relaxation techniques. Exercise would similarly be beneficial.[167,168]

Key learning points

- Fever, chills, and hot flashes are frequently encountered in palliative care patients.

- Fever in patients with cancer should be considered indicative of infection, unless proven otherwise. Neutropenic fever is a medical emergency.

- Fever may be associated with potential metabolic consequences including dehydration and fatigue, which may be especially pronounced in debilitated terminally ill patients.

- Paraneoplastic and drug fevers should be considered in the differential diagnosis of fever.

- Cytokines are implicated in the etiology of fever secondary to infections and paraneoplastic fevers.

- Both fever and hyperthermia result in the elevation of core body temperatures but differ in their pathophysiology and management. Many palliative care patients are on drugs that have the potential to cause hyperthermia.

- Patients should be assessed for night sweats and hot flashes. The latter is widely prevalent in some cancers (breast, prostate) and postmenopausal women and may be associated with significant distress.

- Many nonhormonal therapies are available for consideration for hot flash management.

REFERENCES

1 Seah ST, Low JA, Chan YH. Symptoms and care of dying elderly patients in an acute hospital. *Singapore Med J.* May 2005;46(5):210–214.
2 Hall P, Schroder C, Weaver L. The last 48 hours of life in long-term care: A focused chart audit. *J Am Geriatr Soc.* March 2002;50(3):501–506.
3 McKinlay SM, Jefferys M. The menopausal syndrome. *Br J Prev Soc Med.* May 1974;28(2):108–115.
4 Feldman BM, Voda A, Gronseth E. The prevalence of hot flash and associated variables among perimenopausal women. *Res Nurs Health.* September 1985;8(3):261–268.
5 Couzi RJ, Helzlsouer KJ, Fetting JH. Prevalence of menopausal symptoms among women with a history of breast cancer and attitudes toward estrogen replacement therapy. *J Clin Oncol.* November 1995;13(11):2737–2744.
6 Carpenter JS, Andrykowski MA, Cordova M, Cunningham L, Studts J, McGrath P et al. Hot flashes in postmenopausal women treated for breast carcinoma: Prevalence, severity, correlates, management, and relation to quality of life. *Cancer.* May 1, 1998;82(9):1682–1691.
7 Stedman TL. *Stedman's Medical Dictionary.* 28th edn. Philadelphia, PA: Lippincott Williams & Wilkins; 2006.
8 Kluger MJ. Fever: Role of pyrogens and cryogens. *Physiol Rev.* January 1991;71(1):93–127.
◆ 9 Saper CB. Neurobiological basis of fever. *Ann N Y Acad Sci.* September 29, 1998;856:90–94.
10 Besedovsky HO, del Rey A, Klusman I, Furukawa H, Monge Arditi G, Kabiersch A. Cytokines as modulators of the hypothalamus-pituitary-adrenal axis. *J Steroid Biochem Mol Biol.* 1991;40(4–6):613–618.
11 Breder CD, Dinarello CA, Saper CB. Interleukin-1 immunoreactive innervation of the human hypothalamus. *Science.* April 15, 1988;240(4850):321–324.
12 Sternberg EM. Neural-immune interactions in health and disease. *J Clin Invest.* December 1, 1997;100(11):2641–2647.
13 Dalal S, Zhukovsky DS. Pathophysiology and management of fever. *J Support Oncol.* January 2006;4(1):9–16.
14 Stitt JT. Evidence for the involvement of the organum vasculosum laminae terminalis in the febrile response of rabbits and rats. *J Physiol.* November 1985;368:501–511.
15 Banks WA, Ortiz L, Plotkin SR, Kastin AJ. Human interleukin (IL) 1 alpha, murine IL-1 alpha and murine IL-1 beta are transported from blood to brain in the mouse by a shared saturable mechanism. *J Pharmacol Exp Ther.* December 1991;259(3):988–996.
16 Elmquist JK, Scammell TE, Saper CB. Mechanisms of CNS response to systemic immune challenge: The febrile response. *Trends Neurosci.* December 1997;20(12):565–570.
17 Plata-Salaman CR. Immunoregulators in the nervous system. *Neurosci Biobehav Rev.* Summer 1991;15(2):185–215.
18 Roth J, Conn CA, Kluger MJ, Zeisberger E. Kinetics of systemic and intrahypothalamic IL-6 and tumor necrosis factor during endotoxin fever in guinea pigs. *Am J Physiol.* September 1993;265(3 Part 2):R653–R658.
19 LeMay LG, Vander AJ, Kluger MJ. Role of interleukin 6 in fever in rats. *Am J Physiol.* March 1990;258(3 Part 2):R798–R803.
20 Elmquist JK, Breder CD, Sherin JE, Scammell TE, Hickey WF, Dewitt D et al. Intravenous lipopolysaccharide induces cyclooxygenase 2-like immunoreactivity in rat brain perivascular microglia and meningeal macrophages. *J Comp Neurol.* May 5 1997;381(2):119–129.
21 Li S, Ballou LR, Morham SG, Blatteis CM. Cyclooxygenase-2 mediates the febrile response of mice to interleukin-1beta. *Brain Res.* August 10, 2001;910(1–2):163–173.

22 Rivest S, Lacroix S, Vallieres L, Nadeau S, Zhang J, Laflamme N. How the blood talks to the brain parenchyma and the paraventricular nucleus of the hypothalamus during systemic inflammatory and infectious stimuli. *Proc Soc Exp Biol Med.* January 2000;223(1):22–38.

◆ 23 Blatteis CM, Sehic E. Fever: How may Circulating cyrogens signal the brain? *Physiology.* 1997;12(1):1–9.

24 Li S, Sehic E, Wang Y, Ungar AL, Blatteis CM. Relation between complement and the febrile response of guinea pigs to systemic endotoxin. *Am J Physiol.* December 1999;277(6 Part 2):R1635–R1645.

25 Vizi ES. Receptor-mediated local fine-tuning by noradrenergic innervation of neuroendocrine and immune systems. *Ann N Y Acad Sci.* June 30, 1998;851:388–396.

26 Pizzo PA, Robichaud KJ, Wesley R, Commers JR. Fever in the pediatric and young adult patient with cancer. A prospective study of 1001 episodes. *Medicine (Baltimore).* May 1982;61(3):153–165.

27 Fabiszewski KJ, Volicer B, Volicer L. Effect of antibiotic treatment on outcome of fevers in institutionalized Alzheimer patients. *JAMA.* June 20, 1990;263(23):3168–3172.

28 Volicer L, Seltzer B, Rheaume Y, Karner J, Glennon M, Riley ME et al. Eating difficulties in patients with probable dementia of the Alzheimer type. *J Geriatr Psychiatry Neurol.* October–December 1989;2(4):188–195.

29 Parulkar BG, Barrett DM, Volicer L, Seltzer B, Rheaume Y, Karner J et al. Urinary incontinence in adults. *Surg Clin North Am.* 1988;68(5):945–963.

30 Lipsky BA. Urinary tract infections in men. Epidemiology, pathophysiology, diagnosis, and treatment. *Ann Intern Med.* January 15, 1989;110(2):138–150.

31 Vanderschueren S, Knockaert D, Adriaenssens T, Demey W, Durnez A, Blockmans D et al. From prolonged febrile illness to fever of unknown origin: The challenge continues. *Arch Intern Med.* May 12, 2003;163(9):1033–1041.

32 Chang JC. How to differentiate neoplastic fever from infectious fever in patients with cancer: Usefulness of the naproxen test. *Heart Lung.* March 1987;16(2):122–127.

33 Young L. Fever and septicemia. In: Rubin R, Young L, eds. *Clinical Approach to Infection in the Compromised Host.* 2nd edn. New York: Plenum Medical Book Co.;1995. pp. 75–114.

34 Dinarello CA, Wolff SM. Molecular basis of fever in humans. *Am J Med.* May 1982;72(5):799–819.

35 Kasprisin DO, Yogore MG, Salmassi S, Bolf EC. Blood compounds and transfusion reactions. *Plasma Therapy Transfus Technol.* [Journal]. 1981;2(1):25–29.

36 Milner LV, Butcher K. Transfusion reactions reported after transfusions of red blood cells and of whole blood. *Transfusion.* July–August 1978;18(4):493–495.

37 Huh YO, Lichtiger B. Transfusion reactions in patients with cancer. *Am J Clin Pathol.* February 1987;87(2):253–257.

38 Climent-Peris C, Velez-Rosario R. Immediate transfusion reactions. *P R Health Sci J.* September 2001;20(3):229–235.

39 Decary F, Ferner P, Giavedoni L, Hartman A, Howie R, Kalovsky E et al. An investigation of nonhemolytic transfusion reactions. *Vox Sang.* 1984;46(5):277–285.

40 Goldfinger D, Lowe C. Prevention of adverse reactions to blood transfusion by the administration of saline-washed red blood cells. *Transfusion.* May–June 1981;21(3):277–280.

41 Schned AR, Silver H. The use of microaggregate filtration in the prevention of febrile transfusion reactions. *Transfusion.* November–December 1981;21(6):675–681.

42 Wenz B. Microaggregate blood filtration and the febrile transfusion reaction. A comparative study. *Transfusion.* March–April 1983;23(2):95–98.

43 Hogman CF. Adverse effects: Bacterial contamination(including shelf life). A brief review of bacterial contamination of blood components. *Vox Sang.* 1996;70(S3):78–82.

44 Morel P, Deschaseaux M, Bertrand X, Naegelen C, Talon D. Transfusion-transmitted bacterial infection: Residual risk and perspectives of prevention. *Transfus Clin Biol.* June 2003;10(3):192–200.

45 Blajchman MA, Goldman M. Bacterial contamination of platelet concentrates: Incidence, significance, and prevention. *Semin Hematol.* October 2001;38(4 Suppl 11):20–26.

46 Andreu G, Morel P, Forestier F, Debeir J, Rebibo D, Janvier G et al. Hemovigilance network in France: Organization and analysis of immediate transfusion incident reports from 1994 to 1998. *Transfusion.* October 2002;42(10):1356–1364.

47 Stainsby D, Jones H, Asher D, Atterbury C, Boncinelli A, Brant L et al. Serious hazards of transfusion: A decade of hemovigilance in the UK. *Transfus Med Rev.* October 2006;20(4):273–282.

48 Ness P, Braine H, King K, Barrasso C, Kickler T, Fuller A et al. Single-donor platelets reduce the risk of septic platelet transfusion reactions. *Transfusion.* July 2001;41(7):857–861.

49 Blajchman MA, Ali AM. Bacteria in the blood supply: An overlooked issue in transfusion medicine. From: Nance ST ed. *Blood Safety: Current Challenges.* Bethesda, Maryland: American Association of Blood Banks; 1992. p. xvi, 232 p.

50 Yomtovian R, Lazarus HM, Goodnough LT, Hirschler NV, Morrissey AM, Jacobs MR. A prospective microbiologic surveillance program to detect and prevent the transfusion of bacterially contaminated platelets. *Transfusion.* November–December 1993;33(11):902–909.

51 Soeterboek AM, Welle FH, Marcelis JH, van der Loop CM. Sterility testing of blood products in 1994/1995 by three cooperating blood banks in The Netherlands. *Vox Sang.* 1997;72(1):61–62.

52 Leiby DA, Kerr KL, Campos JM, Dodd RY. A retrospective analysis of microbial contaminants in outdated random-donor platelets from multiple sites. *Transfusion.* March 1997;37(3):259–263.

53 Mackowiak PA, LeMaistre CF. Drug fever: A critical appraisal of conventional concepts. An analysis of 51 episodes in two Dallas hospitals and 97 episodes reported in the English literature. *Ann Intern Med.* May 1987;106(5):728–733.

54 Clements JS, Jr., Peacock JE, Jr. Amphotericin B revisited: Reassessment of toxicity. *Am J Med.* May 1990;88(5N):22N–27N.

55 Quesada JR, Talpaz M, Rios A, Kurzrock R, Gutterman JU. Clinical toxicity of interferons in cancer patients: A review. *J Clin Oncol.* February 1986;4(2):234–243.

56 Ashford RF, McLachlan A, Nelson I, Mughal T, Pickering D. Pyrexia after cisplatin. *Lancet.* September 27, 1980;2(8196):691–692.

57 Shah KA, Greenwald E, Levin J, Rosen N, Zumoff B. Streptozocin-induced eosinophilia and fever: A case report. *Cancer Treat Rep.* June 1982;66(6):1449–1451.

58 Boye J, Elter T, Engert A. An overview of the current clinical use of the anti-CD20 monoclonal antibody rituximab. *Ann Oncol.* April 2003;14(4):520–535.

59 Ishii E, Hara T, Mizuno Y, Ueda K. Vincristine-induced fever in children with leukemia and lymphoma. *Cancer.* February 15, 1988;61(4):660–662.

60 Perry PJ, Wilborn CA. Serotonin syndrome vs neuroleptic malignant syndrome: A contrast of causes, diagnoses, and management. *Ann Clin Psychiatry.* May 2012;24(2):155–162.

61 Styrt B, Sugarman B. Antipyresis and fever. *Arch Intern Med.* August 1990;150(8):1589–1597.

62 Horvath SM, Spurr GB, Hutt BK, Hamilton LH. Metabolic cost of shivering. *J Appl Physiol.* May 1956;8(6):595–602.

◆ 63 Kluger MJ. Is fever beneficial? *Yale J Biol Med.* March–April 1986;59(2):89–95.

64   Mackowiak PA. Fever: Blessing or curse? A unifying hypothesis. *Ann Intern Med.* June 15, 1994;120(12):1037–1040.

65   Alsirafy SA, El Mesidy SM, Abou-Elela EN, Elfaramawy YI. Naproxen test for neoplastic fever may reduce suffering. *J Palliat Med.* May 2011;14(5):665–667.

66   Strickland M, Stovsky E. Fever near the end of life #256. *J Palliat Med.* August 2012;15(8):947–948.

67   Hurley AC, Volicer BJ, Volicer L. Effect of fever-management strategy on the progression of dementia of the Alzheimer type. *Alzheimer Dis Assoc Disord.* Spring 1996;10(1):5–10.

68   Ahronheim JC, Morrison RS, Baskin SA, Morris J, Meier DE. Treatment of the dying in the acute care hospital. Advanced dementia and metastatic cancer. *Arch Intern Med.* October 14, 1996;156(18):2094–2100.

69   Hurley AC, Mahoney M, Volicer L. Comfort care in end-stage dementia: What to do after deciding to do no more?. In: Olson E, Chichin ER, Libow LS, eds. *Springer Series on Ethics, Law, and Aging-Controversies in Ethics in Long-Term Care.* New York: Springer Pub. Co.; 1995. p. xxvii, 155 p.

70   Creechan T, Vollman K, Kravutske ME. Cooling by convection vs cooling by conduction for treatment of fever in critically ill adults. *Am J Crit Care.* January 2001;10(1):52–59.

71   Isaacs SN, Axelrod PI, Lorber B. Antipyretic orders in a university hospital. *Am J Med.* January 1990;88(1):31–35.

72   Rosman N. Febrile convulsions. In: Mackowiak PA, ed. *Fever: Basic Mechanisms and Management.* 2nd edn. Philadelphia, PA: Lippincott-Raven Publishers; 1997. p. xvii, 506 p.

73   Schnaiderman D, Lahat E, Sheefer T, Aladjem M. Antipyretic effectiveness of acetaminophen in febrile seizures: Ongoing prophylaxis versus sporadic usage. *Eur J Pediatr.* September 1993;152(9):747–749.

74   Steele RW, Tanaka PT, Lara RP, Bass JW. Evaluation of sponging and of oral antipyretic therapy to reduce fever. *J Pediatr.* November 1970;77(5):824–829.

75   Forsyth BW, Horwitz RI, Acampora D, Shapiro ED, Viscoli CM, Feinstein AR et al. New epidemiologic evidence confirming that bias does not explain the aspirin/Reye's syndrome association. *JAMA.* May 5, 1989;261(17):2517–2524.

◆ 76   Pizzo PA. Management of fever in patients with cancer and treatment-induced neutropenia. *N Engl J Med.* May 6, 1993;328(18):1323–1332.

77   Pizzo PA. Evaluation of fever in the patient with cancer. *Eur J Cancer Clin Oncol.* 1989;25(Suppl 2):S9–S16.

78   Hughes WT, Armstrong D, Bodey GP, Bow EJ, Brown AE, Calandra T et al. 2002 guidelines for the use of antimicrobial agents in neutropenic patients with cancer. *Clin Infect Dis.* March 15, 2002;34(6):730–751.

79   Walsh TJ, Teppler H, Donowitz GR, Maertens JA, Baden LR, Dmoszynska A et al. Caspofungin versus liposomal amphotericin B for empirical antifungal therapy in patients with persistent fever and neutropenia. *N Engl J Med.* September 30, 2004;351(14):1391–1402.

80   Tsavaris N, Zinelis A, Karabelis A, Beldecos D, Bacojanis C, Milonacis N et al. A randomized trial of the effect of three non-steroid anti-inflammatory agents in ameliorating cancer-induced fever. *J Intern Med.* November 1990;228(5):451–455.

81   Chang JC, Gross HM. Utility of naproxen in the differential diagnosis of fever of undetermined origin in patients with cancer. *Am J Med.* April 1984;76(4):597–603.

82   Chang JC. NSAID test to distinguish between infectious and neoplastic fever in cancer patients. *Postgrad Med.* December 1988;84(8):71–72.

83   Vanderschueren S, Knockaert DC, Peetermans WE, Bobbaers HJ. Lack of value of the naproxen test in the differential diagnosis of prolonged febrile illnesses. *Am J Med.* November 2003;115(7):572–575.

84   Sampaio EP, Sarno EN, Galilly R, Cohn ZA, Kaplan G. Thalidomide selectively inhibits tumor necrosis factor alpha production by stimulated human monocytes. *J Exp Med.* March 1, 1991;173(3):699–703.

85   Sampaio EP, Kaplan G, Miranda A, Nery JA, Miguel CP, Viana SM et al. The influence of thalidomide on the clinical and immunologic manifestation of erythema nodosum leprosum. *J Infect Dis.* August 1993;168(2):408–414.

86   Peuckmann V, Fisch M, Bruera E. Potential novel uses of thalidomide: Focus on palliative care. *Drugs.* August 2000;60(2):273–292.

87   Calder K, Bruera E. Thalidomide for night sweats in patients with advanced cancer. *Palliat Med.* January 2000;14(1):77–78.

88   Iyer CG, Languillon J, Ramanujam K, Tarabini-Castellani G, De las Aguas JT, Bechelli LM et al. WHO co-ordinated short-term double-blind trial with thalidomide in the treatment of acute lepra reactions in male lepromatous patients. *Bull World Health Organ.* 1971;45(6):719–732.

89   King KE, Shirey RS, Thoman SK, Bensen-Kennedy D, Tanz WS, Ness PM. Universal leukoreduction decreases the incidence of febrile nonhemolytic transfusion reactions to RBCs. *Transfusion.* January 2004;44(1):25–29.

90   Pruss A, Kalus U, Radtke H, Koscielny J, Baumann-Baretti B, Balzer D et al. Universal leukodepletion of blood components results in a significant reduction of febrile non-hemolytic but not allergic transfusion reactions. *Transfus Apher Sci.* February 2004;30(1):41–46.

91   Heddle NM, Klama LN, Griffith L, Roberts R, Shukla G, Kelton JG. A prospective study to identify the risk factors associated with acute reactions to platelet and red cell transfusions. *Transfusion.* October 1993;33(10):794–797.

92   Dzik S. Prestorage leukocyte reduction of cellular blood components. *Transfus Sci.* June 1994;15(2):131–139.

93   Heddle NM. Febrile nonhemolytic transfusion reactions to platelets. *Curr Opin Hematol.* November 1995;2(6):478–483.

94   FDA. Procrit Label; Epogen label. FDA; 2007; Warning label. Available from: http://www.accessdata.fda.gov/drugsatfda_docs/label/2007/103234s5122lbl.pdf.

95   Steinbrook R. Erythropoietin, the FDA, and oncology. *N Engl J Med.* June 14, 2007;356(24):2448–2451.

96   Martinsson U, Lundstrom S. The use of blood transfusions and erythropoietin-stimulating agents in Swedish palliative care. *Support Care Cancer.* February 2009;17(2):199–203.

97   Oster HS, Neumann D, Hoffman M, Mittelman M. Erythropoietin: The swinging pendulum. *Leuk Res.* August 2012;36(8):939–944.

98   Walsh TJ, Finberg RW, Arndt C, Hiemenz J, Schwartz C, Bodensteiner D et al. Liposomal amphotericin B for empirical therapy in patients with persistent fever and neutropenia. National Institute of Allergy and Infectious Diseases Mycoses Study Group. *N Engl J Med.* March 11, 1999;340(10):764–771.

99   Dinarello CA, Cannon JG, Wolff SM. New concepts on the pathogenesis of fever. *Rev Infect Dis.* January–February 1988;10(1):168–189.

100 Goodman E, Knochel J. Heat stroke and other forms of hyperthermia. In: Mackowiak PA, ed. *Fever: Basic Mechanisms and Management.* New York: Raven Press; 1991. p. xvi, 366 p.

101 Bhanushali MJ, Tuite PJ. The evaluation and management of patients with neuroleptic malignant syndrome. *Neurol Clin.* May 2004;22(2):389–411.

102 Hadad E, Weinbroum AA, Ben-Abraham R. Drug-induced hyperthermia and muscle rigidity: A practical approach. *Eur J Emerg Med.* June 2003;10(2):149–154.

103 Farver DK. Neuroleptic malignant syndrome induced by atypical antipsychotics. *Expert Opin Drug Saf.* January 2003;2(1):21–35.

104 Kogoj A, Velikonja I. Olanzapine induced neuroleptic malignant syndrome—A case review. *Hum Psychopharmacol.* June 2003;18(4):301–309.

105 Nimmagadda SR, Ryan DH, Atkin SL. Neuroleptic malignant syndrome after venlafaxine. *Lancet.* January 22, 2000;355(9200):289–290.

106 Chan-Tack KM. Neuroleptic malignant syndrome due to promethazine. *South Med J.* October 1999;92(10):1017–1018.

107 Mihara K, Kondo T, Suzuki A, Yasui-Furukori N, Ono S, Sano A et al. Relationship between functional dopamine D2 and D3 receptors gene polymorphisms and neuroleptic malignant syndrome. *Am J Med Genet B Neuropsychiatr Genet.* February 2003;117B(1):57–60.

108 Lichter I, Hunt E. The last 48 hours of life. *J Palliat Care.* Winter 1990;6(4):7–15.

109 Quigley CS, Baines M. Descriptive epidemiology of sweating in a hospice population. *J Palliat Care.* Spring 1997;13(1):22–26.

110 Ventafridda V, De Conno F, Ripamonti C, Gamba A, Tamburini M. Quality-of-life assessment during a palliative care programme. *Ann Oncol.* November 1990;1(6):415–420.

111 Hanks GWC. *Oxford Textbook of Palliative Medicine.* 4th edn. Oxford, New York: Oxford University Press, 2010.

112 Kronenberg F. Hot flashes: Phenomenology, quality of life, and search for treatment options. *Exp Gerontol.* May–August 1994;29(3–4):319–336.

113 Erlik Y, Meldrum DR, Judd HL. Estrogen levels in postmenopausal women with hot flashes. *Obstet Gynecol.* April 1982;59(4):403–407.

114 Chiechi LM, Ferreri R, Granieri M, Bianco G, Berardesca C, Loizzi P. Climacteric syndrome and body-weight. *Clin Exp Obstet Gynecol.* 1997;24(3):163–166.

115 Gold EB, Sternfeld B, Kelsey JL, Brown C, Mouton C, Reame N et al. Relation of demographic and lifestyle factors to symptoms in a multi-racial/ethnic population of women 40–55 years of age. *Am J Epidemiol.* September 1, 2000;152(5):463–473.

116 Fuh JL, Wang SJ, Lu SR, Juang KD, Chiu LM. The Kinmen women-health investigation (KIWI): A menopausal study of a population aged 40–54. *Maturitas.* August 25, 2001;39(2):117–124.

117 Kronenberg F. Hot flashes: Epidemiology and physiology. *Ann N Y Acad Sci.* 1990;592:52–86; discussion 123–133.

118 Hoskin PJ, Ashley S, Yarnold JR. Weight gain after primary surgery for breast cancer—Effect of tamoxifen. *Breast Cancer Res Treat.* 1992;22(2):129–132.

◆119 Loprinzi CL, Zahasky KM, Sloan JA, Novotny PJ, Quella SK. Tamoxifen-induced hot flashes. *Clin Breast Cancer.* April 2000;1(1):52–56.

120 Buchholz NP, Mattarelli G, Buchholz MM. Post-orchiectomy hot flushes. *Eur Urol.* 1994;26(2):120–122.

121 Schow DA, Renfer LG, Rozanski TA, Thompson IM. Prevalence of hot flushes during and after neoadjuvant hormonal therapy for localized prostate cancer. *South Med J.* September 1998;91(9):855–857.

122 Freedman RR, Krell W. Reduced thermoregulatory null zone in postmenopausal women with hot flashes. *Am J Obstet Gynecol.* July 1999;181(1):66–70.

123 Rosenberg J, Larsen SH. Hypothesis: Pathogenesis of postmenopausal hot flush. *Med Hypotheses.* August 1991;35(4):349–350.

124 Freedman RR, Norton D, Woodward S, Cornelissen G. Core body temperature and circadian rhythm of hot flashes in menopausal women. *J Clin Endocrinol Metab.* August 1995;80(8):2354–2358.

125 Berendsen HH. The role of serotonin in hot flushes. *Maturitas.* October 31, 2000;36(3):155–164.

126 Carpenter JS. The Hot Flash Related Daily Interference Scale: A tool for assessing the impact of hot flashes on quality of life following breast cancer. *J Pain Symptom Manage.* December 2001;22(6):979–989.

127 Notelovitz M, Lenihan JP, McDermott M, Kerber IJ, Nanavati N, Arce J. Initial 17beta-estradiol dose for treating vasomotor symptoms. *Obstet Gynecol.* May 2000;95(5):726–731.

128 Miller JI, Ahmann FR. Treatment of castration-induced menopausal symptoms with low dose diethylstilbestrol in men with advanced prostate cancer. *Urology.* December 1992;40(6):499–502.

129 Smith JA, Jr. A prospective comparison of treatments for symptomatic hot flushes following endocrine therapy for carcinoma of the prostate. *J Urol.* July 1994;152(1):132–134.

130 Gerber GS, Zagaja GP, Ray PS, Rukstalis DB. Transdermal estrogen in the treatment of hot flushes in men with prostate cancer. *Urology.* January 2000;55(1):97–101.

●131 Rossouw JE, Anderson GL, Prentice RL, LaCroix AZ, Kooperberg C, Stefanick ML et al. Risks and benefits of estrogen plus progestin in healthy postmenopausal women: Principal results From the Women's Health Initiative randomized controlled trial. *JAMA.* July 17, 2002;288(3):321–333.

132 Li CI, Malone KE, Porter PL, Weiss NS, Tang MT, Cushing-Haugen KL et al. Relationship between long durations and different regimens of hormone therapy and risk of breast cancer. *JAMA.* June 25, 2003;289(24):3254–3263.

133 Loprinzi CL, Michalak JC, Quella SK, O'Fallon JR, Hatfield AK, Nelimark RA et al. Megestrol acetate for the prevention of hot flashes. *N Engl J Med.* August 11, 1994;331(6):347–352.

134 Leonetti HB, Longo S, Anasti JN. Transdermal progesterone cream for vasomotor symptoms and postmenopausal bone loss. *Obstet Gynecol.* August 1999;94(2):225–228.

135 Lobo RA, McCormick W, Singer F, Roy S. Depo-medroxyprogesterone acetate compared with conjugated estrogens for the treatment of postmenopausal women. *Obstet Gynecol.* January 1984;63(1):1–5.

136 Dawson NA, McLeod DG. Dramatic prostate specific antigen decrease in response to discontinuation of megestrol acetate in advanced prostate cancer: Expansion of the antiandrogen withdrawal syndrome. *J Urol.* June 1995;153(6):1946–1947.

137 Wehbe TW, Stein BS, Akerley WL. Prostate-specific antigen response to withdrawal of megestrol acetate in a patient with hormone-refractory prostate cancer. *Mayo Clin Proc.* October 1997;72(10):932–934.

138 Burch PA, Loprinzi CL. Prostate-specific antigen decline after withdrawal of low-dose megestrol acetate. *J Clin Oncol.* March 1999;17(3):1087–1088.

139 Hofseth LJ, Raafat AM, Osuch JR, Pathak DR, Slomski CA, Haslam SZ. Hormone replacement therapy with estrogen or estrogen plus medroxyprogesterone acetate is associated with increased epithelial proliferation in the normal postmenopausal breast. *J Clin Endocrinol Metab.* December 1999;84(12):4559–4565.

140 Isaksson E, Sahlin L, Soderqvist G, von Schoultz E, Masironi B, Wickman M et al. Expression of sex steroid receptors and IGF-1 mRNA in breast tissue—Effects of hormonal treatment. *J Steroid Biochem Mol Biol.* September–October 1999;70(4–6):257–262.

141 Dixon AR, Jackson L, Chan S, Haybittle J, Blamey RW. A randomised trial of second-line hormone vs single agent chemotherapy in tamoxifen resistant advanced breast cancer. *Br J Cancer.* August 1992;66(2):402–404.

142 Egarter C, Huber J, Leikermoser R, Haidbauer R, Pusch H, Fischl F et al. Tibolone versus conjugated estrogens and sequential progestogen in the treatment of climacteric complaints. *Maturitas.* February 1996;23(1):55–62.

143 Ginsburg J, Prelevic G, Butler D, Okolo S. Clinical experience with tibolone (Livial) over 8 years. *Maturitas.* January 1995;21(1):71–76.

144 Kroiss R, Fentiman IS, Helmond FA, Rymer J, Foidart JM, Bundred N et al. The effect of tibolone in postmenopausal women receiving tamoxifen after surgery for breast cancer: A randomised, double-blind, placebo-controlled trial. *BJOG.* February 2005;112(2):228–233.

145 Loprinzi CL, Kugler JW, Sloan JA, Mailliard JA, LaVasseur BI, Barton DL et al. Venlafaxine in management of hot flashes in survivors of breast cancer: A randomised controlled trial. *Lancet.* December 16, 2000;356(9247):2059–2063.

146 Stearns V, Beebe KL, Iyengar M, Dube E. Paroxetine controlled release in the treatment of menopausal hot flashes: A randomized controlled trial. *JAMA.* June 4, 2003;289(21):2827–2834.

147 Loprinzi CL, Sloan JA, Perez EA, Quella SK, Stella PJ, Mailliard JA et al. Phase III evaluation of fluoxetine for treatment of hot flashes. *J Clin Oncol.* March 15, 2002;20(6):1578–1583.

148 Barton DL, Loprinzi CL, Novotny P, Shanafelt T, Sloan J, Wahner-Roedler D et al. Pilot evaluation of citalopram for the relief of hot flashes. *J Support Oncol.* May–June 2003;1(1):47–51.

149 Perez DG, Loprinzi CL, Barton DL, Pockaj BA, Sloan J, Novotny PJ et al. Pilot evaluation of mirtazapine for the treatment of hot flashes. *J Support Oncol.* January–February 2004;2(1):50–56.

150 Stearns V, Johnson MD, Rae JM, Morocho A, Novielli A, Bhargava P et al. Active tamoxifen metabolite plasma concentrations after coadministration of tamoxifen and the selective serotonin reuptake inhibitor paroxetine. *J Natl Cancer Inst.* December 3, 2003;95(23):1758–1764.

151 Guttuso T, Jr., Kurlan R, McDermott MP, Kieburtz K. Gabapentin's effects on hot flashes in postmenopausal women: A randomized controlled trial. *Obstet Gynecol.* February 2003;101(2):337–345.

152 Pandya KJ, Morrow GR, Roscoe JA, Zhao H, Hickok JT, Pajon E et al. Gabapentin for hot flashes in 420 women with breast cancer: A randomised double-blind placebo-controlled trial. *Lancet.* September 3–9, 2005;366(9488):818–824.

153 Loprinzi CL, Dueck AC, Khoyratty BS, Barton DL, Jafar S, Rowland KM, Jr. et al. A phase III randomized, double-blind, placebo-controlled trial of gabapentin in the management of hot flashes in men (N00CB). *Ann Oncol.* March 2009;20(3):542–549.

154 Loprinzi CL, Goldberg RM, O'Fallon JR, Quella SK, Miser AW, Mynderse LA et al. Transdermal clonidine for ameliorating post-orchiectomy hot flashes. *J Urol.* March 1994;151(3):634–636.

155 Pandya KJ, Raubertas RF, Flynn PJ, Hynes HE, Rosenbluth RJ, Kirshner JJ et al. Oral clonidine in postmenopausal patients with breast cancer experiencing tamoxifen-induced hot flashes: A University of Rochester Cancer Center Community Clinical Oncology Program study. *Ann Intern Med.* May 16, 2000;132(10):788–793.

156 Barton DL, Loprinzi CL, Quella SK, Sloan JA, Veeder MH, Egner JR et al. Prospective evaluation of vitamin E for hot flashes in breast cancer survivors. *J Clin Oncol.* February 1998;16(2):495–500.

157 Bergmans MG, Merkus JM, Corbey RS, Schellekens LA, Ubachs JM. Effect of Bellergal Retard on climacteric complaints: A double-blind, placebo-controlled study. *Maturitas.* November 1987;9(3):227–234.

158 Eisenberg DM, Davis RB, Ettner SL, Appel S, Wilkey S, Van Rompay M et al. Trends in alternative medicine use in the United States, 1990–1997: Results of a follow-up national survey. *JAMA.* 11 November, 1998;280(18):1569–1575.

159 Quella SK, Loprinzi CL, Barton DL, Knost JA, Sloan JA, LaVasseur BI et al. Evaluation of soy phytoestrogens for the treatment of hot flashes in breast cancer survivors: A North Central Cancer Treatment Group Trial. *J Clin Oncol.* March 2000;18(5):1068–1074.

160 Van Patten CL, Olivotto IA, Chambers GK, Gelmon KA, Hislop TG, Templeton E et al. Effect of soy phytoestrogens on hot flashes in postmenopausal women with breast cancer: A randomized, controlled clinical trial. *J Clin Oncol.* March 15, 2002;20(6):1449–1455.

161 Taylor M. Botanicals: Medicines and menopause. *Clin Obstet Gynecol.* December 2001;44(4):853–863.

162 Jacobson JS, Troxel AB, Evans J, Klaus L, Vahdat L, Kinne D et al. Randomized trial of black cohosh for the treatment of hot flashes among women with a history of breast cancer. *J Clin Oncol.* May 15, 2001;19(10):2739–2745.

163 Wyon Y, Wijma K, Nedstrand E, Hammar M. A comparison of acupuncture and oral estradiol treatment of vasomotor symptoms in postmenopausal women. *Climacteric.* June 2004;7(2):153–164.

164 Hammar M, Frisk J, Grimas O, Hook M, Spetz AC, Wyon Y. Acupuncture treatment of vasomotor symptoms in men with prostatic carcinoma: A pilot study. *J Urol.* March 1999;161(3):853–856.

165 Irvin JH, Domar AD, Clark C, Zuttermeister PC, Friedman R. The effects of relaxation response training on menopausal symptoms. *J Psychosom Obstet Gynaecol.* December 1996;17(4):202–207.

166 Freedman RR, Woodward S. Behavioral treatment of menopausal hot flushes: Evaluation by ambulatory monitoring. *Am J Obstet Gynecol.* August 1992;167(2):436–439.

167 Morrow PK, Mattair DN, Hortobagyi GN. Hot flashes: A review of pathophysiology and treatment modalities. *Oncologist. [Rev].* 2011;16(11):1658–1664.

168 Luoto R, Moilanen J, Heinonen R, Mikkola T, Raitanen J, Tomas E et al. Effect of aerobic training on hot flushes and quality of life—A randomized controlled trial. *Ann Med.* [Randomized Controlled Trial Research Support, Non-U.S. Gov't]. September 2012;44(6):616–626.

76

Pruritus

KATIE TAYLOR, ANDREW THORNS

INTRODUCTION

Pruritus is defined as "an unpleasant sensation that provokes the desire to scratch." It has a prevalence of 27% in common tumor sites,[1] and in cholestasis, up to 80% of patients may complain of itch.[2] Severe cases cause distress and can be difficult to treat. This chapter will summarize the pathogenesis, causes, and effects of pruritus and will discuss possible treatment options.

PATHOGENESIS OF PRURITUS

The pathogenesis of itch is complex and has not been fully elucidated. Both central and peripheral mechanisms are involved, and a number of mediators are being studied to generate future treatment options. Twycross has suggested a clinical classification based on the understandings of the origins of itch•[3] (Box 76.1).

NEURAL PATHWAYS

The neurons responsible for the sensation of itch are a subset of the large population of polymodal C-nociceptors. They are situated close to the dermal–epidermal junction and comprise about 20% of the C-fiber population in the skin.

The sensation of itch is closely linked to that of pain, and for many years, it was thought that both were transmitted identically. Both are unpleasant sensory experiences; however, pain sensation results in a reflex withdrawal, whereas itch results in a scratch reflex. C fibers that are associated with itch are anatomically identical to those that mediate pain, but there are some important functional differences. The itch C fibers are insensitive to mechanical stimuli and are more sensitive to histamine than those responsible for the sensation of pain.[4] Conduction is 50% slower than for those fibers transmitting pain, and the receptor field is three times larger and more superficial than that associated with pain.[5]

The neural impulse passes via the C fibers to the ipsilateral dorsal root ganglia, and from here to the opposite anterolateral spinothalamic tract, onto the posterolateral ventral thalamic nucleus and through the internal capsule to the somatosensory cortex of the postcentral gyrus. There is a substantial coactivation of the motor areas of the brain, which supports the clinical observation that itch is linked to scratching. There does not appear to be a distinct "itch center."[6]

The sensation of itch can originate at several points on the neural pathway. Activation of the C fibers in the skin/mucous membranes will trigger itch. This type of pruritus is mediated by histamine and therefore generally responsive to treatment with H_1 antihistamines. In the chronic setting, this response diminishes, presumably secondary to desensitization at a central level. Itch can originate at any point along the afferent pathway. This may occur with neural damage locally (e.g., postherpetic neuralgia) or centrally (e.g., a space-occupying lesion).[7,8] This neuropathic itch is not usually H_1 antihistamine responsive. Pruritus may also result from the accumulation of toxins (endogenous or exogenous) in the spinal cord or brain. This type of pruritus is histamine independent. The sensation of itch can be magnified by psychological factors such as stress or anxiety or reduced by training and distraction. It appears that the central inhibitory circuits can be altered, thereby affecting the threshold for detecting pruritogenic stimuli.

Central and peripheral mediators

There are many substances known to be involved in the mediation of itch. Histamine is perhaps the best known of these. It is released from mast cells in response to pruritogenic stimuli and acts on the H_1 receptors of the C fibers in the skin, causing the characteristic wheal and flare reaction specific to histamine-mediated pruritus. Prostaglandins E_2 and H_2 potentiate pruritus via other mediators including histamine,[9] and, in the case of prostaglandin E_2, also directly.[10] Substance P is synthesized in the cell bodies of C fibers and can directly induce itch as well as modulate the sensation. The release of substance P can be stimulated by

Box 76.1 Classification of pruritus based on origin

- Pruritoceptive itch—originating from the skin and transmitted by C fibers, e.g., scabies, urticaria
- Neuropathic itch—originating from disease located along the afferent pathway, e.g., herpes zoster, multiple sclerosis, and brain tumors
- Neurogenic itch—originating centrally without any evidence of neural pathology, e.g., itch caused by cholestasis, which is due to the action of opioid neuropeptides on m-opioid receptors
- Psychogenic itch—as in the delusional state of parasitophobia

tryptase from activated mast cells and neutrophils, and this may increase itch. Other neuropeptides, vasoactive intestinal polypeptide (VIP), and calcitonin gene–related protein (CGRP) are found in the free nerve endings and have been implicated in the mediation of itch. An intradermal injection of acetylcholine causes itch in atopic subjects, but pain in nonatopic subjects,[11] which may explain why some atopic subjects experience itch when sweating.

Opioids are thought to mediate itch at several points in the pathway. Peripherally, opioids cause mast cell degranulation and histamine release, but it is at a spinal level that the role of opioids appears most interesting. They modulate secondary transmission of the itch sensation by stimulating inhibitory signals to afferent neurons. Centrally, opioids have been shown to trigger itch in the laboratory setting by direct action on the floor of the fourth ventricle.

Serotonin induces itch by two mechanisms: indirectly by release of histamine from dermal mast cells, and centrally via a mechanism, which may involve opioid neurotransmitters. Both opioid and serotonin receptors appear to alter the central inhibitory circuits and so adjust the itch threshold.

More detailed reviews on the basic mechanisms of itch are available.[•12]

SCRATCH

Scratch is the natural response to itch. In evolutionary terms, it is likely to have originated when most pruritogens were parasites or insects and served to remove the superficial layers of skin which harbor these.[•13] Itch is linked to the motor response of scratching via a spinal reflex and can be inhibited by cortical centers. Scratching stimulates A fibers adjacent to those conducting itch and the A fibers in turn synapse with inhibitory interneurons, subsequently causing inhibition of C fibers and a reduced sensation of itch. Scratching provides relief for several minutes; it has been postulated that this occurs due to temporary disruption of the circuits in the relay synapses of the spinal cord which otherwise reinforce the itch sensation.

COMPLICATIONS OF PRURITUS

The commonest complication is excoriation that can result in secondary infection. The effects of lack of sleep, social unacceptability, and interference with daily functioning should not be overlooked. One study found depressive symptoms in one-third of patients with generalized pruritus.[14] The power of suggestion can result in itch and learned behavior can quickly develop. The resultant itch–scratch cycle can be hard to break.

ASSESSMENT OF THE PRURITIC PATIENT

Routine assessment involves careful history and examination, particularly noting whether the itch is generalized or localized, and with careful attention to drug history, exacerbating factors, and previous medical history. Examination should involve detailed description of the site and nature of any skin lesions and ideally photographic records. General first-line investigations may include full blood picture, erythrocyte sedimentation rate (ESR), and renal and liver profiles if clinically indicated. Biopsy of any suspicious lesions should be discussed with a dermatologist or dermo-oncologist prior to proceeding.

MEASURING ITCH

The subjective nature of this symptom makes it notoriously difficult to quantify. Two validated questionnaires have been developed, which attempt to assess the qualitative, temporal, and spatial characteristics of itch, based on the long and short forms of the McGill Pain Questionnaire.[6] Monitoring systems have been developed, which provide quantitative data independent of hand/arm movement, and these provide the most reliable assessment method to date.[15]

CAUSES OF PRURITUS IN ADVANCED DISEASE

Table 76.1 summarizes the causes of pruritus that may be relevant in patients with advanced disease. These can be divided into general causes of pruritus and those specifically related to disease. In either case, pruritus may be localized or generalized.

Senile itch is experienced by 50%–70% of those over the age of 70 years. The majority have xerosis and skin atrophy, in others, the cause is unknown. It is best treated with general measures (see the following text) and the application of emollient cream. Pruritus can be iatrogenic, and the following drugs are common culprits: opioids, aspirin, etretinate, amfetamines, and drugs that can cause cholestasis such as erythromycin, hormonal treatment, and phenothiazines.

Iron deficiency with or without anemia can cause pruritus[16] and responds to iron replacement. Pruritus occurs in up to 11%

Table 76.1 *Causes of pruritus*

Localized	Generalized
Dry skin (xerosis)	Primary skin diseases
Infestation, e.g., scabies	Metabolic disorders: Hypothyroidism
Insect bites	and hyperthyroidism, carcinoid
	syndrome: diabetes mellitus and
	insipidus
Candida	Renal disorders: Renal failure with
	uremia
Eczema	Liver disorders: Cholestasis
Contact dermatitis	Infection: HIV, syphilis
Bullous pemphigoid	Hematological disorders: Polycythemia
	vera, iron deficiency anemia
Dermatitis herpetiformis	Neurological disorders:
Urticaria	cerebrovascular accident multiple
	sclerosis, brain abscess/tumors
	Drug-induced (see text)
	Senile pruritus
	Aquagenic
	Psychogenic
Cancer-specific pruritus	
Melanomatosis	Chronic lymphocytic leukemia
Mycosis fungoides	Hodgkin and non-Hodgkin lymphoma
Carcinoma in situ: Vulval, anal	Mycosis fungoides
Paraneoplastic syndrome:	Cutaneous T cell lymphoma
prostatic, rectal/	
Colonic, cervical carcinomas;	Multiple myeloma
glioblastoma	
Metastatic infiltration of skin	Paraneoplastic syndrome: Breast,
	colonic, lung, stomach carcinomas
	and others

of patients with thyrotoxicosis, particularly long-term untreated Grave's disease, and less commonly in hypothyroidism.

Other common causes of pruritus are discussed in the management section.

MANAGEMENT OF PRURITUS

Removal of causative agents (e.g., drugs) and appropriate investigation and treatment of underlying disease are essential first-line measures in the treatment of pruritus. Management can be divided into general and pharmaceutical measures suitable for all causes, and pharmacological measures that are more cause specific. With any intervention for pruritus, a strong placebo response is common.

Evidence for the use of different systemic agents in the treatment of pruritus is limited. In the context of advanced disease, there are few useful trials and the use of many agents remains historical or originates from case reports. This is not to say these agents are not helpful, just that the evidence either confirming or refuting their use is, thus far, unavailable.

General management techniques

These measures are widely accepted as essential although the evidence for their efficacy is largely anecdotal. Exacerbating factors such as heat, dehydration, anxiety, and boredom should be avoided. Particular attention should be paid to measures that keep the skin well hydrated and avoid sweating. Patients should wear light clothes, use fans to maintain a passage of air, take tepid baths or shower avoiding hot water, and use emulsifying ointment or aqueous cream instead of soap. Skin hydration should be maintained with regular use of emollients. Alcohol and spicy foods may worsen itch.

Patients should be advised to gently rub the skin rather than scratching it, and to keep nails short and wear cotton gloves at night to limit the damage to the skin. Sweating may exacerbate itch; the general measures described earlier may help reduce sweating; otherwise, an antimuscarinic agent may be required.

Exposure to ultraviolet (UV) B light may help in cholestatic-, uremic-, and acquired immune deficiency syndrome (AIDS)-related pruritus. Although the nontoxic nature of this treatment makes it an attractive alternative, it may not be a suitable treatment for a very sick patient. The antipruritic effect is thought to be due to a reduction in the vitamin A content of the skin, inhibition of the release of histamine, and inhibition of dermal mast cell proliferation.[17,18]

Sedatives such as benzodiazepines do not relieve itch but may help improve associated anxiety and insomnia.**[19] Behavioral treatments and hypnotherapy may help ease associated psychological issues and break the cycle of itching and scratching.[20] Transcutaneous electronic nerve stimulation (TENS) and acupuncture have been successful in case reports.[21,22]

Topical agents

Topical agents generally provide some relief but may be inconvenient to apply in generalized pruritus, and are probably best reserved for localized symptoms. A number of topical agents have been suggested such as: zinc oxide, calamine, glycerin, and salicylates, but their mechanisms are not understood and their effectiveness is unproved. One double-blind, controlled trial of crotamiton (Eurax®) showed it to be ineffective.**[23] Polidocanol bath oil has been shown to reduce itch in uremia,[24] and 3% polidocanol/5% urea cream has been shown to reduce itch in psoriasis.[25]

Corticosteroid creams may help localized areas of inflamed skin but are not generally indicated for chronic use.[26] Local anesthetic creams can be helpful but may cause skin sensitization. Lidocaine is the least likely to have this effect, but systemic absorption prevents its use over large areas or for prolonged periods. Topical counterirritants such as menthol 0.25%–2% or camphor 1%–3% may be useful.

Capsaicin 0.025% acts by depleting substance P in C fibers on repeated application, reducing pain and itch. It needs to be applied four times a day and has shown benefit in uremic pruritus.[27] Application can cause an initial burning sensation that prohibits widespread application and decreases compliance; for these reasons, it is best reserved for localized pruritus.

Strontium nitrate cream is an effective antipruritic, which may act by selectively blocking C-fiber transmission.[28] Tacrolimus 0.03% ointment has shown some effect in localized pruritus in renal impairment,[29*] as has topical gamma linolenic acid.[30*] Doxepin, a tricyclic antidepressant with potent antihistaminic action now produced in a topical form, has been shown to be effective in atopic dermatitis and chronic urticaria. The topical form has been shown to be less effective than the systemic form.[31] Its place in other causes of pruritus has not been established.

Systemic agents

Choice of systemic agents remains based on limited evidence and theories of action. While the number of placebo-controlled trials has increased clarifying some treatment choices, there are little comparative data to indicate one treatment's effectiveness over another.

Antihistamines are active at either the H_1 or H_2 receptor. H_1 receptor antagonists are often used as the first choice for any form of generalized pruritus; however, there is little evidence for their use other than in urticaria or allergy. The more sedative agents such as chlorphenamine are believed to be more effective either because of a more potent central action or because the sedation itself helps to improve the insomnia caused by the itch. H_2 antihistamines such as cimetidine have been shown to be beneficial in the pruritus associated with lymphoproliferative disorders (see the following text). Doxepin, which acts at H_1 and H_2 receptors, is effective in atopic dermatitis, as discussed earlier.

The 5-hydroxytryptamine 3 ($5\text{-}HT_3$) receptor antagonists showed initial promising results in relieving itch from a number of causes.[32,33**] However, as the research evidence has evolved, their effectiveness has been increasingly brought into doubt.[34,35,36,37]

The serotonin selective reuptake inhibitor (SSRI) paroxetine is helpful in paraneoplastic pruritus, but the effect may only be temporary, lasting about 6 weeks,[38] and may also be associated with initial nausea and vomiting. Paroxetine and fluvoxamine (also an SSRI) have shown a beneficial effect in chronic pruritus of unknown origin.[39*] Another SSRI, sertraline, has some effects in cholestatic pruritus.[40*] Mirtazapine is a norepinephrine and specific serotonin antidepressant, and its actions include blocking H_1, $5\text{-}HT_2$, and $5\text{-}HT_3$ receptors. It has been shown to be a helpful antipruritic agent in cholestasis, uremia, and lymphoma.[41]

Opioid antagonists and kappa-receptor agonists are receiving increasing attention.

Gabapentin appears effective in uremic pruritus though benefit has not been confirmed in cholestatic causes.

Specific management strategies

CANCER-SPECIFIC PRURITUS

Pruritus can be associated with almost any malignancy, complicating the disease in different ways: for example, as a consequence of direct tumor growth, secondary to cholestasis or as a complication of treatment.[42]

Pruritus is commonly associated with hematological malignancies. Pruritus occurs in about 50% of patients with polycythemia rubra vera; in almost 100% of patients with cutaneous T cell lymphoma; and in 30% of patients with Hodgkin disease being more common in the nodular sclerosing subtype with mediastinal mass.[43] Its presence may precede overt disease by up to 5 years.[44]

In pruritus secondary to polycythemia vera, the use of disease-modifying therapy often reduces pruritus and should be considered first[45]; aspirin, paroxetine, and cimetidine have been shown to be helpful.[46**,47,48]

In Hodgkin disease, cimetidine[49] and topical 5% sodium cromoglycate[50] have been reported as helpful. Corticosteroids have been used historically and are felt to be effective, but evidence is lacking. Although cimetidine is an H_2 receptor antagonist, its action is not thought to have a direct antihistaminic effect as it has little effect on itching caused by histamine, but it is thought to be related to its inhibitory action on CYP2D6 liver enzymes that are involved in the synthesis of endogenous opioids and possibly other pruritogens.[51] See Figure 76.1 for a suggested approach to treatment.

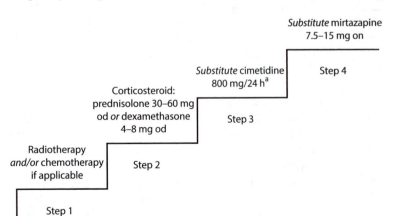

Figure 76.1 *Treatment of pruritus in Hodgkin lymphoma.*
[a]Alternative H_2 receptor antagonists probably equally effective. od, once daily; on, every night. (Redrawn from Twycross, R. and Zylicz, Z., Prog. Palliat. Care, 10, 285, 2002. With permission.)

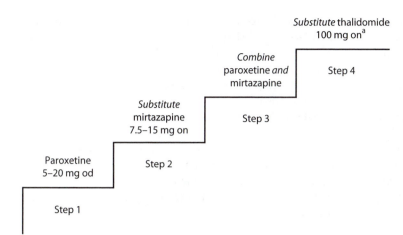

Figure 76.2 *Treatment of paraneoplastic pruritus. ªUndesirable effects include peripheral neuropathy and congenital malformations (shortened or absent limbs). (Redrawn from Twycross, R. and Zylicz, Z., Prog. Palliat. Care, 10, 285, 2002. With permission.)*

Mycosis fungoides often presents in the early stages with pruritic dermatitis that may precede cutaneous lesions by up to 10 years.[52] Tumor-modifying treatments are effective in reducing pruritus, and mycosis fungoides cells are very radiosensitive. Cyclosporin is also effective, but long-term effects of the treatment are currently unevaluated.[53]

Other options suggested in lymphoma are mirtazepine[41] or kappa opioid agonists.[54]

In solid tumors, generalized pruritus may be part of a paraneoplastic syndrome in association with lung, colon, breast, stomach, and prostate primary sites. Localized pruritus can result from gliomas and carcinomas of the cervix, anus and rectum, sigmoid colon, vulva and prostate, which may manifest with pruritus in the related anatomical areas sometimes as the presenting symptom. Itch in Hodgkin disease may appear some years before the tumor is identifiable. However, research has shown that patients with generalized pruritus followed up for 6 years did not have a higher overall incidence of malignancy and that follow-up screening was not warranted.[55]

Paroxetine, an SSRI antidepressant, has been shown to relieve itch in a case series of advanced cancer patients with paraneoplastic itch and in a randomized controlled trial for severe nondermatological pruritus. Its action is probably due to downregulation of $5-HT_3$ receptors, but side effects (nausea, vomiting, and sedation) may limit its use.[38**,56**]

A small study showed that gabapentin was effective and safe in the treatment of IL-2 (interleukin)-induced pruritus for patients undergoing this therapy for metastatic renal cell carcinoma and malignant melanoma.[57*]

A suggested approach to managing paraneoplastic itch is given in Figure 76.2.

OPIOID-INDUCED PRURITUS

Opioids provide good pain control for the majority of patients, and are used frequently in advanced disease. Itch is a well-recognized side effect of opioids although the exact etiology is currently unknown. Pruritus occurs in about 1% of patients on opioids delivered subcutaneously, orally, or intravenously, and up to 90% of patients receiving neuro-axial opioids. Experience suggests that pruritus tends to be generalized in patients on nonspinal opioids, although in children, it is more common in the facial area, particularly the nose. In neuro-axial delivery, the pruritus spreads upward from the level of injection, is commonly maximal in the face, and may be limited to the nose.[58]

Postulated mechanisms include a direct central effect,[59] including serotonin release[60] and a peripheral histamine effect.[61] Although it is suggested that itch is more common with the naturally occurring opioids, the effect is not limited to one class of drug with previous reports of itch with morphine,[62,63] fentanyl,[64] and oxycodone.[65]

Opioid antagonists are useful in reducing pruritus but may reverse the analgesic effect,[66] making them an unhelpful choice of treatment for most patients with advanced disease. There is evidence that using an agonist-antagonist drug such as nalbuphine or pentazocine[67**] can reduce pruritus without compromising analgesic effect.[68] Methylnaltrexone, a selective peripheral opioid receptor antagonist, decreases several side effects of opioids including pruritus[69,70*,71]. Opioid rotation, in particular changing to hydromorphone, may be a more practical solution and may be effective.[63]

Ondansetron has been shown to be useful in opioid-induced itch mainly via the neuro-axial route[72] at traditional antiemetic doses, but this effect has not been supported in later studies.[37]

Mirtazepine and gabapentin used prophylactically before neuro-axial opioids appear to decrease the frequency of itch.[73**,74**]

Antihistamines are only thought to be of benefit in peripherally induced opioid itch.

CHOLESTASIS

Cholestasis may occur in the general population as a result of gallstones, drugs, or intrahepatic disease, as well as obstruction from primary or secondary tumors involving the biliary tree. Pruritus is a common sequela of cholestasis, starting on the palmar and planter surfaces and becoming more generalized. Accumulation of bile salts has long been suspected as an etiological factor, and although it may have a role to play, the evidence for a central mechanism related to increased opioidergic tone and activation of itch centers in the brain is gathering pace.[3] Treatment of cholestatic pruritus with the opioid antagonists naltrexone, naloxone, and nalmefene follows this body of evidence and is successful.[75**,76**,77*,78*] It is interesting to note that opioid withdrawal effects were noted even in opioid-naïve patients with cholestatic pruritus; this may be an effect of high levels of endogenous opioids. Pain may also be a complication of using opioid antagonists for symptom control.[79] These side effects may be avoided by titrating an infusion of naloxone to establish an effective dose before switching to an oral form.[80]

The most effective method of relieving pruritus secondary to cholestasis is to relieve the obstruction. This may be possible by treating the underlying disease with surgery or chemotherapy or high-dose dexamethasone, though the initial treatment of choice is a biliary stent (Figure 76.3), even in the terminally ill.

Cholestyramine binds bile salts in the gut and has traditionally been used for the treatment of cholestatic pruritus, although evidence for benefit is limited to one small, open-label study completed more than 40 years ago.[81*] As a result of this mechanism of action, it is ineffective in complete biliary obstruction. Although often quoted as the first step in management ladders, its use is limited in palliative care, because it is unpalatable and relatively large quantities must be consumed for effect, although helped by mixing with fruit juice. Charcoal has been used along the same therapeutic line, with similar success and similar acceptability problems. Rifampicin has been shown to reduce pruritus in cholestasis.[82**] The mechanism is not clear, but it is thought to interrupt the enterohepatic circulation of bile acids and therefore reduce the impact of bile acids on the metabolic processes of the liver. The presence of severe idiosyncratic side effects in one study requires liver transaminases to be monitored and may limit its use.[83]

Sertraline showed benefit in a small randomized double-blind study[40] Gabapentin showed no benefit in cholestatic pruritus in a double-blind placebo-controlled trial.[84**] Antihistamines are unlikely to be helpful. Treatment with 5-HT$_3$ antagonists was supported by early evidence, but recent robust trials have found little or no benefit.[32**,34**,35**,85**]

The 17-α alkyl androgens have also been used historically with some effect. The action is not fully understood, but the 17-α alkyl androgens are directly toxic to hepatocytes and may limit the capacity of the liver's enkephalin production.[86**] Care should be taken when considering long-term use of 17-α alkyl androgens in patients with years to live as they have the potential to cause masculinization in women and occasional serious liver impairment. Their use in practice has been largely superseded by opioid antagonists and other agents. Other experimental options have been explored including: propofol, S-adenosyl-methionine (SAMe), antioxidants, tetrahydrocannabinol, macrolide antibiotics, plasmapheresis, and albumin dialysis.[87]

CHRONIC RENAL FAILURE

Renal failure may occur as a primary disorder or secondary to a cancer. It is chronic renal failure that is likely to be associated with pruritus. Pruritus may be generalized or limited to the back and the forearm at the site of the arteriovenous shunt.[88] The pathogenesis of pruritus in this setting has not been fully defined but is thought to be multifactorial. The skin of these patients is atrophic and dry,[89] cytokine production in the skin may contribute, and interleukin-1 may cause the release of pruritogens. Mast cells are more numerous in patients with pruritic uremia.[90] Although plasma histamine levels have been shown to be much increased in this group of patients, antihistamines *per se* are ineffectual in improving the pruritus.[91]

Pruritus is reportedly more common in uremic patients receiving dialysis than those who are not, although a recent report of symptoms in patients with stage 5 chronic kidney disease managed without dialysis revealed that more than 80% reported itch in the month before death.[92] High permeability

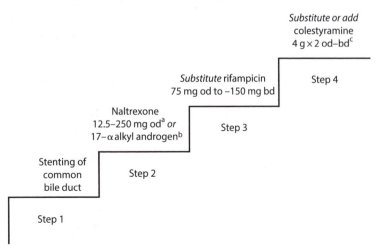

Figure 76.3 *Treatment of cholestatic pruritus. [a]Contraindicated in patients needing opioids for pain relief. [b]e.g. methyltestosterone 25mg sublingual od (not available in UK), danazol 200mg od–tds. [c]Not of benefit in complete large duct biliary obstruction. od, once daily; bd, twice daily; tds, three times daily. (Adapted and redrawn from Twycross, R. and Zylicz, Z., Prog. Palliat. Care, 10, 285, 2002. With permission.)*

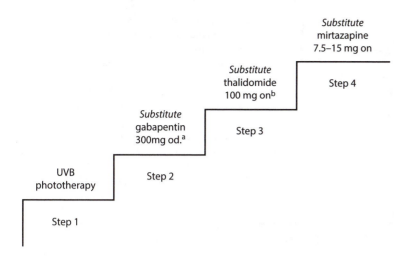

Figure 76.4 *Treatment of uremic pruritus. ªMay be given as 300 mg po post dialysis thrice weekly (From Gunal, A.I. et al., Nephrol. Dial. Transplant., 19(12), 3137, 2004). ᵇUndesirable effects include peripheral neuropathy and congenital malformations (shortened or absent limbs). od, once daily; on, every night. (Adapted and redrawn from Twycross, R. and Zylicz, Z., Prog. Palliat. Care, 10, 285, 2002. With permission.)*

hemodialysis has been shown to be more effective in relieving itch than conventional hemodialysis.[93**]

Pruritus is local in 70% of patients, and for these patients, capsaicin cream can be effective and practical.[26] For generalized pruritus, there appears to be a role for the antiepileptic drugs gabapentin and pregabalin in uremic patients receiving haemodialysis.[94*,95*,96**] The doses studied are similar to those commonly used to treat neuropathic pain.

The efficacy of opioid antagonists is under dispute: opioid antagonists have been found to be effective by some researchers,[97**] and not by others.[33**] A novel kappa-receptor agonist, nalfurafine hydrochloride, improved both itch and sleep disturbance in end-stage renal failure.[98**,99**]

Ondansetron has been used to treat uremic pruritus, but the evidence for success is conflicting.[36**,100]

There is some good evidence of thalidomide having an antipruritic effect in uremia.[101**] Postulated mechanisms for its antipruritic effect include reduction of tumor necrosis factor synthesis by monocytes; anti-inflammatory action; and interference with cytokine production. It has also been shown to be effective in the pruritus of various primary skin conditions, senile pruritus, and primary biliary cirrhosis.[102] UVB phototherapy is established therapy for uremic itch. Its use in palliative care may be limited by the delay of 1–2 months before having an effect.[18]

Other treatments that are being studied for the uremic patients having dialysis include oral cromolyn sodium,[103**] topical 1% pramoxine.[104*] Homeopathic treatments have also been shown to be effective: in one controlled trial patients reported a 49% reduction in pruritus score.[105**] An approach to management is suggested in Figure 76.4.

HIV/AIDS

There are many causes of pruritus in HIV-positive patients,[106] and itch can be the first symptom of disease even in the absence of apparent skin lesions. Pruritus in HIV may be related to cytokine-induced prostaglandin 2 synthesis, and increased plasma cytokine levels are not uncommon in patients with HIV.[107,108] Localized pruritus may occur with peripheral neuropathy.[6] Exposure to UVB light has been shown to be effective.[109] Treatment should relate to the specific cause, but in the absence of an obvious cause, indometacin 25 mg three times daily may be helpful.[3]

CENTRAL LESIONS AND MULTIPLE SCLEROSIS

Historically, pruritus in this group of patients has been treated effectively with antiepileptic drugs such as carbamazepine. Gabapentin may be a better tolerated choice and does not interfere with other medications by inducing liver enzymes.[110] NSAIDS such as ibuprofen may also be helpful.[111]

SUMMARY

Pruritus can be a troublesome symptom in patients with advanced disease and may have a substantial effect on quality of life despite the apparent trivial nature of the symptom relative to a life-limiting diagnosis. Careful history and examination may reveal an easily reversible cause; where this is not the case, symptomatic intervention may be helpful. First and foremost, management should include patient education and lifestyle changes to recognize and avoid triggering factors, and to include important general measures for maximal skin hydration in daily routine. Besides these measures, investigation and treatment of the underlying cause, where possible, is helpful. Topical or systemic medication, appropriate to the cause, should be used when required. The relatively limited etiological understanding of pruritus has hindered logical management, but there is now a more comprehensive body of evidence slowly but surely being created. Development of further useful interventions depends on continued investigation of the complex mechanisms by which pruritus is created, and more detailed evaluation of currently available interventions.

Key learning points

- Pruritus may be directly related to advanced disease (e.g., cancer, multiple sclerosis), indirectly related (e.g., cholestasis, uremia), or associated with the treatment of advanced disease.

- Pruritus may significantly impact on sleep, social acceptance, and daily functioning, and has been shown to be associated with depression.

- Initial management should include patient education and lifestyle changes to encourage identification and avoidance of triggering factors.

- The use of emollients to keep the skin continually hydrated cannot be overemphasized and must continue on a long-term basis. In addition, a large number of other topical agents are available and there is a reasonable evidence base supporting their use.

- Diagnosis of the underlying cause of pruritus is important and treatment of underlying disease will in many cases resolve the pruritus.

- If topical measures and lifestyle changes are not adequate, systemic treatment may be necessary and this chapter provides some evidence-based suggestions for first-, second-, and third-line treatments based on etiology.

- The historical use of histamine antagonists in the treatment of all pruritus has now been modified by the growing evidence base in this area, and these drugs are now only recommended for use in the treatment of urticaria, allergy, and lymphoproliferative pruritus.

REFERENCES

1   Portenoy RK, Thaler HT, Kornblith AB et al. Symptom prevalence, characteristics and distress in a cancer population. *Qual Life Res.* 1994; **3**: 183–189.

2   Connolly CS, Kantor GR, Menduke H. Hepatobiliary pruritus: What are effective treatments? *J Am Acad Dermatol.* 1995; **33**: 801–805.

◆ 3   Twycross R, Greaves MW, Handwerker H et al. Itch: Scratching more than the surface. *Q J Med.* 2003; **96**: 7–26.

4   Schelmz M, Michael K, Weidner C et al. Which nerve fibres mediate the axon reflex flare in human skin? *Neuroreport.* 2000; **11**: 645–648.

5   Schmelz M, Schmidt R, Bickel A et al. Specific C-receptors for itch in human skin. *J Neurosci.* 1997; **17**: 8003–8008.

6   Yosipovitch G, Greaves M, Schmelz M. Itch. *Lancet.* 2003; **361**: 690–694.

7   Oaklander AL, Cohen SP, Raju SV. Intractable postherpetic itch and cutaneous deafferentation after facial shingles. *Pain.* 2002; **96**: 9–12.

8   King CA, Huff FJ, Jorizzo JL. Unilateral neurogenic pruritus: Paroxysmal itching associated with central nervous system lesions. *Ann Intern Med.* 1982; **97**: 222–223.

9   Greaves MW, McDonald-Gibson W. Itch: The role of prostaglandins. *Br Med J.* 1973; **22**: 608–609.

10   Woodward DF, Nieves AL, Hawley SB. et al. The pruritogenic and inflammatory effects of prostanoids in the conjunctiva. *J Ocul Pharmacol Ther.* 1995; **11**: 339–347.

11   Vogelsang M, Heyer G, Hornstein OP. Acetylcholine induces different cutaneous sensations in atopic and non-atopic subjects. *Acta Derm Venereol.* 1995; **75**: 434–436.

◆ 12   Potenzieri C, Undem BJ. Basic mechanisms of itch. *Clin Exp Allergy.* 2011 **42**: 8–19.

◆ 13   Krajnik M, Zylicz Z. Understanding pruritus in systemic disease. *J Pain Symptom Manage.* 2001; **21**: 151–168.

14   Sheehan-Dare RA, Henderson MJ, Cotterill JA. Anxiety and depression in patients with chronic urticaria and generalised pruritus. *Br J Dermatol.* 1990; **123**: 769–774.

15   Molenaar HAJ, Oosting J, Jones EA. Improved device for measuring scratching activity in patients with pruritus. *Med Biol Eng Comput.* 1998; **36**: 220–224.

16   Vickers CF. Iron deficiency pruritus. *JAMA.* 1977; **238**: 129.

17   Szeptietowski JC, Morita A, Tsuji T. Ultraviolet B induces mast cell apoptosis: A hypothetical mechanism of ultraviolet B treatment for uraemic pruritus. *Med Hypotheses.* 2002; **58**: 167–170.

18   Gilchrest BA, Rowe JW, Brown RS et al. Relief of uraemic pruritus with ultraviolet phototherapy. *N Engl Med J.* 1977; **297**: 136–138.

● 19   Ebata T, Izumi H, Aizawa H et al. Effects of nitrazepam on nocturnal scratching in adults with atopic dermatitis: A double blind placebo-controlled crossover study. *Br J Dermatol.* 1998; **138**: 631–634.

20   Pittelkow MR, Loprinzi CL. Pruritus and sweating. In: Doyle D, Hanks GWC, MacDonald N, eds. *Oxford Textbook of Palliative Medicine*, 2nd edn. New York: Oxford University Press, 1998: p. 633.

21   Monk BE. Transcutaneous electronic nerve stimulation in the treatment of generalised pruritus. *Clin Exp Dermatol.* 1993; **18**: 67–68.

22   Bjorna H, Kaada B. Successful treatment of itching and atopic eczema by transcutaneous nerve stimulation. *Acupunct Electrother Res.* 1987; **12**: 101–112.

** 23   Smith EB, King CA, Baker MD. Crotamiton and pruritus. *Int J Dermatol.* 1984; **23**: 684–685.

24   Wasik F, Szeptietowski JC, Szeptietowski T, Weyde W. Relief of uraemic pruritus after balneological therapy with a bath oil containing polidocanol. An open clinical study. *J Dermatol Treat.* 1996; **7**: 231–233.

25   Freitag G, Hoppner T. Results of a postmarketing drug monitoring survey with a polidocanol-urea preparation for dry itching skin. *Curr Med Res Opin.* 1997; **13**: 529–537.

26   Rhiner M, Slatkin NE. Pruritus, Fever and sweats. In: Ferrell BR, Coyle N, eds. *Textbook of Palliative Nursing.* New York: Oxford University Press, **2006**: pp. 345–361.

27   Breneman DL, Cardone JS, Blumsack RF et al. Topical capsaicin for treatment of haemodialysis related pruritus. *J Am Acad Dermatol.* 1992; **26**: 91–94.

28   Zhai H, Hannon W, Hahn, GS, Harper RA et al. Strontium nitrate decreased histamine induced itch magnitude and duration in man. *Dermatology.* 2000; **200**: 244–246.

* 29 Kuypers SR, Claes K, Evenepoel P et al. A prospective proof of concept study of the efficacy of tacrolimus ointment on uraemic pruritus (UP) in patients on chronic dialysis therapy. *Nephrol. Dial. Transplant.* 2004: **19**(7): 1895–1901.

* 30 Chen YC, Chiu WT, Wu MS. Therapeutic effect of topical gamma-linolenic acid on refractory uremic pruritus. *Am J Kidney Dis.* 2006: **48**(1): 69–76.

31 Smith PF, Corelli RL. Doxepin in the management of pruritus associated with allergic cutaneous reactions. *Ann Pharmacother.* 1997; **31**: 633–635.

32 Jones EA, Bergasa NV. Evolving concepts of the pathogenesis and treatment of the pruritus of cholestasis. *Can J Gastroenterol.* 2000; **14**: 33–40.

** 33 Kirschner D, Nagel W, Gugeler N et al. Naltrexone does not relieve uremic pruritus: Results of a randomised, double blind, placebo-controlled study. *J Am Soc Nephrol.* 2000; **11**: 514–519.

** 34 Muller C, Pongratz S, Pidlich J et al. Treatment of pruritus in chronic liver disease with the 5HT3 antagonist ondansetron: A randomised, placebo-controlled double-blind cross over trial. *Eur J Gasterenterol Hepatol.* 1998; **10**: 865–870.

** 35 O'Donohue JW, Haigh C, Williams R. Ondansetron in the treatment of pruritus of cholestasis: A randomised controlled trial. *Gastroenterology.* 1997; **112**: A1349.

** 36 Murphy M, Reaich D, Pai P et al. A randomised, placebo-controlled, double blind trial of ondansetron in renal itch. *Br J Dermatol.* 2001; **145**(Suppl 59): 20–21.

◆ 37 Reich A, Szepietowski JC. Opioid induced pruritus: An update. *Clin Exp Dermatol.* 2009; **35**: 2–6.

38 Zylicz Z, Smits C, Krajnik M. Paroxetine for pruritus in advanced cancer. *J Pain Symptom Manage* 1998; 16: 121–124.

* 39 Stander S, Bockenholt B, Schurmeyer-Horst F et al. Treatment of chronic pruritus with the selective serotonin re-uptake inhibitors paroxetine and fluvoxamine: Results of an open-labelled, two-arm proof-of-concept study. *Acta Dermato-Venerologica* 2009; **89**: 45–51.

* 40 Mayo MJ, Handem I, Saldana S et al. Sertraline as a first-line treatment for cholestatic pruritus. *Hepatology* 2007; **45**: 666–674.

41 Davis MP, Frandsen JL, Walsh D et al. Mirtazapine for pruritus. *J Pain Symptom Manage* 2003; 25: 288–291.

42 Zylicz Z. Neuropathic pruritus. In: Zylicz Z, Twycross R, Jones EA. *Pruritus in Advanced Disease.* Oxford, U.K.: Oxford University Press, 2004.

43 Lober CW. Should the patient with generalized malignancy be evaluated for malignancy? *J Am Acad Dermatol.* 1988; **19**: 350–352.

44 Goldman BD, Koh HK. Pruritus and malignancy. In: Bernhard JD, ed. *Itch Mechanisms and Management of Pruritus.* New York: McGraw-Hill, 1994: pp. 299–319.

◆ 45 Terrifi A. Polycythaemia vera: A comprehensive review and clinical recommendations. *Mayo Clin Proc.* 2003; **78**: 174–194.

46 Jackson N, Burt D, Crocker J, Boughton B. Skin mast cells in polycythameia vera: Relationship to pathogenesis and treatment of pruritus. *Br J Dermatol.* 1987; **116**: 21–29.

47 Terrifi A, Fonseca R. Selective serotonin reuptake inhibitors are effective in the treatment of polycythaemia vera associated pruritus. *Blood.* 2002; **99**: 26–27.

48 Weick JK, Dinovan PB, Najean Y et al. The use of cimetidine for the treatment of pruritus in polycythaemia rubra vera. *Arch Intern Med.* 1982; **142**: 241–242.

49 Aymard JP, Lederlin P, Witz F et al. Cimetidine for pruritus in Hodgkin's Disease. *Br J Med.* 1980; **280**: 151–152.

50 Leven A, Naysmith A, Pickens S et al. Sodium cromoglycate and Hodgkin's disease. *Br J Med.* 1977; **2**: 896.

51 Martinez C, Albet C, Agundez JA et al. Comparative in vitro and in vivo inhibition of cytochrome p450, CYP1A2, CYP2D6 and CYP3A by H2 receptor antagonists. *Clin Pharmacol Ther.* 1999; **65**: 369–376.

52 Pujol RN, Gallardo F, Llistosella E et al. Invisible mycosis fungiodes: A diagnostic challenge. *J Am Acad Dermatol.* 2002; **47**(2 Suppl): S168–S171.

53 Totterman TH, Scheynius A, Killander A et al. Treatment of therapy resistant Sezary syndrome with cyclosporin A: Suppression of pruritus, leukaemic T cell activation markers and tumour mass. *Scand J Haematol.* 1985; **34**: 196–203.

◆ 54 Wang H, Yosipovitch G. New insights into the pathophysiology and treatment of chronic itch in patients with end stage renal disease, chronic liver disease and lymphoma. *Int J Dermatol.* 2010; **49**: 1–11.

55 Paul R, Jansen C. Itch and malignancy prognosis in generalised pruritus: A 6 year follow-up of 125 patients. *J Am Acad Dermatol.* 1987; **16**: 1179–1182.

** 56 Zylicz Z, Krajnik M, van Sorge A, Constantini M. Paroxetine in the treatment of severe non-dermatological pruritus: A randomised controlled trial. *J Pain Symptom Manage.* 2003; **26**: 1105–1112.

* 57 Lee SH, Baig M, Rusciano V, Dutcher JP. Novel management of pruritus in patients treated with IL-2 for metastatic renal cell carcinoma and malignant melanoma. *J Immunotherapy* 2010; **33**(9): 1010–1013.

58 Ballantyne JC, Loach AB, Carr DB. Itching after epidural and spinal opiates. *Pain.* 1988; **33**: 149–160.

59 Stoelting RK. Pharmacology and physiology. In: Capan LM, Miller SM, Turndorf H, eds. *Anaesthetics Practice*, 2nd edn. Philadelphia, PA: Lippincott, 1991.

60 Etches RC. Complications of acute pain management. *Anaesth Clin North Am.* 1992; **10**: 417–433.

61 Larijani G, Goldberg ME, Rogers KH. Treatment of opioid induced pruritus with ondansetron—Report of four patients. *Pharmacotherapy.* 1996; **16**: 958–960.

62 Chaplan S, Duncan SR, Brodsky JB, Brose WG. Morphine and Hydromorphone epidural analgesia. *Anaesthesiology.* 1992; **77**: 1090–1094.

63 Katcher J, Walsh D. Opioid induced itching: Morphine sulfate and hydromorphone hydrochloride. *J Pain Symptom Manage.* 1999; **17**: 70–72.

64 Davies GG, From R. A blinded study using nalbuphine for prevention of pruritus induced by epidural fentanyl. *Anaesthesiology* 1988; **69**: 763–765.

65 Glare P, Walsh TD. Dose ranging study of oxycodone for chronic pain in advanced cancer. *J Clin Oncol* 1993; **11**: 973–978.

66 Wang JJ, Ho ST, Tzeng JI. Comparison of intravenous nalbuphine infusion versus naloxone in the prevention of epidural morphine related side effects. *Reg Anesth Pain Med.* 1998; **23**: 479–484.

** 67 Tamdee D, Charuluxananan S, Punjasawadwong Y et al. A randomized controlled trial of pentazocine versus ondansetron for the treatment of intrathecal morphine-induced pruritus in patients undergoing cesarean delivery. *Anesth Analg.* 2009; **109**(5): 1606–1611.

68 Cohen SE, Ratner EF, Kreitzman TR et al. Nalbuphine is better than naloxone for treatment of side effects after epidural morphine. *Anesth Analg.* 1992; **75**: 747–752.

69 Friedman JD, Dello Buono FA. Opioid antagonists in the treatment of opioid-induced constipation and pruritus. *Ann Pharmacother.* 2001; **35**: 85–91.

* 70 Yuan CS, Foss JF, O'Connor M et al. Efficacy of orally administered methylnaltrexone in decreasing subjective effects after intravenous morphine. *Drug Alcohol Depend.* 1998; **52**: 161–165.

71 Yuan C, Israel RJ. Methylnaltrexone, a novel peripheral opioid receptor antagonist for the treatment of opioid side effects. *Expert Opin Investig Drugs.* 2006; **15**: 541–552.

72 Borgeat A, Stirnemann HR. Ondansetron is effective to treat spinal or epidural morphine-induced pruritus. *Anaesthesiology.* 1999; **90**: 432–436.

** 73 Sheen MJ, Ho ST, Lee CH, Tsung YC, Chang FL, Huang ST. Prophylactic mirtazapine reduces intrathecal morphine-induced pruritus. *Br J Anaesth.* 2008; **101**(5): 711–715.

** 74 Sheen MJ, Ho ST, Lee CH, Tsung YC, Chang FL. Preoperative gabapentin prevents intrathecal morphine-induced pruritus after orthopedic surgery. *Anesth Analg.* 2008; **106**(6): 1868–1872.

** 75 Wolfhagen FH, Sternieri E, Hop WC et al. Oral naltrexone treatment for cholestatic pruritus: A double blind placebo controlled study. *Gastroenterology.* 1997; **113**: 1264–1269.

* 76 Bergasa NV, Talbot TL, Alling DW et al. A controlled trial of naloxone infusions for the pruritus of chronic cholestasis. *Gastroenterology.* 1992; **102**: 544–549.

* 77 Bergasa NV, Talbot TL, Alling DW et al. Oral nalmefene therapy reduces scratching activity due to pruritus of cholestasis: A controlled study. *J Am Acad Dermatol.* 1999; **41**: 431–434.

* 78 Mansour-Ghanaei F, Taheri A, Froutan H et al. Effect of oral naltrexone on pruritus in cholestatic patients. *World J Gastroenterol.* 2006; **12**(7): 1125–1128.

79 McRae CA, Prince MI, Hudson M et al. Pain as a complication of opiate antagonists for symptom control in cholestasis. *Gastroenterology.* 2003; **125**: 591–596.

80 Jones EA, Neuberger J, Bergasa NV. Opiate antagonist therapy for the pruritus of cholestasis: The avoidance of opioid withdrawal-like reactions. *Quart J Med.* 2002; **95**: 547–552.

* 81 Datta DV, Sherlock S. Cholestyramine for long-term relief of the pruritus complicating intrahepatic cholestasis. *Gastroenterology.* 1966; **50**: 323–332.

** 82 Ghent C, Curruthers S. Treatment of pruritus in primary biliary cirrhosis with rifampicin. Results of a double-blind randomised cross-over trial. *Gasterenterology.* 1988; **94**: 488–493.

83 Prince MI, Burt AD, Jones DE. Hepatitis and liver dysfunction with rifampicin therapy for pruritus in primary biliary cirrhosis. *Gut.* 2002; **50**: 436–439.

** 84 Bergasa NV, McGee M, Ginsburg IH et al. Gabapentin in patients with the pruritus of cholestasis: A double blind, randomized, placebo controlled trial. *Hepatology.* 2006; **44**: 1317–1323.

** 85 Jones EA, Molenaar HA, Oosting J. Ondansetron and pruritus in chronic liver disease: A double blind controlled study. *Hepatogastroenterology.* 2007; **54**(76): 1196–1199.

** 86 Bergasa NV, Sabol SL, Yound WS et al. Cholestasis is associated with preproenkephalin mRNA expression in the adult rat liver. *Am J Physiol.* 1995; **268**: G346–G354.

87 Mela M, Mancuso A, Burroughs K. Review article: Pruritus in cholestatic and other liver diseases. *Aliment Pharmacol Ther.* 2003; **17**: 857–870.

88 Szepietowski JC. Selected elements of the pathogenesis of pruritus in haemodialysis patients: My own study. *Med Sci Monitor.* 1996; **2**: 343–347.

89 Young Aw, Sweeney EW, David DS et al. Dermatologic evaluation of pruritus in patients on hemodialysis. *N Y State J Med.* 1973; **73**: 2670–2674.

90 Matsumoto M, Ichimaru K, Horie A. Pruritus and mast cell proliferation of the skin in end stage renal failure. *Clin Nephrol.* 1985; **23**: 285–288.

91 Szepietowski JC, Schwartz RA. Uremic pruritus. In: Demis J, ed. *Clinical Dermatology*, 26th edn. New York: Lippincott, Williams & Wilkins, 1999: Unit 29–2B.

92 Murtagh FE, Addington-Hall J, Edmonds P et al. Symptoms in the month before death for stage 5 chronic kidney disease patients managed without dialysis. *J Pain Symptom Manage.* 2010; **40**(3): 342–352.

** 93 Chen ZJ, Goa G, Tang WX et al. A randomised controlled trial of high permeability haemodialysis against conventional haemodialysis in the treatment of uremic pruritus. *Clin Exp Dermatol.* 2009; **34**(6): 679–683.

* 94 Aperis G, Paliorus C, Zerovos A et al. The use of pregabalin in the treatment of uraemic pruritus in haemodialysis patients. *J Renal Care.* 2010; **36**(4): 180–185.

* 95 Vila T, Gommer J, Scates AC. Role of gabapentin in the treatment of uremic pruritus. *Ann Pharmacother.* 2008; **42**(7): 1080–1084.

** 96 Gunal AI, Ozalp G, Yoldas TK et al. Gabapentin therapy for pruritus in haemodialysis patients: A randomized, placebo-controlled, double-blind trial. *Nephrol Dial Transplant.* 2004; **19**(12): 3137–3139.

** 97 Peer G, Kivity S, Agami O et al. Randomised crossover trial of naltrexone in uraemic pruritus. *Lancet.* 1996; **348**: 1552–1554.

** 98 Wikstrom B, Gellert R, Ladefoged SD et al. Kappa-opioid system in uremic pruritus: Multicenter, randomised, double-blind, placebo-controlled studies. *J Am Soc Nephrology.* 2005; **16**(12): 3742–3747.

** 99 Kumagai H. Ebata T, Takamori K et al. Effect of a novel kappa-receptor agonist, nalfurafine hydrochloride, on severe itch in 337 haemodialysis patients: A Phase III, randomised, double-blind, placebo-controlled study. *Neph Dialysis Transplantation.* 2010; **25**(4): 1251–1257.

100 Balaskas EV, Bamihas HI, Karamouzis M et al. Histamine and serotonin in uremic pruritus: Effect of ondansetron in CAPD-pruritic patients. *Nephron.* 1998; **78**: 395–402.

** 101 Silva SR, Viana PC, Lugon NV et al. Thalidomide for the treatment of uraemic pruritus: A crossover randomised double-blind trial. *Nephron* 1994; **67**: 270–273.

102 Daly BM, Shuster S. Antipruritic action of thalidomide. *Acta Dermatol Venereol.* 2000; **80**: 24–25.

** 103 Vessal G, Sagheb MM, Shilian S et al. Effect of oral cromolyn sodium on CKD-associated pruritus and serum tryptase level: A double-blind placebo-controlled study. *Nephrol Dial Transplant.* 2010; **25**(5): 1541–1547.

* 104 Young TA, Patel TS, Camacho F et al. A pramoxine-based anti-itch lotion is more effective than a control lotion for the treatment of uremic pruritus in adult hemodialysis patients. *J Dermatol Treat.* 2009; **20**(2): 76–81.

** 105 Cavalcanti AM, Rocha LM, Carillo R et al. Effects of homeopathic treatment on pruritus of haemodialysis patients: A randomised placebo-controlled double-blind trial. *Homeopathy.* 2003; **92**: 177–181.

106 Cockerall CJ. The itches of HIV infection and AIDS. In: Bernhard J, ed. *Itch: Mechanisms and Management of Pruritus.* New York: McGraw-Hill, **1994**: pp. 347–365.

107 Smith CJ, Skelton HG, Yeager J et al. Pruritus in HIV-1 disease: Therapy with drugs which may modulate the pattern of immune dysregulation. *Dermatology.* 1997; **195**: 353–358.

108 Breur-McHam JN, Marshall GD, Lewis DE, Duvic M. Distinct Serum Cytokines in AIDS related skin diseases. *Viral Immunol.* 1998; **11**: 215–220.

109 Lim HW, Vallurupalli S, Meola T, Soter NA. UVB phototherapy is an effective treatment for pruitus in patients infected with HIV. *J Am Acad Dermatol.* 1997; **37**: 414–417.

110 Jones EA, ed. *Pruritus in Advanced Disease.* Oxford, U.K.: Oxford University Press, 2004: pp. 117–131.

111 Khan OA. Treatment of paroxysmal symptoms in multiple sclerosis with ibuprofen. *Neurology.* 1994; **44**: 571–572.

112 Twycross R, Zylicz Z. OICPC Therapeutic Highlights. Itch: Scratching more than the surface. *Prog Palliat Care.* 2002; **10**: 285–289.

77

Infections in palliative care

RUDOLPH M. NAVARI, CHRISTOPHER GREEN, MICHELLE L. HANEY, NATHAN L. ROACH

INTRODUCTION

Patients receiving palliative care are at high risk for infections as a result of their underlying disease, poor nutritional state, and/or a direct suppression of the hematological system due to chemotherapy or radiation treatments, viral infection, or corticosteroids [1]. An infectious complication may occur due to an alteration in the phagocytic, cellular, or humoral immunity, an alteration or breach of skin or mucosal defense barriers, indwelling catheters, or a splenectomy. A high index of suspicion, an awareness of the possibility of unusual infectious agents, consideration of the empirical institution of antimicrobials, and constant surveillance of the hematological status of the patients are necessary to provide optimal management of infections in this patient population.

In addition to the high risk of infections, patients in palliative care also experience a high incidence and a wide variety of infections [1–5]. Several retrospective studies have shown that a large number of patients receiving hospice or palliative care are treated with antibiotics for suspected or documented infections [6–13]. The benefits and burdens of the use of antimicrobials in this patient population are topics of much discussion [3,5,10,14]. Prospective studies have suggested that symptom control may be the main objective in the decision to use antimicrobials to treat clinically suspected or documented infections in patients receiving palliative or hospice care [3,5,15,16]. The use of symptom control as the main determinant of whether to use antimicrobials in any given clinical situation is markedly affected, however, by the uncertainty of predicting which patients will achieve symptom relief and which patients will experience only the additional burdens of treatment. Determining whether fever is due to infection, tumor, or other causes, and deciding which symptoms from suspected infections might respond to various antimicrobial interventions can be difficult clinical judgments, particularly in a patient population that has multiple active medical problems and where the goal of treatment is symptom control. These are crucial issues in patients receiving palliative care in that studies have shown that incurably ill patients often receive nonpalliative interventions at the end of life [17].

This chapter will discuss the incidence and the type of infections seen in various palliative care clinical settings and the judicious use of antimicrobials, and will also suggest the use of symptom control as a major criterion for treatment. The chapter concludes by suggesting guidelines for the approach to infections in palliative care.

INCIDENCE AND TYPE OF INFECTIONS

Patients who are receiving palliative care or hospice care have a high frequency of infections due to the underlying disease, the use of indwelling urinary catheters and vascular access devices, as well as the generally poor functional status of the patients, characterized by impaired cognition and immobility. There have been a number of reports on the use of antimicrobials in patients receiving hospice and palliative care [1,3,5,6,7,9,15,16].

Vitetta et al. [6] performed a retrospective chart review on the prevalence of infections in 102 patients (92% with terminal malignant illness) who died after admission to a tertiary care inpatient palliative care unit. Thirty-seven patients were diagnosed with 42 infections. The urinary tract, respiratory tract, blood, skin and subcutaneous tissues, and eyes were the most common sites of infection. *Escherichia coli* was the most common organism. Of the 37 patients, 35 were treated with antibiotics and symptom improvement was noted in half of the patients treated; 2 of 37 patients were not treated with antibiotics due to survival limited to the day of admission. Pereira et al. [7] reported a retrospective chart review of the prevalence of infections in 100 consecutive admissions to a tertiary care palliative care unit. There were 74 infections in 55 patients. The urinary tract, respiratory tract, skin and subcutaneous tissue, blood, and mouth were the most common infection sites. *E. coli*, *Staphylococcus aureus*, and *Enterococcus* were the most common organisms. Twenty-one of the seventy-four infections were not treated, and the reasons for not using antimicrobials were documented in ten patients: very poor general condition, not able to take oral antimicrobials, and refusal of parenteral antimicrobials. The retrospective nature of the study did not allow for an adequate analysis of the symptom response to antibiotic therapy. Homsi et al. [1] reported a retrospective analysis of 393 patients with advanced cancer who were admitted to an acute care palliative medicine unit over an 8-month period. A total of 115 patients had at least one positive bacteriological culture and 100 patients were evaluable. Of these, 66 patients had a urinary tract infection, 31 patients had bacteremia, and 21 patients had pneumonia. *E. coli, Staphylococcus* spp., *Enterococcus*, and *Klebsiella pneumoniae* were cited as the most common organisms. Symptom response was not reported in this study.

Oneschuk et al. [9] retrospectively examined the frequency and types of antibiotics prescribed in the last week of life in three palliative care settings: acute care hospital, tertiary palliative care unit, and hospice inpatient unit. Of 50 patients in each setting, 29 (58%) in the acute care hospital, 26 (52%) in the palliative care unit, and 11 (22%) in the inpatient hospice unit received antibiotics in the last week of life. The types of infection, the specific organisms, and symptom response were not reported. Clayton et al. [15] prospectively studied all patients receiving parenteral antibiotics in a palliative care unit. Of 913 consecutive admissions over a 13-month period, 41 patients received 43 courses of parenteral antibiotics. The most common sites of infection were urinary tract infections (37%), lower respiratory tract infection (26%), and soft tissue/skin infections (16%). The predominant organisms were not reported, and the use of antibiotics was considered "helpful" in 27 of the 43 antibiotics courses (62%).

In a retrospective review of 138 patients in a palliative care unit, Al-Shaqi et al. [13] reported that 63% of patients were receiving antimicrobials during the last week of life. In another retrospective review, Chun et al. [12] reported that 70 of 131 patients receiving palliative care consultation were treated with antimicrobials. Fifty-four of the 70 patients received empiric therapy, primarily for presumed respiratory and urinary tract infections. The effectiveness of the control of symptoms with antimicrobials was not reported in either of these reports.

Lam et al. [11] retrospectively reviewed 87 patients enrolled in a palliative care service over a 6-month period. One hundred seventeen of 120 episodes of infection in 70 patients were treated with antimicrobials. The most frequent sites of infection were chest (52.5%), urinary tract (29.2%), and skin/wound (5%), and dyspnea was associated with a poor prognosis in patients with advanced cancer.

White et al. [3] studied 255 patients with advanced cancer at the time they entered a community-based outpatient hospice and palliative care program. Antimicrobial options were discussed with patients at the time of the initiation of hospice care. Seventy-nine percent of patients chose no use of antimicrobials or symptomatic use only. The use and effectiveness of antimicrobials was prospectively documented during the palliative care period. One hundred seventeen patients had a total of one hundred twenty-nine infections, with the most common sites being urinary tract, respiratory tract, mouth/pharynx, and skin/subcutaneous tissues. The most common organisms in this patient population were *E. coli, S. aureus, Enterococcus* spp., and *K. pneumoniae*. Seventy-seven patients received

antimicrobials, and the use of antimicrobials controlled symptoms in the majority of the urinary tract infections, but were less effective in controlling symptoms of the other sites of infection. Survival was not affected by the patients' choice of whether to use antimicrobials, the prevalence of infections, or the actual use of antimicrobials.

Oh et al. [10] retrospectively reviewed 141 terminal stage cancer patients who were hospitalized for symptom control. One hundred nineteen patients received antibiotics for a clinically suspected infection. Symptomatic improvement in infection related symptoms was achieved in 18 patients (15.1%), with no improvement in 66 patients (55.4%).

Reinbolt et al. [5] prospectively followed 623 outpatient hospice patients with advanced cancer who were treated with antimicrobials for a clinically suspected infection. A complete or partial response of infection-related symptoms was observed in 79% of 265 patients with urinary tract infections, 43% of 221 patients with respiratory tract infections, 46% of 63 patients with oral cavity infections, 41% of 59 patients with skin or subcutaneous infections, and zero of 25 patients with bacteremia. There was no difference in survival in patients with a diagnosed infection compared to those without an infection and no difference in survival in patients who received antimicrobials compared to those who did not receive antimicrobials.

Thai et al. [18] reported on 441 hospitalized advanced cancer patients referred to a palliative care consult service over a 12-month period. Sixteen percent had an episode of sepsis and 23.4% had an organ-related infection; 89.7% received antibiotics. Sepsis and/or organ-related infection reduced overall survival, but a favorable antibiotic response was associated with an increase in survival.

These studies, carried out in a wide variety of palliative care settings, have suggested that 20%–65% of patients receiving palliative care have at least one or more infections that are considered for antimicrobial treatment. The most common clinical conditions are urinary tract infections, upper and lower respiratory tract infections, skin and subcutaneous tissues infections, and a fewer number of patients with bacteremia. The most common organisms are *E. coli, Staphylococcus* spp., *Enterococcus*, and *K. pneumoniae*. Most patients are treated with antimicrobials when an infection is suspected, with varying responses.

EVALUATION OF FEVER

In patients with advanced cancer, fever is common and it may or may not have an infectious etiology. It must be noted that fever may be the only manifestation of an infection in an immunocompromised patient, and there is no pattern of fever, which can be used to definitively rule out an infectious etiology. Fever may also be modified by the use of specific medications such as corticosteroids or nonsteroidal anti-inflammatory agents.

Fever in patients with advanced or terminal cancer must be evaluated in terms of the underlying disease, the specific risk for a local or systemic infection, the urgency for empirical antimicrobial therapy, the presence or absence of neutropenia, and any signs or symptoms, which may suggest a site of infection. Attention should be directed to the most common sites of infection such as the oral cavity, lungs, perirectal area, urinary tract, skin, and soft tissues. In most patients with fever and neutropenia, the initial evaluation does not identify a site of infection.

Depending on the status of the patient at the time of the fever, an initial evaluation may include, in addition to the history and physical examination, a hematological profile, cultures of nose and throat, urine, blood, stool, and cerebrospinal fluid, and radiological evaluation of the chest and sinuses. Whether or not antimicrobials are begun at the time of the initial fever, patients should be carefully reevaluated at least every 24 hours. It must be remembered that in patients with profound and prolonged neutropenia, multiple sites of infection and multiple organisms may be present.

The approach to fever in patients receiving palliative care should be similar to that outlined above, with symptom control, accomplished through a minimum of interventions, as the primary goal. Chen et al. [8] retrospectively studied 535 admissions to a hospice and palliative care unit and identified 93 fever episodes, of which 79 episodes were treated with antibiotics. Although the use of antibiotics appeared to decrease fever-related discomfort, it was not clear that quality of life was improved.

TREATMENT WITH ANTIMICROBIALS

Studies suggest that antimicrobials are initiated in the overwhelming majority (70%–90%) of patients receiving palliative care when they have fever or a suspected or documented infection [1,8]. The response rate to antibiotics appears to be varied with symptom improvement in the majority of patients with urinary tract infections, but symptom improvement in less than half of the patients with infections of other organ systems [3,5,10,16].

The decision-making process in the use of antimicrobials in patients receiving palliative care is highly complex. In most situations, the approach should be individualized for each patient based on the desires of the patient, the goal to control symptoms, and quality of life issues. Issues to be considered include the potential benefit of the use of antimicrobials compared to the potential toxicities that may result from the extent of the investigation of a suspected infection, the number of diagnostic tests to be employed, and the means to be employed to treat a suspected or documented infection. It may be appropriate to treat a fever with an antipyretic alone in a patient whose death is imminent rather than proceed with an extensive laboratory workup and the initiation of antimicrobials. Alternatively, the pain resulting from a urinary tract infection or a symptomatic, localized skin or soft tissue infection may be treated more successfully with both antibiotics and pain medications. For patients receiving hospice care at home or in an institution such as a hospital palliative care unit or a chronic care facility, consideration should be given to initiating oral or parenteral antibiotics based on only clinical indications without the use of laboratory or imaging criteria. Mobilization of the patients for diagnostic interventions may be associated with significant discomfort.

Table 77.1 suggests an approach to the management of common infections in patients receiving palliative care. Patients with uncomplicated urinary tract infections or cystitis can be effectively and inexpensively treated with a 3-day course of oral trimethoprim-sulfamethoxazole or a fluoroquinolone [19]. Acute uncomplicated pyelonephritis can often be managed with a seven-day course of an oral fluoroquinolone [20]. For community-acquired bacterial pneumonia, an oral macrolide (erythromycin, azithromycin, or clarithromycin), doxycycline, or a fluoroquinolone with good antipneumococcal activity (levofloxacin, gatifloxacin, or moxifloxacin)

Table 77.1 *Management of common infections in patients receiving palliative care*

Infection	Signs/symptoms	Antimicrobial(s)	Diagnostic[a]
Urinary tract	Dysuria, fever, frequency, pain	Oral trimethoprim sulfamethoxazole or fluoroquinolone	Urine analysis, culture, and sensitivity
Oral	Fever, mucositis, odynophagia, pain	Fluconazole, nystatin	Mouth swab for culture and sensitivity, endoscopy
Respiratory tract	Cough, dyspnea, fever, sputum production	Oral macrolides (erythromycin, azithromycin, clarithromycin), doxycycline, fluoroquinone (levofloxacin, gatifloxacin, moxifloxacin)	Sputum culture, chest x-ray, bronchoscopy
Skin/subcutaneous	Fever, pain, skin rash/discoloration	Cephalexin, macrolides	Skin culture and sensitivity, blood cultures
Bacteremia	Fever, disorientation, hypotension, tachycardia	Cefotaxime or ceftriaxone	Blood cultures

[a] The decision to use any diagnostic intervention should be evaluated in terms of potential benefit to the patient in symptom control versus the potential toxicities of the diagnostic interventions.

is recommended [21]. An antipneumococcal fluoroquinolone may be added to cover *Legionella*, *Mycoplasma*, and *Chlamydia*. For the management of skin and soft tissue infections, a first- or second-generation cephalosporin or a macrolide is recommended [22]. Vancomycin may be added if there is minimal or no response.

Issues that patients, families, and physicians consider when making decisions concerning the use of a respirator, cardiac resuscitation, dialysis, etc. should, in general, also apply to the use of antimicrobials. Antimicrobial use in patients receiving palliative care may be a part of symptomatic care, may or may not result in prolongation of life, and/or may be associated with symptom-producing interventions such as laboratory testing, venous access, and direct antimicrobial toxicities. The goal of antimicrobial therapy in palliative care is symptom control, in contrast to the goal of decreased morbidity and mortality in acute medical or surgical situations.

White et al. [3] reported that when antimicrobial options were discussed with 255 advanced cancer patients at the time of entrance to a hospice program, 79.2% chose either no antimicrobials or symptomatic use only.

In a survey of patients concerning the use of antibiotics in a palliative care unit, Stiel et al. [4] reported that 286 (63.8%) of 448 patients received antibiotic therapy. Eighty-eight patients had ongoing treatment withdrawn for various reasons, and the outcome of treatment was rated poor in 20%. The initiation of therapy was often decided by physicians only, whereas withdrawing therapy demanded more involvement of other team members. The involvement of patients and family members is essential in the decision to use antibiotics in patients receiving palliative care.

SYMPTOM CONTROL

There has been much discussion in the literature about the use of symptom control as criterion for use of antimicrobials in patients receiving palliative care. However, there have been only a few studies that have evaluated the effects of antimicrobials on the symptoms associated with infections in patients with advanced cancer. Bruera [23] reported a marked improvement in pain with the use of antimicrobials for seven patients with infected, ulcerated head and neck neoplasms. Green et al. [24] described improved symptom control with the use of antibiotics in two patients with advanced cancer. One patient had severe respiratory distress from pneumonia, and one patient had sepsis-induced delirium.

In a retrospective study of 102 patients admitted to a tertiary care palliative care unit, Vitetta et al. [6] reported on antibiotic-induced symptom control in 36 patients. Antibiotic-associated positive symptom response was seen in 8 of 17 patients with urinary tract infections, 3 of 9 patients with respiratory tract infections, 1 of 5 patients with subcutaneous skin infections, and 1 of 5 patients with bacteremia. Clayton et al. [15] reported that the use of parenteral antibiotics was "helpful" (overall condition improved or symptoms and/or signs of infection improved) in 27 of 43 infections in 41 patients in an inpatient palliative care unit. Antibiotic response was seen in 14 of 16 patients with urinary tract infections, 6 of 11 patients with lower respiratory tract infections, 2 of 2 patients with purulent terminal respiratory secretions, 5 of 7 patients with soft tissue/wound infections, and 0 of 7 patients with other suspected infections. The types of infections and the response rates followed a similar pattern to that found in Vitetta et al.'s [6] study, with a somewhat higher response rate possibly due to the use of parenteral rather than oral antibiotics.

Mirhosseini et al. [16] prospectively evaluated the effect of antibiotic treatment on infection-related symptoms in patients with advanced cancer using a questionnaire given to the patients. In 26 patients on a tertiary palliative care unit with 31 episodes of infection, patients reported a statistical significant improvement only in dysuria. Physician assessment revealed only an improvement in cough as statistically significant.

In a prospective study by White et al. [3] of antibiotic choices by patients with advanced cancer receiving outpatient hospice care, antibiotic-associated positive symptom response was seen in 25 of 30 patients with urinary tract infections, 10 of 26 patients with respiratory tract infections, 4 of 9 patients with mouth/pharyngeal infections, 4 of 9 patients with subcutaneous skin infections, and 0 of 3 patients with bacteremia.

In a large prospective study of 1731 advanced cancer patients receiving outpatient hospice care, a complete or partial response of infection-related symptoms was observed in 79% of 265 patients with urinary tract infections, 43% of 221 patients with respiratory tract infections, 46% of 63 patients with oral cavity infections, 41% of 59 patients with skin or subcutaneous infections, and 0 of 25 patients with bacteremia [5].

The types of infections and the responses recorded appear similar in the above studies, despite major differences in the types of palliative care settings. In these studies, it appeared that the majority of the organisms cultured were sensitive to the antimicrobials used, suggesting that the lack of symptom response in some patients may have been due to co-morbid conditions such as an immunocompromised state, malnutrition, the failure of host barriers, decreased level of consciousness or immobility, or the presence of a neoplasm in the symptomatic organ. Regardless of the reason for the lack of symptom response, it is essential that treating clinicians use symptom control as the major criterion for antibiotic use and be aware of the limitations of the use of antimicrobials in this patient population in a palliative care modality.

PATIENT SURVIVAL

Although symptomatic care, and not survival, is the main issue in palliative and hospice care, survival may be an issue for some patients, families, and healthcare professionals.

Survival was not affected by the patients' choice of whether to use antimicrobials, the prevalence of infections, or the actual use of antimicrobials in the study by White et al. [3]. Similarly, in the large study by Reinbolt et al. [5], survival was not affected by the presence of infection or the use of antimicrobials.

Antimicrobial use did not affect survival in patients severely affected with Alzheimer's disease who were treated for fever [25]. In a retrospective study of inpatient hospice patients, a high early mortality followed antibiotic administration [14]. Vitetta et al. [6] and Chen et al. [8], however, showed that terminally ill hospice patients with documented infections treated with antibiotics had a longer median survival. A favorable antibiotic response did increase survival in hospitalized advanced cancer patients with sepsis or organ-related infection [18].

The effect of the use of antimicrobials on survival is important information for patients entering hospice care. This information might strongly influence their choice of whether to receive antimicrobials.

GUIDELINES FOR ANTIBIOTIC USE

Based on the data generated in the current and previous studies, we suggest the following guidelines on the use of antimicrobials in patients with advanced cancer receiving hospice/palliative care:

- On entry into hospice/palliative care, discussions should be held with the patient and family on their wishes in the treatment of infections, just as is done with cardiopulmonary resuscitation, use of a respirator, blood transfusions, etc.
- Strong consideration should be given to symptom control as the major indication for the use of antimicrobials for the treatment of infections. In a previous study [3], 79% of patients chose either no antimicrobials or symptomatic use only.
- Prospective studies [3,5,16] and retrospective studies [6,10] suggest that antimicrobial treatment of urinary tract infections improves symptoms in a large majority of patients, but antimicrobial treatment of respiratory tract infections, mucositis, and skin infections is much less successful in symptom control. Sepsis/bacteremia is poorly controlled by antimicrobials in this patient population [3,5,16].
- Overall survival appears to be unaffected by antimicrobial use [3,5]; there may be some survival benefit in patients with sepsis or organ infections if the infection is sensitive to the employed antimicrobial [18].
- Patients and families should be informed of the effects of antimicrobials on symptom control of various infections and on survival.
- Each patient's specific situation and condition must be evaluated in the decision to employ antimicrobials for a suspected or documented infection.

Key learning points

- Patients in palliative care settings experience a high incidence of infections.
- The most common sites of infection in patients receiving palliative care are the urinary tract, respiratory tract, skin and subcutaneous tissues, mouth, and blood. The most common pathogens are *E. coli*, *Staphylococcus* spp., *Enterococcus*, and *K. pneumoniae*.
- Although the use of antimicrobials improves symptoms in the majority of patients with urinary tract infections, symptom control is less successful with antimicrobial use in infections of the respiratory tract, mouth/pharynx, skin/subcutaneous tissue, or blood.
- Physicians should be aware of the limitations of the use of antimicrobials in patients receiving palliative care.
- Strong consideration should be given to the use of symptom control as the major indication for the use of antimicrobials for the treatment of infections.
- Antimicrobial use has not been shown to significantly affect patients' survival and this information is very valuable to physicians, patients, and caregivers when making decisions about the use of antimicrobials.
- Each patient's specific situation and condition in the palliative care setting must be evaluated in the decision to employ antimicrobials for a suspected or documented infection.

REFERENCES

1 Homsi J, Walsh D, Panta R et al. Infectious complications of advanced cancer. *Support Care Cancer* 2000; **8**: 487–492.
2 Viscoli C. Management of infection in cancer patients: Studies of the EORTC International Antimicrobial Therapy Group (IATG). *Eur J Cancer* 2002; **38**: S82–S87.
3 White PH, Kuhlenschmidt HL, Vancura BG, Navari RM. Antimicrobial use in patients with advanced cancer receiving hospice care. *J Pain Symptom Manage* 2003; **25**: 438–443.
4 Stiel S, Krumm N, Pestinger M et al. Antibiotics in palliative medicine—Results from a prospective epidemiological investigation from the HOPE survey. *Support Care Cancer* 2012; **20**: 325–333.
5 Reinbolt RE, Shenk AM, White PH, Navari RM. Symptomatic treatment of infections in patients with advanced cancer receiving hospice care. *J Pain Symptom Manage* 2005; **30**: 175–182.
6 Vitetta L, Kenner D, Sali A. Bacterial infections in terminally ill hospice patients. *J Pain Symptom Manage* 2000; **20**: 326–334.
7 Pereira J, Watanabe S, Wolch G. A retrospective study of the frequency of infections and patterns of antibiotic utilization on a palliative care unit. *J Pain Symptom Manage* 1998; **16**: 374–381.
8 Chen L, Chou Y, Hsu P, et al. Antibiotic prescription for fever episodes in hospice patients. *Support Care Cancer* 2002; **10**: 538–541.
9 Oneschuk D, Fainsinger R, Demoissac D. Antibiotic use in the last week of life in three different palliative care settings. *J Palliat Care* 2002; **18**: 25–28.
10 Oh DY, Kim JH, Kim DW et al. Antibiotic use during the last days of life in cancer patients. *Eur J Cancer Care* 2006; **15**: 74–79.

11 Lam PT, Chan KS, Tse CY, Leung MW. Retrospective analysis of antibiotic use and survival in advanced cancer patients with infections. *J Pain Symptom Manage* 2005; **30**: 536–543.

12 Chun ED, Rodgers PE, Vitale CA et al. Antimicrobial use among patients receiving palliative care consultation. *Am J Hosp Palliat Med* 2010; **27**: 262–265.

13 Al-Shaqi MA, Alami AH, Al-Zahrani AS et al. The pattern of antimicrobial use for palliative care in-patients during the last week of life. *Am J Hosp Palliat Med* 2012; **29**: 60–63.

14 Brabin E, Allsopp L. How effective are parenteral antibiotics in hospice patients? *Eur J Palliat Care* 2008; **15**: 115–117.

15 Clayton J, Fardell B, Hutton-Potts J et al. Parenteral antibiotics in a palliative care unit: Prospective analysis of current practice. *Palliat Med* 2003; **17**: 44–48.

16 Mirhosseini M, Oneschuk D, Hunter B et al. The role of antibiotics in the management of infection-related symptoms in advanced cancer patients. *J Palliat Care* 2006; **22**: 69–74.

17 Ahronheim JC, Morrison S, Baskin SA et al. Treatment of the dying in the acute care hospital. *Arch Intern Med* 1996; **156**: 2094–2100.

18 Thai V, Lau F, Wolch G et al. Impact of infections on the survival of hospitalized advanced cancer patients. *J Pain Symptom Manage* 2012; **43**: 549–557.

19 Nicolle LE, Bradley SF, Colgan R et al. Infectious Disease Society of America guidelines for the diagnosis and treatment of asymptomatic bacteriuria in adults. *Clin Inf Dis* 2005; **40**: 643–654.

20 Hooton TM, Bradley SF, Cardena DD et al. Diagnosis, prevention, and treatment of catheter-associated urinary tract infections in adults. *Clin Inf Dis* 2010; **50**: 625–663.

21 Mandell LA, Wundernik RC, Anzueto A et al. Infectious Disease Society of America/American Thoracic Society Consensus Guidelines on the management of community-acquired pneumonia in adults. *Clin Inf Dis* 2007; **44**: S27–S72.

22 Stevens DL, Bisno AL, Chambers HF et al. Practive guidelines for the diagnosis and management of skin and soft-tissue infections. *Clin Inf Dis* 2005; **41**: 1373–1406.

23 Bruera E. Intractable pain in patients with advanced head and neck tumors: A possible role of local infection. *Cancer Treat Rep* 1986; **70**: 691–692.

24 Green K, Webster H, Watanabe S, Fainsinger R. Case Report: Management of nosocomial respiratory tract infections in terminally ill cancer patients. *J Palliat Care* 1994; **10**: 31–34.

25 Fabiszewski KJ, Volicer B, Volicer L. Effect of antibiotic treatment on outcome of fevers in institutionalized Alzheimer patients. *JAMA* 1990; **263**: 3168–3172.

78

Pressure ulcers/wounds

KATHRYN G. FROILAND

INTRODUCTION

Skin is an essential organ for physical protection from environmental trauma and for emotional well-being. It functions as a protective barrier providing immunity, thermoregulation, sensation, and synthesis of vitamin D. It performs individual identification and communication roles. Impairment of any of these functions can result in loss of integrity of the skin, which can lead to life-threatening consequences. Age, nutritional status, hydration status, prior sun exposure, current medications, and even the soap used for bathing can affect normal skin function and its ability to heal as breakdown occurs.

Skin breakdown in a patient with cancer can be especially difficult to prevent and treat effectively. Prevention of skin breakdown is essential at all phases of cancer management. The challenges include immunosuppression, infection, edema, prior irradiation of tissue, malnutrition, dehydration, neuropathy, incontinence, and several comorbid conditions (e.g., diabetes mellitus, peripheral vascular disease, autoimmune disorders). These challenges can compromise the ability to heal and may actually prevent healing from occurring. Management of all of these factors must be optimized to progressively heal areas of skin breakdown. Healing often reflects progress in gaining control of the primary cancer disease process. As the cancer becomes resistant to treatment, the potential for skin breakdown increases, and wounds become more difficult to heal.

PATHOPHYSIOLOGY

A pressure ulcer is localized injury to the skin and/or underlying tissue usually over a bony prominence, as a result of pressure, or pressure in combination with shear and/or friction.[1***] The coccyx, sacrum, and heel are most vulnerable, as less soft tissue is present between the bone and skin in these areas than in other areas of the body. Fifty percent of these ulcers develop in the area of the pelvis.[2***] However, they may develop in conjunction with any improperly fitting assistive device. The risk of pressure ulcer formation increases for those who experience atrophy of subcutaneous and muscle tissue layers. Pressure ulcers can be classified in stages that identify tissue layers.

Suspected deep tissue injury: Purple or maroon localized area of discolored intact skin or blood-filled blister due to damage of underlying soft tissue from pressure and/or shear. The area may be preceded by tissue that is painful, firm, mushy, boggy, warmer, or cooler as compared to adjacent tissue.

Stage 1: Intact skin with nonblanchable redness of a localized area usually over a bony prominence. Darkly pigmented skin may not have visible blanching; its color may differ from the surrounding area.

Stage 2: Partial thickness loss of dermis presenting as a shallow open ulcer with a red-pink wound bed, without slough. May also present as an intact or open/ruptured serum-filled blister.

Stage 3: Full thickness tissue loss. Subcutaneous fat may be visible but bone, tendon, or muscle is not exposed. Slough may be present but does not obscure the depth of tissue loss. May include undermining and tunneling.

Stage 4: Full thickness tissue loss with exposed bone, tendon, or muscle. Slough or eschar may be present on some parts of the wound bed. Often include undermining and tunneling.

Unstageable: Full thickness tissue loss in which the base of the ulcer is covered by slough (yellow, tan, gray, green, or brown) and/or eschar (tan, brown, or black) in the wound bed.[1***]

Patients with cancer are at greater risk of pressure ulcer development because they often are older and may have concurrent chronic illnesses. Poorly controlled pain and fatigue may contribute to self-limited mobility during the course of the disease and its treatment. Poor nutritional status is a common finding for patients with cancer, which further impairs their ability to maintain skin integrity and to heal a wound. The situation may be further complicated if the wound is infected or the patient is incontinent.

Friction and shear are extrinsic forces that may exacerbate the effects of pressure on the skin. Friction causes damage to the epidermal and upper dermal layers of the skin caused when two surfaces rub against each other. This may occur when a patient is dragged rather than lifted. Moisture from perspiration or incontinence adds to the force of friction. Shearing force results when friction acts synergistically with gravity. Separation of the skin from underlying structures results when gravity pulls the body downward while resistance from the surface holds the skin in place. Deeper fascia level tissue and blood vessels are primarily affected by shear.[2***]

Although a pressure ulcer can occur at any time during the cancer care continuum, a Kennedy terminal ulcer may develop as a person is dying. These ulcers begin as stage 2 blisters and progress rapidly to stages 3–4 pressure ulcers. They usually occur on the sacral area, are large and superficial, and then change in color from red to yellow, and finally become black. They have been observed most often in older patients rather than in children. The ulcer tends to progress quickly and appears to be a hallmark sign of impending death within 8–24 hours, although some patients have lived up to 2 weeks following the development of the ulceration. Causation may be due to a decline in peripheral perfusion during the dying process. The skin is the largest organ of the body. As the only organ visible to the outside observer, it may reflect the gradual shutdown of function of the internal organs. The ultimate result is multisystem organ failure. Skin organ failure in the form of pressure ulceration over bony prominences occurs over a relatively short period of time and coincides with the patient's death.[3*]

ASSESSMENT AND DIAGNOSIS

Wounds do not exist in isolation. The health-care professional must assess the patient as a whole being to determine the events leading up to the development of a pressure ulcer. This holds true in assessing patients with any type of wound including vascular wounds, diabetic foot ulcers, malignant cutaneous wounds, surgical wounds, burns, or wounds due to trauma. Information on the current status of the underlying cancer disease and its treatment to this point in time is essential. The history of the wound and its management is also necessary for classification and identification of previously unsuccessful treatment strategies. Reasons for delayed healing or progressive deterioration of the wound may be explained by thorough evaluation of the patient's past history and physical status. Remember to position the patient comfortably and medicate if necessary prior to wound assessment and care. Wound assessment and documentation should include the following aspects:

- Anatomical location
- Degree of tissue layer destruction, thickness, and color
- Presence of edema or swelling of tissues
- Length, width, depth, and tunneling using consistent units of measure
- Appearance of the wound bed and surrounding skin
- Drainage and bleeding—specifying amount, color, consistency, odor
- Pain or tenderness of wound and surrounding skin
- Temperature and color of periwound skin[4***]

Wound dimensions can be measured by using a sterile cotton-tipped applicator and a wound measuring guide or ruler. The thumb and forefinger are placed at the point on the applicator that corresponds to the wound's length, width, or depth. Measurements are commonly recorded in centimeters. The depth of tunneling can be measured in the same fashion. The direction of tunneling also can be described. The cotton-tipped applicator is again used to assess the wound for tunneling. The wound is compared to the face of a clock, with 12 o'clock pointing toward the head. Beginning at the 12 o'clock position, progress in a clockwise direction assessing the wound. Document the direction of the existing tunnel(s) according to their corresponding positions on a clock face.[4***] Accurate measurement of the wound serves to describe and then classify the wound.

Potential for further breakdown of the surrounding skin should be assessed so as to plan preventive measures. Excessive dryness, moisture, or nonviable tissue may result in pruritus, pain, and loss of skin integrity. Assessment of the wound for the presence of foreign objects is advised, as these objects may cause infection or delayed healing.

MANAGEMENT

Prevention

A comprehensive program for prevention of the development of pressure ulcers is advised. Monetary savings in the limited use of wound dressings, treatments, or specialized beds, as well as the cost of excess caregiver time, enforces the need for prevention. Any value placed on patient suffering argues for the need for a plan that is comprehensive, but easily implemented.

Risk assessment tools such as the Braden scale or Norton scale for adults, and the Braden Q scale for children, are easy to use and provide basic information useful in developing an individualized plan of care. These scales assess general physical condition, mental status, activity, mobility, incontinence, and nutritional status.[5***]

Following assessment of risk, preventative measures can be implemented and may be helpful in determining reasonable and attainable goals. Basic, but essential, measures include the following:

- Inspecting skin at least daily
- Keeping skin clean and dry
  - Cleanse skin with cleansers or soaps with neutral pH to maintain skin's acid mantle.
  - Apply barrier ointment to protect skin from stool, urine, or perspiration.
  - Consider use of absorbent pads or containment devices for the incontinent patient.
- Preventing friction and shear injuries
  - Use lifting pads and turning sheets when transferring or moving patients.
  - Apply lubricants, thin film dressings, or protectors to heels and elbows.

- Mobilizing patients as tolerated or performing range-of-motion exercises for bedbound patients
- Reducing pressure on tissues
  - Turn and reposition at least every 2 hours.
  - Shift weight if chairbound every 15 min.
  - Avoid positioning on trochanters.
  - Use supports (foam wedges, pillows, heel supports).
  - Off-load heels by placing calves on pillows allowing heels to float above bed surface.[6]***
  - Consider off-loading with a support surface.
  - Avoid massaging skin over bony prominences.[7]**
  - Avoid using foam or rubber rings (i.e., donuts), as they concentrate the intensity of pressure to surrounding tissues.
  - Avoid using sheepskin as it does not relieve pressure.[6]***
- Monitoring nutritional status
  - Assess current and usual weight.
  - Assess history of involuntary weight loss or gain.
  - Assess nutritional intake versus protein, calorie, and fluid needs.
  - Assess appetite.
  - Assess dental health.
  - Assess oral and gastrointestinal history, chewing or swallowing difficulty, and ability to feed him/herself.
  - Assess drug/nutrient interactions.
  - Assess for prior medical/surgical interventions affecting intake or absorption of nutrients.
- Assessing laboratory parameters for nutritional status. Standard measurements of protein status: albumin, transferrin, prealbumin, and total lymphocyte count[8]***

By using an assessment tool for screening, at-risk individuals can be identified early. Incorporating these measures will improve outcomes by reducing the incidence of pressure ulcers and the stress that they incur on the individual and their caregivers.

Treatment

Healing wounds caused by pressure or any other source is the ultimate goal of any treatment plan. However, healing may be unattainable if the patient's cancer disease, effects of treatment, or other medical condition cannot be controlled. Healing may be delayed while the patient is immunosuppressed, malnourished, or infected. Maintaining the wound as is and preventing further deterioration of the wound are realistic goals for a patient with aggressive end-stage disease. Palliation of the symptoms of pain, odor, and itching and managing exudate and bleeding are appropriate goals in this situation.

Prevention strategies of reducing the effects of friction, shear, and pressure must be evaluated and used to prevent further skin breakdown. The patient may become incontinent of urine and/or stool. Establishing a bowel and bladder program may be feasible if the cause can be manipulated. Gentle pH-balanced skin cleansers should be used at each soiling episode. Skin barriers (e.g., creams, ointments, films) may protect and maintain intact skin. Absorbent underpads and diapers should wick moisture away from the skin rather than trapping it against the skin causing maceration. Urinary collection pouches are available for the bedbound female. Condom catheters can be safely used for males. If urinary or fecal incontinence causes contamination or infection of the pressure ulcer, use of an indwelling device is indicated. Indwelling urinary catheters are accessible and easy to care for. Although various types of rectal catheters have been used with considerable morbidity and difficulty, there are several fecal management systems available that have been used successfully in bedbound patients. These devices utilize a rectally placed and secured catheter to collect loose stool. The catheter keeps the wound clean while minimizing pressure to vulnerable bowel mucosa. It is easily inserted and can be maintained in the rectum for several days. Testing of these devices has been done in several acute care settings in patients with various types of wounds. Nosocomial infections have been reduced in high-risk patients.[9]

Good nutrition is essential for maintaining skin integrity and in wound healing. Correcting nutritional deficiencies may or may not be an attainable goal in the palliative care setting. Involving a dietician, nutritionist, and/or nutritional pharmacist in treatment planning is advised. The patient's condition and wishes must be considered when planning to meet nutritional needs. Encouraging consumption of several small meals a day along with protein supplements may be more appealing as the appetite wanes toward end of life.[10]***

Wound care management should be simplified to be comfortable for the patient and achievable for the caregiver. Management techniques must address the following aspects of care:

- Manipulation of the cellular environment
- Prevention or treatment of infection
- Debridement of nonviable tissue
- Promotion of closure of a clean wound
- Protection of wound edges from the effects of excess moisture

Topical wound care is designed to keep the wound moist, clean, warm, and protected from trauma and infection. The choice of an appropriate product(s) depends on

- Amount and character of exudate
- Debridement needs
- Odor control needs
- Compression needs
- Frequency of assessment
- Ease of use by caregiver
- Cost and accessibility

Warmed saline or water can be used as cleansing solutions for chronic wound care. The goal is to clean the wound gently without harming viable tissue. Solution can be applied via soaked gauze sponge or irrigating by pouring solution, using a spray bottle or piston syringe. Irrigation pressure (between 4–15 psi) should be adequate to clean the wound surface without damaging the wound bed or causing it to bleed. A 35 mL. syringe with a 19 gauge needle or angiocatheter produces an 8 psi irrigation pressure stream. Use of commercial wound cleaning products and antiseptic agents is controversial. They require significant dilution to maintain phagocytic function and white blood cell viability. Guidelines can be found online through the National Guidelines Clearinghouse (www.guidelines.gov).[8***] Saline remains acceptable as readily available, comforting, inexpensive, and harmless to the wound bed.

Odor is one of the most distressing symptoms for the patient to cope with. This concern should be addressed even when others cannot detect it. Necrotic tissue, infected tissue, or saturated dressings are sources of odor. There exist several methods of debridement to remove necrotic, devitalized tissue. Surgical or sharp debridement is the fastest method. It is invasive, may require anesthesia, and should not be done if vasculature of the cutaneous tumor places the patient at risk for excessive bleeding. Licensure regulations and institutional policies require that a trained wound care professional perform this type of debridement. Mechanical debridement involves physical force to remove debris and necrotic tissue. It cannot discriminate between viable and nonviable tissue. Although commonly used in the past, wet-to-dry dressings are not recommended as they cause pain, bleeding, and tissue damage upon removal. Enzymatic debridement uses enzymes to dissolve necrotic tissue from the wound. Topical gels and solutions are directly applied to the eschar or applied following scoring of the eschar to allow penetration into the tissue. Autolytic debridement is a process that creates a moist environment allowing the wound bed to rid itself of dead tissue by endogenous proteolytic enzymes and phagocytic cells present in the wound and its drainage. Creation of this environment is achieved by application of an occlusive, semiocclusive, or moisture interactive dressing and/or an autolytic debriding gel directly on to the wound surface. This process is potentially more time-consuming; however, it can be effective and less traumatic than surgical, sharp, or mechanical methods. Biological debridement (larvae/maggot therapy) has resurfaced as a method useful in digesting necrotic tissue and pathogens. Consideration of this method may be appropriate when surgical debridement is not an option.[8***] It is recommended that dry, stable, black eschar on heels should not be debrided if the heel is nontender, nonfluctuant, nonerythematous, and nonsuppurative.[11***]

Chronic wounds are contaminated with surface aerobic pathogens. Wounds may become infected (greater than 10^5 colony-forming units of bacteria) by bacteria that may/may not be normal flora. Odor is associated with anaerobic infection. If infection is suspected, a quantitative culture can be obtained by tissue biopsy or swab culture technique. Use of topical antibiotics is controversial and not supported by clinical research. Systemic antibiotics are warranted if the patient has bacteremia, sepsis, advancing cellulitis, or osteomyelitis.[12***]

Adjunctive therapies utilized in the effort to heal wounds have become available in recent years. Several of these therapies are listed as follows:

- Growth factors
- Electrical stimulation
- Ultrasound
- Electromagnetic therapy

- Noncontact normothermic wound therapy or radiant heat dressing
- Vacuum-assisted wound closure therapy
- Hyperbaric oxygen therapy
  - High-pressure fluid irrigation
  - Ultrasonic mist
  - Ultrasound[8***]

Surgical closure of stage 3 and stage 4 pressure ulcers may be appropriate if the wound does not respond to conservative therapy. This type of intervention is usually reserved for wounds with healing potential.

The shape of the wound and volume of exudate must be matched to the dressing chosen for containment. Changing dressings more than once a day can be burdensome for the caregiver. Painful dressing changes should be avoided by use of contact layer dressings, nonadherent gauze, impregnated gauze, or semipermeable foam dressings. Providing pain medication prior to dressing changes is advised. Alginate, hydrofiber, or foam dressings absorb higher volumes of drainage than hydrocolloids or gauze. Collection of very heavily exudative wound drainage may be accomplished by using a drainable ostomy or wound collection device. These plastic odor-controlling pouches are available in many sizes, have a protective barrier applied to intact surrounding skin, and require changing as infrequently as once a week. Pouches are drained as needed and are less bulky than dressings. Mobility may be facilitated with the use of these products. Charcoal-containing dressings can be used to filter odorous exudate. Silver ion-containing dressings and powders may also be useful in managing odorous and potentially infected wounds. Thousands of wound care products are commercially available. Consultation with a certified wound care specialist is advised for continuity and cost-effective wound care management.

The feasibility of any wound treatment plan must be evaluated and adjusted over time. Consideration of the wound's healing potential, accessibility of therapy, cost, and, most importantly, the patient's wishes and ability to adhere to treatment must be realistically addressed. Management of pain caused by the wound, the removal and application of dressings, and distress caused by seeing the wound must also be acknowledged and resolved. Educating patients and their caregivers in the cause of the wound, its treatment, and in ways to minimize deteriorization must be included in any wound management plan.

Care of a patient with any wound takes time for thorough assessment and ongoing management. Periodic assessment of the wound by health-care providers is necessary, as its characteristics may evolve or the condition and desires of the patient may change. Management goals and treatment plans require review and alteration over time. Patients may present with more than one wound, or more than one type of wound, adding to the complexity of management. Emotional and social issues, pain control, and management of other symptoms of the disease process are challenges that the interdisciplinary palliative care team must address. Of utmost importance, the patients and their families or caregivers need our encouragement, praise, and guidance throughout the course of caring for the wound.

REFERENCES

✶ 1 National Pressure Ulcer Advisory Panel. *Pressure Ulcer Definition and Stages.* Washington, DC: updated 2/2007: http://www.npuap.org.

2 Pieper B. Pressure ulcers: Impact, etiology, and classification. In: Bryant RA, Nix DP, (eds). *Acute & Chronic Wounds: Current Management Concepts,* 4th edn. St. Louis, MO: Elsevier Mosby, 2012: pp. 123–136.

3 Kennedy KL. The Kennedy terminal ulcer. In: Milne CT, Corbett LQ, Dubec DL, (eds). *Wound, Ostomy, and Continence Nursing Secrets.* Philadelphia, PA: Hanley & Belfus, Inc., 2003: pp. 198–199.

4 Hess CT. *Clinical Guide: Skin & Wound Care,* 6th edn. Philadelphia, PA: Wolters Kluwer/Lippincott Williams & Wilkins, 2008: pp. 21–27.

5 Hess CT. *Clinical Guide: Skin & Wound Care,* 6th edn. Philadelphia, PA: Wolters Kluwer/Lippincott Williams & Wilkins, 2008: pp. 35–36.

✶ 6 National Guideline Clearinghouse. Guideline synthesis: Prevention of pressure ulcers. In: *National Guideline Clearinghouse.* Rockville, MD: Agency for Healthcare Research and Quality. December 2006 (revised February 2014). http://www.guideline.gov.

7 Heidrich DE. Skin lesions. In: Kuebler KK, Esper P, (eds). *Palliative Practices from A to Z for the Bedside Clinician.* Pittsburgh, PA: Oncology Nursing Society. 2000: 221–226.

✶ 8 National Guideline Clearinghouse. Guideline Synthesis: Management of pressure ulcers. In: *National Guideline Clearinghouse.* Rockville, MD: Agency for Healthcare Research and Quality. 2006 Dec (revised 2011 January). http://www.guideline.gov.

9 Fecal management systems, 2014. http://www.hollister.com/us/files/pdfs/zassibrochure207.pdf; http://www.convatec.com/flexi-seal-fecal-management-system; http://www.bardmedical.com/DIGNICARE Stool Management System. Accessed May 31, 2012.

10 Langemo D. General principles and approaches to wound prevention and care at end of life: An overview. *Ostomy and Wound Management.* 2012: **58**: 24–34.

11 Black JM, Black SB. Reconstructive surgery. In: Bryant RA and Nix DP, (eds). *Acute & Chronic Wounds: Current Management Concepts,* 4th edn. St. Louis, MO: Elsevier Mosby, 2012: p. 463.

12 Stotts NA. Wound infection: Diagnosis and management. In: Bryant RA and Nix DP, (eds). *Acute & Chronic Wounds: Current Management Concepts,* 4th edn. St. Louis, MO: Elsevier Mosby, 2012: pp. 274–275.

79

Mouth care

FLAVIO FUSCO

INTRODUCTION AND PREVALENCE

In the palliative care patient, oral cavity represents a true "target organ." The mouth plays a fundamental role in many aspects of life: nutrition; hydration; phonation; speech articulation processes; relational and communication activities; and emotional, affective, and sexual relations [1]. Several studies have shown that oral complications and abnormalities of the oral microflora can be found in significant numbers of terminally ill cancer patients, affecting their quality of life. A total of 77 of 99 patients recruited from two Norway palliative care units reported dry mouth, 67% reported mouth pain, and problems with food intake were referred by 56% [2*].

Sweeney and Bagg [3*] studied the prevalence of oral signs and symptoms among a group of 70 terminally ill cancer patients: 68 patients (97%) complained of oral dryness during the day, and 59 patients (84%) complained of oral dryness at night. Oral soreness was reported by 22 patients (31%). Forty-six patients (66%) had difficulty talking, and Thirty-six (51%) reported difficulty eating. Oral mucosal abnormalities were detected in 45 patients (65%), most commonly erythema (20%), coated tongue (20%), atrophic glossitis (17%), angular cheilitis (11%), and pseudomembranous candidiasis (9%). This problem reaches a dramatic evidence in frail population living in poor-resourced settings: a study of 95 children referred for palliative care in Malawi showed that 51% of them had mouth sores and 40% had oral candidiasis [4*].

This chapter describes the major and more frequent oral problems experienced by patients with advanced cancer followed in palliative care programs. Aspects of their management will also be discussed.

INFECTIONS

Fungal and viral infections frequently develop in patients with advanced cancer.

Fungal infections

The most common oral infection is oral candidiasis: high levels of *Candida* have been reported among terminally ill patients, with correspondingly high levels of mucosal disease [5,6*]. Debilitated patients, such as those receiving antibiotics, steroids, cytotoxic therapies, are particularly susceptible to oral candidiasis. Other general factors, such as diabetes mellitus, or predisposing local factors (e.g., poor denture hygiene, presence of xerostomia) are also important in the pathogenesis of oral candidiasis.

There are more than 150 species of *Candida*, but only 10–15 of them are regarded as important pathogens for humans. *Candida albicans* is one of these candidal species, which is found in the oral cavity and responsible for most oral candidal infections.

The *pseudomembranous form* (thrush) is a classic clinical feature, characterized by creamy white, curd-like patches on the tongue and other oral mucosal surfaces. The patches can be removed by scraping and leave a raw, bleeding, and painful surface. Beside the classic lesion, other manifestations include:

- *Acute atrophic candidiasis* or "antibiotic-related stomatitis": This is a nonspecific atrophy of the tongue, associated with burning sensation, dysphagia, and mouth pain.
- *Chronic atrophic candidiasis* (erythematous candidiasis) or "denture sore mouth": This is a chronic inflammatory reaction and epithelial thinning under the dental plates. Dysgeusia is usually present.
- *Angular cheilitis*: This is an inflammatory reaction at the corners of the mouth (not due exclusively to *Candida* but to mixed infection with *Staphylococcus aureus* or, less frequently, beta-hemolytic *Streptococci*). Bleeding may be sometimes present.
- Candida *leukoplakia*, (hyperplasic candidiasis): In this, the lesions are firm, adherent plaques involving the cheek, lips, and tongue. Symptoms are usually absent.

The diagnosis can be made by the clinical appearance of the lesion, by scraping (using either a potassium hydroxide smear or a Gram stain to show masses of hyphae, pseudohyphae, and yeast forms). Other simple methods are swabs, imprint cultures, or culture of oral rinses.

TREATMENT OF ORAL FUNGAL INFECTIONS

Specific antifungal treatment may be provided either topically and systemically.

Nystatin in the form of suspension (100,000 units/mL, 4–6 mL every 6 hours), pastilles, or tablets (100,000 units) is a traditional local treatment. Duration of treatment is usually 10–14 days, but some patients need to continue the treatment for at least 2 weeks after clinical resolution. Miconazole gel is useful for the management of angular cheilitis; it has a weak activity against Gram-positive cocci as well as yeasts [7]. Clotrimazole lozenges (10 mg 5 times a day) are effective and well tolerated in the treatment of oropharyngeal candidiasis forms [8]. Ketoconazole is available in a number of oral and topical forms. The slow therapeutic response, variable absorption, and frequent adverse effects (anorexia, nausea, vomiting, and liver toxicity), all make it a poor choice in patients with advanced cancer. Fluconazole is a triazole with established therapeutic efficacy in candidal infections. It is both an oral and parenteral fungistatic agent that inhibits ergosterol synthesis in yeasts. Fluconazole, 50–100 mg once daily, is one of the most effective treatments of oropharyngeal candidiasis; daily doses of 100–200 mg are recommended for esophageal candidiasis. Extensive clinical studies have demonstrated fluconazole's remarkable efficacy, favorable pharmacokinetics, and reassuring safety profile, all of which have contributed to its widespread use [9,10**]. Itraconazole, structural similar to ketoconazole, has a broader spectrum of action, and it is available in parenteral and oral formulations. To obtain the highest plasma concentration, the tablet is given with food and acidic drinks, whereas the solution is taken in the fasted state.

The most common triazoles-related adverse effects are dose-related nausea, abdominal discomfort, and diarrhea, but symptoms rarely necessitate stopping therapy [11].

Ketoconazole and itraconazole may seriously interact with some of the substrates of CYP3A4. In a double-blind, randomized, three-phase crossover study, Varhe et al. [12**] reported that ketoconazole and itraconazole seriously affect the pharmacokinetics of triazolam and increase the intensity and duration of its effects with potentially hazardous consequences. Azoles have also been implicated in fatal interactions with antihistamines (polymorphic ventricular tachycardia). Caution should be used when fluconazole and methadone are administrated concurrently. [13**,14].

Several studies have showed an emerging high prevalence of non-C. albicans yeasts and azole resistance in the oral flora of patients with advanced cancer: Bagg J et al. [15*] examined the oral mycological flora of 207 patients receiving palliative care. A total of 194 yeasts were isolated, of which 95 (49%) were C. albicans. There was a high prevalence of C. glabrata (47 isolates), of which 34 (72%) were resistant to both fluconazole and itraconazole. Other non-C. albicans species, such as C. parapsilosis, C. kruseii, and, more recently, C. dubliniensis, are less susceptible than C. albicans to fluconazole [16].

In the last years, the echinocandins (caspofungin, micafungin, and anidulafungin) have shown fungicidal activity against most Candida spp., including strains that are fluconazole-resistant [17***]. Posaconazole, a new oral broad-spectrum triazole agent, is active against many species resistant to fluconazole and itraconazole. It is administered as oral suspension, with a favorable toxicity profile and appears to be a promising addition in the antifungal armamentarium [18].

Viral infections

Herpes simplex virus (HSV-1) is the commonest cause of viral infection of the oral mucosa. Herpes viruses are characterized by their ability to establish and maintain latent infections, which can get reactivated. Several stimuli, such as radiotherapy or chemotherapy, can trigger the reactivation of herpes viruses.

Small vesicles usually appear on the pharyngeal and oral mucosa; these rapidly ulcerate and increase in number, often involving the soft palate, buccal mucosa, tongue, and floor of the mouth. Anorexia, fever, mouth pain, and dysphagia may be present. The disease generally runs its course over 10–14 days.

TREATMENT OF ORAL VIRAL INFECTIONS

Acyclovir triphosphate is available as a topical 5% ointment, an intravenous form, and an oral form. In the immunocompromised patients, acyclovir is useful as both treatment and suppression of recurrent mucocutaneous HSV lesions [19**]. Penciclovir, a novel acyclic nucleoside analogue, has demonstrated efficacy against HSV types 1 and 2 and seems to have a pharmacological advantage due to a prolonged half-life of its active form in HSV-infected cells [20,21**].

Al-Waili [22*] carried out an interesting, small, prospective, randomized trial that compared topical application of honey with acyclovir cream in patients with recurrent episodes of labial and genital herpes simplex lesions. For labial herpes, the mean duration of attacks, occurrence of crust, healing time, and pain duration were significantly lower when treated with honey when compared with acyclovir treatment (p < 0,05).

XEROSTOMIA

Xerostomia, defined as the subjective feeling of oral dryness, is one of the five most common symptoms affecting patients with advanced cancer, with a reported prevalence between 30% and

Box 79.1 Main causes of xerostomia in patients with advanced cancer

Related to Cancer Itself

- Head and neck cancer
- Obstruction/compression/destruction of the salivary glands

Related to Dehydration

- Anorexia, poor fluid intake
- Diarrhea, vomiting
- Hemorrhage
- Fever
- Oxygen supply

Related to Treatment

- Radiotherapy
- Oral and jaw surgery
- Drug therapy: Anticholinergics, antihistamines; antihypertensive/diuretics; opioid analgesics; nonsteroidal anti-inflammatory drugs (NSAIDs); corticosteroids; proton pump inhibitors

Related to Concurrent Disorders

- Sjögren syndrome
- Diabetes (mellitus and insipidus)
- Sarcoidosis
- Thyroid dysfunctions
- Anxiety/depression states

substance by its antimicrobial, buffering, and cleansing activities: thus, dental caries and dental erosions are often seen in terminally ill patients [3,24].

MANAGEMENT OF XEROSTOMIA

The primary management of xerostomia involves treatment of underlying cause. Take a detailed treatment history. Discontinuation or substitution of regimens of xerostomic drugs may sometimes be possible. Patients with ill-fitting dentures can be advised to see their dentist: relining of dentures can improve their fit and function and help to lessen oral pain and dryness caused by the lack of support for dentures. Dentate patients should receive preventive or dietary advice, as well as treatment of any caries present.

Current therapy for chronic xerostomia involves the use of salivary substitutes or salivary stimulants. Pilocarpine is a muscarinic agonist, although it does have some effect on the beta-adrenergic receptors in the salivary and sweat glands. There have been a number of double-blind, randomized controlled studies that have shown that pilocarpine is an effective treatment for radiation and drug-induced xerostomia. Davies et al. [27**], in a multicenter, crossover study, compared a mucin-based artificial saliva with oral formulation of pilocarpine hydrochloride in 70 patients with advanced disease and xerostomia. The pilocarpine formulation was found to be more effective than artificial saliva, but it was found to be associated with more side effects such as sweating, lacrimation, and dizziness. Extreme caution in the use of pilocarpine is important due to reported side effects of glaucoma, cardiac disturbances, and sweating. For this reason, other studies explored the possibility to use other saliva stimulants. Davies [28**] carried out a prospective, randomized, open, crossover study comparing a mucin-based artificial saliva with a low-tack, sugar-free chewing gum in the management of xerostomia in 43 patients with advanced cancer. Chewing gum is a saliva stimulant. It produces an increase in salivary flow due to a combination of stimulation of chemo- and mechanoreceptors. In this study, both artificial saliva and chewing gum were effective in the management of xerostomia, but 61% of the patients preferred the chewing gum to the artificial saliva. The use of chewing gum may be limited by the presence of jaw and oral discomfort, headache, and swallowing difficulties.

A variety of saliva substitutes are now commercially available. The substitutes contain different synthetic polymers as thickening agents, for example, carboxymethylcellulose, polyacrylic acid, and xanthan gum, but conflicting results have been reported [1,3,24,29]. Recent developments—still in the experimental stage—include bioactive salivary substitutes and mouthwashes containing antimicrobial peptides to protect the oral tissues against microbial colonization and to suppress and to cure mucosal and gingival inflammation [29].

97% [1,23,24]. Indeed, despite the high prevalence of this distressing symptom—which may contribute to mouth pain and oral infections—there has been relatively little research into this "orphan topic in supportive care" [25].

There are many general causes of xerostomia (Box 79.1), but drug therapies are probably the most important, via a number of different mechanisms: the direct effects include interference with the nerve supply to the salivary glands (e.g., antidepressants), or with the productive capacity of salivary glands (e.g., diuretics, opioids). The indirect effects include imbalance with the normal stimuli to the secretion of saliva [26*].

The effects of xerostomia on patient's symptoms are numerous: the absence of protective effect of saliva on the oral mucosa is a facilitating factor of exogenous bacterial colonization and infections and the loss of lubrification makes swallowing, chewing difficult and painful. Another feature of xerostomia is taste alteration with a subsequent loss of appetite. The sensation of burning, soreness, and dryness sensations may have a considerable effect on speech, with subsequent fall in mood state and relational abilities. Saliva also plays an important role in preventing the loss of tooth

A randomized, controlled trial of standard fractionated radiation with or without amifostine 200 mg/m^2, before each fraction of radiation, was conducted in 315 patients with head and neck cancer. Amifostine administration was associated with a reduced incidence of grade >/= 2 xerostomia over 2 years of follow-up (p = 0.002), an increase in the proportion of patients with meaningful (>0.1 g) unstimulated saliva production at 24 months (p = 0.011), and reduced mouth dryness scores on a patient benefit questionnaire at 24 months (p < 0.001) [30**].

A recent, systematic review was carried out by a task force of the Multinational Association of Supportive Care in Cancer (MASCC) and International Society of Oral Oncology (ISOO) to assess the literature for management strategies and economic impact of salivary gland hypofunction and xerostomia induced by cancer therapies and to determine the quality of evidence-based management recommendations. There was evidence that salivary gland hypofunction and xerostomia induced by cancer therapies can be prevented or symptoms be minimized with intensity-modulated radiation therapy (IMRT), amifostine, muscarinic agonist stimulation, oral mucosal lubricants, acupuncture, and submandibular gland transfer [31***].

CHEMOTHERAPY-/RADIATION-INDUCED STOMATITIS

The oral mucosa is frequently damaged during chemotherapy/radiotherapy in patients with cancer, leading to a high incidence of oral and esophageal mucositis. Patients with mucositis often experience considerable pain and discomfort. The incidence of oral mucositis ranges from 15% to 40% in patients receiving stomatotoxic chemotherapy or radiotherapy, raising to 80% in patients with head and neck cancer [32***].

Raber-Durlacher et al. [33*] reported a retrospective analysis of the incidence and the severity of chemotherapy-associated oral mucositis in 150 patients with various solid tumors. Eighty-seven episodes of mucositis occurred in 47 (31%) patients. Twenty-six patients each experienced only one episode, whereas twenty-one patients had up to eight episodes of mucositis. Multivariate analysis identified the administration of paclitaxel, doxorubicin, or etoposide as an independent risk factor (adjusted rate ratio 8.06, 7.35, and 6.70, respectively), whereas low body mass was associated with a slightly increased risk (adjusted rate ratio 0.92).

Other anticancer drugs, such as alkylating agents, vinca alkaloids, antimetabolites, and antitumor antibiotics, are especially liable to cause stomatitis, and it is important to carefully consider their use in patients with advanced cancer [34].

Both chemotherapy and radiotherapy interfere with cellular mitosis and reduce the regenerative property of the oral mucosa. A poor nutritional status further interferes with mucosal regeneration; oral infections can exacerbate the

mucositis and may lead to systemic infections. If the patient develops both severe mucositis and thrombocytopenia, oral bleeding may occur and this may be difficult to treat.

Direct stomatotoxicity usually is seen 5–7 days after the start of chemotherapy or radiotherapy; in non-immunocompromised patient, oral lesion heals within 2–3 weeks. The most common sites include the buccal, labial, and soft palate mucosa, as well as the floor of the mouth and the ventral surface of the tongue [34].

MANAGEMENT OF CHEMOTHERAPY-/RADIATION-INDUCED STOMATITIS

A Cochrane Review was conducted in 2006 to evaluate the effectiveness of prophylactic agents for oral mucositis in patients receiving treatment, compared to other interventions, placebo, or no treatment. It included 5217 randomized patients. Of the 29 interventions included in trials, 10 showed some evidence of benefit. Only amifostine, antibiotic paste or pastille, hydrolytic enzymes, and ice cubes showed a significant difference when compared with placebo or no treatment in more than one trial. Benzydamine, calcium phosphate, honey, oral care protocols, povidone and zinc sulphate showed some benefit in only one trial [35***]. Topical anesthetics, mixtures (also called cocktails), and mucosal coating agents have been used despite the lack of experimental evidence supporting their efficacy.

In the last 5 years, palifermin, a recombinant humanized keratinocyte growth factor (rHuKGF), has demonstrated an ability to decrease the incidence and duration of mucositis in randomized, placebo-controlled studies and in systematic reviews. The drug seems to be generally well tolerated, but most patients experienced thickening of oral mucosa, flushing, and dysgeusia [36***,37**].

Biswal BM et al. [38**] carried out the first prospective, randomized trial to evaluate the effect of pure natural honey with radiation-induced mucositis. Forty patients undergoing radiotherapy to the head and neck region received topical application of the honey along with radiotherapy or radiotherapy alone. A significant reduction in the symptomatic grade 3–4 mucositis (Radiation/Toxicity Oncology Grading system (RTOG) grading system) was found in the honey-group in respect to controls (p = 0.0005). Another recent Egyptian study tried to evaluate the effect of topical application of honey and a mixture of honey, olive oil-propolis extract, and beeswax (HOPE) in the treatment of oral mucositis in 90 pediatric patients with acute lymphoblastic leukemia and oral mucositis grades 2 and 3. Generally, in both grades of mucositis, honey produced faster healing than either HOPE or controls (p < 0.05) [39**].

The potential analgesic effect of topical morphine, prepared with taste supplements, in treating persistent mucosal pain in palliative care patients, has been explored in two studies. In one study, mouth rinses with morphine were superior to topical lidocaine in treating pain due to chemotherapy-associated mucositis [40*]. In another, randomized, double-blind study, an oral application of 2 per thousand morphine solution in patients suffering from radiotherapy- and/or chemotherapy-induced oral mucositis showed a pain alleviation 1 hour after mouthwash. Duration of pain relief was 123.7 (standard deviation [SD] +/– 98.2) minutes for morphine mouthwash [41**].

ALTERED TASTE SENSATIONS

A reduction (hypogeusia), distortion (dysgeusia), or absence (ageusia) of normal taste sensation is common in patients with cancer, and can be the result of the disease itself and/ or its treatment (drug therapy, chemotherapy, radiotherapy). Between 25% and 50% of patients with cancer are reported to experience taste changes. A recent longitudinal, observational study showed that the prevalence of taste alterations in patients receiving chemotherapy was alarmingly high (69.9%). Patients receiving irinotecan courses reported significantly more taste alterations than patients in other treatment groups [42*]. Taste alterations often start at the beginning of chemotherapy and may persist for weeks or even months beyond its termination [43]. Typically, patients appeared to have difficulty in differentiating sour and bitter tastes, which are affected more than salty and sweet tastes. Women appeared to report greater changes in taste than men [1,44,45]. Zinc deficiency has been linked with abnormalities in taste sensation.

MANAGEMENT OF ALTERED TASTE SENSATIONS

Nonpharmacological treatment includes mouth care, dental hygiene improvement, the withdrawal of drugs that can induce the symptoms, and dietary advice. The urea content in the diet can be reduced by eating white meats and eggs. This masks the bitter taste of food. Food should be eaten cold or at room temperature.

Ripamonti C et al. [46**], in a randomized, double-blind, placebo-controlled trial, described the beneficial effects of oral zinc sulphate tablets (45 mg 3 times a day) in 18 patients with cancer receiving external radiotherapy (ERT) to the head and neck region. One month after ERT was terminated, the patients receiving zinc sulphate had a quicker recovery of taste acuity than those receiving placebo.

A recent, randomized, double-blind, placebo-controlled, pilot trial described the impact of delta-9-tetrahydrocannabinol (THC) on taste and smell (chemosensory) perception in 46 adults with advanced cancer. Compared with placebo, THC-treated patients reported improved (p = 0.026) and enhanced (p < 0.001) chemosensory perception and food "tasted better" (p = 0.04) [47**].

ORAL LESIONS IN HIV/AIDS PATIENTS

Oral candidiasis, hairy leukoplakia, Kaposi sarcoma, necrotizing ulcerative gingivitis, linear gingival erythema, necrotizing ulcerative periodontitis, and oral non-Hodgkin lymphoma are strongly associated with human immunodeficiency virus (HIV) infection and may be present in up to 80% of people with acquired immune deficiency syndrome (AIDS) [48]. These lesions parallel the decline in number of CD4 cells and an increase in viral load. Cross-sectional studies have associated low CD4 lymphocyte count with the presence of oral Kaposi sarcoma, non-Hodgkin lymphoma, and necrotizing ulcerative periodontitis [49*].

Highly active antiretroviral therapy (HAART) has altered the prevalence and incidence of oral mucosal lesions of HIV infection. Although oral candidiasis appears to be the infection more significantly decreased after the introduction of HAART, recent reports show a variation in the prevalence of oral mucosal lesions in different population groups. A cross-sectional estimation of the prevalence of oral mucosal lesions was carried out in 101 HIV-infected ethnic Chinese in Hong Kong. The prevalence of oral mucosal lesions was more common in patients who were classified at baseline as Centers for Disease Control (CDC) C3 category than CDC A2, A3, B2, and B3 (p < 0.05). An overall prevalence of 1.98% was observed for oral Kaposi' sarcoma [50*]. Another study, aimed to determine the therapeutic effects of HAART on the clinical presentations of HIV related oral lesions (HIV-ROLs) in 142 Nigerian adults recruited into the HAART program of an AIDS referral centre, showed that parotid gland enlargement, melanotic hyperpigmentation, and Kaposi's sarcoma were more persistent and had slower response to HAART [51].

HAART may predispose to human papilloma virus infection and potentially increase the risk of later oral squamous cell carcinoma [52*,53]. Regimens based on Protease Inhibitors (PI) may also have adverse effects including oral problems such as paresthesia, taste disturbances, and xerostomia, and may interact with a number of drugs used in oral health care [54].

MANAGEMENT OF ORAL LESIONS IN PATIENTS WITH HIV/AIDS

The grater majority of HIV/AIDS affected people reside today in the developing world and do not have affordable access to HAART and/or conventional antifungal therapy (clotrimazole, fluconazole, and itraconazole). For this reason, some less expensive and more readily available alternatives are being tested: in Malawi, gentian violet was found to be as effective as nystatine for the management of oral candidiasis; topical chlorhexidine, in a pilot-study, also showed promise in the prevention of oral candidiasis in HIV-infected children; the essential oral oil solution of *Melaleuca Artenifolia* (tea tree oil) has been successfully used to treat fluconazole-refractory oropharyngeal candidiasis in AIDS patients [48,55,56]. In poor-resourced limited settings, thalidomide may be a cheap palliative therapy for mucocutaneous pediatric Kaposi sarcoma [48].

OSTEONECROSIS OF THE JAW

Osteonecrosis of the jaw has been shown to be associated with the use of pamidronate and zoledronic acid, two bisphosphonates that inhibit bone resorption and thus bone renewal by suppressing the recruitment and activity of osteoclasts. People at risk include those with multiple myeloma and cancer metastatic to bone who are receiving intravenous bisphosphonates. The risk of developing complication appears to increase with the time of use of the medication [57***,58*].

The predilection for mandibular molar and premolar regions and the infectious conditions that often precede the onset of osteonecrosis support recent pathogenesis theories stating that local inflammation and associated pH changes may trigger the release and activation of nitrogen-containing bisphosphonates, ultimately resulting in necrosis [59*].

Bamias A et al. [60*] studied the incidence, characteristics, and risk factors for the development of osteonecrosis of the jaw among 252 patients with advanced cancer. The incidence increased with time to exposure from 1.5% among patients treated for 4–12 months to 7.7% in those treated for 37–48 months. The cumulative hazard was significantly higher with zoledronic acid compared with pamidronate alone or pamidronate and zoledronic acid sequentially (p < 0.001). In addition, some authors have reported a few cases of osteonecrosis of the jaw in patients taking oral doses of alendronate to treat osteoporosis or osteopenia [61*,62].

Comorbid factors may play a role, such as the presence of diabetes mellitus, the degree of immunosuppression, the use of other medications (chemotherapeutic agents, corticosteroids). Other drug-related risk factors include the use of antiangiogenic agents such as thalidomide and bortezomib in patients with multiple myeloma [63]. Local comorbid factors include oral health status, presence of infection, and the history of radiation therapy.

A survey conducted by the International Myeloma Foundation, in 1203 patients receiving intravenous bisphosphonate therapy for the treatment of myeloma or breast cancer, showed that 81% of the patients with myeloma and 69% of the patients with breast cancer who developed osteonecrosis had underlying dental disease, such as infection, or had a dental extraction, as compared with 33% of the patients who did not develop osteonecrosis [58*].

The most common initial complaint is the sudden presence of intra-oral discomfort and the presence of roughness that may traumatize the oral soft tissues surrounding the area of necrotic bone. The classic clinical features are a growing, painful, and unilateral swelling with jaw pain and difficulty in

---

Box 79.2 Bisphosphonate-associated osteonecrosis of the jaw: Preventive measures

- Clinical dental examination: Comprehensive extraoral and intraoral examination; full-mouth radiographic series plus panoramic radiograph; evaluation of third molars
- Removal of abscessed and nonrestorable teeth
- Restore periodontal health status (pocket elimination, plaque reduction)
- Caries control, elimination of defective restorations
- Oral hygiene and self-care education
- Functional rehabilitation of salvageable dentition (endodontic therapy)
- Properly fitting dentures
- Scheduled periodic follow-up visits

---

chewing and brushing teeth [64]. The mandible and maxilla, with or without oroantral fistulae, are the main areas affected by osteonecrosis.

MANAGEMENT OF OSTEONECROSIS OF THE JAWS

The treatment in patients receiving oral or intravenous bisphosphonate therapy is principally preventive in nature [57***]. Ruggiero et al. [61*], in a case series of 63 patients, reported that despite several treatment modalities, such as minor debridement, major surgical sequestrectomies, partial or complete maxillectomies, and hyperbaric oxygen therapies, no healing occurred in any of the patients treated. For this reason, preventive measures prior to the initiation of intravenous bisphosphonate therapy are of paramount importance, with the dentist and oncologist working collaboratively. In an observational, longitudinal, noncontrolled study of a 43 consecutive patients treated with zoledronate who underwent tooth extractions, the removal of the alveolar bone after the tooth extractions (alveolectomy) and correct antimicrobial prophylaxis (antibiotics and mouthwash) could reduce the risk of occurrence of osteonecrosis [65*].

Box 79.2 summarizes the potential preventive measures in osteonecrosis of the jaw.

There is no scientific evidence to support the discontinuation of bisphosphonate therapy to promote healing of necrotic osseous tissues in the oral cavity [57***].

Systemic antibiotic therapy to control secondary infection and pain may be beneficial and should be administered whenever active infection is present. Antibiotics that have been found useful for osteonecrosis include penicillin or amoxicillin and, in the presence of penicillin-related allergy, clindamycin or erytromycin ethylsuccinate. A 0.12% chlorhexidine antiseptic mouthwash, or minocycline hydrochloride, can be useful for periodontal pockets [66*,67*].

Key learning points

- Oral disturbances are frequently experienced by patients with advanced cancer.

- The most common problems are xerostomia, fungal infections, therapies-related mucositis, and taste disturbances.

- Azoles resistance may become a clinical problem in the treatment of oral fungal infections.

- Improving dental and oral hygiene, good fluid intake, ice chips, and dietary advice are the mainstay of nonpharmacological prophylaxis and treatment of xerostomia, mucositis, and taste alterations in palliative care patients.

- Honey can be a cheaper and worldwide available choice for treating herpes simplex lesions and radiation-induced mucositis.

- In poor-resourced limited-settings, mouth care for people with AIDS is a basic clinical strategy.

- Bisphosphonate-related osteonecrosis of the jaw is a challenging problem in palliative care: Prevention of the osteonecrosis is the best approach to management of this complication.

REFERENCES

● 1 De Conno F, Sbanotto A, Ripamonti C, Ventafridda V. Mouth care. In: Doyle D. et al. (Eds.) *Oxford Textbook of Palliative Medicine*, 3rd edn. Ofxord, U.K.: Oxford University Press, 2004.

● 2 Wilberg P, Hjermstad MJ, Ottesen S, Herlofson BB. Oral health is an important issue in end-of-life cancer care. *Support Care Cancer* March 21, 2012 Epub ahed of print.

◆ 3 Sweeney MP, Bagg J. The mouth and palliative care. *Am J Hosp Palliat Care* 2000 **17** (2): 118–124.

4 Lavy V. Presenting symptoms and signs in children referred for palliative care in Malawi. *Palliat Med* 2007; **21** (4): 333–339.

5 Finlay IG. Oral symptoms and candida in the terminally ill. *Br Med J* 1986; **292**: 592–593.

6 Davies AN, Brailsford SR, Beighton D, Shorthose K, Stevens VC. Oral candidosis in community-based patients with advanced cancer. *J Pain Symptom Manage* 2008; **35** (5): 508–514.

7 Roed-Petersen B. Miconazole in the treatment of oral candidosis. *Int J Oral Surg* 1978; **7**: 558–563.

8 Meunier F, Paesmans M, Autier P. Value of antifungal prophylaxis with antifungal drugs against oropharyngeal candidiasis in cancer patients. *Eur J Cancer* 1994; **30**: 196–199.

9 Meunier F. Fluconazole treatment of fungal infections in the immunocompromized host. *Semin Oncol* 1990; **17** (S6): 19–23.

● 10 Goodman JL, Winston DJ, Greenfield RA et al. A controlled trial of fluconazole to prevent fungal infections in patients undergoing bone marrow tranplantation. *N Engl J Med* 1992; **326**: 845–851.

◆ 11 Perfect JR, Lindsay MH, Drew RH. Adverse drug reactions to systemic antifungals. *Drug Safety* 1992; **7**: 323–363.

● 12 Varhe A, Olkkola KT, Neuvonen PJ. Oral triazolam is potentially hazardous to patients receiving systemic antimycotics ketoconazole or itraconazole. *Clin Pharmacol Ther* 1994; **56**: 601–607.

● 13 Cobb MN, Desai J, Brown LS Jr, Zannikos PN, Rainey PM. The effect of fluconazole on the clinical pharmacokinetics of methadone. *Clin Pharmacol Ther* 1998; **63**: 655–662.

14 Tarumi Y, Pereira J, Watanabe S. Methadone and fluconazole: Respiratory depression by drug interaction. *J Pain Symptom Manage* 2002; **23** (2): 148–153.

● 15 Bagg J, Sweenwy MP, Lewis MAO et al. High prevalence of non-albicans yeasts and detection of anti-fungal resistance in the oral flora of patients with advanced cancer. *Palliat Med* 2003; **17**: 477–481.

16 Davies A, Brailsford S, Broadley K, Beighton D. Resistance amongst yeasts isolated from the oral cavities of patients with advanced cancer. *Palliat Med* 2002; **16**: 527–531.

◆ 17 Sucher AJ, Chahine EB, Balcer HE Echinocandins: The newest class of antifungals *Ann Pharmacother* 2009; **43**: 1647–1657.

18 Rachwalski EJ, Wieczorkiewicz JT, Scheetz MH. Posaconazole: An oral triazole with an extended spectrum of activity *Ann Pharmacother* 2008; **42** (10): 1429–1438.

19 Rooney JF, Straus SE, Manix ML et al. Oral acyclovir to suppress frequently recurrent herpes labialis. A double-blind, placebo controlled trial. *Ann Intern Med* 1993; **118**: 268–272.

20 Schmid-Wendtner MH, Korting HC. Penciclovir cream improved topical treatment for herpes simplex infection. *Skin Pharmacol Physiol* 2004; **17**: 214–218.

21 Raborn GW, Martel AY, Lassonde M et al. Effective treatment of herpes simplex labialis with penciclovir cream: Combined results from two trials. *J Am Dent Assoc* 2002; **133**: 303–309.

22 Al-Waili NS. Topical honey application vs. acyclovir for the treatment of recurrent herpes simplex lesions. *Med Sci Monit* 2004; **10**:MT94–MT98.

23 Ventafridda V, De Conno F, Ripamonti C, Gamba A, Tamburini M. Quality-of-life assessment during a palliative care program. *Ann Oncol* 1990; **1**: 415–420.

24 Sweeney MP, Bagg J, Baxter WP, Aitchinson TC. Oral disease in terminally ill cancer patients with xerostomia. *Oral Oncol* 1998; **34**: 123–126.

25 Senn HJ. Orphan topics in supportive care: How about xerostomia? *Support Care Cancer* 1997; **5**: 261–262.

● 26 Davies AN, Broadley K, Beighton D. Xerostomia in patients with advanced cancer. *J Pain Symptom Manage* 2001; **22**: 820–825.

● 27 Davies AN, Daniels C, Pugh R, Sharma K. A comparison of artificial saliva and pilocarpine in the management of xerostomia in patients with advanced cancer. *Palliat Med* 1998; **12**: 105–111.

● 28 Davies AN. A comparison of artificial saliva and chewing gum in the management of xerostomia in patients with advanced cancer. *Palliat Med* 2000; **14**: 197–203.

29 Vissink A, Burlage FR, Spijkervet FK, Veerman EC, Nieuw Amerongen NV. Prevention and treatment of salivary gland hypofunction related to head and neck radiation therapy and chemotherapy. *Support Cancer Ther* 2004; **1**: 111–118.

30 Wasserman TH, Brizel DM, Henke M et al. Influence of intravenous amifostine on xerostomia, tumour control, and survival after radiotherapy for head-and-neck cancer: 2-year follow-up of a prospective, randomised, phase III trial. *Int J Radiat Oncol Biol Phys* 2005; **63**: 985–990.

◆ 31 Jensen SB, Pedersen AM, Vissink A et al. A systematic review of salivary gland hypofunction and xerostomia induced by cancer therapies: Management strategies and economic impact. *Support Care Cancer* 2010; **18**: 1061–1079.

32 Trotti A, Bellm LA, Epstein JB et al Mucositis incidence, severity and associates outcomes in patients with head and neck cancer receiving radiotherapy with or without chemotherapy: A systematic literature review. *Radiother Oncol* 2003; **66**: 253–262.

33 Raber-Durlacher JE, Weijl NI, Abu Saris M, de Koning B, Zwinderman AH, Osanto S. Oral mucositis in patients treated with chemotherapy for solid tumours: A retrospective analysis of 150 cases. *Support Care Cancer* 2000; **8**: 366–371.

34 Pico JL, Avila-Garavito A, Naccache P. Mucositis: Its occurrence, consequences, and treatment in the oncology setting. *Oncologist* 1998; **3**: 446–451.

35 Worthington HV, Clarkson JE, Eden OB. Interventions for preventing oral mucositis for patients with cancer receiving treatment. *Cochrane Database of Systematic Reviews* 2006; **2**: CD000978.

◆ 36 McDonnell AM, Lenz KL. Palifermin: Role in the prevention of chemotherapy- and radiation-induced mucositis *Ann Pharmacother* 2007; **41**: 86–94.

37 Le QT, Kim HE, Schneider CJ, Muraközy G. Palifermin reduces severe mucositis in definitive chemoradiotherapy of locally advanced head and neck cancer: A randomized, placebo-controlled study. *J Clin Oncol* 2011; **29**: 2808–2814.

● 38 Biswal BM, Zakaria A, Ahmad NM. Topical application of honey in the management of radiation mucositis. A preliminary study. *Support Care Cancer* 2003; **11**: 242–248.

39 Abdulrhman M, Samir El Barbary N, Ahmed Amin D, Saeid Ebrahim R. Honey and a mixture of honey, beeswax, and olive oil-propolis extract in treatment of chemotherapy-induced oral mucositis: A randomized controlled pilot study. *Pediatr Hematol Oncol* 2012; **29**: 285–292.

40 Cerchietti LC, Navigante AH, Korte MW et al. Potential utility of peripheral analgesic properties of morphine in stomatitis-related pain: A pilot study. *Pain* 2003; **105**: 265–273.

41 Vayne-Bossert P, Escher M, deVautibault CG et al. Effect of topical morphine (mouthwash) on oral pain due to chemotherapy- and/or radiotherapy-induced mucositis: A randomized double-blinded study *J Palliat Med* 2010; **13**: 125–128.

42 Zabernigg A, Gamper EA Giesinger JM et al. Taste alterations in cancer patients receiving chemotherapy: A neglected side effect? *The Oncologist* 2010; **15**: 913–920.

43 Bernhardson BM, Tishelman C, Rutqvist LE. Self-reported taste and smell changes during cancer chemotherapy. *Support Care Cancer* 2008; **16**: 275–283.

● 44 Twycross RG and Lack SA. (ed). Taste change. In: *Control of Alimentary Symptoms in Far Advanced Cancer*. Edinburgh, Scotland: Churchill Livingstone, 1986; Vol. **4**: pp. 57–65.

● 45 Ripamonti C, Fulfaro F. Taste disturbance. In: Davies A, Finlay I (eds.) *Oral Care in Advanced Disease*. Oxford, New York: Oxford University Press 2004; pp. 115–124.

46 Ripamonti C, Zecca E, Brunelli C et al. A randomised, controlled clinical trial to evaluate the effects of zinc sulfate on cancer patients with taste alterations caused by head and neck irradiation. *Cancer* 1998; **82**: 1938–1945.

47 Brisbois TD, deKock IH, Watanabe SM et al. Delta-9-tetrahydrocannabinol may palliate altered chemosensory perception in cancer patients: Results of a randomized, double-blind, placebo-controlled pilot trial. *Ann Oncol* 2011; **22**: 2086–2093.

◆ 48 Coogan MM, Greensoan J, Challacombe SJ. Oral lesions in infection with human immunodeficiency virus. *Bull World Health Org* 2005; **83**: 700–706.

49 Glick M, Muzyka BC, Lurie D, Salkin M. Oral manifestation associated with HIV-related disease as markers for immune suppression and AIDS. *Oral Surg Oral Med Oral Pathol* 1994; **77**: 344–349.

50 Perera M, Tsang PC, Samaranayake L, Lee MP, Li P. Prevalence of oral mucosal lesions in adults undergoing highly active antiretroviral therapy in Hong Kong. *J Investig Clin Dent* May 10, 2012. doi: 10.1111/j.2041–1626.2012.00124.x.

51 Taiwo OO, Hassan Z. The impact of Highly Active Antiretroviral Therapy (HAART) on the clinical features of HIV- related oral lesions in Nigeria. *AIDS Res Ther* 2010; **25**: 7–19.

52 Ramirez-Amador V, Esquivel-Pedraza L, Sierra-Madero J, Anaya-Saavedra G, Gonzalez-Ramirez I, Ponce-de-Leon S. The changing clinical spectrum of human immunodeficiency virus (HIV)-related oral lesions in 1,000 consecutive patients. A twelve-year study in referral center in Mexico. *Medicine* 2003; **82**: 39–50.

53 Frezzini C, Leao JC, Porter S. Current trends of HIV disease of the mouth. *J Oral Pathol Med* 2005; **34**: 513–531.

● 54 Porter SR, Scully C. HIV topic update: Protease inhibitor therapy and oral health care. *Oral Dis* 1998; **4**: 159–163.

55 Barasch A, Safford MM, Dapkute-Marcus I, Fine DH. Efficacy of chlorhexidine gluconate rinse for treatment and prevention of oral candidiasis in HIV-infected children: A pilot study. *Oral Surg, Oral Med, Oral Pathol, Oral Radiol Endod* 2004; **97**: 204–207.

56 Vazquez JA, Zawawi AA. Efficacy of alcohol-based and alcohol-free melaleuca oral solution for the treatment of fluconazole-refractory oropharyngeal candidiasis in patients with AIDS. *HIV Clinical Trials* 2002; **3**: 379–385.

● 57 Migliorati CA, Casiglia J, Epstein J, Jacobsen PL, Siegel MA, Woo S-B. Managing the care of patients with bisphosphonates-associated osteonecrosis. An American Academy of Oral Medicine position paper. *J Am Dent Assoc* 2005; **136**: 1658–1668.

58 Durie BGM, Katz M, Crowley J. Osteonecrosis of the jaw and bisphosphonates. *N Eng J Med* 2005; **353**: 99–100.

59 Otto S, Schreyer C, Hafner S, Mast G, Ehrenfeld M, Stürzenbaum S, Pautke C. Bisphosphonate-related osteonecrosis of the jaws—Characteristics, risk factors, clinical features, localization and impact on oncological treatment *J Craniomaxillofac Surg* 2012; **40**: 303–309.

60 Bamias A, Kastritis E, Bamia C et al. Osteonecrosis of the jaw in cancer after treatment with bisphosphonates: Incidence and risk factors. *J Clin Oncol* 2005; **23**: 8580–8587.

61 Ruggiero SL, Mehrotra B, Rosenberg TJ, Engroff SL. Osteonecrosis of the jaw associated with the use of bisphosphonates: A review of 63 cases. *J Oral Maxillofac Surg* 2004; **62**: 527–534.

62 Purcell PM, Boyd IW. Bisphosphonates and osteonecrosis of the jaw. *Med J Aust* 2005; **182**: 417–418.

63 Clerc D, Fermand JP, Mariette X. Treatment of multiple myeloma. *Joint Bone Spine* 2003; **70**: 173–186.

64 Sanna G, Zampino MG, Pelosi G, Nolè F, Goldhirsch A. Jaw vascular bone necrosis associated with long-term use of bisphosphonates. *Ann Oncol* 2005; **16**: 1207–1213.

65 Ferlito S, Puzzo S, Liardo C. Preventive protocol for tooth extractions in patients treated with zoledronate: A case series. *J Oral Maxillofac Surg* 2011; **69**: e1–e4.

66 Migliorati CA, Schubert MM, Peterson DE, Seneda LM. Bisphosphonate-associated osteonecrosis of mandibular and maxillary bone. An emerging oral complication of supportive cancer therapy. *Cancer* 2005; **104**: 83–93.

67 Marx RE, Sawatari Y, Fortin M, Broumand V. Bisphosphonate-induced exposed bone (osteonecrosis/osteopetrosis) of the jaws: Risk factors, recognition, prevention, and treatment. *J Oral Maxillofac Surg* 2005; **63**: 1567–1575.

80

Fistulas

FABIO FULFARO, CARLA IDA RIPAMONTI

FISTULAS

A fistula is an abnormal communication between two digestive organs (internal fistula) or between the skin and a hollow organ (external fistula).[1] Fistulas may be classified according to the amount of the output: low output (<200 mL/24 hour period), moderate output (200–500 mL/day), and high output (>500 mL/day).[2] Fistulas may be single or multiple.[3] In oncological patients, the most frequent causes of fistulas are correlated to cancer (local progression of the disease and/or local relapse) and/or treatments (surgery, radiotherapy, chemotherapy, antiangiogenic biological therapy, locoregional liver tumor ablation, photodynamics, endoscopy, and invasive diagnostic procedures) or both[4–16] (Table 80.1).

The onset of a fistula produces various complications: infection (sepsis), electrolyte imbalance, dehydration, malnutrition, cutaneous lesions, bleeding, delay in oncological treatments, psychosocial problems.

Sepsis is the most frequent cause of death in patients with fistulas.[17] Nutritional status as well as a condition of impaired tissue vascularity may be predisposing factors[18,19] (Table 80.2).

GENERAL PRINCIPLES OF TREATMENT

Prior to planning a treatment, it is important to define the objectives to be achieved.

In advanced cancer patients, treatment will be conservative, whereas for a patient with a longer survival expectancy, a more invasive treatment may be performed. Table 80.3 shows the possible conservative[20–22] and nonconservative treatments.[23,24]

Gastrointestinal fistulas may be classified as external (enterocutaneous fistulas) and internal (communication between hollow organs), or according to the anatomical site of onset: esophageal, gastric and duodenal, pancreatic, enteric, and colonic.[18]

Esophageal fistulas

Esophageal fistulas may be classified as esophagorespiratory (particularly esophagotrachealis) and esophagocardiovascular. As far as the first ones are concerned, most of them are due to esophageal carcinoma (75%) and lung cancer (16%).[25,26]

Literature cites some rare cases due to Hodgkin's disease.[27]

The patient's symptoms may be dysphagia, coughing, aspiration, suffocation, and fever.

Whenever the patient's clinical condition allows it, surgery may be performed[28] with an eventual gastrostomy and/or jejunostomy, the use of metallic stents,[29–31] and/or palliative radiotherapy. Chemotherapy is indicated particularly in the presence of lymphomas.

From a prognostic point of view, patients with esophagorespiratory fistula are at high risk of developing lung abscesses, empyema, and pneumonia ab ingestis.[28]

Esophagocardiovascular fistulas are very rare in cancer patients and also include the aortoesophageal fistula, which is mainly caused by the rupture of a thoracic aneurysm into the esophagus, and the esophagocardiac fistula.[4,28]

Gastric and duodenal fistulas

More than 90% of gastric and duodenal fistulas are a consequence of surgery in those areas.[32] Postoperative fistulas are frequently due to an "anastomotic leak" and abscess formation. Cancers of the transverse colon, stomach, and duodenum are more prone to fistulization. Other rare causes are lymphomas and the placing of pumps for chemotherapy infusion in the gastroduodenal artery.[10] While external fistulas are easily diagnosed, internal fistulas that can cause diarrhea and nutritional deficit are less detectable.

Most postoperative gastrointestinal fistulas heal spontaneously within 4–5 weeks. Factors associated with poor healing or delayed healing include multiple fistulous tracts, malnutrition, acute infection or sepsis, level of serum

Table 80.1 *Causes of fistulas in cancer patients*

Causes correlated to treatments	Surgery
	Radiotherapy
	Chemotherapy
	Photodynamics
	Endoscopy
	Invasive diagnostic procedure
Causes correlated to cancer	Tumoral local progression
	Locoregional relapse of the disease
Mixed causes (correlated to treatments and to cancer)	

Table 80.2 *Frequent complications induced by the fistulas*

Infection → sepsis
Hydro-electrolytic losses
Malnutrition
Skin lesions
Hemorrhages
Delay in oncological treatments
Psychosocial problems

Table 80.3 *General management of fistulas*

Conservative treatment
- Skin care and local disinfection
- Pouching of secretions (particularly gastric and pancreatic)
- Control of odor, delicate fistula areas, use of antibiotics against anaerobic bacteria (metronidazole)
- Control of local itching and pain
- Control of infections (specific antibiotic treatment, care in the use of corticosteroids, RT, and chemotherapy)
- Control of nutrition and electrolytes (particularly in high-output fistulas) and eventual TPN and antisecretory treatments (scopolamine, octreotide)
- Treatment of site-related-symptoms (antiemetic, antispastic, antihemorrhagic, antisecretory, use of vasopressin for urinary incontinence, use of urinary catheters)
- Control of psychological conditions (distortion of body image, isolation, social discomfort).

Nonconservative treatment
- Surgical resection of fistula
- Surgical repair with corrective procedures or with myocutaneous flaps
- Colonic and/or urinary diversion
- Endoscopic treatments with metallic stents

transferrin (unfavorable < 200 mg/dL),[33,34] cancer progression, and previous radiotherapy carried out in the involved areas.[17]

Treatment of gastric and duodenal fistulas may be medical, endoscopic, and/or surgical. Nutritional support[35*] and treatment of infection[36*] are essential in the management of postoperative fistula.

Endoscopically, some authorities have reported obliteration of the fistula tract with adhesive fibrin tissue.[37*] For patients with persistent fistulas and a good performance status, three different surgical approaches are described: (1) exclusion, (2) resection, and (3) "closure of the leak."[32] The exclusion of a fistula is not the treatment of choice and is reserved for the very ill patients. This procedure is carried out with a resection of the diseased segment and an exteriorization of the end parts. In this way, an uncontrolled anastomotic leak is converted into a controlled external fistula. However, procedure of choice is the resection of the anastomotic leak with the formation of a new anastomosis. Major contraindications to this procedure are ischemia or tension on the anastomosis. If resection of the anastomotic leak cannot be performed, then closure of the leak with a serosal patch or roux-en-y anastomosis is the preferred surgical alternative.[32]

Pancreatic fistulas

Pancreatic fistulas are more frequently external and are usually complications due to upper abdominal invasive procedures on the pancreas or surrounding area[38] and occur in 6%–25% of pancreaticoduodenectomies.[39] Fistulas are more frequent during the first postoperative week and present a high level of serum amylase. Internal fistulas, which most commonly involve the peritoneum, are rare. They are usually diagnosed by radiological examination (fistulography, CAT scan), ultrasonography, and/or by endoscopic retrograde cholangiopancreatography (ERCP).[40]

Postoperative external fistulas heal spontaneously in 80% of cases with conservative treatment incorporating skin care, drainage and collection of pancreatic secretion, control of infection, and parenteral nutrition (to reduce pancreatic secretion).[40] Octreotide, in doses of 50–200 mcg tid, has been used in the conservative treatment to reduce GI secretion.[41,42] Many authors suggest the use of subcutaneous injection of octreotide at doses of 50–200 mcg tid according to output.[43] Recently, Barnett et al.[44] have expressed some concern about the use of octreotide in the treatment of pancreatic fistula.

Surgical approaches are reserved for situations of conservative management failure in patients with good performance status and a favorable tumor anatomy.[40] The placement of an endoscopic stent has proved effective in certain studies, but a longer follow-up is necessary to evaluate possible long term complications.[40*] A recent randomized trial has demonstrated the role of external stent drainage to reduce postoperative pancreatic fistula after pancreaticojejunostomy.[45**]

Small bowel and colonic fistulas

Intestinal fistulas are classified as internal, external, or mixed; the most common are external (enterocutaneous).[46] Most of them are a consequence of postoperative complications following surgery on GI cancers with diastasis of the anastomotic wound and damage to the bowel and its vascularization.

The severity of enterocutaneous fistula depends on the site and the amount of secretion: for example, a large volume of secretion and small bowel fistulas can be associated with severe fluid and electrolyte abnormalities and malabsorption. In a series of 25 cancer patients with enterocutaneous fistulas, the most frequent site was the jejunum-ileum, and mortality was correlated to previous radiotherapy, the site, fistula output, and the presence of hypoalbuminemia. In 63% of patients, the presence of a fistula brought about the suspension of any ongoing anticancer treatment.[46] A rare presentation of an enterocutaneous fistula may be subcutaneous emphysema.[47]

Enterocutaneous fistulas may heal spontaneously with adequate supportive therapy including total parenteral nutrition (TPN), prevention and treatment of infective complications (in 70% of these cases). Several studies supported the use of somatostatin analogues to reduce secretion volume, but a recent meta-analysis suggests that somatostatin could be better than analogues in relation to the number of fistulas closed and time to closure.[21,48,49***] The use of TPN allows an adequate fluid intake, normalization of electrolytes as well as catabolic blockage. Factors that negatively influence spontaneous closure of the fistula include the presence of cancer together with sepsis, malnutrition, distal obstruction to the fistula, and the epithelialization of the fistulous tract.[50] Surgery is indicated whenever conservative treatment has not been effective and when the patient's condition allows it.[50*] Recently, a case of enterobiliary fistula following radiofrequency on the liver was observed.[51]

Colonic fistulas, although considered uncommon, can also be classified as external, internal (colocutaneous), and mixed.[52] Among the internal fistulas, the most common are colovesical, followed by colovaginal and coloenteric. The most evident sign of colocutaneous fistulas is the passage of air and feces through an incision in the abdominal wall following surgery. Other signs and symptoms are sepsis, fever, tachycardia, leukocytosis, and pain due to abscess with local peritonitis. Patients with an internal fistula complain of various symptoms according to the viscera involved. Patients with colovesical fistulas frequently complain of cystitis, high fever, shivering, and sweating and, if the fistulous tract is wide, pneumaturia and fecaluria. Patients with colovaginal fistulas suffer from an increase of vaginal secretion, sometimes associated with the passage of feces. Patients with coloenteric fistulas suffer from abdominal pain and abundant diarrhea.[53]

The diagnosis of an internal colovesical fistula is obtained by means of a cystoscopy, for colovaginal fistula by means of a fistulogram and/or a vaginogram, for coloenteric fistula by an abdominal CAT scan with contrast.

Colocutaneous fistulas may be conservatively treated even if the rate of healing is lower than in enteric ones, particularly in the presence of a malignancy or a distal occlusion. Some patients may require a surgical bowel diversion.

In the presence of a malignancy, a partial cystectomy performed together with the sigmoid colon is indicated for colovesical fistulas. Radiotherapy-induced fistulas may be complex and often involve more than one organ, for example, the colon or rectum respectively with the bladder, the vagina, the small bowel, and the skin. These fistulas are more difficult to treat because of the low rate of spontaneous healing and the high rate of relapse.[54*] It is possible to treat coloenteric fistulas with stents.[53*]

HEAD AND NECK FISTULAS

As regards the head and neck cancer patients, the most frequent fistulas are pharyngocutaneous and they are the most common complications resulting from total laryngectomy. It was observed that 12%–16% of the patients undergoing laryngectomy develop fistulas 11–14 days after surgery.[55–57] Although spontaneous fistula closure occurs in two-thirds of the cases, about 20% of the patients have to undergo surgery with direct suture of pharyngeal mucosa or reparative surgery by means of a deltopectoral flap or a pectoralis major myocutaneous flap.[58,59]

Negative prognostic factors that give rise to fistulas can be: hemoglobin levels lower than 12.5 g/dL, concomitant heart pathology, extension of surgery, the surgeon's experience, tumor size, and the use of catgut.[55,60] A randomized study demonstrated the efficacy of arginine-supplemented enteral nutrition in this group of patients.[61]

Previous radiotherapy to the head and neck increases the risk of developing fistulas by 10%–12% and the healing rate is lower.[62,63]

In some groups of patients treated with radiotherapy, the percentage of fistulization increases up to 30% after total laryngectomy with prolonged hospitalization.[64,65]

Some authors suggest using growth factors with the aim of preventing infection and sepsis.[66*] The concomitant use of oxygen therapy and radiotherapy favors neovascularization and prevents fistulas from occurring. Another relatively frequent group of fistulas are the esophagotracheal ones, already described in the paragraph: esophageal fistulas.

Other rarer fistulas are the tracheocutaneous, which are often correlated to a long-term tracheostomy, salivary fistulas,[67] oroantral fistulas,[68] and chylous fistulas.[69]

BRONCHOPLEURIC FISTULAS

Bronchopleuric fistulas are often correlated to pneumonectomy in treating lung cancer.[70] The incidence is about 8%–10%.[71]

Significant risk factors involved in the development of fistulas are preoperative infection, dx pneumonectomy and the presence of subcarenal metastatic lymph nodes, preoperative radiotherapy, and diabetes.

From a pathophysiological view point, it is difficult to preserve bronchial arteries in the dissection of the metastatic subcarenal lymph nodes, which adhere to the bronchial tree.

The bronchial arteries ligature or the protrusion of the bronchial stump in the pleura reduces the blood flow to very low levels, thus favoring fistula development.[71] The most common signs and symptoms are: air in the pleural cavity, dyspnea, front chest pain.[72]

The diagnosis is usually carried out through a bronchoscopy, although, recently, scintigraphic techniques with xenon-133 and technetium-99 m have given good results.[73]

Surgery is the first-choice treatment, whenever possible.[72,74]

However, in the case of fistulas smaller than 3 mm, successful results have been found by means of reparative endoscopy.[74,75] A thorough follow-up in the first 3 months after pneumonectomy is indicated as a preventive measure.[74,75]

GENITOURINARY FISTULAS

The incidence of fistulas in the genitourinary tract is about 2% in cancer patients.

The most frequent causes are: surgery (hysterectomy, prostatectomy, rectal resections, pelvic evisceration,[76,77] radiotherapy on the pelvic organs,[78] and locoregional relapses. Signs and symptoms are characterized by urinary incontinence, pain, and itching at the fistula site, pneumaturia, sometimes fecaluria, GI disorders, hemorrhage, and are often present with psychological distress.[79] For diagnostic aims, the following are often used: CAT, MNR, cystoscopy, charcoaluria, and barium enema.[80–82]

As far as the anatomical site is concerned, the most frequent fistulas in this group of patients are: rectovaginal, enterovesical, vesicovaginal, ureterovaginal, urethrocutaneous, and rectoureteral.

The rarer are the vescicocutaneous, the intraperitoneal chylo, and the vescicouterinos.[83,84]

The rectovaginal and enterovesical fistulas are often the consequence of radiotherapy on the pelvis, with necrosis of the vaginal and rectal walls or hysterectomies.[82,85,86]

Carcinomas of the rectum, uterine cervix, and vagina are those most at risk of fistulaization due to the site and necessary treatments.[87] When the fistula is in the lower part of the rectum, fecal incontinence due to involvement of anal sphincter may be present. Surgical treatment consists of colon or urinary stomia.[88*] Profuse hemorrhages can be controlled by embolization.[89]

Vesicovaginal fistulas are often the outcome of hysterectomies[90] and the two orifices are: 1 cm above the trigone for the bladder and the anterior wall for the vagina.

These fistulas heal using a catheter from 12 to 20 days with a closed drainage to prevent infection.[91]

Ureterovaginal fistulas are often the result of radical hysterectomy via laparotomy. The risk of renal damage should always be taken into consideration and the areas most at risk of fistulaization are: common iliac artery, uterine artery, and sacrouterine ligament. The treatment of the fistulas in these areas is the use of the ureteral catheter of Finney, when possible, or eventually an uretero-neocystostomy may be indicated.[92]

Urethrocutaneous fistulas most frequently concern the prostatic urethra as compared to the bulbar urethra.

The urethrocutaneous fistulas are the result of a perineal prostatectomy, and there is almost always a concomitant prostatic abscess. The cutaneous orifice is usually central and in a preanal area. The urethral orifice is located above the urogenital diaphragm and may reach the bladder.[93]

The urethrorectal fistulas are often associated with carcinoma of the rectum, prostate, and bladder with concomitant abscess. The rectal orifice is suprasphincteric concealed behind a mucosal fold or in the Morgagni cyst.

The urethral orifice is situated in the prostatic urethra.[93]

The vescicocutaneous fistulas, rarer, are often correlated to lesions of the bladder fundus on the laparotomic wound. The cutaneous orifice is suprapubic. Contentive treatment is important in these fistulas.[94,95*] The use of some biological agents such as sunitinib may cause in rare cases fistulization.[96]

CONCLUSIONS

In cancer patients, fistulas are complications to be held in consideration due to delays that can be caused in the treatment of cancer as well as in the worsening of the patients' clinical and psychological conditions. Prior to planning a conservative treatment versus an invasive one, it is mandatory to assess the patient's chances of survival as well as his/her quality of life. Considerable effort should be made by caregivers in order to manage all the different symptoms related to this complication in cancer patients.

REFERENCES

1 Doughty D. Principles of fistula and stoma management. In: Berger A., Portenoy RK, Weissman DE (eds.). *Principles and Practice of Supportive Oncology.* Philadelphia, PA: Lippincott-Raven Publishers, 1998: pp. 285–294.

2 Benson DW, Fisher JE. Fistulas. In: Fischer JE (ed.). *Total Parenteral Nutrition,* 2nd edn. Boston, MA: Little, Brown & CO, 1991: pp. 253–262.

3 Oneschuk D, Bruera E. Successful management of multiple enterocutaneous fistulas in a patient with metastatic colon cancer. *J Pain Symptom Manage* 1997; 14:121–124.

4 Allgaier HP, Schwacha H, Technau K, Blum HE. Fatal esophagoaortic fistula after placement of a self-expanding metal stent in a patient with esophageal carcinoma. *New Engl J Med* 1997; 337:1778.

5 Bonomi P., Faber LP, Warren W et al. Postoperative bronchopulmonary complications in stage III lung cancer patients treated with preoperative paclitaxel-containing chemotherapy and concurrent radiation. *Semin Oncol* 1997; 24 (4 Suppl. 12): S123–S129.

6 Bubenik O, Lopez MJ, Greco AO et al. Gastrosplenic fistula following successful chemotherapy for disseminated histiocytic lymphoma. *Cancer* 1983; 52: 994–996.

7 Hagendoorn J, Schipper ME, Cloïn A et al. A patient with tracheoesophageal fistula and esophageal cancer after radiotherapy. *Nat Rev Gastroenterol Hepatol* 2010;7(12):702–706.

8 Gabrail NY, Harrison BR, and Sunwoo YC. Chemo-irradiation induced aortoesophageal fistula. *J Surg Oncol* 1991; 48: 213–215.

9 Gotlieb WH, Amant F, Advani S et al. Intravenous aflibercept for treatment of recurrent symptomatic malignant ascites in patients with advanced ovarian cancer: A phase 2, randomised, double-blind, placebo-controlled study. *Lancet Oncol* 2012;13(2):154–162.

10 Kernstine KH, Kryjeski SR, Hall LJ et al. Gastroduodenal artery-duodenal fistula: A complication of continuous floxuridine (FUDR) infusion into the gastroduodenal artery. *J Surg Oncol* 1990; 45: 59–62.

11 Luketich JD, Westkaemper J, Sommers KE et al. Bronchoesophagopleural fistula after photodynamic therapy for malignant mesothelioma. *Ann Thorac Surg* 1996; 62: 283–284.

12 Ganapathi AM, Westmoreland T, Tyler D, Mantyh CR. Bevacizumab-associated fistula formation in postoperative colorectal cancer patients. *J Am Coll Surg* 2012;214(4):582–588.

13 Schowengerdt CG. Tracheoesophageal fistula caused by a self-expandin esophageal stent. *Ann Thorac Surg* 1999, 67: 830–831.

14 Pua U, Merkle EM. Case report. Spontaneous cholecystocolic fistula and locoregional liver tumour ablation: A cautionary tale. *Br J Radiol* 2011; 84(1008):243–245.

15 Clavo B, Santana-Rodriguez N, López-Silva SM et al. Persistent PORT-A-CATH®-related fistula and fibrosis in a breast cancer patient successfully treated with local ozone application. *J Pain Symptom Manage* 2012; 43(2):3–6.

16 Yamazaki T, Sakai Y, Hatakeyama K, Hoshiyama Y. Colocutaneous fistula after percutaneous endoscopic gastrostomy in a remnant stomach. *Surg Endoscopy* 1999; 13:280–282.

17 Campos AC, Meguid MM, Coelho JC. Factors influencing outcome in patients with gastrointestinal fistula. *Surg Clin North Am* 1996; 76:1191–1198.

18 Berry SM, Fischer JE. Classification and pathophysiology of enterocutaneous fistulas. *Surg Clin North Am* 1996; 76:1009–1118.

19 Sepehripour S, Papagrigoriadis S. A systematic review of the benefit of total parenteral nutrition in the management of enterocutaneous fistulas. *Minerva Chir* 2010; 65(5):577–585.

20 Dudrick SJ, Maharaj AR, McKelvey AA. Artificial nutritional support in patients with gastrointestinal fistulas. *World J Surg* 1999; 23:570–576.

21 Rahbour G, Siddiqui MR, Ullah MR et al. A meta-analysis of outcomes following use of somatostatin and its analogues for the management of enterocutaneous fistulas. *Ann Surg* 2012; 256(6):946–954.

22 Spiliotis J, Briand D, Gouttebel MC et al. Treatment of fistulas of the gastrointestinal tract with total parenteral nutrition and octreotide in patients with carcinoma. *Surg Gynecol Obstet* 1993; 176:575–580.

23 Ahmed HF, Hussain MA, Grant CE, Wadleigh RG. Closure of tracheoesophageal fistulas with chemotherapy and radiotherapy. *Am J Clin Oncol* 1998; 21:177–179.

24 Cozzaglio L, Farinella E, Coladonato M et al. Current role of surgery in the treatment of digestive fistulas. *Ann Ital Chir* 2010; 81(4):285–294.

25 Reed MF, Mathisen DJ. Tracheoesophageal fistula. *Chest Surg Clin North Am* 2003; 13(2):271–289.

26 Chauhan SS, Long JD. Management of tracheoesophageal fistulas in adults. *Curr Treat Options Gastroenterol* 2004; 7(1):31–40.

27 Tse DG, Summers A, Sanger JR, Haasler GB. Surgical treatment of tracheomediastinal fistula from recurrent Hodgkin's lymphoma. *Ann Thorac Surg* 1999; 67:832–834.

28 Fernando HC, Benfield JR. Surgical management and treatment of esophageal fistula.. *Surg Clin North Am* 1996; 76:1123–1135.

29 Schweigert M, Dubecz A, Beron M et al. Management of anastomotic leakage-induced tracheobronchial fistula following oesophagectomy: The role of endoscopic stent insertion. *Eur J Cardiothorac Surg* 2012; 41(5):74–80.

30 Saxon RR, Morrison KE, Lakin PC et al. Malignant esophageal obstruction and esophagorespiratory fistula: Palliation with a polyethylene-covered Z-stent. *Radiology* 1997; 202: 394–404.

31 Miwa K, Mitsuoka M, Tayama K et al. Successful airway stenting using silicone prosthesis for esophagobronchial fistula. *Chest* 2002; 122(4):1485–1487.

32 Chung MA, Wanebo HJ. Surgical management and treatment of gastric and duodenal fistulas. *Surg Clin North Am* 1996; 76:1137–1145.

33 Kuvshinoff BW, Brodish RJ, McFadden DW, Fischer JE. Serum transferrin as a prognostic indicator of spontaneous closure and mortality in gastrointestinal cutaneous fistulas. *Ann Surg* 1993; 217:615–622.

34 Falconi M, Pederzoli P. The relevance of gastrointestinal fistulae in clinical practice: A review. *Gut* 2001; 49 Suppl 4:2–10.

35 Meguid MM, Campos AC. Nutritional management of patients with gastrointestinal fistulas. *Surg Clin North Am* 1996; 76:1035–1080.

36 Rolandelli R, Roslyn JJ. Surgical management and treatment of sepsis associated with gastrointestinal fistulas. *Surg Clin North Am* 1996; 76: 1111–1122

37 Shand A, Reading S, Ewing J et al. Palliation of malignant gastrocolic fistula by endoscopic human fibrin sealant injection. *E J Gastroenterol Hepatol* 1997; 9:1009–1111.

38 Siewert JR, Bottcher K, Stein HJ et al. Problem of proximal third gastric carcinoma. *World J Surg* 1995; 19:523–531.

39 Jimenez RE, Hawkins WG. Emerging strategies to prevent the development of pancreatic fistula after distal pancreasectomy. *Surgery* 2012; 152:64–70.

40 Ridgeway MG, Stabile BE. Surgical management and treatment of pancreatic fistulas. *Surg Clin North Am* 1996; 76:1159–1173.

41 Kawai M, Kondo S, Yamaue H et al. Predictive risk factors for clinically relevant pancreatic fistula analyzed in 1,239 patients with pancreatic oduodenectomy: Multicenter data collection as a project study of pancreatic surgery by the Japanese society of hepato-biliary-pancreatic surgery. *J Hepatobiliary Pancreat Sci.* 2011; 18(4):601–608.

42 Martineau P, Shwed JA, Denis R. Is octreotide a new hope for enterocutaneous and external pancreatic fistulas closure? *Am J Surg* 1996; 172:386–395.

43 Niv Y, Charash B, Sperber AD, Oren M. Effect of octreotide on gastrostomy, duodenostomy, and cholecystostomy effluents: A physiologic study of fluid and electrolyte balance. *Am J Gastroenterol* 1997; 92:2107–2111.

44 Berberat PO, Friess H, Uhl W, Buchler MW. The role of octreotide in the prevention of complications following pancreatic resection. *Digestion* 1999; 60 (Suppl. 2): 15–22.

45 Barnett SP, Hodul PJ, Creech S et al. Octreotide does not prevent postoperative pancreatic fistula or mortality following pancreaticoduodenectomy. *Am Surg.* 2004; 70(3):222–226.

46 Motoi F, Egawa S, Rikiyama T et al. Randomized clinical trial of external stent drainage of the pancreatic duct to reduce postoperative pancreatic fistula after pancreaticojejunostomy. *Br J Surg* 2012; 99(4):524–531.

47 Chamberlain RS, Kaufman HL, Danforth DN. Enterocutaneous fistula in cancer patients: Etiology, management, outcome, and impact on further treatment. *Am Surg* 1998; 64:1204–1211.

48 Correoso LJ, Mehta R. Subcutaneous emphysema: An uncommon presentation of enterocutaneous fistula. *Am J Hosp Palliat Care* 2003; 20(6):462–464.

49 Stevens P, Foulkes RE, Hartford-Beynon JS, Delicata RJ. Systematic review and meta-analysis of the role of somatostatin and its analogues in the treatment of enterocutaneous fistula. *Eur J Gastroenterol Hepatol.* 2011;23(10): 912–922.

50 Sancho JJ, Di Costanzo J, Nubiola P et al. Randomized double-blind placebo-controlled trial of early octreotide in patients with postoperative enterocutaneous fistula. *Brit J Surg* 1995; 82:638–641.

51 Draus JM Jr, Huss SA, Harty NJ et al. Enterocutaneous fistula: Are treatments improving? *Surgery* 2006; 140(4):570–576.

52 Bessoud B, Doenz F,Qanadli SD et al. Enterobiliary fistula after radiofrequency ablation of liver metastases. *J Vasc Interv Radiol* 2003; 14(12):1581–1584.

◆ 53 Lavery IC. Colonic fistulas. *Surg Clin North Am* 1996; 76:1183–1190.

54 Grunshaw ND, Ball CS, Grunshaw ND, Ball CS. Palliative treatment of an enterorectal fistula with a covered metallic stent. *Cardiovasc Intervent Radiol.* 2001; 24(6):438–440.

55 Levenback C, Gershenson DM, McGehee R. et al. Enterovesical fistula following radiotherapy for gynecologic cancer. *Gynecol Oncol* 1994; 52:296–300.

56 McLean JN, Nicholas C, Duggal P et al. Surgical management of pharyngocutaneous fistula after total laryngectomy. *Ann Plast Surg* 2012; 68(5):442–445.

● 57 Makitie AA, Irish J,Gullane PJ. Pharyngocutaneous fistula. *Curr Opin Otolaryngol Head Neck Surg* 2003; 11(2):78–84.

58 Smith TJ, Burrage KJ, Ganguly P et al. Prevention of postlaryngectomy pharyngocutaneous fistula: The Memorial University experience. *J Otolaryngol* 2003; 32(4):222–225.

59 Chambers PA, Worrall SF. Closure of large orocutaneous fistulas in end-stage malignant disease. *Brit J Oral Maxill Surg* 1994; 32:314–315.

◆ 60 Drezner DA, Cantrell H. Surgical management of tracheocutaneous fistula. Ear, *Nose Throat J* 1998; 77:534–537.

◆ 61 Soylu L, Kiroglu M, Aydogan B. Pharyngocutaneous fistula following laryngectomy. *Head Neck* 1998; 20:22–25.

62 DeLuis DA, Izaola O, Cuellar L et al. A randomized double-blind clinical trial with two different doses of arginine enhanced enteral nutrition in postsurgical cancer patients. *Eur Rev Med Pharmacol Sci.* 2010; 14(11):941–945.

63 Viani L, Stell PM, Dalby JE. Recurrence after radiotherapy for glottic carcinoma. *Cancer* 1991; 67:577–584.

64 Grau C, Johansen LV, Hansen HS, Greisen O, Harbo G, Hansen O, Overgaard J. Salvage laryngectomy and pharyngocutaneous fistulae after primary radiotherapy for head and neck cancer. *Head Neck* 2003; 25(9):711–716.

65 McCombe AW, Jones AS. Radiotherapy and complications of laryngectomy. *J Laryngol Otol* 1993; 107:130–132.

66 Cody DT, Funk GF, Wagner D et al. The use of granulocyte colony stimulating factor to promote wound healing in a neutropenic patient after head and neck surgery. *Head Neck* 1999; 21:172–175.

67 Cavanaugh K, Park A. Postparotidectomy fistula: A different treatment for an old problem. *Intern J Ped Otorhinolaryng* 1999; 47:265–268.

68 Aksungur EH, Apaydin D, Gonlusen G et al. A case of oroantral fistula secondary to malignant fibrous histiocytoma. *Eur J Radiol* 1994; 18:212–213.

69 De Gier HH, Balm AJ, Bruning PF, Gregor RT, Hilgers FJ. Systematic approach to the treatment of chylous leakage after neck dissection. *Head Neck* 1996; 18:347–351.

70 Hollaus PH, Lax F, el-Nashef BB et al. Natural history of bronchopleural fistula after pneumonectomy: A review of 96 cases. *Ann Thorac Surg* 1997; 63:1391–1396.

● 71 Yano T, Yokoyama H, Fukuyama Y et al. The current status of postoperative complications and risk factors after a pulmonary resection for primary lung cancer. A multivariate analysis. *E J Cardiothorac Surg* 1997; 11:445–449.

72 Rodriguez AN, Diaz-Jimenez JP. Malignant respiratory-digestive fistulas. *Curr Opin Pulm Med* 2010; 16(4):329–333.

73 Dutau H, Breen DP, Gomez C, Thomas PA, Vergnon JM. The integrated place of tracheobronchial stents in the multidisciplinary management of large post-pneumonectomy fistulas: Our experience using a novel customised conical self-expandable metallic stent. *Eur J Cardiothorac Surg.* 2011;39(2): 185–189.

74 Raja S, Rice TW, Neumann DR et al. Scintigraphic detection of post-pneumonectomy bronchopleural fistulae. *E J Nucl Med* 1999; 26:215–219.

75 Hollaus PH, Lax F, Janakiev D et al. Endoscopic treatment of postoperative bronchopleural fistula: Experience with 45 cases. *Ann Thorac Surg* 1998; 66:923–927.

◆ 76 Varoli F, Roviaro G, Grignani F et al. Endoscopic treatment of bronchopleural fistulas. *Ann Thorac Surg* 1998; 65:807–809.

◆ 77 Karkhanis P, Patel A, Galaal K. Urinary tract fistulas in radical surgery for cervical cancer: The importance of early diagnosis. *Eur J Surg Oncol* 2012; 38(10):943–947.

78 Magrina JF. Complications of irradiation and radical surgery for gynecologic malignancies. *Obstetr Gynecol Surv* 1993; 48:571–575.

79 Tabakov ID, Slavchev BN Large post-hysterectomy and post-radiation vesicovaginal fistulas: Repair by ileocystoplasty. *J Urol* 2004; 171(1):272–274.

● 80 Bahadursingh AM, Longo WE. Colovaginal fistulas. Etiology and management. *J Reprod Med.* 2003; 48(7:489–495.

81 Blomlie V, Rofstad EK, Trope C, Lien HH. Critical soft tissues of the female pelvis: Serial MR imaging before, during and after radiation therapy. *Radiology* 1997; 203:391–397.

82 Lee BH, Choe DH, Lee HJ et al. Device for occlusion of rectovaginal fistula: Clinical trials. *Radiology* 1997; 203:65–69.

◆ 83 Champagne BJ, McGee F. Rectovaginal fistula. *Surg Clin North Am.* 2010; 90 (1):69–82

◆ 84 Narayanan P, Nobbenhuis M, Reynolds KM et al. Fistulas in malignant gynecologic disease: Etiology, imaging, and management. *Radiographics* 2009; 29(4):1073–1083.

◆ 85 Munoz M, Nelson H, Harrington J et al. Management of acquired rectourinary fistulas: Outcome according to cause. *Dis Colon Rectum* 1998; 41:1230–1238.

86 Pesce F, Righetti R, Rubilotta E, Artibani W. Vesico-crural and vesicorectal fistulas 13 years after radiotherapy for prostate cancer. *J Urol* 2002; 168(5):2118–2119.

◆ 87 Rinnovati A, Milli I, Francalanci R. Entero-vesical fistulae in surgical practice. *Minerva Urol Nefrol* 2002; 54(1):45–49.

88 Fengler SA, Abcarian H. The York Mason approach to repair of iatrogenic rectourinary fistulae. *Am J Surg* 1997; 173:213–217.

89 Dushnitsky T, Ziv Y, Peer A, Halevy A. Embolization—An optional treatment for intractable hemorrhage from a malignant rectovaginal fistula: Report of a case. *Dis Colon Rectum* 1999; 42: 271–273.

90 Langkilde NC, Pless TK, Lundbeck F, Nerstrom B. Surgical repair of vescicovaginal fistulae—A ten-year retrospective study. *Scand J Urol Nephrol* 1999; 33:100–103.

91 Nesrallah LJ, Srougi M, Gittes RF. The O'Conor technique: The gold standard for supratrigonal vesicovaginal fistula repair. *J Urol* 1999; 161:566–568.

◆ 92 Emmert C, Kohler U. Management of genital fistulas in patients with cervical cancer. *Arch Gynecol Obstetr* 1996; 259:19–24.

93   Harpster LE, Rommel FM, Sieber PR et al. The incidence and management of rectal injury associated with radical prostatectomy in a community based urology practice. *J Urol* 1995; 154:1435–1438.

● 94   Turner-Warwick R. Urinary fistulae in the female. In:Walsh PC, Gittes RF, Perlmutter AC, Stanley TA (eds.). *Campbell's Urology*, 5th edn. Philadelphia, PA: W.B. Saunders, 1986: pp. 2718–2738.

95   Dangle PP, Wang WP, Pohar KS. Vesicoenteric, vesicovaginal, vesicocutaneous fistula—An unusual complication with intravesical mitomycin. *Can J Urol* 2008; 15(5):4269–4272.

96   Watanabe K, Otsu S, Morinaga R et al. Vesicocutaneous fistula formation during treatment with sunitinib malate: Case report. *BMC Gastroenterol.* 2010; 1(10):128.

81

Assessment and management of lymphedema

YING GUO, BENEDICT KONZEN

LYMPHEDEMA CLASSIFICATION AND INCIDENCE

Lymphedema is a chronic, progressive, incurable condition, affecting at least 3 million Americans, and 140–250 million patients worldwide. Filariasis, a parasitic infestation, is the most common cause. Lymphedema is an accumulation of lymphatic fluid in the interstitial tissue that causes swelling, most often in the upper or lower extremity(ies), and occasionally in face, neck, trunk, and external genitalia. Lymphedema negatively affects the activities of daily living, vocational, domestic, psychosocial, sexual lives, and quality of life of patients.[1*,2,3*,4*,5*] In addition, it puts patients at increased risk for life-threatening infections and malignancies.[6]

CLASSIFICATION (TABLE 81.1)

Primary lymphedema

Primary lymphedema is caused by a congenital abnormality or dysfunction in the lymphatic system and can be further classified according to age of onset. Primary lymphedema is rare, affecting 1.15 per 100,000 younger than 20 years of age.[7] The congenital form is detected at birth or in the first year of life and may either be sporadic or familial. The onset of lymphedema praecox is between the ages of 1 and 35 years. The onset of lymphedema tarda occurs after 35 years of age.

Alternatively, primary lymphedema can be classified according to the abnormality found in the lymphatics. Thus, it may be aplastic, hypoplastic, or hyperplastic. These terms suggest an abnormality in the development of the lymphatic system. While this is true for congenital lymphedema, cases of later-onset primary lymphedema might be due to an acquired abnormality.

Secondary lymphedema

Secondary lymphedema is edema due to a reduction in lymph flow by an acquired cause. The causes of secondary lymphedema include trauma, recurrent infection, and malignancy and its treatment (*surgery, radiation*). In the developed world, the most common cause of secondary lymphedema is malignancy (including that resulting from cancer treatment). Lymphedema is common in the developing world secondary to infection with the parasitic nematode *Wuchereria bancrofti* (otherwise known as filariasis), making this the most common cause of lymphedema worldwide.[8] Cancer-related lymphedema usually occurs at proximal limb segments (i.e., lymph nodes) due to infection, ligation, malignancy, scar tissue, and radiation therapy.[9] The pelvic and inguinal nodes in the lower extremities and the axillary nodes of the upper extremities are the primary sites of obstruction.

This chapter will be emphasizing on the secondary lymphedema related to cancer and its treatment, which is frequently overlooked. The reported incidence of lymphedema secondary to postmastectomy radiotherapy ranges from 2.4% to 54%.[10*,11*,12–17] The incidence of lower limb lymphedema secondary to gynecological cancer was reported to be 18%.[18*] Lymphedema is uncommon from cancer of the abdominal and pelvic urological organs and their treatment, as a result of rich anastomotic networks and bilaterality of lymphatic drainage from the midline organs. In patients with penile carcinomas, lymph node metastasis is reported in up to 35%[19] and following treatment by groin node dissection, lymphoedema developed in 50%–100% of the patients.[19,20] The incidence and prevalence of lymphoedema in other urological cancers remains largely unknown.[21]

In the pre-Prostate-Specific Antigen era, chronic lymphoedema was reported as a complication of bilateral pelvic lymphadenectomy for prostate cancer in 15 (18%) of 82 patients, 10 of whom had additional radiotherapy.[22] Greskovich et al. reported transient lymphoedema in 2 of 65 patients who underwent a staging lymphadenectomy prior to radiotherapy.[23]

PATHOPHYSIOLOGY

Lymphedema occurs when lymphatic fluid load exceeds the lymphatic transport capacity; an abnormal amount of protein-rich fluid collects in the tissues of the affected area. In most cases, the transport capacity is impaired, but in patients with venous insufficiency, the lymphatic load is increased.

Table 81.1 *Staging of lymphedema*

Stage	Edema	Elevation helps	Pitting	Fibrosis	Acanthosis
0	−	+	−	−	−
1	+	+	±	−	−
2 (early)	+	±	±	−	−
2 (late)	+	−	±	+	−
3	+	−	−	+	+

+, present; −, absent.

The lymphatic drainage system is separate from the general circulatory system and is the conduit for returning tissue fluids to circulation.[24] The superficial lymphatic system begins with initial lymphatics, which are formed from one-layer endothelial cells, overlapping each other but not forming a continuous connection. Each of the cells is attached to the surrounding tissue by anchoring filaments. When there is a change in tissue pressure caused by arterial pulsation, muscle contraction, or respiration, or when the skin is lightly stretched, the anchoring filaments pull on the cells of the initial lymphatics. Because of this, the gap between the cells opens, and fluid drains into the vessels.[25] Initial lymphatics combine to form larger vessels called precollectors and collectors, which in turn lead to the lymph nodes in the axillary and inguinal regions. The collector vessels of the lymphatic system contain smooth muscle and valves to regulate flow.[25] The regional lymph nodes drain fluid from the ipsilateral limb and torso quadrant. Deep lymph nodes are located along major arteries for visceral drainage. Major somatic drainage areas are connected via subcutaneous collateral channels, both anteriorly and posteriorly. Lymph drains from the lower limbs into the lumbar lymphatic trunk, which joins the intestinal lymphatic trunk and cisterna chyli to form the thoracic duct. Lymph returns to the blood circulation at the venous angles, which are formed by the junctures of the internal jugular and subclavian veins. Most of the lymph in the body drains via the thoracic duct, which enters the circulation at the left venous angle. Only the right upper torso, arm, face, and neck drain into circulation on the right side via the right lymphatic duct, which empties into the right subclavian vein.[24] An important function of the lymphatic system is the prevention of infection. The lymphatic system is responsible for picking up excess interstitial water and protein as well as other cells, including bacteria, which can enter the tissue through small cuts or breaks in the skin. Bacteria and other antigens are transported by the lymphatic system from the interstitium to lymphocytes in the lymph nodes, where an immune response may be initiated. Physiologically, most of the interstitial fluid generated daily (18 L) arises from the blood capillaries. Fourteen to sixteen liters subsequently return directly to the venous circulation. The remaining 10%–20%, approximately 2 L per day, passes through lymphatic transport.

Histologically, the reparative process in the traumatized lymphatic vessels after mastectomy demonstrates fibrosis and an accompanying reduction in vessel diameter. With the subsequent ligation or interruption in lymph channels and lymphadenectomy, the body attempts a regenerative process with the formation of collateral circulation. The radiation treatment may lead to fibrosis. Nonirradiated lymph nodes develop compensatory dilated sinuses to handle lymph volume. This may anatomically be associated with a lymph node hyperplasia. If the lymphatic system fails locally, protein subsequently accumulates in the interstitium. If no intervention occurs at this point, fibrosclerosis will follow along with inflammation, scarring, and loss of regional lymphatic integrity.[26]

The frequency with which lymphedema occurs after cancer therapy depends on multiple factors (Box 81.1):

1. The extent of lymphatic system damage. In a study by Kiel in 1996, in the absence of lymph node dissection, the incidence of edema after breast cancer treatment was 21%. With 11–15 nodes removed, edema was present in 27%. With greater than 15 lymph nodes removed, it was 44%.[27] Lymphatics have excellent regenerative capabilities. Even after radical lymph node excision for malignancy, lymphedema does not always happen. When it does occur, it is often a late complication. The reasons for this late development are uncertain, but gradual failure of distal lymphatics, which have to "pump" lymph at a greater pressure through damaged proximal ducts, has been postulated. The transected lymphatics will regenerate after node clearance procedures. If combined with radiotherapy, however, the risk of lymphedema is higher, as fibrous scarring reduces regrowth of ducts. In approximately 10% of cancer patients, the onset of lymphedema heralds local recurrence of tumor or is the result of metastases.[26]

2. The inherent compensatory ability of the lymphatic system. Patient's weight and age may affect the development of lymphedema. Twenty-two percent of breast cancer patients older than 55 were shown to have an increased lymphedema risk when compared to their younger counterparts (14%).[27,28] Comorbidities, such as heart failure, renal insufficiency, and venous insufficiency, may contribute to the

---

Box 81.1 Factors affecting development of cancer-related lymphedema

Extent of lymphatic system damage
- Recurrence of tumor
- Lymph node dissection
- Radiation

Inherent compensatory ability of the lymphatic system
- Age
- Obesity
- Infection
- Heart failure
- Venous insufficiency
- Other factors that affect lymph load

onset and progression of lymphedema. Recurrent cellulitis can further compromise the fluid return. Any situation that causes an increase in lymphatic load can predispose patients to development or worsening of lymphedema. The onset of lymphedema may be provoked in a variety of common situations that occur on a daily basis: muscle fatigue resulting from overuse; vasodilatation following exposure heat; local trauma; vigorous massage; constriction or a "tourniquet effect," which causes swelling distal to that point; or sustained dependency of the limb. Other situations that may increase lymphatic load include airplane flights and higher elevations; these situations involve decreased atmospheric pressure and may result in increased filtration into the tissue from the blood capillaries.

COMMON COMPLICATIONS

1. *Lymph fluid reflux*: Overdistended lymph vessel causes valvular insufficiency and retrograde flow, and patient presents with blister-like formation on the surface of the skin, called lymphatic cysts. Lymphatic cysts, usually located in axillary, cubital, genital, and popliteal area, can easily break open and lead to infection or fistula. Treatment should include prevention of infection.
2. *Muscular skeletal complications*: Lymphedema can lead to muscular skeletal pain, decreased range of motion. Swelling and pain can interfere with mobility and affect the sufferers' perceptions of themselves.[1*]
3. *Infection*: Bacterial and fungal infection are common in stage 2 and 3 lymphedema. Clinical symptoms of cellulites (erysipelas) are fever, erythema, warm, and tenderness. Patients should be treated with either oral or intravenous antibiotics. In general, an antibiotic needs to cover the normal skin flora (i.e., gram-positive cocci) and have good skin penetration. Therapy with an intravenous antibiotic is considered when there is more significant local or systemic infection. Some patients develop chronic infections that may necessitate ongoing antibiotic therapy. Fungal infection causes skin itching, crusting, maceration between the toes, and typical fungal nail changes. Systemic or local antifungal treatment can be used. Recurrence of infection/inflammation indicates reduced local immunity.[29] It is reasonable to emphasize the importance of lymphedema limb care.[30] Decongestive lymphatic therapy (DLT) is contraindicated until infection subsides.
4. *Hyperkeratosis*: Hyperkeratosis presents as thickening of skin and wart-like papillomas. Care must be taken to avoid skin breakdown and infection.
5. *Malignancies*: Lymphangiosarcoma is a rare late complication of lymphedema,[31] also described as Stewart Treves syndrome,[32] and as Milroy disease.[33] In patients with long-standing lymphedema and cellulitis that does not respond to systemic antibiotics, physician should consider a skin biopsy. Treatment is primary radiotherapy, with surgery reserved for patients with discrete, nonmetastatic disease.

DIAGNOSIS

History and physical examination (Box 81.2)

The history should include full medical history, all anticancer therapies, past surgeries, postoperative complications, radiation treatment, the time interval from radiation or surgery to the onset of symptoms, and intervening variables in the presence or severity of symptoms. The quality and behavior of the edema (fluctuation with position, progression over time), and associated symptoms should be assessed. History of trauma or infection should be determined. In addition, information concerning current medications may be important. Edema is not detectable clinically until the interstitial volume exceeds 30% above normal. Postmastectomy and radiation lymphedema initially presents as mild edema in the hand or forearm, often in the dorsal epicondylar region (Figure 81.1A and B). Other complaints related to lymphedema are heaviness or fullness related to the weight of the limb, skin feeling tight, decreased flexibility in the hand, wrist, or ankle, difficulty fitting into clothing in one specific area, or ring/wristwatch/bracelet tightness. Associated clinical features of lower limb lymphoedema include tightness of or inability to wear shoes, itching of the legs or toes, burning sensation in the legs, sleep disturbances, and loss of hair. Ambulation is affected because of the limb size and weight, causing an inability to wear clothing. Activities of daily living, hobby, work, and psychological impact on patient need to be assessed as well.

On exam, the affected limb is swollen with enhanced skin creases, hyperkeratosis, and papillomatosis. Lymphoedema is traditionally described as non-pitting, but in early cases, pitting may be present. Stemmer's sign—inability to pinch the skin at the base of the second toe due to the thickened skin folds—is a useful clinical sign.[34] Cutaneous fungal or bacterial infections are not unusual in patients with lymphatic obstruction. Skin folds should be frequently inspected for ulcers and infections.

Box 81.2 Factors affecting development of cancer-related lymphedema

History
- Medical history (anticancer therapies, past operations, postoperative complications, radiation treatment)
- Edema (onset, fluctuation, progression)
- Associated symptoms
- Infection and trauma
- Function
- Social history
- Psychological impact

Physical examination
- Edema: Skin texture, color, infection, scar; volume
- Neurological examination
- Range of motion

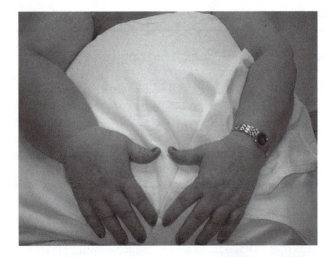

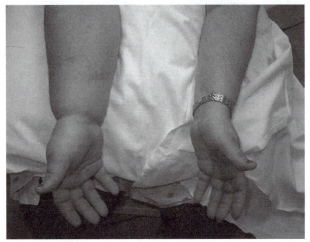

Figure 81.1 *Right upper extremity lymphedema.*

A neurologic examination for possible nerve entrapment and plexus involvement, and range-of-motion of different joints also need to be assessed. In established cases of lymphoedema, the clinical features are diagnostic with no requirement for diagnostic investigations.

Volume and skin condition measurements

The initial assessment of lymphedema and follow-up on the response to treatment should include the measurement of volume and assessment of skin condition.[35] The most commonly used assessment tool involves measuring the contralateral limb circumference at several points along the limb. However, when the disease affects both sides, this type of comparison may not be accurate.[36*] Multiple transverse tapes in a device are placed at 4 cm intervals, can be used to measure circumferences with accuracy, and it is a simple convenient method.[37] Volume can be calculated from surface measurements.[38] The truncal swelling can be measured by skinfold calipers.

This water displacement volumetry, although no longer commonly used, measures limb volume[35] and is more accurate than calculating the leg volume from circumferential measurements with a tape measure.[35]

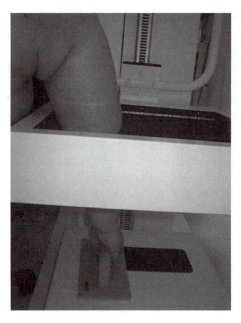

Figure 81.2 *Using optoelectronic pedometer to measure upper extremity volume.*

The optoelectronic pedometer is a validated, reliable, easy-to-use tool for the limb volume measurement [39] (Figure 81.2).

Bioelectrical impedance has been used successfully for the evaluation of swelling in patients with postmastectomy lymphedema[40] and lower extremity lymphedema.[41*]

Skin condition can be measured by recording deformation of tissue by a mass (tonometry) and the step compression method. In lymphedema, the tissue tonicity (degree of tissue resistance to mechanical compression) is either higher or lower compared with the nonedematous leg.[35] Measurement of tissue tonometry is more useful in assessing the response to treatment than in the initial assessment of disease.

Image studies

Lymphangioscintigraphy (LAS) permits high-resolution imaging of peripheral lymphatic vessels and provides insight into lymph flow dynamics. It is indispensable for patients with known or suspected lymphatic circulatory disorders in confirming the diagnosis and delineating the pathogenesis and evolution of lymphedema. In addition, LAS helps evaluate lymphatic truncal anatomy and radiotracer transport. It is also useful in preoperative evaluation, especially for microvascular anastomosis. The procedure involves intradermal injection of a radioactive tracer in the web space in upper or lower extremities, and does not adversely affect the lymphatic vascular endothelium. Radioactive tracers are injected subcutaneously in the web space of the upper or lower extremities; imaging is then performed after 30–60 min to visualize the lymphatic vessels and nodes, lymph node uptake speed, and also measure the rate of lymph transport.[42] Patients with a provisional diagnosis of peripheral lymphatic dysfunction or idiopathic edema should undergo diagnostic LAS to verify diagnostic accuracy, pinpoint the specific abnormality, and help guide subsequent therapy.[43] Conventional oil-contrast lymphography is no longer commonly used, because it is associated with complications such as allergic and inflammatory reactions, pulmonary embolism, and damage to the endothelial lining of the lymphatic vessel.

Magnetic resonance imaging and computed tomography complements LAS in monitoring the progression of cancer. Ultrasonography has proved useful in the setting of filariasis and differential diagnosis of venous obstruction.
Dual x-ray absorptiometry (DEXA) or biphotonic absorptiometry is useful in assessing the chemical component of limb swelling (percentage of fat, water, and lean mass).[44]

DIFFERENTIAL DIAGNOSIS

Lipedema

The clinical features of lipedema (also known as lipomatosis of the leg) include early age of onset, female exclusivity, and positive family history in some patients.[45,46] The clinical signs include elastic symmetrical enlargement of both legs with sparing of the feet.

Deep vein thrombosis and chronic venous disease

Deep vein thrombosis (DVT) results in obstruction to venous flow. The clinical picture is thus one of a swollen, warm, tender extremity. The resulting edema is pitting in nature and is usually much softer than in established lymphedema. Often, there are underlying risk factors, such as recent surgery or immobility, malignancy, a preceding long flight, or thrombophilia. The diagnosis is confirmed with duplex scanning or venography. Treatment is with anticoagulation. Chronic venous stasis results in hyperpigmentation, and varicose veins, and in severe cases, venous ulceration may be more difficult to differentiate from lymphedema. Untreated venous insufficiency can progress into a combined venous/lymphatic disorder, which is treated in the same way as lymphedema.

Heart failure or renal failure

These conditions need proper medical management.[47]

STAGING OF LYMPHEDEMA

Generally, the staging of lymphedema is based on a three-stage scale. However, there is an increasing number of individuals who recognize stage 0. At this stage, swelling is not evident, despite alteration in lymph transport. In stage I, there is an early accumulation of a high protein-laden fluid (versus venous edema) that subsides with limb elevation. Pitting of the extremity may be present. In stage II, limb elevation alone

Table 81.2 *Grading of lymphedema based on severity*

Severity of lymphedema	Volume increase (%)
Minimal	<20
Moderate	20–40
Severe	>40

rarely reduces tissue swelling and pitting is present. In late state II, fibrosis is present and there may or may not be pitting of the extremity. Stage III is characterized by lymphostatic elephantiasis. Pitting is absent, and the trophic skin is characteristically acanthotic with warty overgrowth (Table 81.1).[34] The severity of unilateral lymphedema in each stage can be further assessed by grading system; minimal (less than 20% increase), moderate (20%–40% increase), or severe (more than 40% increase) (Table 81.2).

TREATMENT

As with most chronic problems, the responsibility for managing lymphedema falls on the patient. Education about the etiology of lymphedema and principles for management are the first and most important part of patient care. The management of this condition involves decongesting the reduced lymphatic pathways; encouraging the development of collateral drainage routes and stimulating the function of remaining patent routes the lymphedema control will be long lasting.

The International Society of Lymphology Executive Committee in 2013 revised a consensus document that offered an integrated view of the management of lymphedema.[48] The controversy about the efficacy and application of treatment approaches in different situations still exists.

The most commonly used method is called DLT, also known as combined physical therapy (CPT), complete/complex decongestive therapy (CDT), or complex decongestive physiotherapy (CDP), which involves a two-stage treatment program.[49] In the first phase, intensive every other day physical therapy visits are recommended for a course of 4–6 weeks, although daily treatment is more effective; these treatments usually include: applying and teaching patient manual lymphatic drainage (MLD); multilayer bandaging; care of the skin; exercises to promote lymph drainage. Manual lymphatic drainage (MLD) is a light massage technique used to mobilize lymphatic and reestablish pathways for lymph flow.[50] The multilayer bandaging consists of applying multilayered padding materials and short-stretch (also called low-stretch) bandages repeatedly. The goals of this phase are to reduce the size of the limb, and improve the texture and the health of the skin. In a study by Ko et al.,[51*] 299 patients with both upper and lower extremity lymphedema underwent CDP for 15.9 days. Lymphedema reduction averaged 59.1% after upper extremity CDP and 67.7% in lower extremity treatment. When followed up at 9 months, improvement had been maintained in 86% of patients. These individuals maintained at least 90% of the initial reduction. Incidence of infection also decreased by approximately 50%.[51*] Various outcomes from different studies were due to the skill of the treating therapist, and patient compliance, exercise protocols, duration of the DLT, or number of treatments per week, etc.

DLT may be used palliatively in lymphedema as the result of tumor-obstructing lymphatics. This treatment is usually conducted in conjunction with chemoradiation. In the past, controversy existed as to whether massage and mechanical compression would promote metastasis. In practice, disease is already present and the goal simply is palliation of morbid swelling.[42,51*,52,53]

In the second phase of treatment, patients are usually recommended to wear strong compression hosiery (20–50 mmHg of pressure) to maintain the reduction in swelling; carry out regular daily exercise; perform regular MLD, where possible. The goal of the second phase is to preserve and optimize the improvements gained in the first phase. The role of weight control and regular exercises in the management of lymphoedema is thought to be important.

Relative contraindications to DLT include significant congestive heart failure, acute deep vein thrombosis, acute or untreated infection or inflammation of the affected limb, and active malignancy.

Skin care

Skin care should include routine skin inspection (for ingrown toenails, cuticle integrity, abrasions, bruising, ulcerations, impaired circulation); use of skin emollients; avoidance of extremes in heat and cold including sun exposures. In the clinician's office or hospital setting, blood pressure measurements, venipuncture, or injections should not be undertaken on the affected side. Recent study showed that acupuncture appears safe in lymphoedema related to breast cancer surgery.[54,55]

The patient is counseled on avoiding trauma to the affected region from clothing (brassiere, purse straps). In early pitting stage, many patients benefit from elevating the limb at or above relative heart level overnight. An opinion regarding exercise has changed significantly; recent research showed that slowly progressive exercise is not associated with the development or exacerbation of breast cancer–related lymphedema and can be safely pursued with proper supervision.[56]

Manual lymphatic drainage

MLD is a therapeutic technique used to increase lymph flow. It consists of movement of the therapist's hands over the patient's skin and subcutaneous tissue. The pressure applied is very gentle, and the movements are slow to correspond with the slow lymphatic pulsations. The massage sequence begins at the center of the body and moves to the periphery and from unaffected side to affected side. The rationale for this is that the lymph nodes must be emptied before they can receive more lymph from the periphery. Each maneuver is performed in a distal to proximal direction. Patients and family members or friends can be included in the training of gentle form of self-massage.

Anderson concluded from their study that MLD provided no extra benefit.[57**]

The use of massage (classical massage or effleurage) is not recommended, since it may be excessively vigorous and cause lymphatic vessels damage.

Exercise

When combining with nonelastic compression bandage, it is hypothesized that the contraction of muscle against the elastic bandage, provides increased subcutaneous tissue pressure, and thus encourage movement of interstitial fluid into the lymphatic system.[58]

Compression bandage and compression garment

Wrapping the limb with low-stretch bandages in conjunction with padding and foam provides the ideal type of compression in lymphedema patients. It allows a low resting pressure and a high working pressure during muscle contraction to facilitate lymphatic flow. The bandage accommodates the change of volume overtime and provides "custom-made" compression. However, the disadvantages of this technique are difficult to apply, require training, cumbersome. One study showed compression bandage use prior to compression garment is more effective than compression garment alone.[59**] Once the extremity reaches its smallest obtainable size, a customized low-stretch elastic compression garment can be fitted and used during normal activities. Compression garments provide gradient pressure, ranging from 20 to 60 mmHg. Replacement is needed every 6 months. Proper fitting is necessary to avoid a tourniquet effect.[60,61*] Hornsby investigated the use of hosiery comparing to control and concluded that the results suggest that wearing a compression sleeve is beneficial. Both groups had high dropout rate.[62]

Contraindications to its use would include a concurrent presence of arterial disease, allergy, ulceration, or a painful postphlebitic syndrome.

Pneumatic compression

Controversy exists regarding the use of pneumatic compression pumps. Some schools that support the utilization of pumps generally suggest using relatively low pressures (40 mm of mercury [mmHg] maximum distal pressure) as part of a comprehensive program.[63,64] Pressures greater than 50–60 mmHg may cause injury to lymphatic vessels.[65] The extremity is placed into a long inflatable sleeve that is connected to a pump that inflates the sleeve to a predetermined pressure. External compression therapy is applied with a sequential gradient "pump." Between pump uses, the extremity should be wrapped with elastic compression bandage or have temporary compression garments applied to reduce recurrence of lymph in the extremity. It may take months to obtain a demonstrable reduction in the size of the extremity.[66*]

Surgery

Controversy exists with reference to surgical intervention in the treatment of lymphedema. There are two types of procedures available: excisional procedures (or debulking procedure) with or without skin grafting; and drainage procedures (or microsurgical procedures).

Excisional therapy involves removing a large section of skin and subcutaneous tissue down to the muscle fascia and reapproximating the wound edges. Problems associated with this procedure relate to wound healing. In addition, this method does not treat the underlying problem of lymphatic outflow obstruction. Excisional therapy with skin grafting involves completely degloving the overlying tissue on the affected extremity and split-thickness grafting directly onto the muscular bed. By removing all overlying lymphatic tissue within the dermal and subcutaneous space down to the muscle bed, lymphedema in the area of grafting is no longer a concern. The result is one of marked reduction in the size of the extremity, but any tissue distal to this is left with more exaggerated lymphedema than in the preoperative state. Skin grafts have a 5%–10% incidence of failure. Frequent complications are protracted lymph leak and poor healing.

A drainage procedure intends to drain lymph fluid within the lymphedematous limb into other lymphatic basins or into the venous circulation. These procedures include greater omentum flaps,[67] lymphaticolymphatic bypass,[68,69] microvascular lymph node transfer,[70,71] and lymphovenous shunt.[72,73]

The drainage procedure currently favored for the treatment of limited lymphatic obstruction is a surgical lymphovenous microvascular anastomosis.[74] The lymphovenous shunt operation's effectiveness varies in reports.

Liposuction combined with constant use of compression garment has been reported,[66*,75] but this procedure could potentially damage residual lymphatic and worsen the lymphedema.[76–79]

Drug therapy

No pharmacologic therapy is recommended for the treatment of lymphedema.

Coumarin (5,6-benzo-[(alpha)]-pyrone or 1,2-benzopyrone) and related drugs have been reported to reduce lymphedema, possibly through stimulation of proteolysis by tissue macrophages. In addition to findings that it decreases the pain and discomfort caused by lymphedema, coumarin has been reported to reduce the incidence of cellulitis or lymphangitis and to soften slowly the brawny edema that is often found in conjunction with lymphedema. In 1993, Casley-Smith et al. reported the results of a double-blind, crossover trial of coumarin in 31 women with postmastectomy lymphedema and 21 men and women with lymphedema of the leg of various causes.[80**] Coumarin was reported to be more effective than placebo in reducing the volume of edema fluid in the arm, in reducing skin temperature, and in increasing the softness of the limb tissue. In 1999, Loprinzi et al. studied 140 women

with chronic lymphedema of the ipsilateral arm after treatment for breast cancer. The volumes of the arms at 6 and 12 months were virtually identical, regardless of whether coumarin or placebo was given first, and no significant symptom differences were found in the two treatment groups. Coumarin was well tolerated, except that it resulted in serologic evidence of liver toxicity in 6% of the women.[81**] It appears that at present, there is no drug that will reduce chronic lymphedema and allow the reduction to be maintained.[81**,82***] Antibiotics should be administered when patients develop cellulitis in the affected limb.

Psychosocial support

For a patient with lymphedema, physical and emotional challenges are profound. In a study by Tobin et al., patients with arm edema experienced greater functional impairment, and increased difficulty adjusting to their illness, home life, and personal/familial relationships.[1*] The openly exposed lymphedematous limb is a constant reminder to the patient and the community at large, the occurrence of a cancer, and that the patient is physically different from the norm. As a result, the patient may lose an interest in their dress or general appearance. This loss of self-esteem may also contribute to difficulties with interpersonal relationships, social activities, and intimacy.[83] Efforts may be made to strengthen the women's coping skills, eventually in a multidisciplinary approach by palliative and rehabilitation professionals.

Weight loss

Obesity is a risk factor for developing cancer-related lymphedema, it can also exacerbate existing lymphedema, and therefore, weight reduction has been recommended in lymphedema management. A randomized study had showed the effectiveness of weight reduction.[84]

Key learning points

Definition: Lymphatic fluid exceeds the lymphatic transport capacity.

Classification:
- Primary
- Secondary: Caused by filariasis, cancer, and its treatment, other

Staging: 0,1,2,3

Grading: Mild, moderate, severe

Diagnosis:
- History: Medical and surgical history, edema and associated symptoms, function, psychosocial effect
- Physical Examination:
- Volume (circumference, water displacement volumetry, optoelectronic pedometer, bioelectrical impedance, skinfold calipers)

- Skin (texture, color, tonometry)

Image study:

- LAS
- Magnetic resonance imaging and computed tomography
- Ultrasonography (differential diagnosis of deep venous thrombosis)
- DEXA or biphotonic absorptiometry

Treatment:

- Goal
  - Development of collateral drainage routes, stimulating the function of remaining patent routes
  - Decrease volume and improve skin condition, prevent complications
- Methods
  - Skin care
  - Manual lymphatic drainage
  - Exercise
  - Compression bandaging/compression garment
  - Pneumatic compression
  - Surgery and drug therapy
  - Psychosocial support
  - Weight loss

REFERENCES

1 Tobin MB, Lacey HJ, Meyer L, Mortimer PS. The psychological morbidity of breast cancer-related arm swelling. Psychological morbidity of lymphoedema. *Cancer* 1993; **72**: 3248–3252.

2 Cohen SR, Payne DK, Tunkel RS. Lymphedema: Strategies for management. *Cancer* 2001; **92**(4 Suppl.): 980–987.

3 Velanovich V, Szymanski W. Quality of life of breast cancer patients with lymphedema. *Am J Surg* 1999; **177**: 184–187.

4 Passik SD, McDonald MV. Psychosocial aspects of upper extremity lymphedema in women treated for breast carcinoma. *Cancer* 1998; **83**: 2817–2820.

5 Kwan W, Jackson J, Weir LM et al. Chronic arm morbidity after curative breast cancer treatment: Prevalence and impact on quality of life. *J Clin Oncol* 2002; **20**: 4242–4248.

6 Mortimer PS. The pathophysiology of lymphedema. *Cancer* 1998; **83**: 2798–2802.

7 Smeltzer DM, Stickler GB, Schirger A. Primary lymphedema in children and adolescents: A follow-up study and review. *Pediatrics* 1985; **76**: 206–217.

8 Board J, Harlow W. Lymphoedema 2: Classification, signs, symptoms and diagnosis. *Br J Nurs* 2002; **11**(6): 389–395.

9 Brennan MJ. Lymphedema following the surgical treatment of breast cancer: A review of pathophysiology and treatment. *J Pain Symptom Manage* 1992; **7**(2):110–116.

10 Cambria RA, Gloviczki P, Naessens JM, Wahner HW. Noninvasive evaluation of the lymphatic system with lymphoscintigraphy: A prospective, semiquantitative analysis in 386 extremities. *J Vasc Surg* 1993; **18**: 773–782.

11 Ryttov N, Holm NV, Qvist N, Blichert-Toft M. Influence of adjuvant irradiation on the development of late arm lymphedema and impaired shoulder mobility after mastectomy for carcinoma of the breast. *Acta Oncol* 1988; **27**: 667–670.

12 Ragaz J, Jackson SM, Le N et al. Adjuvant radiotherapy and chemotherapy in node-positive premenopausal women with breast cancer. *N Engl J Med* 1997; **337**: 956–962.

13 Johansson S, Svensson H, Denekamp J. Dose response and latency for radiation-induced fibrosis, edema, and neuropathy in breast cancer patients. *Int J Radiat Oncol Biol Phys* 2002; **52**: 1207–1219.

14 Schunemann H, Willich N. Lymphoedema of the arm after primary treatment of breast cancer. *Anticancer Res* 1998; **18**: 2235–2236.

15 Hinrichs CS, Watroba NL, Rezaishiraz H et al. Lymphedema secondary to postmastectomy radiation: Incidence and risk factors. *Ann Surg Oncol* 2004; **11**(6): 573–580.

16 Hojris I, Andersen J, Overgaard M, Overgaard J. Late treatment-related morbidity in breast cancer patients randomized to postmastectomy radiotherapy and systemic treatment versus systemic treatment alone. *Acta Oncol* 2000; **39**: 355–372.

17 Erickson VS, Pearson ML, Ganz PA et al. Arm edema in breast cancer patients. *J Natl Cancer Inst* 2001; **93**(2): 96–111.

18 Ryan M, Stainton MC, Slaytor EK et al. Aetiology and prevalence of lower limb lymphoedema following treatment for gynaecological cancer. *Aust N Z J Obst Gynaecol* 2003; **43**(2): 148–151.

19 Cabanas RM. An approach for the treatment of penile carcinoma. *Cancer* 1977; **39**: 456–466.

20 Catalona W. Modified inguinal lymphadenectomy for carcinoma of the penis with preservation of saphenous veins: Technique and preliminary results. *J Urol* 1988; **140**: 306–310.

21 Okeke AA, Bates DO, Gillatt DA. Lymphoedema in urological cancer. *Eur Urol* 2004; **45**(1): 18–25.

22 Lieskovsky G, Skinner DG, Weisenburger T. Pelvic lymphadenectomy in the management of carcinoma of the prostate. *J Urol* 1980; **124**: 635–638.

23 Greskovich FJ, Zagars GK, Sherman NE, Johnson DE. Complications following external beam radiation therapy for prostate cancer: An analysis of patients treated with and without staging pelvic lymphadenectomy. *J Urol* 1991; **146**: 798–802.

◆ 24 Brennan MJ, DePompolo RW, Garden FH. Focused review: Postmastectomy lymphedema. *Arch Phys Med Rehabil* 1996; **77**: S74–S80.

25 Szuba A, Rockson SG. Lymphedema: Anatomy, physiology, and pathogenesis. *Vasc Med* 1997; **2**: 321–326.

✶ 26 Weissleder H, Schuchhardt C. Lymphedema in tumor management. In: Weissleder H, Schuchhardt C (eds.). *Lymphedema: Diagnosis and Therapy.* Cologne, Germany: Viavital Verlag GmbH, 2001. pp. 187–213.

27 Kiel KD, Rademacher AW. Early-stage breast cancer: Arm edema after wide-excision and breast irradiation. *Radiology* 1996; **198**: 279–283.

28 Garcia Hidalgo L. Dermatological complications of obesity. *Am J Clin Dermatol* 2002; **3**(7): 497–506.

29 Mallon E, Powell S, Mortimer P, Ryan TJ. Evidence for altered cell-mediated immunity in postmastectomy lymphoedema. *Br J Dermatol* 1997; **137**(6): 928–933.

◆ 30 Badger C, Seers K, Preston N, Mortimer P. Antibiotics/anti-inflammatories for reducing acute inflammatory episodes in lymphoedema of the limbs. *Cochrane Database Syst Rev* 2004; **2**: CD003143.

31 Lewis JM, Wald ER. Lymphedema praecox. *J Pediatr* 1984; **104**: 641–648.

32 Stewart FW, Treves N. Lymphangiosarcoma in postmastectomy lymphedema: A report of six cases in elephantiasis chirurgica. *Cancer* 1948; **1**: 64–81.

33 Brostrom LA, Nilsonne U, Kronberg M, Soderberg G. Lymphangiosarcoma in chronic hereditary oedema (Milroy's disease). *Ann Chir Gynaecol* 1989; **78**: 320–323.

34 Mortimer PS. Investigation and management of lymphoedema. *Vasc Med Rev* 1990; **1**: 1–20.

35 Stanton AW, Badger C, Sitzia J. Non-invasive assessment of the lymphedematous limb. *Lymphology* 2000; **33**(3): 122–135.

36 Berard A, Zuccarelli F. Test–retest reliability study of a new improved Leg-O-meter, the Leg-O meter II, in patients suffering from venous insufficiency of the lower limbs. *Angiology* 2000; **51**: 711–717.

37 Imran D, Mandal A. Measurement of lymphedema using a simple device. *Plast Reconstr Surg* 2004; **113**(1): 456–457.

38 Sitzia J. Volume measurement in lymphoedema treatment: Examination of formulae. *Eur J Cancer Care (Engl)* 1995; **4**: 11–16.

39 Stanton AW, Northfield JW, Holroyd B et al. Validation of an optoelectronic limb volumeter (Perometer). *Lymphology* 1997; **30**(2): 77–97.

40 Ward LC. Regarding Edema and leg volume: Methods of assessment. *Angiology* 2000; **51**: 615–616.

41 Moseley A, Piller N, Carati C. Combined opto-electronic perometry and bioimpedance to measure objectively the effectiveness of a new treatment intervention for chronic secondary leg lymphedema. *Lymphology* 2002; **35**(4): 136–143.

42 Zuther JE. *Lymphedema Management: The Comprehensive Guide for Practitioners.* New York: Thieme, 2005. pp. 68–69.

43 Witte CL, Witte MH, Unger EC et al. Advances in imaging of lymph flow disorders. *Radiographics* 2000; **20**(6): 1697–1719.

✱ 44 Newman AL, et al., *Determining the precision of dual energy x-ray absorptiometry and bioelectric impedance spectroscopy in the assessment of breast cancer-related lymphedema.* Lymphat Res Biol, 2013. 11(2): 104–9.

45 Rudkin GH, Miller TA. Lipedema: A clinical entity distinct from lymphedema. *Plast Reconstr Surg* 1994; **94**: 841–847.

46 Harwood CA, Bull RH, Evans J, Mortimer PS. Lymphatic and venous function in lipoedema. *Br J Dermatol* 1996; **134**: 1–6.

47 Gniadecka M. Localization of dermal edema in lipodermatosclerosis, lymphedema, and cardiac insufficiency. High-frequency ultrasound examination of intradermal echogenicity. *J Am Acad Dermatol* 1996; **35**(1): 37–41.

✱ 48 *The diagnosis and treatment of peripheral lymphedema: 2013 Consensus Document of the International Society of Lymphology.* Lymphology, 2013. **46**(1): 1–11.

49 Casley-Smith JR, Boris M, Weindorf S et al. Treatment for lymphedema of the arm: The Casley-Smith method. *Cancer* 1998; **83**: 2843–2860.

50 Lawenda BD, Mondry TE, Johnstone PA. Lymphedema: A primer on the identification and management of a chronic condition in oncologic treatment. *CA Cancer J Clin* 2009; **59**: 8.

51 Ko DS, Lerner R, Klose G, Cosimi AB. Effective treatment of lymphedema of the extremities. *Arch Surg* 1998; **133**(4): 452–457.

52 Mortimer PS. Managing lymphoedema. *Clin Exp Dermatol* 1995; **20**: 98–110.

53 Foldi E, Foldi M, Weissleder H. Conservative treatment of lymphoedema of the limbs. *Angiology* 1985; **36**(3): 171–180.

54 Cassileth BR, Van Zee KJ, Chan Y et al. A safety and efficacy pilot study of acupuncture for the treatment of chronic lymphoedema. *Acupunct Med* 2011; **29**: 170–172.

55 de Valois, B.A., T.E. Young, and E. Melsome, *Assessing the feasibility of using acupuncture and moxibustion to improve quality of life for cancer survivors with upper body lymphoedema.* Eur J Oncol Nurs, 2012. **16**(3): 301–9.

56 Kwan ML, Cohn JC, Armer JM et al. Exercise in patients with lymphedema: A systematic review of the contemporary literature. *J Cancer Surviv* 2011; **5**: 320–336.

57 Andersen L, Hojris I, Erlandsen M, Andersen J. Treatment of breast-cancer-related lymphedema with or without manual lymphatic drainage—A randomized study. *Acta Oncol* 2000; **39**(3): 399–405.

58 LeDuc O, Peeters A, Bourgeois P. Bandages: Scintigraphic demonstration of its efficacy on colloidal protein reabsorption during muscle activity. In: Nishi M, Uchino S, Yabuki S (eds.). *Progress in Lymphology.* New York: Elsevier Science, 1990. pp. 421–423.

59 Badger CMA, Peacock JL, Mortimer PS. A randomized, controlled, parallel-group clinical trial comparing multilayer bandaging followed by hosiery versus hosiery alone in the treatment of patients with lymphedema of the limb. *Cancer* 2000; **88**: 2832–2837.

60 Bertelli G, Venturini M, Forno G et al. An analysis of prognostic factors in response to conservative treatment of postmastectomy lymphedema. *Surg Gynecol Obstet* 1992; **175**: 455–460.

61 Yasuhara H, Shigematsu H, Muto T. A study of the advantages of elastic stockings for leg lymphedema. *Int Angiol* 1996; **15**: 272–277.

62 Hornsby R. The use of compression to treat lymphoedema. *Prof Nurse* 1995; **11**(2): 127–128.

◆ 63 Brennan MJ, Miller LT. Overview of treatment options and review of the current role and use of compression garments, intermittent pumps, and exercise in the management of lymphedema. *Cancer* 1998; **83**: 2821–2827.

◆ 64 Leduc O, Leduc A; Bourgeois P et al. The physical treatment of upper limb edema. *Cancer* 1998; **83**: 2835–2839.

65 Eliska O, Eliskova M. Lymphedema: Morphology of the lymphatics after manual massage. In: Witte MH, Witte CL (eds.). *Progress in Lymphology.* Zurich, Switzerland: International Society of Lymphology, 1994. pp. 132–135.

66 Pappas CJ, O'Donnell TF Jr. Long-term results of compression treatment for lymphedema. *J Vasc Surg* 1992; **16**: 555–563.

67 Goldsmith HS. Long term evaluation of omental transposition for chronic lymphedema. *Ann Surg* 1974; **180**: 847–849.

68 Baumeister RG, Siuda S. Treatment of lymphedemas by microsurgical lymphatic grafting: What is proved? *Plast Reconstr Surg* 1990; **85**: 64–74.

69 Kleinhans E, Baumeister RG, Hahn D et al. Evaluation of transport kinetics in lymphoscintigraphy: Follow-up study in patients with transplanted lymphatic vessels. *Eur J Nucl Med* 1985; **10**: 349–352.

70 Becker C, Assouad J, Riquet M, Hidden G. Postmastectomy lymphedema: Long-term results following microsurgical lymph node transplantation. *Ann Surg* 2006; **243**: 313–315.

71 Lin CH, Ali R, Chen SC et al. Vascularized groin lymph node transfer using the wrist as a recipient site for management of postmastectomy upper extremity lymphedema. *Plast Reconstr Surg* 2009; **123**: 1265–1275.

72 Campisi C, Davini D, Bellini C et al. Lymphatic microsurgery for the treatment of lymphedema. *Microsurgery* 2006; **26**: 65–69.

73 Koshima I, Inagawa K, Urushibara K, Moriguchi T. Supermicrosurgical lymphaticovenular anastomosis for the treatment of lymphedema in the upper extremities. *J Reconstr Microsurg* 2000; **16**: 437–442.

74 Campisi C. Boccardo F. Lymphedema and microsurgery. *Microsurgery* 2002; **22**(2): 74–80.

75 Brorson H. Liposuction in arm lymphedema treatment. *Scand J Surg* 2003; **92**(4): 287–295.

76 Illouz YG. Body contouring by lipolysis: A 5-year experience with over 3000 cases. *Plast Reconstr Surg* 1983; **72**: 591–597.

77 O'Brien BM, Khazanchi RK, Kumar PA et al. Liposuction in the treatment of lymphoedema; a preliminary report. *Br J Plast Surg* 1989; **42**: 530–533.

78   Brorson H, Svensson H. Liposuction combined with controlled compression therapy reduces arm lymphedema more effectively than controlled compression therapy alone. *Plast Reconstr Surg* 1998; **102**: 1058–1067.

79   Frick A, Hoffmann JN, Baumeister RG, Putz R. Liposuction technique and lymphatic lesions in lower legs: Anatomic study to reduce risks. *Plast Reconstr Surg* 1999; **103**: 1868–1873; discussion 1874–1875.

80   Casley-Smith JR, Morgan RG, Piller NB. Treatment of lymphedema of the arms and legs with 5,6-benzo-(alpha)-pyrone. *N Engl J Med* 1993; **329**: 1158–1163.

81   Loprinzi CL, Kugler JW, Sloan JA et al. Lack of effect of coumarin in women with lymphedema after treatment for breast cancer. *N Engl J Med* 1999; **340**: 346–350.

◆ 82   Badger C, Preston N, Seers K, Mortimer P. Benzo-pyrones for reducing and controlling lymphoedema of the limbs. *Cochrane Database Syst Rev* 2004; **2**: CD003140.

83   Carter BJ. Women's Experiences of Lymphedema. *Oncol Nurs Forum* 1997; **24** (5): 875–882.

84   Shaw C, Mortimer P, Judd PA. A randomized controlled trial of weight reduction as a treatment for breast cancer-related lymphedema. *Cancer* 2007; **110**: 1868–1874.

PART 14

Emergencies in palliative medicine

82

Hypercalcemia

KIMBERSON C. TANCO, PAUL W. WALKER

INTRODUCTION

Hypercalcemia is a common metabolic complication of malignancy and has been termed hypercalcemia of malignancy (HCM), tumor-induced hypercalcemia, and humoral HCM. Hypercalcemia is a metabolic emergency and the most common paraneoplastic syndrome. Signs and symptoms of hypercalcemia may be subtle and can easily be missed unless there is a high index of suspicion.[1] Fortunately, hypercalcemia is readily treatable, and treating it can provide significant patient palliation.[2,3]

EPIDEMIOLOGY

Hypercalcemia is a common metabolic complication of malignant disease. It occurs in up to 30% of cancer patients, and more frequently in advanced stages.[4–8] Malignancy is the most frequent cause of hypercalcemia in the hospital setting, while primary hyperparathyroidism is most common in the community. HCM is more common in certain types of cancers, particularly primary solid tumors of the lung, breast, head and neck, kidney, and ovary. It also occurs preferentially in certain histologies such as squamous cell cancer of the lung compared to adenocarcinomas or small cell lung cancer. However, hypercalcemia should not be discounted in other cancers such as prostate, colon, cervix, and uterus.[1,9–13] Certain hematological malignancies can also present with hypercalcemia, including multiple myeloma.[14–16]

PATHOPHYSIOLOGY

The regulation of calcium levels within the body theoretically is centered on three key organ systems—gastrointestinal (GI) tract, kidneys, and bone. Hypercalcemia results from a combination of any of three main mechanisms, particularly (1) increased calcium absorption from the GI tract; (2) decreased excretion from the kidneys; and (3) enhanced calcium resorption from bone. However, it is a common misconception that bone metastasis is required to cause hypercalcemia.[4] There are two mechanisms of HCM:

- Secretion of parathyroid hormone–related protein (PTHrP), which stimulates osteoclastic bone resorption and calcium reabsorption through the kidneys
- Lytic bone metastases through cytokines released by tumor cells[17]

PTHrP is a 16 kDa peptide, is larger than parathyroid hormone (PTH) and shares a 61% sequence homology with PTH in the first 13 amino acids at the N-terminal.[4,18,19] It has four times the bioactivity of PTH and binds competitively to the PTH receptor.[20] PTHrP is the predominant cause of hypercalcemia in patients with cancer. At least 80% of patients with solid tumors and hypercalcemia have increased serum concentrations of PTHrP. In addition to its humoral effects, PTHrP can also induce local osteolysis around bone metastases, and it appears to be important in the progression of bone metastases in patients with breast carcinoma.[21–24] Other humoral factors secreted by solid and hematologic tumors that are associated with hypercalcemia include IL-1, IL-6, TNF-α, G-CSF, macrophage inflammatory protein-1α, and tumor-induced $1,25(OH)_2D_3$.

The increased calcium level from PTHrP-related secretion and osteolysis diminishes the efficiency of renal elimination of excess calcium. In addition, decreased intravascular volume secondary to hypercalcemia-induced nausea and anorexia results in sodium and calcium resorption through the proximal tubule.

DIFFERENTIAL DIAGNOSIS

Primary hyperparathyroidism and HCM account for greater than 90% of cases.[25–27] Primary hyperparathyroidism accounts for the majority of cases among the general population. The patients usually are relatively well, presenting with vague or little symptoms. In contrast to primary hyperparathyroidism, HCM usually occurs suddenly, resulting in higher calcium levels. Patients with HCM are more symptomatic than individuals with primary hyperparathyroidism, and carry a poor prognosis with a median survival of approximately 6 weeks.[15,21]

CLINICAL MANIFESTATION

The signs and symptoms of hypercalcemia may be subtle and require a high index of suspicion to make the appropriate diagnosis. The severity of symptoms depends on the rate of increase in serum calcium level more than the absolute serum calcium level.[28]

A wide range of multiorgan system changes can be produced. Neurological symptoms range from subtle mental status changes such as changes in concentration, memory, mood and irritability to sedation, stupor, delirium, and coma.[29,30] High symptom expression, including pain, fatigue, insomnia, and drowsiness, can result in cases of delirium, and there should be a low tolerance in testing for hypercalcemia, as it is readily treated and results in palliative symptom control.[31]

Anorexia, nausea, vomiting, and constipation result from decreased smooth muscle contractility, delayed gastric emptying, and slowed intestinal motility. Other gastrointestinal effects include acute pancreatitis and peptic ulcers which occur with long-standing hypercalcemia. The resulting volume contraction from decreased oral intake secondary to nausea, and vomiting can lead to hypotension, tachycardia, mucosal dryness, and altered skin turgor. Furthermore, glomerular filtration is decreased and contributes to renal insufficiency. Polyuria and compensatory polydipsia also result from the impaired ability of the distal nephrons to concentrate urine.[32] Nephrolithiasis may also develop. However, this is less common with HCM since the hypercalcemic state develops rapidly.

Cardiac effects, if they develop, may be the terminal event. Shortened QT intervals, wide T wave, prolonged PR intervals, bradycardia, and arrhythmia result from altered cardiac electrical impulses secondary to the increase in calcium ions.

Due to the relatively rapid elevation in serum calcium in malignancy, the commonly formed mnemonic of "bones, stones, moans, and groans" are rarely seen. These are more associated with chronic elevation in serum calcium (Table 82.1).

Table 82.1 *Clinical manifestations*

Neurological	Concentration changes, memory loss, mood changes, irritability, sedation, delirium, stupor, coma
Gastrointestinal	Anorexia, nausea, vomiting, constipation, acute pancreatitis, peptic ulcers
Renal	Polyuria, polydipsia, nephrolithiasis, dehydration, decreased glomerular filtration, renal insufficiency
Cardiac	Shortened QT, wide T, prolonged PR, bradycardia, hypotension, arrhythmia

LABORATORY EVALUATION

Routine laboratory tests have become standard in cancer patients, and most cases of HCM are found during the asymptomatic phase. The laboratory evaluation for HCM includes serum electrolytes, phosphorus, creatinine, alkaline phosphatase, albumin, and total serum calcium or serum ionized calcium. Measuring creatinine clearance and serum electrolytes is recommended to monitor renal function. The milk alkali syndrome may increase serum bicarbonate. Levels of $1,25(OH)_2D_3$ are elevated in granulomatous disorders such as sarcoidosis and lymphomas.[33]

Measurement of serum ionized calcium should be preferred over total serum calcium levels, because hypoalbuminemia may be associated with low total calcium, but with normal concentration of ionized calcium.[33] Calcium exists in three forms in plasma: bound to albumin and other proteins (~40%), chelated to serum anions (~13%), and as free ionized calcium (~47%).[34,35] Free ionized calcium is the active component of total calcium. A common error is using the uncorrected total serum calcium level, instead of using the corrected or ionized calcium level. Calculations for corrected total serum calcium level adjusted for serum albumin levels are as follows:

- In imperial units: Corrected calcium (mg/dL) = serum calcium + 0.8 mg/dL (4 g/dL - serum albumin)
- In SI Units: Corrected calcium (mmol/L) = serum calcium + 0.2 mmol/L (40 g/L - serum albumin)

TREATMENT

Hydration

Aggressive intravenous rehydration with isotonic saline and close monitoring of volume status is the key initial step in treating hypercalcemia. This helps reverse the vicious cycle of decreased intravascular volume, decreased glomerular filtration, and impaired calcium excretion. Mild hypercalcemia can usually be corrected with outpatient oral rehydration. Monitoring of other electrolytes like potassium and magnesium should also be done as there are usually concurrent electrolyte abnormalities present.[36] Administration of diuretics, such as furosemide, poses risks such as further volume depletion and electrolyte imbalances and is no longer recommended unless there is evidence of fluid overload.[5,37]

Bisphosphonates

The mainstay of treatment is bisphosphonates, which inhibit osteoclastic bone resorption through osteoclastic apoptosis. Due to poor bioavailability of the oral route, parenteral administration is indicated.[38] It usually takes 2–6 days to achieve normal calcium levels. There are two classes of bisphosphonates: nitrogen and non-nitrogen containing.

Common adverse effects from bisphosphonates include hypocalcemia and transient renal insufficiency. Rare side effects include renal failure, jaw osteonecrosis, ocular reactions such as iritis, episcleritis, scleritis, and conjunctivitis. Acute phase reactions include transient fever, malaise, myalgias, bone pain flare, and lymphocytopenia. The acute phase reactions may be lessened with premedication with acetaminophen.

Nitrogen-containing bisphosphonates

Nitrogen-containing bisphosphonates are more potent agents through inhibition of farnesyl diphosphate synthase, resulting in blockage of protein isoprenylation, which is a vital process for osteoclast structural integrity, resulting in apoptosis.[4]

Pamidronate was the first nitrogen-containing agent available clinically and, thus, is also the most thoroughly investigated.[39] A dose–response study found that higher doses of pamidronate, 60–90 mg, have been more effective in achieving normocalcemia.[40,41] This trend has also been found with alendronate in which higher dosages have shown better efficacy.[42] Zoledronate has been found to be more effective than pamidronate in achieving normocalcemia. However, more renal adverse effects have been reported with zoledronate than pamidronate, especially with higher doses and shorter infusion times.[43–45] When renal function is a concern, ibandronate is an alternative, as it has less nephrotoxicity.

Non-nitrogen-containing bisphosphonates

Non-nitrogen-containing bisphosphonates inhibit ATP-dependent intracellular enzymes by incorporating into non-hydrolyzable adenosine triphosphate, which also results in apoptosis.[9]

Etidronate was one of the earliest bisphosphonates to be used clinically. However, due to its low potency and potential effect of inhibiting normal bone mineralization, its use has been relatively anecdotal in the treatment of hypercalcemia.[46,47] Clodronate and pamidronate have been found to have similar efficacy at recommended dosages, with pamidronate having a longer duration of effect.[48,49] Clodronate, a second-generation bisphosphonate, has utility in treating HCM in that it can be administered subcutaneously, which is of particular advantage in palliative settings such as home or hospice facility.[50–52]

Calcitonin

Calcitonin inhibits bone resorption and renal tubular calcium reabsorption. Physiologically, this hormone is secreted from parafollicular or C cells within the thyroid in response to elevated serum calcium levels.[53] Subcutaneous injections have a rapid onset of action, usually in 2–4 hours. However, effect diminishes after 48 hours due to tachyphylaxis, secondary to downregulation of osteoclastic calcitonin receptors.[54] Calcitonin is useful when combined with bisphosphonates, more so in urgent, life-threatening situations because of its rapid effect, while the bisphosphonates have a slower onset of action. Adverse effects include nausea, flushing, abdominal pain, and local irritation at the injection site.

Corticosteroids

Corticosteroids are more effective in treating HCM secondary to steroid-responsive tumors such as lymphoma or myeloma.[41,55] A study by Binstock reported that glucocorticoids prolonged the effective time of treatment with calcitonin by upregulating cell surface calcitonin receptors and therefore may be an effective adjunct to calcitonin administration.[56]

Gallium nitrate

Gallium nitrate accumulates in metabolically active regions of bone where it inhibits osteoclast-mediated bone resorption. It prevents acidification and cell-mediated dissolution of bone material by inhibiting an adenosine triphosphatase–dependent proton pump in the ruffled membrane of the osteoclast.[57] Gallium also inhibits PTH secretion from parathyroid cells in vitro.[58] It has been found to be effective in both PTHrP-mediated and non-PTHrP-mediated hypercalcemia.[59–62] It has been shown to be at least or more effective than pamidronate, etidronate, and calcitonin.[57,63,64] The main concerns with the use of gallium have been nephrotoxicity, hypophosphatemia, nausea, and administration time of 5 days.

RANKL inhibitors

Preliminary data from studies of agents that interfere with the receptor activator of nuclear factor-kB ligand (RANKL) system, which is the molecular pathway that leads to osteoclast recruitment and differentiation, have shown reductions in bone resorption in studies in animals and women with osteoporosis. These agents include recombinant osteoprotegerin and monoclonal antibodies against RANKL, such as denosumab.[6,54,65–67]

Denosumab is a novel agent administered subcutaneously every 4 weeks for the prevention of skeletal-related events (e.g., fracture, spinal cord compression) in patients with cancers metastatic to bone. Its use in HCM is less well studied but promising. The expense of denosumab may be prohibitive as it is more costly than the bisphosphonates.

Other treatments

Results of trials of combining anti-PTHrP antibodies with zoledronic acid have shown to be optimistic so far in decreasing tumor-associated osteoclasts.[68] An additional benefit of increased adipose tissue and muscle weight has also been seen.[69] Tyrosine kinase inhibitors focusing on IL-6 have also been shown in studies to be potential agents in inhibiting osteoclast resorption and treating hypercalcemia.[70,71] A report on a noncalcemic analogue of calcitriol (e.g. 22-oxacalcitriol) suggests its potential to suppress PTHrP gene expression through binding to the vitamin D receptor in HTLV-1 infected cells.[72]

There have been case reports describing the use of long-acting octreotide in controlling hypercalcemia in patients with neuroendocrine tumor and breast cancer.[73,74] Ultrasound-guided

Table 82.2 *Therapeutic dosages*

- IV or SC hydration
  - Isotonic saline ≥ 1–3 L/day
- Bisphosphonates
  - Nitrogen containing
    - Pamidronate 60–90 mg IV
    - Ibandronate 2–6 mg IV
    - Zoledronate 4 mg IV
  - Non-nitrogen containing
    - Clodronate 1500 mg IV or SC single dose or 300 mg IV daily ×
      7–10 days
- Calcitonin 4–8 IU/kg SC/IM q6–12 h
- Corticosteroids
  - Hydrocortisone 100–300 mg/day
  - Dexamethasone 4–12 mg/day
  - Prednisone 25–75 mg/day
- Gallium nitrate 100–200 mg/m^2/day IV over 24 hours × 5 days

percutaneous ethanol injection has been studied in patients with parathyroid carcinoma for palliation, resulting in a transitory decrease in PTH and calcium levels.[75]

The treatments listed above are only temporizing measures. The most effective long-term treatment is still treating the underlying cause, especially in the case of HCM, which is effective antineoplastic intervention. Goals of care should be discussed with the patient and family as hypercalcemia often occurs late in the course of the cancer. Discontinuing medications that can cause hypercalcemia, like thiazides and vitamin D, should not be overlooked (Table 82.2).

Key learning points

- Hypercalcemia is a common, treatable complication of malignant disease.
- Secretion of PTHrP is the predominant cause of hypercalcemia in HCM, even without overt bone metastasis.
- Signs and symptoms may be subtle; a high index of suspicion is required.
- The severity of symptoms depends on the rate of increase in serum calcium levels more than the absolute serum calcium levels.
- The treatment of HCM can result in improved overall palliation.
- Rehydration is a key initial step in the management of HCM.
- Intravenous bisphosphonates are the agents of choice in the treatment of HCM, with nitrogen-containing bisphosphonates being the more potent agents.
- Different novel agents are being investigated in the treatment of hypercalcemia.

REFERENCES

1 Lamy O, Jenzer-Closuit A, Burckhardt P. Hypercalcemia of malignancy: An underdiagnosed and undertreated disease. *J Intern Med* 2001; 250: 73–79.
2 Morita T, Tei Y, Shishido H, Inoue S. Treatable complications of cancer patients referred to an in-patient hospice. *Am J Hosp Palliat Care* 2003; 20: 389–391.
3 Falk S, Fallon M. ABC of palliative care: Emergencies. *BMJ* 1997; 315: 1525–1528.
4 Clines GA, Guise TA. Hypercalcemia of malignancy and basic research on mechanisms responsible for osteolytic and osteoblastic metastasis to bone. *Endocr Relat Cancer* 2005; 12: 549–583.
5 Body JJ. Hypercalcemia of malignancy. *Semin Nephrol* 2004; 24: 48–54.
6 Stewart A. Hypercalcemia associated with cancer. *NEJM* 2005; 352(4): 373–379.
7 Mundy GR, Guise TA. Hypercalcemia of malignancy. *Am J Med* 1997; 103: 134–145.
8 Halfdanarson TR, Hogan WJ, Moynihan TJ. Oncologic emergencies: Diagnosis and treatment. *Mayo Clin Proc* 2006; 81: 835–848.
9 Smith DC, Tucker JA, Trump DL. Hypercalcemia and neuroendocrine carcinoma of the prostate: A report of three cases and a review of the literature. *J Clin Oncol* 1992; 10: 499–505.
10 Matzkin H, Braf Z. Paraneoplastic syndromes associated with prostate carcinoma. *J Urol* 1987; 138: 1129–1133.
11 Mahadevia PS, Ramaswamy A, Greenwald ES, Wollner DI, Markham D. Hypercalcemia in prostatic carcinoma. A report of eight cases. *Arch Intern Med* 1983; 43: 1339–1342.
12 Di Sant'Agnese PA. Neuroendocrine carcinoma of the prostate: The concept 'comes of age'. *Arch Pathol Lab Med* 1988; 112: 1097–1099.
13 Wenk RE, Bhagavan BS, Levy R, Miller D, Weisburger W. Ectopic ACTH, prostatic oat cell carcinoma, and marked hyponatremia. *Cancer* 1977; 40: 773–778.
14 Martin TJ. Hypercalcemia of malignancy. *Clin Rev Bone Mineral Metab* 2002; 1(1): 51–63.
15 Alsirafy SA, Sroor MY, Al-Shahri MZ. Hypercalcemia in advanced head and neck squamous cell carcinoma: Prevalence and impact on palliative care. *J Support Oncol* 2009; 7(5); 154–157.
16 Singer FR. Pathogenesis of hypercalcemia of malignancy. *Semin Oncol* 1991; 18: 4–10.
17 Bayne MC, Illidge TM. Hypercalcaemia, parathyroid hormone-related protein and malignancy. *Clin Oncol* 2001; 13: 372–377.
18 Suva L, Winslow GA, Wettenhall REH et al. A parathyroid hormone-related protein implicated in malignant hypercalcemia; cloning and expression. *Science* 1987; 237: 893–896.
19 Grill V, Body J, Johanson N et al. Parathyroid hormone-related protein: Elevated levels in both humoral hypercalcemia of malignancy and hypercalcemia complicating metstatic breast cancer. *J Clin Endocrinol Metab* 1991; 73: 1309–1315.
20 Karaplis AC, Goltzman D. PTH and PTHrP effects on the skeleton. *Rev Endocr Metab Disord* 2000; 1: 331–341.
21 Strewler GJ. The Physiology of Parathyroid hormone-related protein. *NEJM* 2000; 342: 177–185.
22 Wysolmerski JJ, Broadus AE. Hypercalcemia of malignancy: The central role of parathyroid hormone-related protein. *Annu Rev Med* 1994; 45: 189–200.
23 Guise TA, Yin JJ, Taylor SD et al. Evidence for a causal role of parathyroid hormone-related protein in the pathogenesis of human breast cancer-mediated osteolysis. *J Clin Invest* 1996; 98: 1544–1549.
24 Yin JJ, Selander K, Chirgwin JM et al. TGF-beta signaling blockade inhibits PTHrP secretion by breast cancer cells and bone metastases development. *J Clin Invest* 1999; 103: 197–206.

25   Lafferty FW. Differential diagnosis of hypercalcemia. *J Bone Miner Res* 1991; 6(Suppl. 2): S51.

26   Burtis WJ, Wu TL, Insogna KL, Stewart AF. Humoral hypercalcemia of malignancy. *Ann Intern Med* 1988; 108(3): 454.

27   Ratcliffe WA, Hutchesson AC, Bundred NJ, Ratcliffe JG. Role of assays for parathyroid-hormone-related protein in investigation of hypercalcemia. *Lancet* 1992; 339(8786): 164.

28   Agraharkar M, Dellinger OD, Gangakhedkar AK. Hypercalcemia. Medscape Reference. 2010.

29   Bajorunas DR. Clinical manifestations of cancer-related hypercalcemia. *Semin Oncol* 1990; 17: 16–25.

30   Leboff MS, Mikulee KH. Hypercalcemia: Clinical manifestations, pathogenesis, diagnosis, and management. In Favus MJ (ed.), *Primer on the Metabolic Bone Diseases and Disorders of Mineral Metabolism*, 5th edn. Washington, DC: American Society for Bone and Mineral Research, 2003, pp. 225–229.

31   Solomon B, Schaaf M, Smallridge R. Psychologic symptoms before and after parathyroid surgery. *Am J Med* 1994; 96: 101–106.

32   Delgado-Guay M, Yennurajalingam S, Bruera E. Delirium with severe symptom expression related to hypercalcemia in a patient with advanced cancer: An interdisciplinary approach to treatment. *J Pain Symp Manage* 2008; 36(4): 442–449.

33   Leyland-Jones B. Treatment of cancer-related hypercalcemia: The role of gallium nitrate. *Semin Oncol* 2003; 30(Suppl. 5): 13–19.

34   Basso U, Maruzzo M, Roma A, Camozzi V, Luisetto G, Lumachi F. Malignant hypercalcemia. *Curr Med Chem* 2011; 18: 3462–3467.

35   Clase C, Norman G, Beecroft M, Churchill D. Albumin-corrected calcium and ionized calcium in stable hemodialysis patients. *Nephrol Dial Transplant* 2000; 15: 1841–1846.

36   Riancho J, Arjona R, Sanz J et al. Is the routine measurement of ionized calcium worthwhile in patients with cancer? *Postgrad Med J* 1991; 67: 350–353.

37   Mundy GR. Hypercalcemia of cancer. *N Engl J Med* 1984; 310: 1718–1727.

38   Seccarecia D. Caner-related hypercalcemia. *Can Fam Phys* 2010; 56; 244–246.

39   Hurtado J, Esbrit P. Treatment of malignant hypercalcemia. *Expert Opin Pharmacother* 2002; 3: 521–527.

40   Pecherstorfer M, Brenner K, Niklas Zojer N. Current management strategies for hypercalcemia. *Treat Endocrinol* 2003; 2: 273–292.

41   Thiebaud D, Jaeger P, Jacquet A, Burckhardt P. Dose–response in the treatment of hypercalcemia of malignancy by a single infusion of the bisphosphonate AHPrBP. *J Clin Oncol* 1988; 6: 762–768.

42   Body JJ. Current and future directions in medical therapy: Hypercalcemia. *Cancer* 2000; 88: 3054–3058.

43   Nussbaum SR, Warrell RP, Rude R et al. Dose–response study of alendronate sodium for the treatment of cancer-associated hypercalcemia. *J Clin Oncol* 1993; 11: 1618–1623.

44   Berenson J, Hirschberg R. Safety and convenience of a 15-minute infusion of zoledronic acid. *Oncologist* 2004; 9: 319–329.

45   Perry CM, Figgitt DP. Zoledronic acid: A review of its use in patients with advanced cancer. *Drugs* 2004; 64: 1197–1211.

46   Major P, Lortholary A, Hon J et al. Zoledronic acid is superior to pamidronate in the treatment of hypercalcemia of malignancy: A pooled analysis of two randomized, controlled clinical trials. *J Clin Oncol* 2001; 19: 558–567.

47   Patel S, Lyons A, Hosking D. Drugs used in the treatment of metabolic bone disease. Clinical pharmacology and therapeutic use. *Drugs* 1993; 46: 594–617.

48   Flora A, Hassing GS, Parfitt A, Villanueva A. Comparative skeletal effects of 2 diphosphonates in dogs. *Metab Bone Dis Rel Res* 1980; 2: 389–407.

49   Saunders Y, Ross J, Broadley K, Patel S. Systematic review of bisphosphonates for hypercalcemia of malignancy. *Palliat Med* 2004; 18: 418–431.

50   Purohit O, Radstone C, Anthony C et al. A randomised double-blind comparison of intravenous pamidronate and clodronate in the hypercalcemia of malignancy. *Br J Cancer* 1995; 72: 1289–1293.

51   Roemer-Becuwe C, Vigano A, Romano F, Neumann C, Hanson J, Quan HK, Walker P. Safety of subcutaneous clodronate and efficacy in hypercalcemia of malignancy: A novel route of administration. *J Pain Symptom Manage* September 2003; 26(3):843–848.

52   Walker P, Watanabe S, Lawlor P, Hanson J, Pereira J, Bruera E. Subcutaneous clodronate: A study evaluating efficacy in hypercalcemia of malignancy and local toxicity. *Ann Oncol* September 1997; 8(9): 915–916.

53   Walker P, Watanabe S, Lawlor P, Bruera E. Subcutaneous clodronate. *Lancet* August 1996; 348(9023): 345–346.

54   Becker KL, Snider R, Moore C et al. Calcitonin in extrathyroidal tissues of man. *Acta Endocrinol* 1979; 92: 746–750.

55   Watters J, Gerrard G, Dodwell D. The management of malignant hypercalcemia. *Drugs* 1996; 52: 837–848.

56   Kovacs C, MacDonald S, Chik C, Bruera E. Hypercalcemia of malignancy in the palliative care patient: A treatment strategy. *J Pain Symptom Manage* 1995; 10: 224–232.

57   Binstock ML, Mundy GR. Effect of calcitonin and glucocorticoids in combination on the hypercalcemia of malignancy. *Ann Intern Med* 1980; 93: 269–227.

58   Cvitkovic F, Armand JP, Tubiana-Hulin M, Rossi JF, Warrell RP. Randomized, double-blind, phase II trial of gallium nitrate compared with pamidronate for acute control of cancer-related hypercalcemia. *Cancer J* 2006; 12(1): 47–53.

59   Ridefelt P, Gylfe E, Akerström G, Rastad J. Effects of the antihypercalcemic drugs gallium nitrate and pamidronate on hormone release of pathologic human parathyroid cells. *Surgery* 1995; 117: 56.

60   Warrell RP Jr, Bockman RS, Coonley CJ et al. Gallium nitrate inhibits calcium resorption from bone and is effective treatment for cancer-related hypercalcemia. *J Clin Invest* 1984; 73: 1487.

61   Warrell RP Jr, Israel R, Frisone M et al. Gallium nitrate for acute treatment of cancer-related hypercalcemia. A randomized, double-blind comparison to calcitonin. *Ann Intern Med* 1988; 108: 669.

62   Warrell RP Jr, Murphy WK, Schulman P et al. A randomized double-blind study of gallium nitrate compared with etidronate for acute control of cancer-related hypercalcemia. *J Clin Oncol* 1991; 9: 1467.

63   Cvitkovic F, Armand JP, Tubiana-Hulin M et al. Randomized, double-blind, phase II trial of gallium nitrate compared with pami.

64   Leyland-Jones B. Treatment of cancer-related hypercalcemia: The role of gallium nitrate. *Semin Oncol* 2003; 20: 13–19.

65   Hu MI, Gucalp R, Insogna K, Glezerman I, Lebouleux S, Misiorowski W, Yu B, Ying W, Yeh HS. Denosumab for treatment of hypercalcemia of malignancy in patients with solid tumors or hematological malignancies refractory to IV bisphosphonates: A single-arm multicenter study. *53rd American Society of Hematology Annual Meeting and Exposition*, San Diego, CA; 2011.

66   Study of denosumab in the treatment of hypercalcemia of malignancy in subjects with elevated serum calcium. http://clinicaltrials.gov/show. NCT00896454. 2011.

67   Camozzi V, Luisetto G, Basso SM, Cappelletti P, Tozzoli R, Lumachi F. Treatment of chronic hypercalcemia. *Med Chem* E-pub. 2012.

68   Capparelli C, Kostenuik PJ, Morony S, Starnes C, Weimann B, Van G, Scully S, Qi M, Lacey DL, Dunstan CR. Osteoprotegerin prevents and reverses hypercalcemia in a murine model of humoral hypercalcemia of malignancy. *Cancer Res* 2000; 60(4): 783–787.

69   Yamada T, Muguruma H, Yano S, Ikuta K, Ogino H, Kakiuchi S, Hanibuchi M, Uehara H, Nishioka Y, Sone S. Intensification therapy with anti-parathyroid hormone-related protein antibody plus zoledronic acid for bone metastases of small cell lung cancer cells in severe combined immunodeficient mice. *Mol Cancer Ther* 2009; 8(1): 119–126.

70 Iguchi H, Aramaki Y, Maruta S, Takiguchi S. Effects of anti-parathyroid hormone-related protein monoclonal antibody and osteroprotegerin on PTHrP-producine tumor-induced cachexia in nude mic. *J Bone Miner Metab* 2006; 24(1): 16–19.

71 Yoneda T, Lowe C, Lee CH, Gutierrez G, Niewolna M, Williams PJ, Izbicka E, Uehara Y, Mundy GR. Herbimycin A, a pp60c-src tyrosine kinase inhibitor, inhibits osteoclastic bone resoprtion in vitro and hypercalcemia in vivo. *J Clin Invest* 1993; 91(6): 2791–2795.

72 Moriyama K, Williams PJ, Niewolna M, Dallas MR, Uehara Y, Mundy GR, Yoneda T. Herbimycin A, a tyrosine kinase inhibitor, impairs hypercalcemia associated with a human squamous cancer producing interleukin-6 in nude mice. *J Bone Miner Res* 1996; 11(7): 905–911.

73 Inoue D, Matsumoto T, Ogata E, Ikeda K. 22-Oxacalcitriol, a noncalcemic analogue of calcitriol, suppresses both cell proliferation and parathyroid hormone-related peptide gene expression in human T cell lymphotrophic virus, type I-infected T cells. *J Biol Chem* 1993; 268(22): 16730–16736.

74 Mantzoros CS, Suva LJ, Moses AC, Spark R. Intractable hypercalcaemia due to parathyroid hormone-related peptide secretion by a carcinoid tumour. *Clin Endocrinol* 1997; 46(3): 373–375.

75 Shiba E, Inoue T, Akazawa K, Takai S. Somatostatin analogue treatment for malignant hypercalcemia associated with advanced breast cancer. *Gan To Kagaku Ryoho* 1996; 23(3): 343–347.

76 Montenegro F, Chammas M, Juliano A, Cernea C, Cordero A. Ethanol injection under ultrasound guidance to palliate unresectable parathyroid carcinoma. *Arq Bras Endocrinol Metab* 2008; 52(4): 707–711.

83

Hemorrhage

JEN-YU WEI, SRIRAM YENNURAJALINGAM

INTRODUCTION

Patients in palliative care who have advanced cancers experience a variety of bleeding problems. Bleeding occurs in approximately 10% of patients with advanced cancer [1,2] and manifests as hemoptysis, hematuria, vaginal bleeding, rectal bleeding, hematemesis, melena, or bleeding from tumors fungating through the skin. Hemorrhage is the cause of immediate death ("terminal hemorrhage") in 6%–10% of all cancer patients, and its management poses a challenge to healthcare providers. Many of these patients may require admission to the palliative care unit for intense symptom management, including transfusions and administration of midazolam to manage anxiety and related psychological issues, as hemorrhage is a major source of distress to patients and their families [3].

This chapter focuses on the causes and management of hemorrhage in patients with advanced cancer. We first briefly summarize the pathophysiology of hemorrhage in these patients and then turn to specific bleeding problems (hemoptysis, vaginal bleeding, gastrointestinal hemorrhage, and hematuria) related to certain cancers. We then provide more in-depth discussions of disseminated intravascular coagulation (DIC) and thrombocytopenia and conclude with recommendations for the clinical approach to hemorrhage.

CLINICAL PRESENTATION AND UNDERLYING PATHOPHYSIOLOGY OF BLEEDING IN PATIENTS WITH ADVANCED CANCER

Cancer-caused bleeding may be anatomic, generalized, or combined (Table 83.1). Bleeding may involve damage to local vessels, invasion of vessels, mucositis, a systemic process such as DIC, or abnormalities in platelet number and function. The underlying causes of these abnormalities vary and include liver failure, medications such as anticoagulants, chemotherapy, radiotherapy, surgery, and the cancer itself.

Hemoptysis

Hemoptysis, the coughing up of blood or bloody mucus from the lungs or throat, is a common symptom of bronchial carcinoma, often owing to tumor invasion of intrathoracic vascular structures. Hemoptysis is present in approximately 50% of cancer patients at presentation [4] and may also accompany pulmonary metastasis. Although rare, massive hemoptysis carries a 50% mortality rate if not treated promptly [5]. Although rarely of hemodynamic significance, hemoptysis is a distressing symptom for the patient and an indication for local radiotherapy [6]. In terms of survival, there are no proven advantages in treating asymptomatic patients with inoperable lung cancer. However, some evidence suggests that tumors greater than 10 cm in diameter, whether primary or metastasized, carry a significant risk of hemorrhage, and it has been suggested that patients with such lesions should receive prophylactic treatment for hemoptysis [7].

Surgical resection may be considered for hemoptysis in patients with good performance status, but in advanced cancer, nonsurgical approaches often remain the appropriate first-line treatment [8]. In acute massive hemoptysis, interventions including bronchial stenting and bronchial arterial embolization have shown promising results in case reports [9–12].

Vaginal bleeding

Ninety percent of patients with endometrial cancer report abnormal vaginal bleeding at the time of their diagnosis; however, vaginal bleeding is rarely excessive and can usually be managed conservatively. Occasionally, a patient with a uterine tumor may present with a major hemorrhage requiring immediate resuscitation and vaginal packing before the initiation of urgent treatment to stop the hemorrhage.

Vaginal bleeding in advanced or metastatic cancer may be due to recurrent or locally advanced tumors of the cervix or uterus. Endometrial cancer typically spreads to nearby

Table 83.1 *Etiology of bleeding in cancer patients*

Anatomical
- Local tumor invasion (tumor invasion into blood vessels)
- Tumor surface bleeding (skin wounds, internal bleeding)
- Mucositis (infection, drug-induced, radiation-induced, chemotherapy-related, peptic acid-related, stress)

Generalized
- Platelet disorder (thrombocytopenia or platelet function defects)
- Bone marrow involvement by cancer (hematological malignancies)
- DIC
- Liver failure
- Medications (anticoagulants, aspirin, NSAIDs)
- Concomitant disease (cirrhosis, von Willebrand disease)

Combined
- Local and systemic factors

organs, including local infiltrations of advanced cancers of the bladder and rectum or mucosal deposits along the vaginal wall.

Radiotherapy using either external-beam irradiation or intracavity treatment can help definitively control bleeding. Uterine or other pelvic arterial embolization may be feasible in select cases. Uterine arterial embolization has been used relatively frequently in cases of postpartum hemorrhage and sometimes also in the management of cancer-related vaginal bleeding [47].

Gastrointestinal hemorrhage

Symptomatic gastrointestinal hemorrhage may arise from either the upper or lower gastrointestinal tract and can result in hematemesis and melena or hematochezia. Rectal bleeding occurs in 10%–20% of patients with colorectal cancer. The underlying tumor may be a primary neoplasm arising within the gastrointestinal tract, most commonly from the stomach, large bowel, or rectum, or may be the result of direct invasion of a locally advanced tumor from adjacent structures such as the uterus.

Modest doses of radiation to the bleeding sites will often control the bleeding effectively and durably. Surgery is the treatment of choice in cases of neoplasm-related lower gastrointestinal tract bleeding but is rarely required. In addition to radiotherapy, endoscopic interventions involving thermal coagulation, cryotherapy, mechanical ligation techniques, and local injection of vasoconstricting medications may be used [13,14]. Interventional angiography with transcatheter embolization to control bleeding also has been effective for lower gastrointestinal hemorrhage [13].

Hematuria

Hematuria is a frequent symptom and sign of underlying urological disease. In patients with advanced cancer, hematuria may be secondary to an underlying malignancy, a possibly major coagulation disorder, or a result of interventions such as pelvic irradiation and cyclophosphamide treatment.

Hematuria usually manifests as the passage of brown or red urine or could involve the passage of large clots, clot retention, or colic.

Retained clots require immediate intervention before specific studies are initiated. Upon clinical confirmation of a palpable bladder, resulting from a clot, a complete evacuation can be achieved by inserting a multieyed Robinson catheter (24F or 26F) into the urethra. Once the catheter has passed into the bladder, vigorous irrigation with water or saline using a Toomey syringe will enable removal of all clots [15]. Irrigation of the bladder is uncomfortable and may require analgesia. Unsuccessful initial placement of the catheter or continued bleeding and recurrent obstruction of the irrigating catheter are indications for endoscopic evaluation.

If bleeding is refractory to conservative measures, instillation of 1%–2% alum (potassium or ammonium aluminum sulfate), 1% silver nitrate, or formalin may be tried. However, caution is needed when using alum irrigation in patients with renal insufficiency or s bladder lesions that may allow alum to enter the vascular system, and blood aluminum levels should be monitored in these cases. Formalin instillation is effective but carries a risk of bladder perforation and fibrosis. General or regional anesthesia is usually required to control the pain of formalin instillation [15].

Another treatment option cancer-related hematuria is radiotherapy plus oral tranexamic acid (TA). Bleeding as a result of radiation cystitis may respond to hyperbaric oxygen, and in chronic cases, oral pentosan polysulfate may be used [15].

Laser resection or vaporization is a viable option for bleeding associated with superficial and invasive bladder lesions. A more invasive treatment for the same issue as above is transurethral resection, which may control bleeding more effectively. Embolization or surgical ligation of hypogastric arteries may be required in extreme cases. Cystectomy with urinary diversion should only be considered in patients with good performance status if all other options have failed or are not feasible [16].

DISSEMINATED INTRAVASCULAR COAGULATION

DIC, a systemic process producing both thrombosis and hemorrhage, is initiated by several defined disorders and consists of the following components:

- Exposure of blood to procoagulants such as tissue factor
- Formation of fibrin in the circulation
- Fibrinolysis
- Depletion of clotting factors
- End-organ damage

Common manifestations of acute DIC, in addition to bleeding, include thromboembolism and dysfunction of the kidney, liver, lungs, and central nervous system (CNS). In one series of 118 patients with DIC, the main clinical manifestations were bleeding (64%), renal dysfunction (25%), hepatic dysfunction (19%), respiratory dysfunction (16%), shock (14%), thromboembolism (7%), and CNS involvement (2%) [17].

Petechiae and ecchymoses are common in conjunction with blood oozing from wound sites, intravenous lines, and, in some cases, mucosal surfaces. Such bleeding can be life-threatening if it involves the gastrointestinal tract, lungs, or CNS. In patients who develop DIC after surgical procedures, hemorrhage may develop around indwelling lines, catheters, drains, and tracheostomies, and blood may accumulate in serous cavities.

Malignancy often causes chronic DIC and can also produce acute DIC, particularly in patients with acute promyelocytic leukemia. DIC is often present at the time of diagnosis or soon after the initiation of cytotoxic chemotherapy in patients with this disorder. DIC can cause pulmonary or cerebrovascular hemorrhage in up to 40% of patients with acute promyelocytic leukemia, and some studies have shown early hemorrhagic death in 10%–20% of these patients [18]. Inducing tumor cell differentiation with *all-trans*-retinoic acid can rapidly alleviate the coagulopathy in these cases [18].

Chronic DIC

Compensated or chronic DIC develops when blood is continuously or intermittently exposed to small amounts of tissue factor, and compensatory mechanisms in the liver and bone marrow are largely unable to replenish the resulting depleted coagulation proteins and platelets, respectively. Under these conditions, the patient can be asymptomatic or can have manifestations of venous or arterial thrombosis or both. Patients with chronic DIC may also have minor bleeding from the skin and mucosal membranes.

The most common cause of chronic DIC is malignancies, particularly solid tumors. Venous thrombosis commonly presents as deep venous thrombosis in the extremities or superficial migratory thrombophlebitis (Trousseau syndrome), where arterial thromboses can produce digital ischemia, renal infarction, or stroke. Arterial ischemia can also be due to embolization from nonbacterial thrombotic (marantic) endocarditis.

The diagnosis of acute DIC is suggested by the patient's history (e.g., sepsis, trauma, malignancy), clinical presentation, moderate to severe thrombocytopenia (less than 100,000 platelets/µL), and microangiopathic changes on the peripheral blood smear. The diagnosis is confirmed by the findings of increased thrombin generation (e.g., decreased fibrinogen) and increased fibrinolysis (e.g., elevated fibrin degradation products and D-dimer). The extent of these abnormalities may correlate with the extensiveness of organ involvement. The laboratory values in these studies vary in chronic DIC because a slower-than-normal rate of the consumption of the coagulation factors may be offset by enhanced synthesis of these proteins. In such patients, the diagnosis may be largely based on finding microangiopathy in the peripheral blood smear and increased levels of fibrin degradation products, in particular D-dimer.

Treatment of DIC

Treatment of the underlying disease (e.g., sepsis) is of central importance in controlling acute or chronic DIC. Hemodynamic support is essential, but many patients do not require specific therapy for coagulopathy, because it is either short-term or not severe enough to pose a major risk for bleeding or thrombosis. In select instances, blood component replacement therapy or heparin may be of value, although no controlled studies have shown the definitive benefit of either. In contrast, the administration of antifibrinolytic agents such as ε-aminocaproic acid (EACA) or aprotinin are generally contraindicated, because blockage of the fibrinolytic system may increase the risk of thrombotic complications [19]. DIC associated with acute promyelocytic leukemia responds to treatment with *all-trans*-retinoic acid.

PLATELET TRANSFUSION AND FRESH FROZEN PLASMA

Patients with DIC bleed because of thrombocytopenia and coagulation factor deficiency. There is no evidence to support the administration of platelets and coagulation factors in patients who are not bleeding. However, treatment is justified in patients who have serious bleeding, are at high risk for bleeding (e.g., after surgery), or require invasive procedures.

Patients with marked thrombocytopenia (less than 20,000 platelets/µL) or those with moderate thrombocytopenia (less than 50,000 platelets/µL) and serious bleeding should be given platelet transfusions (1–2 units/10 kg/day). Such patients typically show a less-than-expected rise in platelet count. With respect to replacement therapy, patients who are actively bleeding with a significantly elevated prothrombin time, international normalized ratio (INR), or a fibrinogen concentration less than 50 mg/dL should receive fresh frozen plasma or cryoprecipitate, the latter for fibrinogen replacement. It is preferable to keep the fibrinogen level above 100 mg/dL.

HEPARIN

The administration of heparin or other anticoagulants to interrupt the underlying coagulopathy in DIC would appear to be a logical therapeutic approach. However, no controlled trials indicate a benefit to these anticoagulants, and little evidence suggests that heparin improves organ function [20,21].

THROMBOCYTOPENIA AND HEMORRHAGIC RISK IN PATIENTS WITH CANCER

The most feared complication of thrombocytopenia is intracranial hemorrhage. Research has confirmed that a spontaneous hemorrhage rarely occurs when a patient's platelet count exceeds 50,000/µL, but the risk of bleeding increases considerably as the count falls below 20,000/µL. The direct relationship between the platelet count and bleeding episodes in patients with malignant diseases was first documented in 1962 by Gaydos et al. [22] in patients with acute leukemia. In this study, major bleeding rarely occurred when the platelet count exceeded 20,000/µL, gradually increased as the platelet count ranged between 20,000 and 5,000/µL, and dramatically increased when the platelet count fell below 5,000/µL. In particular, Gaydos et al. observed that bleeding episodes associated with thrombocytopenia frequently follow a decline in platelet count, especially in cases in which the bleeding occurs when platelet counts exceed 5000/µL. Moreover, no intracranial bleeding was observed at a platelet count exceeding 10,000/µL.

Despite these data, Gaydos et al.'s study has been widely misinterpreted and overinterpreted, and for years, it became the practice to administer platelets prophylactically to maintain the platelet count above a level of 20,000/µL [23]. In 1978, Slichter and Harker [24] published a threshold for spontaneous bleeding, as measured by fecal blood loss, at approximately 50,000/µL in patients with aplastic anemia. This finding was confirmed by the randomized study of Solomon et al. [25] showing that patients routinely transfused with platelets at 20,000/µL fared no better than those who were transfused only if they were bleeding or if their platelet count was decreasing rapidly.

The incidence of hemorrhagic complications in patients with solid tumors was first studied by Belt et al. [26] in a cohort of 718 patients receiving myelosuppressive chemotherapeutic agents. Seventy-five patients (10.4%) experienced one or more episodes of hemorrhage. Bleeding was due to tumor invasion in 25 of 75 patients (33.3%) and to DIC in 7 patients (9.3%) and was unrelated to malignant neoplasms or drug treatment in 6 patients (8%). Thirty-seven patients (49.3%) had hemorrhages associated with drug-induced thrombocytopenia. These results confirmed a quantitative relationship between the incidence of hemorrhage and the platelet count for both the group with thrombocytopenia and the group with hemorrhage resulting from all causes. However, the incidence of hemorrhage was low until the platelet count decreased below 10,000/µL, and fatal bleeding was unlikely to occur at platelet counts above 5,000/µL [26].

In 1984, Dutcher et al. [27] reviewed the records of 1274 patients treated between 1972 and 1980 for protocols known to produce significant myelosuppression to evaluate the incidence of thrombocytopenia and bleeding among patients with solid tumors who had been treated intensively with chemotherapy. Of these, 301 patients experienced 5063 days of thrombocytopenia with less than 50,000 platelets/µL and 670 days of severe thrombocytopenia with less than 20,000 platelets/µL. The median number of days with thrombocytopenia was 6 (range: 1–250). There were only 44 episodes of clinically detectable serious bleeding, primarily gastrointestinal (26/44), during thrombocytopenia, and all but 7 episodes first occurred at platelet counts between 20,000 and 50,000/µL. Of these bleeding episodes, 15 were associated with coagulation abnormalities, 24 occurred during serious infection, and 12 occurred at the sites of tumors. Of the 301 patients, 147 (49%) received platelet transfusions. The 86 patients with thrombocytopenia who had CNS tumors showed no evidence of CNS bleeding during thrombocytopenia. Hemorrhagic deaths were uncommon; of the 12 patients who died of bleeding, 7 had normal platelet counts [27].

Ten years after Dutcher et al.'s study, Goldberg et al. [28] retrospectively studied the clinical impact of thrombocytopenia in patients with gynecologic cancer who received chemotherapy.

Thrombocytopenia, defined as a platelet count below 100,000/µL, occurred in 182 of 501 patients (36.3%). No intracranial or life-threatening bleeding occurred in any patient. Of these 182 patients, 139 (76.4%) had no clinical bleeding. Minor bleeding occurred in 34 patients (18.7%) and 44 cycles of chemotherapy (5.4%). Major bleeding occurred in 9 patients (4.9%) and 10 cycles (1.3%). Of the major bleeding, 5 occurred in 49 patients, with platelet counts between 0 and 10,000/µL. Of the 43 patients who received platelet transfusions, 38 (88.3%) had no bleeding. Of the remaining 5 patients, 2 were transfused prophylactically, with no effect. Three major bleeding events occurred in patients with platelet counts that ranged from 11,000 to 20,000/µL, but these were due to chronic instrumentation or trauma. In patients with platelet counts exceeding 20,000/µL, major bleeding occurred only from necrotic metastatic lesions. Therefore, in this study, platelet counts of 10,000/µL were not associated with spontaneous major bleeding [28].

To evaluate the conservative management of chemotherapy-induced thrombocytopenia, prophylactic transfusions were administered only to patients with platelet counts less than 5000/µL. Fanning et al. [29] evaluated 179 episodes of thrombocytopenia in 46 women with gynecologic cancers who were enrolled in 4 dose-intense chemotherapy trials. Of the 179 episodes of thrombocytopenia evaluated, 100 were severe (less than 20,000/µL). None of the 179 episodes of thrombocytopenia resulted in major bleeding, including 70 that occurred in patients with platelet counts below 20,000/µL who were not receiving prophylactic platelet transfusions; 14 of these 70 had platelet counts between 5,000 and 10,000/µL [29].

From these studies, it is evident that the risk of bleeding depends not only on the platelet count but also on the underlying disease, the use of drugs that interfere with platelet function, and complications such as fever, infection, or coagulation defects. Aspirin, nonsteroidal anti-inflammatory drugs (NSAIDs), and some antibiotics such as high-dose penicillin taken by patients with malignant disease may impair platelet function. As a consequence, it is not the absolute platelet count but rather the number of functional platelets that is important for the prevention of bleeding. Despite this conclusion, no studies show that the bleeding time may aid in defining the risk of bleeding.

CLINICAL APPROACH TO HEMORRHAGE (TABLE 83.2)

A broad, open, and inquisitive frame of mind must be used when treating hemorrhage episodes. The patient's history and physical examination should provide important baseline information. Key laboratory tests must be quickly ordered and interpreted. Using these data, one can quickly determine whether the hemorrhagic disorder is congenital or acquired, severe or mild, and progressive or stable. Hemostasis may fail because of the deficiencies of platelets, the plasma coagulation protein system, or endothelial disturbances.

In the palliative setting, many factors must be considered with regard to the management of bleeding. The clinician has

Table 83.2 *Management of hemorrhage*

Identify patients at risk
- General risk factors (hematological cancers, large head and neck cancers or centrally located lung cancers, liver disease, or clotting derangements)
- Thorough history, physical, review of lab and imaging data

Multidisciplinary team discussion and planning
- Preparation and planning
- Involve physicians, nurses, chaplain, social worker, pharmacists, counselors
- Factors to consider include patient's prognosis, performance status, and patient's perceived quality of life and preferences

Level of discussion depends on
- Diagnosis and prognosis based on all current patient data
- Bleeding risk
- Patient's preference
- Available treatment modalities along with associated risks and benefits

General measures
- Apply external pressure if bleeding is visible
- Have dark towels and basins at bedside
- Have equipment available for suctioning at bedside
- Provide psychological support
- Prepare emergency sedative medications that can be given intravenously or subcutaneously quickly

Resuscitative measures
- Fluid resuscitation
- Transfusion of blood products
- Vasopressors if indicated

Specific measures
- Local hemostatic agents
- Radiotherapy
- Surgical interventions
- Interventional arterial embolization
- Systemic treatments (TA, correction of clotting derangements)

to not only consider the underlying cause and the clinical presentation, including the severity and nature of such an event, but also take into account other salient factors, such as the setting of care, availability of various resources, overall disease burden, predicted life expectancy, the patient's overall quality of life, and the wishes of the patient and family. The patients and families facing the prospect or reality of massive bleeding require extensive psychological support.

The choice of treatment modality must balance the risk of aggressive management with increased treatment-related toxicity and with; on the one hand, against the failure to use treatments that have potential symptomatic benefits is on the other. Although the staff providing palliative care can initiate many simple treatments, a definitive approach to hemorrhage management requires an interdisciplinary approach and sometimes the expertise of various specialists.

As an example of the need to set priorities, it is evident that interventional radiology or surgical ligation of the pelvic vessel would be less likely to be considered for a home-bound, cachectic patient who has expressed the desire to

remain at home, particularly if the patient has an estimated life expectancy ranging from a few days to a few weeks. On the other hand, had the same patient presented soon after significant hemorrhaging began, it would have been reasonable to at least consider the aforementioned treatments, particularly if specialists with the required skills and equipment were available. The patients and families facing the prospect or reality of massive bleeding require extensive psychological support.

Management of bleeding

Management of bleeding needs to be individualized and depends on the underlying cause, the likelihood of reversing or controlling the underlying cause, and the burden-to-benefit ratio of the treatment. If the patient's disease burden and life expectancy warrant it, then the management of a bleeding episode consists of general resuscitative measures, such as volume and fluid replacement, and specific measures to stop the bleeding. On the other hand, palliative measures may be most appropriate in end-stage patients.

Appropriate management involves a detailed assessment, including a review of prior bleeding episodes, past illness, psychosocial stressors (including level of family support), and medications such as NSAIDS or anticoagulants. Physical examination should focus on whether the bleeding is focal or occurring at multiple sites. Tests such as a hemogram or a clotting profile may reveal a systemic disease, whereas endoscopic studies or angiography may reveal the site of the bleeding.

LOCAL INTERVENTIONS (TABLE 83.3)

Packing can be used with or without pressure to achieve hemostasis when bleeding originates in the nose, vagina, or rectum. Surgical swabs of various sizes may be used for this purpose.

Table 83.3 *Local measures*

Epinephrine	May be used topically, but its liberal use is discouraged
Prostaglandins E2 and F2	Used in intractable hemorrhagic cystitis
Silver nitrate	Induces chemical cauterization and has been used to control hemorrhages in the bladder and epistaxis
Formalin, 2%–4%	Acts as a chemical cautery and has been used to control intractable rectal and bladder hemorrhaging
Aluminum astringents	An example is 1% alum, which can be delivered by continuous irrigation of the bladder
Sucralfate	Controls cancer-related gastrointestinal bleeding and cutaneous oozing
TA	Controls bleeding when used locally or systemically [33,34]

They can be coated with chemicals that facilitate hemostasis, such as cocaine in nasal packing. Nonadherent dressings should be used.

A variety of hemostatic agents and dressings, mostly designed for surgical procedures, are beneficial for exterior topical use in patients with advanced cancer. Thromboplastin, a natural blood-clotting agent obtained from bovine plasma, is available as a powder for topical preparation [30].

Absorbable gelatin is available as a sterile sponge-like dressing or sterile powder that can be applied dry or saturated with sterile sodium solution and is absorbed within 4–6 weeks. When the gelatin is applied, fibrin is deposited in the interstices of the foam, resulting in the swelling of the sponge, thereby forming a large synthetic clot. When the gelatin is applied to nasal, rectal, or vaginal mucosa, it liquefies within 2–5 days.

Other bioabsorbable topical hemostatic agents include fibrin sealants and oxidized cellulose [31,32]. Fibrin sealants are derived from human plasma and reproduce the final steps in the coagulation pathway to form a clot. The inherent hemostatic activity of absorbable collagen agents provokes a clotting cascade when the bovine-derived mesh comes into contact with blood and forms a clot. Other available hemostatic agents are oxidized cellulose compounds and highly absorbent alginate dressings derived from seaweed. Vasoconstricting or cauterizing agents are used to manage localized capillary-based bleeding.

RADIOTHERAPY

External beam radiotherapy is used to decrease the hemoptysis caused by lung cancer and is effective in 80% of patients [6,7,35,36]. It also controls bleeding in 85% of patients with rectal bleeding and in 60% of those with hematuria from bladder cancer [7,15,37]. Radiotherapy should also be considered for treating bleeding from cancerous lesions in the vagina, skin, rectum, and bladder. Although radiotherapy can be useful in controlling the bleeding in patients with head and neck cancers, many patients have already received the maximal allowable doses of radiotherapy by the time bleeding occurs and cannot receive further radiation. Single or reduced fraction-regimens appear to be as effective as multiple fractions in controlling bleeding. Upper gastrointestinal hemorrhaging from a malignant process is less amenable to radiotherapy.

Embolization may be useful in well-selected patients whose blood vessels are accessible by catheter. The benefits of embolization have been reported in patients with cancers involving the head and neck, pelvis, lung, liver, and gastrointestinal tract [38–50].

Transcutaneous arterial embolization is used to control bleeding in select cases of intractable hemorrhage resulting from advanced pelvic urological malignancies, carotid artery rupture owing to cancer, and spontaneous rupture of hepatocellular carcinoma.

SURGERY

Surgery may be appropriate for select patients deemed fit for the procedure when conservative measures have failed.

Surgery-controlled bleeding was achieved in patients with head and neck cancers who presented with acute or imminent carotid artery rupture and in those with radiation proctitis in whom the bleeding was not controlled by topically applied formalin [51,52].

SYSTEMIC INTERVENTIONS

Vitamin K

Vitamin K (phytonadione, menadiol) may be useful in treating a derangement in vitamin K-dependent coagulation factors, such as factors II, VII, IX, and X, or for treating bleeding in patients with advanced cancer that has been caused by excessive therapy with warfarin. The preferable route of administration would be oral or subcutaneous, but the intravenous route should be considered when rapid correction is required. The recommended doses vary from 2.5 to 10 mg depending on the severity of bleeding [53].

Vasopressin/desmopressin

Vasopressin/desmopressin is a hormone in the posterior pituitary gland that causes splanchnic arteriolar constriction and reduction in portal pressure when it is injected intravenously or intra-arterially. It has been used in a controlled trial to manage bleeding in select patients with upper gastrointestinal bleeding related to a malignancy [54].

Somatostatin analogues

Octreotide, an analogue of somatostatin, has been used in palliative care for reducing secretions in patients with a gastrointestinal obstruction. It also reduces the splanchnic flow and pressure by causing venous dilatation, thereby reducing portal pressure and portal venous flow and may reduce bleeding [55].

Antifibrinolytic agents

TA and EACA are synthetic antifibrinolytic agents that block the binding sites of plasminogen, thereby inhibiting the conversion of plasminogen into plasmin by the tissue plasminogen activator. The end result is decreased lysis of fibrin clots [56,57].

TA and EACA can be administered orally and intravenously. The most common adverse effects of TA and EACA are gastrointestinal in nature (nausea, vomiting, and diarrhea) and occur in 25% of cases [58]. The adverse effects appear to be dose-dependent. Thromboembolism is uncommon [59,60].

ENDOSCOPY (TABLE 83.4)

Endoscopy-based treatments have, for a long time, been used to manage the bleeding from upper gastrointestinal varices, particularly after systemic therapies with agents such as vasopressin or somatostatin analogues have failed [61,62].

TRANSFUSION OF BLOOD PRODUCTS

Transfusions of blood products should be undertaken on a selective basis. There is no scientific basis for the 20,000/μL

Table 83.4 *Endoscopic interventions and their role*

Upper gastrointestinal endoscopy	Uses argon beam plasma coagulation to control bleeding in esophagogastric cancer.
Cystoscopy	Cystoscopic-assisted cautery by either heat or laser probes; has been used in the treatment of hematuria in bladder cancer patients.
Bronchoscopy	In case of hemoptysis, bronchoscopy allows for stenting, ice-cold saline lavages, and/or the use of balloon tamponade, laser photocoagulation, or topical application of thrombin or fibrinogen at the site of the bleeding.
Colonoscopy	Techniques such as bipolar electrocoagulation, heater probe, argon, and Nd:YAG lasers are used to control bleeding in the lower gastrointestinal tract.

cutoff for transfusion. Lassauniere et al. proposed criteria for platelet transfusions in patients with advanced hematological malignancies [63]. These criteria include continuous bleeding of the mouth or gums, epistaxis, extensive and painful hematomas, severe headaches, or recent onset of disturbed vision, as well as continuous bleeding through the gastrointestinal, gynecological, or urinary systems.

Transfusions of fresh frozen plasma are indicated (a) in patients who are bleeding and have specific deficiencies in certain coagulation factors, (b) in patients in whom the effects of warfarin urgently need to be reversed, (c) in patients who require urgent invasive interventions such as thoracentesis or surgery, and (d) with DIC, when appropriate. Transfusions of packed red cells are indicated when anemia resulting from blood loss causes or aggravates symptoms such as fatigue and dyspnea.

The continuation of platelet transfusion in patients with end-stage thrombocytopenia poses an ethical dilemma. Even though the ongoing transfusions may be futile, patients and their families may perceive the cessation of transfusions as the withdrawal of life-sustaining therapy. Sensitive and empathic discussions among patients, their families, the attending physician, and the health team are essential in order to explore their expectations, fears, and concerns and to engage in advanced end-of-life planning while ensuring ongoing support and providing optimal comfort care.

PALLIATIVE MEASURES

General supportive measures should always be applied in cases of massive hemorrhage. Apply external pressure if the source of the bleeding is visible, administer oxygen or place patient in lateral position if possible, and provide psychosocial support to the patients and families. Other measures include using suction and dark towels and basins to decrease the distress from visualization of blood. The medical team should plan before the event by having personal protective equipment such as face shields, dark aprons, and towels readily available.

Hemorrhage can be extremely distressing, and many studies have suggested having prefilled syringes of sedative medications (e.g., midazolam) readily available. The intent of the sedative medication is to alleviate distress. Midazolam is found to be the most commonly recommended drug in this setting in a systematic review on management of terminal hemorrhage by Harris and Noble in 2009 [16]. Midazolam is favored because it is rapid-acting, safe, short-term, and provides some level of retrograde amnesia and, therefore, is less likely to cause harm if the bleeding is not terminal [16]. It is important to debrief and counsel staff and families before and after the event.

CONCLUSION

Massive bleeding, which occurs in 6%–10% of patients in palliative care settings, can be extremely distressing for both the patients and caregivers. These episodes require an individualized approach based on the specific needs of the patient and family, which include the level of distress, the stage of disease, and the expertise available. A multidisciplinary approach that makes use of various modalities may be required. Treatments range from simple hemostatic techniques to more invasive and sophisticated modalities. Minimal management requires the identification of patients at risk and preparatory measures to empower caregivers to deal appropriately with massive bleeding if it occurs.

REFERENCES

1 Smith AM. Emergencies in palliative care. *Ann Acad Med Singapore* 1994;23:186–190.

2 Hoskin P, Makin W (eds.). *Oncology for Palliative Medicine*. Oxford, U.K.: Oxford University Press; 1998. pp. 229–234.

3 Gagnon B, Mancini I, Pereira J, Bruera E. Palliative management of bleeding events in advanced cancer patients. *J Palliat Care* 1998;14:50–54.

4 Devita VT, Hellman S, Rosenberg SA (eds.). *Cancer. Principles and Practice of Oncology*. Philadelphia, PA: JB Lippincott Co.; 1993.

5 Shigemura N, Wan I, Yu S, Wong RH, Hsin M, Thung HK, Lee TW, Wan S, Underwood MJ, Yim A. Multidisciplinary management of life-threatening massive hemoptysis: A 10-year experience. *Ann Thorac Surg* 2009;87:849–853.

6 MRC Lung Cancer Working Party. Inoperable non-small cell lung cancer (NSCLC): A Medical Research Council randomized trial of palliative radiotherapy with two fractions. *Cancer* 1991;63:265–270.

7 Hoskin P. Radiotherapy in symptom management. In D. Doyle, G.Hanks, N.Cherny, & K.Calman (Eds.), *Oxford Text Book of Palliative Medicine*. Oxford, U.K.: Oxford University Press; 2004. pp. 239–255.

8 Andréjak C, Parrot A, Bazelly B, Ancel PY, Djibré M, Khalil A, Grunenwal D, Fartoukh M. Surgical lung resection for severe hemoptysis. *Ann Thorac Surg* 2009;88:1556–1565.

9 Chung IH, Park MH, Kim DH, Jeon GS. Endobronchial stent insertion to manage hemoptysis caused by lung cancer. *Korean Med Sci* 2010;25:1253–1255.

10 Sakr L, Dutau H. Massive hemoptysis: An update on the role of bronchoscopy in diagnosis and management. *Respiration* 2010;80:38–58.

11 Brandes JC, Schmidt E, Yung R. Occlusive endobronchial stent placement as a novel management approach to massive hemoptysis from lung cancer. *J Thorac Oncol* 2008;3:1071–1072.

12 Chun JY, Morgan R, Belli AM. Radiological management of hemoptysis: A comprehensive review of diagnostic imaging and bronchial arterial embolization. *Cardiovasc Intervent Radiol* 2010;33:240–250.

13 Barnert J, Messmann H. Diagnosis and management of lower gastrointestinal bleeding. *Nat Rev Gastroenterol Hepatol* 2009;6:637–646.

14 Shah MB, Schnoll-Sussman F. Cryotherapy to control bleeding in advanced esophageal cancer. *Endoscopy* 2010;42:E46.

15 Wu JN, Meyers FJ, Evans CP. Palliative care in urology. *Surg Clin N Am* 2011;91(2):429–444.

16 Harris DG, Noble SIR. Management of terminal hemorrhage in patients with advanced cancer: A systematic literature review. *J Pain Symptom Manage* 2009;38:913–927.

17 Siegal T, Seligsohn U, Aghai E, Modan M. Clinical and laboratory aspects of disseminated intravascular coagulation (DIC): A study of 118 cases. *Thromb Haemost* 1978;39(1):122–134.

18 Barbui, T, Finazzi, G, Falenga, A. The impact of all-trans-retinoic acid on the coagulopathy of acute promyelocytic leukemia. *Blood* 1998;91(9):3093–3102.

19 Garcia-Avello A, Lorente JA, Cesar-Perez J, Garcia-Frade LJ, Alvarado R, Arevalo JM, Navarro JL, Esteban A. Degree of hypercoagulability and hyperfibrinolysis is related to organ failure and prognosis after burn trauma. *Thromb Res* 1998;89(2):59–64.

20 Feinstein, DI. Diagnosis and management of disseminated intravascular coagulation: The role of heparin therapy. *Blood* 1982;60(2):284–287.

21 Corrigan JJ Jr., Jordan CM. Heparin therapy in septicemia with disseminated intravascular coagulation. Effect on mortality and on correction of hemostatic defects. *N Engl J Med* 1970;283:778–779.

22 Gaydos LA, Freireich EJ, Mantel N. The quantitative relation between platelet count and hemorrhage in patients with acute leukemia. *N Engl J Med* 1962;266:905–909.

23 Ford JM. Should prophylactic platelets be given to patients with acute leukemia? In: Lister TA, Malpas JS (eds.). *Platelet Transfusion*. Baltimore, MD: University Park; 1980. pp. 45–49.

24 Slichter SJ, Harker LA. Thrombocytopenia: Mechanisms and management of defects in platelet production. *Clin Haematol* 1978;7:523–539.

25 Solomon J, Bofenkamp T, Fahey TL, Chillar RK, Beutler E. Platelet prophylaxis in acute non-lymphoblastic leukemia. *Lancet* 1978;1:267.

26 Belt RJ, Leite C, Haas CD, Stephens RL. Incidence of hemorrhagic complications in patients with cancer. *J Am Med Assoc* 1978;239:2571–2574.

27 Dutcher JP, Schiffer CA, Aisner J et al. Incidence of thrombocytopenia and serious hemorrhage among patients with solid tumors. *Cancer* 1984;53:557–562.

28 Goldberg GL, Gibbon DG, Smith HO et al. Clinical impact of chemotherapy-induced thrombocytopenia in patients with gynecologic cancer. *J Clin Oncol* 1994;12:2317–2320.

29 Fanning J, Hilgers RD, Murray KP et al. Conservative management of chemotherapeutic-induced thrombocytopenia in women with gynecologic cancers. *Gynecol Oncol* 1995;59:191–193.

30 Thrombostat. *Compendium of Pharmaceuticals and Specialities*. Ottawa, Ontario, Canada: Canadian Pharmacists Association, 1997;32:1587.

31 Shinkwin CA, Beasley N, Simo R et al. Evaluation of surgical Nu-knit, Merocel and Vaseline gauze nasal packs: A randomized trial. *Rhinology* 1996;34:41–43.

32 Mankad PS, Codispoti M. Role of fibrin sealants in hemostasis. *Am J Surg* 2001;182(Suppl. 2):21S–28S.

33. Waly NG. Local antifibrinolytic treatment with tranexamic acid in hemophilic children undergoing dental extractions. *Egypt Dent J* 1995;41:228–252.

34 Lethaby A, Farguhar C, Cooke I. Antifibrinolytics for heavy menstrual bleeding. *Cochrane Database Syst Rev* 2000;4:CD000249.

35 Brundage MD, Bezjak A, Dixon P, Grimard L, Larochelle M, Warde P, Warr D. The role of palliative thoracic radiotherapy in non-small cell lung cancer. *Can J Oncol* 1996;6(Suppl. 1):25–32.

36 Langendijk JA, ten Velde GP, Aaronson NK, de Jong JM, Muller MJ, Wouters EF. Quality of life after palliative radiotherapy in non-small cell lung cancer: A prospective study. *Int J Radiat Oncol Biol Phys* 2000;47:149–155.

37 Srinivasan V, Brown CH, Turner AG. A comparison of two radiotherapy regimens for the treatment of symptoms from advanced bladder cancer. *Clin Oncol (R Coll Radiol)* 1994;6:11–13.

38 Kvale PA, Simoff M, Prakash UB. Lung cancer. Palliative care. *Chest* 2003;123(Suppl. 1):284S–311S.

39 Patel U, Pattison CW, Raphael M. Management of massive haemoptysis. *Br J Hosp Med* 1994;52:74, 76–78.

40 Bates MC, Shamsham FM. Endovascular management of impending carotid rupture in a patient with advanced head and neck cancer. *J Endovasc Ther* 2003;10:54–57.

41 Sakakibara Y, Kuramoto K, Jikuya T et al. An approach for acute disruption of large arteries in patients with advanced cervical cancer: Endoluminal balloon occlusion technique. *Ann Surg* 1998;227:134–137.

42 Morrissey DD, Andersen PE, Nesbit GM et al. Endovascular management of hemorrhage in patients with head and neck cancer. *Arch Otolaryngol Head Neck Surg* 1997;123:15–19.

43 Nabi G, Sheikh N, Greene D, Marsh R. Therapeutic transcatheter arterial embolization in the management of intractable haemorrhage from pelvic urological malignancies: Preliminary experience and long-term follow-up. *BJU Int* 2003;92:245–247.

44 Wells I. Internal iliac artery embolization in the management of pelvic bleeding. *Clin Radiol* 1996;51:825–827.

45 Yamashita Y, Harada M, Yamamoto H et al. Transcatheter arterial embolization of obstetric and gynecological bleeding: Efficacy and clinical outcome. *Br J Radiol* 1994;67:530–534.

46 Hayes MC, Wilson NM, Page A, Harrison GS. Selective embolization of bladder tumors. *Br J Urol* 1996;78:311–312.

47 Jenkins CN, McIvor J. Survival after embolization of the internal iliac arteries in ten patients with severe haematuria due to recurrent pelvic carcinoma. *Clin Radiol* 1996;51:865–868.

48 Kawaguchi T, Tanaka M, Itano S et al. Successful treatment of bronchial bleeding from invasive pulmonary metastasis of hepatocellular carcinoma: A case report. *Hepatogastroenterology* 2001;48:851–853.

49 Recordare A, Bonariol L, Caratozzolo E, Callegari F, Bruno G, Di Paola F, Bassi N. Management of spontaneous bleeding due to hepatocellular carcinoma. *Minerva Chir* 2002;57:347–356.

50 Srivastava DN, Gandhi D, Julka PK, Tandon RK. Gastrointestinal hemorrhage in hepatocellular carcinoma: Management with transhepatic arterioembolization. *Abdom Imaging* 2000;25:380–384.

51 Yegappan M, Ho YH, Nyam D et al. The surgical management of colorectal complications from irradiation for carcinoma of the cervix. *Ann Acad Med Singapore* 1998;27:627–630.

52 Witz M, Korzets Z, Shnaker A, Lehmann JM, Ophir D. Delayed carotid artery rupture in advanced cervical cancer: A dilemma in emergency management. *Eur Arch Otorhinolaryngol* 2002;259:37–39.

53 Nee R, Doppenschmidt D, Donovan DJ, Andrews TC. Intravenous versus subcutaneous vitamin K1 in reversing excessive oral anticoagulation. *Am J Cardiol* 1999;83:286–288, A6–A7.

54 Allum WH, Brearley S, Wheatley KE et al. Acute haemorrhage from gastric malignancy. *Br J Surg* 1990;77:19–20.

55 Gøtzsche PC, Hróbjartsson A. Somatostatin analogues for acute bleeding oesophageal varices. *Cochrane Database of Systematic Reviews* 2008, Issue 3. Art. No.: CD000193. DOI: 10.1002/14651858.CD000193.pub3.

56   Garewal HS, Durie BG. Anti-fibrinolytic therapy with aminocaproic acid for the control of bleeding in thrombocytopenic patients. *Scand J Haematol* 1985;35:497–500.

57   Fricke W, Alling D, Kimball J, Griffith P, Klein H. Lack of efficacy of tranexamic acid in thrombocytopenic bleeding. *Transfusion* 1991;31:345–348.

58   Herfindal ET, Gourley DR (eds.). *Textbook of Therapeutics: Drug and Disease Management*, 6th edn. Baltimore, MD: Williams and Wilkins; 1996.

59   Hashimoto S, Koike T, Tatewaki W et al. Fatal thromboembolism in acute promyelocytic leukemia during all-trans retinoic acid therapy combined with antifibrinolytic therapy for prophylaxis of hemorrhage. *Leukemia* 1994;8:1113–1115.

60   Woo KS, Tse LK, Woo JL, Vallance-Owen J. Massive pulmonary thromboembolism after tranexamic acid antifibrinolytic therapy. *Br J Clin Pract* 1989;43:465–466.

61   Akhtar K, Byrne JP, Bancewicz J, Attwood SE. Argon beam plasma coagulation in the management of cancers of the esophagus and stomach. *Surg Endosc* 2000;14:1127–1130.

62   Loftus EV, Alexander GL, Ahlquist DA, Balm RK. Endoscopic treatment of major bleeding from advanced gastroduodenal malignant lesions. *Mayo Clin Proc* 1994;69:736–740.

63   Lassauniere JM, Bertolino M, Hunault M et al. Platelet transfusions in advanced hematological malignancies: A position paper. *J Palliat Care* 1996;12:38–41.

84

Spinal cord compression

NORA A. JANJAN, STEPHEN LUTZ, EDWARD CHOW

INTRODUCTION

Approximately half the patients diagnosed with cancer will develop metastatic disease. Over 70% of all cancer patients develop symptoms from either their primary or metastatic disease.[1-5] Prognosis is influenced by the overall metastatic burden and the number and location of the sites involved by disease. When metastases are found also in the lung, liver, and/or central nervous system, the prognosis is especially poor.[6-15]

Spinal cord compression generally results from bone metastases, rather than as a result of leptomeningeal or intramedullary metastases. Prognosis after the development of metastatic disease is important to the type of radiation therapy administered. After bone metastases are diagnosed, the median survivals are 12 months for breast cancer, 6 months with prostate cancer, and 3 months with lung cancer.[7-9] The site of the primary disease and the presence of a solitary metastatic site are predictive of a more prolonged survival.[16-19] The distribution of bone metastases in prostate cancer has prognostic significance. The rate of survival is significantly longer when the metastases are restricted to the pelvis and lumbar spine, and among patients who respond to salvage hormone therapy.[10-12] Any metastatic involvement outside the pelvis and lumbar spine results in lower rates of survival irrespective of response to salvage hormone therapy.

A bone scan index (BSI) has been formulated based on the weighted proportion of tumor involvement in individual bones. The BSI was then related to known prognostic factors and survival in patients with androgen-independent prostate cancer.[13] Using multivariable proportional hazards analyses, only the BSI, age, hemoglobin level, and lactate dehydrogenase level were associated with survival. Survival rates were 18.3 months for a BSI of 1.4%, 15.5 months for a BSI of 1.4%–5.1%, and 8.1 months for a BSI of 5.1%. Elevations in the bone resorption marker N-telopeptide (NTx) have been associated with a 20 times higher risk for the development of a skeletal complications within 3 months, and shorter times to first disease progression and death.[20,21] These identified prognostic factors should be considered, as a surrogate to a staging system for metastatic disease, so that palliative treatment is appropriate to prognosis based on the extent of disease. The prognostic impact of NTx also relates to response to bisphosphonate therapy. The NTx level was lower than 50 nmol/L at 13 weeks in 71% of patients treated with subcutaneous denosumab compared to 29% of patients treated with intravenous [IV] bisphosphonates; the NTx reduction was maintained at 25 weeks in 64% of denosumab versus 37% with IV bisphosphonates. Skeletal events occurred in 8% of the denosumab and 17% of the IV bisphosphonates treated patients.[22]

Bone metastases are the most common cause of cancer-related pain, and over 70% of patients with bone metastases have symptoms. Among hospitalized patients, over 50% of patients experience severe pain due to bone metastases.[4] One of the most important goals in the treatment of bone metastases is to relieve suffering and return the patient to independent function.[23,24] The location of the metastasis influences the type of palliative intervention necessary, especially in weight-bearing bones and bones responsible for ambulation and activities of daily living. Complete pain relief after radiation is achieved in 88% of limb lesions, 73% of spine metastases, and 67% of pelvic metastases.[25] Improved pain control significantly improved overall survival among metastatic lung cancer patients as well as providing better quality of life.[26]

Bone scans are the most sensitive and specific method of detecting bone metastases, but magnetic resonance imaging (MRI) is the best available technique for evaluating the bone marrow, and neoplastic invasion of the vertebrae, the central nervous system, and peripheral nerves.[27-29] In a study of melanoma patients, positron emission tomography (^{18}F-fluorodeoxyglucose PET) also found unsuspected spinal cord compression, later confirmed on MRI.[30] An MRI of the entire spine can accurately identify the level of the disease, including levels where further lesions are identified. Many of these lesions may be currently asymptomatic, but may warrant prophylactic treatment prior to the later development of pain or irreversible symptoms like paralysis. Delineation of metastatic disease to bacterial abscesses (which invades the disk space, where the latter does not), leptomeningeal carcinomatosis (nodular or linear tumor deposits), intradural extramedullary tumors (appearance and enhancement with contrast), and intramedullary metastases (that causes enlargement of the cord) can easily be made with MRI.

Cauda equina syndrome refers to damage to the cauda equina that may be possible due to a number of agents, including cancers. Though primary tumors causing cauda equina syndrome far outnumber those of metastatic origin, improved systemic treatments resulting in improved survival have resulted in spinal metastases and their sequelae to become more common. Similar to metastatic epidural spinal cord compression (MESCC), patients may experience a myriad of symptoms and neurological deficits, including lower back pain, decreased rectal tone and perineal reflexes, bowel and bladder dysfunction, variable amounts of lower-extremity weakness, sciatica, and saddle anesthesia. The investigation of cauda equina syndrome is similar to MESCC, where MRI is the preferred modality. In patients with metastatic disease, management strategies include use of surgery, radiotherapy, and steroids, though the latter two may be preferred with patients having decreased functional status. Bone or other metastases rarely fail to be detected when radiographic diagnosis is pursued. When radiographic confirmation of malignancy is equivocal, bone biopsy should be considered.[31]

Pain, risk for pathological fracture, and spinal cord compression are the most common indications to treat bone metastases with localized therapy including radiation and surgery. Because external beam radiation provides treatment only to a localized symptomatic site of disease, it is frequently used in coordination with systemic therapies such as chemotherapy, hormonal therapy, and bisphosphonates.[32]

PRINCIPLES OF RADIATION THERAPY

Radiotherapy techniques vary considerably based upon the involved and adjacent normal structures. Basic to an understanding of applied techniques and potential morbidity during a course of radiation are the following principles[33]: radiation therapy is delivered in units designated as the Gray. Relating this to the previously used term rad, equivalent doses can be expressed as 1 gray (Gy), 100 centigray (cGy), and 100 rad; 1 rad equals 1 cGy.

Radiation for spinal cord compression is delivered by external beam therapy (linear accelerators, cobalt-60 units) that is administered with a prescribed number of daily fractions over several weeks. A variety of radiation energies and biological characteristics are now available to help localize treatment to the areas at risk and exclude uninvolved normal tissues.

EXTERNAL BEAM IRRADIATION

Included within the classification of external beam radiation are *photons* that are penetrating forms of radiation, and *electrons*, delivering treatment to superficial areas. Other specialized types of external radiation beams are available at only a few centers, and they include *proton beam* therapy (administering radiation with high precision to well-defined small areas of tumor involvement, e.g., pituitary or midbrain lesions) and *neutrons* (used by a few centers to treat bulky unresectable or recurrent tumors). Generally, photons are used to treat spinal cord compression. Occasionally, electron beam therapy is used in children, and proton beam radiation is now becoming available for the treatment of spinal cord tumors at many centers in the United States.

The concept of integral dose relates the amount of radiation deposited to uninvolved normal tissues located between the

Table 84.1 *The concept of integral dose is demonstrated by the following radiation dose distributions for three different energies including cobalt-60, 6 and 18 MeV photons. The [%] represents the percentage of the prescribed dose deposited at that depth of tissue below the skin surface*

Skin surface (cm)	Cobalt-60 (%)	6 MeV (%)	18 MeV (%)
0.5	100	30	25
1.0	98	90	50
1.5	95	100	90
2.0	93	98	96
2.5	90	97	98
3.0	88	95	98
3.5	85	92	100
5.0	80	88	96
10.0	55	68	80

D_{max}, the maximum dose, refers to the depth at which 100% of the prescribed dose is located below the skin surface. The greater the D_{max}, the greater the skin sparing associated with less of an integral dose.

skin surface and tumor; the goal in any radiation plan is to minimize integral dose by selecting the appropriate beam energy (Table 84.1). The D_{max} radiation dose is the depth at which 100% of the prescribed radiation is deposited. Higher-energy photon radiation, for example, 18 MeV photons, reduces integral dose because it deposits more radiation to deeper structures while delivering relatively little radiation to superficial tissues.

Multiple radiation portals, each of which is treated daily, are also routinely used in radiotherapy to reduce integral dose. Table 84.2 gives an example of the impact on integral

Table 84.2 *The impact on integral radiation dose when 200 cGy is prescribed at midline (10 cm depth; patient diameter is 20 cm) from a 6 MeV linear accelerator*

Distance from skin surface [cm]	6 MeV photons [% of prescribed radiation dose]	Radiation Dose [cGy] per fraction [200 cGy per fraction prescribed at 10 cm below the skin surface] using 6MeV photons
0.5	30	88
1.0	90	265
1.5	100	294
2.0	98	288
2.5	97	285
3.0	95	279
3.5	92	270
5.0	88	259
10.0	68	200
15.0	51	150
16.5	48	141
17.5	44	129
18.5	42	123
19.5	40	118

Radiation dose = 200 cGy at 10 cm depth; percentage depth dose = 68%.
Radiation dose at 1.5 cm (D_{max} or 100%) is the radiation dose prescribed/0.68.
Radiation dose at other depths is the D_{max} dose × % isodose (see Table 84.1).

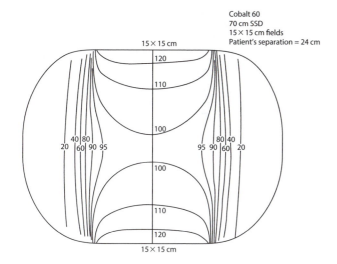

Figure 84.1 *The radiation isodose distribution for a 15 cm × 15 cm radiation field using anterior and posterior (AP and PA) parallel opposed portals with cobalt-60. In this case, the patient has a 24 cm diameter. Each number represents a percentage of the prescribed radiation dose. If 200 cGy was prescribed to the 100% isodose line, then 240 cGy would be delivered to the 120% isodose line near the skin surface and only 180 cGy would be given at the edge of the radiation field at the 90% isodose line.*

radiation dose when 200 cGy is prescribed at 10 cm depth from a 6 MeV linear accelerator. When only the posterior radiation portal is used to deliver radiation in the example, the integral dose is high, because more superficial tissues receive nearly 50% more than the prescribed radiation dose at the site of the tumor located 10 cm below the skin surface; at 1.5 cm from the skin surface, the daily radiation dose is 294 cGy per fraction and the total dose is 5880 cGy as compared to the 200 cGy per fraction and total radiation dose of 4000 cGy at the tumor.

Radiation tolerance is primarily based on the daily radiation dose; as the daily radiation dose increases, the total radiation dose that can be given to normal tissues decreases. Because of this, treatment with a posterior field alone would result in significant side effects due to the high integral dose manifested by skin fibrosis that outlines the radiation field. It is important to realize that giving the first half of the radiation course from the anterior (AP) field alone, and the second half of the radiation course from the posterior (PA) field alone would not reduce radiation side effects. Although the total radiation dose would be more even when using an AP field during the first half and a PA field during the last half of a radiation dose, side effects still may be severe because of the high daily (integral) dose of radiation.

When the radiation is delivered each day from an AP and PA radiation portal, the radiation dose given in the portal is the sum of the radiation dose from each field (Figure 84.1). The integral dose in the case presented decreases significantly the daily administration of both the AP and PA treatment fields because the daily radiation dose throughout the treatment field is within 6% (with a daily dose of 211 cGy per fraction at 16.5 cm below the anterior skin surface) of the prescribed dose of 200 cGy per fraction (Figure 84.2). Likewise, the maximum total radiation dose in the field is 4220 cGy, just 220 cGy more than the prescribed radiation dose at the tumor (Figure 84.3). Newer treatment approaches, like conformal radiation therapy, exploit this relation by treating up to eight different radiation fields each day. Reducing integral dose is a principal concept of radiation treatment planning, because it allows higher radiation doses to the tumor and less radiation to the surrounding normal tissues.

A wide variety of photon energies are available. This allows selective administration of treatment to the tumor and minimizes radiation to uninvolved tissues. As a standard, available photon beam energies range from cobalt-60 to 22 MeV photons. Cobalt-60 delivers 100% of the prescribed radiation dose, indicated as the maximum radiation dose (D_{max}), 0.5 cm below the skin surface; 6 MeV x-rays from a linear accelerator have a D_{max} of 1.5 cm, and 18 MeV photons have a D_{max} of 3.5 cm below the skin. Tissues 0.5 cm below the skin surface treated with

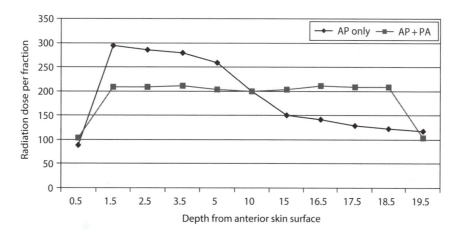

Figure 84.2 *Graphic comparison of the integral radiation dose, defined as the radiation dose deposited between the skin surface and the tumor. In this case, the tumor is 10 cm below the skin surface. If radiation were only given from the anterior treatment portal, the radiation dose to the skin would result in complications because of the high radiation dose per fraction as well as the high total dose of radiation.*

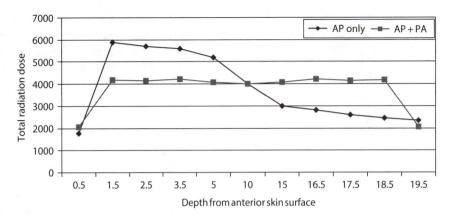

Figure 84.3 *Graphic comparison of the total radiation dose given when a single anterior radiation field is used instead of parallel opposed radiation fields (AP and PA fields) treated every day. With the AP field alone, the skin would receive 30% more radiation than the parallel opposed treatment approach to achieve the same radiation dose at the tumor.*

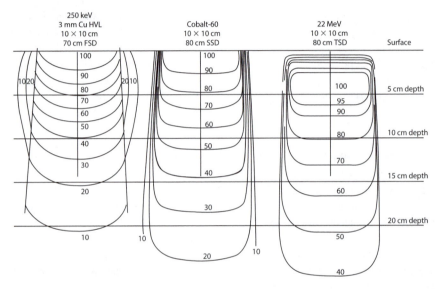

Figure 84.4 *The different radiation isodose distributions for 10 cm × 10 cm radiation fields. The three beams compared include orthovoltage radiation with a 250 keV radiation beam (left), a cobalt-60 unit (middle), and a 22 MeV linear accelerator (right). The 250 keV unit has no skin sparing and little depth of penetration of the radiation beam. The cobalt-60 unit is ideal for treating head and neck cancers in that adequate radiation is given to superficial lymph nodes and scars in the postoperative setting. Because the diameter of the head and neck region is limited, a highly penetrating photon beam is not advisable. Photons of 22 MeV are ideal for deep-seated tumors such as in the pelvis and abdomen because of skin sparing and deep penetration of the photon beams.*

18 MeV photons receive only 30% of the prescribed radiation dose (Figure 84.4). This demonstrates the relation in radiation physics that there is more sparing of superficial structures (skin and subcutaneous tissues) from radiation with higher photon energies even though the beam deeply penetrates into the tissue. In contrast to the 18 MeV linear accelerators currently available, the low radiation energy of orthovoltage radiation ranges between 125 and 250 keV.

Using conventional radiation techniques, radiation for vertebral metastases commonly was prescribed to 5 cm below the skin surface using cobalt-60 or 6 MeV photons. However, mean depths from MRI scans of 20 patients equaled 5.5 cm for the posterior spinal canal, 6.9 cm for the anterior spinal canal, and 9.6 cm for the anterior vertebral body. Based on the radiation dose distributions, a metastatic lesion in the anterior vertebral

body could receive a radiation dose that is significantly lower than that prescribed.[34]

External beam irradiation is administered from specialized machines that emit gamma rays from a housed isotope (cobalt-60) or x-rays (linear accelerators), which are more than 1000 times as powerful as those used in diagnostic radiology, and are generated by electricity. The availability of higher-energy radiation beams and the development of a variety of different radiation energies were critical to the advancement of radiation therapy. These advancements allowed more precise deposition of the radiation in the area of the tumor while sparing surrounding uninvolved normal tissues.

Radiation beams diverge as they penetrate through the body such that the field that exits the body is larger than the field that enters the body. Historically, radiation portals included

1–2 vertebral bodies above and below the involved spinal metastases to avoid having the vertebral metastases at the edge of the radiation beam where the radiation dose is lower [penumbra] and account for potential microscopic involvement of adjacent vertebral bodies. With the more routine specific simulation and positioning techniques now available, local failure in unirradiated adjacent vertebra occurs in less than 5% of patients at 18 months follow-up.[35] If spinal metastases occur near a previously radiated area of the spinal cord, the new radiation field must be matched to the prior radiation field, accounting for the divergence of the radiation beam. Extreme precision is required when administering radiation, especially when the radiation treatment must match a previously radiated segment of the spinal cord.[36,37] A computed tomography (CT) scanner on rails with a linear accelerator is used in this technique to verify the position of the patient immediately before the administration of the radiation treatment; once the patient position is verified on the treatment table by a CT scan, the treatment table is rotated to administer the intensity-modulated radiation therapy (IMRT) treatment (Figure 84.5). Treatment accuracy is within 1 mm of the planned treatment center, and the dose variation in the high-dose region is 2% or less using this CT on rails technique. Five IMRT treatments delivered 30 Gy to the tumor, limiting the spinal cord radiation dose to 10 Gy or less (Figure 84.6).

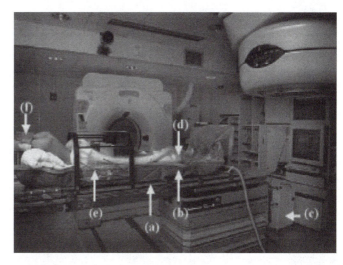

Figure 84.5   *A computed tomography (CT) scanner on rails with a linear accelerator has been used to verify the position of the patient immediately before the administration of the radiation treatment. (a) A carbon fiber base plate; (b) a whole-body vacuum cushion; (c) a vacuum system; (d) a plastic fixation sheet; (e) a stereotactic localizer; and (f) an arm-support system. (Reprinted from* Int. J. Radiat. Oncol. Biol. Phys., *57, Shiu, A.S., Chang, E.L., Ye, J.S. et al., Near-simultaneous CT image–guided stereotactic spinal radiotherapy, 605–613, Copyright 2003, with permission from Elsevier.)*

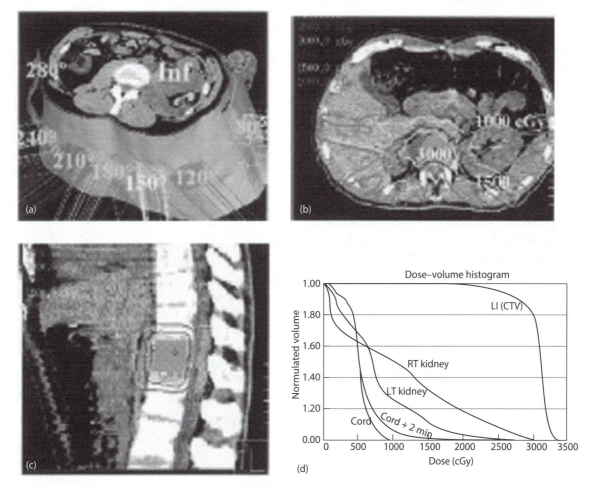

Figure 84.6   *(a–d) Five intensity-modulated radiation therapy (IMRT) treatments delivered 30 Gy to the tumor in the patient in Figure 84.5, limiting the spinal cord radiation dose to 10 Gy or less.*

As a clinical alternative to multiple radiation fractions, a single radiation fraction of 18–24 Gy, has been administered to vertebral metastases either with conformal CT on rails technique or stereotactic radiotherapy. When a large single fraction of radiation is administered, the spinal cord dose is limited to 12–14 Gy, an 89% local tumor control was achieved. Despite achieving an 89% rate of local tumor control, anatomic fracture progression occurred in 39% of patients. Radiographic factors predictive of subsequent fracture progression include metastases located between T10 and the sacrum [fracture 4.6 times more likely], lytic lesions [6.8 times more likely than mixed or sclerotic tumors], and more than 40% tumor infiltration of the vertebral body. Clinical factors predictive of subsequent fracture included higher pain scores and narcotic use, change in Karnofsky performance status (KPS). Posterior vertebral element involvement, bisphosphonate use, kyphosis, and obesity were not significant factors for vertebral fracture. These predictive factors determine high-risk patients who might better benefit from prophylactic vertebroplasty or kyphoplasty.[38]

Stereotactic body radiotherapy (SBT) provides a high dose of photon radiation to a small, well-defined area. Using radiosurgery, the vertebral body can receive 20 Gy while less than 0.5 cm³ of the spinal cord is exposed to 8 Gy of radiation.[39,40] Analysis of unirradiated, reirradiated, and postoperative stereotactic radiosurgery demonstrated local control in over 90% of patients, and improved pain control was reported in approximately 70% of patients.[41] Based on its precise targeting, stereotactic radiosurgery has been used to reirradiate recurrent epidural spinal metastases. Radiation dose depends on the extent of spinal canal involvement; when the tumor does not touch the spinal cord, three 8 Gy fractions are used. For tumors abutting the spinal cord, five 5–6 Gy radiation doses are given. With this approach, median overall survival is 11 months, and median progression-free survival is 9 months, achieving pain relief in 65% and regression of disease or stable tumor in 93% of patients.[42]

Proton beam therapy like SBT, precisely deposits a large amount of radiation to a well-defined volume of tumor while sparing intervening tissues. Precision of proton beam therapy is to the level of the millimeter, requiring exact mapping of the tumor volume and patient positioning. An additional advantage of proton irradiation is the improvement of relative biological effectiveness of this type of radiation because of the characteristic Bragg–Peak distribution of radiation within a narrow volume of tissue (Figure 84.7). Chordomas and localized intracranial tumors, especially around the optic chiasma, have been treated with proton irradiation. Because of its precision, research is ongoing to define further applications of proton therapy, especially in pediatric tumors and previously irradiated recurrent tumors. The primary disadvantage of these techniques is cost.[41]

The clinical status of the patient is accounted for in the treatment setup and in the number of radiation treatments that are prescribed. The radiation dose-fractionation schedule and technique also considers the site and volume irradiated, and the integration of other therapies. Conformal irradiation, IMRT, and proton therapy are all techniques that can better localize radiation dose and reduce side effects, especially in a previously irradiated area.

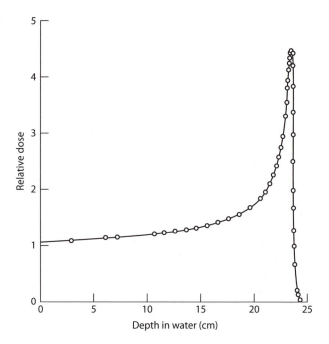

Figure 84.7 *The Bragg–Peak effect in radiation associated with proton radiation. The designated tumor area receives the highest radiation dose, and the surrounding normal tissues are relatively spared. Although currently used to treat intracranial tumors and children, proton radiation may have application in palliative care for the re-treatment of tumors.*

REIRRADIATION

Issues regarding reirradiation are especially important in palliative therapy. Experimental data suggest that acute responding tissues recover from radiation injury in a few months and can tolerate additional radiation therapy. However, there is considerable variability in recovery from radiation among late-reacting tissues such as the spinal cord.[43,44] This recovery depends on the technique used, the organ irradiated, the volume irradiated, the initial total dose of radiation, the radiation dose given with each fraction, and the time interval between the initial and second courses of radiation.[45]

Correlating with existing clinical experience, limited toxicities occur with reirradiation when there is a careful attention to treatment techniques and radiobiological factors. Radiotherapeutic techniques that localize the radiation dose to the recurrent tumor and limit the dose to the surrounding normal tissues allow the reirradiation of recurrent tumors. Techniques include conformal external beam radiation, IMRT, stereotactic body radiotherapy (SBT), and proton therapy.[46,47]

CONFORMAL RADIATION THERAPY/IMRT

Conformal radiation techniques precisely localize the radiation dose using external beam radiation from a linear accelerator. Because very low doses of radiation are given through a number of beams, no one area of normal tissues receives a significant dose of radiation. The tumor, though, is given the sum of the radiation from the beams and receives a high dose of radiation. This technique has allowed high doses of radiation to be given, and has allowed for reirradiation of normal tissues without significant side effects.

IMRT is a form of conformal external beam radiation that even more precisely administers radiation. It is possible to deliver different doses of radiation to specific areas in a single radiation fraction. For example, with IMRT, the center of the tumor may receive 2.20 Gy with each radiation treatment to a total dose of 66 Gy over 30 fractions in 6 weeks, while the periphery of the tumor may receive 2.0 Gy with each radiation treatment to a total dose of 60 Gy. At the same time, the normal tissues within 2 cm of the tumor (clinical tumor volume to account for possible microscopic tumor extension) may receive 1.8 Gy with each radiation treatment to a total dose of 54 Gy. Thus, IMRT provides the radiobiological advantage of giving a high daily dose of radiation localized within a tumor while giving a well-tolerated lower daily dose of radiation to the surrounding tissues at the same time. By localizing high daily and total doses of radiation in the tumor, IMRT is able to kill more cancer cells with higher radiation doses without harming the surrounding tissues. Any shape or configuration of radiation dose, like an hourglass, can be designed with IMRT. Because of these factors, this radiotherapeutic tool is extremely helpful in delivering high radiation doses to inoperable tumors over a shorter period of time, and in treating tumors that recur in a previously irradiated field.

NORMAL TISSUE TOLERANCE WITH RADIATION

A balance is required between the dose required to kill the tumor and the radiation dose tolerated by the normal tissues. The concept of fractionated radiation allows treatment of the cancer while not exceeding the tolerance of the surrounding normal tissues. The four "Rs" of radiation biology are repair of sublethal damage, reoxygenation, repopulation, and reassortment of cells within the cell cycle.[43] These four factors are key to deciding the radiation schedule to optimize tumor regression while minimizing effects to normal tissues.

With fractionated radiation, normal tissues are able to *repair* sublethal radiation effects between treatments. With large daily doses of radiation, a large number of tumor cells are killed, but repair of normal tissues is lower (Figure 84.8). Because the normal tissues are unable to repair the radiation damage of large daily doses of radiation, the total radiation dose that can be given is also much lower.[43]

Equivalent normal tissue effects can be achieved with a variety of radiation treatment schedules. The following clinical radiation schedules are used to treat spine metastases: 2000 cGy is delivered in 5 fractions/400cGy per fraction; 3000 cGy is administered in 10 fractions/300 cGy per fraction; 3500 cGy in 14 fractions/250 cGy per fraction; or 4000 cGy in 20 fractions/200 cGy per fraction. The late radiation effects on the spinal cord would be

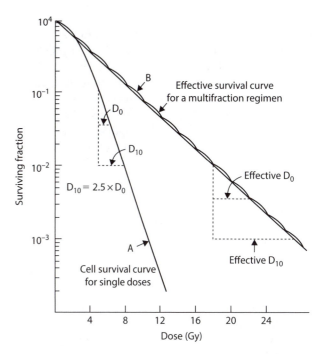

Figure 84.8 *Cell survival curve for single and multiple fraction radiation schedules. A large single dose of radiation, like a single 8 Gy radiation fraction, proportionately kills more tumor cells than equivalent total doses of radiation spread out over multiple fractions, like four 2 Gy fractions, because of repopulation of tumor cells and repair of sublethal damage.*

equal to giving 2800, 3600, and 3900 cGy, respectively, at 200 cGy per fraction. This shows that as the radiation dose per fraction increases, the late radiation toxicities biologically exceed the total radiation dose administered. This effect is more exaggerated as the radiation dose per fraction increases from the standard 200 cGy per fraction.[48] Relating back to the example on integral dose in Table 84.2, administration of 5880 cGy at 294 cGy per fraction would result in severe long-term radiation effects, because this would be biologically equal to a total radiation dose of 7200 cGy at 200 cGy per fraction to a large area of small bowel.[49]

The total dose of radiation necessary to eradicate a tumor is a function of the volume of disease and the number of tumor cells killed with each radiation fraction. The tumor volume is the sum of viable and nonviable cells. In most tumors, the potential number of tumor cells is directly proportional to the tumor volume. In some tumors, for example, soft tissue sarcomas, there is a large necrotic fraction and the rate of cell loss and removal of dead tumor cells from the tumor volume is low. The viable cells may be less responsive to radiation because of the low oxygen tension in the nearby necrotic region. The radiosensitivity of cells also varies during the cell cycle. Cells are most resistant to radiation when they are in the late S phase, and in the late G1/G0 phase. Radiation resistance results from either rapidly proliferating tumors that spend most of their time in S phase or a slowly proliferating tumor where many cells are in G1/G0.

Less total radiation dose is required to control microscopic residual disease than bulk disease. For example, the 2-year rate of local control following radiation alone in the treatment of cervical node metastases in head and neck cancer is directly related to the node diameter and total dose. Using 200 cGy per daily fraction of radiation, over 95% of patients with only microscopic residual cancer achieve tumor control, and over 85% of patients with lymph node diameters of less than 2 cm in size are controlled with a median dose of 6600 cGy. But only 69% of nodes measuring between 2.5 and 3.0 cm are controlled by radiations above 6900 cGy and 59% of nodes larger than 3.5 cm are controlled by radiations above 7000 cGy. Large tumors have a large hypoxic fraction of cells.[43] Hypoxic cells are relatively resistant to radiation effects; it takes three times the dose of radiation to control hypoxic tumors as it does well-oxygenated tumors (Figure 84.9). With fractionated radiation, hypoxic areas are able to reoxygenate to some degree during the course of treatment.

Additionally, tumor cells and normal tissues vary widely in their tolerance to radiation because of cellular repopulation. Radiation doses need to be high enough to kill tumor cells but low enough to allow normal tissues to repair and repopulate. Very low doses of radiation have limited acute effects on normal tissues. No inflammation of the skin or mucosa occurs when the radiation dose is less than 2000 cGy when given in 200 cGy fractions over 2 weeks. But this total dose of radiation

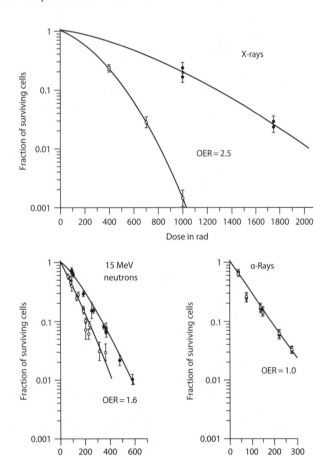

Figure 84.9 *Influence of oxygen on the ability of radiation to kill tumor cells. Open symbols represent hypoxic cells; closed symbols represent oxygenated cells. OER, oxygen enhancement ratio.*

is not sufficient to permanently kill tumor cells due to repopulation of the tumor cells. In the past, a course of radiation was interrupted after 2 weeks of treatment to minimize the side effects of treatment. These so-called split-courses of radiation that allowed repair and repopulation of normal tissues and improved tolerance to radiation have been abandoned, because tumor control rates were compromised by tumor repopulation during the interruption in the treatment.[37,50,51] In fact, tumor repopulation was found during radiobiological evaluations to be accelerated after 2 weeks of radiation because of tumor reoxygenation.

Tolerance to radiation also depends on the type of tissue treated. There are two types of normal tissue:

1. *Acute reacting tissues.* These are rapidly proliferating tissues, for example, mucosal surfaces, and usually develop an inflammatory radiation reaction during the course of treatment.
2. *Late reacting tissues.* Have limited capacity to proliferate or heal injury, for example, brain and spinal cord, liver, and muscle, and generally do not develop a significant inflammatory reaction during the radiation course.

Acute radiation reactions do not predict the extent of late radiation effects. Scar tissue is the most common form of late radiation effect. These effects are similar to those seen in wound healing. The alpha-beta ratio is a calculation that relates to the ability of normal tissues to repair the damage caused by radiation.[43] With low daily doses of radiation over several weeks, more acute radiation effects are seen during the course of radiation. When high daily doses of radiation are given over a short period of time, the most significant radiation side effects occur months to years later after the radiation is completed.

Relating normal tissue tolerance to a 5% risk of a treatment-related complication at 5 years, the tolerance doses (TD 5/5) of each organ have been reported by the National Cancer Institute task force. When the entire organ is treated, the TD 5/5 ranges from 1000 cGy for the eye, to 1750 cGy for the lung, 4500 cGy for the brain, and 7000 cGy for the larynx when the entire organ is treated. Radiation tolerance however is a function of both of the type and the volume of tissue irradiated. When only a third of the organ is irradiated, these values equal 4500 cGy for the lung, 6000 cGy for the brain, and 7900 cGy for the larynx. The normal tissue tolerance for spinal cord is more limited.

RADIATION TOLERANCE OF THE SPINAL CORD

The potential for the development of radiation myelitis with total radiation doses that exceed 40 Gy at 2 Gy per fraction represents the limiting factor in the treatment of large tumor burdens near or involving the spinal canal. Furthermore, the length of spinal cord that needs to be irradiated significantly affects the radiation tolerance of the spinal cord.[52–56] Changes seen in the bone marrow on MRI after palliative radiotherapy initially include decreased cellularity, edema, and hemorrhage followed by fatty replacement and fibrosis. These well-defined changes on MRI after radiotherapy can be distinguished from those seen with progressive disease.[57-59]

Clinical and experimental experience has failed to demonstrate any difference in radiosensitivity in different segments of the spinal cord.[52,55] The risk of radiation myelitis in the cervicothoracic spine is less than 5% when 6000 cGy is administered at 172 cGy per fraction, or 5000 cGy is given with daily fractions of 200 cGy per fraction. Especially among patients who have received chemotherapy or need to have a significant length of spinal cord irradiated, the total dose to the spinal cord is generally limited to 4000 cGy administered at 200 cGy per fraction to minimize any risk of irreversible radiation injury to the spinal cord. A steep curve based on total radiation dose predicts the risk of developing radiation myelopathy; a small increase in total radiation dose can result in a large increased risk for radiation myelopathy.[52,54,56] Re-treatment of a previously irradiated segment of spinal cord results in high risk for radiation-induced myelopathy because other neurological pathways cannot compensate for an injury to a specific level of the spinal cord. Experimental data also have shown that the time course and the extent of long-term recovery from radiation are dependent on the specific type and age of tissue.

The radiation tolerance of the spinal cord can be compromised by prior injury. Difficulty arises in separating traumatic, pathological, and radiotherapeutic injury to spinal cord compression. Vasogenic edema of the spinal cord and nerve roots can be caused by compression injury. Metastatic epidural compression results in vasogenic spinal cord edema, venous hemorrhage, loss of myelin, and ischemia. Other consequences of pathological compression include hemorrhage, loss of myelin, and ischemia.[52-56]

PALLIATIVE RADIATION

With palliative radiation, shorter external beam radiation schedules are generally used that administer a higher radiation dose with each radiation fraction. This is known as

Table 84.3 *Single posterior radiation field delivering 200 cGy at midline (10 cm)*

Depth from posterior skin surface (cm)	Dose from AP	Total dose × 20 fractions
0.5	88 cGy [294 × 0.30]	1760 cGy [88 × 20]
1.5	294 cGy [200/0.68]	5880 cGy [294 × 20]
2.5	285 cGy [294 × 0.97]	5700 cGy [285 × 20]
3.5	279 cGy [294 × 0.92]	5580 cGy [279 × 20]
5.0	259 cGy [294 × 0.88]	5180 cGy [259 × 20]
10.0	200 cGy [294 × 0.68]	4000 cGy [200 × 20]
15.0	150 cGy [294 × 0.51]	3000 cGy [165 × 20]
16.5	141 cGy [294 × 0.48]	2820 cGy [144 × 20]
17.5	129 cGy [294 × 0.44]	2580 cGy [129 × 0]
18.5	123 cGy [294 × 0.42]	2460 cGy [126 × 20]
19.5	118 cGy [294 × 0.40]	2360 cGy [118 × 20]

*hypo*fractionation (Tables 84.3 and 84.4). Tumor cell kill is proportional to the radiation dose that is administered. Therefore, symptomatic relief is more quickly achieved because of the large number of tumor cells that are killed in a short period of time with large daily doses of radiation (see Figure 84.8).

A shorter course of therapy also has a significant impact on quality of life. This short course of treatment not only provides more prompt relief of tumor-related symptoms, but it limits the amount of time needed for the patient to come back and forth for radiation treatments. This is particularly important because the median survival is less than 6 months among patients with poor prognostic factors. However, higher radiation doses, that provide more durable pain relief, are considered warranted for patients with good prognostic factors who require treatment over the spine and other critical sites. It is important to recognize that palliative radiation only results in tumor regression and does not eradicate the tumor. With prolonged survival, the site of metastatic disease may require re-treatment due to regrowth of the tumor.

In contrast to the low daily radiation doses (1.8–2 Gy) given with each treatment during conventional radiation schedules to total radiation doses of 50–60 Gy over 5–6 weeks, large daily radiation fractions are given with hypofractionated radiation

Table 84.4 *Parallel opposed (AP and PA) radiation fields treated each day delivering 200 cGy at midline (10 cm)*

Depth from anterior skin surface (cm)	Dose from AP	Dose from PA	Total dose per fractions (AP + PA)	Total dose × 20 fraction (AP + PA)
0.5	44 cGy [147 × 0.30]	59 cGy [147 × 0.40]	103 cGy	2060 cGy
1.5	147 cGy [100/0.68]	62 cGy [147 × 0.42]	209 cGy	4180 cGy
2.5	143 cGy [147 × 0.97]	65 cGy [147 × 0.44]	208 cGy	4160 cGy
3.5	140 cGy [147 × 0.92]	71 cGy [147 × 0.48]	211 cGy	4220 cGy
5.0	129 cGy [147 × 0.88]	75 cGy [147 × 0.51]	204 cGy	4080 cGy
10.0	100 cGy [147 × 0.68]	100 cGy [147 × 0.68]	200 cGy	4000 cGy
15.0	75 cGy [147 × 0.51]	129 cGy [147 × 0.88]	204 cGy	4080 cGy
16.5	71 cGy [147 × 0.48]	140 cGy [147 × 0.92]	211 cGy	4220 cGy
17.5	65 cGy [147 × 0.44]	143 cGy [147 × 0.97]	208 cGy	4160 cGy
18.5	62 cGy [147 × 0.42]	147 cGy [100/0.68]	209 cGy	4180 cGy
19.5	59 cGy [147 × 0.40]	44 cGy [147 × 0.30]	103 cGy	2060 cGy

schedules used for palliative radiation. Because of normal tissue tolerance to radiation, the total radiation dose that can be administered is low when high doses of radiation are given with each daily fraction. Hypofractionated radiation schedules can range from 2.5 Gy per fraction administered over 3 weeks for a total radiation dose of 35 Gy to a single 8 Gy dose of radiation.[60,61] Most frequently, 30 Gy is administered in 10 fractions over 2 weeks. The decision for the radiation schedule depends on the radiation tolerance of the tissues in the field and the prognosis. The radiation schedule used to relieve symptoms must be indexed to the types of tissues treated, the potential for tumor resection, and overall prognosis. While clinical factors are considered by all radiation oncologists, location of practice, practice type, and country of training, were found to be independently predictive of whether a single 8 Gy radiation dose or 30 Gy over 10 fractions was prescribed in palliative radiation.[62]

Radiopharmaceutical are another systemic option that treats diffuse symptomatic bone metastases. Radiopharmaceuticals, such as strontium-89 or samarium-153, can also be used to treat bone metastases when symptoms recur in a previously irradiated site but are contraindicated with epidural disease because the radiation is deposited directly at the involved area in the bone and the epidural extension is left untreated.[63-68] Radiopharmaceuticals can also act as an adjuvant to localized external beam irradiation and reduce the development of other symptomatic sites of disease.

Control of cancer-related pain with the use of analgesics is imperative to allow comfort during and while awaiting response to antineoplastic interventions. Pain represents a sensitive measure of disease activity. Patients should be closely followed up to ensure control of cancer and treatment-related pain, and to initiate diagnostic studies to determine the cause of persistent, progressive, or recurrent symptoms.

The limited radiation tolerance of the normal tissues, like the spinal cord, that are adjacent to a bone metastasis makes it impossible to administer a large enough dose of radiation to eradicate a measurable volume of tumor. Palliative radiation should result in sufficient tumor regression of critical structures to relieve symptoms. Symptoms that recur after palliative radiation most commonly result from localized regrowth of tumor in the radiation field.

LOCALIZED BONE METASTASES

Radiation of localized bone metastases relieves symptoms and helps prevent spinal cord compression and pathological fractures. There has been much controversy about palliative radiation schedules for localized symptomatic bone metastases. The Radiation Therapy Oncology Group (RTOG) conducted a prospective trial that included a variety of treatment schedules. In order to account for prognosis, patients were stratified on the basis of whether they had a solitary or multiple sites of bony metastases. The initial analysis of the study concluded that low-dose, short-course treatment schedules were as effective as high-dose protracted treatment programs.[69] For solitary bone metastases, there was no difference in the relief of pain when 20 Gy using 4 Gy fractions was compared with 40.5 Gy delivered as 2.7 Gy per fraction. In patients with multiple bone metastases, the following dose schedules were compared: 30 Gy at 3 Gy per fraction, 15 Gy given as 3 Gy per fraction, 20 Gy using 4 Gy per fraction, and 25 Gy using 5 Gy per fraction. No difference was identified in the rates of pain relief between these treatment schedules (Tables 84.5 and 84.6). Partial relief of pain was achieved in 83%, and complete relief occurred in 53% of the patients studied. Over 50% of these patients developed recurrent pain, and 8% of patients developed a pathological fracture.

In a reanalysis of the data, a different definition for complete pain relief was used and excluded the continued administration of analgesics. Using this definition, the relief of pain was significantly related to the number of fractions and the total dose of radiation that was administered.[70] Complete relief of pain was achieved in 55% of patients with solitary bone metastases who received 40.5 Gy at 2.7 Gy per fraction as compared with 37% of patients who received a total dose of 20 Gy given as 4 Gy per fraction. A similar relation was observed in the reanalysis of patients who had multiple bone metastases. Complete relief of pain was achieved in 46% of patients who received 30 Gy at 3 Gy per fraction versus 28% of patients treated to 25 Gy using 5 Gy fractions.

Three important issues are identified from this RTOG experience. First, the results of the reanalysis demonstrate the importance of defining what represents a response to therapy.

Table 84.5 *Different radiation schedules*

Intent	Conventional Curative	Hyperfractionation Curative	Accelerated Curative	Hypofractionation Palliative
No. of fractions per day	1	2 (↑)	1/day for the first 3–4 weeks of XRT (↔) Then 2/day (large field + boost field around the tumor) for the last 1–2 weeks of XRT (↑)	1 (↔)
No. of fractions	25–30	60–70 (↑)	30–35 (↑)	1–15 (↓)
Dose per fraction	1.8–2 Gy	1.2 Gy BID (↓)	1.8–2 Gy to a large field (↔) 1.5 Gy to a boost field (↓)	8 Gy (1 fraction) to 2.5 Gy (15 fractions) (↑)
No. of weeks	5–6	7–9 (↑)	5–6 (↔)	1–3 (↓)
Total radiation dose	45–60 Gy	70–84 Gy (↑)	52–65 Gy (↑)	8–35 Gy (↓)

Arrows represent a comparison to conventional fractionation.

Table 84.6 *Relative relations of radiation dose per fraction, and total dose in a variety of radiation schedules*

Low		High	
Hypofractionation	**Conventional fractionation**	**Hyperfractionation**	**Accelerated fractionation**
20–30 Gy	50–60 Gy	70–80 Gy	55–65 Gy
5–10 fractions	25–30 fractions	60–70 fractions	28–35 fractions
1–2 weeks	5–6 weeks	7–8 weeks	5–6 weeks

When a high dose of radiation is given per fraction, the total dose must be low and given in a small number of fractions.

Second, this revised definition of response showed that the total radiation dose did influence the degree to which the pain was relieved. Third, the RTOG experience identified the amount of time that was needed to experience relief of pain after radiation for bone metastases (Tables 84.7 and 84.8). It is important to note that only half of the patients who were going to respond had relief of symptoms at 2–4 weeks after radiation.[69,70] This underscores the need for continued analgesic support after completing radiation. Consistently, it took 12–20 weeks after radiation to accomplish the maximal level of relief. That period of time may reflect the time needed for reossification.

Pretreatment CT imaging features, such as osseous and soft tissue tumor extent, presence of pathological fracture, vertebral height loss, and kyphosis without neurologic compromise, did not influence pain relief after radiotherapy. Like the RTOG trial, pain relief was 18% at 1 month, 69% at 2 months, and 70% at 3 months even with a pretreatment mean pain severity of 7/10 in another study.[71] Radiographic evidence of recalcification is observed in about a fourth of cases, and in 70% of the time, recalcification is seen within 6 months of completing radiation and other palliative therapies.[72–74] Pretreatment clinical characteristics were evaluated for their influence the level of response. Neuropathic pain is a significant clinical variable, which reduces the response to palliative radiation.[75–77]

The projected length of survival is the critical issue for the prescription of the radiation dose and schedule for palliative radiation. In one study, only 12 of 245 patients were alive at the time of analysis with approximately 50% alive at 6 months, 25% at 1 year, 8% at 2 years, and 3% at 3 years after palliative radiation. For breast cancer patients, the survival rates at these time points after palliative radiation were 60%, 44%, 20%, and 7%, respectively. For prostate cancer, the survival rates were 60% at 6 months, 24% at 1 year, and there were no patients who survived 2 years.[78] In the RTOG trial, the median survival for solitary bone metastases was 36 weeks and was 24 weeks for multiple bone metastases.[69,70]

The RTOG study also demonstrated that the level of pain correlated with prognosis among patients with multiple bone metastases. This survival difference may be an important observation, because unrelieved pain and the resultant sequelae of immobility may contribute to mortality as well as morbidity. Based on recursive partitioning analysis, the predictors of survival among patients with spinal metastases defined 3 prognostic groups. Median overall survival was 21.1 months with the predictors of survival as time from diagnosis was more than 30 months and KPS was more than 70. Median overall survival dropped to 8.7 months either with:

Table 84.7 *Dose–response evaluation from the reanalysis of the RTOG bone metastases protocol*

	Dose/ fx (Gy)	Total dose (Gy)	Tumor dose at 2 Gy/fx	CR (%)	P value
Solitary bone metastases					0.0003
	2.7	40.5	42.9	55	
	4.0	20.0	23.3	37	
Multiple bone metastases					0.0003
	3.0	30	32.5	46	
	3.0	15.0	16.2	36	
	4.0	20.0	23.3	40	
	5.0	25.0	31.25	28	

Source: Boogerd, W., *Radiother. Oncol.*, 40, 5, 1996.
Listed are the dose per fraction (dose/fx), total radiation dose, the radiobiological equivalent dose if administered at 2 Gy/fx, the complete response rate (CR) using the definition that excludes the use of analgesics and that accounts for re-treatment.

Table 84.8 *Percentage of patients who responded to radiation relative to time, designated in weeks after completion of radiation therapy*

Total dose (Gy)	Dose per fraction (Gy)	Tumor dose at 2 Gy/fx	Weeks after radiation therapy (%)			
			<2	2–4	4–12	12–20
Solitary metastasis						
40.5	2.7	42.9	7	29	53	77
20.0	4	23.3	16	50	66	82
Multiple metastasis						
30.0	3	32.5	19	48	73	84
15.0	3	16.2	34	70	84	93
20.0	4	23.3	28	53	75	88
25.0	5	31.25	22	41	72	80

This prospective trial, conducted by the RTOG, randomized radiation dose and number of fractions and stratified the randomization on the basis of solitary or multiple bone metastases.[90,92] Also listed is the radiobiological equivalent dose if administered at 2 Gy per fraction.

(1) a time from diagnosis of greater than 30 months and KPS of less than 70, or (2) a time from diagnosis of less than 30 months and age less than 70 years. The shortest median overall survival of 2.4 months occurred when the time from diagnosis was less than 30 months and age was greater than 70 years.[79]

SPINAL CORD COMPRESSION

The time from the original diagnosis to the development of metastatic spinal disease averages 32 months, and the average time is reported to be 27 months from diagnosis of skeletal metastases to spinal cord compression. Median survival among patients with spinal cord compression ranges between 3 and 7 months, with a 36% probability for a 1-year survival. The vertebral column is involved in metastatic tumor in 40% of patients who die of cancer, and approximately 70% of vertebral metastases involve the thoracic spine, 20% the lumbosacral region, and 10% the cervical spine. From a tumor registry of 121,435 patients, the cumulative probability of at least one episode of spinal cord compression occurring in the last 5 years of life was 2.5%.[82] Additionally, the diagnosis of spinal cord compression was associated with a doubling of the time spent in hospital in the last year of life.

The time between primary tumor diagnosis and development of spinal cord compression is dependent on tumor type with the shortest time associated with lung cancer and the longest time for breast cancer. The demographics of spinal cord compression include 37% of patients had breast cancer, 28% had prostate cancer, 18% lung cancer, and 17% had other solid tumors. Lung cancer patients have the most severe functional deficits from spinal cord compression with more than 50% totally paralyzed while 59% of breast cancer patients remain ambulatory. More severe disturbances in gait occurred when there was a short period of time between the diagnosis of the primary tumor and spinal cord compression was short.[80–85] The mean survival time after the diagnosis of spinal cord compression is 14 months for breast cancer, 12 months in prostate cancer, 6 months in malignant melanoma, and 3 months in lung cancer.[80–82]

In a series of 153 consecutive patients with spinal cord compression, total paralysis was present in 28% of patients presenting for radiation, 20% were able to move their legs but could not walk, 12% were able to walk with assistance, and 40% could walk unassisted. Sensory exam of the legs was normal in 34, slight disturbances were present in 84, and total lack of pain perception occurred in 35 patients. After radiation, 26% were totally paralyzed, 13% were able to move their legs without being able to walk, 11% were able to walk with assistance, and 50% had unassisted gait.[86] Survival in this series was dependent on time from primary tumor diagnosis, ambulatory function at diagnosis and after radiation therapy, and median survival was 3.5 months. The type of primary tumor also has a direct influence on the interval between the diagnosis of the primary tumor and the diagnosis of spinal cord compression due to metastatic disease.[87] However, factors such as age, discharge destination, primary tumor site, other metastases, comorbidities, and hemoglobin and albumin levels had no significant influence on survival time in a study of 60 consecutive patients with metastatic spinal cord compression.[88]

Using a matched pair analysis that compared surgery followed by radiotherapy in 108 patients versus radiotherapy alone in 216 patients for metastatic spinal cord compression, there was no difference in 1-year overall survival rates (47% for surgery and radiotherapy, and 40% for radiotherapy) improvement of motor function (26%) or ambulatory rates (68%). Among nonambulatory patients, 30% of surgery and radiotherapy, and 26% of radiotherapy patients regained ambulatory status.[89] While radiotherapy effectively controls tumor involvement, surgery benefits patients the most, with mechanical collapse of the vertebral elements on neural structures by reinstating anatomic integrity of the spine.

RADIATION SCHEDULE FOR SPINAL CORD COMPRESSION BASED ON PROGNOSIS

The time under radiation needs to be considered as the opportunity cost of palliative treatment.[90] If the median survival of a patient with spinal cord compression is 6 months (180 days), the patient will spend 0.6% of the remaining survival time under radiation treatment when a single fraction of radiation is given. If 10 radiation fractions are given, 8% of the remaining survival and if 20 fractions are prescribed, 16% of the remaining survival will be consumed by radiation therapy. Even if re-treatment with a second single fraction is required, the patient will continue to spend about 1% of the survival time under radiation therapy. For lung cancer patients with a 3-month survival rate, 1% of the remaining time is spent with a single fraction of radiation as compared to 16%, if 10 fractions are given, or 30%, if 20 fractions are prescribed.

A more protracted course of radiation is still used for patients with a more prolonged prognosis who require treatment over the spine and other critical sites. With an actuarial overall survival rate of 85% at 1 year, and 63% at 2 years among selected patients, administration of protracted fractionation for spinal metastases achieved an 88% local control rate at 2 years with long-term pain relief.[91]

With a more limited prognosis, metastatic spinal cord compression has been treated either with a single 8 Gy fraction or five 4 Gy fractions. The median time to recurrence was 6 months among 62 patients with a range of 2–40 months.[83] Re-treatment consisted of another single 8 Gy fraction, or five more fractions of either 3 or 4 Gy. Motor function improved in 40%, and it was stable in an additional 45%; 38% of the nonambulatory patients regained the ability to walk.[92,93] A prospective randomized trial compared the use of 16 Gy in 2 fractions versus 8 Gy in a single fraction for 327 patients with spinal cord compression and life expectancy of less than or equal to 6 months.[94] The ambulation response rate was 69% in the 16 Gy arm and 62% in the 8 Gy arm not significant (NS), with responders maintaining function until death. Nonrandomized data comparing short course regimens of 8 Gy in a single fraction or 20 Gy in 5 fractions versus 30 Gy in 10 fractions, 37.5 Gy in 15 fractions, or 40 Gy in 20 fractions showed identical ambulation response rates, further suggesting that a single 8 Gy dose is a noninferior fractionation scheme for poor prognosis patients with spinal cord compression.[95]

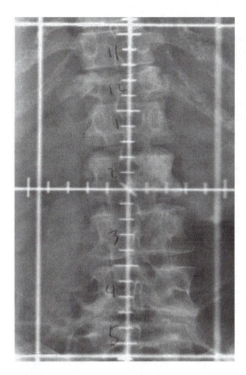

Figure 84.10   *Typical radiation portal to treat disease involvement in the vertebral bodies and epidural region.*

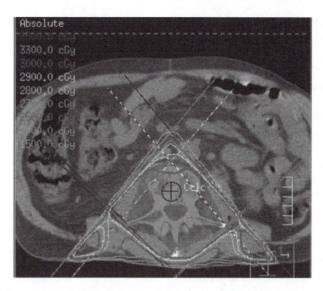

Figure 84.11   *Radiation plan that reduces exit beam and toxicity to adjacent visceral structures.*

The use of a single fraction of radiation provided sufficient tumor regression for neurological improvement while minimizing time under radiation.

Arguments against the use of a single fraction of radiation in patients with a more limited prognosis involve gastrointestinal toxicity from the exit dose of radiation. Using a single posterior radiation field, about two-thirds of the radiation dose causes toxicity as it exits through the esophagus, stomach, and bowel (Figure 84.10). Acute radiation toxicities are a function of the dose per fraction, total dose, and the area and volume of tissue irradiated. If mucosal surfaces like the upper aerodigestive tract, bowel, and bladder can be excluded from the radiation portals, acute radiation side effects can be significantly reduced whether single or multiple fractions are prescribed.[96-104] Gastrointestinal toxicities, like esophagitis, nausea and vomiting, and small bowel toxicity, can be avoided when a high dose of radiation is administered with the use of more conformal radiation that localizes the radiation to the vertebra and minimizing dose to adjacent normal structures (Figure 84.11).

RESPONSE TO RADIATION THERAPY

Pain is the initial symptom in approximately 90% of patients with spinal cord compression, and the development of spinal cord compression is associated with a poor overall prognosis. Paraparesis or paraplegia occurs in over 60%, sensory loss is noted in 70%–80%, and 14%–77% have bladder and/or bowel disturbances.[83,87,105-114] Among 102 consecutive patients with metastatic spinal cord compression, only 51% were fully ambulatory at the time of radiotherapy, and 41% had paraparesis. Median survival was 3.5 months, with normal gait returning in 58%, 2 weeks after completing radiation, and in 71%, 2 months after radiation. No paraplegic patient regained function.[105]

The rate of development of motor symptoms correlates with the possibility of recovering neurological function after radiation therapy. Weakness can signal the rapid progression of symptoms, and 30% of patients with weakness become paraplegic within 1 week. Rapid development of weakness, defined as occurring in less than 2 months, most commonly occurs in lung cancer, whereas breast and prostate cancers can progress more slowly. Neurological deficits can develop within a few hours in up to 20% of patients with spinal cord compression.[80-82,86,87,105,107,109-114] Motor function improved among 86% of patients who had >14-day time to development of symptoms. Only 29% improved when motor deficits developed over 8–14 days before the diagnosis of spinal cord compression. Improvements occurred in only 10% if motor deficits developed over 1–7 days. The severity of weakness at the time that radiation therapy is initiated is the most significant factor for recovery of function. Ninety percent of patients who are ambulatory at presentation will be ambulatory after radiation. Only 13% of paraplegic patients will regain function, particularly if paraplegia is present for more than 24 hours before the initiation of radiation.

The degree and rate of pain relief is also dependent on the level of pain at the time radiation is administered.[86,87,105,107,109-114] Pain relief is accomplished in 73% of patients, and the mean time to pain relief was 35 days in 108 breast cancer patients. Recurrent symptoms at a different spinal level occur in more than three-fourths of patients and within 6 months of radiation.[82]

Without motor impairment, corticosteroids are unnecessary when radiation therapy is administered to relieve pain from vertebral involvement.[115] Elimination of steroids from the standard treatment avoids cortisone side effects, above all, in those patients with diabetes, hypertension, peptic ulcer, and other steroid-sensitive medical problems. However, corticosteroids should be initiated with clinical and/or radiographic evidence of spinal cord compromise prior to the start of radiotherapy to reduce disease-related edema and pain. Oral dexamethasone (4 mg) generally is administered four times daily, but IV dexamethasone should be considered with severe and/or rapid neurological impairment. Experimental studies have shown that high-dose steroids are more effective than lower doses in reversing edema and improving neurological function. Consistent with this are clinical data including a well-designed randomized trial that administered radiation therapy either with high-dose corticosteroids or placebo. In that trial, the group that received corticosteroids was more likely to retain or regain ambulation.[116] Pain relief is also more rapid and complete with high-dose steroids (initial bolus of 100 mg followed by 4 mg dexamethasone four times daily for the duration of radiation therapy) among patients suspected to have spinal cord compression.

The radiation tolerance of the spinal cord can be compromised by prior injury. Difficulty arises in separating the pathological and radiotherapeutic injury to spinal cord compression. Vasogenic edema of the spinal cord and nerve roots can be caused by compression injury. Metastatic epidural compression results in vasogenic spinal cord edema, venous hemorrhage, loss of myelin, and ischemia. Vasogenic edema results in an increased synthesis of prostaglandin E_2, which can be inhibited by steroids or nonsteroidal anti-inflammatory agents. Other consequences of pathological compression include hemorrhage, loss of myelin, and ischemia.[52–54]

A statistically significant improvement in functional outcome occurs with laminectomy and radiotherapy in treatment of epidural spinal cord compression over either modality alone for selected clinical presentations. Laminectomy has been recommended to promptly reduce tumor volume in an attempt to relieve compression and injury of the spinal cord and provide stabilization to the spinal axis. The rate of tumor regression following radiotherapy is too slow in these cases to effect recovery of lost neurologic function, and radiation therapy cannot relieve compression of the spinal column due to vertebral collapse. After radiation alone to treat a partial spinal cord block, 64% of patients regain ambulation, 33% have normalization of sphincter tone, 72% are pain-free, and median survival is 9 months.[80,86,100,103,104,117,118] With a complete spinal cord block, only 27% will have improvement in motor function and 42% will continue to have pain after radiation alone. In paraparetic patients who undergo laminectomy and radiation, 82% regain the ability to walk, 68% have improved sphincter function, and 88% have relief of pain.

Laminectomy is indicated with rapid neurological deterioration, tumor progression in a previously irradiated area, stabilization of the spine, paraplegic patients with limited disease and good probability of survival, and to establish a diagnosis. Adjuvant radiotherapy is often given after laminectomy to treat microscopic residual disease

after neurosurgical intervention.[80,98–100,102–104,117,118] Surgical restoration of the vertebral alignment may be required due to neurologic compromise and pain caused by progressive vertebral collapse. Vertebral collapse may occur due to cancer or vertebral instability after cancer therapy, for example, radiation (Figure 84.12). Appropriate diagnostic studies and intervention should be pursued with persistent pain because the neurological compromise and pain from vertebral instability can be as devastating as that with epidural spinal cord metastases.[103,118] Near-perfect inter- and intraobserver reliability for three categories, stable, potentially unstable, and unstable, was achieved with the spinal instability neoplastic score based on the location and characteristics of the metastatic disease, pain, posterolateral involvement, and vertebral alignment and collapse.[119]

Based on clinical and radiographic grounds, leptomeningeal carcinomatosis must also be considered in the diagnostic evaluation. Leptomeningeal carcinomatosis occurs more commonly than expected. For example, only half of breast cancer patients with leptomeningeal carcinomatosis will be diagnosed before death.[80,85,98,104,111] Radiation therapy is indicated in localized regions of nodular leptomeningeal involvement.[111]

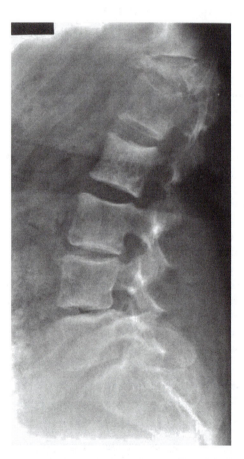

Figure 84.12 *Compression fraction of the 12th thoracic vertebral body following an initial pain-free interval after palliative radiation. Vertebral weakness with rapid tumor regression resulted in the compression fracture that caused recurrent back pain due to spinal instability.*

THERAPEUTIC RECOMMENDATIONS

The primary goals of palliative treatment are to efficiently relieve disease-related symptoms and maintain function while minimizing treatment-related symptoms and time under therapy. Spine metastases cause significant pain and can result in irreversible paralysis. Patients with known vertebral metastases require frequent clinical evaluation to identify any change in symptoms and/or radiographic findings, suggesting risk for spinal cord compromise. Early detection of vertebral compromise is paramount to preventing an oncological emergency with severe pain and neurological compromise from spinal cord compression. Emergent oncological care involves either surgical decompression and/or radiation therapy.

To prevent disease progression resulting in spinal cord compression, radiation should be considered to treat extensive and/or painful vertebral metastases, and with limited asymptomatic epidural involvement. Radiopharmaceuticals, administered by a single injection, are an important option for multifocal bone metastases, especially if symptoms and disease recur in a previously irradiated area in the absence of epidural involvement.

Radiation remains an important modality in palliative care. A number of clinical, prognostic, and therapeutic factors must be considered to determine the most optimal treatment regimen in palliative radiotherapy in general. Especially if there is an associated paraspinal mass, symptoms that persist after palliative radiation should be evaluated to exclude progression of disease in the treated area, and possible extension of disease outside the radiation portal. Pain may also persist due to reduced cortical strength after treatment of spinal metastases that can result in vertebral compression or stress microfractures.

Multiple radiotherapeutic options are available for the treatment of spinal cord compression. Radiobiological principles, the radiation tolerance of adjacent normal tissues, and the clinical condition influence the selection of radiation technique, dose, and fraction size. As a late-reacting tissue, the radiobiological tolerance of the spinal cord to radiation is finite. Technological advances, however, have increased our ability to treat spinal metastases with greater precision, and have allowed consideration of retreatment with radiation to selected patients.

Prevention or early treatment of symptoms is often the most important care administered. The treatment of vertebral metastases and spinal cord compression to prevent or relieve symptoms of pain and paralysis is one of the most important services rendered to cancer patients.

Key learning points

- Spinal cord compression results in significant morbidity, constitutes an oncological emergency, and is associated with a poor overall prognosis.

- Early diagnosis and treatment prevents lasting neurological dysfunction.

- New therapeutic modalities are now available to prevent and treat spinal cord compression.

REFERENCES

1 Cleeland CS, Gonin R, Hatfield AK et al. Pain and its treatment in outpatients with metastatic cancer. *N Engl J Med* 1994; 330: 592–596.

2 Jacox AK, Carr DB, Payne R eds. *Management of Cancer Pain.* Clinical Practice Guideline No. 9. Rockville, MD: Agency for Health Care Policy and Research (AHCPR publication no. 94-0592); 1994.

3 Jacox A, Carr DB, Payne R. New Clinical Practice Guidelines for the management of pain in patients with cancer. *N Engl J Med* 1994; 330: 651–655.

4 Brescia FJ, Portenoy RK, Ryan M et al. Pain, opioid use, and survival in hospitalized patients with advanced cancer. *J Clin Oncol* 1992; 10: 149–155.

5 Dale RG, Jones B. Radiobiologically based assessments of the net costs of fractionated radiotherapy. *Int J Radiat Oncol Biol Phys* 1996; 36: 739–746.

6 Vigano A, Bruera E, Jhangri GS et al. Clinical survival predictors in patients with advanced cancer. *Arch Intern Med* 2000; 160: 861–868.

7 Sherry MM, Greco FA, Johnson DH, Hainsworth JD. Breast cancer with skeletal metastases at initial diagnosis-distinctive clinical characteristics and favorable prognosis. *Cancer* 1986; 58: 178–182.

8 Sherry MM, Greco FA, Johnson DH, Hainsworth JD. Metastatic breast cancer confined to the skeletal system. *Am J Med* 1986; 81: 381–386.

9 Plunkett TA, Smith P, Rubens RD. Risk of complications from bone metastases in breast cancer: Implications for management. *Eur J Cancer* 2000; 36: 476–472.

10 Lai PP, Perez CA, Lockett MA. Prognostic significance of pelvic recurrence and distant metastases in prostate carcinoma following definitive radiotherapy. *Int J Radiat Oncol Biol Phys* 1992; 24: 423–430.

11 Yamashita K, Denno K, Ueda T et al. Prognostic significance of bone metastases in patients with metastatic prostate cancer. *Cancer* 1993; 71: 1297–1302.

12 Knudson G, Grinis G, Lopez-Majano V et al. Bone scan as a stratification variable in advanced prostate cancer. *Cancer* 1991; 68: 316–320.

13 Sabbatini P, Larson SM, Kremer A et al. Prognostic significance of extent of disease in bone in patients with androgen-independent prostate cancer. *J Clin Oncol* 1999; 17: 948–957.

14 Greenwald HP, Bonica JJ, Bergner M. The prevalence of pain in four cancers. *Cancer* 1987; 60: 2563–2569.

15 Borre M, Nerstrom B, Overgaard J. The natural history of prostate carcinoma based on a Danish population treated with no intent to cure. *Cancer* 1997; 80: 917–928.

16 Grabowski CM, Unger JA, Potish RA. Factors predictive of completion of treatment and survival after palliative radiation therapy. *Radiology* 1992; 184: 329–332.

17 Reuben DB, Mor V, Hiris J. Clinical symptoms and length of survival in patients with terminal cancer. *Arch Intern Med* 1988; 148: 1586–1591.

18 Fielding LP, Henson DE. Multiple prognostic factors and outcome analysis in patients with cancer-communication from the American Joint Committee on Cancer. *Cancer* 1993; 71: 2426–2429.

19 Portenoy RK, Miransky J, Thaler HT et al. Pain in ambulatory patients with lung or colon cancer. *Cancer* 1992; 70: 1616–1624.

20 Brown JE, Thomson CS, Ellis SP et al. Bone resorption predicts for skeletal complications in metastatic bone disease. *Br J Cancer* 2003; 89: 2031–2037.

21 Brown J, Cook R, Major P et al. Bone turnover markers as predictors of skeletal complications in prostate cancer, lung cancer and other solid tumors. *J Natl Cancer Inst* 2005; 97: 59.

22 Fizazi K, Lipton A, Mariette X, Body J-J, Rahim Y, Gralow JR, Gao G, Wu L, Sohn W, Jun S. Randomized phase II trial of denosumab in patients with bone metastases from prostate cancer, breast cancer, or other neoplasms after intravenous bisphosphonates. *J Clin Oncol* 2009; 27: 1564–1571.

23 Powers WE, Ratanatharathorn V. Palliation of bone metastases. In: Perez CA, Brady LW, eds. *Principles and Practice of Radiation Oncology*, 3rd edn. Philadelphia, PA: Lippincott Raven, 1998, pp. 2199–2219.

24 Bunting RW, Boublik M, Blevins FT et al. Functional outcome of pathologic fracture secondary to malignant disease in a rehabilitation hospital. *Cancer* 1992; 69: 98–102.

25 Arcangeli G, Micheli A, Arcangeli F et al. The responsiveness of bone metastases to radiotherapy: The effect of site, histology and radiation dose on pain relief. *Radiother Oncol* 1989; 14: 95–101.

26 Temel JS, Greer JA, Muzikansky A et al. Early palliative care for patients with metastatic non-small-cell lung cancer. *N Engl J Med* 2010; 363: 733–742.

27 Steiner RM, Mitchell DG, Rao VM, Schweitzer ME. Magnetic resonance imaging of diffuse bone marrow disease. *Radiol Clin North Am* 1993; 31: 383–409.

28 Algra PR, Bloem JL, Tissing H et al. Detection of vertebral metastases: Comparison between MR imaging and bone scintigraphy. *Radiographics* 1991; 11: 219–232.

29 Le Bihan DJ. Differentiation of benign versus pathologic compression fractures with diffusion-weighted MR imaging: A closer step toward the 'holy grail' of tissue characterization? *Radiology* 1998; 207: 305–307.

30 Francken AB, Hong AM, Fulham MJ et al. Detection of unsuspected spinal cord compression in melanoma patients by 18F-fluorodeoxyglucose-positron emission tomography. *Eur J Surg Oncol* 2005; 31: 197–204.

31 Nielsen OS, Munro AJ, Tannock IF. Bone metastases: Pathophysiology and management policy. *J Clin Oncol* 1991; 9: 509–524.

32 Lutz S, Berk L, Chang E et al. Palliative radiotherapy for bone metastases: An ASTRO evidence-based guideline. *Int J Radiat Oncol Biol Phys* 2011; 79: 965–976.

33 Khan FM. Dose distribution and scatter analysis. In: *The Physics of Radiation Therapy*. Baltimore, MD: Williams and Wilkins, 1984, pp. 157–178.

34 Barton R, Robinson G, Gutierrez E et al. Palliative radiation for vertebral metastases: The effect of variation in prescription parameters on the dose received at depth. *Int J Radiat Oncol Biol Phys* 2002; 52: 1083–1091.

35 Klish DS, Grossman P, Allen PK, Rhines LD, Chang EL. Irradiation of spinal metastases: Should we continue to include one uninvolved vertebral body above and below in the radiation field? *Int J Radiat Oncol Biol Phys* 2011; 81: 1495–1499.

36 Shiu AS, Chang EL, Ye JS et al. Near simultaneous computed tomography image-guided stereotactic spinal radiotherapy: An emerging paradigm for achieving true stereotaxy. *Int J Radiat Oncol Biol Phys* 2003; 57: 605–613.

37 Chang EL, Shiu AS, Lii MF et al. Phase I clinical evaluation of near-simultaneous computed tomographic image-guided stereotactic body radiotherapy for spinal metastases. *Int J Radiat Oncol Biol Phys* 2004; 59: 1288–1294.

38 Rose PS, Laufer I, Boland PJ, Hanover A, Bilsky MH, Yamada J, Lis E. Risk of fracture after single fraction image-guided intensity-modulated radiation therapy to spinal metastases. *J Clin Oncol* 2009; 27: 5075–5079.

39 Gerszten PC, Germanwala AN, Burton SA et al. Combination kyphoplasty and spinal radiosurgery: A new treatment paradigm for pathological fractures. *Neurosurg Focus* 2005; 18: E8.

40 Gerszten PC, Burton SA, Ozhasoglu C et al. Stereotactic radiosurgery for spinal metastases from renal cell carcinoma. *J Neurosurg Spine* 2005; 3: 288–295.

41 Sahgal A, Larson DA, Chang EL. Stereotactic body radiosurgery for spinal metastases: A critical review. *Int J Radiation Oncology Biol Phys* 2008; 71: 652–665.

42 Mahadevan A, Floyd S, Wong E, Jeyapalan S, Groff M, Kasper E. Stereotactic body radiotherapy reirradiation for recurrent epidural spinal metastases. *Int J Radiat Oncol Biol Phys* 2011; 81: 1500–1505.

43 Hall E. Dose–response relationships for normal tissues. In: *Radiobiology for the Radiologist*, 4th edn. Philadelphia, PA: JB Lippincott, 1994, pp. 45–75.

44 Nieder C, Milas L, Ang KK. Tissue tolerance to reirradiation. *Semin Radiat Oncol* 2000; 10: 200–209.

45 Morris DE. Clinical experience with retreatment for palliation. *Semin Radiat Oncol* 2000; 10: 210–221.

46 Mohiuddin M, Marks GM, Lingareddy V, Marks J. Curative surgical resection following reirradiation for recurrent rectal cancer. *Int J Radiat Oncol Biol Phys* 1997; 39: 643–649.

47 Mohiuddin M, Regine WF, Stevens J et al. Combined intraoperative radiation and perioperative chemotherapy for unresectable cancers of the pancreas. *J Clin Oncol* 1995; 13: 2764–2768.

48 Barton M. Tables of equivalent dose in 2 Gy fractions: A simple application of the linear quadratic formula. *Int J Radiat Oncol Biol Phys* 1995; 31: 371–378.

49 Minsky BD, Conti JA, Huang Y, Knopf K. Relationship of acute gastrointestinal toxicity and the volume of irradiated small bowel in patients receiving combined modality therapy for rectal cancer. *J Clin Oncol* 1995; 13: 1409–1416.

50 Cox JD, Pajack TF, Asbell S et al. Interruptions of high-dose radiation therapy decrease long-term survival of favorable patients with unresectable non-small cell carcinoma of the lung: Analysis of 1244 cases from 3 Radiation Therapy Oncology Group (RTOG) trials. *Int J Radiat Oncol Biol Phys* 1993; 27: 493–498.

51 Cox JD, Pajak TF, Marcial VA et al. Interruptions adversely affect local control and survival with hyperfractionated radiation therapy of carcinomas of the upper respiratory and digestive tracts. New evidence for accelerated proliferation from Radiation Therapy Oncology Group Protocol 8313. *Cancer* 1992; 69: 2744–2748.

52 Jeremic B, Djuric L, Mijatovic L. Incidence of radiation myelitis of the cervical spinal cord at doses of 5500 cGy or greater. *Cancer* 1991; 68: 2138–2141.

53 Wen PY, Blanchard KL, Block CC et al. Development of Lhermitte's sign after bone marrow transplantation. *Cancer* 1992; 69: 2262–2266.

54 Powers BE, Thames HD, Gillette SM et al. Volume effects in the irradiated canine spinal cord: Do they exist when the probability of injury is low? *Radiother Oncol* 1998; 46: 297–306.

55 Maranzano E, Bellavita R, Floridi P et al. Radiation induced myelopathy in long-term surviving metastatic spinal cord compression patients after hypofractionated radiotherapy: A clinical and magnetic resonance imaging analysis. *Radiother Oncol* 2001; 60: 281–288.

56 Ridet JL, Pencalet P, Belcram M et al. Effects of spinal cord x-irradiation on the recovery of paraplegic rats. *Exp Neurol* 2000; 161: 1–14.

57 Algra PR, Heimans JJ, Valk J et al. Do metastases in vertebrae begin in the body or the pedicles? Imaging study in 45 patients. *Am J Roentgenol* 1992; 158: 1275–1279.

58 Sugimura H, Kisanuki A, Tamura S et al. Magnetic resonance imaging of bone marrow changes after irradiation. *Investig Radiol* 1994; 29: 35–41.

59 Yankelevitz DF, Henschke C, Knapp PH et al. Effect of radiation therapy on thoracic and lumbar bone marrow: Evaluation with MR imaging. *Am J Roentgenol* 1991; 157: 87–92.

60 Cox JD. Fractionation: A paradigm for clinical research in radiation oncology. *Int J Radiat Oncol Biol Phys* 1987; 13: 1271–1281.

61 Cox JD. Large-dose fractionation (hypofractionation). *Cancer* 1985; 55 (9 Suppl.): 2105–2111.

62 Fairchild A, Barnes E, Ghosh S, Ben-Josef E, Roos D, Hartsell W, Holt T, Wu J, Janjan N, Chow E. International patterns of practice in palliative radiotherapy for painful bone metastases: Evidence-based practice? *Int J Radiat Oncol Biol Phys* 2009; 75: 1501–1510.

63 Porter AT, McEwan AJB, Powe JE et al. Results of a randomized Phase III trial to evaluate the efficacy of Strontium 89 adjuvant to local field external beam irradiation in the management of endocrine resistant metastatic prostate cancer. *Int J Radiat Oncol Biol Phys* 1993; 25: 805–813.

64 Robinson RG, Preston DF, Schiefelbein M, Baxter KG. Strontium 89 therapy for the palliation of pain due to osseous metastases. *JAMA* 1995; 274: 420–424.

65 Serafini AN, Houston SJ, Resche I et al. Palliation of pain associated with metastatic bone cancer using samarium-153 lexidronam: A double-blind placebo-controlled clinical trial. *J Clin Oncol* 1998; 16: 1574–1581.

66 Sciuto R, Maini CL, Tofani A et al. Radiosensitization with low-dose carboplatin enhances pain palliation in radioisotope therapy with strontium-89. *Nucl Med Commun* 1996; 17: 799–804.

67 Alberts AS, Smit BJ, Louw WKA et al. Dose-response relationship and multiple dose efficacy and toxicity of samarium-153-EDTMP in metastatic cancer to bone. *Radiother Oncol* 1997; 43: 175–179.

68 Anderson PM, Wiseman GA, Dispenzieri A et al. High-dose samarium-153 ethylene diamine tetramethylene phosphonate: Low toxicity of skeletal irradiation in patients with osteosarcoma and bone metastases. *J Clin Oncol* 2002; 20: 189–196.

69 Tong D, Gillick L, Hendrickson FR. The palliation of symptomatic osseous metastases-final results of the study by the Radiation Therapy Oncology Group. *Cancer* 1982; 50: 893–899.

70 Blitzer PH. Reanalysis of the RTOG study of the palliation of symptomatic osseous metastasis. *Cancer* 1985; 55: 1468–1472.

71 Mitera G, Probyn L, Ford M et al. Correlation of computed tomography imaging features with pain response in patients with spine metastases after radiation therapy. *Int J Radiat Oncol Biol Phys* 2011; 81: 827–830.

72 Ford HT, Yarnold JR. Radiation therapy—Pain relief and recalcification. In: Stoll BA, Parbhoo S, eds. *Bone Metastases: Monitoring and Treatment*. New York: Raven Press, 1983, pp. 343–354.

73 Hortobagyi GN, Libshitz HI, Seabold JE. Osseous metastases of breast cancer-clinical, biochemical, radiographic, and scintigraphic evaluation of response to therapy. *Cancer* 1984; 53: 577–582.

74 Vogel CL, Schoenfelder J, Shemano I et al. Worsening bone scan in the evaluation of antitumor response during hormonal therapy of breast cancer. *J Clin Oncol* 1995; 13: 1123–1128.

75 Rutten EHJM, Crul BJP, van der Toorn PPG et al. Pain characteristics help to predict the analgesic efficacy of radiotherapy for the treatment of cancer pain. *Pain* 1997; 69: 131–135.

76 Kelly JB, Payne R. Pain syndromes in the cancer patient. *Neurol Clin* 1991; 9: 937–953.

77 Portenoy RK. Cancer pain management. *Semin Oncol* 1993; 20: 19–35.

78 Gaze MN, Kelly CG, Kerr GR et al. Pain relief and quality of life following radiotherapy for bone metastases: A randomised trial of two fractionation schedules. *Radiother Oncol* 1997; 45: 109–116.

79 Chao ST, Koyfman SA, Woody N, Angelov L, Soeder SL, Reddy CA, Rybicki LA, Djemil T, Suh JH. Recursive partitioning analysis index is predictive for overall survival in patients undergoing spine stereotactic body radiation therapy for spinal metastases. *Int J Radiat Oncol Biol Phys* 2012; 82: 1738–1743.

80 Boogerd W, van der Sande JJ, Kroger R. Early diagnosis and treatment of spinal metastases in breast cancer: A prospective study. *J Neurol Neurosurg Psychiatry* 1992; 55: 1188–1193.

81 Bach F, Agerlin N, Sorensen JB et al. Metastatic spinal cord compression secondary to lung cancer. *J Clin Oncol* 1992; 10: 1781–1787.

82 Prie L, Lagarde P, Palussiere J et al. Radiation therapy of spinal metastases in breast cancer: Retrospective analysis of 108 patients. *Cancer/Radiotherapie* 1997; 1: 234–239.

83 Rades D, Stalpers LJA, Veninga T, Hoskin PJ. Spinal reirradiation after short-course RT for Metastatic Spinal Cord Compression. *Int J Radiat Oncol Biol Phys* 2005; 63: 872–875.

84 Rades D, Blach M, Bremer M et al. Prognostic significance of the time of developing motor deficits before radiation therapy in metastatic spinal cord compression: One-year results of a prospective trial. *Int J Radiat Oncol Biol Phys* 2000; 48: 1403–1408.

85 Rades D, Heidenreich F, Karstens JH. Final results of a prospective study of the prognostic value of the time to develop motor deficits before irradiation in metastatic spinal cord compression. *Int J Radiat Oncol Biol Phys* 2002; 53: 975–979.

86 Turner S, Marosszeky B, Timms I, Boyages J. Malignant spinal cord compression: A prospective evaluation. *Int J Radiat Oncol Biol Phys* 1993; 26: 141–146.

87 Helweg-Larsen S, Soelberg Sorensen P, Kreiner S. Prognostic factors in metastatic spinal cord compression: A prospective study using multivariate analysis of variables influencing survival and gait function in 153 patients. *Int J Radiat Oncol Biol Phys* 2000; 46: 1163–1169.

88 Guo Y, Young B, Palmer JL et al. Prognostic factors for survival in metastatic spinal cord compression: A retrospective study in a rehabilitation setting. *Am J Phys Med Rehab* 2003; 82: 665–668.

89 Rades D, Huttenlocher S, Dunst J, Bajrovic A, Karstens JH, Rudat V, Schild SE. Matched pair analysis comparing surgery followed by radiotherapy and radiotherapy alone for metastatic spinal cord compression. *J Clin Oncol* 2010; 28: 3597–3604.

90 Chow E, Coia L, Wu J et al. This house believes that multiple-fraction radiotherapy is a barrier to referral for palliative radiotherapy for bone metastases. *Curr Oncol* 2002; 9: 60–66.

91 Guckenberger M, Goebel J, Wilbert J, Baier K, Richter A, Sweeney RA, Bratengeier K, Flentje M. Clinical outcome of dose-escalated image-guided radiotherapy for spinal metastases. *Int J Radiat Oncol Biol Phys* 2009; 75: 828–835.

92 Milker-Zabel S, Zabel A, Thilmann C et al. Clinical results of retreatment of vertebral bone metastases by stereotactic conformal radiotherapy and intensity-modulated radiotherapy. *Int J Radiat Oncol Biol Phys* 2003; 55: 162–167.

93 Grosu AL, Andratschke N, Nieder C, Molls M. Retreatment of the spinal cord with palliative radiotherapy. *Int J Radiat Oncol Biol Phys* 2002; 52: 1288–1292.

94 Maranzano E, Trippa F, Casale M et al. 8 Gy single-dose radiotherapy is effective in metastatic spinal cord compression: Results of a phase III randomized multicenter Italian trial. 2009; 93: 174–179.

95 Rades D, Stalpers L, Veninga T et al. Evaluation of five radiation schedules and prognostic factors for metastatic spinal cord compression. *J Clin Oncol* 2005; 23: 3366–3375.

96 Chow E, Lutz S, Beyene J. A single fraction for all, or an argument for fractionation tailored to fit the needs of each individual patient with bone metastases? *Int J Radiat Oncol Biol Phys* 2003; 55: 565–567.

97 Haddad P, Wong R, Wilson P et al. Factors influencing the use of single versus multiple fractions of palliative radiotherapy for bone metastases: A 5-yr review and comparison to a survey. *Int J Radiat Oncol Biol Phys* 2003; 57 (Suppl.): S278.

98 Boogerd W, van der Sande JJ. Diagnosis and treatment of spinal cord compression in malignant disease. *Cancer Treat Rev* 1993; 19: 129–150.

99 Byrne TN. Spinal cord compression from epidural metastases. *N Engl J Med* 1992; 327: 614–619.

100 Grant R, Papadopoulos SM, Greenberg HS. Metastatic epidural spinal cord compression. *Neurol Clin* 1991; 9: 825–841.

101 Maranzano E, Latini P, Checcaglini F et al. Radiation therapy in meta-static spinal cord compression—A prospective analysis of 105 consecutive patients. *Cancer* 1991; 67: 1311–1317.

102 Janjan NA. Radiotherapeutic management of spinal metastases. *J Pain Symptom Manage* 1996; 1: 47–56.

103 Loblaw DA, Laperriere NJ. Emergency treatment of malignant extradural spinal cord compression: An evidence-based guideline. *J Clin Oncol* 1998; 16: 1613–1624.

104 Boogerd W. Central nervous system metastasis in breast cancer. *Radiother Oncol* 1996; 40: 5–22.

105 Hoskin PJ, Grover A, Bhana R. Metastatic spinal cord compression: Radiotherapy outcome and dose fractionation. *Radiother Oncol* 2003; 68: 175–180.

106 Bates T, Yarnold JR, Blitzer P et al. Bone metastases consensus statement. *Int J Radiat Oncol Biol Phys* 1992; 23: 215–216.

107 Bates T. A review of local radiotherapy in the treatment of bone metastases and cord compression. *Int J Radiat Oncol Biol Phys* 1992; 23: 217–221.

108 Tow B, Seang BT, Chong TT, Chen J. Predictors for survival in metastases to the spine. *Spine* 2005; 5: 73S.

109 Wada E, Yamamoto T, Furuno M et al. Spinal cord compression secondary to osteoblastic metastasis. *Spine* 1993; 18: 1380–1381.

110 Kim RY, Smith JW, Spencer SA et al. Malignant epidural spinal cord compression associated with a paravertebral mass: Its radiotherapeutic outcome on radiosensitivity. *Int J Radiat Oncol Biol Phys* 1993; 27: 1079–1083.

111 Russi EG, Pergolizzi S, Gaeta M et al. Palliative radiotherapy in lumbosacral carcinomatous neuropathy. *Radiother Oncol* 1993; 26: 172–173.

112 Saarto T, Janes R, Tenhunen M, Kouri M. Palliative radiotherapy in the treatment of skeletal metastases. *Eur J Pain* 2002; 6: 323–330.

113 Loblaw DA, Laperriere NJ, Mackillop WJ. A population-based study of malignant spinal cord compression in Ontario. *Clin Oncol* 2003; 15: 211–217.

114 Altehoefer C, Ghanem N, Hogerle S et al. Comparative detectability of bone metastases and impact on therapy of magnetic resonance imaging and bone scintigraphy in patients with breast cancer. *Eur J Radiol* 2001; 40: 16–23.

115 Maranzano E, Latini P, Beneventi S et al. Radiotherapy without steroids in selected metastatic spinal cord compression patients. A phase II trial. *Am J Clin Oncol* 1996; 19: 179–183.

116 Quinn JA, De Angelis LM. Neurologic emergencies in the cancer patient. *Semin Oncol* 2000; 27: 311–321.

117 Hatrick NC, Lucas JD, Timothy AR, Smith MA. The surgical treatment of metastatic disease of the spine. *Radiother Oncol* 2000; 56: 335–339.

118 Landmann C, Hunig R, Gratzi O. The role of laminectomy in the combined treatment of metastatic spinal cord compression. *Int J Radiat Oncol Biol Phys* 1992; 24: 627–631.

119 Fourney DR, Frangou EM, Ryken TC et al. Spinal instability neoplastic score: An analysis of reliability and validity from the Spine Oncology Study Group. *J Clin Oncol* 2011; 29: 3072–3077.

85

Clinical features and management of superior vena cava syndrome

ÁLVARO SANZ, CARLOS CENTENO

INTRODUCTION

Superior vena cava syndrome (SVCS) results from the impairment of blood flow through the superior vena cava into the right atrium. Traditionally, SVCS has been explained as a medical emergency. However, the majority of cases are due to a subacute progression of the disease and the number of patients who die exclusively from SVCS is low. This translates into a clinical approach that insists on the need of anatomopathologic diagnosis before any specific treatment is started.

ETIOLOGY

The spectrum of underlying conditions associated with SVCS has shifted from a majority of cases caused by infectious diseases about 50 years ago to a preponderance of malignant disorders. Nowadays, one of every three new SVCS cases is due to thrombosis or nonmalignant conditions. It can be explained because of the increased use of intravascular devices as intracava catheters.[1] The most common malignant cause of SVCS is non–small cell lung cancer (NSCLC), followed by small cell lung carcinoma (SCLC) (Table 85.1). Other malignant causes are lymphoma (the most common cause of SVCS in patients less than 50 years old), germ cell tumors, thymoma,[2] and other tumors with direct mediastinal progression (as mesothelioma or esophageal cancer) or those from any other origin that develop metastatic mediastinal lymph nodes and even tumor thrombi.[3]

SVCS results from the compression of the superior vena cava by the tumor arising in the mediastinum or in the right main or upper lobe bronchus or by large-volume mediastinal nodes (most commonly from the right paratracheal or precarinal lymph nodes). The superior vena cava carries blood to the heart from the head, arms, and upper torso. It is formed by the junction of the left and right brachiocephalic veins in the mid-third of the mediastinum and extends caudally for 6–8 cm, coursing anterior to the right main-stem bronchus and insert into right atrium. It is joined posteriorly by the azygos vein as it loops over the right main-stem bronchus. It is a thin-walled vessel and the blood flows with relatively low intravascular pressure in it (2–8 mmHg). Thus, when the superior vena cava is compressed, it leads to an increase in the pressure (to 20–40 mmHg) and it slows or even interrupts local flow. In this case, blood flows through a collateral vascular network to the inferior vena cava or the azygos system. This collateral flow dilates with the time and may accommodate to the flow of the superior vena cava after a few weeks.

The severity of the syndrome depends on the rapidity of onset, the severity of the obstruction, and its location.[4] The more rapid the onset, the more severe the symptoms, because the collateral veins do not have time to distend to accommodate the increased blood flow. If the obstruction is below the entry of the azygos vein, the syndrome is less pronounced, because the azygos system can readily distend to accommodate the shunted blood, allowing a reduction of the venous pressure in the head, arms, and upper torso. If the obstruction is above the entry of the azygos vein, more florid and severe symptoms and signs are seen, because the blood pressure increases in order to return to the heart via the upper abdominal veins and the inferior vena cava.

CLINICAL MANIFESTATIONS

A syndrome is a morbid process characterized by the concurrence of symptoms and signs that are coincident and causally related. SVCS includes both sign and symptoms that have the same origin. The most frequent signs and symptoms that prompt suspicion include swelling of the face, neck, upper trunk and extremities, cyanosis, coughing, venous ingurgitation, hoarseness, and dyspnea (Table 85.2).[5] Most of the symptoms are not SVCS specific. Severe symptoms include neurologic and visual disturbances,[6] dyspnea due to airflow obstruction, or even hemodynamic compromise. Dyspnea, cough, headache, etc., may be caused directly by the tumor that occludes the superior vena cava.

Table 85.1   *Malignant causes of SVCS*

Non–small cell lung cancer	50%
Small cell lung cancer	25%
Lymphoma	10%
Metastatic tumor	<10%
Germ cell tumor	<5%
Thymoma	<5%
Other tumors	<5%

Table 85.2   *Signs and symptoms and in SVCS*

Signs and symptoms of mild or moderate SVCS	
Swelling of the face and neck	80%
Distended neck veins	60%
Distended chest veins	55%
Swelling of the extremities	50%
Dyspnea	50%
Cough	50%
Signs and symptoms of severe SVCS	
Hoarseness/stridor	<5%
Syncope	10%
Headache	10%
Dizziness	<10%
Visual symptoms	<5%
Confusion	<5%

DIAGNOSIS

The first suspicion of SVCS usually came from the patient himself/herself or from proxies who refer a change in personal appearance with swelling and sometimes erythema or cyanosis of face and neck. In severe cases, not only external appearance can be affected as the patient may suffer respiratory and neurologic symptoms and signs as well. After the recognition of symptoms and signs, the initial evaluation should include radiologic studies looking for mediastinal masses and/or thrombosis of the superior vena cava. Computed tomography is very useful to define the presence of masses, the patency of veins, the presence of thrombi, and the anatomy of involved mediastinal nodes.[7,8] It might also assist in radiotherapy planning or act as a baseline for assessment of response to treatment.

First studies orient the diagnosis in a majority of cases to vascular device-induced vein thrombosis or to vein-compression due to local tumor progression. When there is radiological evidence of tumor in the mediastinum, a histological diagnosis should be obtained prior to initiating therapy. Most SVCSs are due to cancer, and treatment will depend on tumor histology.[9] The biopsy specimen of tumor should be taken from the most accessible site. The protocol for biopsy is based on the location of the tumor, the performance status of the patient, and the clinical expertise. It may include bronchoscopy, biopsy of superficial lymph nodes, or needle biopsy of a lung mass or mediastinal nodes using either CT or ultrasound guidance. In a number of patients, more aggressive measures such as mediastinoscopy, mediastinotomy, video-assisted thoracoscopy, or conventional thoracotomy may be required. Complications of such procedures do not seem to be increased because of the presence of SVCS.[10]

Although prompt clinical attention is important, SVCS is rarely a clinical emergency as it usually develops as a subacute process with no sudden progressive development of clinical manifestations, giving time to histological diagnosis.[11] In fact, up to 75% of patients present symptoms and signs for over a week before seeking medical attention.[12] In addition, SVCS is rarely lethal by itself; cancer patients with SVCS (even more, those patients with advanced and refractory tumors) do not die because of this syndrome itself but from the extent of underlying disease. Only in exceptional cases, if tracheal obstruction or cerebral edema are present, SVCS could be considered as an oncological emergency requiring immediate therapy. In the rest, treatment prior to definitive diagnosis does not seem to be justified (Figure 85.1).[13]

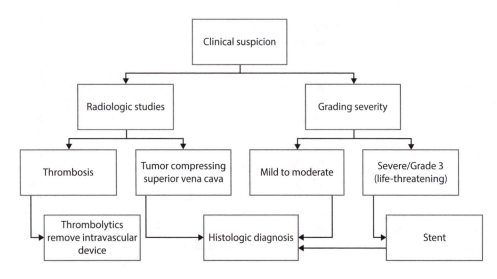

Figure 85.1   *Initial approach to patients with newly diagnosis of SVCS.*

Table 85.3 *Grading system for SVCS*

Grade	Severity	Manifestations
Grade 0	Asymptomatic	Radiographic superior vena cava compromise without signs of symptoms derived
Grade 1	Mild	Edema and/or venous ingurgitation of head and neck, cyanosis
Grade 2	Moderate	Facial edema with a mild compromise of other organs: head and neck movements, dysphagia, dizziness, dyspnea partially related to SVCS
Grade 3	Severe	Cerebral edema with confusion or severe headache, dyspnea or stridor related to laryngeal edema, hemodynamic compromise

Source: Modified from Yu, J.B. et al., *J. Thorac. Oncol.*, 3, 811, 2008.

Recent publications suggest a scoring system to define the severity of SVCS and to design the treatment according to it. It is based on the fact that sign and symptoms that are most frequent (appearing in at least 20% of patients) are usually associated with nonsevere SVCS (Table 85.3). However, it has not been validated prospectively so far.[14]

TREATMENT

A minority of cases, that however nowadays represent an increasing proportion of episodes of SVCS, are induced by the presence of thrombi and implantable venous access system as those used in cancer patients to infuse treatments or pacemakers. In these cases, treatment is directed to solve the thrombus. In many cases, antithrombotic drugs are not efficacious enough and the patient requires that the device be removed.[15]

The treatment of malignant SVCS depends on the cause of the obstruction, the severity of the symptoms, the prognosis of the patient, the availability and expertise in the application of treatments, and the patient's preferences (Figure 85.2).[16] In most patients, the best palliation, measured as symptom control and quality of life and prolonged survival, is achieved by treatment specifically directed against the tumor. Unless airway

obstruction or cerebral edema is present, it appears that the delay of both radiotherapy and chemotherapy until the histological diagnosis does not impair the response of SVCS.

Response to therapy can be assessed both clinically and radiologically. Usually, signs and symptoms that appear initially are those that improve more slowly. Anyway, the evolution of symptoms and signs is not always parallel to the resolution of the obstruction of superior vena cava.[17] Some patients may present clinical improvement of SVCS even when vein patency is not equally improved. Problems derived from vein blood pressure as neck vein ingurgitation or even headache may disappear almost immediately when vein flow is restarted. Facial, cervical, and brachial blood flow may need hours or even days to improve. In patients with persistent flow stop, collateral vessels are present that dilate with time.[18] Signs due to this collateral flow, as varicose veins in torso may remain indefinitely even when SVCS is resolved.

Medical management

Some patients with sufficient collateral blood flow and minimal symptoms may be initially managed by postural maneuvers to increase vein flow pressure and appropriate prevention of further complications such as thrombosis. When the patient develops sufficient collateral circulation, the symptoms and signs may stabilize or improve.

Clinically relevant SVCS can develop in more than 10% of patients with right-sided malignant intrathoracic tumors. In these patients, the treatment directed toward relieving SVCS is commenced at the same time as chemotherapy and/or radiotherapy. In patients with SVCS relapse after the initial antitumor treatment, second-line therapy is hardly successful. In those patients and in patients with poor performance status or who do not want aggressive treatment, palliation of signs and symptoms of SVCS gains relevance as the tumor becomes resistant to treatment.

Palliation of SVCS may be achieved by medical interventions such as postural advice, since a raised head may help blood to flow better through the superior vena cava and collaterals to the heart, and drugs. Steroids (prednisolone or dexamethasone) are frequently used to alleviate respiratory

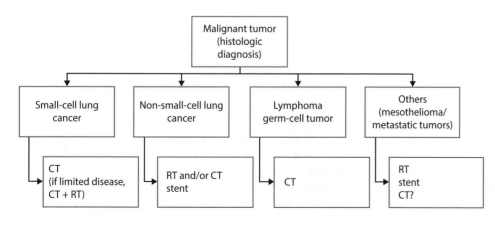

Figure 85.2 *Treatment of malignant SVCS according to histologic diagnosis. (CT: chemotherapy; RT: radiotherapy.)*

compromise[19] and may be useful to prevent radiation-induced inflammatory edema, but there are no definitive data to support their use.[20] Diuretics have been used in the treatment of SCVS but there is no evidence enough to recommend its use and may ultimately lead to complications such as dehydration. Oxygen may palliate dyspnea in some cancer patients with hypoxemia.[21] Low-molecular-weight heparins do not help to palliate those cases of SVCS that are not due to thrombosis, but they may prevent further thrombosis in a cancer patient with slow flow in the vena cava.

Chemotherapy

Chemotherapy is the anticancer treatment of choice in SVCS caused by SCLC, lymphoma, and germ cell tumors. In these cases, SVCS does not appear to be an independent prognostic factor, and its presence should not be used to change the treatment approach. The response rates to chemotherapy in sensitive tumors approach 80%.[22,23] In tumors that are less chemosensitive, such as NSCLC, chemotherapy can relieve SVCS in 60% of the patients.[24,25] Both in SCLC and NSCLC, the proportion of recurrences of SVCS after response to chemotherapy is 20%.

Radiation therapy

When the obstruction of the superior vena cava is caused by a tumor that is or has become refractory to chemotherapy, radiation therapy remains highly effective as a symptomatic treatment.[26,27] Overall, SVCS patients respond to radiotherapy in 60% of NSCLC and 80% of SCLC cases. There are conflicting retrospective data on the benefit of hypofractionating. The scheme will depend on histology, previous therapy, extent of disease, prognosis, and performance status.[28,29] Many fractionation schemes have been used,[30,31] with total doses ranging from 20 Gy in 5 fractions to 50 Gy in 25 fractions. In previously treated patients with short life expectancy and poor performance status, a short-term schedule would be recommended with a total dose of 20–30 Gy or a single-fraction (6–8 Gy).

In lung cancer, there appears to be no distinction between radiotherapy and chemotherapy with regard to the speed of palliation. A proportion of patients receive initially both therapies, because the standard of treatment for newly diagnosed limited-stage SCLC or locally advanced NSCLC (stage III) combines both chemotherapy and local radiotherapy. Median time to response ranges from few days to several weeks.

Stent placement

There is a rapid increase in the use of intravascular expandable stent to treat the occluded superior vena cava.[32–34] This procedure allows immediate restoration of the normal flow with rapid resolution of symptoms.[35,36] Thrombolytic agents such as streptokinase or urokinase can be administered prior to stent insertion.[37] Morbidity following stent insertion is greater if thrombolytics agents are administered, and the relapse rate does not seem to increase when those drugs are not used. In the

same way, there is no agreement on the need for the indication or the duration of anticoagulant or anti-aggregant therapy after stent placement to minimize the probability of re-occlusion. Response rates with intraluminal stenting reaches 95%, with phlebographic resolution in the majority of patients.[38–40] The proportion that relapses following stent placement approaches 10%, frequently due to thrombus within the stent. The use of angioplasty to palliate SVCS is not recommended because of the high probability of relapse.

There is no agreement about the optimal timing of stenting.[41] It is not recommended as a first choice for a majority of patients because of the associated morbidity (5%–10% of patients with complications as thrombus, infections, stent migration, and even vein rupture), and because we can expect some improvement in the SVCS when anticancer therapy is started. For the patients with tumors resistant to treatment as mesothelioma and in the few cases with severe and rapidly progressive SVCS, stent is the most suitable option to solve SVCS. In patients with tumor progression after treatments and with symptoms and signs that are clearly due to SVCS, intraluminal stenting is the recommended option.

Surgery

There are just a few reports on palliative surgery for malignant SVCS. Surgical bypass is more appropriate for patients with a benign obstruction, although it has also been used for some selected patients with malignant obstructions.[42] The indications are limited by the prognosis of patients and the severe complications of the procedure.

Clinical management

In patients with good performance status, several variables have to be considered to select the best treatment. In very sensitive tumors where systemic therapy improves survival and may even result in cure (lymphoma, germ cell tumor, and even limited disease SCLC), conventional systemic and local therapy produces a quick response and improves survival. In these cancers, radiotherapy can be included as part of the protocol to improve local control. In patients with potentially sensitive disease but with poor performance status and/or when cure is not possible chemotherapy, as in extensive-stage SCLC, chemotherapy remains a good palliative resource.[43]

In other tumors where the benefit of chemotherapy is not so impressive, systemic chemotherapy with or without radiotherapy may produce relevant palliation of symptoms in some cases, as in NSCLC. For patients with SVCS due to tumor resistant to chemotherapy, palliative radiotherapy is a good option even in advanced cancer patients with limited prognosis. Stent insertion is a more aggressive approach than single-fraction palliative radiotherapy and is not recommended for patients with very poor survival expectancy. There are no data supporting a particular schedule or timing for the combination of different treatments, in particular, local approaches such as radiotherapy and stents.

Key learning points

- The great majority of cases of SVCS are due to cancer. The second cause is intravascular devices. In the absence of histologic diagnosis, it is advisable that this should be established prior to initiating therapy.

- Most cases of SVCSs tend to improve spontaneously with time as superior vena cava blood flows throughout collateral veins. Emergency treatment is required only in rare cases with cerebral edema or tracheal obstruction.

- SVCS by itself does not modify the prognosis of cancer.

- Anticancer therapies (chemotherapy and/or radiotherapy) are the corner stone of initial treatment of a majority of cancer-induced SVCS.

- Stent insertion provides rapid relief in patients with severe life-threatening SVCS and in those who are or become refractory to anticancer therapy.

REFERENCES

1 Wilson LD, Detterbeck FC, Yahalom J. Superior vena cava syndrome with malignant causes. *N Engl J Med* 2007; **356**: 1862–1869.

2 Pinto Marín A, González Barón M. Superior vena cava syndrome. *Med Clin (Barc)* 2009; **132**: 195–199.

3 Batra S, Doval DC, Batra U et al. Gallbladder cancer with tumor thrombus in the superior vena cava. *Hepatobiliary Pancreat Dis Int* 2010; **9**: 325–328.

4 Yellin A, Rosen A, Reichert N et al. Superior vena cava syndrome. The myth—The facts. *Am Rev Respir Dis* 1990; **141**: 1114–1118.

5 Landis BN, Bohanes P, Kohler R. Superior vena cava syndrome. *CMAJ* 2009; **180**: 355.

6 Barquero-Romero J, López CupidoV, Torrado Sierra O, Valencia Terrón M. Severe ocular symptoms as an initial manifestation of superior vena cava síndrome. *An Med Interna (Madrid)* 2008; **25**: 356–358.

7 Betchtold RE, Wolfman NT, Karstaedt N, Choplin RH. Superior vena caval obstruction: Detection using CT. *Radiology* 1985; **157**: 485–487.

8 Sheth S, Ebert MD, Fishman EK. Superior vena cava obstruction evaluation with MDCT. *AJR* 2010; **194**: 336–346.

9 Bagheri S, Rahim M, Rezaeetalab F et al. Malignant superior vena cava syndrome: Is this a medical emergency? *Ann Thorac Cardiovasc Surg* 2009; **15**: 89–92.

10 Porte H, Metois D, Finzi L et al. Superior vena cava syndrome of malignant origin. Which surgical procedure for which diagnosis? *Eur J Cardiothorac Surg* 2000; 17: 384–388.

11 Gauden SJ. Superior vena cava syndrome induced by bronchogenic carcinoma: Is this an oncologic emergency? *Austral Radiol* 1993; **37**: 363–366.

12 Schraufnagel DE, Hill R, Leech JA, Pare JA. Superior vena caval obstruction. Is it a medical emergency? *Am J Med* 1981; **70**: 1169–1174.

13 Kvale PA, Selecky PA, Prakash UB. Palliative care in lung cancer. ACCP evidence-based clinical practice guidelines (2nd Edition). *Chest* 2007; **132**: 368S–403S.

14 Yu JB, Wilson LD, Detterbeck FC. Superior vena cava syndrome—A proposed classification system and algorithm for management. *J Thorac Oncol* 2008; **3**: 811–814.

15 Stockton PA, Ledson MJ, Walshaw MJ. Persistent superior vena cava syndrome due to totally implantable venous access systems. *J R Soc Med* 2001; **94**: 584–585.

16 Chen JC, Bongard F, Klein SR. A contemporary perspective on superior vena cava syndrome. *Am J Surg* 1990; **160**: 207–211.

17 Ahmann FR. A reassessment of the clinical implications of the superior vena caval syndrome. *J Clin Oncol* 1984; **2**: 961–969.

18 Baker GL, Barnes HJ. Superior vena cava syndrome: Etiology, diagnosis, and treatment. *Am J Crit Care* 1992, 1: 54–64.

19 Rowell NP, Gleeson FV. Steroids, radiotherapy, chemotherapy and stents for superior vena caval obstruction in carcinoma of the bronchus. *Cochrane Database Syst Rev* 2001, Issue 4. Art. No.: CD001316. doi: 10.1002/14651858.CD001316.

20 Ostler PJ, Clarke DP, Watkinson AF, Gaze MN. Superior vena cava obstruction: A modern management strategy. *Clin Oncol (R Coll Radiol)* 1997; **9**: 83–89.

21 Thomas JR, von Gunten CF. Clinical management of dyspnoea. *Lancet Oncol* 2002; **3**: 223–228.

22 Urban T, Lebeau B, Chastang C et al. Superior vena cava syndrome in small cell lung cancer. *Arch Intern Med* 1993; **153**: 384–387.

23 Würschmidt F, Bünemann H, Heilman HP. Small cell lung cancer with and without superior vena cava syndrome: A multivariate analysis of prognostic factors in 408 cases. *Int J Radiat Oncol Biol Phys* 1995; **33**: 77–82.

24 Tanigawa N, Sawada S, Mishima K et al. Clinical outcome of stenting in superior vena cava syndrome associated with malignant tumors. Comparison with conventional treatment. *Acta Radiol* 1998; **39**: 669–674.

25 Pereira JR, Martins SJ, Ikari FK et al. Neoadjuvant chemotherapy versus radiotherapy alone for superior vena cava syndrome (SCVS) due to non small cell lung cancer (NSCLC): Preliminary results of randomized phase II trial. *Eur J Cancer* 1999; **35** (Suppl. 4): 260.

26 Davenport D, Ferree C, Blake D, Raven M. Response of superior vena cava syndrome to radiation therapy. *Cancer* 1976; **38**: 1577–1580.

27 Rodríguez CI, Njo KH, Karim AB. Hypofractionated radiation therapy in the treatment of superior vena cava syndrome. *Lung Cancer* 1993; **10**: 221–228.

28 Levitt SH, Jones TK, Bogardus CR. Treatment of malignant superior vena caval obstruction. A randomized study. *Cancer* 1969; **24**: 447–451.

29 Fisherman WH, Bradfield JS. Superior vena caval syndrome: Response with initial high daily dose irradiation. *South Med J* 1973; **66**: 677–680.

30 Chan RH, Dar AR, Yu E et al. Superior vena cava obstruction in small-cell lung cancer. *Int J Radiat Oncol Biol Phys* 1997; **38**: 384–387.

31 Amstrong BA, Perez CA, Simpson JR, Hederman MA. Role of irradiation in the management of superior vena cava syndrome. *Int J Radiat Oncol Biol Phys* 1987; **13**: 531–539.

32 Lanciego C, Pangua C, Chacón JI et al. Endovascular stenting as the first step in the overall management of malignant superior vena cava syndrome. *AJR* 2009; **193**: 549–558.

33 Hague J, Tippett R. Endovascular techniques in Palliative Care. *Clin Oncol (R Coll Radiol)* 2010; **22**: 771–780.

34 Urruticoechea A, Mesia R, Domínguez J et al. Treatment of malignant superior vena cava syndrome by endovascular stent insertion. Experience on 52 patients with lung cancer. *Lung Cancer* 2004; **43**: 209–214.

35 Nicholson AA, Teles DF, Arnold A et al. Treatment of malignant superior vena cava obstruction: Metal stents or radiation therapy. *J Vasc Intervent Radiol* 1997; **8**: 781–788.

◆ 36   Wilson E, Lynn A, Khan S. Radiological stenting provides effective palliation in malignant central venous obstruction. *Clin Oncol (R Coll Radiol)* 2000; **12**: 331.

● 37   Kee ST, Kinoshita L, Razavi MK et al. Superior vena cava syndrome: Treatment with catheter directed thrombolysis and endovascular stent placement. *Radiology* 1998; **206**: 187–193.

◆ 38   Watkinson AF, Yeow TN, Fraser C. Endovascular stenting to treat obstruction of the superior vena cava. *BMJ* 2008; **336**: 1434–1437.

● 39   Lanciego C, Pangua C, Chacón JI et al. Endovascular stenting as the first step in the overall management of malignant superior vena cava syndrome. *AJR* 2009; **193**: 549–558.

◆ 40   Hague J, Tippett R. Endovascular techniques in Palliative Care. *Clin Oncol (R Coll Radiol)* 2010; **22**: 771–780.

◆ 41   Nicholson AA, Teles DF, Arnold A et al. Treatment of malignant superior vena cava obstruction: Metal stents or radiation therapy. *J Vasc Intervent Radiol* 1997; **8**: 781–788.

● 42   Spaggiari L, Magdeleinat P, Kondoc H et al. Results of superior vena cava resection for lung cancer. Analysis of prognostic factors. *Lung Cancer* 2004; **44**: 339–346.

◆ 43   Bowcock SJ, Shee CD, Rassam SM, Harper PG. Chemotherapy for cancer patients who present late. *BMJ* 2004; **328**: 1430–1432.

86

Acute pain and management*

MELLAR P. DAVIS, PAM GAMIER

INTRODUCTION

Acute pain is a normal reaction to noxious stimuli that alerts individuals to tissue damage and protects them from further tissue damage. Individual pain experiences are controlled by several genetically determined factors, neuroplasticity, and long-term potentiation caused by afferent traffic, which modulates the function of sensory system, psychologic state, and the attributable meaning to the pain. An extreme example of genetically programmed pain involves absence of pain inherited in a mutation of certain sodium channels [1,2]. Loss of pain sensitivity leads to progressive self-inflicted tissue damage while a gain of pain sensitivity limits activity and reduces quality of life.

Acute pain has several presentations: Primary and secondary hypersensitivity, allodynia (pain experienced with non-noxious stimuli), and hyperalgesia (increased pain severity or duration with noxious stimuli), which promotes guarding the affected part, which shields damaged tissues from further injury [3]. The area of secondary hypersensitivity extends beyond the damaged area due to central nervous system (CNS) facilitation through rostral ventromedial medulla to spinal cord nociception input. Acute visceral pain if severe will refer pain to somatic sites, due to convergence of afferent input within the same dorsal horn segment [4].

ACUTE VERSUS CHRONIC PAIN

Acute pain causes a sympathetic response "fight or flight" reaction, whereas chronic pain is associated with very little sweating, tachycardia, and tachypnea and can cause mental dullness and lethargy [5]. Chronic pain is a maladaptive state caused by neuroplastic peripheral and CNS changes, which does not resolve despite resolution of tissue injury. Uncontrolled acute pain will evolve into chronic pain, and hence, severe acute pain is a medical emergency [6–9]. Chronic cancer pain has been classified into various well-recognized syndromes based on location, severity, palliative and exacerbating factors, and referral pattern [3,4,10]. Acute pain is not well classified into syndromes.

ACUTE PAIN SYNDROMES

Acute pain syndromes are variably classified. These syndromes may be the direct result of the cancer, its treatment, complications, or underlying comorbidities. A partial list is provided in Table 86.1.

CELLULAR AND MOLECULAR MECHANISMS OF ACUTE PAIN

Peripheral signals

Transient receptor potential vanilloid (TRPV-1) receptors on unmyelinated C-fibers and poorly myelinated type A-delta fibers are transducers of noxious heat stimuli and activated by capsaicin and temperatures greater than 43°C [3,6]. These channels expressed on unmyelinated neurons with mu receptors are upregulated in neuropathic and bone pain, while mu receptors are downregulated in neuropathic pain. Secondary vanilloid receptors (TRPV-2, 3) are activated by heat intensities at which TRPV-1 are silent (greater than 50°C) and may contribute to pain. These channels are upregulated by inflammatory cytokines and proalgesic mediators (protons, neurotropins, and bradykinins) and hence important mediators of acute inflammatory pain. Sodium and calcium channels, in addition to TRPV channels, are also upregulated by neuropathic damage [11]. TRPM-8 channels are cold-sensitive channels responsive to methanol. These channels are modulated by other channels including voltage-gated sodium and potassium channels and also may contribute to the experience of acute pain [3].

---

* A World Health Organization Demonstration Project in Palliative Medicine.

Table 86.1 *Acute pain syndromes*

Bone metastases

- Joint destruction by tumor
- Pathologic fracture of long bone, vertebral body, pelvis

Visceral cancer

- Bowel obstruction
- Bowel perforation with peritonitis
- Sacral, hypogastric, lumbar, or celiac plexus invasion
- Budd–Chiari syndrome from tumor invasion into hepatic veins
- Mesenteric venous thrombosis
- Hepatic capsular invasion
- Peritoneal carcinomatosis
- Splenic infarct or rupture
- Biliary or renal colic

Thoracic cancer

- Pulmonary artery invasion with infarct
- Bronchopleural fistula from cancer
- Esophageal rupture or fistula to bronchus or tracheal
- Brachial neuropathy
- Cardiac tamponade
- Pleural effusion, implants, and chest wall invasion

Soft tissue and bone cancer or metastases

- Muscle tumor or metastases
- Subcutaneous metastases
- Neurogenic sarcomas or nerve root invasion
- Angiosarcoma or metastatic compression or blood vessels
- Cutaneous metastases, melanoma
- Vertebral and long bone metastases, fracture or collapse

Central or peripheral nervous system

- Brain metastases
- Leptomeningeal metastases
- Intradural or spinal cord metastases

Procedural pain or treatment related pain

- Postoperative pain
- Kyphoplasty
- Radiation induced mucositis, esophagitis, arachnoiditis, enteritis, cystitis, proctitis, skin desquamation
- Chemotherapy endophebitis, extravasations, neuropathy
- Corticosteroid withdrawal arthralgias
- Gonadotropin hormone-related tumor flare
- Hepatic artery embolization
- Portal vein embolization prior to partial hepatectomy
- Embolization of renal bone or soft tissue metastases
- Thoracentesis and chemical pleurodesis
- Pericardiocentesis
- Paracentesis
- Lumbar puncture headache
- Bone marrow biopsy
- Venipuncture
- Wound dressing changes
- Stent placement (gastrointestinal, genitourinary)
- Nephrostomy tube placement
- Transhepatic biliary drainage

(Continued)

Table 86.1 (Continued) *Acute pain syndromes*

Cancer complications

- Pulmonary embolism
- Pneumonia with pleurisy
- Ascending cholangitis
- Venous thrombosis (superficial and deep)
- Decubitus ulcer
- Oral candidiasis, esophagitis, cystitis
- Shingles
- Clostridium enterocolitis
- Pyelonephritis
- Superior vena cava syndrome
- Malignant otitis media
- Typhlitis

Because so many channels and receptors are involved in mediating acute pain, it is unlikely that single analgesic targets will significantly relieve acute pain in all patients [12,13].

Mechanical transducers of pain include acid sense ion channels (ASICs), TRPV-2 and TRPV-4 channels. The ASIC channels are found on unmyelinated fibers in bone marrow and trabecular bone and are in part responsible for bone pain, which frequently has an acid environment due to the accumulation of protons and lactate. Certain potassium channels (KCNK) interact with an ingredient in Szechuan peppercorns. These receptors are found in abundance on C-fibers and A-delta fibers and play a role in acute pain [3].

Another transient receptor potential channel subunit family, TRPA channels, are chemoreceptors that respond to acrolein, teargas, automobile exhaust, and burning vegetation and are known to elicit acute pain [3].

N- and T-type calcium channels on C-fibers are upregulated by pathologic processes such as diabetes neuropathy. Gabapentin targets subunits of the calcium channel (alpha 2-delta-1) and reduces membrane expression of calcium channels and hence reduces neuropathic and bone pain [14,15]. Gabapentin blocks neuroplasticity, synaptogenesis and increases spinal noradrenaline levels, suggesting that the early use of gabapentin is better than starting gabapentin when pain is well established [3,16]. Ziconotide, also an N-type calcium channel blocker, relieves cancer pain when given intrathecally.

Inflammatory signaling molecules (substance P., calcitonin gene related protein, bradykinin, protons, inflammatory cytokines, prostaglandins, and proteases) sensitize certain channels, namely, TRPV1, TRPA1, TRPV-2, TRPV-4, and ASIC, reducing neuron membrane potentials to depolarization [11].

Central mechanisms to acute pain

Central sensitization, initiated by peripheral nociceptor and resulting in spinal-bulbar-spinal facilitated neurotransmission, enhances primary afferent neuron responsiveness through this downward facilitation. The rostral ventromedial medulla area is important to this process. This hypersensitivity can outlast acute injury and continue independent of peripheral nerve input, resulting in maladaptive pain. Low levels of stimulus (usually nonnoxious) maintain neuropathic pain as TPRV-1 channels are upregulated and mu receptors downregulated [4,11]. Long-term potentiation leads to "wind-up" as N-methyl-D-aspartate (NMDA) receptors on wide dynamic range (WDR) neurons in the deeper lamina (V) of the dorsal horn are activated, producing an expanded receptive field and secondary hyperalgesia. The clinical effect of wind-up is not only secondary hyperalgesia but allodynia within the injured [4]. NMDA receptors increase intracellular calcium that in turn activates kinases (protein kinase C and calmodulin-dependent kinase II) to facilitate pain through phosphorylation of ion channels and opioid receptors. A distinct change in somatosensory processing through long-term potentiation and increased membrane excitability can also arise from loss of inhibitory GABA and glycinergic interneurons located in lamina II [17]. Neuroplasticity involving in synapses and dendrites will cause hypersensitization. Activation and proliferation of spinal cord microglia occurs in neuropathic injury and metastatic bone disease [18,19]. Activation occurs over minutes to hours with acute pain [11,17,20–22]. As a result, there are no single defining molecular mechanisms for central sensitization.

The development of central sensitization has important implications. Certain short-acting opioids increase secondary hyperalgesia with acute injury while reducing pain arising from the primary site [23–31]. Certain adjuvant analgesics (lidocaine, clonidine, ketamine, paracoxib, and acetaminophen) reduce secondary hyperalgesia associated with acute pain or caused by short-acting opioids. Buprenorphine uniquely blocks secondary hyperalgesia in contrast to fentanyl, which is primarily analgesic at the site of injury [24,25,32–36].

The clinical implications of central sensitization are several fold. Certain pain phenotypes may not be as responsive to opioids if the pain mechanism is largely due to central sensitization. Little is known about the opioid responsiveness of referred visceral pain [4]. If the central sensitization and long-term potentiation of pain within the spinal cord are the main generators of pain, then interventional nerve blocks will be ineffective [4].

Assessing acute pain and pain responses

Acute pain by default is assessed like chronic pain: by location, quality, referral pattern, and palliative and exacerbating factors, intensity or severity, temporal pattern, and associated symptoms. There is no evidence that directly links timing, frequency, or choice of measure for assessment with timeliness, choice, or safety of treatment in medical patients. There are currently no pain-relevant performance measures in place that can support efforts to enhance pain care in these settings, and research on pain management in nonsurgical, nonmalignant acute pain is sparse [37]. Severity can be measured by a numerical rating scale (NRS), visual analog scale (VAS), categorical scale (CAT), and face scales (for children less than 8 years of age). Meaningful changes in pain severity can be due to active

treatment, placebo responses, and/or nonspecific effects such as recall bias. Nonspecific effects also include the clinical setting, the natural history and fluctuations of pain, altered mood, and the tendency for severe pain to regress toward the mean or be averaged over time [38]. There is moderate variability in individual cut-off points for mild, moderate, and severe pain [39]. As a general rule, severity less than 4 is mild, 5–7 moderate, and greater than 7 severe, on an 11-point numerical scale. As outcomes to pain trials, responses are measured by central tendency (which is either the change in mean or median pain intensity) [40]. Clinically relevant outcome responses are by the number of responders (responders analysis) based on clinically meaningful changes in pain severity. A change in 2 points on an 11-point NRS scale is clinically significant while a change of 10 mm on a VAS is a perceptible pain difference [38,41]. This assumes that pain scales are linear which is more of an assumption been proven. Pain responses were determined by the need for a second rescue dose in breakthrough pain analgesic trials. A 20% reduction in pain intensity was determined to be minimally important clinically, a 30% change was notable improvement, and a 50% reduction substantial improvement [40]. Cumulative responses by central tendency analysis are obtained through measuring changes in pain intensity over time. Differences in pain intensity over time (SPID, sum of pain intensity difference) and pain differences (PD) at separate times are used to compare different treatments [42]. Central tendency differences may reflect a great response in a small number of individuals or little response among the majority. In responder analysis, the cumulative proportion of responders over time provides clinicians with the ability to determine the numbers needed to treat (NNT) to obtain a reduction in pain severity in one individual, which is more meaningful to clinicians than results by the central tendency analysis [43]. The NNT is the inverse of the absolute risk reduction between groups. A 33% reduction in pain intensity is considered a response in breakthrough pain trials, in chronic neuropathic pain trials, and in nonopioid adjuvant trials for neuropathic pain [44]. None of the measures are intended to diagnose the cause of pain and none are perfect across the spectrum of etiologies, pain types, comorbidities, and patient preference. Multiple outcomes should be assessed during treatment: analgesia, improved function, side effects, compliance, patient's satisfaction, and affordability. Since many suffer from breakthrough pain, assessment of rest and dynamic (movement related) pain should be performed independently. Rest pain should be assessed now and over the last 24 hours or over the last week [45].

Management of acute pain

Chronic pain is defined as the pain present for more than 3 months and is largely due to the fact that pain of that duration is unlikely to spontaneously diminish [46]. Acute pain can be anticipatory (procedural), acute or chronic (breakthrough), intermittent without continuous pain, and unstable or reduction in the changing pattern most often associated with cancer complications. Temporal pattern, location, radiating or referral pattern, severity, underlying cause, and response to analgesia and 9 analgesics, all are more important to clinical management than duration (less than 3 months versus greater than 3 months). Implementation of an acute pain service may improve pain and reduce side effects. Staff education and guidelines improve assessment, pain relief, and prescribing analgesics [47–49].

Pharmacologic management of acute pain

There is not one opioid superior to another, but certain opioids are better for particular individuals [50]. The development of parenteral patient-controlled analgesia (PCA) predated the World Health Organization analgesic ladder and provided clinical backdrop to individualization of acute pain management. The fundamental concept of PCA was developed because most individuals wanted to participate in the management of their pain, which was absolutely vital to individualized dosing. With the use of PCA, opioid requirements were found to vary 8–10-fold between patients. In 1963, Roe and colleagues discovered that small intravenous (IV) doses of morphine on a pro re nata (PRN) (when necessary) basis for acute pain severity was more effective than the conventional approach of every 4 hours, weight-based intramuscular morphine [51]. Sechzer and colleagues confirmed that "on patient demand" dosing was superior to every 4 hours dosing [52]. The initial protocol for PCA required frequent assessments by nurses. In 1976, the first commercially available PCA pump became available (Cardiff Palliator) [53]. In general, PCA provides better analgesia than conventional parenteral opioid dosing except in wards with high nurse to patient ratios [45,54]. One of the differences between acute and chronic pain management is that interventional approaches such as epidural or intrathecal analgesia are used more frequently and at least for postoperative pain used frequently as the primary pain management strategy [45,55]. In this way, acute pain management does not follow the WHO analgesic ladder.

Optimizing opioid analgesia requires titration to individual minimal inhibitory concentrations, which differs between individuals but is relatively constant for an individual. Opioids have diverse pharmacokinetic properties that influence dosing strategies for acute pain [56]. There are delays between peak blood concentrations and effective CNS opioid levels. Fentanyl is uniquely sequestered in the lung, which delays CNS levels and differs from alfentanil that is not sequestered [57,58]. Oxycodone and fentanyl are actively transported into the CNS [59,60]. Blood–brain barrier effluxes certain opioids from the CNS, when P-glycoprotein is upregulated and causes opioid "tolerance" seen in animals models [61]. Certain medications block active CNS transporters, potentially reducing CNS opioid levels. Antidepressants, certain antiarrhythmics (mexiletine), and ketamine block oxycodone uptake and potentially reduce analgesia [62]. Verapamil blocks P-glycoprotein efflux and increases CNS levels of P-glycoprotein -dependent opioids [63–66]. Duration of maximal CNS opioid concentrations differs between opioids (2 min for alfentanil and 96 min for

morphine) [56]. Dosing strategies for different opioids should be based on pharmacokinetics. As such, morphine is more suitable than for an upgraded traditional approach to staff administer IV or subcutaneous doses and should have a longer lock-out interval with a PCA compared with lipophilic opioids [56]. Lipophilic opioids such as fentanyl and alfentanil have a more rapid onset and shorter duration of action at least initially than morphine and are more suitable to IV PCA dosing strategies with short lock-out intervals and for incident pain. Buccal, transmucosal, and intranasal lipophilic opioids have a more rapid analgesic onset than immediate release morphine for breakthrough pain and procedure related acute pain, fentanyl have been tailored as a rescue analgesic. Both transmucosal and intranasal routes bypass hepatic first pass clearance. Uniquely, fentanyl half-life increases over time as fat and muscle storage sites become saturated. The frequent use of buccal or intranasal fentanyl leads to delayed opioid toxicity as hepatic clearance becomes rate limiting to fentanyl clearance rather than redistribution [56]. This is the reason for limiting the number of rescue doses per day. Children prefer a "needleless" pain management strategy for procedures or acute pain and prefer intranasal or buccal fentanyl to IV morphine [67,68].

Preventing acute postoperative pain

Individuals with cancer are frequently faced with surgery either to remove the primary or to treat complications related to their cancer. Understanding perioperative acute pain management is important to palliative specialists. Preventive analgesics reduce postoperative pain and opioid requirements through perhaps blunting or preventing central sensitization caused by acute pain [4]. Preemptive opioids without continuation through the operation can lead to central sensitization [69]. Analgesia should begin preoperatively and continue through the operation to the postoperative period of time and is preferred over preemptive opioids prior to surgery alone. Postoperative tissue inflammation upregulates opioid receptors, which improves postoperative opioid responses. Surgery without significant tissue injury or damage generally produces a proportional stimulus–pain response. Pain recedes without central persistent sensitization. Extensive tissue damage generates an afferent barrage through C and A-delta fibers, which activate WDR neurons. Amplification of nociceptive signals (through brain-derived neurotrophic factor release) increases hypersensitivity through spinal-bulbar-spinal facilitation of nociceptive circuits, causing allodynia and secondary hyperalgesia, and can lead to chronic pain that is poorly controlled [70].

The goals of preventive analgesia are to decrease acute pain, prevent neuroplastic changes, which lead to chronic pain, and reduce opioid requirements and opioid-related side effects [71]. Associated with severe postoperative pain are the duration of surgery, high intraoperative opioid doses, and general anesthetics [72]. Nonopioid analgesics such as NSAIDs and adjuvant analgesics, gabapentin, pregabalin, ketamine, lidocaine, bupivicaine, and clonidine reduce postoperative pain and opioid requirements [70,73–78]. Earlier reviews suggested little benefit to the use of adjuvants, but recent reviews report significant benefits to pre-and perioperative gabapentin, ketamine, NSAIDs, and local anesthetics applied to the wound [70,75]. The evidence for ketamine is weak [73,74,77–84].

Adjuvants influence perioperative pain differently. In one study, gabapentin reduced movement-related pain but not the risk of chronic pain; venlafaxine reduced the risk of chronic postoperative pain [85,86]. Overall, when adjuvants are compared for postoperative analgesic outcomes, there is little advantage of one over the other [87,88]. Clinical context will play a significant role in the choice of adjuvant and nonopioid analgesics.

Combinations of adjuvant analgesics may improve acute procedure and postoperative related pain. Gabapentin combined with local anesthetics injected into the surgical wound improves analgesia and reduces the risk of long-term chronic pain compared with gabapentin alone [89,90]. Combinations of gabapentin plus acetaminophen or an NSAID controls acute postoperative pain better than gabapentin or NSAIDs alone [91,92]. Gabapentin, dexamethasone, ketamine, and acetaminophen reduce pain to a greater extent than ketorolac plus acetaminophen [93]. An oral local anesthetic (mexiletine) plus regional block reduces postoperative pain longer than a regional block alone; the combination prevents late onset dysesthesia [94]. Aggressive early multimodality postoperative pain management reduces pain intensity and reduces the risk of chronic pain [95].

Patient-controlled analgesia for acute and postoperative pain

PCA strategies involve a loading dose, demand dose, lockout interval, and background infusion rate (if opioid tolerant preoperatively). A 1 and 4 hours limit on opioid doses is an additional parameter but is rarely used [96]. Subcutaneous PCA opioids are as effective as IV opioids. In the opioid naïve, a background infusion is generally not recommended. The addition of a background infusion to a demand PCA in the opioid naïve does not improve pain relief, sleep or reduce the demand. Loading doses are given in the postoperative acute care unit (PACU). Small but frequent doses (morphine 1 mg or fentanyl 20–40 mcg) are titrated to reduce pain severity to 4 or less on a NRS. Individuals are observed for hemodynamic or respiratory compromise. A common morphine dosing strategy for the opioid naïve is 1 mg bolus as a demand dose with a 6–10 min lockout interval [96]. Hydromorphone doses are 0.2–0.4 mg with the same lockout interval and fentanyl 40 mcg with a 10 min lockout intervals (6 doses per hour). Tramadol demand doses range between 10 and 20 mg with a 5–10 min lockout interval. Demand doses and lockout intervals are adjusted to response [96].

Even with IV PCA in the postoperative setting, the incidence of moderate pain is 35%, 10% will have severe pain [97]. Opioid adverse events are dose related. Nausea is greater with IV PCA than with parenteral morphine or epidural analgesia. Sedation occurs in 24% and is mostly mild. Pruritus occurs in 15%, nausea in 25%, and vomiting in 20% [97]. IV PCA analgesia is associated with a 1%–15% incidence of respiratory

depression despite recommended lockout intervals, cell monitoring is important. Hypotension occurs with less frequency (0.4%) than with epidural analgesia (5.6%) [98].

In general, PCA opioid strategies lead to higher opioid consumption, a greater incidence of pruritus but no difference in other adverse events or hospital stay compared with regular parenteral intermittent opioid injections. Continuous opioid infusions in the opioid naïve are associated with an increased risk of respiratory depression. Transdermal opioids and oral sustained-release opioids should not be used for acute pain management. Neither should transmucosal and intranasal fentanyl in the opioid be naïve. Routine addition of anti-emetics to PCA opioids is unnecessary, nausea and vomiting should be managed as it arises. Postoperative nausea and vomiting can be treated with droperidol, metoclopramide, 5-HT 3 receptor antagonists, corticosteroids, or cyclizine [99]. Opioid-related pruritus responds to naloxone, naltrexone, nalbuphine, droperidol, and 5-HT 3 receptor antagonists [100,101]. PCA systems should include an antisyphon valve and, if used in nondedicated lines, anti-reflux valves.

Managing acute postoperative pain in the opioid tolerant

Opioid tolerant individuals require a distinctly different postoperative opioid dosing strategy than the opioid naïve. Poor pain control and withdrawal symptoms are likely to occur if the same dosing strategies are used as for the opioid naïve. On the preoperative day, patients should be instructed to take their usual chronic opioid dose. A continuous IV opioid infusion or continuous PCA with demand equivalent to the preoperative daily opioid dose is maintained after recovery from anesthesia. This will require conversion of the around-the-clock oral dose to parenteral equivalence [102]. Regional analgesia will help control pain as will epidural analgesia; however, at a minimum, these individuals will need 50% of their preoperative chronic opioid dose to avoid withdrawal since neither regional anesthesia nor epidural analgesia will prevent withdrawal [103]. Demand doses to relieve pain are likely to be 2–4 times greater than those used for the opioid naive. For those on maintenance therapy, methadone or buprenorphine should be continued postoperatively and a short acting potent mu agonist such as morphine, hydromorphone, or fentanyl is used for acute postoperative pain management [103]. Alternatively, the maintenance opioid dose can be divided and given for analgesia. Postoperative pain control in the opioid tolerant may be improved by the addition of low doses of ketamine (0.25–0.5 mg/kg bolus and/or a 1–6 mcg/kg/min infusion) [102,103]. Other adjuvants such as NSAIDs and gabapentinoids should be considered in the perioperative period.

Multimodality analgesia and innovations in managing acute postoperative pain

Single dose extended release epidural morphine lasts 48 hours without the need for an epidural pump. Sustained release epidural morphine reduces perioperative pain associated with knee arthroplasty and cesarean section and is associated with reduced systemic opioid requirements and opioid side effects. However, respiratory depression has been reported with doses of 15 mg or greater [104–106]. Naloxone was needed in 12% of individuals for pruritus or respiratory depression.

Patient-controlled epidural analgesia (PCEA) uses fentanyl or a combination of fentanyl with a local anesthetic such as bupivicaine or ropivacaine for pain control. Compared with continuous epidural analgesia, PCEA side effects and overall analgesic requirements are less. PCEA is superior to IV PCA in controlling pain in the postoperative setting [107]. Thoracic epidural opioid analgesia reduces postoperative complications related to aortic aneurysm repair and thoracic surgery [108]. The addition of a local anesthetic reduces opioid-related side effects and the need for rescue doses. The downside to the combination is an increased incidence of hypotension, pruritus, motor block, and urinary retention [107]. Neuroaxis hydrophilic opioid boluses increase the risk for delayed respiratory depression when compared with fentanyl [109]. Chlorhexidine dressings over the epidural entrance site reduce bacterial colonization better than povidone-iodine [110].

Patient-controlled regional anesthesia uses local anesthetics alone or a combination of local anesthetic and opioid in a regional infusion [111]. Patient-controlled regional analgesia and perineural patient-controlled regional anesthesia allows patients to titrate the local anesthetic to comfort. Patient-controlled regional analgesia results in equivalent to superior analgesia and lowers systemic analgesic requirements compared with continuous infusion regional analgesia [107,111]. In a large review of more than 18,000 patients, PCEA and continuous regional analgesia produced superior analgesia to IV PCA [112]. Intra-articular analgesia using ropivacaine, morphine and ketorolac as a form of regional analgesia results in reduced systemic opioid requirements [111].

Transdermal fentanyl iontophoresis

Electronic currents drive ionic molecules across the stratum corneum to create aqueous pathways through the cutaneous lipid bilayer. Pulses increase transdermal transport of fentanyl by four orders of magnitude [113]. Fentanyl transcutaneous iontophoretic PCA systems deliver 40 mcg by patient activation, which provides 24 hours of analgesia per unit and delivers a maximum of 80 fentanyl doses at a lockout interval of 10 min. Transdermal iontophoresis fentanyl is superior to placebo and equivalent to IV PCA morphine 1 mg demand and a lockout interval of 5 min [114–117].

Bone and joint pain

Bone, joint disorders, and bone metastases are common causes of acute pain. Bone metastases are the most common cause of cancer incident pain.

Nociceptors in joints located in the capsule, ligaments, menisci, periosteum, and subchondral bone are located on the terminals of type IV (unmyelinated) or type III (myelinated with unmyelinated free endings) afferent neurons. Movement generates shear stress on axon membranes that opens gated ion channels [118]. Inflammation decreases firing thresholds and causes peripheral sensitization, wind-up, and secondary hyperalgesia. Synovial fluid volume which is normally 1–4 mL and maintained at subatmospheric pressures, with inflammation and subsequent increased vascular permeability increases to as much as 60 mL or more with pressures up to +20 mmHg [118]. The pressure stimulates mechanical gated ion channels, causing burst firing from afferent neurons. Joint and ligaments have a poor capacity to heal as a result of inflamed joints, and sustained or repeated trauma becomes unstable and develops cartilage erosions, causing osteoarthritis. Pain is experienced with passive joint movement as mechanical gated ion channels are activated. Inflamed and damaged joints release neuroexcitatory peptides (CGRP, SP, and vasoactive intestinal peptide), causing joint pain sensitivity and increased pain at rest as well as with movement. Immunocytes and mast cells in synovium release prostaglandins, which in turn upregulate sodium channels. Nociceptin at low concentrates within the joint sensitizes afferents and at high doses paradoxically reduces sensitization [118]. Voltage gated calcium channels on primary afferents are activated, causing hypersensitization [119]. Gabapentin reduces knee joint pain and bone pain from cancer by blocking alpha-2 delta-1 subunits on primary afferents [120,121]. In animal models, gabapentin also reduces secondary hyperalgesia and referred allodynia by its central actions [122]. Joint disorders in animal models are also associated with neuropathic pain from joint damage, which is responsive to amitriptyline [123,124]. Referred pain from the joint produces muscle soreness, and an extended area of hyperalgesia proximal to the joint [125].

NSAIDs are standard treatment for arthritis, which reduces inflammatory pain and perhaps dampens central sensitization through inhibiting cyclooxygenase, which is a second messenger to NMDA receptors. Topical and systemic NSAIDs and intra-articular corticosteroids block prostaglandin production and reduce muscle soreness related to arthritis. Combining NSAIDs with acetaminophen may be better than either drug alone [126].

Osteolytic and osteoblastic metastases are associated with osteoclast proliferation and bone remodeling. The acid environment within the metastases and increased release of protons stimulates ASIC and TRPV1 channels on afferents [127]. Stromal and tumor and infiltrating immunocytes increase lactate. Bisphosphonates reduce cancer-related skeletal events and bone pain [128]. Bisphosphonates bind to the matrix calcium, and are taken up by osteoclasts by endocytosis that causes osteoclast apoptosis. Long-term bisphosphonates, however, cause complications in a minority due to inhibition of bone repair and remodeling. Complications include fractures of the long bone and osteonecrosis of the jaw [127].

Salmon calcitonin reduces pain from osteoporotic fractures but not from metastases [129,130]. The mechanism of analgesia associated with salmon calcitonin is not known. However, it may be due to changes in descending serotonergic modification on the sensory transmission mediated by C fiber afferents [129,131].

Tumors releases into the stroma receptor activator nuclear factor kappa B ligand (RANKL), which binds to RANKL receptors that regulates osteoclast activity. Denosumab, a fully humanized monoclonal antibody to RANKL, reduces cancer-related bone loss and skeletal events in breast and prostate cancer and myeloma by blocking osteoclast activation [127]. There is presently not known if denosumab relieves pain. Complications related to denosumab are similar to those of bisphosphonates [132,133].

Tumor-infiltrating macrophages, neutrophils, T lymphocytes, and fibroblasts and endothelial cells secrete a number of factors that sensitize afferent neurons. These factors are bradykinins, tumor necrosis factor, endothelin, epidermal growth factor, transforming growth factor-alpha, inflammatory cytokines, and nerve growth factor. Nerve growth factor binds to the receptor TrkA, causing bone pain by upregulating multiple neurotransmitters, sensitizing ion channels, and disinhibiting pronociceptive receptors. Antinerve growth factor antibody therapy reduces bone pain in animal models [127,134]. Recent randomized trials have found that tansumab reduces pain from severe osteoarthritis [135].

Clinically, individuals with pain from bone metastases require higher doses of morphine then individuals with inflammatory pain [136,137]. In mouse models, dose requirements to block cancer bone pain are 10 times those needed to reduce inflammatory pain [22,138]. A characteristic neuropathic "signature" develops in the spinal cord as a result of damage to sensory afferents in bone marrow, trabecular bone, and cortical bone [139]. Spinal cord microglia proliferates ipsilateral to the metastases, which is similar to neuropathic pain [22,138,140]. NSAIDs, opioids, and gabapentin modestly reduce metastatic bone pain [120,141–144]. Loading dose ibandronate is reported to relieve bone pain quickly without impairing renal function [145]. In a randomized trial, parenteral ibandronate reduced bone pain more effectively than pamidronate [146]. In the future, endothelin receptor antagonists, anti-nerve growth factor, and osteoprotegerin (a RANKL blocker) may be found to be effective also [138,147–149].

Acute dosing strategies for acute pain in the emergency department

Three opioids have the most published evidence for managing acute pain in the emergency department: morphine, hydromorphone, and fentanyl [150].

In a randomized, double-blind placebo-controlled trial, IV morphine 0.15 mg/kilogram (kg) was superior to 0.1 mg/kg in adults with acute pain as determined by changes in severity at 60 min [151]. Individuals in this study were opioid naïve. In a randomized double-blind trial, IV morphine 0.05 mg/kg was compared to hydromorphone 0.0075 mg/kg. Response, defined as greater than or equal to 50% reduction in intensity, was the same for both opioids; however, only a minority of participants (45%) responded by 30 min [152]. The authors felt that the dose and strategy were inadequate and a titration strategy was needed.

Morphine 0.1 mg/kg bolus and 3 mg every 5 min was compared with fentanyl 1 mcg/kg and 30 µg every 5 min as needed for severe acute pain (determined by a VAS score greater than 60 mm) [153]. Morphine reduced pain severity to a similar extent as fentanyl (from 83 to 40 mm and 77 to 35 mm at 30 min respectively). Patients rated analgesia good to excellent with equal frequency (62% morphine and 76% fentanyl), and side effects were the same for both opioids.

Morphine 5 mg has been compared with alfentanil 0.5 mg for acute chest pain [154]. Doses were repeated at 2 min intervals as needed, a VAS scale for pain severity was obtained at 2, 4, 6, 10, and 15 min as an outcome measure. Alfentanil resulted in quicker pain relief, and no hemodynamic or respiratory side effects were noted with either opioid.

Two studies reported using a "1 + 1" hydromorphone dosing strategy. In the first study, opioid naive individuals less than 65 years of age with acute pain were treated with 1 and 1 mg of hydromorphone was offered 15 min later if the answer was yes to the question, "Do you want more pain medication?" Adequate analgesia was obtained with the first dose in 77% and an additional 16% responded to the second dose. Eighty-six percent had a 2 point reduction in their NRS by 60 min. Median pain reduction was 6 out of 10 on a NRS. None required naloxone, but 5% had transient oxygen desaturation [155]. In the second study, patients were randomized between the "1 to 1" hydromorphone protocol and a physician-derived dosing standard used in the emergency department was the comparison strategy. Eligibility was the same as in the first study. Patients were assessed at 15, 30, and 60 min, pain intensity differences at 60 min was the primary outcome. The "1 to 1" protocol was superior to the standard dosing regimen with a 1.1 point difference between strategies on a 0–10 NRS, which was statistically significant (95% confidence interval for differences 0.3–1.9).

Fentanyl has been used at the scene of trauma using 0.05–0.1 mcg/kg every 15 min as needed. Patients had moderate-to-severe pain on a NRS scale or a CAT. Fifty-three of sixty-seven had a good response by narrative record review. One hundred twenty-four doses were given (average two doses per patient). No patient had oxygen saturations below 90% [156].

Intranasal fentanyl is a "needleless" pain management strategy. Several studies compared intranasal fentanyl with parenteral morphine for acute pain from bone fractures. Doses were 1–2 mcg/kg (1.5 mcg/kg on average) and repeated if necessary, using 0.5 mcg/kg or 15 mcg repeated at 5–10 min intervals [157,158]. Standard vials of fentanyl (50 mcg/mL) were used for children and administered by the Tory Wolfe mucosal atomizer device (Salt Lake City, Ut, USA) [67]. Fentanyl doses were on average 60 mcg repeated at 5 min prior to arrival at the emergency room. This dosing strategy compared with IV morphine 2.5–5 mg at 5 min intervals as needed provided excellent pain relief [159].

In summary, a reasonable strategy to manage acute pain in the emergency department is to start with 1 mg of parenteral hydromorphone, 5 mg of morphine or 50–100 mcg of fentanyl and reassess 15 min later. If pain is still severe, a second dose is offered. Intranasal fentanyl using 1.5 mcg/kg at 5–10 min intervals for children is a reasonable approach to controlling acute pain.

Breakthrough pain

At least half of the patients with chronic cancer pain experience transient flares of pain (breakthrough pain). The median number of breakthrough episodes is 3–6 per day depending on the series and the average onset to maximum intensity is 3 min. Two-thirds of pain flares are with activity (incident pain). Individuals with breakthrough pain have more severe chronic pain, greater functional impairment, anxiety, and depressed mood [160].

Seventy-four percent of individuals with chronic nonmalignant pain have breakthrough pain. The median number of episodes per day is similar to cancer patients. The time to maximum intensity is 10 min and duration 30–60 min. Sixty-nine percent of episodes are associated with activity [160].

Time to maximum pain intensity is such that oral immediate release morphine, hydromorphone, and oxycodone are unlikely to be of great benefit. Innovations in breakthrough pain management are therefore necessary to successfully reduce intensity of pain in a timely manner. A recent review of the developments in therapeutics for breakthrough pain has been published [161].

Oral transmucosal fentanyl citrate (OTFC) was the first opioid to be specifically licensed for breakthrough pain. High quality randomized studies demonstrate dose proportional responses, superiority over oral immediate release morphine but poor correlations between the effective fentanyl rescue dose and the chronic opioid dose [162,163]. Responses are achieved within 10–15 min; the time to onset of analgesia is close to that of IV morphine [164].

Fentanyl buccal soluble film is a bilayer system, which uses a biodegradable polymer over a fentanyl layer, which is designed to prevent fentanyl from being dissolved in saliva and swallowed [165]. The soluble film rapidly releases fentanyl, and pain relief occurs within 15 min. The dose is empirically titrated to response since there is also a poor correlation between the effective fentanyl rescue dose and the chronic opioid dose [166]. In addition, because of bioavailability differences between the fentanyl lozenge, buccal film, and buccal tablet, conversion from OTFC to buccal fentanyl is not recommended. Pain responses are the same regardless of the opioid used for chronic pain [167]. Drug abuse and misuse were rare in these studies largely due to screening prior to study entrance [168]. Individuals who are appropriate for OTFC, soluble film or buccal tablets must be opioid tolerant, defined as 60 mg of daily morphine or equivalent (30 mg of oxycodone, 8 mg of hydromorphone, or 25 mcg/hour of transdermal fentanyl) per day for 1 week [169]. Serious adverse and fatal events associated with transmucosal (and intranasal fentanyl) are related to improper selection of patients (opioid naïve individuals) and improper dosing (intervals shorter than those recommended in randomized trials). Doses should not be repeated sooner than 4 hours. Patients should be prescribed only one dose strength at a time [169].

Intranasal opioids for cancer breakthrough pain

Drug absorption through the nasal cavity bypasses hepatic clearance [113]. The dose volume must be limited to 150 µL to avoid runoff into nasopharynx. Intranasal fentanyl is 70% bioavailability. To deliver 60 mcg (2 doses in a volume of 150 µL, one per nostril), fentanyl is concentrated to 400 mcg/mL, the parenteral IV solution cannot be used in adults [113]. A single dose of 50 mcg of fentanyl produces rapid analgesia (within 5 min) in postoperative gynecologic patients [170].

Intranasal fentanyl has better bioavailability and shorter onset to action (7 min) than transmucosal fentanyl [171,172]. Fentanyl in pectin and/or chitosan improves nasal absorption. A double-blind randomized trial reported superiority of intranasal fentanyl spray over placebo [173]. In a selective patient population, fentanyl pectin nasal spray was consistently effective in controlling breakthrough pain [174]. Titration is necessary to reach the effective dose; there is a poor relationship to the around-the-clock opioid dose [162,175–177].

In a double-blind, double-dummy crossover study, intranasal compared with IV fentanyl for postoperative pain. Intranasal fentanyl had a delayed time to maximum concentration (13 min) compared with IV fentanyl (6 min). There was also a lower maximum concentration (1.2 versus 2.0 ng/mL), and analgesia was slightly delayed. Duration of pain relief was dose dependent but not route dependent [178].

Intranasal fentanyl has been compared to IV fentanyl in individuals undergoing orthopedic, abdominal, and thyroid surgeries [179]. Intranasal fentanyl doses were 25 mcg and IV PCA doses 17.5 mcg with a lockout interval of 6 min for both. Time to first noticeable reduction in pain intensity was the same for both (21–22 min). Pain intensity was reduced to the same extent (55 to 11 mm by VAS). A 50 mcg intranasal fentanyl dose reduced pain within 5 min of administration [170].

Intranasal sufentanil, in the form of nose drops or spray using the parenteral solutions and a 10–20 mcg dose, is reported to be very effective [180]. Tmax ranges between 15 and 30 min [181]. A dose of 0.05 mcg/kg (average dose to 3.5 mcg) reduced pain to less than 3 on an NRS scale within 20 min in 80% of surgical patients [182].

Nonopioid analgesics and adjuvants for acute pain

NSAIDS have been used for breakthrough pain. Flurbiprofen was reported with some success [183]. NSAIDs are used commonly for postoperative pain management (47% in an Italian survey) [184]. The five commonly used NSAIDS are ketorolac, diclofenac, ibuprofen, ketoprofen, and paracoxib [185]. A novel diclofenac preparation employs hydroxypropyl beta-cyclodextrin solvent, which concentrates diclofenac to a small volume. Half of patients responded to 75 mg of IV diclofenac within 15 min, which was superior to placebo [186]. Diclofenac is superior to ketorolac in managing postoperative pain when side effects were included as outcomes [187]. Diclofenac not only blocks cyclooxygenase but inhibits substance P release, blocks NMDA receptors and ASIC, which may account for the excellent responses [188].

A new IV preparation of ibuprofen has been approved for use during the first 24 hours after surgery; doses are 800 mg every 6 hours. Parenteral ibuprofen reduced morphine requirements by 22% and decreased pain at rest and with movement. Less nausea, vomiting, and constipation were reported than with morphine alone. The main side effect was dizziness that was dose dependent [189].

Acetaminophen, in animal models, is a cox-3 inhibitor and also blocks NMDA receptors, nitric oxide release, and substance P release [190]. Parenteral acetaminophen is available either as the parent drug or the prodrug propacetamol. Propacetamol is converted to acetaminophen by circulating nonspecific esterases [191]. IV acetaminophen was superior to placebo after cardiac surgery [192]. IV acetaminophen 1 g before and 4 and 16 hours after breast surgery reduced morphine requirements by 42% and was superior to placebo. Acetaminophen improved postoperative ambulation compared with metamizol [193]. IV acetaminophen before surgery and every 6 hours after surgery for 24 hours was equivalent to dipyrone and reduced the risk of drug-related renal failure and peptic ulcers.

Tapentadol

Tapentadol is an opioid agonist and a norepinephrine reuptake inhibitor [194]. Tapentadol binds to mu, kappa, and delta opioid receptors. One hundred milligrams is equivalent to 20 mg of oxycodone and 30 mg of morphine (with some individual patient differences). The type of pain influences equivalence [195–197]. Tapentadol has been compared with morphine when treating neuropathic pain. In another randomized trial following bunionectomy, tapentadol 100 mg was equivalent to oxycodone 15 mg, and had less side effects (i.e., reduced constipation) [198].

Gabapentin and pregabalin

Preoperative gabapentin (doses of 300–1200 mg) reduces postoperative pain and morphine requirements by 30%. By meta-regression analysis, benefits were not dose dependent. Both rest- and activity-related pain improves. Opioid side effects are less in part due to reduced morphine requirements. The NNT for less nausea was 25, 6 for less vomiting, and 7 for less urinary retention. Gabapentin side effects include sedation and dizziness, with the number needed to harm (NNH) of 35 for sedation and 12 for dizziness [81,199–203]. The same benefits and side effects are reported with pregabalin [81,199,203,204].

Ketamine

Ketamine is a racemate of R and S enantiomers. In some European countries, S-ketamine is available. Low-dose ketamine improves postoperative analgesia and reduces morphine

requirements [205,206]. Low doses are considered to be less than 1 mg/kg IV bolus and IV infusions are usually given less than 20 mcg/kg/min [80]. Ketamine has been used as bolus doses in the perioperative period, in continuous infusions, by PCA mixed with morphine, by mouth and as a transdermal patch [207–215]. S-ketamine available in Europe is also effective [216–219]. Effective bolus doses of racemate ketamine range from 0.15 to 0.25 mg/kg. Effective continuous infusion doses are in the range of 1.5 mcg/kg/min. A demand PCA of morphine 1 mg and ketamine 5 mg given at 7 min lockout intervals has been reported to be effective in managing postoperative pain [207,210,214]. Transdermal ketamine, 25 mg over 24 hours, is reported to be well absorbed [215]. Transdermal delivery of ketamine was an useful adjuvant to postoperative analgesia after epidural lidocaine blockade [215]. Ketamine reduces nausea and vomiting in the postoperative period, perhaps due to its opioid sparing effects. Ketamine, unlike morphine, does not cause hypotension or respiratory depression, which can be a problem for post-thoracotomy patient and for those on high-dose morphine [210–212,220]. Preemptive and IV infusions of ketamine at the end of surgery (0.3 mg/kg bolus and 0.05 mg/kg/hour during surgery) compared with preemptive gabapentin 1200 mg and placebo reduced postoperative morphine requirements by 35%–42% and was superior to placebo. However, incisional pain at 1, 3, and 6 months was better with gabapentin compared with ketamine [88].

Ketamine infusions (0.1 mg/kg/hour) have been compared with morphine 0.1 mg/kg every 4 hours as needed for acute musculoskeletal trauma. Ketamine resulted in better pain relief and less drowsiness than intermittent morphine. None of the ketamine-treated individuals required supplementary analgesia and were easily mobilized for traction or splints [221].

In a double-blind, randomized placebo-controlled trial involving individuals with severe acute pain (a VAS score of greater than 60 mm on a 100 mm scale), IV morphine 0.1 mg/kg followed by 3 mg every 5 min as needed with or without ketamine 0.2 mg/kg over 10 min IV were compared. Morphine consumption was less with the combination (0.149 versus 0.202 mg/kg); the pain scores were similar at 30 min (34 versus 39 mm by VAS). Side effects with ketamine are hallucinations, dizziness, diplopia, and dysphoria [222].

In a retrospective review of the use of low-dose ketamine (ranging from 0.1 to 0.6 mg/kg) in the emergency department, pain severity was reduced by 54%. Most individuals (91%), however, received an opioid prior to or after ketamine. Eight of 35 individuals failed to respond to ketamine [223].

A randomized control trial compared morphine (0.2 mg/kg) with morphine (0.1 mg/kg) plus ketamine (0.2 mg/kg) prior to hospitalization for acute trauma. Morphine doses needed for analgesia were less with the combination (7 versus 13.5 mg). Pain severity by NRS improved with the combination to a greater extent than to morphine alone (5.4 versus 3.1). Blood pressure increased with ketamine. Side effects occurred in a minority and did not differ between groups [224].

Small doses of ketamine in the opioid tolerant may produce better pain control than escalation of opioid doses.

This strategy reduces the risk of oxygen desaturation, and less opioid is needed to control pain [214,225]. Rotations to methadone plus the addition of 100 mg of ketamine daily improved both rest and movement related pain [226]. In a cohort of patients receiving both intrathecal opioids and high-dose systemic opioids for incident pain, the use of intrathecal boluses of local anesthetics or sublingual ketamine (25 mg) reduced pain within 10 min [227].

Oral ketamine has been used at doses of 0.5 mg/kg twice to three times daily. Responses in those with neuropathic pain on oral opioids and/or antidepressants were seen within 24 hours. Sedation was experienced by a few, which resolved over a week or 2, despite continued ketamine [228].

Retrospective reviews and small cohort studies have found ketamine effective in managing cancer pain [228–231]. In a randomized, double-blind, placebo-controlled trial, ketamine plus morphine did not improve cancer pain compared with morphine alone [232]. There is insufficient evidence to assess the benefits and harms of ketamine as an adjuvant to opioids for the relief of cancer pain [233].

Dexmedetomidine

Dexmedetomidine is a highly selective alpha-2 receptor agonist that avidly binds to alpha-2A adrenergic receptors [234]. Dexmedetomidine activates postsynaptic alpha-2 adrenergic receptors, which hyperpolarize second order afferent neurons, thus inhibiting nociceptive [235]. Dexmedetomidine inhibits adenylyl cyclase, N-type calcium channels and promotes activation of inward rectify potassium channels [234]. Compared with clonidine, dexmedetomidine is more selective and specific for alpha-2 adrenergic receptors [235]. Side effects include hypotension, bradycardia, and sedation, which are a barrier to use the drug on general medical wards.

Dexmedetomidine has been given preemptively at a bolus dose between 1 and 0.5 mcg/kg and 0.4–0.5 mcg/kg/hour infusion. Postoperative opioid requirements and opioid side effects were reduced, analgesia significantly improved. Mild bradycardia and reduced blood pressure occurred but did not lead to dose reduction or discontinuation for most individuals [236–238]. Dexmedetomidine has been combined with morphine in an IV PCA for postoperative pain. Morphine 1 mg and dexmedetomidine 5 mcg with a lockout interval of 5 min were compared to morphine alone. The combination produced a 29% reduction in morphine requirements, as well as reduction in postoperative nausea within the first 24 hours after surgery [239]. Dexmedetomidine, has been used for acute pain in opioid-tolerant individuals admitted to the hospital in severe pain. In a case series, 7 of 11 patients had substantial reductions in opioid doses with dexmedetomidine [240]. Dexmedetomidine, using a loading dose of 0.9–1 mcg/kg over 1 hour and an infusion of 0.3–0.4 mcg/kg/hour, improved pain control and reduced opioid requirements postoperatively. The infusion can be safely done on general medical wards [241]. Dexmedetomidine reduces the

risk of drug-related delirium, preserves sleep architecture, ventilatory drive, decreases sympathetic tone, and reduces postoperative inflammatory responses [242].

Opioid dosing strategies for acute severe pain in cancer

Rapid titration of opioid by parenteral or oral route has been used to treat acute cancer pain. Titration strategies involved boluses at short intervals by clinician or PCA demand only [243]. Morphine and fentanyl are the two most common opioids used by clinicians in managing acute cancer pain. Strategies included the following: (1) IV morphine 10–20 mg over 15 min every 30 min and double the dose if no response after 60 min, (2) IV morphine 1.5 mg every 10 min, (3) IV morphine at 2 mg every 2 min, (4) IV morphine 1 mg every minute for 10 min followed by a 5-min rest, repeat x2 as necessary up to a total of 30 mg of morphine, and (5) fentanyl equivalents from morphine using a ratio of 100 to 1 (oral morphine to parenteral fentanyl). Ten percent of the total daily morphine dose was converted to fentanyl and used IV every 5 min.

A comparison between IV and subcutaneous (sc) opioid dosing strategies has been reported [244]. Dose intervals were 5 min for IV and 30 min for sc opioids. Doses were dependent on total daily morphine or equivalents. If the daily morphine dose was less than 120 mg, then the IV breakthrough dose was 2 mg and the sc dose was 10 mg. If the oral daily morphine dose ranged between 121 and 360 mg/day, then the IV breakthrough dose was 3 mg and sc dose 20 mg. If the oral daily morphine dose ranged between 361 and 600 mg/day, then the IV dose was 4 mg and the sc dose 30 mg. If the daily oral morphine equivalents were greater than 600 mg, then the IV dose was 5 mg and sc dose 40 mg. Adequate analgesia was reached sooner with IV morphine (53 versus 77 min) and at lower doses (18.5 versus 57.9 mg).

Clinician bedside parenteral rapid titration strategies produce pain relief within 1 hour. Evidence is however only from cohort studies and collected case reports, which involved both opioid-naïve and opioid-tolerant individuals [243]. The effective titrated dose was the every 4 hours dose converted to oral equivalents in the opioid naïve. In the opioid tolerant, the titrated dose should be added to the chronic dose to maintain pain control.

Patient-controlled analgesia has been used without titration as a strategy to manage acute pain. Fentanyl 50 mcg or morphine 1 mg with a 5 min lockout interval has been reported [243]. Responses occurred within 6–24 hours. The reason for the delay is the absence of opioid titration to effective pain control. Second, patients not familiar with the PCA device often wait until severe pain to recur before activating the PCA.

Oral morphine dosing strategies involve (1) 10 mg of immediate release every 6 hours increased to 33%–50% every 24 hours for uncontrolled pain; (2) immediate release or sustained release starting with 60 mg daily titrated daily to 90, 120,

180, and 270 mg; and (3) immediate release titrated sequentially at 2–4 hours intervals in a step-dose strategy starting with 5 mg, then 10, 15, 20, 30, 40, 60, 80, 120, 160, and 200 mg. Pain relief occurs within 48 hours if titrated daily, 24 hours if titrated at 4 hours intervals, and 6 hours if titrated at 2 hours intervals [243].

Optimal oral and parenteral dosing strategies for acute severe cancer-related pain are not established with high quality evidence. Recommendations are based often based on expert opinion. Parenteral opioid dosing at frequent intervals using small doses titrated to response produces pain relief quickly usually within 1 hour, whereas PCA dosing without titration and oral dosing strategies take longer to control pain.

The Merito Study, which was recently published, used an opioid titration protocol, which leads to pain control relatively quickly. The dosing strategy consisted of immediate release morphine 5 mg every 4 hours around the clock and every 1 hour as needed in the opioid naïve and 10 mg every 4 hours around the clock and every 1 hour as needed for those on "weak" opioids. Seventy-nine percent achieved pain control within 24 hours and 50% within 8 hours. Pain severity by NRS was initially 7.6 (mean) and decreased to 2.4 (mean) within 3 days. Somnolence was seen in 24%, constipation in 22%, vomiting in 13%, nausea in 10%, and confusion in 7% [245].

A small study by Dr. Khojainova and colleagues added olanzapine (2.5–7.5 mg daily) for patients in a pain crisis on opioids and who were extremely anxious and/or had mild cognitive impairment [246]. Within 24 hours, olanzapine had improved cognition and anxiety and opioid requirements diminished.

Acute neuropathic pain

Acute postoperative neuropathic pain occurs in approximately 1% of individuals; half will have persistent pain at 12 months [247]. Other causes for acute neuropathic pain include chemotherapy (platinum-based, taxanes, vinca alkaloids, thalidomide), nerve root or spinal cord compression, plexopathies from progressive cancers, central poststroke pain syndromes, transverse myelitis, herpes zoster infections, uncontrolled diabetes and multiple sclerosis as well as AIDS associated neuropathy [247]. Trauma to peripheral or CNS is also a major cause of treatment-related acute neuropathic pain.

Amitriptyline used early in the course of an active zoster infection reduced postherpetic neuralgia [248]. Perioperative venlafaxine reduced the risk of developing chronic post-mastectomy pain [249]. A single gabapentin dose of 900 mg reduces acute pain from herpes zoster [250]. Gabapentin also reduced acute pain from burn injuries, which is often neuropathic [251]. Gabapentin with morphine reduced cancer-related neuropathic pain [252,253]. Preemptive venlafaxine reduces oxaliplatin acute neuropathic pain. Fifty milligrams prior to oxaliplatin and 37.5 mg twice daily after oxaliplatin for 10 days was used in 48 patients (27 males, median age: 67.6 years). Most had colorectal cancer (72.9%). Median number of cycles administered at inclusion was 4.5 (mean cumulative oxaliplatin dose: 684.6 mg). Complete pain relief was more frequent in the venlafaxine arm: 31.3% versus 5.3%

for placebo (P = 0.03). Venlafaxine side effects were grade 1–2 nausea (43.1%) and asthenia (39.2%) [254].

Neuropathic injury is associated with upregulation of certain sodium channels, and so it is rational to consider lidocaine either topically or systemically. IV lidocaine reduced pain from partial thickness burns. Alternatively, oral mexilitine may be considered in the management of acute neuropathic injury [255]. Current clinical evidence is subject to the inherent weaknesses of case series or reports. No information is available from the published randomized control trials [256].

Neuropathic injury is associated with activation of NMDA receptors and leads to long-term potentiation of pain. Ketamine infusions have been used to reduce acute neuropathic pain unresponsive to spinal bupivacaine and morphine [257]. Oral ketamine doses start with 100 mg daily, and are titrated by 40 mg until response [258]. A combination of memantine plus a brachial plexus block reduced postoperative phantom pain after acute traumatic upper extremity amputation [259]. Ketamine effectively reduced postherpetic neuralgia in a double-blind randomized crossover trial [260].

IV salmon calcitonin has been used to treat acute neuropathic pain after amputation, phantom limb pain, and complex regional pain syndrome [261,262]. It has been ineffective in complex regional pain syndromes. An IV dose of 200 international units compared to placebo significantly reduced phantom limb pain [263].

SUMMARY

In general, the majority of the evidence for guiding acute pain management is not based on randomized control trials [45]. Treatment is largely based on cohort studies. The exceptions to this are breakthrough pain trials and perioperative analgesics trials, [264]. PCA has been validated in surgical patients and postoperative pain but poorly validated in medical patients [264,265]. Pain improves predictably in the postoperative setting, which allows for routine weaning to oral analgesics. There is not an advantage of one adjuvant analgesic over another in any setting except for fentanyl and breakthrough pain. Gabapentin and nonopioid analgesics added to opioids improve surgical pain. There is less evidence for ketamine. Multidrug adjuvant analgesics combined with an opioid appear to be more efficacious than single adjuvant–opioid combinations in the postoperative setting, but more randomized trials are needed. Regional or spinal opioid–adjuvant(s) drug combinations are more effective than IV PCA for postoperative pain. In the emergence department, bolus hydromorphone, morphine, or fentanyl repeated 15 min later as needed reduces acute pain from trauma in most individuals. Ketamine appears to reduce acute traumatic pain, procedure-related pain and may be helpful in managing acute neuropathic pain. There is little evidence that ketamine is beneficial for cancer pain. For acute neuropathic pain, several adjuvants are beneficial. Single high-dose gabapentin relieves zoster pain quickly and is attractive when combined with opioids but the level of evidence for this is low and needs further validation. Preemptive venlafaxine for acute oxaliplatin neurotoxicity is effective in a randomized study. Individualized therapy and assessment are important to successful management of acute pain. High quality randomized trials are needed to confirm cohort studies and cohort experiences.

REFERENCES

1   Tremblay, J. and P. Hamet, Genetics of pain, opioids, and opioid responsiveness. *Metabolism*, 2010. **59**(Suppl 1): S5–S8.

2   Skeik, N. et al., Severe case and literature review of primary erythromelalgia: Novel SCN9A gene mutation. *Vasc Med*, 2012. **17**(1): 44–49.

3   Basbaum, A.I. et al., Cellular and molecular mechanisms of pain. *Cell*, 2009. **139**(2): 267–284.

4   Coderre, T.J. and J. Katz, Peripheral and central hyperexcitability: Differential signs and symptoms in persistent pain. *Behav Brain Sci*, 1997. **20**(3): 404–419; discussion 435–513.

5   Twycross, R., Cancer pain classification. *Acta Anaesthesiol Scand*, 1997. **41**(1 Pt 2): 141–145.

6   Raphael, J. et al., Cancer pain: Part 1: Pathophysiology; oncological, pharmacological, and psychological treatments: A perspective from the British Pain Society endorsed by the UK Association of Palliative Medicine and the Royal College of General Practitioners. *Pain Med*, 2010. **11**(5): 742–764.

7   Raphael, J. et al., Cancer pain: Part 2: Physical, interventional and complimentary therapies; management in the community; acute, treatment-related and complex cancer pain: A perspective from the British Pain Society endorsed by the UK Association of Palliative Medicine and the Royal College of General Practitioners. *Pain Med*, 2010. **11**(6): 872–896.

8   Fine, P.G., A.W. Burton, and S.D. Passik, Transformation of acute cancer pain to chronic cancer pain syndromes. *J Support Oncol*, 2012. **13**(1):1–4.

9   Sinatra, R., Causes and consequences of inadequate management of acute pain. *Pain Med*, 2010. **11**(12): 1859–1871.

10 Portenoy, R.K., Cancer pain: Pathophysiology and syndromes. *Lancet*, 1992. **339**(8800): 1026–1031.

11 Woolf, C.J. and M.W. Salter, Neuronal plasticity: Increasing the gain in pain. *Science*, 2000. **288**(5472): 1765–1769.

12 Woolf, C.J., Overcoming obstacles to developing new analgesics. *Nat Med*, 2010. **16**(11): 1241–1247.

13 Argoff, C., Mechanisms of pain transmission and pharmacologic management. *Curr Med Res Opin*, 2011. **27**(10): 2019–2031.

14 Gong, H.C. et al., Tissue-specific expression and gabapentin-binding properties of calcium channel alpha2delta subunit subtypes. *J Membr Biol*, 2001. **184**(1): 35–43.

15 Brown, J.P. and N.S. Gee, Cloning and deletion mutagenesis of the alpha2 delta calcium channel subunit from porcine cerebral cortex. Expression of a soluble form of the protein that retains [3H]gabapentin binding activity. *J Biol Chem*, 1998. **273**(39): 25458–25465.

16 Eroglu, C. et al., Gabapentin receptor alpha2delta-1 is a neuronal thrombospondin receptor responsible for excitatory CNS synaptogenesis. *Cell*, 2009. **139**(2): 380–392.

17 Latremoliere, A. and C.J. Woolf, Central sensitization: A generator of pain hypersensitivity by central neural plasticity. *J Pain*, 2009. **10**(9): 895–926.

18 Tsuda, M., K. Inoue, and M.W. Salter, Neuropathic pain and spinal microglia: A big problem from molecules in "small" glia. *Trends Neurosci*, 2005. **28**(2): 101–107.

19 Moss, A. et al., Spinal microglia and neuropathic pain in young rats. *Pain*, 2007. **128**(3): 215–224.

20 Kuner, R., Central mechanisms of pathological pain. *Nat Med*, 2010. **16**(11): 1258–1266.

21 Ren, K. and R. Dubner, Neuron-glia crosstalk gets serious: Role in pain hypersensitivity. *Curr Opin Anaesthesiol*, 2008. **21**(5): 570–579.

22 Luger, N.M. et al., Bone cancer pain: From model to mechanism to therapy. *J Pain Symptom Manage*, 2005. **29**(5 Suppl): S32–S46.

23 Angst, M.S. et al., Short-term infusion of the mu-opioid agonist remifentanil in humans causes hyperalgesia during withdrawal. *Pain*, 2003. **106**(1–2): 49–57.

24 Koppert, W. et al., Differential modulation of remifentanil-induced analgesia and postinfusion hyperalgesia by S-ketamine and clonidine in humans. *Anesthesiology*, 2003. **99**(1): 152–159.

25 Koppert, W. et al., The effects of intradermal fentanyl and ketamine on capsaicin-induced secondary hyperalgesia and flare reaction. *Anesth Analg*, 1999. **89**(6): 1521–1527.

26 Angst, M.S. and J.D. Clark, Opioid-induced hyperalgesia: A qualitative systematic review. *Anesthesiology*, 2006. **104**(3): 570–587.

27 Chu, L.F., M.S. Angst, and D. Clark, Opioid-induced hyperalgesia in humans: Molecular mechanisms and clinical considerations. *Clin J Pain*, 2008. **24**(6): 479–496.

28 Li, X., M.S. Angst, and J.D. Clark, Opioid-induced hyperalgesia and incisional pain. *Anesth Analg*, 2001. **93**(1): 204–209.

29 Gardell, L.R. et al., Opioid receptor-mediated hyperalgesia and antinociceptive tolerance induced by sustained opiate delivery. *Neurosci Lett*, 2006. **396**(1): 44–49.

30 Ossipov, M.H. et al., Antinociceptive and nociceptive actions of opioids. *J Neurobiol*, 2004. **61**(1): 126–148.

31 Vanderah, T.W. et al., Tonic descending facilitation from the rostral ventromedial medulla mediates opioid-induced abnormal pain and antinociceptive tolerance. *J Neurosci*, 2001. **21**(1): 279–286.

32 Koppert, W. et al., The cyclooxygenase isozyme inhibitors parecoxib and paracetamol reduce central hyperalgesia in humans. *Pain*, 2004. **108**(1–2): 148–153.

33 Koppert, W. et al., Different profiles of buprenorphine-induced analgesia and antihyperalgesia in a human pain model. *Pain*, 2005. **118**(1–2): 15–22.

34 Koppert, W. et al., Low-dose lidocaine suppresses experimentally induced hyperalgesia in humans. *Anesthesiology*, 1998. **89**(6): 1345–1353.

35 Koppert, W. et al., Low-dose lidocaine reduces secondary hyperalgesia by a central mode of action. *Pain*, 2000. **85**(1–2): 217–224.

36 Koppert, W. et al., A new model of electrically evoked pain and hyperalgesia in human skin: The effects of intravenous alfentanil, S(+)-ketamine, and lidocaine. *Anesthesiology*, 2001. **95**(2): 395–402.

37 Helfand, M. and M. Freeman, Washington (DC): Department of Veterans Affairs (US); 2008 Apr.

38 Dworkin, R.H. et al., Interpreting the clinical importance of group differences in chronic pain clinical trials: IMMPACT recommendations. *Pain*, 2009. **146**(3): 238–244.

39 Farrar, J.T., Cut-points for the measurement of pain: The choice depends on what you want to study. *Pain*, 2010. **149**(2): 163–164.

40 Farrar, J.T., Advances in clinical research methodology for pain clinical trials. *Nat Med*, 2010. **16**(11): 1284–1293.

41 Farrar, J.T., J.A. Berlin, and B.L. Strom, Clinically important changes in acute pain outcome measures: A validation study. *J Pain Symptom Manage*, 2003. **25**(5): 406–411.

42 Farrar, J.T., What is clinically meaningful: Outcome measures in pain clinical trials. *Clin J Pain*, 2000. **16**(2 Suppl): S106–S112.

43 Farrar, J.T., R.H. Dworkin, and M.B. Max, Use of the cumulative proportion of responders analysis graph to present pain data over a range of cut-off points: Making clinical trial data more understandable. *J Pain Symptom Manage*, 2006. **31**(4): 369–377.

44 Farrar, J.T. et al., The clinical importance of changes in the 0 to 10 numeric rating scale for worst, least, and average pain intensity: Analyses of data from clinical trials of duloxetine in pain disorders. *J Pain*, 2010. **11**(2): 109–118.

45 Macintyre, P.E. and S.M. Walker, The scientific evidence for acute pain treatment. *Curr Opin Anaesthesiol*, 2010. **23**(5): 623–628.

46 Dworkin, R.H. et al., Research design considerations for confirmatory chronic pain clinical trials: IMMPACT recommendations. *Pain*, 2010. **149**(2): 177–193.

47 Ripamonti, C.I., E. Bandieri, and F. Roila, Management of cancer pain: ESMO Clinical Practice Guidelines. *Ann Oncol*, 2011. **22**(Suppl 6): vi69–vi77.

48 Macintyre, P.E., W.B. Runciman, and R.K. Webb, An acute pain service in an Australian teaching hospital: The first year. *Med J Aust*, 1990. **153**(7): 417–421.

49 Walker, S.M. et al., Acute pain management: Current best evidence provides guide for improved practice. *Pain Med*, 2006. **7**(1): 3–5.

50 Caraceni, A. et al., Use of opioid analgesics in the treatment of cancer pain: Evidence-based recommendations from the EAPC. *Lancet Oncol*, 2012. **13**(2): e58–e68.

51 Roe, B.B., Are postoperative narcotics necessary? *Arch Surg*, 1963. **87**: 912–915.

52 Sechzer, P.H., Studies in pain with the analgesic-demand system. *Anesth Analg*, 1971. **50**(1): 1–10.

53 Evans, J.M. et al., Letter: Patient-controlled intravenous narcotic administration during labour. *Lancet*, 1976. **1**(7965): 906–907.

54 Thomas, N., Pain control: Patient and staff perceptions of PCA. *Nurs Stand*, 1993. **7**(28): 37–39.

55 Richman, J.M. and C.L. Wu, Epidural analgesia for postoperative pain. *Anesthesiol Clin North America*, 2005. **23**(1): 125–140.

56 Upton, R.N., T.J. Semple, and P.E. Macintyre, Pharmacokinetic optimisation of opioid treatment in acute pain therapy. *Clin Pharmacokinet*, 1997. **33**(3): 225–244.

57 Waters, C.M. et al., Uptake of fentanyl in pulmonary endothelium. *J Pharmacol Exp Ther*, 1999. **288**(1): 157–163.

58 Henthorn, T.K. et al., Transporter-mediated pulmonary endothelial uptake of fentanyl. *Int J Clin Pharmacol Ther*, 1998. **36**(2): 74–75.

59 Henthorn, T.K. et al., Active transport of fentanyl by the blood-brain barrier. *J Pharmacol Exp Ther*, 1999. **289**(2): 1084–1089.

60 Bostrom, E., U.S. Simonsson, and M. Hammarlund-Udenaes, In vivo blood-brain barrier transport of oxycodone in the rat: Indications for active influx and implications for pharmacokinetics/pharmacodynamics. *Drug Metab Dispos*, 2006. **34**(9): 1624–1631.

61 Aquilante, C.L. et al., Increased brain P-glycoprotein in morphine tolerant rats. *Life Sci*, 2000. **66**(4): PL47–PL51.

62 Nakazawa, Y. et al., Drug-drug interaction between oxycodone and adjuvant analgesics in blood-brain barrier transport and antinociceptive effect. *J Pharm Sci*, 2010. **99**(1): 467–474.

63 Ayrton, A. and P. Morgan, Role of transport proteins in drug absorption, distribution and excretion. *Xenobiotica*, 2001. **31**(8–9): 469–497.

64 Elkiweri, I.A. et al., Competitive substrates for P-glycoprotein and organic anion protein transporters differentially reduce blood organ transport of fentanyl and loperamide: Pharmacokinetics and pharmacodynamics in Sprague-Dawley rats. *Anesth Analg*, 2009. **108**(1): 149–159.

65 Marier, J.F. et al., Enhancing the uptake of dextromethorphan in the CNS of rats by concomitant administration of the P-gp inhibitor verapamil. *Life Sci*, 2005. **77**(23): 2911–2926.

66 Upton, R.N., Cerebral uptake of drugs in humans. *Clin Exp Pharmacol Physiol*, 2007. **34**(8): 695–701.

67 Herd, D. and M. Borland, Intranasal fentanyl paediatric clinical practice guidelines. *Emerg Med Australas*, 2009. **21**(4): 335.

68 Geppetti, P. and S. Benemei, Pain treatment with opioids: Achieving the minimal effective and the minimal interacting dose. *Clin Drug Investig*, 2009. **29**(Suppl 1): 3–16.

69 Dickenson, A.H., Plasticity: Implications for opioid and other pharmacological interventions in specific pain states. *Behav Brain Sci*, 1997. **20**(3): 392–403; discussion 435–513.

70 Dahl, J.B. and S. Moiniche, Pre-emptive analgesia. *Br Med Bull*, 2004. **71**: 13–27.

71 Grape, S. and M.R. Tramer, Do we need preemptive analgesia for the treatment of postoperative pain? *Best Pract Res Clin Anaesthesiol*, 2007. **21**(1): 51–63.

72 Aubrun, F. et al., Predictive factors of severe postoperative pain in the postanesthesia care unit. *Anesth Analg*, 2008. **106**(5): 1535–1541, table of contents.

73 Hariharan, S. et al., The effect of preemptive analgesia in postoperative pain relief—A prospective double-blind randomized study. *Pain Med*, 2009. **10**(1): 49–53.

74 Buvanendran, A. and J.S. Kroin, Multimodal analgesia for controlling acute postoperative pain. *Curr Opin Anaesthesiol*, 2009. **22**(5): 588–593.

75 Katz, J., Pre-emptive analgesia: Evidence, current status and future directions. *Eur J Anaesthesiol Suppl*, 1995. **10**: 8–13.

76 Angst, M.S. and J.D. Clark, Ketamine for managing perioperative pain in opioid-dependent patients with chronic pain: A unique indication? *Anesthesiology*, 2010. **113**(3): 514–515.

77 Straube, S. et al., Single dose oral gabapentin for established acute postoperative pain in adults. *Cochrane Database Syst Rev*, 2010(5): CD008183.

78 Loftus, R.W. et al., Intraoperative ketamine reduces perioperative opiate consumption in opiate-dependent patients with chronic back pain undergoing back surgery. *Anesthesiology*, 2010. **113**(3): 639–646.

79 Ong, C.K. et al., The efficacy of preemptive analgesia for acute postoperative pain management: A meta-analysis. *Anesth Analg*, 2005. **100**(3): 757–773, table of contents.

80 Schmid, R.L., A.N. Sandler, and J. Katz, Use and efficacy of low-dose ketamine in the management of acute postoperative pain: A review of current techniques and outcomes. *Pain*, 1999. **82**(2): 111–125.

81 Tiippana, E.M. et al., Do surgical patients benefit from perioperative gabapentin/pregabalin? A systematic review of efficacy and safety. *Anesth Analg*, 2007. **104**(6): 1545–1556, table of contents.

82 Kong, V.K. and M.G. Irwin, Gabapentin: A multimodal perioperative drug? *Br J Anaesth*, 2007. **99**(6): 775–786.

83 Seib, R.K. and J.E. Paul, Preoperative gabapentin for postoperative analgesia: A meta-analysis. *Can J Anaesth*, 2006. **53**(5): 461–469.

84 Ho, K.Y., T.J. Gan, and A.S. Habib, Gabapentin and postoperative pain—A systematic review of randomized controlled trials. *Pain*, 2006. **126**(1–3): 91–101.

85 Prabhakar, H. et al., The analgesic effects of preemptive gabapentin in patients undergoing surgery for brachial plexus injury—A preliminary study. *J Neurosurg Anesthesiol*, 2007. **19**(4): 235–238.

86 Amr, Y.M. and A.A. Yousef, Evaluation of efficacy of the perioperative administration of Venlafaxine or gabapentin on acute and chronic postmastectomy pain. *Clin J Pain*, 2010. **26**(5): 381–385.

87 Fassoulaki, A. et al., The analgesic effect of gabapentin and mexiletine after breast surgery for cancer. *Anesth Analg*, 2002. **95**(4): 985–991, table of contents.

88 Sen, H. et al., A comparison of gabapentin and ketamine in acute and chronic pain after hysterectomy. *Anesth Analg*, 2009. **109**(5): 1645–1650.

89 Fassoulaki, A. et al., A combination of gabapentin and local anaesthetics attenuates acute and late pain after abdominal hysterectomy. *Eur J Anaesthesiol*, 2007. **24**(6): 521–528.

90   Fassoulaki, A. et al., Multimodal analgesia with gabapentin and local anesthetics prevents acute and chronic pain after breast surgery for cancer. *Anesth Analg*, 2005. **101**(5): 1427–1432.

91   Parsa, A.A. et al., Combined preoperative use of celecoxib and gabapentin in the management of postoperative pain. *Aesthetic Plast Surg*, 2009. **33**(1): 98–103.

92   Durmus, M. et al., The post-operative analgesic effects of a combination of gabapentin and paracetamol in patients undergoing abdominal hysterectomy: A randomized clinical trial. *Acta Anaesthesiol Scand*, 2007. **51**(3): 299–304.

93   Rasmussen, M.L. et al., Multimodal analgesia with gabapentin, ketamine and dexamethasone in combination with paracetamol and ketorolac after hip arthroplasty: A preliminary study. *Eur J Anaesthesiol*, 2010. **27**(4): 324–330.

94   Fassoulaki, A. et al., Regional block and mexiletine: The effect on pain after cancer breast surgery. *Reg Anesth Pain Med*, 2001. **26**(3): 223–228.

95   Kehlet, H., T.S. Jensen, and C.J. Woolf, Persistent postsurgical pain: Risk factors and prevention. *Lancet*, 2006. **367**(9522): 1618–1625.

96   Momeni, M., M. Crucitti, and M. De Kock, Patient-controlled analgesia in the management of postoperative pain. *Drugs*, 2006. **66**(18): 2321–2337.

97   Dolin, S.J., J.N. Cashman, and J.M. Bland, Effectiveness of acute postoperative pain management: I. Evidence from published data. *Br J Anaesth*, 2002. **89**(3): 409–423.

98   Cashman, J.N. and S.J. Dolin, Respiratory and haemodynamic effects of acute postoperative pain management: Evidence from published data. *Br J Anaesth*, 2004. **93**(2): 212–223.

99   Fero, K.E. et al., Pharmacologic management of postoperative nausea and vomiting. *Expert Opin Pharmacother*, 2011. **12**(15): 2283–2296.

100 Dimitriou, V. and G.S. Voyagis, Opioid-induced pruritus: Repeated vs single dose ondansetron administration in preventing pruritus after intrathecal morphine. *Br J Anaesth*, 1999. **83**(5): 822–823.

101 Reich, A. and J.C. Szepietowski, Opioid-induced pruritus: An update. *Clin Exp Dermatol*, 2010. **35**(1): 2–6.

102 Mitra, S. and R.S. Sinatra, Perioperative management of acute pain in the opioid-dependent patient. *Anesthesiology*, 2004. **101**(1): 212–227.

103 Carroll, I.R., M.S. Angst, and J.D. Clark, Management of perioperative pain in patients chronically consuming opioids. *Reg Anesth Pain Med*, 2004. **29**(6): 576–591.

104 Carvalho, B. et al., Single-dose, extended-release epidural morphine (DepoDur) compared to conventional epidural morphine for post-cesarean pain. *Anesth Analg*, 2007. **105**(1): 176–183.

105 Viscusi, E.R., Emerging techniques in the management of acute pain: Epidural analgesia. *Anesth Analg*, 2005. **101**(5 Suppl): S23–S29.

106 Hartrick, C.T. and K.A. Hartrick, Extended-release epidural morphine (DepoDur): Review and safety analysis. *Expert Rev Neurother*, 2008. **8**(11): 1641–1648.

107 Viscusi, E.R., Patient-controlled drug delivery for acute postoperative pain management: A review of current and emerging technologies. *Reg Anesth Pain Med*, 2008. **33**(2): 146–158.

108 Simpson, T. et al., The effects of epidural versus parenteral opioid analgesia on postoperative pain and pulmonary function in adults who have undergone thoracic and abdominal surgery: A critique of research. *Heart Lung*, 1992. **21**(2): 125–138.

109 Etches, R.C., A.N. Sandler, and M.D. Daley, Respiratory depression and spinal opioids. *Can J Anaesth*, 1989. **36**(2): 165–185.

110 Dixon, J.M. and R.L. Carver, Daily chlorhexidine gluconate bathing with impregnated cloths results in statistically significant reduction in central line-associated bloodstream infections. *Am J Infect Control*, 2010. **38**(10): 817–821.

111 Heitz, J.W., T.A. Witkowski, and E.R. Viscusi, New and emerging analgesics and analgesic technologies for acute pain management. *Curr Opin Anaesthesiol*, 2009. **22**(5): 608–617.

112 Popping, D.M. et al., Effectiveness and safety of postoperative pain management: A survey of 18 925 consecutive patients between 1998 and 2006 (2nd revision): A database analysis of prospectively raised data. *Br J Anaesth*, 2008. **101**(6): 832–840.

113 Asenjo, J.F. and K.M. Brecht, Opioids: Other routes for use in recovery room. *Curr Drug Targets*, 2005. **6**(7): 773–779.

114 Viscusi, E.R. et al., Patient-controlled transdermal fentanyl hydrochloride vs intravenous morphine pump for postoperative pain: A randomized controlled trial. *JAMA*, 2004. **291**(11): 1333–1341.

115 Viscusi, E.R. et al., The safety and efficacy of fentanyl iontophoretic transdermal system compared with morphine intravenous patient-controlled analgesia for postoperative pain management: An analysis of pooled data from three randomized, active-controlled clinical studies. *Anesth Analg*, 2007. **105**(5): 1428–1436, table of contents.

116 Viscusi, E.R. et al., An iontophoretic fentanyl patient-activated analgesic delivery system for postoperative pain: A double-blind, placebo-controlled trial. *Anesth Analg*, 2006. **102**(1): 188–194.

117 Mattia, C. and F. Coluzzi, Acute postoperative pain management: Focus on iontophoretic transdermal fentanyl. *Ther Clin Risk Manag*, 2007. **3**(1): 19–27.

118 McDougall, J.J., Arthritis and pain. Neurogenic origin of joint pain. *Arthritis Res Ther*, 2006. **8**(6): 220.

119 Li, C.Y. et al., Calcium channel alpha2delta1 subunit mediates spinal hyperexcitability in pain modulation. *Pain*, 2006. **125**(1–2): 20–34.

120 Caraceni, A. et al., Gabapentin for breakthrough pain due to bone metastases. *Palliat Med*, 2008. **22**(4): 392–393.

121 Donovan-Rodriguez, T., A.H. Dickenson, and C.E. Urch, Gabapentin normalizes spinal neuronal responses that correlate with behavior in a rat model of cancer-induced bone pain. *Anesthesiology*, 2005. **102**(1): 132–140.

122 Fernihough, J. et al., Pain related behaviour in two models of osteoarthritis in the rat knee. *Pain*, 2004. **112**(1–2): 83–93.

123 Ivanavicius, S.P. et al., Structural pathology in a rodent model of osteoarthritis is associated with neuropathic pain: Increased expression of ATF-3 and pharmacological characterisation. *Pain*, 2007. **128**(3): 272–282.

124 Pedulla, E. et al., Neuropathic pain in temporomandibular joint disorders: Case-control analysis by MR imaging. *Am J Neuroradiol*, 2009. **30**(7): 1414–1418.

125 Bajaj, P., T. Graven-Nielsen, and L. Arendt-Nielsen, Osteoarthritis and its association with muscle hyperalgesia: An experimental controlled study. *Pain*, 2001. **93**(2): 107–114.

126 Buescher, J.S., S. Meadows, and J. Saseen, Clinical inquiries. Does acetaminophen and NSAID combined relieve osteoarthritis pain better than either alone? *J Fam Pract*, 2004. **53**(6): 501–503.

127 Jimenez-Andrade, J.M. et al., Bone cancer pain. *Ann N Y Acad Sci*, 2010. **1198**: 173–181.

128 Costa, L., A. Lipton, and R.E. Coleman, Role of bisphosphonates for the management of skeletal complications and bone pain from skeletal metastases. *Support Cancer Ther*, 2006. **3**(3): 143–153.

129 Lyritis, G.P. et al., Analgesic effect of salmon calcitonin suppositories in patients with acute pain due to recent osteoporotic vertebral crush fractures: A prospective double-blind, randomized, placebo-controlled clinical study. *Clin J Pain*, 1999. **15**(4): 284–289.

130 Kadow, C. and J.C. Gingell, Salmon calcitonin for bone pain in patients with metastatic carcinoma of the prostate. A pilot study. *Br J Clin Pract*, 1988. **42**(1): 24–25.

131 Lyritis, G.P. et al., Pain relief from nasal salmon calcitonin in osteoporotic vertebral crush fractures. A double blind, placebo-controlled clinical study. *Acta Orthop Scand Suppl*, 1997. **275**: 112–114.

132 Kyrgidis, A. and K.A. Toulis, Denosumab-related osteonecrosis of the jaws. *Osteoporos Int*, 2011. **22**(1): 369–370.

133 Henry, D.H. et al., Randomized, double-blind study of denosumab versus zoledronic acid in the treatment of bone metastases in patients with advanced cancer (excluding breast and prostate cancer) or multiple myeloma. *J Clin Oncol*, 2011. **29**(9): 1125–1132.

134 Bove, S.E. et al., New advances in musculoskeletal pain. *Brain Res Rev*, 2009. **60**(1): 187–201.

135 Nagashima, H. et al., Preliminary assessment of the safety and efficacy of tanezumab in Japanese patients with moderate to severe osteoarthritis of the knee: A randomized, double-blind, dose-escalation, placebo-controlled study. *Osteoarthritis Cartilage*, 2011. **19**(12): 1405–1412.

136 Mercadante, S., Malignant bone pain: Pathophysiology and treatment. *Pain*, 1997. **69**(1–2): 1–18.

137 Portenoy, R.K., Managing cancer pain poorly responsive to systemic opioid therapy. *Oncology (Williston Park)*, 1999. **13**(5 Suppl 2): 25–29.

138 Halvorson, K.G. et al., Similarities and differences in tumor growth, skeletal remodeling and pain in an osteolytic and osteoblastic model of bone cancer. *Clin J Pain*, 2006. **22**(7): 587–600.

139 Kerba, M. et al., Neuropathic pain features in patients with bone metastases referred for palliative radiotherapy. *J Clin Oncol*, 2010. **28**(33): 4892–4897.

140 Geis, C. et al., Evoked pain behavior and spinal glia activation is dependent on tumor necrosis factor receptor 1 and 2 in a mouse model of bone cancer pain. *Neuroscience*, 2010. **169**(1): 463–474.

141 Heras, P. et al., A comparative study of intravenous ibandronate and pamindronate in patients with bone metastases from breast or lung cancer: Effect on metastatic bone pain. *Am J Ther*, 2011. **18**(5): 340–342.

142 Pecherstorfer, M. and I.J. Diel, Rapid administration of ibandronate does not affect renal functioning: Evidence from clinical studies in metastatic bone disease and hypercalcaemia of malignancy. *Support Care Cancer*, 2004. **12**(12): 877–881.

143 Halvorson, K.G. et al., Intravenous ibandronate rapidly reduces pain, neurochemical indices of central sensitization, tumor burden, and skeletal destruction in a mouse model of bone cancer. *J Pain Symptom Manage*, 2008. **36**(3): 289–303.

144 Diel, I.J. et al., Bone pain reduction in patients with metastatic breast cancer treated with ibandronate-results from a post-marketing surveillance study. *Support Care Cancer*, 2010. **18**(10): 1305–1312.

145 Mancini, I., J.C. Dumon, and J.J. Body, Efficacy and safety of ibandronate in the treatment of opioid-resistant bone pain associated with metastatic bone disease: A pilot study. *J Clin Oncol*, 2004. **22**(17): 3587–3592.

146 Heras, P. et al., A comparative study of intravenous ibandronate and pamindronate in patients with bone metastases from breast or lung cancer: Effect on metastatic bone pain. *Am J Ther*, 2011. **18**(5): 340–342.

147 Luger, N.M. et al., Osteoprotegerin diminishes advanced bone cancer pain. *Cancer Res*, 2001. **61**(10): 4038–4047.

148 McGrath, E.E., OPG/RANKL/RANK pathway as a therapeutic target in cancer. *J Thorac Oncol*, 2011. **6**(9): 1468–1473.

149 Rove, K.O. and E.D. Crawford, Evolution of treatment options for patients with CRPC and bone metastases: Bone-targeted agents that go beyond palliation of symptoms to improve overall survival. *Oncology (Williston Park)*, 2011. **25**(14): 1362–1370, 1375–1381, 1387.

150 Patanwala, A.E., S.M. Keim, and B.L. Erstad, Intravenous opioids for severe acute pain in the emergency department. *Ann Pharmacother*, 2010. **44**(11): 1800–1809.

151 Birnbaum, A. et al., Randomized double-blind placebo-controlled trial of two intravenous morphine dosages (0.10 mg/kg and 0.15 mg/kg) in emergency department patients with moderate to severe acute pain. *Ann Emerg Med*, 2007. **49**(4): 445–453, 453 e1–e2.

152 Chang, A.K. et al., Efficacy and safety profile of a single dose of hydromorphone compared with morphine in older adults with acute, severe pain: A prospective, randomized, double-blind clinical trial. *Am J Geriatr Pharmacother*, 2009. **7**(1): 1–10.

153 Galinski, M. et al., A randomized, double-blind study comparing morphine with fentanyl in prehospital analgesia. *Am J Emerg Med*, 2005. **23**(2): 114–119.

154 Silfvast, T. and L. Saarnivaara, Comparison of alfentanil and morphine in the prehospital treatment of patients with acute ischaemic-type chest pain. *Eur J Emerg Med*, 2001. **8**(4): 275–278.

155 Chang, A.K. et al., Randomized clinical trial comparing a patient-driven titration protocol of intravenous hydromorphone with traditional physician-driven management of emergency department patients with acute severe pain. *Ann Emerg Med*, 2009. **54**(4): 561–567 e2.

156 Thomas, S.H. et al., Fentanyl trauma analgesia use in air medical scene transports. *J Emerg Med*, 2005. **29**(2): 179–187.

157 Borland, M.L., I. Jacobs, and G. Geelhoed, Intranasal fentanyl reduces acute pain in children in the emergency department: A safety and efficacy study. *Emerg Med (Fremantle)*, 2002. **14**(3): 275–280.

158 Borland, M. et al., A randomized controlled trial comparing intranasal fentanyl to intravenous morphine for managing acute pain in children in the emergency department. *Ann Emerg Med*, 2007. **49**(3): 335–340.

159 Rickard, C. et al., A randomized controlled trial of intranasal fentanyl vs intravenous morphine for analgesia in the prehospital setting. *Am J Emerg Med*, 2007. **25**(8): 911–917.

160 Portenoy, R.K., D. Payne, and P. Jacobsen, Breakthrough pain: Characteristics and impact in patients with cancer pain. *Pain*, 1999. **81**(1–2): 129–134.

161 Davis, M.P., Recent development in therapeutics for breakthrough pain. *Expert Rev Neurother*, 2010. **10**(5): 757–773.

162 Grape, S. et al., Formulations of fentanyl for the management of pain. *Drugs*, 2010. **70**(1): 57–72.

163 Coluzzi, P.H. et al., Breakthrough cancer pain: A randomized trial comparing oral transmucosal fentanyl citrate (OTFC) and morphine sulfate immediate release (MSIR). *Pain*, 2001. **91**(1–2): 123–130.

164 Mercadante, S. et al., The use of opioids for breakthrough pain in acute palliative care unit by using doses proportional to opioid basal regimen. *Clin J Pain*, 2010. **26**(4): 306–309.

165 Fentanyl buccal soluble film (Onsolis) for breakthrough cancer pain. *Med Lett Drugs Ther*, 2010. **52**(1336): 30–31.

166 Rauck, R. et al., Fentanyl buccal soluble film (FBSF) for breakthrough pain in patients with cancer: A randomized, double-blind, placebo-controlled study. *Ann Oncol*, 2010. **21**(6): 1308–1314.

167 Mercadante, S., P. Ferrera, and E. Arcuri, The use of fentanyl buccal tablets as breakthrough medication in patients receiving chronic methadone therapy: An open label preliminary study. *Support Care Cancer*, 2011 ;**19**(3):435-8.

168 Passik, S.D. et al., Aberrant drug-related behavior observed during clinical studies involving patients taking chronic opioid therapy for persistent pain and fentanyl buccal tablet for breakthrough pain. *J Pain Symptom Manage*, 2010. [epub ahead of print]

169 Fine, P.G., A. Narayana, and S.D. Passik, Treatment of breakthrough pain with fentanyl buccal tablet in opioid-tolerant patients with chronic pain: Appropriate patient selection and management. *Pain Med*, 2010. **11**(7): 1024–1036.

170 Paech, M.J. et al., A new formulation of nasal fentanyl spray for postoperative analgesia: A pilot study. *Anaesthesia*, 2003. **58**(8): 740–744.

171 Panagiotou, I. and K. Mystakidou, Intranasal fentanyl: From pharmacokinetics and bioavailability to current treatment applications. *Expert Rev Anticancer Ther*, 2010. **10**(7): 1009–1021.

172 Vissers, D. et al., Efficacy of intranasal fentanyl spray versus other opioids for breakthrough pain in cancer. *Curr Med Res Opin*, 2010. **26**(5): 1037–1045.

173 Portenoy, R.K. et al., A multicenter, placebo-controlled, double-blind, multiple-crossover study of Fentanyl Pectin Nasal Spray (FPNS) in the treatment of breakthrough cancer pain. *Pain*, 2010. **151**(3): 617–624.

174 Portenoy, R.K. et al., Long-term safety, tolerability, and consistency of effect of fentanyl pectin nasal spray for breakthrough cancer pain in opioid-tolerant patients. *J Opioid Manag*, 2010. **6**(5): 319–328.

175 Taylor, D. et al., Fentanyl pectin nasal spray in breakthrough cancer pain. *J Support Oncol*, 2010. **8**(4): 184–190.

176 Lossignol, D.A. and C. Dumitrescu, Breakthrough pain: Progress in management. *Curr Opin Oncol*, 2010. **22**(4): 302–306.

177 Hagelberg, N.M. and K.T. Olkkola, Fentanyl for breakthrough cancer pain—What's new? *Pain*, 2010. **151**(3): 565–566.

178 Foster, D. et al., Pharmacokinetics and pharmacodynamics of intranasal versus intravenous fentanyl in patients with pain after oral surgery. *Ann Pharmacother*, 2008. **42**(10): 1380–1387.

179 Toussaint, S. et al., Patient-controlled intranasal analgesia: Effective alternative to intravenous PCA for postoperative pain relief. *Can J Anaesth*, 2000. **47**(4): 299–302.

180 Vercauteren, M. et al., Intranasal sufentanil for pre-operative sedation. *Anaesthesia*, 1988. **43**(4): 270–273.

181 Haynes, G., N.H. Brahen, and H.F. Hill, Plasma sufentanil concentration after intranasal administration to paediatric outpatients. *Can J Anaesth*, 1993. **40**(3): 286.

182 Mathieu, N. et al., Intranasal sufentanil is effective for postoperative analgesia in adults. *Can J Anaesth*, 2006. **53**(1): 60–66.

183 Wu, H. et al., Intravenous flurbiprofen axetil can increase analgesic effect in refractory cancer pain. *J Exp Clin Cancer Res*, 2009. **28**: 33.

184 Nolli, M., G. Apolone, and F. Nicosia, Postoperative analgesia in Italy. National survey on the anaesthetist's beliefs, opinions, behaviour and techniques in postoperative pain control in Italy. *Acta Anaesthesiol Scand*, 1997. **41**(5): 573–580.

185 Allen, S.C. and D. Ravindran, Perioperative use of nonsteroidal anti-inflammatory drugs: Results of a UK regional audit. *Clin Drug Investig*, 2009. **29**(11): 703–711.

186 Leeson, R.M. et al., Dyloject, a novel injectable diclofenac formulation, offers greater safety and efficacy than voltarol for postoperative dental pain. *Reg Anesth Pain Med*, 2007. **32**(4): 303–310.

187 Izquierdo, E. et al., Postoperative analgesia in herniated disk surgery. Comparative study of diclofenac, lysine acetylsalicylate, and ketorolac. *Rev Esp Anestesiol Reanim*, 1995. **42**(8): 316–319.

188 Gan, T.J., Diclofenac: An update on its mechanism of action and safety profile. *Curr Med Res Opin*, 2010. **26**(7): 1715–1731.

189 Southworth, S. et al., A multicenter, randomized, double-blind, placebo-controlled trial of intravenous ibuprofen 400 and 800 mg every 6 hours in the management of postoperative pain. *Clin Ther*, 2009. **31**(9): 1922–1935.

190 Vadivelu, N., S. Mitra, and D. Narayan, Recent advances in postoperative pain management. *Yale J Biol Med*, 2010. **83**(1): 11–25.

191 Duggan, S.T. and L.J. Scott, Intravenous paracetamol (acetaminophen). *Drugs*, 2009. **69**(1): 101–113.

192 Cattabriga, I. et al., Intravenous paracetamol as adjunctive treatment for postoperative pain after cardiac surgery: A double blind randomized controlled trial. *Eur J Cardiothorac Surg*, 2007. **32**(3): 527–531.

193 Ohnesorge, H. et al., Paracetamol versus metamizol in the treatment of postoperative pain after breast surgery: A randomized, controlled trial. *Eur J Anaesthesiol*, 2009. **26**(8): 648–653.

194 Tzschentke, T.M. et al., Tapentadol hydrochloride: A next-generation, centrally acting analgesic with two mechanisms of action in a single molecule. *Drugs Today (Barc)*, 2009. **45**(7): 483–496.

195 Wade, W.E. and W.J. Spruill, Tapentadol hydrochloride: A centrally acting oral analgesic. *Clin Ther*, 2009. **31**(12): 2804–2818.

196 Hartrick, C.T., Tapentadol immediate release for the relief of moderate-to-severe acute pain. *Expert Opin Pharmacother*, 2009. **10**(16): 2687–2696.

197 Hartrick, C. et al., Efficacy and tolerability of tapentadol immediate release and oxycodone HCl immediate release in patients awaiting primary joint replacement surgery for end-stage joint disease: A 10-day, phase III, randomized, double-blind, active- and placebo-controlled study. *Clin Ther*, 2009. **31**(2): 260–271.

198 Daniels, S.E. et al., A randomized, double-blind, phase III study comparing multiple doses of tapentadol IR, oxycodone IR, and placebo for postoperative (bunionectomy) pain. *Curr Med Res Opin*, 2009. **25**(3): 765–776.

199 Dauri, M. et al., Gabapentin and pregabalin for the acute post-operative pain management. A systematic-narrative review of the recent clinical evidences. *Curr Drug Targets*, 2009. **10**(8): 716–733.

200 Hurley, R.W. et al., The analgesic effects of perioperative gabapentin on postoperative pain: A meta-analysis. *Reg Anesth Pain Med*, 2006. **31**(3): 237–247.

201 Peng, P.W., D.N. Wijeysundera, and C.C. Li, Use of gabapentin for perioperative pain control—A meta-analysis. *Pain Res Manag*, 2007. **12**(2): 85–92.

202 Mathiesen, O., S. Moiniche, and J.B. Dahl, Gabapentin and postoperative pain: A qualitative and quantitative systematic review, with focus on procedure. *BMC Anesthesiol*, 2007. **7**: 6.

203 Gilron, I., Gabapentin and pregabalin for chronic neuropathic and early postsurgical pain: Current evidence and future directions. *Curr Opin Anaesthesiol*, 2007. **20**(5): 456–472.

204 Durkin, B., C. Page, and P. Glass, Pregabalin for the treatment of postsurgical pain. *Expert Opin Pharmacother*, 2010. **11**(16): 2751–2758.

205 Geisslinger, G. et al., Pharmacokinetics and pharmacodynamics of ketamine enantiomers in surgical patients using a stereoselective analytical method. *Br J Anaesth*, 1993. **70**(6): 666–671.

206 Bell, R.F. et al., Perioperative ketamine for acute postoperative pain. *Cochrane Database Syst Rev*, 2006(1): CD004603.

207 Adam, F. et al., Small-dose ketamine infusion improves postoperative analgesia and rehabilitation after total knee arthroplasty. *Anesth Analg*, 2005. **100**(2): 475–480.

208 Kwok, R.F. et al., Preoperative ketamine improves postoperative analgesia after gynecologic laparoscopic surgery. *Anesth Analg*, 2004. **98**(4): 1044–1049, table of contents.

209 Heidari, S.M. et al., Effect of oral ketamine on the postoperative pain and analgesic requirement following orthopedic surgery. *Acta Anaesthesiol Taiwan*, 2006. **44**(4): 211–215.

210 Nesher, N. et al., Morphine with adjuvant ketamine vs higher dose of morphine alone for immediate postthoracotomy analgesia. *Chest*, 2009. **136**(1): 245–252.

211 Nesher, N. et al., Ketamine spares morphine consumption after transthoracic lung and heart surgery without adverse hemodynamic effects. *Pharmacol Res*, 2008. **58**(1): 38–44.

212 Kollender, Y. et al., Subanaesthetic ketamine spares postoperative morphine and controls pain better than standard morphine does alone in orthopaedic-oncological patients. *Eur J Cancer*, 2008. **44**(7): 954–962.

213 Subramaniam, K., B. Subramaniam, and R.A. Steinbrook, Ketamine as adjuvant analgesic to opioids: A quantitative and qualitative systematic review. *Anesth Analg*, 2004. **99**(2): 482–495, table of contents.

214 Weinbroum, A.A., A single small dose of postoperative ketamine provides rapid and sustained improvement in morphine analgesia in the presence of morphine-resistant pain. *Anesth Analg*, 2003. **96**(3): 789–795, table of contents.

215 Azevedo, V.M. et al., Transdermal ketamine as an adjuvant for postoperative analgesia after abdominal gynecological surgery using lidocaine epidural blockade. *Anesth Analg*, 2000. **91**(6): 1479–1482.

216 Lahtinen, P. et al., S(+)-ketamine as an analgesic adjunct reduces opioid consumption after cardiac surgery. *Anesth Analg*, 2004. **99**(5): 1295–1301, table of contents.

217 Piper, S.N. et al., Postoperative analgosedation with S(+)-ketamine decreases the incidences of postanesthetic shivering and nausea and vomiting after cardiac surgery. *Med Sci Monit*, 2008. **14**(12): PI59–PI65.

218 Adams, H.A., Ketamine in emergency care: New standard or exclusive alternative?. *Anasthesiol Intensivmed Notfallmed Schmerzther*, 2003. **38**(3): 192–195.

219 Argiriadou, H. et al., Improvement of pain treatment after major abdominal surgery by intravenous S+-ketamine. *Anesth Analg*, 2004. **98**(5): 1413–1418, table of contents.

220 Kronenberg, R.H., Ketamine as an analgesic: Parenteral, oral, rectal, subcutaneous, transdermal and intranasal administration. *J Pain Palliat Care Pharmacother*, 2002. **16**(3): 27–35.

221 Gurnani, A. et al., Analgesia for acute musculoskeletal trauma: Low-dose subcutaneous infusion of ketamine. *Anaesth Intensive Care*, 1996. **24**(1): 32–36.

222 Galinski, M. et al., Management of severe acute pain in emergency settings: Ketamine reduces morphine consumption. *Am J Emerg Med*, 2007. **25**(4): 385–390.

223 Lester, L. et al., Low-dose ketamine for analgesia in the ED: A retrospective case series. *Am J Emerg Med*, 2010. **28**(7): 820–827.

224 Johansson, P., P. Kongstad, and A. Johansson, The effect of combined treatment with morphine sulphate and low-dose ketamine in a prehospital setting. *Scand J Trauma Resusc Emerg Med*, 2009. **17**: 61.

225 Chazan, S. et al., Ketamine for acute and subacute pain in opioid-tolerant patients. *J Opioid Manag*, 2008. **4**(3): 173–180.

226 Mercadante, S. et al., Opioid switching and burst ketamine to improve the opioid response in patients with movement-related pain due to bone metastases. *Clin J Pain*, 2009. **25**(7): 648–649.

227 Mercadante, S. et al., Alternative treatments of breakthrough pain in patients receiving spinal analgesics for cancer pain. *J Pain Symptom Manage*, 2005. **30**(5): 485–491.

228 Kannan, T.R. et al., Oral ketamine as an adjuvant to oral morphine for neuropathic pain in cancer patients. *J Pain Symptom Manage*, 2002. **23**(1): 60–65.

229 Fine, P.G., Low-dose ketamine in the management of opioid nonresponsive terminal cancer pain. *J Pain Symptom Manage*, 1999. **17**(4): 296–300.

230 Jackson, K. et al., "Burst" ketamine for refractory cancer pain: An open-label audit of 39 patients. *J Pain Symptom Manage*, 2001. **22**(4): 834–842.

231 Lossignol, D.A., M. Obiols-Portis, and J.J. Body, Successful use of ketamine for intractable cancer pain. *Support Care Cancer*, 2005. **13**(3): 188–193.

232 Salas, S. et al., Ketamine analgesic effect by continuous intravenous infusion in refractory cancer pain: Considerations about the clinical research in palliative care. *J Palliat Med*, 2012. **15**(3): 287–293.

233 Bell, R., C. Eccleston, and E. Kalso, Ketamine as an adjuvant to opioids for cancer pain. *Cochrane Database Syst Rev*, 2003(1): CD003351.

234 Gertler, R. et al., Dexmedetomidine: A novel sedative-analgesic agent. *Proc (Bayl Univ Med Cent)*, 2001. **14**(1): 13–21.

235 Bekker, A. and M.K. Sturaitis, Dexmedetomidine for neurological surgery. *Neurosurgery*, 2005. **57**(1 Suppl): 1–10; discussion 1–10.

236 Gurbet, A. et al., Intraoperative infusion of dexmedetomidine reduces perioperative analgesic requirements. *Can J Anaesth*, 2006. **53**(7): 646–652.

237 Unlugenc, H. et al., The effect of pre-anaesthetic administration of intravenous dexmedetomidine on postoperative pain in patients receiving patient-controlled morphine. *Eur J Anaesthesiol*, 2005. **22**(5): 386–391.

238 Wahlander, S. et al., A prospective, double-blind, randomized, placebo-controlled study of dexmedetomidine as an adjunct to epidural analgesia after thoracic surgery. *J Cardiothorac Vasc Anesth*, 2005. **19**(5): 630–635.

239 Lin, T.F. et al., Effect of combining dexmedetomidine and morphine for intravenous patient-controlled analgesia. *Br J Anaesth*, 2009. **102**(1): 117–122.

240 Belgrade, M. and S. Hall, Dexmedetomidine infusion for the management of opioid-induced hyperalgesia. *Pain Med*, 2010. **11**(12): 1819–1826.

241 Iwakiri, H. et al., The efficacy of continuous infusion of low dose dexmedetomidine for postoperative patients recovering in general wards. *Eur J Anaesthesiol*, 2012. **29**(5): 251–254.

242 Mantz, J., V. Degos, and C. Laigle, Recent advances in pharmacologic neuroprotection. *Eur J Anaesthesiol*, 2010. **27**(1): 6–10.

243 Davis, M.P., D.E. Weissman, and R.M. Arnold, Opioid dose titration for severe cancer pain: A systematic evidence-based review. *J Palliat Med*, 2004. **7**(3): 462–468.

244 Elsner, F. et al., Intravenous versus subcutaneous morphine titration in patients with persisting exacerbation of cancer pain. *J Palliat Med*, 2005. **8**(4): 743–750.

245 De Conno, F. et al., The MERITO study: A multicentre trial of the analgesic effect and tolerability of normal-release oral morphine during 'titration phase' in patients with cancer pain. *Palliat Med*, 2008. **22**(3): 214–221.

246 Khojainova, N. et al., Olanzapine in the management of cancer pain. *J Pain Symptom Manage*, 2002. **23**(4): 346–350.

247 Gray, P., Acute neuropathic pain: Diagnosis and treatment. *Curr Opin Anaesthesiol*, 2008. **21**(5): 590–595.

248 Bowsher, D., The effects of pre-emptive treatment of postherpetic neuralgia with amitriptyline: A randomized, double-blind, placebo-controlled trial. *J Pain Symptom Manage*, 1997. **13**(6): 327–331.

249 Reuben, S.S., G. Makari-Judson, and S.D. Lurie, Evaluation of efficacy of the perioperative administration of venlafaxine XR in the prevention of postmastectomy pain syndrome. *J Pain Symptom Manage*, 2004. **27**(2): 133–139.

250 Berry, J.D. and K.L. Petersen, A single dose of gabapentin reduces acute pain and allodynia in patients with herpes zoster. *Neurology*, 2005. **65**(3): 444–447.

251 Gray, P., B. Williams, and T. Cramond, Successful use of gabapentin in acute pain management following burn injury: A case series. *Pain Med*, 2008. **9**(3): 371–376.

252 Keskinbora, K., A.F. Pekel, and I. Aydinli, Gabapentin and an opioid combination versus opioid alone for the management of neuropathic cancer pain: A randomized open trial. *J Pain Symptom Manage*, 2007. **34**(2): 183–189.

253 Richardson, P. and L. Mustard, The management of pain in the burns unit. *Burns*, 2009. **35**(7): 921–936.

254 Durand, J.P. et al., Efficacy of venlafaxine for the prevention and relief of oxaliplatin-induced acute neurotoxicity: Results of EFFOX, a randomized, double-blind, placebo-controlled phase III trial. *Ann Oncol*, 2012 Jan; **23**(1):200-205.

255 Dirks, J. et al., The effect of systemic lidocaine on pain and secondary hyperalgesia associated with the heat/capsaicin sensitization model in healthy volunteers. *Anesth Analg*, 2000. **91**(4): 967–972.

256 Wasiak, J. and H. Cleland, Lidocaine for pain relief in burn injured patients. *Cochrane Database Syst Rev*, 2007(3): CD005622.

257 Mercadante, S. et al., Long-term ketamine subcutaneous continuous infusion in neuropathic cancer pain. *J Pain Symptom Manage*, 1995. **10**(7): 564–568.

258 Enarson, M.C., H. Hays, and M.A. Woodroffe, Clinical experience with oral ketamine. *J Pain Symptom Manage*, 1999. **17**(5): 384–386.

259 Schley, M. et al., Continuous brachial plexus blockade in combination with the NMDA receptor antagonist memantine prevents phantom pain in acute traumatic upper limb amputees. *Eur J Pain*, 2007. **11**(3): 299–308.

260 Eide, P.K. et al., Relief of post-herpetic neuralgia with the N-methyl-D-aspartic acid receptor antagonist ketamine: A double-blind, cross-over comparison with morphine and placebo. *Pain*, 1994. **58**(3): 347–354.

261 Simanski, C. et al., Therapy of phantom pain with salmon calcitonin and effect on postoperative patient satisfaction. *Chirurg*, 1999. **70**(6): 674–681.

262 Sahin, F. et al., Efficacy of salmon calcitonin in complex regional pain syndrome (type 1) in addition to physical therapy. *Clin Rheumatol*, 2006. **25**(2): 143–148.

263 Jaeger, H. and C. Maier, Calcitonin in phantom limb pain: A double-blind study. *Pain*, 1992. **48**(1): 21–27.

264 Helfand, M. and M. Freeman, Assessment and management of acute pain in adult medical inpatients: A systematic review. *Pain Med*, 2009. **10**(7): 1183–1199.

265 Block, B.M. et al., Efficacy of postoperative epidural analgesia: A meta-analysis. *JAMA*, 2003. **290**(18): 2455–2463.

87

Suicide

YESNE ALICI, REENA JAISWAL, HAYLEY PESSIN, WILLIAM BREITBART

INTRODUCTION

Suicide is a tragic but often preventable response to the emotional challenges of terminal physical illness. Although it is often assumed that suicide is common in the chronically ill, the fact remains that it is still relatively uncommon.[1***] Suicide in terminal illness may represent a pathologic, and therefore potentially treatable, coping response. The purpose of this chapter is to examine the prevalence of suicide in palliative care settings, factors that contribute to it, and potential interventions both to prevent it as well as to cope with the trauma that completed suicides have on family and significant others.

SUICIDAL IDEATION IN THE TERMINALLY ILL

Suicidal ideation is defined as thoughts of taking one's own life. For most patients, this may only occur as a fleeting consideration they have during particularly distressing moments in their illness. These thoughts may serve as a "steam valve" for ideations often expressed by patients as "no matter how bad things become, I always have a way out." For others, it may occur with more frequency and result in a concrete plan of measures one will take to end their own life. When the latter occurs, it is a psychiatric emergency that can require involuntary hospitalization to protect the individual from self-injury. Because terminally ill patients frequently experience these thoughts, it is important for providers to feel comfortable assessing suicidal ideation in their patients. Table 87.1 provides some suggestions on asking patients about suicidal thoughts.

Published reports have suggested that suicidal ideation is relatively infrequent in illnesses such as cancer and is limited to those who are significantly depressed. Silberfarb et al.[3*] found that only 3 of 146 patients with breast cancer had suicidal thoughts, while none of the 100 cancer patients interviewed in a Finnish study expressed suicidal thoughts.[4*] A study conducted at St. Boniface Hospice in Winnipeg, Canada, demonstrated that only 10 of 44 terminally ill cancer patients were suicidal or desired an early death, and all 10 were suffering from clinical depression.[5*] At Memorial Sloan-Kettering

Cancer Center (MSKCC), suicide risk evaluation accounted for 8.6% of psychiatric consultations, usually requested by staff in response to a patient verbalizing suicidal wishes.[6] Among 185 cancer patients with pain studied at MSKCC, suicidal ideation was found in 17% of the study population.[6] It should be noted that the actual prevalence of suicidal ideation may be considerably higher than these figures suggest, in that patients often disclose these thoughts only after a stable, ongoing physician–patient relationship has been established. It has been our experience that once patients develop such a trusting and safe relationship, they almost universally reveal occasional persistent thoughts of suicide as a means of escaping the threat of being overwhelmed by their illness.

SUICIDE AND TERMINAL ILLNESS

Terminally ill patients are at elevated risk of suicide when compared to the general population. A study done by Hem and colleagues examining data from the Cancer registry of Norway revealed standardized mortality ratios (SMRs) of 1.55 for males and 1.35 for females.[7*] The study also found that risk was greatest in the first months following diagnosis and was significantly increased in male patients with respiratory cancers.[7*] A study by Druss and Pincus examining the relationship between suicide and medical illness found that cancer patients had a 4-fold increase in the likelihood of a suicide attempt.[8*]

A Swedish study of cancer-related suicides revealed that half of all patients who committed suicide had previously conveyed suicidal thoughts or plans to their relatives.[9*] In addition, many of the completed cancer suicides had been preceded by an attempted suicide.[9*] This is consistent with the statistics of suicide in general, which shows that a previous suicide attempt greatly increases the risk of completed suicide.[10*] A family history of suicide is also of increasing relevance in assessing suicide risk.

Factors associated with increased risk of suicide in patients with advanced physical disease[2,6***] are listed in Table 87.2. Patients with advanced illness are at highest risk, perhaps because they are most likely to have such complications

Table 87.1 *Assessing severity of suicidal ideation*

Suicidal ideation	Many patients have passing thoughts of suicide, such as, "If my pain was bad enough, I might..." Have you had thoughts like that? Have you found yourself thinking that you do not want to live or that you would be better off dead?
Suicidal plan	Have you stopped or wanted to stop taking care of yourself? Have you thought about how you would end your life?
Suicidal intent	Do you plan or intend to hurt yourself? What would you do? Do you think you would carry out these plans?

Source: Breitbart, W., Cancer pain and suicide, in: Foley, K.M., Bonica, J.J., Ventafridda, V. (eds.), Advances in Pain Research and Therapy, vol. 16, Raven Press, New York, pp. 399–412, 1990.

Table 87.2 *Factors associated with an increased risk of suicide in patients with advanced illnesses*

- Pain—aspects of suffering
- Advanced illness—poor prognosis
- Depression—hopelessness
- Delirium—disinhibition, poor impulse control, impaired judgment
- Loss of control—helplessness
- Preexisting psychopathology
- Substance/alcohol use disorders (abuse or dependence)
- Personal or family history of suicide attempts
- Fatigue
- Lack of social support—social isolation

such as pain, depression, delirium, and physical disability. Psychiatric disorders including substance use disorders are frequently present in hospitalized patients who are suicidal. A review of consultation data from the psychiatry service at MSKCC revealed that one-third of suicidal cancer patients had a major depression, about 20% suffered from delirium, and 50% were diagnosed as having an adjustment disorder with both anxious and depressed features at the time of evaluation.[2,6***] Delirium and other cognitive disorders place terminally ill patients at risk for suicidality by impairing impulse control and judgment.

Physically ill patients commit suicide most frequently in the advanced stages of disease.[9*,11*,12*,13] Eighty-six percent of suicides studied by Farberow et al.[11*] occurred in the preterminal or terminal stages of illness, despite greatly reduced physical capacity. Poor prognosis and advanced illness usually go hand in hand. It is thus not surprising that in Sweden, those who were expected to die within a matter of months were the most likely to commit suicide. Of 88 cancer suicides, 14 had an uncertain prognosis and 45 had a poor prognosis.[11*] With advancing disease, the incidence of significant cancer pain increases. Uncontrolled pain in cancer patients is a dramatically important risk factor for suicide. The vast majority of cancer suicides in several studies showed

that these patients had severe pain that was often inadequately controlled and poorly tolerated.[9*,11*,12*,13*,14*]

Depression is a factor in 50% of all suicides. Those suffering from depression are at 25 times greater risk of suicide than the general population.[15*,16*] The role depression plays in suicides among the seriously medically ill is equally significant. Approximately 25% of all patients with cancer experience severe depressive symptoms, with about 6% with a major depressive episode.[17*]

Among those with advanced illness and progressively impaired physical function, symptoms of severe depression rise to 77%.[18***] Depression also appears to be important in terms of patient preferences for life-sustaining medical therapy. Ganzini and colleagues reported that among older depressed patients, an increase in desire for life-sustaining medical therapies followed treatment of depression in those subjects who had been initially more severely depressed, more hopeless, and more likely to overestimate the risks and to underestimate the benefits of treatment.[19*] They concluded that whereas patients with mild to moderate depression are unlikely to alter their decisions regarding life-sustaining medical treatment in spite of treatment for their depression, severely depressed patients—particularly those who are hopeless—should be encouraged to defer advance treatment directives. In these patients, decisions about life-sustaining therapy should be discouraged until after treatment of their depression.

Hopelessness is the key variable that links depression and suicide in the general population. Further, hopelessness is a significantly better predictor of completed suicide than is depression alone.[20***] In a study[21*] Chochinov and colleagues demonstrated that hopelessness was correlated more highly with suicidal ideation in terminally ill patients than was the level of depression. With the typical cancer suicide being characterized by advanced illness and poor prognosis, hopelessness is commonly experienced. In Scandinavia, the highest incidence of suicide was found in cancer patients who were offered no further treatment, and no further contact with the healthcare system.[9*,13*] Being left to face illness alone creates a sense of isolation and abandonment that is critical to the development of hopelessness.

Loss of control and a sense of helplessness in the face of one's illness are important factors in suicide vulnerability. Control refers to both the helplessness induced by symptoms or deficits due to the illness or its treatments, as well as the excessive need on the part of some patients to be in control of all aspects of living or dying. Farberow noted that patients who were accepting and adaptable were much less likely to commit suicide than patients who exhibited a need to be in control of even the most minute details of their care.[11**] This need to control may be prominent in some patients and cause distress with little provocation. However, it is not uncommon for illness-related events to induce a great sense of helplessness even in those who are not typically controlling individuals. Impairments or deficits induced by the patient's illness or its treatments often include loss of mobility, paraplegia, loss of bowel and bladder function, amputation, aphonia, sensory loss, and inability to eat or swallow. Most distressing to patients is the sense that they are losing control of their minds, especially when they are confused or sedated by medications. The risk of suicide is increased in patients with such physical impairments, especially when accompanied by psychological distress and disturbed interpersonal relationships due to these deficit factors.[14*]

Fatigue, in the form of emotional, spiritual, financial, familial, communal, and other resource exhaustion, increases the risk of suicide in the seriously physically ill patient.[6] Due to advancements in treatment, illnesses such as cancer now often follow more of a chronic course. Increased survival is accompanied by an increased number of hospitalizations, complications, and expenses. Symptom control thus becomes a prolonged process with frequent advances and setbacks. The dying process also can become extremely long and arduous for all concerned. It is not uncommon for both family members and healthcare providers to withdraw prematurely from the patient under these circumstances. A suicidal patient can thus feel even more isolated and abandoned. The presence of a strong support system for the patient that may act as an external control of suicidal behavior reduces the risk of suicide significantly.

ASSESSMENT AND MANAGEMENT OF THE SUICIDAL PATIENT

Assessment of suicide risk and appropriate intervention are critical. Early and comprehensive psychiatric involvement with high-risk individuals can often avert suicide in the cancer setting. A careful evaluation includes a search for the meaning of suicidal thoughts, as well as an exploration of the seriousness of the risk. The clinician's ability to establish rapport and elicit a patient's thoughts is essential as he or she assesses history, degree of intent, and quality of internal and external controls. The clinician should listen sympathetically, not appearing critical or stating that such thoughts are inappropriate. Allowing the patient to have discussions about suicidal ideation often decreases the risk of suicide. The myth that asking about suicidal thoughts "puts the idea in their head" is one that should be dispelled.[22***] Patients often reconsider and reject the idea of suicide when the physician acknowledges the legitimacy of their option and the need to retain a sense of control over aspects of their death. Once the setting has been made secure, assessment of the relevant mental status and adequacy of pain control can begin. Analgesics, antipsychotics, or antidepressant drugs should be used when appropriate to treat agitation, psychosis, major depression, or pain. Underlying causes of delirium or pain should be addressed specifically when possible. Initiation of a crisis-intervention-oriented psychotherapeutic approach, mobilizing as much of the patient's support system as possible, is important. A close family member or friend should be involved in order to support the patient, provide information, and assist in treatment planning. Psychiatric hospitalization can sometimes be helpful but is usually not desirable in the terminally ill patient.

Thus, the medical hospital or home is the setting in which management most often takes place. Whereas it is appropriate to intervene when medical or psychiatric factors are clearly the driving force in a cancer suicide, there are circumstances when usurping control from the patient and family with overly aggressive intervention may be less helpful. This is most evident in those with advanced illness where comfort and symptom control are the primary concerns.

Ultimately, the palliative care clinician may not be able to prevent all suicides in all terminally ill patients that he or she cares for. The emphasis of intervention should be to aggressively attempt to prevent suicide that is driven by the desperation of uncontrolled physical and psychological symptoms such as uncontrolled pain, unrecognized delirium, and unrecognized and untreated depression. Prolonged suffering caused by poorly controlled symptoms may lead to such desperation, and it is the appropriate role of the palliative care team to provide effective management of physical and psychological symptoms as an alternative to desire for death, suicides, or requests for assisted suicide by their patient. Table 87.3 presents an overview of commonly used suicide assessment questions with terminally ill patients and their families.

Table 87.3 *Questions to ask patients and family when assessing suicide risk*

Acknowledge that these are common thoughts that can be discussed	Most patients with cancer have passing thoughts about suicide, such as "I might do something if it gets bad enough." Have you ever had thoughts like that? Have you had thoughts of not wanting to live? Have you had those thoughts in the past few days?
Assess level of risk	Do you have thoughts about wanting to end your life? How? Do you have a plan? Do you have any strong social support? Do you have pills stockpiled at home? Do you own or have access to a weapon?
Obtain prior history	Have you ever had a psychiatric disorder, suffered from depression, or made a suicide attempt? Is there a family history of suicide?
Identify substance abuse	Have you ever had a problem with alcohol or drugs?
Identify bereavement	Have you lost anyone close to you recently?
Identify medical predictors of risk	Do you have pain that is not being relieved? How long has the disease affected your life? How is your memory and concentration? Do you feel hopeless? What do you plan for the future?

Source: American Psychological Oncology Society, *Quick Reference for Oncology Clinicians: The Psychiatric and Psychological Dimensions of Cancer Symptom Management*, IPOS Press, Charlottesville, VA, 2006.

DESIRE FOR HASTENED DEATH

The desire for hastened death is an issue that may be commonly encountered by the palliative care physician. It may present as a passive wish for death, the decision to forego aggressive therapy that could alter survival outcomes, the decision to discontinue life-prolonging treatment, suicidal ideation or a request for physician-assisted suicide. Breitbart et al.[24*] found that in a hospice setting, 17% of the 92 terminally ill patients evaluated indicated a high desire for hastened death. Chochinov et al. reported that 44.5% of the 200 terminally ill studied reported a fleeting desire for death.[25*] A more persistent wish for hastened death occurred in 8.5% of the sample.[25*] Because of its frequency, being able to identify underlying factors contributing to a patient's desire for hastened death is key for care-providers. Breitbart et al.[24*] found that depression and hopelessness were the strongest predictors of desire for hastened death among terminally ill cancer patients. They were also found to have significantly more pain and less social support when compared to patients without desire for hastened death. Similarly, in 2007, Rodin et al. found that desire for hastened death correlated positively with hopelessness, depression, and physical distress.[26*] Existential concerns such as loss of meaning and purpose, loss of dignity, regret, awareness of incomplete life tasks, and anxiety around what happens after death have been associated with a desire for hastened death. Chochinov et al. found that terminally ill cancer patients with a lowered sense of dignity were more likely to report a loss of will to live.[27*] Terminally ill cancer patients who had low spiritual well-being were more likely to endorse a desire for hastened death, hopelessness, and suicidal ideation based on a study done by McClain and colleagues.[28*]

In summary, common risk factors associated with a desire for hastened death include depression or history of psychiatric illness, hopelessness, physical distress (including pain and symptom burden), poor social support, fear of being a burden to others as well as existential concerns such as loss of meaning and loss of dignity.

REQUESTS FOR ASSISTED SUICIDE

As mentioned in the preceding section, a desire for hastened death may present as a request for physician-assisted suicide. This has become a highly controversial topic in palliative medicine. Several states across the United States (Oregon, Montana and Washington) as well as Switzerland and the Netherlands have legalized physician-assisted suicide for terminally ill patients. A recently published article in *the New England Journal of Medicine* examined attitudes for and against physician-assisted suicide.[29*] Those opposed to it argue that its legalization will alter the fundamental role of the doctor as healer and may place certain more vulnerable communities at risk of abuse, error, and coercion. Advocates argue that allowing patients a legal and socially accepted way of controlling their own death would avoid people having to plan in

secrecy and endure the difficult process alone. They also feel that safeguards, such as a thorough informed consent process and the requirement of an independent second opinion, would protect against most risks.[29*] Since the passing of the Death with Dignity Act (DWDA) in 1997, a total of 1050 people have obtained DWDA prescriptions and 673 have died from ingestion of the medication prescribed.[30] Far more patients talk to their families and physicians regarding the possibility of physician-assisted suicide compared to those terminally ill who actually die using the Death with Dignity Act.[31*] This suggests that even when legally permissible, few patients resort to assisted suicide. Clinicians should allow patients to discuss their wishes for hastened death and physician-assisted suicide in an open, frank manner. Being empathic and nonjudgmental are essential to facilitating these often difficult to discuss issues. Through such conversations, one may be able to identify underlying reasons for such wishes, such as hopelessness or depression and offer appropriate interventions. In a cross-sectional survey of 58 Oregonians who had either requested aid in dying from a physician or contacted an aid in dying advocacy group, Ganzini et al.[32*] found that 15 patients met "caseness" criteria for depression, a diagnosis based on symptoms, as opposed to a constellation of signs and symptoms. Three of the 15 patients met criteria for depression, and all three of the depressed participants died by legal ingestion within two months of the research interview. The authors concluded that most terminally ill Oregonians who receive aid in dying do not have depressive disorders, but the current practice of the DWDA may fail to protect some patients whose choices are influenced by depression.[32*] Breitbart et al. examined depression and desire for hastened death in patients with advanced AIDS.[33*] Patients who were diagnosed with major depressive disorder were placed on antidepressant treatment and assessed weekly for symptoms of depression and desire for hastened death. The results indicated that a patient's desire for hastened death decreased dramatically in patients who responded positively to antidepressant treatment.[33*] A prospective Dutch study of 138 terminally ill cancer patients examined the association between depression and requests for euthanasia. They found that of the 22% of patients, who requested euthanasia, 23% were depressed at baseline and 44% of those depressed requested euthanasia compared to 15% of the nondepressed. The rate of request was 4.1 times greater than that of patients without depression.[34*] Regardless of what one's personal beliefs are on physician-assisted suicide, being able to address treatable symptoms and reduce suffering is at the core of palliative medicine. Clinicians should pay particular attention to underlying depression, hopelessness, and physical distress when such requests are made. In an article on physician-assisted suicide, Dr. Quill suggests that when a terminally ill patient requests assistance in dying, the first step to take is to make sure the person is getting the best possible palliative care. He argues that when applied with skill and expertise, good palliative care can address most, but not always all, end-of-life suffering.[35***] Dr. Breitbart proposed in an editorial on the same matter that the solution to "suffering is the elimination of suffering not the sufferer." Suffering, he

Table 87.4 *Guidelines for the assessment of desire for hastened death and requests for physician-assisted suicide*

Be alert to your own responses	Be aware of how your responses influence discussions
	Monitor your attitude and responses
	Demonstrate positive regard for the patient
	Seek supervision
Be open to hearing concerns	Gently ask about emotional concerns
	Be alert to verbal and nonverbal distress cues
	Encourage expression of feelings
	Actively listen without interrupting
	Discuss desire for death using the patient's words
	Permit sadness, silence, and tears
	Express empathy verbally and nonverbally
	Acknowledge differences in response to illness
Assess contributing factors	Prior psychiatric history
	Prior suicide attempts
	History of alcohol or substance abuse
	Lack of social support
	Feelings of burden
	Family conflict
	Need for additional assistance
	Depression and anxiety
	Existential concerns, loss of meaning and dignity
	Cognitive impairment
	Physical symptoms, especially severe pain
Respond to specific issues	Acknowledge patient or family fears and concerns
	Address modifiable contributing factors
	Recommend interventions
	Develop plan to manage more complicated issues
Conclude discussion	Summarize and review important points
	Clarify patient perceptions
	Provide opportunity for questions
	Assist in facilitating discussion with others
	Provide appropriate referrals
After discussion	Document discussion in medical record
	Communicate with members of the treatment team

Source: Hudson, P.L., Schonfeild, P., Kelly, B. et al., *Palliat. Med.*, 20, 703, 2006.

argues, can be ameliorated by "providing excellent physical, psychological and existential, spiritual interventions in the care of the dying."[36]*** Table 87.4 provides an outline of assessment of desire for hastened death and requests for physician-assisted suicide.

INTERVENTIONS FOR DESPAIR AT THE END OF LIFE

In the past two decades, clinicians working with terminally ill patients have developed psychotherapy techniques targeting factors that contribute to suffering at the end of life. In this section, we will describe interventions that address some of these common factors including spiritual suffering, demoralization, loss of dignity, and loss of meaning.

Spiritual suffering

For some patients, spiritual well-being is felt to be a crucial aspect for coping with terminal illness. Often when faced with dying, patients struggle with questions about their own mortality, the meaning of life, and the existence of a higher power. Some may turn to religion for such answers while others rely on other spiritual beliefs. In their 2003 study examining spiritual well-being in a population of terminally ill hospice patients, McClain and colleagues found that terminally ill patients with a sense of spiritual well-being had some protection against end-of-life despair.[28]* This finding points to the importance of addressing spiritual concerns in the terminally ill. By asking about their spiritual beliefs, assessing the importance of spirituality in patients' lives, exploring whether they belong to a spiritual community, and offering chaplaincy referrals, one may be able to address some of these concerns.

Rousseau[38] outlines an approach for the treatment of spiritual suffering composed of the following steps:

1. Controlling physical symptoms
2. Providing a supportive presence
3. Encouraging life review to assist in recognizing purpose, value, and meaning
4. Exploring guilt, remorse, forgiveness, reconciliation
5. Facilitating religious expression
6. Reframing goals
7. Encourage meditative practices, focus on healing rather than cure

Rousseau has presented an approach to spiritual suffering, which is an interesting blend of basic psychotherapeutic principles. Psychotherapeutic techniques that are particularly adaptive to psychotherapy with the dying such as life narrative and life review are also included. There is an emphasis on facilitating religious expression and confession that in fact may be extremely useful to many patients, but is not applicable to all patients and not necessarily an intervention that many clinicians feel comfortable providing. What Rousseau's work suggests is that novel psychotherapeutic interventions aimed at improving spiritual well-being, sense of meaning and diminishing hopelessness, demoralization, and distress are critically necessary to be further studied and disseminated for provision of best palliative care to the terminally ill.

Demoralization

Kissane[39]*** and colleagues have described a syndrome of demoralization in the terminally ill patient, which consists of a triad of hopelessness, loss of meaning, and existential distress expressed as a desire for death. They argue that this syndrome is distinct from depression because unlike depression, it is not usually associated with anhedonia.

Demoralization is often seen in patients with life-threatening illness, disability, bodily disfigurement, fear, loss of dignity, social isolation, and feelings of being a burden. Kissane and his group describe a treatment approach for demoralization syndrome, which is both multidisciplinary and multimodal. It consists of

- Ensuring continuity of care and active symptom management
- Ensuring dignity in the dying process
- Utilizing various types of psychotherapy to help sustain a sense of meaning, limit cognitive distortions and maintain family relationships (i.e., meaning-based, cognitive-behavioral, interpersonal, and family psychotherapy interventions)
- Using life review and narrative
- Paying attention to spiritual issues
- Using pharmacotherapy for comorbid anxiety, depression, and delirium

The goal of this approach is to restore hope by valuing and affirming the story of their lives, their roles, accomplishments, and sources of fulfillment.[40***]

Loss of dignity

Dignity is defined as the quality or state of being worthy, honored, or esteemed. Dignity therapy, developed by Harvey Chochinov and colleagues, is a therapeutic approach designed to decrease suffering, enhance quality of life, and bolster a sense of dignity for patient's approaching death.[41***] Chochinov et al.[41***] examined how dying patients understand and define the term "dignity," in order to develop a model of dignity in the terminally ill (see Figure 87.1). A semistructured interview was designed to explore how patients cope with their advanced cancer and to detail their perceptions of dignity. Three major categories emerged from

a detailed qualitative analysis, including illness-related concerns (concerns that derive from or are related to the illness itself, and threaten to or actually do impinge on the patient's sense of dignity); dignity-conserving repertoire (internally held qualities or personal approaches or techniques that patients use to bolster or maintain their sense of dignity); and social dignity inventory (social concerns or relationship dynamics that enhance or detract from a patient's sense of dignity). These broad categories and their carefully defined themes and subthemes form the foundation for an emerging model of dignity among the dying. The concept of dignity and the notion of dignity-conserving care offer a way of understanding how patients face advancing terminal illness and present an approach that clinicians can use to explicitly target the maintenance of dignity as a therapeutic objective and principle of bedside care for patients nearing death. In the therapy, patients are invited to discuss issues that matter most or that they would most want remembered. Sessions are transcribed and edited, with a final version that they can bequeath to a loved one. In 2005, Chochinov and colleagues studied 100 terminally ill patients who received dignity therapy: 91% reported feeling satisfied or highly satisfied with the intervention, 86% found it helpful or very helpful, 76% found that it heightened their sense of dignity, 68% indicated that it increased their sense of purpose, 67% reported that it improved sense of meaning, and 47% indicated that dignity therapy increased their will to live.[42*]

Chochinov et al.[43*] reported their findings of the effect of dignity therapy on distress and end-of-life experience in terminally ill patients from a randomized controlled trial. Patients (aged ≥ 18 years) with a terminal prognosis (life expectancy ≤6 months) who were receiving palliative care in a hospital or community setting (hospice or home) in Canada, USA, and Australia were randomly assigned to dignity therapy, client-centered care, or standard palliative care. No significant differences were noted in the distress levels before and after completion of the study in the three

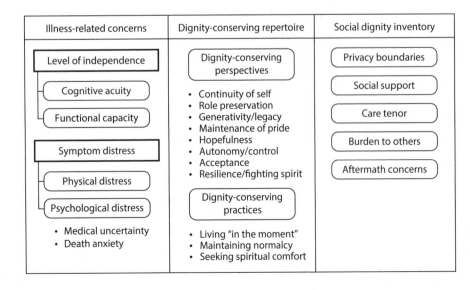

Figure 87.1 *Major dignity categories: Themes and subthemes. (Adapted from Chochinov, H.M. et al., Soc. Sci. Med., 54(3), 433, 2002.)*

groups. For the secondary outcomes, patients reported that dignity therapy was significantly more likely than the other two interventions to have been helpful, improve quality of life, increase sense of dignity, change how their family saw and appreciated them, and be helpful to their family. Dignity therapy was significantly better than client-centered care in improving spiritual well-being, and was significantly better than standard palliative care in terms of lessening sadness or depression; significantly more patients who had received dignity therapy reported that the study group had been satisfactory, compared with those who received standard palliative care. Although the ability of dignity therapy to mitigate outright distress, such as depression, and desire for death or suicidality, has yet to be proven, its benefits in terms of self-reported end-of-life experiences support its clinical application for patients nearing death.

Loss of meaning

Interventions for hopelessness and loss of meaning and purpose in the terminally ill are of particular importance when addressing the issues of desire for death and despair at the end of life. Breitbart et al.[44***] have developed an intervention termed "meaning-centered" psychotherapy for advanced cancer patients; an intervention based on the concepts and principles of Viktor Frankl's writings and logotherapy. Viktor Frankl, a holocaust survivor and psychiatrist, described that the will to meaning is an inherent drive to connect with something greater than one's own needs and through this, one finds meaning and self-transcendence particularly at times of intense psychological and physical suffering.[45] Meaning-centered psychotherapy has aimed at restoring a sense of meaning, peace, and purpose in patients with advanced cancer.[44***] Meaning-centered psychotherapy is a manualized intervention that consists of eight, 90 min weekly sessions. Each session includes didactics, discussion, and experiential exercises focused around particular themes related to meaning and advanced cancer. The session themes include:

Session 1: Concepts and sources of meaning
    *Introductions to interventions and meaning
Session 2: Cancer and meaning
    *Identity—Before and after cancer diagnosis
Session 3: Meaning and historical context of life
    *Life as a living legacy (past)
Session 4: Storytelling, life project
    *Life as a living legacy (present–future)
Session 5: Limitations and finiteness of life
    *Encountering life's limitations
Session 6: Responsibility, creativity, deeds
    *Actively engaging in life (via: creativity and responsibility)
Session 7: Experience, nature, art, humor
    *Connecting with life (via: love, beauty and humor)
Session 8: Termination, goodbyes, hopes for the future
    *Reflections and hopes for the future

In a 2010 study, Breitbart and colleagues found that when compared to supportive group psychotherapy, patients involved in meaning-centered group psychotherapy had significant benefits in areas of spiritual well-being and enhancing a sense of meaning.[46] A later study examining individual meaning-centered psychotherapy found that patients with advanced cancer had clear short-term benefits for spiritual suffering and quality of life when compared to therapeutic massage.[47]

INTERVENTIONS FOR FAMILY MEMBERS FOLLOWING A COMPLETED SUICIDE

When a terminally ill patient chooses to end his or her own life, the treatment team must quickly turn its attention to addressing the needs of the patient's family so as to reduce the chances of complicated bereavement. In order to provide effective support, it is essential that the team is aware of the unique reactions commonly found among suicide survivors. A number of studies have compared the bereavement patterns of suicide survivors and nonsuicide survivors.[48**,49,50*] Findings from these studies indicate that there are several distinguishing themes that arise in suicide bereavement. Foremost among them is the desire for the survivor to make meaning of the suicide, or to answer the question "Why?"[48**,49,51] Van Dongen[52] calls this process "agonizing questioning," given the impossibility of ascertaining the answer from the now deceased. Second, survivors often express feelings of guilt, blame, and responsibility for the death. Often they engage in a struggle to retrace the days and months leading up to the suicide in order to pick up clues that they "missed." Another documented theme is a heightened feeling of rejection or abandonment, which is often accompanied by anger toward the deceased.[48**,49,53**] Finally, perceived feelings of stigmatization, shame, and embarrassment are well documented.[48**,53**] These feelings may be warranted as there is much evidence in the literature showing that suicide survivors are in fact viewed more negatively by others in their social network in comparison with other mourners.[49] One study by Allen et al.[54**] found that individuals bereaved by suicide were viewed as more psychologically disturbed, less likable, more blameworthy, and more in need of professional mental healthcare than those bereaved by other causes. As a result, it is not surprising that these individuals struggle with isolation and lack of social support at a time when it is needed most.

Although the aforementioned themes are likely to arise to some extent in all suicide survivors, some may be more or less likely when the suicide is completed by a terminally ill patient. First, on the positive side, family members of a terminally ill suicide completer may not struggle as restlessly with the meaning of the suicide, particularly if their loved one was in a large amount of physical pain or was somehow physically incapacitated. Second, family members may not feel as much responsibility for the suicide as there is a clear external factor, namely, the terminal illness, to which one can assign blame. Finally, given that the suicide may not be as unexpected among such a population, the family member may have already started the anticipatory grieving process and may not feel as rejected and abandoned as other survivors. On the other hand, although suicide among the terminally ill may be more socially accepted and thus less stigmatizing for the survivor, this group may receive fewer offers of professional support in comparison with other mourners. Additionally, guilt feelings may be more common among this group of survivors as a consequence of the simultaneous feeling of relief they may experience at the end of a possibly long care-giving period.

Armed with an understanding of the key issues for suicide survivors in general, and for survivors of a terminally ill patient's suicide more specifically, the treatment team can now begin to intervene on behalf of the family. First and foremost, the physician and mental health professional on the team should contact the family immediately after hearing of the suicide. This will communicate that the treatment team does not criticize or blame the family, and that they will not abandon the family just because the patient has passed away. Similarly, attempts should be made to attend the funeral memorial services. These acts will serve to diffuse the family's feelings of isolation and stigmatization. Second, attempts should be made to connect the family member to a support group specifically designed for suicide survivors. Jordan[49] argues that groups limited to suicide survivors seem more likely to cohere quickly and to "avoid a replication of the empathic failure that too often occurs for survivors in their larger social networks." Such groups should focus on areas such as facilitating integration of the loss by understanding why and how the suicide occurred, exploring the meaning of the loss for the survivor, and providing space for the expression of all types of feelings, both positive and negative.[51] Effective support groups for suicide survivors should also include a psychoeducational component, which has been found to reduce survivor anxiety and bolster coping strategies.[51] Psychoeducational resources and materials should also be designed to support and educate those in the survivor's support network so as to reduce their negatively held stereotypes about this group of mourners. A third objective of the treatment team should be to encourage the family to engage in a grieving ritual for the survivor. Some cultures restrict the use of traditional grieving rituals, which can leave the survivor with no closure.[51] Developing their own unique ritual can be a liberating experience for the family. Finally, survivors are at risk for increased suicidality of their own, although possibly less so when it is a terminally ill patient that takes his or her own life. Nevertheless, the treatment team should proactively assess the family member's risk, and make an appropriate referral if warranted.

Key learning points

- Suicide is a tragic but often preventable response to terminal illness.

- Terminally ill patients are at elevated risk of suicide when compared to the general population. This is likely due to the increased incidence of distressing symptoms such as depression, physical disability, pain, and cognitive dysfunction. It is far more common for patients to have thoughts of suicide rather than actual intent of committing suicide. For some patients, suicidal thoughts may represent a personal sense of control over the cancer.

- Assessment of suicide risk and appropriate intervention is critical. Early and comprehensive psychiatric involvement with high-risk individuals can often avert suicide in the medical setting.

- Patients who present with a desire for hastened death should be screened for common risk factors such as depression or history of psychiatric illness, hopelessness, physical distress (including pain and symptom burden), poor social support, fear of being a burden to others as well as existential concerns such as loss of meaning and loss of dignity. Studies have shown that when these factors are treated, patients show a decrease in desire for hastened death.

- Physician-assisted suicide remains a controversial topic in palliative care. If the issue should come up with a patient, the physician should be empathic and nonjudgmental, allowing the patient to freely discuss their thoughts. When approached by patients for assistance in dying, the first step should be to provide excellent palliative care.

- Analgesics, antipsychotics, or antidepressant drugs should be used when appropriate to treat any agitation, psychosis, major depression, or pain that are contributing to the patient's suicidal ideation.

- Novel psychotherapeutic interventions aimed at improving spiritual well-being, sense of meaning and diminishing hopelessness, demoralization, and loss of dignity are being studied and disseminated, which may prove effective in reducing suicidal ideation and attempts. Interventions for hopelessness and loss of meaning and purpose in the terminally ill are of particular importance when addressing the issues of desire for death and despair at the end of life.

- In cases of completed suicide, clinicians need to be sensitive to the needs of the patient's family and loved ones. These individuals may require some form of intervention to assist them in coping. Such individuals may also be at a potentially higher risk for suicide themselves.

REFERENCES

◆ 1 Whitlock FA. Suicide and physical illness. In: Roy A (ed.), *Suicide*. Baltimore, MD: Williams & Willkins; 1986. pp. 151–170.

◆ 2 Breitbart W. Cancer pain and suicide. In: Foley KM, Bonica JJ, Ventafridda V (eds.), *Advances in Pain Research and Therapy*, vol. 16. New York: Raven Press; 1990. pp. 399–412.

● 3 Silberfarb PM, Maurer LH, Cronthamel CS. Psychosocial aspects of breast cancer patients during different treatment regimens. *Am J Psychiatry* 1980; 137: 450–455.

● 4 Achte KA, Vanhkouen ML. Cancer and the psyche. *Omega* 1971; 2: 46–56.

● 5 Brown JH, Henteleff P, Barakat S, Rowe JR. Is it normal for terminally ill patients to desire death? *Am J Psychiatry* 1986; 143: 208–211.

◆ 6 Breitbart W. Suicide in cancer patients. *Oncology* 1987; 1: 49.

● 7 Hem E, Loge J, Haldorsen T, Ekeberg, O. Suicide risk in cancer patients from 1960 to 1999. *J Clin Oncol* 2004; 22: 4209–4216.

● 8 Druss B, Pincus H. Suicidal ideation and suicide attempts in general medical illnesses. *Arch Int Med* 2000; 160(10): 1522–1526.

● 9 Bolund C. Suicide and cancer: II. Medical and care factors in suicide by cancer patients in Sweden. 1973–1976. *J Psychosoc Oncol* 1985; 3: 17–30.

● 10 Zweig R, Hinrichsen G. Factors associated with suicide attempts by depressed older adults: A prospective study. *Am J Psychiatry* 1993; 150: 1687–1692.

● 11 Farberow NL, Shneidman ES, Leonard CV. Suicide among general medical and surgical hospital patients with malignant neoplasms. *Med Bull Vet Adm* 1963; MB-9: 1–11.

● 12 Fox BH, Stanek EJ, Boyd SC, Flannery JT. Suicide rates among cancer patients in Connecticut. *J Chronic Dis* 1982; 35: 85–100.

● 13 Louhivuori KA, Hakama J. Risk of suicide among cancer patients. *Am J Epidemiol* 1979; 109: 59–65.

● 14 Farberow NL, Ganzler S, Cuter F, Reynolds D. An eight year survey of hospital suicides. *Suicide Life Threat Behav* 1971; 1: 198–201.

● 15 Robins E, Murphy G, Wilkinson RH Jr et al. Some clinical considerations in the prevention of suicide based on 134 successful suicides. *Am J Public Health* 1950; 49: 888–889.

● 16 Guze S, Robins E. Suicide and primary affective disorders. *Br J Psychiatry* 1970; 117: 437–438.

● 17 Chochinov HMC, Wilson K, Enns M, Lander S. Prevalence of depression in the terminally ill: Effects of diagnostic criteria and symptom threshold judgments. *Am J Psychiatry* 1994; 151: 4.

◆ 18 Breitbart W, Jaramillo JR, Chochinov HM. Palliative and terminal care. In Holland JC et al. (eds.), *Psycho-Oncology*. New York: Oxford University Press; 1998. pp. 437–449.

● 19 Ganzini L, Lec MA, Heintz RT et al. The effect of depression treatment on elderly patients' preferences for life-sustaining medical therapy. *Am J Psychiatry* 1994; 151: 1613–1616.

◆ 20 Beck AT, Kovacs M, Weissman A. Hopelessness and suicidal behavior: An overview. *JAMA* 1975; 234: 1146–1149.

● 21 Chochinov HM, Wilson KG, Enns M, Lander S. Depression, hopelessness, and suicidal ideation in the terminally ill. *Psychosomatics* 1998; 39: 366–370.

◆ 22 Rosenfeld B, Krivo S, Breitbart W et al. Suicide, assisted suicide, and euthanasia in the terminally ill. In Chochinov HM, Breitbart W (eds.), *Handbook of Psychiatry in Palliative Medicine*. New York: Oxford University Press; 2000. pp. 51–62.

◆ 23 American Psychological Oncology Society. *Quick Reference for Oncology Clinicians: The Psychiatric and Psychological Dimensions of Cancer Symptom Management*. Charlottesville, VA: IPOS Press; 2006.

● 24 Breitbart W, Rosenfeld B, Pessin H et al. Depression, hopelessness, and desire for hastened death in terminally ill patients with cancer. *JAMA* 2000; 284 (22): 2907–2911.

● 25 Chochinov HM, Wilson KG, Enns M et al. Desire for death in the terminally ill. *Am J Psych* August 1995; 152(8): 1185–1191.

● 26 Rodin G, Zimmerman C, Rydall A et al. The desire for hastened death in patients with metastatic cancer. *J Pain Symp Manage* 2007; 33(6): 661–675.

● 27 Chochinov HM, Hack T, Hassard T et al. Understanding the will to live in patients nearing death. *Psychosomatics* January–February 2005; 46(1): 7–10.

● 28 McClain CS, Rosenfeld B, Breitbart W. Effect of spiritual well-being on end-of-life despair in terminally-ill cancer patients. *Lancet* May 10, 2003; 361(9369): 1603–1607.

● 29 Bondreau J, Somerville M, Biller-Andorno N. Clinical decisions. Physician-assisted suicide. *NEJM* 2013; 368(15): 1450–1452.

30 http://public.health.oregon.gov/ProviderPartnerResources/ EvaluationResearch/ DeathwithDignityAct/Documents/year15.pdf

● 31 Tolle SW, Tilden VR, Drach LL, Fromme EK, Perrin NA, Hedberg K. Characteristics and proportions of dying Oregonians who personally consider physician-assisted suicide. *J Clini Ethics* 2004; 15: 111–118.

● 32 Ganzini L, Goy ER, Dobscha SK. Prevalence of depression and anxiety in patients requesting physicians aid in dying: Cross sectional survey. *BMJ* October 7, 2008; 337: a1682.

● 33 Breitbart W, Rosenfeld B, Gibson C et al. Impact of treatment for depression on desire for hastened death in patients with advanced AIDS. *Psychosomatics* March–April 2010; 51(2): 98–105. doi: 10.11.

● 34 van der Lee ML, van der Bom JG, Swarte NB et al. Euthanasia and depression: A prospective cohort study among terminally ill cancer patients. *J Clin Oncol* September 20, 2005; 23(27): 6607–6612 [Epub 2005 Aug 22].

◆ 35 Quill T. Physicians should "assist in suicide" when it is appropriate. *J Law Med Ethics* March 2012; 40(1): 57–65.

◆ 36 Breitbart W. Physician-assisted suicide ruling in Montana: Struggling with care of the dying, responsibility and freedom in big sky country. *Palliat Support Care* 2010 March; 8(1): 1–6.

◆ 37 Hudson PL, Schonfeild P, Kelly B et al. Responding to desire to die statements from patients with advanced disease: Recommendations for health professionals. *Palliat Med* 2006; 20: 703–710.

38 Rousseau P. Spirituality and the dying patient. *J Clin Oncol* 2000; 18: 2000–2002.

◆ 39 Kissane D, Clarke DM, Street AF. Demoralization syndrome-a relevant psychiatric diagnosis for palliative care. *J Palliat Care* 2001; 17: 12–21.

◆ 40 Kissane et al., In Chochinov H, Breitbart W (eds.), *Handbook of Psychiatry in Palliative Medicine, Dignity, Meaning and Demoralization: Emerging Paradigms in End-of-Life Care*, 2nd edn. New York: Oxford University Press; 2009. pp. 101–112.

◆ 41 Chochinov HM, Hack T, Hassard T et al. Dignity in the terminally ill: A developing empirical model. *Soc Sci Med* February 2002; 54(3): 433–443.

● 42 Chochinov HM, Hack T, Hassard T et al. Dignity Therapy: A novel psychotherapeutic intervention for patients near the end of life. *J Clin Oncol* 2005; 23: 5520–5525.

● 43 Chochinov HM, Kristjanson LJ, Breitbart W, McClement S, Hack TF, Hassard T, Harlos M. Effect of dignity therapy on distress and end-of-life experience in terminally ill patients: A randomised controlled trial. *Lancet Oncol* August 2011; 12(8): 753–762.

44 Breitbart W, Gibson C, Poppito S, Berg A. Psychotherapeutic interventions at the end of life: A focus on meaning and spirituality. *Can J Psychiatry* 2004; 49: 366–372.

45 Frankl VF. *Man's Search for Meaning*, 4th edn. Boston, MA: Beacon Press; 1959/1992.

46 Breitbart W, Rosenfeld B, Gibson C et al. Meaning-centered group psychotherapy for patients with advanced cancer: A pilot randomized controlled trial. *Psycho-oncology* January 2010; 19 (1): 21–28.

47 Breitbart W, Poppito S, Rosenfeld B et al. Pilot randomized controlled trial for individual meaning-centered psychotherapy for patients with advanced cancer. *J Clin Onc* April 2012; 30 (12): 1304–1309.

48 Bailey SE, Kral MJ, Dunham K. Survivors of suicide do grieve differently: Empirical support for a common sense proposition. *Suicide Life Threat Behav* 1999; 29: 256–272.

49 Jordan JR. Is suicide bereavement different? A reassessment of the literature. *Suicide Life Threat Behav* 2001; 31: 91–103.

● 50 Barrett TW, Scott TB. Suicide bereavement and recovery patterns compared with non-suicide bereavement patterns. *Suicide Life Threat Behav* 1990; 20: 1–15.

51 Barlow CA, Morrison H. Survivors of suicide: Emerging counseling strategies. *J Psychosoc Nurs Mental Health Serv* 2002; 40: 28–39.

52 Van Dongen CJ. Survivors of a family member's suicide: Implications for practice. *Nurse Pract* 1991; 16: 31–36.

● 53 Harwood D, Hawton K, Hope T, Jacoby R. The grief experiences and needs of bereaved relatives and friends of older people dying through suicide: A descriptive and case–control study. *J Affective Disord* 2001; 72: 185–194.

54 Allen BG, Calhoun LG, Cann A, Tedeschi RG. The effects of cause of death on responses to the bereaved: Suicide compared to accidental and natural causes. *Omega* 1993; 28: 39–48.

PART 15

Specific conditions and situations

88

Cancer: Radiotherapy

LULUEL KHAN, EDWARD CHOW, ELIZABETH A. BARNES

INTRODUCTION

Approximately half of all radiotherapy (RT) treatment is given with palliative as opposed to curative intent.[1] The goal of palliative radiotherapy is to use a short treatment schedule to provide effective and durable symptom relief with minimal toxicity.

Radiotherapy is used to treat cancer with ionizing radiation, resulting in damage to cellular DNA (Figure 88.1). Radiotherapy delivery is broadly classified as external beam radiation or brachytherapy. External beam treatment involves high energy gamma rays produced from a linear accelerator, or from a radioactive cobalt source housed within the head of the treatment machine. Brachytherapy involves delivering radiation over a short distance from a radiation source that is placed on or into a body surface, tissue, or cavity. Another form of brachytherapy involves using radioactive isotopes that have affinity to specific tissues, for example, bone or thyroid, and are injected into the blood stream and deposit radiation locally.

When a patient is seen in consultation for palliative radiotherapy, the radiation oncologist takes into consideration tumor factors such as histology and tumor location, and patient factors such as symptom burden and life expectancy to determine whether the treatment is appropriate. Repeat radiotherapy to the same site may be possible depending on the previous treatment parameters (dose and fractionation), time since previous radiotherapy, and the radiation tolerance of structures within the radiotherapy field. As radiotherapy is a local treatment, the objective is to treat the tumor while minimizing dose to surrounding normal tissue. Immobilization of the patient is first required; usually this involves having the patient lie still in the supine position. External beam treatment planning (simulation) involves localizing the tumor clinically if the lesion is superficial or using fluoroscopy or computed tomography (CT) if deep seated. After treatment field planning and radiation dose calculation, the patient then receives treatment from a linear accelerator or cobalt unit in a heavily shielded room.

It is important to remember that the patient must be able to lie still, unattended, on the simulator and treatment tables (which are hard and narrow) for approximately 15 min at a time. This may be difficult for patients who are delirious, orthopneic, or have uncontrolled pain.

The unit of radiation dose is gray (Gy) (0.01 Gy = 1 centigray [cGy]). Typically, one radiotherapy treatment (fraction) is given per day, 5 days a week (Monday through Friday). Large doses per fraction are poorly tolerated and increase the risk of late tissue toxicity. Small doses per fraction delivered over many days are used to take advantage of the observation that cancers have impaired DNA repair as compared with normal tissue. Therefore, during treatment, normal tissue can recover through repair and repopulation, while DNA damage in malignant cells accumulates and is fatal when the cell tries to divide. However, the differential toxicity between cancer and normal tissue is not complete, and normal tissues have a tolerance dose beyond which they are irreversibly damaged. This dose is lower for spinal cord and bowel than muscle and bone. The optimal dose of radiation is one that will produce the maximal probability of tumor control with minimal complications. For symptom palliation, a high total dose is not required; therefore, palliative fractionation schedules can be shorter and use a higher dose per fraction. This serves to minimize patient visits to the cancer center and treatment-related side effects. Commonly used palliative radiotherapy regimens include 800 cGy in a single fraction, 2000 cGy in 5 fractions (400 cGy per fraction), and 3000 cGy in 10 fractions (300 cGy per fraction). Treatment-related side effects are defined as acute (<90 days after treatment start) or late (>90 days). As radiotherapy is a local treatment, apart from fatigue, side effects depend on the area treated. Acute toxicity is self-limiting and tends to resolve within 2 weeks of treatment completion. Late toxicity is usually not a problem in the palliative setting, given the low total radiotherapy doses used and the limited life expectancy of patients with advanced cancer. However, the radiation tolerance of normal tissue such as spinal cord needs to be respected, especially when retreating, as patients can live longer than expected (Table 88.1).

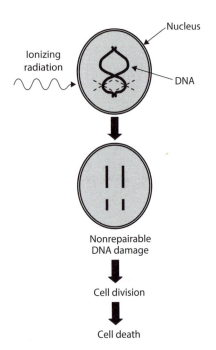

Figure 88.1 *Radiation damaging nuclear DNA resulting in cell death.*

BONE METASTASES

Bone metastases are common in patients with advanced cancer, and are the most common cause of cancer pain.[2] Palliation of bone metastases comprises a significant workload in a radiotherapy department, accounting for 40% of palliative radiotherapy courses.[1] Radiotherapy is used in the management of bone metastases for the relief of bone pain, prevention of impending fractures, and promotion of healing pathological fractures. Radiotherapy remains the gold standard for palliation of painful bone metastases, aiding in effective pain relief and decreasing side effects from increased escalating opioid consumption.[3]

Prophylactic surgical fixation should be considered for good performance status patients with bone lesions at high risk of fracture, as prophylactic surgery is easier to perform than surgery after a pathological fracture, and is associated with better functional outcomes and increased survival.[4]

High-risk lesions include those with >50% cortical destruction of a long bone; femoral lesions >0.25 mm in the neck, subtrochanteric, intertrochanteric, or supracondylar regions; and diffuse lytic involvement of a weight-bearing bone especially if painful.[5*] Postoperative radiotherapy is routinely given and has been shown to improve functional status, decrease pain, and reduce the risk of refracture.[6*] Database analysis found the risk of femoral fracture was most dependent on the amount of axial cortical involvement, and recommended prophylactic fixation for lesions >30 mm, or in nonsurgical candidates, multiple fraction radiotherapy to decrease fracture occurrence.[7**]

The overall and complete pain response rates to bone radiotherapy are 58%–59% and 23%–24%, respectively.[8***] The median time to pain relief is 3 weeks,[9**] and the median duration of pain relief is 12–24 weeks.[8***] Acute toxicity is

Table 88.1 *Tumor sites and symptoms amenable to palliative radiotherapy*

Anatomic site	Symptom
Skeleton	1. Painful bone metastases 2. Spinal cord compression 3. Status post vertebral body decompression 4. Status post fixation of long bone
Brain	1. Neurologic dysfunction 2. Headaches 3. Seizure 4. Status post resection of metastasis
Lung	1. Cough 2. Shortness of breath 3. Hemoptysis 4. Chest pain 5. Postobstructive pneumonia 6. Superior vena cava syndrome
Esophagus	1. Dysphagia 2. Pain
Head and neck	1. Bleeding 2. Pain 3. Dysphagia 4. Shortness of breath 5. Ulceration
Gynecologic	1. Pain 2. Vaginal bleeding 3. Vaginal discharge 4. Obstruction
Genitourinary	1. Hematuria 2. Pain 3. Urinary outlet obstruction
Rectum	1. Pain 2. Rectal bleeding 3. Tenesmus 4. Rectal obstruction
Liver	1. Pain 2. Discomfort 3. Nausea

mild, seen in 10%–17% of patients, and late toxicity is rare (4%).[10**] Toxicity is site specific; for example, acute toxicity from cervical spine radiotherapy can result in dysphagia, thoracic and lumbar spine radiotherapy nausea and vomiting, and pelvic radiotherapy diarrhea. Prophylactic ondansetron can be used to reduce emesis when treating over the epigastrium, lumbothoracic spine, or a large pelvic field.[8***] More recently, the phenomenon of pain flare has been documented. Pain flare is defined as a 2-point increase in the worst pain score (0–10) compared to baseline with no decrease in analgesic intake, or a 25% increase in analgesic intake with no decrease in worst pain score within 10 days following radiotherapy at the index site. Hird et al. reported that 40% incidence of pain flare during and within 10 days following palliative radiotherapy for painful bone metastases.[11**] Corticosteroids have shown promise in early phase trials in decreasing the incidence of pain flare[12*] and a large phase III trial investigating dexamethasone in preventing pain flare after single fraction radiotherapy is ongoing.[13] Re-treatment offers effective palliation, with a response rate of 63%.[14**] Generally, a 4-week interval is given before considering re-treatment, to allow enough time to derive benefit from the first treatment. There is an ongoing international phase III randomized trial of single vs. multiple fractions for re-irradiation of painful bone metastases to determine the optimal dose–fractionation regimen for re-treatment.[15]

Direct comparisons of efficacy between different studies is problematic since a variety of endpoints have been utilized including different pain measurement tools, different data collection time points, and uneven handling of analgesic usage.[16] Meta-analyses by Wu, Sze, and Chow looking at different fractionation schemes have shown no significant difference in overall or complete response rates or duration of pain relief between single and multiple fractions.[15***,16***] Furthermore, no significant differences in quality of life, analgesic use, or acute toxicity were observed. However, the observed re-treatment rates were 2.5 times higher with the use of a single fraction at 20%–25% compared with multiple fraction regimens.[8***,16***]

The optimal palliative radiotherapy treatment regimen is one that provides prompt and effective pain relief with minimal toxicity and patient inconvenience. A single fraction has the advantage of requiring only one treatment visit, which is especially beneficial for patients with poor performance status and those who live at a distance from the center. For patients with longer life expectancy, receiving multiple fractions upfront may avoid the need for re-treatment, and therefore, the choice of fractionation schedule should be discussed with the patient.[17]

Patients with bone metastases often have diffuse bony disease, for which half-body irradiation (HBI) and systemic radionuclides can be useful treatment modalities to simultaneously target all bony lesions. HBI encompasses either the upper half (base of skull to iliac crest) or lower half (iliac crest to ankles) of the body in a single large radiotherapy field.[18**] Single fraction HBI has been shown to provide pain relief in 70%–80% of patients.[19*] The onset of pain relief is quicker than with local radiotherapy, occurring within 24–48 hours, suggesting that cells of the inflammatory response pathway may be the initial target tissue, since tumor cell activities are unlikely to be halted so quickly. The dose delivered is typically a single fraction of 6 Gy to the upper body (reduced dose due to potential for lung toxicity), and 8 Gy to the lower body. HBI is associated with acute gastrointestinal toxicity (nausea, vomiting, diarrhea), thought to be more pronounced with use of a single fraction.[28] Acute toxicity usually requires intravenous fluids and premedication with antiemetics and corticosteroids, and, in some cases, an overnight stay in hospital for observation. Reversible myelosuppression occurs; therefore, sequential treatment of upper and lower body requires a 4–6-week interval for counts to recover.

Systemic radionuclides are deposited at the site of osteoblastic bony metastases, mirroring the uptake seen on bone scan, and emit radiation with a mean range of 3 mm.[20] Radionuclides have been mainly studied in patients with hormone-refractory prostate cancer, as these bone metastases tend to be osteoblastic rather than osteolytic. Patients with lung or breast primaries typically have mixed osteoblastic and osteolytic bone metastases, and therefore, the use of radionuclides is less applicable. Strontium-89 and samarium-153 are the agents most commonly utilized in clinical practice, and can be given in a single intravenous injection on an outpatient basis. Efficacy of the various radionuclides is thought to be similar, although comparative trials have not been conducted. Contraindications for use are fracture, spinal cord compression, lesions with extra-osseous component, renal failure, inadequate hemogram, life expectancy, 2 months, and chemotherapy within 1 month.[20] A randomized trial comparing strontium to local or wide field radiotherapy in patients with metastatic prostate cancer found similar response rates in all arms (65%), and strontium decreased the incidence of new painful sites.[21**] Strontium toxicity consists mainly of reversible myelosuppression, with a decrease in platelet and leukocyte counts of 30%–40% at nadir, occurring at 4–8 weeks.[21**]

BRAIN METASTASES

Brain metastases occur in 20%–40% of cancer patients, most commonly from lung, breast, and gastrointestinal primaries.[22] Brain metastases may cause headache, focal weakness, behavior changes, seizures, speech difficulty, visual changes, and decreased level of consciousness. Most patients with brain metastases will have a short lifespan, and the effects of their intracranial disease commonly contribute to their deaths. Median survival of 1–2 months with corticosteroids alone,[23] and 4–6 months with whole-brain radiotherapy (WBRT) has been reported.[24] Treatment typically consists of corticosteroids to reduce peritumoral edema, followed by WBRT. There is no difference in symptom control among different dose-fractionation regimes as compared with 3000/10 or 2000/5.[25***] The goal of radiotherapy is to provide neurological symptom relief, allow corticosteroid tapering, and possibly improve survival. The acute side effects of treatment include fatigue, alopecia, and erythema of the scalp. Late effects for longer-term survivors include neurocognitive changes, somnolence syndrome, and radiation necrosis. A single brain metastasis is present in 30%–40% of patients.[26] For these patients with good performance status and minimal or no evidence of extracranial disease, surgical excision followed by WBRT has been shown to improve survival over WBRT alone.[27***] Postoperative WBRT after surgical excision of a single metastasis can improve local control.[27***,28****] The addition of a stereotactic radiosurgery boost to WBRT for patients with good performance status has been recently shown to improve survival for patients with a single brain metastasis, and to improve functional autonomy for patients with two to three metastases.[29***]

For selected patients with longer expected survival and one to three brain metastases, there has been interest in the use of stereotactic radiosurgery alone with WBRT or further radiosurgery reserved for salvage. This is partially due to concerns about neurocognitive dysfunction following whole-brain external beam radiotherapy.[30***]

A single institution observational study of all patients receiving WBRT for symptomatic brain metastases found that at 1 month, only 15%–39% of patients benefited from treatment (depending on the criteria used), and 27% died at or soon after 1 month.[31*] This emphasizes the importance of appropriately selecting patients for treatment, as patients with poor performance status and rapidly progressive extracranial disease may not derive a clinical benefit from radiotherapy. A current trial randomizes patients between supportive care and supportive care plus 20 Gy in five fractions to the whole brain for metastatic cancer. The results of this trial will hopefully come to better define the group that would be most likely to benefit from the addition of radiotherapy in this setting.[32]

LUNG CANCER

Lung cancer is one of the most common causes of cancer death worldwide. Non–small cell lung cancer (NSCLC) accounts for 80% of lung cancers, and small cell lung cancer (SCLC) 20%. The latter is typically treated with chemotherapy, given the propensity for widespread dissemination at diagnosis. More than two-thirds of NSCLC patients present with incurable locally advanced or metastatic disease.[33**] The overall prognosis of patients is poor, with a median survival of less than 1 year.

The use of chemotherapy for NSCLC has been increasing over the past two decades, but radiotherapy remains an important treatment modality for patients with predominantly intrathoracic disease, who are unable to receive or decline chemotherapy, or have chemoresistant disease. Thoracic symptoms can be effectively palliated with local radiotherapy, with up to 90% of patients obtaining relief from hemoptysis and chest pain, and up to 65% obtaining relief from cough and dyspnea.[34**] Symptom palliation with radiotherapy has been found to last for over half of the patient's lifetime.[35**] In locally advanced NSCLC patients with asymptomatic pulmonary disease, no advantage has been shown with respect to overall survival, quality of life, or symptom control to immediate vs. delayed thoracic radiotherapy.[36**] For patients with total atelectasis secondary to obstruction of the main-stem bronchus, receiving radiotherapy within 2 weeks of atelectasis results in higher rates of complete re-expansion (71% vs. 23% after 2 weeks).[37*] Intraluminal brachytherapy with a high dose rate applicator can offer effective palliation of symptoms arising from endobronchial disease in one to three fraction outpatient treatments.[38*] This is also a treatment option for patients with endobronchial tumor recurrence who have received maximal doses of external beam radiotherapy.

A meta-analysis of 13 randomized controlled trials of different dose–fractionation schedules for palliation of thoracic symptoms from incurable lung cancer found no significant differences for specific symptom-control end points, although improvement in survival favored higher-dose radiation (≥35 Gy(10)) vs. lower BED.[39***] At 1 year, 26.5% vs. 21.7% of patients were alive in the high- vs. low-dose group. However, dysphagia was more commonly seen

after high-dose radiation. For patients treated with palliative intent, chemotherapy has been shown to improve survival, symptom relief, and quality of life, compared to best supportive care.[40] Whether combining radiotherapy with chemotherapy improves symptom relief or quality of life for selected NSCLC patients is unknown. Systemic symptoms such as fatigue and anorexia are not likely to improve with the addition of radiotherapy aimed at thoracic disease. Radiotherapy to the thorax may in fact worsen fatigue and dysphagia, and it should not be considered worthwhile in these patients. Additionally, those patients with severe dyspnea secondary to severe chronic pulmonary obstructive disease rather than postobstructive causes may suffer worsened rather than improved breathing following radiotherapy.

PELVIC DISEASE

Locally advanced and recurrent pelvic malignancies (i.e., genitourinary, gastrointestinal, and gynecological primaries) can result in many disabling symptoms. These include hemorrhage; necrotic vaginal discharge; local pelvic and neuropathic pain due to adenopathy, invasion of bone and lumbosacral plexus; lower extremity edema; fistula formation; gastrointestinal tract obstruction; and renal failure due to ureteric obstruction.

Effective symptom palliation has been seen following one to three fractions of 10 Gy given 4 weeks apart to the pelvis.[41*,42*,43*] RTOG 7905 (Radiation Therapy Oncology Group) examined combining three fractions with misonidazole (a radiosensitizer) in patients with gynecologic, bowel, and prostate cancers, and found the overall and complete response rate to treatment was 62% and 38%, respectively.[44*] A dose–response relationship has been reported, with repeat fractions giving more effective symptom palliation.[41*,44*] However, RTOG 7905 found three fractions gave a very high rate (49%) of late complications,[44*] while one to two fractions is associated with a late complication rate of 0%–10%.[41*,44*] Given the high complication rate, RTOG 8502 explored using 370 cGy twice a day for 2 days, with a rest interval of 2–4 weeks, repeated three times to a total dose of 440 cGy.[45*] This regimen was associated with a much lower risk of late toxicity (6%), yet gave similar symptom palliation with approximately 50% of patients having complete pain relief, and 90% complete resolution of bleeding or obstruction.[46,47*] As the incidence of late toxicity increases with time, patients with a life expectancy greater than 9 months should receive the second RTOG schedule, or other treatment schedules using lower dose per fraction, or one to two fractions of 10 Gy.

Patients with muscle invasive bladder cancer are typically smokers, older, and often have numerous medical comorbidities. For patients unable to tolerate radical treatment, and for patients with locally advanced incurable disease, palliative radiotherapy with the goal of symptom relief can be given. A large randomized trial was conducted comparing the efficacy and toxicity of two palliative radiotherapy schedules (35 Gy in 10 fractions, and 21 Gy in 3 fractions on alternate days over 1 week).[48**] There was no difference between the two arms, with 68% overall improvement in bladder symptoms at 3 months, median survival of 7.5 months, and late bowel toxicity rate of <1%. Other groups have reported using 5–6-weekly fractions of 6 Gy with effective symptom palliation,[49*,50*] late bowel (2%) and bladder (11%) toxicity was reported in one trial.[49*] Another trial reported that by using 5.75 vs. 6.5 Gy in 6-weekly fractions, the incidence of late bowel toxicity was reduced from 15% to 0%.[51*] Of interest, the radiotherapy treatment volume in these bladder cancer trials consisted of the bladder with a small margin (usually 100 cm³), which was smaller than the volumes treated in the RTOG trials (usually 225 cm³). This may partially explain the higher bowel complication rate seen in the RTOG trials. Using modern CT-based radiation treatment planning to treat the tumor while minimizing bowel and other structures can reduce treatment toxicity and allow for dose escalation.

Para-aortic adenopathy from pelvic primaries can result in lower back pain that can be palliated with local radiotherapy. Recurrent ovarian cancer is typically treated with chemotherapy; however, radiotherapy offers very good symptom palliation with response rates 70%, even in patients with platinum-resistant disease.[52*,53*]

Locally advanced and unresectable rectal cancer can cause severe pelvic pain, bleeding, and bowel obstruction, and palliative resection or diverting colostomy is often recommended. Palliative chemoradiotherapy with concurrent 5-fluorouracil (5-FU) has been shown to provide symptom relief in 94% of patients, and gave a 1-year colostomy-free survival rate of 87%.[54*] This study recommended radiotherapy regimens of 36 Gy/12 fraction/3 weeks, 35 Gy/14 fraction/3 weeks, or 30 Gy/6 fraction/2 weeks. A review addressing the question of the most effective dose fractionation for symptom relief in patients with pelvic recurrence from colorectal or rectal cancer included studies using doses ranging from 1500 to 7000 cGy, but could not provide a definitive answer.[55***]

Locally advanced, hormone-refractory prostate cancer may lead to pain, urinary obstruction, hematuria, and rectal symptoms. Hypofractionated radiotherapy of 20 Gy in five fractions has been shown to provide excellent symptom relief with minimal side effects. Nearly 90% of symptomatic patients treated with this regimen noted partial or complete relief of their symptoms 4 months after completing radiotherapy.[56]

HEAD AND NECK CANCER

Patients with locally advanced head and neck cancer can have many devastating symptoms due to their disease. These include pain, dysphagia, hoarseness, otalgia, and respiratory distress.[57**] Tracheostomy placement may be required to maintain the airway, and patients commonly have malnutrition and may require a feeding tube. Radiotherapy with concurrent chemotherapy can be offered to patients with advanced

inoperable disease with curative intent, but treatment is associated with high rates of acute toxicity, and 3-year survival rates are approximately 40%.[58**]

The "QUAD SHOT" trial in patients with incurable head and neck cancer evaluated 14 Gy in four fractions given over two consecutive days with at least 6 hours intervals. Responders were given a repeat course at 1 and 2 months. Of the 30 patients enrolled, 16 had an objective response, improved quality of life was documented in 44%, and the median survival was nearly 6 months.[59*] Outcomes of this regime were also reported from India on a group of 15 patients with similar results. Thirteen patients had >50% response and received a second course of RT.[60*]

The AIIMS trial enrolled 500 patients and attempted to allow tumor and patient response to radiotherapy determine whether a treatment course should be delivered with palliative or curative intent. Patients with locally advanced and poor prognosis head and neck cancer received 20 Gy in five fractions, and those with >50% tumor regression and whose performance status allowed went on to receive a more conventionally fractionated dose to a total of 70 Gy. About one-third of patients received the full dose and exhibited a median survival of 13 months, while the group receiving 20 Gy in five fractions had a median survival of only about 6 months. The group that received the shorter course still reported had symptom palliation rates of 47%–59% for pain, dysphagia, hoarseness, cough, and otalgia. In this study, the response of the tumor to the initial 20 Gy allowed the treating team to judge the worthiness of a full treatment course.[60**]

ESOPHAGEAL CANCER

More than half of patients with esophageal cancer present with inoperable disease and require palliation of dysphagia.[61] External beam radiotherapy, intraluminal brachytherapy, photodynamic therapy, laser ablation, and stent placement are among the treatment options.[62**] External beam radiotherapy has been shown to be effective in the management of the swallowing difficulties caused by esophageal carcinoma, though radiotherapy is commonly delivered over several weeks and with concurrent chemotherapy.[63**] The value in a prolonged, combined course of therapy in those patients with the poorest performance status and prognosis seems questionable. The time expenditure and cost of external beam radiotherapy may in these cases be inferior to other local modalities such as stent placement or brachytherapy.[64***,65***]

High-dose rate brachytherapy given in one to three fractions palliates dysphagia in 50% of patients, although care needs to be taken with the dose delivered due to the risk of bleeding, and fistula and stricture formation.[66*] A randomized trial comparing a single fraction of brachytherapy with stent placement found dysphagia relief was faster with stent placement, although the overall response was better with brachytherapy.[67**] Higher complication rates were seen with stent placement, and quality-of-life outcomes favored the brachytherapy group. The need for re-intervention was similar in both groups (40%), and there was no difference in median survival. Palliation of dysphagia needs to be individualized based on patient factors, local expertise, and resource availability.

SKIN CANCER

Skin cancers are classified into two main groups: melanoma and nonmelanoma (basal cell and squamous cell carcinoma).[68] Basal and squamous cell carcinomas are common in older patients, and are often seen in sun-exposed areas of the face and limbs. Neglect in older people can lead to patients presenting with large destructive lesions invading surrounding soft tissue and bone. This can result in pain, bleeding, ulceration, and secondary infection. A short course of palliative radiotherapy can reduce bleeding and allow ulcerative lesions to dry out, making dressing changes and nursing care easier.[69] Melanoma is an aggressive disease with high rates of distant metastases. While often considered radiation resistant, palliative radiotherapy does provide effective and durable palliation. Fractional doses of >400 cGy are thought to be more effective than <400 cGy, with response rates of 82% vs. 36%, respectively.[70***] Examples of radiotherapy regimens using high-dose per fraction are 8 Gy days 0–7–21,[71*] and four to five fractions of 6 Gy delivered twice weekly.[70***]

LIVER METASTASES

Lung, breast, and gastrointestinal cancers frequently give rise to liver metastases, and for some patients, the liver may be the only site of disease. In general, systemic therapy is the preferred therapy for liver metastases. However, selected patients with limited involvement of the liver may be suitable for surgical resection, minimally invasive focal ablation, or focal stereotactic radiotherapy delivered with the goal of local control and improving overall survival. In contrast, low-dose whole-liver radiotherapy (WLRT) may be used to palliate symptoms such as pain, discomfort, night sweats, and nausea.

A number of studies have investigated palliative WLRT either alone or combined with systemic therapy. In all studies, WLRT resulted in symptom relief. Pain relief, the most frequently reported endpoint, ranged from 55% to 80% in studies on WLRT alone.[71]

The Radiation Therapy Oncology Group (RTOG) pilot study used dose–fractionation schedules ranging from 21 to 30 Gy in 7–19 fractions to treat 109 patients. Responses were seen for abdominal pain (55%), nausea and vomiting (49%), fever and night sweats (45%), ascites (33%), anorexia (28%), abdominal distension (27%), jaundice (27%), and night sweats/fever (19%), with complete response rates for individual symptoms ranging from 7% to 34%. Performance status improved in 25%. Currently, there is no clinical data indicating that low-dose WLRT offers a survival advantage, and it should be reserved for symptom control. Symptom control can be achieved with hypofractionated WLRT over few fractions with relatively low total doses.

Key learning points

- Local radiotherapy can provide effective palliation of distressing symptoms.
- A short course of radiotherapy (one to five treatments) can be used to minimize treatment-related side effects and limit patient visits to the cancer center.
- A single 8 Gy treatment is recommended for symptomatic relief of uncomplicated bone metastasis, with an expected overall and complete response rate of 60% and 32%, respectively.
- Patients with symptomatic multiple brain metastases and reasonable performance status are recommended to receive WBRT—suggested radiotherapy schedules are 2000 cGy in 5 fractions or 3000 cGy in 10 fractions.
- Radiotherapy can also be used to palliate hemorrhage (hemoptysis, hematuria, vaginal bleeding, infiltrating skin lesions), cough, dyspnea, dysphagia, and pain due to tumor infiltration.
- Radiotherapy can also be used to palliate pain, discomfort, and nausea from liver metastases.

REFERENCES

1 Hoegler D. Radiotherapy for palliation of symptoms in incurable cancer. *Curr Probl Cancer* 1997; 21: 129–183.
2 Mercadante S. Malignant bone pain: Pathophysiology and treatment. *Pain* 1997; 69: 1–18.
3 Arcangeli G, Giovinazzo G, Saracino B et al. Radiation therapy in the management of symptomatic bone metastases: The effect of total dose and histology on pain relief and response duration. *Int J Radiat Oncol Biol Phys* 1998; 42: 1119–1126.
4 Hardman PD, Robb JE, Kerr GR et al. The value of internal fixation and radiotherapy in the management of upper and lower limb bone metastases. *Clin Oncol (R Coll Radiol)* 1992; 4: 244–248.
5 Parrish FF, Murray JA. Surgical treatment for secondary neoplastic fractures. A retrospective study of ninety-six patients. *J Bone Joint Surg (Am)* 1970; 52: 665–686.
6 Townsend PW, Smalley SR, Cozad SC et al. Role of postoperative radiation therapy after stabilization of fractures caused by metastatic disease. *Int J Radiat Oncol Biol Phys* 1995; 31: 43–49.
7 van der Linden YM, Kroon HM, Dijkstra SP et al. Simple radiographic parameter predicts fracturing in metastatic femoral bone lesions: Results from a randomised trial. *Radiother Oncol* 2003; 69: 21–31.
8 Wu JS, Wong R, Johnston M et al. Cancer Care Ontario Practice Guidelines Initiative Supportive Care Group. Meta-analysis of dose-fractionation radiotherapy trials for the palliation of painful bone metastases. *Int J Radiat Oncol Biol Phys* 2003; 55: 594–605.
9 Steenland E, Leer JW, van Houwelingen H et al. The effect of a single fraction compared to multiple fractions on painful bone metastases: A global analysis of the Dutch Bone Metastasis Study. *Radiother Oncol* 1999; 52: 101–109.
10 Hartsell WF, Scott C, Bruner DW et al. Randomized trial of short versus long-course radiotherapy for palliation of painful bone metastases. *J Natl Cancer Inst* 2005; 97: 798–804.

11 Hird A, Chow E, Zhang L et al. Determining the incidence of pain flare following palliative radiotherapy for symptomatic bone metastases: Results from three Canadian cancer centers. *Int J Radiat Oncol Biol Phys* 2009; 75(1): 193–197.

12 Hird A, Zhang L, Holt T et al. Dexamethasone for the prophylaxis of radiation-induced pain flare after palliative radiotherapy for symptomatic bone metastases: A phase II study. *Clin Oncol (R Coll Radiol)* 2009 May; 21(4): 329–335 [Epub 2009 Feb 15].

13 NCIC Clinical Trials Group. Dexamethasone vs Placebo in the prophylaxis of radiation-induced pain flare following palliative radiotherapy for bone metastases. Available at: http://clinicaltrials.gov/ct2/show/NCT01248585, most recently, accessed May 6, 2011.

14 van der Linden YM, Lok JJ, Steenland E et al. Single fraction radiotherapy is efficacious: A further analysis of the Dutch Bone Metastasis Study controlling for the influence of retreatment. *Int J Radiat Oncol Biol Phys* 2004; 59: 528–537.

15 Kachnic L, Berk L. Palliative single-fraction radiation therapy: How much more evidence is needed? *J Natl Cancer Inst* 2005; 97: 786–788.

◆ 16 Chow E, Harris K, Fan G et al. Palliative radiotherapy trials of bone metastases: A systematic review. *J Clin Oncol* 2007; 25: 1423–1436.

17 Shakespeare TP, Lu JJ, Back MF et al. Patient preference for radiotherapy fractionation schedule in the palliation of painful bone metastases. *J Clin Oncol* 2003; 21: 2156–2162.

18 Salazar OM, Sandhu T, da Motta NW, et al. Fractionated half-body irradiation (HBI) for the rapid palliation of widespread, symptomatic, metastatic bone disease: A randomized Phase III trial of the International Atomic Energy Agency (IAEA). *Int J Radiat Oncol Biol Phys* 2001; 50: 765–775.

19 Hoskin PJ, Ford HT, Harmer CL. Hemibody irradiation (HBI) for metastatic bone pain in two histologically distinct groups of patients. *Clin Oncol (R Coll Radiol)* 1989; 1: 67–69.

◆ 20 McEwan AJB. Use of radionuclides for the palliation of bone metastases. *Semin Radiat Oncol* 2000; 10: 103–114.

● 21 Quilty PM, Kirk D, Bolger JJ et al. A comparison of the palliative effects of strontium-89 and external beam radiotherapy in metastatic prostate cancer. *Radiother Oncol* 1994; 31: 33–40.

22 Johnson JD, Young B. Demographics of brain metastasis. *Neurosurg Clin North Am* 1996; 7: 337–344.

◆ 23 Weissman DE. Glucocorticoid treatment for brain metastases and epidural spinal cord compression: A review. *J Clin Oncol* 1988; 6: 543–551.

24 Borgelt B, Gelber R, Kramer S et al. The palliation of brain metastases: Final results of the first two studies of the Radiation Therapy Oncology Group. *Int J Radiat Oncol Biol Phys* 1980; 6: 1–9.

✳ 25 Tsao M, Lloyd N, Wong R et al. Whole Brain Radiotherapy for the treatment of multiple brain metastases. *Cochrane Database Syst Rev* 2012; 4: CD003869.

26 Lohr F, Pirzkall A, Hof H et al. Adjuvant treatment of brain metastases. *Semin Surg Oncol* 2001; 20: 50–56.

● 27 Patchell RA, Tibbs PA, Walsh JW et al. A randomized trial of surgery in the treatment of single metastases to the brain. *N Engl J Med* 1990; 322: 494–500.

◆ 28 Hart M, Grant R, Walker M et al. Surgical resection and whole brain radiation therapy versus whole brain radiation therapy alone for single brain metastases. *Cochrane Database Syst Rev* 2005; 1: CD003292.

◆ 29 Linskey M, Andrews D, Asher A et al. The role of stereotactic radiosurgery in the management of patients with newly diagnosed brain metastases: A systematic review and evidence-based clinical practice guideline. *J Neurooncol* 2010; 96: 45–68.

30 Chang E, Wefel J, Hess K et al. Neurocognition in patients with brain metastases treated with radiosurgery or radiosurgery plus whole-brain irradiation: A randomised controlled trial. *Lancet Oncol* 2009; 1011: 1037–1044.

● 31 Bezjak A, Adam J, Panzarella T et al. Radiotherapy for brain metastases: Defining palliative response. *Radiother Oncol* 2001; 61: 71–76.

32 National Cancer Institute. Dexamethasone and supportive care with or without whole brain radiation therapy in treating patients with non-small cell lung cancer that has spread to the brain and cannot be removed by surgery. Available at: http://www.clinicaltrialssearch.org/dexamethasone-and-supportive-care-with-or-without-wholebrain-radiation-therapy-in-treating-patients-with-non-smallcell-lung-cancer-that-has-spread-to-the-brain-and-cannot-beremoved-by-surgery-nct00403065.html, most recently, accessed May 6, 2011.

● 33 Sundstrom S, Bremnes R, Aasebo U et al. Hypofractionated palliative radiotherapy (17 Gy per two fractions) in advanced non-small cell lung carcinoma is comparable to standard fractionation for symptom control and survival: A national phase III trial. *J Clin Oncol* 2004; 22: 801–810.

◆ 34 Shepherd FA. Chemotherapy for non-small cell lung cancer: Have we reached a new plateau? *Semin Oncol* 1999; 26: 3–11.

● 35 Inoperable non-small-cell lung cancer (NSCLC): A Medical Research Council randomised trial of palliative radiotherapy with two fractions or ten fractions. Report to the Medical Research Council by its Lung Cancer Working Party. *Br J Cancer* 1991; 63: 265–270.

● 36 Falk SJ, Girling DJ, White RJ et al Medical Research Council Lung Cancer Working Party. Immediate versus delayed palliative thoracic radiotherapy in patients with unresectable locally advanced non-small-cell lung cancer and minimal thoracic symptoms: Randomised controlled trial. *BMJ* 2002; 325: 465.

37 Reddy SP, Marks JE. Total atelectasis of the lung secondary to malignant airway obstruction. Response to radiation therapy. *Am J Clin Oncol* 1990; 13: 394–400.

38 Kelly JF, Delclos ME, Morice RC et al. High-dose-rate endobronchial brachytherapy effectively palliates symptoms due to airway tumors: The 10-year M. D. Anderson cancer center experience. *Int J Radiat Oncol Biol Phys* 2000; 48: 697–702.

◆ 39 Fairchild A, Harris K, Barnes E et al. Palliative thoracic radiotherapy for lung cancer: A systematic review. *J Clin Oncol* 2008; 26: 4001–4011.

◆ 40 Socinski MA. The role of chemotherapy in the treatment of unresectable stage III and IV nonsmall cell lung cancer. *Respir Care Clin North Am* 2003; 9: 207–236.

41 Onsrud M, Hagen B, Strickert T. 10-Gy single-fraction pelvic irradiation for palliation and life prolongation in patients with cancer of the cervix and corpus uteri. *Gynecol Oncol* 2001; 82: 167–171.

42 Chafe W, Fowler WC, Currie JL et al. Single-fraction palliative pelvic radiation therapy in gynecologic oncology: 1,000 rads. *Am J Obstet Gynecol* 1984; 148: 701–705.

43 Halle JS, Rosenman JG, Varia MA et al. 1000 cGy single dose palliation for advanced carcinoma of the cervix or endometrium. *Int J Radiat Oncol Biol Phys* 1986; 12: 1947–1950.

● 44 Spanos WJ Jr, Wasserman T, Meoz R et al. Palliation of advanced pelvic malignant disease with large fraction pelvic radiation and misonidazole: Final report of RTOG phase I/II study. *Int J Radiat Oncol Biol Phys* 1987; 13: 1479–1482.

● 45 Spanos W Jr, Guse C, Perez C et al. Phase II study of multiple daily fractionations in the palliation of advanced pelvic malignancies: Preliminary report of RTOG 8502. *Int J Radiat Oncol Biol Phys* 1989; 17: 659–656.

47 Spanos WJ Jr, Pajak TJ, Emami B et al. Radiation palliation of cervical cancer. *J Natl Cancer Inst Monogr* 1996; 21: 127–130.

● 48 Duchesne GM, Bolger JJ, Griffiths GO et al. A randomized trial of hypofractionated schedules of palliative radiotherapy in the management of bladder carcinoma: Results of medical research council trial BA09. *Int J Radiat Oncol Biol Phys* 2000; 47: 379–388.

49 Jose CC, Price A, Norman A et al. Hypofractionated radiotherapy for patients with carcinoma of the bladder. *Clin Oncol (R Coll Radiol)* 1999; 11: 330–333.

50 McLaren DB, Morrey D, Mason MD. Hypofractionated radiotherapy for muscle invasive bladder cancer in the elderly. *Radiother Oncol* 1997; 43: 171–174.

51 Rostom AY, Tahir S, Gershuny AR et al. Once weekly irradiation for carcinoma of the bladder. *Int J Radiat Oncol Biol Phys* 1996; 35: 289–292.

52 Gelblum D, Mychalczak B, Almadrones L et al. Palliative benefit of external-beam radiation in the management of platinum refractory epithelial ovarian carcinoma. *Gynecol Oncol* 1998; 69: 36–41.

53 Tinger A, Waldron T, Peluso N et al. Effective palliative radiation therapy in advanced and recurrent ovarian carcinoma. *Int J Radiat Oncol Biol Phys* 2001; 51: 1256–1263.

● 54 Crane CH, Janjan NA, Abbruzzese JL et al. Effective pelvic symptom control using initial chemoradiation without colostomy in metastatic rectal cancer. *Int J Radiat Oncol Biol Phys* 2001; 49: 107–116.

◆ 55 Wong R, Thomas G, Cummings B et al. In search of a dose–response relationship with radiotherapy in the management of recurrent rectal carcinoma in the pelvis: A systematic review. *Int J Radiat Oncol Biol Phys* 1998; 40: 437–446.

56 Din O, Thanvi N, Ferguson C et al. Palliative prostate radiotherapy for symptomatic advanced prostate cancer. *Radiother Oncol* 2009; 93: 192–196.

● 57 Mohanti BK, Umapathy H, Bahadur S et al. Short course palliative radiotherapy of 20 Gy in 5 fractions for advanced and incurable head and neck cancer: AIIMS study. *Radiother Oncol* 2004; 71: 275–280.

58 Calais G, Bardet E, Sire C et al. Radiotherapy with concomitant weekly docetaxel for Stages III/IV oropharynx carcinoma. Results of the 98-02 GORTEC Phase II trial. *Int J Radiat Oncol Biol Phys* 2004; 58: 161–166.

59 Corry J, Peters LJ, Costa ID et al. The 'QUAD SHOT'—A phase II study of palliative radiotherapy for incurable head and neck cancer. *Radiother Oncol.* 2005; 77: 137–142.

60 Ghoshal S, Chakraborty S, Moudgil N et al. Quad shot: A short but effective schedule for palliative radiation for head and neck carcinoma. *Indian J Palliat Care* 2009 July; 15(2): 137–140.

61 Sagar PM, Gauperaa T, Sue-Ling H et al. An audit of the treatment of cancer of the oesophagus. *Gut* 1994; 35: 941–945.

● 62 Polinder S, Homs MY, Siersema PD, Steyerberg EW, Dutch SIREC Study Group. Cost study of metal stent placement vs single-dose brachytherapy in the palliative treatment of oesophageal cancer. *Br J Cancer* 2004; 90: 2067–2072.

63 Berger B, Belka C. Evidence-based radiation oncology: Oesophagus. *Radiother Oncol.* 2010; 94: 387–388.

64 Sreedharan A, Harris K, Crellin A et al. Interventions for dysphagia in oesophageal cancer. *Cochrane Database Syst Rev* 2009; 4: CD005048.

65 Homs M, Steyerberg E, Eijkenboom W et al. Single-dose brachytherapy versus metal stent placement for the palliation of dysphagia from oesophageal cancer: Multicentre randomised trial. *Lancet* 2004; 364: 1497–1504.

66 Sur RK, Donde B, Levin VC, Mannell A. Fractionated high dose rate intraluminal brachytherapy in palliation of advanced esophageal cancer. *Int J Radiat Oncol Biol Phys* 1998; 40: 447–453.

67 Homs MYV, Essink-Bot M, Borsbom GJJM et al. Quality of life after palliative treatment for oesophageal carcinoma—A prospective comparison between stent placement and single dose brachytherapy. *Eur J Cancer* 2004; 40: 1862–1871.

68 Hoskin P, Makin W. Skin tumours. In: Hoskin P, Makin W (eds.). *Oncology for Palliative Medicine.* Oxford, U.K.: Oxford University Press, 2003. pp. 235–243.

69 Barnes EA, Breen D, Culleton S et al. Palliative radiotherapy for non-melanoma skin cancer. *Clin Oncol(R Coll Radiol)* 2010; 22(10): 844–849.

✳ 70 Ballo MT, Ang KK. Radiotherapy for cutaneous malignant melanoma: Rationale and indications. *Oncology (Huntingt)* 2004; 18: 99–107.

71 Johanson CR, Harwood AR, Cummings BJ, Quirt I. 0-7-21 radiotherapy in nodular melanoma. *Cancer* 1983; 51: 226–232.

◆ 72 Hoyer M, Swaminath A, Bydder S et al. Radiotherapy for liver metastases: A review of evidence. *Int J Radiat Oncol Biol Phys* 2012; 82(3): 1047–1057.

Chemotherapy, hormonal therapy, and targeted agents

DAVID HUI

INTRODUCTION

Chemotherapy was first discovered around the 1940s, with nitrogen mustard being the first systemic agent to be used for cancer treatment.[1] In subsequent years, multiple classes of chemotherapeutic agents have been developed, including alkylating agents, antimetabolites, topoisomerase inhibitors, platinating agents, antimicrotubular agents, and others. Chemotherapeutic agents generally act by damaging deoxyribonucleic acid (DNA) and proteins, and interfering with cell replication. As a result, cytotoxic agents often affect fast-growing cells, which include both cancer and any host tissue with a rapid turnover, such as the bone marrow, gastrointestinal mucosa, and integumentary system.

The recognition that growth of certain malignancies, such as breast, prostate, and endometrial cancers,[2–4] is highly dependent on endogenous hormones led to the development of hormonal therapy. This was initially achieved by surgical removal of the ovaries or testes. Over the past few decades, multiple hormonal medications have been developed for the treatment of hormone-responsive malignancies and include selective estrogen receptor modulators (SERMs), aromatase inhibitors, luteinizing hormone–releasing hormone (LHRH) agonists, antiandrogens, and antiestrogens. These therapies offer effective treatment options for selected patients and are generally better tolerated than chemotherapeutic agents.

With an increased understanding of the molecular basis of cancer, targeted therapies have emerged in late 1990s as a novel class of systemic therapy.[5–7] These agents target specific cellular processes critical for cancer pathogenesis and include growth factor signaling, apoptosis, angiogenesis, and metastasis.[8] Targeted agents can be further classified into (1) monoclonal antibodies directed against a specific molecular target (usually ending with "mab"), (2) tyrosine kinase inhibitors (usually ending with "nib"), and (3) a wide array of other agents working through various mechanisms. Some agents are highly specific for a single molecular target (e.g., most monoclonal antibodies), while others may affect multiple pathways (e.g., sorafenib).[9] The era of personalized cancer medicine involves tailoring targeted therapy based on the cancers' genotype.[10] Because of the higher specificity, targeted agents are generally associated with fewer side effects than chemotherapy.[11]

The increased integration between oncology and palliative care[12] means that more and more patients seen by palliative care are on concurrent antineoplastic therapies, particularly palliative systemic agents. Thus, palliative care specialists should have a good working knowledge of the main risks and benefits associated with these therapies, and the complex decision-making process regarding the use of these agents.

TREATMENT ADMINISTRATION

Over the course of illness, patients may receive several courses (i.e., regimens) of systemic therapy, each consisting of multiple cycles of treatment. A palliative systemic therapy regimen may include a single agent or multiple drugs (e.g., chemotherapy ± targeted agents). Multidrug regimens are generally associated with a higher response rate, albeit at the cost of more toxicities. A majority of chemotherapeutic agents and some targeted agents are administered intravenously every 3–4 weeks, which constitutes one cycle. Other regimens are given orally often on a daily basis with or without a break. In selected circumstances, treatments may be given via the intramuscular, intrathecal, intraperitoneal, or intrahepatic routes.

BENEFITS

Palliative chemotherapy, hormonal therapy, and targeted agents can potentially decrease the tumor mass (i.e., tumor response) and metabolic activity, reduce symptom burden, delay disease progression, and prolong patient survival. Given appropriately,

Table 89.1 *Survival benefit for common palliative systemic therapy regimens*

Cancer type	Regimen	Survival benefit[a]
Stage IV non–small cell lung cancer	First-line chemo + bevacizumab[62]	+2 months
	Second-line docetaxol[63]	+3 months
	Second-/third-line erlotinib[64]	+2 months
Stage IV mesothelioma	Cisplatin/pemetrexed[65]	+3 months
Stage IV pancreatic cancer	First-line gemcitabine[66]	+5–6 weeks
	First-line gemcitabine + erlotinib[67]	+2 weeks
Stage IV colon cancer	Third-line cetuximab[68]	+6 weeks
Stage IV hepatocellular cancer	First-line sorafenib[69]	+3 months
Stage IV renal cell cancer	First-line sunitinib[70]	+6 months[b]
	First-line sorafenib[71]	+2.7 months[b]
	First-line temsirolimus[72]	+3.6 months
Castration-resistant prostate cancer	First-line docetaxel[73]	+2.5 months
	First-/second-line Sipuleucel-T[74]	+4 months
	Second-line cabazitaxel[75]	+2.5 months
	Second-line abiraterone[76]	+4 months

[a] Overall survival unless otherwise specified.

[b] progression free survival.

palliative systemic therapy can be highly effective mainstay or adjuvant therapy for symptom control. Importantly, treatment benefit is highly variable, and tumor response is partly dependent on the cancer's characteristics (e.g., histology, stage, specific mutations), treatment doses, and patient characteristics. In one study, 30 oncologists were asked to rate the reasons for giving palliative chemotherapy to patients with advanced breast cancer. The top three perceived benefits were improvement of activity, symptom relief, and maintenance of hope.[13]

Table 89.1 shows the median survival benefit associated with several palliative systemic therapy regimens. Importantly, not every patient receives the same degree of benefit—some may die earlier as a result of treatment toxicity, while others may derive a prolonged disease control. In general, more resistant disease is associated with a lower response rate and a smaller benefit from systemic therapy.[14]

ADVERSE EFFECTS

Chemotherapy-related side effects

Palliative care specialists should be familiar with the common and severe adverse effects of cancer treatments. The main side effects of chemotherapy can be classified under four major categories: (1) fatigue, (2) nausea and vomiting, (3) effects on fast-growing tissues such as oral mucosa, gastrointestinal tract, skin, and bone marrow, and (4) other agent-specific complications.

Common side effects for various chemotherapeutic agents are listed in Table 89.2. The side-effect profile for chemotherapy differs significantly among regimens. Even among patients receiving the same regimen, the toxicity profile varies depending on the individual's pharmacogenomics, comorbidities, performance status, and adherence to supportive measures.

Careful monitoring, patient education, and prophylactic use of supportive therapies are key to the management of cancer treatment side effects. Patients with severe (e.g., grade 3 or 4) side effects may require chemotherapy dose adjustments, termination of therapy, and/or hospitalization.

CANCER-RELATED FATIGUE

It is the most common complaint associated with cancer treatments.[15] Up to 80%–90% of cancer patients would experience fatigue while on therapy.[16,17] Cancer related fatigue is characteristically not relieved by rest. In addition to physical tiredness, patients may experience neurocognitive changes such as a decrease in short-term memory, inability to concentrate, and drowsiness, commonly known as "chemobrain."[18] The causes of cancer-related fatigue are multifactorial, and may include direct effect of treatment centrally, cytokine dysregulation, autonomic dysfunction, deconditioning, psychological stressors, sleep disturbance, endocrine abnormalities, anemia, electrolyte changes, and other complications.[19] In addition to patient education and management of any reversible causes,[20] both aerobic and resistive physical exercises have been shown to be effective in improving cancer related fatigue.[21] Pharmacologic therapy such as stimulants (e.g., methylphenidate 5 mg PO at 8 am and noon), or corticosteroids (e.g., dexamethasone 4 mg PO twice a day) may also be considered.[22]

CHEMOTHERAPY-INDUCED NAUSEA AND VOMITING

Chemotherapy-induced nausea and vomiting (CINV) is one of the most feared concerns among patients receiving chemotherapy. The pathophysiology of CINV is related to both central and peripheral mechanisms.[23] Centrally, chemotherapeutic agents directly activate the area postrema located in the floor of the

Table 89.2 *Adverse effects of common palliative chemotherapeutic agents*

Chemotherapeutic agents	Myelosuppression	N&V	Alopecia	Selected toxicities
Alkylating agents				
Cyclophosphamide (Cytoxan, IV/PO)	+++	++	++	Hemorrhagic cystitis, mucositis, sterility
Ifosfamide (IV)	+++	+	+++	Hemorrhagic cystitis, neurotoxicity
Melphalan (PO)	++	+	–	Mucositis, sterility
Chlorambucil (PO)	++	–	–	Mucositis, sterility
Bulsulfan (PO)	+++	+	+	Pulmonary
Carmustine (BCNU, IV)	+++	+++	+	Pulmonary, renal, mucositis, diarrhea, hepatotoxicity
Lomustine (CCNU, PO)	+++	++	+	Pulmonary, renal, mucositis, diarrhea, hepatotoxicity
Dacarbazine (DTIC, IV)	++	+++	+	Flu-like symptoms, hepatotoxicity, photo
Temozolomide (PO)	++	++	–	Photosensitivity
Streptozocin (IV)	+	+++	–	Renal, diarrhea, hepatotoxicity, hypoglycemia
Antimetabolites				
Methotrexate (IV/PO)	++	+	–	Mucositis, diarrhea, hepatotoxicity, nephrotoxicity, pulmonary toxicity, neurotoxicity
Pemetrexed (IV)	++	+	–	Mucositis, diarrhea, hand-foot syndrome
Raltitrexed (IV)	++	+	–	Mucositis, diarrhea, hepatotoxicity, fatigue
5-Fluorouracil (IV)	+	+	–	Mucositis, diarrhea, hand-foot syndrome, cerebellar
Capecitabine (Xeloda, PO)	++	+	–	Mucositis, diarrhea, hepatotoxicity, hand-foot, neurotoxicity
Cytosine arabinoside (Ara-C, IV)	+++	++	+	Mucositis, diarrhea, cerebellar
Gemcitabine (IV)	++	++	+	Diarrhea, hepatotoxicity, flu-like, rash
Hydroxyurea (PO, IV)	++	+	–	Mucositis, rash
6-Thioguanine (6-TG, IV)	++	+	–	Mucositis, diarrhea, hepatotoxicity
6-Mercaptopurine (6-MG, IV)	++	+	–	Mucositis, diarrhea, hepatotoxicity
Fludarabine (IV, PO)	++	++	+	Neurotoxicity, AIHA, hepatotoxicity
2-Chlorodeoxyadenosine (Cladribine, IV)	++	+	–	Constipation, fever
Topoisomerase inhibitors				
Doxorubicin (hydroxydaunomycin, IV)	+++	++	+++	Cardiotoxicity
Doxorubicin (liposomal, IV)	++	++	+++	Cardiotoxicity, infusion reaction, hand-foot syndrome
Daunorubicin (IV)	+++	++	+++	Cardiotoxicity
Idarubicin (PO)	+++	++	+++	Cardiotoxicity (less)
Epirubicin (IV)	+++	++	+++	Cardiotoxicity
Mitoxantrone (IV)	++	+	+	Cardiotoxicity, hepatotoxicity
Etoposide (IV/PO)	++	+	+	Neurotoxicity, hepatotoxicity
Topotecan (IV)	+++	++	++	Diarrhea, constipation, fever
Irinotecan (IV)	++	+	++	Diarrhea, constipation, fever
Platinating agents				
Cisplatin (IV)	++	+++	+	Nephrotoxicity, neurotoxicity, ototoxicity
Carboplatin (IV)	++	++	–	Nephrotoxicity, neurotoxicity, ototoxicity (less)
Oxaliplatin (IV)	+	++	–	Neurotoxicity, diarrhea
Antimicrotubular agents				
Vincristine (Oncovin, IV)	–	+	+	Neurotoxicity, constipation
Vinblastine (IV)	++	+	+	Cramps, neurotoxicity, constipation
Vinorelbine (Navelbine, IV)	++	+	+	Neurotoxicity, constipation, diarrhea
Docetaxel (Taxotere, IV)	++	+	+++	Infusion, neurotoxicity, nails, myalgia, arthralgia, edema
Paclitaxel (Taxol, IV)	++	+	+++	Neurotoxicity, nails, myalgia, arthralgia
Cabazitaxel (Jevtana, IV)	++	+	+	Fatigue, diarrhea, back pain, neurotoxicity (mild)

(Continued)

Table 89.2 (Continued)   *Adverse effects of common palliative chemotherapeutic agents*

Chemotherapeutic agents	Myelosuppression	N&V	Alopecia	Selected toxicities
Others				
Bleomycin (IV)	+	++	++	Pulmonary toxicity, hemorrhagic cystitis
Mitomycin C (IV)	+++	+	+	Pulmonary toxicity, HUS, genitourinary irritation

Source: Modified with permission from Hui, D., *Approach to Internal Medicine*, 3rd edn. Springer, New York.

Abbreviations: AIHA, autoimmune hemolytic anemia; HUS, hemolytic uremic syndrome IV, intravenous; PO, oral.

fourth ventricle. Peripheral, chemotherapy damages the gastrointestinal tract, resulting in the release of 5-hydroxytryptamine (5-HT) by enterochromaffin cells lining the mucosa. This then activates the afferent vagal nerve, leading to the release of 5HT3, dopamine, and substance P distally, which subsequently bind to receptors in the nucleus tractus solitarius/area postrema. Efferent signals from the nucleus tractus solitarius/area postrema to the sensory cortex and the central pattern generator in the medulla lead to nausea and vomiting, respectively.

CINV can be classified as acute, delayed, chronic, and anticipatory based on the timing of occurrence: (1) acute CINV occurs within the first 24 hours of chemotherapy administration; (2) delayed CINV occurs in 24–120 hours posttreatment; (3) chronic CINV occurs >120 hours and is less likely to be related to chemotherapy alone; and (4) anticipatory CINV is related to prior bad experience with CINV, with the patient reporting nausea and vomiting 3–4 hours prior to initiation of treatment.

One principle in the management of CINV is the understanding that different chemotherapeutic agents are associated with different risks of CINV, and the prophylactic regimen should differ accordingly. Based on the risk of acute CINV, chemotherapeutic agents are empirically classified as high, moderate, and low emetogenic potential.[24] Patients starting on high emetogenic agents would benefit from prophylactic regimens consisting of NK1 antagonists, 5HT3 antagonists, and corticosteroids. Those on moderately emetogenic agents would require prophylactic use of 5HT3 antagonists and corticosteroids. Patients receiving low emetogenic potential agents may need steroid prophylaxis alone. Antidopaminergic, antihistamines, and anticholinergic agents are useful for treatment of all types of CINV. Benzodiazepines may be appropriate for anticipatory CINV. All patients on chemotherapy should be adequately hydrated and carefully monitored.

MYELOSUPPRESSION

Anemia, neutropenia, and thrombocytopenia are common complications related to chemotherapeutic agents. Patients with severe anemia (i.e., hemoglobin level less than 8.0 g/dL) may benefit from transfusion with packed red blood cells, and the threshold may need to be increased for those with significant cardiac or pulmonary comorbidities. The use of erythropoiesis-stimulating agents, such as epoetin alfa and darbepoetin, in patients with advanced cancer should be discouraged, in light of meta-analysis demonstrating a higher risk of thromboembolism and possible increase in tumor progression and mortality.[25]

Neutropenia (i.e., absolute neutrophil count [ANC] < 1000/mm^3) is common in patients on chemotherapy, and is often not a major concern—patients usually recover their counts prior to the next cycle. However, neutropenic patients who have fever or other signs of infection need to be managed expeditiously because of the risk of overwhelming sepsis.[26,27] All patients on a chemotherapeutic regimen should seek immediate medical assistance and to check their blood count in the event of a fever. Empiric antibiotics and possible hospitalization are warranted.[28] The use of prophylactic granulocyte colony–stimulating factor may be considered for primary or secondary prophylaxis for patients at risk of developing febrile neutropenia.[29]

Thrombocytopenia is generally mild and self-limiting, although patients with platelet count below 10,000/mm^3 may benefit from platelet transfusions. A higher transfusion threshold may be needed for patients with active bleeding, high fever, hyperleukocytosis, rapid decline of platelet count, or coagulation disorders.[30]

ORAL AND INTESTINAL MUCOSITIS

Oral and intestinal mucositis is particularly common among patients with head and neck and gastrointestinal malignancies undergoing chemotherapy treatment. Oral mucositis can be associated with significant pain, dysphagia, dehydration, and weight loss.[31] Similar to the management of CINV, patient education and prophylactic management are key to prevention of oral mucositis.[32,33] Patients should be encouraged to brush their teeth twice daily, floss daily, and use baking soda mouth raise at least four times per day. Topical analgesia, such as lidocaine viscous and xylocaine, may be useful for short-term pain relief. In severe cases, systemic opioids are indicated.

Intestinal mucositis could result in diarrhea, abdominal pain, and dehydration. Diarrhea can usually be controlled with loperamide.[34,35] In severe cases, octreotide may be needed.[36]

OTHER SPECIFIC AGENT SIDE EFFECTS

A detail description of all the agent-specific side effects is beyond the scope of this chapter. Some of the well-documented adverse effects are shown in Table 89.2. Depending on the chemotherapeutic agent, neurotoxicity (e.g., platinums, vinca alkaloids, taxanes),[37,38] cardiotoxicity (e.g., anthracyclines, fluropyrimidines),[39,40] pulmonary toxicity (e.g., bleomycin),[41,42] nephrotoxicity (e.g., cisplatin, methotrexate),[43] and hepatotoxicity[44] may occur. These side effects often occur over weeks or months, but may occasionally be acute in nature. Careful monitoring and anticipatory management are key to minimizing organ damage.

Hormonal agents

Table 89.3 lists the common side effects of various hormonal agents. These include fatigue, hot flashes, mood swings, and sexual dysfunction.[45–47] Aromatase inhibitors may cause myalgia/arthralgia and increase the risk of osteoporosis, while tamoxifen may increase bone mineral density.[48]

HOT FLASHES

Hot flashes occur in a majority of female and male cancer patients on hormonal therapy, and may also occur in individuals who experience premature menopause as a result of cytotoxic therapy. Hot flashes are typically described as episodes with sudden onset of intense heat, sweating, and flushing that last 2–4 min. Potential triggers include stress, anxiety, alcohol, and specific foods. Management of hot flashes includes avoidance of potential triggers, keeping cool, and exercises. Various pharmacologic agents, such as gabapentin, pregabalin, venlafaxine, megestrol, vitamin E, and clonidine, have also been shown to alleviate the effects of hot flashes.[49]

Targeted agents

The number of novel targeted agents is increasing exponentially. As shown in Table 89.4, each agent has its own unique side effects. In general, side effects are related to the agent's mechanism of action. In this section, we shall discuss two classes of agents, epidermal growth factor receptor (EGFR) inhibitors and vascular endothelial growth factor (VEGF) inhibitors, and use them as examples to illustrate some common side effects related to targeted therapy.

INHIBITORS OF EPIDERMAL GROWTH FACTOR RECEPTOR

The EGFR pathway plays a critical role in the tumorigenesis of many malignancies. Monoclonal antibodies (e.g., cetuximab, panitumumab) and tyrosine kinase inhibitors (e.g., erlotinib, gifitinib, and lapatinib) have been developed against EGFR and found to be effective in the treatment of lung, colorectal, and head and neck cancers. Because EGFR is also highly expressed in host keratinocytes and the gastrointestinal mucosa, folliculitis and diarrhea are two common side effects associated with the use of these agents. EGFR rash typically involves the face, chest, and upper back, and occurs after 1–2 weeks of therapy. The rash is papulopustular or macropapular in nature and should be distinguished from acne vulgaris, which has comedones.[50,51] Management of this rash includes prophylactic use

Table 89.3 *Adverse effects of common hormonal therapies*

Hormonal agents	Selected toxicities
LHRH agonists	
Goserelin (Zoladex, IM)	Hot flashes, mood changes, sexual dysfunction, diarrhea, anemia, loss of muscle mass, osteoporosis
Leuprolide (Lupron, IM)	
SERMs	
Tamoxifen (Nolvadex)—SERM (PO)	Hot flashes, mood changes, vaginal dryness/discharge, thromboembolism, hypercalcemia, endometrial cancer
Aromatase inhibitors	
Anastrozole (Arimidex)—nonsteroidal (PO)	Hot flashes, mood changes, arthralgia, vaginal dryness/discharge, osteoporosis
Letrozole (Femara)—nonsteroidal (PO)	Hot flashes, mood changes, arthralgia, vaginal dryness/discharge, osteoporosis
Exemestane (Aromasin)—steroidal (PO)	Hot flashes, mood changes, arthralgia, vaginal dryness/discharge, osteoporosis
Other hormonal agents	
Bicalutamide (Casodex)—antiandrogen (PO)	Hot flashes, mood changes, sexual dysfunction, diarrhea, anemia, loss of muscle mass, osteoporosis
Flutamide (Eulexin)—antiandrogen (PO)	Hot flashes, mood changes, sexual dysfunction, diarrhea, anemia, loss of muscle mass, osteoporosis
Finasteride (Proscar)—α5 reductase inhibitor (PO)	Postural hypotension, sexual dysfunction, dizziness
Megestrol (Megace)—progestin (PO)	Vaginal bleed and irregularities, nausea, weight gain
Fulvestrant (Faslodex)—ER blocker (IM)	Hot flashes, nausea, diarrhea, back pain, pharyngitis
Abiraterone (Zytiga)—CYP17 inhibitor (PO)	Hypokalemia, fluid retention, hypertension

Source: Modified with permission from Hui, D., *Approach to Internal Medicine*, 3rd edn. Springer, New York.

Abbreviations: CYP, cytochrome; ER, estrogen receptor; IM, intramuscular; IV, intravenous; PO, oral.

of topical hydrocortisone, moisturizer, and tetracycline antibiotic (e.g., tetracycline, doxycycline, minocycline), topical steroids, and if necessary, dose adjustments.[52] Other related dermatologic manifestations include xerosis, pruritus, fissures, periungual pyogenic granuloma-like inflammation, paronychia, alopecia, curly/brittle/fine/dark hair, hypertrichosis, and trichomegaly. Ocular changes may also occur, and include dysfunctional tear syndrome, dry eyes, meibomitis, blepharitis, conjunctivitis, corneal erosion, and trichomegaly.[53] Supportive management of EGFR-induced diarrhea is similar to chemotherapy-induced diarrhea (see the preceding text).

Table 89.4 *Adverse effects of common targeted agents*

Targeted agents	Cytopenia	Selected toxicities
Monoclonal antibodies		
Alemtuzumab (Campath)—anti-CD52 (SC/IV)	+++	Infusion, infections (e.g., CMV, HSV, TB, fungal), pancytopenia
Bevacizumab (Avastin)—anti-VEGF (IV)	−	Infusion, HTN, bleed, VTE, perforations, proteinuria, epistaxis, fever
Cetuximab (Erbitux)—anti-EGFR (IV)	−	Rash, diarrhea, abd pain, fatigue, hypomagnesemia, infusion
Gemtuzumab (Mylotarg)—anti-CD33 (IV)	+++	Infusion, N&V, diarrhea, fever, hepatotoxicity
Ipilimumab (Zelboraf)—anti-CTLA-4 (IV)	+	Immune mediated enterocolitis, hepatitis, dermatitis, endocrinopathies, GBS
Panitumumab (Vectibix)—anti-EGFR (IV)	−	Rash, diarrhea, abd pain, fatigue, hypomagnesemia, infusion (fully humanized)
Rituximab (Rituxan)—anti-CD20 (IV)	+	Infusion, cardiac arrhythmia
Trastuzumab (Herceptin)—anti-Her2 (IV)	−	Infusion, cardiomyopathy
Tyrosine kinase inhibitors		
Axitinib (Inlyta)—VEGFR inhibitor (PO)	+	Fatigue, diarrhea, rash, HTN, thrombosis, hypothyroidism,
Crizotinib (Xalkori)—ALK/Met kinase inhibitor (PO)	−	Visual disturbance, nausea, diarrhea, fatigue, edema, hepatotoxicity, pneumonitis
Dasatinib (Sprycel)—bcr/abl, c-kit inhibitor (PO)	++	Effusion, diarrhea, nausea, fatigue, rash, hypophosphatemia
Erlotinib (Tarceva)—EGFR inhibitor (PO)	−	Acneiform rash, diarrhea, mucositis
Gefitinib (Iressa)—EGFR inhibitor (PO)	−	Acneiform rash, diarrhea, mucositis
Imatinib (Gleevec)—bcr/abl, c-kit inhibitor (PO)	+	Periorbital edema, nausea, diarrhea, muscle cramps, bowel perforation, fatigue
Lapatinib (Tykerb)—HER2 and EGFR inhibitor (PO)	−	Acneiform rash, diarrhea, nausea, fatigue, heart failure, pneumonitis
Nilotinib (Tasigna)—bcr/abl, c-kit inhibitor (PO)	++	Effusion, hyperglycemia, hypophosphatemia, QT prolongation, fatigue, rash
Pazopanib (Votrient)—VEGFR inhibitor (PO)	+	Fatigue, diarrhea, HTN, VTE, cardiotoxicity, hypothyroidism, acryl erythema
Sunitinib (Sutent)—VEGFR inhibitor (PO)	+	Fatigue, diarrhea, HTN, VTE, cardiotoxicity, hypothyroidism, acryl erythema
Sorafenib (Nexavar)—VEGFR inhibitor (PO)	+	Fatigue, diarrhea, HTN, VTE, cardiotoxicity, hypothyroidism, acryl erythema
Vemurafenib (Zelboraf)—BRAF inhibitor (PO)	−	Arthralgia, rash, photosensitivity, squamous cell carcinoma, alopecia
Others		
Bortezomib (Velcade)—proteasome inhibitor (IV)	++	GI symptoms, fatigue, cytopenia, peripheral neuropathy
Everolimus (Afinitor)—mTOR inhibitor (IV)	+	Rash, mucositis, fatigue, hyperglycemia, hypophosphatemia, hypertriglyceridemia
Interferon—immune modulatory (IV)	++	Fatigue, fever, myalgia, hepatotoxicity, mood changes
Sipuleucel-T (Provenge)—immunotherapy (IV)	−	Flu-like reaction, nausea, infusion reaction, HTN, stroke
Thalidomide (Thalomid)—antiangiogenic (PO)	++	Sedation, fatigue, constipation, rash, peripheral neuropathy, thromboembolism
Temsirolimus (Torisel)—mTOR inhibitor (IV)	+	Rash, mucositis, fatigue, hyperglycemia, hypophosphatemia, hypertriglyceridemia

Source: Modified with permission from Hui, D., *Approach to Internal Medicine*, 3rd edn. Springer, New York.

Abbreviations: CMV, cytomegalovirus; EGFR, epidermal growth factor receptor; HER2, human epidermal growth factor receptor 2; HSV, herpes simplex virus; HTN, hypertension; IV, intravenous; mTOR, mammalian target of rapamycin; PO, oral; SC, subcutaneous; TB, tuberculosis; VEGFR, vascular endothelial growth factor receptor; VTE, venous thromboembolism.

INHIBITORS OF VASCULAR ENDOTHELIAL GROWTH FACTOR PATHWAY

VEGF antagonists such as bevacizumab interfere with angiogenesis of both cancer and host tissue. Understandably, bevacizumab, a humanized monoclonal antibody against VEGF, is associated various vascular complications, including hypertension, proteinuria, arterial thromboembolism, bleeding, impaired wound healing, and bowel perforation. Similarly, sorafenib and sunitinib, two multikinase inhibitors that affect vascular endothelial growth factor receptor (VEGFR), can result in hypertension, and a slightly elevated risk of thromboembolism, heart failure, and acute coronary syndrome.[54]

Other considerations

Additional complications related to systemic therapy include an increased risk of infections, extravasations, hypersensitivity drug reactions, and catheter-related complications.

Aside from the adverse effects and potential complications, the use of systemic therapy entails frequent clinic visits, blood work, imaging investigations, and significant financial burden associated with medical visits, cancer treatments, and supportive care. A typical cycle of systemic therapy averages thousands of dollars (U.S.$). Furthermore, the pursuit of life-prolonging therapy could potentially delay transition of care for some patients with limited prognosis (i.e., weeks of survival), diverting their precious resources to seeking further cancer treatments rather than planning ahead.

DECISION-MAKING PROCESS

The recommendation for systemic therapy is based on a balance of potential risks and benefits. Factors incorporated into the decision making include cancer biology, treatment history, available clinical evidence, and patient characteristics.[13] The oncologists first need to decide whether treatment should be recommended, and if so, which regimen would be most appropriate. Patients with heavily pretreated disease are less likely to derive a benefit, and those with a poor performance status or significant comorbidities are more likely to experience significant toxicities. Thus, systemic therapy is less likely to be offered to these individuals. Other factors include patient's support system, patient interest, and the oncologist's training and preference.

Commitment to initiating systemic therapy does not mean that the patient needs to finish the planned course of therapy. Instead, the decision for treatment is made one cycle at a time, with careful monitoring throughout treatment. The oncologist usually sees the patient prior to each cycle, and conducts various assessments to assess tumor response and toxicity to ensure that the risk–benefit ratio is still favorable before continuing on with the next cycle. There are three major reasons for stopping treatment prematurely: (1) disease progression while on therapy, (2) severe treatment toxicities, and (3) significant decline in performance status. The palliative care team has an important role working closely with the patient, family, and oncologist to maximize the patient's function, monitor for side effects, and initiate early supportive measures.

SYSTEMIC THERAPY AT THE END OF LIFE

Administration of chemotherapy within the last 14–30 days of life has been established as an important indicator of aggressive quality of end-of-life.[55] At our institution, approximately one in four cancer patients had palliative systemic therapy and one in eight patients had targeted therapy in the last 30 days of life.[56] When a treatment is given to patients so close to death, the benefit is arguably nonexistent. The literature suggests that those patients who are aware of their short prognosis were less likely to choose life-prolonging therapies, particularly when palliative care is involved.[57,58] However, it should be noted that clinicians tend to be overly optimistic in prognostication;[59,60] thus, the use of prognosis as a criterion for systemic therapy eligibility may not be justified.

Instead, performance status is a well-established prognostic and predictive factor.[61] When a patient approaches a Karnofsky

Table 89.5 *Karnofsky performance status*

KPS score (%)	Level of function
100	Normal no complaints; no evidence of disease
90	Able to carry on normal activity; minor signs or symptoms of disease
80	Normal activity with effort; some signs or symptoms of disease
70	Cares for self; unable to carry on normal activity or to do active work
60	Requires occasional assistance, but is able to care for most of his personal needs
50	Requires considerable assistance and frequent medical care
40	Disabled; requires special care and assistance
30	Severely disabled; hospital admission is indicated although death not imminent
20	Very sick; hospital admission necessary; active supportive treatment necessary
10	Moribund; fatal processes progressing rapidly
0	Dead

performance status (KPS) of 40% or less (Table 89.5), he or she is likely not a good candidate for palliative systemic therapies. There are, however, always exceptions to the rule. For instance, a chemotherapy-naïve patient with extensive stage small cell lung cancer may benefit from a treatment trial even if she has a poor performance status because of the high response rate and likely symptom benefit. Close communication with the oncology team and involving them in family conferences can often be helpful when addressing goals of care.

SUMMARY

Systemic therapy consists of chemotherapy, hormonal agents, and various targeted biologic agents. Given with palliative intent, these treatments may help to prolong survival, decrease tumor burden, alleviate symptoms, improve quality of life, and sustain hope. Palliative care specialists and oncologists should collaborate closely to provide patient education, regular monitoring, psychological support, prophylactic measures for treatment-related adverse effects, and early supportive care interventions to maximize patients' quality of life and function while on treatment. Palliative care also has an important role helping patients understand their prognosis, educating them about the risks and benefits of cancer therapies, and facilitating the establishment of goals of care.

REFERENCES

1   Joensuu H. Systemic chemotherapy for cancer: From weapon to treatment. *Lancet Oncol* 2008;9:304.

2   Cheung KL. Endocrine therapy for breast cancer: An overview. *Breast* 2007;16:327–343.

3   Damber JE. Endocrine therapy for prostate cancer. *Acta Oncol* 2005;44:605–609.

4   Emons G, Heyl W. Hormonal treatment of endometrial cancer. *J Cancer Res Clin Oncol* 2000;126:619–623.

5   de Bono JS, Ashworth A. Translating cancer research into targeted therapeutics. *Nature* 2010;467:543–549.

6   Urruticoechea A, Alemany R, Balart J, Villanueva A, Vinals F, Capella G. Recent advances in cancer therapy: An overview. *Curr Pharm Des* 2010;16:3–10.

7   Arias JL. Drug targeting strategies in cancer treatment: An overview. *Mini Rev Med Chem* 2011;11:1–17.

8   Hanahan D, Weinberg RA. Hallmarks of cancer: The next generation. *Cell* 2011;144:646–674.

9   Bergh J. Quo vadis with targeted drugs in the 21st century? *J Clin Oncol* 2009;27:2–5.

10 Dancey JE, Bedard PL, Onetto N, Hudson TJ. The genetic basis for cancer treatment decisions. *Cell* 2012;148:409–420.

11 Dictionary of Cancer Terms: Targeted therapy. National Cancer Institute, 2012. (Accessed March 5, 2012, at http://www.cancer.gov/dictionary?cdrid=270742.)

12 Hui D, Elsayem A, De la Cruz M et al. Availability and integration of palliative care at U.S. cancer centers. *JAMA* 2010;303:1054–1061.

13 Grunfeld EA, Ramirez AJ, Maher EJ et al. Chemotherapy for advanced breast cancer: What influences oncologists' decision-making? *Br J Cancer* 2001;84:1172–1178.

14 Gottesman MM. Mechanisms of cancer drug resistance. *Annu Rev Med* 2002;53:615–627.

15 Weis J. Cancer-related fatigue: Prevalence, assessment and treatment strategies. *Expert Rev Pharmacoecon Outcomes Res* 2011;11:441–446.

16 Yennurajalingam S, Bruera E. Palliative management of fatigue at the close of life: "It feels like my body is just worn out". *JAMA* 2007;297:295–304.

17 Hofman M, Ryan JL, Figueroa-Moseley CD, Jean-Pierre P, Morrow GR. Cancer-related fatigue: The scale of the problem. *The Oncologist* 2007;12 (Suppl 1):4–10.

18 Dutta V. Chemotherapy, neurotoxicity, and cognitive changes in breast cancer. *J Cancer Res Ther* 2011;7:264–269.

19 Ryan JL, Carroll JK, Ryan EP, Mustian KM, Fiscella K, Morrow GR. Mechanisms of cancer-related fatigue. *Oncologist* 2007;12 (Suppl 1):22–34.

20 Mock V, Atkinson A, Barsevick A et al. NCCN practice guidelines for cancer-related fatigue. *Oncology (Williston Park, NY)* 2000;14:151–161.

21 Cramp F, Daniel J. Exercise for the management of cancer-related fatigue in adults. *Cochrane Database Syst Rev England* 2008:CD006145.

22 Minton O, Stone P, Richardson A, Sharpe M, Hotopf M. Drug therapy for the management of cancer related fatigue. *Cochrane Database Syst Rev* 2008;(1):CD006704.

23 Hesketh PJ. Chemotherapy-induced nausea and vomiting. *New England J Med* 2008;358:2482–2494.

24 Naeim A, Dy SM, Lorenz KA, Sanati H, Walling A, Asch SM. Evidence-based recommendations for cancer nausea and vomiting. *J Clin Oncol* 2008;26:3903–3910.

25 Bennett CL, Silver SM, Djulbegovic B et al. Venous thromboembolism and mortality associated with recombinant erythropoietin and darbepoetin administration for the treatment of cancer-associated anemia. *JAMA* 2008;299:914–924.

26 de Naurois J, Novitzky-Basso I, Gill MJ, Marti FM, Cullen MH, Roila F. Management of febrile neutropenia: ESMO clinical practice guidelines. *Ann Oncol* 2010;21 (Suppl 5):v252–v256.

27 Smith TJ, Khatcheressian J, Lyman GH et al. 2006 update of recommendations for the use of white blood cell growth factors: An evidence-based clinical practice guideline. *J Clin Oncol* 2006;24:3187–3205.

28 Freifeld AG, Bow EJ, Sepkowitz KA et al. Clinical practice guideline for the use of antimicrobial agents in neutropenic patients with cancer: 2010 update by the infectious diseases society of america. *Clin Infect Dis* 2011;52:e56–e93.

29 Crawford J, Allen J, Armitage J et al. Myeloid growth factors. *J Natl Compr Canc Netw* 2011;9:914–32.

30 Schiffer CA, Anderson KC, Bennett CL et al. Platelet transfusion for patients with cancer: Clinical practice guidelines of the American Society of Clinical Oncology. *J Clin Oncol* 2001;19:1519–1538.

31 Quinn B, Potting CM, Stone R et al. Guidelines for the assessment of oral mucositis in adult chemotherapy, radiotherapy and haematopoietic stem cell transplant patients. *Eur J Cancer* 2008;44:61–72.

32 Keefe DM, Schubert MM, Elting LS et al. Updated clinical practice guidelines for the prevention and treatment of mucositis. *Cancer* 2007;109:820–831.

33 Peterson DE, Bensadoun RJ, Roila F, Group EGW. Management of oral and gastrointestinal mucositis: ESMO clinical recommendations. *Ann Oncol* 2008;19 (Suppl 2):ii122– ii125.

34 Gibson RJ, Stringer AM. Chemotherapy-induced diarrhoea. *Curr Opin Support Palliat Care* 2009;3:31–35.

35 Wadler S, Benson AB, 3rd, Engelking C et al. Recommended guidelines for the treatment of chemotherapy-induced diarrhea. *J Clin Oncol* 1998;16:3169–3178.

36 Bhattacharya S, Vijayasekar C, Worlding J, Mathew G. Octreotide in chemotherapy induced diarrhoea in colorectal cancer: A review article. *Acta Gastroenterol Belg* 2009;72:289–295.

37 Cavaletti G, Marmiroli P. Chemotherapy-induced peripheral neurotoxicity. *Nat Rev Neurol* 2010;6:657–666.

38 Dropcho EJ. Neurotoxicity of cancer chemotherapy. *Semin Neurol* 2010;30:273–286.

39 Khakoo AY, Liu PP, Force T et al. Cardiotoxicity due to cancer therapy. *Tex Heart Inst J* 2011;38:253–256.

40 Witteles RM, Fowler MB, Telli ML. Chemotherapy-associated cardiotoxicity: How often does it really occur and how can it be prevented? *Heart Fail Clin* 2011;7:333–344.

41 Charpidou AG, Gkiozos I, Tsimpoukis S et al. Therapy-induced toxicity of the lungs: An overview. *Anticancer Res* 2009;29:631–639.

42 Vahid B, Marik PE. Pulmonary complications of novel antineoplastic agents for solid tumors. *Chest* 2008;133:528–538.

43 Kelly RJ, Billemont B, Rixe O. Renal toxicity of targeted therapies. *Target Oncol* 2009;4:121–133.

44 Aloia TA, Fahy BN. Chemotherapy-associated hepatotoxicity: How concerned should we be? *Expert Rev Anticancer Ther* 2010;10:521–527.

45 Grossmann M, Zajac JD. Management of side effects of androgen deprivation therapy. *Endocrinol Metab Clin North Am* 2011;40:655–671, x.

46 Mohile SG, Mustian K, Bylow K, Hall W, Dale W. Management of complications of androgen deprivation therapy in the older man. *Crit Rev Oncol Hematol* 2009;70:235–255.

47 Colleoni M, Giobbie-Harder A. Benefits and adverse effects of endocrine therapy. *Ann Oncol* 2010;21 (Suppl 7):vii107–vii111.

48 Body JJ. Prevention and treatment of side-effects of systemic treatment: Bone loss. *Ann Oncol* 2010;21 (Suppl 7):vii180– vii185.

49 Dalal S, Zhukovsky DS. Pathophysiology and management of hot flashes. *J Support Oncol* 2006;4:315–320, 25.

50 Eng C. Toxic effects and their management: Daily clinical challenges in the treatment of colorectal cancer. *Nat Rev Clin Oncol* 2009;6:207–218.

51 Ricciardi S, Tomao S, de Marinis F. Toxicity of targeted therapy in non-small-cell lung cancer management. *Clin Lung Cancer* 2009;10:28–35.

52 Lacouture ME, Anadkat MJ, Bensadoun RJ et al. Clinical practice guidelines for the prevention and treatment of EGFR inhibitor-associated dermatologic toxicities. *Support Care Cancer* 2011;19:1079–1095.

53 Burtness B, Anadkat M, Basti S et al. NCCN Task Force Report: Management of dermatologic and other toxicities associated with EGFR inhibition in patients with cancer. *J Natl Compr Canc Netw* 2009;7 (Suppl 1):S5–S21; quiz S2–4.

54 Di Lorenzo G, Porta C, Bellmunt J, et al. Toxicities of targeted therapy and their management in kidney cancer. *Eur Urol* 2011;59:526–540.

55 Earle CC, Park ER, Lai B, Weeks JC, Ayanian JZ, Block S. Identifying potential indicators of the quality of end-of-life cancer care from administrative data. *J Clin Oncol* 2003;21:1133–1138.

56 Hui D, Karuturi MS, Tanco KC et al. Targeted agent use in cancer patients at the end-of-life. *J Pain Symptom Manage* July 2013;46(1):1–8.

57 Weeks JC, Cook EF, O'Day SJ et al. Relationship between cancer patients' predictions of prognosis and their treatment preferences. *JAMA* 1998;279:1709–1714.

58 Temel JS, Greer JA, Admane S et al. Longitudinal perceptions of prognosis and goals of therapy in patients with metastatic non-small-cell lung cancer: Results of a randomized study of early palliative care. *J Clin Oncol* 2011;29:2319–2326.

59 Hui D, Kilgore K, Nguyen L et al. The accuracy of probabilistic versus temporal clinician prediction of survival for patients with advanced cancer: A preliminary report. *Oncologist* 2011;16:1642–1648.

60 Lamont EB, Christakis NA. Prognostic disclosure to patients with cancer near the end of life. *Ann Intern Med* 2001;134:1096–1105.

61 Maltoni M, Caraceni A, Brunelli C et al. Prognostic factors in advanced cancer patients: Evidence-based clinical recommendations—A study by the Steering Committee of the European Association for Palliative Care. *J Clin Oncol* 2005;23:6240–6248.

62 Sandler A, Gray R, Perry MC, et al. Paclitaxel-carboplatin alone or with bevacizumab for non-small-cell lung cancer. *N Engl J Med* 2006;355:2542–2550.

63 Shepherd FA, Dancey J, Ramlau R et al. Prospective randomized trial of docetaxel versus best supportive care in patients with non-small-cell lung cancer previously treated with platinum-based chemotherapy. *J Clin Oncol* 2000;18:2095–2103.

64 Shepherd FA, Rodrigues Pereira J, Ciuleanu T et al. Erlotinib in previously treated non-small-cell lung cancer. *N Engl J Med* 2005;353:123–132.

65 Vogelzang NJ, Rusthoven JJ, Symanowski J et al. Phase III study of pemetrexed in combination with cisplatin versus cisplatin alone in patients with malignant pleural mesothelioma. *J Clin Oncol* 2003;21:2636–2644.

66 Burris HA, 3rd, Moore MJ, Andersen J et al. Improvements in survival and clinical benefit with gemcitabine as first-line therapy for patients with advanced pancreas cancer: A randomized trial. *J Clin Oncol* 1997;15:2403–2413.

67 Moore MJ, Goldstein D, Hamm J et al. Erlotinib plus gemcitabine compared with gemcitabine alone in patients with advanced pancreatic cancer: A phase III trial of the National Cancer Institute of Canada Clinical Trials Group. *J Clin Oncol* 2007;25:1960–1966.

68 Jonker DJ, O'Callaghan CJ, Karapetis CS et al. Cetuximab for the treatment of colorectal cancer. *N Engl J Med* 2007;357:2040–2048.

69 Llovet JM, Ricci S, Mazzaferro V et al. Sorafenib in advanced hepatocellular carcinoma. *N Engl J Med* 2008;359:378–390.

70 Motzer RJ, Hutson TE, Tomczak P et al. Sunitinib versus interferon alfa in metastatic renal-cell carcinoma. *N Engl J Med* 2007;356:115–124.

71 Escudier B, Eisen T, Stadler WM et al. Sorafenib in advanced clear-cell renal-cell carcinoma. *N Engl J Med* 2007;356:125–134.

72 Fazio N, Dettori M, Lorizzo K. Temsirolimus for advanced renal-cell carcinoma. *N Engl J Med* 2007;357:1050; author reply -1.

73 Tannock IF, de Wit R, Berry WR et al. Docetaxel plus prednisone or mitoxantrone plus prednisone for advanced prostate cancer. *N Engl J Med* 2004;351:1502–1512.

74 Kantoff PW, Higano CS, Shore ND et al. Sipuleucel-T immunotherapy for castration-resistant prostate cancer. *N Engl J Med* 2010;363:411–422.

75 de Bono JS, Oudard S, Ozguroglu M et al. Prednisone plus cabazitaxel or mitoxantrone for metastatic castration-resistant prostate cancer progressing after docetaxel treatment: A randomised open-label trial. *Lancet* 2010;376:1147–1154.

76 de Bono JS, Logothetis CJ, Molina A et al. Abiraterone and increased survival in metastatic prostate cancer. *N Engl J Med* 2011;364:1995–2005.

90

Physical medicine and rehabilitation

BENEDICT KONZEN, KI Y. SHIN

INTRODUCTION

Some may mistakenly think that the fields of palliative medicine and rehabilitation medicine have divergent goals. Yet, both fields have a common focus in the relief of suffering and the improvement of quality of life. They differ in their historical roots. Palliative medicine grew out of observations made in the care of dying patients in hospice programs. It later grew to include other serious and life-threatening illnesses of uncertain prognosis. Rehabilitation medicine had its roots in restoration of impaired physical and cognitive functioning—"fixed deficits" often incurred as a result of trauma. As a field, it later grew to include patient with progressive acute or chronic deficits, for example, patients with cancer.

The assertion has been made that rehabilitating patients with cancer or other diseases with terminal prognoses is a poor allocation of scarce medical resources. However, when economic and psychological costs are included in the equation, the argument for such treatment is strengthened. In addition to the economic argument, both moral and spiritual arguments can also be made. Every human being values the ability to make decisions, to participate actively in their home, and to have value in the eyes of their peers, family, and community. These needs may become more urgent for the patient with cancer or other serious illness. Rehabilitation medicine and palliative medicine share the goals of permitting a patient the opportunity to reflect on an ongoing life; understand the implication of their disease process as it impacts themselves, their caregiver, family, and friends; and move forward both physically and mentally. Despite illness, the physiatrist's goal is to promote physical functioning; where this is impeded, the physiatrist works with caregiver and family as adjuvant supports. The palliative medicine physician, primarily, and the physiatrist both attempt to reduce the pain, asthenia, fatigue, and symptoms related to ongoing medical treatment, the final goal being living completely and fully—whether that be in a physical, cognitive, or spiritual sense. In this chapter, we will explore the role that rehabilitation medicine plays in the overall care of the palliative medicine patient.

The fields of both physical medicine and palliative care medicine arose out of specific medical care needs. Physical medicine was not formally recognized as a medical specialty until 1950. However, the historical record is long in its documentation of administering physiatric care to patients with mechanical or neurological trauma—often the result of accident or wars. The tenets of physical medicine foster the belief that despite injury, attempts at reestablishing premorbid functioning are not only desirable but, hopefully, obtainable. Palliative medicine seeks to advance all forms of medical care by treating the acute and chronic symptoms of disease. In addition, the field not only focuses on the individual but advances the notion that care requires the additional interaction of spouse, family, acquaintances, and healthcare professionals. Both fields require a host of healthcare professionals—physicians, physician assistants, advance practice nurses, floor nursing, psychologists, and psychology nurses. Equally important are the roles played by case managers, social workers, and chaplains. The healthcare team does not exist independently. There continues to be a daily interchange between these team members. Indeed, team members must be strongly linked in purpose but flexible enough to understand an individual's idiosyncrasies. Cultural diversity, religious belief, language, and perceptions of health, values, success, and disappointment are all unique characteristics in the patient being cared for. The field of physical medicine attempts to restore a prior level of functioning. The physiatrist is aware that family interaction is critical. Neurological injury such as a traumatic brain injury, stroke, or tumor may leave a previously accomplished, mentally adept individual dependent on others. The prior relationship of husband/wife or significant others may be inextricably altered into patient/caregiver roles.

A united team approach of health professionals establishes a support network for ongoing medical care, teaching, and training. Whether in the outpatient clinic setting or on the acute inpatient unit, both rehabilitation and palliative medicine teach patients and their families anticipated and future care needs. As a supervised team, patients and their families can practice new tasks, and troubleshoot and modify unsafe behaviors. In addition, a close-knit team network can promote diversity of ideas as well as solutions. Both fields have a role to play throughout a person's disease state and life. Activity without symptoms of pain, nausea, fatigue, or discomfort will only enhance function. Activities with family and friends help to dissipate isolation and depression. Despite the timeline of a patient's disease, the palliative medicine physician's role remains interactive. Symptom management has both physical and spiritual components. Not only are nausea, fatigue, depression, anxiety, pain, constipation, asthenia addressed, but attempts are also made to assist the patient in coming to terms with both resolved and unresolved issues—including the fear of dying, abandonment, unfulfilled dreams/expectations, and disputes. In essence, both physical medicine and palliative medicine take an integrative look at the components that define us as human: physical, mental, social, and spiritual. When disease intervenes, these two fields attempt to restore a homeostatic balance, with an eventual goal of finding peace after, hopefully, a prosperous life lived.

CANCER FROM THE REHABILITATIONIST'S PERSPECTIVE

In traditional rehabilitation, causes of disability such as stroke, amputation, and brain/spinal cord injury often have a defined deficit. Patients undergo acute treatment. A return to community functioning is often anticipated. In cancer care, initial and ongoing medical treatment is not necessarily curative. The rehabilitationist addresses deficits that may be progressive over time. Traditionally, in rehabilitation medicine, therapies continue until maximal functional improvement has been obtained. However, in a chronic, potentially relapsing disease state such as cancer, the therapist deals with a patient who may have had recent surgery, chemotherapy, and radiation. There may be ongoing functional loss. Despite such losses, it has been shown repeatedly that patients with cancer—even during treatment—benefit from rehabilitation.[1]

Cancer rehabilitation initially arose through the work of three physiatrists, Herbert Dietz, Harold Rusk, and AE Gunn.[2] Financial support was provided by the National Cancer Institute (NCI). Modest gains continued through the 1980s until the focus of the NCI shifted from patient rehabilitation to the cure of cancer.[2] DeLisa[3] further comments on three additional factors limiting the role of cancer rehabilitation:

- Oncologist not being aware of the potential benefits of rehabilitation
- Failure of physiatry residency programs to incorporate cancer rehabilitation into the curriculum
- Trend toward moving rehabilitation from an inpatient service to an outpatient arena

Table 90.1 *Response to inpatient rehabilitation and functional improvement (N = 1019)*

Level achieved	No.
0 (no improvement)	211
1 (slight improvement)	110
2 (moderate improvement)	320
3 (marked improvement)	270
4 (fully independent)	108

Source: Dietz, J.H., *Med. Clin. North Am.*, 53, 607, 1969.

One of the earliest cancer rehabilitationists was Dietz.[4] In 1969, he proposed four goals for the cancer rehabilitationist:

1. Prevent disability whenever possible.
2. Where disability occurs, attempt to restore the individual to the premorbid state of functioning.
3. Institute supports in order to reduce future disability.
4. Palliate to reduce complications, maintain independence, and provide comfort.

Dietz felt that the effects of cancer were wide-reaching, affecting the socioeconomic, vocational, and emotional aspects of an individual's life. Therefore, a team approach initially involving physiatrist, therapists, nursing, and social work was recommended. This has since broadened in scope to also include chaplaincy, case management, speech pathology, pharmacy, medical oncology, surgery, and radiation therapy.[4]

In his initial study, Dietz interviewed 1019 patients with cancer. He devised a scale ranging from 0 to 4 with which to rate the benefit of physical therapy on patients receiving treatment; 0 represented no clinical benefit and 4 represented individuals who were fully independent with no ongoing disability. Of patients being discharged from inpatient rehabilitation, the largest percentage was rated at 2, that is, moderate improvement with an appropriate response to rehabilitative care (Table 90.1).[4] Dietz maintained that rehabilitation care was essential for patients with incurable and terminal disease. Since the overall goal was the maintenance of function and overall range of motion, therapies should be instituted immediately.[4]

A specific study lends further credence to the role of rehabilitation in cancer care. In 1991, O'Toole and Goden investigated functioning in 70 patients with cancer. Of these, 14% were ambulatory at the time of admission to inpatient rehabilitation. At discharge, 80% could ambulate independently. Urinary continence likewise improved from 38% to 87%. However, 3 months after discharge, 33% had either died or were lost to follow-up. Of the remaining 37 patients, 27 had maintained or improved functioning.[5] Of significance in this investigation was O'Toole and Goden's correlation between the Karnofsky performance scale (a measure of functional performance used by oncologists (Box 90.1)) and the Functional Independence Measure (FIM) score (a measure of functioning used by rehabilitationists). The conclusion was that patients with scores as low as 30 (severely disabled, inpatient hospital stay indicated, death not imminent) still were candidates for rehabilitation services.[5]

Box 90.1 Karnofsky scale

- 100—Normal. No complaints; no evidence of disease; able to work.
- 90—Able to carry on normal activity. Minor symptoms; able to work.
- 80—Normal activity with effort. Some symptoms; able to work.
- 70—Cares for self. Unable to carry on normal activity; independent; not able to work.
- 60—Disabled; dependent. Requires occasional assistance; cares for most needs.
- 50—Moderately disabled; dependent. Requires considerable assistance and frequent care.
- 40—Severely disabled; dependent. Requires special care and assistance.
- 30—Severely disabled. Hospitalized, death not imminent.
- 20—Very sick. Active supportive treatment needed.
- 10—Moribund. Fatal processes are rapidly progressing.

Source: Adapted from Karnofsky et al. 1948, taken from www.anapsid.org/cnd/files/karnofskyscale.pdf.[6]

Table 90.2 *Functional Independence Measure (FIM)*

Score range	Interpretation	Patient's effort	In everyday parlance
1	Total assistance	Less than 25%	Completely dependent
2	Maximal assistance	25%–49%	Completely dependent
3	Moderate assistance	50%–74%	Needs hands-on help
4	Minimal contact assist	75%+	Needs minimal hands-on
5	Supervision/ setup	75%+	Needs cues; can do task
6	Modified independent	100%	Completes task without cues but needs assistive device, independent
7	Totally independent	100%	No helper needed, task done safely without device

Source: Functional Independence Measure. Available at www.medfriendly.com/functionalindependencemeasure.html, (accessed June 18, 2006).

FUNCTIONAL AREAS ASSESSED

Functional areas assessed by the FIM (Table 90.2) are eating, grooming, bathing, upper and lower body dressing, toileting, bladder and bowel management, transfers, and locomotion. The FIM scores also assess comprehension, expression, social interaction, problem solving, and memory.

Marciniak et al. from the Rehabilitation Institute of Chicago reviewed 159 patients over a 2-year period and looked at motor function. They found that metastatic disease did not affect functional outcome. Furthermore, radiation therapy was associated with greater functional improvement than when it was not provided or completed before starting rehabilitation.[8] According to Sliwa and Marciniak[1], the most common cause of functional decline in patients with cancer is deconditioning. Prolonged bed rest along with chemotherapy and/or radiation can lead to significant functional limitations. The degree of impairment is based on the duration and degree of immobilization. In general, healthy individuals on complete bed rest exhibit a 1%–1.5% loss in strength per day or 10% per week.[9] Loss of proximal lower extremity strength is often greater than that seen in the upper extremities. This impedes sitting, standing, and ambulation.[10] Urinary calcium excretion increases. Diaphragmatic and intercostal muscle activity is reduced. Maximal oxygen consumption decreases by as much as 15% when healthy individuals resume exercise in an upright position after 10 days of bed rest.[11] Indeed, it may take up to 1 month to reestablish the normal postural response.[11] Healthy young men lose 300–500 mL of plasma volume within the first week of bed rest.[12] As plasma volume declines, blood viscosity increases leading to the risk of deep venous thrombosis.[1] In addition, there may be a hypotensive response. Both stroke volume and cardiac output decline.[12] From a neurological perspective, balance and coordination decline.[13] There may even be sensory deprivation.[14] Effective bladder evacuation is inhibited by recumbency. Inactivity results in impaired colonic function and possibly constipation with anorexia.[1] Lastly, hospitalized patients are at high risk (7.7%) of developing a pressure ulcer as sustained pressure over bony prominences results in ischemic injury.[15]

Neurological impairment in patients with cancer may be an increasing cause of disability. There may be both central and peripheral nerve involvement either by tumor, metastatic disease, side effect of therapy (chemotherapy/radiation), or by concurrent, related issues such as paraneoplastic syndromes, infection, or vasculitis.[1] Intracranial metastases are found in approximately 25% of patients who die from cancer. The origins of these metastases are frequently from lung, breast, and skin.[16,17] In a study of 363 cancer patients with brain metastases, 59% presented with hemiparesis.[18,19] Two recent studies have investigated neurooncological patients who had completed inpatient rehabilitation. Huang et al.[20] noted that there was concordance in functional return and rate of discharge to the community between the brain tumor patients and stroke patients. Indeed, length of stay was shorter for the former. In a second study, O'Dell et al.[21] compared patients with brain tumors and traumatic injuries. With comparable age, gender, and functional admission status, both groups made similar daily functional gains and 82.5% of patients with brain tumors were discharged home. On evaluation of functional status after inpatient rehabilitation, Sherer et al.[22] found that with a mean treatment time of 2.6 months, patients maintained these gains at a mean follow-up time of 8 months.

Of great concern to the rehabilitationist is metastatic disease of the spine. Although direct spinal cord involvement by metastatic tumor is rare, most spinal cord damage is the result of epidural compression by the tumor itself or vertebral body metastases resulting in bony compression. In only a small percentage of vertebral metastatic lesions will symptoms of compression be noted.[1] Many individuals are either asymptomatic or simply present with pain. However, in a study of 211 cancer patients,[23] 74% of individuals with metastatic cord compression were noted to have significant weakness at presentation. Close monitoring of functional status is essential. The involvement of the cervical spine may lead to plegia. Thoracolumbar involvement may lead to paraplegia and a neurogenic bowel/bladder. Typically, in the noncancer patient, this level of injury would still allow an individual to function independently at the wheelchair level. In the case of the oncology patient, however, the activity of the tumor, interrelated surgery/chemotherapy, or radiation—and ensuing comorbidities—may alter the ultimate functional outcome of the cancer patient.[24]

REHABILITATIVE INTERVENTIONS

One of the most important tasks for the rehabilitationist and patient with cancer is the establishment of appropriate goals. Patients vary in their understanding of disease and its implications. Functionally, they will have a unique response to surgical, chemotherapeutic, or radiation treatment. Initial and final expectations of treatment may be diametrically opposed. The rehabilitationist needs to modify general principles of rehabilitation to accommodate for persistent disease and the possibility of imminent or future decline. Challenges unique to patients with cancer would include chemotherapy-induced neuropathies, progressive lymphedema, pathological fractures requiring surgical stabilization, and metastatic disease compromising neurological functioning.[24]

Compensatory strategies in the care of patients with cancer make use of assistive devices. Reachers allow paraparetic, hemiparetic/hemiplegic patients to retrieve objects. Dressing and bathing aids compensate for diminished force and coordination. Orthotics can enhance stability and safety in the patient with motor deficits by protecting and stabilizing joints that are controlled by paretic muscles (e.g., ankle foot orthoses in the treatment of a "drop foot"). In terms of home and community accessing, mobility can be restored with the use of wheelchairs and scooters.[24]

Sensory deficits are often seen in spinal cord compression and leptomeningeal disease (53% and 50%, respectively).[24] Anatomically, they are associated with brachial and lumbosacral plexopathies secondary to tumor encroachment or radiation effect. Chemotherapeutic agents such as cisplatin, vincristine, and taxanes have also been associated with sensory neuropathies. In addition to instruction in compensatory strategies, assistive devices, and the use of orthotic devices, therapists work on enhancing stability by broadening a patient's base of support, enhancing tactile input, and instituting safety awareness of the insensate extremity while further educating patients on the use of alternative senses such as vision.[24]

In a large series of patients with brain metastases, cognitive dysfunction was found in 58%.[18,19] Such deficits can increase caretaker burden, render patients unsafe, and limit effective communication. Deficits arising from neurological tumors include apraxia, alexia, aphasia, and agnosia. Patients may experience inattention, difficulties with concentration, and disturbance in short-term memory. Strategies are limited but may include memory notebooks or computerized prosthetics.[24] In cases of cerebellar dysfunction where ataxia and truncal instability destabilize the patient, therapists use devices with a broad support base such as wide-based quadruped canes, standard walkers, and hemiwalkers.[24]

Discussion continues about what is the most distressing experience among cancer patients, whether it is uncontrolled pain or fatigue. Santiago-Palma and Payne[25] noted that in approximately 70% of patients, fatigue was chronic or was acute during chemoradiation therapy. Specifically, fatigue may be the result of cachexia, infection, anemia, or other metabolic/endocrine disorders.[25] Metastatic disease to the lungs and pleural effusions may result in significant dyspnea with concurrent decline in endurance.[25] In 2001, Winningham[26] identified "cancer-related fatigue syndrome" (CRFS) as the most distressing experience among cancer patients. Winningham looked at fatigue from a metabolic/cellular level. She proposes that fatigue is amenable to rehabilitative efforts. Indeed, treatment for cancer-related fatigue may lie in endurance exercise training. When oxidative metabolism is maximized—as during exercise—there is improvement in muscle mass, plasma volume, pulmonary ventilation/perfusion, cardiac reserve, and a subsequent increased concentration of oxidative muscle enzymes. Interleukin-1 and other myotoxic cytokines are downregulated.[27] Finally, resistance exercise reduces steroid-induced loss of muscle mass.[26] Optimization of oxidative capacity, however, requires sound nutritional support. Even with nutritional intervention in the form of supplements, oral intake may be insufficient. The patient may have alteration to nutrient processing secondary to mechanical (surgical) intervention or cachexia.[28,29]

Pain is a prevalent finding in patients with cancer. In 70%–90% of patients with advanced disease, significant pain is present.[25] From a symptom-control perspective, pain was controlled without excessive sedation in 85%–90% of patients with cancer when the right combination of nonpharmacological techniques, pharmacological therapy, and radiopharmaceuticals were used.[30] Current recommendations suggest the use of nonopioid agents initially for mild pain with the addition of opioids for moderate or severe pain.[30] From the rehabilitationist's perspective, additional useful adjuvant therapy might include massage and heat and cold modalities with certain restrictions. Physical therapy should educate a patient regarding proper seating dynamics, pressure relief, orthotics, assistive equipment, and compensatory strategies.[25]

ROLE OF REHABILITATION IN PALLIATIVE CARE

At first glance, it would appear that the two fields of rehabilitation and palliative care are divergent. Rehabilitation, in the traditional sense, focuses on the restoration of function lost either through illness, trauma, or intervention. Acutely, patients may be cared for in a hospital setting and then transitioned to outpatient services. The expectation is that even with alterations in physical functioning, the patient should reestablish the premorbid level of activity. In contrast, in palliative medicine, the patient is presumed to be in a terminal phase of either an acute or chronic illness. Restoration of physical and cognitive functioning may occur, but is not the overall objective. The goal of palliation becomes assessing symptoms related to the disease state or its subsequent treatment, that is, pain, dyspnea, asthenia, fatigue, cachexia, somnolence, delirium, depression, and constipation, and instituting an appropriate intervention. As an internist, the palliative expert also attempts to maintain a homeostatic balance for the body. Unique to palliative medicine has been the arena of close, dynamic interplay with patients and their families. Whereas most physicians typically distance themselves from talking about dying, coping with illness, and the incorporation of family into this process, the palliative care physician sees this as a prerequisite in the total care of the patient. Discussion of end-of-life issues is viewed merely as a completion of this task.

The role of the cancer rehabilitationist has been modified. Without a clear understanding of the patient's prior health, disease process, prognosis, anticipated limitations based on pharmacological intervention, surgery, radiation, and lastly family and economic supports, the rehabilitationist is unable to completely care for the patient. Therefore, the rehabilitationist dons—in limited fashion—the cloak of the palliative care physician. The goal, however, is maintaining function in the immediate future and preparing for possible future decline. Maintenance of the patient's autonomy in functioning, whether transferring to a chair or to the toilet, is attempted. A close collaboration between both disciplines is essential. In a study of 239 hospice patients, Yoshioka[31] demonstrated that functional improvement occurred in 27% of patients. In another study by Montagnini et al.[32], 18 out of 100 palliative care patients took part in a physical therapy program. In this group, 90% had ongoing deconditioning and pain. Montagnini found that 56% of those undergoing physical therapy demonstrated functional improvement.[32]

The complementary roles of physical medicine and palliative care medicine should be further investigated. Indeed, both disciplines "enable the dying person to live until he dies, at his own maximum potential performing to the limit of his physical and mental capacity with control and independence whenever possible."[33]

Updates

The role of rehabilitation services is constantly evolving. In dealing specifically with the palliative patient, the future brings with it dynamic challenges. With advancements in medical treatment and symptom management, there comes the concern of economic and human costs. Advancements usually portend cost expansion and not contraction. Having outreach is a challenge—providing state-of-the-art resources, meeting the needs of many, and all the while, curtailing inefficiencies in the distribution of services.

Additionally, there is a need for recognition of family members and their contribution to patient care—often placing both patient and caregiver in rather precarious situations related to limitations at home, in nursing services, and with economic flexibility in the workplace. Family leave—while difficult for the employer/employee—may also prove a financial burden to the caregiver and extended family. In a precarious economy, it may be inevitable that family may become further engulfed by the care needs of the loved one. For the patient, there may be limited access to health services (inpatient/outpatient rehabilitation). With financial collapse and tottering human supports, caregiver burnout, frustration, and potentially patient abuse may occur.

The palliative patient often has ongoing rehabilitation needs. In traditional rehabilitation, such patients may no longer qualify under existing precertification processes. As a result, the patient may have to elect a less appealing option of nursing home placement or returning home to an unacceptable social climate—either alone with overwhelmed or ambivalent family members or living with relatives that leads to loss of personal autonomy (now in the confines of a relative's home).

In palliative patients, inpatient rehabilitation often provides an invaluable opportunity. In addition to allowing for physical mobility and attention to self-care tasks, patients also are closely monitored for nutritional status, wound healing, pain, delirium, electrolyte disturbance, anemia, and bowel/bladder irregularities. Once symptoms have been addressed, patients potentially can go back to their former lives. Nursing home is not necessarily the destination of choice.

In the case of the cancer patient, the issues that often are of concern focus on survivorship. Will I be able to return to my prior work, employment, and family unit and remain a viable productive individual? More importantly, if I am unable to return to my work, what safeguards exist so that I can contribute to the family unit?

Increasingly, rehabilitation physicians are called in to assist not only with the day-to-day functioning issues of the patient. For better or worse, we are also required to assist general practitioners with their patients' disability/financial matters. As is often the case in individuals with terminal illness such as end-stage renal disease, cardiopulmonary ailments, and cancer or patients with cardiovascular pathologies resulting in neurological deficits, there is often great confusion as to how to characterize, assess, and quantitate a patient's disability.

All too often, palliative and cancer patients do not fit into a specific equation of disability. An individual may be able to walk and talk, but there may be a number of limitations such as persisting disease, in which constant treatments are being required; restrictions on functioning or danger to not only the patient returning to a prior position but to his colleagues as well, especially in weight-lifting professions; or the operation of mechanical equipment. In these cases, a specialist needs to take an exceptionally detailed history of the patient's past occupational history, understand his prior medical issues, and be able to demonstrate the dangers of treatment-induced medical conditions such as chemotherapy-induced peripheral neuropathy, chemotherapy-induced neurological deficits such as "chemo-brain," or steroid-induced myopathies/neuropathies.

There are many challenges of rehabilitative care in the end-of-life patient. The goal of rehabilitation medicine, however, should never waiver. Experiencing life necessitates maintaining function throughout one's entire life.

CONCLUSION

In general, researchers have yet to look at the overall dynamic of patients with cancer. When a patient presents for initial evaluation to a physician, the overall health and background of the patient is evaluated. Initial presenting complaint, general past medical health, and concurrent medical comorbidities such as cardiopulmonary and endocrine diseases are typically investigated. Emphasis should also be on how patients function in the home, within the family unit, at work, financially, and emotionally—all of these are essential to determine what resources patients will draw upon to combat their illness. If there is no motivation or impetus to get better and if there is a poor support network, negative sense of self-worth, spiritual conflict, or inability to work in trusting union with healthcare workers, the patient is at a marked disadvantage. Correlations have been shown with mood, affect, depression, and the state of one's immune functioning.

Likewise, if a sound relationship of concern, compassion, and investment is not shared by the physician or conveyed in word or action to the patient, medical treatment will not be successful. In terminal disease, the idealistic goal is cure. Cure, however, may not be medically available at this time—despite the best of our scientific endeavors and research protocols. The goal, therefore, is simply and clearly explaining to the patient their disease process, options of optimal care, the true risks and disabilities inherently possible in current treatment regimens, and the promise by healthcare providers of attempting to physically do as little harm as possible in seeking a physical cure wherever possible. When attempts at treatment are exhausted, healthcare workers need to maintain a symptom-relieving role while providing ongoing educational and emotional support to the patient and caregiver.

Key learning points

- Palliative medicine and rehabilitation medicine both aim to restore function. The patient is viewed as a complex individual.

- To understand the patient's psychological, physical, medical, and spiritual dimensions requires an interactive team approach by physician(s), advanced practice nurses, hospital/clinical nursing, psychologist, chaplain, social work, and case manager.

- Physical activity may improve immunological function, cardiorespiratory status, motor ability, and endurance. It may relieve stress and improve symptoms of asthenia, fatigue, dyspnea, anorexia, and constipation.

- Family support is essential in the patient's ongoing medical care and successful transition from hospital to home or hospice setting.

- The goal of both rehabilitation medicine and palliative medicine is restoring autonomy (informed decision making) back to the patient and allowing mental and spiritual clarity.

REFERENCES

1 Sliwa JA, Marciniak C. Physical rehabilitation of the cancer patient [review]. *Cancer Treat Res* 1999; 100: 75–89.
2 Watson PG. Cancer rehabilitation: An overview. *Semin Oncol Nurs* 1992; 8: 167–173.
3 DeLisa JA. A history of cancer rehabilitation. *Cancer* 2001; **92**: 970–974.
4 Dietz JH. Rehabilitation of the cancer patient. *Med Clin North Am* 1969; 53: 607–624.
5 O'Toole DM, Goden AM. Evaluating cancer patients for rehabilitation potential. *West J Med* 1991; 155: 384–387.
6 Karnofsky. Performance status scale definitions rating (%) criteria. Available at www.hospicepatients.org/karnofsky.html, (accessed June 18, 2006).
7 Functional Independence Measure. Available at www.medfriendly.com/functionalindependencemeasure.html, (accessed June 18, 2006).
8 Marciniak CM, James JA, Spill G et al. Functional outcome following rehabilitation of the cancer patient. *Arch Phys Med Rehabil* 1996; 77: 54–57.
9 Muller EA. Influence of training and of inactivity on muscle strength. *Arch Phys Med Rehabil* 1970; 51: 449.
10 Gogin PP, Schneider VS, LeBlaner AD et al. Bed rest effect on extremity muscle torque in healthy men. *Arch Phys Med Rehabil* 1988; 69: 1030–1032.
11 Dietrich JE, Whedon GD, Shon E. Effects of immobilization upon various metabolic and physiologic functions of normal men. *Am J Med* 1948; 4: 3.
12 Hyatt KH, Kamenetsky LG, Smith WM. Extravascular dehydration as an etiologic factor in post-recumbency orthostasis. *Aerosp Med* 1969; 40: 644–650.
13 Taylor HL, Henschel A, Brozek J et al. Effects of bedrest on cardiovascular function and work performance. *J Appl Physiol* 1949; 2: 223.

● 14   Bolin RH. Sensory deprivation: An overview. *Nurs Forum* 1974; 13: 241–258.

● 15   Allman RM, Laprade CA, Noel LB et al. Pressure sores among hospitalized patients. *Ann Intern Med* 1986; 105: 337–342.

● 16   Posner JB. *Intracranial Metastases in Neurologic Complications of Cancer.* Philadelphia, PA: FA Davis, 1995; pp. 77–110.

● 17   Rozenthal JM. Nervous system complications in cancer in current therapy. In: Earlen P, Brain M, eds. *Hematology/Oncology*, Vol. 3. New York: BC Decker, 1998; pp. 314–319.

● 18   Cairncross JG, Kim J-H, Posner JB. Radiation therapy for brain metastases. *Ann Neurol* 1980; 7: 529–541.

◆ 19   Young DF, Posner JP, Chu F et al. Rapid course radiation therapy of cerebral metastases: Results and complications. *Cancer* 1974; 4: 1069–1076.

◆ 20   Huang ME, Cifer DX, Marcus LK. Functional outcome following brain tumor and acute stroke: A comparative analysis. *Arch Phys Med Rehabil* 1998; 79: 1386–1390.

◆ 21   O'Dell MS, Barr K, Spanier P, Warnick R. Functional outcome of inpatient rehabilitation in persons with brain tumors. *Arch Phys Med Rehabil* 1998; 79: 1530–1534.

◆ 22   Sherer M, Meyers CA, Bergloff P. Efficacy of post acute brain injury rehabilitation for patients with primary malignant brain tumors. *Cancer* 2001; 92(4 Suppl): 1049–1052.

● 23   Posner J. *Neurologic Complications of Cancer.* Philadelphia, PA: FA Davis, 1995: p. 118.

● 24   Cheville A. Rehabilitation of patients with advanced cancer. *Cancer* 2001; 92(4 Suppl): 1039–1048.

● 25   Santiago-Palma J, Payne R. Palliative care and rehabilitation. *Cancer* 2001; 92(4 Suppl): 1049–1052.

● 26   Winningham, ML. Strategies for managing cancer related fatigue syndrome: A rehabilitation approach. *Cancer* 2001; 92: 988–997.

◆ 27   Deuster PA, Curale AM. Exercise-induced changes in populations of peripheral blood mononuclear cells. *Med Sci Sports Exerc* 1987; 20: 276–280.

● 28   Easson AM, Hinshaw DB, Johnson DL. The role of tube feeding and total parenteral nutrition in advanced illness. *J Am Coll Surg* 2002; 194: 225–228.

● 29   Olson E, Cristian A. The role of rehabilitation medicine and palliative care in the treatment of patients with end-stage disease. *Phys Med Rehabil Clin North Am* 2005; 16: 285–305.

● 30   Abrahm JL. Update in palliative medicine and end of life care. *Annu Rev Med* 2003; 54: 53–72.

● 31   Yoshioka H. Rehabilitation for the terminal cancer patient. *Am J Phys Med Rehabil* 1994; 73: 199–206.

● 32   Montagnini M, Lodhi M, Born W. The utilization of physical therapy in a palliative care unit. *J Palliat Med* 2003; 6: 11–17.

● 33   Saunders C. Foreword. In: Doyle D, Hanks G, MacDonald N, eds. *Oxford Textbook of Palliative Medicine*, 2nd edn. Oxford, U.K.: Oxford University Press, 1998: pp. v–ix.

91

Integrative and palliative medicine

GABRIEL LOPEZ, RICHARD LEE, LORENZO COHEN

DEFINITIONS: TRADITIONAL, ALTERNATIVE, COMPLEMENTARY, AND INTEGRATIVE MEDICINE

Traditional medicine is defined by the World Health Organization (WHO) as the sum total of knowledge, skills, and practices based on the theories, beliefs, and experiences indigenous to different cultures that are used to maintain health, as well as to prevent, diagnose, improve, or treat physical and mental illnesses.[1] Complementary/alternative medicine (CAM) is defined by the U.S. National Center for Complementary and Alternative Medicine (NCCAM) as a group of diverse medical and health-care systems, practices, and products that are not presently considered as part of conventional medicine.[2] *Complementary medicine* is an approach combining conventional medical therapies with CAM or nonconventional therapies for which there may exist high-quality scientific evidence of safety and effectiveness. *Alternative medicine*, however, is defined as the use of a nonconventional modality for which there is no scientific evidence of efficacy *in place of* conventional medicine.[2] Integrative medicine describes a philosophy of practice using an evidence-based approach to merge conventional and nonconventional therapies. An integrative, interdisciplinary approach advocating open communication between conventional and nonconventional health-care providers can help patients better meet their goals in a safe manner. Nonconventional or CAM therapies have been subdivided into four broad subsections by NCCAM[2] (see Table 91.1).

In palliative care settings, complementary or integrative approaches may be used for managing symptoms and improving quality of life. Integrative oncology uses a comprehensive, personalized, evidence-based, and safe approach to merge conventional and CAM therapies in cancer care, taking into account patients' psychosocial and physical well-being. In this chapter, we will illustrate an integrative approach, using cancer as the disease model, from diagnosis through advanced disease and survivorship (Figure 91.1).

PREVALENCE

The WHO estimates that up to 80% of people in developing countries rely on traditional medicines for their primary health care.[1] People in more developed countries also seek out these medicines and practices assuming that they are effective and may be safer than allopathic medicine because they are natural.[3] A 1997 survey of U.S. adults found CAM use (excluding self-prayer) varied from 32% to 54% among the sociodemographic groups surveyed.[4] A 2002 survey by the U.S. Centers for Disease Control and Prevention (CDC) found that 36% of adults had used CAM therapies (nonprayer) during the past 12 months.[5]

Patients may express interest in nonconventional or CAM therapies for treatment of cancer or its effects or may use them for other chronic conditions. CAM therapies were used by 69% of patients attending six university-based primary care clinics for osteoarthritis, rheumatoid arthritis, or fibromyalgia.[6] A German survey of amyotrophic lateral sclerosis patients revealed CAM use of 54%, with acupuncture most widely used.[7] In a survey of CAM offerings in 300 randomly selected U.S. hospices, 60% of respondents offered complementary therapies, most commonly massage (83%) and music therapy (50%).[8]

An estimated 48%–69% of U.S. patients with cancer use CAM therapies,[9,10] and percentages increase if spiritual practices are included.[10] Complementary therapies are used by 70% of all oncology departments engaged in palliative care in Britain,[11,12] 64% of palliative care units in Japan,[13] and 28% of advanced cancer/palliative care patients in a Canadian community and hospital setting.[14] A survey of five clinics within a U.S. comprehensive cancer care center found that CAM therapies were used by 68.7% of patients (excluding psychotherapy and spiritual practices) and were 11.6 times more likely to be used by patients with distant or unstaged disease.[10] A later survey in the breast and gynecological clinics within that same center found that CAM therapies (defined as herbs, supplements, and mega doses of vitamins) were used by 48% of

Table 91.1 *National Institutes of Health—National Center for Complementary and Alternative Medicine*

CAM categories	Examples
Natural products	Herbal medicines (botanicals)
	Vitamins
	Minerals
	Probiotics
Mind and body medicine	Meditation
	Yoga
	Acupuncture
	Qi gong
	Tai chi
Manipulative and body-based practices	Massage
	Spinal manipulation
	• Chiropractic
	• Osteopathic
	• Physical therapy
Other CAM practices	Whole medical systems
	• Ayurvedic medicine
	• Traditional Chinese medicine
	• Homeopathy
	• Naturopathy
	Energy therapies
	• Magnet therapy
	• Reiki
	• Healing touch
	Movement therapies
	• Feldenkrais method

patients. Statistically significant differences existed by disease status with CAM therapies used by 38% of newly diagnosed patients, 49% of those with recurrence or relapse, and 55% of those in remission.[9]

COMMUNICATION

Provider–patient–caregiver

A nonjudgmental approach to discussion of nonconventional therapies can help develop a comprehensive integrative medicine treatment plan. Deciding whether to recommend a nonconventional therapy or warn against its use may not even be an option for the health-care provider if patients are already using it without the physician's knowledge. The percentage of patients using complementary therapies in cancer centers without telling their physicians has varied from 38% to 60%.[9,10] For this reason, physicians, nurse practitioners, and other palliative care professionals must strive to maintain an inquiring, but nonjudgmental, attitude toward patients concerning nonconventional therapies. Their role is to assist the patient by providing information about the risk and benefits of different treatment options in order to help patients make an informed decision. The ultimate goal is to understand a patient's motivations and ensure that the approach they choose is safe and potentially worth the investment when there is an associated cost with little evidence for efficacy. See Chapter 114 for further discussion regarding strategies for enhancing integrative medicine discussions.

Provider–provider (interdisciplinary)

Opportunities exist to enhance patient care through inclusion of evidence-based modalities that are not part of conventional systems of care. An integrative medicine approach requires effective communication between health-care providers of nonconventional and conventional therapies. Interdisciplinary team meetings are critical settings for the development of patient-centered care plans in palliative care and hospice settings.[15] The inclusion of an integrative medicine practitioner

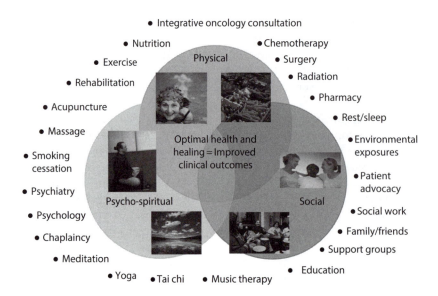

Figure 91.1 *Integrative medicine center model.*

in an interdisciplinary team discussion is one strategy to help identify which nonconventional therapies are most appropriate and safe for the patient. Integrative medicine practitioners can include physicians, midlevel providers, nurses with an integrative medicine focus, and other practitioners already part of most interdisciplinary integrative teams including psychologists, acupuncturists, and massage, art, and music therapists. Clarity of goals of care and open communication between all members of the health-care team is essential to select those approaches most appropriate for the patient. Some nonconventional therapies may be appropriate at the end of life that may not be in the context of a patient with a reversible exacerbation of a chronic disease.

CAM AND SYMPTOM ASSESSMENT

Routine CAM assessment alongside symptom assessment is critical to the ongoing care of patients and ensuring the highest-quality care for patients. For those seeking integrative medicine approaches for the management of their symptoms, this assessment is critical. The Measure Yourself Concerns and Wellbeing (MYCaW) tool asks patients to identify those areas they would most like to discuss during a supportive care consultation and includes CAM concerns.[16] The Edmonton Symptom Assessment Scale (ESAS) is a 10-item symptom assessment tool validated and widely used in the palliative care setting for symptom monitoring in inpatient and outpatient settings.[17] Combining information from the ESAS and MyCAW tools can provide a platform upon which to build an integrative treatment plan and provide information on treatment outcomes after the use of nonconventional therapies. A personalized symptom management strategy utilizing an evidence-based application of conventional and nonconventional therapies can help optimize treatment outcomes.

CAM (NONCONVENTIONAL THERAPIES)

Introduction

Patients may have a variety of motivations for seeking nonconventional therapies, including a desire to improve quality of life and prolong life, boost the immune system, and aid conventional medical treatments.[18] An evidence-based approach to the integration of these nonconventional therapies can help patients develop realistic expectations, optimize safety, and improve outcomes. Natural products, acupuncture, meditation, and music therapy are commonly used nonconventional therapies encountered in a variety of health-care settings (see Table 91.2).[19]

Natural products

QUALITY CONTROL

Herbal products and supplements from different or the same manufacturer may have variable levels of quality and consistency as a result of poor quality control. Widely reported

Table 91.2 *Evidence-based CAM modalities*

Modality	Indication (level of evidence)	Safety considerations
Acupuncture	Pain (1A) Nausea (1A) Xerostomia (1B) Hot flashes (1B) Neuropathy (2C)	Precaution with neutropenia or thrombocytopenia; avoid in limbs with or at risk for lymphedema.
Massage	Pain (1B) Mood disturbance/ anxiety/depression (1B) Constipation (1C) Lymphedema (manual lymphatic drainage)	Encourage use of licensed oncology massage therapist; adjust type and level of massage depth to individual patient; precaution with neutropenia, thrombocytopenia, dysfunctional platelets, recent surgery, or radiation.
Mind body (meditation, yoga, tai chi)	Stress reduction (1B) Mood disturbance/ anxiety (1B) Quality of life improvement (1B) Insomnia (1B)	Risk of injury with movement-based practices (yoga, tai chi); patient with psychiatric disorder or severe anxiety may not tolerate one-on-one or group setting.
Music therapy	Stress reduction (1B) Mood disturbance/ anxiety (1B) Quality of life (1B)	Recommend licensed music therapist.

contamination of natural products has highlighted the need for quality assurance within the herbal industry. The U.S. Food and Drug Administration and the WHO, in consultation with major manufacturers, have proposed guidelines for good manufacturing practices (GMPs). Since most herbs are classified as foods, they are not regulated in the same manner as drugs. Nevertheless, GMPs are being supported by some major producers, natural product companies, and independent nongovernmental groups such as the American Botanical Council,[20] and results of independent laboratory testing are available. ConsumerLab (www.consumerlab.com), for example, tests products according to recognized standards of quality, ingredients claimed on labels, purity, and biological availability.

ORGAN TOXICITY

Botanicals have the potential to cause organ toxicity, including hepatic or renal failure, and increase bleeding risk. Numerous case reports have been published documenting toxicity related to the use of herbal products, including green tea–associated hepatotoxicity.[21] While short-term exposure to hepatotoxins or nephrotoxins present in natural products may lead to transient and reversible organ injury, prolonged exposure can lead to organ failure. A thorough review of potential organ toxicities is warranted when combining prescription drugs with natural products. Early recognition of potentially hepatotoxic or nephrotoxic herbs or supplements can lead to timely discontinuation of potentially dangerous preparations.

Table 91.3   *Recommended websites for evidence-based resources*

Organization/Web site (alphabetical order)	Address/URL
Cochrane Review Organization	www.cochrane.org
ConsumerLab	www.consumerlab.com
Memorial Sloan-Kettering Cancer Center Integrative Medicine Service	http://www.mskcc.org/aboutherbs
NCCAM	http://nccam.nih.gov/
Natural Medicines Comprehensive Database	http://www.naturaldatabase.com/
Natural Standard	http://www.naturalstandard.com/
NCI Office of Cancer Complementary and Alternative Medicine (OCCAM)	http://www.cancer.gov/cam
University of Texas, MD Anderson Cancer Center, Integrative Medicine Program	www.mdanderson.org/ integrativemed

Certain herbs and supplements can result in an increased risk of bleeding by interfering with platelet function, by acting as anticoagulants, or through interactions with anticoagulants. *Ginkgo biloba*, ginseng, green tea, cat's claw, fish oil, and garlic to name a few have all been associated with increased bleeding risk.[22] These agents should be discontinued before surgical procedures and in patients with preexisting bleeding conditions.

DRUG–HERB INTERACTIONS

Vitamins, supplements, or herbal products have the potential to interfere with treatment efficacy, decreasing or increasing therapeutic levels of the active drug. One well-documented example is St. John's wort, an inducer of the cytochrome P450-3A4 hepatic enzyme system. This herb can decrease available drug levels of irinotecan and imatinib, both used for the treatment of a variety of malignancies, leading to poor outcomes.[23,24] St. John's wort can also decrease levels of drugs commonly used in palliative care settings including methadone, haloperidol, benzodiazepines, and mirtazapine, all metabolized by the cytochrome P450-3A4 system. A thorough evaluation of drug–herb interactions is critical, and there are now a number of important resources available to help guide health-care professionals (Table 91.3).

Acupuncture

Acupuncture, a practice with origins in traditional Chinese medicine, may be used for the relief of cancer- or treatment-related symptoms in the appropriately selected patient. The strongest evidence supports the use of acupuncture for relief of pain and nausea, and preliminary data exist for hot flashes, xerostomia, neuropathy, and headaches.[25] The treatment involves insertion of small gauge, sterile, stainless steel needles

into specific points. Although there is a low risk of complications associated with this procedure when practiced by a trained and licensed acupuncturist, it is important to consider the patient's neutrophil count, platelet count, skin integrity, and concurrent use of anticoagulants. As a low-risk, cost-effective treatment option, acupuncture may be a helpful adjunct to conventional treatment for patients suffering from uncontrolled treatment-related side effects or those for whom other treatment approaches have failed.

Massage

Massage is a body-based practice involving the manipulation of body tissues using different techniques and levels of pressure to achieve a therapeutic effect. An integrative approach would support the use of massage for relief of pain,[26,27] anxiety,[26,28] and constipation.[29,30] In the cancer patient, a massage therapist with special training in oncology massage is the best equipped to safely deliver the massage. By taking into account the patient's blood counts and oncologic history, an oncologic massage therapist can maximize safety. Levels of pressure are adjusted from 1 through 5, with a light Level 1 to a deep Level 5 massage[31]. Risk of bruising, bleeding, or injury can be minimized by careful application of pressure, avoiding massage into the deep tissue or bone in selected patients. Caregivers may also benefit from either giving[32] or receiving[33] massage.

Meditation

Meditation is a contemplative practice that may be based on an individual's cultural or religious beliefs, but can also be learned as a technique independent of background. Meditation techniques can be taught through classroom or individual instruction so as to be accessible to patients and caregivers independent of religious or cultural practice. Once learned, meditation techniques can be applied to help with reducing stress and anxiety[34–36] and management of insomnia.[37,38] Focused attention on sound or the breath can help patients enhance their focus and gain a new sense of control over their thoughts and worries. There is increasing interest in the use of meditation for alleviation of cancer-related cognitive deficits.[39] Although there are hundreds of meditation practices throughout the world, consultation with an integrative medicine practitioner can help patients optimize their use of meditation techniques. Some patients may be more successful than others in learning these techniques; for example, those with severe anxiety may not feel comfortable learning meditation in a group setting. Meditation can start as practice used only when needed to relieve anxiety (e.g., during a stressful procedure) or can be incorporated into a daily routine (nightly to calm the mind prior to sleep onset). The duration of meditation is based on the patient's level of comfort with the practice as there is no optimum length or frequency. Patients may also benefit from different movement-based mind–body practices such as yoga, tai chi, or qigong.

Music therapy

Music therapy is the evidence-based use of musical interventions for nonmusical goals, such as to enhance quality of life, manage symptoms, or modify mood. Music therapists receive special training, learning to select the appropriate therapeutic strategy for an individual or group setting. Interventions can include music making, song writing, singing, or listening. Evidence suggests music therapy can help with management of mood disturbances, including anxiety.[40–42] One technique, the ISO-vectoring principle, calls for the music therapist to match the patient's mood with the music tempo; a subsequent increase or decrease in tempo can result in a change in the patient's mood.[43] Patients taught with the ISO principle can learn to develop an individualized musical playlist to change their mood, for relaxation or stimulation. An integrative medicine practitioner can help identify those patients most likely to benefit from consultation with a music therapist.

Key learning points

- Important distinctions exist between *alternative* medicine used in place of conventional treatments and *complementary* medicines, with some evidence supporting the effectiveness of *complementary* medicines used alongside conventional treatments. Integrative medicine aims to create a comprehensive and optimal treatment plan by utilizing all appropriate therapies (both conventional and nonconventional) in an evidence-based approach to improve patient care.

- Many patients engage in some type of CAM modality at some point in their disease trajectory, especially when the disease is advanced. To prevent harm and maximize treatment outcomes, health-care providers, through nonjudgmental inquiry, should take an active role in identifying those patients using or exploring CAM therapies and ensure it is done in a safe manner.

- Inclusion of a colleague with expertise on integrative medicine in an interdisciplinary setting can help identify those CAM modalities most appropriate to a patient's clinical circumstances. A goal-directed approach to inclusion of CAM in a treatment plan can help providers when developing an interdisciplinary symptom management strategy.

REFERENCES

1   World Health Organization traditional medicine strategy: 2014–2023. Published December 2013. 76 pages. ISBN: 978 92 4 150609 0.

2   National Center for Complementary/Alternative Medicine of the National Institutes of Health. What is complementary and alternative medicine? Available at: http://nccam.nih.gov/health/whatiscam. NCCAM Pub No. D347. Date Created October 2008. Accessed July 2 2014. Last updated May 2013.

3   World Health Organization. New WHO guidelines to promote proper use of alternative medicines. 2004; Available at: http://www.who.int/mediacentre/news/releases/2004/pr44/en/index1.html, (accessed July 2, 2014).

4   Eisenberg DM, Davis RB, Ettner SL et al. Trends in alternative medicine use in the United States, 1990–1997: Results of a follow-up national survey. *JAMA* 1998; 280: 1569–1575.

5   Barnes PM, Powell-Griner E, McFann K, Nahin RL. Complementary and alternative medicine use among adults: United States, 2002. Advance Date from Vital and Health Statistics; 2004 (343).

6   Herman CJ, Allen P, Hunt WC et al. Use of complementary therapies among primary care clinic patients with arthritis. *Prevent Chronic Dis* 2004; 1: A12.

7   Wasner M, Klier H, Borasio GD. The use of alternative medicine by patients with amyotrophic lateral sclerosis. *J Neurol Sci* October 15, 2001; 191(1–2): 151–154.

8   Demmer C. A survey of complementary therapy services provided by hospices. *J Palliat Med* 2004; 7(4): 510–516.

9   Navo MA, Phan J, Vaughan C et al. An assessment of the utilization of complementary and alternative medication in women with gynecologic or breast malignancies. *J Clin Oncol* 2004; 22: 671–677.

10 Richardson MA, Sanders T, Palmer JL et al. Complementary/alternative medicine use in a comprehensive cancer center and the implications for oncology. *J Clin Oncol* 2000; 18: 2505–2514.

11 Ernst E. Complementary therapies in palliative cancer care. *Cancer* 2001; 91: 2181–2185.

12 White P. Complementary medicine treatment of cancer: A survey of provision. *Complement Ther Med* 1998; 6: 10–13.

13 Osaka I, Kurihara Y, Tanaka K et al. Attitudes toward and current practice of complementary and alternative medicine in Japanese palliative care units. *J Palliat Med* March 2009; 12(3): 239–244.

14 Oneschuk D, Hanson J, Bruera E. Complementary therapy use: A survey of community- and hospital-based patients with advanced cancer. *Palliat Med* 2000; 14: 432–434.

15 Wiebe LA, VonRoenn JH. Working with a palliative care team. *Cancer J* September–October 2010; 16(5): 488–492.

16 Paterson C, Thomas K, Manasse A, Cooke H, Peace G. Measure Yourself Concerns and Wellbeing (MYCaW): An individualised questionnaire for evaluating outcome in cancer support care that includes complementary therapies. *Complement Ther Med* March 2007; 15(1): 38–45 [Epub 2006 May 3].

17 Bruera E, Kuehn N, Miller MJ, Selmser P, Macmillan K. The Edmonton symptom assessment system (ESAS): A simple method for the assessment of palliative care patients. *J Palliat Care* 1991; 7(2): 6–9.

18 Nahleh Z, Tabbara IA. Complementary and alternative medicine in breast cancer patients. *Palliat Support Care* September 2003; 1(3): 267–273.

19 Deng GE, Frenkel M, Cohen L et al. Evidence-based clinical practice guidelines for integrative oncology: Complementary therapies and botanicals. *J Soc Integr Oncol* Summer 2009; 7(3): 85–120.

20 Blumenthal M, Watts D. FDA issues proposed GMPs for dietary supplements. *HerbalGram: J Am Botanical Council* 2003; 58: 62–65, 80.

21 Mazzanti, G et al. Hepatotoxicity from green tea: A review of the literature and two unpublished cases. *Eur J Pharmacol* 2009; 65(4): 331–341.

22 Ulbricht C, Chao W, Costa D, Rusie-Seamon E, Weissner W, Woods J. Clinical evidence of herb–drug interactions: A systematic review by the natural standard research collaboration. *Curr Drug Metab* December 2008; 9(10): 1063–1120.

23 Mathijssen RHJ, Verweij J, DeBruijn P. Modulation of irinotecan (CPT-11) metabolism by St. John's wort in cancer patients. *American Association for Cancer Research, 93rd Annual Meeting*, San Francisco, CA; April 6–10, 2002.

24 Smith P, Bullock JM, Booker BM, Haas CE, Berenson CS, Jusko WJ. The influence of St. John's wort on the pharmacokinetics and protein binding of imatinib mesylate. *Pharmacotherapy* November 2004; 24(11): 1508–1514.

25 Garcia MK, McQuade J, Haddad R, Patel S, Lee R, Palmer L, Yang P, Cohen L. Systematic review of acupuncture in cancer care: A synthesis of the evidence. *J Clin Oncol* March 1, 2013; 31(7): 952–960.

26 Cassileth BR, Vickers AJ. Massage therapy for symptom control: Outcome study at a major cancer center. *J Pain Symptom Manage* 2004; 28: 244–249.

27 Wilkie DJ, Kampbell J, Cutshall S et al. Effects of massage on pain intensity, analgesics and quality of life in patients with cancer pain: A pilot study of a randomized clinical trial conducted within hospice care delivery. *Hosp J* 2000; 15(3): 31–53.

28 Wilkinson SM, Love SB, Westcombe AM et al. Effectiveness of aromatherapy massage in the management of anxiety and depression in patients with cancer: A multicenter randomized controlled trial. *J Clin Oncol* February 10, 2007; 25(5): 532–539.

29 Lamas K, Lindholm L, Stenlund H, Engstrom B, Jacobsson C. Effects of abdominal massage in the management of constipation—A randomized controlled trial. *Int J Nurs Stud* 2009; 46: 759–767.

30 Sinclair MJ. The use of abdominal massage to treat chronic constipation. *Bodyw Mov Ther* October 2011; 15(4): 436–445 [Epub 2010 August 25].

31 Walton, T. Medical Conditions and Massage Therapy: A Decision Tree Approach. Philadelphia: Wolters Kluwer Health/Lippincott Williams & Wilkins, 2011.

32 Collinge W, Kahn J, Yarnold P, Bauer-Wu S, McCorkle R. Couples and cancer: Feasibility of brief instruction in massage and touch therapy to build caregiver efficacy. *J Soc Integr Oncol* Fall 2007; 5(4): 147–154.

33 Mackereth P, Sylt P, Weinberg A, Campbell G. Chair massage for carers in an acute cancer hospital. *Eur J Oncol Nurs* June 2005; 9(2): 167–179.

34 Speca M, Carlson LE, Goodey E et al. A randomized, wait-list controlled clinical trial: The effect of a mindfulness meditation based stress reduction program on mood and symptoms of stress in cancer outpatients. *Psychosom Med* 2000; 62: 613–622.

35 Carlson LE, Garland SN. Impact of mindfulness-based stress reduction (MBSR) on sleep, mood, stress and fatigue symptoms in cancer outpatients. *Int J Behav Med* 2005; 12: 278–285.

36 Carlson LE, Speca M, Faris P, Patel KD. One year pre-post intervention follow-up of psychological, immune, endocrine and blood pressure outcomes of mindfulness-based stress reduction (MBSR) in breast and prostate cancer outpatients. *Brain Behav Immun* 2007; 21: 1038–1049.

37 Cohen L, Warneke C, Fouladi RT, Rodriguez MA, Chaoul-Reich A. Psychological adjustment and sleep quality in a randomized trial of the effects of a Tibetan yoga intervention in patients with lymphoma. *Cancer* May 15, 2004; 100(10): 2253–2260.

38 Winbush NY, Gross CR, Kreitzer MJ. The effects of mindfulness-based stress reduction on sleep disturbance: A systematic review. *Explore* (NY) 2007; 3: 585–591.

39 Biegler, KA, MA Chaoul, Cohen L. Cancer, cognitive impairment, and meditation. *Acta Oncol* 2009; 8: 18–26.

40 Cassileth, BR, Vickers AJ, Magill LA. Music therapy for mood disturbance during hospitalization for autologous stem cell transplantation: A randomized controlled trial. *Cancer* December 15, 2003; 98(12): 223–229.

41 Bradt J, Dileo C, Grocke D, Magill L. Music interventions for improving psychological and physical outcomes in cancer patients. *Cochrane Database Syst Rev* August 10, 2011; (8): CD006911.

42 Horne-Thompson A, Grocke D. The effect of music therapy on anxiety in patients who are terminally ill. *J Palliat Med* May 2008; 11(4): 582–590.

43 Richardson M, Babiak-Vazquez AE, Frenkel MA. Music therapy in a comprehensive cancer center. *J Soc Integr Oncol* 2008; 6(2): 76–81.

92

Human immunodeficiency virus and palliative care

RICHARD HARDING, ROBERT E. HIRSCHTICK, JAMIE H. VON ROENN

INTRODUCTION

Therapeutic advances in recent years have considerably extended the survival of patients in high-income countries who are infected with the human immunodeficiency virus (HIV).[1*] Those who are able to access and adhere to antiretroviral therapy (ART) are predicted to achieve near-normal life expectancy. Therefore, for many in the world, HIV infection has become a chronic, treatable condition, similar in many ways to congestive heart failure. However, there is still considerable morbidity and mortality associated with HIV infection,[2] and these problems are present throughout the disease trajectory from the point of diagnosis.[3] Moreover, as with congestive heart failure, the trajectory of late-stage illness does not proceed steadily downward but rather follows an irregular course of sudden valleys and surprising peaks.[4,5] Unfortunately, the successes of ART have led HIV medicine away from the core palliative care skills it once offered and as a result have left patients with a burden of distressing yet manageable problems.[6]

Many of the issues faced by people with advanced HIV infection fall within the traditional purview of hospice and palliative care. For example, the palliative care consultation service of a large urban hospital reported the following issues in patients with acquired immune deficiency syndrome (AIDS): pain in 40%, psychosocial issues in 31%, nausea and/or vomiting in 14%, and interpersonal conflicts in 13%.[7] Within a sample of hospice HIV/AIDS patients in two African countries, their most prevalent symptoms were pain (82.6%), feeling sad (75.4%), feeling drowsy (74.1%), worry (73.2%), and lack of energy (71.9%).[8] The most burdensome problems were hunger (36.2%), pain (35.2%), weight loss (27.7%), numbness (26.3%), and lack of energy (25.0%). These data highlight the multidimensional nature of problems, particularly in low- and middle-income countries where the vast burden of HIV disease is found. In such settings, these problems are compounded by other diseases of poverty such as tuberculosis, which may present clinicians with the challenges of managing

polypharmacy. Indeed, among people living with HIV, drug-resistant tuberculosis is a growing public health problem.[9] Therefore, the palliative care approach of family-based care that addresses multidimensional needs is essential where issues such as food security and infection control are present. An understanding of the cultural identities of those groups who have been most affected by HIV is essential when delivering person-centered palliative care, with African patients stressing the importance of spiritual well-being in their construction of quality of life in advanced HIV,[10] injecting drug users facing specific psychosocial problems,[11] and gay men fearing discrimination from hospice providers.[12,13]

Palliative care remains essential alongside treatment. Recent UK data among HIV outpatients have revealed a high symptom burden, with the most common symptoms being lack of energy (70.8%), worry (69.9%), diarrhea (53.6%), sexual dysfunction (53.5%), and pain (53.2%), and that symptom burden was not associated with treatment use.[3] The finding that treatment use does not reduce symptom burden has been reproduced elsewhere.[14]

There are many unique aspects involved in the palliative care of HIV-infected individuals, and HIV/AIDS remains largely a socially unacceptable disease. Infected patients may be shunned by family or friends and suffer physical and emotional isolation as a result.[15] High rates of suicidal ideation are reported,[16] and mental health problems are reported as a major concern for those living with HIV.[17] The comparatively young age at death of HIV-infected patients may exact a toll upon health-care providers. The presence of a homosexual partner may exacerbate friction with family members, especially when major health-care decisions need to be made. The patient may have a history of past or current narcotic abuse, which can challenge not only the prescribing expertise of practitioners but also the limits of their compassion. Finally, many HIV-infected patients, owing to social, cultural, or economic considerations, may be reluctant or unable to access support services and medical resources, including hospice and palliative care programs. For example, African-Americans now comprise the largest group of HIV-infected persons in the United States.[2] However, they are less likely to use hospice and palliative care services than are European Americans.[18] Moreover, physicians are less likely to have discussions about end-of-life issues with African-American AIDS patients than they are with European American AIDS patients.[19]

HIV management has evolved, but many aspects of the patient experience of disease have remained the same: the high burden of physical, psychological, social, and spiritual problems and the life-limiting nature of the disease. Although palliative care has been shown to be effective in improving outcomes for patients,[20] the complexities of palliation alongside treatment, improved life expectancy, and underrecognizing of pain and other symptoms have created a number of barriers to adequate HIV palliative care provision.[21]

SYMPTOM BURDEN

A significant symptom burden is associated with HIV infection throughout the trajectory of disease, although it is greatest in patients with advanced and/or refractory HIV infection.[5,7,22] The high prevalence of pain and other symptoms in patients with HIV and AIDS has been documented since the onset of the epidemic. The etiology of some of the most common symptoms has changed over the course of the epidemic, but the overall prevalence has not. Without the use of highly active antiretroviral therapy (HAART), opportunistic infections account for many symptoms, including headaches with cryptococcal meningitis, wasting and abdominal pain with *Mycobacterium avium* complex (MAC) infection, and blindness from cytomegalovirus (CMV) retinitis. The contribution of opportunistic infections to pain and other symptoms in patients with AIDS has diminished over time as HIV therapy, where available, has become more effective and the frequency of these infections has decreased.

In the pre-HAART era, the most common symptoms in patients with AIDS included weight loss, pain, anorexia, depression, anxiety, cough, dyspnea, fatigue, and diarrhea.[5,7,22] More recent data (1996) from 3000 U.S. patients reported the following as the 10 most common symptoms: constitutional symptoms (fever, sweats, chills) 51%, diarrhea 51%, nausea and anorexia 50%, numbness and tingling/neuropathic pain in the hands and feet 49%, headaches 39%, weight loss 37%, vaginal symptoms 36%, sinus symptoms 35%, visual disturbances 32%, and cough or shortness of breath 30%.[23] Among the recent UK HIV outpatient data cited earlier, a mean of 18 symptoms was reported.[3] Using the same symptom measurement tool among newly diagnosed HIV patients in Uganda with low CD4 counts (>200 cells), the mean total number of symptoms was 14.0, and the ten most common symptoms were pain (76%), weight loss (70%), itching (67%), feeling drowsy/tired (61%), lack of energy (61%), numbness/tingling in hands or feet (57%), cough (53%), skin changes (52%), worry (51%), and lack of appetite (49%). The median number of symptoms was not associated with WHO stage or CD4 count.

PAIN

Pain frequently complicates the course of HIV infection. Often underdiagnosed and undertreated, pain is now more frequently a result of chronic HIV infection and/or medication toxicities than opportunistic infection in the developed world. One longitudinal study found that over a 2-year period, almost 90% of AIDS patients experienced pain and almost 70% experienced continuous pain.[24] Peripheral neuropathy, headache, and abdominal pain are the most common pain syndromes.[24] As described earlier, pain persists in around half of HIV patients irrespective of treatment use.

Neuropathy

Peripheral polyneuropathy develops in about a third to half of patients with AIDS.[23,25,26] The predominant symptoms are pain, paresthesias, and numbness involving the feet and lower legs. The two most common causes of neuropathy are medication induced and HIV induced. These two conditions are indistinguishable clinically. The severity of distal sensory neuropathy induced by HIV is worse in late-stage disease.[27] The antiretroviral medications stavudine (D4T) and didanosine (DDI) are the medications most often associated with painful peripheral neuropathy. Pain may improve or stabilize after discontinuation of these medications but frequently it persists.

Management of peripheral neuropathy in the setting of HIV is similar to that of peripheral neuropathy in general. Gabapentin is the most commonly used medication. It appears to be effective in this setting but most experience is anecdotal. A daily dose of ≥600 mg is required for efficacy.[28***] In a placebo-controlled trial involving diabetics, gabapentin at 900–3600 mg/day was significantly more effective than placebo in reducing pain intensity and quality of life. Dizziness (in 20% of subjects) and sleepiness (in 23%) were the most common adverse effects.[29**] Gabapentin is more effective in reducing pain than in reducing numbness.

Lamotrigine has been studied as a treatment for HIV-associated neuropathy. Simpson et al. found that 11 weeks of lamotrigine was more effective than placebo in reducing neuropathic pain.[30] However, there was no benefit relative to placebo in patients who were no longer taking neurotoxic ART. Hence, lamotrigine may have less relevance in end-of-life care, when neurotoxic ART would likely be discontinued. Rash occurred in 14% of lamotrigine-treated patients, which was not significantly greater than placebo.

Tricyclic antidepressants are inexpensive medications often used for neuropathic pain. However, their frequent adverse effects limit their utility. A controlled trial of amitriptyline showed no benefit and more adverse effects compared with placebo.[31**] Topical capsaicin has also been demonstrated to be ineffective for this indication.[32]

FATIGUE

Fatigue, a highly prevalent symptom in patients with HIV infection, interferes with normal function and quality of life. Leading physiological factors contributing to fatigue in patients with HIV infection include anemia, deconditioning, muscle wasting, involuntary weight loss, hypogonadism, and opportunistic infection. General considerations for the evaluation and treatment of fatigue are outlined in Box 92.1.

Anemia is a well-documented, reversible cause of fatigue. Randomized controlled trials have demonstrated significant improvement in overall quality of life in association with an increase in hematocrit.[33–35] Although health professionals frequently wait until the hemoglobin is 8 g/dL or less to intervene, studies have demonstrated that the incremental increases in quality of life with treatment are highest when hemoglobin is in the range of 11–13 g/dL.[36] The increase in hematocrit has been associated with improvements in energy, activity, and functional level and overall quality of life.

Fatigue has frequently been associated with depression and is a hallmark of major depressive disorders. But treatment of depression, in and of itself, in patients with cancer has not been shown to reverse fatigue.[37**] No similar data are available in the setting of HIV infection. Hormonal abnormalities, such as hypothyroidism and hypogonadism, are readily reversible causes of fatigue. Hypogonadism is the most common endocrine abnormality in patients with HIV infection, with low testosterone

concentrations currently identified in about 15% of HIV-infected men in countries where HAART is available.[38] Changes in exercise or activity pattern, particularly associated with infections or opportunistic infection-related deconditioning, result in decreased activity and performance status and are associated with fatigue regardless of the underlying cause of the deconditioning.

The first step in treatment is the identification of reversible factors that may contribute to fatigue. Common contributing factors, in addition to those given earlier, include pain, sleep disorders, medications, and opportunistic infection. Both pharmacological and nonpharmacological interventions have been evaluated for the treatment of fatigue. Nonpharmacological interventions include exercise programs and maintenance of optimal levels of activity, restorative therapies, sleep therapy, and psychosocial interventions, including stress management, relaxation, and support groups.

The potential utility of psychostimulants for the treatment of HIV-related fatigue is supported by the results of a limited number of trials. A randomized, double-blind, placebo-controlled trial of methylphenidate (up to 60 mg daily), pemoline (150 mg/day), or placebo in patients with AIDS-related fatigue demonstrated an improvement in fatigue with treatment.[39**] Of methylphenidate-, pemoline-, and placebo-treated patients, 41%, 36%, and 15%, respectively, demonstrated improvement in fatigue on self-reported rating scales. Corticosteroids are thought to provide a boost in energy for patients with advanced malignancy, though it is unclear what their role and/or adverse effects might be in patients with chronic viral infection.

GASTROINTESTINAL SYMPTOMS

Diarrhea

Diarrhea is much less common since the introduction of HAART. However, it remains a chronic problem, reported by 28% of HIV-infected individuals who are receiving HAART.[40] Prior to the availability of effective anti-HIV therapy, infection was the most common cause of diarrhea. Now most cases are noninfectious, usually medication related.[41,42*] In one reported cohort, infection was responsible for 53% of cases of chronic diarrhea prior to the availability of HAART. Two years later, after HAART became available, the prevalence of chronic diarrhea was unchanged but infection accounted for only 13% of cases.[42] Many antiretroviral agents, particularly protease inhibitors (PIs), cause diarrhea. The most common infectious causes are CMV, cryptosporidiosis, *Clostridium difficile*, and *Giardia*. The patient's CD4 lymphocyte count (T cell count) is useful in determining the likelihood of certain pathogens. For example, CMV colitis, MAC, and microsporidiosis tend to occur only in patients with CD4 lymphocyte counts lower than $100/mm^3$.

The initial approach to diarrhea in a palliative care situation is to discontinue potential medication culprits (e.g., PIs) and/or initiate nonspecific antidiarrheal therapy such as loperamide. If fever or abdominal pain is present or if initial symptomatic

---

Box 92.1 General considerations for the evaluation and treatment of fatigue

Assessment
- Severity, duration, impact
- Muscle weakness, wasting, somnolence
- Impaired cognitive function, altered mood

Potential Etiologies
- Antiretroviral medications
- Other medications
- Opportunistic infection
- Anemia
- Depression/anxiety disorder
- Cachexia/wasting
- Major organ failure
- Dehydration
- Substance abuse
- Sleep disorder
- Endocrine abnormality
- Deconditioning
- Chronic pain

therapy is unsuccessful, stool studies for ova and parasites and culture and sensitivity for bacterial pathogens, cryptosporidiosis, *C. difficile*, and mycobacteria are warranted. Upper and lower endoscopy with biopsies would be the next step. An extensive workup of this nature would be expected to yield a specific etiological diagnosis in two-thirds of patients.[43,44] Such a workup may not be appropriate in a palliative situation. If the diagnostic workup fails to identify a specific etiology, antimotility agents, such as loperamide, atropine/diphenoxylate, or tincture of opium, can be quite helpful. High doses may be necessary. Subcutaneous octreotide is an effective albeit expensive treatment.[45] Changing antiretroviral agents or discontinuing where appropriate (being mindful of the need for 95% adherence for effective viral suppression and the poor availability of additional combinations of ART once a regimen is no longer effective) may also be helpful.

Nausea

Virtually every anti-HIV medication has the potential to cause nausea. Zidovudine and the PIs are the worst offenders in this regard. Switching anti-HIV medications is the preferred option. In the patient with end-stage infection, stopping anti-HIV therapy altogether is an appropriate step. We have seen many patients who perked up considerably after HAART was discontinued, but only for a period of weeks to a few months.

Oral and esophageal symptoms

Oral candidiasis (thrush) is frequently seen in late-stage infection.[46] It typically appears as white "cottage cheese"-like plaques on buccal, pharyngeal, or lingual mucosa. Less often it manifests as patchy erythema. It may be asymptomatic but frequently is associated with oral discomfort and difficulty swallowing.[47]

Esophageal candidiasis is the most common cause of dysphagia. Concomitant oral thrush is present in approximately 80% of cases.[48] Empirical therapy with oral fluconazole is appropriate for dysphagia, even in the absence of oral thrush. Oral fluconazole is an effective treatment with a 90% response rate.[49**] Extensive use of this drug has fostered the development of resistant strains, particularly in individuals with end-stage AIDS.[50] If fluconazole proves unsuccessful, there may be value in trying oral voriconazole[51] or oral amphotericin suspension.[52] Although the unfavorable side effect profile of IV amphotericin B generally makes it unsuitable in the palliative care setting, once-weekly dosing may be effective and well tolerated in the management of recalcitrant oral and esophageal candidiasis.

Odynophagia (painful swallowing) is usually caused by CMV, herpes simplex virus (HSV), or idiopathic esophageal ulcers.[53] The first two conditions are treated with anti-CMV therapy (e.g., ganciclovir or valganciclovir) and anti-HSV therapy (aciclovir or valaciclovir), respectively. The last condition responds to treatment with oral corticosteroids.

INVOLUNTARY WEIGHT LOSS AND WASTING

Involuntary weight loss, even as little as 5% of premorbid weight, portends a poor prognosis for persons with HIV infection.[54] Weight loss is still common even in the era of HAART.[55] In one cohort of HIV-infected subjects the majority of them receiving HAART, 18% of subjects lost 10% of body weight and 21% lost greater than 5% of body weight. In the Multicenter AIDS Cohort (MACS), an ongoing study of 5622 homosexual and bisexual men at four U.S. sites, the proportion of AIDS diagnoses in which wasting was present increased from 5% in the period between 1988 and 1990 to 18.9% in the time period 1996–1999.[56] Whether or not lipodystrophy (a syndrome of central adiposity and peripheral lipoatrophy) is being misdiagnosed as the wasting syndrome is unclear from current data but needs additional study.

The assessment of patients with HIV-related wasting includes evaluation for opportunistic infections, degree of HIV control, gonadal function, potential adverse effects of medications, gastrointestinal function, symptoms that interfere with oral intake, and psychosocial or financial factors that might contribute to weight loss. Many HIV medications have gastrointestinal side effects.

Endocrine disturbances, particularly gonadal dysfunction, contribute to HIV-related weight loss. Early in the epidemic, and potentially currently, in the absence of HAART, as many as 50% of men with AIDS were hypogonadal. With the availability of HAART, the incidence has dropped to about 15%.[38] Loss of lean body mass and decreased functional status are highly correlated with androgen concentrations in HIV-infected men with hypogonadism and wasting.[57***,58,59] Testosterone therapy in both hypogonadal and eugonadal men increases lean body mass.[57***] A recent meta-analysis of the use of testosterone therapy for the HIV wasting syndrome concluded that testosterone improves lean body mass and weight to a small degree, with the greatest effect seen when testosterone is delivered intramuscularly.[57***]

Anorexia is an important contributor to HIV-related weight loss and was the primary target of early interventions for wasting. Megestrol acetate, a synthetic, orally active progestational agent, has been used widely as an appetite stimulant in patients with advanced cancer.[60**,61**] In patients with AIDS-associated weight loss, treatment with 800 mg/day of megestrol acetate, as compared to placebo, leads to significant improvement in weight, overall sense of well-being, appetite, and caloric intake.[62**,63**] Although generally well tolerated, megestrol acetate may lead to a variety of adverse endocrinological effects. Megestrol acetate, similar to glucocorticoids, suppresses the pituitary–adrenal axis and may cause reversible adrenal suppression, diabetes mellitus, and a steroid withdrawal syndrome.[64,65] In addition, across a broad range of doses, megestrol acetate reduces serum testosterone to castrate levels.[66]

Studies of megestrol acetate for the treatment of cachexia have consistently demonstrated improvement in appetite and weight gain.[60–63] The composition of this weight gain, however, as evaluated by dual energy x-ray absorptiometry, tritiated body water methodologies, or bioimpedance analysis (BIA), is primarily fat mass without a significant increase in lean tissue or edema.[61,67] Dronabinol (delta-9-tetrahydrocannabinol) was first evaluated as an orexigenic agent in patients with cancer-related anorexia and cachexia. A subsequent multicenter, randomized, double-blind, placebo-controlled study of dronabinol, as compared with placebo, demonstrated improved appetite, as measured by a visual analog scale ($P = 0.01$) and improved mood ($P = 0.005$).[68**] There was no significant increase in weight. The dronabinol dose was reduced to 2.5 mg once daily in 18% of patients due to central nervous system toxicity. A four-arm, randomized, pharmacokinetic study evaluated the use of single-agent dronabinol, megestrol acetate, or combination therapy. The addition of dronabinol to megestrol acetate provided no added benefit compared with megestrol acetate treatment alone.[69]

Thalidomide is an inhibitor of tumor necrosis factor (TNF) production by monocytes in vitro. Three placebo-controlled trials of thalidomide in patients with HIV-associated weight loss have demonstrated weight gain with treatment.[70**,71**,72**] In the largest of these trials, thalidomide 100 mg daily for 8 weeks produced a significant weight gain (11.7 kg vs. placebo), about half of which was lean body mass. Anabolic agents offer the potential to improve weight and body composition, ideally by replenishing lean body mass. Two oral anabolic agents, oxandrolone and oxymetholone, have been evaluated in placebo-controlled trials for treatment of HIV wasting.[73**] Oxandrolone led to a sustained increase in weight (mean 11.8 kg) over 14 weeks, while oxymetholone-treated patients gained a mean of 3 kg over 16 weeks.

Resistance training also can increase lean body mass, 1.4–2.1 kg, in asymptomatic HIV-infected men receiving HAART and in eugonadal men with AIDS wasting.[74,75] More dramatic improvements in lean body mass are observed from combination treatment with exercise and an anabolic agent. A randomized controlled trial of testosterone and resistance training stimulated a 4.6 kg gain in lean body mass,[76**] whereas treatment with supraphysiological doses of nandrolone and resistance training resulted in a net weight gain of 2.9 kg.[77]

Growth hormone increases protein synthesis and has anticatabolic, protein-sparing effects. A randomized placebo-controlled study of recombinant growth hormone 0.1 mg/kg/day subcutaneously in patients with AIDS-related weight loss demonstrated increased weight (11.6 kg; $P < 0.0001$) and lean body mass (13 kg; $P < 0.001$) and decreased body fat (21.7 kg; $P < 0.0001$).[78**] Paton et al. evaluated the protein-sparing effects of recombinant human growth hormone in HIV-infected subjects with acute opportunistic infections compared with placebo. Improvement in weight and lean body mass was observed in the treated subjects.[79] This suggests the potential short-term use of growth hormone to prevent or attenuate opportunistic infection-associated wasting. Optimal therapeutic schedules and dosing of growth hormone are unclear, and its cost has limited its use to some degree.

Weight loss remains a clinically and prognostically significant issue for HIV-infected individuals. There is now a large body of knowledge to support the benefits of nutritional counseling, dietary supplements, appetite stimulants, anabolic agents, and an exercise prescription for the treatment of HIV-related weight loss.

DRUG INTERACTIONS

There are many potential drug interactions in the palliative care of HIV-infected individuals. In this regard, the PIs and nonnucleoside reverse transcriptase inhibitors (NNRTIs) are the most problematic. For example, the PI ritonavir is a potent inhibitor of CYP3A4 enzyme of the hepatic cytochrome P450 enzyme system. As a result, ritonavir significantly slows the metabolism of several palliative medications. Ritonavir therapy increases plasma levels and prolongs the duration of activity of benzodiazepines (in particular, midazolam and triazolam), bupropion, and ergot derivatives. These medications should not be used in combination with ritonavir. Furthermore, ritonavir decreases plasma levels of methadone, fentanyl, codeine, and hydrocodone. Increased dosages of these medications may be needed when used concomitantly with ritonavir. Ritonavir is the PI most likely to interact with other medications. Among the remaining PIs, nelfinavir, fosamprenavir, and indinavir are less likely to interact with other drugs. Saquinavir is least likely.[80] Ritonavir is frequently used in a fixed dose combination capsule with another PI, lopinavir (Kaletra). The NNRTIs efavirenz and nevirapine reduce plasma levels of methadone by 35%–50%. An increase in methadone dosage of approximately 20% is required to prevent narcotic withdrawal symptoms when efavirenz is added to a stable methadone regimen. The NNRTI delavirdine increases plasma levels of methadone and amphetamines (see Tables 92.1 and 92.2).

Table 92.1 *Palliative drugs that should not be used concurrently with anti-HIV drugs*

HIV medication	Drugs that should not be coadministered
PIs	Midazolam, triazolam, ergot derivatives, bupropion
NNRTIs	
Delavirdine	Alprazolam, midazolam, triazolam, phenytoin, carbamazepine

HIV, human immunodeficiency virus.

Table 92.2 *Palliative drugs that may require dosage adjustment when given concurrently with anti-HIV drugs*

HIV medication	Drugs requiring dosage adjustment
PIs	Methadone, fentanyl, tramadol, propoxyphene, clonazepam, carbamazepine, nefazodone, SSRI antidepressants, tricyclic antidepressants, amphetamines, dronabinol, risperidone, diazepam, zolpidem, dexamethasone, phenytoin
NNRTIs	
Delavirdine	Methadone, amphetamines
Efavirenz	Methadone, carbamazepine, sertraline
Nevirapine	Methadone

HIV, human immunodeficiency virus; SSRI, selective serotonin reuptake inhibitor.

Alternative therapies are commonly used by people infected with HIV. There is an interaction between St. John's wort and the PI indinavir. St. John's wort induces CYP3A4 and decreases plasma levels of indinavir.[80] Similarly, St. John's wort can affect the metabolism of NNRTIs. Thus, St. John's wort should not be taken by patients who are taking PIs or NNRTIs.

PROGNOSIS

HIV infection and AIDS have become chronic conditions in countries where HAART is available. Without effective ART, the median survival following an AIDS-defining condition is less than 2 years.[81] Now with HAART, it is hoped, and expected, that people with AIDS will live for decades.[1] Rates of HIV-associated death have fallen by 80% in the United States as a result of HAART.[1,2] Since even patients with advanced immunodeficiency may respond to HAART,[82,83**] no patient, regardless of how ill they might appear, should be given a poor prognosis until they have received treatment if it is available.

These improvements have been remarkable. Yet death rates from HIV in the United States have leveled off although AIDS remains the fifth leading cause of death in people aged 24–44 years.[2] African-Americans are disproportionately infected. The combination of longer life expectancy plus 40,000 new infections annually in the United States has yielded an increasing prevalence of the disease.[2]

The modes of AIDS-related death have changed for patients treated with HAART. Although opportunistic infections continue to be the primary cause of death in the developing world, they are much less frequent and are no longer the leading causes of HIV-associated death in countries where HAART is routinely prescribed. Rather, chronic liver disease is now the most common cause of death in people infected with HIV.[84] This is in large part due to coinfection with hepatitis C virus (HCV). It is estimated that 30%–40% of HIV-infected individuals are also infected with HCV.[85] In coinfected individuals, almost half of deaths are due to liver disease. Coinfection with HIV and HCV appears to accelerate the course of both.[86***]

RECOGNITION OF END-STAGE DISEASE

Recognizing the potential for dramatic improvement in health with HAART for patients with previously untreated, advanced HIV disease, how does one recognize the patient who is no longer appropriate for life-sustaining therapy? Virological, clinical characteristics and comorbidities provide useful information. Patients with a history of nonadherence to ART regimens, inability to obtain HAART, and/or highly resistant HIV infection fare poorly. Underlying liver disease, particularly cirrhosis and/or active hepatitis interfering with the ability to deliver effective ART safely, also poses a significant risk for patients' overall longevity.

Refractory malignancy, with or without adequate control of HIV infection, predicts a poor prognosis, as it does in the general population. Similarly, end-stage liver disease, generally secondary to HCV, carries a poor prognosis. For patients whose prognosis is defined by a secondary illness or uncontrolled, refractory HIV infection, withdrawal of HIV medications should at least be considered and discussed at length with the patient. The balance between the potential benefit from HAART versus the burden of continuing to take the medications should be weighed in the context of the patient's goals and comorbidities. As is the case for all patients with chronic and/or progressive illness, constant reassessment of goals, toxicities of therapy, and definitions of quality of life need repeated evaluation and discussion.

MANAGEMENT OPTIONS IN LOW- AND MIDDLE-INCOME COUNTRIES

There has been significant policy, legislative, and practice focus on the availability of opioids for pain relief in sub-Saharan Africa. While significant advances have been made,[87,88] recent evidence has demonstrated availability and supply problems at all steps of the WHO pain ladder for HIV palliative care.[89] Good home-based care in the context of generalized epidemics with poor resources requires innovative solutions with guidance that has been locally driven. A number of guides have been developed for palliative care delivery in sub-Saharan Africa and offer useful alternatives where medicines are not available or prohibitively expensive. An example is Hospice Africa Uganda's Blue Book, which recommends paw-paw seeds for patients with opioid-associated constipation due their laxative action, low cost, and availability, with 5–10 seeds to be chewed initially and increased up to fivefold at night.[90] The high incidence of HIV in low- and middle-income countries also underlines the need for attention to nutrition when assessing a patient's "total palliative care" needs.[91,92] Assisted feeding and nutritional supplements may be an essential component of patient medical management and to optimize immune function. The "Clinical Guide to Palliative and Supportive Care for HIV/AIDS in Sub-Saharan Africa"[93] provides detailed, freely downloadable guidance to all aspects of HIV palliative care delivery in Africa. Importantly, they detail the importance of traditional medicine to people with HIV and the importance of understanding cultural aspects of good patient management. An example of the importance of culture is in assessment, treatment decision making, and advance care planning. Palliative care advocates a person-centered approach, an extension of Western medicine's development in individualized cultures. However, African cultures operate at the community level, and decisions may be more often made collectively rather than individually. Therefore, medical decision making should be made in consultation with the patient's wider family.

Key learning points

- HIV-associated death rates have fallen in developed countries.

- The symptom burden of HIV-infected people remains high, averaging four symptoms per person.

- Anti-HIV medications frequently cause symptoms.

- Fatigue is common and often responds to pharmacotherapy.

- Weight loss is common and often responds to pharmacotherapy.

- Nausea and diarrhea are common and may require discontinuation of anti-HIV therapy.

- Anti-HIV medications frequently interact with palliative medications.

REFERENCES

● 1 Palella FJ, Delaney KM, Moorman AC et al. Declining morbidity and mortality among patients with advanced human immunodeficiency virus infection. *N Engl J Med* 1998; 338: 853–860.
2 Centers for Disease Control and Prevention. *HIV/AIDS Surveillance Report, 2002.* Atlanta, GA: CDC, 2002. Also available at http://www.cdc.gov/hiv/stats/hasrlink.htm, (accessed March 8, 2006).
3 Harding R, Lampe FC, Norwood S et al. Symptoms are highly prevalent among HIV outpatients and associated with poor adherence and unprotected sexual intercourse. *Sex Transm Infect* 2010; 86(7): 520–524.
4 Lynn J. Serving patients who may die soon and their families. *JAMA* 2001; 285: 925–932.
5 Selwyn PA, Forstein M. Overcoming the false dichotomy of curative vs palliative care for late-stage HIV/AIDS. *JAMA* 2003; 290: 806–814.
6 Simms V, Higginson IJ, Harding R. Integration of palliative care throughout HIV disease. *Lancet Infect Dis* 2012; 12(17): 571–575.
7 Selwyn PA, Rivard M, Kappell D et al. Palliative care for AIDS at a large urban teaching hospital: Program description and preliminary outcomes. *J Palliat Med* 2003; 6: 461–474.
8 Harding R, Selman, L, Agupio et al. Prevalence, burden and correlates of physical and psychological symptoms among HIV palliative care patients in sub-Saharan Africa: An international multicentred study. *J Pain Symptom Manage* 2011; 44(1): 1–9.
9 Harding R, Foley K, Connor SR et al. Embracing palliative and end-of-life care in the global response to drug resistant tuberculosis. *Lancet Infect Dis* 2012, in press.
10 Selman L, Higginson IJ, Agupio G et al. Meeting information needs of patients with incurable progressive disease and their families in South Africa and Uganda: Multicentre qualitative study. *Br Med J* 2009; 338: b1326.
11 Pozzi G, Del Borgo C, Del Forno A et al. Psychological discomfort and mental illness in patients with AIDS: Implications for home care. *AIDS Patient Care STDS* 1999; 13(9): 555–564.
12 Harding R, Epiphaniou E, Chidgey-Clark J. Needs, experiences, and preferences of sexual minorities for end-of-life care and palliative care: A systematic review. *J Palliat Med* 2012; 15(5): 602–611.
13 Vermette L, Godin G. Nurses' intentions to provide home care: The impact of AIDS and homosexuality. *AIDS Care* 1996; 8(4): 479–488.
14 Harding R, Molloy T, Easterbrook P et al. Is antiretroviral therapy associated with symptom prevalence and burden? *Int J STD AIDS* 2006; 17 (6): 400–405.
15 Scannell K. *Death of the Good Doctor. Lessons from the Heart of the AIDS Epidemic.* San Francisco, CA: Cleis Press, Inc, 1999.
16 Sherr L, Lampe F, Fisher M et al. Suicidal ideation in UK HIV clinic attenders. *AIDS* 2008; 22(13): 1651–1658.
17 Harding R, Molloy T. Positive futures? The impact of HIV infection on achieving health, wealth and future planning. *AIDS Care* 2008; 20(5): 565–570.
18 Crawley L, Payne R, Bolden J et al. Palliative and end-of-life care in the African American community. *JAMA* 2000; 284: 2518–2521.
19 Curtis JR, Patrick DL, Aldwell E et al. The quality of patient-doctor communication about end-of-life care: A study of patients with advanced AIDS and their primary care clinicians. *AIDS* 1999; 13: 1123–1131.
20 Harding R, Karus D, Easterbrook P et al. Does palliative care improve outcomes for patients with HIV/AIDS? A systematic review of the evidence. *Sex Transm Infect* 2005; 81(1): 5–14.
21 Harding R, Easterbrook P, Higginson IJ et al. Access and equity in HIV/AIDS palliative care: A review of the evidence and responses. *Palliat Med* 2005; 19(3): 251–258.
22 Selwyn PA, Rivard M. Palliative care for AIDS: Challenges and opportunities in the era of highly active anti-retroviral therapy. *J Palliat Med* 2003; 6: 475–487.
23 Mathews W, McCutcheon JA, Asch S et al. National estimates of HIV-related symptom prevalence from the HIV Cost and Services Utilization Study. *Med Care* 2000; 38: 750–762.
24 Frich LM, Borgbjerg FM. Pain and pain treatment in AIDS patients: A longitudinal study. *J Pain Symptom Manage* 2000; 19: 339–347.
25 Schiffito G, McDermott MP, McArthur JC et al. Incidence and risk factors for HIV-associated distal sensory polyneuropathy. *Neurology* 2002; 58: 1764–1768.
26 Hewitt DJ, McDonald M, Portenoy RK et al. Pain syndromes and etiologies in ambulatory AIDS patients. *Pain* 1997; 70: 117–123.
27 Simpson DM, Haidich A-B, Schiffitto GB et al. Severity of HIV-associated neuropathy is associated with plasma HIV-1 RNA levels. *AIDS* 2002; 16: 407–412.
28 Mendell JR, Sahenk Z. Painful sensory neuropathy. *N Engl J Med* 2003; 348: 1243–1255.
29 Backonja M, Beydoun A, Edwards KR et al. Gabapentin for the symptomatic treatment of painful neuropathy in patients with diabetes mellitus: A randomized controlled trial. *JAMA* 1998; 280: 1831–1836.
30 Simpson DM, McArthur JC, Olney R et al. Lamotrigine for HIV-associated painful sensory neuropathies: A placebo-controlled trial. *Neurology* 2003; 60: 1508–1514.
31 Kieburtz K, Simpson D, Yiannoutsos C et al. A randomized trial of amitriptyline and mexiletine for painful neuropathy in HIV infection. AIDS Clinical Trial Group 242 Protocol Team. *Neurology* 1998; 51: 1682–1688.
32 Paice JA, Ferrans CE, Lashley FR et al. Topical capsaicin in the management of HIV-associated peripheral neuropathy. *J Pain Symptom Manage* 2000; 19: 45–52.
33 Abrams DI, Steinhart C, Frascino R. Epoetin alfa therapy for anaemia in HIV-infected patients: Impact on quality of life. *Int J STD AIDS* 2000; 11: 659–665.
34 Grossman H, Bowers P, Leitz G. Once-weekly epoetin alfa (Procrit®) corrects hemoglobin and improves quality of life as effectively as three-times-weekly dosing in HIV + patients [poster ThPeB7381]. In: *Proceedings of the XIV International AIDS Conference (Barcelona).* Stockholm, Sweden: International AIDS Society, 2002.

35 Saag MS, Levine AM, Leitz GJ, Bowers PJ. Once-weekly epoetin alfa increases hemoglobin and improves quality of life in anemic HIV+1 patients [poster]. In: *Proceedings of the 39th Annual Meeting of the Infectious Diseases Society of American (San Francisco)*. Alexandria, VA: Infectious Diseases Society of America, 2001.

36 Crawford J, Cella D, Cleeland CS et al. Relationship between changes in hemoglobin level and quality of life during chemotherapy in anemic cancer patients receiving epoetin alfa therapy. *Cancer* 2002; 95: 888–895.

37 Morrow GR, Hickok JT, Raubertas RF et al. Effect of an SSRI antidepressant on fatigue and depression in 738 cancer patients treated with chemotherapy: A URCC CCOP study [abstract 1531]. *Proc Am Soc Clin Oncol* 2001; 20: 384a.

38 Berger D, Muurshainen N, Witten B et al. Hypogonadism and wasting in the era of HAART in HIV-infected patients. *Program and Abstracts of the XII World AIDS Conference*, June–July 1998, Geneva, Switzerland [abstract 32174].

39 Breitbart W, Rosenfeld B, Kaim M, Funesti-Esch J. A randomized, double-blind, placebo-controlled trial of psychostimulants for the treatment of fatigue in ambulatory patients with human immunodeficiency virus disease. *Arch Intern Med* 2001; 161: 411–420.

40 Knox TA, Spiegelman D, Skinner SC, Gorbach S. Diarrhea and abnormalities of gastrointestinal function in a cohort of men and women with HIV infection. *Am J Gastroenterol* 2000; 95: 3482–3489.

41 Monkemuller KE, Call SA, Lazenby AJ, Wilcox CM. Declining prevalence of opportunistic gastrointestinal disease in the era of combination antiretroviral therapy. *Am J Gastroenterol* 2000; 95: 457–462.

42 Call SA, Heudebert G, Saag M, Wilcox CM. The changing etiology of chronic diarrhea in HIV-infected patients with CD4 cell counts less than 200 cells/mm^3. *Am J Gastroenterol* 2000; 95: 3142–3146.

43 Kartalija M, Sande MA. Diarrhea and AIDS in the era of highly active antiretroviral therapy. *Clin Infect Dis* 1999; 28: 701–707.

44 Wilcox CM, Rabeneck L, Friedman S. AGA technical review: Malnutrition and cachexia, chronic diarrhea, and hepatobiliary disease in patients with human immunodeficiency virus infection. *Gastroenterology* 1996; 111: 1724–1752.

45 Simon DM, Cello JP, Valenzuela J et al. Multicenter trial of octreotide in patients with refractory acquired immunodeficiency syndrome-associated diarrhea. *Gastroenterology* 1995; 108: 1753–1760.

46 Ball SC. Oroesophageal candidiasis in a patient with AIDS. *AIDS Reader* 2004; 14: 289–290, 292.

◆ 47 Vazquez JA, Sobel JD. Mucosal candidiasis. *Infect Dis Clin North America* 2002; 16: 793–820.

48 Wilcox CM, Straub RF, Clark WS. Prospective evaluation of oropharyngeal findings in human immunodeficiency virus-infected patients with esophageal ulceration. *Am J Gastroenterol* 1995; 90: 1938–1941.

49 Phillips P, DeBeule K, Frechette G et al. A double-blind comparison of itraconazole oral solution and fluconazole capsules for the treatment of oropharyngeal candidiasis in patients with AIDS. *Clin Infect Dis* 1998; 26: 1368–1373.

50 Maenza JR, Keruly JC, Moore RD et al. Risk factors for fluconazole-resistant candidiasis in human immunodeficiency virus-infected patients. *J Infect Dis* 1996; 173: 219–225.

51 Ruhnke M, Schmidt-Westhausen A, Trautmann M. In vitro activities of voriconazole (UK-109, 496) against fluconazole-susceptible and -resistant *Candida albicans* isolates from oral cavities of patients with human immunodeficiency virus infection. *Antimicrob Agents Chemother* 1997; 41: 575–577.

52 Nguyen MT, Weiss PJ, LaBarre RC, Wallace MR. Orally administered amphotericin B in the treatment of oral candidiasis in HIV-infected patients caused by azole-resistant *Candida albicans*. *J Acquir Immune Defic Syndr* 1996; 10: 1745–1747.

53 Wilcox CM, Straub RF, Alexander LN, Clark WS. Etiology of esophageal disease in human immunodeficiency virus-infected patients who fail antifungal therapy. *Am J Med* 1996; 101: 599–604.

54 Tang AM, Forrester J, Spiegelman D et al. Weight loss and survival in HIV-positive patients in the era of highly active antiretroviral therapy. *J Acquir Immune Defic Syndr* 2002; 31: 230–236.

55 Wanke C, Silva M, Knox T, Forrester J, Speigelman D, Gorbach S. Weight loss and wasting remain common complications in individuals infected with HIV in the era of highly active antiretroviral therapy. *Clin Infect Dis* 2000; 31: 803–805.

56 Smit E, Skolasky RL, Dobs AS et al. Changes in the incidence and predictors of wasting syndrome related to human immunodeficiency virus infection, 1987–1999. *Am J Epidemiol* 2002; 156: 211–218.

57 Kong A, Edmonds P. Testosterone therapy in HIV wasting syndrome: Systematic review and meta-analysis. *Lancet* 2002; 2: 692–699.

58 Roubenoff R, Wilson IB. Effect of resistance training on self-reported physical functioning in HIV infection. *Med Sci Sports Exerc* 2001; 33: 1811–1817.

59 Schroeder ET, Terk M, Sattler FR. Androgen therapy improves muscle mass and strength but not muscle quality: Results from two studies. *Am J Physiol Endocrinol Metab* 2003; 285: E16–E24.

● 60 Loprinzi CL, Ellison NM, Schaid DJ et al. Controlled trial of megestrol acetate for the treatment of cancer anorexia and cachexia. *J Natl Cancer Inst* 1990; 82: 1127–1132.

61 Loprinzi CL, Michalak JC, Schaid DJ et al. Phase III evaluation of four doses of megestrol acetate as therapy for patients with cancer anorexia and/or cachexia. *J Clin Oncol* 1993; 11: 762–767.

62 Von Roenn JH, Armstrong D, Kotler DP et al. Megestrol acetate in patients with AIDS related cachexia. *Ann Internal Med* 1994; 121: 393–399.

63 Oster MH, Enders SR, Samuels SJ et al. Megestrol acetate in patients with AIDS and cachexia. *Ann Intern Med* 1994; 121: 400–408.

64 Mann M, Koller E, Murgo A et al. Glucocorticoidlike activity of megestrol. *Arch Intern Med* 1997; 157: 1651–1656.

65 Loprinzi CL, Jensen MD, Jiang NS, Schaid DJ. Effect of megestrol acetate on the human pituitary-adrenal axis. *Mayo Clin Proc* 1992; 67: 1160–1162.

66 Engelson ES, Pi-Sunyer FX, Kotler DP. Effects of megestrol acetate therapy on body composition and circulating testosterone concentration in patients with AIDS. *AIDS* 1995; 9: 1107–1108.

67 Eubanks V, Koppersmith N, Wooldridge N et al. Effects of megestrol acetate on weight gain, body composition, and pulmonary function in patients with cystic fibrosis. *J Pediatr* 2002; 140: 439–444.

68 Plasse TF, Gorter RW, Krasnow SH et al. Recent clinical experience with dronabinol. *Pharmacol Biochm Behav* 1991; 40: 695–700.

69 Timpone JG, Wright DJ, Li N et al. The safety and pharmacokinetics of single-agent and combination therapy with megestrol acetate and dronabinol for the treatment of HIV wasting syndrome. *AIDS Res Hum Retroviruses* 1997; 13: 305–315.

70 Kaplan G, Thomas S, Fierer DS et al. Thalidomide for the treatment of AIDS-associated wasting. *AIDS Res Hum Retroviruses* 2000; 16: 1345–1355.

71 Reyes-Teran G, Sierra-Madero JG, Martinez del Cerro V et al. Effects of thalidomide on HIV-associated wasting syndrome: A randomized, double-blind, placebo-controlled clinical trial. *AIDS* 1996; 10: 1501–1507.

72   Klausner JD, Makonkawkeyoon S, Akarasewi P et al. The effect of thalidomide on the pathogenesis of human immunodeficiency virus Type 1 and *M. tuberculosis* infection. *J Acquir Immune Defic Syndr Hum Retrovirol* 1996; 11: 247–257.

73   Hengge UR, Stocks KR, Wiehler H et al. Double-blind, randomized, placebo-controlled phase III trial of oxymetholone for the treatment of HIV wasting. *AIDS* 2003; 17: 699–710.

74   Roubenoff R, McDermott A, Weiss L et al. Short-term progressive resistance training increases strength and lean body mass in adults infected with human immunodeficiency virus. *AIDS* 1999; 13: 231–239.

75   Yarasheski KE, Tebas P, Stanerson B et al. Resistance exercise training reduces hypertriglyceridemia in HIV-infected men treated with antiviral therapy. *J Appl Physiol* 2001; 90: 133–138.

76   Bhasin S, Storer T, Javanbakht M et al. Testosterone replacement and resistance exercise in HIV-infected men with weight loss and low testosterone levels. *JAMA* 2000; 283: 763–770.

77   Sattler F, Jaque S, Schroeder E et al. Effects of pharmacological doses of nandrolone decanoate and progressive resistance training in immunodeficient patients infected with human immunodeficiency virus. *J Clin Endocrinol Metab* 1999; 84: 1268–1276.

● 78   Schambelan M, Mulligan K, Grunfeld C et al. Recombinant human growth hormone in patients with HIV-associated wasting. *Ann Intern Med* 1996; 125: 873–882.

79   Paton N, Newton P, Sharpstone D et al. Short-term growth hormone administration at the time of opportunistic infection in HIV-positive people. *AIDS* 1999; 13: 1195–1202.

◆ 80   Piscitelli SD, Gallicano KD. Interactions among drugs for HIV and opportunistic infections. *N Engl J Med* 2001; 344: 984–996.

81   National Center for HIV, STD, and TB Prevention. AIDS case surveillance data. Available at: www.cdc.gov/hiv, (accessed February 4, 2005).

82   Goodman E. *Living with AIDS: The Lazarus Syndrome.* Baltimore, MD: Baltimore Sun, March 18, 1997, p. 9A.

● 83   Staszewski S, Morales-Ramirez J, Tashima KT et al. Efavirenz plus zidovudine and lamivudine, efavirenz plus indinavir, and indinavir plus zidovudine and lamivudine in the treatment of HIV-1 infection in adults. *N Engl J Med* 1999; 341: 1865–1873.

84   Bica I, McGovern B, Dhar R et al. Increasing mortality due to end-stage liver disease in patients with human immunodeficiency virus infection. *Clin Infect Dis* 2001; 32: 492–497.

85   Monga HK, Rodriguez-Barradas MC, Breaux K et al. Hepatitis C virus infection-related morbidity and mortality among patients with human immunodeficiency virus infection. *Clin Infect Dis* 2001; 33: 240–247.

◆ 86   Sulkowski MS, Thomas DL. Hepatitis C in the HIV-infected person. *Ann Intern Med* 2003; 138: 197–207.

87   Harding R, Foley K, Connor SR et al. Embracing palliative and end-of-life care in the global response to drug resistant tuberculosis. *Lancet Infect Dis* 2012; 12(8): 643–646.

88   Selman L, Higginson IJ, Agupio G et al. Meeting information needs of patients with incurable progressive disease and their families in South Africa and Uganda: Multicentre qualitative study. *Br Med J* 2009; 338: b1326.

89   Harding R, Powell RA, Kiyange F et al. Provision of pain and symptom-relieving drugs for HIV/AIDS in sub-Saharan Africa. *J Pain Symptom Manage* 2010; 40(3): 405–415.

90   Hospice Africa Uganda. Pain and symptom control in the cancer and/or AIDS patient in Uganda and other African countries, 2006; Available at: http://www.hospiceafrica.or.ug/images/attachements/the%20blue%20book%20-%20english.pdf. Accessed 10th June.

91   Gwyther L, Marston J. Dealing with the symptoms of AIDS. In Uys L, Cameron S (eds). Home-based HIV/AIDS Care. Oxford, U.K.: Oxford University Press, 2003. 94–114.

92   Defilippi, K. Dealing with poverty. In Uys L, Cameron S. (eds). *Home-Based HIV/AIDS Care.* Oxford, U.K.: Oxford University Press, 2003. 162–173.

93   FHSSA. A Clinical Guide to Supportive and Palliative Care for HIV/AIDS in Sub-Saharan Africa by Chapter; 2010. Available at: http://www.globalpartnersincare.org/clinical-guide-supportive-and-palliative-care-hivaids-sub-saharan-africa. Accessed 10th June 2014.

93

Neurological diseases

TOBIAS WALBERT

INTRODUCTION

This chapter will focus on the palliative care of adults with the more common progressive neurodegenerative diseases and their caregivers. In addition, stroke will be discussed in some detail due to its high morbidity and prevalence. Detailed discussion of palliative care in children can be found in Chapter 95 and of neoplasms—radiotherapy and chemotherapy—in Chapters 88 and 89, respectively.

Neurological diseases present and progress with great variation. In contrast to patients in many other areas of medicine and especially in oncology, the prognosis and disease trajectory is not always clearly defined. Given the high prevalence of neurological disorders and the fact that a cure or even disease modification remains elusive, proper symptom management and palliation is paramount. The cumulative physical and cognitive morbidities place a high burden on patients and caregivers alike. Despite the different disease trajectories, many more patients die from Parkinson's disease than amyotrophic lateral sclerosis (ALS) each year and just as many die from multiple sclerosis (MS) as from ALS [1]. Studies have showed that dying from cancer is not much different than dying of chronic obstructive pulmonary disease (COPD), congestive heart failure, or stroke [2]. Furthermore, it is documented that people dying from congestive cardiac failure, COPD, and stroke all have unmet health and social needs in the last year of life [3]. Therefore, the application of the principles of specialist palliative care to the management of people with neurological disorders has been supported for some time.

The disease progression of most neurodegenerative disorders cannot be significantly altered; it is therefore all the more important that appropriate palliation of the attendant symptoms and psychological distress is given.

STROKE

Stroke is defined by a sudden onset of a neurologic deficit and caused by an interruption of blood flow to the brain. The lack of oxygen and nutrients and the inability to remove waste products cause brain cells to die quickly. Strokes can be caused by ischemia due to blockage (thrombosis, arterial embolism) or by brain hemorrhage (intracerebral or subarachnoid hemorrhage). Approximately 80% of all strokes are caused by ischemia, while 20% are due to brain hemorrhage.

Stroke is the second most common cause of death and major cause of disability worldwide. In developed countries, the incidence of stroke has declined in recent years. This is due mainly to reductions in risk factors such as hypertension and smoking. However, the overall rate of stroke remains high, and because of the aging population, it is estimated that the burden will increase greatly during the next 20 years [4].

The prevalence of stroke varies in different populations and differs also with age and ethnicity. The Framingham study in the United States estimated that the annual age-adjusted incidence for women was 4.5/1000 and for men 6/1000 [5]. Of these, 60% are atherothrombotic infarctions, 23% cardiac embolisms, 7% subarachnoid hemorrhage, and 7% intracerebral hemorrhage.

The clinical manifestations of stroke are variable due to the brain's complex anatomy and vasculature. Therapeutic options for stroke patients include admission to a specialized stroke unit for possible thrombolysis and acute management of blood pressure and early mobilization. Stroke units have been shown to reduce mortality by approximately 20% and to improve functional outcome by about the same amount [6,7].

Acute management options for acute stroke include treatment with intravenous tissue plasminogen activator within 3–4.5 hours or aspirin within 48 hours of stroke onset. Decompressive surgery for supratentorial malignant hemispheric stroke has shown clinical benefit in trials as well [8]. Even as acute mortality has declined with improved management, the long-term prognosis of stroke remains poor. There are several predictors of functional recovery after stroke: age, previous stroke, consciousness at onset, and urinary continence [9]. Only 25% of stroke patients survive without major disability; 20%–50% of all patients experience some kind of disability with 20%–25% of patients developing poststroke dementia and 10%–30% dying within a year of experiencing a stroke [9].

Only a limited number of studies have assessed the palliative needs of stroke patients and their families [10]. About

25% of stroke patients experience chronic pain [11] such as musculoskeletal pain, central poststroke pain and hemiplegic shoulder pain, painful spasticity, and chronic headaches [3,12]. Other prevalent issues include incontinence; fatigue; psychological conditions such as depression, anxiety, and pseudobulbar affect (emotional incontinence); and advance planning [13].

Palliative care challenges

SYMPTOM CONTROL: PAIN

The pain requirements of patients prior to sustaining a stroke should not be overlooked, particularly when there are communication difficulties following the stroke. The direct result of the stroke may cause several pain syndromes that might interfere with rehabilitation and reduce quality of life. Around 25% of stroke patients experience poststroke pain syndromes such as headaches, central poststroke pain, hemiplegic shoulder pain, painful spasticity, and tension headaches [11,12]. Central poststroke pain is characterized as neuropathic pain starting within weeks to months after the initial stroke. Small studies encouraged the use of the tricyclic antidepressant amitriptyline, lamotrigine, as well as pregabalin. Similar to other neuropathic pain, opioids are not effective, but other standard treatment such as gabapentin or selective noradrenergic receptor inhibitors might be effective [12,14].

Up to 83% of patients without any arm motor function are at risk of developing a "shoulder–hand syndrome" [15]. In this complex regional pain syndrome, the upper limb has reduced movement and appears edematous, blue, painful, and with altered heat and tactile sensations. Early mobilization has been shown to prevent this syndrome. Physical therapy and topical thermal therapies with ice and heat as well as oral analgesics result in temporal pain relief.

PSYCHOSOCIAL CARE: DEPRESSION AND ANXIETY

Poststroke depression is commonly reported. In a Scandinavian study, minor depression was diagnosed in 14% of patients and 26% experienced major depression. The only independent predictors of poststroke depression were found to be a premorbid history of depression and dependency in daily living following stroke. Relatives caring for such patients in the community report that they would have liked more support and those stroke patients who died in hospital are reported as requiring more psychological support in one study [3]. This would suggest a role for palliative care in supporting these patients and their families.

ADVANCE PLANNING/END-OF-LIFE CARE: FEEDING

The dysphagia that necessitates artificial feeding of stroke patients is in itself a poor prognostic indicator [16]. Following a stroke, 30% of conscious patients have impaired swallowing on the day after the stroke, 16% at 1 week, and 2% at 1 month [17]. Given this rapid improvement for a majority of patients, it is important to decide how and when to initiate artificial nutrition. Poor nutrition may predispose to muscle weakness and fatigue, which will impair rehabilitation; it will also predispose the patient to pressure area sores. Therefore, persistent dysphagia may require the insertion of a nasogastric tube or percutaneous gastrostomy. The relative risks and benefits of these two procedures were looked at in a large randomized controlled trial [18].

Unfortunately clear recommendations about the value of early initiation of enteral feeding could not be derived from the study. Although there is no evidence that early initiation of tube feeding will cause harm such as increased risk for pneumonia, there was no significant decrease in mortality or long-term outcomes. Initiating tube feeding with a nasogastric tube was shown to be associated with less mortality and better outcomes than starting early enteral nutrition with PEG tubes.

The input of specialists in palliative care with their experience of end-of-life decision making may be helpful as this issue engenders strong feelings among families and friends of stroke patients.

MULTIPLE SCLEROSIS

MS is the most common of the autoimmune inflammatory demyelinating diseases that share the pathological features of focal areas of degeneration of the myelin sheath that surrounds nervous tissue. It is the most common cause of chronic disability in young adults. The process of demyelination is associated with inflammation, axon degeneration, and then gliosis. While the cause of MS remains unknown, evidence suggests that the disease starts out as an inflammatory autoimmune disorder mediated by autoreactive lymphocytes. The later disease stages are driven by microglial activation and chronic neurodegeneration, which finally result in gliosis. This process leads to a wide range of clinical signs and symptoms [19]. In northern Europe and the United States, the prevalence is about 80–100 per 1,000,000 population. It is roughly twice as common in females as in males and the mean age of onset is around 30 years, with a range of 20–50 years. MS has a variable disease trajectory. About 25% of people affected have relatively benign disease with mild exacerbations from which they make a complete recovery. Unfortunately, 10% of patients develop a rapidly progressive (primary) illness that leads to severe disability relatively quickly [20].

In most patients, the disease follows a relapsing and remitting course with variable degrees of recovery, at least initially, before progressive (secondary) deterioration ensues; 80%–90% of people will convert to secondary progressive MS within 20–25 years of diagnosis. The mortality rate of MS is difficult to determine because of poor data collection and reporting, but it is estimated that the mean age of death of all MS patients in the United States is 58 years, while the national average for all other causes of death in the United States is 71. A longitudinal study from Australia reported the mean age of death as 65 years, 38 years after the time of first symptom onset [21]. Death is most often a result of respiratory disease or infection.

Initially, acute relapses often respond to corticosteroids, most often administered intravenously for 3–5 days. There are a number of immunomodulating therapies available. In addition to interferon-β1a, interferon-β1b, and glatiramer acetate, in recent years, fingolimod (a lymphocyte migration-altering agent) and natalizumab (a recombinant monoclonal antibody directed against alpha-4 integrins) have been approved for the treatment of MS. These treatments have been shown to reduce both attack frequency and the accumulation of plaques within the central nervous system. A number of new disease-modifying agents are scheduled to follow soon; however, there is no cure for MS in the foreseeable future.

AMYOTROPHIC LATERAL SCLEROSIS

ALS is the most common degenerative disorder of the motor neuron system and causes muscle weakness, increasing disability and eventually death within 3–5 years after symptom onset. The prevalence in Europe and the United States ranges between 2.7 and 7.4 cases per 1,000,000 population. Most people are diagnosed after the age of 40 and the incidence increases with each decade thereafter reaching a peak in the 70s [22]. While the familial forms make up 5%–10% of cases, 90%–95% of all cases are of sporadic origin.

ALS is characterized by involvement of upper and lower motor neurons. This manifests itself clinically with fasciculations and slowly progressive paresis of the voluntary muscles coupled with hyperreflexia and spasticity (see also Box 93.1). The sensory system is normal with sparing of eye movements and sphincters in the vast majority of patients. The average prognosis is 3–4 years although there is considerable variation. About 20%–30% of patients present with bulbar symptoms of slurred speech and difficulty in swallowing [23]. Ten percent of patients live more than 10 years. Cognitive function is usually intact although dementia is present in around 2% of patients. While there is no cure for ALS, management of symptoms has evolved significantly over the last 25 years. The American Academy of Neurology has published practice parameters to guide treatment and end-of-life care [24]. The only drug specifically approved for treatment of ALS is riluzole, an antiglutamate agent that has been shown to prolong life by approximately 3–6 months [25].

PARKINSON DISEASE

Parkinson disease (PD) is a progressive neurodegenerative disorder that is defined by depigmentation, neuronal loss, and gliosis, particularly in the substantia nigra. This degeneration results in a decrease of dopamine, an important neurotransmitter. The lack of dopamine leads to major dysregulation in the basal ganglia resulting in a syndrome defined by rest tremor, rigidity, bradykinesia, and postural instability. The diagnosis is made based on clinical observation and the presence of positive response to levodopa or other dopaminergic therapies.

Box 93.1 Symptoms of amyotrophic lateral sclerosis

Direct symptoms

- Muscle atrophy and weakness
- Dyspnea
- Dysphagia
- Dysarthria

Indirect symptoms

- Sleep disturbance
- Pseudobulbar affect
- Sialorrhea
- Pain

The idiopathic form of PD is assumed when no cause of symptomatic Parkinsonism, such as the side effects of medication, can be found. A number of additional symptoms of PD are difficult to improve with drug therapies (Box 93.2).

Younger patients do better than older patients with an expected prognosis of 20–30 years when motor manifestations can be controlled by drugs and neurosurgical procedures such as deep brain stimulation. In particular, older patients may, 5–10 years following diagnosis, begin to experience more difficulties with problems that are not only related to drug-induced on-off periods but also to neuropsychiatric problems. Hallucinations and cognitive decline often herald the onset of diffuse Lewy body disease or dementia with Lewy bodies [26]. Depression is more common in older patients and complicates at least 20% of such cases, rising with increasing age of onset.

Box 93.2 Parkinson disease

Classical motor symptoms

- Tremor
- Rigor
- Akinesis

Typical nonmotor symptoms

- Cognitive dysfunction
- Psychiatric problems
- Autonomic dysfunction
- Bladder symptoms
- Constipation–hypomimia (masklike face)
- Pain
- Sleep disturbance
- Fatigue
- Sialorrhea

Palliative care challenges

SYMPTOM CONTROL

Pain

Thirty to ninety percent of people with MS [27] and up to 75% of people with ALS [28] experience pain, although there is no evidence of sensory involvement in the ALS patients. Musculoskeletal pain is often overlooked in patients with neurodegenerative disorders. It may be the result of immobility in combination with muscle weakness. It is also the result of spasticity, gait disturbance, and poor sitting posture. Joint pain may be exacerbated by the loss of a protective muscle sheath or abnormal tone. Appropriate involvement of physiotherapists and occupational therapists in conjunction with nonsteroidal anti-inflammatory drugs (NSAIDs) can be beneficial. In addition, patients with limited mobility are more prone to develop pain secondary to "skin pressure" and skin breakdown.

ALS and MS patients suffer from neuropathic pain, which is often described as being a burning or shooting sensation, particularly affecting feet and lower extremities. Other unusual sensations, sometimes likened to insects crawling over the skin, can also occur and are due to nerve damage. This type of pain is best treated with neuropathic agents such as amitriptyline, gabapentin, or pregabalin. It has been shown that the combination of an opioid and gabapentin is more effective than either agent on its own [29]. The use of nonpharmacological interventions such as transcutaneous electrical nerve stimulation has been reported to be of benefit on occasion.

In MS, trigeminal neuralgia has an increased prevalence. Recommendations for trigeminal neuralgia include carbamazepine or oxcarbazepine as first-line treatments. Microvascular decompression of the Gasserian ganglion or treatment with stereotactic radiosurgery should be considered for refractory pain; however, trigeminal neuralgia in the setting of MS is less responsive than that of idiopathic origin [30]. Many patients experience more than one if not all of these different pain problems, and the involvement of a palliative care specialist who is experienced in taking a complete and holistic pain history can be appropriate and helpful.

Spasticity

All the neurodegenerative disorders can result in muscle cramps, spasms, and spasticity. In MS, however, spasticity is one of the most typical and debilitating symptoms [27]. Spasticity can lead to pain, spasms, reduced mobility, and limited range of motion as well as contractures. When treating spasticity in a person who is still able to bear weight, special consideration must be given to maintaining muscle tone. The extensor spasm they are experiencing in their lower limbs may be the reason they can still perform weight-bearing activities as it compensates for the loss of strength. Spasticity is also associated with flexor spasm triggered by touch or movement. These spasms can be extremely painful. Any number of preventable stressors such as cold, a full bladder, stretching, overexertion, and infection can initiate spasms and should be avoided.

Oral baclofen, diazepam, dantrolene, and tizanidine are all agents that are equally effective at controlling muscle spasm [31]. Their mechanisms of action vary so treatment can be alternated or combined and titrated until the best clinical effect is achieved. All these drugs can cause sedation and weakness. Baclofen is associated more often with nausea, the benzodiazepines with delirium, and dantrolene with hepatitis. If only a few muscle groups are affected, then local injection of botulinum toxin A has been shown to be helpful [32], especially when combined with postinjection physiotherapy and stretching [33]. Intrathecal baclofen pumps are useful for patients with severe spasticity that is difficult to manage with oral drugs alone. Palliative care is characterized by the systematic and meticulous monitoring of symptoms and their pharmacological management—such expertise could benefit this group of patients.

SALIVARY DROOLING

The inability to swallow one's own saliva may result from a specific bulbar palsy that occurs most commonly in ALS, or it may just be the product of a generally deteriorating swallow as may occur with any of the neurodegenerative disorders. It is a very embarrassing symptom, which causes local soreness and excoriation. Drug therapy is aimed at reducing the amount of saliva produced. The effectiveness of oral medications is generally tried first, but their effectiveness is unproven [24]. Anticholinergic medication such as hyoscine hydrobromide administered either sublingually or transdermally may be of benefit. Other medications such as glycopyrrolate, oral atropine, or amitriptyline can also be useful. For patients who do not respond to oral agents or who have unacceptable side effects, the use of botulinum toxin injected into the parotid and submandibular glands has been shown to be beneficial [34,35]. Low-dose radiotherapy has been used successfully as well [36,37].

Pseudobulbar affect

Pseudobulbar affect (also described as emotional lability or emotional incontinence) describes sudden uncontrollable outbursts of laughter or tearfulness and affects 20%–50% of patients with ALS and has an increased prevalence in MS as well as stroke patients. The combination drug dextromethorphan–quinidine (20 mg/10 mg) has been shown to reduce the frequency and severity of laughing and to improve quality of life in both ALS and MS patients [38].

CONSTIPATION

Bowel and bladder involvement in the late stages of neurodegenerative disorders is inevitable. It is the result of poor gut motility. Constipation may also be exacerbated by poor dietary intake, medication side effects, limited mobility, and decreased intake of fluid for fear of urinary incontinence. When using aperients, an iso-osmolar drug such as polyethylene glycol is preferable to lactulose as iso-osmolar drugs do not cause the same degree of associated flatulence and bloating. Stimulants such as senna or sodium picosulfate may be required. Rigorous bowel management including occasional suppositories is crucial to avoid impaction. Enemata and manual evacuation may become necessary otherwise.

PARENTERAL FEEDING

Many patients with a neurodegenerative disorder will also develop a degree of dysphagia. While less than 50% of patients with MS are estimated to have swallowing problems, more than 50% of patients with PD and the majority of ALS patients develop swallowing deficits [39]. Swallowing difficulties can lead to malnutrition and weight loss, which is identified as a risk factor for survival [40]. Regular assessment of both oral intake and swallow function should be undertaken by a multiprofessional team involving speech and language therapists, dietetic specialists, occupational therapists, and a palliative care specialist.

The goal is to maintain nutrition by the oral route for as long as possible. This period may be extended by appropriate eating aids, neck positioning, and oral food supplements. However, it is important to be aware of the optimal timing for placement of a tube to initiate parenteral feeding. The placement of a percutaneous endoscopic gastrostomy (PEG) tube has been shown to stabilize body weight and might prolong survival in patients [41]. The risks for laryngeal spasm, localized infections, gastric hemorrhage, failure to place a PEG tube, and death due to respiratory arrest increase when the forced vital capacity (FVC) declines below 50%. Patients might reach a point when they are too weak for the placement of a PEG or radiologically inserted feeding tube. They may indeed be too unwell and weak for any parenteral feeding to be appropriate. There are obvious ethical dilemmas involved in making this particular decision [42]. The provision of nutrition to a loved one is a fundamental part of providing care for that person, and the inability to do this can have a very distressing effect on the families of these patients [43]. On the other hand, there is no clear evidence that parenteral feeding increases quality of life in patients with progressive neurodegenerative diseases. Whereas it may be obvious with a patient who has entered the terminal phase of their illness that to proceed with artificial hydration and nutrition is inappropriate, it is a more difficult decision in those with a chronic or even unclear disease trajectory. Therefore, a number of factors should be considered apart from the individual's ability to undergo a placement procedure. There are practical issues about the community and caregiver support that may or may not be available. The patient and their family may hold strong cultural or other beliefs that must be considered. Of paramount importance is whether the benefits of starting feeding outweigh the anticipated burdens (i.e., the likelihood of complications either of the procedure or postprocedure such as pain, hemorrhage, or infection). Advance planning and discussion with or without the writing of a formal advance directive ensures that the wishes of the patient are known. (See Chapter 104 for further details of advance directives.) This further ensures that any decisions are made in the patient's best interests as it encompasses their own assessment of quality of life, well being, and spiritual or religious beliefs. Palliative care specialists have the appropriate experience to be helpful at this stage and to facilitate navigation of this highly individual set of considerations.

RESPIRATORY MANAGEMENT

Neurodegenerative disorders often lead to hypoventilation, which is a common feature of ALS. Most deaths from ALS are caused by respiratory failure. The management of respiratory symptoms in patients with ALS has been extensively reviewed, and consensus guidelines have been published that outline optimal respiratory management [41,44].

An FVC of <50 is frequently associated with respiratory symptoms such as daytime fatigue and somnolence, depression and anxiety, morning headache, reduced appetite and weight loss, disturbed sleep, and nightmares [45]. A further reduction of the FVC to <25%–30% is linked to a significant increase of risk for respiratory failure or sudden death.

Studies have demonstrated that noninvasive positive-pressure ventilation (NIPPV) improves life expectancy and QOL in patients with an FVC of <50 [41,46]. Patients who use NIPPV live an average of several months longer than those who do not. This extended prognosis is, however, in the face of continuing and ongoing disability. In addition to improving survival, NIPPV has been shown to decrease dyspnea, daytime fatigue, and insomnia. These benefits may persist even as the disease continues to progress [47]. Patients with loss of bulbar tone or severe sialorrhea are less likely to benefit from NIPPV [48]. For patients embarking on the use of NIPPV, it is crucial they understand that symptoms of breathlessness can also be palliated by the use of benzodiazepines and opioid drugs and that NIPPV does not preclude their use [49,50]. In addition, respiratory management should include the use of mechanical suction for mucus, mechanical insufflation/exsufflation, and treatment of sialorrhea as outlined earlier.

A discussion should take place detailing the progressive nature of the respiratory muscle weakness and also the tendency to ventilator dependence. The involvement of a palliative professional as part of a multidisciplinary care team to discuss treatment options and to help with the decision-making process is therefore very important.

Key learning points

- There is a need for symptom control, psychosocial support, and help with advance planning and end-of-life decision making in patients with neurodegenerative disorders.

- While there are particular challenges with newly diagnosed patients due to an unpredictable disease course, neurodegenerative disorders in the advanced stages (ALS, end-stage Parkinson's disease, secondary progressive MS) do have a predictable course of progression. Palliative care should be involved early and continuously.

- The central nervous system is complex and many medications act in multiple ways. Many symptoms such as decrease in cognition and increase in fatigue are caused by medications. Set priorities together with the patient and check the medication list frequently—sometimes less is more.

- These patients are prone to fatigue, communication difficulties, and decreased mobility. All of these factors affect their ability to participate in psychosocial support and counseling.

- Cognitive complications of neurodegenerative disorders raise issues around competency in decision making and underscore the importance of early advance planning.

- While there is no cure for neurodegenerative disorders, there are particular treatment options that decrease the burden of symptoms and help to maintain quality of life of patients and caregivers. Many of these interventions require a specific multiprofessional assessment, which should include palliative care.

REFERENCES

1 Elman LB, Houghton DJ, Wu GF, Hurtig HI, Markowitz CE, McCluskey L. Palliative care in amyotrophic lateral sclerosis, Parkinson's disease, and multiple sclerosis. *Journal of Palliative Medicine* 2007;10(2):433–457. Epub 2007/05/03.

2 Addington-Hall J, McCarthy M. Regional study of care for the dying: Methods and sample characteristics. *Palliative Medicine* 1995;9(1):27–35. Epub 1995/01/01.

3 Addington-Hall J, Lay M, Altmann D, McCarthy M. Symptom control, communication with health professionals, and hospital care of stroke patients in the last year of life as reported by surviving family, friends, and officials. *Stroke; a Journal of Cerebral Circulation* 1995;26(12):2242–2248. Epub 1995/12/01.

4 Donnan GA, Fisher M, Macleod M, Davis SM. Stroke. *Lancet* 2008;371(9624):1612–1623. Epub 2008/05/13.

5 Barker WH, Mullooly JP. Stroke in a defined elderly population, 1967–1985. A less lethal and disabling but no less common disease. *Stroke; a Journal of Cerebral Circulation.* 1997;28(2):284–290. Epub 1997/02/01.

6 Indredavik B, Bakke F, Slordahl SA, Rokseth R, Haheim LL. Treatment in a combined acute and rehabilitation stroke unit: Which aspects are most important? *Stroke; a Journal of Cerebral Circulation* 1999;30(5):917–923. Epub 1999/05/07.

7 Cadilhac DA, Ibrahim J, Pearce DC, Ogden KJ, McNeill J, Davis SM et al. Multicenter comparison of processes of care between Stroke Units and conventional care wards in Australia. *Stroke; a Journal of Cerebral Circulation.* 2004;35(5):1035–1040. Epub 2004/04/03.

8 Vahedi K, Hofmeijer J, Juettler E, Vicaut E, George B, Algra A et al. Early decompressive surgery in malignant infarction of the middle cerebral artery: A pooled analysis of three randomised controlled trials. *Lancet Neurology* 2007;6(3):215–222. Epub 2007/02/17.

9 Kwakkel G, Wagenaar RC, Kollen BJ, Lankhorst GJ. Predicting disability in stroke—A critical review of the literature. *Age and Ageing* 1996;25(6):479–489. Epub 1996/11/01.

10 Stevens T, Payne SA, Burton C, Addington-Hall J, Jones A. Palliative care in stroke: A critical review of the literature. *Palliative Medicine* 2007;21(4):323–331. Epub 2007/07/28.

11 Jonsson AC, Lindgren I, Hallstrom B, Norrving B, Lindgren A. Prevalence and intensity of pain after stroke: A population based study focusing on patients' perspectives. *Journal of Neurology, Neurosurgery, and Psychiatry* 2006;77(5):590–595. Epub 2005/12/16.

12 Klit H, Finnerup NB, Jensen TS. Central post-stroke pain: Clinical characteristics, pathophysiology, and management. *Lancet Neurology* 2009;8(9):857–868. Epub 2009/08/15.

13 Creutzfeldt CJ, Holloway RG, Walker M. Symptomatic and palliative care for stroke survivors. *Journal of General Internal Medicine* 2012;27(7):853–860. Epub 2012/01/20.

14 Frese A, Husstedt IW, Ringelstein EB, Evers S. Pharmacologic treatment of central post-stroke pain. *The Clinical Journal of Pain* 2006;22(3):252–260. Epub 2006/03/04.

15 Lindgren I, Jonsson AC, Norrving B, Lindgren A. Shoulder pain after stroke: A prospective population-based study. *Stroke; a Journal of Cerebral Circulation* 2007;38(2):343–348. Epub 2006/12/23.

16 Gordon C, Hewer RL, Wade DT. Dysphagia in acute stroke. *British Medical Journal (Clinical Research Edition)* 1987;295(6595):411–414. Epub 1987/08/15.

17 Barer DH. The natural history and functional consequences of dysphagia after hemispheric stroke. *Journal of Neurology, Neurosurgery, and Psychiatry.* 1989;52(2):236–241. Epub 1989/02/01.

18 Dennis MS, Lewis SC, Warlow C. Effect of timing and method of enteral tube feeding for dysphagic stroke patients (FOOD): A multicentre randomised controlled trial. *Lancet* 2005;365(9461):764–772. Epub 2005/03/01.

19 McDonald WI, Ron MA. Multiple sclerosis: The disease and its manifestations. *Philosophical Transactions of the Royal Society of London Series B, Biological Sciences* 1999;354(1390):1615–1622. Epub 1999/12/22.

20 Lublin FD, Reingold SC. Defining the clinical course of multiple sclerosis: Results of an international survey. National Multiple Sclerosis Society (USA) Advisory Committee on Clinical Trials of New Agents in Multiple Sclerosis. *Neurology* 1996;46(4):907–911. Epub 1996/04/01.

21 Hirst C, Swingler R, Compston DA, Ben-Shlomo Y, Robertson NP. Survival and cause of death in multiple sclerosis: A prospective population-based study. *Journal of Neurology, Neurosurgery, and Psychiatry* 2008;79(9):1016–1021. Epub 2008/02/28.

22 Worms PM. The epidemiology of motor neuron diseases: A review of recent studies. *Journal of the Neurological Sciences* 2001;191(1–2):3–9. Epub 2001/10/26.

23 Li TM, Alberman E, Swash M. Comparison of sporadic and familial disease amongst 580 cases of motor neuron disease. *Journal of Neurology, Neurosurgery, and Psychiatry* 1988;51(6):778–784. Epub 1988/06/01.

24 Miller RG, Jackson CE, Kasarskis EJ, England JD, Forshew D, Johnston W et al. Practice parameter update: The care of the patient with amyotrophic lateral sclerosis: Multidisciplinary care, symptom management, and cognitive/behavioral impairment (an evidence-based review): Report of the Quality Standards Subcommittee of the American Academy of Neurology. *Neurology* 2009;73(15):1227–1233. Epub 2009/10/14.

25 Lacomblez L, Bensimon G, Leigh PN, Guillet P, Meininger V. Dose-ranging study of riluzole in amyotrophic lateral sclerosis. Amyotrophic Lateral Sclerosis/Riluzole Study Group II. *Lancet* 1996;347(9013):1425–1431. Epub 1996/05/25.

26 McKeith IG, Galasko D, Kosaka K, Perry EK, Dickson DW, Hansen LA et al. Consensus guidelines for the clinical and pathologic diagnosis of dementia with Lewy bodies (DLB): Report of the consortium on DLB international workshop. *Neurology* 1996;47(5):1113–1124. Epub 1996/11/01.

27 Thompson AJ, Toosy AT, Ciccarelli O. Pharmacological management of symptoms in multiple sclerosis: Current approaches and future directions. *Lancet Neurology* 2010;9(12):1182–1199. Epub 2010/11/23.

28 O'Brien T, Kelly M, Saunders C. Motor neurone disease: A hospice perspective. *BMJ* 1992;304(6825):471–473. Epub 1992/02/22.

29 Gilron I, Bailey JM, Tu D, Holden RR, Weaver DF, Houlden RL. Morphine, gabapentin, or their combination for neuropathic pain. *The New England Journal of Medicine* 2005;352(13):1324–1334. Epub 2005/04/01.

30 van Kleef M, van Genderen WE, Narouze S, Nurmikko TJ, van Zundert J, Geurts JW et al. 1. Trigeminal neuralgia. *Pain Practice: The Official Journal of World Institute of Pain* 2009;9(4):252–259. Epub 2009/07/22.

31 Shakespeare DT, Boggild M, Young C. Anti-spasticity agents for multiple sclerosis. *Cochrane Database System Review* 2003(4):CD001332. Epub 2003/10/30.

32 Hyman N, Barnes M, Bhakta B, Cozens A, Bakheit M, Kreczy-Kleedorfer B et al. Botulinum toxin (Dysport) treatment of hip adductor spasticity in multiple sclerosis: A prospective, randomised, double blind, placebo controlled, dose ranging study. *Journal of Neurology, Neurosurgery, and Psychiatry* 2000;68(6):707–712. Epub 2000/05/16.

33 Giovannelli M, Borriello G, Castri P, Prosperini L, Pozzilli C. Early physiotherapy after injection of botulinum toxin increases the beneficial effects on spasticity in patients with multiple sclerosis. *Clinical Rehabilitation* 2007;21(4):331–337. Epub 2007/07/07.

34 Lagalla G, Millevolte M, Capecci M, Provinciali L, Ceravolo MG. Long-lasting benefits of botulinum toxin type B in Parkinson's disease-related drooling. *Journal of Neurology* 2009;256(4):563–567. Epub 2009/04/30.

35 Bhatia KP, Munchau A, Brown P. Botulinum toxin is a useful treatment in excessive drooling in saliva. *Journal of Neurology, Neurosurgery, and Psychiatry* 1999;67(5):697. Epub 1999/11/30.

36 Harriman M, Morrison M, Hay J, Revonta M, Eisen A, Lentle B. Use of radiotherapy for control of sialorrhea in patients with amyotrophic lateral sclerosis. *The Journal of Otolaryngology* 2001;30(4):242–245. Epub 2002/01/05.

37 Andersen PM, Gronberg H, Franzen L, Funegard U. External radiation of the parotid glands significantly reduces drooling in patients with motor neurone disease with bulbar paresis. *Journal of the Neurological Sciences* 2001;191(1–2):111–114. Epub 2001/10/26.

38 Pioro EP, Brooks BR, Cummings J, Schiffer R, Thisted RA, Wynn D et al. Dextromethorphan plus ultra low-dose quinidine reduces pseudobulbar affect. *Annals of Neurology* 2010;68(5):693–702. Epub 2010/09/15.

39 Saleem T, Leigh PN, Higginson IJ. Symptom prevalence among people affected by advanced and progressive neurological conditions—A systematic review. *Journal of Palliative Care* 2007;23(4):291–299. Epub 2008/02/07.

40 Desport JC, Preux PM, Truong TC, Vallat JM, Sautereau D, Couratier P. Nutritional status is a prognostic factor for survival in ALS patients. *Neurology* 1999;53(5):1059–1063. Epub 1999/09/25.

41 Miller RG, Jackson CE, Kasarskis EJ, England JD, Forshew D, Johnston W et al. Practice parameter update: The care of the patient with amyotrophic lateral sclerosis: Drug, nutritional, and respiratory therapies (an evidence-based review): Report of the Quality Standards Subcommittee of the American Academy of Neurology. *Neurology* 2009;73(15):1218–1226. Epub 2009/10/14.

42 Huang ZB, Ahronheim JC. Nutrition and hydration in terminally ill patients: An update. *Clinics in Geriatric Medicine* 2000;16(2):313–325. Epub 2000/04/28.

43 Holden CM. Anorexia in the terminally ill cancer patient: The emotional impact on the patient and the family. *The Hospice Journal* 1991;7(3):73–84. Epub 1991/01/01.

44 Andersen PM, Abrahams S, Borasio GD, de Carvalho M, Chio A, Van Damme P et al. EFNS guidelines on the clinical management of amyotrophic lateral sclerosis (MALS)—Revised report of an EFNS task force. *European Journal of Neurology: The Official Journal of the European Federation of Neurological Societies* 2012;19(3):360–375. Epub 2011/09/15.

45 Blackhall LJ. Amyotrophic lateral sclerosis and palliative care: Where we are, and the road ahead. *Muscle and Nerve* 2012;45(3):311–318. Epub 2012/02/16.

46 Ganzini L, Johnston WS, Silveira MJ. The final month of life in patients with ALS. *Neurology* 2002;59(3):428–431. Epub 2002/08/15.

47 Lyall RA, Donaldson N, Fleming T, Wood C, Newsom-Davis I, Polkey MI et al. A prospective study of quality of life in ALS patients treated with noninvasive ventilation. *Neurology* 2001;57(1):153–156. Epub 2001/07/11.

48 Aboussouan LS, Khan SU, Meeker DP, Stelmach K, Mitsumoto H. Effect of noninvasive positive-pressure ventilation on survival in amyotrophic lateral sclerosis. *Annals of Internal Medicine* 1997;127(6):450–453. Epub 1997/10/06.

49 Woodcock AA, Gross ER, Geddes DM. Drug treatment of breathlessness: Contrasting effects of diazepam and promethazine in pink puffers. *British Medical Journal (Clinical Research Edition)* 1981;283(6287):343–346. Epub 1981/08/01.

50 Bruera E, Macmillan K, Pither J, MacDonald RN. Effects of morphine on the dyspnea of terminal cancer patients. *Journal of Pain and Symptom Management* 1990;5(6):341–344. Epub 1990/12/01.

94

End-stage congestive heart failure

KRISTIAN M. BAILEY, MARK T. KEARNEY

INTRODUCTION

Heart failure is the common end point for many cardiac disorders with ischemic heart disease, hypertension, and valvular heart disease being the most frequent causes of left ventricular dysfunction ("pump failure"). Irrespective of the etiology, the resulting clinical picture is similar, with varying degrees of left, right, or biventricular failure. The incidence of heart failure increases with age ranging from 1.4/100,000 person years for those aged under 45 years to 327.6/100,000 person years for those aged over 75 years in the United Kingdom. The lifetime risk of developing heart failure for a person aged 40 years in the United States is approximately 1 in 5 [1].

The clinical course of heart failure is very variable and unpredictable. Patients have stable plateau phases of variable duration punctuated by episodes of decompensation of differing severities, which may precipitate an acute admission to the hospital. As the disease process progresses, the episodes of decompensation typically become more frequent and require longer periods of treatment to reachieve stabilization. The functional status of patients following an episode of decompensation is often less than it was previously. This unpredictability in heart failure makes prognostication for individual patients difficult, and identifying patients entering the final stages of the disease is problematic (Figure 94.1).

Despite advanced heart failure patients having a similar symptom burden to cancer patients [2], access to specialist palliative care services is suboptimal with the latest U.K. National Heart Failure Audit showing less than 4% of patients are referred to specialist palliative care services [3].

Improved treatments for acute cardiac conditions, coupled with an aging population, are resulting in ever increasing numbers of patients living with, and dying of, heart failure. Palliative care physicians are increasingly recognizing the needs of this expanding patient group.

HEART FAILURE DEFINITION

Heart failure is the term used to describe the syndrome that arises from inadequate cardiac output secondary to progressive impairment of heart function. Typically, the term "heart failure" implies left ventricular systolic dysfunction, but a proportion of patients develop the same clinical features despite preserved left ventricular systolic function. There is little correlation between severity of cardiac impairment and symptoms; therefore, heart failure severity is typically classified by functional status. The New York Heart Association (NYHA) classification is most widely used, categorizing patients according to the severity of symptoms at rest and on exertion, and degrees of limitation [4].

CLINICAL COURSE AND PROGNOSIS

Left ventricular dysfunction is usually a progressive problem. An insult to the myocardium, such as an ischemic event, can result in a gradual decline towards ventricular failure irrespective of etiology. Without medical intervention, rarely does left ventricular function improve. In response to insults such as increased pressure load or loss of muscle mass from myocardial infarction, the ventricle undergoes "remodeling," whereby both structural and biochemical changes occur. Activation of the sympathetic nervous system and the renin–angiotensin–aldosterone axis is initially probably adaptive, but in the long term causes progressive worsening of cardiac function and heart failure through multiple mechanisms [5]. Medical therapies (such as angiotensin converting enzyme [ACE] inhibitors) can slow this process, but eventually, worsening left ventricular function leads to the onset of symptoms. The common etiologies of cardiac failure include ischemic heart disease (70%), hypertensive heart disease (15%),

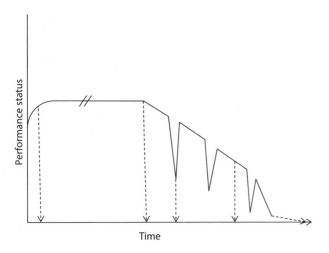

Figure 94.1 *Clinical course of heart failure. There is a plateau phase of variable duration. Decline in functional status is typically characterized by acute decompensations often resulting in hospitalization. A patient's functional status following decompensation is often less than previous. In advanced heart failure, these episodes of decompensation become more frequent and of increasing severity before terminal decline occurs. Death (represented by the dotted arrows) can occur suddenly at any point or as gradual pump failure. This clinical course makes the recognition of patients in the final stages of the disease difficult.*

and valvular heart disease (5%) [6]. Cardiomyopathies and congenital heart disease are less common but remain significant and affect a younger population. Nutritional deficiencies (e.g., beriberi) contribute to cardiac failure in the developing world.

Patients with heart failure are at risk of sudden death, which can occur at any stage during the disease trajectory. Meta-analyses of the early heart failure treatment trials and registries show that between 30% and 50% of patients who die with chronic heart failure do so as a result of sudden death, with approximately 40% dying as a result of progressive pump failure [7,8]. The high incidence of sudden death has led to the development and use of implantable cardioverter defibrillators (ICDs) to treat life-threatening arrhythmias. Sudden death in an ICD-treated population is predictably much lower accounting for less than 10% of all deaths [9]. Increased use of ICDs will in time shift the proportion of heart failure deaths towards progressive pump failure and the attendant difficulties inherent to this process.

The differing trajectories of heart failure patients mean prediction of death, or entering the end-of-life stages, is difficult, thereby meaning that patients are potentially not offered the psychological or medical support they may require. Clinical models have been developed to predict mortality in heart failure patients [10,11], but their usefulness in practice has yet to be determined. Recent evaluation has demonstrated that many end-stage heart failure patients are not identified by these scoring systems [12]. Worsening functional status, as evidenced by the NYHA class, significantly worsens prognosis, with a 1-year mortality of 28% for patients who are NYHA class IV compared to 7% for patients who are NYHA class II [13]. Prediction of death by experienced nursing staff has been shown to be more accurate than some statistical models [14]. This intuitive reasoning by clinical staff has led to the use of the "surprise" question when trying to predict who needs access to specialist palliative care service, that is, "Would you be surprised if this patient were to die in the next 6–12 months?" This intuitive reasoning is aided by factors such as recurrent hospital admissions with worsening heart failure, deteriorating renal function, and refractory symptoms despite optimal therapy.

Once a strategy for determining the terminal stages of heart failure has been found, it will be easier to ensure timely palliative care input and a move away from invasive treatments. Increasingly, centers are exploring combined care, where palliative medicine expertise is combined with standard cardiology care in multidisciplinary clinics. Such a strategy does not require that a point in time be identified where the patient "becomes palliative," but rather that palliative care becomes an early, and integral, part of optimal heart failure management. Increasing community services, particularly heart failure nurse specialists, also helps to aid this transition from treatment to palliation.

HEART FAILURE SYMPTOMS

The level of symptoms experienced by heart failure patients is not proportional to the degree of left ventricular dysfunction. Some patients with extremely poor cardiac function can remain relatively asymptomatic for prolonged periods.

Characteristic symptoms of heart failure include shortness of breath, fatigue, and ankle swelling, but others include depression, poor quality sleep, confusion, short-term memory loss, dizziness, and nausea [15]. As would be expected, the most commonly reported symptom is breathlessness, present in up to 90% of patients [16]. Breathlessness presents either on exertion or at rest, as orthopnea or nocturnal dyspnea. Fatigue is also prevalent (69%) and exaggerated by ankle edema, weight gain/loss, and depression. Depression is very common and yet underdiagnosed and undertreated in those with cardiac failure. Approximately 50% of heart failure patients in a recent study were classed as depressed during a 5.4-year period, with approximately two-thirds of these receiving treatment with antidepressants [17]. Depression has also been linked to increased mortality, increased rates of rehospitalization, and worsening quality of life in those with heart failure [17–19]. It is important to note that cognitive functioning and depression have been noted to worsen during episodes of heart failure decompensation, with some improvement postrecovery, albeit lower than previous levels [20].

Many patients also experience pain in the last 6 months of life (up to 75%) [16]. Chest and joint pains have been reported as common, but often the cause of pain is not specified. In elderly patients, pain may relate to comorbidity rather than to left ventricular failure itself. SUPPORT (Study to Understand Prognoses and Preferences for Outcomes and Risks of Treatments) reported that severe pain in the last 3 days of life occurs at comparable frequencies in heart failure and a number of cancers [21].

Substantial changes occur in the gut as a result of heart failure with hypoperfusion, edema formation, and altered permeability occurring [22]. The altered gut permeability is hypothesized to result in increased absorption of endotoxins with resultant increase in proinflammatory cytokines. Cytokines such as TNF-α not only act as markers of heart failure severity but may in themselves contribute to the progression of myocardial dysfunction [23,24]. This proinflammatory response, coupled with decreased gastrointestinal nutrient absorption, contributes to the development of cardiac cachexia, a well-recognized complication of congestive heart failure. The development of cardiac cachexia confers a poor prognosis with 18-month survival less than 50% [25,26]. It is characterized by a severe wasting process that particularly affects skeletal muscle and promotes exercise intolerance with marked breathlessness and fatigue at low workloads. A comprehensive review of the mechanisms and effects of cachexia in heart failure is out with the scope of this chapter but available elsewhere [27]. The increased cytokines associated with cachexia also contribute to symptoms such as nausea that further exacerbate weight loss.

MEDICAL MANAGEMENT OF HEART FAILURE

Modern heart failure management draws on a broad evidence base, and patients will be receiving polypharmacy with several agents that have been demonstrated to reduce adverse ventricular remodeling and improve prognosis and morbidity. Clear reductions in hospitalizations and mortality have been shown with ACE inhibitors [28–31], beta-blockers [32–34], and aldosterone antagonists [35,36]. Unlike in other end-stage diseases, medications to treat the disorder should not be routinely discontinued, partly due to the difficulty in predicting death, but also as many patients achieve symptomatic relief up to the terminal stages of their disease. In addition to disease-modifying agents, the majority of patients are on loop diuretics and/or thiazide diuretics for symptomatic relief.

The large majority of medical therapies used in heart failure induce a degree of hypotension. If patients are experiencing symptomatic hypotension, then reduction in treatment dosages should be considered. In the absence of severe fluid overload, reductions in diuretics should be considered initially for symptomatic hypotension, whereas in significant fluid overload, reduction in beta-blockers or ACE inhibitors should be considered first.

Diuretics

Loop diuretics are the principal treatment for fluid overload with advanced heart failure patients often on increasing doses. In significant right heart failure with gut edema, absorption of all loop diuretics is reduced [37]; however, there is some evidence that use of bumetanide or torosemide may promote a better diuresis compared to furosemide in these circumstances [38]. During heart failure decompensations, diuretics often need to be given intravenously to overcome poor gut absorption. Intravenous treatment has traditionally required hospital admission for administration of therapy; however, many patients do not wish to spend prolonged periods in the hospital, particularly if they are aware that they are in an advanced stage of their disease. Administration of intravenous diuretics in a community setting has shown to be safe and effective at reducing acute hospital admissions [39]. Increasingly, programs are being developed to deliver intravenous diuretics in the home or hospice environment.

Gaining intravenous access can be problematic and traumatic for preterminal patients. If fluid overload is a significant issue that is not being addressed by oral diuretic therapy, then there is evidence that subcutaneous furosemide can be administered in a safe and effective manner [40]. The subcutaneous route has the additional benefit that hospice staff are more comfortable with administering infusions via this route rather than intravenously.

DEVICE THERAPY FOR HEART FAILURE

Pacemakers and defibrillators

Cardiac mechanical and electrical dysfunction can result in dyssynchronous left and right ventricular contraction, thereby making an impaired ventricle less efficient. The use of biventricular pacemakers to resynchronize ventricular contraction can improve exercise capacity, reduce hospitalizations, and improve prognosis [41–43]. Significant left ventricular dysfunction, particularly secondary to ischemic heart disease, places patients at risk of sudden cardiac death and therefore many patients are offered, and receive, ICDs. ICDs can be implanted in isolation or combined with a biventricular pacemaker.

Biventricular pacemakers should be treated in the same fashion as standard pacemakers for treatment of bradycardias when nearing end of life. Deactivation of the device is not generally indicated and may result in an acute deterioration in symptoms with subsequent added distress to the patient. There may, of course, be patients who feel that their pacemaker is prolonging their death and request deactivation. In these circumstances, it is important to explain that deactivation will not necessarily hasten death and may increase discomfort in the final stages of life. As with all matters, a patient's right to choose must be respected.

Unlike biventricular pacemakers, ICDs do have significant implications when nearing end of life. Patients and doctors rarely discuss deactivation of devices prior to implantation nor is the matter easily addressed as the clinical course progresses. By successfully treating life-threatening arrhythmias, patients are more likely to suffer a progressive decline from cardiac or noncardiac causes. It is important to emphasize to patients that the device can be deactivated when the risk–benefit balance is no longer favorable. Often, patients do not understand that ICDs prevent sudden death thereby making a protracted death more likely. For some patients, the "quality of death" can be as important as length of life when considering ICD management [44]. If patients begin to receive repeated shocks towards the end of life from their device, then this should certainly trigger discussions regarding quality of life and "quality of death" [45].

Discussions regarding deactivation ideally should start prior to implantation. Current American guidelines on device usage encourage physicians to discuss deactivation of devices should a terminal illness arise and advocate the consideration of advance directives to address the issues of device deactivation [46]. All institutions that implant ICDs should have procedures in place for the elective deactivation of devices. Likewise, all involved in the care of terminal patients should have pathways in place to access these facilities.

Left ventricular assist devices

Left ventricular assist devices (LVADs) are being used increasingly in patients with refractory heart failure not responding to standard therapies. These are mechanical pumps that replace the work performed by the left ventricle. Primarily, they are designed to act as a "bridge to transplant," but in some areas, they are beginning to be used as destination therapy due to the shortage of suitable transplant organs.

Assessment of suitability for LVAD therapy is an in-depth process, which assesses not only the physical status of the patient but also their ability to deal psychologically with an intensive treatment plan and all entailed. LVAD therapy has a number of attendant risks including repeated surgery, thrombosis and anticoagulation, and infection. The increasing use as destination therapy means that there will be an increase in the number of patients who deteriorate and approach end of life with LVADs in situ. This brings a number of complex palliative care needs including decisions regarding deactivation of a device that is life supporting. It has been recommended that discussions about patient's wishes in specific situations (e.g., terminal illness) should be held in advance so that the family and medical teams involved are aware of wishes regarding device deactivation. Centers that implant LVADs should adopt a full multidisciplinary approach including experienced palliative care support. This proactive approach aids advance care planning and improves overall care [47].

PALLIATIVE CARE IN TERMINAL CARDIAC FAILURE

A consensus conference convened in the United States in 2003 to define the then current state of "palliative and supportive care in advanced heart failure" acknowledged that symptom palliation in advanced heart failure had simply not been studied [44]. While much has been done to improve access to palliative care, there remains sparse evidence for individual symptom relief strategies. Standard palliative care techniques and practices should be followed.

Opioids are often used to provide symptomatic relief for breathlessness; however, recent data suggest they may be no more effective than placebo when used at the dosages typically prescribed [48]. Opioids do have the additional benefits of improving symptoms of anxiety and pain. Newer therapies such as sildenafil, rolofylline, and nesiritide have failed to show benefit in outcomes in heart failure but may aid with palliation of breathlessness [49].

Patients with cardiac failure are poorly informed about the course of their illness and the purpose of their medications. They often mistake symptoms of their underlying heart failure for side effects of their medication [15]. This occurs because of poor education of patients at and following diagnosis, compounded by barriers to good communication such as fatigue, hypoxia, and confusion. Patients need and want to be better informed regarding their condition and management. Education is a key factor of heart failure care throughout, and this may go someway to relieve symptoms such as anxiety.

Patients with severe heart failure report having to rely heavily on family and friends for help in performing activities of daily living. This provokes feelings of "being a burden." Poor mobility and an inability to leave the house promote isolation. Qualitative studies suggest the majority of patients with severe heart failure have thought about death and find it difficult to discuss with those close to them [50].

Access to hospice care for heart failure patients, while increasing recently, remains low. In 2012, it was reported that only 11.2% of patients in hospice care in the United States had a cardiac condition as a primary diagnosis [51]. As a result, many hospice staff are unfamiliar with the needs of heart failure patients and do not feel confident with caring for them [52].

CONCLUSIONS

Patients with severe cardiac failure represent a highly symptomatic population with a poor overall prognosis who would benefit from palliative care support. Their disease course is unpredictable and this adds to the psychological burden. Over recent years, there has been an increase in palliative care access for heart failure patients, but for many patients, the appropriate expertise and facilities are not available. Good palliative care should start early in the course of treatment to aid the transitional phase to end-of-life care. Collaborative working between cardiologists, primary care services, and palliative care physicians should be encouraged.

Key learning points

- Chronic heart failure is a major health-care issue, and despite contemporary therapies, mortality remains high.

- End-of-life care of patients with chronic heart failure is challenging as prognosis is often difficult to predict.

- Device-based therapies now add to this level of complexity.

- Early involvement of palliative care teams is advisable in patients with chronic heart failure.

REFERENCES

1 Lloyd-Jones DM, Larson MG, Leip EP et al. Lifetime risk for developing congestive heart failure; The Framingham Heart Study. *Circulation* 2002;106:3068–3072.

2 Bekelman DB, Rumsfeld JS, Havranek EP et al. Symptom burden, depression, and spiritual well-being: A comparison of heart failure and advanced cancer patients. *Journal of General Internal Medicine* 2009;24(5):592–598.

3 National Heart Failure Audit 2010. Report for the audit period between April 2009 and March 2010: The NHS Information Centre for Health and Social Care 2010. http://www.hscic.gov.uk/catalogue/PUB02654/nati-hear-fail-audi-2010-rep.pdf

4 The Criteria Committee for the New York Heart Association. *Nomenclature and Criteria for the Diagnosis of Diseases of the Heart and Great Vessels*, 9th edn, Little, Brown, Boston, MA, 1994.

5 Jessup M, Brozena S. Heart failure. *New England Journal of Medicine* 2003;348:2007–2018.

6 McMurray JJ, Stewart S. Epidemiology, aetiology and prognosis of heart failure. *Heart* 2000;83:596–602.

7 Narang R, Cleland JGF, Erhardt L et al. Mode of death in chronic heart failure: A request and proposition for more accurate classification. *European Heart Journal* 1996;17:1390–1403.

8 Mozaffarian D, Anker SD, Anand I et al. Prediction of the mode of death in heart failure: The Seattle heart failure model. *Circulation* 2007;116:392–398.

9 Thijssen J, van Rees JB, Venlet J et al. The mode of death in implantable cardioverter-defibrillator and cardiac resynchronization therapy with defibrillator patients: Results from routine clinical practice. *Heart Rhythm* 2012;9:1605–1612.

10 Levy WC, Mozaffarian D, Linker DT et al. The Seattle heart failure model: Prediction of survival in heart failure. *Circulation* 2006;113:1424–1433.

11 Lee DS, Austin PC, Rouleau JL, Liu PP, Naimark D, Tu JV. Predicting mortality among patients hospitalized for heart failure: Derivation and validation of a clinical model. *JAMA* 2003;290(19):2581–2587.

12 Haga K, Murray S, Reid J et al. Identifying community based chronic heart failure patients in the last year of life: A comparison of the gold standards framework prognostic indicator guide and the Seattle heart failure model. *Heart* [*Comparative Study Research Support, Non-U.S. Gov't*] April 2012;98(7):579–583.

13 Muntwyler J, Abetel G, Gruner C, Follath F. One-year mortality among unselected outpatients with heart failure. *European Heart Journal* 2002;23:1861–1866.

14 Yamokosi LM, Hasselblad V, Moser DK et al. Prediction of rehospitalization and death in severe heart failure by physicians and nurses of the ESCAPE trial. *Journal of Cardiac Failure* 2007;13(1):8–13.

15 Rogers A, Addington-Hall JM, McCoy A et al. A qualitative study of chronic heart failure patients' understanding of their symptoms and drug therapy. *European Journal of Heart Failure* 2002;4:283–287.

16 Nordgren L, Sorenson S. Symptoms experienced in the last six months of life in patients with end stage heart failure. *European Journal of Cardiovascular Nursing* 2003;2:213–217.

17 Diez-Quevedo C, Lupon J, Gonzalez B et al. Depression, antidepressants, and long-term mortality in heart failure. *Int J Cardiol* August 20, 2013;167(4):1217–1225.

18 Jiang W, Alexander J, Christopher E et al. Relationship of depression to increased mortality and rehospitalization in patients with congestive heart failure. *Archives of Internal Medicine* 2001;161(15):1849–1856.

19 Albert NM, Fonarow GC, Abraham WT et al. Depression and clinical outcomes in heart failure: An OPTIMIZE-HF analysis. *American Journal of Medicine* 2009;122(4):366–373.

20 Kindermann I, Fischer D, Karbach J et al. Cognitive function in patients with decompensated heart failure: The Cognitive Impairment in Heart Failure (CogImpair-HF) study. *European Journal of Heart Failure* 2012;14(4):404–413.

21 Lynn J, Teno JM, Phillips RS et al. Perceptions by family members of the dying experience of older and seriously ill patients. SUPPORT Investigators. Study to Understand Prognoses and Preferences for Outcomes and Risks of Treatments. *Annals of Internal Medicine* 1997;126(2):97–106.

22 Romeiro FG, Okoshi K, Zornoff LA, Okoshi MP. Gastrointestinal changes associated to heart failure. *Arquivos Brasileiros de Cardiologia* 2012;98(3):273–277.

23 Bozkhurt B, Kribbs SB, Clubb FJJ, Michael LH, Didenko VV, Hornsby PJ. Pathophysiologically relevant concentrations of tumour necrosis factor alpha promote progressive left ventricular dysfunction and remodelling in rats. *Circulation* 1998;97(14):1382–1391.

24 Yndestad A, Damas JK, Oie E, Ueland T, Gullestad L, Aukrust P. Systemic inflammation in heart failure—The whys and wherefores. *Heart Failure Review* 2006;11(1):83–92.

25 Anker SD, Ponikowski P, Varney S, Chua TP, Clark AL, Webb-Peploe KM. Wasting as an independent risk factor for mortality in chronic heart failure. *Lancet* 1997;349:1050–1053.

26 Anker SD, Negassa A, Coats AJS, Afzal R, Poole-Wilson PA, Cohn JN. Prognostic importance of weight loss in chronic heart failure and the effect of treatment with angiotensin converting enzyme inhibitors: An observational study. *Lancet* 2003;361:1077–1083.

27 Ciciora M, Anker SD, Ronco C. Cardio-renal cachexia syndromes (CRCS): Pathophysiological foundations of a vicious pathological circle. *Journal of Cachexia Sarcopenia and Muscle* 2011;2:135–142.

28 The CONSENSUS Trial Study Group. Effects of enalapril on mortality in severe congestive heart failure. Results of the Cooperative North Scandinavian Enalapril Survival Study (CONSENSUS). *New England Journal of Medicine* 1987;316:1429.

29 Pfeffer MA, Braunwald E, Moye LA. Effect of captopril on mortality and morbidity in patients with left ventricular dysfunction after myocardial infarction. Results of the survival and ventricular enlargement trial. The SAVE Investigators. *New England Journal of Medicine* 1992;327:669.

30 Erhardt L, MacLean A, Ilgenfritz J. Fosinopril attenuates clinical deterioration and improves exercise tolerance in patients with heart failure. Fosinopril Efficacy/Safety Trial (FEST) Study Group. *European Heart Journal* 1995;16:1892.

31 Effect of enalapril on survival in patients with reduced left ventricular function and congestive heart failure. The SOLVD investigators. *New England Journal of Medicine* 1991;325:293–302.

32 Packer M, Fowler MB, Roecker EB et al. Effect of carvedilol on the morbidity of patients with severe chronic heart failure: Results of the carvedilol prospective randomised cumulative survival (COPERNICUS) study. *Circulation* 2002;106:2194.

33 Goldstein S, Fagerberg B, Kjekshus J et al. Metoprolol controlled release/extended release in patients with severe heart failure: Analysis of the experience in the MERIT-HF Study. *Journal of the American College of Cardiology* 2001;38:932.

34 Flather MD, Shibata MC, Coats AJS et al. Randomised trial to determine the effect of nebivolol on mortality and cardiovascular hospital admission in elderly patients with heart failure (SENIORS). *European Heart Journal* 2005;26:215.

35 Pitt B, Zannad F, Remme WJ et al. The effect of spironolactone on morbidity and mortality in patients with severe heart failure. Randomized Aldactone Evaluation Study Investigators. *New England Journal of Medicine* 1999;341:709.

36 Pitt B, Remme WJ, Zannad F et al. Eplerenone, a selective Aldosterone blocker, in patients with left ventricular dysfunction after myocardial infarction. Eplerenone Post-Acute Myocardial Infarction Heart Failure Efficacy and Survival Study Investigators. *New England Journal of Medicine* 2003;348:1309–1321.

37 Brater CD, Day B, Burdette A, Anderson S. Bumetanide and furosemide in heart failure. *Kidney International* 1984;26:183–189.

38 Wargo KA, Banta WM. A comprehensive review of the loop diuretics: Should furosemide be first line? *Annals of Pharmacotherapy* 2009;43(11):1836–1847.

39 Ryder M, Murphy NF, McCaffrey D, O'Loughlin C, Ledwidge M, McDonald K. Outpatient intravenous diuretic therapy; potential for marked reduction in hospitalisations for acute decompensated heart failure. *European Journal of Heart Failure* 2008;10:267–272.

40 Zacharias H, Raw J, Nunn A, Parsons S, Johnson M. Is there a role for subcutaneous furosemide in the community and hospice management of end-stage heart failure? *Palliative Medicine* 2011;25:658–663.

41 Cleland JGF, Daubert J-C, Erdmann E et al. The effect of cardiac resynchronization on morbidity and mortality in heart failure. *New England Journal of Medicine* 2005;352:1539–1549.

42 Bristow MR, Saxon LA, Boehmer J et al. Cardiac-resynchronization therapy with or without an Implantable Defibrillator in advanced chronic heart failure. *New England Journal of Medicine* 2004;350:2140–2150.

43 Abraham WT, Fisher WG, Smith AL et al. Cardiac resynchronization therapy in chronic heart failure. *New England Journal of Medicine* 2002;346:1845–1853.

44 Goodlin SJ, Hauptmann PJ, Arnold R et al. Consensus statement: Palliative and supportive care in heart failure. *Journal of Cardiac Failure* 2004;10:200–209.

45 MacIver J, Rao V, Delgado DH et al. Choices: A study of preferences for end-of-life treatments in patients with advanced heart failure. *Journal of Heart and Lung Transplantation* 2008;27:1002–1007.

46 Epstein AE, DiMarco JP, Ellenbogen KA et al. ACC/AHA/HRS 2008 guidelines for device based therapy of cardiac rhythm abnormalities: A report of the American College of Cardiology/American Heart Association Task Force on Practice Guidelines (Writing committee to revise the ACC/AHA/NASPE 2002 Guideline update for Implantation of Cardiac Pacemakers and antiarrhythmia devices). *Circulation* 2008;117:e350–e408.

47 Swetz KM, Freeman MR, AbouEzzeddine OF et al. Palliative medicine consultation for preparedness planning in patients receiving left ventricular assist devices as destination therapy. *Mayo Clinic Proceedings* [*Case Reports*] June 2011;86(6):493–500.

48 Oxberry SG, Torgerson DJ, Bland JM, Clark AL, Cleland JG, Johnson MJ. Short-term opioids for breathlessness in stable chronic heart failure: A randomized controlled trial. *European Journal of Heart Failure* [*Randomized Controlled Trial Research Support, Non-U.S. Gov't*] September 2011;13(9):1006–1012.

49 Johnson MJ, Oxberry SG. The management of dyspnoea in chronic heart failure. *Current Opinion in Supportive and Palliative Care* [*Review*] June 2010;4(2):63–68.

50 Horne G, Payne S. Removing the boundaries: Palliative care for patients with heart failure. *Palliative Medicine* [*Research Support, Non-U.S. Gov't*] May 2004;18(4):291–296.

51 NHPCO Facts and Figures: Hospice care in America 2013. http://nhcpo.org/sites.default/files/public/Statistics_Research/2013_Facts_Figures.pdf

52 Goodlin SJ, Trupp R, Bernhardt P, Grady KL, Dracup K. Development and evaluation of the "Advanced Heart Failure Clinical Competence Survey": A tool to assess knowledge of heart failure care and self-assessed competence. *Patient Education and Counseling* [*Comparative Study Multicenter Study Research Support, Non-U.S. Gov't*] July 2007;67(1–2):3–10.

95

Palliative care for children

FINELLA CRAIG, JULIE BAYLISS

While the principles of palliative care are similar across all ages, this chapter will address key issues specific to children and young people (CYP). An essential requirement is not only to support the child and family through the disease process but to provide services that nurture each child's ability to participate in childhood, to develop and to achieve their potential.

SPECIFIC ISSUES IN PEDIATRIC PALLIATIVE CARE

The number of CYP requiring palliative care has not been clearly identified and encompasses a broad range of conditions, often rare, familial, unique to childhood, and extending over many years [1]. This, together with a broad geographical distribution, creates unique challenges for the development and sustainability of the funding, resources, and professional skills required to deliver and maintain services.

- CYP are in continuous physical, emotional, and cognitive development, affecting every aspect of their care, from the dosage of medication to communication methods, education, and support. This has implications for professional skill requirement, training, and service delivery.
- Parents legally represent their offspring in clinical, therapeutic, ethical, and social decisions, and professionals must ensure that CYP are appropriately involved in decisions.
- The social and emotional burden for the family is prolonged and complex. Professional carers may also require emotional support.
- Many of the medications used in palliative care have been developed, formulated, and licensed for use in adults and may not be available in appropriate preparations for children. This presents additional challenges for symptom management.
- New challenges are faced as the specific needs of antenatal, neonatal, and adolescent care are emerging.

CHILDREN NEEDING PALLIATIVE CARE

CYP requiring palliative care support can be considered in four broad categories [2]:

1. Life-threatening conditions for which curative treatment may be feasible but can fail
2. Conditions where premature death is inevitable, but where there may be periods of intensive treatment aimed at prolonging life
3. Progressive conditions without curative treatment options, where treatment is exclusively palliative but may extend over many years
4. Irreversible but nonprogressive conditions causing severe disability leading to susceptibility to health complications and likelihood of premature death

Accurate identification of the numbers of children requiring palliative care services has proved difficult, but is likely to be increasing and higher than previously estimated, with a prevalence of 32 per 10,000 population. Numbers may also differ between countries and ethnic groups [3].

NEEDS OF CHILDREN AND THEIR FAMILIES

CYP are in continuous evolution with needs determined by their underlying condition as well as the physical, emotional, and cognitive changes of increasing maturity. Care of the whole family, the needs and dynamics of which will change over time, is essential. Pediatric palliative care services must address the following:

The physical needs of the child, ensuring access to good assessment and management of their symptoms, in the most appropriate setting. Childhood growth and development must be facilitated, helping each child achieve their full potential.

Psychological needs of the child and family, including extended family members.

Social needs, ensuring that CYP and siblings have access to peer groups and age and developmentally appropriate play and leisure activities.

Education, which must be provided in accordance with local statutory requirements and be appropriate to the child's developmental needs.

Spiritual needs should be addressed with respect to the family's religious beliefs and culture. CYP approaching death may not have established their own belief systems and may need support as they explore this.

SUPPORT FOR THE CHILD AND FAMILY

Support begins at diagnosis and continues throughout life, death, and bereavement. All the family, including grandparents, will be affected, but the majority possess considerable strength and resilience to function effectively from day to day. Professionals should be able to identify those at extra risk and in need of additional support [4]. A flexible approach, time to listen, and an understanding and respect for different cultural approaches to illness and death are essential.

At diagnosis

The delivery of the diagnosis has a powerful impact and forms the foundation for communication in the future. Parents, CYP, and siblings can feel overwhelmed as their expectations for the present and future, as well as their day-to-day lifestyle, are disrupted. They may seek lots of information, valuing written information, links to websites, and contact with other parents in similar situations. The sick child faces the trauma of being in hospital and may be particularly confused or frightened if explanations of what is happening are delayed. Some parents may be reluctant to discuss the diagnosis with their child and may need support in considering how best to disclose information.

Living with illness

The family lives with the conflict of maintaining hope and a semblance of day-to-day life despite persistent uncertainty. Heavy nursing needs create a considerable burden of care. Hospital admissions cause practical difficulties of travel, separation, care of siblings, and finance. Parents can experience depression, anxiety, sleep disturbance, and marital discord [5]. They may find it difficult to maintain discipline and boundaries and to balance their time and emotions between the sick child and well siblings.

Supporting the family to maintain as normal a life as possible—maintaining friendships, education, and outside activities—within the confines of the illness is essential. They should be offered assistance with care at home and access to respite, leisure, and social opportunities. Where possible, school attendance should be facilitated, providing normality and structure, with social opportunities and peer group support, in addition to education [6].

Many families, while acknowledging the diagnosis and prognosis, use some avoidance and denial to protect themselves from extremes of emotion. Frequent discussions about the disease may prove burdensome and unhelpful, rather than supportive. Parents may want health professionals to maintain some hope, but this must be expressed with honesty and without raising unrealistic expectations.

Final stages

The proximity of death may be recognized by a gradual and persistent deterioration accompanied by increasing symptoms, or may be more sudden, during an acute episode of illness. The emotional impact can be dramatic for parents, particularly for those who have held a very positive and fighting approach throughout treatment. For others, it is a confirmation of what they have dreaded and known was inevitable.

Families require information and the opportunity to discuss their child's care, to explore their own feelings and express emotions. They may be able to talk to each other openly and offer each other support, but more often, they will cope in different ways. There may be a sense of relief that the uncertainty and suffering will soon be over, which they may feel is abnormal and unacceptable.

Many parents will value the opportunity of talking about what may happen at the moment of death and about the practical details of what to do after their child has died. Some will want to consider and plan the funeral before death, and some young people will want to be involved in planning their own funeral, either with their parents or with support from professionals. Organ or tissue donation may be considered and can be a very positive legacy.

Communicating with children and young people

It is clear that children understand and learn about the illness and its implications whether parents and professionals encourage it or not [7]. A natural reaction of parents is to protect their children by withholding what they perceive as frightening information. It is not unusual for children to *protect* their parents by keeping their worries to themselves.

Throughout their illness, CYP should be given opportunities to seek information and to express their feelings. Communication must be appropriate to their level of understanding about illness and their concept of death, which will be influenced by their age, cognitive level, and previous experiences. Open discussion, allowing the child to control the direction of conversation, is essential, although some children may choose not to seek information or to discuss their concerns despite this opportunity. Expressive media outside language, through play, art, and music, can be hugely beneficial.

Some approaches towards a more open and honest pattern of communication include

- Shifting the emphasis from *telling* to *listening*
- Identifying the child's indirect cues as well as obvious questions
- Discovering the child's fears and fantasies
- Maintaining trust through honesty
- Building up the whole picture gradually

Sibling support

Siblings often feel isolated and excluded as family life is disrupted, parents may have little time for them, and they have fewer opportunities for social activities [6]. They may develop feelings of low self-esteem, anxiety, and depression and may start to resent the sick child. Support should be provided individually, in the family unit and/or with other siblings in a similar situation. They may benefit from being involved in the day-to-day care of the sick child, including planning and attending the funeral.

Bereavement support

Grief following the death of a child is painful and enduring with a depth and persistence that is often underestimated. Parents lose not only their child but also their hopes for the future. It alters the whole family structure and puts additional stress on relationships. Grieving siblings may continue to feel isolated and neglected.

Parents value continuing support from professionals who have known their child, with the opportunity to talk about the child and their grief when others in the community expect them to have come to terms with it. The support provided, initially more frequent and gradually decreasing, will help facilitate the normal tasks of mourning.

KEY ISSUES FOR SYMPTOM MANAGEMENT

The symptoms experienced, principles of symptom management, and medications used in palliative care are similar to adult practice [8]. The main differences lie in the disorders encountered, the assessment of symptoms, routes of administration, doses used, and drug metabolism. Information regarding dosage, benefit, and side effect profile has often been extrapolated from adult data, and some drugs may not be licensed for use in children. However, a body of clinical experience has developed, and guidelines for prescribing have recently been produced by the Association for Paediatric Palliative Medicine (APPM) in the United Kingdom [9]. Our recommendation is that drug dose is determined with reference to this document and local prescribing guidelines, such as (in the United Kingdom) British National Formulary for Children (BNFc) [10].

Assessment of symptoms

The ability of a young person to describe symptoms will vary in relation to their level of understanding, experience, and communication skills. Additional information must be sought from parents and carers and through a variety of techniques, such as play, art, or music therapy or by using symptom assessment tools developed for young people of different ages and developmental levels [11].

Nondrug management: Complementary and alternative therapies

A holistic approach to symptom management is essential as social, psychological, and spiritual concerns impact on the symptom experience. Distraction and relaxation techniques; play, art, and music therapies; and complementary therapies should be available. Some CYP and families may find homeopathy and alternative medicines beneficial.

Basic principles of drug administration

- Involve the young person and family in developing an acceptable and achievable management plan.
- The availability of suitable drug preparations in terms of dose, taste, tablet size, or volume may limit drug choice.
- Avoid complex regimens or large volumes of oral medication.
- If using an oral route, CYP should be allowed to choose between liquids, granules, and tablets. A strong preference for, or aversion to, one preparation may influence the choice of medication used.
- Long-acting preparations, including transdermal patches, are often most convenient and least intrusive.
- Buccal and sublingual routes can be a useful alternative to oral medications, but availability is limited to a few medications and they tend to be short acting.
- Parenteral drugs are usually given by continuous infusion, not as bolus doses.
- Intramuscular drugs are painful and not necessary.
- As a child's condition deteriorates, the treatment plan often has to be simplified, routes of administration altered, and priority given to drugs that contribute most to the child's comfort.

Pain

Where appropriate, the underlying cause of pain should be investigated and treated. Essentially, the drugs used in adult symptom management can also be used in children, although codeine is not generally recommended due to poor response and side effects.

Opioids are appropriate [12]. In young children, metabolism is more rapid than in adults and they may require relatively higher doses, whereas neonates and children under 6 months old require a lower starting dose due to reduced metabolism and increased sensitivity. Respiratory depression is not usually a problem in children with severe pain, and side effects, such as nausea and vomiting, tend to be less frequent. Constipation is common, so laxatives should be prescribed.

Parents may be resistant to the introduction of opioids, fearing they will precipitate their child's death or reduce later options for pain management. Clear explanation and support are essential to avoid the risk of medication being withheld or underreporting of pain.

Neuropathic pain is difficult for children to describe, so knowledge of the underlying disease pathology, combined with clinical judgment and experience, is essential. Where appropriate, interventions such as epidural analgesia and nerve blocks can be used but may be technically difficult due to small size and the need for a general anesthetic.

Nausea and vomiting

Antiemetics should be selected according to their site of action and the presumed cause of vomiting. Overfeeding may be a precipitating factor, particularly if a child is fed via a nasogastric tube or gastrostomy, so a careful history and review of dietary goals is essential.

Vomiting due to gastrointestinal reflux may respond to antireflux medication and/or changes to the feeding regimen, such as the introduction of continuous rather than bolus feeds in those who are fed by nasogastric tube or gastrostomy. In severe reflux, continuous jejunal feeding or surgical management may be indicated.

Seizures

Children with disease involving the central nervous system often develop seizures that require long-term anticonvulsants, adjusted as the seizure pattern changes. Any child at risk of seizures must have a clear management plan that parents and carers can initiate. Palliative care providers may be called upon to assist with managing episodes of status epilepticus that are resistant to conventional drug management, particularly if these are to be managed outside the intensive care environment or at home. While there is little published about the use of subcutaneous phenobarbitone infusions in these situations, our experience is that effective seizure control is often achieved via this method and the child can subsequently be switched to an enteral route.

Respiratory symptoms

Active management of an underlying cause should always be considered. Practical and supportive approaches, such as finding the optimum position and relaxation exercises, may help, alongside symptom management. Some children will find oxygen helpful; others will find the oxygen mask or nasal cannulae too distressing to make the exercise beneficial.

In some CYP with chronic chest diseases or severe muscle weakness, long-term noninvasive respiratory support at night can be beneficial in reducing symptoms and frequency of infections [13].

Secretions

Excess secretions can become problematic for children as they become less able to cough and swallow. Glycopyrronium bromide or hyoscine hydrobromide are helpful, but intermittent suctioning may also be necessary. In terminally ill children, careful positioning and postural drainage may avoid the need for suction.

Anxiety and agitation

Unresolved confusion, fears, and anxieties can lead to increasing agitation as death approaches. Professionals must provide opportunities for children to seek information, clarify misconceptions, and receive support. Medications should only be used as an adjunct to this.

Anemia and bleeding

As death approaches, blood or platelet transfusion is usually indicated only for symptomatic relief. This will require sensitive negotiation, particularly if transfusions have previously been given routinely. Platelet transfusions may continue routinely if there is a risk of florid bleeding. If severe bleeding occurs, dark towels should be used to soak up blood and parents should be trained to administer emergency drugs. These should include an analgesic and sedative, such as morphine and midazolam, which can be given by the buccal route. Parents should be warned that if a large bleed occurs, it is likely to be a terminal event.

Poor nutritional intake

Nutrition is a very emotive issue in pediatrics, as a basic task of parenting is to feed your child.

Children with diseases affecting the central nervous system or causing muscle weakness often have difficulty with chewing and swallowing and are unable to tolerate an oral diet and/or are at risk of aspiration. Assisted feeding, via a nasogastric tube or gastrostomy, is often essential if the feeding difficulty is likely to be prolonged.

Some children may lose their appetite as the disease progresses. Assisted feeding may be appropriate if nutrition is likely to contribute to improved health and/or comfort. Parenteral nutrition should only be introduced if it is likely to be of long-term benefit and will not compromise the quality of the child's remaining life.

At the end stage of a progressive illness, nutritional goals become harder to achieve and large feed volumes may increase nausea, vomiting, and discomfort. If still feeding orally, parents should allow their child to eat small amounts of foods they enjoy whenever they feel like it. If the child has previously been having nasogastric or gastrostomy feeds, the volumes may need to be reduced to those that are more appropriate for a reduced appetite and therefore better tolerated.

PROVIDING SERVICES

CYP must receive good care for their underlying condition, support to participate in a childhood that is as normal as possible, and support to achieve their developmental potential, as well as expert symptom management and palliative care support. Providing a joined-up three-tier service whereby CYP and their families can access universal services (e.g., education and child health), core pediatric and palliative care services (e.g., community nursing), and specialist disease-specific and palliative care services is essential [14]. A key worker, lead professional or care coordinator, should be identified, responsible for coordinating these services.

Models of care

Most families want to be at home for at least some of their care, but some may require residential options, for example, if the emotional or physical burden of care becomes too great or if symptoms become too difficult to manage.

The three main models of home care are the following:

1. *Community-based care*, delivered by community children's nurses, with additional support provided by disease-specific or specialist palliative care services, as well as local pediatricians
2. *Outreach home care from a specialist hospital-based services*, when a specialist team continues to provide care to the child at home, usually in conjunction with services based within the child's community
3. *Outreach home care from a children's hospice*, where expert palliative care support and, in some situations, hands-on nursing care are provided by hospice staff, often in conjunction with other community-based services

Alternatives to care at home include the following:

1. *Hospice care*, where specialist palliative care is delivered in an environment suited to the CYP and family's needs and where holistic support for the whole family is a priority.
2. *Hospital wards* generally focus on acute management and may be inadequately equipped to accommodate and address the holistic needs of the child and family. However, there will be times when hospital interventions are required or where admission is preferable for the child and family.
3. *Inpatient pediatric palliative care units* have been established in some countries providing specialist palliative care support alongside disease-specific treatment.

A single model of care may prove inadequate in terms of availability, flexibility, location, and expertise, so the majority of pediatric programs adopt a combination of different care models, supporting families to access services and to move smoothly from one care setting to another. These *networks* ensure that families have access to advice and support, 24 hours a day, in a location appropriate to their needs.

Neonatal care

Antenatal diagnosis of a lethal condition raises practical and emotional challenges, necessitating support for decision making, planning for the birth, and planning for symptom management [15,16]. Improved survival of neonates with complex care needs demands palliative care provision in the neonatal unit and following discharge.

Adolescent care

Specific challenges arise when adolescent development occurs alongside a life-threatening or life-limiting illness [17]. Providing an appropriate environment for care, delivered by informed professionals, is essential. Transition to adult services, while necessary, can be difficult as many young people with long-term complex care needs may not meet the criteria for adult palliative care services. The development of appropriate services for young adults remains a significant concern.

Intensive care

CYP with complex care needs often have periods of acute life-threatening deterioration, warranting aggressive management in the Intensive Therapy Unit (ITU) [18,19]. The role of palliative care in the ITU is increasingly recognized, including support for ventilation withdrawal in a preferred place of care.

SUMMARY

Palliative care for children poses unique challenges for professionals. Key points to recognize are as follows:

- Childhood is a period of continuous physical, emotional, and cognitive evolution that affects every aspect of care.
- Children must be supported to participate in childhood, to develop and achieve their potential, alongside support for disease progression.
- Holistic support must be provided for the whole family, from diagnosis and into bereavement.
- Communication with children must be appropriate to their level of development and understanding and may require nonverbal techniques.
- Symptom management may be challenging due to the limited availability of appropriate drug preparations, dosage, and licensing arrangements for children.
- Service models must be flexible and well coordinated and enable families to access advice and support, 24 hours a day, in a location appropriate to their needs.

REFERENCES

1   Palliative care for infants, children and young people: The Facts. *European Association of Palliative Care* 2010.

2   Chambers L, Dodd W, McCulloch R, McNamara-Goodger K, Thompson A, Widdas W. A guide to the Development of Children's Palliative Care Services. *ACT (Association for Children's Palliative Care),* 2009. Bristol UK.

3   Fraser LK, Miller M, Hain R, Norman P, Aldridge J, McKinney PA, Parslow RC. Rising national prevalence of life-limiting conditions in children in England. *Pediatrics* 2012; 129: 1–7.

4   Rosenberg AR, Baker KS, Syrjaja K, Wolfe J. Systematic review of psychosocial morbidities among bereaved parents of children with cancer. *Pediatr Blood Cancer* 2012; 58(4): 503–512.

5   Bluebond-Langner M. *In the Shadow of Illness: Parents and Siblings of the Chronically Ill Child.* Princeton, NJ: Princeton University Press, 1996.

6   Craig F, Boden C, Samuel J. Schooling of children with a life-limiting or life-threatening illness. *Eur J Palliat Care* 2012; 19(3): 131–135.

7   Bluebond-Langner M. *The Private Worlds of Dying Children.* Princeton, NJ: Princeton University Press, 1978.

8   Jassal S. Basic symptom control in paediatric palliative care. The Rainbows Children's Hospice Guidelines. *Rainbows Hospice* 2011. www.rainbows.co.uk.

9   Jassal S (ed.). *Association of Paediatric Palliative Medicine Master Formulary.* Bristol, U.K.: ACT, 2012. www.act.org.uk.

10 Paediatric Formulary Committee. BNF for Children (2012), London: *BMJ Group, Pharmaceutical Press and RCPCH Publications;* 2012.

11 Collins J, Byrnes ME, Dunkel IJ, Lapin J, Nadel T et al. The measurement of symptoms in children with cancer. *J Pain Symptom Manage* 2000; 19(5); 363–377.

12 Zernikow B, Michel E, Craig F, Anderson BJ. Paediatric palliative care: The use of opioids for the management of pain. *Pediatr Drugs* 2009; 11(2): 129–151.

13 Collins JJ, Fitzgerald DA. Palliative care and paediatric respiratory medicine. *Paediatr Respir Rev* 2006; 7(4): 281–287.

14 Craft A, Killen S. Palliative care services for children and young people in England: An independent review for the Secretary of State. Department of Health, England, 2007.

15 McNamara-Goodger K. A Neonatal Pathway for Babies with Palliative Care Needs. *ACT (Association for Children's Palliative Care),* 2009. Bristol UK.

16 Palliative Care (supportive and end-of-life care). A framework for clinical practice in perinatal medicine. *British Association of Perinatal Medicine (BAPM)* 2010. www.bapm.org.

17 *The ACT Transition care pathway: A framework for the development of integrated multi-agency care pathways for young people with life-threatening and life-limiting conditions.* ACT, 2007. www.act.org.uk.

18 Ramnarayan P, Craig F, Petros A, Pierce C. Characteristics of deaths occurring in hospitalised children: Changing trends. *J Med Ethics* 2007; 33(5): 255–260.

19 Cottrell S, Edwards F, Harrop E, Lapwood S, McNamara-Goodger K, Thompson A. A Carepathway to Support Extubation within a Children's Palliative Care Frameowrk. *ACT (Association for Children's Palliative Care),* 2011. Bristol UK.

96

Geriatric palliative care

KIMBERSON C. TANCO, MAXINE DE LA CRUZ

INTRODUCTION

Biology of aging

Aging is a part of everyone's life. It is a process that is influenced by environmental and genetic factors and is characterized by a reduced ability to respond to stress and reduced functional reserve as well as an increase in homeostatic imbalance. Changes that occur with aging affect life expectancy and functional capacity and can render an individual more susceptible to disease. As the population ages, the pattern of diseases also changes with increasing cases of chronic diseases such as heart disease, cerebrovascular disease, cancer, dementia, and respiratory diseases. Many older people suffer from several medical comorbidities that contribute to reduced function and death.

Demographics of aging

In the United States and in most parts of the developed world, people over the age of 65 is the most rapidly growing segment of the population.[1] Data from the U.S. Census show that the proportion of the population over age 65 will increase from 13% in 2010 to 20.2% in 2050, and the number of persons over age 65 is expected to increase from approximately 40.2 million in 2010 to an estimated 88.5 million in 2050.[2] Those over age 85 are expected to increase from 5.8 million in 2000 to 19.0 million in 2050. The average life span worldwide is predicted to extend another 10–22 years by 2050.[2] People are living longer as a result in improvement in public health policies and implementation, prevention, and treatment. Such innovations have changed the way health care is delivered to majority of the population greatly causing a reduction in the proportion of deaths in early childhood and early adulthood as well as early detection of preventable diseases and reduction in the complications of chronic medical conditions such as cardiovascular and pulmonary diseases.

Overview of the chapter

In this chapter, we will be discussing the changes that occur with aging along with the challenges in the care of the older individual with terminal illness. Tools that are used to assess specific needs of the geriatric patient will be discussed and its implication on the most appropriate management for such patients.

ASSESSING THE NEEDS OF A GERIATRIC PATIENT

Chronologic age poorly reflects age-related changes that occur. Age of 70 has been identified by experts as a landmark age for which a more comprehensive evaluation of physiologic age using validated tools is recommended. Evaluation of physiologic age is not a simple task, and no single laboratory test or imaging can aid in such determination. The comprehensive geriatric assessment (CGA) is an important tool that provides an estimation of the patient's active life expectancy and functional reserve and identifies resources and provides relevant insight for future needs that may impact the overall therapeutic plan.[3] It involves examination of the patient's function and physical performance, cognition, presence of comorbidities (number and severity), presence of geriatric syndromes, nutrition, polypharmacy, social support, and living environment.[4–6] Findings in CGAs are vital in the clinical discussion on treatment plans for older patients and helpful in determining prognosis without using an arbitrary age cutoff. This also allows for a more holistic approach by physicians to explore other medical issues that may reduce life expectancy and quality of life, by examining both terminal disease and other health issues that may be present. Important questions that may be brought up in therapeutic plan discussions include the following: How will additional treatment alter the prognosis? What is the expected quality of life with or without treatment? What are the patient's goals and priorities? A more truthful discussion about risks and benefits of treatment with the goal of preserving functional independence and acceptable quality of life may be achieved with information from a CGA.

Functional assessment

A patient's functional status is measured using a checklist of activities of daily living (ADLs) and instrumental activities of daily living (IADLs) (Table 96.1) along with objective measurements of physical performance measures including muscle strength testing, walking speed, and the short physical performance scale. Proper assessment will facilitate realistic goals of treatment, expectation of potential recovery, and discharge plans including provisions for appropriate psychosocial support.

Functional impairment involves the inability of an older person to perform daily life activities normally. In the population aged 75 years and older, 75% have limited activities due to functional impairment. Almost 50% require assistance in one or more ADLs in people aged 85 years and older. Up to 25% of community-dwelling older adults have at least one impairment in their IADLs.[4]

Previous studies have shown that functional status is an independent predictor of disability and mortality and frequently associated with poor quality of life and increased utilization and social and health-care services. Impaired ADL is a predictor for functional decline, length of stay, institutionalization, EC visits, response to cancer treatment, and death.[4,7,8] Assessment tools like the Karnofsky Performance Scale or Index and Eastern Cooperative Oncology Group (ECOG) Performance Status Scale are used to predict prognosis in cancer patients.[9,10] Both scales are highly correlated and have predictive validity. ECOG values are followed frequently over the duration of therapy.

Functional impairment affects compliance with medical visits and can contribute to caregiver burden. Referral to social workers or community-based services can reduce caregiver stress and enable continued home care for a longer period of time. Consideration for physical therapy and use of orthotics, wheelchairs, walkers, or other devices can enhance quality of life.[11,12]

Table 96.1 *6 ADLs and 8 IADLs*

ADL	IADL
Using the toilet	Using the telephone
Grooming	Shopping
Feeding	Preparing food
Dressing	Cleaning the house
Ambulating	Laundry
Bathing	Use of transportation
	Taking own medications
	Managing finances

Cognitive assessment

Evaluating cognition is important in assuring good understanding of the disease and adherence to the therapeutic goals and plan. It contributes to difficulty in navigating the health-care system and caregiver distress. Assessment of pain and other symptoms is more difficult in patient with some degree of cognitive impairment. Clinically significant cognitive impairment is seen in about 3% of people aged 65 years and older and may reach 40%–50% of persons aged 90 years or older. Cognitive evaluation is recommended in at risk patients. Common causes of cognitive impairment in the elderly include dementia, delirium, and depression.[13,14]

Assessment tools are available for bedside use including the Folstein's mini–mental state examination (MMSE), the short portable mental status questionnaire, the clock drawing test, the trail making tests A and B, and the time and change test. The MMSE is one of the most widely used and recognized tools. Its strengths include ease of administration and usefulness as a screening tool, which help establish a baseline and monitor for any progress or worsening of cognitive state. The Memorial Delirium Assessment Scale can be administered repeatedly within the same day to allow for objective measurement of changes in delirium severity in response to medical changes or clinical interventions.

Assessment of medical comorbidities

Medical comorbidities are known to increase with age as is associated with reduced life expectancy and risk of morbidity and increase health-care utilization.[15] The Cumulative Illness Rating Score for Geriatrics, Kaplan–Feinstein index, and NIA/NCI cancer and comorbidity measure and the Charlson index are commonly used to estimate comorbidity particularly in the geriatric population. These scales reflect the burden of illness and the cumulative increased likelihood of 1-year mortality and are therefore useful in outlining treatment plans.[16,17] The presence of comorbidities is not predictive of response to chemotherapy[18] but should be taken into account when considering routine cancer screening,[19] treatment decisions,[20] and clinical trial participation.[15] Pathophysiologic effects of aging such as reduced organ function and alteration in body composition should be kept in mind as it may affect therapeutic and toxicity profiles of some medications.

Assessing for geriatric syndromes

Geriatric syndrome is defined as multifactorial health conditions that occur when the accumulated effects of impairments in multiple systems render an older person vulnerable to situational challenges.[21] These include dementia, delirium, falls, incontinence, sensory impairments, sleep disorders, pain, and skin breakdown.

Nutritional assessment

Nutritional status is an independent predictor of mortality and disability in older persons.[22] In frail older patient, assessment of nutritional status is part of routine clinical evaluation. Poor nutritional status can decrease tolerance to chemotherapy and delay tissue recovery from chemotherapy induced injury.

Medication review

A careful review of medications is always recommended as the potential for adverse drug reactions and drug interactions increases with increasing number of medications. Older patients use more than threefold more medications than younger patients as a result of a higher number of concurrent medical conditions.[23] Adverse drug reactions can be caused by polypharmacy as well as physiologic changes in the body.

Assessment of social support

Presence of social support is crucial to safe and effective management of cancer in the older person. Caregivers play a multitude of roles including that of emotional support, assisting in the performance of certain basic physical functions, and advocating for patients by identifying their needs and reactions to therapy. Going to medical or social appointments is usually limited due to difficulties in ambulation or lack of resources for transportation.

Due to a variety of reasons, the geriatric patient may be isolated both physically and socially. Social isolation is defined by a lack of interaction with other people; it denotes feeling of loneliness and lack of genuine communication and companionship.[24] Although older persons can live alone without being socially isolated or feeling lonely, living alone is a leading indicator of the potential for social isolation. Many of these older patients are socially isolated because they have lost several of their family members, friends, and loved ones and also of poverty. Interventions that can reduce social isolation include group interactions in the form of self-help classes, exercise, and skills training have shown to be effective in noncancer settings.[25] Referrals to community support groups or bereavement centers, and if qualified, hospice organizations, can provide needed psychosocial assistance to them.

Spiritual assessment

Elderly patients diagnosed with terminal illness have several unmet needs including existential concerns such as how to continue to have a sense of hope, or to know that their lives were meaningful and purposeful.[26] Providing a safe environment for patients to explore these issues, ponder the meaning of their illness, their suffering, their relationship to God, and their possible death is crucial to good patient care. We have an obligation to assist patients and families in accepting the dying process as a meaningful process of life.

Different interventions have been developed addressing existential distress and enhancing the end-of-life experience of terminally ill patients. Dignity therapy, meaning-centered therapy, supportive–expressive therapy, reflection, and journaling are some of the therapies developed. Dignity therapy is a brief intervention where emphasis is placed on things that matter most in a patient's life or how they most want to be remembered, designed to enhance self-worth and explore life's meaning and purpose.[27,28] Patients reflect on important roles they have held in their lifetime, hopes and dreams that they have achieved or wish for their loved one, and personal legacies they hope to share. Meaning-centered psychotherapy aims to assist patients find meaning in their experiences with illness. Patients contemplate on relationships, experiences, love and beauty as sources of meaning in one's life. Supportive–expressive group therapy is an unstructured group intervention where participants openly support and discuss death and dying. It decreases social isolation by building support among people sharing personal life experiences.[27] Medical providers need to be aware that spirituality is an important aspect of a person's life and belief system and contributes to overall well-being[29] and as such needs to be incorporated in the assessment of patients.

Economic assessment

Financial concern is an important source of stress in older patients with fixed incomes. Financial difficulties also limit them either in transportation expenses or joining social or group programs. It may cause the loss of employment for patient and caregiver and interruptions in academic preparation contributing to significant caregiver burden. Prompt referral to social work to find resources for the patient is recommended.

DEMENTIA AND OTHER GERIATRIC SYNDROMES

Dementia

Dementia is defined as loss of cognitive function affecting one or more domains like memory, cognitive skills (calculation, abstract thinking, or judgment), language, behavior, and thinking. Examples of the more commonly encountered dementias are Alzheimer's disease, vascular dementia, Lewy body dementia, and frontotemporal (Pick's disease) dementia. Other less known include dementia of Parkinson's disease, multiple sclerosis, HIV/AIDS, Lyme disease, chronic alcohol abuse, and brain injuries. Several tools can be used to evaluate cognitive function such as the Folstein's MMSE,[30] Clox 2,[31] Mini-Cog,[32] or word list generation (WLG), for example, letter WLG, "FAS," and category WLG, "animals."

When cognitive impairment is present, health-care proxies should be involved in the decision making with a clear emphasis to explain them the prognosis and clinical course of their cancer in the context of the patient's medical comorbidities, thereby avoiding burdensome interventions.[33]

Delirium

Delirium is a common neuropsychiatric condition that is often seen in frail older patients with severe medical illnesses that is characterized by fluctuating periods of confusion and psychomotor agitation. Frequently, delirium is misdiagnosed as either depression or dementia, especially when it is the hypoactive subtype.[34] When present in the elderly patient, it often is a harbinger of life-threatening illness. Failure to recognize delirium can cause distress in patients and family members and can result in inappropriate management of symptoms.

Risk factors identified for delirium are advanced age, prior cognitive impairment, illness severity, and burden of comorbidities.[34] Etiologies for delirium include dehydration, medications, infections, hypoxia, central nervous system involvement by the cancer, renal failure, and hepatic failure.[34] It is associated with an increased mortality rate.

The intensity of the search for causative factors for delirium and of the treatment strategies used in the end-of-life setting must be individualized, according to the clinical situation and goals of care. Management involves identifying and correcting reversible risk factors and treating the symptoms of delirium. When possible, correction of possible opioid toxicity, dehydration, infection, medication interactions or side effects, and metabolic disturbances may help to reverse delirium. Environmental manipulation strategies such as reorientation, limiting staff changes, and reducing noise stimulation can also be tried. It has been shown that delirium reversibility occurs in about 50% of cases. It is also more commonly observed at the end of life.[35] Antipsychotic medications such as haloperidol, chlorpromazine, olanzapine, and risperidone are the mainstay of treatment.

Depression and anxiety

Depression is common in older adults but is often underrecognized and undertreated. It is estimated to occur in about 36%–50% of patients older than 65. The presentation of depression may be varied and insidious and may be attributed to other comorbid medical conditions. Clinical manifestations are varied and include depressed mood, anhedonia, change in appetite and weight loss, insomnia or hypersomnia, fatigue and difficulty focusing, psychomotor retardation or agitation, preoccupation with somatic symptoms or health status, feelings of worthlessness and hopelessness, or recurrent thoughts of death or suicide. Terminally ill patients at high risk of developing depression include those with a previous history of depression or attempted suicide, history of alcohol or substance abuse, new stressful losses (loss of autonomy, privacy, functional status, family member), use of medications associated with risk of depression (e.g., anticonvulsants, barbiturate, certain B-adrenergic antagonist, digitalis, metoclopramide), poor social support, and advanced disease.

When depression is suspected, search for underlying medical causes may be warranted as this can be easily reversible. Such conditions like thyroid disorders, dementia, anemia, diabetes, or substance abuse must be ruled out. Screening for depression is important as it impacts treatment plan and health-care utilization and overall quality of life. Screening tools commonly used in geriatric patients are the Geriatric Depression Scale, Cornell Scale for Depression in Dementia, Center for Epidemiologic Studies of Depression Scale (CES-D), and Patient Health Questionnaire 9. The two-item scale (PHQ-2) is a sensitive screening tool and is easy to perform. Patients can be asked the following two questions: during the previous 2 weeks, have you often been bothered by feeling down, depressed, or hopeless; and have you often been bothered by having little interest or pleasure in doing things?

The goal of therapy is to improve mood, function, and quality of life regardless of life expectancy. A combination of pharmacotherapy and psychotherapy is most useful.[36] Electroconvulsive therapy is not commonly used at the end of life but is useful in patients with psychotic depression. Pharmacotherapy considerations include drug interaction, anticipated life span, dosage adjustments, and presence of other medical comorbidities. Bicyclic antidepressants (e.g., venlafaxine) and selective serotonin reuptake inhibitors (SSRIs) and serotonin-norepinephrine reuptake inhibitors (SNRIs) are typically well tolerated in the elderly. Fluoxetine and paroxetine are less desirable because of their long half-life and potential anticholinergic effect, which can potentially cause other complications like falls, dizziness, and confusion. Other drugs can be considered particularly if there are coexisting symptoms. One can use mirtazapine for anorexia, trazodone for insomnia, and duloxetine and venlafaxine for neuropathic pain. Tricyclics (TCAs) and monoamine oxidase inhibitors (MAOIs) are not considered first line in geriatric patient because of the strong anticholinergic and sedating effect and their potential to cause orthostatic hypotension, hypertensive crises, ventricular conduction delays, and heart block. Psychostimulants like methylphenidate and modafinil have also been used. Psychotherapy techniques include cognitive-behavioral therapy, life review, and interpersonal psychotherapy.

Anxiety often accompanies the experience of receiving bad news, which may resolve over several days given support from health-care providers, family, and friends. Other uncontrolled symptoms can trigger it as well. Treatment includes counseling as well as addressing possible organic triggers. Caution must be taken when prescribing benzodiazepine in geriatric patients because of its potential for causing.[37]

Urinary incontinence

Incontinence may have significant impact on a patient's quality of life. The prevalence of incontinence in the elderly varies considerably from 15% to 30% in community-dwelling older patients to 50%–60% in nursing home residents.[38] Several conditions can cause incontinence including brain or spinal cord lesions that may interfere with nerve pathways needed for normal micturition.[39,40] Certain medications can exacerbate the symptoms of incontinence adversely affecting quality of life.[41]

A good history and physical examination is essential when a patient presents with urinary incontinence. It is important to differentiate chronic from transient causes such as delirium, urinary tract infections, atrophic vaginitis, use of certain medications (e.g., benzodiazepines, alcohol, diuretics, anticholinergic agents), psychological disorders, endocrine disorders, restricted mobility, and stool impaction.[42] The postvoidal residual (PVR) test studies that measure complete voiding are employed to determine possible causes of incontinence. A PVR > 200 mL suggests detrusor weakness or bladder outlet obstruction. Stress or urge incontinence may be present in PVR > 50 mL.

Polypharmacy

Polypharmacy is defined as the concurrent use of several different medications, including more than one medication from the same drug classification.[43] A study of 282 cancer patients from the Ohio Cancer Incidence Surveillance System (OCISS) showed that polypharmacy was present in more than 22% of patients in this study population.[44] Older patients are especially vulnerable to the risks associated with polypharmacy. Reasons for polypharmacy are multiple comorbidities that require a variety of drugs for proper management, availability of nonprescription medications, the tendency to self-treat, and the rise in so-called natural remedies. Known consequences of polypharmacy are adverse drug reactions, drug interactions, higher medication costs, and noncompliance.

Prevention of polypharmacy is difficult and often is necessary in order to address multiple medical problems. However, it is important to keep in mind certain key points in order to minimize harm to patients. Education and communication are crucial aspects of prevention. Physicians need to be familiar with the Beers Medication list, which is an inventory of drugs that are potentially harmful for the older patients.[37] Communication with other prescribers can result in reduction in medication use as it may eliminate redundancy. Drugs that are not in line with the goals of care for patients should also be discontinued if possible.

SYMPTOM MANAGEMENT IN THE OLDER PATIENT

Older individuals often develop chronic illnesses, which are characterized by long periods of decline, interspersed with partial recovery, and impairment of function. There is a shift from the acute illness model to the chronic, multidisease model that changes the approach to history taking and physical examination and goals of care. They often have an altered presentation of illness including (1) altered mental status and cognitive impairment, (2) altered pain sensation and inability to localize pain, (3) vague symptoms occasionally described in subjective statements such as "he doesn't look right," (4) inability to perform usual activities, (5) falls, (6) dehydration, (7) loss of appetite, and (8) unusual medication reactions.[6] Mental status changes may be caused by drug toxicity, cerebrovascular disease, systemic illness, infection, and substance withdrawal. Instances of altered pain sensation include not noticing incremental increases in pain or a less intense pain experience. Increasing fatigue may be caused by anemia, cardiovascular/pulmonary disease, infections, or endocrine disorders. Older persons are more prone to dehydration due to decreased muscle mass and a resultant lack of intracellular water.

Age-related anatomic and physiologic changes provide additional challenges in the evaluation and management of the elderly. Visual changes and hearing loss may complicate history taking, contribute to social isolation, and may lead to mistakes in following treatment plans. Changes in dentition and decrease in salivary production contribute to dysphagia, anorexia, weight loss, and social isolation through a loss of ability in being able to participate in social groups, which involve food in a majority of the time. Dry mouth can result from medication use and polypharmacy is usually the norm rather than the exception in the elderly. Dermatologic changes, particularly decrease in epidermal, dermal, and subcutaneous fat layers, cause the skin to be more sensitive to minor trauma and also have slower wound healing. Loss of subcutaneous fat may cause more rapid and erratic absorption of medications. Finally, physiologic and pathologic changes in renal and hepatic function are important in medication pharmacokinetics and the utilization of the pharmacological cache.

Elderly individuals are often stereotyped and discriminated against a phenomenon known as ageism, which causes difficulties in symptom assessment. Elderly patients may be at further risk of poor treatment because of an underestimation of their sensitivity to pain and the assumption that they tolerate pain well.[45]

In elderly cancer patients, Barford and D'Olimpio reported a lack of specific guidelines regarding drug selection, dosing, and side effects, which account for changes in aging physiology, pharmacokinetics, and idiosyncratic reactions.[46] Symptom management for basic symptoms such as pain, constipation, fatigue, weakness, nausea and vomiting, mucositis, and nutritional depletion syndromes, such as malabsorption and anorexia/cachexia, is often limited, frequently ineffective, and not evidence-based. Most clinicians have based their therapeutic decisions on individual experience. Validated instruments, such as the ESAS and Faces Pain Scale, help in measuring and providing valuable information regarding the presence and the intensity of a wide range of symptoms.

FAMILY AND CAREGIVER ISSUES

Caregiving for an elderly loved one can be a meaningful exercise as it presents as an opportunity to give thanks and pay back past care and support received. The experiences while caring for a family or friend near the end of life are often the memories remembered during the period of bereavement. It can also be a great source of distress as family caregivers have found themselves providing care with little support in terms of home care services. With advances in medicine, patients are also living longer with chronic illnesses and the provision and duration of care have also increased. Caregivers for the geriatric population are often either adult children with their own families, work responsibilities, and medical conditions or an aged spouse dealing with their own disabilities or illnesses. Caregiving can be a financial burden and may lead to adjustments in work accommodations, including going into work late, leaving early, or taking time off to fulfill their caregiving responsibilities, which all lead to lost wages.

Caregivers may be paid unlicensed or licensed caregivers or informal caregivers comprising family and friends.[47] In the United States, there are at least 43.5 million caregivers aged 18 and over, which is equivalent to 19% of all adults, who provide unpaid care to a family or friend who is age 50 years or older. The average age of the caregivers is 50, while the average age of care recipients is 77. On average, people are caregivers for 4 years, most likely less in the palliative care patient population.

A high proportion of caregiver work involves helping the patient perform ADLs and some IADLs such as assisting with housework and preparing meals. In addition to these, the direct or indirect action of providing medical help and assistance is provided by the informal caregivers to the elderly ill. Caregivers can also involve arranging medical appointments, providing emotional support, and managing financial affairs. Majority of these caregivers are thrust into their roles suddenly and without prior training and complete understanding of their new roles and responsibilities.

Factors that contribute to caregiver burden include age, gender, race, socioeconomic status, disabilities, and location (rural vs. urban areas).[47] Adult children caregivers are more at risk for depressive symptoms than the older spouse caregivers. They are usually expected to juggle multiple roles, which make them prone to exhaustion and fatigue. Missed workdays, decreased productivity, a lack of time for rest and leisure, and a sense of overwhelming burden result. On the other hand, older caregivers may themselves be physically limited or disabled. Furthermore, they may be socially isolated as several friends and family have already died before them, which also adds to their psychological distress and increased depression scores. Older caregivers also more often than not have fixed resources. Females comprise about 65%–70% of caregivers and have been found to have higher caregiver burden than their male counterparts including depressive symptomatology, anxiety, and fear of cancer recurrence.[48,49]

Garlo et al. did not find any significant difference between caregiver burden and type of disease in a study between patients with advanced cancer, heart failure, and COPD.[50] On the other hand, high burden was associated with caregiver's need for greater help with daily tasks suggesting that burden may be a measure of the caregiver's ability to adapt to the caregiving role and their psychological response, rather than the objective tasks needed to care for their loved one. Furthermore, limited social support, social isolation, lack of professional communication with physicians, and concerns about the future of the patient are important aspects of the psychological well-being of the caregiver.

Open communication between patient and caregiver decreases caregiver burden and results in higher levels of perceived support by the patient. However, Andruccioli described that some caregivers feared to be a burden for other relatives involved in the patient's care, while some had a sense of loneliness due to conflicts with other caregivers involved in the patient's care.[51] This results in a protective buffering for each other and may stem from an unwillingness to acknowledge the severity of the patient's disease.

Frequent patient and family meetings with the interdisciplinary team can help develop goals and plan of care. A partnership between the physician, patient, and caregiver would be helpful where the physicians would monitor caregiver function as well as provide information and referrals to caregivers. Health promotion and self-care models are important concepts that have been overlooked from the numerous risk factors and issues prevailing over caregiver burden. Examples of these may include getting enough sleep, nutrition, and exercise, getting proper attention over the caregiver's own medical and psychological illnesses, and maintaining timely routine health checks. In addition, functional coping strategies like maintaining free "self-time," accepting patient's disease progression, having a strong grasp on spirituality, maintaining regular work or hobbies, and being able to emotionally unload to family, friends, and, more importantly, professionals such as chaplains, pastors, counselors, and the palliative care team help buffer against physical and psychological distress. The hospice and palliative care teams can interject and educate the caregivers, which results in valuable support to them. No single intervention is adequate to address all the issues that the family caregivers deal with, but a combination of different interventions including individual and/or family counseling, case management, skills training, environmental modification, and behavior-management strategies would be most effective in reducing caregiver distress.[52] A hospice caregiver support project in where assistance in terms of food, housekeeping, and other services including assistance with ADLs and transportation resulted in a decrease in self-reported stress, and the frequency and number of days of hospice respite benefit used had been shown.[53]

GOAL SETTING AND ADVANCE CARE PLANNING

Advanced care planning consists of various processes that include specifying surrogates; communication with patient, caregivers, and providers; discussing treatment plans and alternatives; incorporating individual values; and formulation of a plan based on these preferences. Advanced directives are specific instructions that are prepared in advance, which guide the medical care of the patient if unable to express directly their health-care choices.

Completion of advance directives is usually more successful when incorporating direct patient–health-care professional interactions, with involvement of repetition and iteration over multiple visits. In contrast, passive education with the use of written materials, such as brochures, was found to be ineffective in increasing the completion rates of advance directives.[54] Patient-centered advance care planning using nonmedical facilitators resulted in identifying and respecting patient's wishes about end-of-life care, improved care from the perspective of the patient and their families, and lowered the risk of stress, anxiety, and depression in the surviving family members.[55] When the patient's family has enough time and preparation for loss, complicated grieving is less likely to occur.

The course of geriatric patients and chronic disease usually involves multiple exacerbations and partial recoveries reflecting a peak and trough pattern. Frequent reassessment of their goals of care must be made to address that it currently conforms to their current wishes. Some conditions need time-limited interventions, with frequent monitoring of its goals of improving quality of life, and if not, then discussions should be made for discontinuing the treatment.

REFERENCES

1   Kinsella K, Velkoff VA. The demographics of aging. *Aging Clin Exp Res* 2002;14(3): 159–169.

2   Vincent GK, Velkoff VA, U.S. Census Bureau. *The Next Four Decades the Older Population in the United States: 2010 to 2050*. Population estimates and projections P25-1138. Washington, DC: U.S. Department of Commerce, Economics and Statistics Administration, U.S. Census Bureau, 2010:1 online resource (14pp.).

3   Solomon DH. Geriatric assessment: Methods for clinical decision making. *JAMA* 1988;259(16): 2450–2452.

4   Fried LP, Guralnik JM. Disability in older adults: Evidence regarding significance, etiology, and risk. *J Am Geriatr Soc* 1997;45(1): 92–100.

5   Cesari M, Onder G, Russo A et al. Comorbidity and physical function: Results from the aging and longevity study in the Sirente geographic area (ilSIRENTE study). *Gerontology* 2006;52(1): 24–32.

6   Balducci L, Colloca G, Cesari M, Gambassi G. Assessment and treatment of elderly patients with cancer. *Surg Oncol* 2010;19(3): 117–123.

7   Wieland D, Hirth V. Comprehensive geriatric assessment. *Cancer Control* 2003;10(6): 454–462.

8   Extermann M. Comprehensive geriatric assessment basics for the cancer professional. *J Oncol Manag* 2003;12(2): 13–17.

9   Ostchega Y, Harris TB, Hirsch R, Parsons VL, Kington R. The prevalence of functional limitations and disability in older persons in the U.S.: Data from the National Health and Nutrition Examination Survey III. *J Am Geriatr Soc* 2000;48(9): 1132–1135.

10   Oken MM, Creech RH, Tormey DC et al. Toxicity and response criteria of the Eastern Cooperative Oncology Group. *Am J Clin Oncol* 1982;5(6): 649–655.

11   Oldervoll LM, Loge JH, Paltiel H et al. The effect of a physical exercise program in palliative care: A phase II study. *J Pain Symptom Manage* 2006;31(5): 421–430.

12   Neuenschwander H, Bruera E, Cavalli F. Matching the clinical function and symptom status with the expectations of patients with advanced cancer, their families, and health care workers. *Support Care Cancer* 1997;5(3): 252–256.

13   Extermann M. Studies of comprehensive geriatric assessment in patients with cancer. *Cancer Control* 2003;10(6): 463–468.

14   Friedrich C, Kolb G, Wedding U, Pientka L. Comprehensive geriatric assessment in the elderly cancer patient. *Onkologie* 2003;26(4): 355–360.

15   Extermann M. Interaction between comorbidity and cancer. *Cancer Control* 2007;14(1): 13–22.

16   Charlson ME, Pompei P, Ales KL, MacKenzie CR. A new method of classifying prognostic comorbidity in longitudinal studies: Development and validation. *J Chronic Dis* 1987;40(5): 373–383.

17   Parmelee PA, Thuras PD, Katz IR, Lawton MP. Validation of the cumulative illness rating scale in a geriatric residential population. *J Am Geriatr Soc* 1995;43(2): 130–137.

18   Maas HA, Janssen-Heijnen ML, Olde Rikkert MG, Machteld Wymenga AN. Comprehensive geriatric assessment and its clinical impact in oncology. *Eur J Cancer* 2007;43(15): 2161–2169.

19   Parnes BL, Smith PC, Conry CM, Domke H. Clinical inquiries. When should we stop mammography screening for breast cancer in elderly women? *J Fam Pract* 2001;50(2): 110–111.

20   Fleming C, Wasson JH, Albertsen PC, Barry MJ, Wennberg JE. A decision analysis of alternative treatment strategies for clinically localized prostate cancer. Prostate Patient Outcomes Research Team. *JAMA* 1993;269(20): 2650–2658.

21   Inouye SK, Studenski S, Tinetti ME, Kuchel GA. Geriatric syndromes: Clinical, research, and policy implications of a core geriatric concept. *J Am Geriatr Soc* 2007;55(5): 780–791.

22   Sharkey JR. The interrelationship of nutritional risk factors, indicators of nutritional risk, and severity of disability among home-delivered meal participants. *Gerontologist* 2002;42(3): 373–380.

23   Carbonin P, Pahor M, Bernabei R, Sgadari A. Is age an independent risk factor of adverse drug reactions in hospitalized medical patients? *J Am Geriatr Soc* 1991;39(11): 1093–1099.

24   Erber R, Wegner DM, Therriault N. On being cool and collected: Mood regulation in anticipation of social interaction. *J Pers Soc Psychol* 1996;70(4): 757–766.

25   Cattan M, Kime N, Bagnall AM. The use of telephone befriending in low level support for socially isolated older people—An evaluation. *Health Soc Care Community* 2011;19(2): 198–206.

26   Bolmsjo I. Existential issues in palliative care—Interviews with cancer patients. *J Palliat Care* 2000;16(2): 20–24.

27   LeMay K, Wilson KG. Treatment of existential distress in life threatening illness: A review of manualized interventions. *Clin Psychol Rev* 2008;28(3): 472–493.

28   Chochinov HM, Kristjanson LJ, Breitbart W et al. Effect of dignity therapy on distress and end-of-life experience in terminally ill patients: A randomised controlled trial. *Lancet Oncol* 2011;12(8): 753–762.

29   Oleckno WA, Blacconiere MJ. Relationship of religiosity to wellness and other health-related behaviors and outcomes. *Psychol Rep* 1991;68(3 Pt 1): 819–826.

30   Folstein MF, Folstein SE, McHugh PR. "Mini-mental state". A practical method for grading the cognitive state of patients for the clinician. *J Psychiatr Res* 1975;12(3): 189–198.

31   Royall DR, Cordes JA, Polk M. CLOX: An executive clock drawing task. *J Neurol Neurosurg Psychiatry* 1998;64(5): 588–594.

32   Borson S, Scanlan J, Brush M, Vitaliano P, Dokmak A. The mini-cog: A cognitive 'vital signs' measure for dementia screening in multi-lingual elderly. *Int J Geriatr Psychiatry* 2000;15(11): 1021–1027.

33   Mitchell SL, Teno JM, Kiely DK et al. The clinical course of advanced dementia. *N Engl J Med* 2009;361(16): 1529–1538.

34   Lawlor PG, Bruera ED. Delirium in patients with advanced cancer. *Hematol Oncol Clin North Am* 2002;16(3): 701–714.

35   Lawlor PG, Gagnon B, Mancini IL et al. Occurrence, causes, and outcome of delirium in patients with advanced cancer: A prospective study. *Arch Intern Med* 2000;160(6): 786–794.

36   Twillman RK, Manetto C. Concurrent psychotherapy and pharmacotherapy in the treatment of depression and anxiety in cancer patients. *Psychooncology* 1998;7(4): 285–290.

37 Fick DM, Cooper JW, Wade WE, Waller JL, Maclean JR, Beers MH. Updating the Beers criteria for potentially inappropriate medication use in older adults: Results of a U.S. consensus panel of experts. *Arch Intern Med* 2003;163(22): 2716–2724.

38 Diokno AC. Epidemiology and psychosocial aspects of incontinence. *Urol Clin North Am* 1995;22(3): 481–485.

39 Voigt JC, Kenefick JS. Sacrococcygeal chordoma presenting with stress incontinence of urine. *S Afr Med J* 1971;45(20): 557.

40 Ehrlich RM, Walsh GO. Urinary incontinence secondary to brain neoplasm. *Urology* 1973;1(3): 249–250.

41 Diokno AC, Brown MB, Herzog AR. Relationship between use of diuretics and continence status in the elderly. *Urology* 1991;38(1): 39–42.

42 Johnson TM, 2nd, Busby-Whitehead J. Diagnostic assessment of geriatric urinary incontinence. *Am J Med Sci* 1997;314(4): 250–256.

43 Tam-McDevitt J. Polypharmacy, aging, and cancer. *Oncology* (Williston Park) 2008;22(9): 1052–1055, discussion 55, 58, 60.

44 Koroukian SM, Beaird H, Madigan E, Diaz M. End-of-life expenditures by Ohio Medicaid beneficiaries dying of cancer. *Health Care Financ Rev* 2006;28(2): 65–80.

45 Pautex S, Berger A, Chatelain C, Herrmann F, Zulian GB. Symptom assessment in elderly cancer patients receiving palliative care. *Crit Rev Oncol Hematol* 2003;47(3): 281–286.

46 Barford KL, D'Olimpio JT. Symptom management in geriatric oncology: Practical treatment considerations and current challenges. *Curr Treat Options Oncol* 2008;9(2–3): 204–214.

47 Hurria A. Geriatric assessment in oncology practice. *J Am Geriatr Soc* 2009;57 Suppl 2: S246–S249.

48 Matthews BA. Role and gender differences in cancer-related distress: A comparison of survivor and caregiver self-reports. *Oncol Nurs Forum* 2003;30(3): 493–499.

49 Akpinar B, Kucukguclu O, Yener G. Effects of gender on burden among caregivers of Alzheimer's patients. *J Nurs Scholarsh* 2011;43(3): 248–254.

50 Garlo K, O'Leary JR, Van Ness PH, Fried TR. Burden in caregivers of older adults with advanced illness. *J Am Geriatr Soc* 2010;58(12): 2315–2322.

51 Andruccioli J, Russo MM, Bruschi A et al. Caregiver evaluation in hospice: Application of a semi-structured interview. *Am J Hosp Palliat Care* 2011;28(6): 393–397.

52 Beach SR, Schulz R, Williamson GM, Miller LS, Weiner MF, Lance CE. Risk factors for potentially harmful informal caregiver behavior. *J Am Geriatr Soc* 2005;53(2): 255–261.

53 Empeno J, Raming NT, Irwin SA, Nelesen RA, Lloyd LS. The hospice caregiver support project: Providing support to reduce caregiver stress. *J Palliat Med* 2011;14(5): 593–597.

54 Ramsaroop SD, Reid MC, Adelman RD. Completing an advance directive in the primary care setting: What do we need for success? *J Am Geriatr Soc* 2007;55(2): 277–283.

55 Detering KM, Hancock AD, Reade MC, Silvester W. The impact of advance care planning on end of life care in elderly patients: Randomised controlled trial. *BMJ* 2010;340: c1345.

97

Advanced chronic obstructive pulmonary disease

GRAEME M. ROCKER, JOANNE YOUNG, J. RANDALL CURTIS

INTRODUCTION

Chronic obstructive pulmonary disease (COPD) is projected to be the third leading cause of death globally by 2020, and prevalence rises while the other medical causes of death in Western society decline.[1-3] Patients with advanced COPD experience a high symptom burden with many feeling breathless all the time.[4] Professional society consensus statements, clinical practice guidelines (CPGs),[5-8] and peer-reviewed literature are promoting more holistic and collaborative approaches to care that address physiological and psychosocial manifestations of chronic respiratory disease and include a palliative dimension. The aim of these efforts is to minimize the suffering and burdens such illnesses place on patients, families, and health-care systems.

A 2012 statement from the American Thoracic Society (ATS) affirms that dyspnea (the cardinal symptom in advanced COPD) is responsible for approximately 50% of tertiary care center admissions.[7] Acute exacerbation of COPD (AECOPD), in many settings, is the most common cause of hospital admission costing an estimated $750 million annually[9] in Canada and approximately $18 billion in the United States.[10] Beyond the significant financial implications, AECOPD not only predicts repeated admissions but also represents an independent risk factor for patient mortality.[11] The increasing burdens that COPD imposes on patients, caregivers, and health-care systems demand significant changes to current models of care. Unless we expedite processes of reform, we will likely fail to deliver the comprehensive care that patients and families need.[12]

Conventional management of COPD has changed little in recent years and professional society guidelines and consensus statements adequately outline standard approaches.[6,13] While these directions are important to follow at all stages of a patient's illness trajectory, this chapter highlights in greater detail some newer understandings and approaches to care for advanced disease. The first section deals with some new information regarding the perception of dyspnea that forms the basis for a rational approach to some innovative treatments, particularly for an advanced disease. The subsequent sections focus on the use of individualized COPD "action plans" (for AECOPD and "dyspnea crises"), the value of engaging patients and their families in meaningful advance care planning (ACP) dialogue, and the efficacy of newer models of care that aim to bridge the gap between chronic disease management and palliative care. The final section reviews the use of opioids as a treatment for dyspnea that is refractory to conventional COPD management.

COPD: SYMPTOM BURDEN

Dyspnea, in simple terms, is the subjective and usually unpleasant experience of discomfort with breathing.[14] For many patients, dyspnea pervades all aspects of their lives. Dyspnea is a significant source of disability, profoundly affecting quality of life. Patients become isolated and often describe themselves as existing rather than living. Dyspnea is nearly universal and, in advanced COPD, is often refractory to conventional treatments.[4,15] The significant physical, emotional, social, and/or spiritual/existential suffering associated with the context of "total dyspnea" has been acknowledged only recently.[7,16]

Dyspnea (like pain) is a multifaceted symptom, which "derives from interactions among physiological, psychological, social and environmental factors, and may induce secondary physiological and behavioral responses,"[7,14] and understanding these various influences is necessary in achieving the goal of effective palliation. The appreciation of a neurobiological basis to dyspnea[17] also offers support for interventions that extend conventional therapies. Similarly, recognition of abnormal muscle physiology and histology[18,19] provides insight into the downward spiral of COPD, the early onset of anaerobic metabolism at low work rates that compounds the intense discomfort felt by patients with hyperinflation,[20] when they breathe close to their total lung capacity.

Functional MRI scanning has provided new insights into the central perception of dyspnea. The amygdala and anterior insular cortex are activated,[7,17] particularly when dyspnea and fear coexist. Fear, anxiety, and panic are common in advanced COPD.[21,22] Anxiolytics seem relatively unhelpful in the management of dyspnea[23,24] but may be useful for treating a coexisting anxiety disorder that can worsen dyspnea symptoms. Cognitive or behavioral therapy can help to treat the combination of anxiety and dyspnea.[25–27] Anxiety has been linked to risk of hospital readmission,[21] to recurrent dyspnea,[28] and to fear of death when dyspnea worsens.[28–30] Fear, anxiety, and panic, when unrecognized, underestimated, and untreated, can cause overwhelming symptoms leading to "dyspnea crises." These crises are defined in a recent ATS consensus statement[31] as a "sustained and severe resting breathing discomfort that occurs in patients with advanced, often life-limiting illness and overwhelms the patient and caregivers' ability to achieve symptom relief." Understanding the components of these crises in individual patients is key to effective management. An example of a patient-specific "action plan" that includes tips for managing "dyspnea crisis" is provided later in this chapter (Figure 97.3).

There are many barriers to effective treatment of impaired psychological function in this patient population; some health-care providers may lack the skills, time, or interest to deal effectively with mental health issues and patients are also reluctant to disclose their symptoms avoiding the additional stigma of a mental health diagnosis. Health-care providers and current systems are simply not well designed or supported for the integration of mental health care into the primary and acute care systems, an important issue to address within health-care reform strategies.[32]

CURRENT APPROACHES TO THE MANAGEMENT OF DYSPNEA IN ADVANCED COPD

The Canadian Thoracic Society (CTS) has recently released a CPG[6] (available via www.copdguidelines.ca) that encapsulates an evidence-based approach to the management of dyspnea (see Figure 97.1).

This CPG[6] builds on the concept of the dyspnea ladder described some years ago[33] and emphasizes a stepwise approach through conventional therapies and nonpharmacological approaches towards palliation with carefully initiated and titrated opioids for refractory dyspnea. In advanced COPD, conventional therapies should be maintained and optimized; however, the symptomatic benefit realized by these biomedical approaches may wane and additional supportive initiatives may be required. The relative social isolation that comes with advanced disease will be one explanation of COPD as an independent risk factor for the development of depression.[34] Effective initiatives need to address not just the physical but also the psychosocial and existential suffering for both patients and caregivers that is so pervasive and damaging.[35,36]

CONVENTIONAL INTERVENTIONS FOR COPD

Inhaled therapy

Inhaled bronchodilator therapy remains a mainstay of treatment and should be optimized as per CPGs.[6,13] Various formulations and delivery devices are available (metered dose inhalers and spacers, dry powder inhalers, or wet nebulizers)

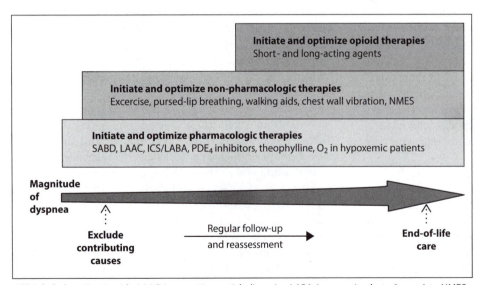

ICS, Inhaled corticosteroids; LAAC, Long-acting anticholinergics; LABA, Long-acting beta-2 agonists; NMES, Neuromuscular electrical stimulation; O₂, Oxygen; PDE₄, Phosphodiesterase 4; SABD, Short-acting bronchodilators

Figure 97.1 Comprehensive approach to management of dyspnea in patients with advanced COPD. (From Marciniuk, D.D. et al., Can. Respir. J., 18(2), 1, 2011.)

and should be tailored to each patient's ability to use them effectively. For most patients with advanced disease, the combination of an "as-needed" short-acting beta-agonist and a long-acting anticholinergic such as daily tiotropium is a standard initial approach. Where a long-acting anticholinergic is unavailable, a short-acting anticholinergic (ipratropium bromide) can be taken by a metered dose inhaler and a spacer with a dosing regimen that might reach a maximum of 4–6 puffs QID. For many patients with advanced COPD, the addition of a combination inhaler containing a long-acting beta-agonist (LABA) and an inhaled corticosteroid (ICS) provides benefit in terms of symptom management and quality of life.[37] Combining a long-acting anticholinergic agent and a LABA/ICS combination has been shown to improve health-related quality of life[37,38]; however, in advanced COPD, we should recognize that these treatments will be limited in what they can achieve.

Systemic therapy

There has been a resurgence of interest in theophylline-like drugs based on anti-inflammatory activities and the reduction of oxidative stress that is increasingly recognized as a feature of COPD.[39] Side effects, however, often outweigh benefits; monitoring of blood levels and risks of drug toxicity through interactions with some antibiotics (e.g., clarithromycin) poses potential limitations to their use.

Phosphodiesterase 4 inhibitors

Phosphodiesterase 4 (PDE_4) inhibitors are the first new therapy for COPD in nearly 20 years. However, initial enthusiasm has been tempered by their side effect profile. PDE_4 inhibitors may be considered in selected patients with advanced disease who have a history of frequent exacerbations and a chronic bronchitis phenotype. PDE_4 inhibitors have been shown to reduce key inflammatory cells and mediators; however, they are not bronchodilators and their effect on dyspnea is modest.[40] The most common adverse effects include diarrhea, nausea, headache, and weight loss and they should be used with caution in cachectic patients and those with a history of mental illness and depression.

Corticosteroids

Global Initiative for Chronic Obstructive Lung Disease (GOLD) statements recommend that systemic steroids not be used over the long term due to significant side effects and lack of compelling data suggesting significant benefit.[41] Nevertheless, despite this lack of data showing efficacy, occasionally, patients feel long-term steroids are helpful in this setting, and for patients approaching terminal stages, clinicians could consider an "n of 1" trial to ensure patients are not denied a reasonable approach that may provide them with improvement in symptom control.

Oxygen therapy

DURING ACUTE EXACERBATIONS OF COPD

The use of oxygen in an AECOPD, especially for patients with baseline hypercarbia, should be carefully controlled. A recent RCT demonstrated an excess mortality in patients treated with uncontrolled oxygen en route to hospital[42] and the dangers of excess use of oxygen have been recognized since the 1960s.[43] It is critically important to choose the appropriate delivery device. The use of nasal prongs should be avoided or limited since it is difficult to monitor the fraction of inspired oxygen (FiO_2) in a distressed patient. The safest approach is to use Venturi masks to supply an FiO_2 of 24% or 28% to maintain an SpO_2 close to 89%. Inappropriately high FiO_2 can cause an increase in $PaCO_2$ by several mechanisms: worsening of V/Q mismatch through reversal of established pulmonary hypoxic vasoconstriction, a lower minute ventilation through reduced hypoxic drive (for some patients), and reverse of the Haldane effect that causes displacement of CO_2 from more oxygenated hemoglobin into plasma.

LONG-TERM OXYGEN THERAPY

For patients who are hypoxemic, long-term oxygen therapy (LTOT) is prescribed for its benefits in reducing morbidity and mortality. Eligibility criteria vary between and within countries. While beneficial for many, LTOT can interfere with self-image, may limit patients to their homes, and thus restricts activities that might otherwise contribute to a better quality of life. While some patients will dislike the technical focus on machines, oxygen readings, or on unacceptable limitations, others adapt and endure benefiting in some cases from improved health-related quality of life.[44]

SUPPLEMENTAL OXYGEN FOR THE MILDLY HYPOXEMIC PATIENT

Based on current evidence,[45,46] oxygen therapy for mild hypoxemia (i.e., $PaO_2 > 55$ without evidence of end-organ damage or $PaO_2 > 60$ with evidence of end-organ damage) cannot be recommended for routine use. Nevertheless, patients and caregivers often request oxygen in this setting and need to be helped to understand that their level of dyspnea does not necessarily equate with "oxygen starvation." An "n of 1" therapeutic trial of oxygen may be indicated in the hospice setting for treatment of patients with persistent dyspnea despite maximal therapy (see other treatments for refractory dyspnea in the following texts).

OTHER TREATMENTS FOR DYSPNEA

Chest wall vibration techniques and neuromuscular electrical stimulation have been shown in some recent RCTS to be promising adjuncts to conventional treatment. They are discussed in more detail in a recent CPG[6] but use in a palliative phase is likely to be limited.

NONPHARMACOLOGICAL APPROACHES: PATIENT SELF-MANAGEMENT EDUCATION FOR COPD

Patient self-management education is a core component of pulmonary rehabilitation programs. Self-management strategies facilitating patients' capacity and motivation have also been the focus of initiatives related to the chronic care model (CCM) described by Wagner.[47] Education can be a stand-alone intervention or one component of a more comprehensive model of care (community- or facility-based) that places patients and families at the center. Such models emphasize the importance of the values, emotions, hopes, and fears of the patients and families rather than the needs of the health-care system. A meta-analysis of self-management education (1066 patients, 8 trials) has confirmed improvements in health status and reduction in hospital admissions.[48] A recent trial of patient self-management for patients with COPD was terminated early due to increased mortality in the intervention cohort.[49] While reasons for increased mortality in this study are unclear, most evidence to date suggests that self-management programs are beneficial. The potential for harm in some circumstances will need further study.

As a generalization, self-management programs tend to include disease-specific education, promotion of healthy lifestyles, and tips on how to save energy and manage emotional symptoms, and they may include the use of an "action plan" that helps patients decide when to initiate antibiotics and/or oral corticosteroids as an early intervention for an impending AECOPD[50–52] to shorten recovery[53] and reduce morbidity and health-care utilization.[54] Professional societies have espoused the use of "action plans" but emphasize the need for *effective* instruction and reinforcement.[8] Recent RCTs in Canada,[55] the United States,[56] and Europe[57] have confirmed the efficacy of action plans within a broader model of self-management. Reductions (~by 40%) in emergency room (ER) visits and hospital readmission rates were similar in the three studies.

PULMONARY REHABILITATION AND INTEGRATED CARE

Pulmonary rehabilitation "is designed to reduce symptoms, optimize functional status, increase participation and reduce health care costs through stabilizing or reversing systemic manifestations of the disease."[58] Exercise is central to pulmonary rehabilitation, reducing both the impact of breathlessness and its incidence through increased fitness and activity and by interrupting the "spiral of disability"[18] (Figure 97.2). Pulmonary rehabilitation is supported by a substantial body of evidence including a Cochrane review[59] testifying to improvements in dyspnea, exercise tolerance, functional capacity, health-related quality of life, and health-care utilization.[54,55] Effects can wane over time[60] and it should be considered early rather than late in the clinical trajectory.[61] Once patients are

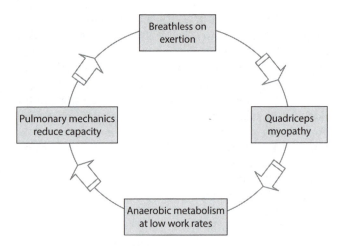

Figure 97.2 *The COPD spiral. (From Polkey, M.I. and Moxham, J., Clin. Med., 6(2), 190, 2006.)*

bed- or chair-bound by severe COPD or suffer dyspnea at rest, opportunities to improve symptoms and function inevitably fade and patients should be referred for pulmonary rehabilitation before this point.

Participants typically attend 6–12 weeks of individualized exercise training, self-management education, nutritional counseling, and psychosocial support. Social aspects of these programs should not be underestimated and some improvements are associated with relief from ongoing anxiety and depression that occurs in the absence of changes in lung function.[62,63] Some advocate for initiating these programs during an acute admission.[64] For the majority of patients with COPD who might not be able to gain access to facility-based programs, Maltais[65] has demonstrated equivalent benefit of home-based pulmonary rehabilitation, a concept that will likely be explored further as a component of more community-based and integrated care.

The ATS defines integrated care as "a continuum of patient-centered services organized as a care delivery value chain for patients with chronic conditions with the goal of achieving the optimal daily functioning and health status for the individual patient and to achieve and maintain the individual's independence and functioning in the community."[8] Hopefully this "value chain of services" will come to include palliative care so discussions about goals of care and ACP will become logical components of this continuum.

GAPS IN CARE

The traditional approach to COPD is often one of treating the AECOPD. The goal is hospital discharge, facilitated by a plan, but not a true "discharge plan" to help the patient reintegrate into and remain within home/community settings. Failing to address the psychosocial dynamics, or needs beyond those of the acute admission, primes patients and the health-care system for failure, with high short-term readmission rates.[21,66,67] Moreover, patients have long been known to hide their symptoms from clinicians who cannot manage them effectively.[68] Clinician ineffectiveness contributes to patients' sense of isolation, helplessness, and frustration.[30,69] The significant mismatches between the care we provide and the care that allows patients to reach more personally meaningful and acceptable goals are a common care gap in COPD.[69]

Acknowledgment of this important gap in care should underpin widespread efforts in favor of a coordinated multidisciplinary approach to effective palliation and support. A systematic review by Adams supports the efficacy of applying Wagner's CCM to COPD.[70] We cannot continue to ignore the many papers describing the sense of isolation, misery, and abandonment of those living with advanced COPD.[22,30,71–73] To overcome the frustration and inadequacies of care, we should be aiming to ensure optimal medical treatment within a more patient-focused approach, one that improves access and is responsive to needs regardless of clinical setting.[74] More efficient use of limited resources[75,76] and improved patient/family satisfaction with care[77] should follow. National support for such strategies are in their infancy in the United States and Canada but further advanced in the United Kingdom where there are clearly delineated standards and appointment of physician leaders with responsibilities in both hospital and community settings.[78]

Examples of an expanded approach were recently described by Booth et al.[79] In Cambridge, United Kingdom, a community-based program, the "Breathlessness Intervention Service" (BIS), focuses on patient-identified needs, symptoms, and concerns of informal carers, a flexible approach responsive to patient and carer(s), education, and support. The BIS is described elsewhere in more detail,[33,79] but the essence of this philosophy is to offer individualized nonpharmacological interventions such as anxiety management (relaxation, visualization, and meditation techniques), positive psychological support, and attention to national guidelines and standards and to COPD research objectives and best practices.[80] Participants indicated the importance they attached to having their concerns addressed.[80]

In Canada, the INSPIRED program in Halifax brings together a new multidisciplinary team of health professionals who visit patients during a hospitalization for an AECOPD and then in their homes to provide evidence-based education[55,56] "action plans," sensitive ACP, and, where necessary, optimal palliative care. In addition to consistently positive participant feedback, ER visits and hospital admissions have been reduced by ~70%.[77] Some patients have benefited from "action plans" that provide step-by-step advice on how to manage recurrent "dyspnea crises" and include using various opioids in these settings, according to circumstance[81] (Figure 97.3). As Booth states, "In health services facing important financial constraints the most cost and clinically effective model may be services like INSPIRED, BIS…that can work with existing teams to transfer a psychologically and psychosocially informed approach to people with early or advanced chronic respiratory illness preventing future morbidity and helping those facing death compassionately."[79]

COMMUNICATION AND ADVANCE CARE PLANNING: AN OPPORTUNITY TO "CARE"

Traditionally, ACP has been envisioned in terms of completing advance directive documents as a way to support and protect patient autonomy for times of potential loss of decision-making capacity. More often than not, discussions around goals of care occur as a clinician-centered "one-shot" effort ("code status" discussion) that often occurs during an illness crisis[82] and in suboptimal settings (the ER or ICU),[83] with potential for an inadequate or erroneous representation of patients' care values/preferences. Prognostic uncertainty, patients' and families' "natural aging" view of declining quality of life in advancing COPD,[84] and increasing institutional pressures (time, personnel, space) militate against continuing the current approach to ACP.

To achieve the goal of informed choice in the context of COPD, clinicians need to provide opportunities for patients, and for those they choose to include, to explore COPD-related current and future uncertainties as manifested in their experiences, hopes, and fears. Incapacitating dyspnea, increasing dependency, isolation-induced social death, perceived stigma, and profound uncertainty-related anxiety experienced by many of these patients and their intimate others indicate the need for ACP that presents the positive aspects of palliation and focuses on *care*.

This type of "caring" improves outcomes for patients and their families and is especially relevant for patients with COPD whose clinicians often hesitate to initiate ACP in a timely way. The barriers to effective ACP[83] are cited as prognostic uncertainty, potential to erode patients' hope, time constraints, and inadequate communication skills.[85–88] These barriers can be overcome and interventions to identify patient-specific barriers and feed this information back to patients and clinicians have improved the occurrence and quality of communication about end-of-life care.[89] Furthermore, many patients desire and/or are open to communication about end-of-life care and ACP[86,88,90] when it is done in a timely, sensitive way, despite clinicians' significant and well-documented concerns.[86,91,92] In a recent review, Patel reaffirms the disease-specific triggers that might signal a time to engage the patient and family in ACP ($FEV_1 < 30\%$, oxygen dependence, one or more hospital admissions in the last year with AECOPD, weight loss/cachexia, decreased functional status, increasing dependence on others, age > 70, and lack of additional therapeutic options).[83] Considerations include provision of noninvasive ventilation (BiPAP) or intubation and conventional mechanical ventilation. Recent publications address the role of noninvasive ventilation and how it may (or may not) fit with patients' overall goals of care.[93,94]

Ultimately, the timing, setting, and manner in which ACP occurs should firmly reflect the needs of the patient and family or substitute decision maker rather than those of health-care providers or institutions. Competence and experience are key; professional discipline, less so. Regardless of who facilitates the discussion, the final step of effective

---

Action plan for shortness of breath (dyspnea)
Created for: [Patient Name ± ID number]
Date: [Insert date plan was created]

A good morning routine to minimize shortness of breath first thing in the morning.

- Take 5 breaths from your incentive spirometer) (slowly open airways). Use 4 times daily as needed.

- Huffing/cough to clear your airway. Do your pursed-lip breathing if this helps.

- Use your blue puffer, gray HandiHaler, and purple puffer as directed (don't forget to use your aerochamber and rinse after your purple puffer). Your blue puffer may be used as often as every four hours as needed.

- Take your long-acting opioid medication [insert name, dose] as directed.

When more short of breath than usual.

- With a slight increase in your shortness of breath at rest (not a result of infection or "crisis"), you can use an extra [insert dose] of your opioid syrup every 1–2 h as needed for "breakthrough" dyspnea between your regular doses.

- For predictable shortness of breath with activity (i.e., getting up, dressed, bathed), time these activities 1/2 hours after your puffers and opioid dosing.

For "crisis" shortness of breath (not due to infection) that comes on suddenly and catches you by surprise:

- Use your hand-held fan and do pursed-lip breathing. Try recovery positions.

- Use 2 puffs of your blue puffer (with aerochamber) or try your nebule instead.

- Adjust oxygen flow from____to____L/min for 10–15 mins only then re-adjust back to____.

- Take your anti-anxiety medication [insert name, doses], 1 tablet under the tongue .

- If not settling, use fentanyl, 12.5 µg, from pre-prepared syringe. Let liquid dissolve under the tongue. Repeat in 10 mins if still not settling and call 911.

For flare-ups of COPD with increased sputum volume and mucky color, use antibiotics and prednisone as per your COPD action plan.

Figure 97.3 *Action plan for shortness of breath.*

patient-centered ACP includes collaborating with physicians and other members of the patient's health-care team so patients' preferences through ACP effectively impact decision making or outcomes. ACP as a patient-centered, ongoing process of adjusting goals of care is much more than a means to an end.[95] It is about improving care throughout the illness trajectory, not just at end of life. Preferences may change after hospitalization,[96] and ACP policies or strategies need to adapt to these changes.

OPIOIDS

An increasing body of evidence supports the use of opioids for refractory dyspnea in patients with advanced COPD. A systematic review in 2002 favored their use for dyspnea (using oral rather than nebulized preparations),[97] but many

of the earlier studies were of limited quality or relevant to real-life experience. While the systematic review conclusion was supported by a subsequent, single, adequately powered, short-term RCT,[98] data on long-term use have only recently become available.[99,100] Long-held biases continue to limit more widespread acceptance by physicians[101] despite recommendations for their use in several recent professional society statements and/or CPGs.[6,102,103] Data from recently completed or ongoing clinical trials are encouraging with benefit outweighing side effects and patients finding them beneficial over the longer term.[99,100] In essence, existing data and clinical experience suggest these medications should be a part of the armamentarium for dyspnea that is not controlled by standard therapy. Our experience through a clinical trial suggests that an initial start low, go slow approach works well[6,99] and helps patients to gain confidence. Often patients are reticent to try opioids, equating them with impending death or fearful of side effects. Sensitive and careful explanations can usually diffuse concerns.[101] Once the daily requirements of an immediate-release preparation (e.g., morphine syrup 1 mg/mL) are established, through a gentle titration schedule, patients can move on to a sustained-release preparation taken daily or twice daily with additional immediate release for "breakthrough" dyspnea. Dyspnea seems to respond to much lower doses of opioids than pain, and if one opioid preparation is not well tolerated, others can be tried. Newer formulations and modes of delivery of fast-acting lipophilic opioids provide new opportunities to incorporate these preparations into patient care plans[15] that seek to provide patients and caregivers with the means to control episodic and frightening dyspnea crises.[81]

CONCLUSIONS

Our health-care systems are faced with the need to care for an aging population significantly burdened with chronic illnesses and frailty.[104,105] As the prevalence of COPD rises, more patients and families will live with the burdens of advanced or "end-stage" COPD than ever before. Within this chapter, we have highlighted some interventions that may help to ease these burdens. We have also provided some concrete examples of models of care that employ interventions and holistic approaches to care that can improve patient and family outcomes. The move towards integrated care approach to COPD will help patients and their families reach informed decisions about care through the trajectory of COPD. Intensive medical treatment focused on increasing survival and holistic, supportive, and palliative approaches focused on quality of life are no longer mutually exclusive within a spectrum of care; the emphasis often simply changes over time. If we truly practice patient-centered care, transitions within this spectrum should occur seamlessly and we will no longer fail our patients "from beginning to end."[106]

REFERENCES

1. Buist AS, McBurnie MA, Vollmer WM, Gillespie S, Burney P, Mannino DM et al. International variation in the prevalence of COPD (the BOLD Study): A population-based prevalence study. *Lancet.* 2007;370(9589):741–750.

2. Jemal A, Ward E, Hao Y, Thun M. Trends in the leading causes of death in the United States, 1970–2002. *JAMA.* 2005;294(10):1255–1259.

3. Mannino DM, Buist AS. Global burden of COPD: Risk factors, prevalence, and future trends. *Lancet.* 2007;370(9589):765–773.

4. Elkington H, White P, Addington-Hall J, Higgs R, Edmonds P. The healthcare needs of chronic obstructive pulmonary disease patients in the last year of life. *Palliat Med.* 2005;19(6):485–491.

5. Hanania NA, Marciniuk DD. A unified front against COPD: Clinical practice guidelines from the American College of Physicians, the American College of Chest Physicians, the American Thoracic Society, and the European Respiratory Society. *Chest.* 2011;140(3):565566.

6. Marciniuk DD, Goodridge D, Hernandez P, Rocker G, Balter M, Bailey P. et al for the Canadian Thoracic Society COPD Committee Dyspnea Expert Working Group. Managing dyspnea in patients with advanced chronic obstructive pulmonary disease: A Canadian Thoracic Society clinical practice guideline. *Can Respir J.* 2011;18(2):1–10.

7. Parshall MB, Schwartzstein RM, Adams L, Banzett RB, Manning HL, Bourbeau J et al. An official American Thoracic Society statement: Update on the mechanisms, assessment, and management of dyspnea. *Am J Respir Crit Care Med.* 2012;185(4):435–452.

8. Nici L, ZuWallack R. An official American Thoracic Society workshop report: The Integrated Care of The COPD Patient. *Proc Am Thorac Soc.* 2012;9(1):9–18.

9. Mittmann N, Kuramoto L, Seung SJ, Haddon JM, Bradley-Kennedy C, Fitzgerald JM. The cost of moderate and severe COPD exacerbations to the Canadian healthcare system. *Respir Med.* 2008;102(3):413421.

10. Mannino DM, Homa DM, Akinbami LJ, Ford ES, Redd SC. Chronic obstructive pulmonary disease surveillance—United States, 1971–2000. *MMWR Surveill Summ.* 2002;51(6):1–16.

11. McGhan R, Radcliff T, Fish R, Sutherland ER, Welsh C, Make B. Predictors of rehospitalization and death after a severe exacerbation of COPD. *Chest.* 2007;132(6):17481755.

12. Rocker GM, Dodek PM, Heyland DK. Toward optimal end-of-life care for patients with advanced chronic obstructive pulmonary disease: Insights from a multicentre study. *Can Respir J.* 2008;15(5):249–254.

13. Qaseem A, Wilt TJ, Weinberger SE, Hanania NA, Criner G, van der Molen T et al. Diagnosis and management of stable chronic obstructive pulmonary disease: A clinical practice guideline update from the American College of Physicians, American College of Chest Physicians, American Thoracic Society, and European Respiratory Society. *Ann Intern Med.* 2011;155(3):179191.

14. Dyspnea. Mechanisms, assessment, and management: A consensus statement. American Thoracic Society. *Am J Respir Crit Care Med.* 1999;159(1):321340.

15. Horton R, Rocker G. Contemporary issues in refractory dyspnoea in advanced chronic obstructive pulmonary disease. *Curr Opin Support Palliat Care.* 2010;4(2):56–62.

16. Abernethy AP, Wheeler JL. Total dyspnoea. *Curr Opin Support Palliat Care.* 2008;2(2):110–113.

17. von Leupoldt A, Sommer T, Kegat S, Baumann HJ, Klose H, Dahme B et al. The unpleasantness of perceived dyspnea is processed in the anterior insula and amygdala. *Am J Respir Crit Care Med.* 2008;177(9):1026–1032.

18. Polkey MI, Moxham J. Attacking the disease spiral in chronic obstructive pulmonary disease. *Clin Med.* 2006;6(2):190–196.

19. Rabinovich RA, Vilaro J. Structural and functional changes of peripheral muscles in chronic obstructive pulmonary disease patients. *Curr Opin Pulm Med.* 2010;16(2):123–133.

20. O'Donnell DE, Webb KA. The major limitation to exercise performance in COPD is dynamic hyperinflation. *J Appl Physiol.* 2008;105(2):753–755; discussion 5–7.

21. Gudmundsson G, Gislason T, Janson C, Lindberg E, Hallin R, Ulrik CS et al. Risk factors for rehospitalisation in COPD: Role of health status, anxiety and depression. *Eur Respir J.* 2005;26(3):414–419.

22. Gore JM, Brophy CJ, Greenstone MA. How well do we care for patients with end stage chronic obstructive pulmonary disease (COPD)? A comparison of palliative care and quality of life in COPD and lung cancer. *Thorax.* 2000;55(12):1000–1006.

23. Rose C, Wallace L, Dickson R, Ayres J, Lehman R, Searle Y et al. The most effective psychologically-based treatments to reduce anxiety and panic in patients with chronic obstructive pulmonary disease (COPD): A systematic review. *Patient Educ Couns.* 2002;47(4):311–318.

24 Simon ST, Higginson IJ, Booth S, Harding R, Bausewein C. Benzodiazepines for the relief of breathlessness in advanced malignant and non-malignant diseases in adults. *Cochrane Database Syst Rev.* (1):CD007354.

25 Eiser N, West C, Evans S, Jeffers A, Quirk F. Effects of psychotherapy in moderately severe COPD: A pilot study. *Eur Respir J.* 1997;10(7):1581–1584.

26 Manning HL. Dyspnea treatment. *Respir Care.* 2000;45(11):1342–1350; discussion 50–54.

27 Smoller JW, Pollack MH, Otto MW, Rosenbaum JF, Kradin RL. Panic anxiety, dyspnea, and respiratory disease. Theoretical and clinical considerations. *Am J Respir Crit Care Med.* 1996;154(1):6–17.

28 Bailey PH. The dyspnea-anxiety-dyspnea cycle—COPD patients' stories of breathlessness: "It's scary/when you can't breathe". *Qual Health Res.* 2004;14(6):760–778.

29 Bailey PH. Death stories: Acute exacerbations of chronic obstructive pulmonary disease. *Qual Health Res.* 2001;11(3):322–338.

30 Booth S, Silvester S, Todd C. Breathlessness in cancer and chronic obstructive pulmonary disease: Using a qualitative approach to describe the experience of patients and carers. *Palliat Support Care.* 2003;1(4):337–344.

31 Mularski RA, Reinke LF, Carrieri-Kohlman V, Fisher MD, Campbell M, Rocker G. et al. An official ATS Workshop report: Assessment and palliative management of dyspnea crisis. *Ann Am Thorac Soc.* October;10(5):S98–S106. PubMed PMID: 24161068. Epub 2013/10/29.

32 Kunik ME, Veazey C, Cully JA, Souchek J, Graham DP, Hopko D et al. COPD education and cognitive behavioral therapy group treatment for clinically significant symptoms of depression and anxiety in COPD patients: A randomized controlled trial. *Psychol Med.* 2008;38(3):385–396.

33 Rocker GM, Sinuff T, Horton R, Hernandez P. Advanced chronic obstructive pulmonary disease: Innovative approaches to palliation. *J Palliat Med.* 2007;10(3):783–797.

34 Schane RE, Woodruff PG, Dinno A, Covinsky KE, Walter LC. Prevalence and risk factors for depressive symptoms in persons with chronic obstructive pulmonary disease. *J Gen Intern Med.* 2008;23(11):1757–1762.

35 Gysels MH, Higginson IJ. Caring for a person in advanced illness and suffering from breathlessness at home: Threats and resources. *Palliat Support Care.* 2009;7(2):153–162.

36 Simpson AC, Young J, Donahue M, Rocker G. A day at a time: Caregiving on the edge in advanced COPD. *Int J Chron Obstruct Pulmon Dis.* 2010;5:141–151.

37 Calverley PM, Anderson JA, Celli B, Ferguson GT, Jenkins C, Jones PW et al. Salmeterol and fluticasone propionate and survival in chronic obstructive pulmonary disease. *N Engl J Med.* 2007;356(8):775–789.

38 Aaron SD, Vandemheen KL, Fergusson D, Maltais F, Bourbeau J, Goldstein R et al. Tiotropium in combination with placebo, salmeterol, or fluticasone-salmeterol for treatment of chronic obstructive pulmonary disease: A randomized trial. *Ann Intern Med.* 2007;146(8):545–555.

39 Barnes PJ. Frontrunners in novel pharmacotherapy of COPD. *Curr Opin Pharmacol.* 2008;8(3):300–307.

40 Global Initiative for Chronic Obstructive Pulmonary Disease. Global strategy for the diagnosis, management, and prevention of chronic obstructive pulmonary disease. Updated 2010. Accessed at www.goldcopd.org on June 5, 2012.

41 Pauwels RA, Buist AS, Calverley PM, Jenkins CR, Hurd SS. Global strategy for the diagnosis, management, and prevention of chronic obstructive pulmonary disease. NHLBI/WHO Global Initiative for Chronic Obstructive Lung Disease (GOLD) Workshop summary. *Am J Respir Crit Care Med.* 2001;163(5):1256–1276.

42 Austin MA, Wills KE, Blizzard L, Walters EH, Wood-Baker R. Effect of high flow oxygen on mortality in chronic obstructive pulmonary disease patients in prehospital setting: Randomised controlled trial. *BMJ.* 2010;341:c5462.

43 Campbell EJ. Respiratory failure: The relation between oxygen concentrations of inspired air and arterial blood. *Lancet.* 1960 Jul 2;2(7140):10–11.

44 Eaton T, Garrett JE, Young P, Fergusson W, Kolbe J, Rudkin S et al. Ambulatory oxygen improves quality of life of COPD patients: A randomised controlled study. *Eur Respir J.* 2002;20(2):306–312.

45 Abernethy AP, McDonald CF, Frith PA, Clark K, Herndon JE, 2nd, Marcello J et al. Effect of palliative oxygen versus room air in relief of breathlessness in patients with refractory dyspnoea: A double-blind, randomised controlled trial. *Lancet.* 2010;376(9743):784–793.

46 Uronis H, McCrory DC, Samsa G, Currow D, Abernethy A. Symptomatic oxygen for non-hypoxaemic chronic obstructive pulmonary disease. *Cochrane Database Syst Rev.* 2011(6):CD006429.

47 Wagner EH. Chronic disease management: What will it take to improve care for chronic illness? *Eff Clin Pract.* 1998;1(1):2–4.

48 Effing T, Monninkhof EM, van der Valk PD, van der Palen J, van Herwaarden CL, Partidge MR et al. Self-management education for patients with chronic obstructive pulmonary disease. *Cochrane Database Syst Rev.* 2007(4):CD002990.

49 Fan VS, Gaziano JM, Lew R, Bourbeau J, Adams SG, Leatherman S et al. A comprehensive care management program to prevent chronic obstructive pulmonary disease hospitalizations: A randomized, controlled trial. *Ann Intern Med.* 2012;156(10):673–683.

50 Bischoff EW, Hamd DH, Sedeno M, Benedetti A, Schermer TR, Bernard S et al. Effects of written action plan adherence on COPD exacerbation recovery. *Thorax.* 2010;66(1):26–31.

51 Trappenburg JC, Koevoets L, de Weert-van Oene GH, Monninkhof EM, Bourbeau J, Troosters T et al. Action Plan to enhance self-management and early detection of exacerbations in COPD patients; a multicenter RCT. *BMC Pulm Med.* 2009;9:52.

52 Walters JA, Turnock AC, Walters EH, Wood-Baker R. Action plans with limited patient education only for exacerbations of chronic obstructive pulmonary disease. *Cochrane Database Syst Rev.* (5):CD005074.

53 Wilkinson TM, Donaldson GC, Hurst JR, Seemungal TA, Wedzicha JA. Early therapy improves outcomes of exacerbations of chronic obstructive pulmonary disease. *Am J Respir Crit Care Med.* 2004;169(12):1298–1303.

54 Bourbeau J, Nault D, Dang-Tan T. Self-management and behaviour modification in COPD. *Patient Educ Couns.* 2004;52(3):271–277.

55 Bourbeau J, Julien M, Maltais F, Rouleau M, Beaupre A, Begin R et al. Reduction of hospital utilization in patients with chronic obstructive pulmonary disease: A disease-specific self-management intervention. *Arch Intern Med.* 2003;163(5):585–591.

56 Rice KL, Dewan N, Bloomfield HE, Grill J, Schult TM, Nelson DB et al. Disease management program for chronic obstructive pulmonary disease: A randomized controlled trial. *Am J Respir Crit Care Med.* 2010;182(7):890–896.

57 Casas A, Troosters T, Garcia-Aymerich J, Roca J, Hernandez C, Alonso A et al. Integrated care prevents hospitalisations for exacerbations in COPD patients. *Eur Respir J.* 2006;28(1):123–130.

58 Nici L, Donner C, Wouters E, Zuwallack R, Ambrosino N, Bourbeau J et al. American Thoracic Society/European Respiratory Society statement on pulmonary rehabilitation. *Am J Respir Crit Care Med.* 2006;173(12):1390–1413.

59 Lacasse Y, Brosseau L, Milne S, Martin S, Wong E, Guyatt GH et al. Pulmonary rehabilitation for chronic obstructive pulmonary disease. *Cochrane Database Syst Rev.* 2002(3):CD003793.

60 Soicher JE, Mayo NE, Gauvin L, Hanley JA, Bernard S, Maltais F et al. Trajectories of endurance activity following pulmonary rehabilitation in COPD patients. *Eur Respir J.* 2011;39(2):272–278.

61 Vogiatzis I, Simoes DC, Stratakos G, Kourepini E, Terzis G, Manta P et al. Effect of pulmonary rehabilitation on muscle remodelling in cachectic patients with COPD. *Eur Respir J.* 2010;36(2):301–310.

62 Harrison SL, Greening NJ, Williams JE, Morgan MD, Steiner MC, Singh SJ. Have we underestimated the efficacy of pulmonary rehabilitation in improving mood? *Respir Med.* 2011;106(6):838–844.

63 Nici L, Lareau S, ZuWallack R. Pulmonary rehabilitation in the treatment of chronic obstructive pulmonary disease. *Am Fam Physician.* 2010;82(6):655–660.

64 Eaton T, Young P, Fergusson W, Moodie L, Zeng I, O'Kane F et al. Does early pulmonary rehabilitation reduce acute health-care utilization in COPD patients admitted with an exacerbation? A randomized controlled study. *Respirology.* 2009;14(2):230–238.

65 Maltais F, Bourbeau J, Shapiro S, Lacasse Y, Perrault H, Baltzan M et al. Effects of home-based pulmonary rehabilitation in patients with chronic obstructive pulmonary disease: A randomized trial. *Ann Intern Med.* 2008;149(12):869–878.

66 Ng TP, Niti M, Tan WC, Cao Z, Ong KC, Eng P. Depressive symptoms and chronic obstructive pulmonary disease: Effect on mortality, hospital readmission, symptom burden, functional status, and quality of life. *Arch Intern Med.* 2007;167(1):60–67.

67 Gruffydd-Jones K, Langley-Johnson C, Dyer C, Badlan K, Ward S. What are the needs of patients following discharge from hospital after an acute exacerbation of chronic obstructive pulmonary disease (COPD)? *Prim Care Respir J.* 2007;16(6):363–368.

68 Roberts DK, Thorne SE, Pearson C. The experience of dyspnea in late-stage cancer. Patients' and nurses' perspectives. *Cancer Nurs.* 1993;16(4):310–320.

69 Simpson AC, Rocker GM. Advanced chronic obstructive pulmonary disease: Rethinking models of care. *QJM.* 2008;101(9):697–704.

70 Adams SG, Smith PK, Allan PF, Anzueto A, Pugh JA, Cornell JE. Systematic review of the chronic care model in chronic obstructive pulmonary disease prevention and management. *Arch Intern Med.* 2007;167(6):551–561.

71 Edmonds P, Karlsen S, Khan S, Addington-Hall J. A comparison of the palliative care needs of patients dying from chronic respiratory diseases and lung cancer. *Palliat Med.* 2001;15(4):287–295.

72 Elkington H, White P, Addington-Hall J, Higgs R, Pettinari C. The last year of life of COPD: A qualitative study of symptoms and services. *Respir Med.* 2004;98(5):439–445.

73 Seamark DA, Blake SD, Seamark CJ, Halpin DM. Living with severe chronic obstructive pulmonary disease (COPD): Perceptions of patients and their carers. An interpretative phenomenological analysis. *Palliat Med.* 2004;18(7):619–625.

74 Gysels M, Higginson IJ. Access to services for patients with chronic obstructive pulmonary disease: The invisibility of breathlessness. *J Pain Symptom Manage.* 2008;36(5):451–460.

75 Morgan MD. Integrated care for COPD. What exactly do we mean? *Chron Respir Dis.* 2008;5(3):131–132.

76 Seemungal TA, Wedzicha JA. Integrated care: A new model for COPD management? *Eur Respir J.* 2006;28(1):4–6.

77 Young J, Simpson AC, Demmons J, Conrad W, Rocker G. Evaluating the impacts of "INSPIRED": A new outreach program for patients and families living with advanced chronic obstructive pulmonary disease (COPD). *Am J Respir Crit Care Med.* 2012;185:A3732.

78 British Thoracic Society/The Primary Care Respiratory Society UK. Improving and Integrating Respiratory Services in the NHS, (accessed June 2012). Available from http//www.impressresp.com, Contract.

79 Booth S, Bausewein C, Rocker G. New models of care for advanced lung disease. *Prog Palliat Care.* 2011;19:254–263.

80 Booth S, Farquhar M, Gysels M, Bausewein C, Higginson IJ. The impact of a breathlessness intervention service (BIS) on the lives of patients with intractable dyspnea: A qualitative phase 1 study. *Palliat Support Care.* 2006;4:287–293.

81 Rocker G. Palliation of Dyspnea. *Chr Resp Dis.* 2012;9(1):49–50.

82 Barnard D. Advance care planning is not about "getting it right". *J Palliat Med.* 2002;5(4):475–481.

83 Patel K, Janssen DJ, Curtis JR. Advance care planning in COPD. *Respirology.* 2012;17(1):72–78.

84 Pinnock H, Kendall M, Murray SA, Worth A, Levack P, Porter M et al. Living and dying with severe chronic obstructive pulmonary disease: Multi-perspective longitudinal qualitative study. *BMJ.* 2011;342:d142.

85 Knauft E, Nielsen EL, Engelberg RA, Patrick DL, Curtis JR. Barriers and facilitators to end-of-life care communication for patients with COPD. *Chest.* 2005;127(6):2188–2196.

86 Goodridge D. People with chronic obstructive pulmonary disease at the end of life: A review of the literature. *Int J Palliat Nurs.* 2006;12(8):390–396.

87 Gott M, Gardiner C, Small N, Payne S, Seamark D, Barnes S et al. Barriers to advance care planning in chronic obstructive pulmonary disease. *Palliat Med.* 2009;23(7):642–648.

88 Spence A, Hasson F, Waldron M, Kernohan WG, McLaughlin D, Watson B et al. Professionals delivering palliative care to people with COPD: Qualitative study. *Palliat Med.* 2009;23(2):126–131.

89 Au DH, Udris EM, Engelberg RA, Diehr PH, Bryson CL, Reinke LF et al. A randomized trial to improve communication about end-of-life care among patients with COPD. *Chest.* 2012;141(3):726–735.

90 Reinke LF, Slatore CG, Uman J, Udris EM, Moss BR, Engelberg RA et al. Patient-clinician communication about end-of-life care topics: Is anyone talking to patients with chronic obstructive pulmonary disease? *J Palliat Med.* 2011;14(8):923–928.

91 Hansen-Flaschen J. Chronic obstructive pulmonary disease: The last year of life. *Respir Care.* 2004;49(1):90–97.

92 Heffner JE. Advance care planning in chronic obstructive pulmonary disease: Barriers and opportunities. *Curr Opin Pulm Med.* 2011;17(2):103–109.

93 Curtis JR, Cook DJ, Sinuff T, White DB, Hill N, Keenan SP et al. Noninvasive positive pressure ventilation in critical and palliative care settings: Understanding the goals of therapy. *Crit Care Med.* 2007;35:932–939.

94 Sinuff T. Noninvasive positive pressure ventilation for acute respiratory failure: What role is there for patients declining intubation or choosing palliation? *Prog Palliat Care.* 2011;19(5):223–229.

95 Sudore RL, Fried TR. Redefining the "planning" in advance care planning: Preparing for end-of-life decision making. *Ann Intern Med.* 2010;153(4):256–261.

96 Janssen DJ, Spruit MA, Schols JM, Cox B, Nawrot TS, Curtis JR et al. Predicting changes in preferences for life-sustaining treatment among patients with advanced chronic organ failure. *Chest.* 2012 141(5):1251–1259.

97 Jennings AL, Davies AN, Higgins JP, Gibbs JS, Broadley KE. A systematic review of the use of opioids in the management of dyspnoea. *Thorax.* 2002;57(11):939–944.

98 Abernethy AP, Currow DC, Frith P, Fazekas BS, McHugh A, Bui C. Randomised, double blind, placebo controlled crossover trial of sustained release morphine for the management of refractory dyspnoea. *BMJ.* 2003;327(7414):523–528.

99 Rocker GM, Simpson AC, Young J, Horton R, Sinuff T, Demmons J, et al. Opioid therapy for refractory dyspnea in patients with advanced chronic obstructive pulmonary disease: Patients' experiences and outcomes. *Canadian Medical Association Open Access Journal.* January 16, 2013;1(1):E27–E36.

100 Currow DC, McDonald C, Oaten S, Kenny B, Allcroft P, Frith P et al. Once-daily opioids for chronic dyspnea: A dose increment and pharmacovigilance study. *J Pain Symptom Manage.* 2011;42(3):388–399.

101 Rocker G, Young J, Donahue M, Farquhar M, Simpson C. Perspectives of patients, family caregivers and physicians about the use of opioids for refractory dyspnea in advanced chronic obstructive pulmonary disease. *CMAJ.* 2012 DOI:101503/cmaj111758. 2012 Apr 23.

102 Lanken PN, Terry PB, Delisser HM, Fahy BF, Hansen-Flaschen J, Heffner JE et al. An official American Thoracic Society clinical policy statement: Palliative care for patients with respiratory diseases and critical illnesses. *Am J Respir Crit Care Med.* 2008;177(8):912–927.

103 Mahler DA, Selecky PA, Harrod CG, Benditt JO, Carrieri-Kohlman V, Curtis JR et al. American College of Chest Physicians consensus statement on the management of dyspnea in patients with advanced lung or heart disease. *Chest.* 2010;137(3):674–691.

104 Lynn J. Palliative care beyond cancer: Reliable comfort and meaningfulness. *BMJ.* 2008;336(7650):958–959.

105 Murray SA, Sheikh A. Palliative care beyond cancer: Care for all at the end of life. *BMJ.* 2008;336(7650):958–959.

106 Partridge MR. Patients with COPD: Do we fail them from beginning to end? *Thorax.* 2003;58(5):373–375.

98

Other infectious diseases: Malaria, rabies, tuberculosis

SUE MARSDEN

INTRODUCTION

Malaria, rabies, and tuberculosis (TB) are diseases from which people die in the developing world.[1–8] They are diseases associated with poverty and therefore are not usually seen as diseases creating palliative care issues for the developed world. Hence, they have received little attention in this regard. Nonetheless, each year, some 1.4 million people die worldwide from TB, more than half a million from malaria, and about 40,000–100,000 die from rabies[1–8]; these are conservative estimates. These three infectious diseases, and others, are all preventable or treatable, and clearly, public health interventions are critically important in this respect. However, while deaths are occurring with unrelieved symptoms and distress as happens daily, management of patients dying with these diseases demands the application of palliative care principles.

MALARIA

Malaria is a life-threatening parasitic disease caused by the genus *Plasmodium*, transmitted by female mosquitoes of the genus *Anopheles*.[1,2] Although malaria has been essentially eliminated from many countries with temperate climates, 40% of the world's population, mostly those living in the developing countries, remain at risk. In 2010, it was estimated that there were 216 million cases of malaria worldwide, and despite a falling mortality since 2000, malaria is still responsible for approximately 600–700,000 deaths each year.[1,2,9–11] Ninety-one percent of these deaths occur in sub-Saharan Africa, with 86% occurring in children under 5 years.[2,9]

Etiology and pathogenesis

Malaria in humans is caused by one of four species of *Plasmodium*: *P. falciparum*, *P. vivax*, *P. ovale*, and *P. malariae*.[1,2] *P. falciparum* causes the highest mortality and is the most

common causative organism in sub-Saharan Africa.[1,2,9] *P. vivax* is more widely distributed and causes mild recurrent disease if the first episode is not treated adequately. *P. ovale* is rare and can also cause recurrent disease.[2] *P. malariae* has scattered distribution, mainly in Africa, and can live in asymptomatic hosts for decades or cause acute illness.[2] It has been associated with membranoproliferative glomerulonephritis and nephrotic syndrome in children.[2,11]

LIFE CYCLE OF THE MALARIAL PARASITE[1,2]

Plasmodium sporozoites are transmitted to humans from the salivary gland of the female *Anopheles* mosquito by injection under the skin. The life cycle in the human host, summarized in Box 98.1, results in some merozoites differentiating into gametocytes. These can then be transferred from an infected human to a biting mosquito. The parasite completes its sexual cycle within the mosquito forming new sporozoites, which are then available to infect another human. *P. vivax* and *P. ovale* can remain dormant in liver parenchyma for months or years and are responsible for recurrent malaria if treatment has not intervened.

PATHOGENESIS

P. falciparum infection is more severe with a higher mortality and thus most likely to be implicated when a patient requires palliative care. It is the only *Plasmodium* causing microvascular disease.[12] As the parasites mature, the infected red blood cells adhere to the endothelial cells in capillaries and postcapillary venules of, significantly, the brain and kidneys but also other organs.[1,13–15] This sequestration leads to a functional microvascular obstruction.[16,17] Cytokines, for example, tumor necrosis factor alpha (TNFα), contribute to the process.[1,18,19]

Lysis of red blood cells occurs leading to acute anemia, as the schizont stage parasites mature. Chronic anemia occurs from lysis and the effect of TNFα.[1,20]

In contrast, *P. vivax* and *P. ovale* do not cause sequestration and hence do not cause the microvascular complications in

Box 98.1 Life cycle of *Plasmodium* in humans[1,2]

Exoerythrocytic and asymptomatic phase of infection

1. Sporozoites reach the blood stream and travel to the liver.

2. Hepatocytes are infected and the asexual sporozoites multiply to a form called schizont containing thousands of merozoites.

3. After 6–16 days, merozoites are liberated into the bloodstream.

Erythrocytic phase

4. The merozoites invade the red blood cells.

5. In the red blood cells, they turn into ring forms, trophozoites, and degrade hemoglobin.

6. Once more, this time within red blood cells, the parasite forms squizonts, which multiply and lyse the red blood cells.

7. Thousands of merozoites are liberated into the blood stream infecting new red blood cells.

8. This process continues with repetitive cycles of red blood cell invasion and lysis resulting in hemolytic anemia.

9. Some merozoites differentiate into gametocytes, the form acquired by female mosquitoes after biting an infected human.

the brain, kidneys, and lungs. However, sickle hemoglobin, which can provide some protection against severe *P. falciparum*, does not protect against those parasites that do not sequester.[1,21]

Prevention

Cooperative public health initiatives aimed at controlling mosquito populations and reducing transmission are critical in preventing malaria, for example, the World Health Organization (WHO) Roll Back Malaria global partnership.[9]

Clinical manifestations[1,2,3,22]

The incubation period after an infectious bite is 8–14 days except for *P. malariae*, which may be 18–42 days. The presentation of uncomplicated malaria is variable and mimics many other infectious diseases. Fever is common and may initially be persistent rather than tertian. Most commonly, there may be general malaise, headache, backache, chills, episodic sweating, and sometimes vomiting and abdominal pain. In young children, there may be nonspecific irritability, refusal to eat, and vomiting. Anemia, jaundice, hepatomegaly, and splenomegaly may follow.

As malaria can mimic a number of other acute illnesses, it is crucial to have a high index of suspicion. It should always be considered in the differential diagnosis of acute febrile illness in endemic areas or in people travelling to these areas. Unless *P. falciparum* infection is diagnosed and treated promptly, deterioration can occur at an alarming rate,

especially in children. Severe malaria may develop with its attendant morbidity and mortality.[23,24] Severe malaria may present with the following:

- CNS dysfunction—clinical manifestations may vary from confusion, delirium, and obtundation to seizures and deep coma. Unrousable coma, not attributable to any other cause in a patient with falciparum malaria, is defined by the WHO as cerebral malaria.
- Hypoglycemia.
- Acidosis.
- Acute renal failure.
- Abnormal bleeding.
- Pulmonary edema.
- Hyperparasitemia—this occurs where more than 5% of red blood cells are infected.

Diagnosis

Microscopic examination of thick and thin blood smears for the parasites is highly sensitive, specific, and economical.[2,3] The thin smear allows identification of the *Plasmodium* species. Rapid diagnostic tests are available, which detect antigens by immunochromatography. They are easy to perform and quick but their sensitivity varies.

Due to the rapid evolution and high mortality of severe malaria, it is crucial to make a rapid diagnosis. Treatment may need to be initiated before laboratory tests are available. For practical purposes and in the environment where severe malaria occurs, this is justified and often necessary.[2]

Treatment

Severe malaria must, if at all possible, be treated aggressively with appropriate antimalarial medications together with general supportive measures and management of organ failures in an intensive care unit.[3] Since 2006, artemisinin-based combination therapies (ACTs) have been replacing failing chloroquine and sulfadoxine–pyrimethamine in *P. falciparum*.[1,3,24–28]

Even with prompt treatment and hospital admission, cerebral malaria may have mortality of more than 20%.[2,3] Sadly, patients often present late and are misdiagnosed. Also, in the environments where severe malaria usually occurs, intensive medical support measures and/or appropriate medications are not available.

Symptom management

As part of the management of malaria, meticulous attention must be paid to all symptoms and emotional support of the patient and family. The goal in the management of malaria is always cure. However, sadly, this is not always possible, and when it is recognized that treatment aimed at aggressive disease is not possible or is futile, palliative care principles clearly assume the primary focus of care.[2]

CENTRAL NERVOUS SYSTEM SYMPTOMS[2]*

Delirium

In the earlier stages of the disease, trajectory attempts must be made to treat any potentially reversible causes of delirium, for example, dehydration, hypoglycemia, urinary retention, and fever. Otherwise the following are important:

Environment. General comfort support measures as always include attention to the physical environment, noise level, presence of family, and quiet music if possible.
Medications. Antipsychotics, for example, haloperidol 2–5 mg every 6 hours and 2–5 mg every 1 hour prn. Rapid titration may be necessary with initial doses given more frequently. Alternative medications are chlorpromazine and levomepromazine.
Sedation. As well as antipsychotics, the patient may require sedation. Diazepam, lorazepam, and midazolam if available should be considered.

Convulsions

Seizure activity requires the use of anticonvulsants, for example, diazepam 10–20 mg intravenously (IV), rectally (PR), or intramuscularly (IM); midazolam 5–10 mg IM/IV/SC or phenobarbital 200 mg SC/IM.

Coma

It is essential to pay careful attention to physical care to maintain skin integrity and maintain hygiene.

PAIN

Severe pain may be the result of increased muscle tone and spasm. Baclofen 5–10 mg SC/IM or diazepam 5–10 mg IM/IV may be given. Opioids may also be required.

FEVER

Fever may be alleviated with oral acetaminophen (paracetamol) in the early stages and may be given rectally if necessary.

OTHER ASPECTS

In addition to good symptom management and personal care of the patient, provision of emotional and spiritual support to the patient and family are important. This can be particularly poignant as the disease presenting earlier is curable and as many of the patients are so young. Both the patient and the family also require clear explanation as to the nature of the disease, prognosis, and symptoms that are being experienced and their management.

RABIES

Rabies is a fatal acute encephalomyelitis and remains one of the most common viral causes of death in developing countries.[4,5,29] It has a mortality approaching 100% in unvaccinated patients. There have been reports of occasional unvaccinated survivors in the last decade in sophisticated intensive care environments, but essentially, it is still considered fatal, and without palliation, death is agonizing.[4,5,30]

Reliable data on the incidence of rabies in humans are scarce. There are estimated 55,000 deaths annually but numbers are likely double this with the vast majority in developing countries.[4–6,31] It is estimated that some 10 million people receive postexposure treatments annually, following bites from animals suspected to have rabies. Unfortunately, most are treated with vaccines carrying a high risk of neurological complications. The incidence of human rabies in developed countries is very low. Some island nations are reported to be rabies free. Most cases in developed countries are from bites from rabid wild animals, for example, bats, foxes, and raccoons. In developing countries, bites from domestic and feral animals, usually dogs, are responsible.[5,6,32] Transmission between humans has only been documented as a result of corneal transplant.[4–6,32]

Etiology and pathogenesis[4–6,32]

Rabies is caused by a *Lyssavirus*, a bullet-shaped, negative-stranded RNA virus, a member of the *Rhabdoviridae* family. It is transmitted via the saliva of infected animals, being introduced by bites, scratches, licks on broken skin, and contact with mucous membranes. After entry through a breach in the skin or mucous membrane, the virus replicates in muscle cells and infects the muscle spindle and subsequently the nerve innervating the spindle. Further replication occurs within these neurons and the virus rapidly spreads centrally toward the central nervous system. Virus is present within dorsal root ganglia within 72 hours of inoculation.

Rabies infection appears to require local viral replication, perhaps to reach a critical load, before nervous system infection occurs.[4,5] Thus, if antirabies immunoglobulin and active immunization are given in time, the virus may be prevented from spread to the nervous system and disease is prevented. Once the virus has entered the peripheral nerve, however, disease is inevitable. After spreading to the spinal cord, the virus spreads throughout the central nervous system and then centrifugally out to the rest of the body via peripheral nerves. High concentration of virus in saliva results from shedding from sensory nerve endings in the oral mucosa as well as replication in salivary glands. The brain in rabies shows an encephalic picture and the spinal cord shows severe inflammation and necrosis.

Prevention[5,6,31,32]

The control of animal rabies is central to the prevention of human disease. Unfortunately, few countries have been able to achieve this. Prophylaxis for domestic animals and humans at high risk together with postexposure treatment for exposed humans is the basis of control. This has reduced the number of human (and animal) rabies in several countries but with a worrying resurgence in parts of Africa,

Asia, and Latin America.[6] In many developing countries, the cost of prevention programs and the cost of controlling feral dog populations remain obstacles and may not achieve political priority.

PREEXPOSURE PROPHYLAXIS[5,6,31,32]

Preexposure prophylaxis (PEP) is usually confined to people at high risk of rabies exposure, for example, veterinarians and laboratory workers. Those caring for patients with rabies should ideally be vaccinated, but in the under-resourced settings that rabies usually occurs, this is prohibitively expensive and vaccination is unlikely to occur. Transmission to health-care workers has *not* been reported and remains a theoretical risk when normal universal infection control measures are observed. This may, of course, be difficult if a patient has uncontrolled aggressive and violent delirium.

The recommended PEP involves a series of three intramuscular or intradermal injections given on days 0, 7, and 21 or 28 with a booster every 2–3 years.

POSTEXPOSURE TREATMENT[6,31,32]

- *First aid.* The most effective mechanism to protect against rabies following a suspicious bite is to vigorously wash and flush the wound with soap and water. Ethanol, iodine, or povidone-iodine solution should be applied.
- *Antirabies immunoglobulin.* This should ideally be applied on the day of the bite (day 0) but can be applied up to day 7. Human immunoglobulin, if available, should be used, or alternatively equine, following a skin test. The immunoglobulin is infiltrated in and around the wound.
- *Vaccination.* This is recommended following a bite from an animal in which rabies is a possibility but may be discontinued if the animal remains healthy for 10 days or is proved at autopsy to be negative for rabies. Purified cell-culture vaccines (CCVs) and embryonic egg-based vaccines (EEVs) are used. There are various vaccination schedules. Reduced intradermal regimens have been found to be effective and less expensive.

Obstacles to treatment

Although postexposure treatment is available, there remain real and heart-rending obstacles to obtaining this. Many patients do not seek treatment through ignorance, fear, folk beliefs, and overwhelming poverty. Education programs are making inroads in some places. An example of this is the national program of the Department of Health in the Philippines encouraging pet owners to have dogs vaccinated and to seek vaccination following a suspicious bite.[5] However, overwhelming poverty and political motivation remain worldwide issues in the eradication of rabies as with many global health problems.

Clinical manifestations[4,5,29]

The incubation period for rabies may be from a few days to several years. The average incubation period is 20–90 days. The time of onset of symptoms depends on the following (Table 98.1):

- The severity of the wound, that is, the depth, size, or multiplicity
- Clothing protection at the site of bite
- The site of wound in relation to the brain, that is, patients with facial bites develop symptoms earlier

The early clinical features are nonspecific influenza-like symptoms and localized paresthesia, pain, and pruritus at the bite site. The later clinical presentation evolves into two forms: the encephalitic (furious) form (in about 80% of patients) or the paralytic (dumb) form.

Table 98.1 *Clinical stages and symptoms of rabies[5]*

Stage	Time period	Symptoms
Incubation period	<30 days (25%) 30–90 days (50%) 90 days–1 year (20%) >1 year (5%)	
Prodromal symptoms	2–10 days	At bite site: paresthesia, pain, and pruritus General: Fever, malaise nausea, vomiting
Acute disease		
Furious (80%)	2–7 days	Hydrophobia Aerophobia Dysphagia Delirium with • Aggression • Disorientation • Hallucinations • Terror • Hyperexcitement • Hypervigilance • Confusion Autonomic dysfunction with • Hypersalivation • Sweating • Priapism Seizures
Dumb (20%)	2–7 days	Ascending flaccid paralysis

Source: Marsden, S.C., Rabies, in: Bruera, E., De Lima, L., Wenk, R., Farr, W., eds., *Palliative Care in the Developing World: Principles and Practice*, IAHPC Press, Houston, TX, pp. 217–226, 2004.

"FURIOUS" RABIES

The features of encephalitic rabies are typically described as hydrophobia—representing an exaggerated irritant reflex of the respiratory tract with laryngeal spasm—episodic hyperactivity, seizures, aerophobia, hyperventilation, and autonomic dysfunction with papillary dilatation, increased salivation, sweating, and occasionally priapism. However, the feature of rabies that is often most distressing for patients, families, and carers is delirium. The features that predominate are aggression, disorientation, hallucinations, overwhelming terror, hyperexcitability, hypervigilance, and confusion.

"DUMB" RABIES

Paralytic rabies is characterized by ascending paralysis resembling Guillain–Barré syndrome.

Outcome

Whatever the initial symptom complex, cardiac arrhythmias and coma intervene and death is inevitable within a few days. Most patients die within 72 hours of the onset of clinical symptoms.

Symptom management

DELIRIUM[5,33–35*]

As in any palliative care situation, the first priority is good symptom management. This in turn allows personal care of the patient and psychosocial and spiritual issues for the patient and family to be addressed. There are few other situations where this is as true as in need for control of the delirium associated with rabies. Rabies patients without appropriate medication often die alone in a locked and barred room, physically restrained, agitated, terrified, paranoid, and with classic hydrophobia and aerophobia. The delirium can be managed with the following:

- Haloperidol 5 mg given hourly subcutaneously (SC) or IM titrated to the desired effect (with a minimum of three doses), followed by regular 4 hourly injections.
- Levomepromazine 25–100 mg every 4–6 hours SC or chlorpromazine 50–100 mg every 4–6 hours IM may be considered as alternatives.
- It may be necessary to add sedation with a benzodiazepine, for example, diazepam or midazolam.

HYDROPHOBIA AND AEROPHOBIA

These do not respond to haloperidol.[33*] Hydrophobia describes, in fact, the exaggerated reflex of the respiratory tract with laryngeal spasm and is not a "phobic" symptom as such. It is more likely to respond to antispasmodics such as diazepam.[4,33*]

SECRETIONS

These have been successfully controlled with diphenhydramine 50–100 mg every 4–6 hours.[5,33–35*] Alternatives that may be considered, if available, are glycopyrrolate or hyoscine butylbromide. Hyoscine hydrobromide should not be used as it may aggravate agitation.

SEIZURE ACTIVITY

This will require the use of anticonvulsants, for example, benzodiazepines, such as diazepam or midazolam, or phenobarbital.

NAUSEA AND VOMITING

Antidopaminergic antipsychotics such as haloperidol and levomepromazine are effective antiemetics. If these are not being used to control delirium then other antiemetics such as metoclopramide may be considered.

FEVER

This is usually a more significant symptom in the prodromal phase and can be managed with paracetamol.

Physical environment

The room in which the patient is cared for should be clean, pleasant, as quiet as possible, and free of drafts. Seating should be available for family.

Family support and communication[5,33–35]

When symptom control is achieved, patient and family can communicate, say their goodbyes, and deal with as much unfinished business as possible in the short remaining time. Staff have an important role in supporting and facilitating this. To support the family, the following are important:

1. Space should be provided close to the patient for the family to rest, talk, and receive support and information.
2. Honest gentle communication concerning the imminence of death should be provided. Emotional support is necessary for the family who are experiencing a sudden loss, often of the family breadwinner. Any practical advice concerning social support services available is important. Most often the family is from a very poor socioeconomic background.
3. Discussion and education concerning transmission of disease and indications for postexposure vaccination. Families need information that the disease is spread by saliva introduced into a wound or mucous membrane. It is not transmitted through touching intact skin. Thus, families need reassurance that it is safe to sit with their dying loved one and that careful contact will not transmit the disease. Postexposure vaccination is recommended for
   a. Sexual partners, due to the possibility of transmission through saliva
   b. Others considered at risk, for example, a contact who has been bitten by the patient or exposed to the saliva of the patient

4. When a rabies patient's symptoms are well controlled, the family may decide to take their loved one home.[5] This may be for purely important economic reasons. It is cheaper to transport a live person than a dead body. It also has obvious emotional and social benefits for patient and family. Families need careful counselling and practical support for this to occur.

Carer education and support[5,33]

All health-care professionals and other carers involved in caring for rabies patients need education regarding the following:

- The facts concerning rabies transmission. In most developing countries, PEP is prohibitively expensive. However, as mentioned earlier, transmission to health-care workers has *not* been reported and remains theoretical and unlikely if normal care and universal infection control rules are followed. Staff attending to patients' personal care should ideally wear protective gown, gloves, and goggles. If good symptom control is achieved, the risk of being bitten or spat at by a patient is minimized.
- The principles of palliative care, emphasizing the pivotal role of good symptom control with *appropriate, adequate, regular* medication.

TUBERCULOSIS

TB is an infectious disease caused by mycobacteria. The histology characteristically consists of granulomas.[7] Infection usually occurs following inhalation of infectious particles into the lungs.[7,8] It then spreads via blood stream, lymphatics, airways, or direct extension. Pulmonary TB is the most common form of the disease constituting 80% of TB infections in developing countries. However, any organ or part of the body can be affected.

Mycobacterium tuberculosis affects nearly a third of the world's population with some 9 million new cases annually. Ninety-five percent TB deaths occur in the developing world. The death rate has been falling steadily, 45% since 1990.[36] The WHO strategy of supervised treatment (TB directly observed treatment short course [DOTS] program) has been successful in this respect. However, there were still 1.4 million deaths in 2010 and mainly in the age group of 15–49 years.[8,36] TB is associated with overcrowding, poverty, malnutrition, alcohol abuse, and an increase in the rate of human immunodeficiency virus (HIV)/acquired immunodeficiency syndrome (AIDS) infection.[7,8] In developed countries, TB had been steadily decreasing until the mid-1980s. With the AIDS epidemic, this decrement had ceased or reversed, again concentrated in underprivileged and low socioeconomic communities in these countries.[7,36–38] However, from 1992 in the United States, the rate has fallen to, in 2007, the lowest in history,[4] while in developing countries, the rate remains high in association with HIV/AIDs.[36]

Pathogenesis and transmission[7,8]

The usual causative organism is *M. tuberculosis*, an aerobic, nonspore-forming acid-fast bacillus, but occasionally, *M. bovine* can also be the cause. Microorganisms are expelled into the air in tiny droplets from an infected patient with pulmonary TB. These dry rapidly, becoming droplet nuclei that harbor the microorganisms and may remain suspended in air for several hours. *M. tuberculosis* can remain alive for up to several hours and even up to 3 years in a closed environment. A close contact may inhale the droplet nuclei, following which bacterial multiplication begins in the terminal airspaces. Initially, the focus is subpleural—in the midlung zone. Macrophages ingest the bacteria and an initial pulmonary Ghon focus is formed. Macrophages may be carried by the lymphatics to regional lymph nodes, where they form the primary complex, and sometimes to distant lymph nodes. However, in an immunocompromised host, they are not retained in the lymph nodes and may spread through the blood stream to other organs. The primary complex itself may progress causing bronchial collapse, erosion of the bronchus and further distal spread, pneumonia and cavitation, or lymphohematogenous dissemination, resulting in miliary TB.

Development of TB is usually arrested at the primary stage by the host's immune system. Hence, healthy well-nourished individuals with an intact immune system do not usually develop the disease, whereas those with a compromised immune system, for example, due to malnutrition or HIV infection, are very likely to develop TB following mycobacterium exposure. Determinants of infection occurring are closeness of contact and infectiousness of the source. Patients with positive smears, that is, direct microscopy positive, are highly infectious. Those with positive findings only on culture, that is, direct microscopy negative, are less infectious.

TB morbidity in a given population, however, is determined by two factors: the risk of infection (e.g., as in overcrowding) and the risk of developing active disease once infected (e.g., as where immune deficiency exists).

Clinical presentation and diagnosis[7,8,39]

In the presence of nonspecific symptoms, TB should always be suspected if occurring in the environment previously described. This is especially so where there are associated sputum-positive family or contacts.

PULMONARY TUBERCULOSIS

The respiratory symptoms of pulmonary TB may be cough; sputum, which may be bloodstained; dyspnea; and chest wall and pleuritic pain.[7,8] Generalized symptoms include weight loss, anorexia, fatigue cachexia, night sweats, and fever.[7,8] Diagnosis is made by direct microscopy of sputum smears (wherever possible, three specimens are collected), sputum culture, and radiography.[7,8,40] Sputum microscopy, however, may detect only 45% of infections.[41] In developing countries, clinical management is hampered by the lack of a simple effective diagnostic test, although new tests and strategies are being developed.[41,42] Since July 2011, 26 countries have been using Xpert MTB/RIF, a rapid molecular test that accurately diagnoses TB and multi-drug-resistant (MDR) TB in about 100 min.[36,43]

COMPLICATIONS[8]

Complications of pulmonary TB include hemoptysis, acute respiratory distress (due to pleural effusion, lung collapse, pneumothorax, or cardiopulmonary insufficiency due to cor pulmonale), and bronchiectasis and/or pulmonary fibrosis.

EXTRAPULMONARY TUBERCULOSIS

TB lymphadenitis and pleuritis are the two most common.[7,8] Others are meningitis, pericarditis, peritonitis, and urogenital and skeletal TB.[7,8] The specific symptoms will depend on the organ involved, for example, chest pain in pleuritis and lymphadenitis, bone pain in skeletal TB, and delirium, seizure activity, headache, vomiting, meningism, focal signs, and coma in TB meningitis.

TUBERCULIN SKIN TESTS

Skin tests such as the Mantoux test reflect exposure to *M. tuberculosis* but have little value in diagnosing clinical disease where TB is common. Especially in adults, a positive test is infrequently followed by disease and a negative test does not exclude disease. It can be useful in young children who have been in contact with infectious persons recently. The diagnosis of TB in children may be difficult and the WHO has developed clear criteria in this respect.[8]

Tuberculosis treatment[7,8,44]

The cornerstone of treatment of TB is appropriate chemotherapy. The usual anti-TB drugs used are isoniazid, rifampicin, pyrazinamide, ethambutol, and streptomycin. For successful treatment, it is essential that the medications are taken

- In appropriate combination
- In the correct dosage
- Regularly
- For a sufficient period to prevent relapse, that is, several months

Unfortunately, these criteria are often not met in environments of poverty and overcrowding[37,44] and patient ignorance of the importance of continued treatment. Inadequately treated TB can be worse than not treating at all due to the emergence of drug-resistant organisms.[8] Therefore, education and counselling of patients, their families, and communities and public health measures are critical in the management of TB.

The implementation of the highly cost-effective DOTS[8,36,45] in 1991 has resulted in cure rates of 95% even in some of the poorest countries. The DOTS strategy uses four different drugs given over 6–8 months, with medications taken under direct observation of health-care workers who continually monitor patients during the course.

Unfortunately, there has been an alarming emergence of MDR-TB organisms in some populations. These can develop when incorrect medications or wrong combinations are given or drugs are not taken for long enough.[8,36,45] Strategies and guidelines continue to be developed to address this problem.[8,46–54]

Tuberculosis prevention

Bacille Calmette–Guérin (BCG) vaccination, using live attenuated vaccine from a strain of *M. bovis*, is used for prevention of TB throughout much of the world. Although evidence is conflicting, it is suggested that BCG vaccination of children will result in 60%–80% decrease in the incidence of TB in a population.[7,8,55–58]

Chemoprophylaxis is used to treat those at risk of developing TB.[7,8,58] It is used for contacts of smear-positive patients and those with depressed immunity in a population where TB is prevalent.[7,8,58]

Palliative care

TB is treatable and every effort must be made to treat and cure the disease even in extremely sick patients.[8] However, when this is no longer achievable, applying palliative care principles is paramount. The focus must include attention to physical, emotional, spiritual, social, and educational needs of the patient and family.

Symptom management

Most patients dying from TB have respiratory and nonspecific symptoms (Box 98.2).[8]

Box 98.2 Symptoms in dying patients with pulmonary tuberculosis

Respiratory symptoms

- Dyspnea
- Cough
- Hemoptysis
- Thoracic pain
- Terminal secretions

General symptoms

- Fatigue
- Cachexia
- Night sweats
- Fever

RESPIRATORY SYMPTOMS

Dyspnea

1. Treat any reversible aspect:
   a. *Pleural effusion*: Drain if feasible
   b. *Associated obstructive airways disease*: Optimal use of bronchodilators and steroids
2. General symptomatic measures:
   a. Supplemental oxygen in the presence of hypoxia.
   b. Airflow using fans or simply open window.
   c. *Opioids*: These reduce the subjective sensation of breathlessness.[59]* If the patient is opioid naïve, a starting dose of oral morphine 5–10 mg every 4 hours or 2.5–5 mg SC every 4 hours with additional as-needed doses available for exacerbations. Patients will still have tachypnea and this needs to be explained to families with reassurance that this in itself is not distressing.[59]
   d. *Benzodiazepines*: Where there are significant anxiety episodes, benzodiazepines could be considered, for example, lorazepam 1 mg prn or diazepam 5–10 mg prn.

Cough

A dry cough is always present in these patients. As the disease progresses, it may become purulent and blood stained. Opioids may be useful, for example, morphine 5–10 mg every 4 hours prn. Inhaled cromoglycate may be useful.

Hemoptysis

Hemoptysis can be a very distressing symptom for both patient and family especially when massive, when it can be the terminal event. The following should be considered:

- In the earlier stages, tranexamic acid 500 mg three times daily, if available, should be considered.
- Dark linen and towels, if available, can reduce the visual impact.
- If massive bleeding and associated choking are possibilities, a short-acting benzodiazepine such as midazolam or lorazepam should be available. In the home situation, a preloaded syringe, for example, of midazolam 5–10 mg, should be made available.

Respiratory secretions

As the patient becomes more unresponsive and secretions accumulate, it is important to counsel the family that the noisy breathing is not distressing for the patient and represents pooling of secretions. It does not indicate that the patient is choking.[52] Medications that may be used to reduce secretions are glycopyrrolate 0.4 mg SC every 4 hours or hyoscine butylbromide 10–20 mg SC every 4–6 hours. Hyoscine hydrobromide should be used with caution as it may cause or aggravate agitation.

NONSPECIFIC SYMPTOMS

Fatigue and cachexia

Fatigue and cachexia are among the most common and severe symptoms in TB. Pain and clinical depression may contribute to fatigue and should be appropriately managed. Antidepressants and psychostimulants, for example, methylphenidate, should be considered.

Patients with anemia may benefit from blood transfusion. Food intake per se is unlikely to resolve the severe weight loss related to TB as cachexia is a syndrome resulting from metabolic abnormalities. However, it may be that cachexia syndrome has been confused with malnutrition in the environment where these patients are dying. Encouraging and extraordinary results have been seen where patients have merely been fed adequately (Starfish Palliative Care Program, personal communication, November 2004, March 2005, July 2005). However, in the presence of true cachexia syndrome, the social value of meals remains important even where the patient is able to take very little. Families need counselling that cachexia is a metabolic consequence of advanced disease.

Night sweats and fever

These are common and unpleasant. Hydration needs to be maintained. Fever can be managed with acetaminophen or nonsteroidal anti-inflammatory medications.

PAIN

Pain is often underreported and undertreated due to reluctance to use analgesics in the presence of dyspnea. Thoracic and skeletal pain is managed with the usual principles of initially using regular nonopioids, for example, acetaminophen, and a nonsteroidal anti-inflammatory, moving to opioids as necessary.

OTHER SYMPTOMS

Less common extrapulmonary TB presentations require symptom management depending on the site. For example, TB meningitis may result in delirium, seizure activity, and coma requiring appropriate attention to these symptoms.

Physical care[8]

Dying TB patients are inevitably wasted, dependent, and often bed bound. They require meticulous attention to skin care and bodily functions to prevent pressure areas and skin excoriation and tears.

Emotional, spiritual, and social needs

The very diagnosis of TB without the knowledge that it is incurable and the patient is now dying will have evoked many emotional issues including fear, grief, anger, and despair. Patients are often in the most productive part of their lives and may be parents and breadwinners. As well as fears for themselves, they may have fears for future support of their families, a sense of uselessness, as well as the stigma attached to the diagnosis.

Patients may see their disease and fate as punishment and this may be inextricably intertwined with spiritual and religious beliefs. Emotional and spiritual counselling and support for both patient and family are thus important. Patients and families may become socially isolated as a result of the diagnosis. The diagnosis has important personal and financial implications. The despair resulting may be compounded by the impoverished, underresourced environments in which patients die from TB, where the aforementioned suggestions made for symptom management of the dying patient are unavailable and/or unaffordable.

These factors, and the public health issue of ensuring that families and contacts are treated and monitored, emphasize the inextricable interconnection between public health medicine and palliative care in the management of TB in developing countries.

Key learning points

- Malaria, rabies, and TB are treatable or preventable diseases that together result in millions of deaths with uncontrolled symptoms in the developing world.

- When it is clear that no disease-orientated treatment is available or no longer possible, palliation of symptoms is paramount. This must not be seen as an excuse to reduce attempts to aggressively treat TB and malaria if at all possible.

- Patients dying of these diseases are often young and in their most productive years. The families' despair and grief needs emotional and social support.

- Public health and palliative care are inextricably linked in the management of these patients, their families, and communities.

REFERENCES

1 Fairhurst RM, Wellems TE. Plasmodium species (malaria). In: Mandell GL, Bennett JE, Dolin R, eds. *Mandell, Douglas and Bennett's Principles and Practice of Infectious Disease*, 7th edn. New York: Churchill Livingstone, 2010: pp. 3437–3462.

● ✱ 2 Villegas MV, Teano R, Zuluaga T, Wenk R. Malaria. In: Bruera E, De Lima L, Wenk R, Farr W, eds. *Palliative Care in the Developing World: Principles and Practice*. Houston, TX: IAHPC Press, 2004: pp. 207–214.

◆ 3 World Health Organization. *Guidelines for the Treatment of Malaria*. 2nd edn. Geneva, Switzerland: WHO, 2010. Available at: http://www.who.int/malaria/publictions/atoz/9789241547925/en. (accessed July 8, 2014).

4 Bassin SL, Rupprecht CE, Bleck TP. Rhabdoviruses. In: Mandell GL, Bennett JE, Dolin R, eds. *Mandell, Douglas and Bennett's Principles and Practice of Infectious Disease*, 7th edn. New York: Churchill Livingstone, 2010: pp. 2249–2263.

● ✱ 5 Marsden SC. Rabies. In: Bruera E, De Lima L, Wenk R, Farr W, eds. *Palliative Care in the Developing World: Principles and Practice*. Houston, TX: IAHPC Press, 2004: pp. 217–226.

6 World Health Organization. Media Centre Fact Sheet No 99. Rabies. September 2011. www.who.int/mediacentre/factsheets/fs099/en.

7 Fitzgerald DW, Sterling T, Haas DW. Mycobacterium tuberculosis. In: Mandell GL, Bennett JE, Dolin R, eds. *Mandell, Douglas and Bennett's Principles and Practice of Infectious Disease*, 7th edn. New York: Churchill Livingstone, 2010: pp. 3129–3176.

● ✱ 8 Clemens E. Tuberculosis. In: Bruera E, De Lima L, Wenk R, Farr W, eds. *Palliative Care in the Developing World: Principles and Practice*. Houston, TX: IAHPC Press, 2004: pp. 187–205.

9 World Health Organization. Roll Back Malaria Partnership. Key malaria facts. Geneva, Switzerland: WHO. Available at: www.rbm.who.int/keyfacts, (accessed June 16, 2012).

10 World Health Organization. World Malaria Report 2013. Geneva, Switzerland: WHO. Available at: http://www.who.int/malaria/publications/world_malaria_report_2013/en/, (accessed July 8, 2014).

11 Kibukamusoke JW, Hutt MSR, Wilks NE. The nephrotic syndrome in Uganda and its association with quartan malaria. *Q J Med* 1967; 36: 393–408.

12 Miller LH, Good MF, Milon G. Malaria pathogenesis. *Science* 1994; 264: 1878–1883.

13 Aikawa M, Iseki M, Barnwell JW et al. The pathology of human cerebral malaria. *Am J Trop Med Hyg* 1990; 43: 30–37.

14 Aikawa M, Rabbege JR, Udeinya IJ et al. Electron microscopy of knobs in Plasmodium falciparum-infected erythrocytes. *J Parasitol* 1983; 69: 435–437.

15 Riganti M, Pongponiratn E, Tegoshi T et al. Human cerebral malaria in Thailand: A clinicopathological correlation. *Immunol Lett* 1990; 25: 199–205.

16 Turner G. Cerebral malaria. *Brain Pathol* 1997; 7: 569–582.

17 Warrell DA, Molyneux ME, Beales PF, eds. Severe and complicated malaria. *Trans R Soc Trop Med Hyg* 1990; 84: 1–65.

18 Grau GE, Tafor TE, Molyneux ME et al. Tumor necrosis factor and disease severity in children with falciparum malaria. *N Engl J Med* 1989; 320: 1586–15891.

19 Kwiatkowski D, Hill AV, Sambou I et al. TNF concentration in fatal cerebral, non-fatal cerebral, and uncomplicated *Plasmodium falciparum* malaria. *Lancet* 1990; 336: 1201–1204.

20 Barnwell JW. Cyto-adherence and sequestration in falciparum malaria. *Exp Parasitol* 1989; 69: 407–412.

21 Friedman JM. Erythrocytic mechanism of sickle cell resistance to malaria. *Proc Natl Acad Sci USA* 1978; 75: 1994–1997.

22 Warrell DA. Clinical features of malaria. In: Gilles HM, Warrell DA, eds. *Bruce-Chwatt's Essential Malariology*, 3rd edn. London, U.K.: Arnold, 1999: pp. 35–49.

23 Jaffar S, Boele van Hensbroek M, Palmer A et al. Predictors of fatal outcome following cerebral malaria. *Am J Trop Med Hyg* 1997; 57: 20–24.

24 World Health Organization. Communicable disease cluster. Severe Falciparum malaria: Prognostic indices in adults. *Trans R Soc Trop Med Hyg* 2000; 94: 11–18.

◆ 25 White NJ. The treatment of malaria. *N Engl J Med* 1996; 335: 800–806.

26 Warrell DA, Looaseesuwan S, Warrell MJ et al. Dexamethasone proves deleterious in cerebral malaria: A double blind clinical trial in 100 comatose patients. *N Engl J Med* 1982; 306: 313–318.

27 Tsai YL, Kregstad DJ. The resurgence of malaria. In: Scheld WM, Craig WA, Hughes JM, eds. *Emerging Infections, Volume 2*. Washington, DC: American Society for Microbiology, 1998: pp. 195–212.

28 White NI, Warrell DA. The management of severe malaria. In: Wernsdorfer WH, McGregor IA, eds. *Principles and Practice of Malariology, Volume 1*. London, U.K.: Churchill Livingstone, 1988: pp. 865–888.

◆ 29 Jackson AC, Warrell MJ, Rupprecht CE et al. Rabies in humans. *Clin Infect Dis* 2003; 36: 60–63.

30 Willoughby Jr RE, Tieves DO, Hoffman GM et al. Survival after treatment of rabies with induction of coma. *N Eng J Med* 2005; 352: 2508–2514.

31 World Health Organization. *WHO Expert Consultation on Rabies. Second Report.* Technical Report Series 982. Geneva, Switzerland: World Health Organization, 2013. Available at http://www.who.int/entity/neglected_diseases/support_to_rabies_elimination_2013/en/, (accessed July 8, 2014)

32 World Health Organization. Rabies vaccines: WHO position paper. *Weekly Epidemiological Record* 2010; 85: 309–320.

● ✳ 33 Marsden SC, Cabanban CR. Rabies: A significant palliative care issue. *Prog Pall Care* 2006; 14(2): 62–67.

34 Dizon MOM, Belandres Jr DC, Marsden SC et al. Palliative care in rabies. In: Abstracts, Posters, 14th International Congress on Care of the Terminally Ill. *J Palliat Care* 2002; 18: 229.

35 Marsden SC. Palliative care in rabies in Manila. Poster, abstract. In: *5th Asia Pacific Hospice Conference Program and Abstracts.* Osaka, Japan: Conference Organizing Committee, 2003: p. 207.

36 World Health Organization. Tuberculosis Fact Sheet No 104. Available at http://www.who.int/mediacentre/factsheets/fs104/en/, (accessed July 8, 2014).

37 Farmer PE. *Infections and Inequalities. The Modern Plagues,* 2nd edn. Berkeley, CA: University of California Press, 2001.

38 Farmer PE. *Pathologies of Power: Health, Human Rights, and the New War on the Poor.* Berkeley, CA: University of California Press, 2002.

39 Davies PDO, Ormerod P, eds. *Case Presentations in Clinical Tuberculosis.* London, U.K.: Arnold, 1999.

40 World Health Organization. Same-day diagnosis of tuberculosis by microscopy: WHO policy statement. Available at: http://www.who.int/tb/publications/2011/tb_microscopy_9789241501606/en/via www.who.int/tb, (accessed July 5, 2014).

41 Guillerm M, Usdin M, Arkinstall J. *Tuberculosis Diagnosis and Drug Sensitivity Testing,* 2006. Geneva, Switzerland: Medicins Sans Frontiers. Available at: http://www.doctorswithoutborders.org/article/tuberculosis-diagnosis-and-drug-sensitivity-testing, (accessed July 8, 2014).

42 World Health Organization. *TB Diagnostics and Laboratory Strengthening.* Available at: http://www.who.int/tb/laboratory/en/. (accessed July 8, 2014).

43 Vassall A, van Kampen S, Sohn H et al. Rapid diagnosis with the Xpert MTB/RIF assay in high burden countries: A cost effectiveness analysis. pmed.1001120 via http://www.ncbi.nlm.nih.gov/pubmed, (accessed July 8, 2014).

44 Farmer PE. Hidden epidemics of tuberculosis. In: *Infectious Disease and Social Inequalities: From Hemispheric Insecurity to Global Cooperation.* A Working Paper of the Latin American Program of the Woodrow Wilson International Center for Scholars. Washington, DC: Wilson Center, 1999: pp. 31–55.

45 World health Organization. *Treatment of Tuberculosis: Guidelines for National Programmes.* 4th edn. Geneva, Switzerland: WHO, 2009. Available at: http://www.who.int/tb/publications/tb_treatmentguidelines/en/index.html, (accessed July 8, 2014).

46 World health Organization. *Guidelines for Surveillance of Drug Resistance in Tuberculosis.* 4th edn. Geneva, Switzerland: WHO. Available at: http://whqlibdoc.who.int/publications/2009/9789241598675_eng.pdf via http://www.who.int/tb/publications/2009/en/, (accessed July 8, 2014).

47 World Health Organization. Guidelines for programmatic management of drug-resistant tuberculosis WHO/HTM/TB2013.2. Geneva Switzerland:WHO. Available at http://www.who.int/tb/challenges/mdr/programmatic_guidelines_for_mdrtb/en/, (accessed July 8, 2014).

48 Farmer PE, Kim J, Mitnick C, Timperi R. Responding to outbreaks of multidrug-resistant tuberculosis: Introducing 'DOTS-Plus'. In: Reichman LB, Hershfield ES, eds. *Tuberculosis: A Comprehensive International Approach,* 2nd edn. New York: Marcell Dekker, 1999: pp. 447–469.

49 Farmer PE, Shin SS, Bayona J et al. Making DOTS-Plus work. In: Bastain I, Portaels F, eds. *Multidrug Resistant Tuberculosis.* Dordrecht, the Netherlands: Kluwer Academic Publishers, 2000: pp. 285–306.

50 Shin SS, Bayona J, Farmer PE. DOTS and DOTS-Plus: Not the only answer. In: Davies PDO, ed. *Clinical Tuberculosis,* 3rd edn. London, U.K.: Arnold, 2003: 211–223.

51 Becerra MC, Freeman J, Bayona J et al. Using treatment failure under effective direct observed short-course chemotherapy programs to identify patients with multi-drug-resistant tuberculosis. *Int J Tuberc Lung Dis* 2000; 4: 108–114.

52 Farmer PE, Furin JJ, Bayona J et al. Management of MDR-TB in resource-poor countries. *Int J Tuberc Lung Dis* 1999; 3: 643–645.

53 Garrett L. *The Coming Plague: Newly Emerging Diseases in a World out of Balance.* New York: Farrar, Strauss and Giroux, 1994.

54 Murray C, Styblo K, Rouillon A. Tuberculosis. In: Jamison DT, Mosley WH, Measham AR, Bodadella JL, eds. *Disease Control Priorities in Developing Countries.* Oxford, U.K.: Oxford University Press, 1993: pp. 233–259.

55 World Health Organization. Tuberculosis vaccines. Geneva, Switzerland:WHO. Avaialble at http://www.who.int/immunization/research/development/tuberculosis/en/, (accessed July 8, 2014).

56 Clemens JD, Chung JH, Feinstein AR. The BCG controversy. A methodological and statistical reappraisal. *JAMA* 1989; 249: 2362–2369.

57 Fine PEM. The BCG story; lessons from the past and implications for the future. *Rev Infect Dis* 1989; 11: 353–359.

58 Hawkridge T. Tuberculosis contacts and prophylaxis. *SAMJ* 2007; 97(10): 998–1000.

59 Elsayem A, Driver LC, Bruera E, eds. *The M.D. Anderson Symptom Control and Palliative Care Handbook,* 2nd edn. Houston, TX: The University of Texas MD Anderson Cancer Centre, 2002.

99

Practical aspects of palliative care delivery in the developing world

LILIANA DE LIMA, ROBERTO WENK

INTRODUCTION

The World Health Report published by the World Health Organization (WHO) indicates that almost 57 million deaths occurred worldwide in 2001. The vast majority of these deaths occurred in developing countries, where over three-fourths of the people in the world live. Infectious diseases such as HIV, malaria, tuberculosis, and respiratory infections caused over half of the cumulative deaths in developing countries.[1]

With the exception of the United States, developed countries registered a decline or no change in population during the last decade, and 99% of population growth took place in developing countries. If this trend continues, by 2050, industrialized nations will record a population increase of only 4%, while the population in developing countries will expand by 55%. For example, countries of Western Asia are expected to gain about 186 million people by 2050.[2] Overall, the world population will reach approximately nine billion by mid-century.

Developing countries will face the burden of this population growth, which will result in greater demand for health care services. With limited funding, inadequate infrastructure, and limited access to preventive and curative measures, more individuals will require palliative care services.

The developing world varies greatly from country to country and region to region. There are a limited number of excellent facilities in developing countries with the latest technology and medications capable of delivering care similar to that of the developed countries, but the majority of the population does not have access to these institutions and are cared for in facilities with limited resources.

Health care initiatives in the developing world must deal with poverty, inadequate infrastructures, poor administrative systems, limited access to medications, bureaucratic and inefficient processes related to the production, importation, and distribution of medications, restrictive laws and regulations related to the prescribing of opioids, insufficient support from national health authorities, low levels of political will to establish palliative care programs,[3–5] and limited education for health care providers.[6] An additional barrier to the implementation of palliative care programs in developing countries is that a majority of health care spending, both public and private, goes to curative efforts.

Patients in extremely resource poor settings pose challenges that need to be taken into account when developing palliative care programs and strategies. Many palliative care initiatives in developing countries have developed as islands of excellence, but they are not well integrated into national health systems, with very limited impact. Palliative care is still not included in the mainstream of care and tends to be delegated to a secondary role with no budget allocation and no reimbursement schemes.

This has resulted in the development and implementation of different models of care. Care is provided by local programs and teams with structural and operational differences shaped by the needs and limitations of each setting rather than by following a set of consistent guidelines. Each one is adapted to its environment and most survive using resources in very unique ways.[7] Sadly, there is evidence that the quality of care during the dying process is poor and that many patients suffer unnecessary pain and symptoms.[8]

In order to adapt to these limitations and the needs of the population, palliative care workers adopt practical measures to provide cost-effective and efficient palliative care to the patients. These include strategies to build and improve capacity, developing tools and resources for education, adopting low-cost treatment measures, developing data management procedures to establish mechanism for quality control and identifying sources of funding to cover the costs of the palliative care services.

Under this framework, the International Association for Hospice and Palliative Care (IAHPC) decided to work on several projects aimed at identifying "essential" components for optimal palliative care provision, including a list of essential medicines in palliative care,[9] an opioid essential prescription package (OEPP),[10] and a list of essential practices in palliative care.[11] This chapter describes these resources as well as cost-effective treatments strategies adopted in Argentina, South Africa, and India, and provides some examples of settings where they have been successful in improving the delivery of palliative care.

TOOLS AND RESOURCES

List of essential practices in palliative care

The objective of this project was to identify, through a consensus process, the essential practices in palliative care, which could be provided by physicians, nurses, and nurse aides working at the primary care level and could be applicable in all socioeconomic settings. To work on this proposal, IAHPC formed a working group that included board members of IAHPC and external advisors from the field. The working group developed a plan of action and methodology that included a Delphi process among 425 health practitioners, primary care providers, and palliative care experts from 63 different countries around the globe, and a ranking survey with representatives from 45 international palliative care and pain relief organizations. Consensus was set at >80% agreement among respondents. After three Delphi rounds with the respondents, the list was finalized.

The list of essential practices in palliative care for health workers working in primary care includes those practices aimed at meeting the most prevalent physical, social, psychological, and spiritual needs of palliative care patients and their families (see Table 99.1).

Opioid essential prescription package

The aim of this study was to determine by consensus the components of an OEPP to be used when initiating a prescription for the control of moderate to severe chronic pain. Palliative care physicians (n = 60) were sampled from the IAHPC membership list to represent a range of countries of varying economic levels and diverse geographical regions. Using a Delphi study method, physicians were asked to rank preferences of drug and dosing schedule for first-line opioid, antiemetic, and laxative for the treatment of adults with chronic pain due to cancer and other life-threatening conditions. Overall response rates after two Delphi survey rounds were 95% (n = 57) and 82% (n = 49), respectively. A consensus (set at ≥75%) was reached to include morphine as first-line opioid at a dose of 5 mg q4h PO. Consensus was reached to include metoclopramide as first-line antiemetic, but there was no consensus on "regular" or "as-needed" administration. No consensus was reached regarding first-line laxative, but a combination of senna and docusate secured 59% agreement. There was consensus (93%) that laxatives should always be given regularly when opioid treatment is started. Further work is needed to establish a recommended dose of metoclopramide and a type and dose of laxative.

Table 99.1   *IAHPC list of essential practices in palliative care*

Symptom/problem management

Identify, evaluate, diagnose, treat, and apply solution measures:
   Bowel function problems with emphasis on constipation and diarrhea
      Delirium
      Dyspnea
      Insomnia
      Nausea and vomiting
      Pain (all types)
      Patient's psychological distress
      Suffering of the relative and/or caregiver
Identify and evaluate—provide support when possible and consider referral for diagnosis, treatment/solution measures:
      Anorexia
      Fatigue
      Patient's spiritual needs
      Family/caregivers grief and bereavement Issues
Other
   Care planning and coordination:
      Develop and implement a plan of care based on the patient's needs, resources available, caregiver's capabilities and skills, community support, etc.
      Provide care in the last days/weeks of life
      Identify, evaluate, and implement solutions to ensure availability and access to medications
   Communication issues:
      Communicate with patient, family and caregivers about diagnosis, prognosis,[a] condition, treatment, symptoms and their management, and last days/weeks care issues
      Provide information and guidance to patients and caregivers according to available resources
      Identify and set priorities with patient and caregivers

[a] The determination of prognosis and safe delivery of this information requires appropriate training and knowledge.

The resulting OEPP is international in scope and is designed to ensure that opioids are better tolerated by reducing adverse effects of opioids, which could lead to more sustained improvements in pain management. Table 99.2 lists the OEPP.

Table 99.2   *IAHPC opioid essential prescription package*

Opioid:
   Morphine, oral, 5 mg every 4 hours.
Laxative:
   Combination of senna and docusate, oral, 8.6 mg/50 mg every 12 hours.
OR:
   Bisacodyl, oral, 5 mg every 12 hours.
Antiemetic:
   Metoclopramide, oral, 10 mg every 4 hours OR as needed.

CAPACITY-BUILDING STRATEGIES

Capacity strengthening is crucial for adopting effective palliative care programs with the ability to reach the majority of the population in need. Many initiatives have been successful largely as a result of the strategies adopted by program leaders that positively influenced the willingness of policy makers to incorporate palliative care in the health care agendas.

Some programs in developed countries, which have been implemented with very significant results, may be applicable and adapted to developing countries. It is a fact that in developing countries, different important governmental as well as nongovernmental palliative care initiatives have emerged in recent years as a result of these capacity-building strategies. But even with these improvements, there are still enormous gaps to be bridged to bring palliative care to those in need.

Community health approach in home care

Given the extent of the problem in developing countries, in which health care resources are severely limited, a community health approach relying extensively on home-based care and community involvement in the provision of care and support is the most cost-effective approach. The community health approach requires team development and networking with actions and tasks by community members, a high level of population coverage, and periodic evaluations for improving the quality dimensions for better program performance in providing palliative care in the patients' homes. In some countries, these palliative care activities are integrated with the ongoing activities of other health care providers, for conditions and diseases such as HIV/AIDS and cancer.[12]

In Kerala, India, neighborhood network palliative care programs have shown exceptionally good success rates. More than 50% coverage for all severely ill patients seem to have been achieved within 2 years of initiation of the project and the district where it was first launched now has an estimated coverage of more than 70%. Involving the local community in all stages, from planning to monitoring, has ensured sustainability of the project. Neighborhood groups locally find the resources to deliver care: 80% of the funds for programs are raised locally. The groups' advocacy role also results in generating support from local government.[13]

In Africa, several model programs are demonstrating the beneficial integration of hospice, and community- and home-based care for people with cancer and HIV/AIDS.[14,15] For example, the South Coast Hospice in KwaZulu-Natal, South Africa, developed an integrated care program in which patients with HIV/AIDS are referred to teams of nurses and trained community caregivers who care for them in their own homes.[16] The program has halved average patient stays at the local hospital, and extended care provided at home costs less than a 2-day stay in the hospital.[17] Hospice Uganda has been successful in implementing a hospice model, which has become part of Uganda's national health care policy. They have been particularly successful in improving access to morphine by establishing a very cost-effective distribution system of inexpensive morphine sulfate preparations.[18]

Volunteers

In settings where the human resource is limited, adopting a volunteers' home-based care program has proven to be useful and practical. Volunteers play an essential role in palliative care and more so in developing countries where limited resources hinder the capacity to hire human resource for end-of-life care.[19,20] Patients in developing countries who are diagnosed with life-threatening conditions are usually sent home with little or no treatment recommendations. By carrying out many of the tasks of the palliative care providers, volunteers from the community become an important and crucial source of support for the patient and the family and, when available, to the palliative care team.[21] In this process, family members are empowered to their highest degree possible in order to ensure continuity of treatment.

Volunteers in palliative care have proven to be efficient in two main areas: direct patient care (feeding, hygiene, administration of medication, patient evaluation, helping in domestic chores such as shopping for food, cleaning house, cooking, etc.) and providing administrative support to the program (administrative and secretarial tasks).

Individuals who are interested in working as volunteers in palliative care need to be carefully selected, trained, and taught about the chores and tasks that they will help with. Figure 99.1 shows the steps of the process to initiate and maintain a volunteer program in palliative care developed and implemented by the Programa Argentino de Medicina Paliativa—Fundacion FEMEBA (PAMPFF).[22]

The following are distinctive practical aspects of the process, which have proven to be effective:

- *Selection*: Careful selection guidelines are aimed to match the required personal skills with the needs of the patient, the family, and the program.[23]
- *Desertion*: Ten percent of the volunteers who have fulfilled the selection criteria abandon the group during the training. Fifteen percent of the volunteers who complete the training abandoned the group after starting the activities.[24] A strategy was designed to solve this problem, and early and late desertion were significantly reduced after including a description of the volunteers' tasks, stories of other volunteers' experiences, and an initial interview with a psychologist.
- *Training*: A comprehensive training program for volunteers is a practical way to maximize the role of the volunteers and to prevent desertion. The training program adopted by PAMPFF is based on other successful initiatives, includes bedside training and spending time with the palliative care team before being sent out to the community.[25] Table 99.3 shows the content areas of the training program used for training volunteers in practical tasks that can make a difference during the care of patients. The guidelines are available in Spanish at http://paliativo-femeba.org/ uploads/2012/4/Entrenamiento%20de%20voluntarios%20 en%20Cuidado%20Paliativo.pdf.

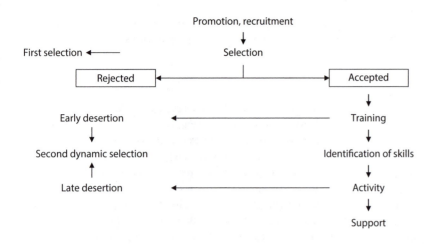

Figure 99.1 *Process to initiate and maintain a volunteer program in palliative care.*

Table 99.3 *Content areas of the volunteer training guidelines*

Self-care techniques
- Proper body mechanics
- Prevention of infections and diseases transmitted by blood and body fluids

Specific techniques to help in activities of daily life:
- Hygiene
- Displacement
- Transfers
- Care of patients with
  - Incontinence
  - Confusion
  - Hearing impairment
  - Visually impairment

Volunteers need to feel that they have the support of the program, the patient, and the family; much of their work is based on reciprocal trust. In order for volunteers to feel comfortable in their role, they must know and feel that their work is crucial and needed, and perceive that the time they spend in care-giving is valuable. The way to achieve this is by investing time in their training while monitoring their work, acknowledging their critical role within the group, and assigning specific roles and tasks.

AVAILABILITY AND ACCESS TO OPIOID ANALGESICS

Pain relief is the cornerstone of palliative care and adequate access and availability of opioid analgesics to all patients in need are crucial.[26] Many countries report an improvement in the availability of different weak and strong opioid analgesics, but their high prices relative to the monthly salaries constitute a barrier to access.[27] A study among developing and developed nations demonstrated that the median cost of opioid medication was twice as high in developing versus developed countries. In U.S. dollars, a 30-day prescription was U.S.$112 in developing countries, compared to U.S.$53 in developed

countries. Cost as percent of GNP per capita per month was 10-fold higher in developing countries where patients have to spend more than a third of their salaries to cover pain therapy. Median cost was 31% of GNP per capita per month in the developing countries, compared to 3% of GNP per capita per month in the developed countries. Half of opioid preparations cost more than 33% of monthly GNP per capita in developing countries compared to only 4% in developed countries. And, there were fewer programs to offset medication costs in developing countries. Only one of the five developing nations (20%) had a subsidization program or socialized medicine, compared to four of seven (57%) of the developed nations.[28]

Probable reasons for the high prices are relative small markets, red tape, bureaucratic procedures, and tax burdens, and thus, large overheads are needed to cover the costs of production, distribution, and sales. Government-imposed cap on the prices of opioids is not a good solution as this may risk the availability of medications, especially in countries with small markets where the operating costs for the pharmaceutical industry are not compensated with the limited sales. In some countries, the only solution is for the health care system to subsidize the opioid analgesics.

Unfortunately, the problem of accessibility does not seem to be a priority for international institutions working to improve pain relief. It is crucial that these organizations initiate claims and requests to governments, the pharmaceutical industry, and health care providers, to help address and solve this problem.

Several hospice and palliative care programs have adopted cost-effective strategies to produce and distribute inexpensive morphine. These include establishing links with local pharmaceutical companies willing to produce the opioid in immediate-release tablets and compound preparations (done by a pharmacist according to the national pharmacopoeia as per the patients' needs) or generic preparations of the following:

1. For oral use: aqueous solutions of morphine (6 mg/cc), oxycodone (3 mg/cc) or methadone (10 mg/cc)
2. For subcutaneous use: micro-pore cold sterilized aqueous solutions of morphine or oxycodone (10 mg/cc). The same can be done with dexamethasone, metoclopramide, hyoscine butylbromide, haloperidol, and others.

3. Hospice Africa Uganda developed a practical way to deliver morphine, reconstituted from powder that has been established for the safe use of opioids for home palliative care as follows[29]:

   a. Using an accurate scale and filtered, powder is weighed and mixed with boiled, filtered water and with bronopol (a preservative).

   b. The solution is mixed in three different strengths and drops of food color added for coding: 1 mg/mL (green), 10 mg/mL (pink), and 20 mg/mL (blue).

   c. The liquid is poured into recycled plastic water bottles. These bottles are washed carefully in the pharmacy before use. The patient or relative receives the morphine from the dispenser.

   d. The patient is provided with a 5 mL syringe without a needle. With the syringe, they are shown how to draw it up, by pouring the liquid into the lid of the bottle that holds about 5 mL.

DATA MANAGEMENT

Data collection and analysis are critical in palliative care to both understand the current levels of quality and measure improvement in care.[30] Also, information facilitates the caring process, especially when several disciplines and different services participate.[31]

Unfortunately, the amount of information available in developing countries on palliative care is very limited and there are no known health systems that systematically collect information on quality of the care they provide.

In countries with financial limitations, it is difficult to secure the support of professional data managers to develop and keep running a system designed to meet the needs of the program. This can lead to quite opposite situations of either collecting burdensome useless data or nothing at all. To establish a cost-effective service, it is important to identify the crucial information to be collected and then develop a data management system based on the needs and existing resources. Several palliative care services have adopted data collection systems with successful results.[32,33]

The following describes one such initiative that was developed by the PAMPFF: After many years of unsuccessful use of a complex electronic health record,[34] the PAMPFF leaders agreed that the culture of data collection was still lacking but that there was a need of a simple system to collect and analyze operational and clinical data to have information on both the patients served and the services provided. After agreement about the need, it was a consensus development process among the program leaders to choose the metrics for common and comparable measures, to take them, and learn from them.[35,36]

Table 99.4 shows the structure of the database and its domains; the data points included represent the core minimum information that the PAMPFF felt should be gathered.

Table 99.4 *Database structure, main domains*

Patient identification
Patient age and gender
Place of residence during the last 6 months
Disease
Health coverage
Responsible caregiver
Location at first consult
Referring service
Reason for referral
Performance status
Physical symptoms
Psychological symptoms
Pain on admission
Pain after 48 hours
Previous opioids
Prescribed opioids
Diagnostic/prognostic information status
Discharge from palliative care
Place of death

Its main characteristics are:

- It was created using the P Hypertext Preprocessor (PHP) general-purpose scripting language and the MySQL open source database.
- It is hosted in the PAMPFF website, all the activity develops on line.
- The information is uploaded twice a month by an external data entry person; he or she is provided with a form with the patients' information. The form is completed in the services with information retrieved from the clinical record.
- Access is restricted with a security system.
- The patient privacy is protected by a secure identification system.
- The analyzed data (tables and figures) is retrieved and displayed easily and can be exported to an Excel worksheet for further analysis with other software applications.
- Participation is entirely voluntary; PAMPFF invites all palliative care services nationwide to take part. Participants are encouraged to capture other data that would be of use in helping to sustain/grow their activity.
- The data is accessible to all participants, but everyone can use only its own; all the data will be used in multicenter projects.

The collected information is grouped in two categories:

Operational metrics: Patient age, patient gender, place of residence, health coverage diagnosis, referring physician/service, location at first consult, reason for consultation, responsible caregiver, reason for discharge from palliative care, place of death, time of referral, length of treatment, survival time

Clinical metrics: Distribution by disease (cancer/non cancer), pain control at 48 hours after starting palliative care, opioid analgesia, reason for discharge from palliative care.

Currently, 4 PAMPFF affiliated services use the database, and during 2011 and 2012, they entered data of more than 1100 patients. Participants meet periodically to identify and fix imperfections, optimize the functionality, and decide what kind automatic generated common information is needed.

The value of the database is twofold: It provides simple operational and clinical data, and increases awareness about the difficulties to obtain reliable data: It demonstrates that data collection and analysis in Argentina is a great challenge.

FUNDING STRATEGIES

With only a few exceptions, palliative care in developing countries is not recognized as a discipline nor is it incorporated within the health system.[37] These result in no budgetary allocation through public funds and the inability to receive reimbursement for services rendered through health insurance programs. Palliative care workers in developing countries are forced to work pro bono or work in other areas and dedicate the remaining hours to palliative care. Programs are forced to look for funding through private pay, donations, and charity from the community in order to cover the cost of operations and the provision of services.

Long-term financing of palliative care is a big challenge, and the mechanisms to finance and sustain the services vary depending on the structure of the team or program.[38] Palliative care programs in developing countries:

- Usually develop with community support
- Are based in donated houses, churches, or community institutions
- Provide services through volunteer work
- Raise funds for nonvolunteer professional fees, medication and supplies from local charity, religious orders, neighbors groups, donations, and sometimes from contracts with local purchasers

These funding mechanisms to sustain palliative care services have proven to be effective in small cities and when servicing a relatively small population base. Patients share similar needs, the amount of resources needed to run the services is small, and it can be offered for locals who establish partnerships with other individuals and institutions with the capacity to raise and/or provide money.

Hospital-based programs delivering care through multidisciplinary teams face tougher challenges to fund their activities. They are more complex, and require a larger infrastructure and more staff members.

Some countries have adopted funding mechanisms that combine efforts from the program and the institution. This joint funding collaboration has worked well in the PAMPFF, and it has provided additional benefits to the program, such as full responsibility over budgetary allocation and the identification of funding sources outside of the health care system. Both strategies have proven to be practical and shield the programs from the pressures and limitations of the health care system.

Palliative care programs and initiatives in developing countries need to identify sources and activities capable of generating funds to support the operational costs of the program. The PAMPFF implemented teaching and educational activities that require registration fees and generate additional revenue and have proven to be a substantial source of funding for the program.

Many other alternatives exist, and programs in each country need to evaluate the resources in the community and the needs in order to develop and implement resource-generating strategies that are successful. Long-term survival is the key to confront critical economic and human resource situations, which interfere with the smooth development of the activity. Economic autonomy requires dedication and labor but guarantees sustainability.

CONCLUSION

Developing countries face two socioeconomic factors that may delay the development of palliative care initiatives: First, the need to constantly adapt to legal, political, economic, and social changes reduces the demand for modifications in the health care system. And second, most of the economic growth registered by developing nations is still not enough to satisfy the social needs of the population. These factors pose financial, organizational, and educational barriers to the development of palliative care. However, the drive to reduce these barriers and generate feasible programs result in the development of practical strategies such as the ones described in this chapter.

The provision of palliative care is far from homogenous, and many developing nations have designed and implemented effective and successful strategies that have proven to help patients and families live a better quality of life until the end. Many of these strategies are not acceptable under the standards of care in developed nations, but a flexible approach is needed in order to be able to help those in need. Home-based care may be the most cost-effective model for adequate access to palliative care in places with limited resources. Provision of effective palliative care for patients and families should rely on the development of home-based palliative care integrated within the existing health care system. Countries should plan to bridge current gaps by building on existing strengths within each country and optimizing available resources. Development of low-cost high coverage approaches and national policy to promote accessibility and drug availability are key components. An understanding of palliative care needs within the community will help to establish broad support from the locals and the health authorities in the countries.

The support that palliative care workers in developed nations may provide to their colleagues in developing countries include the empowerment to generate their own models of care, strengthen their capacity to reach patients and provide care, development of inexpensive medications and design, and application of research to evaluate the effectiveness of their treatment protocols.

REFERENCES

1 The World Health Report 2002. *Reducing Risks, Promoting Healthy Life.* Geneva, Switzerland: WHO, 2002.

2 World Health Organization. *Cities and the Population issue.* 44th World Health Assembly, Technical Discussion 7, background document, Geneva, Switzerland, 1991.

3 De Lima L, Hamzah E. Socioeconomic, cultural and political issues in palliative care. In: *Palliative Care in the Developing World: Principles and Practice.* Bruera E, De Lima L, Wenk R and Farr W (eds.) Houston, TX: IAHPC Press, 2004; 23–37.

4 Rajagopal MR, Mazza D, Lipman AG (eds.). *Pain and Palliative Care in the Developing World and Marginalized Populations: A Global Challenge.* Philadelphia, PA: Haworth Press, 2003.

5 World Health Organization. *Cancer Control Program: Policies and Managerial Guidelines.* Geneva, Switzerland: WHO, 2002.

6 Heber D. New themes in palliative care: Book review. *Social Science and Medicine* 1993; 48: 1301–1303.

7 Bruera E. Palliative care programs in Latin America. *Palliative Medicine* 1992; 6: 182–184.

8 Field D, James N. Where and how people die. In: Clark, D. (ed.) *The Future for Palliative Care: Issues of Policy and Practice.* Philadelphia, PA: Open University Press, 1996; 6–29.

9 De Lima L, Krakauer E, Lorenz K, Praill D, MacDonald N, Doyle D. Ensuring palliative medicine availability: The development of the IAHPC list of essential medicines for palliative care. *Journal of Pain and Symptom Management* 2007; 33(5): 521–526.

10 Vignaroli E, Bennett MI, Nekolaichuk C, De Lima L, Wenk R, Ripamonti CI, Bruera E. Strategic pain management: The identification and development of the IAHPC opioid essential prescription package. *Journal of Palliative Medicine* 2012; 15(2): 186–191.

11 De Lima L, Bennett MI, Murray SA, Hudson P, Doyle D, Bruera E, Granda-Cameron C, Strasser F, Downing J, Wenk R. International Association for Hospice and Palliative Care (IAHPC) list of essential practices in palliative care. *Journal of Pain and Palliative Care Pharmacotherapy* 2012; 26(2): 118–122.

12 Servicio Extremeño de Salud. *Programa Marco de Cuidados Paliativos.* Junta de Extremadura, Consejeria de Sanidad y Consumo: Mérida, España, 2004.

13 Kumar S. Palliative care can be delivered through neighbourhood networks. *British Medical Journal* 2004; 329: 1184.

14 Hardman M. Models of community-based HIV care. *Southern African Journal of HIV Medicine* 2001; 4: 12–13.

15 World Health Organization—Programme on Cancer Control and Department of HIV/AIDS. *A Community Health Approach to Palliative Care for HIV/AIDS and Cancer Patients in Africa.* Geneva, Switzerland: WHO, 2004.

16 Campbell L. Audit of referral of AIDS patients from hospital to an integrated community-based home care programme in Kwazulu-Natal, South Africa. *The Southern African Journal of HIV Medicine*: 2001: 9–11.

17 Diana Fund. *Palliative Care Initiative.* The Diana, Princess of Wales, Memorial Fund Promotional Information, 2001; 2(4): 9–11.

18 Merriman, A. Uganda: Current status of palliative care. *Journal of Pain and Symptom Management* 2002; 24(2), 252–256.

19 Claxton-Oldfield S, Jefferies J, Fawcet C, Wasylkiw L, Claxton-Oldfiel J. Palliative care volunteers: Why do they do it? *Journal of Palliative Care* 2004; 20(2): 78–84.

20 Seibold D, Rossi S, Berteotti C, Soprych S, McQuillan L. Volunteer involvement in a hospice care program. *American Journal of Hospice Care* 1987; 4(2): 43–55.

21 Patchner M, Finn M. Volunteers: The life-line of hospice. *Omega* 1987; 18(2): 135.

22 Jaime E, Wenk R. Diseño y Aplicación de un Programa de Voluntariado en Cuidados Paliativos. In: *Cuidados Paliativos: Guias para el Manejo Clinico* (2ª Edición) E Bruera y L De Lima (eds). International Association for Hospice and Palliative Care y Organización Panamericana de la Salud. Washington, DC: OPS, 2004; 133–136.

23 Lamb D, de St. Aubin T, Foster M. Characteristics of most effective and least effective hospice volunteers. *American Journal of Hospice Care* 1985; 2: 42–45.

24 Black B, Kovacs P. Direct care and indirect care hospice volunteers: Motivations, acceptance, satisfaction, and length of service. *Journal Volunteers Administration* 1996; 14(2): 21–32.

25 National Hospice Organization. Bates IJ, Brand KE (eds.), *Volunteer Training Curriculum.* Arlington, TX: NHO, 1990.

26 World Health Organization. *Ensuring Balance in National Policies on Controlled Substances—Guidance for Availability and Accessibility of Controlled Medicines.* Geneva, Switzerland: WHO, 2011.

27 Wenk R, Bertolino M y Pussetto J. High costs of opioids in Developing countries: An availability barrier that can be overcome. *Journal of Pain and Symptom Management* 2000; 20: 81–82.

28 De Lima L, Sweeney C, Palmer JL, Bruera E. Potent Analgesics are more expensive for patients in developing countries: A comparative study. *Journal of Pain and Palliative Care Pharmacotherapy* 2004; 18: 1.

29 Merriman A, Mwebesa E, Katabira E. *Palliative Medicine: Pain and Symptom Control in the Cancer and/or AIDS Patient in Uganda and Other African Countries ("The Blue Book").* Kampala, Uganda: Hospice Africa Uganda, 2012.

30 Standing Senate Committee on Social Affairs and Technology: Recommendation II. In: *Quality END of Life Care: The Right of Every Canadian: Final Report of the Subcommittee to Update of Life and Death.* Ottawa, Ontario, Canada: Senate of Canada, 2000.

31 Herrera E, Cáceres FL, Rocafort J, Vergeles JM, Villa D. Las tecnologías de la información y comunicación (TICs) son pilar fundamental del proyecto de desarrollo de la sanidad en la Comunidad Autónoma de Extremadura. *Revista Esalud* 2004; 1(1) Retrieved from the Internet in http://www.revistaesalud.com/revistaesalud/index.php.

32 National Council for Palliative Care, Hospice Information Service. *Minimum Data Set for Specialist Palliative Care Services (version 1.2).* London, U.K.: National Council Palliative Care. 1996; Retrieved from the internet on December 30, 2005 from http://www.ncpc.org.uk/policy_unit/mds/data_manual.html.

33 Connor SR, Tecca M, Judi LundPerson J, Teno J. Measuring hospice care: The National Hospice and Palliative Care Organization National Hospice data set. *Journal of Pain and Symptom Management* 2004; 28(4): 316–328.

34 Wenk R, Bertolino M, Minatel M. Recopilación, registro y análisis de información en Cuidados Paliativos. *Medicina Paliativa* 2004; 11(2): 102–106.

35 Weissman DE, Meier DE, Spragens LH. Center to Advance Palliative Care palliative care consultation service metrics: Consensus recommendations. *Journal of Palliative Medicine* 2008; 11(10): 1294–1298.

36 Meier DE, Beresford L. Health systems find opportunities and challenges in palliative care development. *Journal of Palliative Medicine* 2010; 13(4): 387–370.

37 Worldwide Palliative Care Alliance. *Mapping Levels of Palliative Care Development: A Global Update 2011.* London, U.K.: WPCA, 2011.

38 Callaway M, Foley KM, De Lima L, Connor SR, Dix O, Lynch T, Wright M, Clark D. Funding for palliative care programs in developing countries. *Journal of Pain and Symptom Management* 2007; 33(5): 509–513.

100

Prognostic indicators of survival

CATERINA MODONESI, AUGUSTO T. CARACENI, MARCO MALTONI

INTRODUCTION

The three main components of medical intervention are diagnosis, therapy, and prognosis. Of these, prognosis is the least studied aspect in the scientific literature; as a proof of this, a Medline search produced 7,729,769 citations for the term "diagnosis," 6,554,448 for "therapy," and only 1,020,062 for "prognosis" [1]. Physicians do not feel comfortable with the issue of prognosis: a number of surveys on American doctors have highlighted their difficulty in formulating and communicating a prognosis [2*,3***], both tasks considered highly distressing. In this chapter, we strictly focus on foreseeing prognosis from a palliative care point of view, while the issues relating to foretelling will be dealt with elsewhere in the book.

Recent studies show that simultaneous palliative care or early palliative care are effective at any stage of cancer disease. However, palliative care becomes the only clinical approach as the disease progresses [4], leading to specific choices regarding therapeutic programs and appropriate care settings. In the decision-making process, prognosis represents one of the key parameters to be evaluated. Box 100.1 shows the reasons why prognosis prediction is useful.

Many studies have been conducted on prognosis in palliative care, especially for cancer patients, because of the increasing interest shown in this area. We chose to make reference to older papers through their evaluation in recent reviews and to integrate such references with more up-to-date significant original studies. A highly sensitive issue in decision making for cancer patients is that relating to the continuation or abandonment of antiblastic therapy. Recent years have highlighted an increase in the use of chemotherapy during the last months of life, often with higher costs because of the use of new and expensive drugs. [5*,7] Prolonged antiblastic treatment can have a negative effect on both quality of life and survival [15,16**,17***]. If medical oncologists tend to continue anticancer therapies for a long time as the only treatment [18], they move patients to palliative care services only in the last few days of life. This leads to an increased burden in the unmet needs of patients and to less satisfaction and perception of the quality of care received from patients' and families'

point of view [19]. Prolonging chemotherapy in the last weeks of life creates confusion and raises false hopes in terms of potential benefits from treatment [20]. The early introduction of palliative care leads to an improvement in quality of life, mood, and survival [21**].

TERMINAL PHASE AND DISEASE TRAJECTORIES

It is important to remember that prognostic evaluation is influenced by the trajectory of physical functional decline, which varies on the basis of the disease. In advanced cancer, often there is a stabilization or gradual decline in the state of health during the course of years or months, followed by an accelerated decline over a period of weeks or months. Bennett's recent review identified the terminal phase of life as the last 3 months (even though the median survival of cancer patients in most hospice programs is around 30–45 days) [22], characterized by the appearance of symptoms and disabilities that progressively increase the need for access to healthcare services, especially those dedicated to palliative care. Conversely, the trajectory relating to diseases with organ failure (e.g., congestive heart failure, chronic obstructive pulmonary disease [COPD]) is characterized by a progressive decline marked by acute crises from which the individual recovers to the previous or to a slightly worse state of health, until the last crisis occurs. Finally, in the elderly and frail patient, the decline to death is slow and progressive, sometimes taking a few years [23*] (Figure 100.1).

PROGNOSIS IN CANCER PATIENTS

General prognosis in cancer is related to diagnosis, stage of the disease, impact of therapy, comorbidities, and clinical conditions of the patient. However, in advanced disease, patient-related signs and symptoms (performance status [PS], symptoms, metabolic disorders, quality of life, and psychosocial problems) become increasingly important prognostic factors [24] (Figure 100.2).

Box 100.1 Reasons for making a prognosis prediction

An accurate life span evaluation can help

- Cancer specialists to understand when chemotherapy has become futile and is no longer appropriate [5*,6,7,8,9**]

- Medical oncologists, other specialists, and general practitioners to identify the most appropriate health care setting and understand when the time has come to direct patients to a palliative care program [10*]

- Palliative care teams to choose the most suitable palliative care setting (home, inpatient hospice, or acute palliative care unit approach) [11***]

- Palliative care physicians to establish whether the patient's condition is such that he or she is eligible for state reimbursement (when and where this is associated with certain life expectancy conditions) [12,13]

- Researchers to identify a definite population (inception cohort) in which the results of therapeutic actions can be assessed and compared with those from other populations, thus obtaining more accurate information for research design and analysis [14]

- Clinicians to give information on prognosis to both patients and their families to help them to manage practical issues and decision-making correlated with life expectancy

- Patients and families to deal with existential and spiritual end-of-life issues

PROGNOSTIC INDICATORS IN TERMINAL CANCER PATIENTS

Methodologic considerations

Prognostic indicators in cancer patients referred to palliative care programs are generally studied using a set of observations on prognostic variables in series of patients and then assessing the outcome for each patient. Researchers then often use statistical models to evaluate the link between predictors and outcomes. Box 100.2 illustrates the weak points of studies on prognostic factors in advanced and palliative stages of cancer from a methodological point of view.

Information on the prognostic predictivity of different indicators can be gathered from both original studies and from systematic reviews of the literature. Although such reviews were qualitative in the past [25], they have begun to be conducted according to evidence-based medicine directives [3***,11***,26***,27***]. In fact, the quality of studies on prognostic factors in palliative care has improved in recent years and the evidence gathered in this field has increased in terms of both quantity and quality. However, the most appropriate study design when focusing on prognosis is a cohort or case-control study, but the majority of original studies are observational studies, with a moderate level of evidence [28]. Some priorities in prognostication research in palliative care emerging from a consensus workshop are reported in Table 100.1 [29].

Clinical prediction of survival

The clinical prediction of survival (CPS) is one of the most widely studied factors in the literature, with controversial features that characterize its determination [3***,27***,30*]. The main advantages of CPS are its flexibility and rapid adaptability to suit a specific clinical situation. Among its weak points are reports of inaccuracy and subjectivity of the evaluation; a number of studies have highlighted a weak correlation (around 20%–30%) between the evaluation of the physician and actual survival (AS), with a tendency of as much as 60% to overestimate [30*,31*].

According to some physicians, a detection methodology that uses probabilistic prediction is more accurate than simply temporal prediction [32].

Worse accuracy has been linked to a longer physician–patient relationship [30*]. Another element that would seem to be important in CPS determination is the "horizon effect," which sustains that a prediction is more accurate when it is the nearer the event.

No great differences in accuracy have been found among those who prognosticate, while physicians seem to be better predictors initially, nurses become very accurate in the last

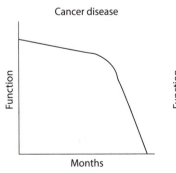

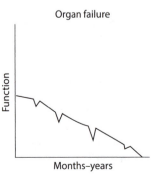

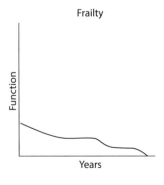

Figure 100.1 *Different trajectories of functional decline approaching death in three clinical situations. (Modified from Lunney, J.R. et al., JAMA, 289, 2387, 2003.)*

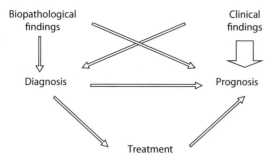

Figure 100.2 *How single factors have a different weight in influencing prognosis in advanced cancer. (Modified from Mackillop, W.J., Differences in prognostication between early and advanced cancer. In Glare, P. and Christakis, N.A. (eds.), Prognosis in Advanced Cancer, Oxford University Press, Oxford, U.K., 2008, pp. 13–23.)*

Box 100.2 Methodological problems of studies on prognostic indicators

- Identification of the inception cohort
- Retrospective cohorts
- Heterogeneous population sampling and setting
- Limited use of multivariate statistical analyses
- Brief description of the statistical methods and insufficient information on the recruitment method and sampling procedures
- Extremely limited use of the training and testing sample method
- Inadequate ratio between the number of variables studied and the number of patients enrolled
- Lack of a systematic procedure, heterogeneity, and selection of the variables studied
- Little attention paid to variables that are becoming increasingly important, for example, comorbidity

---

Table 100.1 *Five priorities in prognostication research emerging from a consensus workshop*

Research question	Rank
How valid are prognostic tools?	1
Can we use prognostic criteria as entry criteria for research?	=2
How do we judge the impact of a prognostic score in clinical practice?	=2
What is the best way of presenting survival data to patients?	4
What is the most user-friendly validated tool?	5

Source: Modified from Stevinson, C. et al., *Palliat. Med.*, 24, 462, 2010.

few days of life, probably because they have closer contact with the patients and are thus able to discern the clinical variations and signs of dying [31*,32,33,34*].

Despite criticism of CPS, it nonetheless correlates significantly with AS and is often considered an independent variable in multivariate analyses of prognostic factors [35*].

Performance status

PS has been studied in great depth and has proven to be an independent prognostic parameter [3***]. It has been assessed using different scales and according to various survey approaches, that is, the Karnofsky performance status (KPS) [36*], activities of daily living (ADL) [37*], Eastern Cooperative Oncology Group (ECOG) PS [38*], and a version of KPS tailored for a palliative setting called the palliative performance scale (PPS) [39*,40].

In general, PS values compatible with low activity indices are more accurate and correlate with low AS, whereas values consistent with high physical functioning are less accurate as early death can occur even when apparently "good" values are registered.

PHYSICAL SIGNS AND SYMPTOMS, AND PSYCHOLOGICAL FACTORS

Several signs and symptoms have been integrated with both CPS and PS to increase their prognostic capability. In 1988, Reuben et al. reported that 5 out of 14 evaluated symptoms retained their prognostic value, which was independent at multivariate analysis [41*]. The symptoms linked to survival included shortness of breath, dry mouth, eating problems or anorexia, difficulty in swallowing, and weight loss. As 4 out of 5 of these symptoms were related to the nutritional state of the patient, a "terminal cancer syndrome" hypothesis was formulated (characterized by a reduction in the functional state of the patient and symptoms of the cancer anorexia-cachexia syndrome [CACS]).

The majority of studies in which the signs and symptoms of CACS were tested reported a significant correlation with worse prognosis in univariate or multivariate analyses [41*,42*,43*]. A negative prognostic correlation was also observed for asthenia [44*]. Other symptoms for which a correlation with negative prognosis has been shown are cognitive failure [40,42*,43*,45*] and dyspnea [11***,35*,38*,39*,41*,42*].

It is still not clear whether the intensity and multiplicity of symptoms worsens prognosis. Factors for which a definite correlation with prognosis has been identified are reported in Table 100.2 [11***,46].

A number of authors have drawn attention to a possible link between quality of life and survival in palliative care populations [30*,47]. In all probability, the prognostic value of multidimensional evaluation tools of quality of life is ascribable to subscales referring to physical symptoms. However, quality of life would seem to be more significant in less advanced phases of disease [40].

BIOLOGICAL FACTORS

Leukocytosis, lymphocytopenia, and C-reactive protein values are the biological parameters with the greatest evidence of prognostic significance [11***,46]. The leukocyte count

Table 100.2 *Prognostic factors according to level of evidence in relation to AS in patients with advanced cancer*

Definite factors	Possible factors
CPS	Patient characteristics: Age, sex, marital status
PS	Tumor characteristics: Primary and secondary sites
Signs and symptoms of CACS: anorexia,	Signs: tachycardia, fever, proteinuria
weight loss, dysphagia, xerostomia	
Other symptoms: delirium, dyspnea	Symptoms: pain, nausea
Biologic factors: leukocytosis, lymphocytopenia, c-reactive protein	Biologic factors: anemia, hypoalbuminemia, prehypoalbuminemia, serum calcium level, serum sodium level, lactate dehydrogenase, and other enzymes
Prognostic scores	Comorbidity

Source: Modified from Maltoni, M. et al., *J. Clin. Oncol.*, 23, 6240, 2005.

Table 100.3 *PaP score*

Prognostic factor		Partial score
Dyspnea	Absent	0
	Present	1
Anorexia	Absent	0
	Present	1.5
KPS	>50	0
	30–40	0
	10–20	2.5
CPS (weeks)	>12	0
	11–12	2.0
	9–10	2.5
	7–8	2.5
	5–6	4.5
	3–4	6.0
	1–2	8.5
Total white blood cell (WBC) count (cell/mm^3)	Normal (4,800–8,500)	0
	High (8,501–11,000)	0.5
	Very high (>11,000)	1.5
Lymphocyte percentage	Normal (20.0–40.0)	0
	Low (12.0–19.9)	1.0
	Very low (0–11.9)	2.5

Total score (sum of partial scores) and expected survival

Risk groups	Total score
A: 30-day survival probability > 70%	0–5.5
B: 30-day survival probability 30%–70%	5.6–11.0
C: 30-day survival probability < 30%	11.1–17.5

Source: Maltoni, M. et al., *J. Pain Symptom Manage.*, 17, 240, 1999.

can, however, be influenced by antiblastic treatments and should thus only be evaluated in patients not receiving chemotherapy or in those a reasonable length of time has passed since the last treatment cycle. It has been reported that the prognostic value of some biological markers, for example, albumin and prealbumin levels, is linked to nutritional status, as evaluated by nutritional index (NI), prognostic nutritional index (PNI), and prognostic inflammatory and nutritional index (PINI) [48]. At multivariate analysis, however, such factors often lose their predictive power if correlated with other, often clinical, nutritional factors, that is, anorexia or weight loss [40].

PROGNOSTIC SCORES

Clinically important prognostic factors can be weighed in relation to statistical parameters and combined to create predictive mathematical models. Such models form the basis of prognostic indices, some of which have been validated for routine use in clinical practice. The palliative prognostic (PaP) score was built and validated on factors identified in an Italian prospective multicenter study of 540 advanced cancer patients with a median survival of 32 days (1–355) [35*,49*]. Parameters considered in the score are symptoms (presence or not of dyspnea and anorexia), poor PS according to KPS,

CPS, and white blood cell abnormalities. The score categories (0–5.5, 6–11, and 11.5–17.5) divide far advanced cancer populations into three iso-prognostic groups with a high >70%, intermediate 30%–70%, and low <30% probability of survival at 30 days (Table 100.3).

The PaP Score was also tested on populations of noncancer patients, retaining its predictive ability [50*]. The peculiarity of the PaP Score is that, as it includes the CPS, it can be used "together with" rather than "instead of" the clinical judgment of the physician [51]. A revised version of the PaP score to which the symptom of delirium was added (D-PaP) [14] has been prospectively tested but shows similar accuracy to that of the original PaP Score [52*].

PPS [53] is a modification of the KPS (Table 100.4) and considers the following variables: ambulation, activity, self-care, oral intake, and level of consciousness. The score is divided into 11 categories ranging from healthy (100%) to death (0%), and patients are grouped into three classes. Although the prognostic capacity of PPS alone has been proven [54*,55,56***], some difficulties may emerge when assessing patients at higher PPS levels because of the exclusively subjective nature of the tool [54*]. This tool has also been incorporated into the Palliative Prognostic Index (PPI).

The PPI was built and internally validated in 1999 by Morita on a Japanese population [43*] to distinguish between patients

Table 100.4 *PPS-version2*

PPS level (%)	Ambulation	Activity and evidence of disease	Self-care	Intake	Conscious level
100	Full	Normal activity and work / No evidence of disease	Full	Normal	Full
90	Full	Normal activity and work / Some evidence of disease	Full	Normal	Full
80	Full	Normal activity and work / Some evidence of disease	Full	Normal or reduced	Full
70	Reduced	Unable to do normal job/work / Significant disease	Full	Normal or reduced	Full
60	Reduced	Unable hobby/house work / Significant disease	Occasional assistance necessary	Normal or reduced	Full or confusion
50	Mainly sit/lie	Unable to do any work / Extensive disease	Considerable assistance required	Normal or reduced	Full or confusion
40	Mainly in bed	Unable to do most activity / Extensive disease	Mainly assistance	Normal or reduced	Full or drowsy ± confusion
30	Totally bed bound	Unable to do any activity / Extensive disease	Total care	Normal or reduced	Full or drowsy ± confusion
20	Totally bed bound	Unable to do any activity / Extensive disease	Total care	Minimal to sips	Full or drowsy ± confusion
10	Totally bed bound	Unable to do any activity / Extensive disease	Total care	Mouth care only	Full or drowsy+/− confusion
0	Death	–	–	–	–

Source: Anderson, F. et al., *J. Palliat. Care*, 12, 5, 1996.

Instructions: PPSv2 level is determined by reading left to right to find a "best horizontal fit." Begin at left column reading downward until current ambulation is determined, then, read across to next and downward until each column is determined. Thus, "leftward" columns take precedence over "rightward" columns.

who have a life expectancy of <3 weeks (PPI > 4.0), between 3 and 6 weeks (PPI 2.1–4.0) and >6 weeks (PPI ≤ 2.0); prognostic factors included are PPS, oral intake, edema, dyspnea at rest, and delirium (Table 100.5).

Some studies comparing different scores have been conducted. Stiel et al. assessed PPI and PaP [33], concluding that both scores yielded similar results, with a better performance in predicting poor prognosis. Tavares et al. reported that PPS alone was less accurate than PaP or PPI, the former slightly more accurate than the latter, but both showing problems in the intermediate prognosis group [57]. Maltoni et al. recently published the results from a prospective multicenter study that compared 4 prognostic scores described in palliative care literature (PaP, D-PaP, PPS, and PPI). All scores showed a statistically significant predictive capacity, and log-rank tests were highly significant ($p < 0.0001$). PaP and its modified version showed a better performance with an accuracy at 30 days of 88.0% for PaP score and 79.6% for D-PaP compared to 72.3% for PPI and <50% for PPS [52*]. The authors concluded that PaP is useful when more accurate prognostication is needed, while the other scores can be used when a rapid and simple evaluation is sufficient.

The literature contains numerous examples of other prognostic scores that have been built and studied [58***], but these tend to be either outdated and no more used or new, and so far invalidated, for example, Bruera's poor prognostic indicator [59*], terminal cancer prognostic score

[60*,51,46], cancer prognostic score [61*,40], Glasgow prognostic score [62], intra-hospital cancer mortality risk model (ICMRM) [63*], Japan palliative oncology study-prognostic index (JPOS-PI) [64*], or prognosis in palliative care study (PiPS) [65*].

Table 100.5 *PPI*

Prognostic factor		Partial score
PPS 10%–20%		4
PPS 30%–50%		2, 5
PPS > 50%		0
Delirium	Present	4
Delirium	Absent	0
Dyspnoea at rest	Present	3, 5
Dyspnoea at rest	Absent	0
Oral intake	Mouthfuls or less	2, 5
Oral intake	Reduced but more than mouthfuls	1
Oral intake	Normal	0
Edema	Present	1
Edema	Absent	0

Total score (sum of partial scores) and expected survival

Risk groups	Total score
A: Greater than 6 weeks	<2, 0
B: 3–6 weeks	2, 0–4
C: Less than 3 weeks	>4, 0

Source: Morita, T. et al., *Support Care Cancer*, 7, 128, 1999.

STRENGTHENING OF PROGNOSTIC ACCURACY ACHIEVED BY THE COMBINED USE OF CPS AND OTHER PROGNOSTIC FACTORS

Some studies have aimed to verify the increase in prognostic accuracy from the combined use of CPS and other prognostic factors with respect to CPS alone. When used in a slightly different population consisting of seriously ill hospitalized adults, the combination of the Study to Understand Prognosis and Preferences for Outcomes and Treatments (SUPPORT) model with physicians' estimates improved both predictive accuracy (receiver operating characteristic [ROC] curve area = 0.82) and capacity to identify patients with a higher probability of survival or death [66*].

Morita et al. [67*] reported that the prognostic accuracy of physicians significantly improved with the combined use of clinical judgment and its PPI, comprising more objective parameters.

Furthermore, in the previously mentioned review by Glare et al. [27***], it emerged that for all the KPS categories identified (<40, 40–50, >50), $R2$ values obtained in 981 patients for CPS alone, other prognostic factors alone, and CPS plus other prognostic factors were as follows: KPS < 40: 0.46, 0.25, 0.50; KPS 40–50: 0.35, 0.15, 0.38; and KPS > 50: 0.24, 0.08, 0.27, respectively.

A recent paper by Gwilliam et al proposed a new score PIPS (prognosis in palliative care study). The "B" version of it, incorporating a blood test, estimated survival better than either physicians (61.5% vs. 52.6% $p = 0.0135$) or nurses (61.5% vs. 52.3%; $p = 0.012$), but was not significantly better than the multiprofessional estimate (61.5% vs. 53.7%; $p = 0.188$) [65*].

Finally, Maltoni et al showed that 30-day prognostic accuracy of CPS alone was 75.6% but 88.0% for the PaP score, indicating that the accuracy of CPS alone was significantly increased when integrating it within the PaP Score [52*].

PROGNOSIS IN NONCANCER PATIENTS

Interest is increasing in the area of prognosis in noncancer patients, as a result of population aging because noncancer diseases are frequent in the elderly. Individuals in the advanced stage of nonneoplastic disease often have needs similar to those of cancer patients. However, the "typical" terminal phase in some noncancer diseases is difficult to identify or may not even exist [23*], making it more complicated for patients to be enrolled in hospice/palliative care programs [68].

Access to hospices can be limited by the fact that, in some countries, reimbursements are only granted if patients can produce certification specifying that they have "a life expectancy of 6 months or less, should the disease take its usual course." The National Hospice Organization (NHO) prognostic guidelines, although published some years ago, may still be useful in predicting prognosis in noncancer patients [12,69*],

even though their accuracy has been criticized, not taking into account the efficacy of modern pharmacologic treatments.

GENERAL PROGNOSTIC INDICATORS IN NONCANCER DISEASES

In October 2011, Salpeter et al. published a systematic review identifying a group of prognostic factors in noncancer diseases that indicate progression toward the end-of-life phase: poor PS, advanced age, malnutrition, comorbid illnesses, organ dysfunction, and hospitalization for acute decompensation. A median survival of 6 months or less was generally associated with the presence of 2–4 of these factors [12,69*,70***].

SPECIFIC PROGNOSTIC INDICATORS IN NONCANCER DISEASES

Heart disease

Unpredictable response to therapy and the specter of sudden cardiac death make the prediction of proximity to death especially difficult in end-stage cardiac disease. In the absence of a precipitating factor, survival normally ranges from 6 months to 4 years. Functional status described according to the New York Heart Association Classification (NYHA) is the most important prognostic factor: class IV, that is, symptoms of congestive heart failure at rest despite optimal treatment with diuretics and vasodilators, is correlated with the worst prognosis.

Factors that contribute to poorer prognoses include a left ventricular ejection fraction of 20% or less, aging, intractability of underlying heart disease, dilated cardiomyopathy, uncontrolled arrhythmia, contractility changes over time, high cardiothoracic ratio measured on a standard chest radiograph, and oxygen consumption [12,69*,71*,70***].

Triggers to evaluate the hypothesis of palliative care include recurring episodes of heart failure within the past 6 months despite optimization of medical therapy, appearance of malignant arrhythmia, frequent or continuous need for intravenous therapy, chronic worsening of quality of life, intractable NYHA stage IV symptoms, and signs of cardiac cachexia [72]. The presence of such events indicates the need for coordination and continuity of care among the various specialists (cardiologists, internists, and palliativists) involved in caring for the patient [73]. Furthermore, the increasing use of implantable cardiac defibrillators (ICDs), resynchronization therapy, and left ventricular assist devices (LVADs) can alter prognosis by modifying disease trajectory.

Numerous clinical scoring systems have been developed in cardiology, some of the most widely used [58***,74***] being heart failure risk scoring system (HFRSS) [75*], Seattle Heart Failure Model [76*], the cardiovascular medicine heart failure (CVM-HF) index [77*], and the cardiac and comorbid conditions HF (3C-HF) score [78*].

Lung disease

Making a prognostic prediction for lung diseases at an advanced stage is extremely difficult. Far advanced COPD is characterized by dyspnea at rest with little or no response to bronchodilators; increased hospitalization or home care visits for respiratory infections or respiratory failure; hypoxemia at rest and on room air; secondary right heart failure, pulmonary heart disease; weight loss >10% in the past 6 months; tachycardia at rest >100 [79].

Forced expiratory volume in one second (FEV1) was considered the main prognostic factor for a long time, but others such as exercise tolerance, pulmonary hyperinflation, systemic manifestations in the cardiovascular area, and exacerbations of the disease have now emerged as further predictors of death [69*,70***,80*,81]. Patients hospitalized following exacerbation of COPD have a median survival of ≤6 mesi when 3 or more of the following factors are present: age >70 years, right heart failure, worsening of functional status, need for home care after discharge from hospital, malnutrition, blood creatinine >2 mg/dL, repeated hospitalization in the previous 2 months, history of intubation, or mechanical ventilation [70***,82].

Dementia

The mean survival rate of patients with dementia ranges from 5 to 8 years, and the "advanced" stage of the disease may last 2 years. Difficulty in formulating a prognosis is one of the obstacles for hospices who accept patients with dementia. The main prognostic indicator is functional status, measured with Functional Assessment STaging (FAST). Stage 7 FAST patients have a mean survival of 6.9 months and a median survival of 4 months [83*]. Other factors include type of dementia (vascular dementia appears to lead to death more rapidly than Alzheimer's disease), age, gender, severity of dementing illness (inability to walk without assistance), and presence of medical complications.

Numerous other prognostic tools have been studied in patients with dementia: dementia prognostic model [84*], minimun data set (MDS) [85**], and survival in Alzheimer's model (SAM) [86*]. Mitchell et al developed the advanced dementia prognostic tool (ADEPT), a risk score to estimate survival in nursing home residents with advanced dementia. This score predicted survival with moderate accuracy and proved better at estimating 6-month mortality than hospice eligibility guidelines simulated with MDS data [87*,88*]. Results showed that survival was lower than 6 months when a patient was hospitalized for an acute illness or admitted to a nursing facility, in association with one of the following conditions: malnutrition, at least one pressure ulcer (bedsore), comorbidities, male >90 years, nasogastric tube, or gastrostomy [70***].

HIV disease

Mortality due to acquired immune deficiency syndrome (AIDS) has substantially improved since the early 1990s. The advent of highly active antiretroviral therapy (HAART), together with treatment of opportunistic infections and symptom palliation, has positively altered the prognosis of a disease that previously led to death within a few months from its diagnosis.

The definition of late-stage HIV can, however, be applied to patients with long-standing symptomatic disease, severe immunosuppression, cumulative morbidity, and failure or inability to tolerate antiretroviral therapy [89]. Consequently, the prognostic validity of some of the traditional prognostic indicators used, for example, CD4 cell count, viral load, specific opportunistic infections, may lessen [23*]. These factors should thus be integrated with more recent ones, for example, noncompliance or nonreaction to HAART, functional deficits (impaired ability to conduct routine activities, cognitive impairment), and/or the existence of other life-threatening conditions predictive of short-term survival, that is, weight loss and neurological abnormalities [89].

Shen et al. reported that age and markers of functional status were more predictive of mortality than traditional HIV prognostic variables [90*]. Despite advances in treatment, AIDS and associated comorbidities remain important causes of death, with a marked decrease in the incidence of some AIDS-defining illnesses such as Kaposi's sarcoma and cerebral lymphoma and an increase in the proportion of deaths from infections not typically associated with AIDS, for example, HCC derived from cirrhosis and HAART-related toxicity.

Amyotrophic lateral sclerosis

Palliative care in amyotrophic lateral sclerosis (ALS) begins when the patient is informed of the diagnosis, provides constant support for the patient throughout the disease, and continues in the intensive care unit after intubation and artificial ventilation until death [91,92]. NHO criteria enable clinicians to predict a survival of <6 months for ALS hospice patients. Such criteria include critically impaired breathing or rapid progression and life-threatening complications, or rapid progression and critical nutritional impairment [12]. The addition of the following parameters would seem to result in a more reliable prognostic evaluation: forced vital capacity (FVC) < 30%, FVC < 60% with a steady decline over past 2–3 months, two other respiratory indicators, or one respiratory and one nutritional indicator [93*]. Advanced age and bulbar beginning forms have also been described as factors of bad prognosis [94,95,96].

Liver disease

Prognostic indicators that are additively negative in end-stage cirrhosis are laboratory indicators of severely altered liver functionality and several clinical conditions (treatment-refractory ascites, spontaneous bacterial peritonitis, hepatorenal syndrome, hepatic encephalopathy refractory to therapies, recurrent variceal bleeding) [69*]. Other factors have also been reported, including malnutrition, muscle wasting, active alcoholism, hepatocellular carcinoma, and

HBsAg positivity [12]. The two most widely used prognostic models developed for decompensated cirrhosis are the Child-Pugh score and the model for end-stage liver disease (MELD) [70***,97,98*]. A prognosis of less than 6 months is estimated for a Child-Pugh score of ≥12 or a MELD score of ≥21 [99]. A 2006 review by Cholongitas et al. reported that general ICU models, that is, acute physiology and chronic health evaluation (APACHE), organ system failure (OSF), and sequential organ failure assessment (SOFA) [100,101***], showed a better performance in cirrhotic populations compared to that of scores designed specifically for the disease [102*,103***].

Renal disease

The Core Curriculum in Nephrology Palliative Care [104] reports that end-stage renal disease (ESRD) patients undergoing dialysis survive a quarter of the time of age-matched patients without renal disease, with an annual mortality rate of 23%. The NHO examines different situations such as ESRD, acute and chronic renal failure, and chronic ambulatory peritoneal dialysis (CAPD) [12]. Laboratory criteria for renal failure, clinical signs, and symptoms associated with renal failure, and comorbid complications that predict early mortality in hospital and patients with acute renal failure are also reported. An independent and graded association between the rate of decline in kidney function and the risk of death has been described [105].

Patients undergoing dialysis have a life expectancy of less than 6 months when this is associated with age >70 years and 2 or more of the following conditions: poor PS, significant comorbidities, malnutrition, resident in a skilled nursing facility, admission to an intensive care unit for an acute illness, or hip fracture with inability to ambulate [70***]. Wong et al.'s observational study showed that the Stoke comorbidity grade (SCG) was an independent prognostic factor in patients who chose not to undergo dialysis [106]. For patients in chronic dialysis who suspend treatment, life expectancy is extremely short, around 7 days.

FUTURE PROGNOSTIC TOOLS

Over the last few years, advances in computer technology have helped to develop, through the application of mathematical models, numerous prediction risk calculators or prognostic models known as web-based prognostic tools [46]. While they can be used for different diseases, they are not specifically designed for palliative or end-of-life phases. Some of the most widely used tools are listed as follows [40,46]:

Prognostigram: http://oto2.wustl.edu/clinepi/prog.html
Prognostat: http://web.his.uvic.ca/research/NET2/index.php o www.victoriahospice.org
Adjuvant! Online for lung, breast and colon cancer: www.adjuvantonline.com

Memorial Sloan Kettering Cancer Centre (MSKCC) nomogram: http://www.mskcc.org
Heart failure models: EFFECT Heart Failure Risk Scoring Scale www.ccort.ca; Seattle Heart Failure Model www.seattleheartfailuremodel.org
HIV/AIDS: antiretroviral (ART) Cohort Collaboration risk calculator: http://www.art-cohort-collaboration.org/

Recently, Feliu et al. have developed and validated a prognostic nomogram specific for terminal ill cancer patients. Five variables (ECOG PS, lactate dehydrogenase levels, lymphocyte levels, albumin levels, and time from initial diagnosis to diagnosis to terminal disease) were retained independent of prognostic factors of survival and formed the basis of the nomogram that predict the probability of survival at 15, 30, and 60 days in terminally ill cancer patients [107].

CONCLUSIONS

Awareness of prognostic indicators can help physicians who do not feel overly confident about making prognoses and find it difficult and stressful [2*]. When communicating a prognosis, ethical, cultural, religious, and psychological issues should borne in mind by carers to avoid causing even greater distress to a gravely ill patient: while patients have a right to be informed, they do not have a duty to be informed.

In conclusion, appropriate use of life expectancy prognostication to improve and personalize the treatment of patients in the advanced and terminal stages of disease can only be achieved if it forms an integral part of a multidisciplinary palliative care program, which holds high the value of life remaining.

Key learning points

- Awareness of prognostic survival indicators helps clinicians in the difficult decision-making process and can lead to better communication with both patients and their families. Prognostication has only a probabilistic value, and this should be taken into consideration when examining the possible course of each individual's illness.

- Trajectories of noncancer chronic disease make prognosis prediction for these diseases more complex than that of the palliative phase of cancer.

- Prognostic indicators in palliative care patients differ from those used for the early and advanced stages.

- CPS is an independent prognostic indicator in palliative care cancer patients. However, as its accuracy is conditioned by a number of restrictions, and it should only be used in conjunction with other, more objective prognostic indicators.

- The following indicators have shown independent prognostic ability in cancer patients: PS, signs and symptoms of CACS, delirium, dyspnea.

- CPS and other prognostic indicators can be included in simple models or prognostic scores. The prognostic ability of CPS increases when it is used "together with" rather than "instead of" clinical judgment.

- Prognostic indicators can also be found in noncancer diseases; some are common to more than one disease (functional status and nutritional status), whereas others are specific to individual diseases.

- The main aim of prognostication is to personalize the treatment of patients when dealing with the severest stage of their disease, while simultaneously continuing to fully consider the individual value of the patient's remaining lifetime.

REFERENCES

1 U.S. National Library of Medicine, National Institutes of Health, PubMedGov. Available at http://www.ncbi.nlm.nih.gov/pubmed. Accessed May 11, 2012.

2 Christakis NA, Iwashyna TJ. Attitude and self-reported practice regarding prognostication in a national sample of internists. *Arch Intern Med* 1998;**158**:2389–2395.

3 Vigano A, Dorgan M, Buckingham J et al. Survival prediction in terminal cancer patients: A systematic review of the medical literature. *Palliat Med* 2000;**14**:363–374.

4 Bruera E, Hui D. Integrating supportive and palliative care in the trajectory of cancer: Establishing goals and models of care. *J Clin Oncol* 2010;**28**:4013–4017.

5 Earle CC, Neville BA, Landrum MB et al. Trends in the aggressiveness of cancer care near the end of life. *J Clin Oncol* 2004;**22**:315–321.

6 Earle CC, Park ER, Lai B et al. Identifying potential indicators of the quality of end-of-life cancer care from administrative data. *J Clin Oncol* 2003;**21**:1133–1138.

7 Earle CC, Landrum MB, Souza JM et al. Aggressiveness of cancer care near the end of life: Is it a quality-of-care issue? *J Clin Oncol* 2008;**26**:3860–3866.

8 Finlay E, Casarett D. Making difficult discussions easier: Using prognosis to facilitate transitions to hospice. *CA Cancer J Clin* 2009;**59**:250–263.

9 Temel JS, Greer JA, Admane S et al. Longitudinal perceptions of prognosis and goals of therapy in patients with metastatic non-small-cell lung cancer: Results of a randomized study of early palliative care. *J Clin Oncol* 2011;**29**:2319–2326.

10 Lamont EB, Christakis NA. Physician factors in the timing of cancer patient referral to hospice palliative care. *Cancer* 2002;**94**:2733–2737.

11 Maltoni M, Caraceni A, Brunelli C et al. Prognostic factors in advanced cancer patients: Evidence-based clinical recommendations—A study by the Steering Committee of the European Association for Palliative Care. *J Clin Oncol* 2005;**23**:6240–6248.

12 Standards and Accreditation Committee, Medical Guidelines Task Force of the National Hospice Organization. *Medical Guidelines for Determining Prognosis in Selected Non-Cancer Diseases*, 2nd edn. Arlington, VA: National Hospice Organization, 1996.

13 Smith JL. Commentary: Why do doctors overestimate? *BMJ* 2000;**320**:472–473.

14 Scarpi E, Maltoni M, Miceli R et al. Survival prediction for terminally ill cancer patients: Revision of palliative prognostic score with incorporation of delirium. *Oncologist* 2011;**16**(12):1793–1799.

15 Saito AM, Landrum MB, Neville BA et al. The effect on survival of continuing chemotherapy to near death. *BMC Palliat Care* 2011;**10**:14.

16 Temel JS, Greer JA, Muzikansky A. Early palliative care for patients with metastatic non-small-cell lung cancer. *N Engl J Med* 2010;**363**:733–742.

17 Salpeter SR, Malter DS, Luo EJ et al. Systematic review of cancer presentations with a median survival of six months or less. *J Palliat Med* 2012;**15**(2):175–185.

18 Andreis F, Rizzi A, Rota L et al. Chemotherapy use at the end of life. A retrospective single centre experience analysis. *Tumori* 2011;**97**:30–34.

19 Teno JM, Shu JE, Casarett D et al. Timing of referral to hospice and quality of care: Length of stay and bereaved family members' perceptions of the timing of hospice referral. *J Pain Symptom Manage* 2007;**34**:120–125.

20 Mack JW, Cook EF, Wolfe J et al. Understanding of prognosis among parents of children with cancer: Parental optimism and the parent-physician interaction. *J Clin Oncol* 2007;**25**:1357–1362.

21 Greer JA, Pirl WF, Jackson VA et al. Effect of early palliative care on chemotherapy use and end-of-life care in patients with metastatic non-small-cell lung cancer. *J Clin Oncol* 2012;**30**(4):394–400.

22 Bennett MI, Davies EA, Higginson IJ. Delivering research in end-of-life care: Problems, pitfalls and future priorities. *Palliat Med* 2010;**24**:456–461.

23 Lunney JR, Lynn J, Foley D et al. Patterns of functional decline at the end of life. *JAMA* 2003;**289**:2387–2392.

24 Mackillop WJ. Differences in prognostication between early and advanced cancer. In: Glare P, Christakis NA (eds.). *Prognosis in Advanced Cancer*. Oxford, U.K.: Oxford University Press, 2008, pp. 13–23.

25 Den Daas N. Estimating length of survival in end-stage cancer: A review of the literature. *J Pain Symptom Manage* 1995;**10**:548–555.

26 Chow E, Harth T, Hruby G et al. How accurate are physicians' clinical predictions of survival and the available prognostic tools in estimating survival times in terminally ill cancer patients? A systematic review. *Clin Oncol* 2001;**13**:209–218.

27 Glare P, Virik K, Jones M et al. A systematic review of physicians' survival predictions in terminally ill cancer patients. *BMJ* 2003;**327**:195–200.

28 Hui D, Parsons HA, Damani S et al. Quantity, design, and scope of the palliative oncology literature. *Oncologist* 2011;**16**(5):694–703.

29 Stevinson C, Preston N, Todd C, Cancer Experiences Collaborative (CECo). Defining priorities in prognostication research: Results of a consensus workshop. *Palliat Med* 2010;**24**:462–468.

30 Christakis NA, Lamont EB. Extent and determinants of error in doctors' prognoses in terminally ill patients: Prospective cohort study. *BMJ* 2000;**320**:469–472.

31 Selby D, Chakraborty A, Lilien T et al. Clinician accuracy when estimating survival duration: The role of the patient's performance status and time-based prognostic categories. *J Pain Symptom Manage* 2011;**42**:578–588.

32 Hui D, Kilgore K, Nguyen L et al. The accuracy of probabilistic versus temporal clinician prediction of survival for patients with advanced cancer: A preliminary report. *Oncologist* 2011;**16**(11):1642–1648.

33 Stiel S, Bertram L, Neuhaus S. Evaluation and comparison of two prognostic scores and the physicians' estimate of survival in terminally ill patients. *Support Care Cancer* 2010;**18**:43–49.

34 Stone CA, Tiernan E, Dooley BA. Prospective validation of the palliative prognostic index in patients with cancer. *J Pain Symptom Manage* 2008;**35**:617–622.

35 Pirovano M, Maltoni M, Nanni O et al. A new palliative prognostic score (PaP Score). A first step for the staging of terminally ill cancer patients. *J Pain Symptom Manage* 1999;**17**:231–239.

36 Maltoni M, Nanni O, Derni S et al. Clinical prediction of survival is more accurate than the Karnofsky performance status in estimating life span of terminally-ill cancer patients. *Eur J Cancer* 1994;**30**:764–766.

37 Schonwetter RS, Robinson BE, Ramirez G. Prognostic factors for survival in terminal lung cancer patients. *J Gen Intern Med* 1994;**9**:366–371.

38 Rosenthal MA, Gebski VJ, Kefford RF, Stuart-Harris RC. Prediction of life-expectancy in hospice patients: Identification of novel prognostic factors. *Palliat Med* 1993;**7**:199–204.

39 Morita T, Tsunoda J, Inoue S, Chihara S. Survival prediction of terminally ill cancer patients by clinical symptoms: Development of a simple indicator. *Jpn J Clin Oncol* 1999;**29**:156–159.

40 Glare P, Sinclair C, Downing M et al. Predicting survival in patients with advanced disease. *Eur J Cancer* 2008;**44**:1146–1156.

41 Reuben DB, Mor V, Hiris J. Clinical symptoms and length of survival in patients with terminal cancer. *Arch Intern Med* 1988;**148**:1586–1591.

42 Maltoni M, Pirovano M, Scarpi E et al. Prediction of survival of patients terminally ill with cancer. Results of an Italian prospective multicentric study. *Cancer* 1995;**75**:2613–2622.

43 Morita T, Tsunoda J, Inoue S, Chihara S. The palliative prognostic index: A scoring system for survival prediction of terminally ill cancer patients. *Support Care Cancer* 1999;**7**:128–133.

44 Viganò A, Bruera E, Jhangri GS et al. Clinical survival predictors in patients with advanced cancer. *Arch Intern Med* 2000;**160**:861–868.

45 Caraceni A, Nanni O, Maltoni M et al. Impact of delirium on short term prognosis of advanced cancer patients. *Cancer* 2000;**89**:1145–1149.

46 Glare P, Sinclair C. Palliative medicine review: Prognostication. *J Palliat Med* 2008;**11**:84–103.

47 Glare PA, Eychmueller S, Mcmahon P. Diagnostic accuracy of the palliative prognostic score in hospitalized patients with advanced cancer. *J Clin Oncol* 2004;**22**:4823–4828. Comparative study.

48 Maltoni M, Amadori D. Prognosis in advanced cancer. *Hematol Oncol Clin North Am* 2002;**16**:715–729.

49 Maltoni M, Nanni O, Pirovano M et al. Successful validation of the palliative prognostic score in terminally ill cancer patients. Italian multicenter study group on palliative care. *J Pain Symptom Manage* 1999;**17**:240–247.

50 Glare P, Eychmueller S, Virik K. The use of the palliative prognostic score in patients with diagnoses other than cancer. *J Pain Symptom Manage* 2003;**26**:883–885.

51 Stone PC, Lund S. Predicting prognosis in patients with advanced cancer. *Ann Oncol* 2007;**18**:971–976.

52 Maltoni M, Scarpi E, Pittureri C et al. Prospective comparison of prognostic scores in palliative care cancer populations. *Oncologist* 2012;**17**(3):446–454.

53 Anderson F, Downing GM, Hill J et al. Palliative performance scale (PPS): A new tool. *J Palliat Care* 1996;**12**:5–11.

54 Lau F, Maida V, Downing M et al. Use of palliative performance scale for end-of-life prognostication in a palliative medicine consultation service. *J Pain Symptom Manage* 2009;**37**:965–972.

55 Olajide O, Hanson L, Usher BM et al. Validation of the palliative performance scale in the acute tertiary care hospital setting. *J Palliat Med* 2007;**10**:111–117.

56 Downing M, Lau F, Lesperance M et al. Meta-analysis of survival prediction with palliative performance scale. *J Palliat Care* 2007;**23**:245–252.

57 Tavares EA. Comparing the accuracy of four methods to predict survival in terminally ill patients referred to a hospital-based palliative medicine team. *Eur J Palliat Care* (Abstracts of the *12th Congress European Association Palliative Care*, Lisbon, Portugal, May 18–21, 2011); Abstract FC1.**5**:48.

58 Lau F, Cloutier-Fisher D, Kuziemsky C et al. A systematic review of prognostic tools for estimating survival time in palliative care. *J Palliat Care* 2007;**23**(2):93–112.

59 Bruera E, Miller MJ, Kuehn N et al. Estimate of survival of patients admitted to a palliative care unit: A prospective study. *J Pain Symptom Manage* 1992;**7**:82–86.

60 Yun HY, Heo Ds, Heo BY et al. Development of terminal cancer prognostic score as an index in terminally ill cancer patients. *Oncol Rep* 2001;**8**:795–800.

61 Chuang RB, Hu WY, Chiu TY, Chen CY. Prediction of survival in terminal cancer patients in Taiwan: Constructing a prognostic scale. *J Pain Symptom Manage* 2004;**28**:115–122.

62 Forrest LM, McMillan DC, McArdle CS et al. Evaluation of cumulative prognostic scores based on the systemic inflammatory response in patients with inoperable non-small-cell lung cancer. *Br J Cancer* 2003;**89**(6):1028–1030.

63 Bozcuk H, Koyuncu E, Yildiz M et al. A simple and accurate prediction model to estimate the intrahospital mortality risk of hospitalised cancer patients. *Int J Clin Pract* 2004;**58**(11):1014–1019.

64 Hyodo I, Morita T, Adachi I et al. Development of a predicting tool for survival of terminally ill cancer patients. *Jpn J Clin Oncol* 2010;**40**:442–448.

65 Gwilliam B, Keeley V, Todd C et al. Development of prognosis in palliative care study (PiPS) predictor models to improve prognostication in advanced cancer: Prospective cohort study. *BMJ* 2011;**343**:d4920.

66 Knaus WA, Harrell FE, Lynn J et al. The SUPPORT prognostic model: Objective estimates of survival for seriously ill hospitalized adults. *Ann Intern Med* 1995;**122**:191–203.

67 Morita T, Tsunoda J, Inoue S, Chihara S. Improved accuracy of physicians' survival prediction for terminally ill cancer patients using the palliative prognostic index. *Palliat Med* 2001;**15**:419–424.

68 Brickner L, Scannell K, Marquet S, Ackerson L. Barriers to hospice care and referrals: Survey of physicians' knowledge, attitudes, and perceptions in a health maintenance organization. *J Palliat Med* 2004;**7**(3):411–418.

69 Fox E, Landrum-McNiff K et al. Evaluation of prognostic criteria for determining hospice eligibility in patients with advanced lung, heart, or liver disease. SUPPORT investigators. Study to Understand Prognoses and Preferences for Outcomes and Risks of Treatments. *JAMA* 1999;**282**:1638–1645.

70 Salpeter SR, Luo EJ, Malter DS, Stuart B. Systematic review of non-cancer presentations with a median survival of 6 months or less. *Am J Med* 2012;**125**(5):512.e1–512.e16.

71 Jaagosild P, Dawson NV, Thomas C et al. Outcome of acute exacerbation of severe congestive heart failure: Quality of life, resource use, and survival. SUPPORT investigators. The Study to Understand Prognosis and Preferences for Outcomes and Risks of Treatment. *Arch Intern Med* 1998;**158**:1081–1089.

72 Jaarsma T, Beattie JM, Ryder M et al. Palliative care in heart failure: A position statement from the palliative care workshop of the Heart Failure Association of the European Society of Cardiology. *Eur J Heart Fail* May 2009;**11**(5):433–443.

✶ ●73 Hunt SA, Abraham WT, Chin MH et al. 2009 focused update incorporated into the ACC/AHA 2005 Guidelines for the Diagnosis and Management of Heart Failure in Adults: A report of the American College of Cardiology Foundation/American Heart Association Task Force on Practice Guidelines: Developed in collaboration with the International Society for Heart and Lung Transplantation. *Circulation* 2009;**119**(14):e391–e479.

◆ 74 Coventry PA, Grande GE, Richards DA, Todd CJ. Prediction of appropriate timing of palliative care for older adults with non-malignant life-threatening disease: A systematic review. *Age Ageing* 2005;**34**(3):218–227.

75 Lee DS, Austin PC, Rouleau JL et al. Predicting mortality among patients hospitalized for heart failure: Derivation and validation of a clinical model. *JAMA* 2003;**290**(19):2581–2587.

76 Levy WC, Mozaffarian D, Linker DT et al. The seattle heart failure model: Prediction of survival in heart failure. *Circulation* 2006;**113**(11):1424–1433.

● 77 Senni M, Santilli G, Parrella P et al. A novel prognostic index to determine the impact of cardiac conditions and co-morbidities on one-year outcome in patients with heart failure. *Am J Cardiol* 2006;**98**(8):1076–1082.

● 78 Senni M, ParrellaP, De Maria R. Predicting heart failure outcome from cardiac and comorbid conditions: The 3C-HF score. *Int J Cardiol* 2013.20;**163**(2):206–11. Epub 2011 Nov 29.

79 Abrahm JL, Hansen-Flaschen J. Hospice care for patients with advanced lung disease. *Chest* 2002;**121**:220–229.

80 Casanova C, Cote T, de Torres JP. Inspiratory total lung capacity ratio predicts mortality in patient with chronic obstructive pulmonary disease. *Am J Respir Crit Care Med* 2005;**171**:591–597,611.

81 Oga T, Nishimura K, Tsukino M. Analysis of the factors related to mortality in chronic obstructive pulmonary disease. Role of exercise capacity and health status. *Am J Resp Crit Care Med* 2003;**167**:544–549.

82 Selecky PA, Elliasson CAH, Hall RI et al. Palliative and end-of-life care for patients with cardiopulmonary diseases: American College of Chest Physicians position statement. *Chest* 2005;**128**:3599–3610.

✶ 83 Luchins DJ, Hanrahan P, Murphy K. Criteria for enrolling dementia patients in hospice. *J Am Geriatr Soc* 1997;**45**:1054–1059.

84 Schonwetter RS, Han B, Small BJ et al. Predictors of six-month survival among patients with dementia: An evaluation of hospice Medicare guidelines. *Am J Hosp Palliat Care* 2003;**20**(2):105–113.

85 Hartmaier SL, Sloane PD, Guess HA et al. Validation of the minimun data set cognitive performance scale: Agreement with the mini-mental state examination. *J Gerontol A Biol Sci Med Sci* 1995;**50**:M128–M133.

86 Paradise M, Walker Z, Cooper C et al. Prediction of survival in Alzheimer's disease the LASER-AD longitudinal study. *Int J Geriatr Psychiat* 2009;**24**(7):739–747.

87 Mitchell SL, Miller SC, Teno JM et al. The advanced dementia prognostic tool: A risk score to estimate survival in nursing home residents with advanced dementia. *J Pain Symptom Manage* 2010;**40**(5):639–651.

88 Mitchell SL, Miller SC, Teno JM et al. Prediction of 6-month survival of nursing home residents with advanced dementia using ADEPT vs hospice eligibility guidelines. *JAMA* 2010;**304**(17):1929–1935.

◆ 89 Selwyin PA, Forstein M. Overcoming the false dichotomy of curative vs palliative care for late-stage HIV/AIDS: "Let me live the way I want to live, until I can't". *JAMA* 2003;**290**:806–814.

90 Shen JM, Blank A, Selwyn PA. Predictors of mortality for patients with advanced disease in an HIV palliative care program. *J Acquir Immune Defic Syndr* 2005;**40**(4):445–447.

◆ 91 Borasio GD, Voltz R. Palliative care in amyotrophic lateral sclerosis. *J Neurol* 1997;**244**(Suppl 4):S11–S17.

◆ 92 Bede P, Oliver D, Stodart J et al. Palliative care in amyotrophic lateral sclerosis: A review of current international guidelines and initiatives. *J Neurol Neurosurg Psychiat* 2011;**82**(4):413–418.

✶ 93 McCluskey L, Houseman G. Medicare hospice referral criteria for patients with amyotrophic lateral sclerosis: A need for improvement. *J Palliat Med* 2004;**7**:47–53.

94 Mandrioli J, Faglioni P, Nichelli P et al. Amyotrophic lateral sclerosis: Prognostic indicators of survival. *Amyotroph Lateral Scler* 2006;**7**(4):211–220.

95 Larrode-Pellicer P, Alberti-González O, Iñiguez-Martínez C et al. Pronostic factors and survival in motor neuron disease. *Neurologia* 2007;**22**(6):362–367.

96 Zoccolella S, Beghi E, Palagano G et al. Analysis of survival and prognostic factors in amyotrophic lateral sclerosis: A population based study. *J Neurol Neurosurg Psychiat* 2008;**79**(1):33–37.

97 Pugh RN, Murray-Lyon IM, Dawson JL et al. Transection of the oesophagus for bleeding oesophageal varices. *Br J Surg* 1973;**60**(8):646–649.

◆ 98 Kamath PS, Wiesner RH, Malinchoc M et al. A model to predict survival in patients with end-stage liver disease. *Hepatology* 2001;**33**(2):464–470.

◆ 99 Kamath PS, Kim WR, Advanced Liver Disease Study Group. The model for end-stage liver disease (MELD). *Hepatology* 2007;**45**(3):797–805.

◆100 Vincent JL, Ferreira F, Moreno R. Scoring systems for assessing organ dysfunction and survival. *Crit Care Clin* 2000;**16**(2):353–366.

◆101 Minne L, Abu-Hanna A, de Jonge E. Evaluation of SOFA-based models for predicting mortality in the ICU: A systematic review. *Crit Care* 2008;**12**(6):R161.

102 Ferreira FL, Bota DP, Bross A et al. Serial evaluation of the SOFA score to predict outcome in critically ill patients. *JAMA* 2001;**286**(14):1754–1758.

◆103 Cholongitas E, Senzolo M, Patch D et al. Review article: Scoring systems for assessing prognosis in critically ill adult cirrhotics. *Aliment Pharmacol Ther* 2006;**24**(3):453–464.

◆104 Moss AH, Holley JL, Davison S et al. Core curriculum in nephrology. Palliative care. *Am J Kidney Dis* 2004;**43**:172–173.

◆105 Al-Aly Z, Cepeda O. Rate of change in kidney function and the risk of death: The case for incorporating the rate of kidney function decline into the CKD staging system. *Nephron Clin Pract* 2011;**119**(2):c179–c185.

106 Wong CF, McCarthy M, Howse ML et al. Factors affecting survival in advanced chronic kidney patients who choose not to receive dialysis. *Ren Fail* 2007;**29**(6):653–659.

107 Feliu J, Jiménez-Gordo AM, Madero R et al. Development and validation of a prognostic nomogram for terminally ill cancer patients. *J Natl Cancer Inst* 2011;**103**(21):1613–1620.

Palliative sedation

Sedation in the context of palliative medicine is the monitored use of medications intended to induce varying degrees of unconsciousness to induce a state of decreased or absent awareness (unconsciousness) in order to relieve the burden of otherwise intractable suffering. The intent is to provide adequate relief of distress [1].

Sedation is controversial insofar as it diminishes capacity: capacity to interact, to function, and, in some cases, to live. In the context of a field of endeavor committed to helping the ill and suffering to live better, there is a potential contradiction of purpose. Sedation for the relief of suffering touches at the most basic conflict of palliative medicine: are we doing "enough" or are we doing "too much." This issue exemplifies the tensions in achieving the dual goals of palliative care: firstly, to relieve suffering and, secondly, to do so in such a manner so as to preserve the moral sensibilities of the patient, the professional carers, and concerned family and friends.

Sedation is used in palliative care in several settings:

1. Transient controlled sedation for noxious procedures
2. Sedation used in end of life weaning from ventilator supports
3. Sedation in the management of refractory symptoms at the end of life
4. Emergency sedation
5. Respite sedation
6. Sedation for psychological or existential suffering

Each of these will be discussed describing the context of application and practical and ethical considerations.

TRANSIENT CONTROLLED SEDATION

Transient controlled sedation is routinely and uncontroversially used to manage the severe pain and anxiety associated with noxious procedures. Sedation enables patients to endure interventions that would otherwise be intolerable. Procedural guidelines exist for transient sedation for noxious procedures [2–5] and in burn care [6]. The depth of sedation required is influenced by the nature of the noxious stimulus,

the level of relief achieved by other concurrent approaches, and individual patient factors. When these techniques are well applied, reports of pain and suffering are infrequent. Since these patients are expected to recover, careful attention is paid to maintaining adequate ventilation, hydration, and nutrition.

Occasionally, transient sedation will be needed for a self-limiting severe exacerbation of pain [7]. In the full anticipation that this will be a reversible intervention, close monitoring of respiratory and homodynamic stability is essential. In one case report, this was achieved with midazolam administered by a patient-controlled analgesia device [7].

SEDATION IN THE MANAGEMENT OF REFRACTORY SYMPTOMS AT THE END OF LIFE (PALLIATIVE SEDATION)

At the end of life, the goals of care may shift and the relief of suffering may predominate over other considerations relating to functional capacity. In this setting, the designation of a symptom as "refractory" may justify the use of induced sedation, particularly since this is the only option that is capable of providing the necessary relief with certainty and speed. Various names have been applied to the issue of sedation in this setting: terminal sedation, palliative sedation, and palliative sedation therapy [8]. Though no single term has achieved universal support, of these options, palliative sedation is generally preferred [9–12].

Symptoms at the end of life

Among patients with advanced cancer, clinical experience suggests that optimal palliative care can effectively manage the symptoms of most cancer patients during most of the course of the disease. Although physical and psychological symptoms cannot be eliminated, they are usually relieved enough to adequately temper the suffering of the patient and family [13–18]. This phase may be referred to as the ambulatory phase of advanced cancer.

As the disease progresses and the end of life approaches, patients commonly suffer more physical and psychological symptoms (including pain) and it often becomes more difficult to achieve adequate relief [19–25]. For some patients, the degree of suffering related to these symptoms may be intolerable. Despite intensified efforts to manage such problems, some patients do not achieve adequate relief and they continue to suffer from inadequately controlled symptoms that may be termed "refractory."

An important study reviewing the data on the prevalence of symptoms in far advanced cancer, AIDS, heart disease, chronic obstructive pulmonary disease (COPD), and renal disease found that breathlessness, pain, and fatigue were a shared common pathway [26].

Refractory symptoms at the end of life

The term "refractory" can be applied to symptoms that cannot be adequately controlled despite aggressive efforts to identify a tolerable therapy that does not compromise consciousness. The diagnostic criteria for the designation of a refractory symptom include that the clinician must perceive that further invasive and noninvasive interventions are either (1) incapable of providing adequate relief, (2) associated with excessive and intolerable acute or chronic morbidity, or (3) unlikely to provide relief within a tolerable time frame [1]. The implication of this designation is that the pain will not be adequately relieved with routine measures and that sedation may be needed to attain adequate relief [1].

Epidemiology of refractory symptoms at the end of life

The prevalence of refractory symptoms at the end of life remains somewhat controversial. Prevalence data reporting the use of sedation in the management of refractory symptoms have been reported in a number of studies over the past 15 years (Table 101.1).

The phenomenology of severe symptoms at the end of life is well studied in patients with malignant and nonmalignant diseases. A comparative analysis of published data on the prevalence of symptoms in far advanced cancer, AIDS, heart disease, COPD, and renal diseases found that breathlessness, pain, and fatigue were a shared common pathway that were the predominant symptoms in over 50% of patients [26]. The use of sedation for the relief of refractory symptoms, particularly dyspnea, is described in end-stage COPD [27], after ventilator weaning [28], in heart failure [29,30], and in motor neuron disease [31,32].

Sedation at the end of life as a clinical dilemma

Persistent severe pain at the end of life challenges the clinician clinically, emotionally, and morally and contributes to the onerous nature of clinical decision-making in this setting. It is useful to recognize both the clinical and the ethical dimensions of this dilemma.

From a moral perspective, there is a major dilemma related to nonmalfeasance. Clinicians want neither to subject severely distressed patients to therapies that provide inadequate relief or excessive morbidity nor to sacrifice conscious function when viable alternatives remain unexplored.

The clinical corollary of this moral dilemma is the need to distinguish a "refractory" pain state from "the difficult situation," which could potentially respond within a tolerable time frame to noninvasive or invasive interventions and yield adequate relief and preserved consciousness without excessive adverse effects. The challenge inherent in this decision-making requires that patients with unrelieved symptoms undergo repeated evaluation prior to progressive application of routine therapies.

Case conference approach to decision-making

Since individual clinician bias can influence decision-making [33,34], a case conference approach is prudent when assessing a challenging case. This conference may involve involving

Table 101.1   *Surveys of the use of sedation in the management of refractory symptoms*

	Year	N	Place	% Sedated for refectory symptoms	References
Ventafridda	1990	120	Home	52	[119]
Fainsinger	1991	100	Inpatient	16	[120]
Morita	1996	143	Hospice	43	[39]
Stone	1997	115	IP and home	26	[121]
Fainsinger	1998	76	IP hospice	30	[53]
Chiu	2001	251	IP palliative care	28	[122]
Muller-Busch	2002	548	IP palliative care	14	[110]
Sykes	2003	237	Hospice	48	[123]
Morita	2004		Multicenter	<10–50	[124]
Kohara	2005	124	IP palliative care	50	[125]
Vitetta	2005	102	Hospice	67	[126]
Rietjens	2008	157	IP palliative care	43	[127]
Maltoni	2009	518	Multicenter	25	[128]
Mercendante	2009	77	IP palliative care	54	[129]

IP = Inpatient

the participation of oncologists, palliative care physicians, specialists from other fields relevant to the prevailing symptom control problem, nurses, social workers, and others. The discussion attempts to clarify the remaining therapeutic options and the goals of care.

Clearly, it is critical that clinicians who are expert in symptom control be involved in the patient evaluation. When local expertise is limited, telephone consultation with physicians who are expert in palliative medicine is strongly encouraged.

Discussing sedation with the patient and their family members

If the clinician perceives that there is no treatment capable of providing adequate relief of intolerable symptoms without compromising interactional function or that the patient would be unable to tolerate specific therapeutic interventions, refractoriness to standard approaches should be acknowledged. In this situation, the clinician should explain that, by virtue of the severity of the problem and the limitations of the available techniques, the goal of providing the needed relief without the use of drugs that may impair conscious state is probably not possible.

The offer of sedation as an available therapeutic option is often received as an empathic acknowledgment of the severity of the degree of patient suffering. The enhanced patient trust in the commitment of the clinician to the relief of suffering may, in itself, influence decision-making, particularly if there are other tasks or life issues that need to be completed before a state of diminished function develops. Indeed, patients can, and often do, decline sedation, acknowledging that symptoms will be unrelieved but secure in the knowledge that if the situation becomes intolerable, this decision can be rescinded. Alternatively, the patient can assert comfort as the paramount consideration and accept the initiation of sedation.

With the hope and knowledge that it may be possible to achieve adequate relief without compromising interactional function, the patient who equally prioritizes comfort and function may elect to pursue only those approaches with modest morbidity, despite a relatively low or indeterminate likelihood of success. As the goals of prolonging survival and optimizing function become increasingly unachievable, priorities often shift. When comfort is the overriding goal of care, and the principal intent of any further intervention is to achieve lasting relief, there may be no tolerable time frame for exploring other therapeutic options. In this situation, interventions of low or indeterminate likelihood of success are often rejected in favor of more certain approaches, even if they may involve impairment of cognitive function or possibly foreshortened duration of survival.

This situation becomes more complicated when the clinician is less certain that the available approaches will fail. Therapeutic decision-making is strongly influenced by the patient's readiness to accept the risk of morbidity and enduring discomfort until adequate relief is achieved. As always, patient evaluation of therapeutic options requires a candid disclosure of the therapeutic options, including information regarding the likelihood of benefit, the procedural morbidity, the risks

of side effects, and the likely time to achieve relief. If these are acceptable to the patient, then further trials of standard therapies should be pursued. If the patient requires relief and either the procedural morbidity, the risks of adverse effects, or the likely time to achieve relief is unacceptable, then refractoriness should be acknowledged and sedation should be offered.

These decisions are usually made by consensus between the clinicians, the patient, and the patient's family. The process of this decision-making is predicated on an understanding of the goals of care for the individual patient. These goals can generally be grouped into three broad categories: (1) prolonging survival, (2) optimizing comfort (physical, psychological, and existential), and (3) optimizing function. The processes of goal prioritization and informed decision-making require candid discussion that clarifies the prevailing clinical predicament and presents the alternative therapeutic options. Other relevant considerations, including existential, ethical, religious, and familial concerns, may benefit from the participation of a religious counselor, social worker, or clinical ethics specialist.

With the patients' consent, it is prudent to involve the family in these discussions. They suffer with the patient and will survive with the memories, pain, and the potential for guilt at not having been effective advocates for their loved one: either because the patient died in unrelieved pain or remorseful that the patient may have been sedated when other options were not given a fair chance.

If it is agreed that sedation is the most humane and appropriate way to control symptoms, it is advisable to ask the patient and family members if they have any specific goals that need to be met prior to starting sedation or if they would appreciate a chaplain/spiritual support prior to starting sedation.

Discussing sedation with the ancillary staff members

Involvement of ancillary staff such as social workers, primary care nurse, psychologist, and other health professionals is a point that cannot be adequately emphasized. Just as cancer is a family illness, so is its management a team effort. Information about who the patient is comes from many sources; the patient and family will find support and connect with different personalities; team involvement allows support for its members, prevents burnout, and helps monitor counter transference issues [35].

Consent and "DNR" status

Consent to the use of sedation acknowledges the primacy of comfort as the dominant goal of care. The initiation of cardiorespiratory resuscitation (CPR) at the time of death is almost always ineffectual in this situation [36–38] and, furthermore, is inconsistent with the agreed goals of care [36,38]. Sedating pharmacotherapy for refractory symptoms at the end of life should not be initiated until a discussion about CPR has taken place with the patient or, if appropriate, with the patient's proxy, and there is agreement that CPR will not be initiated.

Drug administration

The management of sedating pharmacotherapy for refractory symptoms in patients with advanced cancer demands a high level of clinical vigilance. Irrespective of the agent selected, administration initially requires dose titration to achieve adequate relief, followed subsequently by provision of ongoing therapy to ensure maintenance of effect. The depth of sedation that is required to achieve adequate relief is highly variable. In some situations, patients may require only light sedation to achieve adequate relief, and in other situations, particularly at the end of life, deep sedation may be required.

Regular, "around the clock" administration can be maintained by continuous infusion or intermittent bolus. The route of administration can be IV, SC or rectal. In some situations, drugs can be administered via a stoma or gastrostomy. In all cases, provision for emergency bolus therapy to manage breakthrough symptoms is recommended.

Patient monitoring

Once adequate relief is achieved, the parameters for patient monitoring and the role of further dose titration are determined by the goal of care:

1. *When the goal of care is to ensure comfort until death for an imminently dying patient*: In this setting the only salient parameters for ongoing observation are those pertaining to comfort. Symptoms should be assessed until death; observations of pulse, blood pressure, and temperature do not contribute to the goals of care and can be discontinued. Respiratory rate is monitored primarily to ensure absence of respiratory distress and tachypnea. Since downward titration of drug doses places the patient at risk for recurrent distress, in most instances, it is not recommended even as the patient approaches death.

2. *If the patient wishes to be less sedated and dying is not imminent*: In this context comfort, the level of sedation, and routine physiological parameters such as heart rate, blood pressure, and oxygen saturation are monitored. In these cases, the drug should be administered by the lowest effective dose that provides adequate comfort. If physiological parameters are compromised by the sedating medications, doses may need to be adjusted. The depth of sedation necessary to control symptoms varies greatly. For some patients, a state of "conscious sedation," in which they retain the ability to respond to verbal stimuli, may provide adequate relief without total loss of interactive function [39–42]. Some authors have suggested that doses can be titrated down to reestablish lucidity after an agreed interval or for preplanned family interactions [39,42,43]. This, of course, is a potentially unstable situation, and the possibility that lucidity may not be promptly restored or that death may ensue as doses are again escalated should be explained to both the patient and family.

EMERGENCY SEDATION

Context

In some cases, immediately preterminal patients will present with overwhelming symptoms as they are dying. In these situations, emergency decisions will need to be made without recourse to a case conference or even cross consultation. This may occur in the setting of a dying patient with sudden-onset severe dyspnea [44,45], agitated delirium [45,46], and massive bleeding or pain [45]. Care planning that anticipates potential emergencies and response plans can help reduce the stress of emergency decision-making in situations such as these.

Planning

Contingency plans for the management of catastrophic situations should be discussed with the patient and with family members. If the patient is at home, sedating medications should be prepared and a clear plan for emergency administration should be discussed. In situations in which family members or other home carers feel that they would be unable to administer emergency medications, consideration should be given to inpatient care.

Administration

As in the previous scenario, midazolam is recommended as the drug of choice. Initial sedation can be achieved with a bolus of 2.5 mg SC/IV, which can be repeated after 5 min if adequate sedation is not achieved. Once the patient is calm, a subcutaneous or intravenous infusion can be used. In the immediately preterminal patient, the only salient parameters for ongoing observation are those pertaining to comfort. Symptoms should be assessed until death; observations of pulse blood pressure and temperature are superfluous. Respiratory rate is monitored primarily to ensure absence of respiratory distress and tachypnea.

RESPITE SEDATION

Context

In many instances, the notion of refractoriness is relative. Among patients who are not imminently dying, severe emotional and physical fatigue influence the patient's perception of the intolerability of symptoms or of further attempts to alleviate them. Since this may be a reversible phenomenon, sedation is often presented initially as a respite option to provide relief and rest, with a planned restoration of lucidity after an agreed interval. After such respite, some patients will be sufficiently rested to consider further trials of symptomatic therapy [39].

Administration

There are critical differences in the monitoring of sedation in this setting. In addition to the level of sedation, it is essential to monitor routine physiological parameters such as heart rate, blood pressure, and oxygen saturation. In these cases, the sedating agent should be administered by the lowest effective dose that provides adequate comfort. Despite all of these precautions, sedation of this sort is a potentially unstable situation, and the possibility that lucidity may not be promptly restored or that death is among the risks involved should be explained to both the patient and family.

Use of sedation in the management of refractory existential or psychological distress

Sedation in the management of refractory psychological symptoms and existential distress is different from other situations for four major reasons: (1) By virtue of the nature of the symptoms being addressed, it is much more difficult to establish that they are truly refractory; (2) the severity of distress of some of these symptoms may be very dynamic and idiosyncratic and psychological adaptation and coping are common; (3) the standard treatment approaches have low intrinsic morbidity; and (4) the presence of these symptoms does not necessarily indicate a far advanced state of physiological deterioration [47,48].

The European Association of Palliative Care (EAPC) guidelines address this issue with the following caveats [49]:

1. This approach should be reserved for patients in advanced stages of a terminal illness.
2. The designation of such symptoms as refractory should only be done following a period of repeated assessment by clinicians skilled in psychological care who have established a relationship with the patient and his or her family along with trials of routine approaches for anxiety, depression, and existential distress.
3. The evaluation should be made in the context of a multidisciplinary case conference, including representatives from psychiatry, chaplaincy, and ethics, as well as those providing care at the bedside, because of the complexity and frequently multifactorial nature of this situation.
4. In the rare situations that this strategy is indeed appropriate and proportionate to the situation, it should be initiated on a respite basis for 6–24 hours with planned downward titration after a preagreed interval.
5. Only after repeated trials of respite sedation with intensive intermittent therapy have been performed should continuous sedation be considered.

MEDICATIONS USED FOR SEDATION IN PALLIATIVE CARE

The published literature describing the use of sedation in the management of refractory symptoms at the end of life is anecdotal and refers to the use of opioids, neuroleptics, benzodiazepines, barbiturates, and propofol.

Opioids

In the management of pain, an attempt is usually made to first escalate the opioid dose. Although some patients will benefit from this intervention, inadequate sedation or the development of neuroexcitatory side effects, such as myoclonus or agitated delirium, often necessitates the addition of a second agent [50–52].

Benzodiazepines

MIDAZOLAM [39–41, 53–58]

General: Midazolam is the most commonly used agent.
Pharmacology: Water-soluble, short-acting benzodiazepine. Metabolized to a lipophilic compound that rapidly penetrates the central nervous system. Brief duration of action because of rapid redistribution; therefore, administration by continuous infusion is generally required to maintain a sustained effect.
Advantages: Rapid onset. Can be administered IV, SC.
Starting dose: 0.5–1 mg/hour, 1–5 mg as needed.
Usual effective dose: 1–20 mg/hour.
Adverse effects: Paradoxical agitation, respiratory depression, withdrawal if dose is rapidly reduced after continual infusion, tolerance.
Antagonist: Flumazenil

LORAZEPAM

General: Intermediate-acting benzodiazepine that has a peak effect approximately 30 min after intravenous administration. It is less amenable to rapid titration up or down than midazolam, because of its slower pharmacokinetics.
Pharmacology: Elimination is not altered by renal or hepatic dysfunction.
Advantages: Rapid onset. Can be administered IV.
Starting dose: 0.05 mg/kg every 2–4 hours when administered by intermittent bolus.
Adverse effects: Paradoxical agitation, respiratory depression, withdrawal if dose is rapidly reduced after continual infusion, tolerance.
Antagonist: Flumazenil

Neuroleptics/antipsychotics

Neuroleptics may be effective when the patient is manifesting signs and symptoms of delirium. Delirium is an acute confusional state that can be difficult to differentiate from anxiety, yet the distinction is important, because the administration of opioids or benzodiazepines as initial treatment for delirium can worsen the symptom.

LEVOMEPROMAZINE

General: Levomepromazine is an antipsychotic phenothiazine.
Advantages: Rapid onset, antipsychotic effect in cases of delirium, some analgesic effect, can be administered orally or parenterally (IV, SC, or IM).

Starting dose: Stat dose 12.5–25 mg and 50–75 mg continual infusion.

Usual effective dose: 12.5 or 25 mg q8h and q1h prn for breakthrough agitation or up to 300 mg/day continual infusion.

Adverse effects: Orthostatic hypotension, paradoxical agitation, extrapyramidal symptoms, anticholinergic effects.

CHLORPROMAZINE

General: Widely available antipsychotic; can be administered orally, parenterally (IV or IM), and rectally.

Advantages: Antipsychotic effect for delirious patients.

Starting dose: IV or IM 12.5 mg q4–12h, or 3–5 mg/hour IV or 25–100 mg q4–12h PR.

Usual effective dose: Parenteral 37.5–150 mg/day, PR 75–300 mg/day.

Adverse effects: Orthostatic hypotension, paradoxical agitation, extrapyramidal symptoms, anticholinergic effects.

HALOPERIDOL

General: Butyrophenone antipsychotic.

Advantages: Antipsychotic, less sedating than chlorpromazine or methotrimeprazine, can be administered IV, SC, or PO.

Starting dose: For mild delirium, 0.5–1 mg parenterally q4–6h; in cases of severe agitation, start with 2.5 mg with an option to repeat dose in 30 min.

Pharmacodynamics: Slow effect orally, rapid effect parenterally.

Usual effective dose: 5–60 mg/day divided doses or continual infusion.

Adverse effects: Orthostatic hypotension, paradoxical agitation, extrapyramidal symptoms, anticholinergic effects.

Barbiturates and anesthetic agents

Barbiturates and propofol reliably and rapidly cause unconsciousness, and since their mechanism of action differs from the opioids and benzodiazepines, they may be useful in patients who have developed extreme levels of tolerance to these other medications. They do not have analgesic effect; therefore, opioids will probably be necessary for patients with pain.

PHENOBARBITAL

General: Barbiturate [42,43].

Advantages: Rapid onset, anticonvulsant.

Dose: 1–3 mg/kg SQ or IV bolus dose, followed by starting infusion of 0.5 mg/kg/hour.

Usual maintenance dose: 50–100 mg/hour.

Adverse effects: Paradoxical excitement in the elderly, hypotension, nausea and vomiting, Stevens–Johnson syndrome, angioedema, rash, agranulocytosis, thrombocytopenia.

PROPOFOL

General: Propofol is very similar to the short-acting barbiturates, but it has a short duration of action and a very rapid onset [56, 59–62]. These characteristics make it relatively easy to titrate [60].

Dose: In one report, the patient was started on a loading dose of 20 mg, followed by an infusion of 50–70 mg/hour [61].

ETHICAL CONSIDERATIONS

Sedation to relieve otherwise intolerable suffering for patients who are dying as normative practice

There is no distinct ethical problem in the use of sedation to relieve otherwise intolerable suffering for patients who are dying. Rather, the decision-making and application of this therapeutic option represents a continuum of good clinical practice. Good clinical practice is predicated on careful patient evaluation (as previously described) that incorporates assessment of current goals of care. Since all medical treatments involve risks and benefits, each potential option must be evaluated for their potential to achieve the goals of care. Where risks of treatment are involved, the risks must be proportionate to the gravity of the clinical indication. In these deliberations, clinician considerations are guided by an understanding of the goals of care and must be within accepted medical guidelines of beneficence and nonmalfeasance.

Finally, the penultimate decision to act on these considerations depends on informed consent or advanced directive of the patient. In this clinical context, the decision to offer the use of sedation to relieve intolerable suffering to terminally ill patients presents no new ethical problem [63,64].

As with any other high-risk clinical practice, potential for nonbeneficent abuse exists. Adherence to appropriate guidelines and clinical transparency with clear documentation of indications, goals of care, decision-making process, consent, and clinical outcome monitoring are essential.

Despite the potential for shortening life, this approach has been endorsed as acceptable normative practice by legal precedent [65]. In the 1957 English case of *R v Adams*, Justice Devin wrote in his judgment "If the first purpose of medicine, the restoration of health, can no longer be achieved, there is still much for a doctor to do, and he is entitled to do all that is proper and necessary to relieve pain and suffering, even if the measures he takes may incidentally shorten life." He justified this approach rejecting the notion that this is a special defense but rather by endorsing the clinical pragmatist approach that "The cause of death is the illness or the injury, and the proper medical treatment that is administered and that has an incidental effect on determining the exact moment of death is not the cause in any sensible use of the term" [66]. This approach has lent further support when the recent decision of the Supreme Court of the United States rejected a constitutional right that encompasses assisted suicide but endorsed the use of sedation as an extreme form of palliative care in the management of refractory symptoms at the end of life [67].

Problem practices in the use of palliative sedation

There are many ways in which the care of patients can be undermined by the abusive, injudicious, or unskilled use of sedation. Whereas there are very strong data indicating the prevalence of abuse, little is known regarding the prevalence of injudicious or substandard sedation practices.

Abuse of palliative sedation: The most common abuse of sedation occurs when clinicians sedate patients approaching the end of life with the primary goal of hastening the patient's death [68–75]. This has been called "slow euthanasia." Indeed, some physicians administer doses of medication, ostensibly to relieve symptoms, but with a covert intention to hasten death. This may occur by the deliberate use of deep sedation in patients who have no refractory symptoms, or in the deliberate use of doses that far exceed that which is necessary to provide adequate comfort. Excess doses can compromise physiological functions such as spontaneous respiration and hemodynamic stability. These duplicitous practices represent an unacceptable, and often illegal, deviation from normative ethical clinical practice.

Injudicious use of palliative sedation: Injudicious palliative sedation occurs when sedation is applied with the intent of relieving symptoms but in clinical circumstances that are not appropriate. In this situation, sedation is applied with the intent of relieving distress and is carefully titrated to effect, but the indication is inadequate to justify such a radical intervention. The following are representative examples of injudicious use:

1. Instances of inadequate patient assessment in which potentially reversible causes of distress are overlooked [69,76]
2. Situations in which before resorting to sedation, there is a failure to engage clinicians expert in relief of symptoms despite their availability [69,77]
3. The case of an overwhelmed physician resorting to sedation because he is fatigued and frustrated by the care of a complex symptomatic patient [78]
4. Situations in which the demand for sedation is generated by the patient's family and not the patient himself or herself [78]

Injudicious withholding of palliative sedation: Injudicious withholding of sedation in the management of refractory distress occurs when clinicians defer the use of sedation excessively while persisting with other therapeutic options that do not provide adequate relief. Given the subjectivity of refractoriness and the profound interindividual variability of responsiveness to palliative interventions, these assessments are often very difficult to make. Clinicians should be aware of the potential for a "counterphobic determination to treat" whereby

anxiety about having to deal with all of the difficult discussions about sedation and end of life care leads to avoidant behaviors and futile therapeutic trials ultimately resulting in increased patient distress or reservations based on exaggerated concerns about hastening death.

Substandard clinical practice of palliative sedation: This occurs in situations in which sedation is used for an appropriate indication but without the appropriate attention to one or more processes essential to good clinical care. Examples of substandard clinical practices include the following:

1. Inadequate consultation with the patient (if possible), family members, or other staff members to ensure understanding of the indication for the intervention, the goals of the care plan, the anticipated outcomes, and the potential risks
2. Inadequate monitoring of symptom distress or adequacy of relief
3. Inadequate assessment of psychological, spiritual, or social factors that may be contributing to the patient's distress [78]
4. Inadequate monitoring of physiological parameters that may indicate risk of drug overdose (when clinically relevant)
5. Hasty dose escalation of sedative medications without titration to effect and use of minimal effective doses
6. Use of inappropriate medications to achieve sedation (i.e., opioids) [79,80]
7. Inadequate care of the patient's family [78]
8. Inadequate attention to the emotional and spiritual well-being of distressed staff members [78,81]

Distinction from "slow euthanasia"

Some authors argue that although sedation in the relief of uncontrolled symptoms may be justifiable, the concurrent discontinuation of nutrition and hydration does not contribute to patient comfort and almost certainly hastens death by starvation and dehydration. Consequently, they argue that sedation for the management of refractory symptoms is practically the same as "slow euthanasia" [82–85]. This proposition is argued both by opponents to euthanasia, who are concerned about harmful aspects of the practice of forgoing nutrition and hydration [82–86], and also by proponents of elective death who argue that if these acts are morally equivalent, then the more rapid mode of elective death, such as euthanasia or assisted suicide, is more humane and dignified [87,88].

Euthanasia refers to the deliberate termination of the life of a patient by active intervention, at the request of the patient in the setting of otherwise uncontrolled suffering. This is distinct from physician-assisted suicide by the physician that provides the means of suicide and instruction to a patient to facilitate successful suicide.

The use of sedation to relieve otherwise unendurable symptoms at the end of life falls under the rubric of "the provision of a potentially lethal medication for a patient with a narrow therapeutic index." Clearly, this situation may result in the inadvertent foreshortening of the patient's life either by direct action of the drug or as an adverse effect (such as aspiration [89]).

With regard to the concern that sedation routinely incorporates discontinuation of hydration, it is important to reassert that the discontinuation of hydration and nutrition is *not* an essential element to the administration of sedation in the management of refractory symptoms [89]. Furthermore, there are no data to support the assertion that it is "typical" [90] (see section below).

Sedation in the management of refractory symptoms is distinct from euthanasia insofar as (1) the intent of the intervention is to provide symptom relief not to end the life of the suffering patient; (2) the intervention is proportionate to the prevailing symptom, its severity, and the prevailing goals of care; and finally and, most importantly, (3) unlike euthanasia or assisted suicide, the death of the patient is not a criteria for the success of the treatment.

Doctrine of double effect

In cases where a contemplated action has both good effects and bad effects, the doctrine provides an approach to answer the question: "Do the means justify the end?" According to "double effect ethics," an action is permissible if it is not wrong in itself and it does not require that one directly intend the bad result. Double effect ethics assume the integrity of the physician and unambiguous intent and motive.

Classically, five criteria have been described to evaluate the validity of a double effect claim [91]:

1. The action is either morally good or is morally neutral.
2. The undesired yet foreseen untoward result is not directly intended.
3. The good effect is not a direct result of the foreseen untoward effect.
4. The good effect be "proportionate to" the untoward effect.
5. That there be no other way to achieve the desired ends without the untoward effect.

The "doctrine of double effect" is problematic insofar as it does not always apply to the use of sedation in the management of refractory symptoms. When sedation is used to relieve otherwise refractory pain and suffering at the end of life, the intention is to relieve otherwise unendurable suffering. Employing this ethical approach, the untoward consequences that are foreseen include the possibility of foreshortened survival and the loss of interactional function. Indeed, the moral justification of sedation by double effect requires that clinicians make unequivocal claims regarding the undesirability of the possibility of the patient's death. However, since the death of the patient at the end of a long and difficult illness is not always perceived as untoward, there is a significant problem with the application of the double effect justification. Thus, to call the potential for foreshortened survival a "bad

outcome" is problematic insofar as it undermines the essential element of clinician credibility.

It is prudent and appropriate to emphasize that there is no clear evidence that the use of sedation in the relief of refractory symptoms at the end of life foreshortens survival. Ten studies have addressed this issue in the setting of hospice care and the results were recently evaluated in a systematic review [92] that found no difference in overall survival between hospice patients who underwent sedation at the end of life and those who did not. Three studies have addressed this issue on the management of patients with terminal dyspnea after withdrawal of mechanical ventilation [93–95]. These studies found no correlation between level of sedation, dose of sedatives, and duration of survival until death.

Another concern is that since sedation may hasten the death of the patient, the plea of no moral responsibility for foreseen, inevitable untoward outcomes is at best spurious or at worst dishonest [96]. Indeed, the "doctrine of double effect" is not endorsed by all ethical traditions.

Ethical issues regarding nutrition and hydration when patients are sedated

Although sedation is clearly beneficent in terms of providing relief of otherwise intolerable suffering, the beneficence of withdrawal of nutrition and hydration in the already sedated and comfortable patient is not self-evident, and indeed, it may be perceived as harmful. This debate has both medical and ethical dimensions.

Medically, there are little data to support the clinical benefit of hydration or artificial nutrition in the imminently dying or to suggest that it prolongs life or contributes to comfort [97–99]. Ethically, the withdrawal of potentially death deferring treatments (such as hydration) among dying patients is, for some, controversial [82,100]. For reasons of clarity, the issue of sedation must be distinguished from the distinct and separate issue of hydration.

Opinions and practices vary. This variability reflects the heterogeneity of attitudes of the involved clinicians, ethicists, the patient, family, and local norms of good clinical and ethical practice [54]. Individual patient's, family members, and clinicians may regard the continuation of hydration as a nonburdensome, humane, supportive intervention that represents (and may actually constitute) one means of reducing suffering [82,100]. Alternatively, hydration may be viewed as a superfluous impediment to inevitable death that does not contribute to patient comfort or the prevailing goals of care and that can be appropriately withdrawn [101]. Often, the patient will request relief of suffering and give no direction regarding supportive measures. In this circumstance, the family and health-care providers must reach consensus as to what constitutes a morally and personally acceptable approach based on the ethical principles of beneficence, nonmalfeasance, and respect for personhood.

In cases where there are religious or culturally based reservations regarding the discontinuation of nutritional support, it should be maintained unless there is evidence of direct patient harm by the intervention.

CLINICAL PRACTICE GUIDELINES

While acknowledging that specific best practices have not been rigorously developed, procedural guidelines can nonetheless be developed to provide a framework for decision-making and implementation to best promote and protect the interests of patients, their families, and the health-care providers administering care. Sound procedural guidelines, such as checklists, can reduce the risk of adverse outcomes in medicine [102,103].

Guidelines have been, and may be, developed at a national, local, or institutional level. Irrespective, once adopted, they need to be disseminated, opened for discussion, and readily available to clinicians involved in this clinical issue. Many such guidelines have been published [1,12,35,68,78,87,104–118]. Based on a review of these and other guidelines, the EAPC developed a 10-item framework that addresses the key clinical issues in palliative sedation for the management of refractory physical symptoms at the end of life (Table 101.2).

CONCLUSIONS

Sedation is a critically important therapeutic tool of last resort. It enables the clinician to provide relief from intolerable distress when other options are not adequately effective. Because sedation undermines the capacity to interact, it must be used judiciously. Clear indications and guidelines for use are necessary to prevent abuse of this approach to facilitate the deliberate killing of patients, which, while benevolently intended, may have untoward sociological and ethical consequences for palliative care clinicians and the image of palliative medicine as a profession.

Table 101.2 *EAPC developed a 10-item framework for guidelines in palliative sedation*

1. Recommend preemptive discussion of potential role of sedation in end of life care and contingency planning.
2. Describe the indications in which sedation may or should be considered.
3. Describe the necessary evaluation and consultation procedures.
4. Specify consent requirements.
5. Indicate the need to discuss the decision-making process with the patient's family.
6. Present direction for selection of the sedation method.
7. Present direction for dose titration, patient monitoring, and care.
8. Guidance for decisions regarding hydration and nutrition and concomitant medications.
9. The care and informational needs of the patient's family.
10. Care for the medical professionals.

REFERENCES

1 Cherny NI, Portenoy RK. Sedation in the management of refractory symptoms: Guidelines for evaluation and treatment. *Journal of Palliative Care* 1994;10(2):31–38.

2 Godwin SA, Caro DA, Wolf SJ, Jagoda AS, Charles R, Marett BE et al. Clinical policy: Procedural sedation and analgesia in the emergency department. *Annals of Emergency Medicine* 2005;45(2):177–196.

3 Practice Guidelines for Sedation and Analgesia by Non-Anesthesiologists. *Anesthesiology* 2002;96(4):1004–1017.

4 Cote CJ, Wilson S. Guidelines for monitoring and management of pediatric patients during and after sedation for diagnostic and therapeutic procedures: An update. *Pediatrics* 2006;118(6):2587–2602.

5 Waring JP, Baron TH, Hirota WK, Goldstein JL, Jacobson BC, Leighton JA et al. Guidelines for conscious sedation and monitoring during gastrointestinal endoscopy. *Gastrointestinal Endoscopy* 2003;58(3):317–322.

6 Gregoretti C, Decaroli D, Piacevoli Q, Mistretta A, Barzaghi N, Luxardo N et al. Analgo-sedation of patients with burns outside the operating room. *Drugs* 2008;68(17):2427–2443.

7 del Rosario MA, Martin AS, Ortega JJ, Feria M. Temporary sedation with midazolam for control of severe incident pain. *Journal of Pain and Symptom Management* 2001;21(5):439–442.

8 de Graeff A, Dean M. Palliative sedation therapy in the last weeks of life: A literature review and recommendations for standards. *Journal of Palliative Medicine* 2007;10(1):67–85.

9 Rousseau PC. Palliative sedation. *American Journal of Hospice and Palliative Medicine* 2002;19(5):295–297.

10 Jackson WC. Palliative sedation vs. terminal sedation: What's in a name? *American Journal of Hospice Palliative Care* 2002;19(2):81–82.

11 Beel A, McClement SE, Harlos M. Palliative sedation therapy: A review of definitions and usage. *International Journal of Palliative Nursing* 2002;8(4):190–199.

12 Cowan JD, Walsh D. Terminal sedation in palliative medicine—Definition and review of the literature. *Support Care Cancer* 2001;9(6):403–407.

13 Mercadante S. Pain treatment and outcomes for patients with advanced cancer who receive follow-up care at home [see comments]. *Cancer* 1999;85(8):1849–1858.

14 Salisbury C, Bosanquet N, Wilkinson EK, Franks PJ, Kite S, Lorentzon M et al. The impact of different models of specialist palliative care on patients" quality of life: A systematic literature review. *Palliative Medicine* 1999;13(1):3–17.

15 Higginson IJ, Wade AM, McCarthy M. Effectiveness of two palliative support teams. *Journal of Public Health Medicine* 1992;14(1):50–56.

16 Higginson IJ, McGregor AM. The impact of palliative medicine? [editorial]. *Palliative Medicine* 1999;13(4):285–298.

17 Peruselli C, Di Giulio P, Toscani F, Gallucci M, Brunelli C, Costantini M et al. Home palliative care for terminal cancer patients: A survey on the final week of life. *Palliative Medicine* 1999;13(3):233–241.

18 Higginson IJ, Hearn J. A multicenter evaluation of cancer pain control by palliative care teams. *Journal of Pain and Symptom Management* 1997;14(1):29–35.

19 Conill C, Verger E, Henriquez I, Saiz N, Espier M, Lugo F et al. Symptom prevalence in the last week of life. *Journal of Pain and Symptom Management* 1997;14(6):328–331.

20 Storey P. Symptom control in advanced cancer. *Seminars in Oncology* 1994;21(6):748–753.

21 Lichter I, Hunt E. The last 48 hours of life. *Journal of Palliative Care* 1990;6(4):7–15.

22 Johanson GA. Symptom character and prevalence during cancer patients' last days of life. *American Journal of Hospice and Palliative Care* 1991;8(2):6–8, 18.

23   Kutner JS, Bryant LL, Beaty BL, Fairclough DL. Time course and characteristics of symptom distress and quality of life at the end of life. *Journal of Pain and Symptom Management* 2007;34(3):227–236.

24   Tranmer JE, Heyland D, Dudgeon D, Groll D, Squires-Graham M, Coulson K. Measuring the symptom experience of seriously ill cancer and noncancer hospitalized patients near the end of life with the memorial symptom assessment scale. *Journal of Pain and Symptom Management* 2003;25(5):420–429.

25   Kutner JS, Kassner CT, Nowels DE. Symptom burden at the end of life: Hospice providers' perceptions. *Journal of Pain and Symptom Management* 2001;21(6):473–480.

26   Solano JP, Gomes B, Higginson IJ. A comparison of symptom prevalence in far advanced cancer, AIDS, heart disease, chronic obstructive pulmonary disease and renal disease. *Journal of Pain and Symptom Management* 2006;31(1):58–69.

27   Ambrosino N, Simonds A. The clinical management in extremely severe COPD. *Respiratory Medicine* 2007;101(8):1613–1624.

28   Jakob SM, Lubszky S, Friolet R, Rothen HU, Kolarova A, Takala J. Sedation and weaning from mechanical ventilation: Effects of process optimization outside a clinical trial. *Journal of Critical Care* 2007;22(3):219–228.

29   Reisfield GM, Wilson GR. Palliative care issues in heart failure #144. *Journal of Palliative Medicine* 2007;10(1):247–248.

30   Goodlin SJ. Palliative care for end-stage heart failure. *Current Heart Failure Reports* 2005;2(3):155–160.

31   Low JA, Pang WS, Chan DK, Chye R. A palliative care approach to end-stage neurodegenerative conditions. *Annals of the Academy of Medicine Singapore* 2003;32(6):778–784.

32   Elman LB, Houghton DJ, Wu GF, Hurtig HI, Markowitz CE, McCluskey L. Palliative care in amyotrophic lateral sclerosis, Parkinson's disease, and multiple sclerosis. *Journal of Palliative Medicine* 2007;10(2):433–457.

33   Feldman HA, McKinlay JB, Potter DA, Freund KM, Burns RB, Moskowitz MA et al. Nonmedical influences on medical decision making: An experimental technique using videotapes, factorial design, and survey sampling. *Health Services Research* 1997;32(3):343–366.

34   Christakis NA, Asch DA. Biases in how physicians choose to withdraw life support. *Lancet* 1993;342(8872):642–646.

35   Wein S. Sedation in the imminently dying patient. *Oncology (Huntingt)* 2000;14(4):585–592; discussion 592, 597–598, 601.

36   Haines IE, Zalcberg J, Buchanan JD. Not-for-resuscitation orders in cancer patients—Principles of decision-making. *Medical Journal of Australia* 1990;153(4):225–229.

37   Rosner F, Kark PR, Bennett AJ, Buscaglia A, Cassell EJ, Farnsworth PB et al. Medical futility. Committee on Bioethical Issues of the Medical Society of the State of New York. *New York State Journal of Medicine* 1992;92(11):485–488.

38   Marik PE, Zaloga GP. CPR in terminally ill patients? *Resuscitation* 2001;49(1):99–103.

39   Morita T, Inoue S, Chihara S. Sedation for symptom control in Japan: The importance of intermittent use and communication with family members. *Journal of Pain and Symptom Management* 1996;12(1):32–38.

40   Burke AL. Palliative care: An update on "terminal restlessness." *Medical Journal of Australia* 1997;166(1):39–42.

41   Burke AL, Diamond PL, Hulbert J, Yeatman J, Farr EA. Terminal restlessness—Its management and the role of midazolam [see comments]. *Medical Journal of Austalia* 1991;155(7):485–487.

42   Greene WR, Davis WH. Titrated intravenous barbiturates in the control of symptoms in patients with terminal cancer. *Southern Medical Journal* 1991;84(3):332–337.

43   Truog RD, Berde CB, Mitchell C, Grier HE. Barbiturates in the care of the terminally ill. *The New England Journal of Medicine* 1992;327(23):1678–1682.

44   Campbell ML. Terminal dyspnea and respiratory distress. *Critical Care Clinics* 2004;20(3):403–417, viii–ix.

45   Schrijvers D, van Fraeyenhove F. Emergencies in palliative care. *Cancer Journal (Sudbury, Mass.)* 2010;16(5):514–520.

46   Kress JP, Hall JB. Delirium and sedation. *Critical Care Clinics* 2004;20(3):419–33, ix.

47   Rousseau P. Existential distress and palliative sedation. *Anesthesia and Analgesia* 2005;101(2):611–612.

48   Taylor BR, McCann RM. Controlled sedation for physical and existential suffering? *Journal of Palliative Medicine* 2005;8(1):144–147.

49   Cherny NI, Radbruch L. European Association for Palliative Care (EAPC) recommended framework for the use of sedation in palliative care. *Palliative Medicine* 2009;23(7):581–593.

50   Portenoy RK. Continuous intravenous infusion of opioid drugs. *Medical Clinics of North America* 1987;71(2):233–241.

51   Potter JM, Reid DB, Shaw RJ, Hackett P, Hickman PE. Myoclonus associated with treatment with high doses of morphine: The role of supplemental drugs [see comments]. *BMJ* 1989;299(6692):150–153.

52   Dunlop RJ. Excitatory phenomena associated with high dose opioids. *Current Therapy* 1989;30(6):121–123.

53   Fainsinger RL, Landman W, Hoskings M, Bruera E. Sedation for uncontrolled symptoms in a South African hospice. *Journal of Pain and Symptom Management* 1998;16(3):145–152.

54   Chater S, Viola R, Paterson J, Jarvis V. Sedation for intractable distress in the dying—A survey of experts. *Palliative Medicine* 1998;12(4):255–269.

55   Nordt SP, Clark RF. Midazolam: A review of therapeutic uses and toxicity. *Journal of Emergency Medicine* 1997;15(3):357–365.

56   Collins P. Prolonged sedation with midazolam or propofol [letter; comment]. *Critical Care Medicine* 1997;25(3):556–557.

57   Johanson GA. Midazolam in terminal care. *American Journal of Hospice and Palliative Care* 1993;10(1):13–14.

58   Power D, Kearney M. Management of the final 24 hours. *Irish Medical Journal* 1992;85(3):93–95.

59   Tobias JD. Propofol sedation for terminal care in a pediatric patient. *Clinical Pediatrics (Phila)* 1997;36(5):291–293.

60   Krakauer EL, Penson RT, Truog RD, King LA, Chabner BA, Lynch TJ, Jr. Sedation for intractable distress of a dying patient: Acute palliative care and the principle of double effect. *Oncologist* 2000;5(1):53–62.

61   Mercadante S, De Conno F, Ripamonti C. Propofol in terminal care. *Journal of Pain and Symptom Management* 1995;10(8):639–642.

62   Moyle J. The use of propofol in palliative medicine. *Journal of Pain and Symptom Management* 1995;10(8):643–646.

63   Miller FG, Fins JJ, Bacchetta MD. Clinical pragmatism: John Dewey and clinical ethics. *Journal of Contemporary Health Law and Policy* 1996;13(1):27–51.

64   Fins JJ, Bacchetta MD, Miller FG. Clinical pragmatism: A method of moral problem solving. *Kennedy Institute of Ethics Journal* 1997;7:129–145.

65   Gevers S. Terminal sedation: A legal approach. *European Journal of Health Law* 2003;10(4):359–367.

66   Devlin P. *Easing the Passing*. London, U.K.: Bodley Head; 1985.

67   Burt RA. The Supreme Court speaks—Not assisted suicide but a constitutional right to palliative care. *The New England Journal of Medicine* 1997;337(17):1234–1236.

68   Levy MH, Cohen SD. Sedation for the relief of refractory symptoms in the imminently dying: A fine intentional line. *Seminars in Oncology* 2005;32(2):237–246.

69   Hasselaar JG, Reuzel RP, van den Muijsenbergh ME, Koopmans RT, Leget CJ, Crul BJ et al. Dealing with delicate issues in continuous deep sedation. Varying practices among Dutch medical specialists, general practitioners, and nursing home physicians. *Archives of Internal Medicine* 2008;168(5):537–543.

70   Kuhse H, Singer P, Baume P, Clark M, Rickard M. End-of-life deci-sions in Australian medical practice. *Medical Journal of Austalia* 1997;166(4):191–196.

71   Stevens CA, Hassan R. Management of death, dying and euthanasia: Attitudes and practices of medical practitioners in South Australia. *Archives of Internal Medicine* 1994;154(5):575–584.

72   Willems DL, Daniels ER, van der Wal G, van der Maas PJ, Emanuel EJ. Attitudes and practices concerning the end of life: A comparison between physicians from the United States and from The Netherlands [in process citation]. *Archieves of Internal Medicine* 2000;160(1):63–68.

73   Meier DE, Emmons CA, Wallenstein S, Quill T, Morrison RS, Cassel CK. A national survey of physician-assisted suicide and euthanasia in the United States [see comments]. *The New England Journal of Medicine* 1998;338(17):1193–1201.

74   Douglas CD, Kerridge IH, Rainbird KJ, McPhee JR, Hancock L, Spigelman AD. The intention to hasten death: A survey of attitudes and practices of surgeons in Australia. *Medical Journal of Austalia* 2001;175(10):511–515.

75   Rietjens JA, van der Heide A, Vrakking AM, Onwuteaka-Philipsen BD, van der Maas PJ, van der Wal G. Physician reports of terminal seda-tion without hydration or nutrition for patients nearing death in the Netherlands. *Annals of Internal Medicine* 2004;141(3):178–185.

76   Fainsinger RL, De Moissac D, Mancini I, Oneschuk D. Sedation for delir-ium and other symptoms in terminally ill patients in Edmonton. *Journal of Palliative Care* 2000;16(2):5–10.

77   Murray SA, Boyd K, Byock I. Continuous deep sedation in patients near-ing death. *BMJ* 2008;336(7648):781–782.

78   Higgins PC, Altilio T. Palliative sedation: An essential place for clini-cal excellence. *Journal of Social Work in End-of-Life and Palliative Care* 2007;3(4):3–30.

79   Reuzel RP, Hasselaar GJ, Vissers KC, van der Wilt GJ, Groenewoud JM, Crul BJ. Inappropriateness of using opioids for end-stage palliative sedation: A Dutch study. *Palliative Medicine* 2008;22(5):641–646.

80   Hasselaar JG, Reuzel RP, Verhagen SC, de Graeff A, Vissers KC, Crul BJ. Improving prescription in palliative sedation: Compliance with dutch guidelines. *Archives of Internal Medicine* 2007;167(11):1166–1171.

81   Rietjens JA, Hauser J, van der Heide A, Emanuel L. Having a difficult time leaving: Experiences and attitudes of nurses with palliative seda-tion. *Palliative Medicine* 2007;21(7):643–649.

82   Craig GM. On withholding artificial hydration and nutrition from ter-minally ill sedated patients. The debate continues. *Journal of Medical Ethics* 1996;22(3):147–153.

83   Craig GM. On withholding nutrition and hydration in the terminally ill: Has palliative medicine gone too far? [see comments]. *Journal of Medical Ethics* 1994;20(3):139–43; discussion 44–45.

84   Craig G. Is sedation without hydration or nourishment in terminal care lawful? *Medico-Legal Journal* 1994;62(Pt 4):198–201.

85   Orentlicher D. The Supreme Court and physician-assisted suicide—Rejecting assisted suicide but embracing euthanasia. *New England Jounal of Medicine* 1997;337(17):1236–1239.

86   Brody H. Causing, intending, and assisting death. *Journal of Clinical Ethics* 1993;4(2):112–117.

87   Quill TE, Byock IR. Responding to intractable terminal suffering: The role of terminal sedation and voluntary refusal of food and fluids. ACP-ASIM End-of-Life Care Consensus Panel. American College of Physicians-American Society of Internal Medicine. *Annals of Internal Medicine* 2000;132(5):408–414.

88   Quill TE, Lo B, Brock DW. Palliative options of last resort: A compari-son of voluntarily stopping eating and drinking, terminal sedation, physician-assisted suicide, and voluntary active euthanasia. *JAMA* 1997;278(23):2099–2104.

89   Hahn MP. Review of palliative sedation and its distinction from euthanasia and lethal injection. *Journal of Pain and Palliative Care Pharmacotherapy* 2012;26(1):30–39.

90   Sulmasy DP, Ury WA, Ahronheim JC, Siegler M, Kass L, Lantos J et al. Palliative treatment of last resort and assisted suicide. *Annals of Internal Medicine* 2000;133(7):562–563.

91   Boyle J. Medical ethics and double effect: The case of terminal seda-tion. *Theoretical Medicine and Bioethics* 2004;25(1):51–60.

92   Maltoni M, Scarpi E, Rosati M, Derni S, Fabbri L, Martini F et al. Palliative sedation in end-of-life care and survival: A systematic review. *Journal of Clinical Oncology* 2012;30(12):1378–1383.

93   Daly BJ, Thomas D, Dyer MA. Procedures used in withdrawal of mechanical ventilation [see comments]. *American Journal of Critical Care* 1996;5(5):331–338.

94   Campbell ML, Bizek KS, Thill M. Patient responses during rapid ter-minal weaning from mechanical ventilation: A prospective study [see comments]. *Critical Care Medicine* 1999;27(1):73–77.

95   Wilson WC, Smedira NG, Fink C, McDowell JA, Luce JM. Ordering and administration of sedatives and analgesics during the withholding and withdrawal of life support from critically ill patients [see comments]. *JAMA* 1992;267(7):949–953.

96   Quill TE, Dresser R, Brock DW. The rule of double effect—A critique of its role in end-of-life decision making. *The New England Journal of Medicine* 1997;337(24):1768–1771.

97   Ahronheim JC. Nutrition and hydration in the terminal patient. *Clinics in Geriatric Medicine* 1996;12(2):379–391.

98   Barber MD, Fearon KC, Delmore G, Loprinzi CL. Should cancer patients with incurable disease receive parenteral or enteral nutritional sup-port? *European Journal of Cancer* 1998;34(3):279–285.

99   Koshuta MA, Schmitz PJ, Lynn J. Development of an institutional pol-icy on artificial hydration and nutrition. *Kennedy Institute of Ethics Journal* 1991;1(2):133–139; discussion 9–40.

100 Jansen LA, Sulmasy DP. Sedation, alimentation, hydration, and equivo-cation: Careful conversation about care at the end of life. *Annals of Internal Medicine* 2002;136(11):845–849.

101 Ashby M, Stoffell B. Artificial hydration and alimentation at the end of life: A reply to Craig. *Journal of Medical Ethics* 1995;21(3):135–140.

102 Haynes AB, Weiser TG, Berry WR, Lipsitz SR, Breizat AH, Dellinger EP et al. A surgical safety checklist to reduce morbidity and mor-tality in a global population. *The New England Journal of Medicine* 2009;360(5):491–499.

103 Hoffman GM, Nowakowski R, Troshynski TJ, Berens RJ, Weisman SJ. Risk reduction in pediatric procedural sedation by application of an American Academy of Pediatrics/American Society of Anesthesiologists process model. *Pediatrics* 2002;109(2):236–243.

104 Royal Dutch Medical Association Committee on National Guideline for Palliative Sedation. Guideline for palliative seda-tion 2005: Available from http://knmg.artsennet.nl/uri/?uri=AMGATE_6059_100_TICH_R193567276369746.

105 National Hospice and Palliative Care Organization. *Total Sedation: A Hospice and Palliative Care Resource Guide.* Alexandria, VA: NHPCO; 2000.

106 Braun TC, Hagen NA, Clark T. Development of a clinical practice guideline for palliative sedation. *Journal of Palliative Medicine* 2003;6(3):345–350.

107 Morita T, Bito S, Kurihara Y, Uchitomi Y. Development of a clinical guideline for palliative sedation therapy using the delphi method. *Journal of Palliative Medicine* 2005;8(4):716–729.

108 Verkerk M, van Wijlick E, Legemaate J, de Graeff A. A national guide-line for palliative sedation in the Netherlands. *Journal of Pain and Symptom Management* 2007;34(6):666–670.

109 Rousseau P. Palliative sedation in the management of refractory symptoms. *Journal of Supportive Oncology* 2004;2(2):181–186.

110 Muller-Busch HC, Andres I, Jehser T. Sedation in palliative care—A critical analysis of 7 years experience. *BMC Palliative Care* 2003;2(1):2.

111 Cowan JD, Palmer TW. Practical guide to palliative sedation. *Current Oncology Reports* 2002;4(3):242–249.

112 Eisenchlas JH. Palliative sedation. *Current Opinion in Supportive and Palliative Care* 2007;1(3):207–212.

113 Cunningham J. A review of sedation for intractable distress in the dying. *Irish Medical Journal* 2008;101(3):87–90.

114 Hospice and Palliative Care Federation of Massachusetts. *Palliative Sedation Protocol: A Report of the Standards and Best Practices Committee.* Norwood, MA: Hospice and Palliative Care Federation of Massachusetts; 2004.

115 Legemaate J, Verkerk M, van Wijlick E, de Graeff A. Palliative sedation in the Netherlands: Starting-points and contents of a national guideline. *European Journal of Health Law* 2007;14(1):61–73.

116 Lo B, Rubenfeld G. Palliative sedation in dying patients: "we turn to it when everything else hasn't worked." *JAMA* 2005;294(14):1810–1816.

117 Veterans Health Administration National Ethics Committee. The ethics of palliative sedation as a therapy of last resort. *The American Journal of Hospice and Palliative Care* 2006;23(6):483–491.

118 Kirk TW, Mahon MM. National Hospice and Palliative Care Organization (NHPCO) position statement and commentary on the use of palliative sedation in imminently dying terminally ill patients. *Journal of Pain and Symptom Management* 2010;39(5):914–923.

119 Ventafridda V, Ripamonti C, De Conno F, Tamburini M, Cassileth BR. Symptom prevalence and control during cancer patients' last days of life. *Journal of Palliative Care* 1990;6(3):7–11.

120 Fainsinger R, Miller MJ, Bruera E, Hanson J, Maceachern T. Symptom control during the last week of life on a palliative care unit. *Journal of Palliative Care* 1991;7(1):5–11.

121 Stone P, Phillips C, Spruyt O, Waight C. A comparison of the use of sedatives in a hospital support team and in a hospice. *Palliative Medicine* 1997;11(2):140–144.

122 Chiu TY, Hu WY, Lue BH, Cheng SY, Chen CY. Sedation for refractory symptoms of terminal cancer patients in Taiwan. *Journal of Pain and Symptom Management* 2001;21(6):467–472.

123 Sykes N, Thorns A. Sedative use in the last week of life and the implications for end-of-life decision making. *Archives of Internal Medicine* 2003;163(3):341–344.

124 Morita T. Differences in physician-reported practice in palliative sedation therapy. *Support Care Cancer* 2004;28(8):584–592.

125 Kohara H, Ueoka H, Takeyama H, Murakami T, Morita T. Sedation for terminally ill patients with cancer with uncontrollable physical distress. *Journal of Palliative Medicine* 2005;8(1):20–25.

126 Vitetta L, Kenner D, Sali A. Sedation and analgesia-prescribing patterns in terminally ill patients at the end of life. *The American Journal of Hospice and Palliative Care* 2005;22(6):465–473.

127 Rietjens JA, van Zuylen L, van Veluw H, van der Wijk L, van der Heide A, van der Rijt CC. Palliative sedation in a specialized unit for acute palliative care in a cancer hospital: Comparing patients dying with and without palliative sedation. *Journal of Pain and Symptom Management* 2008;36(3):228–234.

128 Maltoni M, Pittureri C, Scarpi E, Piccinini L, Martini F, Turci P et al. Palliative sedation therapy does not hasten death: Results from a prospective multicenter study. *Annals of Oncology* 2009;20(7):1163–1169.

129 Mercadante S, Intravaia G, Villari P, Ferrera P, David F, Casuccio A. Controlled sedation for refractory symptoms in dying patients. *Journal of Pain and Symptom Management* 2009;37(5):771–779.

PART 16

Interdisciplinary issues

102

Physical and occupational therapies in palliative care

HITOSHI OKAMURA, YOSHIYUKI MASUDA, HISAKO TAJIRI

INTRODUCTION

With the current overall survival rate at 50%, cancer is now considered a chronic disease, joining the ranks of other major chronic conditions (cardiovascular disease, lung disease, and dementia) that account for end of life.[1] Treatment of any of these life-threatening diseases, especially in those who are elderly, results in a variety of medical problems, complex functional changes, and a significantly compromised quality of life.[2-4] People with cancer and other serious illnesses require comprehensive care designed to relieve symptoms of pain, fatigue, and weakness during all phases of their disease including pretreatment, treatment, posttreatment, recurrence, and end-of-life phases.[5] Providing that level of comprehensive care requires a team of health professionals who can address both curative care and palliative care issues regardless of where the patient is on the life–death continuum. However, the World Health Organization (WHO) has recognized that it is unrealistic to expect that emerging palliative care needs can be met simply by training a workforce of specialists in palliative care. WHO suggests that expanding the knowledge and skills of health professionals in general is the answer to addressing the increase in health-care needs as individuals begin to live longer.[6] The key to increasing the numbers of health professionals who can improve patient function and quality of life among seriously ill patients and their families is to enhance the awareness and skills of physical therapists and occupational therapists so that they will feel confident in working with palliative patients and their families.

Approaches to cancer patient rehabilitation that take both psychosocial aspects and physical aspects into consideration are important, based on the reported need of "adequately understanding the strong connections between the patients' physical, psychological, and social aspects."[7] Thus, the involvement of representatives of a variety of occupations, including psychologists, clinical psychologists, and nurses, and not just rehabilitation specialists such as physical therapists or occupational therapists, is important for the rehabilitation of cancer patients; thus, multidisciplinary team care is required. However, not many reports on the rehabilitation of cancer patients have appeared since comprehensive research reports on the need for rehabilitation were first published by Lehmann et al.[8] in 1978 and by Harvey et al.[9] in 1982. One reason for this lack of research is that as rehabilitation was originally performed mainly for the purpose of improving and raising the level of activities of daily living (ADLs), there has been little demand from either health-care providers or patients for proactive intervention in cancer care with regard to rehabilitation, which has had the strong image of being intended to improve ADL and return patients to their former lives. In recent years, however, interest has turned to the association between cancer rehabilitation and the increasing numbers of patients who survive for long periods while enduring symptoms caused by cancer or the adverse effects associated with treatment or the association with advances in palliative care.

While physical therapy and occupational therapy are traditionally viewed as rehabilitation interventions, providing rehabilitation services for terminally ill patients is not a new concept. Dietz[10] has classified cancer rehabilitation according to cancer patients' physical and individual needs into four categories: preventive, restorative, supportive, and palliative. Based on these categories, the effectiveness of rehabilitation has been reported for each stage of cancer treatment, from physical rehabilitation during the acute stage of treatment[11***,12***,13,14] to the rehabilitation of physical aspects and psychological aspects during the terminal stage,[15-17] but it remains difficult to claim that cancer rehabilitation is generally acknowledged to be adequate. In view of these situations, Dietz[18] has pointed out the need to focus on a concept of care that asks, "What is the best support that can be provided to enable cancer patients to readapt to society?" DeLisa[19] has also stated that "now that cancer patients' survival rate has increased, attention should be turned to maintaining cancer patients' quality of life and prolonging it." In other words, a shift to an approach that aims to maintain the quality of life of patients at a high level and not just improve their function and prognosis has become necessary.

The benefits of physiotherapy in palliative care were recognized in the United Kingdom in 1978. Shank[20] described the physiotherapist's role as the *relief of discomfort and pain* through the use of massage, exercise, supportive positioning, splinting, and chest physiotherapy and the

Box 102.1 Role of physical/occupational therapy in palliative care

- Help patient determine which activities and roles they can realistically perform.

- Enable the patient to take an active part in establishing goals and treatment priorities.

- Apply physical/occupational therapy interventions to minimize symptoms and optimize functional abilities.

- Assist the patient to find meaning with their available range of activity and occupation considering the interplay between physical, psychological, social, and vocational domains of function.

- Instruct patient regarding methods to maximize function within limits of energy, safety, and capabilities.

- Enhance quality of life at the end of life for the patient and their family.

maintenance/improvement in function through the use of assistive devices, exercise, and retraining. She concluded that the retention of an element of independence could provide the patient with valuable hope and reduced anxiety. About the same time, occupational therapists advocated that good end-of-life care should include not only the management of symptoms but also assistance to make the best of every day. In 1983, Tigges and Sherman[21] described the role of occupational therapists in fostering hospice patients' independence in occupational roles of self-care, work, and leisure as important interventions in coping with feelings of isolation and the loss of independence (Box 102.1).

WHEN TO MAKE REFERRALS

In developed nations, people are living longer and the types of diseases that they are dying from include chronic diseases often associated with musculoskeletal disorders and disabilities. Heart disease, stroke, pulmonary failure, and cancer are recognized as the main causes of death, but comorbid conditions such as arthritis, dementia, and osteoporosis are also contributing to increased levels of disability and the need for additional care.[22] In a study published in the *Journal of the American Medical Association*, clinicians examined the patterns of functional decline at end of life for four types of illness trajectories (cancer death, organ failure death, sudden death, and frailty) and concluded that "end of life care must also serve those who become increasingly frail even without a life-threatening illness."[23*] Additionally, research from WHO indicates that palliative care interventions such as good pain relief, communication, information, and coordinated care from skilled professionals are effective for reducing symptoms and suffering and that these experiences do not differ widely according to disease or across countries.[22] The decision regarding when to begin physical and

occupational therapies for palliative care patients is often based on the need to manage symptoms early during the course of the disease or to improve the quality of life of the patient.

Early referrals for symptom management

The use of palliative care interventions is applicable early during the course of an illness (and not just at the end-of-life stage) to manage distressing clinical complications. Physicians may not consider the benefit of physical and occupational therapies early during the course of cancer or cardiovascular or respiratory diseases; however, preventive interventions offered by these rehabilitation specialists may prevent pain and functional loss during the end-of-life phase of these diseases. Gerber noted that referrals to rehabilitation professionals for cancer patients usually target either specific impairments at an anatomical level (i.e., a loss of range of motion [ROM] or lymphedema) or problems with mobility. However, she recommends earlier referrals to prevent predictable problems associated with medical treatment, such as skin care and exercise to manage connective tissue side effects from radiation.[5]

Recent studies have demonstrated that the benefits of exercise include improvement in mood,[24***] physical capacity,[25***] fatigue,[26***] and quality of life.[27***] Exercise can prevent the loss of strength and functional abilities often associated with a lack of activity or disuse in the cancer population.[28***] Even with bone marrow transplant populations, Demeo[29**] has shown that exercises can be done safely immediately following high-dose chemotherapy and can effectively reduce fatigue, maintain physical performance, and improve hemoglobin levels.

Improvement of quality of life

Quality of life has different meanings for different persons. For measurements of quality of life to be considered valid, the definition of quality of life must be determined based on what the individual identifies it to be at a given point in time.[30] Calman[31] proposed a model for assessing quality of life in which quality of life is defined as the difference (at a particular period in time) between the hopes and expectations of the individual and their present experience. The gap between hopes and realities may be narrowed by improving patients' function through treatment or by reducing their expectations through a better understanding of the limitations imposed by their disease. Using this model, improving quality of life for palliative care patients is a dynamic process that must continually address the ongoing changes in the gap between hope and reality as their disease progresses. Physical therapists and occupational therapists, by the nature of their therapeutic and educational interventions, can and often do assist seriously ill patients to manage this gap between hope and reality.

Nolen and Mock[32] noted that, in addition to the importance of having control over traditional ADL (bathing, dressing, and eating), having functional control over health-care decision making and fulfillment or role expectations are equally

Box 102.2 When physical or occupational therapy is appropriate for palliative patients

- Any patient with a serious illness can benefit from therapy services.
- Physical/occupational therapy can provide specialized treatment of pain, discomfort, and functional loss at any stage of illness.
- Referral is encouraged early in the patient's care to prevent predicable morbidities but can be received at any time, including during and after curative treatment.
- Therapy services can be provided in hospitals, nursing homes, community settings, the patient's home, and the hospice/palliative care unit.

important to patients at the end of life. Occupational therapists can tailor treatments and goals to allow patients to continue to carry out meaningful activities and to fulfill self-identified important life roles. Yoshioka[33*] demonstrated the importance of patient control over health-care decisions in his study of 301 cancer patients who received rehabilitation therapy during their last 6 months of life. Although the mobility and self-care scores improved with therapy in all the participants, the patients and families who received the greatest benefit were those who more actively participated in their rehabilitation and helped to direct their care.

The improvement in quality of life through physical and occupational therapy interventions has been shown to be beneficial at every stage, even during the last days of life (Box 102.2).[34] In a study of 56 cancer patients in Switzerland, the benefits of physical therapy were noted right up to the last 24 hours before death;[35] 79% of the patients received beneficial respiratory management techniques during the 24 hours preceding their death, and 55% received beneficial interventions aimed at improving self-care during the 8 days preceding their death.

GUIDE FOR PHYSICAL/OCCUPATIONAL THERAPY IN PALLIATIVE CARE

Therapeutic goals

Goals should be realistic and should take into consideration numerous interrelated factors such as age, stage/type of disease, social/economic factors, and cognitive abilities. The process of setting appropriate goals is as important as the goals themselves. Although all patients should collaborate in the development of their rehabilitation goals, such collaboration is especially helpful to patients in a palliative care setting, as the process provides a therapeutic outcome of allowing the patient continued control in directing his or her care. Therapists in palliative care settings can encourage patients

to explore what is truly important to them at that point in their life. Collaborative goal setting can also provide an ideal opportunity to assist patients in reframing unrealistic goals in a manner that will match their current medical condition, if necessary.

Therapists' specialized skills

Physical and occupational therapists involved in the care of patients with progressive, debilitating illness or age-associated decline must demonstrate not only well-developed clinical skills but also the ability to communicate effectively, facilitate team interactions, and innovate extemporaneously. They must be sensitive to the emotional needs of the patient and family, as well as the needs of their fellow team members. In more ways than in any other rehabilitation treatment situation, the wants and needs of this patient population should drive the treatment plan. The palliative care therapist must be able to establish a treatment plan focused on comfort and quality of life, rather than on the recovery of normal function.

In the health-care culture, where there is often a general discomfort surrounding the topic of death, physical and occupational therapists traditionally focus on rehabilitation for living. However, in a palliative care setting, therapists must be able to manage their own fears and feelings about serious illness and death to provide effective support to the patients and their families who are facing these issues.[36] Trump[37] advises that to be effective in a palliative care setting, therapists may need to address and sometimes share in patients' and families' intense emotions. Furthermore, when death does occur, the therapist must have appropriate methods for bringing about professional and personal closure to prevent emotional burnout. Foles et al.[38] outline a series of professional and personal activities that promote emotional well-being for the therapist, including the attending of a wake, funeral, or memorial service that allows the therapist to say goodbye to the patient and family. Professional reflection on the outcomes of the therapy provided and reliance on one's own personal/spiritual beliefs and values are essential skills for therapists working in palliative care (Box 102.3).

Box 102.3 Special skills required for therapists working in palliative care

- Effective communication skills: Active listening, empathy, and intuition
- Problem-solving skills and creative approaches to individual needs
- Ability to form compassionate bonds with emotional detachment
- Ability to accept death as a reality but never take away hope

Assessment of functions

An objective assessment of function, which is routinely performed for all patients, allows the implementation of rehabilitation measures to slow, prevent, or remediate performance problems. Physicians and nurses typically evaluate function in patients with cancer using the Karnovsky, Eastern Cooperative Oncology Group (ECOG), or similar rating scales. These scales are not always true indicators of a person's actual physical abilities, as the ratings are usually based on cursory observations of the patient in an artificial environment (a clinic visit) in which they are "stimulated... by the environment, anxiety and expectations."[39] In a small study of patients with non–small cell lung cancer at the Jewish General Hospital in Montreal, Dalzell et al. compared the ECOG performance status (PS) ratings with a global functional score composed of three objective measures of performance. They found that "PS evaluation persistently underestimated the degree of functional disability, as measured by the objective measures."[40*] Cashy and Cella[41*] compared the results of PS assessments for lung cancer patients performed by the physician versus the patient's self-assessment of their function and found that physicians, in general, rated the patients as performing better than the patients rated themselves.

A better indicator of the patient's actual functional abilities is objective tests of observed performance, in which the time or distance is measured. Functional performance tests, such as a 6 min walk, 50 ft fastest speed, and timed sit to stand, have been compared among groups (i.e., cancer, HIV, AIDS, and lower back pain). Although all groups showed an overall decreased performance from normal, the cancer patient group was the lowest performing group.[42*] Lee et al.[43*] evaluated the self-reported fatigue measures and objective functional performances of individuals with lymphoma and recommended that physical performance measures be used in addition to self-reported measures when evaluating the outcomes of rehabilitation.

Physical therapy in actual practice

Giving priority to patients' wishes has become the basis for physical therapy interventions in palliative care, but their content ranges widely, from approaches intended to provide patients with a sense of achievement with regard to feelings of loss of physical strength on bicycle ergometers to supportive interventions by room visits (Box 102.4).[44]

1. *ROM exercises*
   The ROM exercises used in palliative care prioritize ROMs required for the performance of ADL, rather than the expansion of ROMs. Basically, ROM exercises are performed 5 to 10 times so as to understand the patient's normal ROMs (which will differ according to the joint) and not to induce pain. Patients are asked to cooperate with each movement, and care is taken to increase kinesthesia by having the movements accompany voluntary movements produced by muscle contraction. Because of

> ### Box 102.4 Physical therapy interventions in palliative care
>
> - Functional mobility training
> - Therapeutic exercises
> - Dyspnea management
> - Positioning for skin care, comfort, and function
> - Lymphedema control
> - Orthotics
> - Therapeutic modalities (heat, cold, massage, electrical)
> - Caregiver instruction and training

the risk of inducing pathological fractures of long tubular bones when passive ROM exercises impose an external twisting force, guidance is provided so as not to produce any internal rotation or external rotation.

2. *Muscle strength maintenance exercises*
   Muscle fatigue develops very rapidly in patients with disuse syndromes, and for all practical purposes, sometimes patients cannot even perform five repetitions. The resistance or active assistance must be adjusted, while flexion and extension exercises of the lower limbs are being performed so that the patients may experience a sense of achievement. Patients are asked to perform straight leg raises (SLRs, raising the lower limb with the knee in extension) as a means of evaluating the muscle strength of the lower limbs. If a patient can perform SLR without pain or without the action becoming unstable, then there is a strong possibility that the patient will be able to walk.

3. *Approach to antigravity muscle groups*
   Muscle groups that act in opposition to the force of gravity are called antigravity muscle groups, and the term antigravity muscle groups mainly refers to muscle groups of the trunk, the quadriceps femoris muscle, and the triceps surae muscle. Based on the results of research conducted on elderly persons during long-term bed rest and, in recent years, on the weightlessness of astronauts, muscle atrophy is said to progress considerably in the absence of the stimulation of these muscle groups. Thus, training these muscle groups is important, and abdominal muscle exercises, patella setting as quadriceps femoris training, and plantar flexion exercises at the ankle joint, which can be performed even in the supine position, are recommended.

4. *Support for getting out of bed*
   After learning the wishes of patients who tend to stay in bed because of their easy fatigability or lassitude, exercises from the standpoint of providing motivation to get out of bed are also conducted in the rehabilitation room. Even if there is only a brief time for conducting the exercises in the rehabilitation room, patients must be involved in getting out of their bed because this activity is associated with a change in their environment and the accompanying

transfer or sitting. The distance traveled during walking practice should be decided according to how tired the patient feels. Information sharing with the hospital unit should be established, and the time the patient spends out of bed and the amount of daily activity in the hospital unit should be gradually increased. When patients have been spending the whole day in bed, on the other hand, muscle atrophy has often already progressed, their nutritional and respiratory status is likely to poor, and they may tend to feel drowsy. Because of adverse effects such as nausea, pain, or fatigability, each rehabilitation session can often be performed only for a short time. In such situations, passive ROM exercises and active assistive exercises should be performed; in parallel, the bed should be progressively raised until the patient is eventually able to sit on the edge of the bed and to stand up. If the patient becomes able to maintain a sitting position, an attempt may be made to transfer the patient to a reclining wheelchair with assistance, and going for walks around the hospital also becomes possible. Performing physical therapy for patients with generalized wasting is aimed at the recovery of the functions of parts that can be improved and at improving the ADL; at the same time, an understanding of the risks involved is also necessary. When muscle atrophy has progressed, it is important to be careful that physical therapy does not result in lower limb fractures, which tend to occur because of muscle atrophy that has progressed and the absence of weight-bearing activities, or result in a lingering feeling of fatigue, orthostatic hypotension, resistance to exercise, and loss of self-confidence.

5. *General conditioning exercises*

   If patients are capable of walking in the hospital unit, they are instructed in leg stretching exercises that can be performed in a standing position. The leg stretching exercises do not involve particularly difficult movements and consist of "Achilles tendon stretching," "adductor muscle stretching," and "ankle flexibility exercises" while holding onto parallel bars or a hand rail. When the patient is attached to numerous tubes, such as intravenous tubes and monitors, a 4-movement squat–stand exercise that can be done on the spot is performed. In movement 1 of the 4-movement squat–stand exercise, patients squat by slowly flexing their knees from a standing position; in movement 2, patients extend their knees and return to a standing position; in movement 3, patients lift their heels and stand on tiptoe; and in movement 4, patients lower their heels and return to a standing position. This exercise is performed from 5 to 10 times in a rhythmic manner. Because the load increases with the depth of the squat and the number of repetitions can be raised or lowered, the load can be adjusted to the patient's physical strength. This exercise is also very effective with regard to the antigravity muscle groups mentioned earlier.

6. *Use of simple training devices*

   When the lower limb muscles are weak (manual muscle test [MMT], 2–3) and active exercises are unsuitable, devices that facilitate sliding and that are usually used for transfer activities, such as slide boards and transfer slides, can be used. These activities make active exercises possible by reducing the frictional drag caused by gravity. Doing so is linked to the successful experience of being able to move by oneself, and it also provides motivation to continue exercises as so to maintain muscle strength. Using a walker with a load brake to support getting out of bed is also effective for patients with lower limb paresis as a result of spinal metastasis or muscle weakness in their lower limbs because of disuse syndrome. Walkers are used to fulfill the hope that patients in palliative care units express when they say "I want to walk to the toilet," and they are also used with the aim of lessening the burden on nurses involved in providing assistance.

Occupational therapy in actual practice

For patients and families facing problems related to life-threatening illnesses, occupational therapy sets the desired life or work activities as the goal/method, providing spiritual and psychological support as well as support for physical functions. In palliative care, it is important to determine the needs, hopes, and demands of patients and, taking energy allocation into account, to prioritize the approaches. Although this strategy is appropriate when the patient is able to specify his or her needs, hopes, and demands specifically, there may also be many times when it is difficult to confirm their needs because of the physical condition or mental state of the patients themselves. Moreover, there are also times when the patients and their families have no information regarding the possibility of conducting occupational therapy.[45,46] Thus, in addition to the needs that have been elicited, latent needs that are expected to be more important to the patient or family are often hidden. To uncover such latent needs, it is important to also build trusting relationships, to confirm the social background and work history of the patient, and to provide the required information so that occupational therapists may provide support (Box 102.5).

Box 102.5 Occupational therapy interventions in palliative care

- Engagement in meaningful activities that reflect valued roles
- ADL training/adapted techniques
- Energy conservation techniques/fatigue management
- Assessment/training in use of assistive devices and modification of environment
- Group activities (emotional and social benefits)
- Orthotics
- Positioning for skin care, comfort, and function
- Caregiver instruction and training

1. *Reducing physical suffering*
   a. Alleviating lassitude as a result of immobility
   When impaired circulation as a result of immobility causes suffering, such as fatigue or stiffness, it is sometimes possible to alleviate fatigue, stiffness, or pain temporarily by massage, stretching, or ROM exercise, promoting circulation in the muscles around the scapula. Moreover, when respiratory discomfort develops, pain and stiffness often occur because patients must spend more time sitting, and their antigravity muscles, such as the cervical-upper spinal erector spinae muscles, become constantly hypertonic. Heat may be used (with contraindications, such as avoiding the application of heat directly over tumors, kept in mind), and support to promote blood circulation can be performed in an attempt to relax the muscles.
   b. Protecting upper limbs that are difficult to move
   When an upper limb is heavy and difficult to move freely because of brachial plexus paralysis or some other form of paralysis of the upper limb or because of lymphedema or some other type of edema of the upper limb, an attempt should be made to maintain the upper limb in the correct position through the use of an arm sling so as to protect it from hazards, such as wound during housework, and to prevent secondary suffering.
   c. Positioning in a comfortable posture
   Sometimes pain occurs as a result of a tumor metastasizing to the axillary lymph nodes or lymph nodes around the collarbone, with subsequent growth compressing the nerves, or because the tumor has invaded a nerve. Although drug therapy is the mainstay of pain treatment, since the degree of pain likely varies with the position of the shoulder joint or the scapula, methods such as appropriate positioning so that the shoulder joint is unlikely to be subjected to excessive traction should be considered.
   d. Alleviation of suffering and restricted movements as a result of edema during the terminal period
   In patients in the terminal phase of their illness, venous and lymphatic displacement, hypoproteinemia, or paralytic edema tends to develop as a result of advanced cancer. It is also often difficult to improve the edema itself, and because the body movements are limited by the edema and ROMs are limited, these limitations often become causes of patient suffering. It is important to minimize movement limitations by preventing fibrosis around joints and performing ROM exercises to maintain the ROM of major joints.
   e. Preventing contractures
   ROM exercises and positioning to ensure the ROM mainly of the large joints, including the shoulder joint and the hip joint, are important so that contractures do not impede medical care and nursing care.
2. *Maintenance and improvement of ADL and instrumental activities of daily living (IADLs)*
   Even when it is impossible to prevent declines in body functions, sometimes a patient's independence level can be increased by making adjustments to ADL movement methods, making the most of their remaining functions, or introducing long-term care equipment and self-help devices. Movements that the patients can control themselves can be devised. It is also important to devise ways that require minimal amounts of energy and to make adjustments with regard to energy allocation, such as saving energy for other things that the patient wants to do. Some examples are listed in the following.
   a. Modifying the ADL movements of patients in a generalized wasting state
   The overall physical strength of many patients with advanced cancer is depleted, and their ability to continue activities declines as a result of the impact of fatigue or diminished appetite, arising from the deterioration of their respiratory status, anorexia–cachexia syndrome, etc. It has been reported that the comparative "capability ADL" of patients who exhibit these symptoms but do not have motor paralysis or osteoarticular diseases is maintained until about 2 weeks before death, and that the "capability ADL" suddenly becomes difficult around 5 days before death. Movement methods that minimize energy (shortening movement lines, transfer methods that eliminate standing up movements) should be considered in such situations.
   b. Making adjustments to ADL movements according to the degree of bed rest in patients with metastatic bone tumors (bone metastasis) and bone and soft tissue tumors
   Bone and soft tissue metastases account for a large proportion of cancer patients' metastases, and these metastases tend to affect the ADL. Bone metastases have a predilection for the spine, pelvis, ribs, and the proximal portions of the femur and humerus, and fractures tend to occur when the metastases are osteolytic. To prevent pathological fractures, care must be exercised during the early stage so that the sites of the metastases are not exposed to loads or twisting in the direction of rotation, and radiation therapy is often instituted. Whenever a strong possibility of fracture exists, the level of bed rest and "prohibited movements" should be confirmed with a physician as described in the following, and ADL and IADL should be proposed so that such movements do not occur.
   c. Making adjustments to ADL movements for patients with edema (lymphedema or other forms of edema)
   When lymphedema or some other form of edema of the limbs progresses and the skin becomes fibrotic and hard, or when manifestations of hypoproteinemic edema or anasarca develop as the cancer progresses, inadequate flexing of the joints occurs as a secondary manifestation; consequently, the ROMs become limited, and body movements become difficult because of the increased weight of the hands and feet as a result of the edema. When an upper limb is edematous, the movements involved in changing clothes and getting washed become difficult. When a lower limb becomes edematous, the movements involved in changing clothes for the lower

half of the body and washing the lower limbs become difficult, and the movements involved in walking and climbing or descending stairs become difficult. Providing instructions regarding how to make adjustments to aspects of daily living so as not to aggravate lymphedema is important. When multilayer lymphedema bandaging (MLLB) is performed, adjustments to the bandaging may be required so as to facilitate the maintenance of the ADL and IADL and provide motivation, thereby increasing the therapeutic effect and avoiding any reduction in the quality of life, ADL, or IADL during treatment.

3. *Reducing spiritual and psychological distress*
The efficacy of occupational therapy (including rehabilitation) in alleviating spiritual and psychological suffering has long been reported.[47–49] Symptoms, including their spiritual and psychological circumstances, should be identified, and it is important to strictly manage risk and introduce work activities in an individualized and flexible manner to reduce loss experiences, even if only slightly. In addition, when symptoms such as depression, anxiety, or apathy are present, the work task level should be set at a slightly lower to avoid causing fatigue as much as possible, and patients should be carefully observed for signs of fatigue. Tasks can be discontinued before they are completed, attractive tasks should be selected, and consideration should be given to the importance of patients being able to feel a sense of achievement or having a successful experience. Careful supervision of sharp objects, such as scissors and cutters, is also necessary to prevent suicides.

4. *Reducing social distress*
Many patients feel sad as a result of no longer being able to fulfill their roles at work or in the home in the same way that they did before becoming ill (role loss), and they may feel a sense of debt (sense of being a burden) toward being a burden on those around them. Such distress is particularly severe in generations that have many social roles. Methods that enable patients to resume even some of their roles can be a means of dealing with "role loss." When patients are members of what under normal circumstances would be the "caregiver generation," they may feel a sense of being a burden, such as feeling conscience-stricken just because they are receiving nursing care from those around them. If the patient is not experiencing distress, it is better to make adjustments within the scope of the patients' abilities in advance so that they are able to perform their own personal activities (ADLs) with as little assistance as possible.

For example, if a mother says, "I want to make delicious meals for my growing children," adjustments can be made to movements that can be performed in a wheelchair, and self-help devices can be introduced so that they are able to prepare food when they return home. By providing support so that food preparation methods are casually passed on to their children, patients can also play a role in handing down recipes to the next generation. It is also useful to implement group therapy within the facility with the aim of encouraging interpersonal exchanges, enabling a sense of belonging and a sense of connectedness to be achieved, and enabling social roles to be reacquired based on exchanges with other people.

CONCLUSIONS/FUTURE ISSUES

For persons who are at the end-of-life stage, independence or a lack of disability may be defined as the ability to continue to live one's life with dignity, exerting control over one's care and maintaining functional independence in self-care activities as far as reasonably possible. Physical and occupational therapies can facilitate the patient's function at a minimum level of dependence regardless of life expectancy and can improve the quality of survival at the end of life, enabling the patient's life to be as comfortable and productive as possible. Therefore, there is little doubt that quality of life and the quality of the death experience are enhanced when physical and occupational therapists are part of a team of health professions supporting palliative care patients and their families.

However, some patients do not have access to rehabilitation services, either because of their needs that are unrecognized by frontline staff, because of a lack of allied health professionals who are adequately trained in the care of patients with cancer, or because of a lack of high-quality literature evidence. Therefore, it is necessary that all health-care professionals should receive training in rehabilitation needs assessment and that physical or occupational therapists should acquire knowledge about cancer and incorporate established techniques into cancer care. Furthermore, research is needed to explore the role, components, and outcomes of physical and occupational therapies.[50***]

Key learning points

- Rehabilitation interventions should be an integral part of palliative care.

- Physical and occupational therapies enhance function and quality of life for seriously ill people and their families and address their psychological and spiritual needs through meaningful activities.

- Improved care results in meaningful and hopeful end of life.

- Referrals should be made early in the disease to provide symptom management and improve the patient's quality of life.

- Goals of physical and occupational therapies for palliative patients are based upon what is most important to them at the time of evaluation and are continually revised as their priorities change over the trajectory of their disease.

- Therapists use specialized skills to enhance communication, form compassionate bonds, and set goals which are realistic but do not take away hope.

- The measurement of function should be performance based and use objective measures.

- Research is needed to explore the role, components, and outcomes of physical and occupational therapies.

REFERENCES

✳ 1 Lynn J, Adamson DM. *Living Well at the End of Life: Adapting Health Care to Serious Chronic Illness in Old Age.* Santa Monica, CA: RAND White Paper, 2003.

2 Cheville A. American Cancer Society. Cancer rehabilitation in the new millennium: Rehabilitation of patients with advanced cancer. *Cancer* 2001; 92: 1039–1048.

3 Boyd KJ, Murray SA, Kendall M, et al. Living with advanced heart failure: A prospective, community based study of patients and their careers. *Eur J Heart Fail* 2004; 6: 585–589.

4 Horne G, Payne S. Removing the boundaries: Palliative care for patients with heart failure. *Palliat Med* 2004; 18: 291–296.

5 Gerber L. American Cancer Society. Cancer rehabilitation in the new millennium: Cancer rehabilitation into the future. *Cancer* 2001; 92:975–979.

✳ 6 World Health Organization–Europe. *Palliative Care. The Solid Facts.* Geneva, Switzerland: WHO, 2004: pp. 7–32.

◆ 7 Ronson A, Body J. Psychosocial rehabilitation of cancer patients after curative therapy. *Support Care Cancer* 2002; 10: 281–291.

● 8 Lehmann JF, DeLisa JA, Waren CG, deLateur BJ, Bryant PL, Nicholson CG. Cancer rehabilitation: Assessment of need, development and evaluation of a model of care. *Arch Phys Med Rehabil* 1978: 59; 410–419.

● 9 Harvey RF, Jellinek HM, Habeck RV. Cancer rehabilitation: An analysis of 36 program approaches. *JAMA* 1982: 247; 2127–2131.

● 10 Dietz J. Rehabilitation of the cancer patient. *Med Clin North Am* 1969; 53: 607–624.

11 Ibrahim E, Al-Homaidh A. Physical activity and survival after breast cancer diagnosis: Meta-analysis of published studies. *Med Oncol* 2010: (online published).

12 McNeely ML, Campbell K, Ospina M, Rowe BH, Dabbs K, Klassen TP et al. Exercise interventions for upper-limb dysfunction due to breast cancer treatment. *Cochrane Database Syst Rev* 2010: June 16; CD005211.

13 Halle M, Schoenberg MH. Physical activity in the prevention and treatment of colorectal carcinoma. *Dtsch Arztebl Int* 2009: 106; 722–727.

14 van Weert E, Hoekstra-Weebers JE, May AM, Korstjens I, Ros WJ, van der Schans CP. The development of an evidence-based physical self-management rehabilitation programme for cancer survivors. *Patient Educ Couns* 2008: 71; 169–190.

15 Twycross RG. The challenge of palliative care. *Int J Clin Oncol* 2002: 7; 271–278.

16 Cheville A. Rehabilitation of patients with advanced cancer. *Cancer* 2001: 92; 970–974.

17 Santiago-Palma J, Payne R. Palliative care and rehabilitation. *Cancer* 2001: 92; 1049–1052.

18 Dietz J. Rehabilitation of the cancer patients: Its role in the scheme of comprehensive care. *Clin Bull* 1974: 4; 104–107.

19 DeLisa JA. A history of cancer rehabilitation. *Cancer* 2001: 92; 970–974.

20 Shanks R. Physiotherapy in palliative care. *Physiotherapy* 1982; 68: 405–407.

21 Tigges KN, Sherman LM. The treatment of the hospice patient: From occupational history to occupational role. *Am J Occup Ther* 1983; 37: 235–238.

22 Davies E, Higginson I, eds. World Health Organization ––Europe. *Better Palliative Care for Older People.* Geneva, Switzerland: WHO, 2004: 6–37.

● 23 Lunney JR, Lynn J, Foley D et al. Patterns of functional decline at the end of life. *JAMA* 2003; 289: 2387–2392.

24 Craft LL, Vaniterson EH, Helenowski IB, Rademaker AW, Courneya KS. Exercise effects on depressive symptoms in cancer survivors: A systematic review and meta-analysis. *Cancer Epidemiol Biomarkers Prev* 2012; 21: 3–19.

25 McMillan EM, Newhouse IJ. Exercise is an effective treatment modality for reducing cancer-related fatigue and improving physical capacity in cancer patients and survivors: A meta-analysis. *Appl Physiol Nutr Metab* 2011; 36: 892–903.

26 Payne C, Wiffen PJ, Martin S. Interventions for fatigue and weight loss in adults with advanced progressive illness. *Cochrane Database Syst Rev* 2012; 1: CD008427.

27 Fong DY, Ho JW, Hui BP et al. Physical activity for cancer survivors: Meta-analysis of randomised controlled trials. *BMJ* 2012; 344: e70. doi: 10.1136/bmj.e70.

◆ 28 Fialka-Moser V, Crevenna R, Korpan M, Quittan M. Cancer rehabilitation—Particularly with aspects on physical impairments. *J Rehabil Med* 2003; 35: 153–162.

29 Demeo FC, Stieglitz RD, Novelli-Fisher U et al. Effects of physical activity on the fatigue and psychologic status of cancer patients during chemotherapy. *Cancer* 1999; 85: 2273–2277.

30 O'Boyle CA, Waldron D. Quality of life issues in palliative medicine. *J Neurol* 1997; 244: 18–25.

31 Calman KC. Quality of life in cancer patients—An hypothesis. *J Med Ethics* 1984; 10: 124–127.

32 Nolan MT, Mock V. A conceptual framework for end-of-life care: A reconsideration of factors influencing the integrity of the human person. *J Prof Nurs* 2004; 20: 351–360.

● 33 Yoshioka H. Rehabilitation for the terminal cancer patient. *Am J Phys Med Rehabil* 1994; 73: 199–206.

34 Shigemoto K, Abe K, Kaneko F, Okamura H. Assessment of degree of satisfaction of cancer patients and their families with rehabilitation and factors associated with it—Results of a Japanese population. *Disabil Rehabil* 2007: 29; 437–444.

35 Marcant D, Rapin CH. Role of the physiotherapist in palliative care. *J Pain Symptom Manage* 1993; 8: 68–71.

36 Hayes C. General medicine and surgery. In: Hopkins H, Smith H, eds. *Willard and Spackman's Occupational Therapy,* 5th edn. Philadelphia, PA: JB Lippincott Co, 1978: 437.

37 Trump SM. Occupational therapy and hospice: A natural fit. *OT Practice* 2001; 6: 7–11.

38 Foles D, Tigges K, Weisman T. Occupational therapy in hospice home care: Student tutorial. *Am J Occup Ther* 1986; 40: 623–628.

39 Winningham ML, Donovan ES. Fatigue and oncology rehabilitation: An historical perspective. In: Winningham ML, and Barton-Burke M, eds. *Fatigue in Cancer: A Multidimensional Approach.* Sadbury, Ontario, Canada: Jones and Bartlett, 2000: pp. 263–276.

40 Dalzell MA, Kreisman H, Small D, MacDonald N. Is performance status related to functional capacity in patients with non small cell lung cancer (NSCLC). *J Clin Oncol* 2004; 22 (14 Suppl): 7224.

41 Cashy J, Cella D. Discrepancy analysis of patient vs physician assessments of performance status in patients with advanced lung cancer [abstract]. *J Clin Oncol* 2005; 23(16 Suppl): Abs No 8103.

● 42 Simmonds MJ. Physical function in patients with cancer: Psychometric characteristics and clinical usefulness of a physical performance test battery. *J Pain Symptom Manage* 2002; 24: 404–414.

43 Lee JQ, Simmonds MJ, Wang XS, Novy DM. Differences in physical performance in men and women with and without lymphoma. *Arch Phys Med Rehabil* 2003; 84: 1747–1752.

44 Tookman AJ, Hopkins K, Scharpen-von-Heussen. Rehabilitation in palliative medicine. In: Doyle D, Hanks G, Cherny N, Calman K, eds. *Oxford Textbook of Palliative Medicine.* Oxford, U.K.: Oxford University Press, 2005: pp. 1019–1032.

45   Halkett GKB, Ciccarelli M, Keesing S, Aoun S. Occupational therapy in palliative care: Is it under-utilised in western Australia? *Australian Occup Ther J* 2010: 57; 301–309.

46   Kealey P, McIntyre I. An evaluation of the domiciliary occupational therapy service in palliative cancer care in a community trust: A patient and cares perspective. *Eur J Cancer Care* 2005:14; 232–243.

47   Ewer-Smith C, Patterson S. The use of an occupational therapy programme within a palliative care setting. *Eur J Palliat Care* 2002; 9: 30–33.

48   Pizzi MA. Occupational therapy in hospice care. *Am J Occup Ther* 1984: 38; 252–257.

49   Tigges KN, Folts D, Weisman T. The treatment of the hospice patient; from occupational history to occupational role. *Am J Occup Ther* 1983; 37: 235–258.

★ 50   National Institute for Clinical Excellence. *Improving Supportive and Palliative Care for Adults with Cancer: The Manual.* 2004. Available at   http://www.nice.org.uk/nicemedia/live/10893/28816/28816.pdf (last updated: December 29, 2011).

103

Staff stress and burnout in palliative care

MARY L.S. VACHON, LISE FILLION

Working in palliative care (PC) can be challenging, rewarding, and stressful. What happens when clinicians become stressed and/or develop burnout and compassion fatigue? This chapter is divided into four sections. The first provides an overview of stress, burnout, and job engagement, compassion fatigue and compassion satisfaction, and concepts used to describe challenges in PC; presents a model within which to view the research in stress, burnout, and PC; and gives an overview of the extent of the problem. The second identifies the occupational risk factors associated with stress, compassion fatigue, and burnout. The third presents some new approaches to viewing resilience factors including finding meaning and culturing compassion that could be associated with job engagement and compassion satisfaction. The last section reviews some approaches to avoiding and dealing with these issues in PC. The PC research primarily dates from 2000. The concepts come from earlier research as well as current research. Reviews of earlier PC literature can be found elsewhere [1–3].

DEFINITIONS AND AN OVERVIEW OF STRESS AND BURNOUT IN PALLIATIVE CARE

There are a number of concepts used to reflect the distress that caregivers in PC can experience. Of the concepts listed, stress and burnout are the most frequently researched. Compassion fatigue has recently been a topic of research so it is also discussed.

Stress

Much of the current interest in stress subject can be dated to the research of Hans Selye who in 1936 [4] articulated his biological concept of stress as the "general adaptation syndrome," a set of nonspecific physiological reactions to various noxious environmental agents [5].

Antonovsky [6] sees stress as evolving from exposure to stressors. He distinguishes between stressors and routine stimuli. A routine stimulus is seen as being one to which the person can respond more or less automatically. A *stressor* is a demand made by the internal or external environment of an organism that upsets its homeostasis, restoration of which depends on a nonautomatic and not readily available energy-expending action. A routine stimulus can become a stressor under certain circumstances. Whether a stimulus is a stressor depends on the meaning of the stimulus to the person at that point in time and on the repertoire of coping mechanisms readily available. In Antonovsky's model, "stress" refers to the strain that remains "in response to the failure to manage tensions well and to overcome stressors" [7, p. 10].

Stress can be observed at the physiological, psychological, and behavioral levels of analysis [8,9]. It is an ongoing process affected by individual personality factors and environmental variables. The individual is constantly responding to and interacting with the environment, and whether the stress is a benefit or a harm to the individual depends greatly on the individual's cognitive appraisal of the stress and subsequent coping process.

The European Agency for Safety and Health at Work [10] has stated that

> There is increasing consensus around defining work-related stress in terms of the "interactions" between employee and (exposure to hazards in) their work environment. Within this model stress can be said to be experienced when the demands from the work environment exceed the employee's ability to cope with them.

Burnout and job engagement

The term burnout is generally credited to Freudenberger [11,12]. Burnout has been characterized as "the progressive loss of idealism, energy and purpose experienced by people in the helping professions as a result of the conditions of their work" [13, p. 14]. "The root cause of burnout lies in people's need to believe that their life is meaningful, and that the things they do—and consequently they themselves—are important and significant" [14, p. 633].

Christina Maslach, who developed the Maslach Burnout Inventory [15], the most commonly used instrument to measure burnout, together with her colleagues reviewed research in the field of burnout over the first 25 years of the concept's existence [16]. They concluded that burnout is a psychological syndrome in response to chronic interpersonal stressors on the job. The three key dimensions are: (1) overwhelming emotional exhaustion (EE)—the basic *individual stress dimension of* burnout; (2) feelings of cynicism and detachment from the job; depersonalization (DP)—the *interpersonal context* dimension of burnout (referring to a negative, callous, or excessively detached response to various aspects of the job); and (3) a sense of ineffectiveness and lack of personal accomplishment (PA)—the *self-evaluation dimension* of burnout (referring to feelings of incompetence and a lack of achievement and productivity at work [16]).

Job engagement is conceptualized as being the opposite of burnout [17]. It involves energy, involvement, and efficacy. Engagement involves the individual's relationship with work. This includes a sustainable workload, feelings of choice and control, appropriate recognition and reward, a supportive work community, fairness and justice, and meaningful and valued work. Engagement is also characterized by high levels of activation and pleasure [17,18]. Engagement is defined as a persistent, positive-affective-motivational state of fulfillment in employees that is characterized by vigor, dedication, and absorption [17].

Maslach recently distinguished the origins of the two concepts [19]. The concept of burnout "was developed from a grassroots, bottom-up, qualitative approach in which people were asked to describe their work experiences". The core components, emerged from these interviews, as opposed to emerging from related theories and research. Work engagement in contrast,"was originally defined from a theoretical perspective, either as the opposite of burnout [20] or as an independently positive state" [21] [19, p. 48].

Compassion fatigue and compassion satisfaction

Compassion fatigue is described as "'cost of caring' for others in emotional pain that has led helping professionals to abandon their work with traumatized persons" [22, p. 7]. Some researchers consider compassion fatigue to be similar to posttraumatic stress disorder (PTSD), except that it applies to those emotionally affected by the trauma of another (e.g., client or family member) rather than by one's own trauma. Compassion fatigue is also known as secondary or vicarious traumatization [22,23]. In contrast to burnout, the clinician with compassion fatigue can still care and be involved, albeit in a compromised way [24]. However, current measures of compassion fatigue involve measuring burnout as well, so the constructs can get somewhat confusing.

Compassion satisfaction has been defined as "the pleasure you derive from being able to do your work well" [25, p. 12]. It stands in sharp contrast to compassion fatigue, which pertains to the negative effects arising from one's work.

Model of burnout and occupational stress

In reviewing the research, Maslach et al. [16] note previous research in occupational stress focused on the person–environment fit model [26]. More recent research focuses on the degree of match or mismatch between the person and six domains of the job environment. The greater the gap or mismatch between the person and the environment, the greater the likelihood of burnout. The greater the match or fit, the greater the likelihood of engagement with work. Mismatches arise when the process of establishing a psychological contract leaves critical issues unresolved or when the working relationship changes to something that the person finds unacceptable. Six areas of work–life come together in a framework that encompasses the major organizational antecedents of burnout: workload, control, reward, community, fairness, and values. Additional variance in burnout scores over and above job stressors derives from emotion–work variables that require the individual to display or suppress emotions on the job and involve the requirement to be emotionally empathic [16].

Similarly, the French Ministry and a group of international experts [27] suggested defining occupational stress factors around six axes: intensity of work, lack of autonomy, social climate, emotional demand, conflict of values, and safety issues. Integrating these recent findings, we suggest defining occupational stress as a mismatch between the person and the following six areas of occupational risk factors: (1) workload or intensity of work, (2) autonomy (control and reward), (3) social climate (support, communication, and community), (4) emotional demand, (5) values and meaning, and (6) safety.

Burnout arises from chronic mismatches between people and their work settings in some or all of these areas. Preliminary evidence suggests that the area of values and the related concept of meaning of work may play a central mediating role for the other areas [28]. Another study in a university setting found that fairness in the work environment may be the tipping point determining whether people develop job engagement or burnout [29].

Alternatively, people may vary in the extent to which each of the six areas is important to them. Some people may place a higher weight on autonomy than on values, or people may be prepared to tolerate a mismatch regarding workload if they receive praise and good pay, have good relationships with colleagues, and find their work meaningful. The PC literature is reviewed using this framework.

Stress and burnout in palliative care vs. other specialties

A review of the literature of stress in PC over the first quarter century of the movement [1] found many studies reported that staff working in PC had either less burnout and stress than other professionals or experienced no more stress than other healthcare professionals working with seriously ill and/or dying persons. This was confirmed more recently [2,3]. A review of the PC literature from 1999 to 2009 [30] reviewed empirical studies about burnout syndrome in PC nurses and physicians and articles published in Portuguese or foreign/international scientific journals. They concluded that "burnout levels in PC, or in health care settings related to this field, do not seem to be higher than in other contexts" [30, p. 317]. Findings documenting less than anticipated stress or less stress than in colleagues in other specialties have been found in PC physicians in Australia [31], Great Britain [32,33], and Japan [34], as well as nurses in Great Britain [35] and PC staff in New Zealand [36,37].

A recent study by Fillion et al. also confirmed these findings in Quebec nurses working in end-of-life care [38]. Nurses working in hospital settings showed higher stress indicators (higher job demands and efforts) than did nurses working in home care settings. Further comparisons indicated that work stress indicators were higher in nurses working in critical care and oncology units compared with specialized PC units [38, p. 127].

The fact that stress in PC may be less than that in other specialties does not negate the stress that does occur. A study of Senior House Officers in UK hospices [39] found that the median stress score as measured on a visual analog scale was 55 mm (range 0–98 mm). Five respondents (22%) scored for identifiable psychological distress on the GHQ 12. In a recent discussion with a PC colleague, Dr. Monica Branigan [40], she noted that it is difficult to prepare young PC physicians in training for a career in which death is normalized, when they are at an age when death would not be expected to be normalized.

More senior British physicians report stress [32], which appeared to be equal to or greater than that of the oncologists and PC specialists. Up to one-third of consultants and nearly half of General Practitioners (GPs) showed symptoms of stress, which was serious enough to affect their health and impair their ability to provide high-quality care to patients. Much of this stress was due to excessive workloads and lack of control over their workload and work environment.

SOCIODEMOGRAPHIC AND OCCUPATIONAL RISK FACTORS ASSOCIATED WITH STRESS, BURNOUT, AND COMPASSION FATIGUE

Demographic variables

Younger caregivers are more prone to burnout and stress reactions [41], while increased job satisfaction is associated with older age [7,42]. Those with more years of experience were less likely to report stress-related symptoms and burnout [7,43]. Emotional sensitivity and the ability to connect with patients rose after the age of 35 [44]. However, medical residents, 72% of whom were under 30 [45] who were sufficiently attentional to their own needs to engage in self-care activities, were able to care for their patients in a sustainable way with greater compassion, sensitivity, effectiveness, and empathy.

In the large (N = 5704) Physician Worklife Study, female physicians report greater job satisfaction and greater well-being than matched controls [46]. However, the women in that study were 1.6 times more likely to report burnout than men. The odds increased by 12%–15% for each additional 5 hours worked per week over

40 hours. Lack of workplace control predicted burnout in women, but not in men. Women with young children who received support for balancing their lives from their partner, significant other, and colleagues were 40% less likely to report burnout. Kash et al. [41] found those with more responsibility for dependents, either children or elderly parents, reported more stress.

Job home interaction

A model of burnout was tested in a study comparing burnout in two large samples of physicians in the United States (N = 1824) and the Netherlands (N = 1435) [47]. Half the burnout was explained for both samples. Older physicians in the United States felt they had more control than did younger physicians. The study found an adverse impact of academic practice on work control and work–home interference in the United States. Male U.S. physicians described significantly more work control than female U.S. physicians, a sex difference not seen in the Netherlands. For both countries, work control was correlated with job stress and satisfaction, whereas work–home interference was associated with work hours, children, stress, (dis)satisfaction, and burnout. A UK study of specialist registrars in palliative medicine, medical oncology, and clinical oncology [33] also found the "effect of hours of work on personal/family life" is an important stressor for specialists.

Occupational risk factors

WORKLOAD

> The demanding nature of work may come from required time or intensity. Work intensity is expressed in terms of psychosocial risk factors through concepts such as those of "psychological demands" [48] or "effort." [49]
>
> French Ministry of Health [27, p. 85]

The mismatch is often observed when workload and lack of resources interfere with quality of work. Excessive workload exhausts the individual to the extent that recovery becomes difficult. A review of the literature [2] showed that from the early 1970s, there were perceived difficulties with workload and insufficient staff to do the job at hand in both oncology and PC [1–3].

Direct patient care activities have an impact on stress through a heavy workload of complex care, a shortage of staff, and an experienced lack of competence [50]. Nurses working with critically ill and dying children in Hong Kong and Greece felt unable to provide quality care because of the shortage in nursing personnel. This added to their stress [51]. However, in a study of hospice nurses in the United Kingdom, Payne [35] found that despite workload being a frequently reported stressor, it was not related to burnout.

More recently, however, a study of 401 specialist registrars in palliative medicine, medical oncology, and clinical oncology [33] found that one in four had GHQ-12 scores above the threshold indicating possible psychiatric morbidity. The occupational stressor with the highest mean score, and ranking as the highest stressor for all three specialties, was "being overstretched at times." However, significant differences were noted between the three groups in mean scores, with medical oncology having the highest mean. The items with the highest scores appear to relate to the very issue in clinical practice that one might expect these trainees to be concerned about—being competent in the face of conflicting demands on time.

A Canadian study [52] comparing staff in oncology and PC in an oncology center ($N = 60$) found that 63% reported experiencing "a great deal" of stress at work. The top two variables predicting this stress were greater perceived workload and insufficient time to grieve patients' deaths. More than half (52%) felt that their workload negatively affected patient care, and more than 80% felt that it affected their ability to provide emotional support for patients and compassionate end-of-life care. In all, 55% stated that they did not have sufficient time to grieve the death of a patient, and more than 30% felt they did not have enough resources to cope with work-related stress. The actual workplace (PC unit vs. oncology unit) did not predict the degree of perceived distress. Of interest is previous research conducted at the same oncology center more than 30 years earlier. In that study, nurses reported lack of resource personnel, and physicians reported "a tremendous workload imposed by the prevalence of cancer, the increased life expectancy and chronic nature of the disease" [53].

Weissman [54] provides interesting reflections on the PC martyr who believes he or she is both indispensible for managing all patient suffering and responsible to all patients in need. Recognizing that he or she is overworked and under personal stress, the martyr feels helpless to change the situation and feels unappreciated by those in authority, typically hospital administration.

Martyrs [54] are at one extreme end of the bell-shaped curve of how clinicians view their role as a responsible clinician. They devote their entire waking hours to selfless devotion to patient care, typically at the expense of their personal health and relationships with others. Part of the reason for this syndrome is the "rapid uptake of PC services; we generally provide exceptional care fostered by a high degree of internally driven sense of responsibility" [55, p. 1278].

Problems arise "when that sense of responsibility becomes overwhelming, obscuring our sense of self and harming our relationships with those around us. We lose the boundaries necessary for healthy professional and personal relationships [54, p. 1278]. Weissman says it is easy to blame the "system" for failing to provide sufficient resources to lessen the burden on the martyr, but he suggests that the internal drivers of the professional that cause him or her to maintain the state of martyrdom need to be understood and addressed [54, p. 1278]. Similar phenomenon were noted in the early days of PC [3,55].

AUTONOMY, CONTROL, REWARD

Autonomy at work involves the worker as an active actor in work, in participation, in the production of wealth, and in the driving of one's professional life. The "latitude decision" of Karasek's questionnaire [48] includes not only room for flexibility in the work situation but also participation in decision making as well as the use and development of skills and competencies. The notion of autonomy includes the idea of professional development and achievement and the ability to take some pleasure of one's achievements [27].

The mismatch occurs when there is no recognition, low control, or insufficient resources to properly do the work and lack of personal reward at work. Research suggests that restructuring high-demand, low-control jobs may enhance productivity and reduce disability costs [56]. The issue of control is related to lack of efficacy or reduced personal accomplishment. Mismatches often indicate that individuals have insufficient control over the resources necessary to do their work or insufficient authority to pursue the work in what they believe is the most effective manner [20]. Caregivers consistently report having difficulty performing their jobs because of a lack of organizational resources [52,57]. In addition, they report feeling disenfranchised [41] and having an imbalance between their job and their authority.

A Canadian study demonstrated the importance of autonomy and acknowledgment in an occupational stress study with a sample of 209 palliative care nurses. The best predictors of job satisfaction were reward, people-oriented culture, and appropriate workload, whereas the best predictors of emotional distress were reward, professional and emotional demands, and self-efficacy to provide good PC [58]. With a larger and more representative sample ($N = 751$), the same team replicated in part these findings and explained even more satisfaction and distress in adding meaning at work [59] as a mediator between autonomy and satisfaction.

SOCIAL RELATIONSHIP, COMMUNITY BELONGING, AND FAIRNESS

Social relationships at work are the relationships between workers and those between the worker and the employing organization. These social relations must be considered in connection with the concepts of integration (in the sociological sense), justice, and recognition. They were the subject of partial models, which are "social support" [60], "the effort–reward balance" (Siegrist model [49]), and "justice organizational" [27]. Mismatch arises when people lose a sense of personal connection and respect with others in the workplace or with the employing organization. Social support from people with whom one shares praise, comfort, happiness, and humor affirms membership in a group with a shared sense of values [2,3,14,17].

From early in the field of PC, the team was seen simultaneously as being a major stressor, the place where stress was manifest, and the group to whom one turned for support [1,7]. Team communication problems have long been identified as an issue in PC, as in other specialties. These have occurred across time and cultures and have been documented elsewhere [1–3,7,37]. In the European Union, the recognition that there were communication problems between palliative care mobile teams (PCMTs) and hospital staff led to a program of intervention to be discussed in the following [61].

Studying hospice nurses in the United Kingdom, Payne [35] found that dealing with death and dying, inadequate preparation, and workload were slightly more problematic than were conflict with doctors, conflict with other nurses, lack of support, and uncertainty concerning treatment. However, in that study, conflict with staff contributed to both the emotional exhaustion and depersonalization subscales of the Maslach Burnout Inventory. More recently, PC specialist registrars in the United Kingdom were more likely than oncology registrars to report finding stress from low prestige of their specialty and from difficulties with nursing staff [33].

Although teamwork has been seen as being the best, and perhaps only, way of doing PC, some of the assumptions of PC teamwork have come into question [62]. A review of the literature suggests that the effectiveness of multiprofessional teams in delivering PC has never really been addressed [63] and more research is needed to document team functioning, staff well-being, and patients' quality of care. Mutual respect between people is also central to a shared sense of community. Fairness communicates respect and confirms people's self-worth. Fairness in the work environment may be the tipping point determining whether people develop job engagement or burnout [29]. Lack of fairness was perceived in unrealistic expectations of the organization [64].

EMOTIONAL DEMAND

The emotional demands are related to the need to control and shape one's emotions, particularly in order to master and shape those felt by people with whom you interact at work. Having to hide emotions is also demanding. [27]

PC has been recognized as being associated with emotional demands including multiple bereavements and grief, exposure to patients' and families' distress, personal discomfort about suffering, and death [1–3,37,55,64,65].

The mismatch may particularly appear when requirement to display or suppress emotions on the job is challenging and therapeutic relationship, human connections, or empathy could be compromised.

While the literature has been somewhat divided as to whether or not the care of the dying is a major stressor in hospice PC [1–3], research in the burnout area has focused explicitly on emotion–work variables and has found these emotional factors do account for additional variance in burnout scores over and above job stressors [16]. The most problematic stressor reported by UK hospice nurses was "death and dying" [35].

In contrast, a survey of 464 PC staff from a variety of disciplines in New Zealand [36,37] did not identify "death and dying" issues as a major contributor to creating a stressful work environment. Participants reported that these issues were manageable as long as there were sufficient and appropriate organizational support practices, such as acknowledgment of the deaths, the use of rituals, and the availability of debriefing, if required. In fact, under humane conditions,

working with death and dying could even be described as a source of meaning [65,66]. In an in-depth qualitative study of PC nurses ($N = 11$), Vachon et al. [67] found that the connections nurses make with their patients in confronting death can involve both suffering and meaning. They described three patterns of nurses' experience of death confrontation: integrating death, fighting death, and suffering death. While some nurses reported feeling nourished from their contacts with dying patients (empathic resonance), others sometimes experienced feeling frustrated (discordance) or powerless (consonance).

Some situations are particularly difficult and may be considerate to be traumatic exposure and involve compassion fatigue, also known as secondary or vicarious traumatization [22,23]. Compassion fatigue may lead to burnout [23 from 68]. In contrast, when caregivers have developed capacity to cope with suffering, they may experience compassion satisfaction [25] that stands in sharp contrast to compassion fatigue, which pertains to the negative effects arising from one's work.

In a descriptive exploratory study with health-care professionals from two hospice settings, Alkema et al. [69] found that compassion satisfaction was negatively correlated with burnout ($r = -0.612$) and compassion fatigue ($r = -0.300$). Compassion fatigue was negatively related with self-care (excluding physical self-care), suggesting that health-care professionals should integrate self-care strategies into their everyday lives. Further, Alkema et al. found that emotional and spiritual self-care and personal–professional balance were predictive of higher levels of compassion satisfaction. The findings of Alkema et al. [69] can be compared with those of Shanafelt et al. [45] who found that medical residents who engaged in self-care activities were more apt to be empathic with patients.

A large Canadian study of 630 PC workers [70] surveyed clinical, administrative, allied health workers and volunteers and also found a correlation between compassion satisfaction and burnout ($r = -0.531$, $p < 0.001$), between compassion satisfaction and compassion fatigue ($r = -0.208$, $p < 0.001$), and between burnout and compassion fatigue ($r = 0.532$, $p < 0.001$). Respondents were asked which hospice/PC services they usually provided. The top three were

1. Assistance with provision of relief from physical, emotional, and/or spiritual pain or distress
2. Providing psychosocial support to patients and/or families
3. Providing emotional support to other team members

The respondents who provided each of these services reported higher levels of compassion fatigue and burnout and no significant difference in levels of compassion satisfaction compared to those who did not provide the service. One hypothesis was that even staff who did not provide direct clinical care derived compassion satisfaction from their work. Part-time workers had higher compassion satisfaction and lower compassion fatigue and burnout levels compared to full-time workers. Integrative medicine had the highest levels of compassion satisfaction and administration had the lowest. Nurses had the highest compassion fatigue and administration had the lowest. Medicine and nursing had the highest levels of burnout and integrative medicine had the lowest level. Compared with the averages in the existing literature, which utilize the Professional Quality of Life (ProQOL), the respondents in this study had high levels of compassion satisfaction (43.9 vs. top quartile = 42), slightly elevated levels of compassion fatigue (18.6 vs. top quartile = 17), and average levels of burnout (20.8 vs. midpoint = 22). The difference in the strength of the correlation between compassion satisfaction and each of compassion fatigue (−0.208) and burnout (−0.531) support the nascent literature in differentiating between these two constructs. This finding warrants further analysis to understand the causal pathways resulting in compassion fatigue vs. burnout.

Dr. Peter Huggard [71] recently studied compassion fatigue in a self-selected sample of 253 doctors, working in New Zealand and training in a variety of medical specialties. Using the ProQOL instrument, 17.1% of the sample appeared to be at risk for compassion fatigue as indicated by a high score on that subscale of the ProQOL and 19.5% at risk of burnout. These results are similar to those reported in studies of other health professionals.

Some authors question the concept of compassion fatigue. Limitations of this model include an emphasis on a linear direction and dimension for compassion fatigue (either you have it or you don't). This seems antithetical to human behavior responses where individuals may express varying degrees of response [64]. Others ask if compassion can fatigue [72]. These questions will be addressed in the section "Nurturing compassion."

VALUES

Ethical suffering is felt by a person who is asked to act in conflict with professional, social, or personal values. The conflict of values may be associated with an incoherence between workers' beliefs and the aim of the work or its side effects or a pressure to act in opposition to their conscience.

People might feel constrained by their job to do something unethical and not in accord with their own values [27]. Alternatively, there may be a mismatch between their personal career goals and the values of the organization. People can also be caught in conflicting values of the organization, as when there is a discrepancy between a lofty mission statement and actual practice or when the values are in conflict (e.g., high-quality service and cost containment do not always coexist). Staffing problems can lead to not being able to do the job properly, a decrease in quality patient care, and decreased staff morale [64].

An article providing strategies to reduce burnout among oncologists reported that optimization of career fit (balance between personal and professional goals/values) led to increased job satisfaction [73].

When there is a misfit between the values of an individual and the organization, moral distress may result. Moral distress in the workplace occurs when there is an experience of incoherence between one's beliefs and one's actions and possibly also outcomes (i.e., between what one sincerely believes to be right, what one actually does, and

what eventually transpires). Jameton [74] describes moral distress as a situation where "one knows the right thing to do, but institutional constraints make it nearly impossible to pursue the right course of action." Webster and Baylis [75] extend this definition and note that "moral distress may also arise … for one or more of the following reasons: an error in judgment, some personal failing (for example, a weakness or crimp in one's character such as a pattern of 'systemic avoidance'), or other circumstances truly beyond one's control" [75, p. 218].

The concept of moral distress can be seen as being related to the issues of "values," "fairness," and "community" in burnout. Moral distress extends beyond compassion fatigue to involve issues that evolve from ethical conflicts in the treatment of patients and families and may involve vicarious traumatization as caregivers imagine themselves in the value-laden, ethical, and conflictual situations that their patients and family members are experiencing. These situations of moral distress often involve staff members being in conflict with one another [76].

Weissman [77], a PC physician, writes of his team:, who became frustrated working within a system that seemed to be "out of sync" with the needs of both patients and care providers…" and that impedes their ability to meet the needs of the dying, lingered long after each shift. These thoughts and feelings reflect the concept of moral distress, which occurs when the health care professional knows the correct action to take, but institutional or other constraints impede that action. [77, pp. 178–179 in 64].

SAFETY

Finally, safety issues constitute the last occupational factors area. Safety issues include economic uncertainty, unexpected change in tasks, or working conditions. Economic insecurity can come from the risk of losing one's job, associated income reduction, or loss of benefits observed in a more "normal" career pathway [27]. Working conditions can also generate other safety issues. Mismatch occurs when economical and personal safety may be compromised.

Nurses working in a hospice in South Africa were uncomfortable going into some settings, particularly at night. As a group, they explored with administration the option of refusing to go into some areas. The hospice provided them with cell phones. Brainstorming together, the nurses suggested working with the police to alert the police when the nurses were going into a potentially dangerous situation. The nurses asked the police to accompany them if they were really uncomfortable visiting certain areas but felt they should visit for the sake of the patient [78].

Funding issues were reported as problem for many programs [78]. Participants in an Australian study [79] reported that economic pressures resulted in less staff support, competition between services for funding, inadequate funding to provide services in areas of need, lack of support for psychosocial needs including bereavement care, and experienced staff leaving PC.

SUMMARY OF OCCUPATIONAL RISK FACTORS

This section has discussed the concepts of stress, burnout and job engagement, and compassion fatigue and compassion satisfaction as frameworks that have been used to study the experiences of caregivers in PC. Using the work of the French Ministry [27], we have defined occupational stress as a mismatch between the person and the following six areas of occupational risk factors: (1) workload or intensity of work, (2) autonomy (control and reward), (3) social climate (support, communication, and community), (4) emotional demand, (5) values and meaning, and (6) safety. Research from PC has been found to show that there is stress and burnout in each of these areas in the field and compassion fatigue but also compassion satisfaction is found in the area of emotional demand.

RESILIENCE TO STRESS AND BURNOUT

After exploring occupational risk factors, we will now explore factors associated with resilience. Defined as the ability to bounce back or cope successfully despite considerable adversity, Walsh [80] resilience is a commonly held trait that results "from the operation of basic human adaptational systems" [81, p. 227].

When close to 600 caregivers to the critically ill, dying, and bereaved were interviewed and asked what enabled them to continue working in the field, the top coping mechanism was a sense of competence, control, or pleasure in one's work. The next highest coping mechanisms included team philosophy, building, and support; control over aspects of practice; lifestyle management; and a personal philosophy of illness, death, and one's role in life [7].

In a more recent study of 30 PC physicians [82], respondents listed 1–7 strategies (median 4 per respondent) they felt to be important in preventing burnout that were placed in 1 of 13 thematic classes. Physical well-being was the most common strategy reported (60%), followed by professional relationships (57%), taking a transcendental perspective (43%), talking with others (43%), hobbies (40%), clinical variety (37%), personal relationships (37%), and personal boundaries (37%). "Time away" from work (27%), passion for one's work (20%), realistic expectations and use of humor and laughter (13% each), and remembering patients (10%) were cited less frequently.

In a study exploring stress-resilience capacity among pediatric oncologists, researchers found that an optimistic attitude, willingness to discuss existential issues associated with life and death, and high levels of motivation decreased the level of depression and enhanced job satisfaction and resilience [18].

Nurturing compassion

While high levels of empathy and empathic response to a patient's pain, suffering, or traumatic experience were associated with compassion fatigue [22, 83, from 64], concepts of compassion or "exquisite empathy" [84] could be related to the opposite. A Buddhist definition of compassion is "wanting others to be free from suffering." To generate genuine compassion, one needs to realize that one's self is suffering, that an end to suffering is possible, and that other beings similarly want to be free from suffering [85].

In *Mindful Leadership: The 9 Ways to Self-Awareness, Transforming Yourself, and Inspiring Others*, Gonzalez [86] notes that the role of a leader is to be of service. Gonzalez defines a leader as anyone who is in a position to influence others. Dr. Rachel Naomi Remen [87] writes of service as being the role of the health-care professional: "Basically service is about taking life personally, letting the lives that touch yours touch you" (p. 197). She contends that service is a relationship between equals. When you serve, the work itself keeps you from burnout.

Gonzalez [86] says that one of the characteristics of a mindful leader is that he or she is compassionate. Gonzalez defines true compassion as deep caring without attachment. "This is not the same as deep caring with detachment, which would imply an arm's-length relationship that does not touch you, where you could not feel the pain or get hurt in the process of caring" [86, p. 164]. This compassion is caring deeply but not being attached to the outcome. Caregivers do not surprisingly have difficulty with the concept of nonattachment to outcome. Briere, a Buddhist relational psychologist [88], suggests that caregivers may have less difficulty with the issue of nonattachment to outcomes if they frame it as the concept of acceptance. Even though we may do our best as caregivers, things may not turn out the way we would like or think they should.

True compassion with nonattachment to outcome builds resilience and keeps us from burning out. Gonzalez describes mindful leaders as doing their best each and every moment of the day, under the circumstances. They understand the importance and value of self-compassion, because they know that without taking care of themselves, their ability to serve and to perform at a high level is not sustainable [86, p. 7]. Being compassionate requires self-awareness, which can be developed in part through mindfulness meditation. The combination of self-awareness and self-compassion leads us to being aware of when a work situation involves our need to take extra time for ourselves to reflect and grieve. Self-awareness and self-compassion also involve our recognizing that in order to continue to be involved in this type of service, we need to be aware of our own ongoing needs for self-care. Shanafelt et al. [45] found that medical residents who were sufficiently attentional to their own needs to engage in self-care activities, including relationships, work attitudes, religious/spiritual practice, personal philosophies, and strategies related to job–life balance, were able to care for their patients in a sustainable way with greater compassion, sensitivity, effectiveness, and empathy. Neuroscience research has shown that part of the brain that is connected to our ability to connect to our own physical processes (the insular cortex) is associated with the ability to be attuned to the somatic and affective processes of others. So, by paying attention and caring for our own needs, we are better able to care for the needs of others [89].

True compassion does not involve the ego, as such, if one is practicing true compassion one does not fatigue.

Dr. Lisa Marr [72], a PC physician, says "to say compassion can fatigue assumes that there is a limited well of compassion in each of us. Once it is used up, either we must replenish the well, or move along without it, devoid of our compassion, or with impaired compassion" [72, p. 739]. She says compassion isn't a static state, nor is it work or a label. We are not 'compassionate people' or 'not compassionate people'. Compassion manifests itself in each moment-if we are truly engaged in that moment, not focusing on ourselves or worrying about where I should or could be at that moment, but truly engaged in the interaction with the other person, then compassion cannot fatigue, and frankly burnout is less likely to occur [72, p. 739].

Harrison and Westwood [84] found that exemplary therapists who thrived in their work with traumatized clients, including PC patients and their families, utilized "exquisite empathy," which they defined as "highly present, sensitively attuned, well-boundaried, heartfelt empathic engagement." These therapists were "invigorated rather than depleted by their intimate professional connections with traumatized clients" [84, p. 213] and protected against compassion fatigue and burnout. This idea, which has also been referred to as *bidirectionality* [90], refutes the commonly held notion that being empathic to dying patients must lead to emotional depletion [22]. The practice of exquisite empathy is facilitated by clinician self-awareness [84], which was identified in another study as the most important factor in psychologists functioning well in the face of personal and professional stressors [91 from 68].

The compassionate care of the dying and bereaved requires the ability to give of oneself without being destroyed in the process. Learning how to do this takes time and requires that the caregiver come to know himself or herself intimately, knowing what may trigger a sense of loss and grief and how to best care for oneself in order that one can grieve appropriately and move on with caring for others [92]. The subtitle of Kearney et al.'s [68] article on self-care for physicians in end-of-life care is "Being Connected ... A Key to My Survival." As caregivers, it is crucial that we are "connected" to ourselves, others in our personal life, our patients, and perhaps the transcendent, if we are going to be able to survive and thrive in our work with the dying and bereaved. Organizations have a role to help caregivers with the grief that accumulates as a result of their work, but we also have a responsibility to care for ourselves.

Kearney et al. [68] note that effective self-awareness involves a combination of self-knowledge and development of *dual awareness*, a stance that permits the clinician to simultaneously attend to and monitor the needs of the patient, the work environment, and his or her own subjective experience. When caregivers do not have self-awareness, they are more likely to

> lose perspective, experience more stress in interactions with their work environment, experience empathy as a liability, and have a greater likelihood of compassion fatigue and burnout ... Physicians with burnout who use self-care without self-awareness may feel as though they are drowning and barely able to come up for air, whereas self-care with self-awareness is like learning to breathe underwater. [68, p. 1160]

Summary

Caregivers who have developed self-care strategies promote resilience and decrease the risk of burnout. Marr [72] warns, however, that developing a self-care strategy that involves simply focusing on oneself such that one is going through the day wanting to get to one's "real life" does not work. Self-care strategies involve self-care, optimism, support from others, willingness and ability to confront challenging issues, and connectedness. True compassion may well increase resilience, keeping us from burnout and not fatiguing. Exquisite empathy involving self-care as well as boundaries is associated with being able to continue in this work.

INTERVENTIONS TO PREVENT OR DECREASE STRESS AND BURNOUT

This last section focuses on literature demonstrating interventions to prevent or decrease stress and burnout in PC. An overview of interventions to decrease occupational risk factors applied to different setting is first presented. Descriptions of interventions to decrease occupational risk factors and increase resilience in oncology and PC follow. This area of research is still limited and mostly aimed at reducing risks factors. Finally, mindfulness interventions designed for health providers are briefly introduced and discussed in terms of their relevance for oncology and PC settings.

Interventions to decrease occupational risk factors in health-care settings

A meta-analysis of 48 occupational stress-reducing interventions ($N = 3736$ participants) [93] categorized the studies as cognitive-behavioral interventions, relaxation techniques, multimodal programs (emphasizing both active and passive coping skills), and organization-focused interventions. A small but significant overall effect was found. Cognitive-behavioral and multimodal interventions had a moderate effect, a small effect was found for relaxation, and the effect size for organization-focused intervention was nonsignificant. Cognitive-behavioral interventions appeared to be effective in improving perceived quality of work–life, enhancing psychological resources and responses, and reducing complaints. Multimodal programs showed similar effects; however, they appeared to be ineffective in increasing psychological resources and responses. The authors note that there is a marginally significant effect of job status on treatment outcome—those who appeared to have more job control had a better response to the interventions. The authors urge caution here because job status was inferred. They suggest that the relatively large effect of cognitive-behavioral interventions in those with higher job control may be because employees profit most when they are provided with individual coping skills in a job that allows them to use these skills. The lack of effect of organization-focused interventions was attributed to a variety of factors.

In the domain of oncology, literature reviews provide a global picture of interventions focusing either at the occupational level or at the individual one. Mimura and Griffeths [94] conducted a systematic review of the literature from 1999 forward addressing nursing stress management. In this review, they examined stress management interventions and evaluation of change in individual stress levels as measured by instruments with established validity. The results of their review indicate that the self-care program components that appear to be effective (limitations include few controlled studies and small samples) include relaxation training, social support, cognitive techniques, exercise, and music The studies selected were mostly focusing at reducing individual risk factors.

Similarly, in 2005, Sherman et al. [95] also conducted a literature review including studies aimed at reducing stress at both the organizational and individual levels. At the organizational level, few interventions were properly assessed. The studies reviewed involved providing adequate staffing or reducing workload, increasing staff autonomy and control over scheduling, enhancing teamwork and reducing interprofessional conflicts, improving space and facilities, and increasing personal days/vacation time. At the individual level, more interventions were reviewed including emotional support (support groups, grief/bereavement workshops), stress management (healthy lifestyle and self-care strategies), improving communication skills, finding meaning at work, and humor. Earlier, stress related to communicating bad news was identified as a significant stress [96,97]. Sherman et al. [95] noted that training in communication skills, particularly as related to breaking bad news, and transitions from acute treatment to PC constituted a growing literature. For example, Fallowfield et al. [98] showed improvement in the communication skills of oncologists, which persisted over a 12-month period [99]. Razavi et al. [100] found that communication skills training for oncology nurses had a significant effect on attitudes, especially those related to self-concept, and occupational stress related to inadequate preparation.

Patients who interacted with Belgian physicians who had a communications skills course [101] reported higher scores related to their physicians' understanding of their disease. Australian oncologists [102] who attended communication skills workshop valued the training highly, but it did not decrease their stress and burnout scores, which were lower than those reported, elsewhere at the beginning of the study [96].

More recently, Barth and Lannen [103] conducted a meta-analysis on communication training in oncology (CTO). They selected 13 trials, 10 with no specific intervention in the control group. Results showed a moderate effect of CTO on communication behavior: ES = 0.54. Three trials compared basic training courses with more extensive training courses and showed a small additional effect on communication skills (ES = 0.37). Studies investigating participants' attitudes ES = 0.35 and patient outcomes ES = 0.13 (trend) confirmed this effect. They concluded that communication training of health professionals is a promising approach to change communication behaviors and attitudes. Patients might also benefit from specifically trained health professionals, but strong studies are lacking.

Other additional intervention studies have documented stress reduction or burnout prevention. At the organizational level, LeBlanc et al. [104] conducted a quasi-experimental study among staff of 29 oncology wards on effects of a team-based burnout intervention program combining a staff support group with a participatory action research approach. Nine wards were randomly selected to participate in the program. Before the program started (Time 1), directly after the program ended (Time 2), and 6 months later (Time 3), study participants filled out a questionnaire on their work situation and well-being. Results of multilevel analyses showed that staff in the experimental wards experienced significantly less emotional exhaustion at both Time 2 and Time 3 and less depersonalization at Time 2, compared with the control wards. Changes in burnout levels were significantly related to changes in the perception of job characteristics over time.

At the individual level, although often using a group format, several efforts were devoted at facilitating emotional and grieving process and active coping from the beginning of the hospice movement, many hospices and PC units have offered support groups for their staff. These groups can be specific for nurses or can include any member of the interdisciplinary team (e.g., doctors, chaplain, volunteers). Support groups allow participants to share work-related affective experiences and discuss clinical management of patients. Such groups were described but not tested as being effective in decreasing stress. For example, a descriptive evaluation on emotional support provision of a Support Group for Junior Doctors Working in Palliative Medicine was conducted [105]. The group includes case study discussion. Participants found it helpful through sharing clinical experiences, establishing relationships, having a confidential forum for discussion, and having protected time set aside for the group.

Another type of group intervention to support PC professionals focused on creativity and self-care [106]. It was aiming at encouraging caregivers to discover their own resources through creativity and play. The intervention consists of a one-day workshop including three modalities: journal writing, art therapy, and music therapy. At the end of the day, participants discuss their experience. Participants reported appreciating the opportunity to take time for themselves and to share their experience in PC with other caregivers. A pre–post decrease on burnout was also associated with the participation to an art therapy group in a pilot study with oncology staff [107].

These strategies and interventions can help caregivers cope with some occupational risk factors specific to PC but present limitations. For instance, strategies that could more specifically address death and dying, suffering of the patient and the family, and other existential issues (i.e., meaning-making coping strategies) and dimensions that are crucial in end-of-life care giving [108] were not directly addressed in any of these interventions. Additionally, rewards and benefits associated with accompanying end-of-life patients, an experience frequently reported by nurses as satisfying, were not used in the therapeutic process (e.g., self-awareness and finding meaning). The workplace positive elements (i.e., rewards and benefits) could stimulate nurses to find meaning in their work and, consequently, enhance their well-being and job satisfaction [109].

Focusing more directly on PC issues, some more recent training programs on enhancing a variety of competencies were documented. For instance, Kravit et al. [110] developed and evaluated a psychoeducational program for 248 nurses in oncology that assists nurses who work in high-stress areas to develop personalized stress management plans that rely on the use of adaptive coping strategies to reduce stress and cultivate a meaning-based resilience focusing on setting creative and achievable goals and maintain positive mood. They report preliminary data on feasibility and acceptability.

With a goal of improving the interaction between PCMTs and the hospital staff with whom they interact [61], the European Union recognizing the full range of convictions held by persons in a hospital setting, the concept of PC/terminal care has been bolstered by the concept of *continuous care*. Continuous care tends to *articulate* curative and palliative procedures focusing on the holistic care of patients and their family:

> 'Promoting the integration of continuous care in the hospital' intends to identify the challenges in integrating continuous care through an inventory and analysis of the activity of palliative care mobile teams in several countries of Europe (p. 4). Competencies for PCMTs have been derived, and three educational programs were undertaken and evaluated.

Meier et al. [111] proposed an approach to physician awareness that involves identifying and working with emotions that may affect patient care. This involves looking at physician, situational, and patient risk factors that can lead to physician feelings and thus influence patient care. The steps include the following: Identify the factors that predispose to emotions that might affect patient care; monitor for signs (behavioral) and symptoms (feelings) of emotions; name and accept the emotion; identify possible sources of the emotion; respond constructively to the emotion; step back from the situation to gain perspective; identify behaviors resulting from the feeling; consider implications and consequences of behaviors; think through alternative outcomes for patients according to different behaviors.; and consult a trusted professional colleague.

Also targeting to specifically cope with emotional demands, as well as meaning-based coping and grieving issues, Macpherson [112] used a mixed-methods single-group descriptive repeated-measures study examined peer-supported storytelling for grieving pediatric oncology nurses. The study aims were to examine (1) the support exchanged in storytelling sessions, (2) the impact of storytelling sessions on nurses' grief, (3) the impact of storytelling sessions on nurses' meaning making, and (4) the content of sessions. Participating had an impact on their meaning making, and the explicit session focus on making sense of and identifying benefit in their experiences was particularly helpful. There was a significant positive correlation between participant report of number of special patient deaths during career and impact of sessions on grief.

Similarly, writing in a reflective and emotionally expressive way could also constitute an intervention that enhances coping with emotional demands and grieving processes. Narratives and written emotional expression have been demonstrated to promote reflection and empathic engagement in physicians. A feasibility study [113] of a narrative intervention conducted with an interdisciplinary group of health-care professionals in pediatric oncology also demonstrated promising effects on perspective taking, empathy, and teamwork [114].

Wessel and colleagues [115,117,118] integrated reflective narratives into the practice of palliative care education for nurses. The narrative reflection allowed the nurses to document meaningful experiences in end-of-life care situations. . The education content included goals of end-of-life care; overview of pain control, symptom management, and nutrition at end of life; access to ethics resource services, and communication techniques; and issues of spirituality, grief, and bereavement. Significant decrease of death anxiety was observed. However, no significant change in nurse's attitudes toward caring for dying patients and their family members was reported.

Aiming at developing knowledge and coping with existential issues or competencies building in spiritual care could also contribute to improve ways to cope with emotional demands and reduce stress. Whitehead et al. [119] evaluated the impact of the end-of-life nursing education consortium at the institutional level on death anxiety, concerns about dying, and knowledge of the dying process. Participants in the experimental group significantly improved their knowledge of the dying process at posttest and 12 months. However, no differences between experimental and control were noticed on death anxiety and concerns about dying suggesting that education is not enough to enhance spiritual care competencies.

Using a pretest–posttest design, Wasner et al. [120] evaluated the effects of spiritual care training for PC professionals on spiritual quality of life, self-transcendence, and level of religiosity. The training "Wisdom and Compassion in Care for the Dying" was delivered in a 3.5-day format, based on Tibetan Buddhist traditions and techniques of active and compassionate listening, contemplation, and meditation. Spirituality increased significantly after the training and still after 6 months. Self-transcendence increased significantly after the training but not after 6 months. Level of religiosity did not change significantly over time.

Following the development of meaning-centered interventions (MCIs) to address emotional demands and existential issues encountered in PC [121], the authors designed an experimental study (randomized waiting-list design, Fillion et al. [122]) to test its effectiveness. The intervention applied didactic and process-oriented strategies, including guided reflections, experiential exercises, and didactics on themes of Viktor Frankl's logotherapy [123]. Spirituality (using the same tool by Wasner et al. [120]), well-being, and satisfaction at work (general index and perception of benefits of working in PC) were measured at pretest, posttest, and 3 months follow-up. PC nurses in the experimental group reported more perceived benefits of working in PC after the intervention and at follow-up. Spirituality and well-being remained, however, unaffected. Selection bias was suggested to explain the null findings (participants recruited were healthy workers—had higher spirituality at pretest than in Wasner et al. [120] post scores, for instance). Improving access to the intervention and recruitment strategy was recommended to reach all nurses. Documenting more in depth the benefits perceived was also proposed. Two qualitative studies were designed to better understand the beneficial effect on the MCI. From the first study conducted with 11 PC nurses [123], two essential themes emerged. MCI expanded nurses' spiritual and existential awareness by increasing their awareness of life's finiteness, opening them up to new meanings and purposes of suffering, having them become more aware of sources of meaning and purpose in life, and having them access a state of mindfulness. The second essential theme was the group's containing function for nurses. The group process allowed nurses to develop a shared language to talk about their spiritual and existential experience and experience validation through sharing their experience with peers.

In the second study, Leung et al. [124] used also an interpretative phenomenology approach with 14 nurses working in bone marrow transplants unit. The MCI seemed to inspire participants to engage more with patients and their suffering. Three subthemes reflected this influence: (a) greater awareness of boundaries between their personal and professional involvement, (b) enhanced empathy from an awareness of a shared mortality, and (c) elevated hope when nurses linked patients' suffering with meaning. The qualitative studies also suggested the integration of a self-care component to the MCI, such as mindfulness stress reduction techniques to further self-awareness, self-care, and self-regulation of emotion.

The recommendation of complementing MCI with mindfulness is in line with the being with dying intervention (BWD [125,126]). The premise of BWD, which is based on the development of mindfulness and receptive attention through contemplative practice, is that cultivating stability of mind and emotions enables clinicians to respond to others and themselves with compassion. In a survey, Rushton et al. [127] described the impact of

BWD: Professional Training Program in Contemplative End-of-Life Care on the participants: Nurses, physicians, social workers, chaplains. Ninety-five BWD participants completed an anonymous online survey; 40 completed a confidential open-ended telephone interview. Form the qualitative analyses of the interviews, four main themes emerged: the power of presence, cultivating balanced compassion, recognizing grief, and the importance of self-care. The interviewees considered BWD's contemplative and reflective practices meaningful, useful, and valuable and reported that BWD provided skills, attitudes, behaviors, and tools to change how they worked with the dying and bereaved.

Other studies conducted with health-care providers are giving some support to the usefulness of mindfulness in the context of PC. Rooted in Buddhism and westernized by Jon Kabat-Zinn at the University of Massachusetts Medical Center, mindfulness-based stress reduction (MBSR) is a structured therapy package combing mindfulness-based meditation (MBM) with yoga. It consists of an 8-week course in which participants meet once a week for a 2.5 hours session and one 8 hours session per day. Kabat-Zinn and colleagues have taught MBSR to medicals for over two decades.

Pre- and postdesign quantitative research on medical and premedical students who participated in an MBSR program demonstrated positive effects on self-report measures of psychological symptoms such as anxiety and depression, as well as increased ratings of empathy and spirituality. MBSR is also therapeutic for health-care providers, enhancing their interactions with patients (for reviews, see Refs. [128,129]). A brief format was piloted by Mackenzie et al. [130] with nurses and nurse aides. In comparison with 14 waiting-list control participants, 16 participants in the mindfulness intervention experienced significant improvements in burnout symptoms, relaxation, and life satisfaction. The authors concluded that mindfulness training is a promising method for helping those in the nursing profession to manage stress, even when provided in a brief format.

In summary, several interventions to decrease occupational risk factors were described and offered potential foundations upon which to build. Combining organizational and individual factors notably to improve team functioning and increase access to supportive interventions is also emerging as a promising area. For most of the studies reported, however, except for communication skill areas, lack of scientific protocol or very small sample was described. Lack on consensual selection of outcomes also limited comparison among studies. For the communication area, these programs tend to improve staff confidence and attitudes toward comprehensive care, but limited documentation and nonsignificant potential benefits in terms of burnout or job satisfaction were noticed. There still is a need for longitudinal, multivariate studies to examine changes over time in levels of burnout and distress in various practice areas, for example, medical oncology, radiotherapy, and terminal care. To extend our understanding of risk and resilience factors, inclusion of positive (e.g., benefits, compassion, empathy, meaning at work, satisfaction, vitality) and associated outcomes such as provider health status, staff turnover, and quality of care indices are suitable.

REFERENCES

1 Vachon MLS. Staff stress in palliative/hospice care: A review. *Palliat Med* 1995;**9**:91–122.

2 Vachon MLS, Sherwood C. Staff stress and burnout. In: A.M. Berger, J.L. Shuster, J.H. Von Roenn (eds.). *Principles and Practice of Palliative Care and Supportive Oncology.* Philadelphia, PA: Lippincott, Williams & Wilkins, 2007, pp. 667–683.

3 Vachon MLS. Four decades of selected research in hospice/palliative care: Have the stressors changed? In: I. Renzenbrink (ed.). *Caregiver Stress and Staff Support in Illness, Dying, and Bereavement.* Oxford, U.K.: Oxford University Press, 2011, pp. 1–24.

4 Selye H. *Stress without Distress.* Philadelphia, PA: Lippincott, 1974.

5 Selye H. *The Stress of Life.* New York: McGraw-Hill, 1956.

6 Antonovsky A. *Health, Stress and Coping.* San Francisco, CA: Jossey-Bass, 1979.

7 Vachon MLS. *Occupational Stress in the Care of the Critically Ill, the Dying and the Bereaved.* New York: Hemisphere Press, 1987.

8   Lazarus RS, Cohen J, Folkman S. Psychological stress and adaptation: Some unresolved issues. In: H. Selye (ed.). *Selye's Guide to Stress Research*, Vol. 1. New York: Von Nostrand Reinhold, 1980, pp. 90–117.

9   Lazarus R, Launier R. Stress related transactions between person and environment. In: L. Pervin, M. Lewis (eds.). *Perspectives in International Psychology*. New York: Plenum, 1978, pp. 287–327.

10 European Agency for Safety and Health at Work. *Safety at Work*, 2000. http://agency.osha.eu.int/publications/factsheets/8/en/facts8_en.pdf. (Accessed 23 June 2014).

11 Freudenberger HJ. Staff burnout. *J Soc Issues* 1974;**30**:159–165.

12 Freudenberger HJ, Richelson G. *Burn Out: The High Cost of High Achievement*. New York: Anchor Press, 1980.

13 Edelwich J, Brodsky A. *Burn-out: Stages of Disillusionment in the Helping Professions*. New York: Springer, 1980.

14 Pines AM. Burnout: An existential perspective. In: W. Schaufeli, C. Maslach, T. Marek (eds.). *Professional Burnout*. Washington, DC: Taylor & Francis, 1993.

15 Maslach C, Jackson SE. *The Maslach Burnout Inventory* (*Manual*), 2nd edn. Palo Alto, CA: Consulting Psychologists Press, 1986.

16 Maslach C, Schaufeli WB, Leiter MP. Job burnout. *Annu Rev Psychol* 2001;**52**:397–422.

17 Maslach C. Job burnout: New directions in research and interventions. *Curr Direct Psychol Sci* 2003;**13**:189–192.

18 Stenmarker M, Palmerus K, Marky I. Life satisfaction of Swedish pediatric oncologists: The role of personality, work-related aspects and emotional distress. *Pediatr Blood Cancer* 2009;**53**:1308–1314.

19 Maslach C. Engagement research: Some thoughts from a burnout perspective. *Eur J Work Organ Psychol* 2011;**20**(1):47–52.

20 Maslach C, Leiter M. *The Truth about Burnout: How Organizations Cause Personal Stress and What to Do about It*. San Francisco, CA: Jossey-Bass, 1997.

21 Schaufeli WB, Salanova M, González-Romá V, Bakker AB. The measurement of engagement and burnout: A two sample confirmatory factor analytic approach. *J Happiness Stud* 2002;**3**:71–92.

22 Figley C. *Compassion Fatigue: Coping with Secondary Traumatic Stress Disorder in Those Who Treat the Traumatized*. New York: Brunner-Routledge, 1995.

23 Figley CR (ed.). *Treating Compassion Fatigue*. New York: Brunner-Routledge, 2002.

24 Garfield C, Spring C, Ober D. *Sometimes My Heart Goes Numb: Caring in a Time of AIDS*. San Francisco, CA: Jossey-Bass, 1995.

25 Stamm B. *The Concise Manual for the Professional Quality of Life Scale: The ProQOL*. Pocatello, ID: ProQOL.org, 2009.

26 French JRP, Rodgers W, Cobb S. Adjustment as person-environment fit. In: G.V. Coelho, D.A. Hamburg, E. Adams (eds.). *Coping and Adaptation*. New York: Basic Books, 1974, pp. 316–333.

27 Collège d'expertise sur le suivi des risques psychosociaux au travail. Rapport faisant suite à la demande du Ministre du travail, de l'emploi et de la santé. *Mesurer les facteurs psychosociaux de risque au travail pour les maîtriser*, 2011. www.college-risquespsychosociaux-travail.fr

28 Jourdain G, Chenevert D. Job demands—Resources, burnout and intention to leave the nursing profession: A questionnaire survey. *Int J Nurs Stud* 2010;**47**:709–722.

29 Maslach C, Leiter M. Early predictors of job burnout and engagement. *J Appl Psychol* 2008;**93**:498–512.

30 Pereira SM, Fonsecal AM, Carvalho AN. Burnout in palliative care: A systematic review. *Nurs Ethics* 2011;**18**(3) 317–326.

31 Dunwoodie DA, Auret K. Psychological morbidity and burnout in palliative care doctors in Western Australia. *Int Med J* 2007;**37**:693–698.

32 Beecham L. BMA warns of stress suffered by senior doctors. *BMJ* July 1, 2000;**321**(7252):56.

33 Berman R, Campbell M, Makin W et al. Occupational stress in palliative medicine, medical oncology and clinical oncology specialist registrars. *Clin Med* 2007;**7**:235–242.

34 Asai M, Morita T, Akechi T et al. Burnout and psychiatric morbidity among physicians engaged in end-of-life care for cancer patients: A cross-sectional nationwide survey in Japan. *Psycho-Oncology* 2007;**16**:421–428.

35 Payne N. Occupational stressors and coping as determinants of burnout in female hospice nurses. *J Adv Nurs* 2001;**33**:396–405.

36 Huggard J. A national survey of the support needs of interprofessional hospice staff in Aotearoa/New Zealand. Unpublished Master's Thesis, University of Auckland, Auckland, New Zealand, 2008.

37 Vachon MLS, Huggard J. The experience of the nurse in end-of-life care in the 21st century: Mentoring the next generation. In: B.R. Ferrell, N. Coyle (eds.). *Textbook of Palliative Nursing*, 3rd edn. Oxford, U.K.: Oxford University Press, 2010, pp. 1131–1156.

38 Fillion L, Desbiens JF, Truchon M, Dallaire C, Roch G. Le stress au travail chez les infirmières en soins palliatifs selon le milieu de pratique. *Psycho-Oncologie* 2011;**5**(2):127–136 (article in French with abstract in English).

39 Lloyd Williams M. Senior house officers' experience of a six month post in a hospice. *Med Educ* January 2002;**36**(1):45–48.

40 Branigan M. Personal communication to MLS Vachon.

41 Kash KM, Holland JC, Breitbart W, Berenson S, Dougherty J, Ouelette-Kobasa S, Lesko L. Stress and burnout in oncology. *Oncology* 2000;**14**:1621–1637.

42 Wetterneck TB, Linzer M, McMurray JE, Douglas J, Schwartz MD, Bigby J, Gerrity MS, Pathman DE, Karlson D, Rhodes E. Worklife and satisfaction of general internists. *Arch Int Med* 2002;**162**:649–656.

43 Whippen DA, Zuckerman EL, Anderson JW, Kamin DY, Holland JC. Burnout in the practice of oncology: Results of a follow-up survey. *J Clin Oncol* 2004;**22**(14S):6053.

44 Gambles M, Wilkinson S, Dissanayake C. What are you like? A personality profile of cancer and palliative care nurses in the United Kingdom. *Cancer Nurs* 2003;**26**:97–104.

45 Shanafelt T, West C, Zhan X et al. Relationship between increased personal well-being and enhanced empathy among internal medicine residents. *J Gen Intern Med* 2005;**20**:559–564.

46 McMurray JE, Linzer M, Konrad TR, Douglas J, Shugerman R, Nelson K, for the SGIM Career Satisfaction Study Group. The work lives of women physicians: Results from the physician work life study. *J Gen Intern Med* 2000;**15**:372–380.

47 Linzer M, Visser MR, Oort FJ, Smets EMA, McMurray JE, de Haes HCJM, for the Society of General Internal Medicine (SGIM) Career Satisfaction Study Group (CSSG) [Association of Professors of Medicine]. Predicting and preventing physician burnout: Results from the United States and the Netherlands. *Am J Med* August 1, 2001;**111**:170–175.

48 Karasek RA. Job demands, job decision latitude and mental strain: Implications for job redesign. *Admin Sci Quarterly* 1979;**24**:285–308.

49 Siegrist J, Peter R, Junge A, Cremer P, Seidel D. Low status control, high effort at work and ischemic heart disease: Prospective evidence from blue-collar men. *Soc Sci Med* 1990;**31**:1127–1134.

50 van Staa AL, Visser A, van der Zouwe N. Caring for caregivers: Experiences and evaluation of interventions for a palliative care team. *Patient Educ Couns* 2000;**41**:93–105.

51 Papadatou D, Martinson IM, Chung P, Man MN. Caring for dying children: A comparative study of nurses' experiences in Greece and Hong Kong. *Cancer Nurs* 2001;**24**(5):402–412.

52 Dougherty E, Pierce B, Ma C et al. Factors associated with work stress and professional satisfaction in oncology staff. *Am J Hosp Palliat Med* 2009;**26**:105–111.

53 Vachon M, Lyall W, Freeman S. Measurement and management of stress in health professionals working with advanced cancer patients. *Death Educ* 1978;**1**:365–375.

54 Weissman, D. Martyrs in palliative care. *J Palliat Med* 2011;**14**(12):1278–1279.

55 Vachon MLS. Reflections on the history of occupational stress in hospice/palliative care. In: I.B. Corless, Z. Foster (eds.). *The Hospice Heritage: Celebrating Our Future.* New York: The Hayworth Press, Inc., 1999, pp. 229–246. Published simultaneously as *The Hospice Journal* 14:3/4, 1999.

56 Yandrick RM. High demand low control. *Behav Healthc Tomorrow* 1997;**6**(3):40–44.

57 Grunfeld E, Whelan TJ, Zitzelsberger, Willan AR, Montesanto B, Evans WK. Cancer care workers in Ontario: Prevalence of burnout, job stress and job satisfaction. *JAMC* 2000;**163**:166–169.

58 Fillion L, Tremblay I, Truchon M et al. Job satisfaction and emotional distress among nurses providing palliative care: Empirical evidence for an integrative occupational stress-model. *Int J Stress Manag* 2007;**14**(1):1–25.

59 Fillion L, Truchon M, L'Heureux M, Dallaire C, Langlois L, Bellemare M, Dupuis, R. To improve services and care at the end of life; Understanding the impact of workplace satisfaction and well-being of nurses. Rapport R-794, Montréal, IRSST, 2013. http://www.irsst.qc.ca/-projet-vers-l-amelioration-des-services-et-des-soins-de-fin-de-vie-mieux-comprendre-l-impact-du-milieu-de-travail-sur-la-satisfaction-et-le-bien-etre-des-0099-6050.html

60 Johnson JV, Hall EM. Job strain, work place social support, and cardiovascular disease: A cross-sectional study of a random sample of the Swedish Working population. *Am J Public Heath* 1988;**78**:1336–1342.

61 European Commission. *Promoting the Development and Integration of Palliative Care Mobile Support Teams in the Hospital.* Brussels, Belgium: Directorate-General for Research Food Quality and Safety, 2004.

62 Speck P (ed.). *Teamwork in Palliative Care: Fulfilling or Frustrating?* Oxford, U.K.: Oxford University Press, 2006.

63 Munroe B, Speck P. Team effectiveness. In: P. Speck (ed.). *Teamwork in Palliative Care: Fulfilling or Frustrating?* Oxford, U.K.: Oxford University Press, 2006, pp. 201–209.

64 Sabo BA, Vachon MLS. Care of professional caregivers. In: M.P. Davis, P.C. Feyer, P. Ortner, C. Zimmerman (eds.). *Supportive Oncology.* Philadelphia, PA: Elsevier, 2011, pp. 575–589.

65 Fillion L, Saint-Laurent L, Rousseau N. Les stresseurs liés à la pratique infirmière en soins palliatifs: les points de vue des infirmières. *Les Cahiers de Soins Palliatifs* 2003;**4**(1):5–40.

66 Fillion L, Saint-Laurent L. Les conditions favorables liées à la pratique infirmière en soins palliatifs: les points de vue des infirmières. *Les Cahiers de Soins Palliatifs* 2003;**4**(2):5–42.

67 Vachon M, Fillion L, Achille M. Death confrontation, spiritual–existential experience and caring attitudes in palliative care nurses: An interpretative phenomenological analysis. *Qual Res Psychol* 2012;**9**(2):151–172.

68 Kearney MK, Weininger RB, Vachon MLS, Mount BM, Harrison RL. Self-care of physicians caring for patients at the end of life: "Being Connected ... A Key to My Survival". *JAMA* 2009;**301**:1155–1164.

69 Alkema K, Linton J, Davies R. A study of the relationship between self-care, compassion satisfaction, compassion fatigue, and burnout among hospice workers. *J Soc Work End-of-Life Palliat Care* 2008;**4**:101–119.

70 Slocum-Gori S, Hemsworth D, Chan WWY, Carson A, Kazanjian A. Understanding compassion satisfaction, compassion fatigue and burnout: A survey of the hospice palliative care workforce. *Palliat Med* 2011;27(2):172–178, doi:10.1177/0269216311431311. (Accessed online 23 May 2012).

71 Huggard P, Dixon R. "Tired of Caring": The impact of caring on resident doctors. *Australas J Disaster Trauma Stud* 2011;**3**:105–111.

72 Marr L. Can compassion fatigue? *J Palliat Med* 2007;**12**(8):739–740.

73 Shanafelt T, Chung H, White H et al. Shaping your career to maximize personal satisfaction in the practice of oncology. *J Clin Oncol* 2006;**24**:4020–4026.

74 Jameton A. *Nursing Practice: The Ethical Issues.* Englewood Cliffs, NJ: Prentice Hall, 1984.

75 Webster GC, Baylis FE. Moral residue. In: S.B. Rubin, L. Zoloth (eds.). *Margin of Error: The Ethics of Mistakes in the Practice of Medicine.* Hagerstown, MD: University Publishing Group, 2000.

76 Vachon MLS. Reflections on compassion, suffering and occupational stress. In: J. Malpas, N. Lickiss (eds.). *Perspectives on Human Suffering.* Dordrecht, the Netherlands: Springer, 2012, pp. 317–331.

77 Weissman DE. Moral distress in palliative care. *J Palliat Med* 2009;**12**:865–866.

78 Vachon MLS. The nurse's role: The world of palliative care nursing. In: B. Ferrell, N. Coyle (eds.). *The Oxford Textbook of Palliative Nursing.* New York: Oxford University Press, 2001, pp. 647–662.

79 Webster J, Kristjanson LJ. "But isn't it depressing?" The Vitality of palliative care. *J Palliat Care* 2002;**18**(1):15–24.

80 Walsh F. *Strengthening Family Resilience.* New York: Guilford Press, 2006.

81 Masten A. Ordinary magic: Resilience processes in development. *Am Psychol* 2001;**56**:227–238.

82 Swetz KM, Harrington SE, Matsuyama RK, Shanafelt TD, Lyckholm LJ. Strategies for avoiding burnout in hospice and palliative medicine: Peer advice for physicians on achieving longevity and fulfillment. *J Palliat Med* 2009;**12**:773–777.

83 Adams R, Boscarino J, Figley C. Compassion fatigue and psychosocial distress among social workers: A validation study. *Am J Orthopsychiatry* 2006;**76**:103–108.

84 Harrison R, Westwood M. Preventing vicarious traumatisation of mental health therapists: Identifying protective practices. *Psychother Theory Res Pract Train* 2009;**46**:203–219.

85 Rinpoche LZ. A view on Buddhism: Compassion and bodhicitta. www.viewonbuddhism.org. (Accessed 17 April 2014).

86 Gonzalez M. *Mindful Leadership: The 9 Ways to Self-awareness, Transforming Yourself and Inspiring Others.* San Francisco, CA: Jossey-Bass, 2012.

87 Remen RN. *My Grandfather's Blessings.* New York: Riverhead Books, 2000.

88 Briere J. Personal communication to MLS Vachon, June 1, 2012.

89 Halifax J. A heuristic model of enactive compassion. *Curr Opin Support Palliat Care* 2012;**6**:228–235.

90 Katz R. When our personal selves influence our professional work: An introduction to emotions of counter transference in end-of-life care. In: R. Katz, T. Johnson (eds.). *When Professionals Weep: Emotional and Counter Transference Responses in End-of-Life Care.* New York: Routledge, 2006, pp. 3–12.

91 Coster JS, Schwebel M. Well-functioning in professional psychologists. *Prof Psychol Res Pract* 1997;**28**:5–13.

92 Vachon MLS. Caring for the professional caregivers: Before and after the death. In: K.J. Doka (ed.). *Living with Grief: Before and After the Death.* Washington, DC: Hospice Foundation of America, 2007, pp. 311–330.

93 van der Klink JJL, Blonk RWB, Schene AH, van Dijk FJH. The benefits of intervention for work-related stress. *Am J Public Health* 2001;**91**:270–276.

94 Mimura C, Griffeths P. The effectiveness of current approaches to work place stress management in the nursing profession: An evidence based literature review. *Occup Environ Med* 2003;**60**:10–15.

95   Sherman AC, Edwards D., Simonton S. Mehta P. Caregiver stress and burnout in an oncology unit. *Palliat Support Care* March 2006;**4**(1):65–80.

96   Vachon MLS. Oncology staff stress and related interventions. In: J.C. Holland, W.S. Breitbart, P.B. Jacobsen, M.S. Lederberg, M.J. Loscalzo, R. McCorkle (eds.). *Psycho-Oncology*, 2nd edn. New York: Oxford University Press, 2010, pp. 575–581.

97   Vachon MLS, Müeller M. Burnout and symptoms of stress. In: W. Breitbart, H.M. Cochinov (eds.). *Handbook of Psychiatry in Palliative Medicine*. New York: Oxford University Press, 2009, pp. 559–625.

98   Fallowfield L, Jenkins V, Farewell V, Saul J, Duffy Am Eves R. Efficacy of a cancer research UK communication skills training model for oncologists: A randomized controlled trial. *Lancet* 2002;**359**:650–656.

99   Fallowfield L, Jenkins V, Farewell V, Solis-Trapala J. Enduring impact of communication skills training: Results of a 12-month follow-up. *Br J Cancer* 2003;**89**:1445–1449.

100 Razavi D, Delvaux N, Marchal S, Bredart A, Farvacques C, Paesmans M. The effects of a 24-h psychological training program on attitudes, communication skills and occupational stress in oncology: A randomized study. *Eur J Cancer* 1993;**29A**:1858–1863.

101 Razavi D, Merckaert I, Marchal S, Libert Y, Delvaux N, Boniver J, Etienne A-M, Klastersky J, Reynaert C, Scalliet P. How to optimize physicians' communication skills in cancer care: Results of a randomized study assessing the usefulness of post training consolidation workshops. *J Clin Oncol* 2003;**21**:3141–3149.

102 Butow P, Cockburn J, Girgis A, Bowman D, Schofield P, D'Este C, Stojanovski E, Tattersall MHN, and the CUES Team. Increasing oncologists skills in eliciting and responding to emotional cues: Evaluation of a communication skills training program. *Psycho-Oncology* 2008;**17**:209–218.

103 Barth J, Lannen P. Efficacy of communication skills training courses in oncology: A systematic review and meta-analysis. *Ann Oncol* 2001;**22**:1030–1040.

104 LeBlanc PM, Hox JJ, Schaufeli WB, Taris TW. Take Care!: The evaluation of a team-based burnout intervention program for oncology care providers. *J Appl Psychol* 2007;**92**:213–227.

105 Feld J, Heyse-Moore L. An evaluation of a support group for junior doctors working in palliative medicine. *Am J Hospice Palliat Med* 2006;**23**(4):287–296.

106 Murrant GM, Rykov M, Amonite D, Loynd M. Creativity and self-care for caregivers. *J Palliat Care* 2000;**16**(2):44–49.

107 Italia S, Favara-Scacco C, Di Cataldo A, Russo G. Evaluation and art therapy treatment of the burnout syndrome in oncology units. *Psycho-Oncology* 2008;**17**:676–680.

108 Park CL, Folkman S. Meaning in the context of stress and coping. *Rev General Psychol* 1997;**1**(2):115–144.

109 Fillion L, Tremblay I, Truchon M, Côté D, Struthers CW, Dupuis R. Job satisfaction and emotional distress among nurses providing palliative care: Empirical evidence for an integrative occupational stress-model. *Int J Stress Manage* 2007;**14**(1):1–25.

110 Kravit K, McAllister-Black R, Grant M, Kirk C. Self-care strategies for nurses: A psycho-educational intervention for stress reduction and the prevention of burnout. *Appl Nurs Res* 2010;**23**:130–138.

111 Meier DE, Back AL, Morrison RS. The inner life of physicians and care of the seriously ill. *JAMA* 2001;**286**:3007–3014.

112 Macpherson CF. Peer-supported storytelling for grieving pediatric nurses. *J Pediatric Oncol Nurs* 2008;**25**:148–163.

113 Brady D, Corbie-Smith G, Branch W. "What's important to you?": The use of narratives to promote self-reflection and to understand the experiences of medical residents. *Ann Int Med* 2002;**137**:220–223.

114 Sands SA, Stanley P, Charon R. Pediatric narrative oncology: Interprofessional training to promote empathy, build teams, and prevent burnout. *J Support Oncol* 2008;**6**(7):307–312.

115 Wessel EM, Rutledge DN. Home care and hospice nurses' attitude toward death and caring for the dying. *J Hospice Palliat Nurs* 2005;**7**(4):212–217.

116 Rogers S, Badgi A, Gomez C. Educational interventions in end-of-life care: Part I. An educational intervention responding to the moral distress of NICU Nurses provided by an ethics consultation team. *Adv Neonatal Care* 2008;**8**(1):56–65.

117 Wessel EM, Garon M. Introducing reflective narratives into palliative care home care education. *Home Health Nurse* 2005;**23**:516–522.

118 Whitehead PB, Anderson ES, Redican KJ, Stratton R. Studying the effects of the end-of-life nursing education consortium at the institutional level. *J Hospice Palliat Care Nurs* 2010;**12**(3):184–193.

119 Wasner M, Longaker C, Borasio GD. Effects of spiritual care training for palliative care professionals. *Palliat Med* 2005;**19**:99–104.

120 Fillion L, Dupuis R, Tremblay I, de Grace G-R, Breitbart W. Enhancing meaning in palliative care practice: A meaning-centered intervention to promote job satisfaction. *Palliat Support Care* 2006;**4**:333–344.

121 Fillion L, Duval S, Dumont S, Gagnon P, Tremblay I, Bairati I, Breitbart W. Impact of a meaning-centered intervention on job satisfaction and on quality of life among palliative care nurses. *Psycho-Oncology* 2009;**18**:1300–1310.

122 Frankl VE. Logotherapy and the challenge of suffering. *Rev Existential Psychol Psychiatry* 1987;**20**:1–3.

123 Vachon M, Fillion L, Achille M, Duval S, Leung D. An awakening experience: An interpretive phenomenological analysis of the effects of a meaning-centered intervention shared amongst palliative care nurses. *Qualit Res Psychol* 2011;**8**(1):66–80.

124 Leung D, Fillion L, Howell D, Duval S, Brown J, Rodin G. Meaning in bone marrow transplant nurses' work: Experiences before and after a 'meaning-centered' intervention. *Cancer Nurs*, in press.

125 Halifax J. *Being with Dying: Cultivating Compassion and Fearlessness in the Presence of Death*. Boston, MA: Shambala, 2008.

126 Halifax, J. (2013) Being with dying: Experiences in end-of-life-care. In: T. Singer & M. Bolz (Eds.) *Compassion: Bridging practice and Science* ebook. (pp. 108–120). Munich, Germany: Max Planck Society.

127 Rushton CH, Sellers DE, Heller KS, Spring B, Dossey BM, Halifax J. Impact of a contemplative end-of-life training program: Being with dying. *Palliat Support Care* 2009;**7**:405–414.

128 Irving JA, Dobkin PL, Park J. Cultivating mindfulness in health care professionals: A review of empirical studies of mindfulness-based stress reduction (MBSR). *Complement Therap Clin Pract* 2009;**15**:61–66.

129 Praissman S. Mindfulness-based stress reduction: A literature review and clinician's guide. *J Am Acad Nurse Pract* 2008;**20**:212–216.

130 Mackenzie CS, Poulin PA, Carlson RS. A brief mindfulness-based stress reduction intervention for nurses and nurse aides. *Appl Nurs Res* 2006;**19**:105–109.

104

Communication in palliative care

JOSEPHINE M. CLAYTON, MARTIN H.N. TATTERSALL

INTRODUCTION

Communication has been identified by patients and their families as one of the most important aspects of care for patients living with an advanced life-limiting illness [1–5]. For health professionals working in specialist palliative care, communication is a core and required skill. Indeed, it has been argued that use of words and interactional skills are the tools of palliative care or palliative medicine, much like surgical skills are the procedure for surgeons [6].

In this chapter, we review the importance of communication skills, provide recommendations for communicating with patients and their families in palliative care settings, and discuss the importance of palliative care health professionals receiving formal training in communication skills.

WHY COMMUNICATION IS SO IMPORTANT

Communication has been defined as the "imparting of knowledge or exchanging of information, ideas and feelings" [7]. When health professionals communicate effectively, they are more likely to understand and address the issues that are important for the individual patient, and patients are more likely to understand their medical problems and treatment options [8]. Moreover, effective communication can reduce patient anxiety and distress [9] and increase satisfaction with the consultation [10].

Six key functions of clinician–patient communication have been identified by the U.S. National Cancer Institute monograph [11] on patient-centered communication:

- Exchanging information
- Making decisions
- Fostering healing relationships
- Enabling patient-centered self-management
- Managing uncertainty
- Responding to emotions

While communication in palliative care shares many of the general features of communication in other health-care settings, the fear and uncertainty associated with an advanced life-limiting illness adds a greater emotional element to the interaction and thus communication assumes an even greater significance.

Studies of actual communication during physician–clinician discussions in palliative and end-of-life care suggest that there is a need for improvement in this area. There is a tendency for physicians to focus on medical or technical aspects during consultations, and there is room for improvement of physicians' listening skills and ability to respond to patients' emotion during sensitive discussions [12].

HOW TO COMMUNICATE IN PALLIATIVE CARE

Preparation for the consultation

It is important to be able to provide consistent, accurate, and sensitive information relevant to the person's circumstances during a palliative care consultation. Hence, before seeing the patient, it is important to ascertain the reason for the referral and how much the person has been told about their illness and any concerns of the health-care team about this patient and their family/caregivers. It is important to be clear about the clinical details by reviewing patient's clinical records and investigation results and to understand what the patient has been told about their referral to palliative care. As needed, consult with the referring health-care professionals for up-to-date knowledge about the patients' underlying illness and available remaining treatment options. Mentally preparing for the consultation is important to ensure that you are able to fully attend to the patient during the consultation.

Establishing an effective clinician–patient relationship

A good clinician–patient relationship is the cornerstone to effective communication in palliative care [1,4]. Attributes of a good doctor–clinician relationship include mutual trust, care, respect, honesty, empathy, support, and partnership, as well as the patients' confidence in their clinicians' professional competence [13,14]. It is important that the clinician create an atmosphere where the patient is treated as a "whole person" and that the patient feels that the clinician is interested in and sensitive to their problems and feelings [8].

Trust can be developed using an empathic, patient-centered style [15]. Good generic communication skills advocated in all health-care settings are a foundation, including eye contact (where culturally appropriate), appropriate body language such as an open posture, sitting close to the patient, and showing compassion in a warm and respectful manner [16].

Introducing yourself as a palliative care clinician

Referral to specialist palliative care services may evoke an emotional response in patients and their families, for example, fears of impending death, helplessness, and abandonment [16]. Hence, the initial palliative care consultation should include eliciting the patients' understanding about their referral to palliative care and a sensitive explanation of the role of specialist palliative care services. We recommend being open and honest and using the term "palliative care" explicitly when introducing yourself. The exception may be when the team is concerned that the patient will react negatively to the concept of palliative care or the patient was not told the context of your consultation. Preferably, even if delayed, the term "palliative care" should be used by the end of the initial consultation. The referral to palliative care is best expressed in a way that emphasizes nonabandonment from referring clinicians. In addition, the role of palliative care should be framed in a positive way relevant to the person's situation. Further recommendations and examples of phrases for introducing yourself as a palliative care clinician are shown in Table 104.1.

Eliciting patient concerns and negotiating an agenda for the consultation

Prior to imparting information, it is important that palliative care clinicians actively listen to the patient and elicit their full list of concerns [8,17,18]. The extent to which patients' concerns have been disclosed and resolved has been found to be associated with the likelihood of subsequent depression and anxiety [19]. When clinicians elicit "patients' perceptions of the problems and reactions, and the impact on their daily lives, patients feel more satisfied and comply better with offered advice and medication" [20]. Clinicians cannot assume that patients will volunteer all of their concerns. Studies in palliative care and oncology settings show that a substantial number of patients' concerns remain undisclosed in practice [21,22]. Patients may be reluctant to disclose their psychosocial and other more sensitive concerns and believe these are an inevitable part of their illness, for which nothing can be done [18]. Furthermore, patients may perceive their concerns to be embarrassing or abnormal and/or be concerned about burdening their health professionals, whom they see as busy people. Therefore, physicians and nurses need to encourage and facilitate patient disclosure of their psychosocial and other sensitive concerns.

To elicit concerns, ask open questions such as "What are the main things worrying you?" and "Is there anything else troubling you?" Active listening involves attending to the patient fully and observing both their verbal and nonverbal communication while allowing the patient to complete statements without interrupting prematurely as well as making comments encouraging the patient to go on (e.g., "go on" or "tell

Table 104.1 *Introducing yourself as a palliative care clinician*

Recommendation	Useful phrases
• Raise the topic by being both honest and open, using the term "palliative care" explicitly.	"I work closely with the other doctors and nurses caring for you. The aim of palliative care is to ensure that at all stages of your illness, you are kept as comfortable as possible, regardless of what is happening to you (cancer, heart, or lungs)."
• Clarify and correct misconceptions about palliative care services (particularly that it is not solely for people who are dying or associated with imminent death).	"What does the term palliative care mean to you?" "Many people have either not heard of 'palliative care' or associate it with dying in the very near future." Then respond to the patient's cues. "It might be useful for you if I explain what palliative care is really all about." "Have you had any experiences with others receiving palliative care?"
• Discuss the role of the palliative care team, emphasizing expertise in symptom management as well as a wide range of support services, assistance with quality of life, and support for family/partner/children.	"Our palliative care team are able to provide you with extra support; this includes pain control and the control of other symptoms resulting from your illness." "Palliative care includes a whole range of clinicians who can help support you and your family at this time."
• Explain that the patient can be linked up with the palliative care team at the same time as receiving treatments directed at the underlying disease (e.g., chemotherapy).	"Our team/service often works very closely with the (name of team) while people are receiving treatment X, to optimize symptom management and support."
• Explain that the patient will still be followed up by the primary health-care team (e.g., GP, generalist nurse) and/or the primary specialist (e.g., oncologist, respiratory physician) where applicable.	"I will work closely with Dr. X. Dr. X will still be your main doctor, but we will work together to ensure that you are as comfortable as possible."

Source: Data from Clayton, J.M. et al., *Med. J. Aust.,* 186(12), S77, 2007. Copyright *Medical Journal of Australia.* Reproduced with permission.

me more"). The next step is to clarify that you have understood the patient correctly and understand what is most troubling them, by reflecting back what you think they have said. If there is a long list of concerns, you may wish to ask them to rank those that are most troubling them.

Negotiating an agenda involves acknowledging the patient's key concerns, as well as outlining yours, and then mutually agreeing on the most important things to be discussed during the consultation.

Responding to emotions

One of the key communication skills for palliative care clinicians is responding to negative emotions from patients and their families. When providers respond empathically to such emotions, patients report lower distress [23,24] and higher quality of life [24]. Even brief expressions of empathy may reduce patient anxiety [25]. It is therefore important to be attentive to emotional cues from patients and their families during palliative care consultations. One way to open discussions about emotions is to ask an open question with an emotional focus. For example, "How do you feel about what we have discussed?" It is helpful to think about accepting and validating emotions, rather than feeling you have to "solve the problem." Many emotions in the palliative care setting reflect matters that cannot be solved. Some strategies for responding to emotions are shown in Table 104.2.

Discussing prognosis and end-of-life issues

One of the most difficult and frequent communication tasks in palliative care settings is discussing prognosis and end-of-life issues with patients and their family members [26]. Pertinent information about these topics is essential if patients with a life-limiting illness and their caregivers are to participate in decisions about their care, set goals and priorities, and

Table 104.2 *Strategies for exploring and responding to patients' and family members' emotions during palliative care consultations*

- *Normalize or validate*: e.g., "it's very understanding that you would be upset by this" or "this is a really tough situation"
- *Name or acknowledge the emotion*: e.g., "you seem angry"
- Seek to understand the emotion: e.g., "what upsets you the most about this?"
- *Nonverbal acknowledgement*: e.g., gesture or touch where culturally appropriate
- *Encourage expression*: e.g., "Tell me more ..."
- *Summary and reflect back*: e.g., "If I understand you correctly, you are angry because ..."
- *Praise adaptive coping*: e.g., "I really admire the way you have been there for your mother during her illness"; "that takes enormous courage"
- Silence

Source: Data from Levin, T.T. and Weiner, J.S., End of life communication training, in: Kissane, D., Bultz, B., Butow, P., Finlay, I. eds., *Handbook of Communication in Oncology and Palliative Care*, Oxford University Press, New York, 2010; Smith, R.C., *Patient-Centered Interviewing: An Evidence-Based Method*, Lippincott Williams & Wilkins, Philadelphia, PA, 2002.

prepare for their death and its aftermath. Clinicians need to provide information in a way that allows patients and their families to be informed to the level that they wish about their health situation and treatment options, assists them to deal with the emotional impact of a life-limiting illness and to cope with their situation, and helps them to make appropriate decisions. Furthermore, open discussion about prognosis and end-of-life issues has been associated with increased patient satisfaction and sense of control, reduced patient depression and anxiety, reduced use of aggressive treatments in the final days of the patient's life, and improved outcomes for bereaved carers [26–29].

General recommendations from evidence-based clinical practice guidelines for discussing prognosis and end-of-life issues with patients with life-limiting illnesses and their families are shown in Table 104.3.

CLARIFYING PATIENT AND CAREGIVER UNDERSTANDING AND INFORMATION NEEDS

Prior to providing any new information about prognosis and end-of-life issues, it is very important to first clarify the person's understanding of their health situation. This helps to establish a common ground from which to start the discussion.

Likewise, it is important to first explore what information the person would like to know. There is evidence that clinicians are not good at predicting patients' preferences for information [26].

In Western countries, numerous studies have documented that most English-speaking patients with serious illnesses prefer to be fully informed about a variety of topics including diagnosis, prognosis, and treatment options [30–32]. However, not all patients want extensive information about their illness or prognosis [33,34], and some patients may experience conflict between wanting to know and fearing bad news [32]. For example, while most patients in Western cultures want to be informed that their lifespan will be limited by their illness, some patients do not want to be provided with the likely time frame [26].

Patients' information needs may be strongly influenced by their countries' culture and also by the different cultures within countries. Patients from some cultures may prefer nondisclosure or disclosure negotiated through the family especially when life expectancy is short [35,36]. However, the evidence for this is conflicting with other studies suggesting that the majority of people from certain non-Western countries still want to be fully informed about their diagnosis and prognosis [37,38].

Other factors may influence patients' preferences for information. Higher levels of information tend to be desired by patients who are younger, are female, come from a higher socioeconomic background, and are better educated [26]. Patients' may also desire less detailed information over time as their illness progresses [31,39], while caregivers may want more information especially as the person's death approaches [26]. However, it is not possible to make assumptions about individuals' information preferences based on their demographic characteristics or cultural background [16]. It is important therefore to clarify with the individual and their family about their information

Table 104.3 *Summary of recommendations for communicating prognosis and end-of-life issues with patients with advanced life-limiting illnesses and their families, the PREPARED framework*

P   *Prepare for the discussion*, where possible:
- Confirm pathological diagnosis and investigation results before initiating discussion.
- Try to ensure privacy and uninterrupted time for discussion.
- Negotiate who should be present during the discussion.

R   *Relate to the person*:
- Develop rapport.
- Show empathy, care, and compassion during the entire consultation.

E   *Elicit patient and caregiver understanding and information preferences*:
- Identify the reason for this consultation and elicit the patient's expectations.
- Clarify the patient's or caregiver's understanding of their situation and establish how much detail and what they want to know.
- Consider cultural and contextual factors influencing information preferences.

P   *Provide information* tailored to the individual needs of both patients and their families:
- Offer to discuss what to expect, in a sensitive manner, giving the patient the option not to discuss it.
- Pace information to the patient's information preferences, understanding, and circumstances.
- Use clear, jargon-free, understandable language.
- Explain the uncertainty, limitations, and unreliability of prognostic and end-of-life information.
- Avoid being too exact with time frames unless in the last few days.
- Consider the caregiver's distinct information needs, which may require a separate meeting with the caregiver (provided the patient, if mentally competent, gives consent).
- Try to ensure consistency of information and approach provided to different family members and the patient and from different clinical team members.

A   *Acknowledge emotions and concerns*:
- Explore and acknowledge the patient's and caregiver's fears and concerns and their emotional reaction to the discussion.
- Respond to the patient's or caregiver's distress regarding the discussion, where applicable.

R   (Foster) *Realistic hope* (e.g., peaceful death, support):
- Be honest without being blunt or giving more detailed information than desired by the patient.
- Do not give misleading or false information to try to positively influence a patient's hope.
- Reassure that support, treatments, and resources are available to control pain and other symptoms, but avoid premature reassurance.
- Explore and facilitate realistic goals and wishes and ways of coping on a day-to-day basis, where appropriate.

(Continued)

Table 104.3 *(Continued)* *Summary of recommendations for communicating prognosis and end-of-life issues with patients with advanced life-limiting illnesses and their families, the PREPARED framework*

E   *Encourage questions* and further discussions:
- Encourage questions and information clarification; be prepared to repeat explanations.
- Check understanding of what has been discussed and if the information provided meets the patient's and caregiver's needs.
- Leave the door open for topics to be discussed again in the future.

D   *Document*:
- Write a summary of what has been discussed in the medical record.
- Speak or write to other key health-care providers involved in the patient's care. As a minimum, this should include the patient's general practitioner.

Source: Data from Clayton, J.M. et al., *Med. J. Aust.*, 186(12), S77, 2007. Copyright *Medical Journal of Australia*. Reproduced with permission.

needs and to tailor the information provided, as preferences for the amount, type, and timing of information vary.

DISCUSSING GOALS OF CARE AT THE END OF LIFE

The ability to discuss goals of care with patients with life-limiting illnesses and/or with their substitute decision makers (when the patient is no longer competent to make decisions) is a core skill for palliative care clinicians. The opportunity and/or need to discuss this with patients and their families may arise in either an emerging clinical situation or as part of advanced care planning.

It is beyond the scope of this chapter to outline specific recommendations for a wide range of prognostic and end-of-life discussions, although such recommendations together with example phrases are provided in evidence-based clinical practice guidelines published by our group [16]. In the following, we provide a general framework for discussion about goals of care at the end of life with patients with advanced life-limiting illnesses and/or their families:

- Ensure the patient or family understand the medical situation to the level that they wish: see the PREPARED framework in Table 104.3.
- *Assess the patient's and/or the family's readiness to talk about what's next or future care*: sensitively offer to discuss the topic. While it is important to be proactive about initiating advance care planning discussions, it is also important to give the patient the option not to discuss it or to defer the discussion to another time if they prefer. If the patient does not currently wish to discuss this topic, raise it again when the person's condition or situation changes. Some patients may prefer their families to be involved in such discussions on their behalf. Ideally, it is helpful to include both the patient and their key family members/ substitute decision makers in such discussions. The latter approach has been shown to improve the effectiveness of advance care planning discussions [16].

- *Before discussing any specific treatment options, explore the patients' values, goals, and priorities* regarding their remaining life and treatment of their illness, as well as their fears and wishes regarding the future. Some sample questions for eliciting patient's understanding, values, goals, and priorities during goals of care discussions are shown in Table 104.4.
- Frame discussions about goals of end-of-life care around the persons' goals/wishes/concerns wherever feasible.
- If there is a need to discuss specific treatment options (e.g., CPR), it may be helpful to first check the person's understanding of the likely outcomes of such treatment(s), then provide further clarification as required.
- If there are appropriate treatment options relevant to the persons' clinical situation, discuss their burden versus benefits.
- If particular interventions, like CPR, would be considered medically inappropriate by the attending physician or treating team, *do not ask the patient or their family "what do you want done"* [40–42] when the person arrests/dies, as this creates an inappropriate burden of choice for the person and/or their family.
- Rather, *offer to make a recommendation* in order to share the burden of decision making near the end of life [40–42]. This involves proposing a treatment plan that is appropriate to the persons' clinical situation and that meets the patient's goals (wherever feasible), then asking for feedback from the patient and/or their family about your proposal.
- If a decision is made to limit future life-prolonging interventions, it is important to *emphasize the available support throughout the dying process* as well reassuring the

Table 104.4 *Example questions for goals of care and advanced care planning discussions*

- What is your understanding of your health situation and what is likely to happen in the future?
- What is most important to you now (or regarding your care in the future)? What aspects of your life do you most value and enjoy?
- When you look at the future,
  - What do you hope for?
  - What concerns you?
- Do you have any thoughts about how you would like to be cared for in the future if you became more unwell?
  - How would you want decisions regarding your medical treatment to be made?
  - Is there a specific person that you would like us to speak to?
- Is there anything that you worry about happening?
  - What would you "not" want to happen to you in terms of your care?
  - Are there any situations where you would regard life-prolonging treatments to be overly burdensome?
- Is there anything else you would like our team to know about your values and priorities in order to take the best care of you?

Source: Data from Clayton, J.M. et al., *Med. J. Aust.*, 186(12), S77, 2007.

person and their family that the health-care team will do everything they can to maximize the person's comfort.
- *Remember to respond to emotions* throughout the discussion (see Table 104.2).

Discussions about advance care planning or goals of care at the end of life ideally can be thought of as a process that unfolds over many conversations and that evolves as the person's illness progresses [40]. Preferably, such discussions should be commenced early after the diagnosis of a life-limiting illness. A hypothetical question can be a very useful way of gently initiating advance care planning discussions for patients who are still very focussed on disease-specific treatments for their underlying illness. For example, *"While we are hoping that things will go well with this treatment, if by some chance you didn't get better, what would be most important to you?"*

FACILITATING HOPE WHEN HAVING END-OF-LIFE DISCUSSIONS

Patients, caregivers, and health-care professionals have identified hope as an integral component of end-of-life discussions, yet this can be challenging [43]. Some ways of facilitating hope during end-of-life discussions are shown in Table 104.3. It is important to balance honesty with hope and empathy. In some studies, patients perceived that hope could be facilitated by health professionals "being there" and treating them as a whole person [43]. It is helpful to recognize a spectrum of hope and that patients may simultaneously hope for a cure as well as acknowledge the terminal nature of their illness. Phrases such as "we can prepare for the worst while hoping for the best" may be useful. When patients ask for treatments that you do not think will be beneficial, the use of an "I wish" statement can allow the clinician to align themselves with the patient, be supportive, as well as be honest [44]. For example, "I wish that treatment would help but I am concerned that in your case it would make you more unwell."

IMPORTANCE OF COMMUNICATION SKILLS TRAINING

Health professional communication skills do not reliably improve with experience alone. Communication skills training interventions, especially involving workshops lasting 3 days or more, have been consistently shown in randomized studies to improve communication behaviors among clinicians [45,46***]. Specific communication modules regarding transitions to a palliative care approach and discussion of end-of-life issues have been developed and evaluated. For example, Back et al. [47*] developed a 4-day workshop on end-of-life communication skills designed for specialist medical oncology trainees from the United States. The workshop was evaluated with 115 participants using audiotaped standardized patient encounters pre-/postcompletion of the training. Postworkshop, participants acquired a mean of 5.5 skills in breaking bad news ($P < 0.001$) and 4.4 skills in transitioning to palliative care ($P < 0.001$) compared with baseline. Participants' skills significantly improved in nearly all of the individual skill items assessed.

In Australia and New Zealand, a 3-day intensive communication skills workshop has been specifically designed for doctors specializing in palliative care [48*]. The workshop has been run annually since 2008. Sixty-one participants have completed the training with significant improvements ($P > 0.001$) in participants' confidence in communication that was sustained at 3 months. The education committee and specialist advisory committee for the Australasian Chapter of Palliative Medicine have recommended that the course now become a compulsory part of training in palliative medicine in Australia and New Zealand, as well as an optional continuing professional development activity for specialists already practicing in palliative medicine. Shorter training interventions on end-of-life communication have also been developed and evaluated for resident medical officers reporting improvements in participants' skills after completion of the intervention [49–51*].

Given the importance of communication skills to palliative care practice, we encourage all health professionals wishing to specialize in palliative care practice to participate in formal communication skills training. Further research is needed to assess the impact of communication skills training relevant to palliative care practice on outcomes for patients and their families [52].

Key learning points

- Communication has been identified by patients and their families as one of the most important aspects of medical care at the end of life.

- Most patients and their families, at least in Western countries, have high needs for information, but not all patients want detailed information about their condition at all stages of their illness, hence the importance of tailoring information provision to individual needs.

- When discussing sensitive topics with patients and their families, a key skill for clinicians is to acknowledge and respond to emotions.

- When discussing goals of end-of-life care, explore the patients' (and/or family members') understanding of their situation, their values and priorities, fears, and concerns prior to discussing specific treatment options.

- If a decision is made to limit future life-prolonging interventions, it is important to emphasize the available support throughout the dying process.

- Communication skills training has been found to improve clinicians' communication behaviors.

REFERENCES

● 1 Steinhauser KE, Christakis NA, Clipp EC, McNeilly M, McIntyre L, Tulsky JA. Factors considered important at the end-of-life by patients, physicians and other care providers. *JAMA* 2000; 284: 2476–2482.

2 Curtis JR, Wenrich MD, Carline JD et al. Understanding physicians' skills at providing end-of-life care perspectives of patients, families, and health care workers. *J Gen Intern Med* 2001; 16: 41–49.

3 Steinhauser KE, Clipp EC, McNeilly M et al. In search of a good death: Observations of patients, families, and providers. *Ann Intern Med* 2000; 132: 825–832.

4 Wenrich MD, Curtis JR, Shannon SE et al. Communicating with dying patients within the spectrum of medical care from terminal diagnosis to death. *Arch Intern Med* 2001; 161: 868–874.

5 Tong E, McGraw SA, Dobihal E et al. What is a good death? Minority and non-minority perspectives. *J Palliat Care* 2003; 19: 168–175.

6 Hanson LC. Communication is our procedure. *J Palliat Med* 2011; 14(10): 1084–1085.

7 Wilkinson S. Schering Plough clinical lecture communication: It makes a difference. *Cancer Nurs* 1999; 22: 17–20.

8 Maguire P, Pitceathly C. Key communication skills and how to acquire them. *BMJ* 2002; 325: 697–700.

9 Roberts CS, Cox CE, Reintgen DS, Baile WF, Gibertini M. Influence of physician communication on newly diagnosed breast patients' psychologic adjustment and decision-making. *Cancer* 1994; 74: 336–341.

10 Kaplan SH, Ware JE. The patients' role in healthcare and quality assessment. In: Goldfield N, Nash DB (eds). *Providing Quality Care*. Ann Arbor, MI, Health Administration Press, 1995; pp. 25–27.

◆ 11 Epstein RM, Street RL. *Patient-Centered Communication in Cancer Care: Promoting Healing and Reducing Suffering*. Publication No. 07-6225. Bethesda, MD: National Institutes of Health; 2007.

◆ 12 Fine E, Reid MC, Shengelia R, Adelman RD. Directly observed patient-physician discussions in palliative and end-of-life care: A systematic review of the literature. *J Palliat Med* 2010; 13: 595–603.

13 Henman MJ, Butow PN, Brown RF et al. Lay constructions of decision-making in cancer. *Psychooncology* 2002; 11: 295–306.

14 Wright EB, Holcombe C, Salmon P. Doctors' communication of trust, care, and respect in breast cancer: Qualitative study. *BMJ* 2004; 328: 864–867.

15 Tulsky JA. Beyond advance directives: Importance of communication skills at the end of life. *JAMA* 2005; 294: 359–365.

★ 16 Clayton JM, Hancock KM, Butow PN, Tattersall MHN, Currow DC. Clinical practice guidelines for communicating prognosis and end-of-life issues with adults in the advanced stages of a life-limiting illness, and their caregivers. *Med J Aust* 2007; 186 (12): S77–S108.

17 Makoul G. Essential elements of communication in medical encounters: The Kalamazoo consensus statement. *Acad Med* 2001; 76: 390–393.

18 Arora NK. Interacting with cancer patients: The significance of physicians' communication behaviour. *Soc Sci Med* 2003; 57: 791–806.

19 Parle M, Jones B, Maguire P. Maladaptive coping and affective disorders among cancer patients. *Psychol Med* 1996; 26: 735–744.

20 Maguire P. Improving communication with cancer patients. *Eur J Cancer* 2000; 35: 2058–2065.

21 Heaven CM, Maguire P. Disclosure of concerns by hospice patients and their identification by nurses. *Palliat Med* 1997; 11: 283–290.

22 Stewart F, Walker A, Maguire P. Psychiatric and social morbidity in women treated for cancer of the cervix. Report to the Cancer Research Campaign, 1988

23 Butow PN, Kazemi JN, Beeney LJ, Griffin AM, Dunn SM, Tattersall MH (1996) When the diagnosis is cancer: Patient communication experiences and preferences. *Cancer* 77:2630–2637.

24 Zachariae R, Pedersen CG, Jensen AB, Ehrnrooth E, Rossen PB, von der Maase H. Association of perceived physician communication style with patient satisfaction, distress, cancer-related self-efficacy, and perceived control over the disease. *Br J Cancer* 2003; 88:658–665.

25 Fogarty LA, Curbow BA, Wingard JR et al. Can 40 seconds of compassion reduce patient anxiety? *J Clin Oncol* 1999; 17(1): 371–379.

◆ 26 Parker S, Clayton JM, Hancock K, Walder S, Butow P, Carrick S, Currow D, Ghersi D, Glare P, Hagerty R, Tattersall M. A systematic review of prognostic/end-of-life communication with adults in the advanced stages of a life-limiting illness: Patient/caregiver preferences for the content, style and timing of information. *J Pain Symptom Manage* 2007; 34 (1): 81–93.

◆ 27 Innes S, Payne S. Advanced cancer patients' prognostic information preferences: A review. *Palliat Med* 2009; 23: 29–39.

● 28 Wright AA. Keating NL. Balboni TA. Matulonis UA. Block SD. Prigerson HG. Place of death: Correlations with quality of life of patients with cancer and predictors of bereaved caregivers' mental health. *J Clin Oncol* 2010; 28(29):4457–4464.

◆ 29 Trice ED. Prigerson HG. Communication in end-stage cancer: Review of the literature and future research. *J Health Commun* 2009; 14 Suppl 1:95–108.

30 Jenkins V, Fallowfield L, Saul J. Information needs of patients with cancer: Results from a large study in UK cancer centres. *Br J Cancer* 2001; 84: 48–51.

31 Butow PN, Maclean M, Dunn SM et al. The dynamics of change: Cancer patients' preferences for information, involvement and support. *Ann Oncol* 1997; 8: 857–863.

● 32 Kutner JS, Steiner JF, Corbett KK et al. Information needs in terminal illness. *Soc Sci Med* 1999; 48: 1341–1352.

33 Leydon GM, Boulton M, Moynihan C, Jones A, Mossman J, Boudioni M et al. Cancer patients' information needs and information seeking behaviour: In depth interview study. *BMJ* 2000; 320: 909–913.

34 Friis LS, Elverdam B, Schmidt KG. The patient's perspective: A qualitative study of acute myeloid leukaemia patients' need for information and their information-seeking behaviour. *Support Care Cancer* 2003; 11: 162–170.

35 Huang X, Butow PN, Meiser M et al. Communicating in a multicultural society: The needs of Chinese cancer patients in Australia. *Aust N Z J Med* 1999; 29: 207–213.

36 Goldstein D, Thewes B, Butow P. Communicating in a multicultural society II: Greek community attitudes towards cancer in Australia. *Intern Med J* 2002; 32: 289–296.

37 Fielding R, Hung J. Preferences for information and involvement in decisions during cancer care among a Hong Kong Chinese population. *Psychooncology* 1996; 5: 321–329.

38 Yun YH, Lee CG, Kim SY, Lee SW, Heo DS, Kim JS et al. The attitudes of cancer patients and their families toward the disclosure of terminal illness. *J Clin Oncol* 2004; 22: 307–314.

● 39 Kirk P, Kirk I, Kristjanson LJ. What do patients receiving palliative care for cancer and their families want to be told? A Canadian and Australian qualitative study. *BMJ* 2004; 328: 1343–1347.

40 Levin TT, Weiner JS. End of life communication training. In: Kissane D, Bultz B, Butow P, Finlay I (eds). *Handbook of Communication in Oncology and Palliative Care*. New York: Oxford University Press; 2010: 215–227.

41 Jackson VA, Mack J, Matsuyama R, Lakoma MD, Sullivan AM, Arnold RM, Weeks JC, Block SD. A qualitative study of oncologists' approaches to end-of-life care. *J Palliat Med* 2008, 11(6): 893–906.

42 Pantilat S. Communicating with seriously ill patients. *JAMA* 2009; 301 (12): 1279–1281.

◆ 43 Clayton JM, Hancock K, Parker S et al. Sustaining hope when communicating with terminally ill patients and their families: A systematic review. *Psychooncology* 2008; 17 (7): 641–659.

◆ 44 Back AL. Anderson WG. Bunch L. Marr LA. Wallace JA. Yang HB. Arnold RM. Communication about cancer near the end of life. *Cancer* 2008; 13(7 Suppl):1897–1910.

◆ 45 Rao JK, Anderson LA, Inui TS et al. Communications interventions make a differences in conversations between physicians and patients: A systematic review of the evidence. *Med Care* 2007; 45: 340–349.

◆ 46 Barth J, Lannen P. Efficacy of communication skills training courses in oncology: A systematic review of the review and meta-analysis. *Ann Oncol* 2011; 22: 1030–1040

● 47 Back AL, Arnold RM, Baile WF et al. Efficacy of communication skills training for giving bad news and discussing transitions to palliative care. *Arch Intern Med* 2007; 167: 453–460.

48 Clayton JM, Adler JL, O'Callaghan A, Martin P, Hynson J, Butow PN, Powell RC, Arnold RM, Tulsky JA, Back AL. Intensive communication skills teaching for specialist training in Palliative Medicine: Development and evaluation of an experiential workshop. *J Palliat Med* 2012; 15 (5): 585–591.

49 Szmuilowicz E, el-Jawahri A, Chiappetta L et al. Improving residents' end-of-life communication skills with a short retreat: A randomized controlled trial. *J Palliat Med* 2010; 13: 439–452.

50 Alexander SC, Keitz SA, Sloane R et al. A controlled trial of a short course to improve residents' communication with patients at the end of life. *Acad Med* 2006; 81: 1008–1012.

51 Clayton JM, Butow PN, Waters A et al. Evaluation of a novel individualized communication-skills training intervention to improve doctors' confidence and skills in end-of-life communication. *Palliat Med* 2013, 27: 236–243.

◆ 52 Uitterhoeve RJ, Bensing JM, Grol RP et al. The effect of communication skills training on patient outcomes in cancer care: A systematic review of the literature. *Eur J Cancer Care* 2009; 19: 442–457.

53 Smith RC. *Patient-Centered Interviewing: An Evidence-Based Method*. Philadelphia, PA: Lippincott Williams & Wilkins; 2002.

105

Spiritual care

MARVIN OMAR DELGADO-GUAY

INTRODUCTION

Spirituality is recognized as a factor that contributes to health in many people and is an important component in the care of patients with life-threatening illnesses, such as cancer and congestive heart failure [1–4]. Spiritual and religious beliefs can affect the way patients cope with their illnesses creating distress and worsening the burden of the illness [1,5]. The concept of spirituality is found in all cultures and societies. Its meaning is not limited to participation in organized religion, but is rather much broader than that encompassing a belief in God, family, naturalism, rationalism, humanism, and even the arts [1,5–9]. Spirituality is a dimension of personhood, a part of our being, and religion is a construct of human making, which enables the conceptualization and expression of spirituality [10,11]. A key goal of palliative care services is to alleviate patient suffering. Suffering is a biopsychosocial, multidimensional construct that includes physical, emotional, as well as spiritual pain. The spirituality and religiosity field is important to consider when we evaluate patients with advanced and terminal illness, because it can influence coping strategies and quality of life. The presence of spiritual pain can be an important component of the patients with chronic or acute pain and other physical and psychological symptoms [12]. Spiritual care is an important part of health care, especially when facing the crisis of advanced cancer and at the end of life. When spiritual needs and spiritual distress are not addressed, patients are at risk of depression and reduced sense of spiritual meaning and peace [13] and dignity [14]. The purpose of this chapter is to provide an overview about the role of spirituality and religiosity in advanced illness patients' way of coping and the importance to provide a comprehensive spiritual assessment and spiritual care in an interdisciplinary team work setting, such as palliative care.

SPIRITUALITY AND RELIGIOSITY

Many authors have highlighted the considerable overlap and the distinct characteristics of religion and spirituality [11,15–17]. Main themes encompass a relationship with a God, spiritual being, higher power, or reality greater than the self (not of the self); transcendence or connectedness unrelated to a belief in a higher being; existential, not of the material world; meaning and purpose in life; life force of the person, integrating aspect of the person; and a combination of multiple themes [9,18]. Spirituality can be defined as "the aspect of humanity that refers to the way individuals seek and express meaning and purpose and the way they experience their connectedness to the moment, to self, to others, to nature, and to the significant or sacred" [1]. The spirituality is a dimension of personhood, a part of our being, while religion is a construct of human making, which enables the conceptualization and expression of spirituality [11]; this encompasses structured belief systems that address spiritual issues, often with a code of ethical behavior and philosophy [17]. Religious rituals enact and manifest the meaning of the sacred; they establish shared meaning, foster belonging, and bridge the boundary between the personal and the social [17].

Both religious practices and spiritual beliefs are common in the United States [19,20]. Gallup [20] reported in 2000–2001 that religion/spirituality was noted as "very important" by 60% of Americans aged 50–64, 67% of those aged 65–74, and 75% of those aged 75 and older.

50%–95% patients living with cancer consider spirituality/religion an important part of their life [21–25]. Many also report the need for a sense of connectedness or spirituality [6,26–30]. It has also been documented that those who report greater religiosity/spirituality also report more adaptive coping styles and a better quality of life [8,26,31–35]. Thus, in the context of coping with a life-threatening illness such as cancer, one possibility is that spiritual well-being may serve as a buffer against depression, hopelessness, and desire for death in patients with advanced disease [21,30,36]. Another possibility is that greater spirituality/religiosity is associated with more negative religious coping (illness as a consequence of God's punishment), which can lead to distress and decreased quality of life and suffering [7,37,38].

In a cohort of advanced cancer patients evaluated in the palliative care outpatient clinic, almost all of them considered themselves spiritual (98%) and religious (98%). The patients also reported that spirituality and/or religiosity help them cope with their illness (99%), as a source of strength (100%), and have a positive impact on their physical (69%) and emotional (84%) symptoms [12]. Also, advanced cancer patients expressed their inner strength and meaning of life in terms of the divine (through praying, hope, faith, communication with God) in 76%, in terms of their own value as human beings in 17%, and in terms of their relationships to others (family members, friends, and partners) in 7% [39].

Different models of spirituality have been developed for a health-care context. Farran and her colleagues proposed one that use a functional definition of spirituality operating through seven major dimensions such as belief and meaning, authority and guidance, and ritual and practice. These dimensions are set within a context of universal events and experiences (such as health, illness, pain, and suffering), which provide the possibility for expanded or limited spiritual functioning and spiritual growth [40]. Models of spirituality have been developed explicitly for palliative care. Kellehear's descriptive model is focused on the need of patients to find meaning beyond their suffering through situational, moral–biographical, and religious transcendence [41]. Also, Wright proposes an inclusive model of spirituality based on a synthesis of ideas that includes activities of "transcending," "connecting," "finding meaning," and "becoming" that operate through the dimensions of the self, others, and the cosmos [42].

Spirituality is lived and experienced in the lives of patients with life-limiting conditions and also in their caregivers. That allows them to cope with different situations in their life and respond to them either with or without distress or suffering (Figure 105.1).

Spirituality serves several purposes in different stages of life, which is similar to the concept of different needs and conflicts associated with different ages [43]. In addition, Fowler recognized six stages of faith and also recognized the fact that individual development may stop at any stage [44,45]:

1. Intuitive–projective faith (ages 2–7 years): When child becomes aware of God
2. Mythic–literal faith (ages 7–12 years): When family-specified perspectives and meanings of morals and God are internalized
3. Synthetic–conventional faith (adolescence onward): When faith is accepted without critical evaluation
4. Individuative–reflective faith: When an individual's own belief is critically examined and reconstructed
5. Conjunctive faith (midlife and beyond): When disillusionment with that belief system sets in and one is caught between it and openness to other religious traditions
6. Universalizing faith (late life): Brings oneness with the power of being or divinity; willingness to promote justice in the world and fellowship with others, regardless of their faith stage or religious tradition

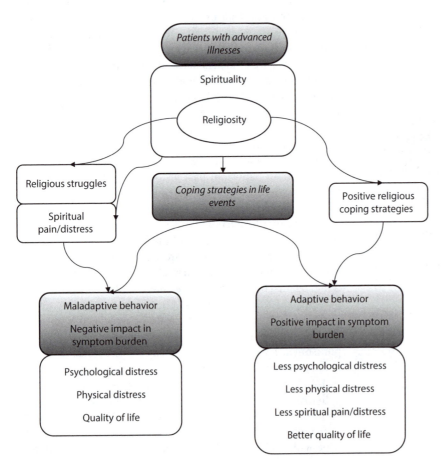

Figure 105.1 *Spirituality and religiosity as a lived experience in coping strategies and their impact in symptom distress and quality of life in patients with advanced illnesses.*

The theories of faith development emphasize faith development in late life after completion of all developmental cognitive stages. Spirituality is a lifelong developmental task, lasting until death [46,47].

Dying is no longer a part of human daily consciousness or an accepted final event of life. The continuing advances of medical technology have altered attitudes toward dying. The dying stage in our life can be experienced as the most profound event of our life experience. Dying begins when the facts of life are finally recognized, communicated, and accepted [48]. Older people tend to think about dying and death more than any other age group [49].

The fear of dying is considered as the most prevalent emotion. The findings about the relationship of age and fear of dying are mixed [50,51]. Other emotions linked to death and dying are hope and the continuity of hope [52], the feeling of loss (e.g., of control, competence, independence, people, or dreams for the future) [53], loneliness [54], dignity/integrity [55], forgiveness [56], and love [57]. As a society, we shy away from death and the idea of termination. In recent years, research has led people toward greater awareness and an increase of interest in the dying process and death. Spirituality and storytelling can be used as resources in aging successfully and in dying given the constraints of the modern-day Western culture [58].

The end of life can be a spiritual crisis, and having a sense of spirituality has been identified as an important coping resource. A needs assessment can identify the specific services and assistance the patient most desires and is a first step in designing needs-tailored interventions [59].

SPIRITUAL NEEDS AND SPIRITUAL/EXISTENTIAL CONCERNS IN PATIENTS WITH ADVANCED ILLNESS AND THEIR CAREGIVERS

Spiritual needs should be met in an individualized reciprocal process. Patients like conversations that allow them to set the pace and agenda. Patients selected simple questions such as "What principles do you live by?" "Do you have a personal faith?" "Have you ever prayed about your situation?" as useful ways to start discussions.

The words patients use to communicate the perceptions of their end-of-life needs reveal how important it is to assess the dynamics of patient–clinician communication [59,60].

It is important to recognize also that patients who have spiritual distress and thus need spiritual care are the least likely to ask for it [61].

Although the importance of religion and spirituality in coping with cancer and other diseases is high for many people and well documented, health-care providers and medical institutions often do not do a good job of attending to this dimension of the patient's care [62]. It has been reported that over 70% of cancer patients said that their spiritual needs were minimally or not at all supported by the medical system [9]. Most importantly is that attention to religious/spiritual issues has been shown to have a significant influence on several important indicators of quality care. Several studies have documented the positive relationship between meeting spiritual needs and patient satisfaction [63,64]. Several other findings suggest that attention to spiritual needs improves quality of life [4] and reduces use of aggressive care at the end of life [65].

It was reported in a sample of 248 ethnically diverse, urban cancer patients that 75% had at least one spiritual need. 51% of these patients wanted help to overcome their fears, 42% in finding hope, and 40% in finding meaning. Hispanics and African-American patients more frequently endorsed spiritual needs than Caucasians [66].

In another study of patients at an outpatient cancer clinic, 73% reported at least one spiritual need [64]. In a study by Delgado-Guay et al. [39], among a palliative care population, 44% of advanced patients reported experiencing "spiritual pain." Patients with spiritual pain had significantly lower self-perceived religiosity and spiritual quality of life. Likewise, in a study by Alcorn et al. [67] of advanced cancer patients receiving palliative radiation therapy, 85% identified one or more spiritual issues with a median of 4 issues per patient among 14 spiritual issues assessed. Key spiritual issues among patients included "seeking a closer connection with God or one's faith," 54%; "seeking forgiveness (of oneself or others)," 47%; and "feeling abandoned by God," 28%. Surprisingly, among the 22% of patients who said that religion/spirituality was "not important" to their cancer experience, two-thirds had at least one spiritual issue and 40% reported four or more spiritual issues.

It is important also to notice that caregivers of patients of advanced illnesses have spiritual needs/concerns and suffering.

Concerns about spiritual issues also arise in the caregiver population. Previous studies have shown that caregivers who are facing significant physical, social, and emotional hardships rely heavily on their faith to cope with these burdens [68].

Persons who take responsibility for caregiving are engaging in "meaning-making" activities by expressing important values such as hope, dignity, togetherness, involvement, and continuity and demonstrating their desire to strengthen family ties and deepen personal growth [69]. People who are more religious feel more positively about their role as caregivers, get along better with those for whom they provide care, and express less caregiver distress [70]. Faith communities foster belief systems of responsibility and compassion that are likely to help caregivers doing the emotionally difficult work of caring for others [69]. Because spirituality provides caregivers hope and sustenance and helps them express themselves more fully during difficult times of change, feel the presence of a greater power, practice rituals, be one with nature, and interact with family and friends [71]. Although caregivers have reported that their satisfaction in the spirituality and meaning domains increased over time, they might be less satisfied during the bereavement period [72], most likely because their spiritual needs have not been optimally addressed during the dying phase [71,73]. Caregivers' quality of life might decrease in direct proportion to declines in the patient's functioning and health and increases in the patient's need for care and the intensity of his or her symptoms and distress [74].

There is a high prevalence of spiritual needs/concerns among patients facing life-threatening diseases and their caregivers, particularly among ethnic minorities, and that even among patients who do not consider themselves religious/spiritual, spiritual needs remain frequent. It is extremely important to explore, assess, and support their spiritual needs/concerns and work as a team to decrease suffering and improve their quality of life.

Spiritual assessment is a conversation in which the patient is encouraged to tell and explore their spiritual story. As in spiritual screening, there are several options in the literature for taking a spiritual history. It is to be patient centered and guided by the extent to which the patient chooses to disclose *his or her* spiritual needs.

There are several tools available for taking a spiritual history, including the Systems of Belief Inventory-15R [75], brief measure of religious coping [76], functional assessment of chronic illness therapy-spiritual well-being [77,78], SPIRITual History [79], HOPE [80], and FICA (Faith, Importance, Community, Address in care) Spiritual History [81]. Some of these instruments are intended primarily for research, whereas the others have been used primarily in the clinical setting for nonchaplain clinicians.

The FICA tool developed at the George Washington Institute for Spirituality and Health (Table 105.1) has been tested and validated [81]. It is recommended that it be incorporated into the social history section of the overall history and physical. In incorporating this area into a history, providers should be conscious of not imposing their own beliefs on the patient or trying to answer any questions or concerns that the patient may have

in this area. Such questions and concerns should be referred to a professional chaplain. They also should be clear that this process does not oblige them to discuss their own beliefs and practices. The main goal of this process is to understand the role of spiritual and religious beliefs and practices in the patient's life and the role they play in coping with illness. As in the screening, a basic goal of the history is to diagnose spiritual distress, which should be referred to the professional chaplain [62,82]. Through active listening, a relationship between the patients and the provider and/or the professional chaplain is established. The chaplain then extracts themes and issues from the story to explore further with the patient. These themes might include meaning, making God as judge versus God as comforter, grief, despair, and forgiveness. This assessment should result in a spiritual care plan that is fully integrated into the patient's and family's total plan of care, which should be communicated to the rest of the treatment team [82].

PROVIDING SPIRITUAL CARE TO PATIENTS WITH ADVANCED ILLNESS AND THEIR CAREGIVER IN DISTRESS

The process of good spiritual care involves all health-care professionals and mimics the process for other domains of care. Patients have stated that all health-care professionals should be able to assess and provide spiritual care. The process is built around the premise that spiritual care, like all other domains of care, should focus on quickly identifying and attending to distress in this domain. Thus, the interdisciplinary palliative care model of spiritual care proposes inclusion of the spiritual domain in the overall screening and history-taking process as well as a full spiritual assessment by the professional chaplain as needed. Again, the generalist/specialist model presumes the professional chaplain as the specialist [62]. The plan should include the spiritual care interventions for all members of the health-care team.

Developing interventions will raise awareness of the dying process and, ultimately, result in a more peaceful experience. These interventions will likely improve the experience of death and dying for the patient and their families in various medical settings, such as palliative care, hospice, long-term care, and primary care settings [1,9].

Spiritual care is an essential domain of quality palliative care [1,4]. Studies have consistently indicated the desire of patients with serious illness and end-of-life concerns to have spirituality included in their care [7,9]. While there is an emerging scholarly body of literature to support the inclusion of spiritual care as part of a biopsychosocial–spiritual approach to health care [9], palliative care programs are working for strategies for effecting institutional change and resources to assist in improving the delivery of spiritual care [83,84].

One of the issues that often arises with regard to spiritual care is that, even when teams accept the necessity of participation in spiritual screening and history taking; they are uncomfortable taking on any role in the delivery of spiritual

Table 105.1   *FICA tool*

FICA tool	Questions
F—Faith, belief, meaning	Do you consider yourself spiritual or religious? Do you have spiritual beliefs that help you cope with stress? What gives your life meaning?
I—Importance and influence	What importance does your faith or belief have in your life? On a scale of 0 (not important) to 5 (very important), how would you rate the importance of faith/belief in your life? Have your beliefs influenced you in how you handle stress? What role do your beliefs plan in your health-care decision making?
C—Community	Are you a part of a spiritual or religious community? Is this of support to you and how? Is there a group of people you really love or who are important to you?
A—Address in care	How would you like your health-care provider to use this information about your spirituality as they care for you?

care itself. However, the provision of spiritual care is shared by all members of the team in the same way that documentation of spiritual need is shared. It is important to remember that taking time with a patient and being empathetic and compassionate is spiritual care. Any staff member can take the time to listen to a patient's story, to listen to a patient's angst, and to be a compassionate presence with that patient. Many times this is all that the patient asks. The patient is not looking for answers. What is spoken as a spiritual question is most often not a question at all but an expression of spiritual pain.

Practitioners who are personally uncomfortable with religious/spirituality should respectfully identify if a patient has spiritual needs and then refer the patient to chaplaincy or clergy. This approach, however, might best be understood as what is minimally appropriate in spiritual care rather than its gold standard [84–88].

Pastoral care of the dying and the bereaved is a core activity for all parish clergy. It was reported that the majority of clergy perceived the need for further training in this area. Clergy training colleges, although offering placements to clergy within pastoral care settings, were constrained by the amount of time given to this area during clergy training. The training in care of the dying and the bereaved (including communication skills) should be part of the core curriculum within clergy training colleges and regularly revisited by all those who provide continual ministerial training for clergy [84,87].

SPIRITUAL INTERVENTIONS

Spiritual interventions can be understood as therapeutic strategies that incorporate a spiritual or religious dimension as a central component of the intervention. This practice advocates for a holistic view of health. Spirituality is interwoven in the therapeutic process and cannot be separated from it [89].

Religious or spiritual activities can be practiced through the continuum of care to help support persons with life-threatening illness. Religious interventions are more structured, cognitive, denominational, external, ritualistic, and public, whereas spiritual interventions are more cross-cultural, affective, transcendent, and experiential. Interventions should be agreed with the patient and tailored to their worldly perspectives to help them during an illness or crisis [90]. Spiritual interventions are contraindicated in cases of psychotic illnesses when dealing with poor "ego boundaries" or when a patient does not want to participate [90,91].

Prayer is a powerful form of coping that helps people physically and mentally. Nearly 60% of Americans report praying daily [92]. Prayer is a communication or conversation with divine powers or a "higher self." Prayer is practiced by all Western theistic religions and several of the Eastern traditions (e.g., Hinduism, Sikhism, Buddhism, and Taoism). Group prayer is associated with a greater well-being and happiness, while solitary prayer is associated with depression and loneliness [93].

Worship and religious rituals are encouraged by most religions. It is important to recognize that potentially therapeutic elements of worship include music, aesthetic surroundings, rituals, prayer and contemplation, and opportunities to socialize with others [94]. Bibliotherapy involves the use of literature to help gain insight into feelings and behaviors and to assist with positive coping. All major world religions have a text that their followers view as holy and use as a source of comfort, wisdom, and guidance [95,96].

In medical settings, forgiveness and repentance are within the purview of a pastoral counselor and clergyperson. Both prayer and bibliotherapy with sacred writings must be consistent with patients' needs and requests [84,95].

Meditation produces the sense of calm, limited thought and attention. Meditation is widely used as an alternative therapy for physical ailments [97]. Meditation, essentially, is a physiological state of reduced metabolic activity that elicits physical and mental relaxation and is reported to enhance psychological balance and emotional stability [97]. Meditation involves either the narrowing or focusing of the attention on internal events, such as breathing, an object, one point in space or a mantra (in Buddhist or yoga practices), or expanding the attention nonjudgmentally on moment-to-moment experiences and observing thoughts and feelings from a metacognitive awareness state (mindful meditation, vipassana, and Zen Buddhist practices) [97,98] While evidence is not yet definitive, preliminary studies suggest health benefits of meditation for improved reaction time, creativity, and comprehension [97].

Ethical considerations should be taken into account when practicing or recommending spiritual interventions by healthcare professionals, to avoid promoting self-interest or imposing personal beliefs on patients via linking religious practices to better health outcomes; acknowledging limitations of current research into the effects of spirituality on health and, most importantly, respecting patients boundaries and beliefs by obtaining their informed consent to share their spiritual history and choosing spiritual interventions should be recognized [97].

Cognitive–behavioral therapy (CBT) represents a unique category of psychological interventions based on scientific models of human behavior, cognition, and emotion. CBT intends to directly reduce distress, target symptoms, reevaluate thinking, and promote helpful behavioral responses. Cognitive interventions refer to how patients create meaning about symptoms, situations, and events in their lives, as well as beliefs about themselves, others, and the world. CBT and psychodynamic therapy are the most commonly used psychotherapeutic treatments of mental disorders in adults. There is evidence from randomized controlled studies that CBT is an efficacious treatment of many mental disorders, especially depression and anxiety [99]. Provision of spiritually oriented or spiritually attuned approaches to psychodynamic psychotherapy pays especial attention to the roles religious beliefs, God representations, and spirituality play in the psychic world and health of the patient [99].

Psychotherapies involving religiosity and spirituality offer spiritual benefits to the patients that with emotional distress. The patients receiving these therapies improve on spiritual outcomes more than patients in alternate therapy [100]. For patients and contexts in which spiritual outcomes are highly valued, spirituality and religiosity psychotherapy can be considered a treatment of choice [100]. Importantly also is that the incorporation of religiosity and spirituality should follow the desires and needs of the patients. There is limited research about the impact of spiritually modified cognitive therapy on patients with spiritual pain/distress in the palliative care setting.

The psychodynamic approach to spirituality goes beyond sole consideration of consciously held religious beliefs and practices. This therapy plays attention on understanding the person's experience of their relationship to the transcendent realities. This might provide insight into the ways they relate to themselves and to others [101].

Another important intervention is the religiously oriented mindfulness-based cognitive therapy [101]. This therapy has been aimed at helping patients suffering from depression or anxiety disorders to relate to their experience in a new way, always placing particular emphasis of religious and spiritual aspects of the patient [102]. In this therapy, the patients are taught to experience their thoughts, feelings, and sensations in an accepting manner, helping them to develop a new mode of mind in which they "recognize and disengage from mind states characterized by self-perpetuating patterns of ruminative, negative thought. This involves moving from a focus on content to a focus on process, away from cognitive therapy's emphasis on changing the content of negative thinking, toward attending to the way all experience is processed" [102].

The patients receiving this type of cognitive therapy learn to develop an action plan to prevent relapse of depressive symptoms over the course of treatment. This action plan consists of three phases: (1) take a breathing space and decenter from unpleasant emotions and maladaptive thoughts, (2) choose a practice that is helpful for grounding the person in the present, and (3) take action that gives a sense of pleasure or mastery and break the activity down into smaller parts [102]. At the same time, the practice of gratitude therapy could provide a heightened well-being over time [103].

Future spiritual interventions that aim to enhance coping and improve quality of life of patients with life-threatening illness and their caregivers must consider spiritual diversity and develop targeted programs that offer choices of health care based on individual spiritual beliefs, thus creating a basis for biopsychospiritual personalized approach of care. Future research should test culturally appropriate interventions tailored to the needs of different populations, which combine methods demonstrated to be effective in reducing stress and improving well-being and coping.

Another priority in the development of this biopsychospiritual personalized approach is the training of health-care professionals in assessing and integrating spirituality into health care and the active participation also of a trained chaplain to be involved in the care of patients with complex spiritual suffering.

It will be important to continue to develop interdisciplinary training programs through a comprehensive curriculum for medical schools, schools of nursing and social work, allied health, and clinical pastoral programs.

A comprehensive multidimensional model that combines psychological, social, genetic, and neurobiological factors, based on previous research and theory, is needed to guide future research in the area of spirituality in patients with life-threatening illness and their caregivers.

Key learning points

- Religion and spirituality play an important role in coping with disease-related symptoms, improve quality of life, and impact medical decision making near death.
- Many patients report spiritual concerns and needs arising within illness.
- Many patients desire spiritual care from medical providers but its provision remains infrequent.
- Existential and spiritual suffering is among the most debilitating conditions in end-of-life care and yet it lacks a clear definition, concept, effective assessment, and measurement.
- Spiritual assessment of patients and families ranges from spiritual screening, taking spiritual history, and in-depth spiritual assessment, of active listening to patient's story and/or using specific measurement tools.
- There are various tools and measurement techniques developed and validated, but no consensus on standardized processes yet across palliative care settings.
- Family caregivers may experience typical patterns of spiritual well-being and distress in parallel with patients.
- Future research is needed to better understand the role of medical professionals in spiritual care provision.
- Open-ended questions always.
- Asking for everything doesn't mean to give any and all invasive treatment.
- Several interventions can be provided; the spiritual care is part of the all members of the team.
- Integrative care with multidisciplinary approaches, to provide a touch of hope and a touch of love to decrease suffering and to improve the quality of life of patients and families in distress.

REFERENCES

1 Puchalski C, Ferrel B, Virani R et al. Improving the quality of spiritual care as a dimension of palliative care: The report of the consensus conference. *J Palliat Med* 2009;10:885–904.
2 Puchalski C, Dorff R, Hendi I. Spirituality, religion, and healing in palliative care. *Clin Geriatr Med* 2004;20:689–714.
3 National Cancer Institute: Spirituality in cancer care. 2012. http://www.nci.nih.gov/cancertopics/pdq/supportivecare/spirituality/ September 2012. Last accessed May 2013.

4   The National Consensus Project for Quality Palliative Care Clinical Practice Guidelines for Quality Palliative Care 3rd edition 2013. Accessed May 2013.

5   Pargament KI, Koenig HG, Tarakeshwar N, Hahn J. Religious coping methods as predictors of psychological, physical and spiritual outcomes among medically ill elderly patients: A two year longitudinal study. *J Health Psychol* 2004;9:713–730.

6   Hinshaw D. Spiritual issues at the end of life. *Clin Fam Practice* 2004;6:423–440.

7   Puchalski C. Spirituality in health: The role of spirituality in critical care. *Crit Care Clin* 2004;20:487–504.

8   Chochinov H, Cann B. Interventions to enhance the spiritual aspects of dying. *J Palliat Med* 2005;8:S103–S115.

9   Balboni T, Vanderwerker L, Block S et al. Religiousness and spiritual support among advanced cancer patients and associations with end-of-life treatment preferences and quality of life. *J Clin Oncol* 2007;25:550–560.

10 Puchalski C, Romer A. Taking a spiritual history allows clinicians to understand patients more fully. *J Palliat Med* 2000; 3:129–137.

11 Kearney M, Mount B. Spiritual care of the dying patient. In: Chochinov H., Breitbart W (eds). *Handbook of Psychiatry in Palliative Medicine.* New York: Oxford University Press, 2000, pp. 357–373.

12 Delgado-Guay MO, Hui D, Parsons HA, Govan K, De la Cruz M, Thorney S, Bruera E. Spirituality, religiosity, and spiritual pain in advanced cancer patients. *J Pain Symptom Manage.* 2011;41(6):986–994.

13 Pearce MJ, Coan AD, Herndon JE, Koenig HG, Abernethy AP. Unmet spiritual care needs impact emotional and spiritual well-being in advanced cancer patients. *Support Care Cancer* 2012;20(10):2269–2276.

14 Thompson GN, Chochinov HM. Dignity-based approaches in the care of terminally ill patients, *Curr Opin Support Palliat Care* 2008;2:49–53.

15 Koenig H., McCullough M., Larson D. *Handbook of Religion and Health.* Oxford, U.K.: Oxford University Press, 2001.

16 McGrath P. Creating a language for "spiritual pain" through research: A beginning. *Support Care Cancer* 2002;10:637–646.

17 Rousseau P. Spirituality and the dying patient. *J Clin Oncol* 2000;18:2000–2002.

18 Unruh A, Versnel J, Kerr N. Spirituality unplugged: A review of commonalities and contentions, and a resolution. *Can J Occup The* 2002;69:5–19.

19 Koenig H, George L, Titus P. Religion, spirituality, and health in medically ill hospitalized older patients. *J Am Geriatr Soc* 2004;52:554–562.

20 Gallup G. Gallup Tuesday Briefing. June 2, 2002 (on-line). Available at http://www.gallup.com/poll/6124/Religiosity-Cycle.aspx

21 Roberts J, Brown D, Elkins T et al. Factors influencing views of patients with gynecologic cancer about end-of-life decisions. *AM J Obst Gynecol* 1997;176:166–172.

22 Jenkins R, Pargament K. Religion and spirituality as resources for coping with cancer. *J Psychosoc Oncol* 1995;13:51–74.

23 Gail T., Cornblat M. Breast cancer survivors give voice: A qualitative analysis of spiritual factors in long-term adjustment. *Psychooncology* 2002;11:524–535.

24 True G, Phipps E, Braitman L et al. Treatment preferences and advance care planning at the end of life: The role of ethnicity and spiritual coping in cancer patients. *Ann Behav Med* 2005;30:174–179.

25 Kappeli S. Religious dimensions of suffering from and coping with cancer: A comparative study of Jewish and Christian patients. *Gynecol Oncol-* 2005;99:S135–S136.

26 McClain C, Rosenfeld B, Breitbart W. Effect of spiritual well-being on end-of-life despair in terminally-ill cancer patients. *Lancet* 2003;361:1603–1607.

27 Kuin A, Deliens L. Spiritual issues in palliative care consultations in the Netherlands. *Palliat Med* 2006;20:585–592.

28 Moadel A, Morgan C, Fatone A, et al: Seeking meaning and hope: Self-reported spiritual and existential needs among an ethically-diverse cancer patient population. *Psychooncology* 1999;8:378–385.

29 Holmes S, Rabow M, Dibble S. Screening the soul: Communication regarding spiritual concerns among primary care physicians and seriously ill patients approaching the end of life. *Am J Hosp Palliat Care* 2006;23:25–33.

30 Grant E, Murray S, Kendall M et al. Spiritual issues and needs: Perspectives from patients with advanced cancer and nonmalignant disease—A qualitative study. *Palliat Support Care* 2004;2:371–378.

31 Nelson C, Rosenfeld B, Breitbart W et al. Spirituality, religion, and depression in the terminally ill. *Psychosomatics* 2002;43:213–220.

32 Cotton S, Levine E, Fitzpatrick C et al. Exploring the relationships among spiritual well being, quality of life, and psychological adjustment in women with breast cancer. *Psychooncology* 1999;8:429–438.

33 Tarakeshwar N, Vanderwerker L, Paulk E et al. Religious coping is associated with the quality of life of patients with advanced cancer. *J Palliat Med* 2006;9:646–657.

34 Brady M, Peterman A, Fitchett G et al. A case for including spirituality in quality of life measurement in oncology. *Psychooncology* 1999;8:417–428.

35 Simon C, Crowther M. The stage-specific role of spirituality among African American Christian women throughout the breast cancer experience. *Cultur Divers Ethnic Minor Psychol* 2007;13:26–34.

36 Breitbart W, Rosenfeld B, Pessin H et al. Depression, hopelessness, and desire for death in terminally ill patients with cancer. *JAMA* 2000;284:2907–2911.

37 Hills J, Paice J, Cameron J et al. Spirituality and distress in palliative care consultation. *J Palliat Med* 2005;8:782–788.

38 Sherman A, Simonton S, Latif U et al. Religious struggle and religious comfort in response to illness: Health outcomes among stem cell transplant patients. *J Behav Med* 2005;28:359–367.

39 Delgado-Guay MO, Parsons HA, Hui D et al. Spirituality: An expression of Inner Strength and Meaning of life in patients with advanced cancer (ACAP) and their caregivers in the Palliative Care Setting. Poster Presentation in EAPC 2011: Athens, Greece.

40 Farran CJ, Fitchett G, Quiring-Emblen JD et al. Development of a model for spiritual assessment and intervention. *J Relig Health* 1989; 28(3):185–194.

41 Kellehear A. Spirituality and palliative care: A model of needs. *Palliat Med* 2000; 14(2):149–155.

42 Wright M. Hospice care and models of spirituality. *Eur J Palliat Care* 2004;11:75–78.

43 Erikson EH. *Childhood and Society*, 2nd edn. New York: Norton, 1963.

44 Fowler JW. *Stages of Faith: The Psychology of Human Development and the Quest for Meaning.* California: Harper & Row, 1981.

45 Fowler JW. *Weaving the New Creation: Stages of Faith and the Public Church.* California: Harper & Row, 1991.

46 Koenig H. *Aging and God.* New York: The Haworth Pastoral Press, 1994.

47 Moberg DO. *Aging and Spirituality: Spiritual Dimensions of Aging Theory, Research, Practice, and Policy.* New York: The Haworth Press, Inc., 2001.

48 Kastenbaum RJ. *Death, Society, and Human Experience*, 3rd edn. Columbus OH (ed.). New York: Charles E Merrill Publishing Company, 1986;100–120.

49 Blesky JK. *The Psychology of Aging*, 2nd edn. Belmont, CA: Brooks/Cole Publishing Company, 1990.

50 Feifel H, Branscomb AB. Who's afraid of death? *J Abnorm. Psychol* 1973;81:282–288.

51 Templer DI. Death anxiety as related to depression and health of retired persons. *J Gerontol* 1997;26:521–523.

52 Kalish R. *Death, Grief, and Caring Relationships*, 2nd edn. Belmont, CA: Brooks/Cole Publishing Company, 1985.

53 Bianchi EC. *Aging as a Spiritual Journey.* New York: Crossroad Publishing Company, 1982.

54 Feifel H. *New Meanings of Death.* New York: McGraw-Hill Book Company, 1977.

55 Johnson R. Forgiveness: Our bridge to peace. *Liguorian* 1992;80:44–45.

56 Thibault JM. *A Deepening Love Affair: The Gift of God in Later Life*. TX: Upper Room Books, 1993.

57 Fischer K. *Winter Grace*. TX: Upper Room Books, 1998.

58 Schenck DP, Roscoe LA. In search of a good death. *J. Med. Humanit* 2009;30:61–72.

59 Lunder U, Furlan M, Simonic A. Spiritual needs assessments and measurements. *Curr Opin Support Palliat Care*, 2011;5(3):273–278.

60 Arnold BL. Mapping hospice patients' perception and verbal communication of end-of-life needs: An exploratory mixed methods inquiry. *BMC Palliat Care* 2011;10:1.

61 Fitchett G, Risk JL. Screening for spiritual struggle. *J Pastoral Care Couns* 2009;62(1, 2):1–12.

62 Handzo, G., Spiritual care for palliative patients. *Curr Probl Cancer* 2011;35(6):365–371.

63 Williams JA et al. Attention to inpatients' religious and spiritual concerns: predictors and association with patient satisfaction. *J Gen Intern Med* 2011;26(11):1265–1271.

64 Astrow AB et al. Is failure to meet spiritual needs associated with cancer patients' perceptions of quality of care and their satisfaction with care? *J Clin Oncol* 2007;25(36):5753–5757.

65 Balboni TA et al. Provision of spiritual care to patients with advanced cancer: Associations with medical care and quality of life near death. *J Clin Oncol* 2010;28(3):445–452.

66 Moadel A, Morgan C, Fatone A et al. Seeking meaning and hope: Self-reported spiritual and existential needs among an ethnically-diverse cancer patient population. *Psychooncology* 1999;8:378–385.

67 Alcorn SR, Balboni MJ, Prigerson HG et al. 'If God wanted me yesterday, I wouldn't be here today': Religious and spiritual themes in patients' experiences of advanced cancer. *J Palliat Med* 2010;13:581–588.

68 Weaver AJ, Flannelly KJ. The role of religion/spirituality for cancer patients and their caregivers. *South Med J* 2004;97(12):1210–1214.

69 Sand L, Olsson M, Strang P. What are motives of family members who take responsibility in palliative care? *Mortality* 2010;15:64–80.

70 Kim Y, Wellisch DK, Spillers RL, Crammer C. Psychological distress of female cancer caregivers: effects of type of cancer and caregivers' spirituality. *Support Care Cancer* 2007;15:1367–1374.

71 Pierce LL, Steiner V, Havens H, Tormoehlen K. Spirituality expressed by caregivers of stroke survivors. *West J Nurs Res* 2008;30(5):606–619.

72 Heyland DK, Frank C, Tranmer J et al. Satisfaction with end-of-life care: A longitudinal study of patients and their family caregivers in the last months of life. *J Palliat Care* 2009;25:245–256.

73 Rosenbaum JL, Smith JR, Zollfrank R. Neonatal end-of life spiritual support care. *J Perinat Neonatal Nurs* 2011;25:61–69.

74 Stajduhar KI, Funk L, Toye C et al. Part 1. Home-based family caregiving at the end of life: A comprehensive review of published quantitative research (1998–2008). *Palliat Med* 2010;24:573–593.

75 Holland JC, Kash KM, Passik S et al. A brief spiritual beliefs inventory for use in quality of life re-search in life-threatening illness. *Psychooncology* 1998;7:460–469.

76 Pargament KI, Smith BW, Koenig HG, Perez L. Patterns of positive and negative religious coping with major life stressors. *J Sci Study Relig* 1998;37:710–724.

77 Brady MJ, Peterman AH, Fitchett G, Mo M, Cella D. A case for including spirituality in quality of life measurement in oncology. *Psychooncology* 1999;8:417–428.

78 Cella DF, Tulsky DS, Gray G et al. The functional assessment of cancer therapy scale: Development and validation of the general measure. *J Clin Oncol* 1993;11:570–579.

79 Maugans TA. The spiritual history. *Arch Fam Med* 1996;5:11–16.

80 Anandarajah G, Hight E. Spirituality and medical practice: Using the hope questions as a practical tool for spiritual assessment. *Am Fam Physician* 2001;63:81–89.

81 Borneman T, Ferrell B, Puchalski C. Evaluation of the FICA tool for spiritual assessment. *J Pain Symptom Manag* 2010;20(2):163–173.

82 Fitchett G, Canada AL. The role of religion/spirituality in coping with cancer: Evidence, assessment, and intervention. In: Holland JC (ed.). *Psycho-Oncology*, 2nd edn. New York: Oxford University Press, 2010. pp. 440–446.

83 Otis-Green, S, Ferrel B, Bomeman T, Puchalski C, Uman G, Garcia A. Integrating spiritual care within palliative care: An overview of nine demonstration projects. *J Palliat Med* 2012;15:154–162.

84 El Nawawi NM, Balboni MJ, Balboni TA. Palliative care and spiritual care: The crucial role of spiritual care in the care of patients with advanced illness. *Curr Opin Support Palliat Care* 2012, *Curr Opin Support Palliat Care* 2012;6(2):269–274.

85 Lo B, Kates LW, Ruston D et al. Responding to requests regarding prayer and religious ceremonies by patients near the end of life and their families. *J Palliat Med* 2003;6:409–415.

86 Sulmasy DP. Spirituality, religion, and clinical care. *Chest* 2009;135:1634–1642.

87 Lloyd-Williams M, Cobb M, Shiels C, Taylor F. How well trained are clergy in care of the dying patient and bereavement support? *J Pain Symptom Manage* 2006;32:44–51.

88 Balboni MJ, Babar A, Dillinger J et al. 'It depends': Viewpoints of patients, physicians, and nurses on patient-practitioner prayer in the setting of advanced cancer. *J Pain Symptom Manag* 2011;41:836–847.

89 Brown O, Elkonin D, Naicker S. The use of religion and spirituality in psychotherapy: Enablers and barriers. *J Relig Health* 2013;52(4):1131–1146.

90 Yoon DP, Lee EK: The impact of religiousness, spirituality, and social support on psychological well-being among older adults in rural areas. *J Gerontol Soc Work* 2007;48:281–298.

91 Richards PS, Bergin AE. A *Spiritual Strategy for Counseling and Psychotherapy*. Washington, DC : American Psychological Association Press, 1997.

92 Boehnlein JK. *Psychiatry and Religion: The Convergence of Mind and Spirit*. Washington, DC: American Psychiatric Press, 2000.

93 Poloma MM, Pendleton BF. The effects of prayer and prayer experience on measures of general well-being. *J Psychol Theol* 1991;19:71–83.

94 Benson H. *Timeless Healing: The Power and Biology of Belief*. New York: The Gale Group, 1997.

95 Woll ML, Hinshaw DB, Pawlik TM. Spirituality and religion in the care of surgical oncology patients with life-threatening or advanced illnesses. *Ann Surg Oncol* 2008;15(11):3048–3057.

96 Jarvis GK, Northcott HC. Religion and differences in morbidity and mortality. *Soc Sci Med* 1987;25:813–824.

97 Candy B, Jones L, Varagunam M, Speck P, Tookman A, King M. Spiritual and religious interventions for well-being of adults in the terminal phase of disease. *Cochrane Database Syst Rev* 2012, Issue 5. Art. No.: CD007544. DOI:10.1002/14651858.CD007544.pub2.

98 Ivanovski B, Malhi GS. The psychological and neurophysiological concomitants of mindfulness forms of meditation. *Acta Neuropsychiatr* 2007;19;76–91.

99 Leichsenring F, Hiller W, Weissberg M, Leibing E. Cognitive–behavioral therapy and psychodynamic psychotherapy: Techniques, efficacy, and indications. *Am J Psychother* 2006;60(3):233–259.

100 Worthington EL, Hook JH, McDaniel MA. Religion and spirituality. *J Clin Psychol* 2011;In Session 67:204–214.

101 Shafranske EP. Spiritually oriented psychodynamic psychotherapy. *J Clin Psycho* 2009:In session 65:147–157.

102 Hathaway W, Tan e. religiously oriented mindfulness-based cognitive therapy. *J Clin Psychol* 2009;In Session 65: 158–171.

103 Emmons RA, McCullough ME. Counting blessings versus burdens: An experimental investigation of gratitude and subjective well-being in daily life. *J Person and Soc Psychol* 2003;84:377–389.

106

Family caregivers

RONY DEV, MARY DEV

INTRODUCTION

Psychosocial support for both patients and their family is at the foundation of palliative care. The World Health Organization (WHO) defines palliative care "as an approach that improves the quality of life of patients and their families facing the problem associated with life-threatening illness, through the prevention and relief of suffering by means of early identification and impeccable assessment and treatment of pain and other problems, physical, psychosocial and spiritual" [1]. In addition to relieving the unnecessary suffering of patients, an interdisciplinary palliative care team should provide psychosocial support for family caregivers who may be overwhelmed with the care of chronically ill patients and may themselves have a difficult time coping with the burden of caregiving. In addition, palliative care emphasizes the need to support family caregivers not only during the illness stage but also while grieving the death of a loved one.

The definition of family is open ended and should be defined by the patient. One definition of family developed by the Canadian Palliative Care Association is "…those closest to the patient in knowledge care and affection. This includes the biological family, the family of acquisition (related by marriage/contract), and the family of choice and friends (not related biologically, by marriage/contract)" [2]. Family caregivers are often classified as primary or secondary. Primary caregivers are defined as those who provide the majority of unpaid care, while secondary caregivers either provide the minority of unpaid care or split the care with another family member [3]. The primary caregivers, who voluntarily or involuntarily assume the responsibility of caregiving, often carry the greatest burden [4,5] and have been branded the "hidden patient" [6]. In the majority of cases, the primary caregiver is the spouse, partner, parent, or adult child. In some cases, friends or even neighbors may carry the burden of caregiving. Recent studies suggest that the caregiving burden is distributed not just on the primary caregiver but often to family/community networks of carers who collectively provide the majority of care [7].

The following chapter will outline the distress that family caregivers may experience and the support that palliative care health-care professional can provide to alleviate caregiver distress. Research examining family caregivers has identified distress of caregiving, which can be overwhelming and result in burnout, and the importance of meeting the information needs of both patients and their family; noted the practical burden of day-to-day care of frail chronically ill patients; and emphasized the need for culturally sensitive care at the end of life. The majority of caregiver research involves the care of patients with dementia or cancer but can be applicable for caregivers of patients with other chronic life-threatening illness.

CAREGIVER DISTRESS

The burden of caregiving for aged, demented, or cancer patients or other chronic illnesses can be overwhelming. Modern medicine has been successful in treating acute illnesses and increasing the life span of the general population; however, it has been less successful in improving the functional ability of patients afflicted with chronic illnesses [8]. Most terminally ill people when surveyed often prefer to live at home [9,10] as opposed to institutions, such as nursing homes, resulting in family caregivers providing the majority of care [11,12]. Family caregiver's responsibilities may include the following: shopping and preparing food; assisting a patient with eating and administering their medications at the appropriate time; bathing and grooming the patient; providing financial support and paying the bills; managing medical problems, coordinating care, and contacting health-care providers in emergencies; and supporting the psychological well-being of a loved one.

Positive aspects of caregiving have been reported [13,14] and include the opportunity to "give back" to loved ones [15]. Often, family caregivers view with pride their ability to provide care [16], and a survey of family caregivers conducted in the United States reported increased personal strength and opportunities for growth when providing care for a loved one [17].

Although there are positive aspects associated with the act of caregiving, distress from the burden of providing care can lead to a combination of physical and emotional distress [18]. Caregiver burden has been defined as the distress that family caregivers experience as a result of providing care, which is different from other emotional responses, such as depression or anxiety [19,20]. Caregiver distress that impacts upon physical, psychological, social, and financial well-being can be perceived as "burdensome" [21] and may result in caregiver burnout. The level of caregiver distress was noted to have a close association with caregiving outcomes, even being a better predictor than the functional status of the patient being cared for [22,23]. Even in cancer patients who have survived their illness, a recent systematic review of patients and their spouses reported a high frequency of anxiety in both, with some studies reporting higher anxiety in spouses than cancer survivors [24].

Major contributors to caregiver distress include the following: a caregiver's loss of independence secondary to the responsibilities of caregiving, time constraints that may result in social isolation, and an unpredictable trajectory of illness or rapid deterioration of a patient's condition [25] results in increased distress. In addition, a primary caregiver's social network, spiritual support, as well as financial resources may also contribute to the level of caregiver distress [26–29]. Recent research indicates that the perceived strength of social support was more important than the actual size of a caregiver's social network with regard to caregiver outcomes [30]. In addition, family caregivers who can recruit extended family and friends to provide assistance with caregiving were more likely to have loved ones supported at home until death [7].

In a study of 96 patients with advanced cancer, the primary caregivers' psychological burden was found to have a greater impact than the physical burden of caregiving [31]. Most primary caregivers were found to have increased anxiety that was significantly higher than the norm during the late phase of palliative care [31]. Primary caregivers displayed increased levels of anxiety and depression from the initiation of the palliative phase to the start of the terminal stage of a patient's life; however, only 15 of 84 primary caregivers (18%) completed psychological assessments at the start of the terminal stage [32]. Of note, female primary caregivers experienced more psychological morbidity and strain than male caregivers when patients were in the palliative phase [33]. For family caregivers of patients with dementia, a Brazilian study identified the strongest association with caregiver distress with the duration of the caregiver role, the degree of kinship between the patient and the caregiver, and the patient's neuropsychiatric symptoms [34].

The transition from curative treatment to palliative care often elicits a strong emotional response in both patients and their family. During this emotional transition, the degree of caregiver distress depends on multiple factors including their understanding of options for further treatment and symptom management, the coping abilities of caregivers, and the capability of caregivers to navigate a fragmented health-care network [35]. Previous studies [36–38] have revealed an increased feeling of helplessness among caregivers, which was associated with the progression of a patient's illness, the degree of struggle undergone to obtain needed medical services, and the inability of caregivers to relieve a patient's pain and discomfort. Of note, the caregiver burden was shown to escalate during the final 3 months of the life of a chronically ill patient [39]. In the last days of life, family caregivers may hold vigil at the patient's bedside, often providing emotional and spiritual support. In this critical period of time, family caregivers may develop emotional exhaustion resulting in caregiver burnout.

CAREGIVER BURNOUT

The burden of caregiving is often carried by the primary caregiver, and responsibilities are often not shared with other family members [40]. Often, the family caregivers lack positive feedback from the patient, as well as from society, which may contribute to a sense of low self-accomplishment [41]. Burnout, a psychosocial syndrome initially characterized in the workplace, can occur in family caregivers who have poor coping mechanisms or dysfunctional families with limited support from the community. Burnout is characterized by the following: emotional exhaustion, depersonalization, and feelings of decrease personal accomplishment [42].

Burnout has been well studied in the workplace, often in health-care settings involving paid caregivers. However, a growing number of studies exist—mainly of family caregivers of patients with dementia—which indicate the presence of family caregiver burnout [43–45]. In these studies, predictors of burnout for the family caregiver include restrictions in social life, indicators of poor health or comorbidities, and a negative outlook regarding the role of being a family caregiver. In a recent study, caregiver burnout and depression were the most significant factors associated with a caregiver's poor quality of life [46].

Interventions that reduce the distress of family caregivers have not been well researched, and limited evidence exists on how to best support the "hidden patient." A family caregiver's self-esteem, confidence in caregiving, and amount of social network including family support have been shown to alleviate the distress of caregivers and enhance their ability to provide care [47,48]. Feeling prepared for the role of a caregiver of a critically ill patient has been a critical factor associated with caregiver outcomes, and psychoeducational interventions should aim to improve caregiver's preparedness to care [49]. In addition, caregiver groups with peer support may help alleviate distress. In a small qualitative study of family caregivers of patient's with dementia, support groups with peer volunteers helped family caregivers feel that they were "not alone" in their experiences and emotions, facilitated their ability to talk freely about the difficult experiences of caregiving, and increased their caregiving capability by learning how other caregivers cope, which was reported to be helpful [50].

The palliative care team, by treating patients and their family as a "unit of care," is able to assess the distress level of family caregivers. Assessment for symptoms of depression, social isolation, or emotional exhaustion is critical when evaluating a family caregiver. It is critical that health-care providers be vigilant for caregiver burnout since assessments of family caregivers may only occur during brief or sporadic visits [6].

When meeting with the family, palliative health-care providers should emphasize the burden to caregiving and stress the importance of self-care for family caregivers. In addition, secondary caregivers can be recruited to assist the primary caregiver who may be overwhelmed. Practical education about wound care, how to safely mobilize patients, or the management of surgical drains and other medical devices may be provided to multiple family members in order to recruit help for the primary caregiver. Caregiving tasks that are taxing are often perceived as manageable by health-care providers since they are executed in a detached and impersonal manner [51]; however, caregiving tasks that appear manageable to health-care providers may be difficult for family caregivers who are emotionally attached to the patient and inexperienced with caregiving. It is important to understand that family caregivers may need more education than a paid health-care provider in order to have the confidence to perform the tasks correctly. Positive reinforcement by the health-care team of the care provided by family caregivers may alleviate some distress.

More research is needed in evaluating interventions to decrease caregiver distress and burnout. Research should focus on identifying caregivers at risk of burnout and interventions that target increasing caregiver resources, their perception of support, and ability to cope with the burden of caregiving.

BARRIERS TO COMMUNICATION WITH FAMILY MEMBER

Vachon identified multiple barriers related to family communication that can be summarized by three key problematic areas including concealing feelings, information exchange, and coping with helplessness [52].

Families of critically ill patients often will conceal feelings in order to shield their loved one from emotional suffering. Hinton studied couples coping with the terminal phase of cancer and identified the following barriers to communication: (1) consciously concealing negative feelings in order to maintain a positive attitude, (2) patients minimizing symptoms to avoid burdening their primary caregivers, and (3) patients and family members avoiding discussions of the patient's illness to maintain an optimistic outlook [53]. In the last stages of life, patients and family often need increased support from health-care providers to prevail over these barriers. Issues of death may overwhelm patients and their family caregivers who may have little experience with the dying process. Health-care providers need to encourage caregivers to express concealed emotions and be an empathetic audience willing to take the time to listen.

For critically ill patients and their family, guidelines for therapeutic communication to promote psychological well-being include the following: health-care professionals actively listening and displaying empathy; clinicians providing information about current illness and options for treatment as well as what to expect in the future; and patients and family member being encouraged to express their emotions in a safe environment [54]. In addition, studies have shown that to improve

communication, clinicians should also spend more time listening than speaking, express nonabandonment, ensure discussions are patient centered, be more accessible, and avoid missed opportunities to provide emotional support and give information to family members [55–60].

INFORMATION NEEDS OF FAMILY CAREGIVERS

In addition to concealed feelings, family caregivers may not have adequate information to provide high-quality end-of-life care. The lack of information may exacerbate the distress level of the family caregivers. For example, commonly held deficiencies with respect to pain management including fear of respiratory depression, drug tolerance, or addiction may lead to inadequate (or even excessive) opioid administration. Inadequate communication with family caregivers can result in additional distress (stress, anxiety, and dissatisfaction) due to unmet information needs, lack of knowledge and understanding, lack of shared decision making, conflict with staff and among family members, as well as lack of trust in health-care providers [61].

Family caregivers often mediate interactions between the patient and health-care provider and act as a patient advocate. If they feel that they have not provided the best possible care for their loved one, distress in the family caregiver can escalate.

In a recent study examining the quality of palliative care, researchers showed a high family satisfaction with the care provided to dying cancer patients with the highest level of satisfaction with the following: nurse availability, hospital bed availability, coordination of care, and clinicians' attention to symptom control including pain relief; however, family members had low satisfaction with the following interventions—family conferences conducted to discuss the patient's illness and information provided regarding medication side effects, a patient's prognosis, pain management, and tests [62]. It is critical that the interdisciplinary team answer the questions of both patients and their family caregivers. Individual members of the palliative care team should be utilized, such as the pharmacist who may be deployed to review the indications, side effects, and how to safely administer the patient's medications as well as a social worker who can assist with expressive supportive counseling.

Studies show that end-of-life discussions improve a patient's understanding of their prognosis and increase enrollment in hospice care [63]. A prospective, longitudinal, cohort study revealed that frequency of end-of-life discussions varied at different medical institutions, which was attributed to their unique institutional cultures, and increased when patients had a lower performance status and a higher symptom burden [64]. In addition, end-of-life discussions were not associated with increased patient psychological distress but were associated with fewer aggressive medical treatments (i.e., mechanical ventilation, resuscitation, admission into an intensive care unit [ICU]). Patients who had end-of-life discussions initiated by health-care providers were more likely to enroll in hospice with improvements in quality of life, and bereaved caregivers who participated were less likely to have symptoms of anxiety or depression after a patient has died [64].

Qualitative studies have revealed variable degree of information needs [65–67] for patients and family caregivers that are often divergent as the patient's illness progresses. A study involving focus groups consisting of 19 patients with advanced cancer and 24 caregivers has revealed that caregivers have distinct information needs concerning end-of-life issues and prognosis, which often differ from the needs of patients [65]. Patient surveys reveal that one in five patients with terminal cancer would prefer not to discuss prognosis [66]. Preferences for information may change over time, and requests for information by patients with terminal cancer often decline as their illness progresses [67]. It is critical for health-care providers, prior to discussing issues such as prognosis with a critically ill patient, to ask what the patient and family already know and what questions they would like to be answered before providing information regarding end of life.

Open and regular communication is critical to meet the information needs of patients and family caregivers. Medical information may have to be repeated with care to avoid using medical terminology. Written material, question prompt lists [68], and consultations recorded with audiocassettes or digital devices can increase satisfaction with information exchange [69]. Written summaries and recordings of the consultation can be used to communicate with family members who are not able to physically be with the patient at the time of the meeting.

In addition, family caregivers report difficulty accessing medical information, often are overloaded with too much information or too little information, and often themselves are reluctant to interrupt busy health-care providers and ask questions [70,71]. Health-care providers may lack the ability to break bad news such as a poor prognosis [72] or when they do, often use medical jargon, which is difficult for patients and family to understand. A recent study reported that when oncologists communicate information in an optimistic manner regarding the benefits of chemotherapy, they are rated as better communicators by patients and their family [73]. Patients and family preference for an optimistic message may reinforce avoidance of discussing bad news and honest disclosure of information such as a poor prognosis.

FAMILY CONFERENCES

Family conferences have been championed by palliative care providers as a useful clinical tool to improve information exchange between health-care providers and a patient's family. A family conference is defined as a "meeting which involves a patient and their family members, including the primary caregiver, and healthcare professionals (defined as physicians, nurses, a social worker, case manager, and the chaplain) in discussions concerning cancer treatment, optimal symptom management, prognostication, advanced directives, and discharge planning" [74,75]. Currently, a paucity of research

exists evaluating the impact of family conferences on clinical outcomes including patient and caregivers' satisfaction with information giving and assessments of quality palliative care (i.e., hospice enrollment, bereavement outcomes) in the palliative care setting.

Guidelines [76,77] on conducting family meetings have been developed and are based on expert opinion and qualitative studies and extrapolated from studies of conferences conducted in ICUs. Pilot work investigating the benefits of family meetings using clinical guidelines proved useful and reduced the information needs of family caregivers [78]; however, further testing via a controlled trial with a larger sample size was recommended. In a pilot study, Hudson examined 19 family meetings revealing that caregivers found them to be useful and reduced their information needs [78]. In the same study, benefits of family meetings for participants included meeting the health-care team, providing a forum to ask questions and obtain information, clarifying goals of care, and allowing them to express feelings and mediate differences within the family [78].

In a prospective study of 140 family meetings in a palliative care unit, family conferences were found to have a high frequency of emotional expression by cancer patients and their family members and frequently involved discussions regarding a patient's goals of care, information regarding prognosis, and how to manage symptoms, but less frequently regarding issues of the well-being of the family caregiver, advanced directives, and what symptoms to expect at the end of life [79]. Of note, patient participation in the family conference was associated with discussions regarding prognosis and what dying patients may experience to less likely occur [79].

In addition, patients who participate in a family conference often misunderstand and are unable to recall what was discussed during the meetings including issues such as prognosis [80]. In a recent study, 60% of dying patients did not recall end-of-life discussions that had recently been conducted [64]. Interestingly, patients with lower functional status and increase symptom burden had a higher recollection of these discussions [64]. Currently, it is unclear if critically ill patients are able to grasp the information provided to them during family meetings and more research is needed.

FAMILY CONFERENCES IN THE ICU SETTING

Researchers have observed that in an ICU, a family conference improves communication between health-care providers and a patient's family [54–59,81]. Studies on family conferences in the ICU setting have shown improvements in communication [54–59], reductions in the burden of bereavement [82], and even reductions in the length of stay [83]. Of note, studies of end-of-life conferences in the ICU setting often lack active participation by patients in the meetings, which was noted to be less than 5% [82,84], since patients are often too critically ill, intubated, or too sedated.

In the ICU setting, a landmark trial [82] using the mnemonic VALUE (V, value and appreciate what family members say; A, acknowledge the family member's emotions; L, listen; U, understand who the patient is as a person by asking open-ended questions; and E, elicit questions from all family members) [85] to provide consistency of therapeutic communication in family conferences led to measurable benefits including decreased posttraumatic stress disorder, anxiety, and depression.

PAIN, SYMPTOM MANAGEMENT, AND PRACTICAL CONCERNS OF FAMILY CAREGIVERS

Chronically ill patients, such as those with advanced cancer, may experience severe physical and psychosocial symptoms, including pain, dyspnea, fatigue, anorexia/cachexia, depression, and sleep disorders [86,87], which are often inadequately treated [88,89]. The management of pain is reported to be a major concern of family caring for patients with a life-threatening illness and [36,90,91] uncontrolled pain at the end of life and can result in distress and feelings of guilt or helplessness in family caregivers [92] and lead to the transfer of patients from the home setting to the hospital.

It is not uncommon for family caregivers to fear the use of opioids secondary to concerns of addiction or side effects such as respiratory depression, which can increase the difficulty in controlling pain in the home setting. Unfortunately, they are limited well-designed trials of interventions addressing caregiver's ability to manage symptoms, including pain control, at the end of life. After-hours telephone and videophone services have been studied and found to be simple, effective, and valued by patients and family caregivers who could access these services even when they were not in close proximity to a hospital [93–95]. Educational programs administered in the patient's home consisting of a diary recording the intensity of pain and administration of opioids, video demonstration of how to safely transfer patients without pain, and education pamphlet describing the proper use of opioids resulted in improved administration of pain medications and confidence in caregivers [36]. Home care nurses who provide paid assistance with caregiving and emotional support for both patients and the primary caregiver were reported to be a valuable source of information [70], as well as having 24 hours access to a health-care provider [96]. In another study where caregivers participated via videophone in hospice interdisciplinary team meetings as opposed to nonparticipation, there was a significant increase in the discussion regarding pain management in the meetings [97]. The only well-designed, double-blinded, randomized, controlled trial examining caregiver-guided pain interventions including educational information about pain management and a cognitive–behavioral pain coping strategy for caregivers reported that caregivers had an increased sense of confidence in managing pain, but unfortunately, the patient's pain level was not significantly reduced [98].

Dyspnea, sensation of shortness of breath, is a common symptom in patients with cancer, heart failure, and lung disorders such as chronic obstructive pulmonary disease. Dyspnea not only results in distress for patients but impacts their caregiver's quality of life [99]. Breathlessness has been reported to be associated with low family well-being and increased likelihood of death in the hospital setting for cancer patients [100]. The caregiver burden of patients with dyspnea was higher than patients without shortness of breath [101] and noted to be the most common symptoms of palliative care appropriate patients who presented to the emergency department [102]. Interventions targeting caregivers of patients with dyspnea need to be developed in order to maintain better control of symptoms and prevent caregiver burnout.

Loss of appetite is a common symptom at the end of life and can result in distress in family caregivers. A recent study surveying the impact of poor oral intake among bereaved caregivers has recommended interventions to decrease the sense of helplessness and guilt associated with a loved one losing weight such as providing education on hydration and nutrition at the end of life and emotional support to family caregivers [103]. Health-care providers need to educate family caregivers that weight loss secondary to an illness is not equivalent to starvation and difficult to reverse, stress the pleasure of tasting small bites of food over attempting to increase caloric intake, and emphasize the need to participate in the social aspects of eating at the dinner table with the family. Unfortunately, a qualitative study involving bereaved family caregivers highlights the limited communication provided to families regarding nutrition at the end of life [104].

Practical information provided by health-care providers on administration of medications, feeding, dressing, and bathing patients to family caregivers can also be helpful. Family caregivers often take over many roles, which may have been previously assigned to the patient, such as managing the household finances, working to provide income for the family, or coordinating the schedule and care of the children. Role reversal may lead to distress for both patients and their primary caregiver if they are unable to adapt to their new responsibilities.

In addition, the financial burden of caregiving can add to the distress faced by the family of a chronically ill patient. In many countries, medical care has been migrating from the hospital setting to an outpatient/home setting, which results in patients and their family being responsible for a larger share of health-care costs. Families often have to sell assets, borrow money, or work additional jobs in order to meet the financial costs of health care [104]. In the United States, approximately 42 million family caregivers are providing unpaid assistance for ill patients with an estimated economic value of $450 million [105]. It is not uncommon for families frequently declare bankruptcy in order to escape the financial burden they accumulate when one member develops an illness. In one study conducted in Australia, family caregivers had to forgo work or work fewer hours in order to provide care for a loved one [106]. In a study conducted in Canada, unpaid caregiving was the largest cost for providing care at the end of life with monthly costs increasing exponentially with proximity to death [107].

Often, there are limited or no resources available for patients and their family, which forces patients to choose from continuing their medications versus using their income to pay for food or other essentials. Health-care providers can assess the financial burden for patients and identify resources available to lessen the cost of care to some degree. One simple intervention is to review a patient's medications and substitute more affordable medication for expensive drugs or even eliminate unnecessary medications that have been ineffective at controlling symptoms or found to be unnecessary.

When the caregiving responsibilities become overwhelming, respite services are indicated. By admitting patients temporarily to a hospital or inpatient hospice or by providing assistance at home at night, family caregivers are relieved briefly from the burden of caregiving and allowed to rest and reenergize. Family caregivers often are deprived of sleep [108], and research examining a community-based night respite service for critically ill cancer patients reported positive outcomes including more patients dying at home, family caregivers being able to manage patients at home, and reduced overall costs secondary to less patients being hospitalized [109].

In the last days of life, distress often escalates for both patients and their family caregivers. Family caregivers have expressed fears concerning providing care when patients are at the end of life and at the actively dying stage and appreciate knowing the signs of imminent death [110–112]. Preparing family caregivers for the last stages of life can lessen the emotional distress of witnessing the actively dying stage and normalize the process so as not too confuse signs of death with symptoms of increased pain or shortness of breath. For instance, the "death rattle" or signs of agonal breathing may be perceived by family members that the patient is short of breath. In addition to the appropriate medical interventions to control symptoms when indicated, health-care providers should provide reassurance and clarification of what is a normal or an expected sign associated with the actively dying stage.

COPING OF FAMILY CAREGIVERS

Family members of patients with a chronic illness will encounter caregiver distress and psychological symptoms including anticipatory grief and experience bereavement after the death of a loved one. Family caregivers rely on coping mechanism during this stressful period in their lives. Coping has been defined as "a person's cognitive and behavioral efforts to manage (reduce, minimize, master, or tolerate) the internal and external demands of the person-environment transaction that is appraised as taxing or exceeding the person's resources" [113].

To help with caring for a patient with a chronic illness, various coping strategies used by family caregivers such as reliance on social support, rationalization, and acceptance have been identified [114]. Other coping strategies noted in one recent study include distraction, mental stimulation, disengagement from stressful thoughts, and viewing the positive aspects of caregiving [115]. In one study, a positive coping strategy identified as "taking one day at a time" was noted to be helpful in managing the uncertainty about the future [116]. Other positive coping strategies include accepting responsibility, planful

problem solving, and positive reappraisal [47,113]. Some evidence indicates that positive coping strategies prevent depression in the caregiver and are noted to be associated with a better functional status of the patient [117,118].

Family caregivers engaging in negative expectation coping that included excessive worrying, expecting the worst, taking tension out on others, or perceiving that they were poorly coping with the caregiving role were more likely to experience a sense of entrapment in their responsibilities as a caregiver and emotional fatigue [119]. In the same study, these negative expectation coping strategies were associated with symptoms of anxiety, guilt, and depression, while positive coping mechanisms such as hoping for improvement, finding purpose, setting goals, and taking one step at a time were associated with less emotional exhaustion.

Interventions to support the psychosocial well-being of family caregivers can be organized as educational approaches, skills training to develop effective coping strategies and problem-solving skills, and therapeutic counseling [120]. Promising interventions include counseling sessions with caregivers that stress problem-solving approaches to manage the responsibilities of caregiving, techniques to enhance communication between patient and caregiver, and emphasis on the self-care of the family caregiver [121]. Another more recent trial that showed significant benefits for family caregivers involves five 2 hours home visits by a psychologist, two 30 min sessions over the telephone, and a follow-up telephone session at 6 months with both patient and primary caregiver [122]. Session involved meeting the information needs of the primary caregiver, interventions directed an enhancing a patient's body image, and techniques for both patient and caregiver to improve coping and problem-solving skills [122]. More studies are needed in examining interventions for primary caregivers that examine their ability to reduce family caregiver distress and prevent burnout.

FAMILY FUNCTIONING AND CULTURAL SENSITIVITY

Families who have open and effective communication prior to the development of an illness have been reported to cope and function better than families who have difficulty communicating with each other [123]. In addition, caring for patients with a chronic illness may cause family conflict resulting in less support from family or friends, which only exacerbates the distress of the primary caregiver [124]. Care of a chronically ill patient requires availability of caregivers throughout the day and night. The primary caregiver in a dysfunctional family may be unable to recruit or persuade other family members to assist in the role as a secondary caregiver. Also if the goals of care differ between the patient and individuals within the family, conflict can develop resulting in patients having to align themselves with one family member over another. In addition, studies have shown that poor family function results in an increased burden of bereavement after the patient has died [125,126], and family-focused grief therapy may be indicated for dysfunctional families in order for them to accept the loss of a loved one [127].

Health-care professionals working with family members of chronically ill patients must also be mindful of the cultural and ethnic diversity of values as they communicate with and provide psychosocial support to critically ill patients and their family. Culture and acculturation can influence attitudes, beliefs, preferences, and behaviors with respect to health care. Issues regarding disclosure of medical information, gender-determined role restrictions for caregivers, intergenerational shifts in values, and acceptance of the psychosocial sequelae of a chronic illness may vary across different cultures.

In the United States and other Western European countries, there has been a shift in the ethical framework for communication during the end of life towards an emphasis on patient autonomy and full disclosure of information. In contrast, non-Western cultures emphasize the ethical principle of nonmaleficence and feel that honest disclosure regarding death and end-of-life issues will result in more harm than good for the patient. Research has emphasized three areas of end-of-life care that cultural attitudes, which if not taken into consideration, may result in patient and family distress and include breaking "bad news," decision-making preferences for medical care, and willingness to complete advanced directives and acceptance of end-of-life care. In addition to being mindful of cultural beliefs of particular ethnic groups, health-care providers need to be aware that compared to whites of European descent, ethnic minorities exhibit a greater degree of variability in their cultural views and preferences [128].

In order to communicate medical information effectively and ensure a high degree of patient and family satisfaction, health-care providers need to be cognizant of a patient and families' acceptance of "truth telling." In many countries, health-care professionals will conceal a patient's diagnosis or a poor prognosis from patients and communicate bad news only to their family. For example, in many Asian cultures, it is felt to be unacceptably cruel to inform a cancer diagnosis to a patient [129,130]. Also recent Bosnian immigrants to America reported a preference for Bosnian physicians who indirectly communicate the seriousness of an illness as opposed to American physicians whose blunt truth telling was perceived to be unnecessarily harsh [131]. In addition, some cultures believe that the acknowledgment of impending death may become a self-fulfilling prophecy [132]. Native Americans, for example, will emphasize thinking and speaking in a "positive way" [133], which may result in conflict and distrust of health-care providers who are open and honest regarding a diagnosis or a poor prognosis. In cases where patients and family request nondisclosure, clinician can offer to divulge the diagnosis and treatment options in order to respect cultural norms but also allow the patient to refuse medical information and direct communication to either their family, friend, or confidant responsible for the medical decision making [134].

In addition, medical jargon or terminology that obscures the seriousness of a diagnosis is often used by physicians outside the United States. Japanese and African physicians have been reported to use terms including "growth," "mass," "blood disease," or "unclean tissue," rather than disclosing that the patient has cancer [129]. In the United States, family members of patients from minority groups may also conceal information by intentionally not translating the diagnosis or accurate treatment information to the patient [135], which emphasizes the need for a professional medical translator when communicating end-of-life issues to a non-English speaking patient [136].

Decisional role preferences may vary across cultures and ethnic groups. In the United States, patient autonomy takes precedence as long as a patient has cognitive function or is not impaired by a psychiatric illness or medication. In minority groups, alternative models of decision making are emphasized and include family based, physician based, and shared physician and family based [28]. For African-American families, a recent systematic review emphasized the preference for family-centered decision making [137]. As compared to African-Americans, non-Hispanic white patients preferred to be more exclusive with family member participation in end-of-life discussions [138]. In the same study, African-American had a preference for greater spiritual support and protection of life at all costs, while non-Hispanic whites favored more medical information, valued information regarding the cost of treatment, and had more concerns concerning maintaining their quality of life [138].

Mexican-Americans, as compared to individuals of European descent, prefer that family members, rather than the patient, have decision-making power regarding end-of-life issues such as requesting life support [133]. In one recent study, Hispanic-American patients preferred a higher degree of patient autonomy than Hispanic-Latin Americans; however, the majority in each group favored a shared decision making, family-centered approach to decisions regarding end-of-life care [139]. These findings highlight the process of acculturation of Hispanic-American immigrants whose decisional role preferences may often quickly shift. Even among a specific ethnic group, variations in preferences for end-of-life care may exist, and health-care providers need to assess for these preferences and then communicate information in a culturally sensitive way.

In addition, many cultural groups have a high degree of respect and admiration for physicians. Pakistani physicians often are adopted into family unit, which allows them to participate in sensitive end-of-life discussions [140]. In Russia, physicians, rather than patients, have been reported to make decisions regarding continuing life support [141]. In addition, Eastern European immigrants preferred physicians who took a paternalistic approach to decision making and cited that physicians are the experts and should be the ones with the knowledge to make difficult medical decision, which reduces the burden on the family [131].

Research also shows significant discrepancies to end-of-life care within different ethnic groups. Asians, African-Americans, and Hispanics have lower rates of advanced directive completion [142,143]. Low rates of completion of advanced directives could be attributed to distrust of the health-care system, disparities in health-care delivery, or cultural preferences regarding death [144]. Also African-American patients were less likely to accept DNR status, more likely than white patients to change DNR status to a more aggressive treatment plan [145], and less likely to enroll in hospice care [27]. By obtaining a better understanding of a patient and family's cultural views and decision-making preferences, health-care providers can apply a culturally sensitive approach to end-of-life care.

CONCLUSIONS

Distress is not uncommon for family caregivers of patients with chronic illnesses. Family caregivers are often unpaid, are underappreciated, and lack the support of health-care providers resulting in emotional exhaustion and burnout. Multiple factors contribute to the distress of the family caregiver, and palliative care professional should be able to assess and intervene to diminish the suffering experienced by both patients and their caregivers. Health-care professional providing timely and appropriate medical information can give the family caregiver the confidence to provide end-of-life care and encourage caregivers to express emotions to lessen the psychological distress that accompanies the role of being a caregiver, and identifying successful coping strategies allows caregivers to handle the responsibilities of caring for a critically ill spouse, parent, friend, or child. Interventions, such as peer support groups, emphasis on the importance of self-care, and education directed to increasing the confidence of the primary caregiver, show potential in decreasing caregiver distress, and more studies are needed to identify and treat the burden facing family caregivers.

Key learning points

- Psychosocial support for both patients and their family is at the foundation of palliative care.
- The definition of family is open ended and should be defined by the patient.
- Although there are positive aspects associated with the act of caregiving, distress from the burden of providing care can lead to a combination of physical and emotional distress.
- Research reveals increased feeling of helplessness among family caregivers, which was associated with the progression of a patient's illness, the degree of struggle undergone to obtain needed medical services, and the inability of caregivers to relieve a patient's pain and discomfort.
- Predictors of caregiver burnout for the family caregiver include restrictions in social life, indicators of poor health or comorbidities, and a negative outlook regarding the role of being a family caregiver.
- A family caregiver's self-esteem, confidence in caregiving, and amount of social network including family support have been shown to alleviate the distress of caregivers and enhance their ability to provide care.

- Barriers related to family communication that can be summarized by three key problematic areas include concealing feelings, information exchange, and coping with helplessness.
- Preliminary studies of family conferences were found to be useful and an emotional experience for both patients and their family members.
- Benefits of family conferences for participants included meeting the health-care team, providing a forum to ask questions and obtain information, and allowing for the clarification of the goals of care.
- The management of pain is reported to be a major concern of family caring for patients with a life-threatening illness.
- Educational programs administered in the patient's home consisting of a diary recording the intensity of pain and administration of opioids, video demonstration of how to safely transfer patients without pain, and education pamphlet describing the proper use of opioids resulted in improved administration of pain medications and confidence in caregivers.
- After-hours telephone and videophone services have been found to be simple, effective, and valued by patients and family caregivers in meeting their information needs and can be accessed even when they were not in close proximity to a hospital.
- Respite services either in a facility or provided at home during the night for family caregivers allow for temporary relief from the burden of caregiving.
- Family caregivers have expressed fears concerning providing care when patients are at the end of life and the actively dying stage and appreciate knowing the signs of imminent death.
- Promising interventions to help support family caregivers include counseling sessions that stress problem-solving approaches to manage the responsibilities of caregiving, techniques to enhance communication between patient and caregiver, and emphasis on the self-care of caregivers.
- Health-care professionals working with family members of chronically ill patients must also be mindful of the cultural and ethnic diversity of values as they communicate with and provide psychosocial support to critically ill patients and their family.

ACKNOWLEDGMENT

The authors would like to acknowledge Linda J. Kristjanson for her previous work on the family care chapter in the first edition.

REFERENCES

1 www.who.int/cancer/palliative/definition/en/
2 Canadian Palliative Care Association. Standards for palliative care provision: Canadian palliative care association, Ottawa, 1998.
3 Longacre ML. Cancer caregivers information needs and resource preferences. *J Cancer Educ* 2013;28(2):297–305.

4 Brody EM. The Donald P. Kent Memorial Lecture. Patient care as normative family stress. *Gerontologist* 1985;25(1):19–29.

5 Bass DM, Noekler LS. The influence of family caregivers on elders' use of in-home services: An expanded conceptual framework. *J Health Soc Behav* 1987;28(2):184–196.

6 Kristjanson LJ, Aoun S. Palliative care for families: Remembering the hidden patients. *Can J Psychiatry* 2004;49(6):359–365.

7 Burns CM, Abernethy AP, Dal Grande E, Currow DC. Uncovering an invisible network of direct caregivers at the end of life: A population study. *Palliat Med* 2013;27(7):608–615.

8 Mitchell JM, Kemp BJ. Quality of life in assisted home living. *J Gerontol B Psychol Sci* 2000;55(2):117–127.

9 Tang ST, McCorkle R. Determinants of congruence between the preferred and actual place of death for terminally ill cancer patients. *J Palliat Care* 2003;19(4):230–237.

10 Hunt RW, Fazekas BS, Luke CG, Roder DM. Where patients with cancer die in South Australia, 1990–1999: A population-based review. *Med J Aust* 2001;175(10):526–529.

11 Noekler LS, Bass DM. Home care for elderly persons: Linkages between formal and informal caregivers. *J Gerontol* 1989;44(2):S63–S70.

12 John R, Hennessy CH, Dyeson TB, Garrett MD. Toward the conceptualization and measurement of caregiver burden among Pueblo Indian family caregivers. *Gerontologist* 2001;41:210–219.

13 Lawton M, Moss M, Kleban MH, Glicksman A, Rovine M. A two-factor model of caregiving appraisal and psychological well-being. *J Gerontol* 1991;46:181–189.

14 Young RF. Elders, families, and illness. *J Aging Stud* 1994;8(1):1–15.

15 Merz EM, Consedine NS. The association of family support and wellbeing in later life depends on adult attachment style. *Attach Hum Dev* 2009;11(2):203–221.

16 Grbick C, Parker D, Maddocks I. The emotions and coping strategies of caregivers of family members with a terminal cancer. *J Palliat Care* 2001;17(1):30–36.

17 Kim Y, Schulz R, Carver CS. Benefit-finding in the cancer caregiving experience. *Psycosom Med* 2007;69(3):283–291.

18 Foley KL, Tung HJ, Mutran EJ. Self-gain and self-loss among African American and white caregivers. *J Gerontol B Psychol Sci Soc Sci* 2002;57(1):S14–S25.

19 Ferrel B, Mazanec P. Family Caregiver. In: Hurria A, Balducci L., eds. *Geriatric Oncology: Treatment, Assessment, and Management.* Springer, New York, 2009, pp. 135–155.

20 Montgomery RV, Gonyea J, Hooyman N. Caregiving and the experience of subjective and objective burden. *Fam Relat* 1985;34(1):19–26.

21 Aneshensel CS, Pearlin LI, Schuler RH. Stress, role captivity, and the cessation of caregiving. *J Health Soc Behav* 1993;34(1):54–70.

22 Colerick EF, George LK. Predictors of institutionalization among caregivers of patients with Alzheimer's disease. *J Am Geriatr Soc* 1986;34(7):493–498.

23 Hills GA. Caregivers of the elderly: Hidden patients and health team members. *Top Geriatr Rehabil* 1998;14(1):1–8.

24 Mitchell AJ, Ferguson DW, Gill J, Paul J, Symonds P. Depression and anxiety in long-term cancer survivors compared with spouses and healthy controls: A systematic review and meta-analysis. *Lancet Oncol* 2013;14:721–732.

25 Braithwaite VA. *Bound to Care.* Allen Unwin, Sydney, New South Wales, Australia, 1992.

26 Field MJ, Cassell CK., eds. *Approaching Death: Improving Care at the End of Life.* Institute of Medicine Committee on Care at the End of Life, National Academy Press, Washington, DC, 1997.

27 McKinley ED, Garrett JM, Evans AT, Danis M. Differences in end-of-life decision making among black and white ambulatory cancer patients. *J Gen Intern Med* 1996;11(11):651–656.

28 Hern HE, Koenig BA, Moore LJ, Marshall PA. The difference that culture can make in end-of-life decision making. *Camb Q Healthc Ethics* 1998;7(1):27–40.

29 Pearce MJ, Singer JL, Prigerson HG. Religious coping among caregivers in terminally ill patients, main effects on psychosocial mediators. *J Health Psychol* 2006;11(5):743–759.

30 Burton AM, Sautter JM, Tulsky JA et al. Burden and well-being among a diverse sample of cancer, congestive heart failure, and chronic obstructive pulmonary disease caregivers. *J Pain Symptom Manage* 2012;44(3):410–420.

31 Grov EK, Dahl AA, Moum T, Fossa SD. Anxiety, depression, and quality of life in caregivers of patients with cancer in late palliative phase. *Ann Oncol* 2005;16(7):1185–1191.

32 Grunfeld E, Coyle D, Whelan T et al. Family caregiver burden: Results of a longitudinal study of breast cancer patients and their principal caregivers. *Can Med Assoc J* 2004;170(12):795–801.

33 Payne S, Smith P, Dean S. Identifying the concerns of informal carers in palliative care. *Palliat Med* 1999;13(1):37–44.

34 Garrido R, Menezed PR. Impact on caregivers of elderly patients with dementia treated at a psychogeriatric service. *Rev Saude Publica* 2004;28(6):835–841.

35 LoBiondo-Wood G, Williams L, Kouzekanani K, McGhee C. Family adaptation to a child's transplant: Pretransplant phase. *Prog Transplant* 2000;10(2):81–87.

36 Oldham L, Kristjanson LJ. Development of a pain management programme for family carers of advanced cancer patients. *Int J Palliat Nurs* 2004;10(2):91–99.

37 Perreault A, Fothergill-Bourbonnais F, Fiset V. The experience of family members caring for a dying loved one. *Int J Palliat Nurs* 2004;10(3):133–143.

38 Andershed B. Relatives in end-of-life care. Part 1: A systematic review of the literature from the five last years, January 1999–February 2004. *J Clin Nurs* 2006;15(9):1158–1169.

39 Brazil K, Bedard M, Willison K, Hode M. Caregiving and its impact on families of the terminally ill. *Aging Ment Health* 2003;7(5):376–382.

40 Schulz R, Martire LM. Family caregiving of person with dementia: Prevalence, health effects, and support strategies. *Am J Geriatr Psychiatry* 2004;12(3):240–249.

41 Hubbell L, Hubbell K. The burnout risk for male caregivers providing care to spouses afflicted with Alzheimer's disease. *J Health Hum Serv Adm* 2002;25:115–132.

42 von Kanel R. The burnout syndrome: A medical perspective. *Praxis (Bern)* 1994;97(9):477–487.

43 Almberg B, Grafstrom M, Winblad B. Caring for a demented elderly person—Burden and burnout among caregiving relatives. *J Adv Nurs* 1997;25(1):109–116.

44 Truzzi A, Valente L, Ulstein I, Engelhardt E, Laks J, Engedal K. Burnout in familial caregivers of patients with dementia. *Rev Bras Psiquiatr* 2012;34(4):404–412.

45 Takai M, Takahashi M, Iwamitsu Y et al. The experience of burnout among home caregivers of patients with dementia: Relations to depression and quality of life. *Arch Gerontol Geriatr* 2009;49(1):e1–e5.

46 Takai M, Takahashi M, Iwamitsu Y, Oishi S, Miyaoka H. Subjective experiences of family caregivers of patients with dementia as predictive factors of quality of life. *Psychogeriatrics* 2011;11(2):98–104.

47 Pearlin LI, Mullan JT, Semple SJ, Skaff MM. Caregiving and the stress process: An overview of concepts and their measures. *Gerontologist* 1990;30(5):583–594.

48 Braithwaite V. Contextual or general stress outcomes: Making choices through caregiving. *Gerontologist* 2000;40(6):706–717.

49 Henriksson A, Arestedt K. Exploring factors and caregiver outcomes associated with feelings of preparedness for caregiving in family caregivers in palliative care: A correlational, cross-sectional study. *Palliat Med* 2013;27(7):639–646.

50 Greenwood N, Habibi R, Mackenzie A, Drennan V, Easton N. Peer support for carers: A qualitative investigation of the experiences of carers and peer volunteers. *Am J Alzheimers Dis Other Demen* 2013;28(6):617–626. June 30. (Epub ahead of print).

51 Maslach C, Schaufeli WB, Leiter MP. Job burnout. *Annu Rev Psychol* 2001;52:397–422.

52 Vachon MLS. Emotional problems in palliative medicine: Patient, family, and professional. In: Doyle D, Hanks GWC, MacDonald N, eds. *Oxford Textbook of Palliative Medicine.* Oxford University Press, Oxford, U.K., 1993, pp. 575–605.

53 Hinton J. Sharing or withholding awareness of dying between husband and wife. *J Psychosom Res* 1981;25(5):337–343.

54 National Breast Cancer Center. *Clinical Practice Guidelines for the Psychosocial Care of Adults with Cancer.* National Health and Medical Research Council, Canberra, Australian Capital Territory, Australia, 2003.

55 Stapleton RD, Engelberg RA, Wenrich MD, Goss CH, Curtis JR. Clinician statements and family satisfaction with family conferences in the intensive care unit. *Crit Care Med* 2006;34(6):1679–1685.

56 West HF, Engelberg RA, Wenrich MD, Curtis JR. Expressions of non-abandonment during the intensive care unit family conference. *J Palliat Med* 2005;8(4):797–807.

57 Curtis JR, Engelberg RA, Wenrich MD, Shannon SE, Treece PD, Rubenfeld GD. Missed opportunities during family conferences about end-of-life care in the intensive care unit. *Am J Respir Crit Care Med* 2005;171(8):844–849.

58 McDonagh JR, Elliott TB, Engelberg RA, Treece PD, Shannon SE, Rubenfeld GD, Patrick DL, Curtis JR. Family satisfaction with family conferences about end-of-life care in the intensive care unit: Increased proportion of family speech is associated with increased satisfaction. *Crit Care Med* 2004;32(7):1484–1488.

59 Curtis JR. Communicating about end-of-life care with patients and families in the intensive care unit. *Crit Care Clin* 2004;20(3):363–380.

60 Lilly CM, De Meo DL, Sonna LA, Haley KJ, Massaro AF, Wallace RF, Cody S. An intensive communication intervention for the critically ill. *Am J Med* 2000;109(6):469–475.

61 Boyle DK, Miller PA, Forbes-Thompson SA. Communication and end-of-life care in the intensive care unit: Patient, family, and clinician outcomes. *Crit Care Nurs Q* 2005;28(4):302–316.

62 Ringdal G, Jordhoy M, Kaasa S. Measuring quality of palliative care: Psychometric properties of the FAMCARE Scale. *Qual Life Res* 2003;12:167–176.

63 Prigerson HG. Socialization to dying: Social determinants of death acknowledgement and treatment among terminally ill geriatric patients. *J Health Soc Behav* 1992;33(4):378–395.

64 Wright A, Zhang B, Ray A et al. Association between end-of-life discussions, patient mental health, medical care near death, and caregiver bereavement adjustment. *JAMA* 2008;300(14):1665–1673.

65 Clayton JM, Butow PN, Tattersall MH The needs of terminally ill cancer patients versus those of caregivers for information regarding prognosis and end-of-life issues. *Cancer* 2005;103(9):1957–1964.

66 Hagerty R, Butow P, Ellis P et al. Cancer patients' preferences for communication in the metastatic setting. *J Clin Oncol* 2004;22:1721–1730.

67 Butow PN, Maclean M, Dunn SM et al. The dynamics of change: Cancer patients' preferences for information, involvement and support. *Ann Oncol* 1997;8:857–863.

68 Clayton JM, Butow PN, Tattersall MH et al. Randomized controlled trial of a prompt list to help advanced cancer patients and their caregivers to ask questions about prognosis and end-of-life care. *J Clin Oncol* 2007;25(6):715.

69 Tattersall MH, Butow PN, Griffin AM, Dunn SM. The take-home message: Patients prefer consultation audiotapes to summary letters. *J Clin Oncol* 1994;12(6):1305.

70 Kristjanson LJ. Caring for families of people with cancer: Evidence and interventions. *Cancer Forum* 2004;28(3):13–15.

71 Northouse PG, Northouse LL. Communication and cancer: Issues confronting patients, health professionals, and family members. *J Psychosoc Oncol* 1998;5(3):17–46.

72 Szmuilowicz E, el-Jawahri A, Chiappetta L, Kamdar M, Block S. Improving residents' end-of-life communication skills with a short retreat: A randomized controlled trial. *J Palliat Med* 2010;13(4):439–452.

73 Weeks JC, Catalano PJ, Cronin A et al. Patients' expectations about effects of chemotherapy for advanced cancer. *N Engl J Med* 2012;367:1616–1625.

74 Moneymaker K. The family conference. *J Palliat Med* 2005;8(1):157.

75 Hansen P, Cornish P, Kayser K. Family conferences as forums for decision making in hospital settings. *Soc Work Health Care* 1998;27(3):57–74.

76 Hudson P, Quinn K, Hanlon B, Aranda S. Family meetings in palliative care: Multidisciplinary clinical practice guidelines. *BMC Palliat Care* 2008;7:12.

77 Clayton JM, Hancock KM, Butow PN et al. Clinical practice guidelines for communication prognosis and end-of-life issues with adults in the advanced stages of a life-limiting illness, and their caregivers. *Med J Aust* 2006;186(12 Suppl):S77–S108.

78 Hudson P, Thomas T, Quinn K. Family meetings in palliative care: Are they effective? *Palliat Med* 2009;23(2):150–157.

79 Dev R, Coulson L, Del Fabbro E et al. A prospective study of family conferences: Effects of patient presence on emotional expression and end-of-life discussions. *J Pain Symptom Manage* 2013;46(4): 536–545. March 15.

80 Hagerty RG, Butow PN, Ellis PM et al. Communicating with realism and hope: Incurable cancer patient's views on the disclosure of prognosis. *J Clin Oncol* 2005;23(6):1278–1288.

81 Curtis JR, Patrick DL, Shannon SE, Treece PD, Engelberg RA, Rubenfeld GD. The family conference as a focus to improve communication about end-of-life care in the intensive care unit: Opportunities for improvement. *Crit Care Med* 2001;29(2 Suppl):N26–N33.

82 Lautrette A, Darmon M, Megarbane B et al. A communication strategy and brochure for relatives of patients dying in the ICU. *N Engl J Med* 2007;356(5):469–478.

83 Ahrens T, Yancey V, Kollef M. Improving family communications at the end of life: Implications for length of stay in the intensive care unit and resource use. *Am J Crit Care* 2003;12(4):317–334.

84 Luce JM. Making decision about the forgoing of life-sustaining therapy. *Am J Respir Crit Care Med* 1997;156:1715–1718.

85 Curtis JF, Patrick DL, Shannon SE et al. The family conference as a focus to improve communication about end-of-life care in the intensive care unit: Opportunities for improvement. *Crit Care Med* 2001;29(2 Suppl):N26–N33.

86 Trask PC, Griffith KA. The identification of empirically derived cancer patient subgroups using psychosocial variables. *J Psychosom Res* 2004;57:287–295.

87 Walsh D, Donnelly S, Rybicki L. The symptoms of advanced cancer: Relationship to age, gender, and performance status in 1,000 patients. *Support Care Cancer* 2000;8(3):175–190.

88 Lynn J, Teno JM, Phillips RS, Wu AW, Desbiens N, Harrold J, Claessens MT, Wenger N, Kreling B, Connors AF Jr. Perceptions by family members of the dying experience of older and seriously ill patients. SUPPORT investigators. Study to understand prognoses and preferences for outcomes and risks of treatments. *Ann Intern Med* 1997;126(2):97–106.

89 Teno JM, Clarridge BR, Casey V, Welch LC, Wetle T, Shield R, Mor V. Family perspectives on end-of-life care at the last place of care. *JAMA* 2004;291(1):88–93.

90 Bucher JA, Trostle GB, Moore, M. Family reports of cancer pain, pain relief and prescription access. *Cancer Pract* 1999;7(2):71–77.

91 Ferrel B. Pain observed: The experience of pain from the family caregiver's perspectives. *Clin Geriatr Med* 2001;17(3):595–609.

92 Ferrel B, Rhiner M, Cohen MZ, Grant M. Pain as a metaphor for illness. Part I: Impact of cancer pain on family caregivers. *Oncol Nurs Forum* 1991;18(8):1303–1309.

93 Bradford N, Irving H, Smith AC, Pedersen LA, Herbert A. Palliative care afterhours: A review of a phone support service. *J Pediatr Oncol Nurs* 2012;29(3):141–150.

94 Hudson P, Trauer T, Kelly B et al. Reducing the psychological distress of family caregivers of home-based palliative care patients: Short-term effects from a randomized controlled trial. *Psychooncology* 2013;22(9):1987–1993.

95 Demiris G, Parker Oliver D, Wittenberg-Lyles E et al. A non-inferiority trial of a problem-solving intervention for hospice caregivers: In person versus videophone. *J Palliat Med* 2012;15(6):653–660.

96 Kristjanson LJ. Quality of terminal care: Salient indicators identified by families. *J Palliat Care* 1989;5:21–28.

97 Oliver D, Demiris G, Wittenberg-Lyles E et al. Caregiver participation in hospice interdisciplinary team meetings via videophone technology: A pilot study to improve pain management. *Am J Hosp Palliat Care* 2010;27(7):465–473.

98 Keefe F, Ahles T, Sutton L et al. Partner-guided cancer pain management at the end of life: A preliminary study. *J Pain Symptom Manage* 2005;29(3):263–272.

99 Booth S, Silvester S, Todd C. Breathlessness in cancer and chronic obstructive pulmonary disease: Using a qualitative approach to describe the experience of patients and carers. *Palliat Support Care* 2003;1(4):337–344.

100 Edmonds P, Higginson I, Altmann D et al. Is the presence of dyspnea a risk factor for morbidity in cancer patients? *J Pain Symptom Manage* 2000;19(1):15–22.

101 Emanuel EJ, Fairclough DL, Slutsman J et al. Understanding economic and other burdens of terminal illness: The experience of patients and their caregivers. *Ann Intern Med* 2000;132(6):451–459.

102 Beynon T, Gomes B, Murtagh FE et al. How common are palliative care needs among older people who die in the emergency department? *Emerg Med J* 2011;28(6):491–495.

103 Yamagishi A, Morita T, Miyashita M et al. The care strategy for families of terminally ill cancer patients who become unable to take nourishment orally: Recommendations from a nationwide survey of bereaved family members' experiences. *J Pain Symptom Manage* 2010;40(5):671–683.

104 Raijmakers NJH, Clark JB, van Zuylen L, Allan SG, van der Heide A. Bereaved relatives' perspectives of the patient's oral intake towards the end of life: A qualitative study. *Palliat Med* 2013;27(7):665–672.

105 Feinberg L, Reinhard SC, Houseer A, Choula R. *Valuing the Invaluable: 2011 Update the Growing Contributions and Costs of Family Caregiving.* American Association of Retired Persons Public Policy Institute, Washington, DC, 2011.

106 Schofield HL, Herman HE, Bloch S, Howe A, Singh B. A profile of Australian family caregivers: Diversity of roles and circumstances. *Aust N Z J Public Health* 1997;21(1):59–66.

107 Chai H, Guerriere DN, Zagorski B, Coyte PC. The magnitude, share and determinants of unpaid care costs for home-based palliative care service provision in Toronto, Canada. *Health Soc Care Community* 2013;22(1):30–39, June 12. (Epub ahead of print).

108 Bramwell L, MacKenzie J, Laschinger H, Cameron N. Need for overnight respite for primary caregivers of hospice clients. *Cancer Nurs* 1995;18(5):337–343.

109 Kristjanson LJ, Cousins K, White K, Andrews L et al. Evaluation of a night respite community palliative care service. *Int J Palliat Nurs* 2004;10(2):84–90.

110 Krsitjanson LJ, Hudson P, Oldham L. Working with families in palliative care. In: Aranda S, O'Connor M, eds. *Palliative Care Nursing: A Guide to Practice.* (2nd edn.) AUSMED publications, Melbourne, Victoria, Australia, 2003.

111 Grbich C, Parker D, Maddocks I. Communication and information needs of caregivers of adult family members at diagnosis and during treatment of terminal cancer. *Prog Palliat Care* 2000;8(6):345–350.

112 Vachon M. Psychosocial needs of patients and families. *J Palliat Care* 1998;14(3):49–56.

113 Folkman S, Lazarus RS, Dunkel-Schetter C, DeLongis A, Gruen RJ. Dynamics of a stressful encounter: Cognitive appraisal, coping, and encounter outcomes. *J Pers Soc Psychol* 1986;50:992–1003.

114 Hull MM. Coping strategies of family caregivers in hospice home care. *Oncol Nurs Forum* 1992;19(8):1179–1187.

115 Epiphaniou E, Hamilton D, Bridger S et al. Adjusting to the caregiving role: The importance of coping and support. *Int J Palliat Nurs* 2012;18(11):541–545.

116 Higginson IJ, Wade AM, McCarthy M. Effectiveness of two palliative support teams. *J Public Health Med* 1992;14(1):50–56.

117 Carter PA, Acton GJ. Personality and coping: Predictors of depression and sleep problems among caregivers of individuals who have cancer. *J Gerontol Nurs* 2006;32:45–53.

118 Schumacher KL, Dodd MJ, Paul SM. The stress process in family caregivers of persons receiving chemotherapy. *Res Nurs Health* 1993;16:395–404.

119 Gaugler JE, Eppinger A, King J, Sanberg T, Regine WF. Coping and its effects on cancer caregiving. *Support Care Cancer* 2013;21:385–395.

120 Northouse LL, Katapodi MC, Song L, Zhang L, Mood DW. Interventions with family caregivers of cancer patients: Meta-analysis of randomized trials. *CA Cancer J Clin* 2010;60:317–339.

121 Blanchard C, Toseland R, McCallion P. The effects of a problem-solving intervention with spouses of cancer patients. *J Psychosoc Oncol* 1996;14:1–21.

122 Scott JL, Halford WK, Ward BG. United we stand? The effects of a coupling-coping intervention on adjustment to early stage breast or gynecological cancer. *J Consult Clin Psychol* 2004;72:1122–1135.

123 Kissane DW, Bloch S. Family grief. *Br J Psychiatry* 1994;164:728–740.

124 Charlesworth G, Shepstone L, Wilson E et al. Befriending carers of people with dementia: Randomized controlled trial. *BMJ* 2008;336(7656):1295–1297.

125 Kissane DW, Bloch S, Burns WI, McKenzie DP, Posterino M. Psychological morbidity in the families of patients with cancer. *Psychooncology* 1994;347–356.

126 Kissane DW, Bloch S, Burns WI, Patrick JD, Wallace CS, McKenzie DP. Perceptions of family functioning and cancer. *Psychooncology* 1994;3:259–269.

127 Kissane DW, McKenzie M, Bloch S et al. Family focused grief therapy: A randomized, controlled trial in palliative care and bereavement. *Am J Psychiatry* 2006;163(7):L1208–L1218.

128 Blackhall LJ, Murph ST, Frank G, Michel V, Azen S. Ethnicity and attitudes toward patient autonomy. *JAMA* 1995;274:820–825.

129 Holland JL, Geary N, Marchini A, Tross S. An international survey of physician attitudes and practice in regard to revealing the diagnosis of cancer. *Cancer Invest* 1987;5:151–154.

130 Matsumura S, Bito S, Liu H, Kahn K, Fukuhara S, Kagawa-Singer M et al. Acculturation of attitudes toward end-of-life care: A cross-cultural survey of Japanese American and Japanese. *J Gen Intern Med* 2002;17:531–539.

131 Searight HR, Gafford J. "It's like playing with your destiny": Bosnian immigrants' views of advance directives and end-of-life decision-making. *J Immigr Health* 2005;7(3):195–203.

132 Liu JM, Lin WC, Chen YM, Wu HW, Yao NS, Chen LT et al. The status of the do-not-resuscitate order in Chinese clinical trial patients in a cancer centre. *J Med Ethics* 1999;25:309–314.

133 Carrese JA, Rhodes LA. Western bioethics on the Navajo reservation. Benefit or harm? *JAMA* 1995;274:826–829.

134 Freedman B. Offering truth. One ethical approach to the uninformed cancer patient. *Arch Intern Med* 1993;153:572–576.

135 Kaufert JM, Putsch RW. Communication through interpreters in healthcare; ethical dilemmas arising from differences in class, culture, language, and power. *J Clin Ethics* 1997;8:71–87.

136 Herndon E, Joyce L. Getting the most from language interpreters. *Fam Pract Manag* 2004;11:37–40.

137 Wicher CP, Meeker MA. What influences African American end-of-life preferences? *J Health Care Poor Underserved* 2012;23:28–58.

138 Shrank WH, Kutner JS, Richardson T, Mulaski RA, Fischer S, Kagawa-Singer M. Focus group findings about the influence of culture on communication preferences in end-of-life care. *J Gen Intern Med* 2005;20(8):703–709.

139 Yennurajalingam S, Noguera A, Parson HA et al. A multicenter survey of Hispanic caregiver preferences for patient decision control in the United States and Latin America. *Palliat Med* 2013;27(7):692–698.

140 Moazam F. Families, patients, and physicians in medical decision-making: A Pakistani perspective. *Hasting Cent Rep* 2000;30:28–37.

141 Karakuzon M. Russia. In: Crippen D, Kilcullen JK, Kelly DF, eds. *Three Patients: International Perspectives on Intensive Care at the End-of-Life*. Kluwer Academic Publishers, Boston, MA, 2002, pp. 67–72.

142 Pietch JH, Braun KL. Autonomy, advance directives, and the patient self-determination act. In: Braun K, Pietsch JH, Blanchette PL, eds. *Cultural Issues in End-of-Life Decision Making*. Sage, Thousand Oaks, CA, 2000, pp. 37–53.

143 Baker ME. Economic, political and ethnic influences on end-of-life decision-making: A decade in review. *J Health Soc Policy* 2002;14:27–39.

144 Ersek M, Kagawa-Singer M, Barnes D, Blackhall L, Koenig BA. Multicultural considerations in use of advance directives. *Oncol Nurs Forum* 1998;25:1683–1690.

145 Tulsky JA, Casssileth BR, Bennett CL. The effect of ethnicity on ICU use and DNR orders in hospitalized AIDS patients. *J Clin Ethics* 1997;8:150–157.

107

Bereavement

VICTORIA H. RAVEIS

INTRODUCTION

Although bereavement and loss are familiar occurrences in palliative care, an appreciation of what constitutes grief and an understanding of the special circumstances of bereavement in the palliative care setting may aid clinicians in attending to the needs and preferences of families during this period of impending loss. As a universal occurrence, bereavement can also be a particularly potent and stressful life event. The death of someone significant represents a multifaceted challenge for the survivors. They must adapt to the social and economic readjustments emerging from this event and come to terms with changes in self-identity resulting from their loss while dealing with the psychological and physiological reactions engendered by the death.[1] Mourning is the expression of grief and represents the process of coming to terms with this loss. Although bereavement can predispose people to physical and mental illness, precipitate illness and death, and aggravate existing illness, most individuals are resilient and adjust to their loss in time.[2,3***,4***] A small proportion of the bereaved, approximately 10%–20%, experience debilitating grief reactions of such severity and chronicity that specialist care is warranted.[2,5***,6***]

BEREAVEMENT IN PALLIATIVE CARE

The terminal period of an illness can be an extremely stressful time for the families of dying patients. Although bereavement is usually the specific event that precipitates the mourning process, for deaths that occur in the context of palliative care, a variety of circumstances occurring prior to the death are likely to impact survivors' grief.

Illness-related losses need to be mourned. When death is preceded by a chronic illness, grieving is inexorably tied up with mourning the losses experienced during the course of an illness. These losses include altered relationships, changes in lifestyle, the forfeit of future dreams that will never be realized, as well as losses related to illness-induced changes (e.g., progressive debilitation, increasing dependence, cognitive decline, and excessive pain).[7,8*]

Caregiving demands may complicate recovery from bereavement. Families are commonly involved in the provision of emotional and practical assistance to their ill family members in palliative care situations. While the benefits to the patient of familial caregiving are readily apparent, this care provision is not without cost to the carer.[9***] Financial stress, neglect of their own health, physical and psychological exhaustion from providing care, and the social isolation resulting from restricting outside activities to carry out caregiving responsibilities are some of the routine consequences families endure.[10*] Carers with multiple stresses, high illness-related burdens, and limited support are at increased risk of adverse bereavement outcomes.[8*,11***]

Anticipatory grief. Anticipatory grief refers to the process whereby survivors rehearse the bereaved role and initiate working through the emotional changes associated with a death.[7] It is generally thought that anticipatory grief mitigates the intensity of the grief reaction following the actual death, leaving the survivor less vulnerable to maladaptive reactions. Palliative care situations enable families to be forewarned about an impending death, permitting preparation for the loss. The evidence on the adaptive value of being forewarned that a death will occur is inconsistent.[11***,12***]

Some investigations have shown that the bereaved who have had an opportunity for anticipatory grief adjust better to their loss,[13***,14] while other research has not demonstrated any benefit.[15] The development of premature grief, whereby family members socially and emotionally withdraw from the dying patient in advance of the death, can result in the bereaved experiencing guilt postdeath over having abandoned their dying relative.[16] Forewarning of a death does not ensure that individuals are prepared for the actual occurrence. The circumstances leading up to the death may adversely impact the extent to which the bereaved are capable of being able to prepare themselves for the loss. A long and protracted illness, or one marked by multiple losses or intensive caregiving demands in which carers direct all their energy and attention toward tending to the patient, may impede the bereaved's ability to initiate preparations for the death and deplete personal resources for coping with the loss.[10*,13***,17] A review of the limited literature on preparedness and bereavement outcomes documented that lack of preparedness for the death was associated with adverse grief outcomes.[11***]

Experiencing death. In Western society, dying is "medicalized" and the family is generally distanced from death.[18] Death in a home setting is unfamiliar. With the provision of palliative care, families are intimately exposed to the dying process. Anticipating its occurrence and the resultant responsibility associated with this event can induce considerable distress and anxiety. Families worry that they will be unable to address their relative's potential suffering at the end and express concern that they will be unable to cope with the challenges of being "in charge" during this dying event.[10*]

OVERVIEW OF THE GRIEF PROCESS

Freud's seminal essay on *Mourning and Melancholia* provided the foundation for contemporary understanding of grief and bereavement.[19] His work conceptualized mourning as a prolonged inner struggle to adapt to and accept an irreversible loss. Two comprehensive theoretical models have informed current approaches to bereavement and grief therapy. Worden's task of mourning[1] delineates four tasks that define the mourning process. The bereaved needs to (1) accept the reality of the loss (i.e., face the reality that the person is dead and will not return and that reunion is impossible); (2) process the pain of grief (i.e., acknowledge and work through the emotional and behavioral pain associated with the loss); (3) adjust to a world without the deceased, a task that involves external adjustments (i.e., coming to terms with living alone, facing an empty house, and managing finances alone), internal adjustments (i.e., adjusting to one's own altered sense of self), and spiritual adjustments (i.e., making accommodations in basic beliefs and one's sense of the world); and (4) find an enduring connection with the deceased in the midst of embarking on a new life (i.e., finding an appropriate place for the deceased in their emotional lives that will enable them go on living effectively in the world). Not necessarily performed in sequence, overlap and revisiting of tasks can occur.

Stroebe and Schut's dual process model of coping with bereavement[20] represents an integrative approach to describing the ways bereaved individuals come to terms with a significant loss. It posits that the bereaved undertake both loss- and restoration-oriented coping. Loss orientation refers to dealing with or processing some aspect of the loss experience itself, particularly relating to the deceased. Restoration orientation focuses on the secondary sources of stress that the bereaved need to deal with, such as changes in financial status or social loneliness, for example, bereavement tasks outlined earlier.[5***] The dual process model also introduces a third concept—oscillation. Coping with bereavement is posited to be a dynamic process, one in which individuals confront their loss some of the time and at other times avoid such confrontation. Oscillation is necessary to provide a balance to this process and prevent the adverse mental and physical costs that can arise with unremitted grieving.

Bereavement specialists and cross-cultural researchers[18,21] note that understanding of the grief process has been strongly influenced by Western thought. Its applicability to non-Western societies merits reflection, given the fundamental world-view differences in how death is perceived in different cultures. For example, in Asian cultures, through practices such as ancestor worship, death represents a transition to a different state in which deceased relatives remain important participants in the world of the living and communication is still considered possible.[22] The dual process model accommodates individual, situational, and cultural variations in coping with bereavement.[20] The tasks of mourning model also acknowledges that although mourning is universal, people do not grieve in the same way.[1] As the approach and adaptation process are not held to a fixed pattern, the model implicitly takes account of cultural nuances and societal influences.

DURATION OF GRIEF

Although there is considerable variability in the temporal course at which individuals integrate their loss into their lives, grief-related distress is generally most intense during the first year following the loss. The clinical and epidemiological literature support that in Western societies, after a period of acute grief, most bereaved individuals gradually return to a normal level of functioning 1–2 years after their loss.[5***,16,23] Societal mores can also influence the duration of grief. For example, Taiwanese cultural ideology proscribes "one man per lifetime" and widows are expected to grieve for the rest of their lives.[22]

MANIFESTATIONS OF GRIEF

Immediately following a death, bereaved individuals are usually in a state of shock. They feel numb and experience disbelief over the event, even when the death has been anticipated, as in palliative care.[10*] Cognitions may be impacted and the bereaved may experience a sense of confusion and have difficulty concentrating. During this acute mourning period, individuals can experience a variety of psychological and physiological reactions of varying intensity and duration.[1] The most commonly expressed emotions include shock, numbness, sadness, anxiety, loneliness, fatigue, anger, relief, and guilt. Bereaved individuals often report somatic complaints as well, such as weakness, lethargy, loss of appetite, tightness in the throat or chest, shortness of breath, and sleeplessness. Such reactions are not necessarily indicative of a psychiatric problem or a physical disorder and should not be pathologized. They are normal manifestations of acute grief. Although grief reactions are universally experienced, the emotional and behavioral responses to a loss are culturally bound. In some societies, wailing, unrestrained crying, self-mutilation, or prostration may be a common and acceptable means of expressing grief[18] but regarded as indicative of an intense or severe grief reaction by other cultural groups.

NORMAL AND COMPLICATED OR PROLONGED GRIEF

Lindemann's landmark study of bereavement,[24] following the Cocoanut Grove nightclub fire, focused attention on the intensity and trajectory of expressed grief and introduced the distinction between normal and pathological grief responses, attributes central to understanding the course and outcome of the bereavement process. Most bereaved individuals are able to adjust to their loss over time and return to a level of functioning normal for their society and culture. Nonetheless, for a minority of the bereaved individuals, approximately 10%–20%, bereavement is not a transient life crisis.[2,5***,6***] Unable to integrate the loss into their lives, these individuals experience a severe, protracted emotional reaction that impairs everyday functioning. Current understanding of the grief process characterizes grief that is chronic, intense, disabling, and persisting beyond a period considered adaptive as indicative of complicated grief.[25*,26] This emotional response is also known as prolonged grief disorder (PGD).[23]

VULNERABILITY FACTORS FOR ADVERSE BEREAVEMENT OUTCOMES

The clinical and research literature on bereavement suggests a constellation of situational, interpersonal, and individual factors that affect the course and outcome of the grieving process, influence the risk of mental and physical consequences following the loss, and increase the risk of complicated grief.[4***,26,27***,28***,29***] Described in the following are some of the factors present in palliative care situations.

Protracted illness. The bereaved whose loved one suffered a long, lingering illness adjust more poorly to bereavement than those whose loved one died after a short illness.[30***] This may reflect the impact of providing informal support and care during an extended illness and the stresses of having lived with a protracted illness course.[10*,13***]

Disease course. Terminal conditions that impact patients' functioning and quality of life, such as severe, chronic pain or dementia, are difficult and stressful for family members to witness. Their distress is exacerbated by feeling helpless in alleviating or managing these conditions and worrying over future escalation.[13***,31*]

Stigmatized death. When death is from an illness that is stigmatized, such as HIV/AIDS, or associated with unhealthy or socially unacceptable lifestyles, such as alcoholism or drug abuse, the family may be less open about the cause of death or the circumstances leading up to the event.[32*] As a consequence, the bereaved's naturally occurring support systems may be less forthcoming. The family may also experience conflicting emotions or encounter difficulty resolving their feelings about the deceased. In communicable illnesses such as HIV/AIDS, the bereaved may be infected as well or may be dealing with multiple deaths or advanced disease of other family members.[33*]

Nature of the loss. The death of a spouse is considered to be one of the most stressful life events. A high level of dependency or an ambivalent relationship (feelings of love/hate, need/resentment) between the deceased and the bereaved often culminates in a severe grief reaction and difficulty in accepting and resolving the loss.[27***,28***] Ambiguous loss, the physical presence but psychological loss of a loved one, characteristic of the situation faced by dementia carers has been shown to increase the risk of complicated grief.[13***]

Life circumstances. Vulnerability for a poor postdeath adjustment is increased by additional severe stresses concurrent to the bereavement, such as multiple losses or life changes.[1,34] Deficits in social support or restricted social resources can also contribute to adverse grief outcomes.[27***] Limited financial resources predeath or declining income as a consequence of the death can also precipitate problems in the grieving process.[35*] Widowhood can have especially adverse economic, social, and psychological ramifications for older adults.[36]

Individual characteristics. The bereaved's preexisting physical health condition, history of substance abuse, and/or premorbid mental illness[1] can contribute to adverse bereavement outcomes. Personality characteristics, such as low self-esteem or a low internal sense of control, are also associated with increased distress postdeath. In Western societies, men are at higher risk for bereavement-related mortality; women experience more affective distress.[11***,27***]

HEALTH CONSEQUENCES OF BEREAVEMENT

A variety of physical and psychological health consequences have been associated with bereavement. The recently bereaved have been shown to display an increased incidence of depressive symptoms, somatic complaints, and insomnia, as well as experiencing changes in their endocrine, immune, and cardiovascular systems. Higher rates of utilization of medical and mental health-care services (i.e., increased hospitalizations, prescribed drug use, and physician and mental health clinician visits) have also been observed in the early weeks and months after loss compared to nonbereaved samples.[4***] Persons experiencing complicated grief are at heightened risk for serious mental and physical health problems and may also engage in behaviors injurious to their health, such as alcohol or substance abuse.[23,26,28***]

PRINCIPLES OF BEREAVEMENT SUPPORT IN PALLIATIVE CARE

Palliative care offers the health-care practitioner multiple opportunities to attend to the well-being of affected family members. The provision of compassionate care during this stressful period may facilitate families' grieving process and reduce adverse bereavement consequences. Five broad principles of bereavement support can be readily applied in palliative care situations: (1) view the patient and family as one unit of care; (2) enable open discussion of illness and death-related concerns; (3) provide emotional support; (4) facilitate practical assistance; and (5) respect cultural, ethnic, and religious practices.

View patient and family as one unit of care. The terminal illness period is stressful to the family. Patients and families should be viewed as one unit of care.[31*] Clinicians are in contact with families during this period of heightened vulnerability. Attending to the informational, emotional, and practical support needs of the family may make the dying experience less stressful for the family, facilitate their grieving, and reduce their risk of adverse bereavement outcomes.[37] As a secondary benefit, addressing family members' needs during this period can facilitate their remaining engaged in the patient's care provision.

Enable open discussion of illness and death-related concerns. Attending to families' concerns about the patient's condition and care, and providing reassurance that appropriate therapeutic and ameliorative measures are being utilized, can comfort families and reduce later recriminations. Enabling open communication, discussion of emerging concerns, and providing guidance as to what to expect during the dying process can avert the development of future regrets, facilitating families' grieving process.[17]

Provide emotional support. Supporting families in their grief during the terminal phase of the illness is also important in facilitating adjustment after the death. In palliative care, most families are aware of the nature of their relative's condition and its prognosis. Families can experience anger, sadness, regret, resentment, guilt, or anxiety over the illness, the burdens and responsibilities they are required to assume, and the impending death.[31*] They may also feel isolated and alone. Families need to be supported in expressing their feelings and concerns and be reassured that these feelings are normal.[17]

A family's contact with the clinical care team often ceases with the patient's death. For many families, this is a significant loss. Its impact can be lessened by a condolence note or brief sympathy call from a member of the care team. Anniversaries of the death or important family events are also times when grief is intensified.[38] A follow-up note or call from the team on these occasions may be beneficial.

Facilitate practical assistance. Families often become very involved in the dying patient's care, neglecting their own health and setting unreasonable expectations of what they personally should accomplish. It is common for families to be fearful about leaving the patient for any length of time, curtailing outside activities, and cutting themselves off from their broader social network.[10*] Clinicians may need to encourage family members to respect and attend to their own needs or actively support accepting help from relatives and friends. Families may also require guidance and aid in following through with a dying patient's care preferences.

Respect cultural, ethnic, and religious practices. Bereavement takes place within a social context in which rituals and customs provide for a sanctioned public articulation of private distress. When individuals are prevented from performing such activities, their mourning process is adversely impacted.[39***] Institutional policies that limit children's visiting rights, restrict the number of visitors in a room, or

bar the performance of religious and cultural ceremonies can impede families from carrying out specific practices required at death. Terminal illness provides forewarning of the death. This affords the care team opportunity to become aware of and address any particular needs and requirements associated with specific mourning customs and rituals.

Bereavement resources, programs, and treatments

Consensus-based hospice and palliative care practice standards and policies specify having in place an organized program of bereavement services available to families appropriate to their needs, preferences, and culture, beginning during the terminal period and continuing after the death.[40,41] Use in these settings of valid, reliable tools that differentiate between resilient and at-risk individuals ensures that bereavement support is offered appropriate to individual need.[42***,43]

Supportive services. Bereavement-related supportive services are provided in a variety of treatment modalities and venues. The duration of these various bereavement services can range from a single session or meeting to ongoing programs, initiated during the terminal illness period and continued postdeath. Apart from the bereavement services available through hospice and palliative care settings, community groups, churches, and charitable organizations, such as Cruse Bereavement Care in Great Britain, also sponsor a range of bereavement support resources. Support or counseling may be delivered individually or through a group session by mental health clinicians or other trained professionals. Some programs use trained volunteers supported by professionals. These services help normalize the bereaved's experiences while also supporting their grief. Self-help groups and peer-to-peer support resources, such as the Widowed Persons Service in the United States, involve bereaved individuals offering friendship and empathy of shared status to help each other in their grief and adjustment to their loss. Virtual communities of support, available through the Internet, such as GriefNet, provide individuals with another resource when coping with loss.[44]

Psychotherapeutic interventions. Most bereaved individuals will not require psychotherapy or specialized grief therapy.[1] However, palliative care settings provide the opportunity to initiate preventive interventions in advance of the death with those individuals identified as being at high risk for adverse bereavement outcomes.[11***,45] Family-focused grief therapy (FFGT), a preventive intervention, has been found to be effective in reducing bereavement-related distress and depression by optimizing in the predeath period a family's relational functioning, mutual support, and sharing of grief.[37] A recent meta-analysis of randomized controlled trials initiated to treat bereaved individuals experiencing complicated grief supports the efficacy of post-death psychotherapeutic interventions in diminishing the symptoms of complicated grief and facilitating the normal grieving process.[46***] Complicated grief treatment (CGT), a psychotherapeutic intervention that has received empirical support in randomized trials, focuses on removing the psychological and social impediments that prevent the natural progression of the grief process.[47**]

Pharmacologic therapies. Pharmacological interventions are not clinically indicated for most bereaved individuals. The emotional expression of grief following a loss is a normal and natural aspect of the grieving process. In some clinical situations, antidepressants, tranquilizers, and sedatives have been prescribed to remediate severe and debilitating bereavement-related reactions that impede functioning.[45] Such use, however, warrants discretion. If initiated early in the bereavement period, pharmacological treatment could interfere with the natural grieving process.[6***] A systematic review of case–control studies demonstrated that a beneficial pharmacologic treatment effect on depression and sleep quality in bereaved samples persisted only while the subjects received the medication.[48***] This review noted further that there was no demonstrated treatment impact on the bereaved's resolution of grief. Although the evidence base is sparse, clinical reports and limited research studies on the pharmacological management of bereavement-related depression suggest that the efficacy of pharmacological treatments for complicated grief merits further scientific investigation.[49] An ongoing multisite randomized controlled trial in the United States is exploring the utility of using a serotonin-active antidepressant in combination with CGT, a psychotherapy program that has demonstrated beneficial outcomes with complicated grief.[50,51]

CONCLUSIONS

Although there may be considerable individual variation in the experience and expression of grief, grieving is a normal, natural response to a significant loss. Understanding of the grief process has been substantially influenced by Western thought. Consequently, clinicians should be careful to not ascribe pathological or abnormal labels to mourning responses when the cultural meaning or appropriateness of these actions is not well understood. Clinicians involved in palliative care are in contact with families at a point of heightened vulnerability. The provision of emotional support and compassionate care by the health-care team during this stressful period may facilitate families' grieving process and reduce adverse bereavement consequences.

Grief specialists advise,[45] supported by clinical evidence,[3***,6***,48***] that clinical interventions are not necessary for most bereaved individuals, as the cognitive and emotional responses generally abate over time. Consensus opinion is that such an approach may do more harm than good, impeding the activation of the bereaved's natural support systems and disrupting the pattern of the normal grieving.[3***,4***] About 10%–20% of individuals experience grief reactions of such severity or chronicity that necessitate professional intervention. An understanding and appreciation of the normal grief process, along with an awareness of the individual and situational factors that may complicate mourning, will aid clinicians in determining those instances when specialist evaluation is indicated. As Raphael et al.[45] succinctly state: "There can be *no justification for routine intervention* for bereaved persons in terms of therapeutic modalities—either psychotherapeutic or pharmacological—because grief is not a disease" [p. 587].

Key learning points

- Grief is universally experienced; it is not a disease.
- Grief is expressed with a constellation of psychological and physiological reactions.
- Grieving is a process, most bereaved adapt to the loss over time.
- Normal grief and mourning practices reflect cultural and ideological belief systems.
- Benefits of anticipatory grief are mitigated by care provision, illness duration, and cause of death.
- Patients and families should be viewed as a unit of care.
- Attending to carers' needs and preferences during the terminal phase of illness can support their grieving process.
- Facilitating culturally appropriate death rites and mourning practices benefits the bereaved.
- Bereavement can predispose some people to physical and mental illness and precipitate death.
- Complicated grief, present in a small proportion of bereaved, warrants therapeutic treatment.

REFERENCES

1 Worden JW. *Grief Counseling and Grief Therapy: A Handbook for the Mental Health Practitioner.* 4th edn. New York: Springer; 2009.
2 Bonanno GA, Boerner K, Wortman CB. Trajectories of grieving. In: Stroebe MS, Hansson RO, Schut H, Stroebe W. (eds.) *Handbook of Bereavement Research and Practice: Advances in Theory and Intervention.* Washington, DC: American Psychological Association; 2008. pp. 287–307.
3 Stroebe W, Schut H, Stroebe MS. Grief work, disclosure and counseling: Do they help the bereaved? *Clinical Psychology Review.* 2005; 25(4): 395–414.
4 Stroebe M, Schut H, Stroebe W. Health outcomes of bereavement. *Lancet.* 2007; 370(9603): 1960–1973.
5 Bonanno GA, Kaltman S. The varieties of grief experience. *Clinical Psychology Review.* 2001; 21(5): 705–734.
6 Schut H, Stroebe MS. Interventions to enhance adaptation to bereavement. *Journal of Palliative Medicine.* 2005; 8(Suppl 1): S140–S147.
7 Rando TA. Understanding and facilitating anticipatory grief in the loved ones of the dying. In: Rando TA (ed.) *Loss & Anticipatory Grief.* Lexington, MA: Lexington Books; 1986. pp. 97–130.
8 Schulz R, Beach SR, Lind B, Martire LM, Zdaniuk B, Hirsch C et al. Involvement in caregiving and adjustment to death of a spouse: Findings from the Caregiver Health Effects Study. *Journal of the American Medical Association.* 2001; 285(24): 3123–3129.
9 Williams AL, McCorkle R. Cancer family caregivers during the palliative, hospice, and bereavement phases: A review of the descriptive psychosocial literature. *Palliative and Supportive Care.* 2011; 9(3): 313–3225.
10 Raveis VH. Psychosocial impact of spousal caregiving at the end-of-life: Challenges and consequences. *The Gerontologist.* 2004; 44(Special Issue 1): 191–192.

11   Schulz R, Boerner K, Herbert RS. Caregiving and bereavement. In: Stroebe MS, Hansson RO, Schut H, Stroebe W. (eds.) *Handbook of Bereavement Research and Practice: Advances in Theory and Intervention*. Washington, DC: American Psychological Association; 2008. pp. 265–285.

12   Siegel K, Weinstein L. Anticipatory grief reconsidered. *Journal of Psychosocial Oncology*. 1983; 1(2): 61–73.

13   Chan D, Livingston G, Jones L, Sampson EL. Grief reaction in dementia carers: A systematic review. *International Journal of Geriatric Psychiatry*. 2013; 28(1): 1–17.

14   Parkes CM, Weiss RS. *Recovery from Bereavement*. New York: Basic Books; 1983.

15   Dessonville-Hill C, Thompson LW, Gallagher D. The role of anticipatory bereavement in older women's adjustment to widowhood. *Gerontologist*. 1988; 28(6): 792–796.

16   Zisook S. Understanding and managing bereavement in palliative care. In: Chochinov HM, Breitbart W. (eds.) *Handbook of Psychiatry in Palliative Medicine*. New York: Oxford University Press; 2000. pp. 321–334.

17   Raveis VH. Facilitating older spouses adjustment to widowhood: A preventive intervention program. *Social Work in Health Care*. 1999; 29(4): 12–32.

18   Laungani P, Young B. Conclusions 1: Implications for practice and policy. In: Parkes CM, Young B, Laungani P. (eds.) *Death and Bereavement across Cultures*. London, U.K.: Routledge; 1997. pp. 218–232.

● 19   Freud S. Mourning and melancholia. In: Strachey J. (ed.) *The Standard Edition of the Complete Psychological Works of Sigmund Freud*, Volume XIV. London: Hogarth Press; 1957; 243–258.

● 20   Stroebe M, Schut H. The dual process model of coping with bereavement: Rationale and description. *Death Studies*. 1999; 23(3): 197–224.

21   Klass D. Continuing bonds in the resolution of grief in Japan and North American. *American Behavioral Scientist*. 2001; 44(5): 742–763.

22   Hsu MT, Kahn DL, Yee DH, Lee WL. Recovery through reconnection: A cultural design for family bereavement in Taiwan. *Death Studies*. 2004; 28(8): 761–786.

● 23   Prigerson HG, Horowitz MJ, Jacobs SC, Parkes CM, Aslan M, Goodkin K et al. Prolonged grief disorder: Psychometric validation of criteria proposed for DSM-V and ICD-11. *PLoS Medicine*. 2009; 6(8): e1000121.

● 24   Lindemann E. Symptomatology and management of acute grief. *American Journal of Psychiatry*. 1944; 101(2): 141–148.

25   Bonanno GA, Neria Y, Mancini A, Coifman KG, Litz B, Insel B. Is there more to complicate grief than depression and posttraumatic stress disorder? A test of incremental validity. *Journal of Abnormal Psychology*. 2007; 116(2): 342–351.

◆ 26   Lichtenthal WG, Cruess DG, Prigerson GH. A case for establishing complicated grief as a distinct mental disorder in *DSM-V*. *Clinical Psychology Review*. 2004; 24(6): 637–662.

27   Burke LA, Neimeyer RA. Prospective risk factors for complicated grief: A review of the empirical literature. In: Stroebe M, Schut H, van den Bout J. (eds.) *Complicated Grief: Scientific Foundations for Health Care Professionals*. New York: Routledge; 2013. pp. 145–160.

28   Lobb EA, Kristjanson LJ, Aoun SM, Monterosso L, Halkett GKB, Davies A. Predictors of complicated grief: A systematic review of empirical studies. *Death Studies*. 2013; 34: 673–698.

29   Hudson P, Remedios C, Zordan R, Thomas, K, Clifton, D, Crewdson, M et al. *Clinical Practice Guidelines for the Psychosocial and Bereavement Support of Family Caregivers of Palliative Care Patients*. Melbourne, Australia: Centre for Palliative Care, St. Vincent's Hospital Melbourne; 2010.

30   Sanders CM. Effects of sudden vs. chronic illness death on bereavement outcome. *Omega—Journal of Death and Dying*. 1982-1983; 13(3): 227–241.

31   Raveis VH, Pretter S. Existential plight of adult daughters following their mother's breast cancer diagnosis. *Psycho-Oncology*. 2005; 14(1): 49–60.

32   Houck JA. A comparison of grief reactions in cancer, HIV/AIDS, and suicide bereavement. *Journal of HIV/AIDS & Social Services*. 2007; 6(3): 97–112.

33   Raveis VH, Siegel K. Impact of caregiving on informal or familial caregivers. *AIDS Patient Care and STDs*. 1991; 5(1): 39–43.

34   Sanders C. *Grief: The mourning after dealing with adult bereavement*. New York: John Wiley & Sons; 1989.

35   Galatzer-Levy I, Bonanno GA. Beyond normality in the study of bereavement: Heterogeneity in depression outcomes following loss in older adults. *Social Science & Medicine*. 2012; 74(12): 1987–1994.

36   Carr D. Factors that influence late-life bereavement: Considering data from the changing lives of older couples study. In: Stroebe MS, Hansson RO, Schut H, Stroebe W. (eds.) *Handbook of Bereavement Research and Practice: Advances in Theory and Intervention*. Washington, DC: American Psychological Association; 2008. pp. 417–440.

37   Kissane DW, Lichtenthal WG. Family focused grief therapy: From palliative care into bereavement. In: Stroebe MS, Hansson RO, Schut H, Stroebe W. (eds.) *Handbook of Bereavement Research and Practice: Advances in Theory and Intervention*. Washington, DC: American Psychological Association; 2008. pp. 485–510.

● 38   Raphael B. *The Anatomy of Bereavement*. New York: Basic Books, 1983.

39   Firth S. Approaches to death in Hindu and Sikh communities in Britain. In: Dickenson D, Johnson M, Katz JS. (eds.) *Death, Dying and Bereavement*. London, U.K.: Sage Publications; 2000. pp. 28–34.

✱ 40   National Consensus Project for Quality Palliative Care. *Clinical Practice Guidelines for Quality Palliative Care*. 3rd edn. Available at: http://www.nationalconsensusproject.org/NCP_Clinical_Practice_Guidelines_3rd_Edition.pdf, (accessed September 26, 2013).

✱ 41   Hudson P, Remedios C, Zordan R, Thomas K, Clifton D, Crewdson M et al. Guidelines for the psychosocial and bereavement support of family caregivers of palliative care patients. *Journal of Palliative Medicine*. 2012; 15(6): 696–702.

42   Agnew A, Manktelow R, Taylor B, Jones L. Bereavement needs assessment in specialist palliative care: A review of the literature. *Palliative Medicine*. 2010; 24(1): 46–59.

✱ 43   National Institute for Clinical Excellence (NICE). *Improving Supportive and Palliative Care for Adults with Cancer*. Available at: http://www.nice.org.uk/nicemedia/live/10893/28816/28816.pdf, [accessed September 26, 2013].

44   Lynn C, Rath A. GriefNet: Creating and maintaining an internet bereavement community. In: Sofka CJ, Cupit IN, Gilbert KR. (eds.) *Dying, Death, and Grief in an Online Universe*. New York: Springer; 2012. pp. 87–102.

45   Raphael B, Minkov C, Dobson M. Psychotherapeutic and pharmacological intervention for bereaved persons. In: Stroebe MS, Hansson RO, Stroebe W, Schut H. (eds.) *Handbook of Bereavement Research: Consequences, Coping, and Cure*. Washington, DC: American Psychological Association; 2001. pp. 587–612.

46   Wittouck C, Van Autreve S, De Jaegere E, Portzky G, van Heeringen K. The prevention and treatment of complicated grief: A meta-analysis. *Clinical Psychology Review*. 2011; 31(1): 69–78.

47   Shear MK, Frank E, Houck PR, Reynolds CF. Treatment of complicated grief: A randomized controlled trial. *The Journal of the American Medical Association*. 2005; 293(21): 2601–2608.

48   Forte A, Hill M, Pazder R, Feudtner C. Bereavement care interventions: A systematic review. *BMC Palliative Care*. 2004; 3: 3.

49   Bui E, Nadal-Viens M, Simon NM. Pharmacological approaches to the treatment of complicated grief: Rationale and a brief review of the literature. *Dialogues in Clinical Neuroscience*. 2012; 14(2): 149–157.

50   Shear MK. Complicated grief treatment: The theory, practice and outcomes. *Bereavement Care*. 2010; 29(3): 10–14.

51   ClinicalTrials.gov. *A Study of Medication with or without Psychotherapy for Complicated Grief (HEAL)*. Available at: http://clinialtrials.gov/ct2/show/NT01179568, [accessed September 20, 2013].

108

Children of palliative care patients

ESTELA BEALE

INTRODUCTION

The children of palliative care patients present unique challenges for the palliative care professional. Until very recently, this group of children represented a hidden high-risk group whose needs were often minimized or overlooked by overwhelmed parents and were unknown to most of the medical staff. The reasons for the neglect of this population varied. A belief among parents and caretakers that children are generally resilient and that they will adapt to their circumstances was prevalent. Also, parents and caretakers sometimes voiced the belief that children, particularly younger ones, do not really understand what is going on (Kastenbaum, 1967; Pettle and Britten, 1995; Spinetta, 1974; Stambrook and Parker, 1987) and, therefore, it was best not to discuss the situation with them. Consequently, the children did not receive the attention they needed at this critical time.

Over the past 10 years, research on childhood bereavement has increased, drawing attention to the need to provide intervention for children of palliative care patients (Christ, 2000b; Christ and Christ, 2006; Hames, 2003; Karns, 2002; Kornreich et al., 2008). The short- and long-term effects of the bereavement process of these children may be considerably mitigated by early intervention during the parent's terminal phase (Christ and Christ, 2006; Dunning, 2006; Kennedy and McIntyre, 2008; Kornreich et al., 2008; Popplestone-Helm and Helm, 2009).

Many factors must be taken into consideration in determining the best way to help a child cope with their parent's terminal condition and adjust to the idea and subsequent reality of their parent's death. Effective intervention must be appropriate to the developmental age of the child. Other critical factors that strongly influence children at this time are their relationship to the well parent, family characteristics, and the stability of their home environment, among others (Christ and Christ, 2006; Haine et al., 2008; Schmitt et al., 2008).

A patient with terminal cancer presents the palliative care professional with a unique set of situations that can create severe distress in children, due to the dramatic fluctuations of the patient's symptoms. The potential of an extensive terminal phase with increasing physical and mental deterioration can exacerbate the family's stress.

Communicating the bad news of a cancer diagnosis is difficult enough for doctors (Buckman, 1984; Butow et al., 2002; Fallowfield and Jenkins, 1999; Maguire, 1999), so it is not surprising that parents dying of cancer, who are coming to terms with the existential issues surrounding dying, are often at a loss as to when, how, and what to tell their children about cancer and death. It often falls to a member of the palliative care team to advise and assist the parents in comforting and communicating with the children at this critical time.

The research and clinical experience of a wide range of medical professionals from many countries and cultures is providing a foundation to assist us in developing effective interventions for the children of palliative care patients. This chapter reviews the research concerning the main issues that affect these children and the types of interventions that appear most promising.

FACTORS INFLUENCING A CHILD'S RESPONSE TO A TERMINALLY ILL

Parent

DEVELOPMENTAL AGE

Throughout the last several decades, developmental theorists have tried to understand the impact of parental loss on a young child. The attachment theory was first espoused by Bowlby (1980) who, in groundbreaking research, demonstrated that when primates are separated from the mother early in life, their reaction escalates from a state of protest to miasmas and death. Since then, other researchers have confirmed the instinctual roots of attachment, which assures the safety of infants who use intuitive behaviors to engage their caretakers and to guarantee their caretaker's presence and attentiveness. Infants do not recognize death, feelings of separation, or loss. However, they react usually with behavioral and physical changes such as increased quietness, listlessness, unresponsiveness, weight loss, and changes in sleep patterns. In other words, there is increased deregulation of physical functions.

Internalization of primary caretakers is a process that becomes established by the time the child is 2 or 3 years of age. Once this process of internalization is accomplished, the child can sustain prolonged separations yet retain the memory of the parent. For the child to be able to obtain optimal emotional, social, and psychosexual maturity, a predictable, caring environment is required. Separation from the primary caretaker produces anxiety, which is manifested differently depending on the child's developmental stage and is exacerbated by a terminal illness. While toddlers age two to three do not understand the concept of death, they have definite reactions shown by generalized distress, disturbances in sleep, and temper tantrums among others. By 3–5 years of age, comprehension has increased but there is still a tendency to rely on magical thinking. The idea of permanence is not present, so it is difficult to understand the finality of death (Black, 1998; Christ and Christ, 2006; Hames, 2003).

By 5 years of age, most children can distinguish between separation and death. At this point, some characteristics of personality are most likely established. In addition, a variety of other factors will now influence the child's development, such as the relationship to the well parent, the family structure, and the child's general social circumstances, as well as genetic makeup. These children often become overprotective of the well parent and may withhold showing them any signs of distress. At the death of the parent, it is characteristic of this age group for there to be increased activity, often resulting in behavioral problems (Black, 1998).

Several lines of research have indicated that children from 5 to 11 years old should be informed that the parent is terminally ill and should be told what to expect (Elizur and Kaffman, 1983; Hilden et al., 2000; Kroll et al., 1998; Pfeffer et al., 2000; Sourkes, 1992; Waechter, 1971). A study by Christ and Christ (2006), which included children in three different developmental groupings, 3–5, 6–8, and 9–11 years, suggests that children in all of these age groups be informed of their parent's illness in a manner appropriate to their developmental age.

Developmental factors also shape the adolescent's response to the terminal illness of a parent. Support by health professionals, coping strategies, and the adolescents' own mastery of adaptive tasks are posed by the terminal phase of the parent's illness. Open communication between parents and children is of utmost importance (Christ et al., 2002). Often, the parent's illness creates the need for greater assistance in the home that clashes with the adolescent's developmental tasks of withdrawing and achieving autonomy and emotional independence from the parents. Adolescent's inconsistent behavior and mood swings typically become exaggerated under the stress of a parent's illness. The adolescent's advanced cognitive abilities may lead to more intense grief than that of younger children due to their increased ability to comprehend the enduring consequences of death. Some adolescents experience prolonged emotional disturbance during the parent's illness and for several years after the parent's death. These adolescents tend to exhibit severe depression, alcohol and/or drug abuse, refusal to attend school, and oftentimes suicidal ideation (Christ, 2000a; Christ et al., 1994; Clark et al., 1994; Dehlin and Mertensson, 2009).

Researchers studying the impact of development on children's response to terminal illness and death of a parent have reported the emergence of behavioral patterns (Christ and Christ, 2006). Further clarification of such patterns could help the clinician determine more effective age-specific interventions.

SITUATIONAL FACTORS

The role of situational factors that can affect a child's response and adjustment to the death of a parent has been gaining attention among researchers. Christ and Christ (2006) provide a list of situational factors that they categorize as either risk factors or protective factors that may mediate the coping of bereaved children. The risk factors they cite that may hinder the child's bereavement process include concurrent stressful life events, a negative or nonsupportive relationship with the surviving caregiver, a poor relationship with the parent who died, low self-esteem, preexisting mental health problems in the adolescent or the surviving parent or caregiver, and circumstances of the death, such as violent or traumatic death.

They identified protective factors that may help mitigate the child's bereavement process, including having a relationship with the surviving parent or caregiver characterized by open communication, warmth, and positive experiences; surviving parent able to sustain parenting competence; feeling accepted by peers and other adults, such as relatives and teachers; higher socioeconomic status; religiousness; intellectual and social competence; and the opportunity to express thoughts and feelings about the deceased parent and have them validated by others.

Among these factors, the most consistently identified mediating variables are the quality of the relationship with the surviving parent or caregiver and their competence in parenting bereaved children (Baker et al., 1992; Buxbaum, 2001; Christ, 2002; Christ et al., 2002; Hahn et al., 1997; Raveis et al., 1999; Siegel et al., 1996).

Haine et al. (2008) group situational factors as either malleable risk and protective factors or nonmalleable factors. Malleable risk and protective factors include increasing self-esteem, increasing child adaptive control beliefs, improving child coping skills, supporting adaptive expression of emotion that the child wishes to express, facilitating a positive parent–child relationship, parental warmth, parent–child communication, effective discipline, reducing parental distress, increasing positive family interactions, and reducing child exposure to negative life events.

Nonmalleable factors include children's developmental level, child gender, cause and type of death, time since the death, and cultural background (Haine et al., 2008; Sandler et al., 1999, 2003; Wolchik et al., 2008; Worden and Silverman, 1996; Zambelli and DeRosa, 1992).

COMMUNICATION

The ability of the parents to engage in open communication with their children is a key mediating factor that can be addressed during early intervention that can positively influence the child's response to a terminally ill parent (Forest et al., 2006; Kennedy and Lloyd-Williams, 2009).

Hilden et al. (2000) found that when given the opportunity to communicate, children can conquer their fears as well as express their love in the terminal phase of a parent's illness and that honesty is indeed the best policy with children of all ages. In this way, the reality of the situation, no matter how awful it is, can be shared in an open manner. Trying to protect children from knowledge about what is really happening often confuses the child even more than circumstances alone and escalates concerns about events that are beyond their control. A study conducted by Pfeffer et al. (2000) reported that the children in their sample were likely either denying or reluctant to acknowledge problems in the emotional domains assessed, for reasons that were directly or indirectly related to the loss of their parent. For example, they may have been reluctant to acknowledge their own feelings of depression for fear that doing so would upset other family members. However, reports of bereaved parents regarding their children's psychological distress and symptoms of depression reported lower levels than found in the children's reports of their own distress and psychiatric symptomatology. Bereaved parents may be so overwhelmed by their own grief and mourning that they are not fully aware of the level of distress of their children, or they may not be able to cope with their children's psychologically distressed states. There should be no curtain of silence drawn around the child's worst fears.

Kornreich et al. (2008) report that parents can minimize their child's distress by maintaining open communication throughout the diagnosis, treatment, and recovery processes. Furthermore, an informative, timely, and supportive response from a multidisciplinary health-care team can successfully reduce stressors and guide the child through the experience.

Studies provide support for the belief that anxiety diminishes when a child is given opportunities to discuss his fears. Providing the child with understanding, acceptance of his feelings, and conveyance of permission to discuss any aspect of the parent's illness can decrease feelings of isolation and alienation. Waechter (1971) points out the striking dichotomy between the child's degree of awareness of the prognosis, as inferred from his imaginative stories, and the parent's belief about the child's degree of awareness of the parent's prognosis. This dichotomy suggests that knowledge is communicated to the child by the changes that he encounters in his total environment after the diagnosis is made and by his perceptiveness of various nonverbal clues. This disparity may result in a deepening isolation that is exacerbated when the child becomes aware of the evasiveness that meets expressions of his concern.

Children who are forewarned of the imminence and inevitability of death have lower levels of anxiety than those who are not, even children within the same family. Children and adolescents report that they value open communication with both parents about the illness and death, and research suggests that it

helps them during their bereavement (Christ et al., 2005; Raveis et al., 1999). Family communication about the parent's illness is one of the focuses of parent-guidance intervention programs (Siegel et al., 1990).

The practitioner needs to be aware that some children may need specialized help in recovering from depression and other symptoms that are associated with bereavement. Several studies specifically related to parents dying of cancer reiterate the importance of communication between parents and children and provide support for the claim that parents underestimate the impact of a terminal illness on their children. The results suggest that emotional restraint in the surviving parent made it difficult for the child to express feelings. This led to a sense of intensified loneliness and increased anxiety and confusion. The ability of bereaved children to report grieving emotions correlated significantly with improved functioning (Christ and Christ, 2006; Elizur and Kaffman, 1983; Kranzler et al., 1990; Moore et al., 2010).

SHORT- AND LONG-TERM EFFECTS OF CHILDHOOD BEREAVEMENT

There has been some progress in assessing the short-term effects of the bereavement process in children. The Family Bereavement Program (FBP) at Arizona State University uses a theoretical model to study which factors are critical for the effect that bereavement of parental death has on psychological functioning. Factors targeted by the intervention included parental demoralization, negative life events, parental warmth, and stable positive events in the family.

The program involved separate groups for caregivers, adolescents, and children, which were designed to change potentially modifiable risk and protective factors for bereaved children. The evaluation involved random assignment of 156 families (244 children and adolescents) to the FBP or a self-study condition. Families participated in assessments at pretest, posttest, and 11-month follow-up. Results indicated that the FBP led to improved parenting, coping, and caregiver mental health and to reductions in stressful events at posttest (Sandler et al., 2003).

A study by Kwok et al. (2005) used a multirater, multimethod measurement model of positive parenting to study 214 bereaved children ages 7–16 and their surviving parent or current caregiver. The authors reported a correlation between the surviving parent's ability to express warmth and consistent discipline with the parentally bereaved children's mental health problems. They believe this model has implications for understanding the development of mental health problems of parentally bereaved children.

Cerel et al. (2006) interviewed 360 parent-bereaved children (ages 6–17) over a 2-year period after the death of a parent. They reported that the children who are at most risk of depression and overall psychopathology were those who experienced depression in combination with parental depression or in the context of other family stressors.

Studies regarding the long-term effects of childhood parental loss have been inconsistent or inconclusive. The evidence from many of these studies provides mixed evidence for the changes in psychological symptoms of bereaved children. Some of the studies indicate a significant difference in depression and suicide in adults bereaved in childhood, while other studies show no significant difference in this group. There are several reasons for these inconsistencies, which range from nonrepresentative samples and small sample sizes to the use of a wide range of data collection methodologies, all of which make it difficult to compare otherwise similar studies.

INTERVENTIONS FOR THE CHILDREN OF PALLIATIVE CARE PATIENTS

Educational programs and guidelines have been developed to help parents and clinicians communicate with children about the ill parent's situation and impending death, and support programs for children of palliative care patients have grown substantially (Giesberg and Verdonck-de leeuw, 2010; Mondanaro, 2005; Popplestone-Helm and Helm, 2009; Saunders, 1996; Sweetland, 2005; Turner, 2004; Turner and Clavarino, 2007). However, there are still few qualitative and even fewer quantitative studies focused on interventions for the children of palliative care patients (Karns, 2002; Kennedy and McIntyre, 2008; Rauch and Durant, 2003).

A study by Sivesind and Beale (2002) showed a high percentage of children of a terminally ill parent sought reassurance, and most of them considered themselves to be caregivers of their dying parent. A strong wish to do everything possible to keep the parent alive was triggered. It also appeared that while the child was lost in frenetic activity, he or she was not faced with as much anxiety and grief as might otherwise occur. In contrast to the standard account (Matthews, 1989) of developmental stages, small children demonstrated a remarkable awareness of the parent's medical condition and its implications. Disruptive behavior alternated with some desperate attempts to be helpful. The helpfulness was always associated with the wish to help the parent get better. These findings are consistent with the findings of Siegel et al. (1996). The latency age group tended to present academic difficulties, which the parents related to the disruptions caused by the cancer. The children, whose families were secure, provided enough stability for the children to free themselves from the worries of the illness and continue with their day-to-day life. Those where financial or family problems prevailed felt much more burdened by the implications of the illness. The children from this group attached themselves to the therapist, recognizing him or her as one trustworthy person in their life. Results of this study suggest that children with dying parents manifest significant distress as well as a greater understanding of their parent's illness than it is usually suspected. Three types of interventions were found to be useful: normalization for both patient and

family (50%), expressive–supportive counseling (100%), and occasional cognitive reframing (35%).

Hahn et al. (1997) developed a parent-guidance mode of communicating the parent's terminal illness to children to try to positively affect the children's adjustment process to the terminal illness and death of a parent due to cancer. The specific goals of the intervention were to facilitate the competence of the parents and increase communication among the family members about the illness and impending death. The intervention consisted of 3 hours of providing information, advice, and communication training to both of the parents. The authors report that this model seems promising and points to the importance of a standardized intervention for children with a terminally ill parent.

Christ (2000b) developed a psychoeducational intervention to facilitate the adjustment of children to the terminal illness and subsequent death of a parent. The intervention emphasized a parent-guidance approach. As part of this intervention, a telephone supportive intervention was also developed as a control condition. The goal of this intervention was to maintain contact with the well parent between psychological evaluations, to provide referrals to community based therapists or support groups when such a referral was requested, or to appropriate hospital personnel when questions such as uncertainty about planned treatment procedures, billing, or untoward reactions of the ill parent were raised by the well parent. Since the data generated by this intervention were insufficient for qualitative analyses, only data from families who participated in the psychoeducational intervention were used for the qualitative arm of the analyses. Based on clinical experience, the interventions started during the terminal illness. The researchers found that the family member's responses differed substantially during the terminal stage of the illness from responses following the death. "This clinical experience was confirmed by the quantitative analyses of depression and anxiety measures that indicated that children were significantly more anxious and depressed during the pre-death period than at the end of the reconstitution stage." A typical psychoeducational parent- guidance intervention spanned about 14 months and included six or more 60–90 min therapeutic interviews during the terminal stage of the illness and six or more after the death. The therapeutic engagement was emphasized during the second interview. It was the family's option to include the patient in these interviews. At each meeting, ways of handling problems with the children were discussed. A separate interview was then done with each child. This was followed by an informing interview with the parent(s) in whom the parent(s) was given an assessment of the children's adaptation to the illness. A family interview that included the well parent and all of the children in that family was then done and was followed by two or more biweekly to monthly parent interviews. Beginning 2–4 weeks after the death of the parent, a similar schedule of interviews was followed. Additional child and/or family interviews were scheduled as requested. After the final interview, the social worker initiated bimonthly to monthly telephone contacts with the surviving parent until the final postdeath psychological assessment was completed about

14 months after the death of the parent. Additional telephone contacts were scheduled if significant family crises emerged during the psychologist's final assessment or the social worker's final telephone contact. Finally, if necessary, individual parent, child, and/or family sessions were offered.

Christ et al. (2005) conducted a second psychoeducational intervention program involving 184 families over a 12-month period. The research team reported that "children in the parent-guidance intervention reported greater reduction in trait anxiety and greater improvement in their perceptions of the surviving parent's competence and communication, a primary goal of the intervention."

Dr. Paula Rauch is the founder of a parent-guidance program at Massachusetts General Hospital called "Parenting at a Challenging Time" (PACT). The program provides individual and group parenting support by child psychiatrists and psychologists for cancer patients, their spouses, and children. Of the program, Dr. Rauch says, "I tell parents, – because it's true – that they are the experts on their children… My role is to be a co-pilot navigating with them the unfamiliar waters of a life threatening illness." Through lessons learned from this program for adults with cancer, Dr. Rauch has developed a series of guiding principles for clinicians who are supporting children of parent's facing cancer (Rauch, 2000; Rauch and Durant, 2003; Rauch et al., 2002, 2003; Swick and Rauch, 2006).

Children between the ages of 5 and 18 participated in a support program for families with a parent who had terminal cancer (Bugge and Helseth, 2008). The goals of the intervention were to increase the children's understanding of the situation, to encourage them to talk about the ill parent, and to be assured there were people there to help them. Evaluation of the program was based on in-depth interviews with the children. The researchers reported that the intervention helped the children cope as the parent transitioned into palliative care.

A study by Lewis et al. (2006) reports on the impact of a short-term program on mothers' and children's adjustment to the mother's diagnosis of breast cancer. Research reveals that both mothers and children have elevated distress attributed to cancer, struggle with how to talk about and deal with the impact of the cancer, and fear the mother will die. The Enhancing Connections Program (ECP) was developed to reduce this cancer-related distress and morbidity. The program involves five, 1-hour educational counseling sessions delivered at 2-week intervals by specially trained clinicians. Thirteen households were recruited within 7.5 months of the mother's diagnosis with early-stage breast cancer. Impact was evaluated within a single group design using data obtained from standardized questionnaires with established reliability and validity. Results revealed significant improvements in the mother's depressed mood, anxiety, and self-confidence to assist her child (mother report). There were also significant decreases in the child's behavioral problems (mother and father report), the child's cancer-related worries (child report), and the child's anxiety/depressed mood (mother and father report) (Lewis, 2011).

Support for more research studies focused on developing effective intervention programs for children who have a parent with terminal cancer are slowly gaining ground. There is hope that these efforts will yield more effective intervention strategies for these children.

CONCLUSIONS

The literature on children whose parents die of cancer is abundant. However, most of these studies focus on the process of bereavement. Only a few research studies have focused on children experiencing the terminal phase of their ill parent. The difference in the time of the intervention notwithstanding, several themes emerge: (1) the ability of the surviving parent to meet the needs of the child is crucial for the child's well-being; (2) a child's increased anxiety is directly correlated with a lack of information about his parent's cancer diagnosis; (3) anxiety increases when information is available but there is no opportunity for discussion with the child; (4) children of parents who die of cancer are at a higher risk for psychological problems; (5) previous family history affects the child's bereavement process; (6) meeting with a mental health professional can provide the child with a supportive adult who can clarify confusing thoughts and allay painful feeling and also serve as a model for family discussions; (7) the professionals involved in this type of work need to maintain a clear understanding of their motivation for this work, as well as being attuned to the impact that serving this population may have on their lives.

It is important to remember that making recommendations to families in such a situation is difficult. There is no clear-cut solution for dealing with a family's reaction to terminal cancer. When a parent is dying of cancer, discussions among parents, children, and all other adult caretakers are important. However, these discussions are part of a process that should begin when the patient is first aware of his terminal condition. This may coincide with his referral to a palliative care team. The mental health professional should contact the family at this entry point and establish a connection. An assessment of the parent's adaptation to the illness and of the family and other support systems is very important. The children should be assessed independently to determine developmental age, level of information, adaptation to the critical situation, understanding of the facts, and wishes and fantasies about the future. Finally, the interventions have to take place before despair or resignation sets in so that there is enough motivation to accomplish a higher level of communication and possibly resolution of conflicts before death is imminent.

Interventions for children of palliative care patients and their families have two different aspects: the structure of the meetings and the content. The structure determines where the meeting takes place, when it happens, who is present, and how long it takes. The site should be comfortable, quiet, and relatively private to avoid distractions or interruptions.

The family and the professional should meet when the patient first enters the palliative care service. Ideally, the ill parent will be conscious and have enough energy to be able to connect with the children as well as continue to participate in whatever limited way in their lives. Time should be sufficient so the meeting is not ended prematurely. The professional acts as a consultant to the family by promoting disclosure, clarifying the goals of the meeting, and eliciting information from the different participants, especially the children.

The content of the meeting is determined by the discussion, which is not arbitrarily confined to this situation but uses this time to revisit events. It is of primary importance to explore the information, speculations, and conclusions that the children have reached so far. This provides a springboard for clarifications, providing more information and beginning a discussion of the ill parent's prognosis. When this is a new information to a child, he will need time to react and possibly talk about feelings. It is also important to pay attention to the child's tolerance for information and pace the discussion based on the child's ability to absorb. The child may not want to hear or continue the discussion. The challenge is to know how much to push without assaulting the child with unwelcome facts and when to back off and wait.

This discussion is personal, intimate, and private, requiring a great deal of acceptance and support. The professional will model this through empathetic statements and reassurance. This is a time when the expressions of love, regret for the truncated life, gratitude, and reassurance of unending memory will solidify the bonds and, paradoxically, facilitate the ability to let go. Because this is a very personal and intimate subject, parents are ideally the ones to have this conversation with the child. However, parents are so often burdened with the weight of the illness and all of their other responsibilities that they are not able to take on this task. As previously stated, the two parents, or just the well parent with a professional assistant, may create the optimal situation to clarify issues, provide reassurance, intensify trust and attachment, and prepare the child for the final farewell.

ISSUES FOR THE FUTURE

Over the past decade, there has been a substantial increase in research in the area of childhood bereavement, both in the United States and internationally. These research studies, theories, intervention strategies, support programs, and guidelines are providing a body of knowledge and clinical experience from which we hope to develop more effective intervention strategies for the children of palliative care patients.

The complexity of developing and evaluating psychosocial intervention programs for these children has led to efforts to bridge the gap between the knowledge gained from the quantitative studies and qualitative studies. A literature review by Niemela et al. (2010) indicated a lack of valid psychosocial preventive intervention methods focusing on children with parental cancer and highlighted the need of intervention research with controlled study designs and long follow-up periods. The authors believe that by refining the practice-based experiences with scientific research evidence, it is possible to move to the next level in providing effective psychosocial support and prevention of mental health problems for children living in families with parental cancer.

Christ and Christ (2006) propose three research directions for the twenty-first century, which they believe show promise for obtaining more specific and less confusing and contradictory findings:

1. Studying developmentally homogeneous subgroups of children and the differing effects of different types of deaths
2. Conducting longer-term prospective studies that include critical experiences (e.g., terminal stage in predictable deaths, later responses) that may clarify different outcomes
3. Combining qualitative and quantitative analytic approaches to provide a way to understand the realistic complexity of the area and populations under study

There are many difficulties associated with framing these types of studies. However, there is general agreement among investigators that early intervention for children of palliative care patients is important for the child's bereavement process and ultimate adjustment to life.

As the terminal phase of cancer becomes extended and, thus, the length of palliative care, it is becoming increasingly important to be able to provide effective early interventions for the children of palliative care patients.

Key learning points

- The child's reaction to the ill parent will be affected by the quality of the relationship to the well parent as well as the family integration.

- For the child of a terminal cancer patient, increased anxiety will correlate with confusion about the parent's condition.

- Communication is a process that should begin when the parent enters the palliative care service.

- Anxiety increases when there are no avenues for supportive discussions.

- Previous family history as well as the social and financial conditions will affect the child's adjustment to the parent's illness and ultimate death.

- Children of parents who die of cancer are at a higher risk for psychological problems.

- Meeting with a mental health professional can provide opportunities for discussions as well as a model for family communication.

REFERENCES

Baker, J.E., Sedney, M.A., Gross, E. (1992). Psychological tasks for bereaved children. *Am. J. Orthopsychatr.* 61(1), 105–116.

Black, D. (1998). Coping with loss: Bereavement in childhood. *BMR*, 316:931–933.

Bowlby, J. (1980). *Attachment and Loss: Sadness and Depression.* Vol. 3. New York: Basic Books; pp. 252–259.

Breier, A., Kelsoe., J.R., Jr., Kirwin, P.D. (1988). Early parental loss and development of adult psychopathology. *Arch. Gen. Psychiatry*, 987–993.

Buckman, R. (1984). Breaking bad news: Why is it still so difficult? *Br. Med. J. (Clin. Res. Ed.)*, 1597–1599.

Bugge, K.E., Helseth, S. (2008). Children's experiences of participation in a family support program when their parent has incurable cancer. *Cancer Nurs.* 31(6), 426–434.

Butow, P.N., Brown, R.F., Cogar, S. (2002). Oncologists' reactions to cancer patients' verbal clues. *Psycho-Oncology*, 447–458.

Buxbaum, L., Brant, J.M. (2001). When a parent dies from cancer. *Clin. J. Oncol. Nurs.* 5(4):135–140.

Cerel, J., Fristad, M.A., Verducci, J. et al. (2006). Childhood bereavement: Psychopathology in the 2 years post parental death. *J. Am. Acad. Child Adolesc. Psychiatry.* 45:683–690.

Christ, G.H. (2000a). Impact of development on children's mourning. *Cancer Pract.* 8(2):72–81.

Christ, G.H. (2000b). *Healing Children's Grief: Surviving a Parent's Death from Cancer.* New York: Oxford University Press.

Christ, G.H., Christ, A.E. (2006). Current approaches to helping children cope with a parent's terminal illness. *CA Cancer J. Clin.* 56:197–212.

Christ, G.H., Siegel, K., Christ, A.E. (2002). Adolescent grief: "It never hit me until it actually happened." *JAMA.* 288:1269–1278.

Christ, G.H., Siegel, K., Karus, D., Christ, A.E. (2005). Evaluation of a bereavement intervention. *Social Work End-of-Life Palliat. Care.* 1:57–81.

Christ, G.H., Siegel, K., Sperber, D. (1994). Impact of parent terminal cancer on adolescents. *Am. J. Orthopsychiatry.* 64(4):604–613.

Clark, D.C., Pynoos, R.S., Goebel, A.E. (1994). Mechanisms and processes of adolescent bereavement. In: Haggerty, R.J., Sherrod, L.R., Garmezy, N., Rutter, M. (eds.) *Stress, Risk and Resilience in Children and Adolescents: Processes, Mechanisms, and Interventions.* New York: Cambridge University Press, pp. 100–146.

Dehlin, L., Mertensson, R.G. (2009). Adolescents' experiences of a parent's serious illness and death. *Palliat. Support. Care.* 7(1):13–25.

Dunning, S. (2006). As a young child's parent dies: Conceptualizing and constructing preventive interventions. *Clin. Social Work J.* 34(4):499–514.

Elizur, E., Kaffman, M. (1983). Factors influencing the severity of childhood bereavement reactions. *Am. J. Orthopsychiatry.* 53:668–676.

Fallowfield, L., Jenkins, V. (1999). Effective communication skills are the key to good cancer care. *Eur. J. Cancer.* 1592–1597.

Forrest, G., Plumb, C., Ziebland, S., Stein, A. (2006). Breast cancer in the family—Children's perceptions of their mother's cancer and its initial treatment: Qualitative study. *BMJ.* 332:998.

Giesberg, J., Verdonck-de leeuw, M. (2010). Coping with parental cancer: Web-based peer support in children. *Psycho-Oncology.* 19(8):887–892.

Hahn, D., Kaats, E., Stutterheim, A., Aalders, C., de Best, A., Vessies, T., Uiterwaal, J., van Weezel, L. (1997). Facilitation of children's adjustment to the terminal illness and death of a parent due to cancer. *Eur. J. Cancer, Abstract.* 33(1008):339.

Haine, R.A., Ayers, T.S., Sandler, I.N., Wolchik, S.A. (2008). Evidence-based practices for parentally bereaved children and their families. *Prof. Psychol. Res. Pract.* 39(2):113–112.

Hames, C. (2003). Helping infants and toddlers when a family member dies. *J. Hosp. Palliat. Nurs.* 5(2):103–112.

Hilden, J.M., Watterson, J., Chrastek, J. (2000). Tell the children. *J. Clin. Oncol.* 3193–3195.

Karns, J.T. (2002). Children's understanding of death. *J. Clin. Activ. Assign. Handouts Psychother. Pract.* 2(1):43–50.

Kastenbaum, R. (1967). The child's understanding of death: How does it develop? Explaining death to children. In: Grollman, E. (ed.) Boston, MA: Beacon Press, pp. 89–108.

Kennedy, K.C., McIntyre, R. (2008). Supporting children and families facing the death of a parent: Part 2. *Int. J. Palliat. Nurs.* 14(5):230–237.

Kennedy, V.L., Lloyd-Williams, M. (2009). How children cope when a parent has advanced cancer. *Psycho-Oncology.* 18(8):886–892.

Kornreich, D., Harriet Mannheim, H., Axelrod, D. (2008). How children live with parental cancer. *Prim. Psychiatry.* 15(10):64–70.

Kranzler, E.M., Shaffer, D., Wasserman, G., Davies, M. (1990). Early childhood bereavement. *J. Am. Acad. Child Adolesc. Psychiatry.* 29:513–520.

Kroll, L., Barnes, J., Jones, A.L. (1998). Cancer in parents: Telling children. *BMJ.* 880.

Kwok, O.M., Haine, R., Sandler, I. (2005). Positive parenting as a mediator of the relations between parental psychological distress and mental health problems of parentally bereaved children. *J. Clin. Child Adolesc. Psychol.* 34:260–271.

Lewis, F.M. (2011). Therapy for parental cancer and dependent children. In: Watson, M., Kissane, D.W (eds.) *Handbook of Psychotherapy in Cancer Care.*

Lewis, F.M., Casey, S.M., Brandt, P.A., Shands, M.E., Zahlis, E.H. (2006). The enhancing connections program: Pilot study of a cognitive-behavioral intervention for mothers and children affected by breast cancer. *Psychooncology.* 15(6):486–497.

Maguire, P. (1999). Improving communication with cancer patients. *Eur. J. Cancer.* 1415–1422.

Matthews, G.B. (1989). Children's conceptions of illness and death. In: Kopelman, L.M., Moskop, J.C. (eds.) *Children and Health Care: Moral and Social Issues.* Boston, MA: Kluwer Academic Publishers, pp. 133–146.

Mondanaro, J. (2005). Interfacing music therapy with other arts modalities to address anticipatory grief and bereavement in pediatrics. In: Dileo, C., Loewy, J.V. (eds.) *Music Therapy at the End of Life.* Cherry Hill, NJ: Jeffrey Books, pp. 25–32.

Moore, C.W., Pengelly, M., Rauch, P.K. (2010). Communicating with children when a parent is dying. In: Kissane, D., Bultz, B., Butow, P., Finlay, I. (eds.) *Handbook of Communication in Cancer and Palliative Care.* New York: Oxford University Press, pp. 557–572.

Niemela, M., Hakko, H., Rasanen, S. (2010). A systematic narrative review of the studies on structured child-centered interventions for families with a parent with cancer. *Psychooncology.* 19:451–461.

Pettle, S.A., Britten, C.M. (1995). Talking with children about death and dying. *Child: Care Health Develop.* 395–404.

Pfeffer, C.R., Karus, D., Siegel, K. (2000). Child survivors of parental death from cancer or suicide: Depressive and behavioral outcomes. *Psycho-Oncology.* 1–10.

Popplestone-Helm, S.V., Helm, D.P. (2009). Setting up a support group for children and their well carers who have a significant adult with a life-threatening illness. *Int. J. Palliat. Nurs.* 15(5):214.

Rauch, P. (2000). Comment: Supporting the child within the family. *J. Clin. Ethics.* 11:169–170.

Rauch, P., Muriel, A., Cassem, N. (2002). The art of oncology: When the tumor is not the target. Parents with cancer: Who's looking after the children? *J. Clin. Oncol.* 21:4399–4402.

Rauch, P., Muriel, A., Cassem, N. (2003). Parents with cancer: Who's looking after the children? *J. Clin. Oncol.* 21(9):(Suppl):117–121.

Rauch, P.K., Durant, S. (2003). Helping children cope with a parent's cancer. In: Stern, T., Sekeres, M. (eds.) *Facing Cancer: A Complete Guide for People with Cancer, Their Families, and Caregivers.* New York: McGraw-Hill Professional, pp. 125–136.

Raveis, V.H., Siegel, K., Karus, D. (1999). Children's psychological distress following the death of a parent. *J. Youth Adolesc.* 28(21):165–180.

Sandler, I.N., Ayers, T.S., Wolchik, S.A., Siegel, K., Karus, D. (1999). Children's psychological distress following the death of a parent. *J. Youth Adolesc.* 28:165–180.

Sandler, I.N., Ayers, T. S., Wolchik, S.A., Tein, J.-Y., Kwok, O.-M., Haine, R.A., Twohey-Jacobs, J. et al. (2003). The Family Bereavement Program: Efficacy evaluation of a theory-based prevention program for parentally bereaved children and adolescents. *J. Consult. Clin. Psychol.* 71:587.

Saunders, J. (1996). Innovations in practice: Anticipatory grief work with children. *Br. J. Commun. Health Nurs.* 1(2):103–106.

Schmitt, F., Piha, J., Helenius, H., Baldus, C., Kienbacher, C., Steck, B., Thastum, M., Watson, M., Romer, G. (2008). Multinational study of cancer patients and their children: Factors associated with family functioning. *J. Clin. Oncol.* 26(36):5877–5883.

Siegel, K., Karus, D., Raveis, V.H. (1996). Adjustment of children facing the death of a parent due to cancer. *J. Am. Acad. Child Adolesc. Psychiatry.* 35:442–450.

Siegel, K., Mesagno, R., Christ, G.H. (1990). A preventive program for bereaved children. *Am. J. Orthopsychiatry,* 60:168–175.

Sivesind, D.M., Beale, E. (2002). Children of terminally ill cancer patients: Findings of psychosocial assessment and counseling. *ASCO Annual Meetings, Abstract* No: 1441.

Sourkes, B.M. (1992). The child with a life threatening illness. In: Brandell, J. (ed.) *Countertransference in Psychotherapy with Children and Adolescents,* New York: Jason Aronson, pp. 267–284.

Spinetta, J.J. (1974). The dying child's awareness of death: A review. *Psychol. Bull.* 256–260.

Stambrook, M., Parker, K.C.H. (1987). The development of the concept of death in childhood: A review of the literature. *Merrill-Palmer Quart.* 133–157.

Sweetland, C. (2005). The palliative care nurse's role in supporting the adolescent child of a dying patient. *Int. J. Palliat. Nurs.* 11(6):294–298.

Swick, S.D., Rauch, P.K. (2006). Children facing the death of a parent: The experiences of a parent guidance program at the Massachusetts general hospital cancer center. *Child Adolesc. Psychiatr. Clin. N. Am.* 15(3):779–794.

Turner, J. (2004). Children's and family needs of young women with advanced breast cancer: A review. *Palliat. Support. Care.* 2:55–64.

Turner, J., Clavarino, A. (2007). Development of a resource for parents with advanced cancer: What do parents want? *Palliat. Support. Care.* 5(2):135–145.

Waechter, E.H. (1971). Children's awareness of fatal illness. *Am. J. Nurs.* 1168–1172.

Wolchik, S.A., Ma, Y., Tein, J.-Y., Sandler, I.N., Ayers, T.S. (2008). Parentally bereaved children's grief: Self-system beliefs as mediators of the relations between grief and stressors and caregiver-child relationship quality. *Death Stud.* 32(7):597–620.

Worden, J.W., Silverman, P.R. (1996). Parental death and the adjustment of school-age children. *Omega,* 33, 91–102.

Zambelli, G.C., DeRosa, A.P. (1992). Bereavement support groups for school age children: Theory, intervention and case example. *Am. J. Orthopsychiatry.* 62(4):484–493.

PART 17

The assessment and management of effects of medical treatments

109

Chemotherapy- and radiotherapy-induced emesis

JOSEPH ARTHUR

INTRODUCTION

Nausea is described as an unpleasant subjective feeling of the urge to vomit and manifested by autonomic symptoms such as tachycardia, pallor, salivation, and flushing. It may or may not be associated with vomiting. Vomiting or emesis is the act of forcefully expelling stomach contents through the mouth with the combined actions of the abdominal muscles, diaphragm, and the opening of the gastric cardia. Nausea and vomiting are common symptoms encountered in the palliative care setting. These are quite distressing and tend to have a profound negative impact on a patient's quality of life [1]. The field of palliative care is more familiar with the chronic forms of nausea and vomiting of multifactorial etiologies, including underlying advanced disease process, medications, constipation, mechanical bowel obstruction, and autonomic failure [2]. Chemotherapy- and radiotherapy-induced emesis (CRIE) is, however, not well known among palliative care specialists. It is important that the palliative care specialists become aware of and gain a good understanding of these symptoms. Palliative care has traditionally been seen as a sequential specialty to which patients are referred at the very late stage of their illness. However, it has now evolved into a significant and integral part of holistic patient care, and continues to do so at a steady rate. These days, many healthcare professionals tend to utilize palliative care services early in the course of the disease trajectories of the appropriate patients. This is because they are becoming increasingly aware of the importance and benefits of early referral of patients to the palliative care and supportive care services. In view of this, the patient population on the inpatient palliative care services and the outpatient palliative care clinics is expected to eventually comprise patients with a broader symptom profile, including chemotherapy- and radiotherapy-induced nausea and vomiting.

Providing good patient quality of life is a predominant focus and goal of palliative care providers. Overall, about 70%–80% of patients receiving chemotherapy experience nausea and vomiting [3]. This negatively impacts their ability to care for themselves, eat, and carry out other activities of daily living. This may lead to patients becoming hesitant to pursue subsequent cycles of treatment, and they may sometimes delay or even decline further treatment [4]. Good control of CRIE is an effective way of ensuring good quality of life in patients undergoing chemotherapy and radiotherapy treatment. Studies have shown that oncology physicians and nurses tend to wrongly perceive and underestimate the incidence and severity of chemotherapy-induced nausea and vomiting (CINV) in patients. This may lead to inadequate treatment of these symptoms [5].

CLASSIFICATION OF CINV

Acute CINV: This usually occurs within the first 24 hours after chemotherapy administration. Control of acute CINV seems to minimize the severity of the delayed form. It peaks within the first 4 hours, reaches a peak within the first 4–10 hours, and begins to subside by 12–24 hours [6].

Delayed CINV: This usually occurs after the first 24 hours of chemotherapy administration and may last for as long as 5–7 days, with a peak occurring 48–72 hours after drug administration [7–10,15]. It is relatively more difficult to treat than acute CINV.

Anticipatory CINV: This occurs before the second or later course of chemotherapy. It is a learned or conditioned response in patients who had an unpleasant experience of poorly managed nausea and vomiting during previous cycles of chemotherapy. It is usually triggered by sensory stimuli such as the sights, sounds, smells, and tactile experiences associated with the therapy, and it appears to have a strong psychological component. Good management of the patient's earlier courses of chemotherapy seems to be the most effective way to prevent CINV (Table 109.1).

Table 109.1 *National Cancer Institute's common terminology criteria for adverse events: Nausea and vomiting*

Nausea

Grade 1	Loss of appetite without change in eating habits
Grade 2	Decreased oral intake without significant weight loss, dehydration, or malnutrition
Grade 3	Insufficient oral caloric or fluid intake; tube feeding, TPN, or hospitalization indicated

Vomiting

Grade 1	1–2 episodes (separated by 5 min) in 24 hours
Grade 2	3–5 episodes (separated by 5 min) in 24 hours
Grade 3	≥6 episodes (separated by 5 min) in 24 hours; tube feeding, TPN, or hospitalization indicated
Grade 4	Life-threatening consequences; urgent intervention required
Grade 5	Death

Source: http://www.cancer.gov/cancertopics/pdq/supportivecare/nausea/
HealthProfessional/page1

PATHOPHYSIOLOGY

Generally, vomiting occurs when a group of neurons in the medulla oblongata called the vomiting center is activated. The vomiting center is located in the medulla and is activated when it receives afferent neuronal impulses from predominantly four main areas of the body: the chemoreceptor trigger zone (CTZ), the gastrointestinal tract, the cerebral cortex, and the vestibular apparatus. The CTZ, located in the floor of the fourth ventricle, does not have a true blood–brain barrier. It is therefore accessible to emetogenic substances and senses changes in the concentrations of drugs, chemical agents, and metabolites in the bloodstream [6]. The gastrointestinal tract can also activate the vomiting center indirectly via the CTZ. When mechanoreceptors located in the muscle wall of the gut are stimulated by contraction and distension and chemoreceptors located in the mucosa of the gut are stimulated by chemical irritants, they send visceral vagal afferent signals to the CTZ for onward transmission to the vomiting center (Figure 109.1).

Various neurotransmitters are known to mediate the transmission of impulses to the CTZ and the vomiting center. The major ones are serotonin, which act on the

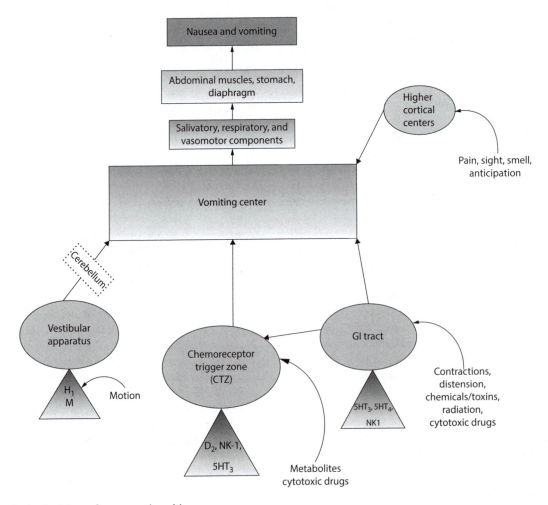

Figure 109.1 *Pathophysiology of nausea and vomiting.*

serotonin-3(5-HT3) receptors, dopamine, which act on dopamine-2(D2) receptors, and substance P, which act on natural killer-1(NK-1) receptors [9] Others include histamine and acetylcholine, which act on the histaminic and muscarinic receptors, respectively [10,11]. These are prominent in motion sickness–related vomiting.

The gastrointestinal tract is one of the organs that are in a constant state of regeneration and repair and thus is very vulnerable to the effects of chemotherapy, including nausea and vomiting. Chemotherapy is known to cause vomiting by stimulating the enterochromaffin cells lining the gastrointestinal tract to release serotonin in response to cell damage [27]. Serotonin binds to serotonin-3 receptors in the gastrointestinal tract, which then send impulses directly to the vomiting center. Substance P, which is colocalized with serotonin in the enterochromaffin cells, is also released either in response to increased serotonin levels or in response to the toxic effects of chemotherapy medications. It is known that acute CINV is mediated by both serotonin and substance P, whereas the delayed phase is primarily mediated by substance P. The gastrointestinal tract can also stimulate the vomiting center indirectly through the CTZ as already mentioned earlier.

RISK FACTORS FOR CINV

The incidence and severity of the symptoms vary depending on the individual and the type of chemotherapy being administrated. It has been found that heavy alcohol users tend to have less vomiting. History of nausea and vomiting associated with previous exposure to chemotherapy, or even from other causes such as motion sickness and pregnancy, may predict a high likelihood of CINV with new chemotherapy treatment [10,16]. The emetogenic potential of each chemotherapy agent is additive when given concomitantly instead of sequentially (Table 109.2).

Different chemotherapy agents have different emetogenic potentials. Examples of highly emetogenic agents include cisplatin, cyclophosphamide (>1500 mg/m^2), dacarbazine, pentostatin, and dactinomycin. Examples of moderately emtogenic agents include cyclophosphamide (<1500 mg/m^2), carboplatin, doxorubicin, irinotecan, oxaliplatin, and clofarabine. Most other agents, including targeted therapy agents, are of either low or minimal emetogenic potential.

CINV is treated by four main classes of medications: D2 receptor antagonists, 5-HT3 receptor antagonists, NK-1 receptor antagonists, and corticosteroids. Benzodiazepines are also sometimes used as adjunctive medications.

1. *Dopamine-2 (D2) receptor antagonists.* They work centrally to block dopamine receptors in the CTZ and the vomiting center [6]. Examples of the three classes of drugs include butyrophenones (e.g., droperidol), phenothiazines (e.g., prochlorperazine), and substituted benzamides (e.g., metoclopramide) [13]. Known side effects include extrapyramidal symptoms, restlessness, and CNS depression. Metoclopramide is unique among this class because it blocks dopamine receptors both centrally in the CTZ and peripherally in the gastrointestinal tract. It also acts as a prokinetic agent, thereby increasing gut motility. At high doses, it is also capable of blocking serotonin receptors. It is actually one of the early agents shown to significantly decrease the volume and frequency of CINV when given at high intravenous doses [32–34]. Reports of potential extrapyramidal side effects were minor even at high doses. Drowsiness and diarrhea are the common side effects of metoclopramide.

2. *5-Hydroxytryptamine-3 (5-HT3) receptor antagonists.* These act both centrally and peripherally by binding to 5-HT3 receptors in the CTZ and the gastrointestinal tract [6,12]. Examples include dolasetron, granisetron, ondansetron, which are first-generation 5 HT3 receptor antagonists, and palonosetron (IV only), a second-generation 5 HT3 receptor antagonist. These agents are comparably safe and effective for CINV when used at equivalent doses [17]. However, palonosetron is found to be superior to the first-generation agents mainly because it has a significantly longer half-life (about 40 hours, 10 times longer than first-generation antagonists), has a very high binding affinity, is highly selective to the 5-HT3 receptors (with little effect on other receptors), and has an exceptional safety profile [18]. The major side effects are constipation and headache [17,19].

3. *Neurokinin-1 (NK-1) receptor antagonists.* These work by blocking the NK-1 receptors in the CNS. They are a relatively new class of antiemetic medications and have been shown to be very effective in the prevention and control of delayed CINV when combined with other standard antiemetic agents [20]. Examples include aprepitant and fosaprepitant. Fosaprepitant is a prodrug of aprepitant and is administered intravenously [21]. Dizziness, anorexia, diarrhea, and nausea are the most common side effects.

4. *Corticosteroids.* The mechanisms of action are unknown, but it is believed that they work through multiple actions. They are believed to decrease nausea and vomiting by interfering with prostaglandin synthesis. They are also thought to decrease serotonin production in the central nervous system (CNS). A third possible action is that they

Table 109.2 *Risk factors for CINV*

Factor	Effect
Age > 50 years	↑
Female gender	↑
Alcohol use	↓
Previous experience with nausea and/or Vomiting with pregnancy or motion sickness	↑
Anxiety	↑
Emetogenic potential of the chemotherapeutic agent	↑
Low social functioning	↑

reduce the permeability of the blood–brain barrier and may therefore limit the penetration of emetogenic agents to the brain or reduce chemotherapy or radiation-induced brain edema [6]. Common side effects include fluid retention, anxiety, insomnia, gastrointestinal upset, and immunosuppression.

5. *Benzodiazepines.* Their mechanism of action in managing CINV is unclear, but their sedative, anxiolytic, and amnesic properties have been implicated. They are particularly useful in treating anticipatory CINV [26,22]. Examples include lorazepam and diazepam. Common side effects include dizziness, sedation, confusion, and fatigue.

6. *Novel agents under investigation*: Researchers are currently actively looking into the use of several medications for CINV, including netupitant, a selective NK-1 receptor antagonist with potential long-lasting antiemetic activity (ClinicalTrials.gov identifier: NCT01339260); carbamazepine, an anticonvulsant and mood-stabilizing medication mainly used to treat epilepsy, bipolar disorder and trigeminal neuralgia (ClinicalTrials.gov identifier: NCT 01581918); gabapentin, originally developed as an anticonvulsant but currently being used mainly for painful neuropathy, postherpetic neuralgia and migraines (ClinicalTrials.gov identifier: NCT 00880191); and olanzapine, an antipsychotic known to bind to a wide variety of receptors, including dopaminergic, serotonergic, histaminic, and muscarinic receptors [26].

Nonpharmacological interventions

Studies have shown the effect of family relationships on patients' experience during cancer treatment. Among women, it was found that increased conflict within the family was associated with an increased severity of anticipatory nausea. Also, among younger adults, increased family conflict was associated with an increased duration of post-treatment nausea and greater severity of anticipatory nausea [28]. Psychosocial interventions such as cognitive behavioral therapy, increase in general social support, and the Multiple Family Discussion Group, a program that encourages the consideration of multiple points of view, have been found to be effective in helping patients during their chemotherapy treatment experience [27]. Other nonpharmacological interventions such as relaxation techniques, systematic desensitization, and hypnosis may be useful. Anticipatory CINV particularly responds well to behavioral interventions [23–25,14].

RADIOTHERAPY-INDUCED NAUSEA AND VOMITING

Radiotherapy-induced nausea and vomiting (RINV) is also common among cancer patients just like CINV. It presents with a latent period after the radiation, followed by a period of nausea and vomiting lasting about 6 hours with a subsequent gradual resolution, but may sometimes last up to 24 hours [29].

The rapidly dividing cells of the gastrointestinal tract are very sensitive to radiation. The radiation treatment damages the enterochromaffin cells of the gastrointestinal mucosa, thereby causing the release of serotonin. Serotonin then binds to receptors on the vagal afferent nerves. These then send impulses to the vomiting center of the brain, thereby causing vomiting, similar to the pathway described in CINV.

The severity of the symptoms is determined by the location of the radiation field, the size of the radiation field, and the dose of radiation given. The most recent clinical practice guideline by the American Society of Clinical Oncology classified the emetic risk of radiation therapy as high, moderate, low, or minimal based on the site of the radiation therapy. Sites with high emetic risk include total body irradiation and total nodal irradiation. Sites with moderate risk include upper abdomen, upper body irradiation, and half-body irradiation. Sites with low emetic risk include the cranium, craniospinal region, head and neck, lower thorax region, and the pelvis. Sites with minimal risk include the extremities and breast [30].

RECOMMENDED TREATMENT REGIMENS FOR CINV AND RINV

Because of the multifactorial etiologies for CINV and radiation-induced emesis, it is believed that no single medication will be completely effective and combination therapies are therefore recommended. It is also always important to evaluate the patient for other common causes of nausea and vomiting such as opioids, constipation, bowel obstruction, and metabolic derangements. What follows are some recommended treatment regimens based on the most recent clinical practice guideline update by the American Society of Clinical Oncology [31] (Table 109.3).

CLINICAL PEARLS ON THE TREATMENT APPROACH

- For highly emetogenic chemotherapy regimens, the three-drug combination of an NK-1 antagonist, 5-HT3 antagonist, and dexamethasone is recommended.
- For moderately emetogenic chemotherapy regimens, palonosetron is the preferred 5-HT3 antagonist. It should be combined with a corticosteroid. If palonosetron is unavailable, a first-generation 5-HT3 serotonin receptor antagonist may be substituted, preferably granisetron or ondansetron.
- For combination chemotherapy regimens, antiemetic treatment should be given based on the agent with the highest emetogenicity.
- Pediatric patients receiving either highly or moderately emetogenic chemotherapy should be treated with a 5-HT3 antagonist. A higher weight-based dosing may be required. A corticosteroid should be added to the regimen.

Table 109.3 *Antiemetic dosing based on the emetogenicity of the chemotherapeutic agent*

	NK_1 antagonist	5-HT3 antagonist	Corticosteroid
Highly emetogenic	Aprepitant oral on days 1–3 OR Fosaprepitant IV on day 1	Granisetron oral or IV on day 1 OR Ondansetron oral or IV on day 1 OR Palonosetron oral or IV on day 1 OR Dolasetron oral on day 1 OR Tropisetron oral or IV on day 1 OR Ramosetron IV day 1	Dexamethasone oral or IV on days 1–3 and/or 4
Moderately emetogenic		Palonosetron oral or IV on day 1. If unavailable, then give Granisetron oral or IV on day 1 OR Ondansetron oral or IV on day 1 OR Dolasetron oral on day 1 OR Tropisetron oral or IV on day 1 OR Ramosetron IV day 1	Dexamethasone oral or IV on days 1–3
Lowly emetogenic			Dexamethasone oral or IV on days 1–3
Minimally emetogenic	Antiemetic agents are given only on an as-needed basis		

Source: Lee, V.H. et al., *Int. J. Radiat. Oncol. Biol. Phys.*, 84(1), 176, 2012.

- For highly emetogenic radiation therapy, a 5-HT3 antagonist before each fraction and at least 24 hours after completion, plus a 5-day course of dexamethasone, is recommended.
- For moderately emetogenic radiation therapy, a 5-HT3 antagonist before each fraction is also recommended, but a 5-day course of dexamethasone is optional.
- For lowly emetogenic radiation therapy, a 5-HT3 antagonist alone as either prophylaxis or rescue is

recommended. Antiemetic medication should continue until completion of radiotherapy if a patient develops radiation-induced nausea and vomiting during the course of treatment.

- For minimally emetogenic radiation therapy, a dopamine receptor antagonist alone or 5-HT3 antagonist as rescue therapy is recommended. Antiemetic medication should continue until completion of radiotherapy if a patient develops radiation-induced nausea and vomiting during the course of treatment.
- If the patient is receiving combination chemoradiotherapy, antiemetic therapy is given based on the emetogenicity of chemotherapy, unless the emetic risk of radiation therapy is higher.
- Lorazepam or diphenhydramine are useful adjunctive medications to antiemetic drugs but are not recommended as single-agent antiemetics.
- If nausea and vomiting persist despite optimal prophylaxis, a comprehensive review and reevaluation is recommended. This should include the emetic risk, disease status, concurrent illnesses, medications, and other possible causes of emesis. Ensure that the best regimen is being administered for the degree of emetogenicity. It is also recommended to consider adding a benzodiazepine, a dopamine antagonist like olanzapine, or substituting high-dose intravenous metoclopramide for the 5-HT3 antagonist.

REFERENCES

1 Chan A, Low XH, Yap KY. Assessment of the relationship between adherence with antiemetic drug therapy and control of nausea and vomiting in breast cancer patients receiving anthracycline-based chemotherapy. *J Manage Care Pharm*. 2012;18(5):385–394. PubMed PMID: 22663171.

2 Hanks G, Cherny N, Christakis N, Fallon M, Kaasa S, Portenoy R. *Oxford Textbook of Palliative Medicine*. 4th edn.

3 Grunberg SM. Chemotherapy-induced nausea and vomiting: Prevention, detection, and treatment—How are we doing? *J Support Oncol*. 2004;2(1 Suppl 1):1–10.

4 Bloechl-Daum B, Deuson RR, Marvos P et al. Delayed nausea and vomiting continue to reduce patient's quality of life after highly and moderately emetogenic chemotherapy despite antiemetic treatment. *J Clin Oncol* 2006;24:4472–4478.

5 Grunberg SM, Hansen M, Deuson R, Mavros P. Incidence and impact of nausea/vomiting with modern antiemetics: Perception vs. reality. In: *Program/Proceedings of the 38th Annual Meeting of the American Society of Clinical Oncology*; May 18–21, 2002; Orlando, FL. Abstract 996. National Comprehensive Cancer Network. *NCCN Antiemesis Practice Guidelines. Oncology* 1997;11:57–89.

6 Veyrat-Follet C, Farinotti R, Palmer JL. Physiology of chemotherapy-induced emesis and antiemetic therapy. Predictive models for evaluation of new compounds.

7 Herrstedt J, Rapoport B, Warr D et al. Acute emesis: Moderately emetogenic chemotherapy. *Support Care Cancer* 2011;19(Suppl 1):S15–S23.

8 Hesketh PJ, Van Belle S, Aapro M et al. Differential involvement of neurotransmitters through the time course of cisplatin-induced emesis as revealed by therapy with specific receptor antagonists. *Eur J Cancer* 2003;39:1074–1080.

9   ASHP therapeutic guidelines on the pharmacologic management of nausea and vomiting in adult and pediatric patients receiving chemotherapy or radiation therapy or undergoing surgery. *Am J Health Syst Pharm* 1999;56:729–764.

10 Grunberg SM, Hesketh PJ. Control of chemotherapy- induced emesis. *N Engl J Med* 1993;329:1790–1796.

11 Balfour JA, Goa KL. Dolasetron: A review of its pharmacology and therapeutic potential in the management of nausea and vomiting induced by chemotherapy, radiotherapy, or surgery. *Drugs* 1997;54:273–298.

12 Kovac AL. Benefits and risks of newer treatments for chemotherapy-induced and postoperative nausea and vomiting. *Drug Saf* 2003;26:227–259.

13 Kovac AL. Prevention and treatment of postoperative nausea and vomiting. *Drugs* 2000;59:213–243.

14 Hofman M, Morrow GR, Roscoe JA et al. Cancer patients' expectations of experiencing treatment-related side effects: A University of Rochester Cancer Center-Community Clinical Oncology Program study of 938 patients from community practices. *Cancer* 2004;101:851–785.

15 Kris MG, Gralla RJ, Clark RA et al. Incidence, course, and severity of delayed nausea and vomiting following the administration of high dose cisplatin. *J Clin Oncol* 1985;3:1379–1384.

16 Roscoe JA, Morrow GR, Hickok JT et al. Biobehavioral factors in chemotherapy-induced nausea and vomiting. *J Natl Compr Canc Netw* 2004;2:501–508.

17 Aloxi (palonosetron HCl injection). *Prescribing Information.* Bloomington, MI: MGI Pharma Inc; 2003.

18 Poli-Bigelli S, Rodrigues-Pereira J, Carides AD et al., for the Aprepitant Protocol 054 Study Group. Addition of the neurokinin-1 receptor antagonist aprepitant to standard antiemetic therapy improves control of chemotherapy-induced nausea and vomiting: Results from a randomized, double-blind, placebo-controlled trial in Latin America. *Cancer* 2003;97:3090–3098.

19 Navari RM. Palonosetron for the prevention of chemotherapy-induced nausea and vomiting in patients with cancer. *Future Oncol* 2010;6:1073–1084.

20 Hesketh PJ, Grunberg SM, Gralla RJ et al. The oral neurokinin-1 antagonist aprepitant for the prevention of chemotherapy-induced nausea and vomiting: A multinational, randomized, double-blind, placebo-controlled trial in patients receiving high-dose cisplatin—The Aprepitant Protocol 052 Study Group. *J Clin Oncol* 2003;21:4112.

21 Stewart OJ. Cancer therapy, vomiting, and antiemetics. *Can J Physiol Pharmacol* 1990;68:304–313.

22 Roscoe JA, Morrow GR, Aapro MS et al. Anticipatory nausea and vomiting. *Support Care Cancer* 2011;19:1533–1538.

23 Colagiuri B, Roscoe JA, Morrow GR et al. How do patient expectancies, quality of life, and postchemotherapy nausea interrelate? *Cancer* 2008;113:654–661.

24 Hickok JT, Roscoe JA, Morrow GR. The role of patients' expectations in the development of anticipatory nausea related to chemotherapy for cancer. *J Pain Symptom Manage* 2001;22:843–850.

25 Figueroa-Moseley C, Jean-Pierre P, Roscoe JA et al. Behavioral interventions in treating anticipatory nausea and vomiting. *J Natl Compr Canc Netw* 2007;5:44–50.

26 Danjoux CE, Rider WD, Fitzpatrick PJ. The acute radiation syndrome. A memorial to William Michael Court-Brown. *Clin Radiol* 1979;30:581–584.

27 Janelsins MC, Tejani MA, Kamen C, Peoples AR, Mustian KM, Morrow GR. Current pharmacotherapy for chemotherapy-induced nausea and vomiting in cancer patients. *Expert Opin Pharmacother.* 2013;14(6):757–766.

28 Kim Y, Morrow GR. Changes in family relationships affect the development of chemotherapy- related nausea symptoms. *Support Care Cancer* 2003;11:171–177.

29 Horiot JC. Prophylaxis versus treatment: Is there a better way to manage radiotherapy-induced nausea and vomiting? *Int J Radiat Oncol Biol Phys* 2004;15:1018–1025.

30 Lee VH, Ng SC, Leung TW, Au GK, Kwong DL. Dosimetric predictors of radiation-induced acute nausea and vomiting in IMRT for nasopharyngeal cancer. *Int J Radiat Oncol Biol Phys.* 2012;84(1):176–182. doi: 10.1016/j.ijrobp.2011.10.010. Epub January 13, 2012. PubMed PMID: 22245210.

31 Basch E, Prestrud AA, Hesketh PJ et al. Antiemetics: American Society of Clinical Oncology clinical practice guideline update. *J. Oncol. Pract.* 7(6):395–398.

32 Gralla RJ, Itri LM, Pisko SE, Squillante AE, Kelsen DP, Braun DW Jr, Bordin LA, Braun TJ, Young CW. Antiemetic efficacy of high-dose metoclopramide: Randomized trials with placebo and prochlorperazine in patients with chemotherapy-induced nausea and vomiting. *N Engl J Med.* 1981;305(16):905–909. PubMed PMID: 7024807.

33 Bruera E, Michaud M, Partington J, Brenneis C, Paterson AH, MacDonald RN. Continuous subcutaneous (CS) infusion of metoclopramide (MCP) using a plastic disposable infusor for the treatment of chemotherapy-induced emesis. *J Pain Symptom Manage.* 1988;3(2):105–107.

34 Bruera E, MacDonald N, Brenneis C, Simpson I, LeGatt D. Metoclopramide infusion with a disposable portable pump. *Ann Intern Med.* 1986;104(6):896.

35 http://www.cancer.gov/cancertopics/pdq/supportivecare/nausea/HealthProfessional/page1

110

Neutropenic fever

HIROSHI ISHIGURO, HARUMI GOMI

RISK FACTORS FOR INFECTION IN CANCER PATIENTS

Despite the progress made in supportive care in oncology, infection is a very common, and occasionally serious, problem. The following factors increase the susceptibility of cancer patients to infection.[1]

Local factors

Local factors that obstruct or disrupt normal anatomic barriers play an important role in infections occurring in cancer patients. Pneumonia and abscess can develop distal to obstruction of the major bronchi and respond poorly to antibiotic therapy. Obstruction of the biliary tract can result in ascending cholangitis. Urinary tract infections are common in patients with genitourinary tumors that obstruct the ureter or bladder neck, causing retention of urine. In such cases, one or more of the microorganisms colonizing the site of obstruction generally cause the infection. Mucosal surfaces (particularly of the gastrointestinal mucosa) damaged by antineoplastic chemotherapy frequently provide a portal of entry for pathogens. Radiation also causes local tissue damage, which can predispose to secondary infection.[1]

Neutropenia

Both the degree and the duration of neutropenia are risk factors for infection, and bacteremias can develop during the episodes of severe and/or prolonged neutropenia (>1 week). Patients with neutropenia often fail to develop the characteristic signs and symptoms of infection due to their impaired ability to mount an adequate inflammatory response. Common sites of infection in patients with neutropenia include the lung, oropharynx, blood, urinary tract, skin and soft tissues, including the perirectal area. Infections are generally caused by organisms colonizing the patient (Table 110.1).[1]

Cellular immune dysfunction

Cell-mediated immunity plays a primary role in protecting against intracellular pathogens (Table 110.1). In addition, T lymphocytes impact on practically all aspects of immunity. Patients with Hodgkin's disease and chronic/acute lymphocytic leukemia have impaired cell-mediated immunity. Immunosuppressive therapy with cyclosporine, tacrolimus, azathioprine, corticosteroids, or some cytotoxic agents (fludarabine and other purine analogues) causes cellular immunity dysfunction. Radiation therapy results in depression of cell-mediated immunity lasting several months.[1]

Humoral immune dysfunction

B lymphocytes are responsible for antibody production. In disorders such as multiple myeloma, Waldenström macroglobulinemia, and the various "heavy-chain diseases," overproduction of a specific subcomponent of an immunoglobulin occurs due to malignant proliferation of plasma cells or their precursors, which in turn results in low levels of normal immunoglobulins. Patients are then especially susceptible to infection by encapsulated organisms such as *Streptococcus pneumoniae* and *Haemophilus influenzae* because specific opsonizing antibodies are diminished (Table 110.1).[1]

Foreign bodies

Foreign bodies such as urinary and venous catheters can damage or circumvent normal anatomic barriers, thereby facilitating the entry of microorganisms into tissues and the bloodstream. Prosthetic devices such as stents can be infected.[1]

PREVENTION OF NEUTROPENIC FEVER

Patients with generalized malignancy, transplant recipients, and patients being treated with immunosuppressive or radiation therapy are all considered to have altered immunocompetence.[2]

Table 110.1 *Defects in host defense mechanisms and common pathogens*

Neutropenia	Gram-positive cocci, gram-negative bacilli, fungus (*Candida, Aspergillus*)
Cellular immune dysfunction	*Pneumocystis, Cryptococcus, Mycobacterium, Toxoplasma, Listeria, Cryptosporidium, Candida, Cytomegalovirus*
Humoral immune dysfunction	Encapsulated organisms (*Streptococcus pneumonia, Haemophilus influenzae, Neisseria meningitidis*)

Source: Data from Rolston, V.I.K. and Bodey, P.G., Infection in patients with cancer, in: Hong, K.W., Bast, Jr. C.R., Hait, N.W., Kufe, W.D., Pollock, E.R., Weichselbaum, R.R., Holland, F.J., Frei, III E. (eds.), *Holland-Frei Cancer Medicine*, 8th edn., pp. 1921–1940, McGraw Hill, London, U.K., 2009.

Controlling local factors

It is often possible to prevent serious infection by proactive control of the aforementioned local factors.[1]

- Consider radiation therapy for obstructive pneumonia due to mass.
- For patients with cholelithiasis, cholecystectomy may be indicated depending on the risk for acute cholecystitis.
- Since the placement of a foreign body such as a urinary or venous catheter can be a port of entry for bacterial pathogens, consider removing them.
- Poor oral hygiene or incompletely erupted wisdom tooth can be the source of periodontitis during profound neutropenia. Provide advice on improving oral hygiene and, when necessary, consult a specialist regarding tooth extraction before starting intensive chemotherapy.
- Consider draining pleural effusion to prevent infection, which is occasionally difficult to control.

Vaccinations

Pneumococcal polysaccharide vaccine is currently recommended by the Centers for Disease Control and Prevention for patients between 18 and 65 years of age with asplenia, HIV infection, or generalized malignancy, as well as those under immunosuppressive chemotherapy or corticosteroid therapy or who have received organ or bone marrow transplant.[2] Whenever feasible, a single dose of the vaccine should be administered to these patients at least 2 weeks before starting cytotoxic or immunosuppressive therapy if they have not been previously vaccinated or if their previous vaccine history is unknown; otherwise, they are considered unprotected.[3] A recent study demonstrated that a 13-valent conjugate pneumococcal vaccine (PCV13) had superior antibody response among adults over 50 years of age compared with a 23-valent polysaccharide vaccine (PPSV23).[4]

Influenza infections in immunocompromised cancer patients are often associated with hospitalizations, delays in potentially life-saving chemotherapy, and occasionally death. Annual vaccination against influenza with the inactivated virus—not intranasal live influenza vaccine—is currently recommended. The guidelines also recommend annual immunization with the inactivated virus for all healthcare professionals and household members or caregivers of cancer patients.[3]

Antibacterial prophylaxis

Fluoroquinolone prophylaxis should be considered for patients at high risk for prolonged and profound neutropenia (absolute neutrophil count [ANC] ≤ 100 cells/μL (mm³) for >7 days). Levofloxacin has superior activity against certain gram-positive pathogens to ciprofloxacin. Antibacterial prophylaxis is not routinely recommended for low-risk patients with severe neutropenia expected to last <7 days due to possible adverse effects of drugs (e.g., rash, gastrointestinal intolerance) and selection of resistant pathogens. Since fluoroquinolones are categorized as a "concentration-dependent" agent in antibacterial activity, a dose of 500 mg once daily is recommended.[3,5,6**]

Prophylactic use of granulocyte–colony stimulating factors (G-CSF)

It is important to evaluate the risk for chemotherapy-induced neutropenic fever prior to the first cycle. The risk assessment should include not only the chemotherapeutic regimen (dose and schedule) but also patient risk factors. Based on the results, patients are designated high risk (>20% risk of neutropenic fever), intermediate risk (10%–20% risk), or low risk (<10% risk). Treatment intent should also be considered since patients with neutropenic complications in the preceding cycle and without dose reduction are also considered to be at high risk.[7]

Primary prophylaxis involves the use of a G-CSF beginning in the first cycle of treatment. For "dose-dense" regimens, G-CSFs are required. Clinical trial data support the use of G-CSF when the risk of neutropenic fever is ≥20%. Adjuvant treatment of early-stage breast cancer with TAC or FEC100 or the use of CHOP in older patients with aggressive non-Hodgkin's lymphoma are examples. G-CSF should be given 24–72 hours after the administration of chemotherapy and should be continued until an ANC of at least 2 to 3 × 10³ cells/μL (mm³). In adults, the recommended G-CSF dose is 5 μg/kg/day for filgrastim. For a longer-acting G-CSF, a single injection of pegfilgrastim 6 mg (a lower dose was shown to be as effective in certain populations), given 1–3 days after administration of chemotherapy, is sufficient per chemotherapy cycle.[7,8] A recent study showed that less frequent G-CSF dosing is as effective as daily G-CSF and is associated with less bone pain.[9] However, since this finding is for patients in whom G-CSF is not routinely indicated, the efficacy of less frequent G-CSF dosing has not been definitively proven.

Secondary prophylaxis involves the use of G-CSF to prevent neutropenic fever or chemotherapy dose modifications in a subsequent chemotherapy cycle in patients who have experienced neutropenic complications in an earlier course (e.g., beginning in the second or later cycle of treatment). Secondary prophylaxis is recommended for patients in whom a reduced dose could compromise disease-free or overall survival or treatment outcome. In many clinical situations, dose reduction or delay may be a reasonable alternative.[8]

MANAGEMENT OF NEUTROPENIC FEVER

Definition of neutropenic fever

The definitions of neutropenic fever are consistent among those given by the Infectious Disease Society of America (IDSA), National Comprehensive Cancer Network (NCCN), and the U.S. Food and Drug Administration (FDA) for evaluating antimicrobial therapy for neutropenic fever. Fever is defined as a single oral temperature measurement of $\geq 38.3°C$ (101°F) or oral temperature of $\geq 38.0°C$ (100.4°F) sustained over a 1 hour period. Use of axillary temperature may not accurately reflect core body temperature, and rectal temperature measurement may cause mucosal damage that can facilitate the entry of colonizing bacteria. Neutropenia is defined as ANC < 500 cells/μL (mm³) or ANC < 1000 cells/μL (mm³) with a predicted decline to <500 cells/μL (mm³) over the next 48 hours. Profound neutropenia is defined as ANC < 100 cells/μL (mm³); a manually read blood smear is required to confirm this.[3,5]

Evaluation of patients with neutropenic fever

Neutropenic fever is a true medical emergency. Without timely administration of proper antibiotics, sepsis syndrome and even death might occur. The education of patients and family members as well as appropriate initial management is of critical importance.[10] The initial evaluation should focus on determining the potential sites and causative organisms of infection and assessing the patient's risk for an infection-related complication. Since signs and symptoms of inflammation are often subtle or absent in neutropenic patients, the physical examination requires a careful search in the most commonly infected areas such as the skin (e.g., sites of previous procedures or catheters), oropharynx, alimentary tract, lungs, and perineum.[3,5]

An initial laboratory/radiology evaluation should include a complete blood count with differential analysis and a blood chemistry test for liver function (e.g., total bilirubin, albumin, ALT, AST) and renal function (e.g., blood urea nitrogen, creatinine, electrolytes). These tests should be repeated at least every 3 days. Chest radiographs should be taken for all patients with respiratory signs or symptoms since pneumonia during neutropenia can progress rapidly; radiographic findings may be absent however.[3,5]

At least two sets (one aerobic and one anaerobic blood culture bottles, 10 mL each) of blood culture specimens should be obtained, as a sufficient volume of blood must be cultured in order to detect bloodstream infection. The sensitivity of two blood culture sets is 80%–90% for bloodstream pathogens.[3,5] Skin preparation with an alcohol solution of 0.5% chlorhexidine is more efficacious than skin preparation with an aqueous solution of 10% povidone-iodine in reducing contamination of blood culture (1.4% vs. 3.3%; odds ratio, 0.40; 95% confidence

interval [CI], 0.21–0.75).[11**] Routine cultures from various sites are rarely helpful in the absence of clinical signs and symptoms. Culture of urine samples is indicated if signs or symptoms of urinary tract infection exist, a urinary catheter is in place or urinalysis is abnormal. Sputum samples for routine bacterial culture are indicated if the patient has a productive cough, although neutropenic patients with pulmonary infiltrates frequently cannot produce sputum. For patients with pulmonary infiltrates on imaging, a more invasive approach such as bronchoscopy with bronchoalveolar lavage may occasionally be needed for a microbiological diagnosis.[3,5] For patients with a central venous catheter, it is recommended that one set from a peripheral vein and one set from each catheter lumen be obtained during the initial evaluation of fever.[3,5] A useful diagnostic tool for central line–associated bloodstream infection is the differential time to positivity of blood cultures performed on specimens drawn simultaneously through the catheters and peripheral vein with >85% sensitivity and >90% specificity when a cut-off of 120 min is used.[12]

In patients with diarrhea, a stool specimen should be evaluated for *Clostridium difficile*. Since enzyme immunoassay (EIA) testing for *C. difficile* toxin A and B is less sensitive than the cell cytotoxin assay, confirmation of *C. difficile* infection should involve a two-step strategy: recommended is EIA detection of glutamate dehydrogenase (GDH) as initial screening, and, if positive, the cell cytotoxicity assay or toxigenic culture as the confirmatory test. Sending a stool specimen for bacterial pathogen culture is of limited value in most developed countries due to the time and costs involved; nevertheless, stool culture is the most sensitive test for *C. difficile* infection.[13] Other diagnostic test includes polymerase chain reaction (PCR) of toxin, which is more expensive.

Initial management of neutropenic fever

At presentation of neutropenic fever, risk assessment for complications should be performed. This may determine the type of empirical antibiotics (oral vs. intravenous therapy) and needs for inpatient care. With use of the Multinational Association of Supportive Care in Cancer (MASCC) scoring system (Table 110.2), all high-risk patients (MASCC score < 21)

Table 110.2 *Multinational Association of Supportive Care in Cancer risk-index score*

Characteristics	Weight
Burden of illness	
No or mild symptoms	5
Moderate symptoms	3
No hypotension	5
No chronic obstructive pulmonary disease	4
Solid tumor or no previous fungal infection	4
No dehydration	3
Outpatient status	3
Age < 60 years	2

Source: Data from Klastersky, J. et al., *J. Clin. Oncol.*, 18, 3038, 2000.

should be initially admitted to the hospital for empirical intravenous (IV) antibiotics therapy. Carefully selected low-risk patients (MASCC score ≥ 21) may be candidates for oral and/or outpatient empirical antibiotic therapy.[14***]

Historically, gram-negative bacteria have been the most common pathogens detected in neutropenic patients, but recently these have been overtaken by gram-positive cocci, especially *Staphylococcus aureus*, *S. epidermidis* and Streptococcal species, due to increased use of chemotherapeutic agents that cause mucositis, increased use of central venous catheters, and the use of prophylactic agents against gram-negative bacteria.[5] However, gram-negative bacteremias are associated with higher mortality than gram-positive bacteremias (5% vs. 18%).[15*] Since *Pseudomonas aeruginosa* especially is associated with a high mortality rate, initial empirical antibiotic coverage for *P. aeruginosa* is essential.[5,10]

Only carefully selected adult patients with neutropenic fever who are at low risk for complications may be treated initially with oral antibiotics. Ciprofloxacin should not be used as empirical monotherapy because it has less activity against gram-positive cocci.[16**] Although levofloxacin has better activity for gram-positive organisms, there are insufficient data to recommend fluoroquinolone monotherapy for this indication. Outcomes for low-risk patients treated with an empirical oral combination of ciprofloxacin and amoxicillin-clavulanate were comparable to those treated with IV antibiotic regimens.[17**,18**]

Ciprofloxacin 500–750 mg orally every 12 hours and amoxicillin-clavulanate 500 mg orally every 8 hours.[3]

Remaining high-risk patients require hospitalization for IV empirical antibiotics therapy. As monotherapy, antipseudomonal beta-lactam agents such as cefepime, carbapenems (imipenem-cilastatin or meropenem), or piperacillin-tazobactam are recommended.[3] Local institutional bacterial susceptibilities, which are determined by antibiogram, should be considered when selecting the empirical antibiotic regimen. Ceftazidime is no longer a reliable agent because of its decreasing potency against gram-negative organisms and its poor activity against many gram-positive organisms.[5]

For concentration-dependent killing agents (e.g., fluoroquinolone and aminoglycosides), the higher the ratio of the concentration to the minimum inhibitory concentration (MIC), the greater the killing occurs. On the other hand, for time-dependent (concentration-independent) killing agents (e.g., penicillins, cephalosporins, aztreonam, macrolides, clindamycin), the time during which the serum drug concentration is greater than the MIC is important.[19] What follows are the NCCN guideline–recommended dosages[3]:

- Cefepime 2 g IV every 8 hours
- Imipenem-cilastatin 500 mg IV every 6 hours
- Meropenem 1 g (2 g for meningitis) IV every 8 hours
- Piperacillin-tazobactam 4.5 g IV every 6 hours

Since aminoglycoside use carries a risk for renal and otic toxicity, it should not be routinely added to standard initial empirical therapy, except in patients at high risk for *Pseudomonas* infection such as those with a history of previous *Pseudomonas* infections or presence of ecthyma gangrenosum.[5] Once-daily dosing of aminoglycoside may lower renal toxicity compared with multiple daily dosing (or shorter interval dosing).[19]

Vancomycin is not recommended for an initial antibiotic regimen due to the risk for emergence of vancomycin-resistant organisms.[3] Randomized studies comparing empirical regimens with or without vancomycin as the initial empirical regimen have shown no significant reduction in overall mortality.[20**,21***] The addition of vancomycin was also found to be associated with increased renal and dermatological adverse events. When a single set of blood cultures is positive for coagulase negative staphylococci (the most commonly identified cause of bacteremia in neutropenic patients) and a second set is negative, it should be generally considered as contaminant. There is usually no urgent need to start treatment with vancomycin, and it should be reserved for the specific clinical indications listed next[3,5,10]:

- Hemodynamic instability
- Radiographically documented pneumonia
- Positive blood culture for gram-positive bacteria, before available identification and susceptibility
- Clinically apparent, serious catheter-related infection
- Skin or soft tissue infection
- Colonization with methicillin-resistant *S. aureus*, vancomycin-resistant enterococcus or penicillin-resistant *S. pneumoniae*
- Risk factors for viridans group streptococcal bacteremia such as severe mucositis and prophylaxis with fluoroquinolones or trimethoprim/sulfamethoxazole

A vancomycin loading dose of 25–30 mg/kg (based on actual body weight) is used to achieve the target trough serum concentration rapidly and is followed by a daily dose of 15–20 mg/kg every 8–12 hours (not to exceed 2 g per dose) for most patients with normal renal function. Trough serum concentration is the most accurate and practical method for monitoring efficacy, and a serum concentration of 15–20 mg/L is recommended in complicated infections.[22] Vancomycin should be discontinued within 2–3 days if susceptible bacteria are not recovered.[3,5]

Catheter-related infections

Infections caused by S. *aureus*, *P. aeruginosa*, fungi or mycobacteria or by tunnel or port pocket site infection, septic thrombosis, endocarditis, hypodynamic instability, or persistent bloodstream infection despite ≥72 hours of appropriate antibiotics all require removal of catheters and the addition of vancomycin. For infections caused by coagulase-negative staphylococci, the catheter may be retained with the administration of vancomycin through the infected catheter lumen.[3,5]

Reassessment

After 2–4 days of initial empirical antibiotics therapy, reassessment should be performed. Since it takes 2–7 days (median, 5 days) for patients with neutropenic fever to defervesce with appropriate initial antibiotics therapy, persistent fever alone in stable patients is rarely an indication to alter the antibiotic regimen. Modification of the initial empiric antibiotic therapy should occur based on new clinical and/or microbiological findings and not on recurrent or persistent fever alone, unless the patients are clinically unstable.[3,5]

Patients with unexplained fever who are responding to initial empirical therapy should be maintained on that initial regimen until ANC recovers to ≥500 cells/μL (mm³) and antibiotics can be discontinued once they become afebrile for at least 24 hours. Lower-risk patients can be switched to oral antibiotics until their neutropenia resolves. A switch from one empirical monotherapy to another or the addition of an aminoglycoside or vancomycin to the treatment regimen is not generally useful for persistent fever in asymptomatic and hemodynamically stable patients.[3,5]

For recurrent or persistent fever >3 days in duration despite empirical antibiotic therapy, a search must be made for an infection source and should include an additional set of blood cultures and symptom-directed diagnostic tests, and a reassessment should be made of their antimicrobial therapy. For documented infections, the duration of antibiotic therapy should be guided by the infections identified. Pneumonia and most bacterial bloodstream or soft tissue infections require 10–14 days of appropriate antibiotic therapy, at least until ANC recovers to ≥500 cells/mm³.[3,5]

Antifungal therapy

Empirical antifungal therapy should be considered for patients with persistent or recurrent fever after 4–7 days of antibiotics and whose duration of neutropenia is expected to be >7 days because clinical examination and cultures are not sensitive enough for early detection of fungal infections. Because *Candida* species are ubiquitous colonizers of human mucosal surfaces and they can cause bloodstream infection with mucosal barrier breakdown, fluconazole prophylaxis significantly reduces the incidence of invasive *Candida* infections in certain high-risk patients who have not received prior antifungal prophylaxis. Patients with profound neutropenia (≤100 cells/μL (mm³)) lasting longer than 10–15 days are at risk for invasive mold infection, such as aspergillosis. Fluconazole lacks any activity against mold infections, and infections by azole-resistant strains may also occur. Empirical antifungal therapy with antimold coverage is indicated in such cases.[3,5]

In a subset of patients who are stable, have no clinical or chest/sinus CT signs of fungal infections, have a negative serological assay for invasive fungal infections, and show no recovery of fungi from any body site, preemptive antifungal management is an alternative to empirical antifungal therapy. This has been made possible by advances in the early detection of fungal infections, such as with the serum test for fungal antigen or DNA, and advances in high-resolution chest CT. Antifungal therapy should be instituted if there are any signs of invasive fungal infections.[3,5]

Therapeutic use of G-CSF

Compared with prophylactic use, there is less evidence to support the therapeutic use of G-CSF in patients with neutropenic fever. A meta-analysis showed no improvement in overall survival with therapeutic use of G-CSF, although a shorter length of hospitalization (hospitalization rate 0.63; 95% CI 0.49–0.82) was seen.[23***] Therapeutic use of G-CSF in nonfebrile neutropenic patients is not recommended since it does not even improve a clinically important endpoint.[24**]

Key learning points

- Risk factors for infection in cancer patients include local factors, neutropenia, cellular and/or humoral immune dysfunction, and presence of foreign bodies.

- Some risk factors are controllable to prevent neutropenic fever.

- Routine vaccination against pneumococcus and influenza is advised.

- Prophylactic use of antibiotics and granulocyte-colony stimulating factor is indicated in certain situations.

- Source of infection and risks for complications should be evaluated in patients with neutropenic fever.

- Proper use of antibiotics is important.

REFERENCES

1 Rolston VIK, Bodey PG. Infection in patients with cancer. In: Hong KW, Bast Jr CR, Hait NW, Kufe WD, Pollock ER, Weichselbaum RR, Holland FJ, Frei III E (eds.) *Holland–Frei Cancer Medicine*, 8th edn. London, U.K.: McGraw Hill, 2009: pp. 1921–1940.

◆ 2 Centers for Diseases Control and Prevention. General Recommendations on Immunization: Recommendations of the Advisory Committee on Immunization Practice (ACIP). *MMWR Recomm Rep* 2011; **60**: 1–64.

◆ 3 Prevention and Treatment of Cancer-Related Infections, NCCN Clinical Practice Guidelines in Oncology™-v.2. 2011. Accessed March 6, 2012.

4 Paradiso PR. Pneumococcal conjugate vaccine for adults: A new paradigm. *Clin Infect Dis* 2012; **55**: 259–264.

◆ 5 Freifeld AG, Bow EJ, Sepkowitz KA et al. Clinical practice guideline for the use of antimicrobial agents in neutropenic patients with cancer: 2010 update by the Infectious Diseases Society of America. *Clin Infect Dis* 2011; **52**: e56–e93.

● 6 Bucaneve G, Micozzi A, Menichetti F et al. Levofloxacin to prevent bacterial infection in patients with cancer and neutropenia. *New Engl J Med* 2005; **353**: 977–987.

◆ 7 Myeloid Growth Factors, NCCN Clinical Practice Guidelines in Oncology™-v.1. 2012. Accessed March 14, 2012.

◆ 8 Smith TJ, Khatcheressian J, Lyman GH et al. 2006 update of recommendations for the use of white blood cell growth factors: An evidence-based clinical practice guideline. *J Clin Oncol* 2006; **24**: 3187–3205.

9   Papaldo P, Lopez M, Marolla P et al. Impact of five prophylactic fil-grastim schedules on hematologic toxicity in early breast cancer patients treated with epirubicin and cyclophosphamide. *J Clin Oncol* 2005; **23**: 6908–6918.

10 Yeung JS, Escalante C. Oncologic emergency. In: Hong KW, Bast Jr CR, Hait NW, Kufe WD, Pollock ER, Weichselbaum RR, Holland FJ, Frei III E (eds.) Holland-Frei Cancer Medicine, 8th edn. London, U.K.: McGraw Hill, 2009: pp. 1941–1962.

● 11 Mimoz O, Karim A, Mercat A et al. Chlorhexidine compared with povidone-iodine as skin preparation before blood culture. A random-ized, controlled trial. *Ann Intern Med* 1999; **131**: 834–837.

● 12 Gaur AH, Flynn PM, Giannini MA et al. Difference in time to detec-tion: A simple method to differentiate catheter-related from non-catheter-related bloodstream infection in immunocompromised pediatric patients. *Clin Infect Dis* 2003; **37**: 469–475.

◆ 13 Cohen SH, Gerding DN, Johnson S et al. Clinical Practice Guidelines for *Clostridium difficile* Infection in Adults: 2010 Update by the Society for Healthcare Epidemiology of America (SHEA) and the Infectious Diseases Society of America (IDSA). *Infect Control Hosp Epidemiol* 2010; **31**: 431–455.

● 14 Klastersky J, Paesmans M, Rubenstein EB et al. The Multinational Association for Supportive Care in Cancer risk index: A multinational scoring system for identifying low-risk febrile neutropenic cancer patients. *J Clin Oncol* 2000; **18**: 3038–3051.

15 Klastersky J, Ameye L, Maertens J et al. Bacteraemia in febrile neu-tropenic cancer patients. *Int J Antimicrob Agents* 2007; **30** Supp 1: S51–S59.

16 Meunier F, Zinner SH, Gaya H et al. Prospective randomized evalu-ation of ciprofloxacin versus piperacillin plus amikacin for empiric antibiotic therapy of febrile granulocytopenic cancer patients with lymphomas and solid tumors. The European Organization for Research on Treatment of Cancer International Antimicrobial Therapy Cooperative Group. *Antimicrob Agents Chemother* 1991; **35**: 873–878.

● 17 Kern WV, Cometta A, De Bock R et al. Oral versus intravenous empiri-cal antimicrobial therapy for fever in patients with granulocytopenia who are receiving cancer chemotherapy. International Antimicrobial Therapy Cooperative Group of the European Organization for Research and Treatment of Cancer. *New Engl J Med* 1999; **341**: 312–318.

● 18 Freifeld A, Marchigiani D, Walsh T et al. A double-blind comparison of empirical oral and intravenous antibiotic therapy for low-risk febrile patients with neutropenia during cancer chemotherapy. *New Engl J Med* 1999; **341**: 305–311.

19 Mandell LG BE, Dolin R, eds. *Mandel, Douglas, and Bennett's Principals and Practice of Infectious Disease*, 7th edn. London, U.K.: Churchill Livingstone, Elsevier; 2010.

20 Vancomycin added to empirical combination antibiotic therapy for fever in granulocytopenic cancer patients. European Organization for Research and Treatment of Cancer (EORTC) International Antimicrobial Therapy Cooperative Group and the National Cancer Institute of Canada-Clinical Trials Group. *J Infect Dis* 1991; **163**: 951–958.

21 Paul M, Borok S, Fraser A et al. Empirical antibiotics against Gram-positive infections for febrile neutropenia: Systematic review and meta-analysis of randomized controlled trials. *J Antimicrob Chemother* 2005; **55**: 436–444.

◆ 22 Martin JH, Norris R, Barras M et al. Therapeutic monitoring of vanco-mycin in adult patients: A consensus review of the American Society of Health-System Pharmacists, the Infectious Diseases Society of America, and the Society Of Infectious Diseases Pharmacists. *Clin Biochem Rev* 2010; **31**: 21–24.

● 23 Clark OA, Lyman GH, Castro AA et al. Colony-stimulating factors for chemotherapy-induced febrile neutropenia: A meta-analysis of randomized controlled trials. *J Clin Oncol* 2005; **23**: 4198–4214.

● 24 Hartmann LC, Tschetter LK, Habermann TM et al. Granulocyte col-ony-stimulating factor in severe chemotherapy-induced afebrile neutropenia. *New Engl J Med* 1997; **336**: 1776–1780.

111

Anemia-related fatigue

TOSHIYUKI KITANO, AKIFUMI TAKAORI-KONDO

ANEMIA

Anemia is the state in which there are insufficient red blood cells in the bloodstream, resulting in insufficient oxygen delivery to tissues causing a variety of symptoms, and restricting daily activities in severe cases. Mechanisms causing anemia can be classified into three categories, namely, deficient red cell production in the bone marrow, increased red cell destruction (hemolysis), and loss of red cells from the vasculature (hemorrhage). These three mechanisms often coexist in actual clinical settings.

Anemia is often classified according to red cell indices (Table 111.1). Microcytic anemia involves cases with low mean hemoglobin volume (MCV). Anemia with normal MCV is called normocytic anemia, whereas anemia with increased MCV is called macrocytic anemia. This classification is useful because it often indicates the underlying pathophysiological mechanisms of anemia.

The causes of normocytic anemia include diverse processes such as acute bleeding, hypothyroidism, and bone marrow failure. Macrocytic anemia is often caused by the disturbances of nucleic acid metabolism, for example, vitamin B12 or folate deficiency, and treatment with folate antagonists and other antimetabolites. Hemolytic anemia with increased reticulocyte count usually manifests with mild macrocytosis. Iron deficiency is the leading cause of microcytic anemia. Anemia of chronic disorders, resulting from disturbed iron metabolism caused by inflammatory processes, often manifests as microcytic anemia [1,2]. Thalassemia, caused by genetic impairments of globin synthesis, is another condition resulting in microcytic anemia.

Causes of cancer-related anemia

Cancer can cause anemia by inducing hemorrhage, and patients with gastrointestinal cancer often present with anemia. Extensive metastasis to bone marrow, with or without bone marrow necrosis, is another direct consequence of cancer resulting in anemia. Cancer can also cause anemia by other indirect mechanisms. Immune hemolytic anemia caused by autoantibody to red cells is a complication sometimes seen in lymphoid and other malignancies. Hemolytic anemia may be caused by some drugs used in cancer treatment. In patients treated with erythropoiesis-stimulating agents (ESAs), antibodies to erythropoietin are produced in rare circumstances, leading to pure red cell aplasia [3].

Cancer is a prothrombotic state, and thrombus formation in microvasculature can cause direct mechanical destruction of red blood cells leading to anemia, as seen in disseminated intravascular coagulation (DIC), thrombotic thrombocytopenic purpura (TTP), and hemolytic-uremic syndrome (HUS).

Treatments of cancer are other significant causes of anemia in cancer patients. Direct suppression of hematopoiesis by chemotherapeutic agents and radiation is one of the most common causes of anemia in cancer patients [4]. HUS is a rare but well-known complication of some chemotherapeutic agents, such as mitomycin C [5].

Anemia seen in cancer and other chronic inflammatory disorders often exhibits no clear causes and is called anemia of chronic disorders. Deranged iron metabolism caused by chronic inflammation is now thought to be the cause of this mysterious anemia [1,2].

Epidemiology of anemia in cancer patients

Anemia is one of the most common complications of cancer. A prospective survey of adult cancer patients conducted in Europe [6] reported that, among 14,520 patients with available data, 39.3% presented with anemia at enrollment. Among patients not receiving cancer treatment at enrollment, 31.7% were already anemic. During the survey with an enrollment period of 7 months and maximal follow-up of 6 months, 67.0% of patients were anemic at some point. Furthermore, among 2,732 patients not anemic at enrollment and who received some treatment for cancer during the survey with sufficient follow-up data, 53.7% developed anemia. A similar study from Australia [7] reported 35% prevalence of anemia at study entrance, and 37% incidence during the 6-month survey period. Patients receiving cancer chemotherapy are reported to be at even higher risk of anemia [4].

Table 111.1 *Classification of anemia according to red cell indices*

	Examples
Microcytic anemia (MCV ≤ 80)	Iron deficiency Anemia of chronic disorders Thalassemia Sideroblastic anemia
Normocytic anemia (80 < MCV ≤ 100)	Renal insufficiency Anemia of chronic disorders Hypothyroidism Aplastic anemia Pure red cell aplasia
Macrocytic anemia (MCV > 100)	Vitamin B12 deficiency Folate deficiency Hemolytic anemia Liver cirrhosis

Significance of anemia in cancer patients

Not only causing distressing symptoms that limit the daily activities of cancer patients, patients with anemia were reported to have shorter survival than nonanemic patients [8,9]. According to a review, anemic patients have higher relative risk of death than nonanemic patients: 19% higher risk in lung cancer, 75% in head and neck cancer, 47% in prostate cancer, and 67% in lymphoma [8]. It is not clear whether anemia itself has some survival disadvantages or is merely a surrogate marker for other adverse prognostic factors such as advanced disease or more aggressive disease in cancer patients.

ANEMIA AND FATIGUE

Fatigue is another very common symptom of cancer. In a cross-sectional study comparing advanced cancer patients no longer receiving chemotherapy or radiotherapy with age and sex-matched volunteers without cancer, it was reported that 75% of cancer patients experienced severe fatigue defined as fatigue greater than that experienced by 95% of control subjects [10]. Fatigue has often been under-recognized by the health professionals and undertreated. In a study using a questionnaire on patients attending outpatient department, fatigue was reported to affect 58% and compromised their daily activities, whereas pain and nausea/vomiting affected 22% and 19%, respectively. Fatigue was reported by a majority of patients to be the factor that affected their everyday life the most. Fifty-two percent of those patients with fatigue never reported their fatigue to their doctors. Of note in this study is the fact that only 14% received any treatment for fatigue [11].

Anemia and fatigue often coexist, and since fatigue is generally thought to be a symptom of anemia, treating anemia in patients with fatigue may improve the fatigue symptoms. However, the relationship between anemia and fatigue is not simple. In a population-based study examining the relationships between hemoglobin level and various symptoms in women, severity of fatigue did not show a significant correlation with hemoglobin level, at least in those with mild-to-moderate anemia (hemoglobin levels between 8 and 12), indicating that correcting anemia might not work to improve fatigue [12]. Supporting this, the administration of iron to anemic patients in their study did not improve fatigue and other symptoms, whereas serum iron and hemoglobin increased compared with those given placebo [12]. Since most cases of anemia in this study must have resulted from iron deficiency in otherwise healthy individuals, the generalizability of these findings to patients in palliative situations where the causes of anemia are multifactorial should be evaluated carefully.

Some reports with recently developed quality of life (QOL) questionnaires have shown the existence of an association of QOL scores with hemoglobin levels in cancer patients. In a report of a community-based study on 4382 anemic cancer patients receiving chemotherapy treated with ESA, hemoglobin level and QOL measures show direct correlations, and it has been suggested that up until a hemoglobin level of 12–13 g/dL is reached, QOL score continues to improve [13]. In a study using the Functional Assessment of Chronic Illness Therapy (FACIT) fatigue questionnaire to compare QOL in cancer patients and that in the general population, the QOL score of cancer patients with anemia was lower than that of cancer patients without anemia. The QOL score of the general population was better than that of cancer patients. Although the severity of anemia and the QOL score did show a statistically significant association, the distributions of QOL score almost overlapped, and the strength of the association between hemoglobin level and the score did not seem to be very strong [14]. In a study aimed at identifying factors associated with fatigue in cancer patients, hemoglobin level showed only a moderate association with fatigue [15]. Although QOL scores may be better than absolute hemoglobin levels alone in assessing the severity of fatigue, other studies have argued against the presence of a simple relationship between absolute hemoglobin level and fatigue [16,17].

There are still other problems in assessing fatigue using QOL questionnaires. Fallowfield et al. reported results of multivariate regression analysis of cancer patients treated with ESA [18]. In this study, QOL scores of patients with progressive disease deteriorated significantly, regardless of hemoglobin level.

From these studies, we must conclude that it is difficult to estimate the effect of anemia on the severity of fatigue only from blood hemoglobin level, and the absolute value of hemoglobin level would not be very suitable in guiding the treatment for fatigue-related anemia. QOL questionnaires, although probably more promising in reflecting the effects of anemia on fatigue than absolute blood hemoglobin levels, still require further research to delineate their precise roles in optimizing care for fatigue-related anemia.

TREATMENT OF ANEMIA

In the assessment of anemic patients, treatable causes should be sought first. Nutrient deficiencies, such as iron, vitamin B12, or folate deficiencies, are easily correctable once identified. Anemia in patients with chronic renal failure is usually caused by insufficiency in renal erythropoietin production, and ESAs are effective in treating those patients. Bleeding and drugs are other potentially correctable causes of anemia.

Anemia complicating a majority of patients with chronic disorders such as cancer is caused by intrinsic abnormalities in iron metabolism, and no specific treatments are known [1,2]. In cancer patients, chemotherapy and radiation therapy often cause bone marrow suppression, resulting in anemia. In those situations in which treatable causes of anemia are not present, blood transfusion and ESAs may be treatment options.

Blood transfusion

Infusing red blood cells from compatible donors is a rapid and reliable means of correcting anemia. Red blood cell transfusion is usually the treatment of choice in symptomatic patients with severe anemia. However, the treatment effect of blood transfusion is only transient, and repeated red cell transfusions for chronic anemia pose the risk of iron overload. Furthermore, there is still some risk of blood-borne viral and other infections [19,20]. Allergic reactions and transfusion-related lung injury are other potentially serious complications of blood transfusions. Risks of volume overload must be considered in frail patients.

Who should receive transfusions?

In general medical settings, red cell transfusion is not recommended for patients with a hemoglobin concentration greater than 10 g/dL [20***, 21***]. Red cell transfusions are indicated in symptomatic patients with hemoglobin level lower than 10 g/dL. In stable anemic patients, restrictive strategies of transfusion only when hemoglobin levels fall below 6–8 g/dL are recommended. These guidelines are based on randomized controlled trials demonstrating no clinical benefits of a higher transfusion trigger level of hemoglobin.

In palliative care settings, there is no consensus over indications and optimal hemoglobin level at which transfusion should be considered. There are studies showing QOL benefits of red cell transfusion in terminally ill cancer patients. For example, in a prospective study of 91 patients receiving palliative care with a median hemoglobin level of 7.9 g/dL (range 4.9–10.7), transfusion resulted in improved VAS scores of well-being, strength, and breathing 2 and 14 days after transfusion [22*]. In another study assessing the effect of transfusion on fatigue using the Functional Assessment of Cancer Therapy fatigue subscale (FACT-F) and the Brief Fatigue Inventory (BFI) questionnaires in 30 cancer patients receiving palliative care with a mean hemoglobin level of 7.96 g/dL before transfusion, both QOL scores improved significantly 3 days after transfusion. When responders and nonresponders were compared, no difference in baseline characteristics was found [23*]. Although both studies were small in size without control patients and the results should be interpreted cautiously, red cell transfusions in terminally ill cancer patients may help to improve or maintain their QOL.

On the other hand, in a randomized trial comparing two different target hemoglobin levels (10 and 12 g/dL) in patients with advanced gastric cancer receiving chemotherapy, maintaining a higher hemoglobin level with transfusion did not translate into better QOL scores [24*].

High interindividual variability has been reported between hemoglobin levels and QOL scores. In a randomized trial on the effect of epoetin beta in severely anemic patients with hematological malignancies, a change in FACT-anemia scores correlated with final hemoglobin level, but the distribution was widely scattered [16]. Similar results were obtained in a study assessing the relationships between hemoglobin concentration and QOL scores among patients attending outpatient oncology units [17].

Thus, effects of anemia and transfusion on fatigue and QOL seem to differ according to patients' conditions or treatments they are undergoing as well as absolute blood hemoglobin concentrations. At the moment, it might not be possible to define precise trigger and target hemoglobin levels for blood transfusion in patients receiving palliative care. Carefully designed studies are required to clarify the benefits and harms of blood transfusion in palliative care settings.

Erythropoiesis–stimulating agents

ESAs are another treatment option in anemic patients. As has been mentioned, they are the treatment of choice for patients with anemia caused by chronic renal insufficiency. However, an optimal target hemoglobin level has not been firmly established. In randomized controlled trials, higher target hemoglobin levels of 13–14 g/dL resulted in higher mortality and risks of thromboembolic events than lower hemoglobin targets [25–27**]. The U.S. Food and Drug Administration labeling states that ESAs should be considered in chronic renal failure patients with hemoglobin concentration of less than 10 g/dL and should be used to reduce the need for blood transfusions.

Although ESAs have been widely used in cancer patients, reports suggesting possible negative effects of ESAs on survival [28**, 29**] prompted reappraisal of the impact of ESAs on survival in cancer patients. A recent meta-analysis pointed out that ESAs increase the risk for thromboembolic events and death in cancer patients [30***]. Although ESAs reduced the need for red cell transfusion and positive effects on QOL were suggested, their roles in cancer patients are now thought to be limited. At present, only patients receiving myelosuppressive chemotherapy without curative intent are thought to be candidates for treatment with ESAs in the field of oncology [31***]. When treating cancer patients with ESAs, the fact that ESAs are effective in only 50%–60% of patients and require several weeks to exert their effects [32] should also be considered, besides the risks already mentioned.

Key learning points

- Anemia and fatigue are prevalent in palliative care settings and often coexist.

- The relationship between anemia and fatigue is not simple.

- Treating anemia may improve fatigue in some patients.

- Roles of blood transfusion and erythropoiesis stimulating agents in palliative care are controversial and require further research.

REFERENCES

1. Weiss G, Goodnough LT. Anemia of chronic disease. *The New England Journal of Medicine*. 2005;352(10):1011–1023.

2. Cullis JO. Diagnosis and management of anaemia of chronic disease: Current status. *British Journal of Haematology*. 2011;154(3):289–300.

3. Bennett CL, Luminari S, Nissenson AR, Tallman MS, Klinge SA, McWilliams N et al. Pure red-cell aplasia and epoetin therapy. *The New England Journal of Medicine*. 2004;351(14):1403–1408.

4. Groopman JE, Itri LM. Chemotherapy-induced anemia in adults: Incidence and treatment. *Journal of the National Cancer Institute*. 1999;91(19):1616–1634.

5. Moake JL. Thrombotic microangiopathies. *The New England Journal of Medicine*. 2002;347(8):589–600.

6. Ludwig H, Van Belle S, Barrett-Lee P, Birgegard G, Bokemeyer C, Gascon P et al. The European Cancer Anaemia Survey (ECAS): A large, multinational, prospective survey defining the prevalence, incidence, and treatment of anaemia in cancer patients. *European Journal of Cancer (Oxford, England: 1990)*. 2004;40(15):2293–2306.

7. Seshadri T, Prince HM, Bell DR, Coughlin PB, James PP, Richardson GE et al. The Australian Cancer Anaemia Survey: A snapshot of anaemia in adult patients with cancer. *The Medical journal of Australia*. 2005;182(9):453–457.

8. Caro JJ, Salas M, Ward A, Goss G. Anemia as an independent prognostic factor for survival in patients with cancer: A systemic, quantitative review. Cancer. 2001;91(12):2214–2221.

9. Knight K, Wade S, Balducci L. Prevalence and outcomes of anemia in cancer: A systematic review of the literature. *The American Journal of Medicine*. 2004;116 (Suppl 7A):11S–26S.

10. Stone P, Hardy J, Broadley K, Tookman AJ, Kurowska A, A'Hern R. Fatigue in advanced cancer: A prospective controlled cross-sectional study. *British Journal of Cancer*. 1999;79(9–10):1479–1486.

11. Stone P, Richardson A, Ream E, Smith AG, Kerr DJ, Kearney N. Cancer-related fatigue: Inevitable, unimportant and untreatable? Results of a multi-centre patient survey. Cancer Fatigue Forum. *Annals of Oncology*. 2000;11(8):971–975.

12. Elwood PC, Waters WE, Greene WJ, Sweetnam P, Wood MM. Symptoms and circulating haemoglobin level. *Journal of Chronic Diseases*. 1969;21(9):615–628.

13. Crawford J, Cella D, Cleeland CS, Cremieux PY, Demetri GD, Sarokhan BJ et al. Relationship between changes in hemoglobin level and quality of life during chemotherapy in anemic cancer patients receiving epoetin alfa therapy. *Cancer*. 2002;95(4):888–895.

14. Cella D, Lai JS, Chang CH, Peterman A, Slavin M. Fatigue in cancer patients compared with fatigue in the general United States population. *Cancer*. 2002;94(2):528–538.

15. Minton O, Strasser F, Radbruch L, Stone P. Identification of factors associated with fatigue in advanced cancer: A subset analysis of the European palliative care research collaborative computerized symptom assessment data set. *Journal of Pain and Symptom Management*. 2012;43(2):226–235.

16. Osterborg A, Brandberg Y. Relationship between changes in hemoglobin level and quality of life during chemotherapy in anemic cancer patients receiving epoetin alfa therapy. *Cancer*. 2003;97(12):3125–3126; author reply 6–7.

17. Bremberg ER, Brandberg Y, Hising C, Friesland S, Eksborg S. Anemia and quality of life including anemia-related symptoms in patients with solid tumors in clinical practice. *Medical Oncology (Northwood, London, England)*. 2007;24(1):95–102.

18. Fallowfield L, Gagnon D, Zagari M, Cella D, Bresnahan B, Littlewood TJ et al. Multivariate regression analyses of data from a randomised, double-blind, placebo-controlled study confirm quality of life benefit of epoetin alfa in patients receiving non-platinum chemotherapy. *British Journal of Cancer*. 2002;87(12):1341–1353.

19. Blajchman MA, Vamvakas EC. The continuing risk of transfusion-transmitted infections. *The New England Journal of Medicine*. 2006;355(13):1303–1305.

20. Carson JL, Grossman BJ, Kleinman S, Tinmouth AT, Marques MB, Fung MK et al. Red blood cell transfusion: A clinical practice guideline from the AABB*. *Annals of Internal Medicine*. 2012;157(1):49–58.

21. Ferraris VA, Brown JR, Despotis GJ, Hammon JW, Reece TB, Saha SP et al. 2011 update to the Society of Thoracic Surgeons and the Society of Cardiovascular Anesthesiologists blood conservation clinical practice guidelines. *The Annals of Thoracic Surgery*. 2011;91(3):944–982.

22. Gleeson C, Spencer D. Blood transfusion and its benefits in palliative care. *Palliative Medicine*. 1995;9(4):307–313.

23. Brown E, Hurlow A, Rahman A, Closs SJ, Bennett MI. Assessment of fatigue after blood transfusion in palliative care patients: A feasibility study. *Journal of Palliative Medicine*. 2010;13(11):1327–1330.

24. Park SH, Nam E, Bang SM, Cho EK, Shin DB, Lee JH. A randomized trial of anemia correction with two different hemoglobin targets in the first-line chemotherapy of advanced gastric cancer. *Cancer Chemotherapy and Pharmacology*. 2008;62(1):1–9.

25. Besarab A, Bolton WK, Browne JK, Egrie JC, Nissenson AR, Okamoto DM et al. The effects of normal as compared with low hematocrit values in patients with cardiac disease who are receiving hemodialysis and epoetin. *The New England Journal of Medicine*. 1998;339(9):584–590.

26. Singh AK, Szczech L, Tang KL, Barnhart H, Sapp S, Wolfson M et al. Correction of anemia with epoetin alfa in chronic kidney disease. *The New England Journal of Medicine*. 2006;355(20):2085–2098.

27. Pfeffer MA, Burdmann EA, Chen CY, Cooper ME, de Zeeuw D, Eckardt KU et al. A trial of darbepoetin alfa in type 2 diabetes and chronic kidney disease. *The New England Journal of Medicine*. 2009;361(21):2019–2032.

28. Henke M, Laszig R, Rube C, Schafer U, Haase KD, Schilcher B et al. Erythropoietin to treat head and neck cancer patients with anaemia undergoing radiotherapy: Randomised, double-blind, placebo-controlled trial. *Lancet*. 2003;362(9392):1255–1260.

● 29   Leyland-Jones B, Semiglazov V, Pawlicki M, Pienkowski T, Tjulandin S, Manikhas G et al. Maintaining normal hemoglobin levels with epoetin alfa in mainly nonanemic patients with metastatic breast cancer receiving first-line chemotherapy: A survival study. Journal of Clinical Oncology. 2005;23(25):5960–5972.

◆ 30   Tonia T, Mettler A, Robert N, Schwarzer G, Seidenfeld J, Weingart O et al. Erythropoietin or darbepoetin for patients with cancer. *Cochrane Database of Systematic Reviews* (Online). 2012;12:CD003407.

◆ 31   Rizzo JD, Brouwers M, Hurley P, Seidenfeld J, Arcasoy MO, Spivak JL et al. American Society of Hematology/American Society of Clinical Oncology clinical practice guideline update on the use of epoetin and darbepoetin in adult patients with cancer. *Blood.* 2010;116(20):4045–4059.

32   Demetri GD. Anaemia and its functional consequences in cancer patients: Current challenges in management and prospects for improving therapy. *British Journal of Cancer.* 2001;84 (Suppl 1):31–37.

112

Platelets and bleeding: Thrombosis risks

YUKIKO MORI

DEFINITIONS

Platelets are released from megakaryocytes, and the major regulator of platelet production is the hormone thrombopoietin (TPO), which is synthesized in the liver. Platelets have an average circulation lifespan of 7–10 days. Approximately one-third of the platelets reside in the spleen, and this number increases in proportion to spleen size [1]. The normal platelet count in adults is 150,000–450,000 μL^{-1} [2].

PLATELET DISORDERS

Thrombocytopenia

Thrombocytopenia is defined as a platelet count <150,000 μL^{-1}, keeping in mind that 2.5% of the normal population will have a platelet count below this number [2]. Thrombocytopenia results from one or more of the following three processes: (1) decreased bone marrow production; (2) sequestration, usually in an enlarged spleen; and (3) increased platelet destruction [1]. Production disorders are inherited or acquired. A reduction in platelet count by 50%, while still in the normal range, may herald severe clinical problems and require active follow-up. A "safe" platelet count is an imprecise concept, varying from disorder to disorder and even between patients with the same disorder. Regardless, surgical bleeding due solely to a reduction in the number of platelets does not generally occur until the platelet count drops below 50,000 μL^{-1}, and clinical or spontaneous bleeding does not occur until the platelet count is <10,000–20,000 μL^{-1}.

Pseudothrombocytopenia

During the evaluation of a patient with thrombocytopenia, it is imperative to validate the platelet count to exclude the possibility of spurious thrombocytopenia or pseudothrombocytopenia and to confirm thrombocytopenia's existence. Reviewing a peripheral blood smear is a key step for ruling out pseudothrombocytopenia.

Pseudothrombocytopenia is a relatively uncommon phenomenon caused by ex vivo agglutination of platelets. As a result of platelet clumping, platelet counts reported by automated counters may be much lower than the actual count in the blood because these devices cannot differentiate platelet clumps from individual cells. Approximately 0.1% of normal subjects have EDTA-dependent agglutinins, which can lead to platelet clumping, spurious thrombocytopenia, and spurious leukocytosis. This is thought to result from a "naturally occurring" platelet autoantibody directed against a normally concealed epitope on the platelet membrane glycoprotein (GP) IIb/IIIa, which is exposed by EDTA-induced dissociation of GP IIb/IIIa [2]. Pseudothrombocytopenia subsequently occurs because EDTA is the anticoagulant employed in the tubes used for routine complete blood counts. Pseudothrombocytopenia can also occur after the administration of the murine monoclonal antibody abciximab, which is directed against the GP IIb/IIIa receptor [3]. If a low platelet count is obtained in EDTA-anticoagulated blood, a blood smear can be evaluated and a platelet count can be determined in blood collected into sodium citrate or heparin, or ideally, a smear of freshly obtained unanticoagulated blood, such as that from a fingerstick, can be examined [1].

THROMBOCYTOPENIA RESULTING FROM IMPAIRED PLATELET PRODUCTION

Platelet production by the bone marrow can be impaired when the marrow is suppressed or damaged. In almost all disorders caused by marrow suppression or damage, production of both white and red cells is also affected.

Infection-induced thrombocytopenia

Many viral and bacterial infections result in thrombocytopenia. This may or may not be associated with laboratory evidence of disseminated intravascular coagulation (DIC), which is most commonly seen in patients with systemic infections with gram-negative bacteria. Infection can affect platelet production and platelet survival. Certain infectious agents, such as the human immunodeficiency virus (HIV), are capable of damaging megakaryocytes directly [4,5].

Chemotherapy- and radiation therapy–induced thrombocytopenia

The hematopoietic system appears to recover promptly after doses of chemotherapy and radiotherapy. However, heavily treated patients have a reduced tolerance to additional therapy, showing lower nadirs for blood counts, particularly platelets [4].

Nutritional deficiencies and alcohol- induced thrombocytopenia

Thrombocytopenia sometimes occurs in patients with megaloblastic anemia resulting from vitamin B12 deficiency and/or folic acid deficiency. Vitamin B12 deficiency is usually due to inadequate absorption associated with pernicious anemia or is secondary to gastric disease. In contrast, folic acid deficiency is generally attributable to an inadequate diet and/or alcoholism. Both deficiencies are known to coexist in some patients with malabsorption [6]. Besides folic acid deficiency, thrombocytopenia in alcoholic patients almost always results from liver cirrhosis with thyroid peroxidase deficiency and also from congestive splenomegaly. In some cases, thrombocytopenia results from direct marrow suppression by alcohol [4,7–10].

THROMBOCYTOPENIA RESULTING FROM ACCELERATED PLATELET DESTRUCTION

Immune thrombocytopenic purpura

Immune thrombocytopenic purpura (ITP) is an acquired disorder leading to immune-mediated destruction of platelets and potential inhibition of platelet release from megakaryocytes. Only two criteria are required to make this diagnosis [11–13]:

1. Presence of isolated thrombocytopenia—The remainder of the complete blood count, including examination of the peripheral blood smear, is entirely normal.
2. Absence of clinically apparent associated conditions—Patients with these associated conditions are described as having "secondary immune thrombocytopenia" [11,12].

Laboratory testing for antibodies is usually ineffective due to low sensitivity and specificity. The peripheral blood smear may show large platelets with otherwise normal morphology. Depending on the bleeding history, iron-deficiency anemia may be present. Laboratory testing is performed to evaluate for secondary ITP and should include testing for HIV infection and hepatitis C, serologic testing for systemic lupus erythematosus (SLE), serum protein electrophoresis and immunoglobulin levels to potentially detect hypogammaglobulinemia, IgA deficiency, or monoclonal gammopathy, and if anemia is present, direct antiglobulin testing (Coomb's test) to rule out combined autoimmune hemolytic anemia with ITP (Evans's syndrome) [1]. Major bleeding is rare in patients with ITP and occurs primarily in those with platelet counts <10,000 μL^{-1} [11].

The goal for ITP treatment is to provide a safe platelet count to prevent major bleeding rather than to return the platelet count to normal [12,14,15]. Initial treatment of patients without significant bleeding symptoms, severe thrombocytopenia (<5000 μL^{-1}), or signs of impeding bleeding can be instituted using single agents,

such as predonine. For patients with severe ITP and/or symptoms of bleeding, hospital admission and combined modality therapy are given using high-dose corticosteroid with intravenous gamma globulin (IVg) or anti-D (in appropriate patients) immunoglobulin therapy. Splenectomy is recommended for patients who fail to respond to corticosteroid therapy, whereas thrombopoietin receptor agonist is recommended for patients at risk of bleeding who relapse after splenectomy or who fail to respond to at least one other therapy. Rituximab may be considered for patients at risk of bleeding who have failed one-line therapy such as corticosteroids, IVg, or splenectomy [16]. Unnecessary treatment should be avoided for asymptomatic patients with mild-to-moderate thrombocytopenia (i.e., platelet count > 30,000 μL^{-1}).

Drug-induced thrombocytopenia

Many drugs have been associated with thrombocytopenia; in particular, numerous cytotoxic drugs used in chemotherapy induce thrombocytopenia as a result of bone marrow suppression. Commonly used drugs known to cause isolated thrombocytopenia are listed in Table 112.1 [1,17]. However, all drugs should be treated as suspect in a patient exhibiting thrombocytopenia without an apparent cause and should be stopped or substituted if possible.

Table 112.1 *List of drugs known to cause drug-induced thrombocytopenia*

Drug
Abciximab
Acetaminophen
Acyclovir
Aminosalicylic acid
Amiodarone
Amphotericin B
Ampicillin
Carbamazepine
Chlorpropamide
Danazol
Diatrizoate meglumine (Hypaque Meglumine)
Diclofenac
Digoxin
Eptifibatide
Hydrochlorothiazide
Ibuprofen
Levamisole
Octreotide
Phenytoin
Quinine
Rifampin
Tamoxifen
Tirofiban
Trimethoprim/sulfamethoxazole
Vancomycin

Source: Adapted from Dan Longo, et al., *Harrison's Principles of Internal Medicine,* 18th edn., 2011. McGraw-Hill Professional.

Heparin-induced thrombocytopenia

Heparin-induced thrombocytopenia (HIT) is described as a reduction in platelet count of >50% or a decrease to <150,000 µL^{-1} during heparin use, typically 5–10 days after its initiation [18,19]. Therefore, it is imperative to recognize HIT, given its possible complication of paradoxical life-threatening thromboembolus formation. There are two types of HIT: type I and type II.

HIT type I is a benign condition characterized by a mild transient decrease in platelet count not associated with immune formation or increased risk of thrombosis. HIT type II is an immune-mediated phenomenon that causes a drop in platelets and puts patients at risk of developing significant thrombosis. Examples of complications secondary to HIT type II include deep vein thrombosis (DVT), myocardial infarction, stroke, pulmonary embolus (PE), limb gangrene or acute limb ischemia, organ infarction, and cerebral sinus thrombus [19].

HIT type II results from antibody formation against a complex of platelet-specific protein platelet factor 4 (PF4) and heparin. Many patients exposed to heparin develop antibodies to heparin/PF4 but do not appear to have adverse consequences. A fraction of those who develop antibodies develop thrombocytopenia, and a portion of those develop HIT and thrombosis. HIT can occur following exposure to low-molecular-weight (LMW) heparin, as well as unfractionated heparin, although it is more common with the latter (0.2% vs. 2.6%) [18].

The 4 Ts—thrombocytopenia, timing of platelet count fall, thrombosis or other complications, and other causes for thrombocytopenia—is a pretest clinical scoring system that may be utilized for determining the probability of HIT when suspected in a patient (Table 112.2) [20]. Combining the 4 Ts with a diagnostic test is recommended to help reduce inappropriate switches from heparin to more expensive medications as a result of false positives in diagnosing HIT. A score of 0–3 points gives a low pretest probability of HIT, 4–5 points is intermediate, and 6–8 points gives a high probability of HIT [19,21].

Due to the risk of life-threatening thromboembolism formation, it is imperative to treat HIT as soon as it is diagnosed. The first step is to discontinue all exposure to heparin-containing products, including catheters coated with heparin. Aside from stopping heparin use, treatment with a direct thrombin inhibitor such as lepirudin, bivalirudin, or argatroban is necessary as there is an increased risk of developing thrombosis. When transitioning to warfarin, current recommendations are to start warfarin once the platelet count has plateaued above 150,000 µL^{-1} [22], and the transition should occur after the patient has been adequately anticoagulated [23]. Warfarin treatment is initiated in patients who are in need of long-term anticoagulation with a goal international normalized ratio (INR) of 2–3 [24]. Situations that may require long-term anticoagulation include patients with a history of HIT and the sustained presence of antibodies [24] and those at risk of future thrombus formation. Platelet transfusion should be used in patients with HIT and severe thrombocytopenia, only when bleeding or during an invasive procedure with a high risk of bleeding [22].

Thrombotic thrombocytopenic purpura and hemolytic uremic syndrome

Thrombotic thrombocytopenic purpura (TTP) and hemolytic uremic syndrome (HUS) are acute syndromes with abnormalities in multiple organ systems and show evidence of microangiopathic hemolytic anemia and thrombocytopenia.

TTP is defined by the following: (1) thrombocytopenia, (2) microangiopathic hemolytic anemia, and (3) no alternative explanations [25,26]. TTP is an appropriate diagnostic term for adults who fulfill these diagnostic criteria, whether or not neurologic or renal abnormalities are present. HUS is a syndrome characterized by acute renal failure, microangiopathic hemolytic anemia, and thrombocytopenia [1], and is seen predominantly in children.

The pathogenesis of inherited and idiopathic TTP is related to a deficiency of, or antibody to, ADAMTS13, a metalloprotease that cleaves von Willebrand's factor.

Although many causes of TTP-HUS are idiopathic, a variety of causes in ADAMTS13 deficiency have been identified, for example, shiga toxin–producing *Escherichia coli*, disseminated malignancy, and drug-induced (e.g., quinine, anticancer drugs, and immunosuppressive agents) [27].

Table 112.2 *The 4Ts scoring system for determining HIT probability*

The 4Ts	2 Points	1 Point	0 Points
Thrombocytopenia	Platelet count >50% and nadir >20 × 10^9 L^{-1}	Platelet count 30%–50% or nadir 10–19 × 10^9 L^{-1}	Platelet count <30% or nadir <10 × 10^9 L^{-1}
Timing of platelet count fall	At day 5–10 or fall within 1 day if heparin used within 30 days	Not clear about timing between 5 and 10 days or after 10 days or within 1 day with prior heparin exposure within 30–100 days	Platelet count fall <4 days without recent exposure
Thrombosis/other complications	Confirmed thrombosis, skin necrosis	Progressive/recurrent thrombosis, erythematous skin lesions, or suspected thrombosis not yet proven	None
Presence of alternative diagnosis	None	Possible	Definite

The mainstay therapy for adult TTP-HUS is plasma exchange, which should be initiated even if there is some uncertainty about the diagnosis of TTP-HUS, as it is considered that the potential dangers of rapid deterioration from TTP-HUS exceed the significant risks of plasma exchange treatment [27–31]. If an alternative diagnosis is subsequently discovered (e.g., systemic infection, disseminated malignancy, or malignant hypertension), plasma exchange should then be stopped. On the other hand, medication-related TTP may be secondary to antibody formation or direct endothelial toxicity, and, in this case, withdrawal or reduction in the dose of endothelial toxic agents may decrease microangiopathy [1].

With regard to plasma infusion, the superior efficacy of plasma exchange compared with plasma infusion alone for the treatment of TTP-HUS in adults has been demonstrated [25,32]. Platelet transfusion may lead to new or worsening neurological symptoms and to acute renal failure, presumably due to the production of new or expanding microvascular thrombi as infused platelets are consumed [32,33].

Thrombocytosis

The threshold for clinically significant thrombocytosis varies among patients, and the exact definition of thrombocytosis also varies across reports in the literature, although a platelet count of $\geq 450,000\ \mu L^{-1}$ is a generally accepted value [34]. Thrombocytosis has a multitude of potential etiologies, and thus evaluation of a patient with thrombocytosis requires careful consideration of patient history, comorbid conditions, other hematological parameters, and past platelet counts. In general, causes of thrombocytosis can be described as spurious, reactive, or clonal in nature (Table 112.3) [35]. Patients presenting with an elevated platelet count should be evaluated for underlying inflammation or malignancy, and iron deficiency should be ruled out [1]. Reactive thrombocytosis is generally considered a self-limited process that resolves with resolution of the underlying disorder when possible. The risk of thrombotic complications with reactive thrombocytosis is felt to be low as 1.6% of patients with reactive thrombocytosis in a large case series experienced thrombotic complications [36]. A paradoxical risk of bleeding has been noted in patients with thrombocytosis, especially extreme thrombocytosis [37,38], and bleeding in this setting is usually mucocutaneous in nature. Because of this lack of thrombotic risk as well as a theoretical risk of paradoxical bleeding, no antiplatelet therapy is recommended for reactive thrombocytosis, even for extreme thrombocytosis [39].

THROMBOSIS

Venous thromboembolism (VTE) is a common cause of morbidity and mortality in patients with cancer. Patients with cancer carry a risk of VTE four- to sevenfold higher than patients without cancer, and on average 15% of patients develop DVT or PE during the clinical course of their cancer [40–42]. Clinical suspicion for VTE should reflect the totality of the patient's risk

Table 112.3 *Causes of thrombocytosis*

Primary	Secondary	Spurious
Essential thrombocythemia	Infection	Microspherocytes (e.g., severe burns)
Polycythemia vera	Inflammation	Cryoglobulinemia
Primary myelofibrosis	Tissue damage	Neoplastic cell cytoplasmic fragments
Myelodysplasia with del(5q)	Hyposplenism	Schistocytes
Refractory anemia with ring sideroblasts associated with marked thrombocytosis	Postoperative	Bacteria
Chronic myeloid leukemia	Hemorrhage	Pappenheimer bodies
Chronic myelomonocytic leukemia	Iron deficiency	
Atypical chronic myeloid leukemia	Malignancy	
MDS/MPN-U	Hemolysis Drug therapy (e.g., corticosteroids, adrenaline) Cytokine administration (e.g., thrombopoietin) Rebound following myelosuppressive chemotherapy	

profile, including age, primary cancer site, histologic type and stage, recent major surgery, trauma, hospitalization or serious medical illness, immobility, and use of chemotherapy, radiotherapy, hormone or erythropoietic stimulatory agents, as well as the presence of thrombophilia or a past history of VTE [43]. Common and well-established risk factors for thrombosis are listed in Table 112.4 [44].

The signs and symptoms of VTE are evident in a number of clinical conditions. Therefore, clinical prediction rules (CPRs) have been developed to quantitatively assess the pretest probability of VTE. The most widely used CPRs are the Wells DVT and PE models (Tables 112.5 and 112.6) [45–47]. D-dimer testing is also commonly used for diagnosis of thrombosis. Carrier and colleagues found that a low or unlikely score on the Wells CPR and a negative D-dimer result were associated with negative predictive values of 100% (95% CI 70%–100%) and 100% (95% CI 83%–100%), respectively. However, these strategies were of limited utility in cancer patients because 94% (using the low/moderate/high version of the Wells DVT CPR) or 88% (using the unlikely/likely version of the Wells DVT CPR) of patients required additional testing due to the high prevalence of elevated D-dimer levels or clinical findings associated

Table 112.4 *Risk factors for thrombocytosis*

Surgery
Trauma
Venous catheters
Prolonged bed rest
Plaster cast
Long haul travel
Malignancy
Chemotherapy
Pregnancy
Puerperium
Oral contraceptives
Hormone replacement therapy
Obesity
Infection
Inflammatory disease
Smoking
Lupus anticoagulant
Genetic factors

with VTE in patients with cancer [48]. The results of these studies indicate that objective imaging techniques (e.g., venous ultrasound, contrast-enhanced computed tomography (CT), magnetic resonance venography, and CT angiography) remain the cornerstone for diagnosis of VTE in patients with cancer.

Treatment of nonmassive venous thrombosis consists of the following three phases: initial phase, early maintenance phase, and long-term secondary prevention phase. LMW heparin,

Table 112.5 *Wells's clinical deep vein thrombosis model*

Clinical characteristic	Score
Active cancer (patient receiving treatment for cancer within 6 months or currently receiving palliative treatment)	1
Paralysis, paresis, or recent plaster cast immobilization of a lower extremity	1
Recently bedridden for 3 days or more, or major surgery within the previous 12 weeks requiring general or regional anesthesia	1
Localized tenderness along the distribution of the deep venous system	1
Entire leg swollen	1
Calf swelling at least 3 cm more than the asymptomatic side (measured 10 cm below the tibial tuberosity)	1
Pitting edema confined to the symptomatic leg	1
Collateral superficial veins (nonvaricose)	1
Previously documented deep vein thrombosis	1
Alternative diagnosis at least as likely as deep vein thrombosis	−2

A score of <2 indicates unlikely deep vein thrombosis.
A score of ≥2 points indicates likely deep vein thrombosis.

Table 112.6 *Wells's clinical pulmonary embolism model*

Clinical characteristic	Score
Active cancer (patient receiving treatment for cancer within 6 months or currently receiving palliative treatment)	1
Surgery or bedridden for 3 days or more during the past 4 weeks	1.5
History of deep venous thrombosis or pulmonary embolism	1.5
Hemoptysis	1
Heart rate >100 beats per minute	1.5
Pulmonary embolism judged to be the most likely diagnosis	3
Clinical signs and symptoms compatible with deep venous thrombosis	3

A score of >4 indicates likely pulmonary embolism.

unfractionated intravenous heparin, adjusted-dose or fixed dose subcutaneous heparin, and subcutaneous fondaparinux are commonly used for initial treatment. Compared with unfractionated heparin (UFH), LMW heparin and fondaparinux offer major benefits of convenient dosing, facilitation of outpatient treatment, and lower incidence of heparin-induced thrombocytopenia. In the early maintenance phase, vitamin K antagonist (VKA) is commonly used. Administration of heparin or fondaparinux should overlap for at least 5 days with administration of VKA. The parenteral drug can be stopped when the anticoagulant concentration induced by the VKA has reached an INR of 2.0. Treatment with VKA needs close monitoring using the INR; the targeted therapeutic level is 2.5 (range 2.0–3.0). VKA is also used for long-term secondary prevention (target INR 2.0–3.0) [49].

Prophylaxis is of paramount importance because VTE is difficult to detect and imposes an excessive medical and economic burden. Mechanical and pharmacological measures often succeed in preventing VTE. In some reports including meta-analysis, UFH, LMW heparin, and fondaparinux have all been shown to be superior to placebo for preventing VTE in hospitalized and immobilized patients [50–54].

Mechanical methods for the prevention of VTE are primary indicated in patients at high risk of bleeding [55], such as in the case of peptic ulcer or intracranial hemorrhage. Intermittent pneumatic compression, graduated compression stockings, and venous foot pumps are commonly used for mechanical thrombophylaxis [56].

REFERENCES

1 Dan Longo, Anthony Fauci, Dennis Kasper, Stephen Hauser, J. Jameson, Joseph Loscalzo. *Harrison's Principles of Internal Medicine*, 18th edn., 2011. McGraw-Hill Professional.
2 Lindaw SA, George LN. Approach to the adult patient with thrombocytopenia. Up to date. http://www.uptodate.com. Accessed June 2012.

3   Sane DC, Damaraju LV, Topol EJ et al. Occurrence and clinical significance of pseudothrombocytopenia during abciximab therapy. *J Am Coll Cardiol.* 2000;36(1):75–83.

4   Kaushansky K, Lichtman MA, Beutler E et al. *Williams Hematology,* 8th edn. McGrawHill, New York, 2010.

5   Zucker-Franklin D, Cao YZ. Megakaryocytes of human immunodeficiency virus-infected individuals express viral RNA. *Proc Natl Acad Sci U S A.* 1989;86(14):5595–5599.

6   Schrier SL. Etiology and clinical manifestations of vitamin B12 and folic acid deficiency. Up to date. http://www.uptodate.com. Accessed June 2012.

7   Latvala J, Parkkila S, Niemelä O. Excess alcohol consumption is common in patients with cytopenia: Studies in blood and bone marrow cells. *Alcohol Clin Exp Res.* 2004;28(4):619–624.

8   Sullivan LW, Adams WH, Liu YK. Induction of thrombocytopenia by thrombopheresis in man: Patterns of recovery in normal subjects during ethanol ingestion and abstinence. *Blood.* 1977;49(2):197–207.

9   Michot F, Gut J. Alcohol-induced bone marrow damage. A bone marrow study in alcohol-dependent individuals. *Acta Haematol.* 1987;78(4):252–257.

10 Wolber EM, Jelkmann W. Thrombopoietin: The novel hepatic hormone. *News Physiol Sci.* 2002;17:6–10.

11 George JN. Clinical manifestations and diagnosis of immune (idiopathic) thrombocytopenic purpura in adults. Up to date. http://www.uptodate.com/. Accessed June 2012.

12 Rodeghiero F, Stasi R, Gernsheimer T et al. Standardization of terminology, definitions and outcome criteria in immune thrombocytopenic purpura of adults and children: Report from an international working group. *Blood.* 2009;113(11):2386.

13 Provan DR, Newland AC, Blanchette VS et al. International consensus report on the investigation and management of primary immune thrombocytopenia. *Blood.* 2010;115(2):168.

14 George JN, Woolf SH, Raskob GE et al. Idiopathic thrombocytopenic purpura: A practice guideline developed by explicit methods for the American Society of Hematology. *Blood.* 1996;88(1):3–40.

15 Toltl LJ, Arnold DM. Pathophysiology and management of chronic immune thrombocytopenia: Focusing on what matters. *Br J Haematol.* 2011;152(1):52–60.

16 Neunert C. The American Society of Hematology 2011 evidence-based guideline for immune thrombocytopenia. *Blood.* 2011;117(16):4190–4207.

17 James N. George. http://moon.ouhsc.edu/jgeorge.

18 Martel N, Lee J, Wells PS. Risk for heparin-induced thrombocytopenia with unfractionated and low-molecular-weight heparin thromboprophylaxis: A metaanalysis. *Blood.* 2005;106:2710–2715.

19 Bambrah RK, Pham DC, Zaiden R et al. Heparin-induced thrombocytopenia. *Clin Adv Hematol Oncol.* 2011;9(8):594–599.

20 Lo GK, Juhl D, Warkentin TE et al. Evaluation of pretest clinical score (4Ts) for the diagnosis of heparin-induced thrombocytopenia in two clinical settings. *J Thromb Haemost.* 2006;4(4):759–765.

21 Coutre S. Heparin-induced thrombocytopenia. Up to date. www.uptodate.com. Accessed June 2012.

22 Linkins LA, Dans AL, Moores LK et al. Treatment and prevention of heparin-induced thrombocytopenia: Antithrombotic therapy and prevention of thrombosis, 9th ed: American college of chest physicians evidence-based clinical practice guidelines. *Chest* 2012;141:e495S–e530S.

23 Hursting MJ, Lewis BE, Macfarlane DE. Transitioning from argatroban to warfarin therapy in patients with heparin-induced thrombocytopenia. *Clin Appl Thromb Hemost.* 2005;11:279–287.

24 Dager WE, Dougherty JA, Nguyen PH et al. Heparin-induced thrombocytopenia: Treatment options and special considerations. *Pharmacotherapy.* 2007;27:564–587.

25 Rock GA, Shumak KH, Buskard NA et al. Comparison of plasma exchange with plasma infusion in the treatment of thrombotic thrombocytopenic purpura. *N Engl J Med.* 1991;325:393–397.

26 George JN. Thrombotic thrombocytopenic purpura. *N Engl J Med* 2006;354:1927–1935.

27 George JN. How I treat patients with thrombotic thrombocytopenic purpura. *Blood.* 2010;118(20):4060–4069.

28 Kaplan AA, George JN. Treatment of thrombotic thrombocytopenic purpura-hemolytic uremic syndrome in adults. Up to date. http://www.uptodate.com. Accessed June 2012.

29 Moake JL. Thrombotic microangiopathies. *N Engl J Med.* 2002;347(8):589–600.

30 Rizvi MA, Vesely SK, George JN et al. Complications of plasma exchange in 71 consecutive patients treated for clinically suspected thrombotic thrombocytopenic purpura-hemolytic-uremic syndrome. *Transfusion.* 2000;40(8):896–901.

31 Nguyen L, Terrell DR, Duvall D et al. Complications of plasma exchange in patients treated for thrombotic thrombocytopenic purpura. IV. An additional study of 43 consecutive patients, 2005 to 2008. *Transfusion.* 2009;49(2):392–394.

32 Bell WR, Braine HG, Ness PM et al. Improved survival in thrombotic thrombocytopenic purpura-hemolytic uremic syndrome. Clinical experience in 108 patients. *N Engl J Med.* 1991;325(6):398–403.

33 Andre AK, George JN. Treatment of thrombotic thrombocytopenic purpura-hemolytic uremic syndrome in adults. Up to date. http://www.uptodate.com. Accessed June 2012.

34 Skoda RC. Thrombocytosis. *Hematol—Am Soc Hematol Educ Program.* 2009;2009:159–167.

35 Harrison CN, Bareford D, Butt N et al. Guideline for investigation and management of adults and children presenting with a thrombocytosis. *Br J Haematol.* 2010;149(3):352–375.

36 Griesshammer M, Bangerter M, Sauer T et al. Aetiology and clinical significance of thrombocytosis: Analysis of 732 patients with an elevated platelet count. *J Intern Med.* 1999;245(3):295–300.

37 Buss DH, Stuart JJ, Lipscomb GE. The incidence of thrombotic and hemorrhagic disorders in association with extreme thrombocytosis: An analysis of 129 cases. *Am J Hematol.* 1985;20(4):365–372.

38 Chistolini A, Mazzucconi MG, Ferrari A et al. Essential thrombocythemia: A retrospective study on the clinical course of 100 patients. *Haematologica.* 1990;75(6):537–540.

39 Bleeker JS, Hogan WJ. Thrombocytosis: Diagnostic evaluation, thrombotic risk stratification, and risk-based management strategies. *Thrombosis.* 2011;2011:536062.

40 Heit JA, Silverstein MD, Mohr DN et al. Risk factors for deep vein thrombosis and pulmonary embolism: A population-based case-control study. *Arch Intern Med.* 2000;160:809–815.

41 Blom JW, Doggen CJ, Osanto S et al. Malignancies, prothrombotic mutations, and the risk of venous thrombosis. *JAMA* 2005;293:715–722.

42 Deitcher SR. Cancer and thrombosis: Mechanisms and treatment. *J Thromb Thrombolysis.* 2003;16:21–31.

43 Streiff MB. Diagnosis and initial treatment of venous thromboembolism in patients with cancer. *J Clin Oncol.* 2009;27(29):4889–4894.

44 Reitsma PH, Versteeg HH, Middeldorp S. Mechanistic view of risk factors for venous thromboembolism. *Arterioscler Thromb Vasc Biol.* 2012;32(3):563–568.

45 Kearon C, Ginsberg JS, Douketis J et al. An evaluation of D-dimer in the diagnosis of pulmonary embolism: A randomized trial. *Ann Intern Med.* 2006;144:812–821.

46 Wells PS, Anderson DR, Rodger M et al. Evaluation of D-dimer in the diagnosis of suspected deep-vein thrombosis. *N Engl J Med.* 2003;349:1227–1235.

47 van Belle A, Buller HR, Huisman MV et al. Effectiveness of managing suspected pulmonary embolism using an algorithm combining clinical probability, D-dimer testing, and computed tomography. *JAMA.* 2006;295:172–179.

48 Carrier M, Lee AY, Bates SM et al. Accuracy and usefulness of a clinical prediction rule and D-dimer testing in excluding deep vein thrombosis in cancer patients. *Thromb Res.* 2008;123:177–183.

49 Goldhaber SZ, Bounameaux H. Pulmonary embolism and deep vein thrombosis. *Lancet.* 2012;379:1835–1846.

50 Dentali FJ, Douketis D, Gianni M et al. Meta-analysis: Anticoagulant prophylaxis to prevent symptomatic venous thromboembolism in hospitalized medical patients. *Ann Intern Med.* 2007;146(4):278–288.

51 Wein L, Wein S, Haas SJ et al. Pharmacological venous thromboembolism prophylaxis in hospitalized medical patients: A meta-analysis of randomized controlled trials. *Arch Intern Med.* 2007;167(14):1476–1486.

52 Själander A, Jansson JH, Bergqvist D et al. Efficacy and safety of anticoagulant prophylaxis to prevent venous thromboembolism in acutely ill medical inpatients: A meta-analysis. *J Intern Med.* 2008;263(1):52–60.

53 Mismetti P, Laporte-Simitsidis S, Tardy B et al. Prevention of venous thromboembolism in internal medicine with unfractionated or low-molecular-weight heparins: A meta-analysis of randomised clinical trials. *Thromb Haemost.* 2000;83(1):14–19.

54 Bump GM, Dandu M, Kaufman SR et al. How complete is the evidence for thromboembolism prophylaxis in general medicine patients? A meta-analysis of randomized controlled trials. *J Hosp Med.* 2009;4(5):289–297.

55 Geerts WH, Bergqvist D, Pineo GF. Prevention of venous thromboembolism: American college of Chest Physicians Evidence-based Clinical Practice Guideline (8th edition). *Chest.* 2008;133(6 Suppl.):381S–453S.

56 Pineo GF. Prevention of venous thromboembolic disease in medical patients. Up to date. http://www.uptodate.com. Accessed June 2012.

113

Integrative medicine in palliative care

ROBERT ALAN BONAKDAR, ERMINIA GUARNERI, DAVID C. LEOPOLD

INTRODUCTION AND OVERVIEW

Integrative medicine (IM) and complementary and alternative medicine (CAM) as defined in the following have become an increasingly popular avenue of treatment for patients in the palliative care setting. Because many of these treatments traditionally have not been prescribed or recommended by healthcare providers, there is often an unfortunate lack of discussion and coordination of care. The following chapter provides an evidence-based overview of common treatments as well as insight into the prevalence, rationale, and approach to the patient who is considering these therapies.

Definition and background

The definition of CAM has evolved recently with the current NIH Center for Complementary and Alternative Medicine (NCCAM) categories and definitions presented in Tables 113.1 and 113.2.[1] Previously, CAM was defined as therapies not taught as part of medical school training. This is no longer relevant as more than 60% of the nation's allopathic medical schools were providing some level of instruction in CAM as of 1998.[2] This definition has also evolved as clinicians and hospitals are increasingly incorporating selected evidence-based CAM options into mainstream care in a practice known as integrative medicine. Also as detailed in the following, the vast majority of patients receive these therapies in conjunction with and not as alternatives to conventional care. Thus, for consistency, the term CAM will be used to describe the specific therapies discussed with the understanding that IM better describes the totality of how these treatments are used in a palliative care setting.

Integrative and palliative medicine: The crossroads of optimized, cost–effective care

IM, in addition to the NCCAM definition, is further defined by various key principles. These are as noted in Table 113.3 alongside those of palliative care. Similarities in their guiding principles are notable across current definitions.[3,4] In addition to

being patient-centered, these models of care have been shown to be cost-effective as well as linked improved satisfaction with care.[5] Experts familiar with both fields have argued that the principles of IM lend themselves well to those commonly accepted in the field of palliative care.

> If we accept the argument that palliative care is ethically desirable and that all patients are entitled to palliative services regardless of a terminal diagnosis, it follows that it needs to be integrated across a wide range of healthcare services ... Complementary and alternative medicine (CAM) therapies are ... useful and necessary components of palliative care. If we as a society look beyond separating cures and palliation, we will come closer to incorporating compassionate care throughout the disease process.[6]

Implicit in this discussion is that the integration of services throughout the care process is true both in the setting of cancer as well as other conditions for which integrative palliative care is well suited. One well-elucidated example is in the treatment of congestive heart failure. Figure 113.1 illustrates how palliative care may be viewed in the continuum of comprehensive heart failure care.[7]

Prevalence and predictors of use

CAM in general has become popular over the last several decades. Total CAM usage was reported in one third of the population in 1990 and increased to 42% by 1997. This represented 628 million office visits and $27 million spent, which far exceeded out-of-pocket expenditure for all conventional care as well as the 328 million visits to primary care providers in the same year. Usage of CAM specifically by cancer patients varies widely based on the therapies examined, definition of use, and population surveyed. These surveys demonstrate a range of use extending from less than one-third of the population to >90% of those surveyed as well as spanning all five realms of CAM as defined by NCCAM.[8] In several meta-analyses, CAM use appeared to average approximately one-half of those surveyed. Among the most commonly utilized treatments were dietary supplements. In one survey of patients with head and neck cancers, herbs were used by 47% followed

Table 113.1 *Definitions and categories of complementary and alternative medicine/integrative medicine*

Complementary and alternative medicine: A group of diverse medical and health care interventions, practices, products, or disciplines that are not generally considered part of conventional medicine.
Complementary medicine: Interventions used in conjunction with conventional medicine.
Alternative medicine: Intervention used in place of conventional medicine.
Integrative medicine: Combines treatments from conventional medicine and CAM for which there is some high-quality evidence of safety and effectiveness.
Categories:

1. *Alternative medical systems*: Systems of care based on unifying health paradigms, which may incorporate individual treatments including those noted in the following categories. Examples: traditional Chinese medicine (TCM), ayurveda, naturopathy, and homeopathy.
2. Biologically based therapies (see examples from category 2–5 in Table 113.2)
3. Manipulative and body-based methods
4. Mind–body interventions
5. Energy therapies (biofield therapies)

Source: Beider, S., *Evid Based Complement Altern. Med.*, 2(2), 227, 2005.

by herbal teas by 23% and vitamin/mineral preparations by 12%.[9] Other studies looking at hospitalized patients and those entering clinical trials, where supplement use may be more scrutinized, reported supplement use at 63%–73%.[10,11] Figure 113.2 provides an overview of the large variety of supplements utilized in this setting as noted in a survey of 573 cancer patients of various diagnoses, of whom 83.6% reported some types of dietary supplements use.[12]

Additionally, most estimates demonstrate an increasing trend in the usage of CAM. In a survey comparing CAM use in women with breast cancer, there was an increase in use from 62% in 1998 to 80% in 2005, with 41% noting use in a specific attempt to manage their breast cancer. Concomitantly, there were increases seen with the use of CAM products and visits to CAM practitioners. The authors of this survey, including the faculty of the University of Michigan Comprehensive Cancer Center, stated that "CAM use can no longer be regarded as an 'alternative' or unusual approach to managing breast cancer."[13] Although there is debate about what therapies should or should not be included in these surveys, what remains is that a significant and increasing portion of cancer patients are considering or utilizing CAM modalities as components of their integrative approach to cancer. Unfortunately, there are still many questions regarding the discussion and coordination of CAM therapies, as discussed in the following, that remain challenging.

Epidemiology

The predictors and rationale for the use of CAM in palliative care has been described in several surveys. Palliative care

patients utilizing CAM are more likely to be females who are younger, married, more highly educated, insured, and involved in a support group.[14–16] Additionally, in some surveys, utilizers tend to be more symptomatic than nonutilizers.[17–19] Interestingly, these rate and predictors of use appear to be similar to those found with other chronic conditions. This was confirmed in a study that found no significant difference in trends related to visits to CAM providers between cancer and coronary heart disease patients.[20]

The health values of persons considering CAM are also quite important to consider. Those who are involved in "active coping behaviors" such as greater physical activity tend to view CAM use in a similar manner.[21] Several surveys also demonstrate that those with a more "holistic outlook" wish to utilize complementary methods that may take this viewpoint into consideration.[22] Although there has been speculation that CAM use is a sign of dissatisfaction with conventional care, the more prevalent view is that CAM is used as an adjunct to optimize care. In fact, dissatisfaction with conventional care did not predict the use of CAM in a previous national survey, and fewer than 5% of CAM users did so in isolation from conventional care. Most CAM users state that their motivations for CAM use give them more control over their healthcare, and up to 80% report substantial benefit from its use.[23,24] As a corollary, CAM users have been noted to have more frequent relationships with a primary care physician and have regular physician follow-up and good compliance with recommended preventative health behaviors such as regular mammography.[25]

Regulation

The regulation of CAM varies with the type of modality, the training of practitioners, and state laws. As an example, acupuncture done by a licensed acupuncturist (LAc) or physician acupuncturist in the same state is regulated differently based on the state board of oriental medicine, medical board, or department of consumer affairs. The level of training and oversight for acupuncture varies widely by state, and the referring clinician should guide patients in confirming the CAM practitioner's credentials and certification whenever possible. Verification of licensure can be obtained by initially contacting the state's medical board, department of consumer affairs/protection, or therapy-specific national certification body with resources listed in Table 113.4.

Dietary supplements are governed according to the Dietary Supplement Health and Education Act (DSHEA) of 1994. Unlike prescription medications that must proceed through multiphase trials to gain premarketing approval from the Food and Drug Administration (FDA), supplements (with established ingredients) are not required to have safety, efficacy, or bioavailability data prior to marketing.[26] Ensuring these important qualities, along with having a clear and truthful label, is mainly the responsibility of the manufacturer. Because of many factors, the role of the FDA often begins after

Table 113.2   *Definition of common CAM modalities*

Biologically based therapies
Therapies that modify nutrient intake either through dietary intervention or supplementation. Typically categorized as vitamin/mineral or nonvitamin nonmineral supplements

Vitamin and mineral supplements	Vitamins (i.e., vitamin D) are organic substances (made by plants or animals). Minerals (i.e., calcium) are elements that come from the earth, soil, and water and are absorbed by plants. Animals and humans absorb minerals from the plants they eat. Vitamins and minerals are nutrients that your body needs to grow and develop normally.

Nonvitamin nonmineral supplements:

Herbal/botanical supplement	An herb (also called a botanical) is a plant or plant part used for its scent, flavor, and/or therapeutic properties. An herbal supplement is a type of dietary supplement that contains herbs, either alone or in mixtures.
Other dietary supplements	Dietary supplements (i.e., glucosamine, fish oil) which are neither plant derived nor primarily vitamin-/mineral-based supplements

Manipulative and body-based practices
Manipulative and body-based practices focus primarily on the structures and systems of the body, including the bones and joints, soft tissues, and circulatory and lymphatic systems.

Spinal manipulation	Technique performed by chiropractors and by other health care professionals such as physical therapists, osteopathic physicians, and some conventional medical doctors. Practitioners use their hands or a device to apply a controlled force to a joint of the spine, moving it beyond its passive range of motion; the amount of force applied depends on the form of manipulation used. Spinal manipulation is among the treatment options used by people with low-back pain—a very common condition that can be difficult to treat.
Massage therapy	Various techniques in which therapists press, rub, and otherwise manipulate the muscles and other soft tissues of the body. People use massage for a variety of health-related purposes, including to relieve pain, rehabilitate sports injuries, reduce stress, increase relaxation, address anxiety and depression, and aid general well-being.

Energy/biofield therapies
A diverse group of therapies that involve the transfer of human and nonhuman energy. These may be divided based on the type of energy (electrical, magnetic, light, etc.) as well as practitioner-based energy therapies (subtle energy)

Acupuncture	A family of procedures involving the stimulation of specific points on the body using a variety of techniques, such as penetrating the skin with needles that are then manipulated by hand or electrical stimulation. It is one of the key components of TCM and is among the oldest healing practices in the world. American practices of acupuncture incorporate medical traditions from China, Japan, Korea, and other countries.
Qi gong	An ancient Chinese discipline combining the use of gentle physical movements, mental focus, and deep breathing directed toward specific parts of the body.
Healing touch	Healing touch is a biofield therapy that encompasses a group of noninvasive techniques that utilize the hands to clear, energize, and balance the human and environmental energy fields. Healing touch was developed as a nursing continuing education program by Janet Mentgen, RN, BSN.
Reiki	Healing practice that originated in Japan. Reiki practitioners place their hands lightly on or just above the person receiving treatment, with the goal of facilitating the person's own healing response.
Therapeutic touch	It is a noninvasive method of healing that was derived from an ancient "laying on of hands" technique.
Aromatherapy	The use of fragrances and essences from plants to affect or alter a person's mood or behavior and to facilitate physical, mental, and emotional well-being. The chemicals comprising essential oils in plants have a host of therapeutic properties and have been used historically in Africa, Asia, and India. It is often used in conjunction with massage.

Mind–body therapies
Practices focused on the interactions among the brain, mind, body, and behavior, with the intent to use the mind to affect physical functioning and promote health. Many complementary health practices embody this concept as listed earlier and may be predominately movement- (yoga, tai chi) or behaviorally based.

Yoga	Healthcare practice that combines physical postures, breathing techniques, and meditation or relaxation. People use yoga as part of a general health regimen and also for a variety of health conditions.
Tai Chi	Practice that originated in China as a martial art and is sometimes referred to as "moving meditation"—practitioners move their bodies slowly, gently, and with awareness, while breathing deeply.

(Continued)

Table 113.2 (Continued) *Definition of common CAM modalities*

Cognitive behavior therapies	The application of modern theories of learning and conditioning in the treatment of behavior disorders. Techniques include cognitive therapy, biofeedback, relaxation techniques, and meditation. Some examples are noted in the following.
Biofeedback	Biofeedback uses simple electronic devices to teach clients how to consciously regulate bodily functions, such as breathing, heart rate, and blood pressure, in order to improve overall health.
Hypnosis	A state of increased receptivity to suggestion and direction, initially induced by the influence of another person.
Imagery	The use of mental images produced by the imagination (a form of psychotherapy). It can be classified by the modality of its content: visual, verbal, auditory, olfactory, tactile, gustatory, or kinesthetic. Common themes derive from nature imagery (e.g., forests and mountains), water imagery (e.g., brooks and oceans), travel imagery, etc. Imagery is often used to help patients cope with other diseases. Imagery often forms a part of hypnosis, relaxation techniques, and behavior therapy.
Cognitive coping strategies	Attempt to alter patterns of negative thoughts and dysfunctional attitudes to foster more healthy and adaptive thoughts, emotions, and actions. Major classes include external focus of attention, neutral imaginings, pleasant imaginings, dramatized coping, rhythmic cognitive activity, and pain acknowledging. They emphasize the basic components: education, skills acquisition, cognitive and behavioral rehearsal, and generalization and maintenance.
Relaxation techniques	The use of muscular relaxation and breathing techniques and activities in treatment to reduce feelings of tension. Often used in conjunction with imagery techniques.
Art and music therapy	The use of art and music as an adjunctive therapy in the treatment of neurologic, mental, or behavioral disorders.

Source: Beider, S., *Evid Based Complement Altern. Med.*, 2(2), 227, 2005.

Table 113.3 *Definition and principles of palliative and integrative care*

WHO definition of palliative care[6]	Bravewell definition of integrative medicine[6]
Palliative care is an approach that improves the quality of life of patients and their families facing the problem associated with life-threatening illness, through the prevention and relief of suffering by means of early identification and impeccable assessment and treatment of pain and other problems, physical, psychosocial, and spiritual. Palliative care:	IM is an approach to care that puts the patient at the center and addresses the full range of physical, emotional, mental, social, spiritual, and environmental influences that affect a person's health. Employing a personalized strategy that considers the patient's unique conditions, needs, and circumstances, IM uses the most appropriate interventions from an array of scientific disciplines to heal illness and disease and help people regain and maintain optimal health.
Defining principles/characteristics: • Provides relief from pain and other distressing symptoms • Affirms life and regards dying as a normal process • Intends neither to hasten nor postpone death • Integrates the psychological and spiritual aspects of patient care • Offers a support system to help patients live as actively as possible until death • Offers a support system to help the family cope during the patients illness and in their own bereavement • Uses a team approach to address the needs of patients and their families, including bereavement counseling, if indicated • Will enhance quality of life and may also positively influence the course of illness • Is applicable early in the course of illness, in conjunction with other therapies that are intended to prolong life, such as chemotherapy or radiation therapy, and includes those investigations needed to better understand and manage distressing clinical complications.	Defining principles/characteristics • The patient and practitioner are partners in the healing process. • All factors that influence health, wellness, and disease are taken into consideration, including body, mind, spirit, and community. • Providers use all healing sciences to facilitate the body's innate healing response. • Effective interventions that are natural and less invasive are used whenever possible. • Good medicine is based in good science. It is inquiry-driven and open to new paradigms. • Alongside the concept of treatment, the broader concepts of health promotion and the prevention of illness are paramount. • The care is personalized to best address the individual's unique conditions, needs, and circumstances. • Practitioners of IM exemplify its principles and commit themselves to self-exploration and self-development.

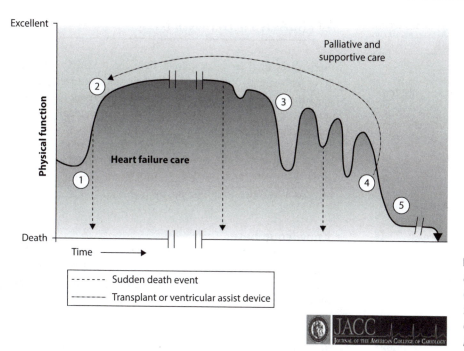

Figure 113.1 *Schematic depiction of comprehensive heart failure care. (From Goodlin, S.J., Palliative care in congestive heart failure, J. Am. Coll. Cardiol., 54(5), 386, 2009. Copyright 2009 American College of Cardiology Foundation.)*

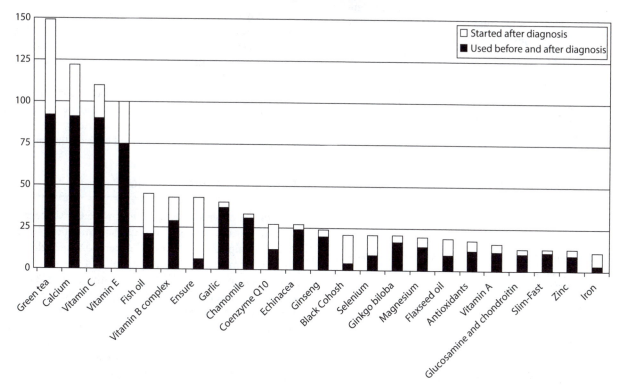

Figure 113.2 *Specific dietary supplements,* other than multivitamins, used after cancer diagnosis by 10 or more participants. *Participants could select multiple items. (From Ferrucci, L.M. et al., J. Altern. Complement Med., 15(6), 673, 2009.).*

a supplement is marketed as it monitors safety and label claims. The FDA must utilize adverse drug reports and product analysis to prove that a supplement poses significant health risks.[27,28] One well-publicized case in the setting of cancer was the herbal compound PC-SPES that was popular with prostate cancer patients. After reports and confirmation of contaminants, it was taken off the market in 2002, raising questions regarding the proper regulation of dietary supplements.

Since then, two more recent regulatory measures have also been enacted. The 2007 Dietary Supplement and Non-Prescription Drug Consumer Protection Act (S. 3546), which mandates the reporting of serious adverse events to the FDA and has allowed for improved monitoring and enforcement. In addition, the FDA has published guidelines for good manufacturing practices (GMPs) for dietary supplements in 2007 that are now required by all manufacturers.[29] The passage of these

Table 113.4 *Regulation resources for complementary and alternative medicine*

Organization/agency	Website
Federation of State Medical Boards	http://www.fsmb.org/m_pub.html
American Academy of Medical Acupuncture	http://www.medicalacupuncture.org
The National Certification Commission for Acupuncture and Oriental Medicine	http://www.nccaom.org/
American Chiropractic Association	http://www.acatoday.org
The National Certification Board for Therapeutic Massage and Bodywork	http://www.ncbtmb.com

acts has allowed increased enforcement of GMPs at several levels of manufacturing and distribution.[30]

In addition to governmental oversight, several independent agencies offer testing and monitoring services that allow manufacturers to demonstrate their adherence to regulatory standards. Those that pass inspection may carry an independent "seal of approval" on their label and advertising. Several of the government and independent agencies currently involved in testing are listed in Table 113.5. Clinicians should become familiar with well-regulated and well-researched brands for the supplements that are likely to be discussed with patients.

Table 113.5 *Governmental and independent regulatory agencies*

Agency	Website
Governmental	
FDA Medwatch Program for collecting adverse reactions to prescription and over the counter (OTC) medications as well as dietary supplements	www.fda.gov/medwatch
Federal Trade Commission (FTC) site for submitting complaints on false or misleading advertising	www.ftc.gov/ftc/complaint.htm
American Association of Poison Control Centers for reporting and management of adverse effects	www.poison.org or (800)222–1222
Independent labs providing supplement testing	
The ConsumerlabProduct Review	www.Consumerlab.com
Dietary Supplement Verification Program (DSVP) through the United States Pharmacopeia (USP)	www.uspverified.org
NSF	www.NSF.ORG/consumer/dietary_supplements

APPROACH TO THE PATIENT

Regardless of their particular beliefs about CAM, clinicians have an ethical obligation to discuss and counsel patients regarding treatment alternatives. The interaction between patients and clinicians regarding CAM use typically creates a less than optimal environment for the coordination of care. This situation is linked to several factors that are reviewed in the following, including patient and clinician CAM knowledge base, level of CAM discussion, and management strategies such as charting and follow-up.

Knowledge base

The knowledge base of the average clinician and the consumer regarding CAM is suboptimal to poor. The clearest example of this is found in the dietary supplement literature. Physician surveys have found that physicians may have an insufficient general understanding of commonly utilized supplements as well as their safety and interaction profiles, which may negatively influence the likelihood of discussion.[31,32] Similarly, consumers and patients tend to have misconceptions regarding product claims and efficacy. As pointed by a previous Harris Poll, the majority of respondents believed that the government provided a higher level of premarket regulation than is actually required as well as the belief that claims for safety or effectiveness required scientific support.[33] This level of regulatory trust may provide a scenario for a decreased perceived need for clinician guidance that is described in the following.

Clinician–patient discussion

One of the other key deficiencies in the CAM scenario is the level of clinician–patient discussion. In 2006, NCCAM and AARP completed a survey of Americans over the age of 50 that confirmed that 77% of patient had not discussed CAM with their physician.[34] More recently, in the 2011 version of the same survey, 67% of respondents had not discussed the topic of CAM with their provider.[35] For patients in the palliative care setting, the level of discussion appears to be somewhat improved at >50% disclosure rate, which appears to be dependent on the clinic setting and patient comfort with the clinician.[16,36] Unfortunately, although the level of discussion is improved compared to other patient encounters, the disclosure of CAM use in a palliative consultation is associated with pre- and postconsultation anxiety.[37] Overall, although the percentage appears to be improving, there are still many encounters in which neither the patient nor the clinician introduces the topic.[38] More concerning is the fact that if a patient is hospitalized by a specialist, CAM use is not identified up to 88% of the time.[39]

It is important to understand why patients do not discuss CAM use. Surveys indicate that factors such as anticipation of a negative or disinterested clinician response as well as belief that the clinician will not provide useful information motivate nondisclosure.[36] However, most important may be clinician inquiry, because patients demonstrate increasing willingness to disclose CAM use, but only if asked by a clinician directly.[40] Unfortunately, a survey of physicians found that few of those surveyed felt comfortable discussing CAM with their patients. One of the major reasons for this lack of comfort was related to a need to improve one's knowledge base regarding CAM (84% of responders). It is hypothesized that with improved education and tools regarding CAM and the importance of discussion, physicians may be more willing to discuss and counsel patients.[41] One effort that has been launched by NCCAM to improve the level of discussion has been the "Time to Talk" Campaign, which provides patient and clinician resources to increase the level of dialogue.[42]

Implications and resources in palliative care

As the preceding discussion points out, the level of CAM discussion in those receiving palliative care appears to be suboptimal, especially keeping in mind the potential level of interaction between CAM and conventional therapies during active treatment. As the conclusion of Juraskova et al.'s study on the communication between oncologists and breast cancer patients points out,

> CAM discussions during initial consultations between early-stage breast cancer patients and oncologists appear to be limited and linked with higher patient anxiety before and after the consultation. These findings indicate that doctors require further education about CAM therapies and supplements as well as guidance in how to raise and effectively discuss CAM issues with concern for their safety while balancing respect for the patients' beliefs.[37]

In order to support this important dialogue, the first comprehensive guidelines for discussing CAM in a palliative care setting have been recently developed. These guidelines are summarized in Table 113.6.

In addition to these guidelines, there are a number of resources available to clinicians interested in better understanding

Table 113.6 *Guidelines for discussion of CAM in a palliative care setting*

1. Elicit the person's understanding of their situation
2. Respect cultural and linguistic diversity and different epistemological framework
3. Ask questions about CAM use at critical points in the illness trajectory
4. Explore details and actively listen
5. Respond to the person's emotional state
6. Discuss relevant concerns while respecting the person's beliefs
7. Provide balanced, evidence-based advice
8. Summarize discussions
9. Document the discussion
10. Monitor and follow-up

Source: Beider, S., *Evid Based Complement Altern. Med.*, 2(2), 227, 2005.

IM /CAM as a means of improving patient communication and care. These resources are listed in Table 113.7 and include print and online information on the evidence-based use of CAM as well as continuing medical education courses available to clinicians.

CAM AND INTEGRATIVE MEDICINE INTERVENTIONS

The following section will review specific IM interventions that have been evaluated primarily in a palliative care setting. This review will include the role of these interventions in common palliative care scenarios, including nutritional support, symptom management, and quality of life. The summary of recommendation related to these interventions is noted in Table 113.8 and is derived primarily from the referenced meta-analyses, systematic reviews, and the best available controlled trials if no reviews are available.

Nutritional and dietary supplement overview

Although a number of dietary supplements, such as green tea (*Camellia sinensis*), turmeric (*Curcuma longa*), and vitamin D have typically been examined in regard to prevention, there is less available evidence in the palliative care setting.[43,44] This review will focus on interventions that have been most extensively evaluated in the palliative care setting, including general nutritional support, oral nutrient supplementation, omega-3 fatty acids, and ginger. The discussion of nutritional supplements beyond these is available elsewhere.[45]

General nutritional considerations are quite relevant in the palliative care setting. Malnourishment and weight loss can be common occurrences from various sources related to the background condition, comorbidities, treatment, and related outcomes. Because it is not uncommon for patients to have changes in appetite, gastrointestinal function, and mucosal integrity, all of which combine to decrease the ability to maintain proper nutritional status, the role of nutritional monitoring and counseling is integral. In several palliative care trials, the importance of dietary counseling has been demonstrated. Garg et al., in their systematic review of nutritional support for head and neck cancer patients receiving radiotherapy, found that nutritional status appeared to be maintained or improved when dietary counseling is provided.[46***]

In addition to general counseling, oral nutritional supplementation (ONS) is often considered to maintain nutritional status and decrease macro- or micronutrient deficiencies. Elia et al. provided a systematic review on the role of ONS.[47***] Although no difference in mortality was noted, in patients undergoing radiotherapy, ONS significantly increased dietary intake (381 kcal/day, 95% CI 193–569 in 3 RCTs) compared to routine care. Additionally, Baldwin et al., in their systematic review, found that ONS in malnourished patients with cancer had a beneficial effect on several aspects related to quality of life, including emotional functioning, dyspnea, loss of appetite, and global QOL.[48***]

Table 113.7   *Selected integrative medicine/CAM resources*

Organizations/institutes

- Society for Integrative Oncology (www.integrativeonc.org) is a multidisciplinary organization of professionals dedicated to studying and facilitating the cancer treatment and recovery process through the use of evidence-based, comprehensive, integrative healthcare.
- The NCCAM (http://nccam.nih.gov). Overview of CAM fields as well as information on clinical trials and patient education materials.

Internet

- The NCCAM (http://nccam.nih.gov) Overview of CAM fields as well as information on clinical trials and patient education materials.
- American Cancer Society Guidelines on Exercise: Summary of the ACS Guidelines on Nutrition and Physical Activity. Accessed at http://www.cancer.org on May 30, 2012.
- American Cancer Society Guidelines for Using Complementary and Alternative Methods. Accessed at http://www.cancer.org on May 30, 2012.
- National Cancer Institute Questions and Answers About Complementary and Alternative Medicine in Cancer Treatment. Accessed at http://www.cancer.gov on May 30, 2012.
- CAM on PubMed (http://nccam.nih.gov/research/camonpubmed). Focused search on PubMed for articles related to CAM, can be further designed for particular conditions or therapies.
- Cochrane Library (www.cochrane.org). Collection of systematic reviews with a Complementary Medicine Field.[6]
- NIH Office of Dietary Supplements and International Bibliographic Information on Dietary Supplements (IBIDS) (http://ods.od.nih.gov). Collaborative database of available abstract on dietary supplements.
- FDA Division of Dietary Supplement (http://vm:cfsan.fda.gov/~dms/supplmnt/html). Discussion of dietary supplement regulation, including a list of recalls and warnings.
- Natural Medicines Comprehensive Database (www.naturaldatabase.com). An extensive collection of supplement information, including uses, indication, efficacy, and adverse effects with a drug interaction checker.

Peer-reviewed information for patients

- MedlinePlus CAM page: (http://www.nlm.nih.gov/medlineplus/complementaryandalternativemedicine.html),
- The NCCAM (www.nccam.nih.gov) NIH clearinghouse of government-funded initiatives in CAM, including research, fellowships, grants, and patient education materials, including cancer treatments: http://nccam.nih.gov/health/cancer/camcancer.htm.
- Natural Medicine Comprehensive Database patient handouts (www.naturaldatabase.com).

The essential fatty acids comprise a group of lipids that must be acquired from exogenous sources, most often plants or animals that have ingested plants rich in omega-3 fatty acids (e.g., grasses, algae). Most commonly, with key fatty acid components Eicosapentaenoic Acid and Docosahexaenoic Acid (EPA/DHA) as derived from fish oil have been evaluated for their potential benefit in the setting of palliative care. One area of interest has been adjunctive use with first-line chemotherapy in patients with advanced non–small cell lung cancer. In a recent trial (n = 46), subjects in the fish oil group had an increased response rate and greater clinical benefit compared with the chemotherapy-only group (60.0% vs 25.8%, P =.008; 80.0% vs 41.9%, P =.02, respectively).[49***] There was also a nonsignificant trend toward increased 1-year survival (60.0% vs 38.7%; P =.15). Elias et al. in their systematic review of EPA-specific O3FAs in patients undergoing bone marrow transplant (BMT) found that "improvements in survival, complications and inflammatory markers".[47***] However, in the non-BMT setting, they found inconsistent positive benefit on quality of life and survival.

GINGER (*ZINGIBER SPP.*)

Ginger (*Zingiber officinale*) has been utilized for over 2500 years in traditional Chinese, ayurvedic (Indian), and Tibetan medicine for rheumatological, gastrointestinal, and oncological

conditions. A number of active ingredients have been isolated from the ginger plant, including the gingeroles, which exert direct anti-inflammatory activity, as well as galanolactones, which have serotonin receptor activity and likely modulate gastrointestinal and anti-inflammatory actions. Additionally, animal studies have demonstrated that some ginger subspecies have documented cyclooxygenase-2 (COX-2) and Prostaglandin E2 (PGE2) inhibitory activities, which may be relevant to the palliative care setting.[50,51]

In clinical trials, ginger has been utilized mostly for nausea, and a systematic review for this use in all settings demonstrated benefit.[52***] In the palliative care setting, ginger, typically at 1 g/day, has demonstrated benefit in several trials in the setting of postoperative and chemotherapy-associated nausea.[53**54**55**]

Acupuncture

Acupuncture is a component of TCM and is typically defined as the therapeutic utilization of fine needles at specific body points. Acupuncture is traditionally used in conjunction with other TCM treatments (Chinese herbal medicine, acupressure, moxibustion) that are collectively used to correct physiologic or energetic dysfunction. Because acupuncture has been the most popular and translatable

Table 113.8 *Summary of recommendation for integrative therapies evaluated in systematic reviews in the palliative care setting*

Intervention	Specific setting	Outcome	Notes
Weight loss/malnourishment			
Dietary counseling for weight loss (+)	HNSCC receiving radiotherapy	Nutritional status (+)	Nutritional status appeared to be maintained or improved with dietary counseling.[6]
ONS	Prevention of weight loss/ malnutrition during chemotherapy	Increase dietary intake (+)	In patients undergoing radiotherapy, meta-analysis showed that ONS significantly increases dietary intake (381 kcal/day, 95% CI 193–569 in 3 RCTs) compared to routine care.[6]
		Mortality (–)	There was also no difference in mortality between ONS and routine care in patients undergoing chemotherapy/radiotherapy (OR 1.00, 95% CI 0.62–1.61 in 4 RCTs) or surgery (OR 2.44, 95% CI 0.75–7.95 in 4 RCTs). (Elia as mentioned earlier)[6]
ONS	Cancer-related malnourishment	Quality of life emotional Global QOL (+) Functioning (+) Dyspnea (+) Loss of appetite (+)	Nutritional intervention had a beneficial effect on some aspects of QOL (emotional functioning, dyspnea, loss of appetite, and global QOL) but had no effect on mortality (RR = 1.06, 95% CI = 0.92–1.22, P =.43; I(2) = 0%; P(heterogeneity) =.56).[6]
		Mortality (–)	As mentioned earlier
O3FAs (EPA)	Nutritional support during BMT_	Survival (+) Complications (+) Inflammatory markers (+)	Individual studies of EPA supplementation as capsules showed improvements in survival, complications, and inflammatory markers in patients undergoing BMT [6]
O3FAs (EPA)	Palliative care (non-BMT)	Survival (+/–)	EPA-enriched ONS or capsules, there were inconsistent positive effects on survival and quality of life. (Elias as mentioned earlier)
O3FAs (EPA)	Cancer-related surgery	Survival (–)	In those undergoing surgery, EPA-enriched ETF had no effect. (Elias)
O3FAs	Cancer-related surgery	Length of hospital stay (+)	Supplementation in surgical oncology may reduce the length of hospital stay.[6]
Pain			
Acupuncture		+/–	See detailed description in Table 113.9
TENS		Pain reduction (+/–)	The results of this updated systematic review remain inconclusive due to a lack of suitable RCTs[6]
Biofield therapies	Various	Pain reduction (+)	Beider[6]
Mind–Body therapies	Various techniques	Pain reduction (+)	Beider[6]
Oral Mucositis (OM)			
LLLT red (630–670 nm) and infrared (780–830 nm)		Risk, duration, severity of OM (+)	LLLT reduced risk of oral mucositis with RR 2.45 [CI 1.85–3.18], reduced duration, severity of oral mucositis and reduced number of days with oral mucositis (4.38 days, P = 0.0009). Pain-relieving effect based on the Cohen scale was at 1.22 (CI 0.19–2.25).[6]
Chemotherapy-induced nausea or vomiting			
Acu-therapies		All methods: V: Incidence (+) V: Severity (+/–) N Severity (–)	Overall, acupuncture point stimulation of all methods combined reduced the incidence of acute vomiting (RR = 0.82; 95% CI 0.69–0.99; P = 0.04), but not acute or delayed nausea severity compared to control.

(Continued)

Table 113.8 (*Continued*) *Summary of recommendation for integrative therapies evaluated in systematic reviews in the palliative care setting*

Intervention	Specific setting	Outcome	Notes
Electroacupuncture		Acute vomiting (+)	Electroacupuncture reduced the proportion of acute vomiting (RR = 0.76; 95% CI 0.60 to 0.97; P = 0.02), but manual acupuncture did not.
Manual acupuncture		Acute vomiting (−)	
Acupressure		Acute N severity (+) Acute V (−)	Acupressure reduced mean acute nausea severity (SMD = −0.19; 95% CI −0.37 to −0.01; P = 0.04) but not acute vomiting or delayed symptoms.
TCM		Various (+/−)	Chinese medicinal herbs, when used together with chemotherapy, may offer some benefit to breast cancer patients in terms of bone marrow improvement and quality of life, but the evidence is too limited to make any confident conclusions.[6]
Breathlessness/ DOE			
Neuroelectrical muscle stimulation (NMES)	Advanced stages of malignant and nonmalignant diseases[a]	+	There was a high strength of evidence that NMES ... could relieve breathlessness.[6]
Acupuncture		+[a]	There is a low strength of evidence that acupuncture/acupressure is helpful (as mentioned earlier and recent RCT=[6]
Exercise/PA		+	Beider[6]
Fatigue			
Biofield therapies		+/−	
Exercise/PA		+	Beider[6]
Psychological distress			
Massage/aromatherapy		+	Massage and aromatherapy massage confer short-term benefits on psychological well-being, with the effect on anxiety supported by limited evidence.[6]
Mind–body therapies, various	Anxiety Mood disturbance	(+)	Mind–body modalities are recommended as part of a multidisciplinary approach to reduce anxiety, mood disturbances, or chronic pain. Grade of recommendation, 1B[6]
Meditation (MBSR)		Mood Disturbance (+) Overall QOL (+) Stress (+) Sleep quality (+)	Beider[6]
Hypnotherapy	Symptoms control in the terminally ill	+/−	Beider[6]
Exercise/PA		Anxiety (+) Stress (+) Depression (+) Insomnia (+)	Beider[6]

Symbols and abbreviations: (+), Predominately supports use in the setting for the specified outcome; (−), Does not support use in the setting for the specified outcome; (+/−), Nonsignificant or inconsistent evidence in the setting.

Abbreviations: BMT, bone marrow transplant; COPD, chronic obstructive pulmonary disease; EPA, eicosapentaenoic acid as an active component of omega-3 fatty acids; ETF, enteral tube feeding; HNSCC, squamous cell carcinoma of the head and neck; LLLT, low-level laser therapy; MBSR, mindfulness-based stress reduction; O3FAs, omega-3 fatty acids–related supplementation including ONS; ONS, oral nutritional supplements; TCM, traditional Chinese medicine; TENS, transcutaneous electrical nerve stimulation.

[a] Most studies in the setting of COPD

component of TCM, it has received increasing attention regarding its mechanism and potential efficacy in various conditions. The mechanism for acupuncture's benefits stems from potential local tissue, spinal cord, and cortical effects. The strongest evidence appears to focus on frequency-dependent increase of endomorphin-1, beta endorphin, encephalin, and serotonin levels after acupuncture, which may be partially reversal with naloxone[56–58]

The clinical efficacy of acupuncture in palliative care is variable and appears to be based on several factors, such as the condition being treated and the specific methodology employed, including treatment protocol and randomization. The most extensive condition-based review of the cancer-related scenarios for which acupuncture has been employed was published by the Harvard Medical School faculty and the Dana-Farber Cancer Institute faculty as noted in Table 113.9. They conclude, "Recent advances in acupuncture clinical research suggest that acupuncture may provide clinical benefit for cancer patients with treatment-related side effects such as nausea and vomiting, post operative pain, cancer related pain, chemotherapy-induced leukopenia, post chemotherapy fatigue, xerostomia, and possibly insomnia, anxiety and quality of life (QOL)." However, they note, "...Clinical research on acupuncture in cancer care is a new and challenging field in oncology. The results of clinical research will continue to provide us with clinically relevant answers for patients and oncologists."[59***]

In the setting of noncancer-related palliative care, there have been a number of trials examining the use of acupuncture. One example is the use of acupuncture for dyspnea on exertion (DOE), which is common in those with advanced chronic obstructive pulmonary disease (COPD). In a recent 12-week trial of acupuncture in addition to convention care, those receiving adjunctive care demonstrated clinically relevant improvements in DOE (Borg scale), nutrition status (including BMI), airflow obstruction, exercise capacity, and health-related quality of life.[60**] Overall, more research is needed to confirm the benefit of acupuncture and related techniques in a palliative care setting. However, because of its relative safety and potential benefit, acupuncture should be considered for a therapeutic trial based on participatory decision making, especially in the setting of nonresponsive symptoms.

Biostimulation

Biostimulation refers to the application of light, electrical, magnetic, or subtle energy for therapeutic purposes. Several biostimulation methods, such as ultrasound or transcutaneous electrical nerve stimulation (TENS), have become standard practice, especially in the treatment of musculoskeletal rehabilitation. The majority of biostimulation types continue to be considered CAM, and the most common are referred in the following.

LOW LEVEL LASER THERAPY

Low-level laser therapy (LLLT) refers to the application of low-intensity monochromatic wavelengths of light typically for the treatment of pain and inflammatory conditions. The intensity of the treatment is below that which is used for laser in other medical setting such as surgical or dermatological applications and thus is also referred to as "cold laser." Although LLLT has been used for several decades in Europe, the mechanism for LLLT has not been fully elucidated. It appears to be a nonthermal, photochemical cellular reaction that may provide anti-inflammatory and tissue-healing effects.

Several recent controlled trials have attempted to examine the role of LLLT in palliative care, especially in the setting of chemoradiotherapy-induced oral mucositis. One of larger recent trials was done by Gautam et al. using low-level helium neon laser. In this trial of 121 subjects, the incidence of severe oral mucositis in the laser group versus placebo was significantly reduced (29% vs. 89%, $p < 0.001$) as were associated pain (18% vs. 71%, $p < 0.001$), opioid analgesic use (7% vs. 21%, $p < 0.001$), and need for total parental nutrition (TPN) (30% vs. 39% $p = 0.039$) significantly less in laser than placebo group patients with no significant side effects noted.[61**] These finding are similar to those found in a recent reviews on the subject, which notes that LLLT "reduced risk of oral mucositis with relative risk (RR) 2.45 [confidence interval (CI) 1.85–3.18], reduced duration, severity of oral mucositis and reduced number of days with oral mucositis (4.38 days, $P = 0.0009$). Risk reduction appears similar between the red (630–670 nm) and infrared (780–830 nm) LLLT utilized and pain-relieving effect based on the Cohen scale was at 1.22 (CI 0.19–2.25)."[62***] Based on the strong safety profile, these studies lend support to the use of well-established LLLT protocols and equipment to reduce the burden of this condition.

BIOFIELD THERAPIES

Biofield therapies are typically referred to as practices that involve the balancingor exchange of subtle energies. Typically, practices in this category include healing touch, therapeutic touch, reiki, and qi gong with definition as noted in Table 113.2. Based on the preliminary level of research in this area, a recent review[63***] provided the following conclusions:

- Cancer-related pain (four studies): "Studies thus far suggest moderate (level 2) evidence for biofield therapies to reduce acute pain in cancer. Currently, there is little evidence for longer-term pain outcomes in cancer, and it is unclear whether biofield therapies offer benefit over other modalities (such as massage) on pain in cancer."

Table 113.9   *Clinical trials and systematic review of acupuncture use in clinical cancer care (2001–2007)[6]*

Clinical conditions	Author and study design	Major outcome	Reported adverse events	Study population features
Chemotherapy-induced nausea & vomiting	Roscoe et al.[9] Randomized controlled multicenter trial (n = 739)	Patients in the acupressure group experienced less nausea on the day treatment compared to controls (p < 0.05).	No adverse events were discussed.	85% breast cancer, 10% hematologic neoplasms patients undergoing chemotherapy
Postoperative nausea and vomiting	Gan et al.[41] RCT (n = 77) (electroacupoint stimulation, ondansetron versus placebo)	The complete response rate was 77% vs. 64% and 42% (p = 0.01); electroacupoint stimulation is more effective in controlling nausea.	No difference in adverse events rate among groups	Patients undergoing major breast surgery
Cancer pain	Alimi et al.[11] Randomized, blinded, controlled trial (n = 90)	Pain intensity deceased by 36% at 2 months from baseline in the study group (p < 0.0001)	No infection was reported; no other adverse events were reported	Patients with chronic peripheral or central neuropathic pain arising after cancer treatment
Postoperative Pain	Mehling et al.[58] RCT (n = 138)	Patients in the massage and acupuncture group with usual care experienced a decrease of 1.4 points on a pain scale (p = 0.038).	No adverse events were discussed.	Patients undergoing cancer-related surgery. including breast, bladder, and prostate and ovarian cancers
Postthoracotomy wound pain	Wong et al.[57] RCT (n = 27) (electroacupuncture vs. sham acupuncture)	A trend for lower visual analogue scale pain score in the electroacupuncture group was observed. Postoperative morphine use was significantly lower in electroacupuncture group (p < 0.05).	No adverse reactions related to acupuncture were observed.	Patients with operable non–small cell lung carcinoma
Hot flashes	Deng et al.[69] RCT (n = 72) (true acupuncture versus sham acupuncture)	True acupuncture was associated with 0.8 fewer hot flashes per day than sham (p = 0.3).	Very minor slight bleeding and bruising at the needle cite were reported.	Breast cancer patients
Vasomotor symptoms (hot flashes) and psychological well-being	Nedstrand et al.[70] RCT (electroacupuncture vs. applied relaxation) (n = 38)	Longitudinally, patients in the electroacupuncture group experienced a decrease of hot flashes >50% at 12 weeks and at 6 months follow-up.	No adverse event were discussed.	Patients treated for breast cancer
Chemotherapy-induced leukopenia	Lu et al.[12] Systematic review on RCTs (n = 682)	WBC counts in study group was significantly higher than that in control group (p < 0.05).	No adverse effects were discussed.	Patients with non–small cell lung cancer or nasopharynx cancer undergoing chemotherapy
Postchemotherapy fatigue	Vickers et al.[13] Uncontrolled prospective study (n = 37)	The mean improvement from baseline fatigue score was 31.3% (95% CI: 20.6%–41.5%).	No adverse events were reported.	Cancer patients who had completed cytotoxic chemotherapy at least 3 weeks previously but complained of persisting fatigue.
Radiation-induced xerostomia	Johnstone et al.[15] Uncontrolled prospective study (n = 50)	Response rate as improvement of 10% or better from baseline xerostomia inventory (XI) was 70%; 48% of patients received benefit of 10 points or more on the XI.	No adverse effects were reported.	Patients with pilocarpine-resistant xerostomia after radiotherapy for head and neck cancer

Source: Beider, S., *Evid Based Complement Altern. Med.*, 2(2), 227, 2005.

- Fatigue (five studies): "Taken together, these five studies suggest conflicting (level 4) evidence for biofield therapies' effects on reducing fatigue."
- Quality of life (three studies): "Suggests conflicting (level 4) evidence for biofield therapies' impact on quality of life for cancer patients; certainly more studies are needed to clarify these initial findings."

Overall, the reviewers note the positive evidence for these therapies in the area of pain with increasing need for trials to determine potential benefit in other areas of palliative care.

ELECTRICAL STIMULATION

Various types of electrical stimulation have been employed in palliative care. These have been utilized in both conventional (i.e., stimulation of the area of dysfunction) and acupuncture-like (AL) set-up (i.e., stimulation to acupuncture points). Although there is evidence in focused settings, such as the use of acupoint stimulation to improve dyspnea, the majority of evidence regarding the use of electrostimlation is difficult to interpret.[64***]

MAGNETIC STIMULATION

Magnets, typically simple static or pulsed, are often touted as helpful agents in the setting of cancer. Unfortunately, there are numerous claims made in this arena with very little proof of efficacy. Small trials that have been done have largely been negative.[65*] Interestingly, more advanced research is examining the therapeutic benefit of magnetic therapy at the cellular level: "Magnetic attraction between cells and tumors may provide a valuable method by which adoptively transferred cells are forced into tumors in significantly greater numbers than is possible by relying on natural cell trafficking; however, the level of therapeutic efficacy remains to be tested..."[66] Further research is anticipated to understand the potential role of magnetic stimulation in this setting. Until then, the use of over-the-counter magnetic devices in the setting of palliative care is discouraged.

Mind–body/manipulative interventions

The importance of psychological distress in palliative care cannot be overstated. The palliative care setting may be exacerbated by psychological or physiological stressors, and these stressors may, to some extent, be involved in additional symptomatology. As interventions, in general, multiple mind–body techniques have previously been shown to effectively lower physiological stress.[67] In addition to intrinsic

benefits, stress management techniques, meditation, biofeedback, exercise, and prayer are potential means for controlling mood and improving compliance with other palliative care options. One of the most complete summaries of IM in palliative care is provided by the American College of Chest Physicians (ACCP) evidence-based clinical practice guidelines for *complementary therapies and integrative oncology in lung cancer*, which notes as follows: *Specifically mind-body therapies such as meditation/MBSR, yoga, hypnosis and massage have all been studied in controlled trials in a palliative care setting and demonstrated consistent benefit.*[68***] However, not all trials have been positive that illustrates the importance of finding therapists with appropriate training in the area as well as focus on specific symptoms that may be likely to show improvement during a therapeutic trial.[69***]

Exercise and physical activity

Attention to the potential role of exercise in the palliative care setting has increased substantially in recent years. What was previously thought to be helpful in the preventative or recovery stages is now more routinely provided in advance cancer and other palliative settings. This is based on increasing research in the setting, which has elucidated symptomatic benefit. Albrecht et al. in their systematic review of physical activity in advanced-stage cancer, note as follows:

> Research has shown that, for people with cancer (including advanced-stage cancer), exercise can decrease anxiety, stress, and depression while improving levels of pain, fatigue, shortness of breath, constipation, and insomnia. People diagnosed with cancer should discuss with their oncologist safe, easy ways they can incorporate exercise into their daily lives.[70**]

The role of the physician in encouraging patients to become physically active is well established, though unfortunately too often underutilized.[71] When physicians initiated discussion of exercise, the discussion was four times as likely to occur, with strong impact on the subsequent follow-through for an exercise prescription.[72] Several of the exercise resources noted in Table 113.7 may be utilized to support the discussion and utilization of exercise in this setting.

OTHER INTERVENTIONS FOR THE PATIENT AND FAMILY: WHAT'S THE EVIDENCE?

A host of additional interventions, which are often considered CAM, should be kept in mind as they may play an important role in patients and families coping with the palliative care setting. This is best summarized in Kongsgaard et al.'s article: *Evidence-based medicine works best when there is evidence: challenges in palliative medicine when randomized controlled trials are not possible.*

Although we must exercise caution in making definitive claims from uncontrolled trial data, limitations in performing controlled trials should neither preclude the use of findings from well-designed nonrandomized controlled trials nor, more importantly, deprive patients of potentially effective treatments.[73]

The lack of evidence for certain therapies is also notable regarding the utilization and benefit of therapies for families and caregivers. Although more research is certainly needed, recent research has found that the offering of selected therapies, such as massage, can benefit families who are caring for those in a palliative care setting.[74*] Thus, clinicians who are caring for palliative care patients should be cognizant of the limitation of evidence for both patients and caregivers and tailor treatment based on the available evidence, individual preference, clinical experience and knowledge of the therapies, and therapists involved.

CONCLUSION

As IM and palliative care expand their role in various healthcare settings, it is interesting to observe their parallel and overlapping paths. We can observe that they both play a strong role in better understanding the optimal care of patients and their families. Beyond economic or evidence-based discussion, which are both relevant, it is prudent to understand that in many cases, we are discussing a philosophy that intersects with medicine. This is best summarized by Beider as follows:

> Integrated palliative care can be part of a philosophical movement in healthcare to see the patient and their suffering as inter-related in a dynamic exchange process that continuously influences health and well-being. In this regard the patient, family and care team are also integrated in an ongoing attempt to individualize and optimize care.[6]

Key learning points

1. *CAM is utilized in some form by a significant portion of palliative care patients.*

2. *Most patients will not discuss CAM use or preferences unless asked specifically by a clinician.*

3. *CAM use is strongly linked to health beliefs and is most commonly used in conjunction with conventional care.*

4. *Asking patients and families about their current or potential use of CAM is important for*

   a. Avoiding harmful or unproven therapies

   b. Coordinating therapies that have some evidence of benefit

   c. Reviewing therapies that have equivocal evidence but whose safety profile makes them worthy of a therapeutic trial, especially in the setting of refractory symptomatology

REFERENCES

1   NIH Center for Complementary and Alternative Medicine (NCCAM Accessed at http://nccam.nih.gov/health/whatiscam/#sup2 on 10.23.06.

2   Wetzel MS, Eisenberg DM, Kaptchuk TJ. Courses involving complementary and alternative medicine at U.S. medical schools. *JAMA.* 1998;280(9):784–787.

3   *National Cancer Control Programmes: Policies and Managerial Guidelines,* 2nd edn. Geneva, Switzerland, World Health Organization, 2002. accessed on May 24, 2012 at: http://www.who.int/cancer/palliative/definition/en/.

4   Guarneri E, Horrigan BJ, Pechura CM. The efficacy and cost effectiveness of integrative medicine: Aa review of the medical and corporate literature. Explore (NY). September–October 2010;6(5):308–312.

5   Comprehensive, Integrated Palliative Care Reduces Costs and Improves Satisfaction Among Patients and Their Families Within a Large Health System as part of the Agency for Healthcare Research and Quality (AHRQ) Health Innovations Exchange accessed on May 30, 2012 at http://www.innovations.ahrq.gov/content.aspx?id=263.

6   Beider S. An ethical argument for integrated palliative care. *Evid Based Complement Alternat Med.* June 2005;2(2):227–231.

7   Goodlin SJ. Palliative care in congestive heart failure. *J Am Coll Cardiol.* July 2009 28;54(5):386–396.

8   Yates JS, Mustian KM, Morrow GR, Gillies LJ, Padmanaban D, Atkins JN, Issell B, Kirshner JJ, Colman LK. Prevalence of complementary and alternative medicine use in cancer patients during treatment. *Support Care Cancer.* 2005;13(10):806–811.

9   Molassiotis A, Ozden G, Platin N et al. Complementary and alternative medicine use in patients with head and neck cancers in Europe. *Eur J Cancer Care (Engl)* 2006;15(1):19–24.

10 Gupta D, Lis CG, Birdsall TC, Grutsch JF. The use of dietary supplements in a community hospital comprehensive cancer center: Implications for conventional cancer care. *Support Care Cancer* 2005;13(11):912–929.

11 Sparber A, Bauer L, Curt G et al. Use of complementary medicine by adult patients participating in cancer clinical trials. *Oncol Nurs Forum* 2000;27(4):623–630.

12 Ferrucci LM, McCorkle R, Smith T, Stein KD, Cartmel B. Factors related to the use of dietary supplements by cancer survivors. *J Altern Complement Med.* June 2009;15(6):673–680.

13 Boon HS, Olatunde F, Zick SM. Trends in complementary/alternative medicine use by breast cancer survivors: Comparing survey data from 1998 and 2005. *BMC Womens Health.* 2007;7:4.

14 Verhoef MJ, Balneaves LG, Boon HS, Vroegindewey A. Reasons for and characteristics associated with complementary and alternative medicine use among adult cancer patients: A systematic review. *Integr Cancer Ther.* 2005;4(4):274–286.

15 Cassileth BR, Vickers AJ. High prevalence of complementary and alternative medicine use among cancer patients: Implications for research and clinical care. *J Clin Oncol.* April 2005 20;23(12):2590–2592.

16 Wanchai A, Armer JM, Stewart BR. Complementary and alternative medicine use among women with breast cancer: A systematic review. *Clin J Oncol Nurs.* August 2010;14(4):E45–E55

17 Rakovitch E, Pignol JP, Chartier C, Ezer M, Verma S, Dranitsaris G, Clemons M. Complementary and alternative medicine use is associated with an increased perception of breast cancer risk and death. *Breast Cancer Res Treat.* 2005;90(2):139–148. doi: 10.1007/s10549-004-3779-1.

18 Hlubocky FJ, Ratain MJ, Wen M, Daugherty CK. Complementary and alternative medicine among advanced cancer patients enrolled on phase I trials: A study of prognosis, quality of life, and preferences for decision making. *J Clin Oncol.* 2007;25(5):548–554.

19 Helyer LK, Chin S, Chui BK, Fitzgerald B, Verma S, Rakovitch E, Dranitsaris G, Clemons M. The use of complementary and alternative medicines among patients with locally advanced breast cancer—A descriptive study. *BMC Cancer.* 2006;6:39.

20 Kristoffersen AE, Norheim AJ, Fønnebø VM. Any difference? Use of a CAM provider among cancer patients, coronary heart disease (CHD) patients and individuals with no cancer/CHD. *BMC Complement Altern Med.* January 12, 2012;12:1.

21 Astin, JA, Why patients use alternative medicine: Results of a national study. *JAM.A.* 1998; 279(19):1548–1553.

22 Furnham A, Bhagrath R, A comparison of health beliefs and behaviours of clients of orthodox and complementary medicine. *Br J Clin Psychol.* 1993; 32:237.

23 Astin, J.A. (1998), As above

24 Druss BG, Rosenheck RA. Association between use of unconventional therapies and conventional medical services. *JAMA.* August 18, 1999;282(7):651–656.

25 Astin, J.A. et al., Complementary and alternative medicine use among elderly persons: One-year analysis of a Blue Shield Medicare supplement. *J Gerontol A Biol Sci Med Sci.* 2000;55(1):M4–M9.

26 FDA Dietary Supplements Overiew. Accessed on May 23, 2012 at http://www.fda.gov/food/dietarysupplements/default.htm.

27 Federal Drug Administration press release: FDA announces plans to prohibit sales of dietary supplements containing Ephedra Dec. 30, 2003. Accessed at http://www.fda.gov/oc/initiatives/ephedra/december2003/. Accessed on May 1, 2004.

28 Federal Drug Administration Medwatch Press Release. 2002 Safety Alert - SPES, PC SPES, June 5, 2002. Accessed on May 1, 2004 at http://www.fda.gov/medwatch/SAFETY/2002/spes_press2.htm.

29 FDA Issues Dietary Supplements Final Rule accessed at http://www.fda.gov/bbs/topics/NEWS/2007/NEW01657.html on June 22, 2007.

30 FDA inspections, compliance, enforcement, and criminal investigations. Accessed on May 23, 2012 at: http://www.fda.gov/ICECI/EnforcementActions/WarningLetters/ucm262443.htm

31 Ashar BH, Rice TN, Sisson SD. Physicians' understanding of the regulation of dietary supplements. *Arch Intern Med.* May 14, 2007;167(9):966–969.

32 Kemper KJ, Gardiner P, Gobble J, Woods C. Expertise about herbs and dietary supplements among diverse health professionals. *BMC Complement Altern Med.* April 2006;286:15.

33 Harris Interactive. Widespread ignorance of regulation and labeling of vitamins, minerals and food supplements, according to a national Harris interactive survey. Accessed on May 23, 2012 at http://www.harrisinteractive.com/news/printerfriend/index.asp?NewsID=560].

34 Complementary and alternative medicine: What people aged 50 and older discuss with their health care providers, 2006. Accessed on May 23, 2012 at http://assets.aarp.org/rgcenter/health/cam_2007.pdf.

35 Complementary and alternative medicine: What people aged 50 and older discuss with their health care providers, April, 2011. Accessed on May 23, 2012 at http://assets.aarp.org/rgcenter/health/complementary-alternative-medicine-nccam.pdf.

36 Adler SR, Fosket JR. Disclosing complementary and alternative medicine use in the medical encounter: A qualitative study in women with breast cancer. *J FamPract.* June 1999;48(6):453–458.

37 Juraskova I, Hegedus L, Butow P, Smith A, Schofield P. Discussing complementary therapy use with early-stage breast cancer patients: Exploring the communication gap. *Integr Cancer Ther.* June 2010;9(2):168–176.

38 Wold RS, Wayne SJ, Waters DL, Baumgartner RN. Behaviors underlying the use of nonvitamin nonmineral dietary supplements in a healthy elderly cohort. *J Nutr Health Aging.* January–February 2007;11(1):3–7.

39 Azaz-Livshits, T. et al., Use of complementary alternative medicine in patients admitted to internal medicine wards. *Int J Clin Pharmacol Ther.* December 2002;40(12):539–547.

40 Hansrud, D.D. et al., Underreporting the use of dietary supplements and nonprescription medication among patients undergoing a periodic health examination. *Mayo Clin Proc.* 1999;74:443–447.

41 Corbin-Winslow, L. et al., Physicians want education about CAM to enhance communication with their patients. *Arch Intern Med.* 2002;162 (10):1176–1181.

42 NCCAM time to talk campaign. Access on May 23, 2012 at http://nccam.nih.gov/timetotalk.

43 Registered clinical trials in the setting of turmeric and cancer. Accessed on May 30, 2012 at http://clinicaltrials.gov/ct2/results?term=turmeric±cancer.

44 Davies AA, Davey Smith G, Harbord R, Bekkering GE, Sterne JA, Beynon R, Thomas S. Nutritional interventions and outcome in patients with cancer or preinvasive lesions: Systematic review. *J Natl Cancer Inst.* July 19, 2006;98(14):961–973.

45 Hardy ML. Dietary supplement use in cancer care: Help or harm. *Hematol Oncol Clin North Am.* August 2008;22(4):581–617, vii.

46 Garg S, Yoo J, Winquist E. Nutritional support for head and neck cancer patients receiving radiotherapy: A systematic review. *Support Care Cancer.* June 2010;18(6):667–677.

47 Elia M, Van Bokhorst-de van der Schueren MA, Garvey J, Goedhart A, Lundholm K,Nitenberg G, Stratton RJ. Enteral (oral or tube administration) nutritional support and eicosapentaenoic acid in patients with cancer: A systematic review. *Int J Oncol.* January 2006;28(1):5–23.

48 Baldwin C, Spiro A, Ahern R, Emery PW. Oral nutritional interventions in malnourished patients with cancer: A systematic review and meta-analysis. *J Natl Cancer Inst.* March 7, 2012;104(5):371–385.

49 Murphy RA, Mourtzakis M, Chu QS, Baracos VE, Reiman T, Mazurak VC. Supplementation with fish oil increases first-line chemotherapy efficacy in patients with advanced nonsmall cell lung cancer. *Cancer.* August 15, 2011;117(16):3774–3780.

50 Murakami, A. Zerumbone, a Southeast Asian ginger sesquiterpene, markedly suppresses free radical generation, proinflammatory protein production, and cancer cell proliferation accompanied by apoptosis: The alpha, beta-unsaturated carbonyl group is a prerequisite. *Carcinogenesis.* 2002;23(5):795–802.

51 Thomson, M., The use of ginger (Zingiber officinale Rosc.) as a potential anti-inflammatory and antithrombotic agent. *Prostaglandins Leukot Essent Fatty Acids.* 2002;67(6):475–478.

52 Ernst E, Pittler MH. Efficacy of ginger for nausea and vomiting: A systematic review of randomized clinical trials. *Br J Anaesth.* March 2000;84(3):367–371.

53 Nanthakomon T, Pongrojpaw D. The efficacy of ginger in prevention of postoperative nauseaand vomiting after major gynecologic surgery. *J Med Assoc Thai* 2006;89(Suppl 4):S130–S136.

54 Manusirivithaya S, Sripramote M, Tangjitgamol S et al. Antiemetic effect of ginger ingynecologic oncology patients receiving cisplatin. *Int J Gynecol Cancer* 2004;14(6):1063–1069.

55 Levine ME, Gillis MG, Koch SY, Voss AC, Stern RM, Koch KL. Protein and ginger for the treatment of chemotherapy-induced delayed nausea. *J Altern Complement Med.* June 2008;14(5):545–551.

56 Cabyoglu MT, Ergene N, Tan U. The mechanism of acupuncture and clinical applications. *Int J Neurosci.* February 2006;116(2):115–125.

57 White P. A background to acupuncture and its use in chronic painful musculoskeletal conditions. *J R Soc Health.* September 2006;126(5):219–227.

58 Staud R, Price DD. Mechanisms of acupuncture analgesia for clinical and experimental pain. *Exp Rev Neurother.* May 2006;6(5):661–667.

59 Lu W, Dean-Clower E, Doherty-Gilman A, Rosenthal DS. The value of acupuncture in cancer care. *Hematol Oncol Clin North Am.* August 2008;22(4):631–648, viii.

60 Suzuki M, Muro S, Ando Y, Omori T, Shiota T, Endo K, Sato S, Aihara K, Matsumoto M, Suzuki S, Itotani R, Ishitoko M, Hara Y, Takemura M, Ueda T, Kagioka H, Hirabayashi M, Fukui M, Mishima M. A randomized, placebo-controlled trial of acupuncture in patients with chronic obstructive pulmonary disease (COPD): The COPD-acupuncture trial (CAT). *Arch Intern Med.* June 11, 2012;172(11):878–886.

61 Gautam AP, Fernandes DJ, Vidyasagar MS, Maiya GA. Low level helium neon laser therapy for chemoradiotherapy induced oral mucositis in oral cancer patients—A randomized controlled trial. *Oral Oncol.* April 11, 2012;48:893–897.

62 Bensadoun RJ, Nair RG. Low-level laser therapy in the prevention and treatment of cancer therapy-induced mucositis: 2012 state of the art based on literature review and meta-analysis. *Curr Opin Oncol.* 2012;24(4):363–370.

63 Jain S, Mills PJ. Biofield therapies: Helpful or full of hype? A best evidence synthesis. *Int J Behav Med.* March 2010;17(1):1–16. Review. Erratum in: *Int J Behav Med.* March 2011;18(1):79–82.

64 Hurlow A, Bennett MI, Robb KA, Johnson MI, Simpson KH, Oxberry SG. Transcutaneous electric nerve stimulation (TENS) for cancer pain in adults. *Cochrane Database Syst Rev.* March 14, 2012;3:CD006276.

65 Carpenter JS, Wells N, Lambert B, Watson P, Slayton T, Chak B, Hepworth JT, Worthington WB. A pilot study of magnetic therapy for hot flashes after breastcancer. *Cancer Nurs.* April 2002;25(2):104–109.

66 Kaluza K, Vile RG. Magnetic cells for cancer therapy: Adopting magnets forcell-based cancer therapies. *Gene Ther.* December 2008;15(23):1511–1512.

67 Devine EC, Westlake SK. The effects of psychoeducational care provided to adults with cancer: Meta-analysis of 116 studies. *Oncol Nurs Forum.* October 1995;22(9):1369–1381.

68 Cassileth BR, Deng GE, Gomez JE, Johnstone PA, Kumar N, Vickers AJ; American College of Chest Physicians. Complementary therapies and integrative oncology in lung cancer: ACCP evidence-based clinical practice guidelines, 2nd edn. *Chest.* September 2007;132(Suppl 3):340S–354S.

69 Rajasekaran M, Edmonds PM, Higginson IL. Systematic review of hypnotherapy for treating symptoms in terminally ill adult cancer patients. *Palliat Med.* July 2005;19(5):418–426.

70 Speed-Andrews AE, Courneya KS. Effects of exercise on quality of life and prognosis in cancer survivors. *Curr Sports Med Rep.* July–August 2009;8(4):176–181.

71 Andersen RE et al. Encouraging patients to become more physically active: The physician's role. *Ann Int Med.* 1997;127:395–400.

72 Iversen MD et al. How rheumatologists and patients with rheumatoid arthritis discuss exercise and the influence of discussions on exercise prescriptions. *Arthistis Rhem* February 15, 2004;51(1): 63–72.

73 Kongsgaard UE, Werner MU. Evidence-based medicine works best when there is evidence: Challenges in palliative medicine when randomized controlled trials are not possible. *J Pain Palliat Care Pharmacother.* 2009;23(1):48–50.

74 Cronfalk BS, Ternestedt BM, Strang P. Soft tissue massage: Early intervention for relatives whose family members died in palliative cancer care. *J Clin Nurs.* April 2010;19(7–8):1040–1048.

114

Alternative medicine: The approach to the patient wanting to go to Tijuana

RICHARD LEE, GABRIEL LOPEZ, DANIEL EPNER, MICHAEL FISCH

INTRODUCTION

Practicing clinicians are commonly asked about the use of complementary and alternative medicine (CAM) for a wide range of ailments. Among patients with life-threatening diseases with limited treatments or chronic conditions with refractory symptoms despite conventional medicines, CAM approaches seem very appealing. Patients near the end of life are especially attracted to unconventional therapies that claim dramatic result with no side effects. The allure of these treatments is too strong for patients to ignore despite the potentially high costs including financial, emotional, time, and energy. Thus, the physician is often involved in discussions about alternative therapies and may even be asked to assist with their implementation. Although physicians may consider such discussions a waste of time, patients are interested in their physicians' opinion about the topic as a trusted source. When patients are told new information about the potential harms of herbs, the majority would either stop the herb or talk with their physician about it.[1] Because patients seek information from their physicians and value this discussion, this chapter focuses on providing the practicing physician a framework in which to have discussions with patients wanting to pursue unproven complementary or alternative therapies. Please refer to the previous chapter on integrative medicine for background information about this topic.

IMPORTANCE OF THE DOCTOR–PATIENT RELATIONSHIP IN DISCUSSING CAM

When beginning a discussion with a patient interested in alternative therapies, an evaluation of the doctor–patient relationship (DPR) is absolutely necessary. The strength of this relationship will assist the healthcare professional and help inform the discussion. Sir William Osler, a Canadian physician often described as "The Father of Modern Medicine,"

remarked, "Care more for the individual patient than for the special features of the disease… Put yourself in his place… The kindly word, the cheerful greeting, the sympathetic look—these the patient understands."[2] Because CAM therapies are inherently controversial and discussing them may strain the DPR, strengthening and maintaining this relationship is important.

Communication, trust, decision making, and the establishment of care goals are critical components contributing to a successful interaction. We propose the doctor-patient-health model (Figure 114.1) as a framework for interacting with patients. It creates a common point from which to think about the DPR and can be modified as each clinician considers appropriate. This model provides key checkpoints for any potential discussion with patients in which different opinions may exist.

When the topic arises about alternative therapies, physicians may unintentionally express an immediate strong negative response or show apprehension about a topic they have limited knowledge. The following responses to a patient may seem harmless:

"Oh that nonsense"
"You're not really thinking about taking that are you?"

These types of responses have the potential for weakening the DPR. Instead, one practical approach when the topic arises is to re-assure the patient that you are:

1. Interested in discussing the topic—"Sounds interesting, let's talk about this."
2. Invested in the best outcome possible for the patient—"I want to help you feel better."
3. Willing to provide appropriate support no matter what the patients decides, even if it is in opposition to the medical advice you provide. In many instances, this involves emotional support.—"No matter what you decide, I'm here to help you in the best way possible as your physician."
"I can see you are scared and anxious about this diagnosis; please tell me more about how you are feeling."

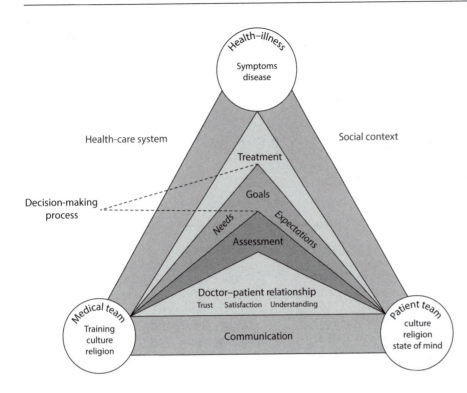

Figure 114.1 *Doctor-patient-health model.*

This sends a clear message to the patient that you, as the physician, are committed to their health and well-being and will not abandon them even if there is a difference of opinion. Additionally, by providing these statements at the beginning of the conversation about alternative therapies, the patient understands that a disagreement about the benefits of an alternative therapy does not equate to abandonment. The idea of abandonment is poisonous to the DPR. Showing commitment in your role as a physician to help the patient will strengthen the bond between clinician and patient.[3]

PATIENT–CLINICIAN COMMUNICATION REGARDING COMPLEMENTARY AND ALTERNATIVE THERAPIES

Clinicians must understand their patients' health concerns or their "state of illness," as described by Cassell.[4] To understand their patients' health concerns, clinicians must be able to communicate effectively. The clinician, patient, and health-illness anchor the DPR, and through this relationship, the healing process begins. Clinicians, through their words and nonverbal actions, can alleviate their patients' anxieties and fears, providing the hope of help.

A discussion about CAM therapies can be a challenge for health care professionals who typically have limited knowledge of this area. When physicians are faced with unfamiliar information about CAM therapies, they may feel "de-skilled" by being forced outside their medical specialty, and this discomfort can lead to defensiveness and a breakdown in communication with the patient. At the same time,

patients can become frustrated if they cannot discuss CAM with their physician. This bilateral frustration can result in a communication gap, which damages the DPR. Physicians should be receptive to patient inquiries and aware of subtle, nonverbal messages to create an environment in which patients can openly discuss potential CAM choices.[5,6] Research indicates that neither adult nor pediatric patients receive sufficient information or discuss CAM therapies with physicians, pharmacists, nurses, or CAM practitioners.[7,8] The most common reason patients state for not bringing up the topic of CAM (even if they have questions or are taking CAM) is that it never came up in the discussion or no one asked them. Thus, patients believe it is unimportant. Patients may also fear that the topic will be received with indifference or dismissed without discussion,[6,9] and health care professionals may fear being unable to respond to questions or may shy away from initiating a time-consuming discussion. As a result, it is estimated that upwards of 70% of patients are taking complementary medicines without informing any member of their health care team.[10,11] This lack of discussion is of concern, because biologically based therapies such as herbs may interact with medical treatments.

It is the health care professional's responsibility to ask patients about their use of complementary medicines.[12] Communication is crucial to gathering information, addressing patient emotions, and assisting patients in decisions about medical care. Optimally, the discussion should take place before the patient starts using a CAM treatment whether it is a nutritional supplement, mind-body therapy, or other CAM approach. A number of strategies can be used to increase the chance of a worthwhile dialogue. One approach is to include the topic of CAM as part of a new patient assessment. For example, when asking about medications, physicians should inquire about everything the patient ingests—including over-the-counter products, vitamins, minerals, herbs, and diet. Physicians may consider having the patients bring in the actual bottles of herbs and supplements for evaluation. When asking about a patient's past medical history, a question about other healthcare professionals involved in their care is a natural transition to learn if they have visited with naturopathic or chiropractic practitioners. These inquiries send a message to your patient that you are interested and open to discussing the topic of CAM therapies.

If the topic of CAM arises, clinicians need to develop an empathic communication strategy that addresses patients' needs while maintaining the health care professional's understanding of the current state of the science. The strategy needs to balance clinical objectivity and bonding with the patient so that it can benefit both parties. One important strategy is an exploratory approach—to ask why they are interested in CAM therapies. Fear and anxiety are commonly involved in a patient's decision to pursue CAM therapies. Acknowledging these fears is an important aspect of empathic responses. If a patients states, "I'm really scared about my diagnosis and what is going to happen." Instead of immediately replying with a way to fix the situation with a treatment, first consider an empathic response.

This situation must be very scary (or frustrating) for you.

By addressing patients emotional states, they often become much more open to hearing what you have to say about the topics of CAM and thus an important first step to consider.

Research indicates many fixed factors are related to CAM use (those unable to change easily) such as age, gender, socioeconomic status, stage of disease, prior treatments, accessibility of CAM therapies, and inability to access health care.[13] Flexible factors include opinions about conventional treatments and CAM therapies including efficacy and side effects, loss of control, and unmet needs such as untreated symptoms. Often times when asked why, the patient will indicate that a family member or friend is driving this process. An exploratory approach will help direct the discussion to the most important topics.

Because of the threat posed by a serious illness and the uncertain outcome of treatment, most patients seek information about their disease and its treatment to make an informed decision.[14] Patients need reliable information and an opportunity to openly discuss CAM therapies. However, the complexity of commercial CAM products and the science, if it exists, behind their use commonly leads to confusion among patients. Patient–physician communication should not be unilateral, but rather an interactive process in which both parties create an environment of understanding.[15] This open dialogue may require your willingness to consult with other health care professionals.[16] Involvement of a CAM practitioner can complicate communication because of a triangular relationship: patient–physician, patient–CAM practitioner, and the physician–CAM practitioner. A productive and fruitful communication process requires all three relationships to be in contact.[17] A willingness to talk

with involved CAM practitioners shows your commitment to work collaboratively and provide the best care.

Another key issue to consider is the patient's expectations from the DPR especially if they come from a different cultural background. Western physicians often diagnose "disease" as a biological process, while patients experience an "illness" a culturally based and personal interpretation of symptoms resulting from the disease process. CAM therapies may actually be more effective at addressing patient's needs and improving their experience by decreasing their symptom burden. The danger lies in the realm where "feeling better" subjectively does not necessarily correlate with "getting better" objectively. Openly expressing a desire to learn about a patient's religious and cultural beliefs will acknowledge your knowledge gap and willingness to include these important issues into the decision-making process.[18] When clinicians communicate empathetically and effectively, patients will often leave the encounter feeling better, regardless of the medical decisions made.

DECISION MAKING AND GOALS OF CARE

Today, most patients expect to be part of the decision-making process. Shared decision making between the clinician and patient helps create a sense of control for patients, which has been cited as a reason for pursuing CAM.[19] Whereas some patients may demand to be the final decision maker in their care, other patients may prefer a more passive role, allowing the physician to direct therapy. In either case, the personalized approach provides patients with a sense of ease about their goals of care and medical decisions. By utilizing a shared decision-making process and assessing goals of care, physicians have an opportunity to address common reasons why patients seek CAM therapies: sense of control and unmet needs. Having patients and family play an active role in decision making and treatment planning can provide patients with a sense of empowerment and responsibility, leading to a more powerful therapeutic relationship. Although the clinical endpoint may remain the same, all parties experience an enhanced sense of success and satisfaction.

Creating and agreeing upon goals of care is crucial when evaluating CAM therapies. Many physicians have increasingly demanding schedules in which clinical visits are restricted to discussing treatment decisions. However, by avoiding the process of creating common goals of care, the discussion regarding the most appropriate treatments is limited as it will be difficult to evaluate which therapies provide the highest chance of achieving the goals. Conversations focused only on treatment often fail to address the unspoken needs of patients in the realm of psychological, social, and spiritual dimensions of care. For some patients, the unmet needs may be more of a priority than the treatment of the disease.

For instance, if a patient with cancer brings up the topic of acupuncture, the natural reaction might be that acupuncture has no role in treating cancer—this would be correct if acupuncture was used to cure the cancer. However, if the patient's goal was to treat pain or nausea, strong evidence exists that acupuncture is a reasonable treatment option. It may be equally important for patients to discuss the treatment of symptoms or other goals for which the patient might be seeking alternative therapies. An open discussion regarding needs and goals of care will help both the physician and patient place treatment options in the appropriate context.

In this example, the discussion of goals highlighted an unmet need and emphasizes the importance of a comprehensive assessment. Engel's biopsychosocial model of healthcare, first published in *Science* more than 30 years ago, describes the domains of patient care and their importance in the treatment of all patients.[9] If clinicians do not address these needs, their patients may seek out other treatments for these symptoms, including complementary or alternative medicine. Although some of these therapies, such as massage, are considered harmless, others, such as the use of dietary supplements or herbal remedies, may have significant potential for harm. Without comprehensive assessment and appropriate attention given to all their needs—including the nonbiological ones—patients may perceive gaps in their care. By addressing the topic of goals, the physician may discover additional needs and goals beyond treating the disease.

Creating realistic goals is important as unrealistic expectations will in all likelihood lead to future dissatisfaction. In the preceding example, acupuncture for pain or nausea is likely to help, but rarely is the benefit such that acupuncture can be used alone or resolves the symptoms entirely. Although physicians realize the limitations of modern medical treatment, it is still common for some physicians to be overconfident in their ability to treat a disease. While it is appropriate to commit to striving on the patient's behalf under all circumstances, clinicians must acknowledge that the promise to cure cannot always be guaranteed. The higher the patient's expectations, the higher their degree of disappointment when the course of care does not go as expected. These types of disappointments may drive patients to seek alternative medicines. Clinicians should always be cautious of making promises when setting goals. In some instances, CAM practitioners may contribute to unrealistic expectations by not informing patients about realistic risks and benefits. This situation may benefit from contacting the CAM provider to discuss the patient's case. Creating realistic goals provides patients with an opportunity to plan accordingly for the future. For patients, in whom a prolonged course over several years is likely, a process of assessment, goal setting, and treatment followed by reassessment and modification of goals and treatments is likely the most effective method for attaining optimal clinical outcomes.

TREATMENT PLANNING

Treatment planning, including the evaluation of alternative therapies, is by far the most difficult aspect of any discussion of CAM. As with any treatment discussion, clinicians should consider informed decision making in which patients are educated about the risks and benefits. However, in the discussion of CAM therapies, it is often the physician rather than the CAM practitioner that informs the patient about the risks and benefits of the CAM therapies in question. In addition to the risk and benefits of any therapy, this discussion should also include the current clinical evidence, cost (financial, time, resources, etc.), and feasibility. A helpful place to start the discussion is to set the core principles in evaluating all treatment options. For some patients, it may focus on treatment efficacy, and for others, it may focus on maintaining quality of life. Principles you may want to include are evidence-based medicine, personalized approach, and safety. A discussion of reliable information should also be included. When beginning such a discussion, consider asking the patient what they understand about the CAM therapy in question or how they decided upon which therapies to pursue. You may find the patient may share some common beliefs, and stating you agree with some of their statements is always a positive way to start a conversation.

While evidence-based thinking is fundamental to contemporary medical practice, patients often do not base their decisions in the same scientific processes. Understanding evidence-based medicine can be challenging for patients. A physician's failure to recognize this difference interferes with their ability to discuss CAM in a manner that patients will understand. Whether hearing a second hand story from a friend, watching story on the evening news, or reading about a phase III clinical trial—these sources of information often have the same influence on patients. The physician can help create a common understanding of reliable information by taking time to explain the different levels of evidence. For example, emphasizing that research conducted in human patients is the gold standard because it provides the most reliable information about the risks and benefits for patients. This distinction helps provide patients with a framework in which to interpret different types of information.

Reviewing the risks and benefits

The common belief by patients that "natural" means a product or therapy is safe needs to be addressed with education. Some herbs and supplements have been associated with multiple drug interactions,[20] as well as increased health risks such as organ toxicity. Many CAM therapies can potentially cause adverse outcomes, and are thus a major concern among health care professionals. Nonbiologically based CAM therapies, such as massage or acupuncture, often have minimal risks when performed by trained health professionals. In contrast, herbs and supplements should be considered more similar to prescription medications in that they have the potential to have powerful effects on the natural biological processes of the body. This is especially true when natural plants are processed into concentrated powders, liquids, or pills. The pathways by which CAM therapies may lead to negative clinical outcomes include metabolic interactions, treatment interactions, direct organ toxicity, direct biological effects on the disease process, and unregulated manufacturing of biologically based CAM. Even the quality of herbs and supplements can be variable. Studies show as much as 50% of products do not contain the amount indicated on the product label.

Patients are commonly unaware of the differences between United States Food and Drug Administration (FDA)–approved medications (which require evidence of efficacy, safety, and quality control manufacturing) and supplements, which are governed not by the FDA but by the Dietary Supplement Health and Education Act (DSHEA) of 1994. Supplements under this legislation are exempt from the same scrutiny the FDA imposes on medications; furthermore, these supplements are not intended to treat, prevent, or cure diseases.

While most CAM therapies may become a financial burden, as most are not covered by insurance, there are other hidden costs. Others include the delay of potentially curative treatments, which, if used too late, will have diminished benefit. Perhaps the most important for those patients with limited prognosis is time and energy. Imagine a terminally ill patient desires to go to another country to pursue an untested CAM therapy for 2 months. In addition to the cost of the actual therapy, the patient will need to spend time, energy, and money to travel and spend time in a foreign country. Would these 2 months be best spent with family and friends or in a hospital setting away from the patient's strongest psychosocial support? Would the patient feel comfortable dying in a foreign hospital away from family and friends if an unexpected medical emergency occurred? These types of questions must be asked in order to have a full discussion about the potential outcomes of pursuing CAM therapies.

Unfortunately, for many CAM therapies, no reliable clinical data exist to inform the discussion about risks and benefits. With this in mind, it is important to acknowledge that three potential outcomes are possible: beneficial, harmful, or no effect on the goals of care. The estimate of promising treatments that look helpful in preclinical studies that actually are found to be clinically helpful is in the range of 10% or less. Patients will often argue that because these therapies are nonpatentable or have no profit-driven company to fund the research, none of the CAM therapies will have good clinical research. Reminding patients that many of our commonly used medications are derived from plants including aspirin, morphine, antibiotics, and even chemotherapies can help counter these false claims perpetuated by the CAM industry. With regard to research, dozens of clinical trials have been funded by the government to research areas such as fish oil, acupuncture, and vitamins, with some results being positive and others negative. This type of myth needs to be addressed by facts. For instance, the supplement industry is estimated to be a 30 billion dollar industry. Most of these same companies are almost all entirely profit driven and do not support clinical research of their own products. These facts may help patients view their beliefs in a different light.

Discussions about the use of CAM therapies can be time consuming and draining for the physician. Unless an urgent deadline exists, providing patients enough time to process the information is always helpful and plan for follow-up in 1–2 weeks. Another important strategy is to offer other options that help them achieve their goals. Patients commonly ignore the most natural approaches to their needs such as fatigue or insomnia. Good evidence exists that physical activity can improve fatigue levels, and growing research shows that sleep hygiene and yoga meditation can improve sleep quality. Many would consider these approaches more natural than taking a processed pill. If questions still exist, offer to investigate the topic or refer them to a specialist.

Accepting patient choices: Respecting autonomy

Despite your efforts to inform patients about the risks of CAM therapies and encouragement to pursue the safe evidence-based options, some patients will still wish to pursue CAM therapies. One should not feel any sense of failure or shame. Often time patients may have strongly held emotions or beliefs about certain therapies. Just as Jehovah's witnesses generally refuse blood transfusions, we should not feel our job is to change their beliefs. Instead, we should still aim to provide them with the best care possible within the limits provided by the patient. The next decision will be what type of follow-up plan is needed to evaluate for safety and efficacy. Unlike Western trained physicians, CAM practitioners may not incorporate appropriate follow-up assessments for safety and efficacy. Discuss with the patient what potential risks exist and how it would be best to monitor for these. In addition, it is useful to decide prior to the treatment the goals and criteria for success or failure of the CAM therapy within a certain time frame. Without well-defined criteria for success, these types of CAM therapies could be continued indefinitely without any clear benefit. For instance, if a young, paraplegic man decides to pursue an alternative therapy to improve his paralysis, consider simple tests for improvement such as his ability to move his feet within 3 months. Creating a follow-up plan serves to help keep the patient safe and minimizes the duration of ineffective treatment. This strategy provides an avenue for the patient to return to the physician to seek further help if ultimately these CAM treatments prove to be ineffective. Otherwise, patients without a follow-up plan may feel abandoned and, when these CAM treatments fail, are too embarrassed to return to see the physician for further medical care.

Lastly consider other reliable resources for guidance such as the National Center for Complementary and Alternative Medicine website (http://nccam.nih.gov). This site has a library of information for physicians and patients. As the field of integrative medicine develops, a growing number of physicians have training in an evidence-based approach to CAM and consultation with appropriately trained clinicians at an academic center could prove interesting to a patient.

SUMMARY

Discussing with patients the use of unproven CAM therapies can be a daunting task, especially for physicians with limited knowledge about the field. Begin with creating a strong DPR built upon excellent communication. At the onset, clearly state your interest in discussing the topic of CAM therapies, interest in treating their medical condition in the best way possible, and commitment to helping them even if they choose different options from what is recommended. From this foundation, clinicians should proceed with an open-minded, empathetic, comprehensive assessment of the patient as a person. Inquiring why patients are seeking these therapies may uncover unmet needs of the patient including emotional support. Establish realistic goals of care through a shared decision-making process. As the discussion proceeds to evaluating different CAM treatments, be sure patients understand what is meant by reliable information. Review the topics of risks, benefits, and costs—especially time and energy to the patient. Ultimately if the patient chooses to pursue unproven CAM therapies despite your best advice, protect the patient from further harm by formulating a follow-up plan that will assess safety and efficacy in the context of the goals established. Because many of the unproven CAM therapies will eventually fail, the time and energy spent constructing a strong DPR will foster a clear path for the patient to return to receive further medical care from a trusted and reliable health professional.

REFERENCES

1 McCune JS, Hatfield AJ, Blackburn AA et al.: Potential of chemotherapy-herb interactions in adult cancer patients. *Support Care Cancer* 12:454–462, 2004.

2 Cushing H: *The Life of Sir William Osler.* Oxford, U.K., The Clarendon Press, 1925.

3 Epner DE, Ravi V, Baile WF: When patients and families feel abandoned. *Support Care Cancer* 19:1713–1717, 2011.

4 Eric J Cassell. Making the patient better—Whatever the outcome. *J Support Oncol* 5(2):58, 2007.

5 Kao GD, Devine P: Use of complementary health practices by prostate carcinoma patients undergoing radiation therapy. *Cancer* 88:615–619, 2000.

6 Tasaki K, Maskarinec G, Shumay DM et al.: Communication between physicians and cancer patients about complementary and alternative medicine: Exploring patients' perspectives.[see comment]. *Psycho-Oncology* 11:212–220, 2002.

7 Friedman T, Slayton WB, Allen LS et al.: Use of alternative therapies for children with cancer. *Pediatrics* 100:E1, 1997.

8 Swisher EM, Cohn DE, Goff BA et al.: Use of complementary and alternative medicine among women with gynecologic cancers. *Gynecol Oncol* 84:363–367, 2002.

9 Wyatt GK, Friedman LL, Given CW et al.: Complementary therapy use among older cancer patients. *Cancer Pract* 7:136–144, 1999.

10 Richardson MA, Sanders T, Palmer JL et al.: Complementary/alternative medicine use in a comprehensive cancer center and the implications for oncology. *J Clin Oncol* 18:2505–2514, 2000.

11 Robinson A, McGrail MR: Disclosure of CAM use to medical practitioners: A review of qualitative and quantitative studies. *Complement Ther Med* 12:90–98, 2004.

12 Sugarman J, Burk L: Physicians' ethical obligations regarding alternative medicine. *JAMA* 280:1623–1625, 1998.

13 Boon H, Brown JB, Gavin A et al.: Men with prostate cancer: Making decisions about complementary/alternative medicine. *Med Decis Making* 23:471–479, 2003.

14 Jenkins V, Fallowfield L, Saul J: Information needs of patients with cancer: Results from a large study in UK cancer centres. *Br J Cancer* 84:48–51, 2001.

15 Epner DE, Baile WF: Wooden's pyramid: Building a hierarchy of skills for successful communication. *Med Teach* 33:39–43, 2011.

16 Cohen L, Cohen MH, Kirkwood C et al.: Discussing complementary therapies in an oncology setting. *J Soc Integr Oncol* 5:18–24, 2007.

17 Frenkel M, Ben-Arye E: Communicating with patients about the use of complementary and integrative medicine in cancer care, in Cohen L, Markman M (eds): *Incorporating Complementary Medicine into Conventional Cancer Care.* Totowa, NJ, Humana Press, 2008, pp. 33–46.

18 Epner DE, Baile WF: Patient-centered care: The key to cultural competence. *Ann Oncol* 23 Suppl 3:33–42, 2012.

19 Richardson MA, Masse LC, Nanny K et al.: Discrepant views of oncologists and cancer patients on complementary/alternative medicine. *Supportive Care Cancer* 12:797–804, 2004.

20 Ulbricht C, Chao W, Costa D et al.: Clinical evidence of herb-drug interactions: A systematic review by the natural standard research collaboration. *Curr Drug Metab* 9:1063–1120, 2008.

115

Side effects of radiation therapy

ALYSA FAIRCHILD, ELIZABETH A. BARNES

RADIOTHERAPY AND RADIOBIOLOGY BASICS

Radiation therapy (RT) is a cornerstone of cancer treatment. Approximately half of all patients will receive RT, delivered with either radical or palliative intent, at some point during the course of their disease [1]. The goals of palliative RT are to provide durable and timely symptom relief while minimizing toxicity, resource utilization, and the number of visits to the cancer centre [2]. Secondary aims include tumor regression and short recovery time [3]. Palliative RT may also prophylactically address an area with a high likelihood of becoming symptomatic in future.

Patients who are not likely to benefit from palliative RT, especially those who are not likely to complete the prescribed course, should not be offered treatment [4]. In one retrospective series of 153 patients receiving palliative-intent RT to various sites, treatment was terminated prematurely in 12% due to clinical deterioration, lack of efficacy, or death [5]. It can take 3–6 weeks to see maximal benefit in many circumstances [6]. However, two recent studies described patient cohorts who survived <12 weeks after receiving single-fraction (SF) palliative RT, with response rates of 45% at a median of 2 weeks [7] and 70% at 1 month [8]. Additionally, hemibody RT relieves bony pain within 24–28 hours [9]. However, there are clinical settings in which RT should be omitted entirely in favor of supportive care, described in the excellent review by Lutz et al. [4].

The etiology of a symptom should be clearly understood before radiation treatment is undertaken. Otherwise, palliative RT might be ineffective or actually worsen quality of life (QoL). For example, breathing might actually deteriorate after RT if dyspnea is not due to lung cancer but primarily to underlying COPD [10]. Moreover, RT is not expected to reverse obstruction of a tubular organ caused by postoperative stricture or significantly improve systemic symptoms such as fatigue or anorexia [4].

Tumors do not have to be completely eradicated in order to improve symptoms, and therefore, doses lower than that required for total lesion ablation are used in palliative situations [11]. The optimal RT schedule balances administering a high enough dose to achieve the desired treatment goal, while not delivering so much as to result in significant side effects [12]. There are many circumstances where SFs have been proven efficacious; without assurances of improved outcomes, multifraction (MF) RT increases the burden of both overall treatment time and transportation on patients and their caregivers [6]. If insufficient dose is delivered, however, disease progression (and its attendant symptoms) may occur, and this risk usually outweighs the potential increased side effect profile of higher dose palliative RT.

Factors that contribute to RT toxicity include volume irradiated, total dose (TD), dose per day (fraction size), concurrent systemic therapy, and radiosensitivity of neighboring normal tissues [13]. Patient factors may also affect the likelihood of toxicity (e.g., aging-associated decreases in bone marrow reserve). The predictable side effects of RT, similar to those of chemotherapy, should probably not be described as "complications." This term does apply, however, if side effects are significant enough to interfere with planned treatment, or are unexpected [13].

Acute RT side effects, generally self-limited, are mainly influenced by TD and overall treatment time [6]. They tend to be cumulative, may peak after the RT is finished, and are usually controllable with conservative measures [4]. They are most prominent in tissues with rapid cell turnover such as skin and GI tract. Functional cells are lost as part of normal tissue turnover, and compensatory stem cell proliferation leads to resolution of symptoms. "Acute" is generally 3 months or less after completion of treatment, although they most commonly occur hours, days, or weeks following RT. As RT is a localized treatment modality, potential side effects are site specific, the only exception being fatigue [10].

Generally, palliative RT is delivered using a higher dose per fraction than would be used in a curative-intent course, which correlates with a risk of late, rather than acute, damage to normal tissues [6]. Large fraction sizes may provide faster onset of relief in some situations, such as tumor-related bleeding [14]. Although the possibility of late toxicity must be considered, many patients will not live long enough to be at risk [10]. However, care needs to be taken especially when considering re-treating the same site as physicians are generally poor at survival estimation [2]. Late side effects are less common and almost always permanent, in comparison to acute side effects that occur more often and are usually reversible. Fibrosis, atrophy, and neural and vascular damage are examples of late RT effects. Evaluation and reporting of long-term toxicity after palliative RT is limited by the short median survival of patients with incurable malignancy [12,15].

While side effects are divided along timelines for clinical reporting, they share a common ongoing molecular process [16]. Irradiation causes ionization events and free radical production, resulting in DNA damage during mitosis, and cell death occurs by apoptosis. The pathogenesis of late radiation injury begins immediately after radiation exposure with activation of a cytokine cascade [17]. Fibrinogenesis, the most extensively studied etiology, can be considered as a dysfunctional wound healing response with the upregulation of pro-inflammatory cytokines and growth factors [18].

SIDE EFFECTS OF PALLIATIVE RADIOTHERAPY

General

There is no evidence that incidence or severity of side effects correlates with eventual response to treatment. Degree of toxicity does not usually correlate with pre-RT symptom

burden. For selected acute side effects and their incidence, see Table 115.1. Management suggestions are found in Table 115.2, and late side effect information is given in Table 115.3.

Fatigue

Up to 80% of patients undergoing RT complain of fatigue, the causes of which are poorly understood [19,20]. RT-related fatigue may be exacerbated by anemia, sleep disorders, psychological issues, chemotherapy, or hormonal disturbances [19]. Fatigue may occur with RT treatment of any site [21] and generally improves on its own after a variable time interval. No agent has been yet validated against fatigue related to cancer or cancer treatment, although many have been tried (methylphenidate, modafinil, and guarana) [19,22–24].

Hematologic

Hematologic side effects are usually mild and transient, but myelosuppression may occur if the treatment portals are large, TD is moderate to high, and a significant proportion of marrow is included, especially in heavily pretreated patients [25]. After hemi-body irradiation (HBI), for example, pancytopenia is transient and reaches a nadir at day 10, but counts can remain low for weeks. Counts should be monitored until recovery, however, as patients may be at risk for neutropenic sepsis [20].

Table 115.1   *Acute and subacute side effects*

Acute

Irradiated site	Toxicity	Incidence	Selected references
Bone	Pain flare	SF—7%–39%; MF—3%–41%	[26,53]
Bone	Emesis	30%–32%	[54]
Head and neck	Skin erythema	Mild—37%[b]–52%[a]	[3,55]
Head and neck	Mucositis	Mild or moderate—44%[a]–63%[b]	[3,55]
Head and neck	Xerostomia	Mild or moderate—74%[a]–88%[b]	[3,55]
Head and neck[b]	Dysphagia	Mild or moderate—75%	[55]
Breast	Moist desquamation	14%	[56]
Gastric	Nausea/emesis	Mild or moderate—12%–28%	[15]
Gastric	Hepatic enzyme abnormalities	Mild—3%	[12]
Gastric	Anemia	Mild—73%, Moderate—14%,	[12,15]
Gastric	Anorexia	Mild or moderate—12%–57%	[12,15]
Lung[c]	Esophagitis	Mild—34% Moderate or severe—10%	[57]

Subacute

Irradiated site	Toxicity	Incidence	Selected references
Whole brain	Somnolence syndrome	Not specified	[24]
Lung	Pneumonitis	2%–4%	[32]

MF, multifraction; SF, single fraction.
[a]Quad shot = 14 Gy/4 fractions BID for 2 days repeated at 4 weekly intervals a maximum of 3 times.
[b]Hypo trial = 30 Gy/5 twice per week, ≥ 3 day apart with an optional further 6 Gy boost.
[c]High-dose palliation delivered via split course. Sites irradiated with multifraction courses unless indicated.

Table 115.2 *Management of acute side effects*

Symptom/Sign	Management suggestions	Reference
Fatigue	• Supervised exercise program	[58]
Desquamation	• Good hygiene Dressings Topical steroids Silver sulfadiazine	[10]
Mucositis	• Dietary modifications Oral rinses—sodium bicarbonate Antifungals—mycostatin Analgesics in elixir form, viscous xylocaine, "Pink Lady." benzydamine mouthwash Sucralfate suspension Fluid supplementation and electrolyte correction	[10,25]
Esophagitis	• Similar to mucositis Analgesics in elixir form Treatment of associated acid reflux Fluid supplementation and electrolyte correction	[13,34]
Pneumonitis	• Prednisone 60–100 mg/day in divided doses	[13]
Nausea/Emesis	• Antiemetics H_2 blockers Fluid supplementation and electrolyte correction	[34]
Gastritis	• Antacids H_2 blockers Antiemetics Fluid supplementation and electrolyte correction Analgesics	[34]
Enteritis	• Fluid supplementation and electrolyte correction Antidiarrheals once *C. difficle* ruled out Antiemetics Dietary modifications (low residue, low fat, lactose-free) Octreotide Steroids	[34]
Proctitis	• Sitz baths Local measures—hydrocortisone acetate/zinc sulfate, phenylephrine hydrochloride	[10]
Increased intracranial pressure	• Dexamethasone 4–16 mg/day in divided doses	[24]

Skin and bone

Skin toxicity may also occur with treatment of any site, but is limited to the RT fields, and usually consists of mild erythema, pruritis, or dryness [10,21]. Higher dose to skin may result in desquamation that should be treated similar to sunburns [10]. Alopecia will occur in the irradiated region after 1–2 weeks, and regrowth may take up to 3 months although may not occur at all depending on TD. Increased or decreased skin pigmentation may be seen within the RT fields. Late fibrosis or dermal atrophy can lead to scarring and telangiectasia [13].

Pain flare is a self-limited worsening of pain in the treated bone metastasis occurring within a week of commencing RT. Its incidence varies from 3% to 44%, and it lasts for a median of 3 days [6]. The proportion of patients experiencing pain flare may be higher after large, SF versus multiple, smaller fractions [26]. Pain flare is usually managed by adjusting pain medications. Corticosteroids have shown promise in early phase trials at decreasing pain flare incidence. A large phase III trial investigating dexamethasone in preventing pain flare is underway. Otherwise acute toxicity is mild. There is conflicting evidence as to whether nausea, emesis, or diarrhea is worse after higher dose treatment [6].

Although reossification does occur, bone weakened by disease will not be strengthened immediately by RT and may in fact be weakened temporarily [27]. Post-RT fractures within the treatment field have been reported in up to 18% of patients [25]. In the three bone metastases meta-analyses,

Table 115.3 *Late side effects*

Irradiated site	Symptom	Incidence	Timeline	Selected references
Bone	Fracture	SF—2%–5% MF—0.5%–18%	Median time to fracture: SF—7 weeks; MF—20 weeks	[31,54]
Breast	Skin (cosmetic effects)	11%	—	[56]
Esophagus[c]	Dysphagia[a]	5%	—	[33]
Thorax	Pneumonitis	2%	—	[59]
Thorax	Osteoradionecrosis	2%	—	[59]
Thorax	Myelopathy	0.7%–3%	—	[59,60]
Whole brain	RT necrosis	Not specified	6–24 months	[24]
Whole brain	Dementia[b]	0%–11%[a]	At 12 months	[61]

MF, multifraction; SF, single fraction.

[a] Not related to tumor progression/recurrence.

[b] All patients with dementia received nonstandard RT due to either fraction size or concurrent radiosensitizer.

[c] 40 Gy/20 fractions BID, ≥6 hours apart, 5 day/week. Sites irradiated with multifraction courses unless indicated.

there were no significant differences found in pathologic fracture rates after SF versus MF regimens (2%–3%) [28–30]. Late toxicity was rare (4%) in both arms of the RTOG 9714 trial [31].

Head and neck

RT to the mucosa of the head and neck may induce mucositis causing odynophagia, dysphagia, dry mouth, taste changes, and pain [21]. Secondary infections should be treated.

Thorax

A meta-analysis of 13 randomized controlled trials each evaluating dose-fractionation schedules for palliation of thoracic symptoms from incurable lung cancer included 3473 patients [32]. Dysphagia secondary to esophagitis was the most common acute side effect described. Physician-assessed dysphagia was more common after higher versus lower RT dose (20.5% vs 14.9%; p = 0.01); pooling of patient self-report data could not be performed [32]. In one of the reviewed trials, for example, the incidence of severe dysphagia rose from 5% at baseline to 40% during treatment and then back to 5% approximately 1 month after RT completion. Dysphagia can lead to complications such as malnutrition, dehydration, and aspiration [33].

Other acute toxicities of thoracic RT include anorexia, nausea, and lethargy, which tend to resolve by 8 weeks [33]. Pericarditis or pericardial effusion may occur but is often asymptomatic [13]. Palliative thoracic RT may also cause sub-acute pneumonitis, a pneumonia-like illness typically occurring 4–12 weeks after treatment completion [13]. Pneumonitis affected 3.6% of patients after higher dose RT compared with 1.8% of patients who received lower dose in the meta-analysis (p = 0.68) [32]. Symptoms include acute worsening of dyspnea, cough, and low-grade fever, with signs of wheeze, rub, or consolidation. Imaging may lag symptoms. Chest x-ray typically reveals diffuse haziness, loss of the vascular pattern, confluent consolidation, or pleural effusion in the RT field. CT demonstrates patchy or generalized consolidation [13].

RT delivered to any tubular structure, such as the esophagus, can result in late effects of stricture, perforation, submucosal fibrosis, mucosal atrophy, stenosis, ulceration, or fistula [13,34]. Pulmonary fibrosis evolves over 6–24 months after treatment, causing worsening dyspnea and cough. Chest x-rays show streaky opacification, volume loss, and pleural thickening; historically, demarcation of RT field borders was seen. Treatment is supportive with no intervention of proven benefit [13].

Abdomen and pelvis

Irradiation of the liver, stomach, intestine, or pancreas may induce nausea and emesis within hours of the first RT fraction [34]. Malaise and anorexia are very common, affecting up to ¾ of patients receiving gastric RT [12]. Approximately 1/3 of patients experience some degree of nausea, especially with large RT volumes [20]. Prophylactic oral antiemetic (e.g., ondansetron) should be offered 45–60 min prior to each fraction and continued on an as-needed basis between fractions. RT to the stomach can also result in abdominal pain from gastritis, and less commonly reduced acid secretion resulting in dyspepsia and ulcers [34].

Diarrhea related to enteritis can occur when the small or large intestine or rectum is in the radiation path [21]. This is manifested by abdominal cramping, pain, frequent loose stools, and occasionally bleeding [25]. For patients already taking laxatives, these should be temporarily held.

Along with diarrhea, RT to the prostate or rectum may induce hematuria, hematochezia, tenesmus, or urgency [34,35]. RT cystitis often responds to increased fluid intake and analgesics, but coexistent infection should be ruled out [10].

Similar to intrathoracic structures, late effects of RT to abdominal or pelvic viscera may include bleeding, obstruction, ulcers, strictures, fibrosis, ischemia, or fistula [34]. For rectal side effects, as an example, analgesics, suppositories, steroid enemas, locally applied formulations, and surgical and endoscopic procedures can be considered [34].

CNS

Partial or whole brain RT-induced edema often exacerbates preexisting neurologic symptoms and increases intracranial pressure [24]. Patients with symptomatic brain metastases routinely receive steroids prior to initiation of whole brain RT (WBRT), which is tapered after RT completion. Acute side effects of WBRT include fatigue, alopecia, and scalp erythema in the majority of patients. Less common effects are otitis externa, nausea, and headache. Late effects for longer-term survivors include neurocognitive changes, somnolence syndrome, and RT necrosis.

The degree of impact of WBRT on neurocognitive decline is debatable, as prospective studies have shown that the majority of patients with brain metastases have preexisting neurocognitive deficits at baseline [36,37]. The impact of these neurocognitive changes following RT must be considered in relation to the risk of untreated tumor also causing loss of mental and physical abilities [6,38].The degree of tumor control achieved with WBRT appears to be positively correlated with preservation of cognition [39].

Stereotactic radiosurgery is being more commonly used in the management of brain metastases with the goals of increasing local tumor control, improving survival, and decreasing side effects compared to WBRT. Acute side effects include short-term exacerbation of neurologic symptoms and seizures. Late side effects are uncommon (<5% incidence) and include edema, necrosis, and worsening of preexisting neurologic symptoms or development of new deficits [40].

IMPACT OF TECHNOLOGY ON TOXICITY

RT from different eras is not directly comparable in terms of likelihood of toxicity: older techniques using two-dimensional (2D) planning and lower energy machines such as cobalt-60 are much more likely to cause side effects than modern advanced technologies [15]. For example, the lower energy of cobalt-60 photons delivered a higher proportion of dose to the skin, increasing the incidence of superficial (skin/subcutaneous/ bone) acute and late toxicities. Most hypothetical gains with newer technologies such as intensity-modulated RT (IMRT) and tomotherapy relate to decreased volumes of critical tissue irradiated [34,35]. One series of 57 patients treated with palliative-intent IMRT with a median dose of 20 Gy/5 reported more homogeneous tumor doses and less irradiation of adjacent normal tissues [41]. Whether this translates into definitive clinical benefits such as decreased frequency or severity of side effects remains to be seen. Any potential gains, however, may be outweighed by cost, resource use, need for specialized equipment, and laborious setup and treatment.

SUPPORTIVE CARE DURING AND AFTER PALLIATIVE RADIOTHERAPY

The RT treatment position is, with few exceptions, supine. Supportive care should be provided to maximize comfort with both transportation and RT positioning, such as premedication for breakthrough pain, oxygen for orthopnea, and anxiolytics for anxiety. Reversible issues should be addressed prior to referral; for example, patients with delirium may not be able to lie still for treatment planning and delivery, and those with severe dyspnea or cough may not be able to tolerate being supine. For patients with incident pain, transfer on and off the simulation and treatment couches can be problematic, and short-acting opioids may be required prior to movement [42]. Pretreatment optimization of baseline status and QoL should be considered.

Patients should be warned about the incidence and timeline of predictable RT side effects, and prophylaxis should be instituted when possible. The temporary exacerbation of baseline symptoms due to RT-induced edema may transiently worsen QoL during treatment. For example, up to 40% will experience pain flare subsequent to RT for bone metastasis; in general, patients informed of the possibility are not concerned by this experience [43]. Dexamethasone has been used to prevent RT-induced side effects including nausea, emesis, and worsening of neurologic symptoms. It is routinely given to patients with symptomatic brain metastases and spinal cord compression at presentation. Dexamethasone is presently being investigated for prevention of pain flare after SF RT for bone metastasis. However, it has an extensive side effect profile that must also be addressed. Additionally, 5HT3 antagonists +/– dexamethasone are recommended for prophylaxis of nausea and vomiting when treating the upper abdomen and can be considered when treating the pelvis and lower thorax [44].

Evaluation of RT toxicity, especially when identical to a preexisting tumor-induced symptom, is challenging. Do not assume that symptom worsening after treatment is due to RT toxicity. Tumor progression must always be ruled out before ascribing worsening symptoms to toxicity. Patients should be monitored for evolution of RT response and resolution of side effects so that analgesics and other medications can be appropriately titrated.

TOXICITY MANAGEMENT IN DEVELOPING COUNTRIES

Symptoms from disease and toxicity from treatment may be more difficult to manage in countries where supportive care lags behind. Deandrea et al. reviewed 26 studies investigating adequacy of cancer pain management. After adjusting for potential confounders, year of publication, European or Asian country of study origin, low gross national income per capita, and setting of care were each associated with a higher likelihood of undertreatment [45]. Additionally, health care provider knowledge varies with geographic location, with fears about risk of addiction to opioids, for example, reported most commonly by physicians from Asia [46,47].

Barriers to adequate symptom management include under-reporting, poor compliance, maladaptive beliefs, lack of education, and poor access to specialized care. Poor communication with providers may be due to language barrier [46,47]. Sociocultural factors can influence a patient's illness experience and interpretation of symptom questions [48]. Patients who are illiterate or who cannot tell time cannot be expected to comply with around-the-clock medication dosing or complete pain diaries. Patients may not have the means to travel to regional hospitals. Stigma associated with specific medications influences adherence [46]. Additional challenges for patients in developing countries include cost and availability of medications [46,47], and lack of access to RT facilities and palliative care specialists [47].

An International Atomic Energy Agency publication illustrates differences in management in resource-poor countries [48]. Rosenblatt et al. reported a prospective multicentre randomized clinical trial that accrued 219 patients from Brazil, China, Croatia, India, South Africa, and Sudan investigating palliation of esophageal obstruction. Lack of available imaging infrastructure resulted in patients being understaged at study entry, and toxicity was not radiologically investigated. Discovery of late side effects was incidental at the time of follow-up endoscopy. RT was delivered with cobalt-60 in 85% of patients and 98% of RT was planned 2D. Actuarial dilatation rate was 20% at 400 days, with a 25% rate of fistula, 15% stent, 10% stricture rates, and 3% treatment-related deaths [48].

Choice of a clinically appropriate palliative RT schedule is especially important for patients in rural communities where protracted treatment would remove patients from their support systems for an extended period. Several cancer centers in Canada and other countries have developed a rapid access-type program for palliative RT, where patient consultation, treatment planning, and delivery can be performed on the same day [49–51]. Patients with uncomplicated painful bone metastases, who only require a single treatment, therefore need only one visit to the cancer centre. Other institutions have gone a step further, developing a program where treatment planning and delivery can be done in a single session on the treatment unit, without even moving patients between machines [52].

CONCLUSIONS

Palliative RT can relieve symptoms from locally advanced or metastatic disease. Acute side effects of treatment are typically mild and of limited duration, and long-term side effects are usually not a significant consideration given a population with limited life expectancy. Symptom relief, toxicity, and patient-rated QoL are important components in the equation evaluating whether RT provides good palliation [3]. Concerns regarding treatment-related morbidity must be weighed against baseline symptoms and likelihood of benefit from palliative RT [38].

Key learning points

- Acute side effects are generally mild, well-tolerated, self-limited, and occur within 3 months of radiation.

- Patients with incurable malignancy do not usually live long enough to be at risk for late side effects.

- The predictable side effects of palliative radiotherapy should be prevented when possible to avoid deterioration in QoL.

- Do not assume that symptom worsening after radiotherapy is due to treatment-related toxicity; other etiologies, such as tumor progression, must be ruled out.

REFERENCES

1 Ringborg U, Bergqvist D, Brorsson B et al. The Swedish Council on Technology Assessment in Health Care systematic overview of radiotherapy for cancer including a prospective survey of radiotherapy practice in Sweden 2001—Summary and conclusions. *Acta Oncol* 2003;42:357–365.

2 Chow E, Wong R, Hruby G et al. Prospective patient-based assessment of effectiveness of palliative radiotherapy for bone metastases in an outpatient radiotherapy clinic. *Radiother Oncol* 2001;61:77–82.

3 Corry J, Peters L, D'Costa I et al. The 'QUAD SHOT': A phase II study of palliative radiotherapy for incurable head and neck cancer. *Radiother Oncol* 2005;77:137–142.

4 Lutz S, Korytko T, Nguyen J et al. Palliative radiotherapy: When is it worth it and when is it not? *Cancer J* 2010;16(5):473–482.

5 Van Oorschot B, Schuler M, Simon A et al. Patterns of care and course of symptoms in palliative radiotherapy. *Strah und Onkol* 2011;187:461–466.

6 Lutz S, Chow E, Hartsell W, Konski A. A review of hypofractionated palliative radiotherapy. *Cancer* 2007;109:1462–1470.

7 Meeuse J, van der Linden Y, van Tienhoven G et al. Efficacy of radiotherapy for painful bone metastases during the last 12 weeks of life. *Cancer* 2010;116(11):2716–2725.

8 Dennis K, Wong K, Zhang L et al. Palliative radiotherapy for bone metastases in the last 3 months of life: Worthwhile or futile? *Clin Oncol* 2011;23(10):709–715.

9 Qasim M. Half body irradiation in metastatic carcinomas. *Clin Radiol* 1981;32:215–219.

10 Samant R, Gooi A. Radiotherapy basics for family physicians: Potential tool for symptom relief. *Can Fam Physician* 2005;51:1496–1501.

11 Kirkbride P, Barton R. Palliative radiation therapy. *J Pall Med* 1999;2(1):87–97.

12 Sun J, Sun Y, Zeng Z et al. Consideration of the role of radiotherapy for abdominal lymph node metastases in patients with recurrent gastric cancer. *Int J Radiat Oncol Biol Phys* 2010;77(2):384–391.

13 Spiro S, Douse J, Read C, Janes S. Complications of lung cancer treatment. *Semin Respir Crit Care Med* 2008;29:302–318.

14 Smith S, Koh W. Palliative radiation therapy for gynaecological malignancies. *Best Pract Res Clin Obstet Gynaecol* 2001;15(2):265–278.

15 Tey J, Back M, Shakespeare T et al. The role of palliative radiation therapy in symptomatic locally advanced gastric cancer. *Int J Radiat Oncol Biol Phys* 2007;67(2):385–388.

16 Stone H, Coleman C, Anscher M, McBride W. Effects of radiation on normal tissue: Consequences and mechanisms. *Lancet Oncol* 2003;4:529–536.

17 Rubin P, Johnston C, Williams J et al. A perpetual cascade of cytokines postirradiation leads to pulmonary fibrosis. *Int J Radiat Oncol Biol Phys* 1995;33:99–109.

18 Martin M, Lefaix J, Delanian S. TGF-β1 and radiation fibrosis: A master switch and a specific therapeutic target? *Int J Radiat Oncol Biol Phys* 2000;47:277–290.

19 Miranda V, Trufelli D, Santos J et al. Effectivness of guarana (Paullinia cupana) for postradiation fatigue and depression: Results of a pilot double-blind randomized study. *J Altern Complement Med* 2009;15(4):431–433.

20 Bashir F, Parry J, Windsor P. Use of a modified hemi-body irradiation technique for metastatic carcinoma of the prostate: Report of a 10-year experience. *Clin Oncol* 2008;20:591–598.

21 Tanner C. Palliative radiation therapy for cancer. *J Pall Med* 2011;14(5):672–673.

22 Bruera E, Driver L, Valero V et al. Patient controlled methylphenidate for cancer-related fatigue: A randomized controlled trial. *Proc Am Soc Clin Oncol* 2005;23:740S.

23 Morrow G, Gillis L, Hickok J et al. The positive effect of the psychostimulant modafinil on fatigue from cancer that persists after treatment is completed. *Proc Am Soc Clin Oncol* 2005;23:732S.

24 Taillibert S, Delattre JY. Palliative care in patients with brain metastases. *Curr Opin Oncol* 2005;17:588–592.

25 Frassica D. General principles of external beam radiation therapy for skeletal metastases. *Clin Orthop Relat Res* 2003;415S:S158–S164.

** 26 Roos D, Turner S, O'Brien P et al. Randomized trial of 8Gy in 1 versus 20Gy in 5 fractions of radiotherapy for neuropathic pain due to bone metastases (TROG 96.05). *Radiother Oncol* 2005;75:54–63.

27 Dijkstra S, Wiggers T, van Geel B et al. Impending and actual pathological fractures in patients with bone metastases of the long bones. A retrospective study of 233 surgically treated fractures. *Eur J Surg* 1994;160:535–542.

*** 28 Chow E, Harris K, Fan G et al. Palliative radiotherapy trials for bone metastases: A systematic review. *J Clin Oncol* 2007;25:1423–1436.

*** 29 Sze W, Shelley M, Held I et al. Palliation of metastatic bone pain: Single fraction versus multifraction radiotherapy—A systematic review of randomized trials. *Clin Oncol* 2003;15:345–352.

*** 30 Wu J, Wong R, Johnston M et al. Meta-analysis of dose-fractionation radiotherapy trials for the palliation of painful bone metastases. *In J Radiat Oncol Biol Phys* 2003;55:594–605.

** 31 Hartsell W, Konski A, Scott C et al. Randomized trial of short versus long-course radiotherapy for palliation of painful bone metastases. *J Natl Cancer Inst* 2005;97:798–804.

*** 32 Fairchild A, Harris K, Barnes E et al. Palliative thoracic radiotherapy for lung cancer: A systematic review. *J Clin Oncol* 2009;26(24):4001–4011.

33 Kassam Z, Wong R, Ringash J et al. A phase I/II study to evaluate the toxicity and efficacy of accelerated fractionation radiotherapy for the palliation of dysphagia from carcinoma of the esophagus. *Clin Oncol* 2008;20:53–60.

34 Howell D. The role of radiation therapy in the palliation of gastrointestinal malignancies. *Gastroenterol Clin North Am* 2006;35:125–130.

35 Din O, Thanvi N, Ferguson C, Kirkbride P. Palliative prostate radiotherapy for symptomatic advanced prostate cancer. *Radiother Oncol* 2009;93:192–196.

36 Chang E, Wefel J, Major M et al. A pilot study of neurocognitive function in patients with one to three new brain metastases initially treated with stereotactic radiosurgery alone. *Neurosurgery* 2007;60:277–283.

37 ááMeyers C, Smith J, Bezjak A et al. Neurocognitive function and progression in patients with brain metastases treated with whole-brain radiation and motexafin gadolinium: Results of a randomized phase III trial. *J Clin Oncol* 2004;22:157–165.

38 Oldenburg N. The role of palliative radiation in the management of brain, spinal cord, and bone metastases. *Med Health R I* 2006;89(2):59–62.

39 Li J, Bentzen S, Renschler M, Mehta MP. Regression after whole-brain radiation therapy for brain metastases correlates with survival and improved neurocognitive function. *J Clin Oncol* 2007;25:1260–1266.

◆ 40 Suh J. Stereotactic radiosurgery for the management of brain metastases. *N Engl J Med.* 2010;362(12):1119–1127.

41 Samant R, Gerig L, Montgomery L et al. High-technology palliative radiotherapy using image-guided intensity-modulated radiotherapy. *Clin Oncol* 2008;20:718–720.

42 Danjoux C, Franssen E, Chow E et al. Sublingual fentanyl citrate for control of breakthrough pain in patients referred for palliative radiotherapy. *Curr Oncol* 2003;11(1):3–7.

43 Chow E, Prescutti R, Nguyen J et al. Bone metastases and quality of life. *J Pain Manage* 2010;4(1):117–131.

* 44 Roila F, Herrstedt J, Aapro M et al. Guideline update for MASCC and ESMO in the prevention of chemotherapy and radiotherapy-induced nausea and vomiting: Results of the Perugia consensus conference. *Ann Oncol* 2010;21(Suppl 5):v232–v243.

*** 45 Deandrea S, Montanari M, Moja L, Apolone G. Prevalence of undertreatment in cancer pain. A review of published literature. *Ann Oncol* 2008;19(12):1985–1991.

46 Davis M, Walsh D. Epidemiology of cancer pain and factors influencing poor pain control. *Am J Hosp Pall Med* 2004;21(2):137–142.

47 Koshy R, Rhodes D, Devi S, Grossman S. Cancer pain management in developing countries: A mosaic of complex issues resulting in inadequate analgesia. *Support Care Cancer* 1998;6:430–437.

** 48 Rosenblatt E, Jones G, Sur R et al. Adding external beam to intra-luminal brachytherapy improves palliation in obstructive squamous cell esophageal cancer: A prospective multi-centre randomized trial of the International Atomic Energy Agency. *Radiother Oncol* 2010;97:488–494.

49 Danjoux C, Chow E, Drossos A et al. An innovative rapid response radiotherapy program to reduce waiting time for palliative radiotherapy. *Support Care Cancer* 2006;14(1):38–43.

50 Fairchild A, Pituskin E, Rose B et al. The rapid access palliative radiotherapy program: Blueprint for initiation of a one-stop multidisciplinary bone metastases clinic. *Support Care Cancer* 2009;17(2):163–170.

51 Wu J, Monk G, Clark T et al. Palliative radiotherapy improves pain and reduces functional interference in patients with painful bone metastases: A quality assurance study. *Clin Oncol* 2006;18(7):539–544.

52 Létourneau D, Keller H, Sharpe M, Jaffray D. Integral test phantom for dosimetric quality assurance of image guided and intensity modulated stereotactic radiotherapy. *Med Phys* 2007;34(5):1842–1849.

53 Hird A, Chow E, Zhang L et al. Determining the incidence of pain flare following palliative radiotherapy for symptomatic bone metastases: Results from three Canadian cancer centres. *Int J Radiat Oncol Biol Phys* 2009;75:193–197.

54 Steenland E, Leer J, van Houwelingen et al. The effect of a single fraction compared to multiple fractions on painful bone metastases: A global analysis of the dutch bone metastasis study. *Radiother Oncol* 1999;52:101–109.

55 Porceddu S, Rosser B, Burmeister B et al. Hypofractionated radiotherapy for the palliation of advanced head and neck cancer in patients unsuitable for curative treatment—"Hypo Trial". *Radiother Oncol* 2007;85:456–462.

56 Dulley L, Li S, Ah-See M. Efficacy of hypofractionated palliative radiotherapy in locally advanced breast cancer. *Clin Oncol* 2011;23:S35–S36, Abstr P29.

57 Metcalfe S, Milano M, Bylund K et al. Split-course palliative radiotherapy for advanced non-small cell lung cancer. *J Thorac Oncol* 2010;5(2):185–190.

58 Rorth M, Andersen C, Quist M et al. Health benefits of a multidimensional exercise program for cancer patients undergoing chemotherapy. *Proc Am Soc Clin Oncol* 2005;23:731S.

59 Quddus A, Kerr G, Price A, Gregor A. Long-term survival in patients with non-small cell lung cancer treated with palliative radiotherapy. *Clin Oncol* 2001;13:95–98.

60 Macbeth F, Wheldon T, Girling T et al. Radiation myelopathy: Estimates of risk in 1048 patients in three randomized trials of palliative radiotherapy for non-small cell lung cancer. *Clin Oncol* 1996;8:176–81.

61 DeAngelis L, Delattre JY, Posner J. Radiation-induced dementia in patients cured of brain metastases. *Neurology* 1989;39:789–786.

116

Cardiac and pulmonary toxicities of treatments

MARIEBERTA VIDAL

Cardiac and pulmonary toxicities are complications that can severely affect the quality of life of cancer patients. These days, with the development of novel treatments, patients' expectancy of life might be longer despite advanced disease. In palliative care, the recognition of these toxicities is important in view to be able to control better the patient's symptoms. Especially when palliative care is introduced early in the disease process, manifestation of toxicities of treatments can be a significant cause of distress for patients. We will review the cardiac and pulmonary toxicities associated to antineoplastic treatments, their presentations, and treatments.

CARDIAC TOXICITIES

Cardiovascular toxicity is a potential complication for cancer patients undergoing treatment. Several drugs including anthracyclines and other biological agents have been associated with short- and long-term cardiac complications, some of them irreversible. Target therapy agents are still considered better tolerated and less toxic than the classic chemotherapy, but still worrisome complications have been described. The severity of some therapies depends on the existence of underlying cardiac problems, immediate and cumulative doses, site of action of the drug, and method of administration. It is important to be aware of these complications as they might present immediately during the administration of the agent or even months or years after treatments. Because these complications can present as symptoms that can affect the quality of life of the patients, the palliative care team should be aware of them.

Each chemotherapy has unique cardiac effects and can also increase the toxicity of other agents when used together. In a patient that also undergoes radiation, this toxicity is even higher. The toxicities from radiation will be explained in another chapter.

Antitumor antibiotics

The most commonly implicated agents in cardiac toxicities are anthracyclines like doxorubicin, daunorubicin, idarubicin,

epirubicin, and related compounds like mitoxantrone. When these drugs were initially used, the myelosuppression was the limiting factor. These days, with more supportive measures, patients are able to tolerate this treatment that causes toxicities from the cumulative exposure to these treatments for longer periods.

The cardiac toxicities can be acute or chronic. Acute or subacute cardiotoxicity, which can occur anytime from treatment initiation to several weeks after termination, may present as electrocardiographic abnormalities like nonspecific ST segment and T wave abnormalities, arrhythmia, ventricular dysfunction, an increase in plasma brain natriuretic peptide (BNP), or a pericarditis-myocarditis syndrome. These events are rare and seldom of clinical importance since they usually resolve within a week. Late effects are usually seen as the development of cardiomyopathy. Chronic anthracycline-related cardiotoxicity typically presents within a year after the termination of chemotherapy. The peak time for the appearance of symptoms of heart failure is about 3 months after the last anthracycline dose. The patient who develops late toxicity has a high mortality rate. Mitoxantrone has also been associated with mild cardiotoxicity similar to the other anthracyclines.

Mitomycin has been associated with cardiomyopathy, especially when given with or after an anthracycline. Bleomycin has been associated with several different forms of cardiotoxicity including pericarditis, substernal chest pain, coronary artery disease, myocardial ischemia, and infarction. Treatment is mainly supportive.

Antimetabolites

5-fluorouracil is the second most common cause of chemotherapy-related cardiotoxicity, after anthracyclines. The most common cardiac symptom due to 5-FU is the ischemic syndrome, that varies from angina to myocardial infarction. Multiple mechanisms have been proposed, including coronary artery vasospasm, endothelial injury, and a transient stress-induced cardiomyopathy. Risk appears to be related to the method of 5-FU administration, the presence of coronary artery disease, and the use of concurrent radiation or anthracyclines. Cardiac symptoms usually resolve with termination of 5-FU treatment and the implementation of antianginal treatment. Capecitabine is a fluoropyrimidine that is metabolized to 5-FU, this one is considered to be less toxic.

Fludarabine is a purine antagonist used in hematologic malignancies. It has been reported to cause hypotension and chest pain. In addition, the combination of fludarabine and melphalan has been associated with severe cardiac toxicity in at least seven cases when used as the conditioning agent for bone marrow transplantation. The use of either agent alone in high doses has only rarely been associated with cardiac toxicity. Pentostatin (2′-deoxycoformycin) and cladribine (2-chlorodeoxyadenosine) are additional purine antagonists also used in hematologic malignancies. Both have rarely been reported to cause ischemia and heart failure. Methotrexate is not considered cardiac toxic, but there are rare reports of syncope, myocardial infarction, supraventricular and ventricular arrhythmias associated with it. Cytarabine has been associated with multiple cases of pericarditis. This can progress to pericardial effusion and cardiac tamponade. Corticosteroid therapy may be beneficial in the treatment of this complication.

Alkylating agents

Cyclophosphamide is usually used for several solid tumors and lymphomas and has been associated with an acute cardiomyopathy that is associated with high doses and not related to cumulative dose. The incidence of cardiotoxicity may be particularly high in patients receiving cyclophosphamide as part of a program of high-dose chemotherapy followed by autologous stem cell rescue. Subsequent cardiac events can include hemorrhagic myopericarditis resulting in pericardial effusions, tamponade, and death, typically within the first week after treatment. Most pericardial effusions can be treated with glucocorticoids and analgesics without serious sequelae. These complications may be due to endothelial capillary damage.

Ifosfamide has been associated with arrhythmias, ST-T wave changes, and heart failure in a dose-related manner. These cardiac complications, when symptomatic, are generally reversible with medical management. Cardiotoxicity due to cisplatin can be manifested by supraventricular tachycardia, bradycardia, ST-T wave changes, left bundle branch block, acute ischemic events, myocardial infarction, and ischemic cardiomyopathy. This toxicity may be related to electrolyte abnormalities secondary to cisplatin-induced nephrotoxicity. Laboratory testing is important in these patients. Cisplatin can cause late cardiovascular complications even after more than 10 years of exposure.

Antimicrotubule agents

Vinca alkaloids have been associated with hypertension, myocardial ischemia, and infarction, and other vaso-occlusive complications. These complications have been reported most commonly with vinblastine, but have also been described with vincristine and vinorelbine. Bradycardia and heart block are the most frequently described cardiac effects of paclitaxel, although these usually are asymptomatic.

Paclitaxel can cause sinus bradycardia, heart block, premature ventricular contractions, and ventricular tachycardia. Cardiomyopathy is reported when paclitaxel is combined with doxorubicin. Heart failure has developed in up to 20% of patients treated with paclitaxel plus doxorubicin.

Eribulin mesylate has been associated with QTc changes. EKG monitoring in patients who have heart failure or bradyarrhythmias or who are receiving drugs that can prolong QTc interval should be carried out.

Monoclonal antibodies

Monoclonal antibodies infusions commonly cause hypotension due to the increased release of cytokinase as well as dyspnea, fever, hypoxia or death. Trastuzumab is a monoclonal that has been associated with the development of a cardiomyopathy that is typically manifested by an asymptomatic decrease in the left ventricular ejection fraction (LVEF) and less commonly by clinical heart failure. Previous or concurrent anthracycline use and age greater than 50 years are the strongest risk factors for development of trastuzumab-related cardiotoxicity. Trastuzumab cardiac complications are usually reversible in many patients and respond to standard treatment for heart failure.

Rituximab, a monoclonal antibody used to treat a variety of malignant and benign hematologic conditions, can cause arrhythmias and angina during the first infusion. Administration of IV fluids, vasopressors, bronchodilators, dyphenidramine, and acetaminophen are usually effective. Heart failure associated with bevacizumab has been sporadically reported, but ischemic cardiac events and severe hypertension are increased.

Alemtuzumab therapy used for hematologic malignancies is associated with a significant risk of heart failure and/or arrhythmias. Cetuximab used to treat refractory metastatic colorectal cancer was noticed to cause a range of cardiac events when combined with 5-FU; it is not clear that all of these events can be attributed exclusively to the 5-FU.

Cytokines

The toxicities of cytokines are generally not due to a direct cytotoxic effect of the drugs, but rather reflect alterations of cellular physiology. Interferon-alfa (IFNa) is used in the treatment of many types of cancer. The cardiovascular side effects of IFNa include myocardial ischemia, atrial and ventricular arrhythmias, hypertension, or hypotension. Prolonged administration of IFNa has been associated with cardiomyopathy, manifested by a depressed ejection fraction and heart failure. The cardiomyopathy was reversible upon cessation of IFNa infusion in some but not all.

In the case of interleukin-2 (IL-2), a capillary leak syndrome has been associated with increased vascular permeability and hypotension. This results in cardiovascular symptoms similar to those of septic shock, with an increased heart rate and cardiac output and a decrease in systemic peripheral resistance.

These symptoms are partially responsive to fluid replacement therapy, but patients often require vasopressors as well.

Tyrosine kinase inhibitors

Sorafenib and sunitinib are orally active multitargeted tyrosine kinase (TK) inhibitors that are used for the treatment of multiple solid tumors; both drugs have been associated with a small but definite risk of cardiotoxicity. In addition to declines in LVEF and clinical heart failure, reported ECG changes have included changes in rhythm, conduction disturbance, change in axis or QRS amplitude, ST or T wave changes, and QTc prolongation with sunitinib.

Imatinib is used in the treatment of chronic myeloid leukemia and was associated with the development of heart failure. Nilotinib, dasatinib, crizotinib, vandetanib, and vemurafenib have been associated with QTc prolongation. The FDA-approved manufacturer's labeling recommends avoiding the drug in patients with congenital long QT syndrome and that patients with heart failure, bradyarrhythmias, electrolyte abnormalities, or who are taking other medications known to prolong the QTc interval undergo periodic monitoring with electrocardiograms and serum electrolytes.

Miscellaneous agents

Etoposide mainly is used for refractory testicular tumors and has been linked to the development of myocardial infarction and vasospastic angina in several case reports.

All-trans retinoic acid (ATRA) is used to treat acute promyelocytic leukemia. Approximately 10%–15% of patients develop the retinoic acid syndrome, which can cause fever, dyspnea, hypotension, pericardial effusions and myocardial ischemia/infarction.

Arsenictrioxide is used to treat relapsed acute promyelocytic leukemia and commonly causes ECG abnormalities. It can cause QT prolongation in more than 50% of patients. Other associated complications are sinus tachycardia, nonspecific ST changes, and torsades de pointes.

Diethylstilbestrol (DES) is a synthetic estrogen that was used to treat advanced prostate cancer and breast cancer. Multiple studies demonstrated an increased risk of cardiovascular death in patients treated with DES. This agent is no longer commercially available in the United States.

Serotonin antagonists are often used during chemotherapy as antiemetics. They have some potential for cardiac complications. Clinical trials in healthy subjects and patients undergoing chemotherapy have demonstrated transient asymptomatic ECG changes, like increases in PR interval, QRS complex duration, and QTc interval after administration of ondansetron, granisetron, or dolasetron (Table 116.1).

Management

Cancer patients receiving chemotherapy have an increased risk of developing cardiovascular complications, and the risk is even greater if there is a known history of heart disease. The

Table 116.1 *Cardiac toxicities associated to antineoplastic treatments*

Cardiovascular syndrome	Agents
Ischemia	5-FU
	Cisplatin
	Capecitabine
	IL-2
Cardiomyopathy	Anthracyclines
	Mitoxantrone
	Cyclophosphamide
	Transtuxumab
	Ifosmamide
	ATRA
Hypotension	Etoposide
	Paclitaxel
	Alemtuzumab
	Ceftuximab
	Rituximab
	IL-2
	Interferon
	ATRA
	Homoharingtonine
Hypertension	Bevacizumab
	Cisplatinin
QT prolongation	Sorafenib, sunitib, crizotinib, dasatinib, nilotinib
	Arsenic trioxide

majority of the cardiac toxicities can be managed by removing the offending agent. In the event of ischemia, the standard acute coronary syndrome measures should be followed. Patients with chemotherapy-induced cardiomyopathy usually respond to CHF treatment, and some improvement has been seen after the use of beta-blockers and ace inhibitors. Symptoms of dyspnea and chest pain can be controlled with supplemental oxygen, diuretics, and opioids.

PULMONARY TOXICITIES

Pulmonary toxicities can develop in approximately 10%–20% of all patients treated with antineoplastic agents. The high prevalence can be explained by the increased blood supply in the lungs, leading to greater exposure to potentially harmful antineoplastic agents compared to other organs. Even though the pathogenesis of anticancer agent–induced lung injury is not well understood, most toxic effects are thought to result from direct cytotoxicity. Similar to patients with cardiovascular toxicities, the patients that have been exposed to radiation are at a higher risk of developing pulmonary complications.

The clinical presentation of pulmonary toxicities varies and can also be difficult to differentiate from other pulmonary clinical syndromes. The majority of clinical trials do not report the details of pulmonary toxicity, and literature reports may describe pulmonary toxicity based upon clinical or radiographic criteria like acute lung injury, pneumonitis, noncardiogenic pulmonary edema, acute respiratory distress syndrome, or other pathologic findings.

Most of the time, the symptoms are nonspecific including cough, dyspnea, low-grade fever, and hypoxemia. Physical examination might reveal bibasilar crackles, but it is often normal. Wheezing is rare but, when present, suggests a hypersensitivity mechanism with a component of bronchoconstriction. The presence of a rash can suggest hypersensitivity to a drug, such as drug-induced hypersensitivity (DIHS), also known as drug rash with eosinophilia and systemic symptoms (DRESS).

The time of presentation is also variable, it might present early during the first cycle of therapy or with subsequent treatments. Most regimens now also include more than one agent that makes it more difficult to identify the cause for the symptoms.

Bleomycin

Bleomycin pulmonary toxicities can present as subacute progressive pulmonary fibrosis, hypersensitivity pneumonitis, and organizing pneumonia. The risk of bleomycin-induced lung toxicity appears to be higher in older patients and those with renal insufficiency. The onset of clinical manifestations usually occurs subacutely between 1 and 6 months after bleomycin treatment but may occur during therapy or more than 6 months following of exposure. Symptoms include nonproductive cough, dyspnea, pleuritic or substernal chest pain, fever, tachypnea, crackles, lung restriction, and hypoxemia. Discontinuation of bleomycin permanently is recommended. Initially, it was thought that the administration of high inspired fractions of oxygen may exacerbate the pulmonary toxicity. Now the suggestion is to carefully titrate any supplemental oxygen to provide only enough oxygen to keep oxygen saturation at 89%–92%.

Taxanes

Taxanes pulmonary toxicities can present as an acute infusion reaction or subacute diffuse interstitial pneumonitis. Taxanes-induced pulmonary toxicity needs to be considered in the differential diagnosis when patients receiving these agents develop respiratory symptoms. Treatment is generally supportive with discontinuation of the drug. The use of glucocorticoids is recommended.

Docetaxel has been associated with fluid retention that is attributed to capillary leakage. The usual initial symptom is peripheral edema and eventually pleural effusions and pulmonary edema. For these patients, glucocorticoid premedication and diuretics is helpful.

Molecular target therapy

Molecular targeted therapies have been associated with pulmonary toxicities. Anti-EGFR agents like gefitinib and erlotinib are used in the treatment of advanced non–small cell lung cancer. Patient treated with both agents can develop lung toxicity, usually within the first few months of treatment. The risk is higher in patients with preexisting lung disease and in smokers. About one-third of patients who develop interstitial lung disease while being treated with gefitinib die of this complication.

Treatment is largely supportive, with immediate drug discontinuation, administration of supplemental oxygen, empiric antibiotics, and mechanical ventilation as clinically indicated. Systemic glucocorticoids are usually recommended.

Imatinib's lung toxicities are related to fluid retention, but peripheral and periorbital edema are more frequent than pleural or pericardial effusions and pulmonary edema.

Rare cases of acute pneumonia with and without eosinophilic infiltrates and subacute interstitial pneumonitis are reported.

Dasatinib has been associated with the highest frequency of pulmonary side effects. During treatment with dasatinib, pleural, pulmonary, vascular, and lung parenchymal abnormalities can develop. Pleural effusions are more commonly seen in patients treated with dasatinib than with imatinib and may be bilateral or unilateral. Case reports describe reversible pulmonary arterial hypertension (PAH) in patients treated with dasatinib. Patients usually present with fatigue, dyspnea on exertion, tachypnea, and peripheral edema, up to 2 years after treatment.

Crizotinib is used for the treatment of advanced non-small cell lung cancer and has been associated with severe, life threatening or fatal pneumonitis in 1.6% of patients. Permanent discontinuation is advised in the event of treatment-related pneumonitis.

Several complications have been associated with the use of bevacizumab like hemorrhage, tracheoesophageal (TE) fistula, and thromboembolic disease. Tumor cavitation and bleeding complications have been observed rarely with the use of sunitinib and sorafenib for NSCLC. However, pulmonary hemorrhage has not been described in patients receiving either drug for other malignancies.

Dyspnea and cough have been reported with sunitinib. In a review of the drug, severe dyspnea was seen in 19% of patients and cough in 13%. Rare cases of pulmonary toxicity with dyspnea, cough, and fever have been reported in patients receiving sorafenib (Table 116.2).

Table 116.2 *Other agents*

Agent	Associated pulmonary toxicity
Cetuximab	Infusion reaction (brochospasm)
Transtuzumab	Infusion reaction, subacute interstitial pneumonia, organizing pneumonia
Rituximab	Infusion reaction, pulmonary parenchymal toxicity is uncommon
Everolimus, Temsirolimus	Pneumonitis

Treatment

The treatment of antineoplastic pulmonary toxicity includes drug discontinuation, glucocorticoid therapy, and supportive care. The decision to initiate glucocorticoid therapy usually depends on the severity and rapidity of worsening of pulmonary impairment. When considering the option of systemic glucocorticoid, it is important to exclude an infectious etiology. Supportive care may include supplemental oxygen, inhaled bronchodilating medications, and opioids. Oxygen has been helpful for patients who are hypoxemic at rest or with minimal exertion. In patients who have distressing dyspnea, systemic opioids are recommended to improve comfort.

REFERENCES

1 Floyd JD, Nguyen DT, Lobins RL et al. Cardio toxicity of cancer therapy. *J Clin Oncol* 2005; 23: 7685.

2 Monsuez JJ, Charniot JC, Vignat N, Artigou JY. Cardiac side-effects of cancer chemotherapy. *Int J Cardiol* 2010; 144: 3.

3 Smith LA, Cornelius VR, Plummer CJ et al. Cardiotoxicity of anthracycline agents for the treatment of cancer: Systematic review and meta-analysis of randomised controlled trials. *BMC Cancer* 2010; 10: 337.

4 Carver JR, Shapiro CL, Ng A et al. American Society of Clinical Oncology clinical evidence review on the ongoing care of adult cancer survivors: Cardiac and pulmonary late effects. *J Clin Oncol* 2007; 25: 3991.

5 Folkman J. Tumorangiogenesis: Therapeutic implications. *N Engl J Med* 1971; 285: 1182.

6 Yeh ETH, Tong AT et al. Cardiovascular complications of cancer therapy, Diagnosis pathogenesis and management. *Circulation* 2004; 109: 3122–3131.

7 Ozkan M, Dweik RA, Ahmad M. Drug-induced lung disease. *Cleve Clin J Med* 2001; 68: 782.

8 Rosenow EC III, Limper AH. Drug-induced pulmonary disease. *Semin Respir Infect* 1995; 10: 86.

9 Snyder LS, Hertz MI. Cytotoxicdrug-induced lung injury. *Semin Respir Infect* 1988; 3: 217.

10 Vahid B, Marik PE. Pulmonary complications of novel antineoplastic agents for solid tumors. *Chest* 2008; 133: 528.

11 Classen DC, Pestotnik SL, Evans RS, Burke JP. Computerized surveillance of adverse drug events in hospital patients. *JAMA* 1991; 266: 2847.

12 Pai VB, Nahata MC. Cardiotoxicity of chemotherapeutic agents: Incidence, treatment and prevention. *Drug Saf* 2000; 22: 263–302.

13 Cranston JM, Crockett A, Currow D. Oxygen therapy for dyspnoea in adults. *Cochrane Database Syst Rev* 2008; 16: CD004769.

14 Bruera E, deStoutz N, Velasco-Leiva A et al. Effects of oxygen on dyspnoea in hypoxaemic terminal-cancer patients. *Lancet* 1993; 342: 13.

117

Oral complications of cancer therapies

SIRI BEIER JENSEN, DEBORAH P. SAUNDERS

INTRODUCTION

Cancer therapy commonly causes oral complications of significant morbidity and may have a severe impact on the patient's quality of life during treatment or appear as late oral complications following treatment (Figure 117.1). The oral complications vary in pattern, duration, intensity, and number for cancer chemotherapy, head and neck radiation therapy, targeted therapies, and hematopoietic stem cell transplantation.[1] Not every patient will develop every complication; however, it is characteristic that oral complications often appear concurrently and a cancer patient may experience oral mucositis, oral pain, oral fungal or viral infection, salivary gland hypofunction/xerostomia, and dysgeusia at the same time (Figure 117.2).[2] Combined oral complications commonly lead to dysphagia (swallowing dysfunction) in cancer patients (Figure 117.1).[3]

Oral complications associated with cancer chemotherapy and radiation therapy result from complex interactions among multiple factors. For example, therapy-related toxicity to the oral mucosa can be exacerbated by colonizing oral microflora when local and systemic immune functions are concurrently compromised.

The understanding of the mechanisms associated with oral complications continues to increase. Unfortunately, there are no universally effective agents or protocols to prevent toxicity. Thus, the current approach to reduce the frequency and severity of oral complications in cancer patients is the elimination of preexisting dental/periapical, periodontal, and mucosal infections; institution of comprehensive oral hygiene protocols; reduction of factors that may compromise oral mucosal integrity (e.g., physical trauma to oral tissues); and prompt diagnosis of developing oral complications during and after cancer treatment with adequate alleviation and treatment.

It is of importance that a multidisciplinary team collaborates closely with the patient to assess, prevent, and treat oral complications in a regular, systematic way.

This chapter provides a concise overview of oral complications associated with cancer therapies and the principles of management (Figure 117.3). The focus is on the adult cancer population. The palliative oral care in patients with advanced cancers and terminally ill cancer patients is discussed in detail in Chapter 79.

BASIC ORAL CARE

The principles of basic oral care apply to all cancer patients in order to decrease the incidence and severity of oral complications during and after cancer therapies.

Poor oral health has been associated with increased incidence and severity of oral complications in cancer patients; hence, the adoption of an aggressive approach is needed to stabilize oral care before treatment.[4,5] Initiating a program of effective oral hygiene with emphasis on maximizing patient compliance on a continuing basis, early detection of oral lesions, and appropriate nutritional intake are important pretreatment interventions.

The involvement of a dental team experienced with oral oncology may reduce the risk of oral complications via either direct examination of the patient or in consultation with the community-based dentist. Ideally, this examination should be performed at least one month before the start of cancer treatment to permit adequate healing from required invasive oral procedures.[6***] In order for the dentist to assess the risk of oral complications, the oncology team must provide the underlying oncologic disease, current hematologic status, present medications, and any other underlying medical conditions. In turn, the dentist can provide the oral and dental status and required pretreatment with anticipated healing times if dental extractions are necessary.

Oral care during cancer therapies can be divided into the following sections: oral decontamination, oral moisturization, and management of bleeding and pain. This was originally conceptualized for the management of mucositis but can be adapted to other oral complications.[7]

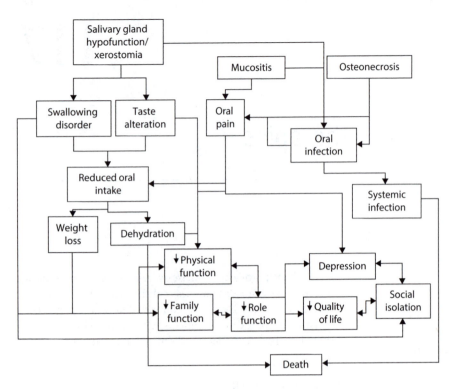

Figure 117.1   *Relationships among oral complications of cancer and cancer therapies. (Modified from* Dent. Clin. North Am., *52, Elting, L.S., Avritscher, E.B., Cooksley, C.D. et al., Psychosocial and economic impact of cancer, 231–252, Copyright 2008, with permission from Elsevier.)*

Oral decontamination

Routine oral hygiene includes toothbrushing two to three times a day with a soft nylon-bristled brush. Dental flossing is recommended once daily with instruction on atraumatic technique and modifications as needed. Fluoridated and phosphate-/calcium-containing pastes are recommended for use as tolerated. The use of a bland rinse composed of 0.9% saline or 0.5% sodium bicarbonate is beneficial for decontamination but also allows debridement of the tissues and neutralizes pH. This can easily be prepared by the patient by mixing 1 tsp salt, 1 tsp baking soda in 1 liter of water. The frequency of rinsing depends on the oral status of the patient, starting at every 4–6 hours up to every hour

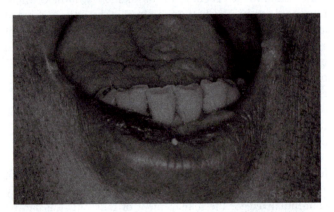

Figure 117.2   *Cancer patient (solid tumor) during chemotherapy presenting with viral (tongue), fungal (corners of the mouth), and bacterial (gingival) infections, oral mucositis (lower lip), and oral pain with overlying xerostomia and salivary gland hypofunction.*

as needed. Antimicrobial rinses such as 0.12% chlorhexidine gluconate may be applied with the frequency of use based on the capability of maintaining other routine oral hygiene and the severity of periodontal disease.[8]

Oral moisturization

Alleviation of xerostomia includes frequent sipping or spraying of the oral cavity with water, the use of saliva substitutes (e.g., oral rinses, sprays, or gels), or the stimulation of saliva production from intact salivary glandular tissues (see "Dry mouth" section and Figure 117.3).[9]*** The use of bland rinses, as noted in the section on oral decontamination, also provides moisturization.

Lip care encompasses lubrication to prevent cracking. Petroleum-based products are discouraged due to their anhydrous nature while wax and oil-based products such as lanolin and bees wax are better replacements.

Management of bleeding

Periodontal infection (gingivitis and periodontitis) increases the risk for oral bleeding; healthy gingival tissues do not bleed unless traumatized. It is not uncommon for oncology patients to be told specifically not to use toothbrushes and dental floss when their platelet counts drop below 40,000/mm³. This is generally poor advice unless there are extenuating circumstances. Discontinuation of routine oral hygiene increases the risk of infection that not only promotes bleeding but also increases the risk of local and systemic infection (Figure 117.1). Bleeding can be controlled with adequate periodontal care (see "Oral

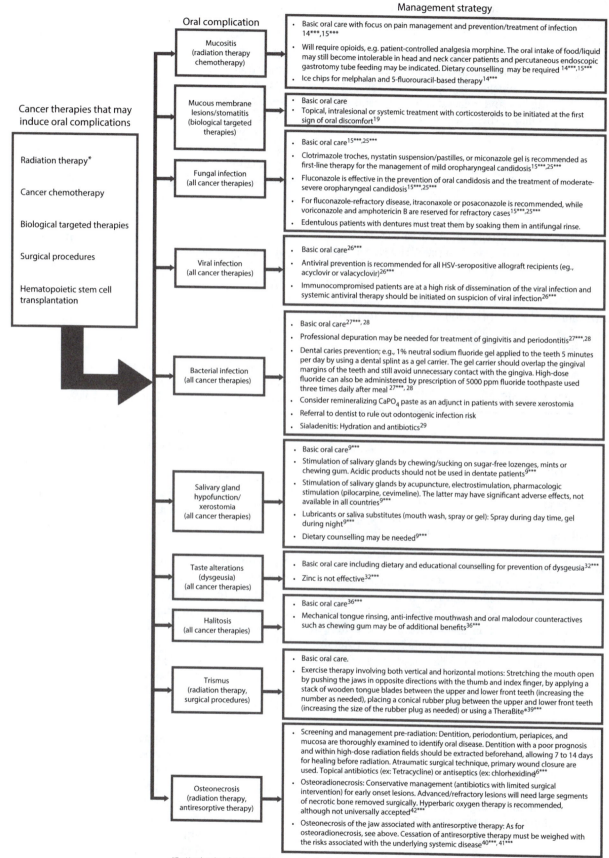

Figure 117.3   *Management strategies of oral complications of cancer therapies*

decontamination" section). If prolonged bleeding (>2 min) occurs, periodontal care should be discontinued and the oncologist consulted.

The management of oral bleeds revolves around the use of vasoconstrictors, clot-forming agents, and tissue protectants, which include the use of epinephrine, topical thrombin and/or hemostatic collagen agents, and mucosal adherent agents such as cyanoacrylate products, which help seal sites and protect organized clots.[10]

Oral pain

Pain management must be directed at the severity of pain. The World Health Organization (WHO) pain relief ladder is a three-step strategy for managing pain in cancer patients.[11] The lowest dose of strong opioids (step 3 in the WHO ladder) may be chosen instead of weak opioids for better pain control.[12] Depending on the severity of mucositis, topical anesthetic rinses can be used to allow for continuity of oral care and food intake with comfort.[13] Patient-controlled analgesia morphine has been well documented as the treatment of choice for severe pain secondary to mucositis.[14***,15***]

ORAL COMPLICATIONS

Oral mucositis

Oral mucositis is the consequence of complex biological events arising in the epithelium and the submucosa induced by cancer chemotherapy and radiation therapy.[16] Due to arrest of epithelial proliferation, mucosal atrophy and erythema appears followed by ulceration and subsequently healing after cancer therapy. Oral mucositis ulcerations are commonly colonized with bacteria contributing to the mucositis development. The oral mucosal damage is strongly related to the chemotherapy regimen and doses, or the radiation dose, volume of irradiated tissue, and fractionation regimen. Thus, more than 50% of patients undergoing radiation therapy for head and neck cancer and some chemotherapy conditioning regimens/total body irradiation conditioning prior to hematopoietic stem cell transplantation will develop oral mucositis, while other chemotherapy regimens (e.g., cyclic moderate-dose chemotherapy for the treatment of solid cancers) will be at a lower risk of less than 50% of developing oral mucositis.

Oral mucositis primarily affects the soft palate, floor of the mouth, buccal mucosa, lateral margins, and ventral surface of the tongue and lips. For radiation therapy, the first clinical signs of mucositis are erythema, epithelial sloughing, and oral discomfort occurring at the end of the first week (days 7–14) of a conventional 7-week radiation protocol (2 Gy/day, five times a week). Ulceration and severe pain will occur during the second or third week and persist during the radiation schedule. Healing will generally be complete within 2–4 weeks after radiation. For chemotherapy-induced oral mucositis, the clinical signs begin within 5 days after the drug administration

with the ulcerative phase lasting for 7–10 days and healing within 3 weeks. The timing of the ulcerative phase usually precedes the nadir of the neutropenic phase of some treatments placing patients at risk for infection. Generally, there is a risk of infection of the damaged oral mucosa with fungi, bacterial pathogens, or viruses and this may further provide a portal for systemic infection (Figure 117.1).

Late mucous membrane changes characterized by epithelial atrophy, telangiectasia, loss of deeper capillary vessels, and fibrosis in the submucosa may be permanently present following radiation therapy, leaving the oral mucosa susceptible to infection and secondary trauma. See "Basic Oral Care" section and Figure 117.3 for management strategies.[14***]

Oral mucous membrane lesions/stomatitis induced by targeted therapies

Oral ulcerations are a frequent side effect of some targeted therapies, here among the multitargeted tyrosine kinase inhibitors and mammalian target of rapamycin inhibitors.

The clinical signs resemble aphthous stomatitis, and it may cause treatment delay or interruption due to pain. The lesions appear within few days after administration of the drug and resolve in approximately 1 week. They are characterized by distinct, ovoid, superficial, well-demarcated ulcerations with a central gray area surrounded by an erythematous halo and are localized on the movable oral/oropharyngeal mucosa while not presenting on the keratinized mucosa of the hard palate, gingiva, or dorsum of the tongue. The pathogenesis is assumed to be similar to aphthous stomatitis. Patients who develop these lesions may be more likely to have nonspecific cutaneous rashes and acneiform dermatitis but not gastrointestinal adverse effects.[17,18] See "Basic Oral Care" section and Figure 117.3 for management strategies.[19]

Oral fungal infections

Candidosis, the most commonly occurring oral fungal infection of the immunocompromised patient, is usually caused by *Candida albicans*. Local predisposing factors to oral candidosis are salivary gland dysfunction, chronic local irritants (dentures, smoking, high sugar intake), and asthma steroid inhalers. Immunosuppressed cancer patients are at risk for spread to the oropharyngeal regions and to the systemic circulation, which can be fatal (Figure 117.1).[20]

Oral candidosis has a number of clinical presentations: (1) pseudomembranous candidosis (thrush) presenting as white curd-like pseudomembranes, which can be removed with some pressure, leaving behind an erythematous mucosa, (2) chronic hyperplastic candidosis presenting as hyperkeratotic white patches, which cannot be removed by scraping, (3) erythematous candidosis presenting as intensely red inflamed areas of the oral mucosa, often under a denture or following antibiotic therapy, and (4) angular cheilitis presenting as erythema, fissuring, and crusting of the lip commissures.[20–22] Oral candidosis can be asymptomatic; however, erythematous candidosis is often associated with a burning sensation of the mouth,[23] while involvement of the dorsal tongue may lead to diffuse loss of filiform papillae, leading to a "bald" and red appearance, often accompanied by discomfort and taste changes. Pseudomembranous candidosis may be accompanied by burning pain, taste changes when eating, and a foul taste when not eating.[24]

The prevalence of oral candidosis is 37% during head and neck radiation therapy and 38% during chemotherapy.[25***]

In general, topical agents are considered preferable to systemic agents due to lower risk of side effects and drug interactions. However, recent studies present an inconsistent picture of the efficacy of topical agents in patients receiving cancer therapy.[25***] Troches/pastilles require saliva to dissolve, and hyposalivation is a frequent problem, especially in patients receiving head and neck radiation therapy. In addition, troches/pastilles can be traumatic to patients who have significant oral mucositis. Most formulations of troches/pastilles also contain sugar, which is not desirable from a caries prevention standpoint. Studies on the efficacy of systemic agents for antifungal prophylaxis provide a more consistent result.[25***] The use of systemic agents may be limited by their side effects and drug interactions while the emergence of resistant species is also an important concern. See "Basic Oral Care" section and Figure 117.3 for management strategies.[24***,15***]

Oral viral infections

Viral reactivation or de novo viral infections affecting the oral cavity or the perioral region are frequent complications of cancer therapies. Herpes simplex virus (HSV) infection is the most common viral infection of the oral mucosa followed by other Herpesviridae: for example, varicella zoster virus, Epstein-Bar virus, and cytomegalovirus.

Infection is characterized by the appearance of small vesicles on the oral mucosa (e.g., the gingival, tongue, buccal, and palatal mucosa), as well as the vermillion border rapidly developing ulceration and extensive confluent lesions. The lesions may cause significant morbidity in cancer patients, inducing severe pain, which makes the intake of fluid and food difficult, fever, cervical lymphadenopathy, and malaise (Figure 117.1). Immunocompromised patients primarily treated for hematologic malignancies are at a greater risk of oral and perioral viral infections, while the risk is found to be low in patients treated with radiation therapy for head and neck cancer. However, there is a significant increase in prevalence in the head and neck cancer patients if they are treated with combined radiation and chemotherapy regimens.[26***] See "Basic oral Care" section and Figure 117.3 for management strategies.[26***]

Oral bacterial infections

Cancer patients are disposed to oral bacterial infection due to impaired oral hygiene, development of oral mucositis, immunosuppression, and salivary gland hypofunction.

Bacterial infections of the periodontal tissues are characterized by erythema and edema of the marginal gingiva that becomes loosely attached and bleeds easily with toothbrushing or food intake. In a longer perspective, periodontitis can develop if the inflammation spreads deeper into the connective tissues supporting the tooth and patients may experience loosening of the teeth/tooth loss. Dental caries is a multifactorial disease also of infectious character; in particular, head and neck cancer patients suffering from hyposalivation are at high risk of rapidly progressive caries.[27***] Gingivitis, periodontitis, and dental caries are all associated with the accumulation of bacterial plaque on the teeth. Thus, prevention of oral bacterial infections aims at reducing the colonization of both normal and pathogenic bacteria (see "Basic Oral Care" section).[28] Furthermore, dental caries can be prevented by administration of high-dose fluorides (Figure 117.3).

Salivary glands may become acutely infected (bacterial sialadenitis), particularly in cancer patients suffering from low salivary flow rate as this allows for retrograde microbial colonization of the salivary gland duct. It is characterized by painful swelling of a single salivary gland, primarily the parotid, and a purulent discharge may be expressed from the duct orifice in conjunction with fever, malaise, and cervical lymphadenopathy.[29]

Undiagnosed or nontreated bacterial infections of the oral tissues may develop into additional severe complications (Figure 117.1 and "Oral mucositis" section). Dental periapical and periodontal infections increase the risk of osteomyelitis in the immunocompromised patient or osteoradionecrosis (ORN) in the irradiated head and neck cancer patient (see "Osteonecrosis" section). Special precaution regarding diagnosis of bacterial infections should be taken in the immunocompromised patient since the classical signs of inflammation/infection may be indistinct and bacteremia/sepsis can be a life-threatening complication. See "Basic Oral Care" section and Figure 117.3 for management strategies.[27***,28,29]

Dry mouth

Salivary gland hypofunction (reduced saliva flow rate) and xerostomia (subjective feeling of oral dryness) may be induced by cancer therapies including irradiation (i.e., irradiation in head and neck cancer, total body irradiation in hematopoietic stem cell transplantation, and radioactive iodine in thyroid cancer), cancer chemotherapy, and surgical trauma to salivary gland tissue. Xerostomia has been found to be the most common late adverse effect of radiation therapy in head and neck cancer patients. Irradiation of salivary glands manifests in a loss of saliva secretion within the first week of radiation treatment with a continuous decrease to barely measurable saliva flow rate. A second phase of deterioration may be noted up to 3 months after completion of radiation therapy, where after saliva secretion from spared gland tissue has the potential to gradually recover over time (e.g., within 1–2 years).[30]

Regarding chemotherapy, temporarily decreased saliva secretion and xerostomia have been reported in high- and moderate-dose chemotherapy for hematological malignancies and solid tumors, likely to resolve within 6 months to one year after treatment.[31] Comorbidities, daily intake of xerogenic medication (e.g., antiemetics, opioids, antihypertensives, diuretics, antidepressives), and dehydration may aggravate salivary gland hypofunction. Graft-versus-host disease (GVHD) is an autoimmune-like complication induced by the production of antibodies against the host of an allograft bone marrow transplant or peripheral blood stem cell transplant. GVHD may result in significantly decreased salivary flow rate and xerostomia.

Salivary gland hypofunction increases the risk of dental caries, dental erosion, mucosal trauma, oral candidosis, and mucosal soreness/pain. Oral functions may also be impaired, that is, speech, taste, chewing, and swallowing, and further manifested in inadequate food intake (Figure 117.1).

The management of salivary gland hypofunction and xerostomia induced by cancer therapies is symptomatic by stimulation of the residual secretory capacity of the salivary glands or by application of oral mucosal lubricants/saliva substitutes.[9***] See Figure 117.3 for management strategies.[9***]

Taste alterations

Taste alterations often occur with radiation therapy and chemotherapy and can appear as hypogeusia (reduction in taste sensation), dysgeusia (distorted taste sensation; e.g., bitter, metallic, salty or unpleasant), or hypergeusia (heightened taste sensation) (Figure 117.1).[32***] During radiation therapy of head and neck cancer, alteration of taste sensation initiates after 1 week of treatment and persists throughout the entire treatment period whereafter it resolves within a few months after radiation therapy.[33] Antineoplastic drugs are also associated with taste alterations that can be attributed to either a direct damage of the gustatory cells or the salivary secretion of the antineoplastic drug into the oral cavity.[34] The taste alterations induced by antineoplastic drugs usually resolve within a few months following the cancer treatment. However, some patients may experience that the taste alterations persists, which may be attributed to other aggravating factors: for example, salivary gland hypofunction, oral infections, poor oral hygiene, drug intake, zinc deficiency, gastrointestinal reflux, or damage to sensory taste nerves as sequelae from cancer surgery.[32***] See "Basic Oral Care" section and Figure 117.3 for management strategies.[32***]

Halitosis

Halitosis (oral malodor) in cancer patients may be due to impaired oral hygiene and consequently accumulation of microbial plaque on teeth, dorsum of the tongue, gingival crevices, and periodontal pockets.[35] Further aggravating factors are tumor growth/tissue necrosis, oral mucositis, oral infection, salivary gland hypofunction, and accumulation of food debris. See "Basic Oral Care" section and Figure 117.3 for management strategies.[36***] The etiology of halitosis may also be systemic, for example, lung infections, sinusitis, gastrointestinal disease, and hepatic or renal disease. Halitosis can largely be reduced by meticulous oral hygiene procedures.[36***]

Trismus

Trismus (severely restricted mouth opening) is frequent in head and neck cancer patients. Tumor growth into the temporomandibular joint/masticatory muscles and surgical procedures may be the cause. Radiation therapy may also cause trismus by inducing fibrosis of the temporomandibular joint or oral soft tissues. Radiation-induced trismus may begin by the end of the radiation schedule or any time following cancer treatment. The frequency and severity is somewhat unpredictable and may increase slowly over several months or the progression may arrest.[37] After radiation therapy of the head and neck region, mouth opening decreases by 18% on average compared to before cancer treatment.[38] Trismus may severely impact food intake, compromise oral hygiene, and cause difficulty in speaking.

Regarding management, it is of outmost importance to measure mouth opening regularly to evaluate the degree of trismus and to initiate exercise therapy to prevent it, although the evidence for effectiveness of exercise therapy is limited.[39] See Figure 117.3 for management strategies.[39***]

Osteonecrosis

Osteonecrosis is defined as "necrosis of bone due to obstruction of its blood supply." Osteonecrosis of the jaw (ONJ) can result from radiation therapy of the head and neck, long-term corticosteroid therapy, herpes zoster virus infection in immunocompromised patients, antiresorbative medications, uncontrolled infections, and major trauma; however, idiopathic cases can also occur. ONJ associated with antiresorptive therapy (ARONJ) deserves distinction from other causes.[40***,41***]

The risk of ORN is directly related to radiation dose and volume of tissue irradiated. The unilateral vascular supply to each half of the mandible results in postradiation ORN most frequently involving the mandible, compared with the maxilla. Presenting clinical features include pain, diminished or complete loss of sensation, fistula drainage, and infection.

Patients who have received high-dose radiation to the head and neck are at lifelong risk for ORN, with an overall risk of approximately 15%. Ideally, postradiation management of ORN is based on prevention that begins with comprehensive oral and dental care before radiation therapy. The following prevalence has been reported for ORN; conventional radiation therapy 7%, intensity-modulated radiation therapy 5%, chemoradiation therapy 7%, and brachytherapy 5%.[42***] See Figure 117.3 for management strategies.[42***]

Due to the high bone turnover rate in the jaws, bisphosphonates are particularly concentrated within the alveolar processes. Bisphosphonates remain in bone and their effect to decrease bone resorption markers can be detected many months later.[43,44] Unlike bisphosphonates, medications composed of human monoclonal antibodies (denosumab) do not become incorporated into bone.[45] This plays an important role in assessing long-term risk for ARONJ. Signs and symptoms of a bony event can mimic that of common oral and odontogenic conditions. Since invasive oral surgery is contraindicated in this situation, a misdiagnosis can lead to ONJ secondary to extraction.[41] See Figure 117.3 for management strategies.[40***,41***]

Key learning points

- A variety of oral complications of cancer therapies often appear concurrently, which complicates the differential diagnosis and management.

- Implementation of stringent basic oral care is of the outmost importance during cancer therapy.

- A multidisciplinary team, including dental professionals, is required to work closely with the patient in order to adequately assess, prevent, and treat oral complications of cancer therapy with a regular and systematic approach.

- Special precaution is needed for the immunocompromised patient since the classical signs of inflammation/infection may be vague and the development of bacteremia/sepsis can be a life-threatening complication.

REFERENCES

1   Dreizen S. Oral complications of cancer therapies. Description and incidence of oral complications. *NCI Monogr.* 1990; **9**: 11–15.

2   Brennan MT, Spijkervet FK, Elting LS. Systematic reviews and guidelines for oral complications of cancer therapies: Current challenges and future opportunities. *Support Care Cancer.* 2010; **18**: 977–978.

3   Raber-Durlacher JE, Brennan MT, Verdonck-de Leeuw IM et al. Swallowing dysfunction in cancer patients. *Support Care Cancer.* 2012; **20**: 433–443.

4   Sonis ST, Woods PD, White BA. Oral complications of cancer therapies. Pretreatment oral assessment. *NCI Monogr.* 1990; **9**: 29–32.

5   Epstein JB. Infection prevention in bone marrow transplantation and radiation patients. *NCI Monogr.* 1990; 73–85.

6   Stevenson-Moore P, Saunders D, Epstein J. Pretreatment screening and management. In: Davies AN, Epstein JB (eds). *Oral Complications of Cancer and its Management*, 1st edn. Oxford, U.K.: Oxford University Press, 2010: pp. 35–42.

◆ 7   Trotti A, Bellm LA, Epstein JB et al. Mucositis incidence, severity and associated outcomes in patients with head and neck cancer receiving radiotherapy with or without chemotherapy: A systematic literature review. *Radiother Oncol.* 2003; **66**: 253–262.

8   Sweeney P, Davies A. Oral hygiene. In: Davies AN, Epstein JB (eds). *Oral Complications of Cancer and its Management*, 1st edn. Oxford, U.K.: Oxford University Press, 2010: pp. 43–51.

◆ 9   Jensen SB, Pedersen AML, Vissink A et al. A systematic review of salivary gland hypofunction and xerostomia induced by cancer therapies: Management strategies and economic impact. *Support Care Cancer.* 2010; **18**: 1061–1079.

10   Schubert MM, Peterson DE. Oral complications of hematopoietic cell transplantation. In: Appelbaum FR, Forman SJ, Negrin RS, Blume KG (eds). *Thomas' Hematopoietic Cell Transplantation: Stem Cell Transplantation*, 4th edn. Oxford, U.K.: Wiley-Blackwell, 2009: pp. 1589–1607.

11   Meuser T, Pietruck C, Radbruch L et al. Symptoms during cancer pain treatment following WHO-guidelines: A longitudinal follow-up study of symptom prevalence, severity and etiology. *Pain.* 2001; **93**: 247–257.

12   Eisenberg E, Marinangeli F, Birkhahn J et al. Time to modify the WHO analgesic ladder? *Pain Clinical Updates.* 2005; **13**: 1–4.

◆ 13   Epstein JB, Hong C, Logan RM et al. A systematic review of orofacial pain in patients receiving cancer therapy. *Support Care Cancer.* 2010; **18**: 1023–1031.

◆ 14   Lalla RV, Bowen J, Barasch A et al; Mucositis Guidelines Leadership Group of the Multinational Association of Supportive Care in Cancer and International Society of Oral Oncology (MASCC/ISOO). MASCC/ISOO clinical practice guidelines for the management of mucositis secondary to cancer therapy. *Cancer.* 2014; **120**: 1453–1461.

◆ 15   Saunders DP, Epstein JB, Elad S et al; Mucositis Study Group of the Multinational Association of Supportive Care in Cancer/International Society of Oral Oncology (MASCC/ISOO). Systematic review of antimicrobials, mucosal coating agents, anesthetics, and analgesics for the management of oral mucositis in cancer patients. *Support Care Cancer.* 2013; **21**: 3191–3207.

16   Sonis ST. Oral mucositis. *Anticancer Drugs.* 2011; **22**: 607–612.

● 17   Sonis S, Treister N, Chawla S et al. Preliminary characterization of oral lesions associated with inhibitors of mammalian target of rapamycin in cancer patients. *Cancer.* 2010; **116**: 210–215.

18   Boers-Doets CB, Epstein JB, Raber-Durlacher JE et al. Oral adverse events associated with tyrosine kinase and mammalian target of rapamycin inhibitors in renal cell carcinoma: A structured literature review. *Oncologist.* 2012; **17**: 135–144.

19   Pilotte AP, Hohos MB, Polson KM et al. Managing stomatitis in patients treated with Mammalian target of rapamycin inhibitors. *Clin J Oncol Nurs.* 2011; **15**: E83–E89.

20   Epstein JB, Vickars L, Spinelli J, Reece D. Efficacy of chlorhexidine and nystatin rinses in prevention of oral complications in leukemia and bone marrow transplantation. *Oral Surg Oral Med Oral Pathol.* 1992; **73**: 682–689.

21   Epstein JB, Freilich MM, Le ND. Risk factors for oropharyngeal candidiasis in patients who receive radiation therapy for malignant conditions of the head and neck. *Oral Surg Oral Med Oral Pathol.* 1993; **76**: 169–174.

22   Nicolatou-Galitis O, Velegraki A, Sotiropoulou-Lontou A et al. Effect of fluconazole antifungal prophylaxis on oral mucositis in head and neck cancer patients receiving radiotherapy. *Support Care Cancer.* 2006; **14**: 44–51.

23   Terai H, Shimahara M. Tongue pain: Burning mouth syndrome vs Candida-associated lesion. *Oral Dis.* 2007; **13**: 440–442.

24   Sakashita S, Takayama K, Nishioka K, Katoh T. Taste disorders in healthy "carriers" and "non-carriers" of Candida albicans and in patients with candidosis of the tongue. *J Dermatol.* 2004; **31**: 890–897.

◆ 25   Lalla RV, Latortue MC, Hong CH et al. A systematic review of oral fungal infections in patients receiving cancer therapy. *Support Care Cancer.* 2010; **18**: 985–992.

◆ 26   Elad S, Zadik Y, Hewson I, et al. A systematic review of viral infections associated with oral involvement in cancer patients: A spotlight on Herpesviridea. *Support Care Cancer.* 2010; **18**: 993–1006.

◆ 27   Hong CH, Napenas JJ, Hodgson BD, et al. A systematic review of dental disease in patients undergoing cancer therapy. *Support Care Cancer.* 2010; **18**: 1007–1021.

28   Chow A. Oral bacterial infections. In: Davies AN, Epstein JB (eds). *Oral Complications of Cancer and its Management*, 1st edn. Oxford, U.K.: Oxford University Press, 2010: pp. 185–193.

29   Jensen SB, Pedersen AML, Nauntofte B. The causes of dry mouth: A broad panoply. Other causes of dry mouth: The list is endless. In: Sreebny LM, Vissink A (eds). *Dry Mouth—The Malevolent Symptom: A Clinical Guide*, 1st edn. Ames, IA: Wiley-Blackwell, 2010: pp. 158–181.

30 Vissink A, Mitchell JB, Baum BJ et al. Clinical management of salivary gland hypofunction and xerostomia in head and neck cancer patients: Successes and barriers. *Int J Radiat Oncol Biol Phys.* 2010; **78**: 983–991.

◆ 31 Jensen SB, Pedersen AML, Vissink A et al. A systematic review of salivary gland hypofunction and xerostomia induced by cancer therapies: Prevalence, severity and impact on quality of life. *Support Care Cancer.* 2010; **18**: 1039–1060.

◆ 32 Hovan AJ, Williams PM, Stevenson-Moore P et al. A systematic review of dysgeusia induced by cancer therapies. *Support Care Cancer.* 2010; **18**: 1081–1087.

33 Mossman K, Shatzman A, Chencharick J. Long-term effects of radiotherapy on taste and salivary function in man. *Int J Radiat Oncol Biol Phys.* 1982; **8**: 991–997.

34 Wickham RS, Rehwaldt M, Kefer C et al. Taste changes experienced by patients receiving chemotherapy. *Oncol Nurs Forum.* 1999; **26**: 697–706.

35 Porter SR, Scully C. Oral malodour (halitosis). *BMJ.* 2006; **333**: 632–635.

36 Scully C, Greenman J. Halitology (breath odour: aetiopathogenesis and management). *Oral Dis.* 2012; **18**: 333–345.

◆ 37 Bensadoun RJ, Riesenbeck D, Lockhart PB et al. A systematic review of trismus induced by cancer therapies in head and neck cancer patients. *Support Care Cancer.* 2010; **18**: 1033–1038.

38 Goldstein M, Maxymiw WG, Cummings BJ, Wood RE. The effects of antitumor irradiation on mandibular opening and mobility: A prospective study of 58 patients. *Oral Surg Oral Med Oral Pathol Oral Radiol Endod.* 1999; **88**: 365–373.

39 Dijkstra P, Roodenburg J. Trismus. In: Davies AN, Epstein JB (eds). *Oral Complications of Cancer and its Management*, 1st edn. Oxford, U.K.: Oxford University Press, 2010: pp. 99–116.

★ 40 Migliorati CA, Casiglia J, Epstein J et al. Managing the care of patients with bisphosphonate-associated osteonecrosis: An American Academy of Oral Medicine position paper. *J Am Dent Assoc.* 2005; **136**: 1658–1668.

41 Hellstein JW, Adler RA, Edwards B et al. Managing the care of patients receiving antiresorptive therapy for prevention and treatment of osteoporosis: Executive summary of recommendations from the American Dental Association Council on Scientific Affairs. *J Am Dent Assoc.* 2011; **142**: 1243–1251.

◆ 42 Peterson DE, Doerr W, Hovan A et al. Osteoradionecrosis in cancer patients: The evidence base for treatment-dependent frequency, current management strategies, and future studies. *Support Care Cancer.* 2010; **18**: 1089–1098.

43 Ravn P, Weiss SR, Rodriguez-Portales JA et al. Alendronate in early postmenopausal women: Effects on bone mass during long-term treatment and after withdrawal. Alendronate Osteoporosis Prevention Study Group. *J Clin Endocrinol Metab.* 2000; **85**: 1492–1497.

44 Johnson DA, Williams MI, Petkov VI, Adler RA. Zoledronic acid treatment of osteoporosis: Effects in men. *Endocr Pract.* 2010; **16**: 960–967.

45 Lewiecki EM. RANK ligand inhibition with denosumab for the management of osteoporosis. *Expert Opin Biol Ther.* 2006; **6**: 1041–1050.

118

Dermatologic side effects

JEN-YU WEI

INTRODUCTION

Survival rates in cancer have improved drastically over the last two decades with enhancements in treatment options for many types of malignancies. However, these treatments are accompanied by an array of dermatological and mucosal side effects that can negatively affect quality of life. Although these side effects are rarely life threatening, the symptoms can reduce a cancer patient's ability to tolerate treatment and may impact morbidity and mortality.

Skin problems in palliative cancer patients can be from a manifestation of metastatic malignancy, drug reactions to treatment, metabolic derangements caused by the neoplasm, infections, exacerbation of a previously existing skin condition, and nutritional disorder, or from paraneoplastic syndromes.

In this chapter, we will review the common dermatologic side effects associated with different modalities of nonsurgical cancer treatment and discuss the management of these side effects.

SYSTEMIC CHEMOTHERAPY

Effective management of mucocutaneous side effects of systemic cancer therapy requires the clinician to be knowledgeable about the common skin reactions associated with the drugs the patient is receiving. In certain instances, diagnosis may be difficult because the clinician must also be familiar with the cutaneous manifestations of certain cancers, as well as the dermatologic effects of other forms of cancer treatments.

The common types of toxicities seen in the skin, hair, nails, and mucous membranes from conventional systemic chemotherapeutic treatments and targeted therapies are discussed here.

Alopecia

Alopecia is the most common type of dermatologic complication associated with cancer treatment. It often has a negative emotional impact on patients receiving cancer treatment, even leading some patients to refuse treatment.[1] A wide range of cytotoxic agents can cause alopecia and most commonly affects scalp hair, although axillary and pubic hair and even the eyebrows and eyelashes may be lost as well. Cytotoxic agents attack rapidly dividing cells, including the hair matrix cells, and lead to hair loss from anagen effluvium or by thinning of the hair shaft that results in increased breakage.[2-4] The ability of individual agents to cause hair loss appears to be dependent upon the route, dose, and schedule of drug administration. Hair loss can occur soon after initiation of treatment, as is typically the case for high-dose regimens used in the setting of stem cell transplantation, or it may be gradually lost over a period of several weeks, as often occurs with the use of cyclic chemotherapy regimens.[3]

Chemotherapy-induced hair loss is usually completely reversible since the cytotoxic effects of the drugs do not destroy the ability of the stem cells that are responsible for hair regrowth. Hair follicles usually resume hair growth within weeks after completion of cancer treatment. It is not uncommon for new hair to take on different characteristics. Certain drugs such as methotrexate may induce hair hyperpigmentation, resulting in a darker hair color that alternates with normal hair color in bands, a feature known as the "flag sign."[4] Cyclophosphamide can also induce hair color changes.[5,6]

There are limited interventions for the prevention and management of chemotherapy-induced alopecia. Topical minoxidil and other biological agents, as well as techniques such as scalp tourniquet and scalp hypothermia intended to decrease drug delivery to the scalp hair bulbs, have been studied. However, there is lack of evidence on the efficacy of these interventions on the prevention and treatment of chemotherapy-induced alopecia.[2,7] Management of this side effect includes proper scalp and hair care. Reassurance should be provided, as permanent hair loss is rare.

NAIL CHANGES

Common chemotherapy-related nail effects include color changes, onycholysis, and inflammatory nail reactions. A common nonspecific nail finding associated with severe illness and treatment is Beau's lines (a horizontal depression in the nail plate that can occur in both the fingernails and toenails).[8] Nail hyperpigmentation is common and occurs more frequently in dark-skinned patients.[6] Treatment is primarily supportive and should include patient reassurance about the fact that these nail changes will dissipate after discontinuation of chemotherapy as new nails grow out. Nail changes are primarily a cosmetic issue in most cases. However, inflammatory nail changes such as acute exudative paronychia should be monitored closely, as these conditions can lead to subungual abscess formation.[9]

PIGMENTATION CHANGES

Chemotherapy-induced pigmentation changes can involve the hair, skin, nails, and mucous membranes. Common causative agents for this side effect include the alkylating agents and antitumor antibiotics.[6] The distribution of these skin changes can be localized or diffuse. Most of the pigmentation changes resolve with drug cessation, although some may be permanent. For example, cyclophosphamide-induced gingival margin hyperpigmentation is usually permanent.[6] Busulfan can induce a generalized darkening of the skin, causing what is known as the "busulfan tan," which can mimic Addison's disease.[10,11] Appropriate workup including laboratory investigations of adrenocorticotropic hormone (ACTH) and melanocyte-stimulating hormone (MSH) should be pursued to rule out adrenal insufficiency. Fluorouracil induced hyperpigmentation reaction that may be diffuse, local (in sun-exposed areas), serpentine, or mucosal (tongue and conjunctiva). Extrinsic factors such as occlusion with adhesive tape and trauma, combined with chemotherapy, can lead to localized hyperpigmentation. For example, 5-FU, thiotepa, ifosfamide, and docetaxel may cause skin pigmentary changes at the site where adhesive tape was applied.[6] Cisplatin, hydroxyurea, and bleomycin also cause skin color changes at sites of trauma or pressure.[6]

EXTRAVASATION INJURIES

Extravasation skin reaction occurs when a drug escapes into the extravascular space, either by leakage from a vessel or by direct infiltration, into the subcutaneous tissues.[12] Extravasation injuries are rare; some drugs cause benign reactions, while others can lead to devastating tissue injuries. Cytotoxic agents cause extravasation injuries via *irritant* and *vesicant* reaction. Irritant drugs cause inflammatory reaction, with aching, burning, tightness, pain, and phlebitis at the needle insertion site or along the veins. This type of reaction usually causes only a short period of discomfort for the patient without long-term sequelae. Vesicant cytotoxic drugs can cause tissue necrosis with a more severe and/or lasting injury in severe cases.[13–15] Prevention of this side effect by carefully choosing the site for drug administration is important.

When extravasation occurs, the drug infusion should be discontinued immediately. The use of antidotes, such as sodium bicarbonate, topical dimethylsulfoxide (DMSO), sodium thiosulfate, hyaluronidase, and corticosteroids, is controversial.[15,16]

HYPERSENSITIVITY REACTIONS

Almost all chemotherapeutic drugs can cause hypersensitivity reactions via type I, II, III, or IV immune-mediated allergy.[6,17] The platinum drugs (cisplatin, oxaliplatin, carboplatin) cause classic type I IgE-type reactions characterized by urticaria, pruritus, angioedema, and other symptoms of anaphylaxis post infusion. Taxane (paclitaxel, docetaxel)-related reactions are generally non–IgE mediated.[18] Premedication with antihistamines and corticosteroids appears to help decrease the frequency.[18] Skin testing may be useful for diagnosis and discontinuation of the causative drug in most cases is warranted.

PHOTOSENSITIVITY

A variety of chemotherapeutic drugs have been associated with increased sensitivity to ultraviolet (UV) light. This often presents as a sunburn-like eruption in sun-exposed areas characterized by pain, swelling, and erythema. Blistering may occur in severe cases. A large variety of chemotherapy agents can induce photosensitivity; the drugs that are well known to cause this side effect include dacarbazine, fluorouracil, tegafur, doxorubicin, and methotrexate.[6,9] Some of these eruptions may resolve with hyperpigmentation that may linger for months. The offending drug should be discontinued. Preventive measures such as wearing sunscreen and protective clothing, and avoiding sunlight, should be taken during treatment and for at least 2 weeks after cessation of drug.[6] Symptomatic management with cold compresses over the photosensitive area, along with topical steroids and systemic antihistamines, may decrease discomfort.[6]

ACRAL ERYTHEMA (HAND AND FOOT SYNDROME)

It is also known as palmar–plantar erythrodysesthesia. Many cytotoxic drugs can cause this effect, with most common offending agents being 5-FU, cytarabine, and pegylated liposomal doxorubicin.[6,9,19–21] Multitargeted tyrosine kinase (TK) inhibitors such as sorafenib and sunitinib that target angiogenesis are also associated with a high incidence of a hand–foot skin reaction.[38,40,41] It initially causes a tingling sensation in the palms and/or soles, followed by painful erythema in the palms, soles, and fingers. The affected areas eventually form blisters and desquamation follows. This syndrome can be a dose-limiting side effect for many chemotherapy drugs.

Management involves prevention of superinfection and pain management until resolution, which is typically within weeks after discontinuation of the drug.[20]

ORAL MUCOSITIS

Chemotherapy and/or radiation therapy can cause damage to the integrity and function of the epithelium lining the entire gastrointestinal tract. The oral cavity is most commonly affected, although it has the potential to affect the entire alimentary tract, leading to a range of symptoms to include oral ulcerations, dysphagia and odynophagia, gastritis, diarrhea, and malabsorption. Oral mucositis affects about 35%–40% of the patients receiving chemotherapy.[22–24] The severity of mucositis is affected by many factors, including patient tolerance and susceptibility and the drug, dose, and route and frequency of administration.[6] Almost all of the conventional chemotherapeutic drugs have the potential to cause oral mucositis, but the ones that are associated with high frequencies of oral mucositis include 5-FU, cytarabine, doxorubicin, capecitabine, bleomycin, etoposide, and methotrexate.[17] The existence of pretreatment dental disease is a risk factor for chemotherapy-induced oral mucositis. Younger patients also appear to be at greater risk for this toxicity perhaps due to higher mitotic oral epithelial activity.[25]

Oral cytotoxic effects from chemotherapy start shortly after the initiation of the drug regimen and peak around day 7 of therapy. Symptoms range from mild subjective soreness in the mouth with or without clinical findings to severe erosive mucositis characterized by ulcerations, intense pain, and oftentimes the inability to eat or drink. The World Health Organization and the National Cancer Institute both have mucositis grading scales incorporating both subjective and objective findings that are widely used. Severe, high-grade mucositis may necessitate dose reduction in drug therapy. Oral mucositis is self-limited; it usually resolves within 1–2 weeks after chemotherapy.

Superinfection with viral, fungal, or bacterial etiologies in chemotherapy-induced oral mucositis should not be missed; septicemia is a concern as the disrupted oral mucosal barrier serves as a source of entry for many pathogens.[25] Candida albicans is the most common organism that causes superinfection of chemo- and/or radiation-induced oral mucositis. Topical treatment with nystatin or clotrimazole is usually effective. Oral fluconazole should be used if the patient cannot tolerate topical therapy. Refractory candida infections may require parenteral antifungal treatment.

Reactivation of HSV may lead to a more severe and prolonged course of oral mucositis during chemotherapy. Vesicular lesions may not always be evident; diagnosis requires high level of suspicion in patients who presents with unusually severe symptoms and clinical findings on exam and acquisition of viral cultures. Treatment with parenteral or oral antiviral drugs should be started in patients with high symptom burden who are HSV-1 seropositive while viral cultures are pending. HSV-1 seropositive patients undergoing induction chemotherapy or those who are receiving high-dose chemotherapy after hematopoietic cell transplants should be given prophylactic antivirals because these treatments are associated with high HSV-1 reactivation rates.[26]

Good dental oral and dental hygiene should be maintained during treatment with cytotoxic agents with oral toxicities. The use of mouth rinses containing supersaturated calcium phosphate is widely popular, but currently there is conflicting evidence to support its use in clinical practice for the treatment of oral mucositis.[27–30] Chlorhexidine mouth rinses are also widely used, but the efficacy of this intervention is uncertain.[31,32] Diluted hydrogen peroxide could also be used with for debridement; it should be used with caution because overuse may delay healing. Povidone-iodine, NaCl 0.9%, water salt soda solution, and chamomile mouthwash also show conflicting results in terms of their efficacy.[33] Granulocyte/macrophage colony-stimulating factor (GM-CSF) has not been shown to have significant benefit in preventing mucositis. Topical lidocaine is frequently used in combination with a coating or cleansing agent. Systemic opioids may be required for severe pain associated with oral mucositis.

TARGETED THERAPIES

Collectively, antineoplastic drugs that target the molecular abnormalities in certain cancers are known as targeted therapies. This class of drugs includes epidermal growth factor receptor (EGFR) inhibitors, small-molecule TK inhibitors, and other monoclonal antibodies that target molecules other than EGFR.

Papulopustular (acneiform) eruption is the most common cutaneous complications in patients receiving EGFR inhibitors.[34–37] These skin lesions typically erupt during the first week of treatment over the face, chest, and extremities, sparing the palms and soles. The presence of these skin changes does not warrant discontinuation of therapy. Patients should be monitored for secondary skin infections. Associated symptoms such as pain and pruritus should be treated to improve quality of life. There is a paucity of data on treatment options for this EGFR-inhibitor-induced side effect; mild skin care and photoprotection is recommended.[13,37–40]

In addition to skin rashes, anti-EGFR drugs commonly cause paronychial inflammation. Secondary infections of these nail changes are common; antiseptic creams and drying pastes have been reported to be useful to prevent infection of the nail fold.[13,40] Other treatment options include topical or intralesional corticosteroids, oral antibiotics, and/or electrodessication for larger lesions.[40]

TK inhibitors exert their antineoplastic activity on kinase pathways. Common skin reactions include exanthematous papular lesions, especially with imatinib, which is widely used in the treatment for a variety of tumor types.

Other mucocutaneous reactions from targeted therapies include hand–foot syndrome, oral mucositis, xerosis, pruritus, alopecia, and other types of hair changes.[37,40-45]

RADIATION-ASSOCIATED DERMATOLOGIC TOXICITIES

There are two types of radiation-related skin toxicities, including radiation recall and radiation enhancement. In both types of radiation-induced skin toxicities, the skin changes are characterized by painful erythema, swelling, and desquamation. In severe cases, affected areas may exhibit ulcerations and even tissue necrosis.

Radiation recall dermatitis affects previously irradiated areas, occurring most commonly with chemotherapy. Many drugs have been associated with this side effect, particularly the antitumor antibiotics.[46] The interval between drug administration and presentation of radiation recall dermatitis is variable. Management should include symptom control such as treating pain with analgesic medications and prevention of secondary infections. Avoidance of irritants, UV light, and trauma should be recommended.

Radiation enhancement injury occurs when a radiation-sensitizing chemotherapeutic drug is given together or within 1 week of radiation treatment. Management is similar to that for radiation recall dermatitis.

A wide variety of topical agents are used in clinical practice for the prevention and management of radiation-induced skin reactions. Some of the common remedies include topical corticosteroids, hyaluronic acid, sucralfate, calendula, Cavilon cream (3M, St. Paul, Minnesota), and silver leaf dressing. Currently, there is lack of evidence to support the benefits of topical agents in clinical practice.[47,48]

CONCLUSION

Dermatologic skin reactions associated with cancer treatment are rarely life threatening. Moreover, the majority of these side effects are self-limited and short-lived. However, these side effects can have a major impact on quality of life. Accurate diagnosis and appropriate management of these skin conditions and their associated symptoms is pertinent, as this can greatly improve the cancer patient's physical and emotional well-being.

REFERENCES

1   Hesketh PJ, Batchelor D, Golant M et al. Chemotherapy-induced alopecia: Psychosocial impact and therapeutic approaches. *Support Care Cancer* August 2004;12(8):543–549.

2   Chon SY, Champion RW, Geddes ER et al. Chemotherapy-induced alopecia. *J Am Acad Dermatol* July 2012;67(1):e37–e47.

3   Dorr VJ. A practitioner's guide to cancer-related alopecia. *Semin Oncol* 1998;25(5):562.

4   Wheeland RG, Burgdorf WH, Humphrey GB. The flag sign of chemotherapy. *Cancer* 1983;51(8):1356.

5   Ramot Y, Sinclair RD, Zlotogorski A. Regrowth of black hair in two red-haired alopecia areata patients. *Australas J Dermatol* November 2013;53(4):e91–e92.

6   Susser WS, Whitaker-Worth DL, Grant-Kels JM. Mucocutaneous reactions to chemotherapy. *J Am Acad Dermatol* March 1999;40(3):367–398.

7   Trueb RM. Chemotherapy-induced alopecia. *Curr Opin Support Palliat Care* December 2010;4(4):281–284.

8   Dreno B. Mucocutaneous side effects of chemotherapy. *Biomed Pharmacother* 1990;44(3):163–167.

9   Payne AS, James WD, Weiss RB. Dermatologic toxicity of chemotherapeutic agents. *Semin Oncol* 2006;33(1):86.

10 Harrold BP. Syndrome resembling Addison's disease following prolonged treatment with Busulphan. *Br Med J* February 19, 1966;1(5485):463–464.

11 Sprunt JG, Rizza CR. Pigmentation and busulphan therapy. *Br Med J* March 1966;1(5489):736–737.

12 Fischer D, Knobf M, Durivage H. *The Cancer Therapy Handbook*. St. Louis, MO: Mosby;1991;Vol. 7:pp. 43–47.

13 Langer SW. Extravasation of chemotherapy. *Curr Oncol Rep* 2010;12(4):242–246.

14 Hahn JC, Shaftritz AB. Chemotherapy extravasation injuries. *J Hand Surg Am* February 2012;37(2):360–362.

15 Schulmeister L. Extravasation management: Clinical update. *Semin Oncol Nurs* February 2011;27(1):82–90.

16 Wengstrom Y, Margulie A, European Oncology Nursing Society Task Force. European Oncology Nursing Society extravasation guidelines. *Eur J Oncol Nurs* September 2008;12(4):357–361.

17 Huang V, Anadkat M. Dermatologic manifestations of cytotoxic therapy. *Dermatol Ther* July–August 2011;24(4):401–410.

18 Lee C, Gianos M, Klaustermeyer WB. Diagnosis and management of hypersensitivity reactions to chemotherapy agents. *Ann Allergy Asthma Immunol* 2009;102(3):179–187; quiz 187–189, 222.

19 Baack BR, Burgdorf WH. Chemotherapy-induced acral erythema. *J Am Acad Dermatol* March 1991;24(3):457–461.

20 Degen A, Alter M, Schenck F et al. The hand-foot-syndrome associated with medical tumor therapy—Classification and management. *J Dtsch Dermatol Ges* September 2010;8(9):652–661. Epub May 6, 2010.

21 Farr KP, Safwat A. Palmar-plantar erythrodysesthesia associated with chemotherapy and its treatment. *Case Rep Oncol* 2011;4(1):229–235. Epub April 11, 2011.

22 Sonis ST. The pathobiology of mucositis. *Nat Rev Cancer* 2004;4(4):277.

23 Sonis ST, Elting LS, Keefe D et al. Perspectives on cancer therapy-induced mucosal injury: Pathogenesis, measurement, epidemiology, and consequences for patients. *Cancer* 2004;100(9 Suppl):1995.

24 Keefe DM, Schubert MM, Elting LS et al. Updated clinical practice guidelines for the prevention and treatment of mucositis. *Cancer* 2007;109(5):820.

25 Sonis ST, Sonis AL, Lieberman A. Oral complications in patients receiving treatment for malignancies other than of the head and neck. *J Am Dent Assoc* 1978;97 (3):468.

26 Whitley RJ, Gnann JW Jr. Acyclovir: A decade later. *N Engl J Med* 1992;327(11):782.

27 Lembrecht M, Mercier C, Geussens Y et al. The effect of a supersaturated calcium phosphate mouth rinse on the development of oral mucositis on head and neck cancer patients treated with (chemo)radiation: A single-center, randomized, prospective study of a calcium phosphate mouth rinse + standard of care versus standard of care. *Support Care Cancer* Epub May 18, 2013.

28 Papas AS, Clark RE, Martuscelli G et al. A prospective, randomized trial for the prevention of mucositis in patients undergoing hematopoietic stem cell transplantation. *Bone Marrow Transplant* 2003;31(8):705.

29 Markiewicz M, Dzierzak-Mietla M, Frankiewicz A et al. Treating oral mucositis with a supersaturated calcium phosphate rinse: Comparison with control in patients undergoing allogeneic hematopoietic stem cell transplantation. *Support Care Cancer* September 2012;20(9):2223–2239. Epub June 27, 2012.

30 Clarkson JE, Worthington HV, Furness S et al. Interventions for treating oral mucositis for patients with cancer receiving treatment. *Cochrane Database Syst Rev* August 4, 2010;(8):CD001973.

31 Ferretti GA, Ash RC, Brown AT et al. Control of oral mucositis and candidiasis in marrow transplantation: A prospective, double-blind trial of chlorhexidine digluconate oral rinse. *Bone Marrow Transplant* 1988;3(5):483.

32 Sorensen JB, Skovsgaard T, Bork E et al. Double-blind, placebo-controlled, randomized study of chlorhexidine prophylaxis for 5-fluorouracil-based chemotherapy-induced oral mucositis with nonblinded randomized comparison to oral cooling (cryotherapy) in gastrointestinal malignancies. *Cancer* 2008;112(7):1600.

33 Potting CM, Uitterhoeve R, Op Reimer WS et al. The effectiveness of commonly used mouthwashes for the prevention of chemotherapy-induced oral mucositis: A systematic review. *Eur J Cancer Care (Engl)* December 2006;15(5):431–439.

34 Fabbrocini G, Cameli N, Romano MC et al. Chemotherapy and skin reactions. *J Exp Clin Cancer Res* May 28, 2012;31:50.

35 Dreno B, Bensadoun RJ, Humbert P et al. Algorithm for dermocosmetic use in the management of cutaneous side-effects associated with targeted therapy in oncology. *J Eur Acad Dermatol Venereol* February 1, 2013.

36 Jacot W, Bessis D, Jorda E et al. Acneiform eruption induced by epidermal growth factor receptor inhibitors in patients with solid tumours. *Br J Dermatol* 2004;151(1):238.

37 Balagula Y, Garbe C, Myskowski PL et al. Clinical presentation and management of dermatological toxicities of epidermal growth factor receptor inhibitors. *Int J Dermatol* February 2011;50(2):129–146.

38 Gridell C, Malone P, Amoroso D et al. Clinical significance and treatment of skin rash from erlotinib in non-small cell lung cancer patients: Results of an Experts Panel Meeting. *Crit Rev Oncol Hematol* May 2008;66(2):155–162.

39 Grande R, Narducci F, Bianchetti S et al. Pre-emptive skin toxicity treatment for anti-EGFR drugs: Evaluation of efficacy of skin moisturizers and lymecycline. A phase II study. *Support Care Cancer* June 2013;21(6):1691–1695. Epub January 13, 2013.

40 Wu PA, Balagula Y, Lacouture ME, Anadkat MJ. Prophylaxis and treatment of dermatologic adverse events from epidermal growth factor receptor inhibitors. *Curr Opin Oncol* July 2011;23(4):343–351.

41 Van Doorn R, Kirtschig G, Scheffer E et al. Follicular and epidermal alterations in patients treated with ZD1839 (Iressa), an inhibitor of the epidermal growth factor receptor. *Br J Dermatol* 2002;147(3):598.

42 Lipworth AD, Robert C, Zhu AX. Hand-foot syndrome (hand-foot skin reaction, palmar-plantar erythrodysesthesia): Focus on sorafenib and sunitinib. *Oncology* 2009;77(5):257–271. Epub November 16, 2009.

43 Papaetis GS, Syrigos KN. Sunitinib: A multitargeted receptor tyrosine kinase inhibitor in the era of molecular cancer therapies. *BioDrugs* 2009;23(6):377–389.

44 Lacouture ME, Reilly LM, Gerami P et al. Hand foot skin reaction in cancer patients treated with the multikinase inhibitors sorafenib and sunitinib. *Ann Oncol* 2008;19(11):1955.

45 Chu D, Lacouture ME, Fillos T et al. Risk of hand-foot skin reaction with sorafenib: A systematic review and meta-analysis. *Acta Oncol* 2008;47(2):176.

46 Camidge R, Price A. Characterizing the phenomenon of radiation recall dermatitis. *Radiother Oncol* 2001;59(3):237.

47 Kumar S, Juresic E, Barton M et al. Management of skin toxicity during radiation therapy: A review of the evidence. *J Med Imaging Radiat Oncol* June 2010;54(3):264–279.

48 Zhang Y, Zhang S, Shao X. Topical agent therapy for prevention and treatment of radiodermatitis: A meta-analysis. *Support Care Cancer* April 2013;21(4):1025–1031.

119

Peripheral neuropathy and neurotoxicity

IVO W. TREMONT-LUKATS, PEDRO GARCIARENA

WHY IS THIS TOPIC IMPORTANT?

The toxicity of drugs on the peripheral nervous system (PNS) is a huge problem for many persons treated with chemotherapy. Patients may be weak, dropping objects, or stumbling and falling; they may not feel touch, pain, temperature, or other sensory modalities; or if they do, sensation is abnormal and many times painful. Damage includes not only sensory and motor fibers but autonomic pathways as well, affecting orthostasis, sweating, skin trophy, peristalsis, urination, and sexual function. The severity of symptoms often will force the treating physician to reduce the dose or to stop the offending drug, compromising any potential therapeutic benefit. With this burden, the performance status (PS) of many of these patients declines, depression and anxiety increase, and all wonder what is worse, the remedy or the disease.

In the following sections, we will present the tools necessary to understand and approach this problem, aiming at helping these patients recover as much and as soon as possible. Although many neurologists prefer the term polyneuropathy, throughout the text, the keyword peripheral neuropathy will have the same meaning. Because chemotherapy triggers this condition, a common term in the literature is chemotherapy-induced peripheral neuropathy (CIPN). CIPN is a common, underdiagnosed, underreported, and undertreated problem in cancer patients. CIPN can interfere with activities of daily living (ADLs), with a negative effect on quality of life (QoL). Patients with CIPN cost more to treat (approximately $18,000 on average, in 2012) and use more resources (outpatient visits and hospital days) than patients without CIPN [1]. The causative drugs, the pattern, and the time course are known but our knowledge about the pathophysiology, the long-term prognosis, and how best to prevent and treat CIPN is a work in progress.

LINK BETWEEN CHEMOTHERAPY AND PERIPHERAL NERVE

The chemotherapy drugs that cause CIPN are too large to penetrate an intact blood–brain barrier. A variant of this barrier in the PNS, the blood–nerve barrier, is permeable to these molecules, which accumulate and bind to axons and dorsal root ganglion (DRG) cells (Figure 119.1). The result is damage of microtubules, interference with axonal transport, and mitochondrial death. Current research points to a contributory role of cytokines (IL-6 and IL-8) and the matrix metalloproteinases MMP2, MMP3, and MMP24 in the pathogenesis of peripheral nerve injury by chemotherapy [2]. There is also evidence from animal models of paclitaxel-induced neuropathy that the reactive oxygen species superoxide radical O_2^- and hydroxyl radical OH^-, by-products of the mitochondrial oxidative phosphorylation, are key mediators in neuropathic pain [3]. Although myelin can be a target of chemotherapy drugs, it seems this is more a consequence of the axonal damage than a direct attack on Schwann cells [4].

ONCE UPON A TIME

Cisplatin and vincristine were for years the classic references of neurotoxic drugs. The list has grown and now includes other cytotoxic drugs (Tables 119.1 and 119.2). With the exception of oxaliplatin, all these agents cause a similar pattern of injury and clinical course, with subtle differences helpful to remember in the neurological evaluation of these patients. There are covariates that dictate how soon CIPN can start, how severe it can be, and how difficult it is to recover: Age, preexisting neuropathies (e.g., diabetes and hereditary motor sensory neuropathies), nutritional status, and PS (Figure 119.2).

WHAT IS IMPORTANT IN THE ASSESSMENT OF CIPN?

A clinical evaluation that determines what symptoms, location, severity, onset, time course, concomitants, and aggravating and attenuating factors will lead us to the severity of damage, that is, what ADLs are affected by CIPN. A neurological exam will only corroborate this assessment. We can diagnose this condition without any of the scales used to diagnose and grade CINP in clinical trials. For illustration purposes,

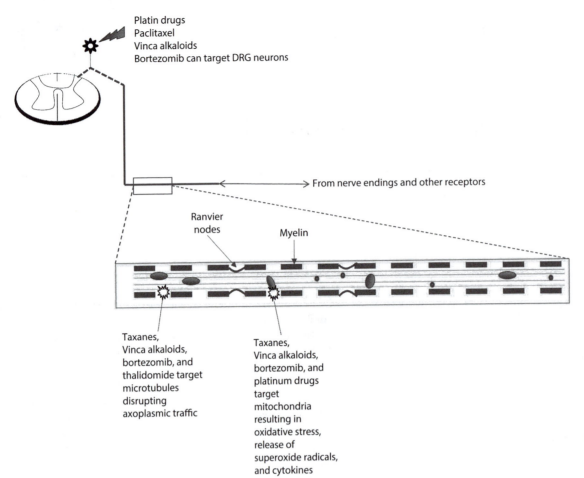

Platin drugs
Paclitaxel
Vinca alkaloids
Bortezomib can target DRG neurons

From nerve endings and other receptors

Ranvier nodes

Myelin

Taxanes, Vinca alkaloids, bortezomib, and thalidomide target microtubules disrupting axoplasmic traffic

Taxanes, Vinca alkaloids, bortezomib, and platinum drugs target mitochondria resulting in oxidative stress, release of superoxide radicals, and cytokines

Figure 119.1 *The link between chemotherapy and peripheral nerve.*

Table 119.3 shows the Common Toxicity Criteria for Adverse Effects (CTCAE) in its latest version as an example of such scales. However, there is nothing wrong in using these tools, especially those that deal with QoL and ADLs like the Patient Neuropathy Questionnaire (PNQ) [5] and the Chemotherapy Induced Neurotoxicity Questionnaire (CINQ) [6]. Nerve conduction velocity studies, electromyography, and quantitative sensory tests are not helpful in the diagnosis and management of CIPN, because of inconsistency, low correlation, and low acceptance rates of patients to undergo some of these tests. The nerve biopsy could be useful in excluding other conditions, but it does not add anything in CIPN.

CIPN IS EQUAL TO AXONOPATHY, NEURONOPATHY, OR BOTH

We have found useful in clinical practice the diagnostic classification of CIPN discussed by Hausheer and others [5]. Patients with axonal injury (*axonopathy*) present with the typical, well-known pattern of length-dependent, sensorimotor polyneuropathy. The initial location is in the toes and feet with proximal progression to include hands and more proximal segments in some cases. The onset is subacute and gradual, and the progression is predictable. *It is the most common presentation of CIPN.*

Neuronopathy is the result of direct damage to DRG cells. Patients with neuronopathy also have a pattern of length-dependent sensorimotor polyneuropathy with a more rapid onset and deterioration. Symptoms can start simultaneously or almost in feet and hands and may involve also cranial nerves. There is diffuse loss of deep-tendon reflexes. There is no anatomic progression like in axonopathy; it is not gradual but persistent and permanent because the damage to DRG cells is irreversible. Weakness is mild, if it is present. *When motor symptoms and findings predominate or coexist with sensory symptoms, it is not a neuronopathy, and probably it is not even CIPN.*

PREVENTION OF CIPN

Prevention is the best strategy against CIPN, but until now there is no intervention convincingly effective to prevent it. Vitamin E, intravenous infusions of calcium and magnesium, glutathione, glutamine, *N*-acetylcysteine, oxcarbazepine, amifostine, and xaliproden have been tested with conflicting results, as others have reviewed [7,8]. A Cochrane systemic review of interventions for preventing neuropathy by cisplatin and other platin compounds concluded that "At present, the data are insufficient to conclude that any of the

Table 119.1 *Classic chemotherapy drugs that can cause CINP[a,c]*

Family (member drugs)	Pathophysiology	Clinical course	Type of neuropathy	Recovery
Platinum (cisplatin, carboplatin, oxaliplatin)	Unclear. Disruption of axonal transport with intact myelin; direct cytotoxic damage to DRG cells also possible	*Onset*: Between cycles 1–6. Mostly gradual but it can be rapid if DRG cells are affected. Oxaliplatin may have two distinct phases: one is acute, transient, and exacerbated by cold (85%–95% of patients); the other is chronic, persistent paresthesias (16%–20% of patients). *Symptoms*: sensory. Weakness, Lhermitte phenomenon, and dysautonomia are much less frequent. Patients treated with oxaliplatin characteristically have perioral or pharyngeal paresthesias, dysphagia, and myotonia. Hypo- or areflexia. *Location*: Symmetric, stocking-glove pattern. May improve if drug is stopped but can worsen for 3–4 more months before stabilization.	Axonal for most cases; neuronopathy due to direct damage of DRG cells in others	80% of those treated with cisplatin and carboplatin may recover within 8 months. Oxaliplatin, 80% probability of improvement within 4–6 months; 50% of patients improve within 13 weeks of stopping the drug.
Taxanes (paclitaxel, docetaxel, cabazitaxel, and nanoparticle albumin formulation of paclitaxel Abraxane®)	Unclear. Disruption of axoplasmic traffic; direct damage to DRG cell	*Onset*: Within 24–72 h of administration. Toxicity is dose cumulative, with no differences in dosing schedules. Four times more likely with paclitaxel than docetaxel. Probability of neuropathy: 60%–80%. Symptoms can disappear spontaneously after stopping the drug. *Symptoms*: Similar to cisplatin; predominantly sensory; motor and autonomic less frequent. *Location*: Similar to cisplatin.	Axonal. Similar to cisplatin	Reversible, but timing is variable (weeks to months). The probability of recovery with docetaxel seems higher than for paclitaxel (>90%). Total recovery only possible for a minority (about 15%), but most others report only mild symptoms with no disruption of ADLs [12].
Vinca alkaloids (vincristine, vinorelbine, vinblastine)	Disruption of axonal flow	*Onset*: Probability of CIPN with vinblastine or vinorelbine is much lower than vincristine. Cumulative dose is proportional to risk of CIPN (6–8 mg of total dose). Probability is highest 2–3 weeks after injection. Severe weakness before reaching this threshold should alert to subclinical, preexisting neuropathy. *Course*: Mostly subacute onset but gradual course. *Symptoms*: Paresthesias, similar to cisplatin and taxanes; motor symptoms are more frequent; patients have weakness of foot and hand extensors. Ankle areflexia is an early sign of neuropathy. Dysautonomia and mononeuropathies can also occur. *Location*: Similar to cisplatin and taxanes.	Axonal	Partial or complete 1–3 months after end of treatment. Some patients do not recover.
Miscellaneous (etoposide, Ara-C, procarbazine, gemcitabine)[b]	Unknown	*Onset*: Gradual. *Course*: Slowly progressive. *Symptoms*: Similar to cisplatin and others *Location*: Similar to cisplatin.	Unknown	Recovery is possible, but very little is known.

CINP, chemotherapy-induced neuropathy; DRG, dorsal root ganglion.

[a] This table is a schematic outline trying to synthesize information. It is not a substitute for detailed, thorough descriptions or reviews on this topic. Most quantitative data are estimates but are valid data for clinicians to use in assessments and decision making.

[b] The probability of CIPN with these drugs is low, but there have been case reports in the literature linking these drugs to CIPN [13,14]. It is very difficult to attribute CIPN to etoposide or gemcitabine since both are mostly used in combination with well-known neurotoxic drugs.

[c] In our clinical experience, there are always outliers that do not fit conventional descriptions. We have seen patients with bilateral but asymmetric sensory symptoms, with or without concurrent weakness. Those patients with motor symptoms and signs only or as a predominant feature have other conditions that need to be identified for proper management; in this respect, we agree with others [5].

Table 119.2   *Other chemotherapy drugs that cause CIPN*

Family (drug members)	Pathophysiology	Clinical course	Type of neuropathy	Recovery
Antiangiogenic (thalidomide)	Unknown. Probably axonal injury	Slow, generally after months of treatment. Overall probability of neuropathy: 30%. Risk is higher if treatment lasts longer. No clear dose-cumulative effect. Paresthesias in hands and feet can be painful; sometimes symptoms appear after drug is stopped.	Sensorimotor, axonal, length-dependent neuropathy.	Expected partial or total recovery in up to 50% of patients.
Proteasome inhibitors (bortezomib)	Unknown	Gradual, progressive onset. Probability of neuropathy: 40%. Sensory symptoms, paresthesias, neuropathic pain. Minor weakness possible. Dose reductions or interruptions can improve or resolve symptoms.	Similar to thalidomide.	Resolution or improvement of symptoms in 70% of patients, after a median time of 1.5 months.
Epothilones (ixabepilone)	Unknown	Symptoms can appear after first treatment, with gradual course. paresthesias are common; some patients can have autonomic symptoms. Probability of grade 3–4 neuropathy: up to 24%.	Sensory polyneuropathy, not well characterized yet.	Improvement and resolution of symptoms possible after dose adjustments or discontinuation of the drug within a median of 1.5 months.
Halichondrin B analogues (eribulin mesylate)	Unknown	Overall probability of CIPN: 35% seen in phase III studies.	Sensory polyneuropathy. It has not been studied well yet.	Possible after dose reduction or interruption.
Purine nucleoside analogues (nelarabine)	Unknown	Neurotoxicity is dose limiting. Probability of developing neuropathy: 21%. Patients report paresthesias, neuropathic pain in limbs, and sensory ataxia [15,16].	Not studied.	Recovery is possible once the drug is stopped. For safety, nelarabine should be stopped if patients develop grade 2 or higher neuropathy.

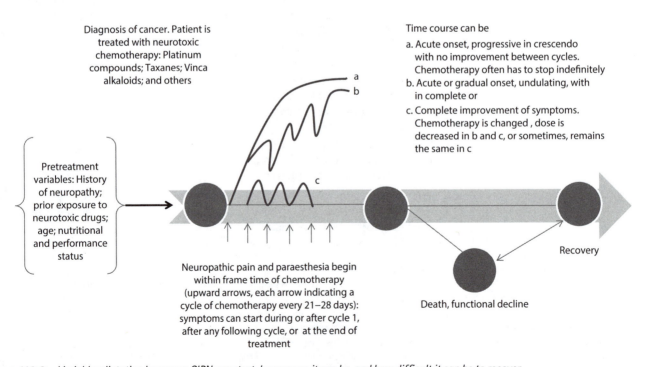

Figure 119.2   *Variables dictating how soon CIPN can start, how severe it can be, and how difficult it can be to recover.*

Table 119.3   *National Cancer Institute (NCI) CTCAE v.4.03*

Neuropathy	Grade 1	Grade 2	Grade 3	Grade 4	Grade 5
Sensory	Asymptomatic; loss of DTRs or paresthesias[a]	Paresthesias, moderate intensity, limiting instrumental ADL	Severe symptoms, limiting self-care ADL	Life-threatening consequences; urgent intervention indicated	Death
Motor	Asymptomatic; clinical or diagnostic observations only. Interventions not indicated	Moderate symptoms, limiting instrumental ADL	Severe symptoms; limiting self-care ADL	Life-threatening consequences; urgent intervention indicated	Death

DTR, deep-tendon reflexes; ADLs, activities of daily living.

[a] A liberal interpretation here is that in grade 1 neuropathy, patients can have paresthesias and therefore they are no longer asymptomatic. However, the intensity is mild and there is no interference at all with ADL.

purported chemoprotective agents (acetylcysteine, amifostine, calcium and magnesium, diethyldithiocarbamate, glutathione, Org 2766, oxcarbazepine, or Vitamin E) prevent or limit the neurotoxicity of platin drugs among human patients" [9]. Therefore, we do not recommend any of these drugs for prevention until adequate and more definitive data are available.

TREATMENT OF CIPN

The treatment of CIPN is symptomatic. The best intervention currently is to change to a different chemotherapy drug or to stop the drug until satisfactory improvement or resolution with reintroduction using a lower dose level. It is possible to relieve pain using any of the drugs listed in Table 119.4.

Table 119.4   *Drugs for pain in CIPN*

Drug class	Starting dose	How to titrate	Max dose	Comments
Tricyclics (amitriptyline, nortriptyline, desipramine)	25 mg at bedtime.	By 25 mg or less every week as tolerated.	150–175 mg daily.	May need to start with 10 mg daily in patients 60 years or older.
SSNRI (duloxetine, venlafaxine)	30 mg daily (duloxetine); 75 mg once daily (venlafaxine).	Increase by 30 mg each week.	60 mg twice daily (duloxetine); 150 mg daily (venlafaxine). Higher doses are ineffective.	Nausea and anticholinergic effects can limit treatment success or satisfaction.
Calcium channel α-2-δ ligands (gabapentin, pregabalin)	100 mg three times daily; 300 mg three times daily in younger patients (gabapentin); 50 mg three times daily or 75 mg twice daily (pregabalin).	Gabapentin: Increase by 300 mg every week; pregabalin: Increase by 75 mg weekly.	Gabapentin: 3600 mg daily. Higher doses do not benefit; pregabalin: 600 mg daily in two or three divided doses.	Dizziness, somnolence, and weight gain are limiting side effects.
Local anesthetics (lidocaine)	5% topical lidocaine as a transdermal patch q12h for 12h daily.	No titration.	—	IV lidocaine is used very little in clinical practice (cumbersome; requires cardiac monitoring), despite good evidence of efficacy [17].
Opioids (morphine, hydromorphone; oxycodone; methadone)	7.5–30 mg morphine orally every 4 hours around the clock, with 10% of total daily dose given as needed every 2 hours; use conversion doses for other opioids.	Titration is possible every 24–48 hours; follow specific titration and conversion guidelines.	There is no maximum dose; patients have different dose requirements.	Use with stool softeners and antiemetic. Opioid switch is a good strategy to circumvent adverse effects. Avoid meperidine. Patients with renal failure have less risk of toxicity with hydromorphone and methadone.
Synthetic opioids (tramadol)	50 mg orally once to three times daily.	Increase by 50 mg weekly or more frequently as tolerated.	100 mg orally up to four times daily.	Good evidence that it is effective to treat neuropathic pain [18].

SSNRI, selective serotonin and noradrenergic reuptake inhibitors.

Some patients require more than one drug. Unfortunately, symptoms like numbness can still be distressing and they do not respond to any treatment. One of the drugs most often used to treat CIPN is gabapentin, although a double-masked, placebo-controlled study with random allocation found gabapentin was no better than placebo [10]. Of all drugs listed in Table 119.4, the best evidence has come from a small double-blinded, placebo-controlled trial with random allocation of venlafaxine to prevent and treat oxaliplatin-induced acute neurotoxicity, the EFFOX trial [11]. This study was a hybrid of prevention and treatment; 24 patients allocated to the treatment group took 50 mg of venlafaxine 24 hours before the first dose of oxaliplatin and then 37.5 mg twice daily of extended-release venlafaxine from days 2 through 11 of every cycle. The placebo group, 24 patients, was treated identically with placebo. Patients treated with venlafaxine had more relief from cold-triggered pain, worst daily pain, and pins-and-needles symptoms and a less decline in ADL than patients treated with placebo. More patients in the venlafaxine arm reported a greater than 50% relief in pain (69%), compared with placebo (26%, P = 0.02). Also, 31% of patients treated with venlafaxine had complete relief of acute neurotoxicity versus 5.3% in the control group (P = 0.03). The study was closed early due to low accrual rate and the expiration of the study drug. Despite such drawbacks, these data are encouraging, and in the future, other trials could test the effectiveness of venlafaxine for CINP.

REFERENCES

1 Pike CT, Birnbaum HG, Muehlenbein CE, Pohl GM, Natale RB. Healthcare costs and workloss burden of patients with chemotherapy-associated peripheral neuropathy in breast, ovarian, head and neck, and nonsmall cell lung cancer. *Chemotherapy Research and Practice* 2012;2012:913848.
2 Wang XM, Lehky TJ, Brell JM, Dorsey SG. Discovering cytokines as targets for chemotherapy-induced painful peripheral neuropathy. *Cytokine* 2012;59(1):3–9.
3 Fidanboylu M, Griffiths LA, Flatters SJ. Global inhibition of reactive oxygen species (ROS) inhibits paclitaxel-induced painful peripheral neuropathy. *PLoS One* 2011;6(9):e25212. Epub 2011 Sept 26.
4 Gilardini A, Avila RL, Oggioni N, Rodriguez-Menendez V, Bossi M, Canta A et al. Myelin structure is unaltered in chemotherapy-induced peripheral neuropathy. *Neurotoxicology* 2012;33(1):1–7.
5 Hausheer FH, Schilsky RL, Bain S, Berghorn EJ, Lieberman F. Diagnosis, management, and evaluation of chemotherapy-induced peripheral neuropathy. *Seminars in Oncology* 2006;33(1):15–49. Epub 2006 Feb 14.
6 Driessen CM, de Kleine-Bolt KM, Vingerhoets AJ, Mols F, Vreugdenhil G. Assessing the impact of chemotherapy-induced peripheral neurotoxicity on the quality of life of cancer patients: The introduction of a new measure. *Supportive Care in Cancer* 2012;20(4):877–881. Epub 2011 Dec 14.
7 Beijers AJ, Jongen JL, Vreugdenhil G. Chemotherapy-induced neurotoxicity: The value of neuroprotective strategies. *The Netherlands Journal of Medicine* 2012;70(1):18–25. Epub 2012 Jan 25.
8 Paice JA. Clinical challenges: Chemotherapy-induced peripheral neuropathy. *Seminars in Oncology Nursing* 2009;25(2 Suppl. 1):S8–S19. Epub 2009 May 19.
9 Albers JW, Chaudhry V, Cavaletti G, Donehower RC. Interventions for preventing neuropathy caused by cisplatin and related compounds. *Cochrane Database System Review* 2011;(2):CD005228. Epub 2011 Feb 18.
10 Loprinzi CL, Kugler JW, Barton DL, Dueck AC, Tschetter LK, Nelimark RA et al. Phase III trial of gabapentin alone or in conjunction with an antidepressant in the management of hot flashes in women who have inadequate control with an antidepressant alone: NCCTG N03C5. *Journal of Clinical Oncology* 2007;25(3):308–312. Epub 2006 Dec 6.
11 Durand JP, Deplanque G, Montheil V, Gornet JM, Scotte F, Mir O et al. Efficacy of venlafaxine for the prevention and relief of oxaliplatin-induced acute neurotoxicity: Results of EFFOX, a randomized, double-blind, placebo-controlled phase III trial. *Annals of Oncology* 2012;23(1):200–205. Epub 2011 Mar 24.
12 Osmani K, Vignes S, Aissi M, Wade F, Milani P, Levy BI et al. Taxane-induced peripheral neuropathy has good long-term prognosis: A 1- to 13-year evaluation. *Journal of Neurology* 2012;259(9):1936–1943.
13 Dormann AJ, Grunewald T, Wigginghaus B, Huchzermeyer H. Gemcitabine-associated autonomic neuropathy. *Lancet* 1998;351(9103):644. Epub 1998 Mar 21.
14 Imrie KR, Couture F, Turner CC, Sutcliffe SB, Keating A. Peripheral neuropathy following high-dose etoposide and autologous bone marrow transplantation. *Bone Marrow Transplant* 1994;13(1):77–79. Epub 1994 Jan 1.
15 Reilly KM, Kisor DF. Profile of nelarabine: Use in the treatment of T-cell acute lymphoblastic leukemia. *OncoTargets and Therapy* 2009;2:219–228. Epub 2009 Jan 1.
16 Roecker AM, Stockert A, Kisor DF. Nelarabine in the treatment of refractory T-cell malignancies. *Clinical Medicine Insights Oncology* 2010;4:133–141. Epub 2010 Dec 15.
17 Tremont-Lukats IW, Challapalli V, McNicol ED, Lau J, Carr DB. Systemic administration of local anesthetics to relieve neuropathic pain: A systematic review and meta-analysis. *Anesthesia and Analgesia* 2005;101(6):1738–1749.
18 Arbaiza D, Vidal O. Tramadol in the treatment of neuropathic cancer pain: A double-blind, placebo-controlled study. *Clinical Drug Investigation* 2007;27(1):75–83. Epub 2006 Dec 21.

120

Sex and sexuality

MARY K. HUGHES

INTRODUCTION

Palliative care is an approach that improves the quality of life of patients and their families facing problems associated with life-threatening illness [1]. While living with cancer, a person experiences numerous assaults on his or her quality of life. Sexuality is an important quality of life issue for everyone, regardless of age or health status. According to Thaler-DeMers, all cancers can impact sexuality and intimacy [2]. Schover reports sexuality to be one of the first elements of daily living disrupted by a cancer diagnosis and in 2008 found that unlike other side effects of cancer and its treatments, these problems do not tend to resolve after several years of disease-free survival [3]. Often, the innate desire to express and experience sexual and emotional closeness is abruptly and irreversibly changed by the cancer diagnosis and/or its treatments [4]. All patients regardless of age, sexual orientation, marital status, or life circumstances should have the opportunity to discuss sexual matters with their health-care professional [5]. But it is not easy to talk about despite living in a culture that is saturated with overtly sexual images, graphic lyrics, and explicit advertising [6].

The main difference between taking a history about a sexual problem and an ordinary medical history is the level of embarrassment and discomfort of the patient and the health-care provider [7]. A discussion of sexual changes can begin by acknowledging the sexual changes brought about by cancer or treatment of the cancer [2]. Sexual changes after treatment is not routinely addressed or only barely touched on despite patients having significant needs for education, support, and practical help with managing them. Maslow described sexual activity to be a basic need on his hierarchy of needs, while love and connection to others was at a higher level [8]. Everyone has a lifelong need for touch and emotional connection to others regardless of current relationship status [9]. Physical touching changes with cancer. Often, the partner becomes the caregiver, changing dressings and managing drains and wounds, and intimate touching decreases and becomes treatment related. Sexual intercourse is not the defining characteristic of a person's sexuality; a sexual relationship includes the need to be touched and held along with closeness and tenderness [10,11].

SEXUALITY

Masters and Johnson [12] describe the human sexual response cycle that begins with libido or the desire for sexual activity. Gregorie reports that men are more attracted to visual sexual stimuli, whereas women are more attracted to auditory and written material, particularly stimuli associated within the context of a loving and positive relationship [13]. Women aren't linear in their sexual response but more circular and may experience sexual excitement before they have a desire for sexual activity [14]. Sexuality is a broad term including social, emotional, and physical components [15]. It is not just genitals or gender but includes body image, love of self and others, relating to others, and pleasure. It is genetically endowed, phenotypically embodied, and hormonally nurtured, is not age related, but is matured by experience, and can't be destroyed despite what is done to a person. Sexuality includes affection, sexual orientation, sexual activity, eroticism, reproduction, intimacy, and gender roles and encompasses feelings of trust [16,17]. Sexual excitement is the phase where the penis becomes rigid enough to use (erection), and in the female, the vagina lubricates and enlarges in depth and width, and the clitoris enlarges [18,19]. Orgasm is the height of sexual pleasure and the release of sexual tension. The penis emits semen through muscular spasms and there are rhythmic contractions of the vagina and the cervix lifts up out of the vaginal vault. The last phase of the cycle is the resolution phase where the genitals return to their normal, nonexcited state. During this phase, there is an evaluation of the sexual experience as well as relaxation and contentment [20]. The refractory period, where the genitals are resistant to sexual stimulation, happens during this stage. In males, this period can be a matter of minutes in youth but take days in older men or with certain medications or with medical conditions like cancer.

Expressions of sexuality include style of dress, values and attitudes, as well as hugging, touching, kissing, acting out scenarios/fantasies, sex toys, masturbation, sexual intercourse, and oral genital stimulation, either alone or with others [9,17,21]. Sexual behaviors may involve oral, vaginal, and/or anal penetration [30]. Sexual behavior is influenced by religious beliefs, age, education, level of comfort with one's body and physical functioning, experiences of sexual abuse and trauma, their partner's wishes, and comfort level with one's own sexual orientation and gender identity [22,23].

SEXUAL DYSFUNCTION

Sexual dysfunction is failure of any aspect of the sexual response cycle to function properly. Goldstein et al. report that sexual dysfunction is 90% psychological and 75% physiological so there can be a lot of overlap between the two causes [24]. When a person with cancer has sexual dysfunction, it is usually physiological. Causes of sexual dysfunction include psychosocial/interpersonal stressors, medical illness, depressive illness, medication, and sexual disorders (DSM-IV) [25]. What constitutes a sexual problem?

- Physiological dysfunction
- Altered experiences
- Own perceptions and beliefs
- Partner's perceptions and expectations
- Altered circumstances
- Past experiences [13]

Most often, sexual dysfunction in people with cancer is treatment related due to changes in physiological, psychological, and social dimensions of sexuality and disruption in one or more phases of the sexual response cycle [9,26]. As early as 1981 [27], Derogatis and Kourlesis reported that the majority of patients have sexual problems after cancer treatment. Thaler-DeMers [2] reports that treatment decisions made at the time of diagnosis impact interpersonal relationships, sexuality, and reproductive capacity of all cancer survivors. Radiation and surgery can have long-lasting effects on sexuality due to chronic pain, scarring, and body image issues. Other than chemotherapy, biologic agents, and hormones, there are numerous medications that can have sexual side effects that range from decreased desire to difficulty reaching orgasm. Many of these medications are used in palliative care and include

- Neurotransmitters
- Stimulants
- Hallucinogens
- Sedatives
- Narcotics
- Anxiolytics
- Anticholinergics
- Antipsychotics
- Lipid-lowering drugs
- H_2 antagonists
- Many antidepressants
- Phenothiazines
- Antihypertensives
- Recreational drugs
- Alcohol
- Herbals and vitamins
- SPECIFIC serotonin reuptake inhibitors (SSRIs)
- Anticonvulsants [14,28–31]

It should be remembered that sexual dysfunction is not an all-or-nothing phenomena but occurs on a continuum in terms of frequency and severity. Comorbidity of sexual dysfunction is common. Gregorie reports that almost half the men with low libido also have another sexual dysfunction, and 20% of men with erectile dysfunction (ED) have low libido [13]. The patient's partner and their relationship probably have a more profound effect on sexual health than on any other aspect of health.

Table 120.1 describes sexual effects of menopause [32–40].

Menopausal symptoms can be very distressing to women and interfere with sexuality because of the changes in her body [41]. These changes happen gradually in women without cancer,

Table 120.1 *Menopausal symptoms*

Menopausal symptoms	Sexual effects
Vaginal dryness and atrophy	Painful intercourse
Decreased vaginal ridges	Decreased friction on the vagina
Labia minora and vulvar atrophy	Painful intercourse, decreased arousal
Hot flashes	Decreased libido and arousal and difficulty having an orgasm, hard to remain physically close
Change in body aroma	Decreased libido and arousal
Decreased clitoral sensation	Decreased arousal and longer time to achieve orgasm
Insomnia	Fatigue
Joint pain and decreased muscle mass	Harder to engage in sexual activities due to pain
Irritability, mood swings	Lower libido and arousal; partner doesn't know what to expect
Decreased bone density	Fear of fractures with sexual activity
Skin and hair changes	Poor body image, decreased libido, altered sense of sexual self
Migraine headaches	Decreased libido
Stature loss	Poor body image
Decreased sexual hair	Poor body image, less cushioning during sex, altered sense of sexual self
Increased urinary tract infections	Painful intercourse
Vaginal itching	Painful intercourse
Loss of tissue elasticity	Painful intercourse
Infertility	Change in body image
Urogenital atrophy	Dyspareunia, vaginal dryness, decreased libido, frequent urinary tract infections
Mood swings	May be worse with aromatase inhibitors, decreased libido

which gives them time to adjust and enjoy sexual activity 5–10 years longer with fewer sexual problems than women with cancer who rapidly experience menopause [42,43]. One should note that while dyspareunia assumes pain with penile–vaginal intercourse, it may be a source of distress as well for women with same-sex partners, where touch and/or finger or object penetration is uncomfortable [44]. Katz [45] found that physical appearance was important in gay culture and having a partner show that acceptance of treatment- or disease-related physical changes was comforting. A study by Katz found that homophobia does not affect current cancer care experiences of gay and lesbian patients, and health-care providers accepted the support of the patient's same-sex partners [45]. Often, the health-care practitioner does not know the sexual orientation or gender identity of their patients [21]. Dibble et al. found that because of heterosexism, those who do not share a heterosexual orientation may have difficult lives especially when they are ill [21]. Heterosexism is the belief that heterosexuality is the only "normal" option for relationships [21]. Most of the research on the effects of cancer and its treatment on sexuality has been limited to heterosexual women or women assumed to be heterosexual [46].

Case study: Ms. A was a 42-year-old partnered Caucasian female being treated with chemotherapy for Stage II left breast cancer. She had very little side effects from her chemotherapy and when asked about her sexual changes replied that she would like to be intimate with her female partner, but didn't know if it would be safe. She was given information about dental dams that provide a latex barrier when used during oral sexual activities with females. On her next visit, she reported that she and her partner were quite pleased with using the dental dam.

Many people have adopted a pattern of sexual behavior before their diagnosis and attempt to return to it after treatment. If they experience discomfort or failure to function as before, they will stop trying and feel they cannot enjoy sexual activity [47]. Couples who are cancer survivors and are in a stressful relationship with an unsupportive partner tend to have more distress that can lead to avoidant coping behaviors and avoid talking about difficult issues including sexuality [48]. During the time of treatment, the cancer experience encourages a more intimate and intense interpersonal relationship, but there are few studies that have attempted any type of psychosocial intervention to assist survivors in integrating the cancer experience into their personal life [2].

Case study: Mr. B was a 54-year-old married Caucasian male with rectal cancer and had a colostomy and successful treatment for it. He reported that he and his wife had been less sexually active before his treatment, but felt they had a close relationship. Now, several years after his treatment, they are still not having any sexual activity despite his successful use of sildenafil (Viagra®). He masturbates but reports this is not as satisfying emotionally as sexual intercourse with his wife. He is very disappointed and has attempted discussing this with her, but she is postmenopausal and is not interested nor will she accompany him on his visits to me. He is very discouraged and reports that the marriage is strong in every other area except sexually.

SEXUAL ASSESSMENT

Regardless of one's role in providing care to patients, most practitioners do not have experience discussing sexuality and intimacy in a frank, direct, and authentic manner [6]. Annon's PLISSIT model can provide a framework for doing a sexual assessment [49]. It has four components: P, permission; LI, limited information; SS, specific suggestions; and IT, intensive therapy. The practitioner gives the patient permission (P) to think about cancer and sexuality at the same time by asking, "What sexuality changes have you noticed since your cancer?" which lets them know that they aren't the only ones to experience sexuality changes. By asking open-ended questions, the health-care provider is better able to get a thoughtful response from the patient [50]. Giving them time to answer is important. Try to remain relaxed with good eye contact to let them know that you are interested in this area of their lives. Addressing sexuality issues early on in the assessment and treatment of the patient allows the practitioner to open up a line of communication with the patient so that these issues can be addressed as they come up in the future [50].

INTERVENTIONS

Giving the patient limited information (LI) about side effects from treatments by saying, "Sometimes people notice sexuality changes when they get this treatment," lets them know that you are comfortable talking about sexuality issues. One of the first steps toward sexual rehabilitation is sex education Describing specific suggestions (SS) such as books to read, lubricants, and positions to use can offer them help with the problem. Table 120.2 lists other suggestions [51,52].

Some patients are in difficult relationships, which only get worse with cancer treatment and need intensive therapy (IT) from a marital or a sex therapist. Having a list of those resources in the community can be helpful to the patient. Schover reports that patients often prefer to receive information from a member of the health-care team instead of being sent to a sex specialist [53]. Giving referrals depends on the patient's needs and who may benefit from specialized assistance. Table 120.3 describes some of these referrals [41,45,54–56].

Interventions for sexual dysfunction resulting from cancer treatment can be limited because of the hormone status of the tumor. Women with estrogen-receptive positive breast cancer are often unable to use any estrogen products, while some oncologists give them the go-ahead to use an estrogen vaginal ring, vaginal creams, or tablets. A study reported that use of vaginal estradiol tablet was associated with a rise in systemic estradiol levels that reverses estrogen suppression achieved by aromatase inhibitors and should be avoided [35].

Case study: Mrs. C is a 39-year-old married African-American female who had a left modified radical mastectomy after chemotherapy for estrogen-receptive, progestin-receptive breast cancer. She was started on tamoxifen after 6 weeks of radiation treatments. She and her husband had an active sex

Table 120.2 *Interventions for alibido and sexual arousal*

Suggestion	Example
Vaginal dilator	Different sizes to find comfortable fit with partner or to be able to tolerate gynecological examination. Use lubrication with dilator.
Using erotica	Videos, magazines.
Vaginal lubricants and moisturizers	Water-soluble or silicone-based lubricants for sexual activity, Replens® moisturizer for vaginal health and comfort. Extra virgin olive oil, almond oil, or coconut oil may be used as a lubricant since they have no petroleum products in them and last longer than other lubricants.
Videos	Better Sex Videos®, an inexpensive, graphic, but tastefully done option.
Contraceptive options	Oral contraceptives may not be an option; use barrier protection such as condoms, female condoms, and diaphragms.
Planning for sexual activity	Take medications to control symptoms 30 min before encounter.
	Schedule encounters when energy is highest.
Communicating more openly about sexual needs	Tell partner what feels good; when sexual desire is highest.
Exploring one's own body	Finding out new erogenous zones, pleasuring self.
Safer sexual practices	If not in committed relationship, use barrier protection.
Different means of sexual expression	Oral–genital activity, different sexual positions, erotic devices (toys).
Better symptom control	Take medications for pain, nausea, and diarrhea as needed.
Using erotic devices	Vibrators can enhance sexual activity.
Sensate focus	Focuses on receiver's pleasure, no genital activity, uses all of the senses.
Planned sexual encounters rather than random one	Takes pressure off each other when knowing that sexual activity will take place on a schedule they chose.

Table 120.3 *Interventions and referral sources for sexual dysfunction*

Treatment	Example
PDE5 inhibitors	Tadalafil, vardenafil, sildenafil.
Penile implants	Genitourinary specialist referral.
Penile injections	Alprostadil.
Penile suppositories	Alprostadil.
Vacuum erection device	Need prescription.
Fertility specialists	Both male and female.
EROS-CT for women	Vacuum device for female (need prescription).
Physical therapist (PT) for pelvic floor exercises	PT must have specialized training.
Reconstructive surgery	Plastic surgeon, dentists, wound–ostomy nurses.
Breast implants	Plastic surgeon.
Hormone therapy	Endocrinology.
Psychosexual therapy	Sexual therapist.
Lymphedema	PT with specialized training.
Vaginal dilators	Need prescription. Different sizes and use vaginal lubrication with them.
Testosterone	Improves men's libido; off label for women.
L-arginine	Amino acid in oral tablet form that does not raise estrogen levels of females. Anecdotally, it improves sexual arousal.

life before her cancer treatment with sexual encounters five to seven times weekly and she would like to resume it, but not at that level since her libido is very low. This is creating problems in her marriage since her husband considers her cured after 2 years of treatment. They have two children so have weekly planned date nights to give them time for the relationship. She accommodates her husband with sexual activity on those nights, but is really not interested in doing this. Off-label testosterone was suggested and she checked it out with her oncologist who told her that it might increase her estrogen level, but she still wanted to try it. She was given testosterone gel that she uses every other day and reports that it has vastly improved her libido and she and her husband are sexually active three to four times a week.

CONCLUSION

The Institute of Medicine report, *From Cancer Patient to Survivor: Lost in Transition*, recommends intervention for consequences of cancer and its treatment including sexual side effects [57]. Palliative care can address these side effects as they treat other side effects the patient experiences. By legitimizing the topic of sexuality from the onset of patient assessment, practitioners support patients who then find it easier to raise issues of sexuality as they evolve. According to Taylor and Davis, sexual well-being includes participation in sexual activity, satisfaction with sexual experiences, and sexual function [58]. Recognizing the importance of sexual well-being for the patient can prompt the practitioner to include a sexual assessment on all patients. The patient will realize that the practitioner is interested in all aspects of his or her quality of life.

SUMMARY

- Define sexuality.
- How cancer affects sexuality.
- Using Annon's PLISSIT model to do a sexual assessment.
- How menopause affects sexuality.
- Interventions to safely improve sexuality.

REFERENCES

1   World Health Organization. Palliative care, 2012. Available at: http://www.who.int/cancer/palliative/definition/en/, accessed August 1, 2012.

2   Thaler-DeMers D. Intimacy issues: Sexuality, fertility, and relationships. *Seminars in Oncology Nursing* 2001;**17**:255–262.

3   Schover L, Montague D, Lakin M. Sexual problems. In: Devita VT, Hellman S, Rosenberg SA (eds.), *Cancer: Principles and Practices of Oncology*, 5th edn. Philadelphia, PA: Lippincott-Raven; 1997, pp. 2857–2871.

4   Lee JJ. Sexual dysfunction after hematopoietic stem cell transplantation. *Oncology Nursing Forum* 2011;**38**(4):409–412. Online article: www.ons.org. Accessed 2012 Mar 8.

5   Leiblum SR, Baume RM, Croog SH. The sexual functioning of elderly hypertensive women. *Journal of Sex and Marital Therapy* 1994;**20**:259–270.

6   Bober SL. From the guest editor: Out in the open: Addressing sexual health after cancer. *Cancer Journal* 2009;**15**:13–14.

7   Tomlinson JM. Talking a sexual history. In: Tomlinson JM (ed.), *ABC of Sexual Health*, 2nd edn. Malden, MA: Blackwell Publishing, Inc; 2005, pp. 13–16.

8   Maslow A. A theory of human motivation. *Psychological Review* 1943;**50**:370–396.

9   Tierney DK. Sexuality: A quality-of-life issue for cancer survivors. *Seminars in Oncology Nursing* 2008;**24**:71–79.

10 Shell JA. Sexuality. In: Carroll-Johnson R, Gorman L, Bush N (eds.), *Oncology Nursing*. St. Louis, MO: Mosby; 2007, pp. 546–564.

11 Stausmire JM. Sexuality at the end of life. *American Journal of Hospice and Palliative Care* 2004;**21**:33–39.

12 Masters WH, Johnson VE. *Human Sexual Response*, 1st edn. Boston, MA: Little Brown; 1966.

13 Gregoire A. Male sexual problems. In: Tomlinson JM (ed.), *ABC of Sexual Health*, 2nd edn. Malden, MA: Blackwell Publishing, Inc; 2005, pp. 37–39.

14 Basson R. Human sex-response cycles. *Journal of Sex and Marital Therapy* 2001;**27**:33–43.

15 Southard NZ, Keller J. The importance of assessing sexuality: A patient prospective. *Clinical Journal of Oncology Nursing* 2009;**13**:213–217.

16 Krebs L. What should I say? Talking with patients about sexuality issues. *Clinical Journal of Oncology Nursing* 2006;**10**:313–315.

17 Wilmoth MC. Life after cancer: What does sexuality have to do with it? 2006 Mara Mogensen Flaherty Memorial Lectureship. *Oncology Nursing Forum* 2006;**33**:905–910.

18 Kandeel FR, Koussa VK, Swerdloff RS. Male sexual function and its disorders: Physiology, pathophysiology, clinical investigation, and treatment. *Endocrinology Review* 2001;**22**:342–388.

19 Schiavi RC, Segraves RT. The biology of sexual function. *Psychiatric Clinics of North America* 1995;**18**:7–23.

20 Gallo-Silver L. The sexual rehabilitation of persons with cancer. *Cancer Practice* 2000;**8**:10–15.

21 Dibble S, Eliason MJ, Dejoseph JF, Chinn P. Sexual issues in special populations: Lesbian and gay individuals. *Seminars in Oncology Nursing* 2008;**24**:127–130.

22 Dibble SL, Eliason MJ, Christiansen MA. Chronic illness care for lesbian, gay, and bisexual individuals. *Nursing Clinics of North America* 2007;**42**:655–674; viii.

23 Bruner DW. Quality of life: Sexuality issues for cancer patients. Paper presented at the *NCCN Conference*, Hollywood, FL, February 2005.

24 Goldstein, I, Meston CM Davis, S & Traish, A. Future directions. In: *Women's Sexual Function and Dysfunction: Study, Diagnosis, and Treatment*. London, U.K.: Taylor & Francis; 2007, pp. 745–748.

25 American Psychiatric Association. *Diagnostic and Statistical Manual of Mental Disorders: DSM-IV-TR*. Washington, DC: American Psychiatric Association; 2000.

26 Schover L. Reproductive complications and sexual dysfunction in cancer survivors. In: Ganz PA (ed.), *Cancer Survivorship: Today and Tomorrow*. New York: Springer; 2007, pp. 251–271.

27 Derogatis LR, Kourlesis SM. An approach to evaluation of sexual problems in the cancer patient. *CA: A Cancer Journal of Clinicians* 1981;**31**:46–50.

28 Galbraith ME, Crighton F. Alterations of sexual function in men with cancer. *Seminars in Oncology Nursing* 2008;**24**:102–114.

29 Crenshaw TL, Goldberg JP (eds.). *Sexual Pharmacology: Drugs That Effect Sexual Functioning*. New York: WW Norton; 1996.

30 Sadock V. Psychotropic drugs and sexual dysfunction. *Primary Psychiatry* 1995;**4**:16–17.

31 Montejo-Gonzalez AL, Llorca G, Izquierdo JA et al. SSRI-induced sexual dysfunction: Fluoxetine, paroxetine, sertraline, and fluvoxamine in a prospective, multicenter, and descriptive clinical study of 344 patients. *Journal of Sex and Marital Therapy* 1997;**23**:176–194.

32 Holland JC, Greenberg DB, Hughes MK. *Gynecological Cancer, Quick Reference for Oncology Clinicians: The Psychiatric and Psychological Dimensions of Cancer Symptom Management*. Charlottesville, VA: IPOS Press; 2006, pp. 128–134.

33 Holland JC, Greenberg DB, Hughes MK. *Sexual Dysfunction, Quick Reference for Oncology Clinicians: The Psychiatric and Psychological Dimensions of Cancer Symptom Management*. Charlottesville, VA: IPOS Press; 2006, pp. 90–96.

34 Stein KD, Jacobsen PB, Hann DM, Greenberg H, Lyman G. Impact of hot flashes on quality of life among postmenopausal women being treated for breast cancer. *Journal of Pain and Symptom Management* 2000;**19**:436–445.

35 Kendall A, Dowsett M, Folkerd E, Smith I. Caution: Vaginal estradiol appears to be contraindicated in postmenopausal women on adjuvant aromatase inhibitors. *Annals of Oncology* 2006;**17**:584–587.

36 Gupta P, Sturdee DW, Palin SL et al. Menopausal symptoms in women treated for breast cancer: The prevalence and severity of symptoms and their perceived effects on quality of life. *Climacteric* 2006;**9**(1):49–58.

37 Santoro N. The menopause transition. *American Journal of Medicine* 2005;**118**(12B):85–135.

38 Lester JL, Bernhard LA. Urogenital atrophy in breast cancer survivors. *Oncology Nursing Forum* 2009;**36**(6):693–698.

39 Barton D, Wilwerding M, Carpenter L, Loprinzi C. Libido as part of sexuality in female cancer survivors. *Oncology Nursing Forum* 2004;**3**:599–609.

40 Wilmoth MC. The aftermath of breast cancer: An altered sexual self. *Cancer Nursing* 2001;**24**:278–286.

41 Hughes MK. Alterations of sexual function in women with cancer. *Seminars in Oncology Nursing* 2008;**24**:91–101.

42 Conde DM, Pinto-Neto AM, Cabello C, Sa DS, Costa-Paiva L, Martinez EZ. Menopause symptoms and quality of life in women aged 45 to 65 years with and without breast cancer. *Menopause* 2005;**12**(4):436–443.

43 Fobair P, Stewart SL, Chang S, D'Onofrio C, Banks PJ, Bloom JR. Body image and sexual problems in young women with breast cancer. *Psycho-Oncology* 2006;**15**:579–594.

44 Rosenbaum TY. Managing postmenopausal dyspareunia: Beyond hormone therapy. *Female Patient* 2006;**31**:1–5.

45 Katz A. Gay and lesbian patients with cancer. *Oncology Nursing Forum* 2009;**36**:203–207.

46 Boehmer U, Potter J, Bowen DJ. Sexual functioning after cancer in sexual minority women. *Cancer Journal* 2009;**15**:65–69.

47 Andersen BL. In sickness and in health: Maintaining intimacy after breast cancer recurrence. *Cancer Journal* 2009;**15**:70–73.

48 Manne SL, Ostroff J, Winkel G, Grana G, Fox K. Partner unsupportive responses, avoidant coping, and distress among women with early stage breast cancer: Patient and partner perspectives. *Health Psychology* 2005;**24**:635–641.

49 Annon JS. The PLISSIT model: A proposed conceptual scheme for the behavioral treatment of sexual problems. *Journal of Sexual Education Therapy* 1976;**2**:1–15.

50 Hughes MK. Sexuality and the cancer survivor: A silent coexistence. *Cancer Nursing* 2000;**23**:477–482.

51 Hughes MK. Sexuality changes in the cancer patient: M.D. Anderson case reports and review. *Nursing Interview Oncology* 1996;**8**:15–18.

52 Masters WH, Johnson VE, Kolodny RC. *Human Sexuality*. New York: HarperCollins; 1992.

53 Schover LR. Sexual rehabilitation after treatment for prostate cancer. *Cancer* 1993;**71**:1024–1030.

54 Guirguis WR. Oral treatment of erectile dysfunction: From herbal remedies to designer drugs. *Journal of Sex and Marital Therapy* 1998;**24**:69–73.

55 Padma-Nathan H, Hellstrom WJ, Kaiser FE et al. Treatment of men with erectile dysfunction with transurethral alprostadil. Medicated Urethral System for Erection (MUSE) Study Group. *New England Journal of Medicine* 1997;**336**:1–7.

56 Albaugh JA. Intracavernosal injection algorithm. *Urologic Nursing* 2006;**26**:449–453.

57 Hewitt M, Greenfield S, Stovall E. *From Cancer Patient to Cancer Survivor: Lost in Transition. Institute of Medicine.* Washington, DC: National Academies Press; 2005.

58 Taylor B, Davis S. The extended PLISIT model for addressing the sexual wellbeing of individuals with an acquired disability or chronic illness. *Sexuality and Disability* 2007;**25**:135–139.

121

Managing communication challenges with patients and families

ANTHONY L. BACK

INTRODUCTION

In the setting of approaching a patient and family about palliative care, some of the most challenging encounters involve strong emotions.[1-3] For a clinician, the value of recognizing emotions—as when patients are angry, demanding, chaotic, or shut down—is for the clinician to recognize that these emotions need to be dealt with first.[4] These emotions are not epiphenomena—they are central to navigating the encounter.

The second large category of communication challenges for palliative care clinicians goes beyond emotion, however, and involves how patients see the world. This second type of communication challenge typically presents as a patient who is difficult to engage. For these patients and families, this chapter will describe a series of issues often called "cultural issues,"[5,6] but here we will focus on "worldview mismatches." The term worldview mismatches describes encounters when clinicians meet patients and families who see illness and medical care in a very different perspective, and these different perspectives, if not detected and understood, can lead to serious problems. The classic description of this kind of problem is in Anne Fadiman's book describing a Hmong child, her family, and their physicians (http://www.amazon.com/Spirit-Catches-You-Fall-Down-ebook/dp/B003OYIA9M).

COMMUNICATION CHALLENGES INVOLVING STRONG EMOTIONS

For this category of challenges, the chapter focuses on patients or families with strong emotions that present serious challenges for clinicians—patients who are angry, or demanding, or belligerent. This list is not exhaustive, but covers the critical skills a palliative care clinician needs. It is worth noting that even a glimpse of these emotions is important as many people conceal their emotions—which are then visible in facial expressions that appear briefly, or in body postures, or in tone of voice—and in addition, clinicians tend to miss cues—so detecting even one cue about the following emotions is worth following up on. There is a growing literature that describes whether clinician responds to emotional cues,[7] and empirical studies to date demonstrate that responding to emotion is a learnable skill[8,9] and that increases in responding to emotional cues are associated with increased patient trust[8] and increased information recall.[10]

Angry patient or family

How it presents. The emotional cues that signify anger involve facial grimaces, increased voice volume and higher pitch, and gestures involving the upper body (someone who looks ready to throw a punch or hold off something with their hands and arms).

What makes anger challenging is that it often triggers clinician feelings of low self-worth ("I didn't do this quite right, I could have done better...thus I deserve this anger"). If the clinician is triggered in this way, the negative self-talk can lead to the clinician becoming ineffectual. Another kind of pitfall in talking to an angry person is becoming angry yourself. Strong emotions tend to have an infectious quality, as our affective brain systems can mirror those around us. But if the clinician returns the patient's or families' anger, a shouting match may ensue.[11]

How to deal with it. The most important thing about anger is to acknowledge it without intensifying it. Thus, in acknowledging the anger, it is worth choosing an emotion word that understates the intensity of the emotion. For example, the clinician may feel that a family member is furious; but rather than say "You are furious," the clinician will choose to say "You're very concerned about when the test will be done." The acknowledgment should be scaled with the intensity of the patient's emotion. If the anger is less evident, a clinician could simply comment on what they observed directly: "I hear something in your voice there—what is it?"

What really helps in dealing with anger is to enable the anger to subside enough so that the angry person can explain to you what they are angry about. This requires some emotional self-regulation on the part of the clinician—the clinician has to be able to notice and manage his or her own instinctual reactions and reply in a thoughtful and intentional way. This exchange of patient anger for a thoughtful clinician response will usually result in gradual de-escalation of the emotion. Very often sadness will be the emotion underneath the anger.

What you need to watch for is a person who has trouble controlling his or her own emotions. For a small subset of patients, anger can turn into a vicious spiral that acknowledgement will not de-escalate. If this proves to be the case, and acknowledgement results in an increasing spiral of anger, it is time to switch to emotional containment (Dealing with belligerent behavior).

Table: Dealing with anger

1. Notice the anger (an internal step: "The reason this man is repeating the same point over is because he is angry about what happened").
2. Verbally acknowledge the anger ("I hear that you are concerned about x").
3. Offer a chance for the person to explain their anger—what's their story ("Tell me what you have experienced/observed").
4. Listen to the patient or families' story without trying to modify it or defend your behavior or your clinic's behavior ("It's helpful for me to hear it from your point of view").
5. Explain that you can see how your actions may have contributed (even inadvertently) to the anger (in some circumstances, an apology is worth considering)—there is an aspect of personal responsibility in this ("I can see that when I was late to this meeting that it made you feel like we didn't care").
6. Show your willingness to name and address the real issue ("I'm ready to try to make this situation better for you").
7. Create with the patient/family a plan that responds to the issue that triggered the anger.

A final point: You are modeling emotional self-regulation and you may be providing the scaffold for some self-regulation—the idea being that you can have the emotion but not let it run away with you—not ignoring it yet not letting it run your life.

Demanding patient or family member

How it presents: Demanding patients insist on a particular medical outcome or process. The emotion that is presented may be anxiety that something go as they wish, a threatening tone or posture, dogged repetition, or sarcasm. The request is often repeated over and over, with escalating emotional intensity.

What makes demanding patients and families challenging: Insisting on a particular outcome provokes clinicians to want

to confront them and push back—about why they can't have what they want. Demanding patients and families want to control the clinician or the illness in some way, and their frustration and ultimately exhaustion can be palpable. Sometimes their demanding behavior masks an underlying fear that the clinical team is giving up on the patient, and the demanding behavior is an attempt to keep the clinician involved (although it can have the opposite effect).[12–14]

How to deal with it: Re-articulate the demand in a way that captures the hope and omits the threat—"What I'm hearing is that you are hoping for is…." This re-articulation is a kind of reframing that shifts the focus towards what the patient and family would like to accomplish and away from a simple act of control. What really helps here is to demonstrate that you understand their hopes, that you are working on their behalf, and that you are not disengaging from them or the clinical problem. To the degree that you can turn your response into a series of discrete steps, you help make your action visible to them and manageable for you. The pitfall is to simply try to please them by acceding to all their demands and ending up in never-ending sequences of fulfilling their impulses (which may or may not actually move their hopes forward). In the act of discussing what you can do concretely, you are helping the patient and family understand what they can expect from you realistically, and you are modeling an accepting stance a difficult situation that still looks for actionable steps that can be taken.

What you need to watch for is that underlying anxiety that drives demanding behavior is recognized and treated. Once anxiety is triggered, patients can start to pull many different topics into their field of anxiety, and this free-floating anxiety requires its own approach—a useful start is a direct acknowledgment of the anxiety ("It seems like you are worried about a number of things").[15] Finally, demanding patients also induce clinicians to insist that they can make no guarantees, because the demands seem like things that cannot be fulfilled—but insisting on what you cannot do tends to seem defensive and places the focus on your limitations rather than their hopes.

Table: Dealing with demanding behaviors

1. Notice the demand (internal step: "They keep bringing up the same thing, I hope you have something for me").
2. Re-articulate the demand as a hope ("I hear that you are hoping for…"). Reinforce the importance of the hope ("This hope is really important for you, I can see that").
3. Explain in concrete ways how you are working on their behalf of their hopes ("Here is something I can do to help with this issue").
4. Acknowledge underlying issues like anxiety ("It seems like you are really worried, is that true?").
5. Establish milestones that you can both agree to ("Here's what you can expect from me…" or "Here's what I will do next, and when I will get back to you").

BELLIGERENT PATIENT OR FAMILY MEMBER

How it presents: These patients and families have very strong emotions that seem volatile and out of control and seem to intensify if acknowledged. These individuals tend to have intense emotions; they are easily triggered and, once triggered, take a long time to settle down. The time course of their emotions is quicker to start and slower to finish than for many others.

What makes belligerent patient and families hard: The training that palliative care clinicians have to empathize with patients and families, to talk about emotions, and to acknowledge them may backfire for this subset of individuals. For these people, talking about emotions and directing attention to them may intensify emotions and trigger their volatility in ways they are unable to control.[16]

How to deal with it: Here you need to provide containment, usually in the form of behavioral suggestions about what to do next. So rather than talk about emotion, which shifts the patient's focus to emotion and makes it more volatile, try shifting the patient to behaviors that will help get the emotion under control. ("Why don't you sit down for a few minutes, let's put this discussion on hold. I'll come back in 15 minutes and we'll talk about what to do next, ok?")

What really helps is to provide structure (I prefer to think about creating safe structure rather than setting boundaries because it shifts the clinician's focus to identifying what the clinician can do to encourage patient or family behaviors that we can engage with constructively).

Note that a pitfall for dealing with these patients is to say to yourself, "I'll hang in there until they do [x], then I'll stop!" But note that for you to behave "as usual" and then to suddenly change does not set the stage for reinforcing behavior from the patient or family that you want. Remember that the patient is experiencing chaos and is usually not intentional in their actions or expressions of emotion. Clinicians can help guide patients and families by identifying what they've done that is constructive. You do not want a patient to find, for example, that throwing a temper tantrum to result in getting their way—what you've inadvertently done is reinforce the tantrum.

Table: Dealing with belligerent behavior

1. Notice the chaos and volatility.
2. Realize that you are going to need to shift from empathizing to containment. Shift (from emotion talk) to behavior talk ("Let's sit down and take a little break from this issue").
3. Think of alternative behaviors that you can reinforce. Provide reinforcement by offering re-engagement ("I will be back in 15 minutes and if you are calmer then we'll continue this discussion").
4. Expect the belligerent behavior to recur multiple times before it improves.

COMMUNICATION CHALLENGES INVOLVING WORLDVIEW MISMATCHES

There are other times when a patient and family don't seem to interact with us in the usual way. The encounter leaves us puzzled. For example, the patient and family seem extremely agreeable, are very quiet, don't have a lot of questions, and are not disagreeing—but later, we find out that they don't follow through with what we thought we had discussed and agreed upon. It's tempting to just throw up our hands, and often these patients and families are seen as not adherent, not cooperative, and frustrating. And the real issue is usually not explicitly named by the patient. These encounters frustrate clinicians—because what is said explicitly does not seem to capture what the patient and family really think. Their actions suggest that they are operating in a different way.

A useful way to think about these instances is to consider that our "usual medical interactions" aren't making sense to them and that they may be operating from a different set of assumptions. In the United States, for example, most clinicians approach patients with the following assumptions. They assume that scientific biomedical knowledge is the most important way of understanding the human body and human health. They assume that biomedical tests can detect abnormalities in health status that explain the patient's symptomatic complaints. They assume that many of those abnormalities can be treated with specific interventions like medicine or surgery. They assume that the patient will want to make all decisions about their body and that individual choice and control are paramount. They assume that the family is in a supporting role and does not make decisions unless the patient is so sick that they no longer have decisional capacity. They assume that patients want scientific information and that decision making is a rational process of weighing benefits and burdens.[17] Put this way, of course, it is obvious that many patients and families do not completely share these assumptions. But in the rush of day-to-day practice, it is easy to start the conversation in a way that the assumptions are taken for granted. The result is what I will call in this chapter a "worldview mismatch." What I mean by the term "worldview mismatch" is a situation in which the patient and clinician do not share important assumptions that shape what medical care would be considered best. These worldview mismatches are, in a certain way, cultural differences. However, many recommendations about cultural difference emphasize learning specific cultural beliefs, and my own experience is that these catalogs of culturally specific recommendations can create as many problems as they solve. Thus here, I have selected three worldview mismatches that have special relevance to palliative care practice.

Mismatch: Individual or group?

What this mismatch involves: This mismatch is when a clinician views a medical decision as best made by the patient's individual preferences, but the patient and family view that decision as defined by social norms. For example, an elderly Korean woman has metastatic cancer and the oncologist wishes to talk about whether she wishes to focus on extending life (with more chemotherapy) or quality of life (thus stopping chemotherapy). The oncologist finds the patient vague and noncommittal, although pleasant. The patient does not say, "Do what you think is best," but turns to look at her daughter for most issues. The oncologist discusses the decision and feels that the patient doesn't know what she wants or doesn't quite understand the issues. So the oncologist makes a recommendation to stop chemo, to which the patient nods politely. The oncologist thinks that a decision has been made to stop chemotherapy and focus on comfort care. The following day, the patient's son calls the oncologist's office, asking when more chemotherapy could start. The oncologist, now confused, calls the palliative care consultant.

What happened? The oncologist assumed that the patient would be the one to make this medical decision about whether or not more chemotherapy should be done. The patient did not explicitly object to the oncologist's recommendation.

What can the palliative care consultant can do? The palliative care consultant talks to the patient and finds the patient also to be polite yet noncommittal. The consultant notes this discrepancy between what the patient presents and the actions the family has taken. The palliative care consultant hypothesizes that a worldview mismatch may be operating.[18] So the consultant asks both the patient and the son, separately, the following question: How does your family make medical decisions? The patient says, "We all talk." The son says, "It is my responsibility as the first-born son. I am the one charged with this responsibility."[19]

At this point, a palliative care clinician can easily become distracted trying to explain to the son why the decision making should be done differently, using the U.S. biomedical model. But as with many worldview issues, pushing patients to make a decision in a way she does not feel is the "right" way is likely to be futile. It is better to understand the family's process and respect it. The patient may genuinely wish for the son to make the decision. The clinician could then confirm with the patient that this is how the decision ought to be made.

This can result in a situation in which the clinician feels that the best course of treatment is not being chosen, because the patient's and family's values conflict with the clinician's values. The clinician then faces an internal decision about how to proceed. There is no one right course of action in these situations. However, a useful approach is for the clinician to clarify her understanding of the situation explicitly, and one of the most useful techniques to use here is to try to explain the situation and your quandary to a thoughtful colleague who will spend more time listening to you than giving you advice.

Mismatch: Science or spirit?

What this mismatch involves. This mismatch occurs when a clinician assumes that clinical decisions should be made using a biomedical paradigm, but the patient and family view decision making as a matter of spiritual power. By spiritual power, I mean that patients and families feel that what happens to them is influenced or even determined by a higher power and that individual human decisions have a limited impact on ultimate outcomes. For example, a Latino gentleman has congestive heart failure, and the cardiologist wishes to discuss turning off a defibrillator. The cardiologist asks what the patient considers important, and the patient replies that his hope and faith rest in God. The cardiologist presses with a question about how the defibrillator could create problems at the time of death, and the patient responds to all these questions by saying that God will tell him when it is time to talk about this. The cardiologist, frustrated, feels that the patient is at best evasive and at worst rejecting his medical expertise.

What happened? The cardiologist assumed that the patient would see the scientific data about problems occurring at the end of life if defibrillators are not turned off as the major consideration about decision making. But the patient thinks about the end of life as something that cannot be planned and that a higher power will "take care of," thus feeling that arrangements about defibrillators are not an important issue.[20]

What can the palliative care consultant do? The palliative consultant recognizes the worldview problem and begins with a broad question: What caused this illness? The patient replies that he believes it is a spiritual problem that he has been working on. The palliative care consultant, now understanding more about the patient's illness beliefs, can begin to find a language that can bridge the patient's spirituality and the cardiologist's clinical science. In the end, the palliative care consultant arranges for the patient to speak to a minister in the patient's faith tradition who reinforces that God's will is separate from medical decisions, and the consultant also recommends to the cardiologist that he explain to the patient that he respects the patient's faith and tells the patient that the best thing to do now with the defibrillator is to turn it off. The patient nods in assent.

It would be easy for the palliative care consultant to become distracted trying to explain to the patient how medical decision making works. If the consultant felt that he had to have the patient's ok to proceed with a recommendation, the consultant could offer that the patient could hear the medical reasoning so the patient could choose or hear a recommendation about what the cardiologist thought would be best for him in his particular situation. But trying to convince the patient that he must make a biomedical decision may not prove useful.

An important internal step can be to reflect on what role the clinical team should play with a patient who wishes to take a very-high-level view of the biomedical considerations in decision making.

Mismatch: Explicit or indirect?

What this mismatch involves. This mismatch occurs when clinicians assume that an explicit discussion about prognosis is required for a patient and family to make preparations for dying. Clinicians tend to assume, from their biomedical perspective, that a discussion of prognosis is a logical preparatory step for discussing advance care plans, and moreover clinicians may assume that discussing prognosis will motivate patients and families to discuss end-of-life preparation. However, patients and families do not necessarily view biomedical information about prognosis, in the form of statistical probabilities, as motivational. For example, a Native American man with end-stage liver disease has been in the hospital after an episode of bleeding varices, and the hepatologist explains that another episode is very likely and could result in death. The patient and family nod politely and begin to talk about preparations for discharge. The hepatologist, frustrated that they do not seem willing to engage in discussions about prognosis or advance care plans, calls for a palliative care consultant.

What happened? The hepatologist assumed that the patient would see planning for death as an important consideration for future care. But the patient and family had another belief that they did not articulate directly to the hepatologist—that discussing death explicitly will make it happen, that the act of speaking something can play a role in its occurrence.[21]

What can the palliative care consultant do? The palliative care consultant recognizes that the hepatologist's usual practice of discussing death explicitly is mismatched with the patient's belief that death should not be discussed explicitly but can be acknowledged indirectly. The palliative care consultant can then ask a more foundational question to the patient and family: "How does your family handle a serious medical issue such as the one you have just experienced?" The consultant suggests an arrangement where the patient names a trusted family member to help with biomedical issues, so that the patient himself can concentrate on the spiritual work that he needs to do with the native healer given his serious condition. In this way, the patient's worldview can be respected and medical decisions still be made that respect the patient's beliefs.

A pitfall in this situation is for the consultant to continue to question this family arrangement and reconstruct this decision at every visit. In my experience, most families will bring the patient back into the decision making at some point, when they feel that they understand the situation in a way that they can explain to the patient. Often, the major concern for the family is that the patient not be treated to medical facts that they feel are brutal. In addition, in many of these situations, death is acknowledged and prepared for in ways that acknowledge death but do not name it explicitly. By continuing to ask "How does your family talk about this illness," the consultant can gradually unearth the language that the patient and family feel is most genuine.

The physician and anthropologist Arthur Kleinman devised a set of questions to use when worldview mismatches may be involved. While they may seem at first glance extraordinarily basic, they can be amazingly useful to construct a path with a patient and family when a complex worldview mismatch is involved.

Table: Questions for patients and families with a different worldview

1. What do you think caused your problem?
2. Why do you think it started when it did?
3. What do you think your sickness does to you? How does it work?
4. How severe is your sickness?
5. What kind of treatment do you think you should receive?
6. What are the most important results you hope to receive from this treatment?
7. What are the chief problems your sickness causes for you?
8. What do you fear most about your sickness?
9. How do you and your family decide what to do about this?

In summary, communication challenges often stem from strong emotions and from mismatches in worldviews. Palliative care clinicians can nonetheless maintain engagement in these challenging situations by using these introductory frameworks.

REFERENCES

1   Back, A., Arnold, R., and Tulsky, J. *Mastering Communication with Seriously Ill Patients: Balancing Honesty with Empathy and Hope.* Cambridge University Press, Cambridge, U.K., 2009. Available at: http://books.google.com/books?hl=en&lr=&id=2LKJr8VCQoMC&oi=fnd&pg=PA11&dq=-back+arnold+tulsky&ots=QNSrQ6VECz&sig=-Y9Itgf56H9fx1oP3FoFM-3H-WM. Accessed today July 23, 2014.
2   Parker, S. M. et al. A systematic review of prognostic/end-of-life communication with adults in the advanced stages of a life-limiting illness: Patient/caregiver preferences for the content, style, and timing of information. *J. Pain Symptom Manage.* **34**, 81–93 (2007).
3   Evans, W. G., Tulsky, J. A., Back, A. L., and Arnold, R. M. Communication at times of transitions: How to help patients cope with loss and re-define hope. *Cancer J.* **12**, 417–424 (2006).
4   Quill, T. E. Recognizing and adjusting to barriers in doctor-patient communication. *Ann. Intern. Med.* **111**, 51–57 (1989).
5   Barclay, J. S., Blackhall, L. J., and Tulsky, J. A. Communication strategies and cultural issues in the delivery of bad news. *J. Palliat. Med.* **10**, 958–977 (2007).
6   Kagawa-Singer, M. and Blackhall, L. J. Negotiating cross-cultural issues at the end of life. *JAMA* **286**, 2993–3001 (2001).
7   Finset, A. and Mjaaland, T. A. The medical consultation viewed as a value chain: A neurobehavioral approach to emotion regulation in doctor–patient interaction. *Patient Educ. Couns.* **74**, 323–330 (2009).
8   Tulsky, J. A. et al. Enhancing communication between oncologists and patients with a computer-based training program a randomized trial. *Ann. Intern. Med.* **155**, 593–601 (2011).
9   Butow, P. et al. Increasing oncologists' skills in eliciting and responding to emotional cues: Evaluation of a communication skills training program. *Psychooncology* **17**, 209–218 (2008).
10 Jansen, J. et al. Emotional and informational patient cues: The impact of nurses' responses on recall. *Patient Educ. Couns.* **79**, 218–224 (2010).
11 Lang, F. and Young, V. K. Responding effectively to patient anger directed at the physician. *Fam. Med.* **34**, 331–336 (2002).
12 Haas, L. J., Leiser, J. P., Magill, M. K., and Sanyer, O. N. Management of the difficult patient. *Am. Fam. Physician* **72**, 2063–2068 (2005).
13 Steinmetz, D. and Tabenkin, H. The 'difficult patient' as perceived by family physicians. *Fam. Pract.* **18**, 495–500 (2001).
14 Levinson, W., Stiles, W. B., Inui, T. S., and Engle, R. Physician frustration in communicating with patients. *Med. Care* **31**, 285–295 (1993).
15 Waxer, P. H. Nonverbal cues for anxiety: An examination of emotional leakage. *J. Abnorm. Psychol.* **86**, 306 (1977).

16 Back, A. L. and Arnold, R. M. 'Isn't there anything more you can do?':
    When empathic statements work, and when they don't. *J. Palliat. Med.*
    16(11), 1429–1432 (2013).

17 Hern, H. E., Koenig, B. A., Moore, L. J., and Marshall, P. A. The difference
    that culture can make in end-of-life decisionmaking. *Camb. Q. Healthc.*
    Ethics **7**, 27–40 (1998).

18 Bowman, K. W. and Singer, P. A. Chinese seniors' perspectives on end-
    of-life decisions. *Soc. Sci. Med.* **53**, 455–464 (2001).

19 Frank, G. et al. A discourse of relationships in bioethics: Patient auton-
    omy and end-of-life decision making among elderly Korean Americans.
    Med. Anthropol. Q. **12**, 403–423 (1998).

20 Born, W., Greiner, K. A., Sylvia, E., Butler, J., and Ahluwalia, J. S.
    Knowledge, attitudes, and beliefs about end-of-life care among inner-
    city African Americans and Latinos. *J. Palliat. Med.* **7**, 247–256 (2004).

21 Carrese, J. A. and Rhodes, L. A. Western bioethics on the Navajo reserva-
    tion. Benefit or harm? *JAMA* **274**, 826–829 (1995).

Supportive and palliative care for patients with HIV infection

ELIZABETH J. CHUANG, PETER A. SELWYN

INTRODUCTION

The fields of HIV medicine and palliative care have both seen dramatic changes over the past 20 years. Prior to 1996, when the era of highly active antiretroviral therapy (HAART) began, care for patients with AIDS consisted of symptom management and support, while patients rapidly declined and died [1]. The field of palliative care similarly was focused mainly on treating symptoms at or near the end of life. In fact, palliative care grew and developed in some geographic locations where AIDS was concentrated due to the advent of the disease.

As HIV infection became a chronic disease rather than a rapidly fatal one, palliative care and HIV treatment became less intertwined [2]. The widespread dissemination of HAART in developed countries led to a precipitous decline in mortality for HIV-infected patients [3]. As a result, the number of people living with HIV for long periods of time has increased dramatically [4] (Figure 122.1). In the United States, an estimated one million people are currently living with HIV infection, a population that is rapidly aging; by 2015, more than half of people living with HIV will be over the age of 50 [5]. As this population grows, it will be increasingly important to understand how HIV modifies the natural aging process.

Over the same time period, the field of palliative care has broadened, as it became more apparent that patients with complex chronic diseases can benefit from palliative interventions throughout the course of their disease, not just at the very late stages [6,7]. Early palliative care has been shown to prolong life in patients with cancer [8] and to improve quality of life in patients with chronic diseases such as CHF and chronic obstructive pulmonary disease (COPD), which often have an uncertain prognosis and variable course [9]. Definitive research is still needed on whether early palliative care can similarly improve outcomes for patients with HIV infection [10], though clinical experience suggests that this is often the case.

Palliative interventions can decrease the symptom burden of patients initiating treatment [11], provide psychosocial and spiritual support, and improve care coordination, all of which are likely to improve antiretroviral adherence and therefore survival [2]. Adherence to HAART treatment is of the utmost importance for increasing survival for patients living with HIV. Newer guidelines indicate that most if not all patients with HIV infection should be started on HAART at the time of diagnosis (Table 122.1).

In order to optimize benefit from early HAART, patients must be retained in care reliably for years. In addition, though more generally tolerable and with a lower pill burden than earlier regimens, antiretroviral medications still can cause significant toxicity, particularly over the long periods of time in which patients are exposed to these lifelong therapies (Table 122.2). Even small lapses in medication compliance can lead to drug resistance and ultimately progression of disease. HIV practitioners have long employed strategies to assist patients in continuing with HAART, including peer support, assistance with medication regimens, and frequent follow-up. However, excellent pain and symptom management can also play an important role in treatment retention in chronic disease. No one would have predicted this in the 1980s, but in the current phase of the AIDS epidemic, palliative care involvement may be as important in supporting engagement and adherence with antiretroviral therapy (ART) as in helping with the challenges of end-of-life care.

Demographic shifts in the HIV-infected population include not only aging of the population but also a shift from a disease that affected all ethnicities and socioeconomic strata in the beginning of the epidemic to what is now largely a disease of poor and socially disadvantaged groups. In the United States, Blacks represent 13% of the population, but 44% of persons living with HIV, and Hispanic populations are also disproportionately affected [12]. Sixty-seven percent of people living with HIV live in Africa [13]. In developing countries, as well as in underserved populations in developed countries,

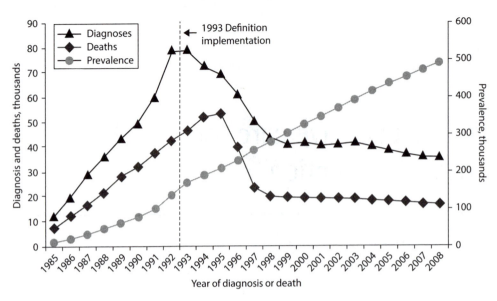

Figure 122.1 *AIDS diagnosis, death, and persons living with AIDS, 1985–2008, United States, and 6 U.S. dependent areas. (From Centers for Disease Control and Prevention, MMWR, 60, 689, 2011, available at: http://www.cdc.gov/mmwr/pdf/wk/mm6021.pdf, Accessed June 6, 2014).*

Table 122.1   Recommendation on initiating ART and first-line treatment regimens for HIV infection

Consensus panel recommendations on initiating ART in treatment-naïve patients

- ART is recommended for all HIV-infected individuals to reduce the risk of disease progression.
  The strength and evidence for this recommendation vary by pretreatment CD4 cell count: CD4 count <350 cells/mm³ (AI); CD4 count 350–500 cells/mm³ (AII); CD4 count >500 cells/mm³ (BIII).
- ART also is recommended for HIV-infected individuals for the prevention of transmission of HIV.
  The strength and evidence for this recommendation vary by transmission risks: perinatal transmission (AI); heterosexual transmission (AI); other transmission risk groups (AIII).
- Patients starting ART should be willing and able to commit to treatment and understand the benefits and risks of therapy and the importance of adherence (AIII). Patients may choose to postpone therapy, and providers, on a case-by-case basis, may elect to defer therapy on the basis of clinical and/or psychosocial factors.

Rating of recommendations: A = strong; B = moderate; C = optional

Rating of evidence: I = data from randomized controlled trials; II = data from well-designed nonrandomized trials or observational cohort studies with long-term clinical outcomes; III = expert opinion

Recommended first-line treatment regimens for HIV infection

	Agents	Pills/day	Dosing schedule
Nonnucleoside reverse transcriptase inhibitor (NNRTI)-based	Tenofovir + emtricitabine + efavirenz	1	qd
Protease inhibitor (PI)-based	Tenofovir + emtricitabine + atazanavir/ritonavir	3	qd
	Tenofovir + emtricitabine + darunavir/ritonavir	3	qd
Integrase strand transfer inhibitor (INSTI)-based	Tenofovir + emtricitabine + raltegravir	3	bid

Source: Panel on Antiretroviral Guidelines for Adults and Adolescents, Guidelines for the use of antiretroviral agents in HIV-1-infected adults and adolescents, Department of Health and Human Services, Washington, DC, August 2013, available at: http://aidsinfo.nih.gov/contentfiles/lvguidelines/adultandadolescentgl.pdf, accessed September 13, 2013.

palliative care services can and should be provided alongside disease-specific therapy [11] and must not substitute for effective HAART [14].

As the population of people living with HIV has aged, the prevalence of comorbid conditions such as non-AIDS-defining cancers, COPD, CHF, and liver disease has increased

dramatically. Care of HIV-infected patients is now likely to require input from multiple specialties such as cardiology and geriatrics, potentially leading to increased fragmentation of care.

Although HIV infection is no longer rapidly fatal, HIV-infected patients continue to face significant stigma in both developing and developed countries. In addition, the cohort

Table 122.2   *Classes of antiretrovirals and cumulative toxicities*

Antiretroviral classes	Toxicities
Nucleoside Reverse Transcriptase Inhibitors (NRTIs)	
Stavudine (d4T)	Peripheral neuropathy, lipoatrophy, pancreatitis, lactic acidosis, hepatic steatosis
Didanosine (ddI)	Pancreatitis, peripheral neuropathy, nausea/vomiting
Zidovudine (AZT)	Anemia, headache, nausea
Tenofovir (TDF)	Renal insufficiency, Fanconi syndrome, decreased bone mineralization, nausea, flatulence
Abacavir (ABC)	Hypersensitivity reaction,[a] myocardial infarction (studies conflicted but should be used with caution in individuals at risk for myocardial infarction)
Lamivudine (3TC)	Minimal toxicity
Emtricitabine (FTC)	Minimal toxicity, hyperpigmentation/skin discoloration
Protease Inhibitors (PIs)	
Lopinavir/ritonavir (LPV/RTV)	Diarrhea, nausea, hyperlipidemia, hyperglycemia, pancreatitis
Atazanavir (ATV)	Indirect hyperbilirubinemia, rare cardiac conduction abnormalities (PR prolongation), hyperlipidemia, hyperglycemia, fat maldistribution
Ritonavir (RTV)	Nausea, vomiting, diarrhea, abdominal pain, fatigue, taste perversion, hepatotoxicity, headache, hyperlipidemia, hyperglycemia, fat maldistribution, circumoral paresthesia
Darunavir (DRV)	Rash, hepatotoxicity, hyperlipidemia, hyperglycemia, diarrhea nausea, fat maldistribution
Fosamprenavir (FAPV)	Rash, diarrhea, nausea, headache, hyperlipidemia, hyperglycemia, fat maldistribution, transaminase elevation
Nonnucleoside Reverse Transcriptase Inhibitors (NNRTIs)	
Entecavir (ETV)	Rash, nausea
Rilpivirine (RPV)	Rash, depression, insomnia, headache
Efavirenz (EFV)	Rash, neuropsychotic symptoms, transaminase elevation; teratogenic in nonhuman primates
Nevirapine (NVP)	Rash, hepatotoxicity (increased risk in women with CD4 counts >250 cells/mm^3, and in men with CD4 counts >400/mm^3)
Fusion Inhibitors	
Enfuvirtide (INN)	Injection site pain and reactions
Integrase Strand Transfer Inhibitors (INSTIs)	
Raltegravir (RAL)	Headache, nausea, diarrhea
Elvitegravir (EVG)	Headache, nausea, diarrhea, back pain

Source: Panel on Antiretroviral Guidelines for Adults and Adolescents, Guidelines for the use of antiretroviral agents in HIV-1-infected adults and adolescents, Department of Health and Human Services, Washington, DC, August 2013, available at: http://aidsinfo.nih.gov/contentfiles/lvguidelines/adultandadolescentgl.pdf, accessed September 13, 2013.

of older patients living with HIV experienced the loss of many of their peers who succumbed to AIDS in the early days of the epidemic. These factors contribute to the higher prevalence of social isolation in HIV-infected patients and can complicate advance care planning. Despite the obvious need for advanced care planning in HIV-infected patients, practitioners are less likely to broach these subjects with HIV-infected patients compared to patients living with other chronic diseases [15].

Principles of palliative care, including a holistic approach to patient care, excellent pain, and symptom management, focus on patient-centered goals of care and psychosocial and spiritual support, and open and honest discussion about end-of-life preferences can offer many benefits to patients living with HIV infection and its related comorbidities throughout the course of the disease [16].

EARLY TREATMENT

U.S. guidelines have recently been updated to recommend initiating HAART in nearly all patients with HIV infection [17] (Table 122.1). The "Panel on Antiretroviral Guidelines for Adults and Adolescents" strongly recommends initiating treatment in patients with a CD4 count of ≤500 cells/mm^3 and has an only slightly less emphatic recommendation to begin HAART in patients with CD4 counts >500 cells/mm^3. In patients presenting with opportunistic infections (OIs), treatment should ideally be initiated within the first 2 weeks of treatment for the OI [18]. The WHO recently also recommended starting HAART when the CD4 count falls below 500 cells/mm^3 for most people and earlier in certain high-transmission-risk groups [19]. These changes mean that more people will be taking antiretrovirals (with their accompanying side effects) for longer periods of time, usually decades.

Palliative assessment and interventions for HIV-infected patients should begin at the time of presentation for care. Historically, the term "asymptomatic" HIV infection has referred to disease without clinical manifestations of OIs. However, it is clear that patients living with HIV infection experience a high symptom burden whether or not they have initiated HAART and at all different levels of virologic activity as measured by CD4 count and viral load [20]. At the time of presentation to medical care, symptom burden may be particularly high. Common symptoms include tiredness, weight loss, fever, skin problems, cough, diarrhea, and pruritus [21]. Psychological burden is high, including anxiety and depression, and "shock" and fear after initial diagnosis [21]. In sub-Saharan Africa, symptom burden may be particularly high at time of presentation since patients are unlikely to seek testing until they are in the advanced stages of immunosuppression [22]. In many cases, control of symptoms of advanced immunosuppression is best achieved in the long term by initiating HAART. However, many other effective symptom-focused treatments can be offered in the short term to alleviate immediate suffering. Eliciting these symptoms and addressing them effectively can help establish trust and develop the strong patient–clinician relationship necessary to sustain treatment adherence over a long period of time.

IMMUNE RECONSTITUTION INFLAMMATORY SYNDROME

Patients with OIs at the initiation of therapy are at risk for developing the immune reconstitution inflammatory syndrome (IRIS) during early ART [23–26]. This syndrome is due to the rapidly recovering host inflammatory reaction against the antigens of the OI [23]. IRIS can occur in up to 25% of patients with mycobacterial, fungal, or viral OIs and may worsen symptoms of a known OI or unmask a previously unrecognized OI [23]. IRIS occurs most commonly in the setting of *Mycobacterium avium* complex (MAC), tuberculosis (TB), and cryptococcal infections [18]. IRIS should be suspected if there is worsening of symptoms of an OI that was previously improving with effective treatment and if there is evidence of effectiveness of HAART including a rise in CD4 count or a decrease in HIV viral load. Since there is no confirmatory test for IRIS, other causes for deterioration such as new OIs, drug resistance (e.g., rifampicin-resistant TB), or drug reaction should be ruled out.

The symptom burden of IRIS depends on the severity and the nature of the underlying OI. Neurological, pulmonary, and dermatological symptoms are common. If IRIS is not recognized and managed aggressively, it can be fatal. The cornerstones of treatment for IRIS are corticosteroids and nonsteroidal anti-inflammatory drugs (NSAIDs). NSAIDs are usually used in milder IRIS and should be used with caution in patients with preexisting renal disease and patients taking tenofovir.

Lumbar puncture is an important intervention to decrease intracranial pressure in patients with cryptococcal infection and IRIS [18]. IRIS may persist for months in many patients. Therefore, adverse effects of corticosteroid use can be expected including local infections like HSV and oral candidiasis, hyperglycemia, hypertension and fluid retention, cushingoid features, and psychiatric disorders such as mania or depression [23]. Pain is common in patients with IRIS and should be treated with analgesics, including opiates in severe cases. Fever and nausea may respond to simple antipyretics and antiemetics [27]. It is important to provide intense symptomatic and emotional support during IRIS and to explain the risks of IRIS clearly to patients initiating HAART to ensure future compliance. These clinical issues all are reflective of how timely palliative symptom management can enhance outcomes, improve quality of life, and potentially support adherence with ART in patients with IRIS.

CHRONIC PHASE

The chronic phase of HIV infection can be expected to last decades for patients with adequate access to HAART. In developed countries, the median life expectancy for those living with HIV is now >70 years [5]. Many patients do not experience OIs for much of the duration of their disease; however, patients being treated for HIV infection in the outpatient setting still have a high symptom burden whether or not their disease is well controlled [20,28]. Although HAART regimens have become less burdensome over the years, side effects are still experienced at some point in treatment by the majority of patients. Pain and other physical and psychological symptoms remain strikingly common in HIV-infected patients [29], and symptom burden approaches or exceeds that of patients with late-stage cancer [30,31]. Symptom burden is similar in diverse settings including various populations within the United States [28,29,32,33], Europe [33], and sub-Saharan Africa [30,34–37], although many HIV-infected individuals living in developing countries experience the added burden of hunger [30,35]. Almost half of these patients have pain, and more than 50% of those reporting pain have moderate to severe pain. Patients reported a median of 8–9 physical or psychological symptoms [28,29]. Common physical symptoms included fatigue, numbness and tingling, drowsiness, sweats, cough, dry mouth, diarrhea, and sexual dysfunction [28,29,31,33]. Common psychological symptoms included worry, feeling sad, difficulty sleeping, and irritability [28,29,31,33].

Symptom-directed treatment is essential alongside disease-modifying treatment for HIV. Impeccable adherence to HAART is essential to prevent progression of HIV disease [38]. In developed nations, patients with high symptom burdens may have lower adherence to HAART [33,39–42], both related to the symptoms themselves (e.g., nausea, diarrhea) and also possibly in part because ongoing symptoms may erode the patient's belief in the efficacy of ART [39]. In sub-Saharan Africa, high rates of medication adherence, generally within a supervised therapy setting, have been reported overall, and the negative association between symptom burden and adherence has not been replicated [37]. However, as HAART becomes more routine in sub-Saharan Africa, patterns of adherence may change. Studies are conflicting about whether patients on HAART experience more or less symptom burden compared with patients not on HAART [20,31], which may be related to improved side-effect profiles of newer drugs [43]. However, it is clear that in both on and off treatment, patients with HIV infection can report high levels of distressing symptoms. Uncontrolled side effects of HAART may necessitate changes in drug regimens that leave fewer options open over years of treatment [33]. This underscores the importance of careful symptom assessment and management in patients on ART. A more thorough description of the clinical management of specific symptoms in HIV disease is presented in Chapter 92.

AGING WITH HIV

As noted earlier, with people living longer with HIV infection, many are now facing the challenges aging with the disease. Due to increased life expectancy on HAART and due to increased incidence of new HIV infection among older adults, by 2015, more than half of people living with HIV in the United States will be over the age of 50, and studies in sub-Saharan Africa suggest that the population of HIV-infected people in developing nations is experiencing a similar demographic shift [5,44]. Evidence is accumulating that the chronic HIV infection and its associated chronic low-grade inflammation and prolonged treatment for HIV accelerate the aging process [5,45]. In addition, older people living with HIV belong to a cohort that is more likely to have been exposed to prolonged viremia during the pre-HAART era and more likely to have been exposed to older, more toxic antiretroviral regimens [46]. Newly infected older adults may also suffer from delayed diagnosis due to low clinical suspicion among providers, thus exposing them to risks from uncontrolled HIV infection.

Frailty is a concept from the field of geriatrics that encompasses the "excess vulnerability to stressors, with reduced ability to maintain or regain homeostasis after a destabilizing event [47]," which is a hallmark of biological (rather than chronological) aging [48]. Frailty is typically measured by criteria that include unintentional weight loss, self-reported exhaustion and low physical activity, weak grip strength, and slow walking time. Evidence is accumulating that frailty occurs at a younger age in patients with HIV infection [48,49]. Low functional status in patients with HIV infection is associated with loss of bone and muscle mass [50].

Osteoporosis and osteopenia are disorders of reduced bone density associated with aging, particularly in older women. Osteoporosis confers a risk of fracture and contributes to frailty in elderly individuals. HIV-infected people have more than three times the odds of having osteopenia or osteoporosis compared with uninfected controls, and risk is related to treatment with HAART, particularly protease inhibitors [51].

Loss of bone density may be exacerbated by concurrent heroin use and hepatitis C virus (HCV) infection [52]. This higher prevalence of osteoporosis and osteopenia confers a greater risk of fragility fractures on people living with HIV [53,54].

Neurocognitive decline is not typically included as a component of frailty in studies of aging; however, it is another hallmark of aging that reduces physical functioning and increases vulnerability in aging populations. The prevalence of neurocognitive disorders in HIV-infected individuals is expected to increase 5- to 10-fold by 2030 [55]. In one study, the functional brain demands in HIV-infected patients were similar to uninfected patients 15–20 years older [56]. HIV-associated neurocognitive disorders (HANDs) refer to a group of disorders related to HIV penetration into the CNS that include mental slowing, difficulty with sequential tasks, easy distraction, difficulties with learning and memory, and difficulties with motor coordination and gait [46]. Although HAART is protective against HAND, effective antiretroviral treatment has not completely eliminated it [57], in part because many antiretrovirals have poor penetration into the CNS [55]. HIV-associated dementia may also occur in newly infected older individuals if diagnosis is delayed. As the HIV-infected population ages, other neurodegenerative diseases such as Alzheimer's disease, cerebrovascular diseases such as vascular dementia and ischemic stroke, and Parkinson's disease will become more prevalent as well. Evidence is unclear as to whether HIV infection is associated with greater risk for these diseases; however, there have been some reports of increased protein deposition in the brain in HIV-infected patients, suggesting a link to Alzheimer's disease. Multiple reports have indicated that chronic HIV infection is a proinflammatory state with associated hypercoagulability and increased risk for cerebrovascular disease [57]. Palliative care practitioners have accumulated expertise in treating individuals with advanced dementia. Principles of care for these individuals include weighing risks and benefits of medical treatments carefully in light of relative contributions to quality of life compared with burdens of medical interventions. Palliative care providers can lend expertise in medical decision-making that promotes dignity and autonomy for these patients at the end of life.

CHRONIC COMORBIDITIES

In addition to "accelerated aging" or premature development of syndromes associated with aging, many more HIV-infected people are also now living with major comorbid conditions (Table 122.3) [58]. In fact, >50% of deaths in HIV-infected individuals are from "non-AIDS" conditions [59,60]. The prevalence of comorbidities in HIV-infected individuals depends on a number of factors, including age, health behaviors, CD4 count, and HIV treatment history [59]. Comorbid cardiovascular disease, lung disease, liver disease, and renal disease as well as non-AIDS-defining malignancies and substance abuse are important contributors to the overall morbidity and decreased health-related quality of life and physical functioning

Table 122.3 *Comorbidities by age in cohort of patients in U.S. Veteran Administration System with chronic HIV infection*

Comorbidity (%)	Age 40–49 years n = 14,561 (%)	Age 50–59 years n = 7,225 (%)	Age ≥ 60 years n = 3,112 (%)
Any medical disease	39	53	66
Hypertension	20	30	45
Diabetes	8	12	21
Vascular disease	6	11	23
Pulmonary disease	8	11	16
Liver disease	13	17	7
Renal disease	3	4	6

Source: Goulet, J.L. et al., *Clin. Infect. Dis.*, 45(12), 1593, 2007.

in the HIV-infected population (Table 122.3) [5,58–63]. Polypharmacy is a particular problem for HIV-infected patients with multiple comorbidities, and there are little data to help clinicians weigh risks and benefits of multiple therapies in these patients [64].

Cardiovascular disease is prevalent in the HIV-infected population due to normal aging, established risk factors such as smoking and hypertension [65], and disease-specific risks. HIV infection itself is a proinflammatory state that leads to increased risk for cardiovascular events, and controlling HIV infection may be an important risk-modifying intervention [66]. A recent study showed that HIV infection conferred a 50% increase in risk of acute myocardial infarction even when controlling for traditional risk factors [67]. Although controlling HIV infection is an important preventive measure, choice of antiretrovirals is also important. Protease inhibitor treatment is associated with elevated lipid levels, insulin resistance, and increased risk for cardiovascular events [68,69]. Abacavir use increases the risk of cardiovascular events, most likely through a proinflammatory mechanism [63]. Further research should focus on optimizing preventive measures for patients with HIV. Controlling risk factors such as hyperlipidemia and smoking is likely at least as important in HIV-infected people as in uninfected people [70]; however, there may be nuances to treatment that must be worked out for the HIV-infected population. For example, statin use may be associated with increased risk of peripheral neuropathy in HIV-infected individuals, and this may have important implications for adherence [71].

In addition to opportunistic lung infections such as *Pneumocystis jirovecii* pneumonia, bacterial pneumonia and TB can cause respiratory disease in patients with higher CD4 counts while on HAART. HIV infection in both the pre- and post-HAART eras also poses an independent risk for development of COPD and emphysema [72]. HIV-infected people have

higher rates of smoking, and the deleterious effects of smoking appear to be synergistic with HIV disease itself, causing even greater mortality and morbidity in smokers with HIV compared to smokers without HIV [73].

HIV-infected adults commonly have comorbid liver disease, partly because of high rates of hepatitis C in the population of IV drug users in developed countries and higher rates of heavy alcohol use in HIV-infected populations. Risk for liver disease is further exacerbated by HIV infection itself. Coinfected individuals progress more rapidly to fibrosis, increased HCV viral load and persistence, end-stage liver disease, and death [63,74]. In fact, end-stage liver disease is a major cause of death in HIV-infected individuals. Consistent use of HAART can have a protective effect, and screening for and treatment of HCV in HIV-infected individuals should be part of routine HIV care. Coinfection is associated with increased symptom burden including abdominal pain, mental status change, and bleeding risk, which are all important areas for palliative intervention.

HIV infection is linked to renal disease, particularly in African-American patients, through an unknown mechanism [63]. In the pre-HAART era, HIV-associated nephropathy, HIV-associated immune complex kidney disease, and thrombotic microangiopathy were common. In the HAART era, treatment-related nephrotoxicity, particularly from the use of tenofovir and indinavir, has become an issue. There is evidence that even in the HAART era, the risk of renal disease persists [75]. The risk of progressing to chronic renal disease over time is similar in HIV-infected patients to patients with diabetes [76]. Lessons learned from the experiences of palliative providers can assist in open and sensitive discussion about when to initiate and stop hemodialysis.

The HAART era has changed the spectrum of malignancy in patients living with HIV infection. Although AIDS-defining cancers such as Kaposi's sarcoma and non-Hodgkin lymphoma remain important, many patients are now also developing cancers not traditionally associated with AIDS, such as lung cancer, skin cancer, hepatocellular cancer, Hodgkin's lymphoma, and HPV-related cancers such as anal cancer, penile cancer, cervical cancer, and vulvar and vaginal cancer [77]. The elevated risk for HCV-, EBV-, and HPV-related cancers appears to be related to immune deregulation in addition to behavioral risk factors [77,78]. Lower CD4+ T cell count is strongly associated with the risk of developing non-AIDS-associated cancer, and a similar risk for cancer is present in chronically immunosuppressed transplant recipients, suggesting immune dysfunction as an important part of the pathogenesis [63]. Although many people living with HIV are current or former smokers, HIV infection itself seems to act synergistically to elevate the risk of lung cancer. Anal cancer is a particularly prevalent cancer in people living with HIV [79,80] and can present specific challenges to patients and clinicians. Anal cancer tends to be very painful and to require high-level symptom management, particularly as the disease progresses. Pain can be related to both tumor burden and to radiation therapy for the disease. Stigmatization of sexual behavior and vulnerable patient groups (e.g., transgendered people) add particularly to the emotional burden of living with anal cancer.

In developed nations, injection drug use remains an important risk factor for contracting HIV. Continued misuse of opioids can place patients at greater risk for hepatitis B and C coinfection, hypogonadism, osteoporosis, malnutrition, and decreased physical activity [52]. Substance abuse is also linked to poor adherence to HAART and greater mortality [81]. In addition to substance use, other psychiatric conditions are among the most common comorbidities in the population of people living with HIV, with a prevalence of anxiety and depression of almost 50% in this group. Anxiety and depression are strong predictors of poor adherence to HAART [81], and treatment with psychotropic medication can improve adherence [82]. Although HAART treatment itself may improve psychiatric comorbidities, it is imperative and in fact lifesaving to adequately treat underlying mood disorders in this population.

The chronic phase of HIV infection is now characterized by complex interactions between HIV infection, multiple comorbid conditions, and aging (Table 122.4). As HIV-infected patients live longer, the field of HIV medicine

Table 122.4 *Interrelated challenges of chronic HIV infection in the HAART^a era: biologic, clinical, and social factors*

Biologic/pathophysiologic factors
Chronic inflammation
Oxidative stress
Immune dysfunction
Microbial translocation
Hypercoagulability
Immune senescence

Clinical factors/comorbidities
Cumulative medication toxicity
Polypharmacy
Accelerated aging/frailty
Comorbidities
    Cardiovascular
    Renal
    Hepatic
    Metabolic
    Pulmonary
    Neurocognitive
    Coinfections
        hepB, hepC, HPV
    Malignancies

Social/behavioral factors
Psychosocial distress
Social isolation
Marginalized populations
Unsafe environments
Stigma

^a HAART, highly active antiretroviral therapy.

must expand beyond the traditional focus on markers of HIV disease such as CD4 count and viral load [59]. This may will be a particular challenge in developing countries where clinics created for the treatment of HIV lack access to resources to diagnose and treat other comorbid conditions, such as lipid-lowering drugs for cardiovascular disease or rehabilitative services for patients with functional decline [83]. In addition to improvements in infrastructure, adoption of principles of palliative care including holistic patient care, an interdisciplinary approach and care coordination can be applied to the field of HIV medicine to help meet these new challenges.

PSYCHOSOCIAL DISTRESS

The aging HIV-infected cohort is also at increased risk for psychosocial distress [84]. In the United States, many HIV-infected individuals face the dual stigma associated with both HIV disease and homophobia. Some HIV-infected older gay men may have withdrawn from their biological families and may be lacking this support during the aging process. Many of these individuals have created families of choice or supportive social networks; however, those infected early in the epidemic may have lost many friends and their partners to AIDS. Support groups and outreach programs may be geared more towards LGBT youth, and some older HIV-infected patients may find their support systems shrinking at a time when they are in need of material and emotional assistance. In the United States, the bulk of custodial care for older adults is performed by informal (i.e., unpaid) caregivers, who are often family members. The lack of informal caregivers for patients aging with HIV is likely to become a pressing issue in the near future [85]. In HIV-infected patients with injection drug use, support networks and family relationships may be strained due to the behaviors accompanying addiction. HIV-infected individuals also still experience significant discrimination from healthcare providers within the health-care system. Similar stigma is an important isolating factor in developing countries as well.

As these individuals near the end of life, specific problems may arise. Many patients may have never disclosed their HIV status to their biological families [85], making end-of-life decision-making strained and difficult. Important interventions include clarifying advanced directives and naming health-care agents well in advance of terminal illness and providing support and counseling to patients who may be interested in reconciling with family members prior to the terminal phase of illness. Psychosocial support can help patients come to terms with emotional rifts caused by prior traumatizing societal rejections and ease the transition towards end of life. Encouraging self-acceptance, generativity or giving back to the community and society, and rational living through engaging formal and informal support systems may improve resilience [84]. Patients may be encouraged to reconnect with faith communities or explore spirituality. Those who were rejected by their childhood faith communities may be able to find similar faith communities that have a more accepting view of same-sex partnerships and people living with AIDS. A sensitive exploration of spiritual beliefs may aid patients in finding support and fulfillment prior to terminal illness.

HIV INFECTION AT THE END OF LIFE

Prognostication in HIV has traditionally rested on markers of HIV disease such as CD4 count, viral load, and AIDS-defining conditions. However, given that many HIV-infected individuals will die of other causes, a broader approach to prognostication near the end of life is needed [59]. The Veterans Aging Cohort Study risk index is the first attempt at improving prognostication in the increasingly complex HIV-infected population [59]. HIV-infected patients with malignancies may have a similar prognosis compared with non-HIV-infected individuals with the same malignancy [86]. For patients with serious comorbidities such as non-HIV-associated malignancies or COPD, use of prognostic indicators for these diseases may be more appropriate.

As patients near the end of life, weighing the continued use of HAART is an important clinical problem. If a patient's life expectancy is limited to weeks to months from comorbid cancer, cardiovascular, pulmonary, liver, or renal disease, clinicians must weigh the benefits and burdens of continuing HAART carefully. Pill burden and side effects may outweigh any benefit that can be expected in this case. However, discontinuing HAART may have its own risks even in patients nearing the end of life. If patients are at imminent risk for developing uncomfortable infectious complications such as oral candidiasis, HSV, or infectious lung disease, for example, continuation of HAART may maintain a better quality of life. Continuing HAART in patients with MDR TB may also help prevent the spread of the disease to others. Finally, clinicians must remain aware of the "Lazarus effect." For patients who appear to be imminently dying from AIDS-related causes who have not had an adequate trial of HAART, initiating antiretrovirals may cause a rapid reversal of the disease process, allowing them years of additional life. This has important implications for prognostication and discussions pertaining to goals of care.

CONCLUSIONS

The field of HIV medicine is becoming more complex as treatment options expand, life expectancy is improved, and HIV-infected individuals live long enough to accumulate more comorbidities. Early palliative care can help manage symptoms and psychosocial stressors to promote adherence to treatment and well-being during the early and chronic phases of HIV disease. Palliative care should be provided alongside disease-specific therapy in both developed and developing countries. Clinicians should strive to provide the best possible comprehensive care regardless of setting. The changing landscape of chronic care and end-of-life challenges for HIV-infected individuals provides new avenues for research and development of best practices and indeed reinforces the importance of reintegrating palliative care into the mainstream of HIV care.

REFERENCES

1 Selwyn P. Palliative care for patients with human immunodeficiency virus/acquired immune deficiency syndrome. *Journal of Palliative Medicine.* 2005;8(6):1248–1268.

2 Simms V, Higginson IJ, Harding R. Integration of palliative care throughout HIV disease. *Lancet Infectious Diseases.* 2012;12:571–575.

3 Centers for Disease Control and Prevention HIV surveillance report, vol. 23, 2011 [cited 6/2/2013]. Available from: http://www.cdc.gov/hiv/topics/surveillance/resources/reports/. Accessed June 6, 2014.

4 Chu C, Selwyn PA. An epidemic in evolution: The need for new models of HIV care in the chronic disease era. *Journal of Urban Health: Bulletin of the New York Academy of Medicine.* 2011;88(3):556–566.

5 High KP, Brennan-Ing M, Clifford DB, Cohen MH, Currier J, Deeks SG et al. HIV and aging: State of knowledge and areas of critical need for research. A report to the NIH Office of AIDS Research by the HIV and Aging Working Group. *Journal of Acquired Immune Deficiency Syndrome.* 2012;60:S1–S18.

6 Eti S. Palliative care: An evolving field in medicine. *Primary Care.* 2011;38(2):159–171.

7 Kelley AS, Meier DE. Palliative care—A shifting paradigm. *New England Journal of Medicine.* 2010;363:781–782.

8 Temel J, Greer J, Muzikansky A. Early palliative care for patients with metastatic non-small-cell lung cancer. *New England Journal of Medicine.* 2010;363:733–742.

9 Bekelman DB, Nowels CT, Retrum JH, Allen LA, Shakar S, Hutt E et al. Giving voice to patients' and family caregivers' needs in chronic heart failure: Implications for palliative care programs. *Journal of Palliative Medicine.* 2011;14(12):1317–1324.

10 Harding R, Karus D, Easterbrook P, Raveis VH, Higginson IJ, Marconi K. Does palliative care improve outcomes for patients with HIV/AIDS? A systematic review of the evidence. *Sexually Transmitted Infections.* 2005;81:5–14.

11 Harding R, Simms V, Alexander C, Collins K, Combo E, Memiah P et al. Can palliative care integrated within HIV outpatient settings improve pain and symptom control in a low-income country? A prospective, longitudinal, controlled intervention evaluation. *AIDS Care.* 2013;25(7):795–804.

12 Centers for Disease Control and Prevention. Monitoring selected national HIV prevention and care objectives by using HIV surveillance data—United States and 6 U.S. dependent areas—2010. HIV surveillance supplemental report, vol. 17(no. 3, part A). enters for Disease Control and Prevention, Atlanta, GA, 2012.

13 WHO. Data on the size of the HIV/AIDS epidemic: Data by WHO region. WHO, Geneva, Switzerland, 2013 [June 26, 2013]. Available from: http://apps.who.int/gho/data/node.main.619?lang=en. Accessed June 26, 2014.

14 Selwyn P. Palliative care and social justice. *Journal of Pain and Symptom Management.* 2008;36(5):513–515.

15 Wenger N, Kanouse D, Collins R, Liu H, Schuser M, Gifford A. End-of-life discussions and preferences among persons with HIV. *Journal of the American Medical Association.* 2001;285(22):2880–2887.

16 Greenberg B, McCorkle R, Vlahov D, Selwyn P. Palliative care for HIV disease in the era of highly active antiretroviral therapy. *Journal of Urban Health: Bulletin of the New York Academy of Medicine.* 2000;77(2):150–165.

17 Panel on Antiretroviral Guidelines for Adults and Adolescents. Guidelines for the use of antiretroviral agents in HIV-1-infected adults and adolescents. Department of Health and Human Services, Washington, DC, August 2013. Available from: http://www.aidsinfo.nih.gov/contentfiles/lvguidelines/adultandadolescentgl.pdf, accessed September 13, 2013.

18 Grant PM, Zolopa AR. When to start ART in the setting of acute AIDS-related opportunistic infections: The time is now! *Current HIV/AIDS Reports*. 2012;9:251–258.

19 WHO. Consolidated guidelines on the use of antiretroviral drugs for treating and preventing HIV infection: Recommendations for a public health approach. August 2013. Available from: http://www.who.int/hiv/pub/guidelines/arv2013/download/en/index.html. Accessed June 6, 2014.

20 Willard S, Holzemer WL, Wantland DJ, Cuca YP, Kirksey KM, Portillo CJ et al. Does "asymptomatic" mean without symptoms for those living with HIV infection? *AIDS Care: Psychological and Socio-Medical Aspects of AIDS/HIV*. 2009;21(3):322–328.

21 Simms VM, Higginson IJ, Harding R. What palliative care-related problems do patients experience at HIV diagnosis? A systematic review of the evidence. *Journal of Pain and Symptom Management*. 2011;42(5):734–753.

22 Wakeham K, Harding R, Bamukama-Namakoola D, Levin J, Kissa J, Parkes-Ratanshi R et al. Symptom burden in HIV-infected adults at time of HIV diagnosis in rural Uganda. *Journal of Palliative Medicine*. 2010;13(4):375–380.

23 Meintjes G, Scriven J, Marais S. Management of the immune reconstitution inflammatory syndrome. *Current HIV/AIDS Reports*. 2012;9(3):238–250. Epub 2012 Sept.

24 Martin-Blondel G, Mars LT, Liblau RS. Pathogenesis of the immune reconstitution inflammatory syndrome in HIV-infected patients. *Current Opinion in Infectious Diseases*. 2012;25(3):312–320. Epub 2012 June.

25 Huis in 't Veld D, Sun HY, Hung CC, Colebunders R. The immune reconstitution inflammatory syndrome related to HIV co-infections: A review. *European Journal of Clinical Microbiology & Infectious Diseases*. 2012;31(6):919–927. Epub 2012 June.

26 Lorent N, Conesa-Botella A, Colebunders R. The immune reconstitution inflammatory syndrome and antiretroviral therapy. *British Journal of Hospital Medicine*. 2010;71(12):691–697. Epub 2010 Dec 8.

27 Marais S, Wilkinson RJ, Pepper DJ, Meintjes G. Management of patients with the immune reconstitution inflammatory syndrome. *Current HIV/AIDS Reports*. 2009;6:162–171.

28 Lee KA, Gay C, Portillo CJ, Coggins T, Davis H, Pullinger CR et al. Symptom experience in HIV-infected adults: A function of demographic and clinical characteristics. *Journal of Pain and Symptom Management*. 2009;38(6):882–893.

29 Merlin J, Cen L, Praestgaard A, Turner M, Obando A, Alpert C. Pain and physical and psychological symptoms in ambulatory HIV patients in the current treatment era. *Journal of Pain and Symptom Management*. 2012;43(3):638–645.

30 Peltzer K, Phaswana-Mafuya N. The symptom experience of people living with HIV and AIDS in the Eastern Cape, South Africa. *BMC Health Services Research*. 2008;8:271.

31 Harding R, Molloy T, Easterbrook P, Frame K, Higginson IJ. Is antiretroviral therapy associated with symptom prevalence and burden? *International Journal of STD & AIDS*. 2006;17:400–405.

32 Silverberg M, Jacobson L, French A, Witt M, Gange S. Age and racial/ethnic differences in the prevalence of reported symptoms in human immunodeficiency virus-infected persons on antiretroviral therapy. *Journal of Pain and Symptom Management*. 2009;38(2):197–207.

33 Harding R, Lampe F, Norwood S, Date H, Clucas C, Fisher M. Symptoms are highly prevalent among HIV outpatients and associated with poor adherence and unprotected sexual intercourse. *Sexually Transmitted Infections*. 2010;86(7):520–524.

34 Farrant L, Gwyther L, Dinat N, Mmoledi K, Hatta N, Harding R. The prevalence and burden of pain and other symptoms among South Africans attending HAART clinics. *South African Medical Journal*. 2012;102(6):499–500.

35 Harding R, Selman L, Agupio G, Dinat N, Downing J, Gwyther L et al. Prevalence, burden, and correlates of physical and psychological symptoms among HIV palliative care patients in sub-Saharan Africa: An international multicenter study. *Journal of Pain and Symptom Management*. 2012;44(1):1–9.

36 Namisango E, Harding R, Atuhaire L, Ddungu H, Katabira E, Muwanika FR et al. Pain among ambulatory HIV/AIDS patients: Multicenter study of prevalence, intensity, associated factors and effect. *The Journal of Pain*. 2012;13(7):704–713.

37 Bhengu BR, Ncama BP, McInerney PA, Wantland DJ, Nicholas PK, Corless IB et al. Symptoms experienced by HIV-infected individuals on antiretroviral therapy in KwaZulu-Natal, South Africa. *Applied Nursing Research*. 2011;24:1–9.

38 Gonzalez JS, Pnedo FJ, Llabre MM, Duran RE, Antoni MH, Schneiderman N et al. Physical symptoms, beliefs about medications, negative mood, and long-term HIV medication adherence. *Annals of Behavioral Medicine*. 2007;34(1):46–55.

39 Gay C, Portillo CJ, Kelly R, Coggins T, Davis H, Aouizerat BE et al. Self-reported medication adherence and symptom experience in adults with HIV. *Journal of the Association of Nurses in AIDS Care*. 2011;22(4):256–268.

40 Gonzalez J, Batchelder A, Psaros C, Safren S. Depression and HIV/AIDS treatment nonadherence: A review and meta-analysis. *Journal of Acquired Immune Deficiency Syndrome*. 2011;58(2):181–187.

41 Al-Dakkak I, Patel S, McCann E, Gadkari A, Prajapati G, Maiese EM. The impact of specific HIV treatment-related adverse events on adherence to antiretroviral therapy: A systematic review and meta-analysis. *AIDS Care: Psychological and Socio-Medical Aspects of AIDS/HIV*. 2013;25(4):400–414.

42 Ammassari A, Murri R, Pezzotti P, Trotta MP, Ravasio L, Longis PD et al. Self-reported symptoms and medication side effects influence adherence to highly active antiretroviral therapy in persons with HIV infection. *Journal of Acquired Immune Deficiency Syndrome*. 2001;28:445–449.

43 Edelman EJ, Gordon K, Rodriguez-Barradas MC, Justice AC. Patient-reported symptoms on the antiretroviral regimen efavirenz/emtricitabine/tenofovir. *AIDS Patient Care and STDs*. 2012;26(6):312–319.

44 Negin J, Barnighausen T, Lundgren JD, Mills EJ. Aging with HIV in Africa: The challenges of living longer. *AIDS*. 2012;26(Suppl. 1):S1–S5.

45 Capeau J. Premature aging and premature age-related comorbidities in HIV-infected patients: Facts and hypotheses. *Clinical Infectious Diseases*. 2011;53(11):1127–1129.

46 Wendelken LA, Valcour V. Impact of HIV and aging on neuropsychological function. *Journal of Neurovirology*. 2012;18:256–263.

47 Walston J, Hadley EC, Ferrucci L et al. Research agenda for frailty in older adults: Toward a better understanding of physiology and etiology: Summary from the American Geriatrics Society/National Institute on Aging Research Conference on Frailty in Older Adults. *Journal of the American Geriatric Society*. 2006;54:991–1001.

48 Onen N, Overton E. A review of premature frailty in HIV-infected persons; another manifestation of HIV-related accelerated aging. *Current Aging Science*. 2011;4(1):33–41.

49 Desquilbet L, Jacobson LP, Fried LP, Phair JP, Jamieson BD, Holloway M et al. HIV-1 infection is associated with an earlier occurrence of a phenotype related to frailty. *Journal of Gerontology*. 2007;67(11):1279–1286.

50 Erlandson KM, Allshouse AA, Jankowski CM, MaWhinney S, Kohrt WM, Campbell TB. Functional impairment is associated with low bone and muscle mass among persons aging with HIV infection. *Journal of Acquired Immune Deficiency Syndrome*. 2013;63:209–215.

51   Brown TT, Qaqish RB. Antiretroviral therapy and the prevalence of osteopenia and osteoporosis: A meta-analytic review. *AIDS*. 2006;20:2165–2174.

52   Sharma A, Flom PL, Weedon J, Klein RS. Prospective study of bone mineral density changes in aging men with or at risk for HIV infection. *AIDS*. 2010;24:2337–2345.

53   Triant V, Brown T, Lee H, Grinspoon S. Fracture prevalence among human immunodeficiency virus (HIV)-infected versus non-HIV-infected patients in a large U.S. healthcare system. *The Journal of Clinical Endocrinology and Metabolism*. 2008;93(9):3499–3504.

54   Womack J, Goulet J, Gilbert C, Brandt C, Chang C, Gulanski B. Increased risk of fragility fractures among HIV infected compared to uninfected male veterans. *PLoS One*. 2011;6(2):e17217.

55   Mateen FJ, Mills EJ. Aging and HIV-related cognitive loss. *Journal of American Medical Association*. 2012;308(4):349–350.

56   Ances BM, Vaida F, Yeh MJ, Liang CL, Buxton RB, Letendre S et al. HIV infection and aging independently affect brain function as measured by functional magnetic resonance imaging. *The Journal of Infectious Diseases*. 2010;201:336–340.

57   Cruse B, Cysique LA, Markus R, Brew BJ. Cerebrovascular disease in HIV-infected individuals in the era of highly active antiretroviral therapy. *Journal of Neurovirology*. 2012;18:264–276.

58   Goulet JL, Fultz SL, Rimland D, Butt A, Gibert C, Rodriguez-Barradas M et al. Aging and infectious diseases: Do patterns of comorbidity vary by HIV status, age, and HIV severity? *Clinical Infectious Diseases*. 2007;45(12):1593–1601. Epub 2008 Dec 15.

59   Justice AC. HIV and aging: Time for a new paradigm. *Current HIV/AIDS Reports*. 2010;7:69–76.

60   Marin B, Thiebaut R, Bucher HC, Rondeau V, Costagliola D, Dorrucci M et al. Non-AIDS-defining deaths and immunodeficiency in the era of combination antiretroviral therapy. *AIDS*. 2009;23:1743–1753.

61   Oursler KK, Goulet JL, Crystal S, Justice AC, Crothers K, Butt AA et al. Association of age and comorbidity with physical function in HIV-infected and uninfected patients: Results from the veterans aging cohort study. *AIDS Patient Care and STDs*. 2011;25(1):13–20.

62   Rodriguez-Penney AT, Iudicello JE, Riggs PK, Doyle K, Ellis RJ, Letendre SL et al. Co-morbidities in persons infected with HIV: Increased burden with older age and negative effects on health-related quality of life. *AIDS Patient Care and STDs*. 2013;27(1):5–16.

63   Deeks S, Phillips A. HIV infection, antiretroviral treatment, ageing and non-AIDS related morbidity. *British Medical Journal*. 2009;338:a3172.

64   Justice AC, Braithwaite RS. Lessons learned from the first wave of aging with HIV. *AIDS*. 2012;26(Suppl. 1):S11–S18.

65   Glass T, Ungesedhapand C, Wlbers M, Weber R, Vernazza O, Rickenbach M. Prevalence of risk factors for cardiovascular disease in HIV-infected patients over time: The Swiss HIV Cohort Study. *HIV Medicine*. 2006;7(6):404–410.

66   Guaraldi G, Zona S, Alexopoulos N, Orlando G, Carli F, Ligabue G et al. Coronary aging in HIV-infected patients. *Clinical Infectious Diseases*. 2009;49:1756–1762.

67   Freiberg MS, Chang C-CH, Kuller LH, Skanderson M, Lowy E, Kraemer KL et al. HIV infection and the risk of acute myocardial infarction. *JAMA Internal Medicine*. 2013;173(8):614–622.

68   Kuritzkaes D, Currier J. Cardiovascular risk factors and antiretroviral therapy. *New England Journal of Medicine*. 2003;348(8):679–680.

69   Friis-Moller N, Reiss P, Sabin C, Weer R, Monforte A, El-Sadr W. Class of antiretroviral drugs and the risk of myocardial infarction. *New England Journal of Medicine*. 2007;356(17):1723–1735.

70   Petoumenos K, Worm S, Reiss P, Wit Sd, Monforte AdA, Sabin C. Rates of cardiovascular disease following smoking cessation in patients with HIV infection: Results from the D:A:D: Study. *HIV Medicine*. 2011;12(7):412–421.

71   Evans S, Ellis R, Chen H, Yeh T, Lee A, Schifitto G. Peripheral neuropathy in HIV: Prevalence and risk factors. *AIDS*. 2011;25(7):919–928.

72   Madeddu G, Fois A, Calia G, Babudieri S, Soddu V, Becciu F. Chronic obstructive pulmonary disease: An emerging comorbidity in HIV-infected patients in the HAART era? *Infection*. 2013; 41(2):347–353. Epub 2012 Sept 13.

73   Crothers K, Goulet JL, Rodriguez-Barradas MC, Gilbert CL, Oursler KAK, Goetz MB et al. Impact of cigarette smoking on mortality in HIV-positive and HIV-negative veterans. *AIDS Education and Prevention*. 2009;21(Suppl. A):40–53.

74   Operskalski E, Kovacs A. HIV/HCV co-infection: Pathogenesis, clinical complications, treatment and new therapeutic technologies. *Current HIV/AIDS Reports*. 2011;8(1):12–22.

75   Izzedine H, Deray G. The nephrologist in the HAART era. *AIDS*. 2007;21(4):409–421.

76   Medapalli RK, Parikh CR, Gordon K, Brown ST, Butt AA, Gilbert CL et al. Comorbid diabetes and the risk of progressive chronic kidney disease in HIV-infected adults: Data from the Veterans Aging Cohort Study. *Journal of Acquired Immune Deficiency Syndrome*. 2012;60:393–399.

77   Dubrow R, Silverberg M, Park L, Crothers K, Justic A. HIV infection, aging, and immune function: Implications for cancer risk and prevention. *Current Opinion in Oncology*. 2012;24(5):506–516.

78   Silverberg MJ, Chao C, Leyden WA, Xu L, Tang B, Horberg MA et al. HIV infection and the risk of cancers with and without a known infectious cause. *AIDS*. 2009;23:2337–2345.

79   Bedimo R, McGinnis K, Dunlap M, Rodriguez-Barradas M, Justice A. Incidence of non-AIDS-defining malignancies in HIV-infected versus noninfected patients in the HAART era: Impact of immunosuppression. *Journal of Acquired Immune Deficiency Syndrome*. 2009;52(2):203–208.

80   Piketty C, Selinger-eneman H, Grabar S, Duvivier C, Bonmarchand M, Abramowwitz L. Marked increase in the incidence of invasive anal cancer among HIV-infected patients despite treatment with combination antiretroviral therapy. *AIDS*. 2008;22(10):1203–1211.

81   Ammassari A, Antinori A, Aloisi MS, Trotta MP, Murri R, Bartoli L et al. Depressive symptoms, neurocognitive impairment, and adherence to highly active antiretroviral therapy among HIV-infected persons. *Psychosomatics*. 2004;45:394–402.

82   Dalessandro M, Conti M, Gambi F, Falasca K, Doyle R, Conti P. Antidepressant therapy can improve adherence to antiretroviral regimens among HIV-infected and depressed patients. *Journal of Clinical Psychopharmacology*. 2007;27(1):58–61.

83   Mills E, Barnighausen T, Negin J. HIV and aging—Preparing for the challenges ahead. *New England Journal of Medicine*. 2012;366(14):1270–1273.

84   Emlet CA, Tozay S, Raveis VH. "I'm not going to die from the AIDS": Resilience in aging with HIV disease. *The Gerontologist*. 2010;51(1):101–111.

85   Shippy RA, Karpiak SE. The aging HIV/AIDS population: Fragile social networks. *Aging and Mental Health*. 2005;9(3):246–254.

86   Biggar R, Engels E, Ly S, Kahn A, Shymura M, Sackoff J. Survival after cancer diagnosis in persons with AIDS. *Journal of Acquired Immune Deficiency Syndrome*. 2005;39(3):293–299.

87   Centers for Disease Control and Prevention. HIV surveillance—United States, 1981–2008. *MMWR* 2011;60:689–693. Available at: http://www.cdc.gov/mmwr/pdf/wk/mm6021.pdf

123

Implantable cardiac devices

LAURA J. MORRISON

INTRODUCTION

For an expanding number of patients with advanced or end-stage heart failure (HF), new technology in the form of implantable cardiac devices can be lifesaving and increase quality of life. Device therapy indications continue to increase.[1-3] This chapter will discuss implantable cardiac devices including standard pacemakers or those with cardiac resynchronization therapy (CRT), implantable cardioverter defibrillators (ICDs), and ventricular assist devices (VADs). Survival and quality of life may improve significantly for years in many patients receiving an implantable cardiac device through improved symptom management and function. However, all HF patients will eventually die of either their cardiac disease or another terminal condition. Mortality rates for patients with pacemakers and ICDs are still 5%–20% per year translating to tens of thousands of deaths annually.[4] Similarly, while survival continues to improve for VAD patients, mortality rates remain high.[5] Implantable devices can also change the character of a patient's dying and death to include painful shocks[6] or a more prolonged course of symptoms and morbidity before death.[7,8] In other words, these devices can both play a palliative role in advanced HF and alter life in unpleasant ways. A patient may become dependent on a device for survival or symptom relief, become immobile or unable to leave an institutional setting due to debility or complications, and require surgery for upgrades or replacements of devices and parts. In summary, depending on a patient's clinical picture and goals, the prolonged HF course with an implanted device may be for better or worse.

Compared to new advances and indications for implantable cardiac devices, device management for patients experiencing clinical decline or approaching death has received little attention.[9-11] Despite more than 30 years of ICD use in developed countries, 2005 U.S. practice guidelines for HF were the first to encourage consideration of deactivation for end-stage HF patients.[12] Taking time to educate and consider possible outcomes for these devices can be challenging when an HF patient deteriorates rapidly and VAD implantation means

life or death. Patients, families, and health-care providers may find themselves in very complex situations if goals or quality of life later changes. They may question whether and how to discontinue one or more of these devices. Clarifying expectations, goals, and treatment options as a person's course evolves is one potential role for palliative care. This chapter aims to fill the information void in this area by describing the course of advanced HF and the role of pacemakers, CRT, ICDs, and VADs. The management and deactivation of these devices will be highlighted with practical and ethical considerations emphasizing a palliative care framework.

HEART FAILURE

HF refers to a decrease in the heart's ability to pump enough blood to meet the metabolic demands of the body. The failure may be due to structural or functional abnormalities leading to impaired contraction (HF with reduced ejection fraction), relaxation (HF with preserved ejection fraction), or both. An advanced state of HF implies that an individual experiences fatigue, dyspnea, or other symptoms at rest due to hypoperfusion despite maximal medical therapy.

Cardiovascular disease burden

U.S. 2012 statistics indicate an adult prevalence rate for HF of 2.4%, greater than 11.5% for those over 80, and an annual incidence approaching 10 per 1000 for those older than 65.[13] These statistics are in line with other developed countries (approximate prevalence of 1%–2% and incidence of 5–10 per 1000 persons per year).[14-19] Approximately half of all people diagnosed with HF will die within 5 years.[13] This is similar whether ejection fraction is preserved or reduced.[20] This mortality rate is similar to, if not higher than, that for many common cancers combined.[21] As new treatments in developed nations have slowed disease progression and demographics have shifted to an older population, the prevalence of patients with advanced disease continues to increase.[19,22]

Similar figures for HF are more difficult to identify for developing parts of the world,[14,19,23] particularly Africa.[19] Worldwide, cardiovascular disease, specifically ischemic cardiomyopathy, is becoming more prevalent as countries progress with socioeconomic development and control infectious causes of death.[23,24] In 2001, cardiovascular disease ranked third in causes of death in developing countries, accounting for 25% of all deaths.[23] More recently, it ranks first globally accounting for 30% of worldwide deaths.[25] Citizens live longer when improved nutritional status and health-care access allow HF to eventually surface.[23,24] In Africa and Asia, rheumatic heart disease continues to be a prominent cause of HF, often manifested by valvular disease.[26,27] With hypertension, dilated and peripartum cardiomyopathy are also prevalent in Africa, with an incidence of 1 in 100 to 1 in 1000 deliveries for the latter.[23,26] Chagas disease remains a significant cause of HF in South and Central America, largely through conduction system abnormalities.[19,23]

HF severity is categorized with different systems of classification. The New York Heart Association (NYHA) Classes I–IV categorize HF based on symptom severity and functional level. Class I indicates no symptoms or functional impairment, while Class IV reflects significant symptoms at rest with severe limitations. The American College of Cardiology (ACC)/American Heart Association (AHA) system stages HF based on disease burden and severity (Figure 123.1[28]). Stage A is high risk without disease or symptoms, and Stage D is advanced disease with refractory symptoms requiring specialized interventions or hospice care. Figure 123.1 represents an overlap of these classifications with a sequential approach to

interventions.[28] The NYHA classification is the more widely used and has been the basis for many randomized study designs.[29] Although HF survival and symptom severity have a direct relationship, the correlation between symptoms and ventricular function is less clear.[30]

Clinical guidelines exist for an evidence-based approach to HF management.[29,31–33] These now support end-of-life care discussions of options, including hospice care, and planning for Stage D HF patients[31] and specific triggers for palliative care involvement.[29] Some organizations have even created specific statements on the role of palliative care in HF.[34,35] In the last decade, palliative care has become a recognized component of high-quality care for HF.

The use of implantable cardiac devices creates potential challenges in the provision of palliative care for HF patients. These devices represent significant advances in technology that go beyond routine medical therapy for HF. As HF progresses, patients may face increasing symptom burdens and/or increased risk for sudden cardiac death (SCD). Ideally, all these devices improve quality of life and extend survival for a given HF patient. However, lack of clarity around patient goals and an evolving landscape of illness with exacerbations, complications, and progression of disease may eventually result in a device becoming less appropriate for someone. Repeated assessments of therapeutic benefits versus burdens are critical for high-quality HF care.

Additional challenges for palliative care providers working with implantable cardiac devices include screening for the presence of pacemakers and ICDs (e.g., an ICD or pacemaker may not be readily apparent on exam or history taking) and keeping

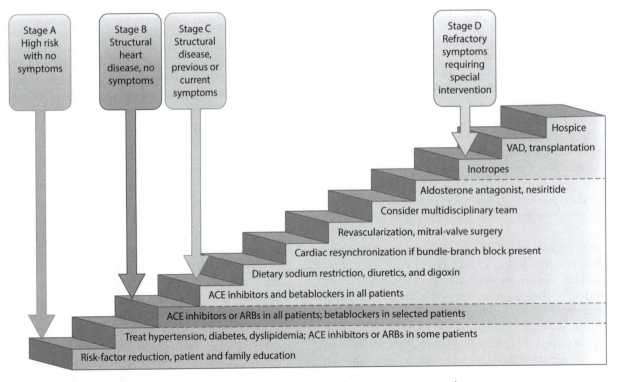

Figure 123.1 *Stages of HF. (Adapted from Jessup, M. and Brozena, S., N. Engl. J. Med., 348, p. 2013, 2003.)*

up to date as new technologies evolve (e.g., future ICDs may respond differently to magnet application). Research on these devices has not yet focused on how best to manage deactivation or withdrawal when this is indicated. The available expertise and education in this area is, thus, limited. Similarly, collaboration between clinicians involved in the management of patients with devices is recommended; however, clarification of roles and responsibilities can be difficult, especially with differing views on who should initiate discussions and actual deactivations.[36,37]

Pacemakers

A pacemaker is an implantable pulse generator powered by a battery that senses a heart's native rhythm and sends out appropriate pacing impulses through a lead. The first pacemaker was implanted in the 1950s. Early devices were large, requiring extended surgery and recovery. Today, smaller devices are implanted in the anterior chest or upper abdomen during outpatient procedures (see Figure 123.2b). Pacemakers and ICDs both run on lithium batteries, now lasting 5–10 years. Approximately 900,000 pacemakers were implanted, and 330,000 replaced worldwide in 2009 with 61 countries contributing data to a world survey.[38] The United States led implantations with 225,567 (767 new per million population), while Germany had the highest number of new implants per million at 927.[38] Of note, most countries increased implantations over 2005 figures,[38] and most pacemakers were implanted in people 65 and older.[13,38]

WORLDWIDE ACCESS

Although pacemakers are implanted in many countries, access to pacemakers for the underserved in developing countries is especially limited. The need is clear. Estimates indicate more than one million people die annually due to lack of access to a pacemaker.[25] Pacemaker reuse initiatives have been implemented in different parts of the world over many years with some success.[25,39–42] Legal, ethical, logistical, and safety concerns, mainly around infection rates, continue to bring challenges in these programs.[39,43–46] Palliative care providers in developing countries may, thus, find themselves advocating for someone to receive a pacemaker or face device management issues near the end of life.

PACEMAKER INDICATIONS, ADVANCES, AND CRT

Early pacemakers helped people with complete heart block continue living and with symptomatic bradyarrhythmias increase function. Today, patients in these groups are considered pacemaker dependent if they have an absolute need for a pacemaker generated heartbeat (atrial or ventricular) to prevent symptoms or prolong life. Although the majority of pacemakers are still placed for bradyarrhythmias, pacemakers can also be used to address tachyarrhythmias with antitachycardia pacing and advanced HF with resynchronization therapy. Over time, pacemakers have progressed from fixed rate, single-chamber devices to dual chamber and now biventricular devices.

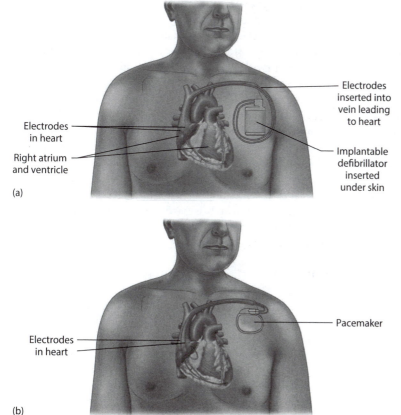

Figure 123.2 *An Implantable Cardioverter-Defibrillator (ICD) and Pacemaker. (a) ICD in the upper chest. (b) Pacemaker in the upper chest.*

Biventricular pacing technology has opened the way to the development of CRT. Many people with HF have left ventricular dyssynchrony, or delayed interventricular electrical activation and ventricular coordination, which further decreases the mechanical efficiency of an already challenged heart. Left bundle branch block is a prominent example of such a ventricular conduction delay. CRT allows for the right and left ventricles to be better coordinated for optimal contraction to create improved hemodynamic heart function and perfusion. In landmark randomized controlled trials, CRT has been shown to increase functional status, exercise capacity, and quality of life in NYHA Class III and IV HF patients, while decreasing all-cause morbidity, mortality, and hospitalizations.[3,47,48] Mortality appears to decrease further when CRT is combined with ICD therapy,[48] but longer follow-up is needed for confirmation.[49] Some studies have even shown structural remodeling with improved ejection fractions and left ventricular volumes.[50,51] Thus, for many patients with moderate to severe HF, CRT may serve a distinctly palliative role in improving quality of life while also increasing survival. Interestingly, the literature documents a lack of CRT efficacy for approximately 30% of those receiving CRT.[3]

To the untrained eye, a single, dual-chamber, or CRT pacemaker will grossly appear the same in a patient as an ICD. New models continue to advance technically with decreasing size and increasing function. Most devices today have potential for myriad pacing and defibrillation functions and require interrogation to reveal settings and therapeutic capacity. Nonetheless, a chest radiograph could suggest the presence of traditional or biventricular lead placement. For any device, regular follow-up with an electrophysiologist to monitor device function and delivered therapy is optimal.[52] It is also standard practice to give a device recipient a wallet identification card that indicates the make, model, and implanting physician. This helps a health-care provider more quickly identify necessary equipment for interrogation or reprogramming of a device.

Cardiology organizations in developed regions of the world provide intermittently updated device-based guidelines for pacemaker implantation.[53,54] Along with evolving indications for sinus node dysfunction, atrioventricular and chronic bifascicular block, neurocardiogenic syncope, and tachyarrhythmias, the ACC/AHA/Heart Rhythm Society 2008 adult guidelines recommend CRT with or without defibrillator therapy for those with severe systolic HF (left ventricular ejection fraction [LVEF] ≤35% and QRS interval ≥120 ms) and NYHA Class III or ambulatory IV.[54] The European Society of Cardiology (ESC) 2010 guidelines for device therapy in HF also support CRT for this same group and present additional considerations for Class I and II patients.[53] On a global level, 2009 survey data indicate high-degree atrioventricular block and sick sinus syndrome as the most common pacemaker indications.[38] At present, CRT is mostly limited to developed countries due to cost, lack of trained professionals and cardiology centers, and less access to newer technology in developing countries.

In summary, pacemakers may have a role in improving troublesome symptoms and function in advanced HF, especially when CRT is indicated and available. This palliative role may be accompanied by clearly prolonged survival in those with complete heart block. As a health-care provider follows an HF patient over time, a core focus should be to reassess whether the pacemaker continues to match that patient's unique goals. Complex issues can arise, and educating patients, family members, and health-care providers from the beginning is important.

In examining the risk/benefit profile for a pacemaker/CRT, the potential burdens include device complications, regular follow-up, and eventual battery replacement. Aside from these standard elements, the burden is less clear. Studies show that health-care providers perceive a relatively low burden of this device, especially when compared to an ICD and potential shocking.[55–57] As a result, there is often less acknowledgement of the option to deactivate a pacemaker later in a patient's course. In some cases, however, a patient or legal surrogate may perceive a burden of suffering from a prolonged poor, undesirable quality of life. Late-stage dementia is an increasingly common scenario where goals may change as a person's function declines with or without HF.[58,59] Patients judged to be pacemaker dependent with complete heart block may even decide for device deactivation with anticipation of SCD.[60] Thus, even with a low physical device burden, a patients' perceived burden may vary dramatically. Recent consensus guidelines identify fear of prolonged dying, loss of control and dignity, and existential suffering as other potentially relevant considerations.[7]

Whether pacemakers prolong life during dying has been debated. Berger[9] suggested pacemakers may stand in the way of the natural dying process. Others indicate that systemic events in the dying process eventually overwhelm individual organs like the heart, creating a nonfunctioning pacemaker.[61,62] This is supported by a study that found participants who had ICDs deactivated near the end of life had similar survival whether pacing was turned off or left intact.[10] Importantly, the effect of pacemaker deactivation on symptoms remains a concern. Unless someone has complete heart block, deactivation is unlikely to lead to painless SCD.[59] Experts indicate that a symptomatic bradycardia is the most likely result with potential worsening of HF symptoms.[61,63] Although palliative care measures can manage these symptoms, experts recommend pacemaker continuation,[10,61] specifically antibradycardic and CRT pacing.[64] Research is needed in this domain, especially for those receiving CRT and the 30% for whom CRT is less effective, as use expands.

ICDs

The first ICD was successfully implanted in 1980, an extension of the original battery-powered generator and lead pacemaker technology. ICDs are designed to prevent SCD by using defibrillation, delivery of a high-energy shock, to convert a lethal tachyarrhythmia to a stable normal rhythm. Modern ICD devices include pacing functions and are almost indistinguishable from a pacemaker device on physical examination (ICDs are slightly larger) (see Figure 123.2a). When a tachyarrhythmia is sensed, the device will either provide antitachycardia pacing, cardioversion, or defibrillation. Only device interrogation will reveal its programming and recent activity.

ICD use has expanded rapidly as new populations who benefit from this technology are identified.[65,66] In 2009, approximately 278,000 ICDs were implanted, and 132,000 replaced worldwide.[38] The United States led here, as well, with 133,262 implants and 434 new implants per million people.[38] The majority of ICDs were also placed in those 65 and older.[13] Compared to 2005 survey data, almost all countries had an exponential rate of implant increase, and use of biventricular ICDs increased.[38] Like pacemakers, ICDs are far underutilized in developing countries,[38] and logistical, legal, ethical, and safety issues exist around potential ICD reuse.[43] Initiatives to facilitate ICD reuse exist[67,68] but lag behind those promoting pacemakers as the most basic, needed electrophysiological intervention for symptomatic bradycardia.[25,42]

ICD INDICATIONS AND ADVANCES

ICDs have a role in both primary and secondary prevention of SCD. Attention to secondary prevention led the initial technology push as physicians aimed to prevent SCD in those already suffering a prior cardiac arrest or sustained ventricular tachycardia (VT). More recently, however, efforts to prevent a first cardiac arrest have identified expanded "at-risk" groups that may benefit from defibrillator therapy. In particular, ICDs have been shown to significantly increase survival in those with LVEF 30%–35% with prior myocardial infarction or nonischemic cardiomyopathy.[65,69,70] Compared to standard antiarrhythmic pharmacotherapy, mortality reductions with ICDs have been in the range of 23%–55%.[71]

Per U.S. guidelines, ICDs are indicated for secondary prevention in prior cardiac arrest, sustained VT, or syncope with significant ventricular arrhythmia.[54] For a primary prevention indication, ESC and U.S. guidelines recommend that a person have a predicted 1-year survival, be on optimal medical management, and be ambulatory.[53,54] An ICD should be considered for someone with NYHA Class II, III, or IV with ejection fraction ≤35% and mainly combined with CRT.[53,54] The U.S. guidelines are more comprehensive and detailed around indications for different characteristics like ischemic versus nonischemic HF.[54] Interestingly, earlier U.S. guidelines from 2002 specifically identified terminal illness with prognosis of 6 months or less as a contraindication to ICD therapy, citing limited benefit for such a patient.[72]

Of note, a wearable cardioverter defibrillator (WCD) is now available in the United States, Europe, and slowly other countries, with expanding indications. The U.S. Food and Drug Administration (FDA) approved the device for adults in December 2001.[73] Use in children is being studied.[74] The device consists of two parts: a lightweight vest garment that detects arrhythmias and delivers shocks and a monitor with battery pack worn at the waist or by shoulder strap that records the cardiac rhythm. It is a self-contained device requiring no bystander assistance. Guidelines indicate WCDs should be considered for people at temporary high risk of SCD, those with ischemic or nonischemic cardiomyopathy or postmyocardial

infarction with or without revascularization, and those who are not able to have immediate ICD support or heart transplant.[75] Studies show similar survival to ICDs and favorable patient tolerability.[76] Although WCDs are not implanted devices, similar management challenges may arise for palliative care clinicians taking care of patients with them.

In contrast to pacemakers, the burden versus benefit breakdown for ICDs is better defined. In advanced HF, an ICD may transition a patient's course from SCD to a prolonged course of HF. At a basic level, when preventing SCD no longer aligns with a person's goals or device burdens outweigh benefits, consideration for deactivation should occur. Potential device complications, routine care and monitoring, and battery replacement are also standard burdens for ICDs. From a palliative perspective, it is significant that the intended effect of the ICD, defibrillation, can become a clear source of suffering.[77] ICD shocks can cause patient and family distress and are not consistent with dignity or comfort care near the end of life.[6,61,78–81] A person touching the patient at the time of shocking may experience mild discomfort from a small current. For some patients, even appropriate shocks produce suffering through pain,[82–84] anxiety,[85] fear, and depression.[82,86,87,88] More shocks may negatively impact quality of life measures.[89] Only recently has a state-of-the-science report sought to improve the identification and care of psychosocial distress in ICD patients and their families.[90] Our ability to predict whether a dying patient will receive ICD shocks is limited, and our accuracy poorly defined,[92] but dying patients are likely to experience arrhythmias from electrolyte disturbances, hypoxia, and sepsis.[10] In the setting of an arrhythmia, ICD deactivation may allow for a painless SCD.[61,63] However, while patients and families should be prepared for the possibility of immediate SCD after ICD deactivation, this appears to be rare and different from the complete heart block situation for pacemakers. It is clearly important for ICD patients to undergo a comprehensive informed consent process and have intermittent opportunities to reevaluate the appropriateness of the device over time.[77]

PACEMAKER AND ICD COSTS AND COMPLICATIONS

Cost is an important consideration with implantable cardiac devices as it pertains to the benefit versus harm analysis for patients in different settings. Kirkpatrick et al.[43] indicate 2009 estimated device costs as follows: pacemaker pulse generator $2,500–$3,000 with leads at $800–$1,000 each compared to ICD generator $20,000–$40,000 with leads at $10,000 or more. Baman et al.[92] state that with associated costs, a device implantation may cost as much as $55,000. An ICD battery replacement procedure in the hospital may cost nearly $50,000.[93]

Pacemaker and ICD complications, while decreasing markedly over time, are similar and add an additional consideration for patient decision making. ICDs have more complexity with defibrillation therapy and thus additional complications. Implant mortality is low, usually measured as death at 30 days after procedure.[94] One study of resuscitated patients showed 2.4% 30-day mortality for those with ICDs compared to 3.5% for those on antiarrhythmic medication instead.[95] Surgical device complications, including infection rates of 1%–2%, may lead to additional surgery.[52] Hematoma, seroma, pneumothorax, hardware connection problems, and device erosion within cardiac or soft tissue, especially with cachexia, are other potential complications.[52] Lead dislodgement, malfunction, or fracture may lead to ineffective pacing therapy and inappropriate shocking from ICDs and again additional surgery. Frequent, and inappropriate, shocks are the most common complication of ICD implantation.[52] In the MADIT trial,[65] patients in the ICD group had lead problems and nonfatal infections requiring surgery at a combined rate of 2.5% and a slightly higher rate of new or worsened HF than those in the conventional therapy group. Persons with either device may also experience malfunctions from electric current or magnetic field exposures (e.g., MRI testing, surgical cautery, cell phone use near device), thus potentially limiting these activity and procedural options.[52] Finally, leading device manufacturers have released multiple advisories and recalls for pacemakers and ICDs malfunctions since 2005, affecting well over 100,000 devices in 2005 alone.[96] It can be difficult for patients and clinicians to determine whether the risk of device malfunction or complication from device replacement is higher.[1] One study suggests these can be high-stake decisions as complications occur even when replacements are performed by experienced hands.[96]

Palliative care role for pacemaker and ICD management

National medical organizations have begun to provide more guidance around pacemaker and ICD management and deactivation. Two 2010 documents from the United States[7] and Europe[64] provide overlapping consensus on the management of implantable cardiac devices in patients near the end of life or requesting withdrawal of device therapy. These are comprehensive with input from palliative care clinicians and serve as a detailed roadmap for a palliative care approach to device management. In addition, an earlier U.S. and European guideline on implantable cardiac device monitoring includes a detailed section on device management and ethical issues.[62] Lastly, a 2012 scientific statement details the role of shared decision making in device management.[5]

COMMUNICATION

Widespread agreement exists on the importance of an ongoing conversation about goals of care between clinicians and patients with pacemakers and ICDs. The complexity of the prolonged course of advanced HF and these devices makes this imperative. The discussion ideally starts at preimplantation with a robust informed consent process that includes advance care planning (ACP) and education about current and future therapeutic options like device deactivation.[7,9,10,56,57,64] Evidence indicates that device deactivation and other end-of-life implications are not routinely included in implantation informed consent.[97,98] The shared decision-making model, one grounded in patient autonomy, patient centeredness, and informed consent where both patient and clinician share information, has been suggested to guide this communication.[5,99] This model emphasizes the clinician role in making

sure patients and families have adequate understanding of the medical context[100] and complexity of potential tradeoffs.[101] For example, if a patient is receiving a device with both pacing and ICD functions, an understanding of the benefits and burdens and potential consequences of each function would need to be achieved. This is a proactive approach that empowers the patient's examination of benefits and harms, options, and consequences, along the continuum of device management, to arrive at the best decision for the patient. Since patient preferences can change over time with disease progression,[102] the serial and iterative aspect is key. Effective communication is timely and overall focused on patient's goals and values, allowing informed consent to be optimized and undesirable outcomes minimized. Clinician consultation with colleagues may define specific facts or options and promote clarity. Goal discussions often focus on symptoms, function, and quality of life, as well as aspects of dependency, control, and dignity. Once goals are clarified, treatment options can be negotiated to find the best patient fit. Evidence suggests such proactive communication can benefit patients and their families.[103] The ultimate outcome of shared decision making for an advanced HF patient would be a patient-driven, comprehensive end-of-life plan, including preferences for device management.[5]

ACP is a process widely accepted in the United States that promotes patient identification of goals and preferences for future health needs and a legal surrogate for decision making in case of incapacitation (ACP source). It ideally includes completion of written advance directives, a living will (for personal health-care goals and preferences) and designation of a legal surrogate, and documentation in the medical record. Perhaps more importantly, with or without written document completion, it should encourage directed discussions of identified patient goals, values, and preferences with family members or a legal surrogate. ACP should be included as a key part of communication for implantable cardiac device management from preimplantation counseling onward. This discussion could be triggered by the acknowledgement that device deactivation may be appropriate at a future point and the course ahead is uncertain. Given most ICD patients have never considered the role of their device at end of life,[43] ACP for this population appears limited at present. Nonetheless, those ICD patients engaged in ACP and those with earlier device deactivation have received fewer shocks at the end of life.[10] A specific statement about device deactivation in a living will is encouraged[7] but is rare in practice, even among ICD patients with advance directives.[105,106]

Many experts recommend event triggers for clinicians to initiate these serial conversations with patients so that opportunities for updating patient wishes and preferences are not missed[7] (see Table 123.1). In addition to preimplantation, increased ICD firing, progression of cardiac disease with repeated hospitalizations, consideration of a new therapy, major change in medical condition or diagnosis of another terminal disease, battery replacement, transition to do not attempt resuscitation (DNAR) status, and imminent death are possible triggers. An annual HF visit should also have a structured review of all current and potential therapies for

Table 123.1 *Goals of care conversations for implantable cardiac devices—Triggers, content, and phrasing*

Timing of conversation	Points to be covered	Helpful phrases to consider
Prior to implantation	Clear discussion of the benefits and burdens of the devices Brief discussion of potential future limitations or burdensome aspects of device therapy Encourage patients to have some form of advanced directive Inform of options to deactivate in the future	"It seems clear at this point that this device is in your best interest, but you should know at some point if you become very ill, from your heart disease or another process you develop in the future, the burden of this device may outweigh its benefit. While that point is hopeful a long way off, you should know that turning off your defibrillator is an option."
After an episode of increased or repeated firings from ICD	Discussion of possible alternatives, including adjusting medications, adjusting device settings, and cardiac procedures to reduce future shocks in context of goals of care	"I know that your device caused you some recent discomfort and that you were quiet distressed. Let's see if we can find a correctable reason why this may be happening and discuss options to decrease the number of firings."
Progression of cardiac disease and/ or secondary disease process	Reevaluation of benefits and burdens of device Assessment of functional status, quality of life, and symptoms Referral to palliative and supportive care services	"It appears as though your heart disease is worsening. We should really talk about your thoughts and questions about your illness at this point and see if your goals have changed at all."
When patient/surrogate chooses a do not resuscitate order	Reevaluation of benefits and burdens of device Exploration of patient's understanding of device and how he or she conceptualizes it with regard to external Defibrillation Referral to palliative care or supportive services	"Now that we've established that you would not want resuscitation in the event your heart was to go into an abnormal pattern of beating, we should reconsider the role of your device. In many ways, it is also a form of resuscitation. Tell me your understanding of the device and let's talk about how it fits into the larger goals for your medical care at this point."
Patients at end of life	Reevaluation of benefits and burdens of devices Discussion of option of deactivation addressed with all patients, though deactivation *not* required	"I think at this point, we need to reevaluate what your [device] is doing for you, positively and negatively. Given how advanced your disease is, we need to discuss whether to make sense to keep it active. I know this may be upsetting to talk about, but can you tell me your thoughts at this point?"

Sources: Adapted from Lampert R, Hayes DL, Annas GJ et al. Expert Consensus Statement on the Management of Cardiovascular Implantable Electronic Devices (CIEDs) in patients nearing end of life or requesting withdrawal of therapy. *Heart Rhythm.* 2010;7(7):1008–1026.

anticipated or unanticipated events.[5] More general discussion triggers for advanced HF may also be relevant for those with devices.[5,29]

Pacemaker and ICD deactivation

Experts suggest two potential scenarios for pacemaker or ICD withdrawal[62]: (1) patient's quality of life has diminished or is poor due to ICD shocking or decline of overall condition due to coexisting diseases, or (2) patient's death is approaching and the device is no longer of benefit. Given these provide only a general framework; decisions for device deactivation should be tailored in all cases to the individual patient and relevant circumstances. Table 123.2 suggests a general protocol. Again, this is ideally a shared decision-making process with the clinician providing directive guidance based on the patient's expressed goals and the patient and physician arriving at a mutual decision.[5] Deactivation is to be undertaken only after careful planning and thorough investigation of a patient's clinical circumstance is completed, all other options are considered, verbal informed consent is obtained from

the patient or legal surrogate with family involvement, and ideally, all those involved in active medical care, including the interdisciplinary team, are informed. Coordination and communication of responsibilities between all team members is crucial to facilitate a smooth process for everyone.

Anticipatory symptom assessment and management should also be in place. Continuation of prior symptom-related medications may or may not be appropriate. Premedication for symptoms such as pain or dyspnea (opioids), anxiety (anxiolytics), or delirium (neuroleptics) should be considered.[7] If SCD is predicted or if painful, unwanted shocks are already happening, sedation prior to discontinuation may be indicated and desired by patient or legal surrogate. Nonpharmacologic interventions should always be optimized, for example, fan for dyspnea.

In all cases, clinicians will want to continue to assess the patient before, during, and after deactivation for symptoms or distress with the ability to quickly administer medications. Prior to deactivation, clearly labeled syringes of opioids or sedatives can be prepared for urgent administration and dose titration as needed. For example, three syringes containing

Table 123.2   *Implantable Cardiac Device Deactivation—A Stepwise Approach for Clinicians*

Level of Intervention	Communication and Documentation	Details
I. Initial approach	Pre-implantation or preliminary discussion	• Present deactivation option well in advance of need to • Patient, legal surrogate, family members, caregivers

II. Indications of patient's declining condition
• Progressive cardiac dysfunction
• Progressive secondary disease (e.g. malignancy, dementia)
• Poor quality of life
• Catastrophic device complications
	More detailed and continuing discussion	• Discuss benefits/risks of deactivation
		• Explore medical, ethical, legal, religious cultural aspects
		• Discuss deactivation of
		  • Pacemaker functions
		  • ICD therapies
		  • Alert and/or remote monitoring
		  • VAD functions

III. Patient or legal surrogate desires device deactivation	Ethical or legal consultation helpful for clarification in some cases	• Document in chart:
		  • Clinician's perception of patient's cognitive and psychological state, including confirmation of patient's decision-making competence
		  • Informed consent of patient or legal surrogate, including situation specific uncertainty in survival or timing of death outcomes
		  • Resuscitation status
		  • Communication with the patient's family
		• Clarify optimal timing, sequence of events, and presence of supportive individuals, including family, for deactivation based on patient or legal surrogate preferences and practical aspects (e.g. family member arriving next day)

IV(a). Deactivation – immediate death (death in seconds to minutes) unlikely	Details of device reprogramming should always be reviewed and documented by physician	• A suitably trained person performs deactivation upon the express, written order of a physician • Provide active symptom management
IV(b). Deactivation – immediate death anticipated	Optimally performed by a physician	• Perform active symptom management and care for imminent death, if occurs

Practical points: Pacemaker
- Consider device interrogation in advance to determine function and likely deactivation outcome
- Determine approach to continuation or discontinuation of other life-sustaining therapies, including resuscitation status

Practical points: ICD
- Consider device interrogation in advance to determine function and likely deactivation outcome
- Determine approach to continuation or discontinuation of other life-sustaining therapies, including resuscitation status
- Use magnet if inappropriate shocks and not able to deactivate

Practical points: VAD
- Think of VAD deactivation as analogous to ventilator withdrawal
- Determine approach to continuation or discontinuation of other life-sustaining therapies as they relate to timing and goals around VAD deactivation (VAD is often last therapy to be stopped)
- If active ICD is present, deactivate in advance of VAD deactivation
- Confirm Do Not Attempt Resuscitation Status
- Discuss palliative sedation, as indicated by circumstances, with patient and/or family/legal surrogate
- Have pre-deactivation meeting to specify team roles and responsibilities, in detail, and to clarify expectations and concerns with bedside RN, respiratory therapist, perfusionist, clergy, social worker, and all other involved staff
- Have pre-deactivation meeting with patient or legal surrogate and involved family to clarify plan, expectations, and concerns
- Confirm needed expertise is present for deactivation of specific VAD device (mechanism for deactivation and silencing of alarms with appropriate sequence of events) to minimize anxiety for all present
- If pre-medication appropriate, administer prior to deactivation with reassessment to ensure adequate circulation and efficacy
- Silence alarms and discontinue all non-symptom directed monitoring
- Have a back-up "quiet container" in case alarm will not silence (e.g. large hazard box with foam or pillows)

morphine 10 mg each and three syringes containing midazolam 10 mg each might be individually labeled and on a bedside table. If the patient is already receiving opioids, equianalgesic calculations should be made, and appropriate bolus doses determined beforehand. If the patient has been taking benzodiazepines, an alternative sedative such as a barbiturate or propofol may be considered because of tolerance. If available, involvement of an interdisciplinary palliative care team may facilitate additional support for clinicians, patient, and family along with expertise in complex communication and symptom management for therapy withdrawal or end-of-life situations. Psychiatry, ethics consultation, and legal counsel are not required unless there is an institutional policy or a clinical question. Deactivation is an accepted medical procedure.

Pacemaker deactivation implies the device is turned off or reprogrammed to be nonfunctional in treating bradycardia. ICD, or defibrillator, deactivation, by contrast, means the device is reprogrammed to no longer treat tachyarrhythmias; pacing activity may continue or not depending on the clinical decision. Documentation in the medical record is standard of care in all cases. Details of expert recommendations for this vary but may include confirmation of the decision and decision-making capacity, components of informed consent, therapies to be deactivated, and family notification. Patient, surrogate, or witness signatures may be required by institutional policies but are not legal requirements.[7,62,107,108] The presence of the physician, or another clinician with appropriate expertise, at the bedside during a device withdrawal is encouraged and may be required for deactivation in a patient with complete heart block.[62,108] In any case, continued clinician involvement and caring is critical following device deactivation to avoid any sense of abandonment. Depending on the patient and resource situation, device deactivation may occur in a hospital or residential setting; thereafter, a transition to another level of care may be appropriate and should be made as smoothly as possible.

The withdrawal of an ICD or pacemaker can be carried out painlessly with the device undisturbed in the patient. With time to plan, the patient's device identification card can facilitate arrival of the correct manufacturer-specific computer. Contacting the implanting physician and/or obtaining an overpenetrated anteroposterior chest radiograph to see the identification code on the device are other means to discover the specific manufacturer. In an emergency situation, all devices will stop functioning if a circular magnet is placed or taped directly over the device (see more detail on this situation in the following).

When possible, prior to device deactivation, it can be helpful to know the original device indication and to interrogate the device with the same computer for current function to anticipate the deactivation outcome. In the case where a patient may have complete heart block, this is especially important. Counseling, education, support, and medication can then be in place for a sudden death. Otherwise, as with discontinuation of ventilators, it is not wise to predict certain death following deactivation. Unanticipated escape rhythms may emerge that sustain enough cardiac contractility and blood pressure to sustain life. Specific counseling around uncertainty in the deactivation

outcome is critical; standardization in the determination of device functioning, especially for pacemaker dependency, is lacking and may result in variable outcomes.[60,108]

In almost all settings, a medical order for device deactivation will be required. The order and medical record should reflect which therapies are to be withdrawn or continued (e.g., "discontinue all tachyarrhythmia therapies" for an ICD[108]). Most commonly, a physician or industry-employed allied professional (IEAP) uses a manufacturer-specific computer transdermally over the device to reprogram it. If present, it is often appropriate to discontinue rhythm monitoring at this time. If an IEAP is involved, this person works directly under physician supervision.[7]

Practical concerns

Once device deactivation has been performed, the patient and family will need support adjusting to the outcome. Whether this is death, continued uncertainty or slow decline, or no tangible physical change, attentive care with tailored updates and interdisciplinary team support is appropriate. If death occurs, in addition to compassionate death care, education to families about device function may be helpful, namely, that pacemakers do not continue to function after death. Family members, friends, and other formal caregivers can safely touch an ICD patient without being shocked. In the case of cremation, both devices will be removed after death to prevent battery explosion.

While technically possible, scheduling device therapy withdrawal may be difficult to coordinate for a patient at home, in a hospice unit,[109] or even in a hospital,[79,80] due to lack of equipment and expertise availability or infrequency with which this occurs. Clinician continuity and responsibility may be hard to define with multiple physicians involved, lack of training and research around these scenarios, and lack of facilitating protocols or institutional memory. This fragmented care is a potential challenge for patients with a device near end of life. Physician advocacy is frequently able to overcome such barriers if there is time and confidence. No matter the scenario, the physician in charge of a patient's care will want to contact clinicians or IEAPs to organize a device withdrawal. Whether medical staff or IEAPs perform the actual deactivation can vary; a European survey[110] indicates medical staff predominate, while U.S. surveys[55,108] suggest a dominant role for IEAPs. The same European survey explored the idea of safe remote deactivation with high physician disapproval.[110] Increased research, innovation, and education are needed to create optimal facilitation of device withdrawals for patients who have made this decision.

If urgent deactivation of an ICD is needed in a dying patient, a strong doughnut-shaped magnet placed transdermally over the device should stop the shocking and/or specifically programmed pacing immediately. In many hospice and palliative care settings, such magnets are available and specifically carried by home visit nurses. The default bradycardic pacing function (typically HR < 60) will continue. If the magnet is removed, the tachyarrhythmia sensing and shocking may resume. Some investigators suggest that household objects with magnetic fields, like cell phones, refrigerator magnets, speakers, and laptop computers, may also be effective in stopping ICD shocks in an emergency.[109] A more passive approach to deactivation of either device is the decision to not replace a battery or defective part. More than 25,000 ICD replacement procedures alone occur in the United States annually.[111] Experts recommend a triggered reevaluation of patient's projected survival, quality of life, and goals prior to any replacement procedure.[112] In a resource poor setting, achieving part replacement may be more challenging, and the option to forego replacement may be more prominent.

Consideration of pacemaker and ICD deactivation can also arise in the pediatric realm. Though increasing in number, most recent statistics suggest that less than 2% of all pacemaker and ICD implantations occur in minors.[13] In general, ethical principles and considerations for the clinical approach are similar to the situation for adults. However, the added challenge is determining the minor's degree of autonomy and decisional capacity. While the child's relevant prior experience and developmental stage will contribute to this determination,[7] the guiding concern must always be the best interest of the child (UN).[113]

Authors, IEAPs, and clinicians have called for institutional protocols and guidelines for pacemaker and ICD deactivation in order to improve quality and standardization.[6,10,56,57,108] Hospice and palliative care clinicians indicate a dearth of protocols in their institutions.[57] Any health-care setting that may have a patient with a pacemaker or ICD with comfort care goals or nearing the end of life should have a device management policy.[7] Hospices, where dying is more likely, need to ensure devices are identified on patient admission and conversations occur to identify patient's goals and allow appropriate management. One study indicates that most hospices are receiving patients with ICDs and almost 60% report a patient being shocked within the last year, but only 10% of hospices have protocols.[114] Comprehensive device management includes coordinated care across all settings, including hospice, that communicates and supports patient care goals.

Practices and attitudes in pacemaker and ICD deactivation

In the realm of implantable cardiac devices, most attention to date has focused on device development, indications, and implantation training. The ethics and practices of device deactivation have received less.[7,9,36,55,57,115] However, decisions about continuing or deactivating these devices near the end of life arise[6,55,58,60,78–81,116,117] and will become more common globally with the aging population and expanding indications for device implantation. Multiple U.S. surveys demonstrate that clinicians display attitudinal and practice differences for pacemaker and ICD deactivation, feeling less comfortable with pacemaker deactivation.[4,55–57,118,119] IEAPs[108] and cardiology society consensus statements also express this.[7,60,64] Cardiology nurses also describe a perceived difference between withholding and withdrawing these devices.[119]

Most clinicians agree that ICD deactivation in terminally ill patients with informed consent is ethical.[55–57,110,119] However, clinicians report low rates of personal experience in the actual procedure of deactivating a device.[36,55,57,110] When performed, ICD deactivation occurs very late in the clinical course, hours to days before death.[6] Despite the overall consensus on ethics and procedure, clinicians still struggle emotionally with this issue.[4] In one study of HF professionals, 22% had refused requests for pacemaker deactivation and 6% for ICD deactivation.[55] Clinicians appear more comfortable with deactivation as a patient's death appears more imminent.[56,110] Physicians acknowledge that although discussions of the deactivation option should occur, they rarely do.[37,110,120] These attitudes and practices cross physician specialties, representing primary care doctors and even electrophysiologists, as do the multiple potential obstacles to discussions.

Inadequate knowledge is one potential barrier.[4,6,56,115] A surprising number of physicians are unaware that ICD shocks can be painful, 38% in one study[56] and 41% in another,[115] or that deactivation is an option, 9%.[36] Some appear overconfident in their ability to predict which patients will be shocked.[91] Other known obstacles are the internal nature of the ICD (less visible reminder), less developed patient–physician relationships, discomfort with discussing death, and ethical concerns.[6,120] Some doctors believe this discussion is not their responsibility and should be initiated by another physician or the patient instead.[36] It is clearly problematic when subspecialists defer responsibility to generalists who may have limited knowledge and experience.[36] Doctors also assume that patients are aware of the deactivation option.[36,91] In fact, research suggests most patients are not aware; instead, they report few prior discussions, have mixed responses to these discussions, and may desire a guiding physician role in deactivation decisions.[85,121–123] While prior studies have suggested patient reluctance to consider ICD deactivation even with frequent shocking[122] or terminal cancer,[124] a more recent study suggests that after receiving ICD benefit and burden information, 70% of patients would request deactivation in at least one of five common end-of-life scenarios.[125]

Fortunately, our experience is growing, and the medical literature continues to expand. New consensus statements on pacemaker and ICD end-of-life management now exist.[7,61,64] Experts and clinicians emphasize the need for clinician and patient education and earlier discussions.[11,57,115,118,119] Despite this expanding base of support, the perception persists that a systematic approach to device deactivation is lacking.[62,110]

Ethical and legal considerations

The emotions surrounding pacemaker and ICD deactivation continue to trigger ongoing discussion as evidenced by a steady flow of literature on this topic. There is broad medical and legal consensus in the United States and many western countries for the right of a patient with decision-making capacity, terminal or not, or a legal surrogate, to request the withdrawal of any life-sustaining therapy, implantable cardiac device or other, and for the physician obligation to respect these wishes.[7,62,104,126–129] This extends to support for a patient's ability to determine one's own acceptable quality of life as a result or in spite of possible medical therapies.[130] No specific medical therapy has a unique ethical or legal status,[7] and withholding or withdrawing a therapy is ethically equivalent.[55] Moreover, when a patient dies after device deactivation, the death is attributed to the underlying disease process, or lethal pathophysiology, not device withdrawal.[7,172] The death certificate should be completed in accordance with this approach. This consensus is derived from a western tradition of medical ethics where patient autonomy (the patient's right to self-determination), beneficence (promoting good to a patient), and nonmaleficence (avoiding harm to a patient) are central.[131] In this paradigm, when a clinician deactivates a device, the intent is to relieve or prevent the patient's burden and suffering, not to achieve death (assisted death). Of note, although years of case law in the United States support this consensus approach to device deactivation, the particular case of implantable cardiac device withdrawal has not yet come before the U.S. courts.[107,118]

Informed consent is a critical element allowing a patient with decision-making capacity to weigh benefits and burdens, understand options and consequences, and make a decision in line with personal goals and values.[127] Ethically and legally, clinicians are bound to ensure patients are informed participants in clinical decision making.[7,104] In the case of a patient without decision-making capacity, a legal surrogate, as determined by an advance directive or legal hierarchy, is encouraged to use substituted judgment to act on a patient's known wishes (these wishes may come from an advance directive) or, if unknown, to make a decision based on the patient's best interest. A surrogate has the legal status of a capacitated patient but is never to base a decision solely on one's own preferences.

Knowing that an option is considered ethical in principle is different from actually writing an order or reprogramming a device with one's own hand. For some, device deactivation brings up concerns about euthanasia and physician-assisted suicide even though this is unambiguously rejected by authorities.[7,62,172] Nevertheless, studies demonstrate different perceptions.

Euthanasia is defined as intentionally causing the death of someone very sick or dying; physician-assisted suicide occurs when a physician helps a patient take his or her own life, most commonly by prescribing a lethal medication the patient then takes.[131] One study reports 11% and 1% of clinicians, respectively, indicate pacemaker and ICD deactivation are euthanasia with similar, slightly lower figures for physician-assisted suicide.[55] In one group of ICD patients, 26% equated deactivation with assisted suicide.[121] When deactivation will likely lead to immediate death, that is, a pacemaker patient has complete heart block, these actions can seem more active in assisting the path to dying. In one group of medical and legal professionals and patients, 30% considered deactivation in a pacemaker-dependent patient to be physician-assisted death or euthanasia.[118] Most device IEAPs and cardiology nurses[119]

report much greater discomfort with deactivation in a pacemaker-dependent patient, and some device companies prevent technician participation in these cases.[108] IEAPs report feeling uncomfortable, experiencing moral distress, and needing training around emotional aspects of deactivation.[108] For these clinicians and technicians, the support of a responsible physician, interdisciplinary team members, an ethics committee, or palliative care team may be helpful.[7]

Conscientious objection is a well-accepted ethical concept and relevant option in this situation. Any clinician or IEAP in this situation has the option to not participate in deactivation. However, he or she or their supervisor is obligated to provide another able clinician to perform the task in a timely fashion.[7,104,132] For instance, IEAPs report often setting up the reprogramming of a device for deactivation but having a physician or nurse push the button.[108]

Individual clinicians, patients, or family members may disagree with this widespread acceptance of device deactivation or follow a different ethical framework. Varied viewpoints, religious precepts, cultures, and values will be encountered and should be explored and respected.[118] Two authors[133] have recently argued that by replacing a native body function, pacemakers and VADs create a new lethal pathophysiology when withdrawn, not a return to the underlying one. For them, withdrawal in these cases is not equivalent to withholding therapy and represents assisted suicide. Natural death comes only when a noncardiac lethal pathophysiology intervenes. Specific opposition to this viewpoint has been expressed with questioning of an ethical framework that would create an even larger population of those dying a prolonged death from HF.[134] Above all, this alternative viewpoint highlights the importance of preimplantation counseling and informed consent for patients receiving these devices. In another example, two groups have expressed concerns about physicians making unilateral decisions to deactivate ICDs without appropriate consideration of circumstances (e.g., interpreting a DNAR status to mean ICD deactivation). Both suggest implantation changes the nature of a device to a status between body part and medical device, implying a greater emphasis toward patient decisional ownership.[135,136] Legal and ethical precedents support that all life-sustaining therapies, whether of longer or shorter duration, integrated into the body, or permanently taking over a vital function, are of equal status and may be withdrawn, emphasizing the patient's decisional role.[137]

Globally, wherever one is, it is imperative to be aware of local palliative and end-of-life care practices, culture, faiths, viewpoints, etc., as they potentially bear on device deactivation. Both U.S. and European experts emphasize the pluralistic traditions encountered by clinicians in their settings and the need for sensitivity and awareness.[7,64] For example, legal practices and politics of advance directives vary greatly by culture, country, and within countries. Not all countries, including some in Europe,[7] have advance directive legislation or pursue this framework of expression. In the United States, 95% of patients in one study supported the concept of a device-specific advance directive.[121] Even if advance directives exist, the interpretation or application may vary.[7] As a result, accepted palliative care practices in the literature, or in more developed countries, may be more or less relevant and accepted in other parts of the world. Not surprisingly, pacemaker deactivation is less consistently supported in Europe than in the United States and less so than ICD deactivation.[55] In fact, pacemaker deactivation is illegal in some European countries.[7] Ideally, an ethical consensus can prevail.

The manner in which decisions around patient cardiopulmonary resuscitation are handled at the end of life should also be expected to vary globally. The presence of an ICD creates further complexity. Some espouse that a patient's transition to DNAR status should imply ICD deactivation—equating both types of defibrillation.[105,138] Clinician opinion on this varies greatly as demonstrated by three surveys with combined agreement and disagreement at 19%–63% and 25%–66%, respectively.[55,56,115] A study of ICD patients also indicated a lack of consensus with 22% disagreement.[121] Wilkoff et al.[62] agree with ICD deactivation for DNAR status in most cases but specify patients may benefit from continued ICD therapy if (1) the arrhythmias reflect the primary cardiac condition (vs. a different irreversible process) and (2) the patient agrees that ICD therapy confers meaningful improved survival and quality of life.

Lack of consensus also exists around ICD management in hospice. In one study, 46% of ICD patients supported deactivation in hospice and 32% did not. Thirty percent of HF professionals agreed that hospices should require ICD deactivation on admission.[55] Many advocate that a patient's transition to DNAR status[56,138] or hospice[114] should be a trigger to consider deactivation of an ICD.

VADs

With the increasing prevalence of HF, technological innovation has focused on mechanical and surgical approaches to complement medical management. The first human heart transplant was performed in 1967. With further advances, survival rates have increased to nearly 50% at 10 years for heart recipients.[139] This is the best overall treatment option for advanced HF patients who are eligible for transplant. However, many patients will die waiting for a heart. Less than 1% of those eligible will receive a heart transplant since available organs remain scarce.[140] Thus, other efforts have focused on developing a total artificial heart (TAH). The first human TAH was implanted in 1984, but poor survival and prevalent safety issues were barriers.[141] TAH technology continues to advance but remains limited clinically. In this realm of mechanical circulatory support (MCS) technology, VADs were developed as a temporary bridge for survival to more advanced HF therapies like transplant.

A VAD is a mechanical pump that does the work of the left or right ventricle or both to restore normal hemodynamic parameters and perfusion for the body in advanced HF. Early VADs were transcutaneous, or extracorporeal, but most modern devices are now surgically implanted, or intracorporeal, aside from the power source. The pump mechanism may generate a pulsatile or continuous flow depending on the device model. Left ventricular assist devices (LVADs) pull blood from the left ventricle into the ascending aorta via two surgical conduits and the pumping device that sits within the abdominal wall. A third conduit, the driveline, attaches the LVAD to an external power source through a person's abdominal wall (see Figure 123.3). In 1994, the U.S. FDA approved an LVAD as bridge therapy to heart transplantation, and the first wearable device was used.[141]

Right ventricular assist devices (RVADs) are typically used less often and more for short-term support after cardiac surgery or to treat increased pulmonary pressures. Blood is pumped from the right ventricle to the pulmonary artery. A biventricular assist device (BIVAD) combines an LVAD and RVAD but is distinctly different from a TAH.

VAD indications and advances

Indications for VAD therapy have expanded since the early 1990s due to improving outcomes. Prior to the emergence of VADs, medical management, CRT, and ICDs were the maximal interventions short of transplant or TAH for those symptomatic and dying of advanced HF. Three common VAD pathways are currently defined: bridge to transplantation (BTT), destination therapy (DT), and bridge to recovery (BTR). Survival and duration of VAD use in all three depend on the strategy of support at time of VAD implant, timing of implant, medical comorbidities, and patient age, among other factors.[142] BTT indicates a person who is a heart transplant candidate but is not likely to survive to receive a transplant without VAD support. U.S. registry data indicate average 1- and 2-year actuarial survival for BTT exceeds 80% and 70%, respectively.[143] DT is for someone with advanced HF who is not a transplant candidate but could benefit from VAD support. In 2002, the U.S. FDA approved LVADs for DT.[140] The 2001 REMATCH study[144] drew increased attention to this category. It demonstrated dramatically improved survival and quality of life in patients with LVADs when compared to medical therapy for those not transplant eligible.[144] Average 1- and 2-year survival was 52% and 23% for those with LVADs compared to 25% and 8%, respectively, for those receiving medical management; health-related quality of life was also superior at 1 year for the LVAD group.[144] Other studies on DT have shown similar or better outcomes,[145–148] including a more recent average 1-year survival figure of 74%[142] and a predicted 2-year survival of 87% at a different center.[149] Overall, VAD patients have survival rates of 80% at 1 year and 70% at 2 years, with the DT pathway having a slightly higher risk of mortality versus BT.[150]

The BTR indication is rare and usually begins with a BTT or DT pathway. The native heart recovers adequate function to have VAD explantation and survival without heart transplant. Multiple institutions have now reported such cases.[151–155] Despite the compelling evidence of recovery in some cases, overall rates for achieving successful VAD explantation are

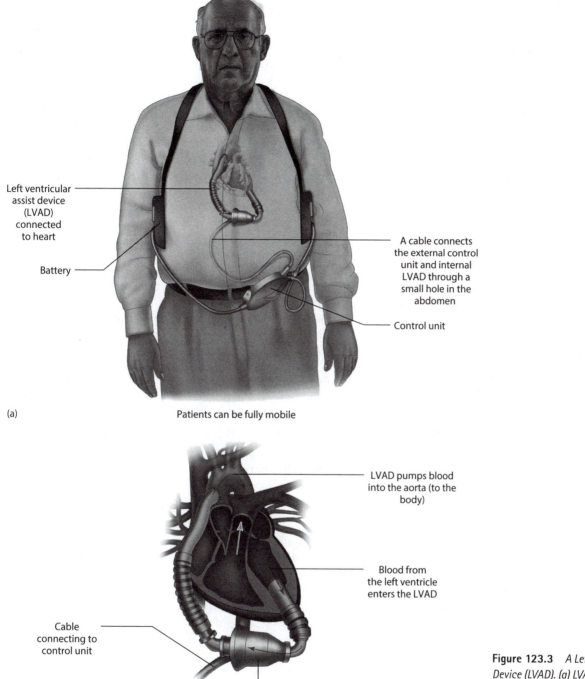

(a)   Patients can be fully mobile

(b)   Heart is shown in cross section

Left ventricular
assist device
(LVAD)
connected
to heart

Battery

A cable connects
the external control
unit and internal
LVAD through a
small hole in the
abdomen

Control unit

LVAD pumps blood
into the aorta (to the
body)

Blood from
the left ventricle
enters the LVAD

Cable
connecting to
control unit

LVAD

Figure 123.3 *A Left Ventricular Assist Device (LVAD). (a) LVAD in mobile patient. (b) Heart in cross section with LVAD. (Adapted from http://www.nhlbi.nih.gov/health/health-topics/topics/vad/.)*

low at 5%–24% in different case series.[154] Interestingly, a recent study suggests comparable outcomes for BTR and BTT VAD pathways with a suggestion that a portion of transplants may be avoidable in the future.[155]

As with other cardiac technologies, VAD use is primarily limited to more developed nations. High costs, the need for tertiary HF centers, and ideally cardiac transplant programs remain barriers to global VAD access.[29] In the United States, FDA-approved VAD use is prospectively monitored by the

Interagency Registry for Mechanically Assisted Circulatory Support (INTERMACS).[156] The Pediatric Mechanically Assisted Circulatory Support (PEDIMACS) Registry[157] was created in late 2012 to capture similar data unique to those younger than 19 years old. The International Society for Heart and Lung Transplantation (ISHLT)[158] recently announced an international effort, ISHLT Mechanical Assist Circulatory Support (IMACS) Registry, which will eventually include current databases from Europe, Asia, and other locations.[159]

At present, international VAD data are not readily available. Prior 2005 data from an earlier MCS database included four European countries, Canada, Israel, and Singapore in addition to the United States.[160] As a surrogate VAD marker, ISHLT cardiac transplant centers are growing in number and most prevalent in North America and Europe followed by Australasia and South America; very few transplants are noted in Africa.[158] INTERMACS reports data from 131 U.S. hospitals as of June 2012.[156] From June 2006 to June 2012, 6274 patients received a primary LVAD or BIVAD with those on a BTT strategy decreasing from 40% to 21% during this timeframe and DT increasing from 18% to 44%.[150] Patient numbers remain low for BTR in the same period; the TAH population represents less than 3% of devices in 2008–2012.[150] Despite improving survival statistics as mentioned earlier, one in five of these adult patients still dies within 2 years.[150] During this same timeframe, 72 pediatric patients received some form of MCS.[150]

The ESC, ACC Foundation/AHA, Canadian Cardiovascular Society (CCS), and Australian guidelines support VAD use for BTT and more recently DT with an emphasis on appropriate patient selection.[29,31–33,53] Interestingly, ESC and CCS guidelines outline additional VAD pathways for consideration; bridge to decision (BTD) is for VAD use in an imminently dying patient, so further evaluation of options can be completed, and bridge to candidacy (BTC) is used to allow an ineligible patient to recover enough end-organ function to become transplant eligible.[29] Importantly, the ability to follow guidelines in a given country may be limited by payment mechanisms. For instance, the National Health Service currently limits use of VADs in the United Kingdom to BTT or BTR, but payment extension to DT is being debated.[161] In addition to these recognized VAD pathways, early INTERMACS data have been used to define seven clinical patient profiles of those being considered for VAD therapy.[162] These profiles reflect the subsets of patients in NYHA Classes III and IV, spanning the spectrum of Profile 1, critical cardiogenic shock, and Profile 2, progressive decline, to Profile 7, advanced NYHA Class III symptoms. Interestingly, INTERMACS data have already documented a shift to LVAD implantation earlier in the HF trajectory. First-year (2006–2007) data indicated 42% of VAD recipients were Profile 1, decreasing to 28% by year 3[163] and 16% by year 5.[150]

Over time, VAD innovation has led to smaller devices, greater patient mobility, improved safety, more dependable access to a power source, more advanced surgical approaches, and a transition from pulsatile to continuous flow devices (now 95% of implanted VADs)[150] with improved survival.[142,149] Advances leading to smaller devices have even led to a recent pediatric VAD trial in children 16 and younger.[164] Progress toward the goal of a totally implantable device continues.[141] Today, LVADs are frequently used in the developed world with potential for mobility and independence at home.

VAD COSTS AND COMPLICATIONS

Few publications address LVAD costs, but 2001 figures report average device cost at $67,085, initial implantation hospitalization at $141,287, and total first-year costs at $222,460,

comparable to a heart transplant.[165] More recent figures from Norway indicate two device costs of $32,000 (2005–2009) and $58,000 (2009–2011) and average costs for the "LVAD phase" from implantation to hospital discharge of $378,450 and $346,403, respectively.[166]

VADs can clearly have a palliative role in advanced HF. Survival can usually be extended along with potential improvement in symptoms and function. If all goes well, the palliative framework may even shift to one of survivorship with DT as permanent palliation. However, for some, these gains are balanced by the potential serious complications, treatment burden, and high mortality. Thirty to 90-day mortality for LVAD implantation is 14%–27%.[167] Early risks include multiorgan system failure, bleeding, air embolism, and right HF, while later threats are typically thromboembolism, infection, and device failure.[141,168] Infection rates range from 30% to 40% and thromboembolic or hemorrhagic stroke from 10% to 30%.[169] In one trial, 35% of devices had a malfunction at 2 years (REMATCH). Intensive care, including chronic renal replacement, ventilator support, and other cardiac supports like ICDs, may be necessary and results in an extended course with critical illness.[170] If death occurs, sepsis, multiorgan system failure, stroke, and right HF are common causes.[145] In less acute circumstances, the burden of device alarms, reliance on a power supply, increased anxiety, early satiety and anorexia from device size in the abdomen,[169] altered mobility, and other medical complications, like pressure ulcers, may be central for a patient and family.

Palliative care role for VAD management

COMMUNICATION

As with pacemakers and ICDs, communication and the shared decision-making model[5] are critical and recommended for clinicians and patients starting at preimplantation for VAD.[5,8] Many experts are now recommending early involvement of palliative care teams in the VAD course to facilitate this aspect of care with other interdisciplinary care domains.[5,8,167,171,172] The realm of MCS device technology is very complex, and the decision for which specific device/model to use may even be difficult for clinicians.[173] The clinician role in facilitating patient understanding around this even greater level of medical complexity is more challenging but crucial in introducing and revisiting the possibility of VAD withdrawal. Achieving adequate informed consent for implantation may be a true test,[170] especially when emergent events remove or weaken a patient's decision-making capacity.

Although VAD programs have structured processes for patient selection and implantation, the steps may blur when all want an imminently dying patient to live.[167,174] The value of longitudinal communication and shared decision making upstream for all advanced HF patients in just this situation cannot be overemphasized. Serial communications to revisit VAD patient goals, values, and preferences in alignment with cardiac disease status, current and potential therapies, and other medical conditions should occur regularly. One study found that less than 50% of patients with LVADs had advance directives, and of those, none specifically mentioned LVAD end-of-life wishes.[175] ACP should thus be fully integrated using the "hope for the best, plan for the worst" approach and emphasizing clinician continuity.[5] Triggers for these discussions, similar to those previously (see Table 123.1), are also suggested. For VADs, new serious complications like stroke or renal failure, the need for additional life support measures, and loss of eligibility for heart transplantation would be other potential triggers for proactive communication.

Recent research has suggested improved ACP, end-of-life planning, symptom management, and holistic care with palliative care team involvement for potential or current VAD patients.[176] One group of investigators[8] has proposed a model for proactive palliative medicine consultation for VAD patients termed "preparedness planning." It begins prior to implantation and continues longitudinally for the entire patient course with a focus on serial conversations around patient goals in line with the patient's disease progression. The approach to ACP and communication is tailored specifically to VAD patients and families. Others have emphasized a detailed informed consent process specific to VADs with similar emphasis.[167,174,177]

VAD withdrawal

When VAD benefits no longer outweigh burdens for a patient or meet a patient's goals, withdrawal of the VAD should be considered. Whether the VAD is BTT or DT, the grim prognosis of advanced HF has worsened. Routine VAD withdrawal is not invasive and does not require surgery. As with pacemakers and ICDs, great preparation and coordination is required. Decision making and planning should be clearly documented in the medical record. Beyond appropriate clarification of the goals of care, technical aspects should be clarified with the whole team, including technicians or perfusionists, in line with an optimal end-of-life setting for the patient and family. Involvement of an interdisciplinary palliative care team is ideal to address whole person care for the patient and family.

Education for all involved about expectations for the order and flow of events is important. Average time to death after VAD withdrawal was about 20 min in one study[171] and 1 day or less in another.[172] Comparison has been made to an endotracheal ventilator withdrawal scenario.[5] Thus, families should be counseled to prepare for a very short timeframe of minutes with the caveat that one of hours or longer is possible. Very rarely, a patient's native heart function may be stronger than anticipated and allow for brief stabilization, perhaps even transition to another site of care. VAD patients may be receiving other life-prolonging therapies, like mechanical ventilation or hemodialysis, and the potential for deactivation of these devices needs to be clarified and prioritized. ICDs, if present, should be deactivated in preparation for VAD withdrawal. Resuscitation status will likely need clarification with updating of paperwork to allow natural death during VAD withdrawal.

Symptom assessment before, during, and after the withdrawal will focus on dyspnea, anxiety, and pain from the anticipated decrease in cardiovascular support. The medications to be ordered and immediately available at the bedside do not differ from those needed for pacemakers and ICDs. Premedication with opioids and anxiolytics before VAD withdrawal should be strongly considered to ensure adequate circulation of medications prior to decreased cardiac function. Dosing is based on medications already in use and symptoms prior to withdrawal. This planning will ideally be discussed with the patient or family based on anticipated distress and medication effects. Some patients may request sedation during the procedure, while others may not.

A recommended checklist of steps for VAD withdrawal is provided for guidance (see Table 123.2). Once family members are present and ready, a device technician can plan for alarm silencing. Heart, blood pressure, and pulse oximetry monitors should be turned off. The technician can then turn off the device; this is generally an act of unplugging the power source. Physician presence is needed for the duration if the timeframe is short, or until the patient appears clinically stable, particularly for continued assessment, reassurance, and education. When a last breath is taken, standard death pronouncement and postdeath care are conducted with device again left in place. The VAD may be removed later during preparation of the body depending on chosen rituals.

Practical concerns

When patients have a good functional outcome with VAD therapy, they can often leave the hospital setting. More and more patients are living at home or in nursing facility settings[178] with their devices. When their medical status changes and the decision is made for VAD withdrawal, patients may also wish to die in these settings.[5] While there is no medical, ethical, or legal barrier to this, practical considerations, like physician expertise, may be a challenge. As with pacemakers and ICDs, physician leadership in coordinating events and achieving the technical support and appropriate interdisciplinary team may be difficult to organize outside a hospital.

Practice and attitudes in VAD withdrawal

Attention to VAD management near the end of life has been limited to date[180] though HF specialists are expected to be competent in VAD withdrawal.[181] Cases of VAD withdrawal occur and are becoming more common.[177,182] In two groups of nearly 70 VAD patients, 24%[171] and 21%[172] requested device withdrawal. Evidence suggests that new or worsening comorbidities serve as a primary trigger for patient or clinician consideration of LVAD withdrawal, specifically sepsis, stroke, cancer, renal failure, and pump failure.[171]

Research is needed to better document current practices and attitudes among clinicians, patients, and families; define standards of practice; and explore quality of end-of-life care and caregiver burden.[167] Some institutions have a more structured, proactive approach to defining VAD patient wishes and decisions near end of life and facilitating a smooth withdrawal process.[8,171] Many do not. In one program review of 20 VAD patients who died,[171] 11 died at home, 8 in the hospital, and 1 in a nursing home. All were offered hospice and/or palliative care support and noted to have appropriate symptom management at time of death. Seventeen chose to turn off their device, while 3 continued the VAD until death, another 2–5 months. In another review of 14 VAD patients,[172] 12 died in the hospital and 2 in hospice units. Two patients made their own decisions for withdrawal, and surrogates acted for the other 12.

Ethical and legal considerations

Despite some who disagree, broad consensus supports decisions for VAD withdrawal in the same way that other life-sustaining measures may be discontinued.[5,172,174,177] Informed consent and symptom control to prevent physical suffering are part of this ethical framework. For some, the newness of the technology may lead to questioning the ethics of VAD withdrawal. As with the aforementioned discussion of pacemakers and ICDs, some may object to VAD withdrawal based on characteristics of the device (being surgically implanted and taking over an essential physiologic function) or a perceived overlap with assisted suicide and euthanasia.[172] Some specifically struggle with the extent to which the LVAD changes the physiology of the dying process once turned off.[177] Personal beliefs and emotions may also differ from the ethical consensus. Conscientious objection is always an option for clinicians and technicians. Cultural, religious, and legal differences around the world may also affect the option of VAD withdrawal. Palliative care and ethics committee involvement is encouraged when clinicians, patients, or families struggle with these dilemmas.[172,174]

Ethical concerns may also arise before VAD withdrawal, or if withdrawal is not pursued, when a patient is judged to be receiving more burden than benefit from a VAD. Of course, this is the common situation for those considering VAD withdrawal as earlier. Some have termed this condition "destination nowhere" reflecting prolonged suffering without improvement in a DT VAD course.[183] All involved may develop distress over the ongoing VAD support if patient suffering continues. The recognition of this ethically complex endpoint has led some to advocate for more stringent processes for selection of and communication with potential DT VAD patients.[174,183] Excluding patients from DT who do not have the capacity to voluntarily consent and those in whom implantation would be rushed to prevent imminent death has been proposed.[174]

CONCLUSION

The landscape of advanced HF management continues to evolve rapidly with advancing technology. Implantable cardiac devices, pacemakers, ICDs, and VADs, in particular, have created exciting opportunities for improved patient quality of life, function, and survival. These devices have a clear role in the palliative realm. However, they do not prevent death or disability.

Although they may change the course of a patient's illness in a positive way, they may also adversely affect a patient with complications and adverse events. Devices may worsen a patient's dying and death by prolonging the course and increasing suffering. Even in the best scenario, the role of a given device will be temporary as that person ages and eventually dies.

A palliative approach will include shared decision making with attention to informed consent and ACP processes starting at preimplantation. This extends into serial points of continued communication and reassessment of device appropriateness over a patient's lifetime. Routine checkups and specific events, like a new terminal diagnosis, progressing noncardiac illness, or the need for battery replacement, should trigger such reviews. If and when the decision is made to deactivate or withdraw a device, a structured palliative approach to informed consent, communication, education, coordination, symptom management, and the spiritual, social, and emotional needs of the patient/family/team is essential. Palliative care specialty level expertise is expanding in this area, but the literature is limited. Helpful resources are available.

ACKNOWLEDGMENT

The author wishes to thank Dr. Nathan E. Goldstein for his advice on chapter development and Drs. George A. Taffet and Miguel Valderrabano for their suggestions with chapter edits.

REFERENCES

1 Goldberger Z and Lampert R. Implantable cardioverter–defibrillators: Expanding indications and technologies. *J Am Med Assoc.* 2006;295(7):809–818.

2 Kusumoto FM and Goldschlager N. Device therapy for cardiac arrhythmias. *J Am Med Assoc.* 2002;287(14):1848–1852.

3 Linde C, Ellenbogen K, and McAlister FA. Cardiac resynchronization therapy (CRT): Clinical trials, guidelines, and target populations. *Heart Rhythm.* 2012;9(Suppl. 8):S3–S13.

4 Kramer DB, Kesselheim AS, Brock DW, and Maisel WH. Ethical and legal views of physicians regarding deactivation of cardiac implantable electrical devices: A quantitative assessment. *Heart Rhythm.* 2010;7:1537–1542.

5 Allen LA, Stevenson LW, Grady KL et al. Decision making in advanced heart failure: A scientific statement from the American Heart Association. *Circulation.* 2012;125(15):1928–1952.

6 Goldstein NE, Lampert R, Bradley E, Lynn J, and Krumholz HM. Management of implantable cardioverter defibrillators in end-of-life care. *Ann Intern Med.* 2004;141(11):835–838.

7 Lampert R, Hayes DL, Annas GJ et al. Expert Consensus Statement on the Management of Cardiovascular Implantable Electronic Devices (CIEDs) in patients nearing end of life or requesting withdrawal of therapy. *Heart Rhythm.* 2010;7(7):1008–1026.

8 Swetz KM, Freeman MR, Abou Ezzeddine OF, Carter KA, Boilson BA, Ottenberg AL, Park SJ, and Mueller PS. Palliative medicine consultation for preparedness planning in patients receiving left ventricular assist devices as destination therapy. *Mayo Clin Proc.* 2011;86(6):493–500.

9   Berger JT. Ethics of deactivating implanted cardioverter defibrillators. *Ann Intern Med.* 2005;142(8):631–634.

10 Lewis WR, Luebke DL, Johnson NJ, Harrington MD, Costantini O, and Aulisio MP. Withdrawing implantable defibrillator shock therapy in terminally ill patients. *Am J Med.* 2006;119(10):892–896.

11 Sinclair CT. Implantable cardioverter-defibrillators and complications [letter]. *N Engl J Med.* 2004;350(7):734–735.

12 Hunt SA, Abraham WT, Casey DE Jr. et al. ACC/AHA 2005 guideline update for the diagnosis and management of chronic heart failure in the adult: A report of the American College of Cardiology/American Heart Association Task Force on Practice Guidelines (Writing Committee to Update the 2001 Guidelines for the Evaluation and Management of Heart Failure). *J Am Coll Cardiol.* 2005;46:e1–e82.

13 Roger VL, Go AS, Lloyd-Jones DM et al. Heart disease and stroke statistics–2012 update: A report from the American Heart Association. *Circulation.* 2012;125:e2–e220.

14 Mosterd A and Hoes AW. Clinical epidemiology of heart failure. *Heart.* 2007;93:1137–1146.

15 Mosterd A, Hoes AW, de Bruyne MC et al. Prevalence of heart failure and left ventricular dysfunction in the general population; The Rotterdam Study. *Eur Heart J.* 1999;20(6):447–455.

16 Cowie MR, Wood DA, Coats AJ et al. Incidence and aetiology of heart failure; a population-based study. *Eur Heart J.* 1999;20(6):421–428.

17 Cost B, Grobbee DE, Van der Schoot-van Venrooy J et al. Chapter 5: Incidence and risk factors of heart failure. pp. 47–64. *In Thesis: Heart Failure in the Elderly.* 2000.

18 Bleumink GS, Knetsch AM, Sturkenboom MC et al. Quantifying the heart failure epidemic: Prevalence, incidence rate, lifetime risk and prognosis of heart failure The Rotterdam Study. *Eur Heart J.* 2004;25(18):1614–1619.

19 World Heart Failure Society. Heart failure worldwide facts and figures. http://www.worldheartfailure.org/index.php?item=75. Last accessed: February 3, 2013.

20 Bhatia RS, Tu JV, Lee DS, Austin PC, Fang J, Haouzi A, Gong Y, and Liu PP. Outcome of heart failure with preserved ejection fraction in a population based study. *N Engl J Med.* 2006;355(3):260–269.

21 Stewart S, Ekman I, Ekman T, Oden A, and Rosengren A. Population impact of heart failure and the most common forms of cancer: A study of 1 162 309 hospital cases in Sweden (1988 to 2004). *Circ Cardiovasc Qual Outcomes.* 2010;3:573–580.

22 Cubbon RM, Gale CP, Kearney LC et al. Changing characteristics and mode of death associated with chronic heart failure caused by left ventricular systolic dysfunction: A study across therapeutic eras. *Circ Heart Fail.* 2011;4:396–403.

23 Mendez GF and Cowie MR. The epidemiological features of heart failure in developing countries: A review of the literature. *Int J Cardiol.* 2001;80:213–219.

24 Callow AD. Cardiovascular disease 2005–The global picture. *Vasc Pharmacol.* 2006;45:302–307.

25 Baman TS, Kirkpatrick JN, Romero J et al. Pacemaker reuse: An initiative to alleviate the burden of symptomatic bradyarrhythmia in impoverished nations around the world. *Circulation.* 2010;122:1649–1656.

26 Sliwa K, Damasceno A, and Mayosi BM. Epidemiology and etiology of cardiomyopathy in Africa. *Circulation.* 2005;112(23):3577–3583. (No stats on developing countries).

27 Marijon E, Mirabel M, Celermajer DS, and Jouven X. Rheumatic heart disease. *Lancet.* 2012;379:953–964.

28 Jessup M and Brozena S. Heart failure. *N Engl J Med.* 2003;348:2007–2018.

29 McMurray JJ, Adamopoulos S, Anker SD et al. ESC guidelines for the diagnosis and treatment of acute and chronic heart failure 2012: The task force for the diagnosis and treatment of acute and chronic heart failure 2012 of the European Society of Cardiology. Developed in collaboration with the Heart Failure Association (HFA) of the ESC. *Eur J Heart Fail.* 2012;14(8):803–869.

30 Chen J, Normand SL, Wang Y, and Krumholz HM. National and regional trends in heart failure hospitalization and mortality rates for Medicare beneficiaries, 1998–2008. *J Am Med Assoc.* 2011;306:1669–1678.

31 Jessup M, Abraham WT, Casey DE et al. 2009 Focused update: ACCF/AHA guidelines for the diagnosis and management of heart failure in adults: A report of the American College of Cardiology Foundation/American Heart Association Task Force on Practice Guidelines. *Circulation.* 2009;119(14):1977–2016.

32 McKelvie RS, Moe GW, Cheung A et al. The 2011 Canadian Cardiovascular Society heart failure management guidelines update: Focus on sleep apnea, renal dysfunction, mechanical circulatory support, and palliative care. *Can J Cardiol.* 2011;27(3):319–338.

33 National Heart Foundation of Australia and the Cardiac Society of Australia and New Zealand (Chronic Heart Failure Guidelines Expert Writing Panel). Guidelines for the prevention, detection and management of chronic heart failure in Australia. Heart Foundation, New South Wales, Australia, Updated July 2011.

34 Jaarsma T, Beattie JM, Ryder M et al. Palliative care in heart failure: A position statement from the palliative care workshop of the Heart Failure Association of the European Society of Cardiology. *Eur J Heart Fail.* 2009;11:433–443.

35 Goodlin SJ, Hauptman PJ, Arnold R et al. Consensus statement: Palliative and supportive care in advanced heart failure. *J Card Fail.* 2004;10:200–209.

36 Kelley AS, Mehta SS, and Reid MC. Management of patients with ICDs at the end of life (EOL): A qualitative study. *Am J Hosp Palliat Care.* January 2008–December 2009;25(6):440–446.

37 Hauptman PJ, Swindle J, Hussain Z, Biener L, and Burroughs TE. Physician attitudes toward end-stage heart failure: A national survey. *Am J Med.* 2008;121(2):127–135.

38 Mond HG and Proclemer A. The 11th world survey of cardiac pacing and implantable cardioverter-defibrillators: Calendar year 2009–A World Society of Arrhythmia's Project. *Pacing Clin Electrophysiol.* 2011;34:1013–1027.

39 Groh WJ. You shouldn't take it with you: Postmortem device reuse. *Heart Rhythm.* 2012;9:215–216.

40 Bogáts G, Kovács G, and Rudas L. Postmortem device reuse. *Heart Rhythm.* 2012;9(6):e15.

41 Yusuf SW. Letter by Yusuf regarding article, "Pacemaker reuse: An initiative to alleviate the burden of symptomatic bradyarrhythmia in impoverished nations around the world". *Circulation.* 2011;123(24):e637.

42 Rydén L. Re-use of devices in cardiology. Report from a Policy Conference at the European Heart House. *Eur Heart J.* 1998;19:1628–1631.

43 Kirkpatrick JN, Papini C, Baman TS, Khota K, Eagle KA, Verdino RJ, and Caplan AL. Reuse of pacemakers and defibrillators in developing countries: Logistical, legal, and ethical barriers and solutions. *Heart Rhythm.* 2010;7:1623–1627.

44 Aragam KG, Baman TS, Kirkpatrick JN, Goldman EB, Brown AC, Crawford T, Oral H, and Eagle KA. The ethics of pacemaker reuse: Might the best be the enemy of the good? *Heart.* 2011;97(24):2005–2006.

45 Baman TS, Meier P, Romero J, Gakenheimer L, Kirkpatrick JN, Sovitch P, Oral H, and Eagle KA. Safety of pacemaker reuse: A meta-analysis with implications for underserved nations. *Circ Arrhythm Electrophysiol.* 2011;4:318–323.

46 Boal BH, Escher DJW, Furman S et al. Report of the policy conference on pacemaker reuse sponsored by the North American Society of Pacing and Electrophysiology. *J Am Coll Cardiol.* 1985;5(3):808–810.

47 Cleland JGF, Daubert JC, Erdmann E et al. The effect of cardiac resyn-chronization on morbidity and mortality in heart failure. *N Engl J Med.* 2005;352:1539–1549.

48 Bristow MR, Saxon LA, Boehmer J et al. Cardiac-resynchronization therapy with or without an implantable defibrillator in advanced chronic heart failure. *N Engl J Med.* 2004;350(21):2140–2150.

49 Rosanio S, Schwarz ER, Vitarelli A, Zarraga IG, Kunapuli S, Ware DL, Birnbaum Y, Tuero E, and Uretsky BF. Sudden death prophylaxis in heart failure. *Int J Cardiol.* 2007;119(3):291–296.

50 Abraham WT, Fisher WG, Smith AL et al. Cardiac resynchronization in chronic heart failure. *N Engl J Med.* 2002;346:1845–1853.

51 Ghio S, Freemantle N, Scelsi L et al. Long-term left ventricular reverse remodeling with cardiac resynchronization therapy: Results from the CARE-HF trial. *Eur Heart J.* 2009;22:480–488.

52 DiMarco JP. Implantable cardioverter–defibrillators. *N Engl J Med.* 2003;349:1836–1847.

53 Dickstein K, Vardas PE, Auricchio A et al. 2010 Focused guidelines on device therapy in heart failure: An update of the 2008 ESC guide-lines for the diagnosis and treatment of acute and chronic heart failure and the 2007 ESC guidelines for cardiac synchronization therapy. Developed with the special contribution of the Heart Failure Association and the European Heart Rhythm Association. *Eur Heart J.* 2010;31(21):2677–2687. Epub 2010 Aug 27.

54 Epstein AE, DiMarco JP, Ellenbogen KA et al. Executive summary: A report of the American College of Cardiology/American Heart Association Task Force on Practice Guidelines (Writing Committee to Revise the ACC/AHA/NASPE 2002 Guideline Update for Implantation of Cardiac Pacemakers and Antiarrhythmia Devices). *Heart Rhythm.* 2008;5(6):e1–e62.

55 Mueller PS, Jenkins SM, Bramstedt KA, and Hayes DL. Deactivating implanted cardiac devices in terminally ill patients: Practices and atti-tudes. *Pacing Clin Electrophysiol.* 2008;31(5):560–568.

56 Kelley AS, Reid MC, Miller DH, Fins JJ, and Lachs MS. Implantable cardioverter defibrillator at end-of-life: A physician survey. *Am Heart J.* 2009;157:702–708.

57 Morrison LJ, Calvin AO, Nora H, and Porter Storey C Jr. Managing car-diac devices near the end of life: A survey of hospice and palliative care providers. *Am J Hosp Palliat Care.* 2010;8:545–551.

58 Rhymes JA, McCullough LB, Luchi RJ, Teasdale TA, and Wilson N. Withdrawing very low-burden interventions in chronically ill patients. *J Am Med Assoc.* 2000;283(8):1061–1063.

59 Harrington MD, Luebke DL, Lewis WR, Aulisio MP, and Johnson NJ. Cardiac pacemakers at the end of life #111. *J Palliat Med.* 2005;8(5):1055–1056.

60 Whitlock SN, Goldberg IP, and Singh JP. Is pacemaker deactivation at the end of life unique? A case study and ethical analysis. *J Palliat Med.* 2011;14(10):1184–1188.

61 Braun TC, Hagen NA, Hatfield RE, and Wyse DG. Cardiac pacemak-ers and implantable defibrillators in terminal care. *J Pain Symptom Manage.* 1999;18(2):126–131.

62 Wilkoff BL, Auricchio A, Brugada J et al. HRS/EHRA Expert Consensus on the Monitoring of Cardiovascular Implantable Electronic Devices (CIEDs): Description of techniques, indications, personnel, frequency, ethical considerations: Developed in partnership with the Heart Rhythm Society (HRS) and the European Heart Rhythm Association (EHRA); and in col-laboration with the American College of Cardiology (ACC), the American Heart Association (AHA), the European Society of Cardiology (ESC), the Heart Failure Association of ESC (HFA), and the Heart Failure Society of America (HFSA). Endorsed by the Heart Rhythm Society, the European Heart Rhythm Association (a registered branch of the ESC), the American College of Cardiology, the American Heart Association. *Europace.* 2008;10:707–725.

63 Ballentine JM. Pacemaker and defibrillator deactivation in competent hospice patients: An ethical consideration. *Am J Hosp Palliat Care.* 2005;22(1):14–19.

64 Padeletti L, Arnar DO, Boncinelli L et al. EHRA Expert consensus state-ment on the management of cardiovascular implantable electronic devices in patients nearing end of life or requesting withdrawal of therapy. *Europace.* 2010;12(10):1480–1489.

65 Moss AJ, Zareba W, Hall WJ, Klein H, Wilber DJ, Cannom DS, Daubert JP, Higgins SL, Brown MW, and Andrews ML. Prophylactic implantation of a defibrillator in patients with myocardial infarction and reduced ejection fraction. *N Engl J Med.* 2002;346:877–883.

66 CMS. National coverage determination for implantable automatic defi-brillators (20.4) document. http://www.cms.gov/medicare-coverage-database/details/ncd-details.aspx?NCDId=110&ncdver=3&NCAId=39&ver=11&NcaName=Implantable+Cardioverter+Defibrillators+(ICDs)&CoverageSelection=National&KeyWord=ICD&KeyWordLookUp=Title&KeyWordSearchType=And&bc=gAAAABAACAAAAA%3d%3d&. Accessed February 3, 2013.

67 Baman TS and Eagle KA. Cardiac device reutilization: Is it time to "go green" in underserved countries? *Pacing Clin Electrophysiol.* 2011;34(6):651–652.

68 Pavri BB, Lokhandwala Y, Kulkarni GV, Shah M, Kantharia BK, and Mascarenhas DA. Reuse of explanted, resterilized implant-able cardioverter-defibrillators: A cohort study. *Ann Intern Med.* 2012;157(8):542–548.

69 Kadish A, Dyer A, Daubert JP et al. Prophylactic defibrillator implan-tation in patients with nonischemic cardiomyopathy. *N Engl J Med.* 2004;350:2151–2158.

70 Bardy GH, Lee KL, Mark DB et al. Amiodarone or implantable car-dioverter-defibrillator for congestive heart failure. *N Engl J Med.* 2005;352:225–237.

71 Zipes DP, Camm AJ, Borggrefe M et al. ACC/AHA/ESC 2006 guidelines for management of patients with ventricular arrhythmias and the pre-vention of sudden cardiac death: A report of the American College of Cardiology/American Heart Association Task Force and the European Society of Cardiology Committee for Practice Guidelines (Writing Committee to Develop Guidelines for Management of Patients With Ventricular Arrhythmias and the Prevention of Sudden Cardiac Death). *J Am Coll Cardiol.* 2006;48(5):e247–e346.

72 Gregoratos G, Abrams A, Epstein AE et al. ACC/AHA/NASPE 2002 guideline update for implantation of cardiac pacemakers and anti-arrhythmia devices: Summary article: A report of the American College of Cardiology/American Heart Association Task Force on Practice Guidelines (AHA/ACC/NASPE Committee to Update the 1998 Pacemaker Guidelines). *Circulation.* 2002;106:2145–2161.

73 United States Food and Drug Administration. Wearable cardio-verter defibrillator approval. http://www.fda.gov/MedicalDevices/ProductsandMedicalProcedures/DeviceApprovalsandClearances/Recently-ApprovedDevices/ucm083949.htm. Accessed February 3, 2013.

74 Everitt MD and Saarel EV. Use of the wearable external cardiac defi-brillator in children. *Pacing Clin Electrophysiol.* 2010;33(6):742–746.

75 Heart Rhythm Society. Sudden cardiac death primary preven-tion protocols, 2012 (Version 2; Revised: 9/10/2012; Review date: 9/10/2013). http://www.hrsonline.org/News/Sudden-Cardiac-Arrest-SCA-Awareness/SCA-Provider-Resources/SCD-Primary-Prevention-Protocols#axzz2JCnZ8RU7. Accessed February 3, 2013.

76 Klein HU, Meltendorf U, Reek S et al. Bridging a temporary high risk of sudden arrhythmic death. Experience with the wearable cardioverter defibrillator (WCD). *Pacing Clin Electrophysiol.* 2010;33(3):353–367.

77 Withell B. Patient consent and implantable cardioverter defi-brillators: Some palliative care implications. *Int J Palliat Nurs.* 2006;12(10):470–475.

78   Grassman D. EOL considerations in defibrillator deactivation. *Am J Hosp Palliat Care*. 2005;22(3):179–180. (Author response Ballentine-No truly informed consent).

79   Nambisan V and Chao D. Dying and defibrillation: A shocking experience. *Palliat Med*. 2004;18(5):482–483.

80   Looi YC. And it can go on and on and on. *J Pain Symptom Manage*. 2006;31:1–2.

81   Basta LL and Jennings TR. Ethical issues in the management of geriatric cardiac patients: A patient asks to put an end to the nightmare of living with a lifesaving AICD. *Am J Geriatr Cardiol*. 2002;11(5):326–327.

82   Sears SF, Shea JB, and Conti JB. How to respond to an ICD shock. *Circulation*. 2005;111(23):e380–e382.

83   Ahmad M, Bloomstein L, Roelke M, Berstein A, and Parsonnet V. Patients' attitudes toward implanted defibrillator shocks. *Pacing Clin Electrophysiol*. 2000;23(6):934–938.

84   Pelletier D, Gallagher R, Mitten-Lewis S, McKinley S, and Squire J. Australian implantable cardiac defibrillator recipients: Quality-of-life issues. *Int J Nurs Pract*. 2002;8(2):68–74.

85   Goldstein NE, Mehta D, Siddiqui S et al. "That's like an act of suicide": Patients' attitudes toward deactivation of implantable defibrillators. *J Gen Intern Med*. 2008;23(Suppl. 1):7–12.

86   Eckert M and Jones T. How does an implantable cardioverter defibrillator (ICD) affect the lives of patients and their families? *Int J Nurs Pract*. 2002;8(3):152–157.

87   Freedenberg V, Thomas SA, and Friedmann E. Anxiety and depression in implanted cardioverter-defibrillator recipients and heart failure: A review. *Heart Fail Clin*. 2011;7(1):59–68. Review.

88   Jeffrey K. Preventing sudden cardiac death: The implantable defibrillator. In: *Machines in Our Hearts: The Cardiac Pacemaker, the Implantable Defibrillator, and American Health Care*. The Johns Hopkins University Press, Baltimore, MD, 2001, Chapter 10.

89   Irvine J, Dorian P, Baker B et al. Quality of life in the Canadian implantable defibrillator study (CIDS). *Am Heart J*. 2002;144:282–289.

90   Dunbar SB, Dougherty CM, Sears SF et al. Educational and psychological interventions to improve outcomes for recipients of implantable cardioverter defibrillators and their families: A scientific statement from the American Heart Association. *Circulation*. 2012;126(17):2146–2172.

91   Goldstein NE, Bradley E, Zeidman J, Mehta D, and Morrison RS. Barriers to conversations about deactivation of implantable defibrillators in seriously ill patients: Results of a nationwide survey comparing cardiology specialists to primary care physicians. *J Am Coll Cardiol*. 2009;54(4):371–373.

92   Baman TS, Crawford T, Sovitch P et al. Feasibility of postmortem device acquisition for potential reuse in underserved nations. *Heart Rhythm*. 2012;9:211–214.

93   Tan ZS. The limits of life. *J Am Geriatr Soc*. 2012;60(4):786–787.

94   Glikson M and Friedman PA. The implantable cardioverter defibrillator. *Lancet*. 2001;357(9262):1107–1117.

95   A comparison of antiarrhythmic-drug therapy with implantable defibrillators in patients resuscitated from near-fatal ventricular arrhythmias: The Antiarrhythmics versus Implantable Defibrillators (AVID) Investigators. *N Engl J Med*. 1997;337:1576–1583.

96   Costea A, Rardon DP, Padanilam BJ, Fogel RI, and Prystowsky EN. Complications associated with generator replacement in response to device advisories. *J Cardiovasc Electrophysiol*. 2008;19(3):266–269.

97   Luderitz B and C Wolpert. The patient's informed consent for pacemakers and ICD implantation: How to write and how to explain it. *Z Kardiol*. 2003;92(5):377–383.

98   Niewald A, Broxterman J, Rosell T, and Rigler S. Documented consent process for implantable cardioverter-defibrillators and implications for end-of-life care in older adults. *J Med Ethics*. 2013;39(2):94–97.

99   Lampert R. Quality of life and end-of-life issues for older patients with implanted cardiac rhythm devices. *Clin Geriatr Med*. 2012;28(4):693–702.

100   Frosch DL and Kaplan RM. Shared decision making in clinical medicine: Past research and future directions. *Am J Prev Med*. 1999;17:285–294.

101   Elwyn G, Edwards A, Kinnersley P, and Grol R. Shared decision making and the concept of equipoise: The competences of involving patients in healthcare choices. *Br J Gen Pract*. 2000;50:892–899.

102   Fried TR, Byers AL, Gallo WT et al. Prospective study of health status preferences and changes in preferences over time in older adults. *Arch Intern Med*. 2006;166(8):890–895.

103   Wright AA, Zhang B, Ray A et al. Associations between end-of-life discussions, patient mental health, medical care near death, and caregiver bereavement adjustment. *J Am Med Assoc*. 2008;300(14):1665–1673.

104   Ethics, Professionalism, and Human Rights Committee. American College of Physicians (ACP) Ethics Manual: Sixth edition. *Ann Intern Med*. 2012;156(1):73–101.

105   Berger JT, Gorski M, and Cohen T. Advance health planning and treatment preferences among recipients of implantable cardioverter defibrillators: An exploratory study. *J Clin Ethics*. 2006;17(1):72–78.

106   Tajouri TH, Ottenberg AL, Hayes DL, and Mueller PS. The use of advance directives among patients with implantable cardioverter defibrillators. *Pacing Clin Electrophysiol*. 2012;35(5):567–573.

107   McGeary A and Eldergill A. Medicolegal issues arising when pacemaker and implantable cardioverter defibrillator devices are deactivated in terminally ill patients. *Med Sci Law*. 2010;50:40–44.

108   Mueller PS, Ottenberg AL, Hayes DL, and Koenig BA. I felt like the angel of death ": Role conflicts and moral distress among allied professionals employed by the U.S. cardiovascular implantable electronic device industry. *J Interv Card Electrophysiol*. 2011;32(3):253–261.

109   Beets MT and Forringer E. Urgent implantable cardioverter defibrillator deactivation by unconventional means. *J Pain Symptom Manage*. 2011;42(6):941–945.

110   Marinskis G, van Erven L and EHRA Scientific Initiatives Committee. Deactivation of implanted cardioverter-defibrillators at the end of life: Results of the EHRA survey. *Europace*. 2010;12:1176–1177.

111   Hammill SC, Kremers MS, Kadish AH et al. Review of the ICD Registry's third year, expansion to include lead data and pediatric ICD procedures, and role for measuring performance. *Heart Rhythm*. 2009;6:1397–1401.

112   Kramer DB, Buxton AE, Zimetbaum PJ. Time for a change—A new approach to ICD replacement. *N Engl J Med*. 2012;366(4):291–293.

113   United Nations. Convention on the Rights of the Child. No. GA res.44/25, annex, 44 UN GAOR Supp.(No.49) at 167, U.N. Doc. A/44/49 (1989). 1989.

114   Goldstein N, Carlson M, Livote E, and Kutner JS. Brief communication: Management of implantable cardioverter-defibrillators in hospice: A nationwide survey. *Ann Intern Med*. 2010;152(5):296–299.

115   Sherazi S, Daubert JP, Block RC et al. Physicians' preferences and attitudes about end-of-life care in patients with an implantable cardioverter-defibrillator. *Mayo Clin Proc*. 2008;83:1139–1141.

116   Reitemeier PJ, Derse AR, and Spike J. Retiring the pacemaker. *Hastings Cent Rep*. 1997;27(1):24.

117   Powell T. Life imitates work [A Piece of My Mind]. *J Am Med Assoc*. 2011;305(6):542–543.

118   Kapa S, Mueller PS, Hayes DL, and Asirvatham SJ. Perspectives on withdrawing pacemaker and implantable cardioverter-defibrillator therapies at end of life: Results of a survey of medical and legal professionals and patients. *Mayo Clin Proc*. 2010;85:981–990.

119 Kramer DB, Ottenberg AL, Gerhardson S, Mueller LA, Kaufman SR, Koenig BA, and Mueller PS. "Just Because We Can Doesn't Mean We Should": Views of nurses on deactivation of pacemakers and implantable cardioverter-defibrillators. *J Interv Card Electrophysiol.* 2011;32(3):243–252.

120 Goldstein NE, Mehta D, Teitelbaum E, Bradley EH, and Morrison RS. "It's like crossing a bridge": Complexities preventing physicians from discussing deactivation of implantable defibrillators at the end of life. *J Gen Intern Med.* 2008;23(Suppl. 1):2–6.

121 Kirkpatrick JN, Gottlieb M, Sehgal P, Patel R, and Verdino RJ. Deactivation of implantable cardioverter defibrillators in terminal illness and end of life care. *Am J Cardiol.* 2012;109(1):91–94.

122 Raphael CE, Koa-Wing M, Stain N, Wright I, Francis DP, and Kanagaratnam P. Implantable cardioverter-defibrillator recipient attitudes towards device deactivation: How much do patients want to know? *Pacing Clin Electrophysiol.* 2011;34(12):1628–1633.

123 Herman D, Stros P, Curila K, Kebza V, and Osmancik P. Deactivation of implantable cardioverter-defibrillators: Results of patient surveys. *Europace.* 2013;15(7):963–969 Epub 2013 Feb 27.

124 Kobza R and Erne P. End-of-life decisions in ICD patients with malignant tumors. *Pacing Clin Electrophysiol.* 2007;30(7):845–849.

125 Dodson JA, Fried TR, Van Ness PH, Goldstein NE, Lampert R. Patient preferences for deactivation of implantable cardioverter-defibrillators. *JAMA Intern Med.* 2013;173(5):377–379.

126 Furrow B, Greaney T, Johnson H, Jost T, and Schwartz R. Bioethics health care law and ethics. In: *Life and Death Decisions: Principles of Autonomy and Beneficence.* St. Paul, MN: West Group, 2001, pp. 246–263.

127 Annas GJ. *The Rights of Patients: The Authoritative ACLU Guide to the Rights of Patients,* 3rd edn. New York: New York University Press, 2004.

128 Pellegrino ED. Decisions to withdraw life-sustaining treatment: A moral algorithm. *J Am Med Assoc.* 2000;283:1065–1067.

129 AMA 1996. *AMA Code of Medical Ethics: Policy on End of Life Care: Opinion E-2.20.* Chicago, IL: AMA Press, 1996.

130 Gostin LO. Deciding life and death in the courtroom. From Quinlan to Cruzan, Glucksberg, and Vacco—A brief history and analysis of constitutional protection of the "right to die." *J Am Med Assoc.* 1997;278:1523–1528.

131 Beauchamp TL and Childress JF. *Principles of Biomedical Ethics,* 6th edn. New York: Oxford University Press, 2008.

132 AMA Council on Ethical and Judicial Affairs. Physician objection to treatment and individual patient discrimination: CEJA report 6-A-07. Chicago, IL: AMA Press, 2007.

133 Rady MY and Verheijde JL. When is deactivating an implanted cardiac device physician-assisted death? Appraisal of the lethal pathophysiology and mode of death. *J Palliat Med.* 2011;14(10):1086–1088.

134 Stuart B. On deactivating cardiovascular implanted electronic devices (CIEDs): Let our people go. *J Palliat Med.* 2001;14(10):1089–1090.

135 Paola FA and Walker RM. Deactivating the implantable cardioverter defibrillator: A biofixture analysis. *South Med J.* 2000;93:20–23.

136 England R, England T, and Coggon J. The ethical and legal implications of deactivating an implantable cardioverter-defibrillator in a patient with terminal cancer. *J Med Ethics.* 2007;33:538–540.

137 Sulmasy DP. Within you/without you: Biotechnology, ontology, and ethics. *J Gen Intern Med.* 2008;23(Suppl. 1):69–72.

138 Morrison LJ and Sinclair CT. Next-of-kin responses and do-not-resuscitate implications for implantable cardioverter defibrillators [letter]. *Ann Intern Med.* 2005;142(8):676–677.

139 Hertz MI, Taylor DO, Trulock EP, Boucek MM, Mohacsi PJ, Edwards LB, and Keck BM. The registry of the International Society for Heart and Lung Transplantation: Nineteenth Official Report—2002. *J Heart Lung Transplant.* 2002;21:950–970.

140 Ferris H and Hunt S. Destination ventricular assist devices for heart failure. Fast facts and concepts. *J Palliat Med.* 2009;12(10):956–957. Available at: http://www.eperc.mcw.edu/fastfact/ff_205.htm.

141 Goldstein DJ, Oz MC, and Rose EA. Implantable left ventricular assist devices. *N Engl J Med.* 1998;339(21):1522–1533.

142 Goldstein NE, May CW, and Meier DE. Comprehensive care for mechanical circulatory support: A new frontier for synergy with palliative care. *Circ Heart Fail.* 2011;4(4):519–527.

143 Kirklin JK, Naftel DC, Kormos RL, Stevenson LW, Pagani FD, Miller MA, Baldwin JT, and Young JB. The Fourth INTERMACS Annual Report: 4,000 implants and counting. *J Heart Lung Transplant.* 2012;31(2):117–126.

144 Rose EA, Gellins AC, Moskowitz AJ et al. Long-term use of a left ventricular assist device for end stage heart failure. *N Engl J Med.* 2001;345:1435–1443.

145 Lietz K, Long JW, Kfoury AG et al. Outcomes of left ventricular assist device implantation as destination therapy in the post-REMATCH era: Implications for patient selection. *Circulation.* 2007;116(5):497–505.

146 Long JW, Healy AH, Rasmusson BY et al. Improving outcomes with long-term "destination" therapy using left ventricular assist devices. *J Thorac Cardiovasc Surg.* 2008;135(6):1353–1360.

147 Park SJ, Tector A, Piccioni W et al. Left ventricular assist devices as destination therapy: A new look at survival. *J Thorac Cardiovasc Surg.* 2005;129:1464.

148 Slaughter MS, Rogers JG, Milano CA et al. Advanced heart failure treated with continuous-flow left ventricular assist device. *N Engl J Med.* 2009;361(23):2241–2251.

149 Pamboukian SV, Tallaj JA, Brown RN et al. Improvement in 2-year survival for ventricular assist device patients after implementation of an intensive surveillance protocol. *J Heart Lung Transplant.* 2011;30(8):879–887.

150 Kirklin JK, Naftel DC, Kormos RL, Stevenson LW, Pagani FD, Miller MA, Timothy Baldwin J, Young JB. Fifth INTERMACS annual report: Risk factor analysis from more than 6,000 mechanical circulatory support patients. *J Heart Lung Transplant.* 2013;32(2):141–156.

151 Levin HR, Oz MC, Chen JM, Packer M, Rose EA, and Burkhoff D. Reversal of chronic ventricular dilation in patients with end-stage cardiomyopathy by prolonged mechanical unloading. *Circulation.* 1995;91:2717–2720.

152 Muller J, Wallukat G, Weng Y-G et al. Weaning from mechanical cardiac support in patients with idiopathic dilated cardiomyopathy. *Circulation.* 1997;96:542–549.

153 Simon MA, Kormos RL, Murali S et al. Myocardial recovery using ventricular assist devices: Prevalence, clinical characteristics, and outcomes. *Circulation.* 2005;112(Suppl.):I-32–I-36.

154 Birks EJ, Tansley PD, Hardy J, George RS, Bowles CT, Burke M, Banner NR, Khaghani A, and Yacoub MH. Left ventricular assist device and drug therapy for the reversal of heart failure. *N Engl J Med.* 2006;355(18):1873–1884.

155 Birks EJ, George RS, Firouzi A, Wright G, Bahrami T, Yacoub MH, and Khaghani A. Long-term outcomes of patients bridged to recovery versus patients bridged to transplantation. *J Thorac Cardiovasc Surg.* 2012;144(1):190–196. Epub 2012 Apr 11.

156 Interagency Registry for Mechanically Assisted Circulatory Support (INTERMACS). http://www.uab.edu/intermacs. Accessed February 3, 2013.

157 Pediatric Mechanically Assisted Circulatory Support (PEDIMACS) Registry. http://www.uab.edu/intermacs/pedimacs. Accessed February 3, 2013.

158 International Society for Heart & Lung (ISHLT) Transplantation Transplant Registry. http://www.ishlt.org/registries/quarterlyDataReport.asp. Accessed February 3, 2013.

159 Kirklin JK, Mehra MR. The dawn of the ISHLT Mechanical Assisted Circulatory Support (IMACS) Registry: Fulfilling our mission. *J Heart Lung Transplant.* 2012;31(2):115–116.

160 Deng MC, Edwards LB, Hertz MI, Rowe AW, and Kormos RL. Mechanical Circulatory Support device database of the International Society for Heart and Lung Transplantation: Third annual report—2005. *J Heart Lung Transplant.* 2005;24(9):1182–1187.

161 Macgowan GA, Parry G, Schueler S, and Hasan A. The decline in heart transplantation in the UK. *Br Med J.* 2011;342:d2483. doi: 10.1136/bmj.d2483.

162 Stevenson LW, Pagani FD, Young JB, Jessup M, Miller L, Kormos RL, Naftel DC, Ulisney K, Desvigne-Nickens P, and Kirklin JK. INTERMACS profiles of advanced heart failure: The current picture. *J Heart Lung Transplant.* 2009;28(6):535–541.

163 Miller MA, Ulisney K, and Baldwin JT. INTERMACS (Interagency Registry for Mechanically Assisted Circulatory Support): A new paradigm for translating registry data into clinical practice. *J Am Coll Cardiol.* 2010;56(9):738–740.

164 Fraser CD Jr., Jaquiss RD, Rosenthal DN et al. Prospective trial of a pediatric ventricular assist device. *N Engl J Med.* 2012;367(6):532–541.

165 Moskowitz AJ, Rose EA, and Gelijns AC. The cost of long-term LVAD implantation. *Ann Thorac Surg.* 2001;71:195–198.

166 Mishra V, Fiane AE, Geiran O, Sørensen G, Khushi I, and Hagen TP. Hospital costs fell as numbers of LVADs were increasing: Experiences from Oslo University Hospital. *J Cardiothorac Surg.* 2012;7:76.

167 Rizzieri AG, Verheijde JL, Rady MY, and McGregor JL. Ethical challenges with the left ventricular assist device as a destination therapy. *Philos Ethics Humanit Med.* 2008;3:20.

168 Bogaev RC, Pamboukian SV, Moore SA, Chen L, John R, Boyle AJ, Sundareswaran KS, Farrar DJ, and Frazier OH. Comparison of outcomes in women versus men using a continuous-flow left ventricular assist device as a bridge to transplantation. *J Heart Lung Transplant.* 2011;30:515–522.

169 Stevenson LW and Shekar P. Ventricular assist devices for durable support. *Circulation.* 2005;112:e111–e115.

170 Raiten JM and Neuman MD. If only I had known: On choice and uncertainty in the ICU. *N Engl J Med.* 367;19:1779–1781.

171 Brush S, Budge D, Alharethi R et al. End-of-life decision making and implementation in recipients of a destination left ventricular assist device. *J Heart Lung Transplant.* 2010;29:1337–1341.

172 Mueller PS, Swetz KM, Freeman MR, Carter KA, Crowley ME, Severson CJ, Park SJ, and Sulmasy DP. Ethical analysis of withdrawing ventricular assist device support. *Mayo Clin Proc.* 2010;85(9):791–797.

173 Baughman KL and Jarcho JA. Bridge to life—Cardiac mechanical support. *N Engl J Med.* 2007;357(9):846–849.

174 Dudzinski DM. Ethics guidelines for destination therapy. *Ann Thorac Surg.* 81(4):1185–1188.

175 Swetz KM, Mueller PS, Ottenberg AL, Dib C, Freeman MR, and Sulmasy DP. The use of advance directives among patients with left ventricular assist devices. *Hosp Pract (Minneap).* 2011;39(1):78–84.

176 Schwarz ER, Baraghoush A, Morrissey RP, Shah AB, Shinde AM, Phan A, and Bharadwaj P. Pilot study of palliative care consultation in patients with advanced heart failure referred for cardiac transplantation. *J Palliat Med.* 2012;15(1):12–15.

177 Bramstedt KA and Wenger NS. When withdrawal of life-sustaining care does more than allow death to take its course: The dilemma of left ventricular assist devices. *J Heart Lung Transplant.* 2001;20:544–548.

178 Gafford E and Swetz K. Hospice and palliative care consultant's guide to Ventricular Assist Devices (VADs). *American Academy of Hospice and Palliative Medicine Annual Assembly,* Denver, CO, March 8, 2012.

179 Goldberg RJ, Kaplan LA, and Boucher LJ. New biotechnology in long-term care: Left ventricular assist devices. *J Am Med Dir Assoc.* 2006;7(5):319–321.

180 Landzaat LH, Sinclair CT, and Rosielle DA. Continuous-flow left ventricular assist device [letter]. *N Engl J Med.* 2010;362(12):1149.

181 Francis GS, Greenberg BH, Hsu DT et al. ACCF/AHA/ACP/HFSA/ISHLT 2010 clinical competence statement on management of patients with advanced heart failure and cardiac transplant: Are port of the ACCF/AHA/ACP Task Force on Clinical Competence and Training. *J Am Coll Cardiol.* 2010;56(5):424–453.

182 MacIver J and Ross HJ. Withdrawal of ventricular assist device support. *J Palliat Care.* 2005;21(3):151–156.

183 Bramstedt KA. Destination no where: A potential dilemma with ventricular assist devices. *ASAIO J.* 2008;54(1):1–2.

184 Wiegand DL and Kalowes P. Withdrawal of cardiac medications and devices. *AACN Adv Crit Care.* 2007;18(4):415–425.

185 Gafford EF, Luckhardt AJ, and Swetz KM. Deactivation of a left ventricular assist device at the end of life #269. *Palliat Med.* 2013;16(8):980–982.

124

Supportive care for patients with advanced chronic kidney disease

SARA N. DAVISON

INTRODUCTION

Chronic kidney disease (CKD) is defined as abnormalities of kidney structure or function, present for a minimum of 3 months, with implications for health.[1] It is classified based on cause, glomerular filtration rate (GFR), and albuminuria category (Table 124.1). Stage 5 CKD is also known as end-stage renal disease (ESRD), in which patients will ultimately require renal replacement therapy in the form of either dialysis or a kidney transplant to sustain life.

Patients with advanced CKD are typically elderly: the average age of those starting chronic dialysis in most developed countries is approximately 65 years, and patients over the age of 75 are the fastest-growing incident cohort of dialysis patients.[2] As CKD advances, patients typically experience numerous, complex comorbidities (e.g., heart disease, diabetes, geriatric syndromes), high symptom burden, and substantial emotional and spiritual suffering. Even for patients who elect to start dialysis, the mortality rate is extremely high at 20%–25%/year, rivaling that of AIDS and most cancers (Table 124.2). Incident dialysis patients aged 65–74 years have a survival probability of ~50% at 2 years and patients aged ≥75 years ~50% at 1 year.[2] In North America and several European countries, approximately 15%–25% of the annual mortality results from decisions to discontinue dialysis, representing the second leading cause of death after cardiovascular disease.

There is growing recognition that people with advanced CKD have tremendous palliative care needs and require excellent care towards the end of life. Early integration of palliative care into renal care is essential to optimize symptom control, to facilitate advance care planning, and to ease transitions at the end of life.[3] Providing high-quality palliative care to patients with advanced CKD has the potential to improve markedly patient outcomes.[4] It needs a systematic approach, probably best delivered through the combined expertise of nephrology professionals, family- or community-based professionals, and specialist hospice or palliative care providers, relevant training, and dedicated resources.[5]

WHICH CKD PATIENTS NEED PALLIATIVE/SUPPORTIVE CARE?

Not all CKD patients require palliative care. However, most patients will transition eventually to a trajectory of progressive functional decline associated with complex clusters of physical and psychological symptoms. Predicting and understanding patients' needs aid in timely and effective planning of palliative services. At a minimum, those at high risk for death within the next year and those experiencing significant suffering, whether physical, psychosocial, or spiritual, should have a palliative care assessment. Table 124.3 outlines CKD patients most likely to benefit from palliative and supportive care services.

Determining prognosis in patients with advanced CKD

Illness trajectories are particularly heterogeneous among CKD patients,[6*,7*] and predicting survival is difficult. However, to facilitate informed decisions about ongoing care, especially starting, withholding, or withdrawing dialysis, current clinical guidelines recommend that all patients with stage 5 CKD receive patient-specific estimates of prognosis.[5] Factors associated with poor prognosis are summarized in Table 124.3. Age is a powerful risk factor for death (Table 124.2), with incident dialysis patients in most developed countries having remaining lifetimes that are on average one-fourth as long as nondialysis patients of the same age and gender. Serum albumin level, both at baseline and during the course of dialysis treatment, is a consistent and strong predictor of death.[5,8*] Poor functional status is highly predictive of early death (relative risk ranges of 1.5–3), and the inability to transfer and falls are particularly indicative of a poor prognosis.[5,9*,10*,11*] Measures of functional status used in CKD include mobility impairment, Karnofsky scale, Gutman functional status, activities of daily living, and the Medical Outcomes Study 36-item Short Form (SF-36). Comorbidity is one of the most important determinants of outcome in CKD patients. Scoring systems range from simply noting the presence of at least one

Table 124.1   *Kidney disease: Improving global outcomes (KDIGO) classification of CKD*

Stage	Description	GFR (mL/min/1.73 m²)ᵃ
1	Normal or high	≥90
2	Mildly decreased	60–89
3a	Mildly to moderately decreased	45–59
3b	Moderately to severely decreased	30–44
4	Severely decreased	15–29
5	Kidney failure	<15

Source: Data from KDIGO, *Clinical Practice Guideline for the Evaluation and Management of Chronic Kidney Disease*, Nature Publishing Group, New York, 2013.

ᵃ GFR is estimated (eGFR) from serum creatinine (Cr) using the 2012 CKD-EPI creatinine–cystatin C equation. (1) GFR can also be estimated by creatinine clearance (CrCl) using the Cockroft–Gault formula: CrCl = (140 − age) × (weight in kg)/(72 × serum creatinine in mg/dL) × 0.85 for women.

Table 124.2   *Unadjusted survival probabilities (%) for incidentᵃ dialysis patients based on age[2]*

Age	1 year	2 years	3 years	5 years	10 years
40–49	89.6	81.6	73.5	61.9	37.7
50–59	86.2	75.9	65.4	49.5	21.8
60–64	83.0	69.6	58.3	38.1	12.3
65–69	79.1	63.1	50.8	30.7	6.4
70–79	71.2	53.5	39.0	20.2	2.7
80+	60.5	40.8	25.7	9.6	0.9

ᵃ Incident cohorts are determined at the time of ESRD initiation (dialysis or renal transplantation) with 60-day stable modality and 90-day survival.

comorbid illness to grading the comorbidity burden such as with the Charlson comorbidity index (Table 124.4).[12,13*] The most consistent comorbidities that predict less than a 12-month survival are New York Heart Association class IV heart failure, moderate to severe chronic obstructive pulmonary disease, severe peripheral vascular disease, and dementia.[14*,15*,16*,17*] One of the most simple and useful clinical tools to identify dialysis patients at high risk for early mortality is the "surprise question" (SQ)—*Would you be surprised if this patient were to die in the next 12 months?* The SQ identifies dialysis patients with higher comorbidity scores and lower performance status and who are 3.5 times more likely to die within 1 year.[18*]

Unlike the oncology literature, there are only a small number of studies that attempt to combine prognostic factors into clinically useful prognostic tools. Perhaps one of the most promising prognostic models for prevalent hemodialysis patients combines estimations from the presence of peripheral vascular disease and dementia, with the SQ and the more traditional risk factors of age and serum albumin.[19*] The area under the curve for this prognostic model's prediction of 6-month mortality was 0.87 (95% CI 0.82–0.92) in a derivation cohort of 512 prevalent hemodialysis patients and 0.80 (95% CI 0.73–0.88) in a validation cohort of 514 prevalent hemodialysis patients. The model also predicts 12- and 18-month mortality although the

Table 124.3   *Patients most likely to benefit from palliative and supportive care*

- High mortality risk within the next year.
  - Managed conservatively (without dialysis) with an eGFR < 10 mL/min/1.73 m² over the past 3 months.
  - Advanced age.
  - Answer "no" to the SQ "Would you be surprised if the patient died within the next 12 months?"
  - Functional decline.
  - Serum albumin < 3.5 g/dL (associated with ~ 50% 1-year mortality)
  - High comorbidity score (e.g., modified Charlson comorbidity index > 8, associated with ~ 50% 1-year mortality) (12).
  - Prognostic models may also be used.
- Experiencing significant suffering, whether physical, emotional, psychosocial, or spiritual.
- Considering withdrawal from dialysis or conservative management without dialysis.
  - Whenever possible, referrals should be before withdrawal of dialysis as aspects of management such as care at home may need considerable advanced planning.
- Difficulty with end-of-life decision making and determining goals of care.
- Patient request.

Table 124.4   *Scoring for the modified Charlson comorbidity index[12]*

Points

1 point each for coronary artery disease, congestive heart failure, peripheral vascular disease, dementia, chronic pulmonary disease, connective tissue disorder, peptic ulcer disease, mild liver disease, diabetes

1 point for every decade over 40 (e.g., a 64-year-old would receive 3 points)

2 points each for hemiplegia, moderate to severe renal disease (including being on dialysis), diabetes with end-organ damage, cancer (including leukemia or lymphoma)

3 points for moderate to severe liver disease

6 points each for metastatic solid tumor, AIDS

Score Totals	Low score (≤3)	Moderate (4–5)	High (6–7)	Very high (≥8)
Annual Mortality Rate	3%	13%	27%	49%

accuracy of these predictions has yet to be described. The simplicity of the model, however, allows for easy integration into routine dialysis care with limited staff and no patient burden. Unlike other models, this prognostic system has been converted into user-friendly applications that are available free online and for handheld devices[20] (last accessed on July 16, 2012).

DECISION MAKING REGARDING DIALYSIS

A recently updated clinical practice guideline on the initiation of and withdrawal from dialysis recommends a shared decision-making process between nephrology staff and the patient, taking into account the patient's overall prognosis and goals of care.[2] In patients where dialysis affords no tangible benefits and may negatively affect their quality of life, conservative management (foregoing the initiation of dialysis) with palliative care is appropriate.

Conservative management

Dialysis is generally associated with survival and quality-of-life benefits. However, in some patients with poor prognostic factors, initiation of dialysis confers neither a quality-of-life nor a survival advantage and in fact may be associated with accelerated rates of functional and/or cognitive decline and high early mortality.[2] Patients residing in long-term care facilities at the time of dialysis initiation have an especially poor outcome.[21*] Using retrospective administrative data, it was reported that by 12 months after starting dialysis, 87% of long-term care residents ≥75 years had died or had functional decline; only 1 in 8 had maintained functional status. Some elderly patients managed conservatively without chronic dialysis may live almost or as long as patients who elect to start dialysis therapy, with more days spent outside the dialysis unit or hospital.[22*,23*,24*,25*] Conservative care focuses on slowing the decline in renal function, actively managing symptoms, facilitating advance care planning, and providing appropriate palliative care.[26] Conservatively managed patients can remain stable for long periods of time: deciding to not start chronic dialysis does not mean imminent death.

For patients with limited benefit and considerable burden of dialysis, conservative management may be more appropriate and better aligned with patient-derived goals of care. Situations in which it is appropriate to withhold initiation of dialysis are outlined in Table 124.5.

Withdrawal of dialysis

Once dialysis is initiated, the dialysis team works closely with patients to evaluate regularly the utility of dialysis. It is a widely accepted practice in most countries to stop dialysis when it is no longer achieving a meaningful goal for the patient. Approximately 25% of deaths in dialysis patients in North America and many European countries are preceded by a decision to stop dialysis.[27] Authoritative psychiatry and nephrology opinion supports the notion that patients who choose to forgo dialysis are neither psychopathological nor suicidal even though depression may be present.[28] When a patient asks to withdraw from dialysis, it is important to explore their reasons. Treatable factors might contribute to their desire to stop dialysis. These may include inadequate social support; concerns with being a burden to loved ones; inadequately treated depression, anxiety, pain, and other physical or psychological symptoms (including spiritual and existential suffering); or dissatisfaction with dialysis itself (e.g., modality, time commitment, or setting of treatment). Offer to evaluate and treat these concerns and consider a time-limited trial to see if their quality of life can be improved. However, once a clinician feels a patient or surrogate is making a fully informed choice that is consistent with a patient's values and goals, that decision

Table 124.5 *Decision making in withholding initiation of or withdrawing dialysis[5]*

Categories of Patients to Consider Withholding the Initiation of Dialysis[a]

1. Medical condition that precludes the technical process of dialysis because the patient is unable to cooperate (e.g., advanced dementia patient who pulls out dialysis needles) or because the patient's condition is too unstable (e.g., severe hypotension)
2. Terminal illness from nonrenal causes (acknowledging that some may perceive benefit from and choose to undergo dialysis)
3. Those over the age of 75 who meet two or more of the following very poor prognosis criteria:
   - Clinicians' response of "No, I would not be surprised" to the SQ
   - High comorbidity score
   - Significantly impaired functional status (e.g., Karnofsky performance status score <40)
   - Severe chronic malnutrition (e.g., serum albumin <2.5 g/dL)

Categories of Patients to Consider Withdrawing Dialysis[a]

1. Patients with decision-making capacity, who are being fully informed and making voluntary choices, refuse dialysis or request that dialysis be discontinued.
2. Patients who no longer possess decision-making capacity who have previously indicated refusal of dialysis
3. Patients who no longer possess decision-making capacity and whose properly appointed legal agents refuse dialysis or request that it be discontinued based on patient's best interests
   - Decision making in the preceding three scenarios usually involves the following reasons:
     a. Dialysis is no longer serving to substantially prolong life or is only prolonging a patient's death (e.g., a patient dying from advanced cancer or multiorgan system failure).
     b. The burdens of dialysis and its complications outweigh its life-prolonging benefits to a patient (i.e., it is not able to restore a patient to an acceptable quality of life as assessed by the patient or his or her surrogate decision maker).
4. Irreversible, profound neurological impairment such that the patient lacks signs of thought, sensation, purposeful behavior, and awareness of self and environment.

[a] Palliative care is an integral part of the decision to forgo dialysis, and attention to patient comfort and quality of life while dying must be addressed directly, including referral to a hospice program when appropriate and where available.

should be honored. Situations where it is appropriate to consider stopping dialysis are outlined in Table 124.5.

Once dialysis is stopped, patients have an average survival of 8–10 days. Palliative care should work closely with the renal team to provide optimal symptom control along with end-of-life preparations. Suggestions for the treatment of common uremic symptoms can be seen in Table 124.6. The United Kingdom has established renal specific terminal symptom algorithms as part of the Liverpool Care Pathway, an integrated care pathway designed to care for patients in their last days of life across health-care settings.[29] These are accessible easily online.[30]

Table 124.6 *Symptom management in advanced CKD*[a]

Shortness of breath[b]	• Oxygen, positioning, calm environment. • Opioids. • Combining low-dose opioid with midazolam may be effective if low-dose opioids alone are inadequate. • For the occasional patient who has a residual urine output of >100 mL/day, high-dose diuretics can be used (e.g., furosemide 120 mg BID). • Ultrafiltration using dialysis is not usually recommended after stopping dialysis, as it can be distressing for patients/family to see the patient back on a therapy, which appears similar to hemodialysis.

Anxiety, agitation, restlessness	• Haloperidol may lower the seizure threshold and metabolites are excreted in the urine and feces so it is recommended to dose at half the typical starting dose.
	• Benzodiazepines (short-acting) do not accumulate in CKD; however, clinical experience supports starting with very low doses.
	   1. Lorazepam 0.5–1.0 mg po or s/L
	   2. Midazolam 1.25–2.5 mg s/c q 2–4 h and titrated according to effect

Restless legs	• Gabapentin 100–300 mg daily is effective but becomes too toxic once dialysis is stopped. • Clonazepam 0.5–2.0 mg bid (associated with drowsiness). • Clonidine 0.1–0.2 mg bid.
Muscle cramps	• Quinine sulfate 300 mg before dialysis or daily. It accumulates rapidly once dialysis is stopped and should be discontinued. • Clonazepam and other benzodiazepines.
Nausea	• Metoclopramide (low doses starting at 5 mg bid) or domperidone is effective for gastroparesis. • Haloperidol 0.5–1.5 mg PRN is effective for uremia-induced nausea; often sedating in the context of uremia. • Ondansetron is less sedating and does not accumulate in kidney failure.
Pruritus	• Gabapentin becomes too toxic once dialysis is stopped. • Emollients: Hydrourea cream. • Ondansetron. • Antihistamines may be beneficial in some.

[a] Anticipatory prescribing should be undertaken to ensure that in the last hours and days of life, there is no delay responding to a symptom if it occurs. As a general rule, if three or more doses of PRN medication are required, then consider a subcutaneous syringe driver to deliver a continuous infusion over 24 hours.
[b] Sodium restriction is the mainstay of treatment for patients to maintain euvolemia.

SYMPTOM MANAGEMENT IN ADVANCED CKD

Symptom prevalence and screening

Patients with advanced CKD are among the most symptomatic of any chronic disease group. The number and severity of symptoms, whether treated with dialysis or managed conservatively, is similar to that reported by many cancer patients in palliative care settings.[31*,32*,33*] The most frequently reported moderate to severe symptoms are tiredness (74%), decreased well-being (60%), pain (50%), anorexia (49%), and pruritus (46%).[31*] Insomnia is also distressing for many patients and has been reported by 50%–90% of dialysis patients.[34] Many of these patients have specific primary sleep disorders such as sleep apnea, periodic leg movement disorder, and restless legs syndrome. Symptoms of depression affect approximately 25% of dialysis patients.[35] Symptom burden accounts for up to 39% of the impairment in CKD patients' quality of life (31), and a change in symptom burden is associated with up to a 46% change in quality of life.[36*,37*] Unfortunately, pain and other symptoms are underrecognized[38*] and undertreated[39*] in CKD.

Clearly symptom assessment and management is a fundamental component of quality CKD care. A clinically relevant and valid symptom assessment should be completed systematically for all patients at regular intervals. There are three global symptom scores, which have been adapted and validated specifically for use in those with CKD and can be downloaded from the Internet:

1. The Edmonton Symptom Assessment System Revised Renal (ESAS-r: Renal)[31*,37*,40*]
2. The renal Palliative care (or Patient) Outcome Scale—symptom module (POS renal)[33*,41*]
3. The dialysis symptom index (DSI)[42]

Epidemiology of pain in CKD

Approximately 50% of patients with stage 5 CKD, regardless of age, whether treated with dialysis or cared for conservatively, experience chronic pain.[33*,43*,44*,45*] Up to 82% of patients report their pain as moderate or severe.[43*] Even in the last days of life following withdrawal of dialysis, pain is present in 42% of patients.[46*] Dialysis patients with chronic pain are two to three times more likely to suffer from depression and insomnia than patients without chronic pain.[47*] CKD patients typically experience chronic pain in the context of multiple other symptoms and end-of-life issues, all of which interfere markedly with psychosocial and physical coping strategies.

Causes of pain in CKD are diverse and often multifactorial. Pain may be due to comorbidity (e.g., diabetic neuropathy, peripheral vascular disease), the primary renal disease (e.g., polycystic kidney disease), and disease consequent upon kidney failure itself (e.g., renal osteodystrophy, calciphylaxis, dialysis-related amyloidosis [DRA]) or related to the dialysis procedure (e.g., ischemic neuropathies from arteriovenous fistulae, dialysis-related cramping). Table 124.7 describes some of the painful syndromes encountered almost exclusively in patients with advanced CKD.

Pharmacologic management of pain in CKD

This has been reviewed in detail elsewhere.[3] The high incidence of comorbidity, polypharmacy, and an elderly population complicate pain management due to increased risk of

Table 124.7 *Painful syndromes associated with CKD*

Syndrome	Pathophysiology	Clinical presentation	Diagnosis	Treatment
Renal osteodystrophy[71]	Bone disease occurs early in the course of CKD and worsens with decline in kidney function. By the time dialysis is initiated, nearly all patients are affected. There are three types of renal bone diseases that are collectively referred to as renal osteodystrophy.		Radiographs provide important information. Recommended sites are the hands, shoulder, skull, spine, and pelvis. However, radiographic findings will not conclusively establish the type of bone disease; bone biopsy is the gold standard for diagnosis but is not done routinely.	Normalization of serum calcium, phosphorous, parathyroid hormone, and vitamin D levels.
a. *Osteitis fibrosa*	Increased bone turnover due to secondary hyperparathyroidism affecting ∼ 20% of dialysis patients.	Bone and joint pain on exertion in skeletal sites subject to biomechanical stress. Associated with calcium phosphate precipitation in arteries, joints, soft tissues, and the viscera leading to red-eye syndrome, proximal myopathy, ruptured tendons, pseudogout, pseudoclubbing, and calciphylaxis.	Radiographic findings may occur before clinical signs and symptoms and include subperiosteal resorption and resorptive loss of acral bone (e.g., terminal phalanges, distal ends of clavicles, and skull), resorption within cortical bone (leading to longitudinal striation), endosteal resorption (leading to cortical thinning), brown tumors, and osteosclerosis in the upper and lower thirds of the vertebra ("rugger jersey spine").	
b. *Osteomalacia*	Decreased bone turnover and an increased volume of unmineralized bone (osteoid), usually due to aluminum deposition from aluminum in dialysis water and aluminum-containing phosphate binders. With the avoidance of aluminum, there has been a marked decrease in the incidence of pure osteomalacia in CKD in developed countries.	Pain at rest, localized pain, pathologic fractures, and bone deformities.	Pathologic fractures and bone deformities.	Avoid aluminum.
Adynamic bone disease[72]	Decreased bone turnover due to an excess suppression of parathyroid hormone induced by the use of vitamin D. Affects 20%–60% of dialysis patients depending upon geography. In contrast to osteomalacia, there is no increase in unmineralized bone.	Bone and joint pain, both at rest and with exertion, fractures, and skeletal deformities.	Unlike osteitis fibrosa, radiographic changes (pathologic fractures and bone deformities) usually appear after clinical signs and symptoms.	

(Continued)

Table 124.7 (Continued) *Painful syndromes associated with CKD*

Syndrome	Pathophysiology	Clinical presentation	Diagnosis	Treatment
Dialysis-related amyloidosis (DRA)[73]	Deposition of amyloid in bone, joints, and synovium in long-term dialysis patients. Clinical prevalence is zero at 5 years, ~50% at 12 years, and almost 100% by 20 years.	Swollen painful joints, carpal tunnel, spondyloarthropathy, and pathologic fractures	Characteristic x-ray picture of multiple bone cysts (typically at the ends of long bones) that contain amyloid and enlarge with time. They may be mistaken for the brown tumors seen in osteitis fibrosa. DRA can be confirmed by synovial biopsy or aspirate of joint to detect amyloid. Extra-articular tissues can also be sampled for DRA, e.g., subcutaneous fat pad aspiration, rectal submucosal biopsy, and 2-D echocardiography. Skin biopsy, in contrast, is generally negative. Ultrasonography may be of use in DRA of the shoulder. It can detect increased rotator cuff thickness and a thickened synovial sheath of the long head of the biceps.	Analgesics help with periarticular and bone pain. However, since DRA is a progressive disease, early surgical correction of complications such as carpal tunnel syndrome is warranted.
Calciphylaxis (calcific uremic arteriolopathy [CUA])[74]	A syndrome of small vessel vascular calcification thrombosis and skin necrosis. The rate has been reported as high as 4.5/100 patient-years.	Painful livedo reticularis that progresses to painful ulcers and eschar formation. Mortality is high, especially once lesions become ulcerated.	There is no diagnostic laboratory test for CUA. Characteristic ischemic skin lesions usually suggest the diagnosis. X-rays may exhibit ectopic calcification of the soft tissue. Diagnosis can be confirmed by skin biopsy. Ulceration, however, often develops at the site of the biopsy within 2 to 6 weeks. Most cases can be confirmed by bone scan showing abnormal uptake in areas of calcium deposition.	No definitive treatments are available. Serum calcium, phosphorous, and parathyroid hormone levels should be normalized. A trial of steroids can be undertaken for nonulcerating disease. Aggressive systemic antibiotics and repeated debridement of necrotic tissue are required. Hyperbaric oxygen therapy may be helpful. Even with aggressive therapy, up to 60%–89% of patients die from sepsis.

| Polycystic kidney disease (PCKD)[75] | The pathophysiology of pain in PKCD has been reviewed elsewhere (76). Pain afflicts about 60% of patients. | Infected cysts can lead to diffuse unilateral or bilateral pain associated with fever. Cyst rupture causes acute, localized pain with or without hematuria. Pain usually resolves spontaneously over 2–7 days. Hemorrhage into a larger cyst can cause referred pain to the abdomen or shoulder. Kidney stones occur in 20%–30% of patients. Chronic pain may result from the following: (a) enlarged cysts causing increased abdominal girth leading to lumbar lordosis and accelerated degenerative changes in the spine and (b) cysts that may also compress surrounding tissues or distend the renal capsule causing steady, well-localized pain (often anterior abdominal rather than lower back) that is often exacerbated by standing and walking. | Because cysts may not communicate with the urinary tract, urine cultures may be negative. | Antibiotics with good cyst-penetrating ability such as trimethoprim–sulfamethoxazole, metronidazole, and fluoroquinolones are typically required for infected cysts. Renal prostaglandins may be a major contributing factor in renal colic: NSAIDs, therefore, can be very effective for the management of acute pain and used with or without opioids. Because of the compressed and distorted renal calices, ureteroscopy and extracorporeal shock wave lithotripsy are more difficult and may not be as efficacious for nephrolithiasis. If conservative measures fail to produce adequate pain relief, surgical intervention such as laparoscopic cyst decortication (unroofing and collapse of cysts) and marsupialization may be required. This is typically reserved for patients with severe pain attributed to cysts >5 cm in diameter. For occasional patients with or approaching ESRD, nephrectomy may be the only option for pain control. |

Table 124.8 *Analgesic use in advanced CKD*

Recommended

Acetaminophen: Maximum daily dose of 3.2 g/day. In high-risk patients, limit the maximal dose to 2.6 g/day (chronic stable liver disease, alcoholics, and malnourished patients).

Hydromorphone: Hydromorphome-3-glucuronide (a toxic metabolite) accumulates without dialysis; therefore, this may not be an appropriate analgesic for patients with stage 5 CKD *not* on dialysis.

Fentanyl patch.

Methadone.

Buprenorphine patch: Limited experience in CKD, but pharmacokinetics appears minimally altered. It might be difficult to antagonize with opioid antagonists. Care should be taken when used with benzodiazepines.

Gabapentin: Titrate slowly; doses up to 300 mg/day are generally safe but monitor for side effects (nystagmus, ataxia, tremor, somnolence, and reduced level of consciousness).

Use with Caution

Oxycodone: Limited pharmacokinetic evidence for safety in ESRD.

Tramadol: Sustained-release tablets *not* recommended in dialysis patients. Maximum dose 150 mg/day. Risk of seizure with higher doses in ESRD.

Nortriptyline/desipramine: TCA antidepressants are alternatives to gabapentin; however, they have more adverse effects.

Do not use codeine, morphine, meperidine, propoxyphene.

Morphine, codeine, meperidine, and propoxyphene have neurotoxic metabolites that are renally excreted and that accumulate in CKD and may cause toxicity.

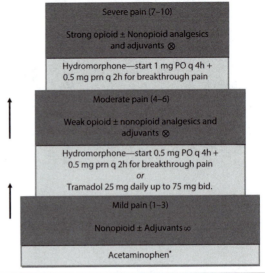

Figure 124.1 *Adapted WHO analgesic ladder for patients with advanced CKD*

toxicity and adverse effects of analgesics. Probably the largest obstacle, however, is the altered pharmacokinetics and pharmacodynamics of analgesics in advanced kidney failure and the increased risk for toxicity. This has led to a reluctance of health-care providers to prescribe analgesics, especially opioids. The Dialysis Outcomes and Practice Patterns Study (DOPPS) compared analgesic use in 1997–2000 for 3749 patients in 142 U.S. facilities.[39*] The percentage of patients using any analgesic decreased from 30% to 24%. Narcotic use decreased from 18% to less than 15%, acetaminophen use decreased from 11% to 6%, and 74% of patients with pain that interfered with work had no analgesic prescription. Table 124.8 summarizes appropriate analgesic selection in CKD. Data, however, remain limited with these opioids and the evidence is anecdotal at best.

An adapted World Health Organization (WHO) analgesic ladder that takes into account the altered pharmacokinetics of analgesics in severe kidney failure should be used to treat chronic pain in advanced CKD. An example can be seen in Figure 124.1. In view of the potential for toxicity, short-acting rather than long-acting preparations should be used until stable pain relief has been achieved. Naloxone, an opioid receptor antagonist, is metabolized in the liver with little excreted unchanged in urine, and no dosage alteration is required in CKD. However, it should be remembered that prolonged

dosing may be needed to counteract the accumulation of opioid metabolites in CKD patients.

WHO analgesic ladder

Step 1: Acetaminophen is considered the nonnarcotic analgesic of choice for mild to moderate pain in CKD patients.[48] It is metabolized by the liver with only 2%–5% excreted unchanged in the urine and does not require dose adjustment in CKD. Nonsteroidal anti-inflammatory drugs (NSAIDs) can be used in conjunction with acetaminophen, but their use in CKD is best reserved for specific indications of acute pain such as gout or renal colic. The risks of NSAIDs include irreversible reduction in GFR for those who still have residual renal function[49] and an increased risk of gastrointestinal bleeding, and studies have suggested that there might be an increased risk of myocardial infarction.[50***]

Step 2: Very few step 2 opioids are appropriate for use in advanced CKD. The active metabolites of codeine are renally excreted and accumulate in patients with renal impairment[51*] and can cause prolonged narcosis and respiratory depression, even at trivial doses.[52,53*] This appears to be an idiosyncratic phenomenon with some patients able to tolerate regular doses of codeine for prolonged periods without experiencing toxicity. For this reason, codeine is not recommended for chronic use in patients with advanced CKD. Oxycodone is metabolized in the liver to noroxycodone and oxymorphone, both of which accumulate in dialysis patients.[54] A single case study reported that oxycodone and its metabolites were reduced by dialysis, but without loss of analgesia.[55] However, another case report demonstrated respiratory depression in a dialysis patient who received 5 mg of oxycodone six times a day for 8 days. The patient needed a 4-day naloxone infusion.[56] There are no long-term studies of chronic use of oxycodone in CKD, and the conflicting case reports mean there is insufficient evidence currently for a recommendation. Tramadol, a centrally acting analgesic, may induce fewer opioid adverse effects for a given level of analgesia compared with traditional opioids.[57] Since 90% of tramadol and its metabolites are excreted in the urine, dose adjustments are required in patients with CKD.

Step 3: Morphine is extensively metabolized to the active metabolites morphine-3-glucuronide (M3G) and morphine-6-glucuronide (M6G), both of which rapidly accumulate and cause significant toxicity in patients with CKD[58]: morphine is therefore not recommended. A retrospective audit suggests that hydromorphone is better tolerated than morphine when normal release preparations are used.[59] Hydromorphone is rapidly metabolized in the liver to the active metabolite hydromorphone-3-glucuronide (H3G), which is excreted in the urine. The only pharmacokinetic data in advanced CKD showed that although H3G accumulated between hemodialysis treatments in 12 anuric patients, it appeared to be removed effectively during hemodialysis.[60] These patients had been taking a mean daily dose of 20 mg for a mean of 9 months. However, due to the accumulation of H3G, hydromorphone may not be as effective or as well tolerated in conservatively managed patients or during the final days of life following withdrawal from dialysis. Methadone may be more effective for neuropathic pain than other strong opioids because of its NMDA receptor antagonism. Methadone has high oral bioavailability and is extensively distributed in the tissues where it accumulates with repeated dosing. Slow release from the reservoirs in the tissues can result in prolonged pharmacological action of up to 60 hours.[61] It is excreted mainly in the feces, with metabolism into pharmacologically inactive metabolites primarily in the liver, although ~20% is excreted unchanged in the urine. It does not appear to be removed by dialysis,[62*,63*] but in anuric patients, it appears to be exclusively excreted in feces with no accumulation in plasma.[62] These factors suggest that methadone may be an appropriate analgesic for use in CKD. Fentanyl is rapidly metabolized in the liver, with only 5%–10% excreted unchanged in the urine. Its metabolites are considered to be inactive. There does not appear to be clinically significant accumulation of fentanyl when administered to patients with renal impairment.[64*,65*,66*] Transdermal preparations have been used successfully in patients with CKD. Buprenorphine can also be administered via a transdermal patch. It is metabolized by the liver with little unchanged drug found in the urine.[67] The two major metabolites, buprenorphine-3-glucuronide (B3G) and norbuprenorphine, are excreted in the urine and accumulate in CKD. However, B3G is inactive with no analgesic properties. Norbuprenorphine is a less potent analgesic than buprenorphine; the clinical relevance of which is thought to be limited as it does not readily cross the blood–brain barrier. However, it is not known if this remains the case in the presence of uremia.[68*]

In short-term use of transdermal buprenorphine in 10 dialysis patients, buprenorphine levels were not reduced by dialysis.[69] However, norbuprenorphine was only detectable above 0.05 ng/mL in three patients. The median buprenorphine dose was 52.5 µg/hour. There are no data on long-term use. Given the minimal changes in kinetics in renal failure, it may be a potentially useful analgesic in CKD. Meperidine (pethidine) is metabolized in the liver mainly to norpethidine, which has twice the proconvulsive activity as its parent compound and accumulates in patients with renal impairment.[70] It should be avoided in CKD patients.

Patients with CKD have extensive and unique end-of-life care considerations and needs. Identifying CKD patients likely to benefit from palliative and supportive care services should be a priority in all nephrology programs. Further research is required on symptom management, prognostication, especially of conservatively managed patients, and anticipated changes in functional status and quality of life with the initiation of dialysis, especially in the frail elderly, in order to provide quality care at the end of life for patients with advanced CKD.

REFERENCES

✱ 1 KDIGO. *Clinical Practice Guideline for the Evaluation and Management of Chronic Kidney Disease.* New York: Nature Publishing Group, 2013.

   2 U.S. Renal Data System. USRDS 2010 annual data report: Atlas of end-stage renal disease in the United States. Bethesda, MD: National Institutes of Health, National Institute of Diabetes and Digestive and Kidney Diseases, 2010.

◆ 3 Chambers EJ, Brown E, Germain M. *Supportive Care for the Renal Patient.* Oxford, England: Oxford University Press, 2010.

   4 Germain MJ, Kurella M, Davison SN. Palliative care in CKD: The earlier the better. *Am J Kidney Dis* 2011;57(3):378–380.

✱ 5 Renal Physicians Association. *Shared Decision Making in the Appropriate Initiation of and Withdrawal from Dialysis,* 2nd ed. Rockville, MD: Renal Physicians Association, 2010.

   6 Lunney JR, Lynn J, Foley DJ, Lipson S, Guralnik JM. Patterns of functional decline at the end of life. *JAMA* 2003;289(18):2387–2392.

   7 Gill TM, Gahbauer EA, Han L, Allore HG. Trajectories of disability in the last year of life. *N Engl J Med* 2010;362(13):1173–1180.

   8 Pifer TB, McCullough KP, Port FK, Goodkin DA, Maroni BJ, Held PJ et al. Mortality risk in hemodialysis patients and changes in nutritional indicators: DOPPS. *Kidney Int* 2002;62(6):2238–2245.

   9 Johansen KL, Chertow GM, Jin C, Kutner NG. Significance of frailty among dialysis patients. *J Am Soc Nephrol* 2007;18(11):2960–2967.

  10 Mauri JM, Cleries M, Vela E, Catalan RR. Design and validation of a model to predict early mortality in haemodialysis patients. *Nephrol Dial Transplant* 2008;23(5):1690–1696.

  11 Li M, Tomlinson G, Naglie G, Cook WL, Jassal SV. Geriatric comorbidities, such as falls, confer an independent mortality risk to elderly dialysis patients. *Nephrol Dial Transplant* 2008;23(4):1396–1400.

● 12 Beddhu S, Bruns FJ, Saul M, Seddon P, Zeidel ML. A simple comorbidity scale predicts clinical outcomes and costs in dialysis patients. *Am J Med* 2000;108(8):609–613.

  13 Hemmelgarn BR, Manns BJ, Quan H, Ghali WA. Adapting the Charlson comorbidity index for use in patients with ESRD. *Am J Kidney Dis* 2003;42(1):125–132.

14 Rajagopalan S, Dellegrottaglie S, Furniss AL, Gillespie BW, Satayathum S, Lameire N et al. Peripheral arterial disease in patients with end-stage renal disease: Observations from the dialysis outcomes and practice patterns study (DOPPS). *Circulation* 2006;114(18):1914–1922.

15 Rakowski DA, Caillard S, Agodoa LY, Abbott KC. Dementia as a predictor of mortality in dialysis patients. *Clin J Am Soc Nephrol* 2006;1(5):1000–1005.

16 Kurella M, Mapes DL, Port FK, Chertow GM. Correlates and outcomes of dementia among dialysis patients: The dialysis outcomes and practice patterns study. *Nephrol Dial Transplant* 2006;21:2543–2548.

17 Postorino M, Marino C, Tripepi G, Zoccali C. Prognostic value of the New York Heart Association classification in end-stage renal disease. *Nephrol Dial Transplant* 2007;22(5):1377–1382.

18 Moss AH, Ganjoo J, Sharma S, Gansor J, Senft S, Weaner B et al. Utility of the "surprise" question to identify dialysis patients with high mortality. *Clin J Am Soc Nephrol* 2008;3(5):1379–1384.

19 Cohen LM, Ruthazer R, Moss AH, Germain MJ. Predicting six-month mortality for patients who are on maintenance hemodialysis. *Clin J Am Soc Nephrol* 2010;5(1):72–79.

20 Cohen LM, Ruthazer R, Moss AH, Germain MJ. Predicting 6 month mortality on hemodialysis, 2010. www.qxmd.com/calculate-online/nephrology/predicting-6-month-mortality-on-hemodialysis. Last accessed July 16, 2012.

21 Tamura MK, Covinsky K, Chertow G, Yaffe K, Landefeld C, McCulloch C. Functional status of elderly adults before and after initiation of dialysis. *N Engl J Med* 2009;361(16):1539–1547.

22 Murtagh FE, Marsh JE, Donohoe P, Ekbal NJ, Sheerin NS, Harris FE. Dialysis or not? A comparative survival study of patients over 75 years with chronic kidney disease stage 5. *Nephrol Dial Transplant* 2007;22(7):1955–1962.

23 Smith C, Da Silva-Gane M, Chandna S, Warwicker P, Greenwood R, Farrington K. Choosing not to dialyse: Evaluation of planned non-dialytic management in a cohort of patients with end-stage renal failure. *Nephron Clin Pract* 2003;95(2):c40–c46.

24 Chandna SM, Da Silva-Gane M, Marshall C, Warwicker P, Greenwood RN, Farrington K. Survival of elderly patients with stage 5 CKD: Comparison of conservative management and renal replacement therapy. *Nephrol Dial Transplant* 2010;26(5):1608–1614.

25 Carson RC, Juszczak M, Davenport A, Burns A. Is maximum conservative management an equivalent treatment option to dialysis for elderly patients with significant comorbid disease? *Clin J Am Soc Nephrol* 2009;4(10):1611–1619.

26 Burgess E. Conservative treatment to slow deterioration of renal function: Evidence-based recommendations. *Kidney Int Suppl* 1999;70:s17–s25.

27 Murtagh F, Cohen LM, Germain MJ. Dialysis discontinuation: Quo vadis? *Adv Chronic Kidney Dis* 2007;14(4):379–401.

28 Cohen LM, Bostwick JM, Mirot A, Garb J, Braden G, Germain M. A psychiatric perspective of dialysis discontinuation. *J Palliat Med* 2007;10(6):1262–1265.

29 The Marie Curie Palliative Care Institute. Liverpool care pathway. http://www.mcpcil.org.uk/service-innovation-and-improvement-division/lcp.aspx, Accessed June 04, 2014.

30 Douglas C, Murtagh FE, Chambers EJ, Howse M, Ellershaw J. Symptom management for the adult patient dying with advanced chronic kidney disease: A review of the literature and development of evidence-based guidelines by a United Kingdom Expert Consensus Group. *Palliat Med* 2009;23(2):103–110.

31 Davison SN, Jhangri GS, Johnson JA. Cross-sectional validity of a modified Edmonton symptom assessment system in dialysis patients: A simple assessment of symptom burden. *Kidney Int* 2006;69(9):1621–1625.

32 Saini T, Murtagh FE, Dupont PJ, McKinnon PM, Hatfield P, Saunders Y. Comparative pilot study of symptoms and quality of life in cancer patients and patients with end stage renal disease. *Palliat Med* 2006;20(6):631–636.

33 Murphy EL, Murtagh FE, Carey I, Sheerin NS. Understanding symptoms in patients with advanced chronic kidney disease managed without dialysis: Use of a short patient-completed assessment tool. *Nephron Clin Pract* 2008;111(1):c74–c80.

34 Kosmadakis GC, Medcalf JF. Sleep disorders in dialysis patients. *Int J Artif Organs* 2008;31(11):919–927.

35 Zalai D, Szeifert L, Novak M. Psychological distress and depression in patients with chronic kidney disease. *Semin Dial* 2012;25(4):428–438.

36 Davison SN, Jhangri GS. Impact of pain and symptom burden on the health-related quality of life of hemodialysis patients. *J Pain Symptom Manage* 2010;39(3):477–485.

37 Davison SN, Jhangri GS, Johnson JA. Longitudinal validation of a modified Edmonton symptom assessment system (ESAS) in haemodialysis patients. *Nephrol Dial Transplant* 2006;21(11):3189–3195.

38 Weisbord SD, Fried LF, Mor MK, Resnick AL, Unruh ML, Palevsky PM et al. Renal provider recognition of symptoms in patients on maintenance hemodialysis. *Clin J Am Soc Nephrol* 2007;2(5):960–967.

39 Bailie GR, Mason NA, Bragg-Gresham JL, Gillespie BW, Young EW. Analgesic prescription patterns among hemodialysis patients in the DOPPS: Potential for underprescription. *Kidney Int* 2004;65(6):2419–2425.

40 Davison SN, Jhangri JS. Edmonton Symptom Assessment System Revised: Renal (ESAS-r: Renal) 2013. http://www.albertahealthservices.ca/ps-1022201-narp-tools-esas.pdf. Last accessed June 04, 2013.

41 Palliative care outcome scale. London, U.K.: Cicely Saunders Institute, King's College London. http://pos-pal.org/index.php. Last accessed January 18, 2013.

42 Weisbord SD, Fried LF, Arnold RM, Rotondi AJ, Fine MJ, Levenson DJ et al. Development of a symptom assessment instrument for chronic hemodialysis patients: The Dialysis Symptom Index. *J Pain Symptom Manage* 2004;27(3):226–240.

43 Davison SN. Pain in hemodialysis patients: Prevalence, cause, severity, and management. *Am J Kidney Dis* 2003;42(6):1239–1247.

44 Weisbord SD, Fried LF, Arnold RM, Fine MJ, Levenson DJ, Peterson RA et al. Prevalence, severity, and importance of physical and emotional symptoms in chronic hemodialysis patients. *J Am Soc Nephrol* 2005;16(8):2487–2494.

45 Abdel-Kader K, Unruh ML, Weisbord SD. Symptom burden, depression, and quality of life in chronic and end-stage kidney disease. *Clin J Am Soc Nephrol* 2009;4(6):1057–1064.

46 Chater S, Davison SN, Germain MJ, Cohen LM. Withdrawal from dialysis: A palliative care perspective. *Clin Nephrol* 2006;66(5):364–372.

47 Davison SN, Jhangri GS. The impact of chronic pain on depression, sleep, and the desire to withdraw from dialysis in hemodialysis patients. *J Pain Symptom Manage* 2005;30(5):465–473.

48 Kurella M, Bennett WM, Chertow GM. Analgesia in patients with ESRD: A review of available evidence. *Am J Kidney Dis* 2003;42(2):217–228.

49 Shankel SW, Johnson DC, Clark PS, Shankel TL, O'Neil WM, Jr. Acute renal failure and glomerulopathy caused by nonsteroidal anti-inflammatory drugs. *Arch Intern Med* 1992;152(5):986–990.

◆ 50 Chen YF, Jobanputra P, Barton P, Bryan S, Fry-Smith A, Harris G et al. Cyclooxygenase-2 selective non-steroidal anti-inflammatory drugs (etodolac, meloxicam, celecoxib, rofecoxib, etoricoxib, valdecoxib and lumiracoxib) for osteoarthritis and rheumatoid arthritis: A systematic review and economic evaluation. *Health Technol Assess* 2008;12(11):1–278, iii.

51 Guay DR, Awni WM, Findlay JW, Halstenson CE, ABRAHAM PA, Opsahl JA et al. Pharmacokinetics and pharmacodynamics of codeine in end-stage renal disease. *Clin Pharmacol Ther* 1988;43(1):63–71.

52 Davies G, Kingswood C, Street M. Pharmacokinetics of opioids in renal dysfunction. *Clin Pharmacokinet* 1996;31(6):410–422.

53 Barnes JN, Goodwin FJ. Dihydrocodeine narcosis in renal failure. *Br Med J (Clin Res Ed)* 1983;286(6363):438–439.

54 Kirvela M, Lindgren L, Seppala T, Olkkola KT. The Pharmacokinetics of Oxycodone in uremic patients undergoing renal transplantation. *J Clin Anesth* 1996;8:13–18.

55 Lee MA, Leng M, Cooper RM. Measurements of plasma oxycodone, noroxycodone and oxymorphone levels in a patient with bilateral nephrectomy who is undergoing haemodialysis. *Palliat Med* 2005;192413(3):259–260.

56 Foral PA, Ineck JR, Nystrom KK. Oxycodone accumulation in a hemodialysis patient. *South Med J* 2007;100(2):212–214.

57 Scott LJ, Perry CM. Tramadol: A review of its use in perioperative pain. *Drugs* 2000;60(1):139–176.

58 Hanna MH, D'Costa F, Peat SJ, Fung C, Venkat N, Zilkha TR. Morphine-6-glucuronide disposition in renal impairment. *Br J Anaesth* 1993;70:511–514.

59 Lee MA, Leng ME, Tiernan EJ. Retrospective study of the use of hydromorphone in palliative care patients with normal and abnormal urea and creatinine. *Palliat Med* 2001;15:26–34.

60 Davison SN, Mayo P. Pain management in chronic kidney disease: The pharmacokinetics and pharmacodynamics of hydromorphone and hydromorphone-3-glucuronide in hemodialysis patients. *J Opioid Manage* 2008;4(6):335, 339–336, 344.

61 Fainsinger R, Schoeller T, Bruera E. Methadone in the management of cancer pain: A review. *Pain* 1993;52(2):137–147.

62 Kreek MJ, Schecter AJ, Gutjahr CL, Hecht M. Methadone use in patients with chronic renal disease. *Drug Alcohol Depend* 1980;5:197–205.

63 Furlan V, Hafi A, Dessalles MC, Bouchez J, Charpentier B, Taburet AM. Methadone is poorly removed by haemodialysis. *Nephrol Dial Transplant* 1999;14(1):254–255.

64 Koehntop DE, Rodman JH. Fentanyl pharmacokinetics in patients undergoing renal transplantation. *Pharmacotherapy* 1997;17(4):745–752.

65 Bower S. Plasma protein binding of fentanyl: The effect of hyperlipoproteinaemia and chronic renal failure. *J Pharm Pharmacol* 1982;34:102–106.

66 Mercadante S, Caligara M, Sapio M, Serretta R, Lodi F. Subcutaneous fentanyl infusion in a patient with bowel obstruction and renal failure. *J Pain Sympt Manage* 1997;13:241–244.

67 Hand CW, Sear JW, Uppington J, Ball MJ, McQuay HJ, Moore RA. Buprenorphine disposition in patients with renal impairment: Single and continuous dosing, with special reference to metabolites. *Br J Anaesth* March 1990;64(3):276–282.

68 Ohtani M, Kotaki H, Sawada Y, Iga T. Comparative analysis of buprenorphine- and norbuprenorphine-induced analgesic effects based on pharmacokinetic-pharmacodynamic modeling. *J Pharmacol Exp Ther* February 1 1995;272(2):505–510.

69 Filitz J, Griessinger N, Sittl R, Likar R, Schuttler J, Koppert W. Effects of intermittent hemodialysis on buprenorphine and norbuprenorphine plasma concentrations in chronic pain patients treated with transdermal buprenorphine. *Eur J Pain* November 2006;10(8):743–748.

70 Szeto HH, Inturrisi CE, Houde R, Saal S, Cheigh J, Reidenberg MM. Accumulation of normeperidine, an active metabolite of meperidine, in patients with renal failure or cancer. *Ann Int Med* 1977;86(6):738–741.

71 Martin KJ, Olgaard K, Coburn JW, Coen GM, Fukagawa M, Langman C et al. Diagnosis, assessment, and treatment of bone turnover abnormalities in renal osteodystrophy. *Am J Kidney Dis* March 2004;43(3):558–565.

72 Coen G. Adynamic bone disease: An update and overview. *J Nephrol* March 2005;18(2):117–122.

● 73 Koch KM. Dialysis-related amyloidosis. *Kidney Int* May 1992;41(5):1416–1429.

74 Fine A, Zacharias J. Calciphylaxis is usually non-ulcerating: Risk factors, outcome and therapy. *Kidney Int* June 2002;61(6):2210–2217.

● 75 Bajwa Z, Gupta S, Warfield C, Steinman T. Pain management in polycystic kidney disease. *Kidney Int* 2001;60:1631–1644.

125

Palliative care in the emergency department

TRAVIS DeVADER, TAMMIE QUEST

INTRODUCTION

The emergency department (ED) remains the entry point to the health-care system for many patients. The specialty of emergency medicine (EM) was developed with the intent to rapidly assess patients and quickly initiate life-sustaining measures in an effort to improve morbidity and mortality. As such, the mentality of emergency physicians has been to "save first and ask questions later." This model of emergency care served the population well prior to the burden that severe, life-limiting chronic diseases have placed on the EDs as well as the health-care system as a whole. In 2006 alone, there was less than a 1% increase in cancer diagnoses but a 20% increase in ED visits for cancer patients.[1]

The culture of EM has slowly begun to change. EM was 1 of 10 specialties that petitioned for the recognition of hospice and palliative medicine as a subspecialty.[2] Leaders in the field of EM also collaborated to begin educating more emergency providers in the core content of palliative care via the Education in Palliative and End-of-Life Care for Emergency Medicine (EPEC-EM).[3] EPEC-EM has trained over 150 emergency providers including physicians, social workers, and chaplains in palliative care skills necessary in the ED.

NEW ERA OF INTEGRATION

Palliative care providers increasingly have begun to view the ED as a place to begin to provide palliative care for patients with serious illness in addition to other units in the hospital, just as the ED is beginning to assess how palliative care is best incorporated into the environment. Studies have shown that 35%–56% of ED deaths are secondary to incurable chronic illnesses in which death is the expected outcome.[4,5] Delay in palliative care interventions to include goals of care assessment, symptom control, or consultation may have unintended costs to the patient, their family, and the health-care system as a whole.[6] However, the ideal model of delivery of palliative care interventions in the ED remains unknown. Since both EM and palliative medicine are relatively new specialties, little is known regarding the best use of palliative medicine subspecialty service in the ED and which patient populations stand to gain most from a subspecialty collaboration of the two fields.

This chapter is meant to serve as an introduction to the field of ED palliative care. The culture and attitudes of the ED and its practitioners are explored. Models of providing palliative care in the ED are identified as well as identifying ED patients that may best be served by a palliative medicine consultant in the ED. ED utilization by seriously ill patients is reviewed as well as methods to decrease unnecessary and unwanted ED visits in the final days of life. The use of advance directives in the ED population and their usefulness for the emergency provider is identified, and barriers to providing palliative care in the ED are explored.

CHANGING CULTURE

EM remains a rescue-oriented culture in the context of an increasingly chronically ill population that will reach a point where rescue and reversal of illness is not possible. Up to one third of ED deaths are due to the effects of chronic disease.[7] Consistent with previous studies, a recent study from Australia notes that nearly 70% of patients who died made at least one visit to the ED prior to death with the mean number of ED visits at 1.9 per patient.[8,9] A convenience sample study of 50 elderly adults with chronic medical conditions found that over half of the patients had unmet needs in the areas of physical symptom management, financial need, mental health needs, and lacking access to care with the mean quality of life reported as 3.62 on the McGill index.[10] While there has been one successful pilot program using volunteers to provide the family with bereavement care both during and after the ED visit, this is not the norm.[11] ED use within the last 2 weeks of life has been determined to be a marker of poor quality of life. Thus, research has been conducted to try and identify those patients who are at risk for making an ED visit. For patients with all diagnoses, weight loss, decrease in cognition, male gender, and overnight admission to a hospital within the previous 2 weeks have been identified as risk factors for making an ED visit.[12] In a study of hospice patients with end-stage cardiac disease, patients were less likely to make an ED visit if they had a DNR in place, were older and Caucasian, had greater frequencies of home visits by nurses and chaplains, had medication compliance, were taking morphine sulfate, had caregivers in the home, and had an emergency kit in the home.[13] For men with prostate cancer, receiving hospice services was associated with significantly less ED visits.[14]

Increasingly, there is a recognized need to assess in the ED the risks and benefits of an intervention, assess the presence of an advance care plan, and assess distressing symptoms in lieu of illness reversal. Under multiple demands for care delivery, ED clinicians question the feasibility of establishing advanced care plans in the ED as well as doubt their skill sets to provide palliative care in the ED despite calls from national societies to provide such care.[15–17] While those practicing EM see the utility in providing palliative care, only 10% of EM residents described palliative care in the ED as desirable and feasible.[15]

GAPS IN TRAINING

Consistent with the perceptions of EM as a medicolegal-focused specialty,[18] EM residents reported receiving the most training in the legalities of end-of-life care and advance directives and little training in symptom management.[19] Less than half of participating EM residents reported receiving formal training in pain management and managing the imminently dying patient while less than 55% reported receiving training in managing the hospice patient and withholding and withdrawing life-sustaining therapies.[20] Despite doubts, several studies have begun to show the feasibility of palliative care in the emergency setting that have shown the ability to identify patients with palliative care needs including those that would benefit from a hospice model of care and subspecialty[21] consultation with no significant increase in ED length of stay.[22]

ROLE OF EDUCATION

Part of the challenge of integrating palliative care into the ED has been lack of formal education in palliative care principles. Core competencies in palliative care have been identified for the practicing emergency physician (Table 125.1).[2] Educating EM trainees in core palliative care skills even briefly may have an impact. In one study, 4 hours of devoted lecture to key concepts in palliative care for the emergency physician have been shown to improve EM residents' comfort level with discussing end-of-life care with ED patients and families, and an 88% increase in referrals to inpatient hospice care was noted.[23]

ED patients who ultimately receive a palliative care consultation most often have the chief complaint of shortness of breath followed by neurological complaints such as weakness. Most patients had an Emergency Severity Index of Level 2 (Level 1 is most critical and Level 5 is least critical). Only 14%–17% of these patients presented to the ED with a DNR order in place.[24] If the ED visit was made during the last 2 weeks of life, 72% of the time the patient was admitted, and 77% of the admitted patients subsequently died in the acute care setting.[25]

Table 125.1 *Twelve palliative care skills that all EM physicians should learn*

Twelve palliative care skills for the EM physician
Psychosocial skills
Communicate bad news.
Resuscitate the terminally ill with family members present.
Plan advanced care.
Medical skills
Assess illness trajectory.
Formulate a prognosis.
Manage pain and nonpain symptoms.
Manage the imminently dying.
Manage the dying child.
Withdrawal and withholding of care.
Systems-based skills
Manage hospice patients and palliative care system referrals.
Understand ethical and legal issues pertinent to end-of-life care.
Cultural and spiritual skills
Display spiritual and cultural competency.

Source: Quest, T.E. et al., *Ann. Emerg. Med.*, 54, 94, 2009.

MODELS OF EMERGENCY PALLIATIVE CARE

Currently, there is no ideal model identified of providing palliative care in the ED setting. There are success stories using each model, and the model used in any particular community is usually dictated by the availability of local resources.[26] Common models of care include (1) traditional consultation of the palliative care subspecialty service, (2) a focus on primary palliative care by the ED clinicians or in rare circumstances, (3) provision of palliative care by a subspecialty trained emergency physician trained in hospice and palliative medicine, or (4) links to community palliative care resources such as community hospice care.

A model that has been proposed but not yet validated is to define early goal-directed therapy for palliative care in the ED. Presumably, EDs could identify early therapies needed for patients' overall comfort and symptom control and ensure that these goals are at least started, if not met, in the ED.[27] EDs across the country already use early goal-directed therapies in a number of emergency situations including acute myocardial infarction, acute coronary syndrome, pneumonia, sepsis, and stroke. Using an "early goal-directed therapy" approach that is already familiar to the emergency clinician may improve compliance.[28]

AVOIDING ED TRANSFER OF TERMINALLY ILL PATIENTS

Given the fact that ED transfers in the last week of life and the ED as a place of death are viewed as poor quality of life and quality of death indicators, respectively, much effort has been given to avoiding ED transfers in terminally ill patients. Just as the ED has examined how it can improve the care of these patients,[29] primary and palliative care has focused on how to avoid unnecessary ED visits.

One of the reasons cited by terminally ill patients for ED utilization is lack of access to care.[30] The data on whether intense primary care can avoid unnecessary ED visits are mixed. It appears that just having a primary care provider is not sufficient to avoid ED utilization. Those patients who experienced a high degree of continuity with the same primary care provider were almost four times less likely to utilize the ED; however, patients who had access to primary care but did not have a high degree of continuity with the same provider were much more likely to utilize the ED.[31]

An area of great concern for emergency physicians is the number of ED visits made by those patients in residential nursing facilities. Urgent transfers to the ED when a patient is dying are often avoidable and unwanted by patients.[32] Reasons for transfer of the residential nursing patient to the ED include the following: (1) transfer to the ED is initiated only after all other potential options have been exhausted by facility staff; (2) inadequate staffing leads to increased demands on staff that may not be adequately trained; (3) primary care providers were not timely in answering pages so staff felt obligated to transfer the patient if the condition continued to deteriorate; and (4) residential care staff felt pressured by families of patients to "do something."[33]

ED utilization in long-term care is complex. Patients enrolled in an integrated service model of palliative care were less likely to utilize the ED. However, although the results were statistically significant, there was only a 6% reduction in ED utilization resulting in 29% of patients enrolled in the service making at least one visit to the ED.[34] Ontario, Canada, introduced a $115.5 million end-of-life care strategy that spanned 3 years. The overarching goal of the initiative was to keep terminally ill patients in the home care setting thus avoiding placing demand on the acute care system. Unfortunately, results one year after the start of the initiative show that ED utilization among terminally ill patients held steady at 16%.[35]

SERIOUS ILLNESS TRAJECTORIES FOR ED PATIENTS

The first step in identifying who might be appropriate for palliative care in the ED begins with identifying patients who are in need. With the acknowledgment that palliative care is appropriate at any point in a serious illness trajectory, in the emergency care setting making sure that patients with the highest intensity of palliative care needs, those at the end of life, this may be an appropriate population of focus. There is an under recognition by emergency clinicians that patients are on an end-of-life trajectory prior to the "last hours of living." In an effort to describe the end-of-life pathway for emergency clinicians, two overarching trajectories toward end of life have been identified in the context of the ED: the spectacular and subtacular death trajectories. The spectacular death is a

death that is often unanticipated or unexpected and requires the mobilization of resources. Examples include fulminant traumatic illness (e.g., motor vehicle collision) or sudden medical illness (e.g., acute myocardial infarction or cerebral vascular event) in which a team of clinicians employ massive resuscitative efforts to reverse sudden illness. The subtacular death is described as a patient whose death is anticipated or expected by the ED staff or where the patient could have goals of care and an advance care plan in place that may prevent the heroics of the spectacular route.[36]

The spectacular and subtacular death categories can then be divided further into disease-specific end-of-life trajectories: (1) disseminated cancer, (2) frailty—often those in long-term care, (3) organ failure, (4) sudden death, and (5) others (which includes infectious etiologies). Many patients on a subtacular trajectory could benefit from ED-based and subspecialty palliative care interventions. Whichever the trajectory, palliative care needs are high in these populations with high rates of pain and ICU utilization.[37] The recognition of an end-of-life trajectory in patients allows for palliative care needs to be assessed and addressed earlier.

WHY PATIENTS PRESENT TO THE ED WITH SERIOUS ILLNESS

Often times, the emergency clinician may be left wondering why a patient who is seriously chronically or terminally ill returns repeatedly to the emergency care system—particularly when receiving hospice care. Reasons include symptom burden, difficulty with outpatient care access, financial barriers of the uninsured or underinsured, miscommunication with the primary clinician, and mixed messages by the primary care provider particularly when prognosis was unclear.[30] When patients presented to the ED for symptom management issues, typically, patients were advised to go to the ED by other clinical caregivers, and/or the patient and caregiver either felt unprepared to manage the symptom at home or felt that the symptom could not be managed at home. During ED visits, patients and caregivers have noted a lack of communication between the emergency clinicians and the primary care clinician as well as lack of communication about what happens during the ED stay. Lack of care coordination leads to increased anxiety on the part of both the patient and caregiver.[38]

The ED itself presents a unique communication challenge for patients and families who may be reluctant to communicate their needs to the ED. While patients state in interviews that they do not wish for aggressive end-of-life care,[30] only 12.5% make this request known to emergency staff.[4] The ED is not the ideal place of death due to lack of privacy, staff shortages, and inexperience of the staff in managing patients at the end of life.[39] Yet despite making preferences known for no ED transfer or hospitalization at the time of death, it often happens.[32] Care of the dying has been shown to improve with end-of-life order sets, and these order sets have also been shown to improve clinician communication with patients and their families.[40]

MISSED OPPORTUNITIES FOR CARING

When palliative care is globally defined as optimal physical, spiritual, psychological, and social support and practically implemented in the form of providing relief from pain and nonpain symptoms, hydration, mouth care, repositioning for comfort, and providing emotional support to the patient and family, it has been shown that only half of the patients who die in the ED get this level of care. Specifically, 55% of patients received analgesia, 51% of patients and families received emotional support, 35% received mouth care, 33% received repositioning and relief from anxiety, and 24% received emotional support.[41] It appears that a large focus of ED nursing staff is preparing the body for viewing after death and allowing family adequate time for viewing[42] in addition to self-care in terms of debriefing[43] as opposed to symptom management.

ROLE OF ADVANCE DIRECTIVES AND THE ADVANCE CARE PLAN

Caring for a terminally ill patient without advance care plans in place continues to be a source of frustration for many emergency physicians. Unfortunately, the rate of documented advance care plans remains low. The National Center for Health Statistics reports that 28% of home care patients, 65% of nursing home residents, and 88% of discharged hospice patients have at least one documented advance care plan on record with patients aged 85 years and older having the highest percentage of documentation.[44] Fifty-six percent of nursing home patients had a DNR order compared with 7% for home care patients.[44] Thus, large numbers of patients elect not to express wishes in the form of formal advance care plans. Approximately, 30% of ED patients have expressed their desire not to have advance directives in place.[45] The reasons given for not wanting to form an advance directive include always wanting to have aggressive life-sustaining treatment, fear of not getting enough or proper treatment if an advance directive was in place, and fear of being allowed to die.[45] Emergency physicians have reported difficulty in interpreting advance directives in the middle of an emergent visit but have also reported being able to contact family in 90% of the cases in which they felt family input was important.[46,47] Obtaining timely information continues to be a problem for emergency physicians, and they have requested that residential nursing facilities standardized communication of advance directives and include the date when the information was last updated with the patient.[48]

Surveys of ED patients have shown varying levels of utilization and understanding of advance care plans. Only 22%–27% of ED patients have formal advance directives, and of those who have advance directives, only 23% brought them to the ED at the time of their visit.[49–51] Factors associated with higher rates of documented advance care plans are presence of a primary care physician, advanced age, and having a life-threatening disease or considering yourself as very ill.[49–51] Historically, emergency clinicians have felt that initiating an ED DNR order or enforcing an advance directive is outside of the scope of practice[52,53]; attitudes are changing. Patients and families are receptive in the ED setting regarding advance care planning. When families were contacted about a patient's advance directive or code status, 85% of those conversations led to a DNR order in the ED, and 97% of the families contacted felt that it was appropriate for the emergency clinician to contact them and have the conversation regardless of the decision that was made.[54]

PEDIATRIC PALLIATIVE CARE IN THE ED

To this point, all of the data have focused on adults with terminal illnesses. The field of pediatric palliative care is in its infancy with even less data available than for adults. The field of emergency palliative care for children is nonexistent, but there are data available for children who died in the ED. Of all children who died, most died at home while 14% died in the ED with the rate climbing to 22% if the child was not hospitalized in the last week of life.[55] Interestingly, children with cancer composed less than half of ED deaths. Children with cardiovascular disorders were six times more likely to die in the ED, those children with metabolic and genetic disorders were five times more likely to die in the ED, and children with neuromuscular disorders were four times more likely to die in the ED.[55]

BARRIERS TO EMERGENCY PALLIATIVE CARE

Identified barriers to providing palliative care in the ED include lack of education of emergency clinicians in the key concepts in palliative care, lack of knowledge of available resources, time constraints of the ED, challenges of the physician–patient relationship, family dynamics, overstepping the traditional role of the ED, and legal concerns and comfort level of the treating physician (Table 125.2).[23,56] Research into providing palliative care in the ED is evolving. Research to date has focused on what patients can best be served by providing palliative care in the ED, what the ideal role of the emergency physician should be, how providing palliative care in the ED affects healthcare utilization, and educating emergency providers on the fundamentals of palliative care.[57]

CONCLUSION

The integration of palliative care in the emergency setting is a rapidly evolving field. EM and palliative care clinicians alike increasingly see the benefits of providing palliative care in the ED. The model of EM is focused on providing the right level of care for the right patient at the right time for the life stage of the patient. As the field evolves, barriers to providing palliative care in the ED will be overcome. Future research will

Table 125.2 *Perceived barriers to providing palliative care in the ED*

Theme	Barrier	Opportunity
Time constraints	Slow palliative care response time in busy environment of the ED.	Time constraints discourage providers from providing supportive care.
Knowledge of available services	Palliative care services and availability vary widely across communities.	Providers can cultivate new relationships to provide better care to patients.
Lack of education and training in end-of-life care	Limited understanding of palliative care.	Recognized need for provider education.
Challenges of the physician–patient relationship	Need for explicit criteria for consultation.	Including family is complex and time-consuming.
Family dynamics	May not arrive with the patient in the ED or may be fractured in terms of care plan.	Goals of care conference can alleviate family concerns and facilitate a united plan of care.
Personal comfort level of the treating physician	Aggressive care decreases risk of lawsuits.	Palliative approach is right for the patient.
Role of the ED	Primary care's role to discuss goals of care; patients and families expect aggressive care; little sense of patient ownership.	Emergency patients have true palliative care needs.

Sources: Adapted from DeVader, T.E. and Jeanmonod, R., *J. Palliat. Med.*, 15, 510, 2012; Grudzen, C.R. et al., *J. Pain Symptom Manage.*, 43, 1, 2012.

focus on the impact that providing palliative care in the ED has on health-care utilization, quality of life, and quality of death. Just as EM was born out of the necessity to quickly diagnose and treat patients with emergent life-threatening conditions, it will continue to evolve to be able to provide the necessary quality palliative and end-of-life care that an aging chronically ill population needs and deserves.

REFERENCES

1 Pitts SR, Niska RW, Xu J et al. National hospital ambulatory medical care survey: 2006 emergency department summary. *Natl Health Stat Rep* 2008;6(7):1–38.

2 Quest TE, Marco CA, Derse AR. Hospice and palliative medicine: New subspecialty, new opportunities. *Ann Emerg Med* 2009;54:94–102.

3 EPEC. *EPEC for Emergency Medicine*. Chicago, IL: Northwestern University, 2011.

4 Tardy B, Venet C, Zeni F et al. Death of terminally ill patients on a stretcher in the emergency department: A French speciality? *Intensive Care Med* 2002;28:1625–1628.

5 Beynon T, Gomes B, Murtagh FE et al. How common are palliative care needs among older people who die in the emergency department? *Emerg Med J* 2011;28:491–495.

6 DeVader TE, Albrecht R, Reiter M. Initiating palliative care in the emergency department. *J Emerg Med* 2012;43:803–810.

7 Kompanje EJ. The worst is yet to come. Many elderly patients with chronic terminal illnesses will eventually die in the emergency department. *Intensive Care Med* 2010;36:732–734.

8 Rosenwax LK, McNamara BA, Murray K et al. Hospital and emergency department use in the last year of life: A baseline for future modifications to end-of-life care. *Med J Aust* 2011;194:570–573.

9 Katelaris AG. Time to rethink end-of-life care. *Med J Aust* 2011;194:563.

10 Grudzen CR, Richardson LD, Morrison M et al. Palliative care needs of seriously ill, older adults presenting to the emergency department. *Acad Emerg Med* 2010;17:1253–1257.

11 Ting SM, Li P, Lau FL et al. Acute bereavement care in the emergency department: Does the professional-supported volunteers model work? *Eur J Emerg Med* 1999;6:237–243.

12 Brink P, Partanen L. Emergency department use among end-of-life home care clients. *J Palliat Care* 2011;27:224–228.

13 Schonwetter RS, Clark LD, Leedy SA et al. Predicting emergency room visits and hospitalizations among hospice patients with cardiac disease. *J Palliat Med* 2008;11:1142–1150.

14 Bergman J, Kwan L, Fink A et al. Hospice and emergency room use by disadvantaged men dying of prostate cancer. *J Urol* 2009;181:2084–2089.

15 Smith AK, Fisher J, Schonberg MA et al. Am I doing the right thing? Provider perspectives on improving palliative care in the emergency department. *Ann Emerg Med* 2009;54:86–93, e81.

16 American College of Emergency Physicians. Ethical issues in emergency department care at the end of life. *Ann Emerg Med* 2006;47:302.

17 Rosen P. Let the emergency department do it—A simple solution to a complex problem. *J Emerg Med* 1991;9(Suppl. 1):75–77.

18 George JE. Law and the ED nurse: The terminally ill emergency patient. *J Emerg Nurs* 1984;10:333–334.

19 Meo N, Hwang U, Morrison RS. Resident perceptions of palliative care training in the emergency department. *J Palliat Med* 2011;14:548–555.

20 Lamba S, Pound A, Rella JG et al. Emergency medicine resident education in palliative care: A needs assessment. *J Palliat Med* 2012;15:516–520.

21 Waugh DG. Palliative care project in the emergency department. *J Palliat Med* 2010;13:936.

22 Mahony SO, Blank A, Simpson J et al. Preliminary report of a palliative care and case management project in an emergency department for chronically ill elderly patients. *J Urban Health* 2008;85:443–451.

23 DeVader TE, Jeanmonod R. The effect of education in hospice and palliative care on emergency medicine residents' knowledge and referral patterns. *J Palliat Med* 2012;15:510–515.

24 Grudzen CR, Hwang U, Cohen JA et al. Characteristics of emergency department patients who receive a palliative care consultation. *J Palliat Med* 2012;15:396–399.

25 Barbera L, Taylor C, Dudgeon D. Why do patients with cancer visit the emergency department near the end of life? *Can Med Assoc J* 2010;182:563–568.

26 Grudzen CR, Stone SC, Morrison RS. The palliative care model for emergency department patients with advanced illness. *J Palliat Med* 2011;14:945–950.

27 Lamba S. Early goal-directed palliative therapy in the emergency department: A step to move palliative care upstream. *J Palliat Med* 2009;12:767.

28 Stone S, Rodriguez L, Calder K. Lack of pain assessment for patients with cancer presenting to the emergency department with pain complaints: Can we improve with a simple intervention? *J Palliat Med* 2006;9:7–9.

29 Pines JM, Asplin BR. Conference proceedings-improving the quality and efficiency of emergency care across the continuum: A systems approach. *Acad Emerg Med* 2011;18:655–661.

30 Grudzen CR, Stone SC, Mohanty SA et al. I want to be taking my own last breath: Patients' reflections on illness when presenting to the emergency department at the end of life. *J Palliat Med* 2011;14:293–296.

31 Burge F, Lawson B, Johnston G. Family physician continuity of care and emergency department use in end-of-life cancer care. *Med Care* 2003;41:992–1001.

32 Purdy W. Nursing home to emergency room? The troubling last transfer. *Hastings Cent Rep* 2002;32:46–48.

33 Arendts G, Reibel T, Codde J et al. Can transfers from residential aged care facilities to the emergency department be avoided through improved primary care services? Data from qualitative interviews. *Australas J Ageing* 2010;29:61–65.

34 Lawson BJ, Burge FI, McIntyre P et al. Can the introduction of an integrated service model to an existing comprehensive palliative care service impact emergency department visits among enrolled patients? *J Palliat Med* 2009;12:245–252.

35 Seow H, Barbera L, Howell D et al. Did Ontario's end-of-life care strategy reduce acute care service use? *Healthc Q* 2010;13:93–100.

36 Bailey C, Murphy R, Porock D. Trajectories of end-of-life care in the emergency department. *Ann Emerg Med* 2011;57:362–369.

37 Lamba S, Nagurka R, Murano T et al. Early identification of dying trajectories in emergency department patients: Potential impact on hospital care. *J Palliat Med* 2012;15:392–395.

38 Smith AK, Schonberg MA, Fisher J et al. Emergency department experiences of acutely symptomatic patients with terminal illness and their family caregivers. *J Pain Symptom Manage* 2010;39:972–981.

39 Clarke R. Improving end-of-life care in emergency departments. *Emerg Nurse* 2008;16:34–37.

40 Paterson BC, Duncan R, Conway R et al. Introduction of the Liverpool Care Pathway for end of life care to emergency medicine. *Emerg Med J* 2009;26:777–779.

41 Le Conte P, Riochet D, Batard E et al. Death in emergency departments: A multicenter cross-sectional survey with analysis of withholding and withdrawing life support. *Intensive Care Med* 2010;36:765–772.

42 Beckstrand RL, Smith MD, Heaston S et al. Emergency nurses' perceptions of size, frequency, and magnitude of obstacles and supportive behaviors in end-of-life care. *J Emerg Nurs* 2008;34:290–300.

43 Norton CK, Hobson G, Kulm E. Palliative and end-of-life care in the emergency department: Guidelines for nurses. *J Emerg Nurs* 2011;37:240–245.

44 Jones AL, Moss AJ, Harris-Kojetin LD. Use of advance directives in long-term care populations. *NCHS Data Brief* 2011;(54):1–8.

45 Taylor DM, Ugoni AM, Cameron PA et al. Advance directives and emergency department patients: Ownership rates and perceptions of use. *Intern Med J* 2003;33:586–592.

46 Lahn M, Friedman B, Bijur P et al. Advance directives in skilled nursing facility residents transferred to emergency departments. *Acad Emerg Med* 2001;8:1158–1162.

47 Weinick RM, Wilcox SR, Park ER et al. Use of advance directives for nursing home residents in the emergency department. *Am J Hosp Palliat Care* 2008;25:179–183.

48 Pauls MA, Singer PA, Dubinsky I. Communicating advance directives from long-term care facilities to emergency departments. *J Emerg Med* 2001;21:83–89.

49 Llovera I, Mandel FS, Ryan JG et al. Are emergency department patients thinking about advance directives? *Acad Emerg Med* 1997;4:976–980.

50 Llovera I, Ward MF, Ryan JG et al. Why don't emergency department patients have advance directives? *Acad Emerg Med* 1999;6:1054–1060.

51 Ishihara KK, Wrenn K, Wright SW et al. Advance directives in the emergency department: Too few, too late. *Acad Emerg Med* 1996;3:50–53.

52 Thewes J. Playing with fire: Advance directives in the emergency department. *Acad Emerg Med* 1997;4:83–84.

53 Ritchie KS, Rubenstein EB, Valentine AD. Do-not-resuscitate orders in the emergency department. *Am J Med* 1992;93:586–587.

54 Balentine J, Gaeta T, Rao N et al. Emergency department do-not-attempt-resuscitation orders: Next-of-kin response to the emergency physician. *Acad Emerg Med* 1996;3:54–57.

55 Guertin MH, Cote-Brisson L, Major D et al. Factors associated with death in the emergency department among children dying of complex chronic conditions: Population-based study. *J Palliat Med* 2009;12:819–825.

56 Grudzen CR, Richardson LD, Hopper SS et al. Does palliative care have a future in the emergency department? Discussions with attending emergency physicians. *J Pain Symptom Manage* 2012;43:1–9.

57 Quest TE, Asplin BR, Cairns CB et al. Research priorities for palliative and end-of-life care in the emergency setting. *Acad Emerg Med* 2011;18:e70–e76.

126

Symptom control in stem-cell transplantation: A multidisciplinary palliative care team approach

ERIC ROELAND, WILLIAM MITCHELL, CAROLYN MULRONEY, KATHRYN THORNBERRY,
RABIA ATAYEE, JOSEPH MA, HEATHER HERMAN

INTRODUCTION

For the past three decades, bone marrow transplantation has been used to treat children and adults with otherwise incurable malignant disorders, certain inherited diseases, and immune system disorders. Bone marrow harvest was the original method for acquiring hematopoietic blood stem cells from related or unrelated donors or autologous transplantation. Today, stem-cell sources also include mobilized blood stem cells and umbilical cord cells. Therefore, the term "hematopoietic stem-cell transplantation" or more simply "stem-cell transplantation" (SCT) is now used to encompass these additional sources instead of the term "bone marrow transplantation." Despite the growing number of stem-cell sources, the basic goal remains unchanged: to replace or supplement host hematopoietic stem cells with donor cells.

Patients are frequently offered SCT, a treatment with significant morbidity and mortality, at the same time they are adjusting to the diagnosis of a fatal malignancy. Extensive teaching and information about the SCT treatment is provided in spoken and/or written form, so that the patient knows the nature of his or her treatment, its risks and benefits, and possible outcomes. The preparative treatment prior to transplant is used to treat the underlying disease in the case of malignant disorders as well as to suppress the immune system so that the transplanted cells will be accepted. The patient must accept the possibility of severe systems related to treatment. They will also very likely experience prolonged periods of isolation while the transplanted hematopoietic stem cells engraft, potential infections while their immune system recovers, and complications such as graft-versus-host disease (GVHD). Despite all of this, there is still the possibility of recurrence of their disease. Even with the extensive efforts related to informed consent, no patient can fully understand the information when he or she is primarily focused on the potential cure. It should be expected that the patient's understanding of the ordeal of SCT treatment changes throughout the process and retrospective dissatisfaction with initially presented information is common [1].

This shift in patient perspective after transplant can be significantly improved by addressing the combination of physical, social, psychological, emotional, and spiritual stressors that the patient and family endure. Invasive medical procedures, distressing physical symptoms, social isolation, uncertainty regarding outcomes, changes in body image, and lost sense of control all increase vulnerability and suffering in these patients [2]. Improving these multidimensional features of suffering will enhance the experience for everyone involved, including the patient, family, and SCT team.

Based on our experience at an academic adult inpatient SCT unit, we review and summarize the management of physical, psychological, social, and spiritual symptoms that frequently occur in the course of SCT and offer an approach to their management. We will describe approaches to patients receiving autologous or allogeneic SCT. Although the prevalence, spectrum, and severity of symptoms differ between these two types, the approach to symptom management is the same.

SCT process

Relieving the suffering associated with SCT begins with an understanding of the patient experience throughout the SCT process. While patterns in treatment regimens and symptoms exist, the experience of the patient undergoing SCT is unique. Additionally, given the increasing availability of alternate donors as well as the increasing applications and ability for this procedure to be performed at many centers further emphasizes the need for more practitioners to understand the needs of these patients. Although it is important to know the diagnosis, pretransplant comorbidities, source of donor cells (matched related vs. unrelated donor), time to transplant, source of stem cells (bone marrow, peripheral blood, or cord blood), type of transplant (autologous vs. allogeneic), degree of histocompatibility of donor cells, conditioning regimens (myeloablative vs. nonmyeloablative regimens), and complications (GVHD, opportunistic infections, and sinusoidal obstruction syndrome), it is equally important to know the patient's understanding of the process. Furthermore, beyond physical health, each patient is unique with regard to personality and psychological well-being. For example, understanding how each patient copes with stress prior to transplant and exploring these coping strategies provides insight on how the patient will cope with the SCT process. The assessment should address the patient's premorbid psychiatric state, past adaptation to stressors, history of adherence with treatment, substance abuse history, and level of social support, including community- and faith-based support systems [3]. It has been demonstrated that pretransplant variables in cognitive beliefs, affect, and social support contribute 21%–40% of posttransplant psychosocial outcomes [4]. Therefore, prompt evaluation is necessary as the period of greatest emotional distress and vulnerability occurs after initial admission to the hospital for transplant [2].

SCT culture

The commitment to improve SCT with regard to its science and outcomes has a positive and significant effect on the ability of nurses and physicians to routinely interact with patients. In order to avoid caregiver burnout, each SCT professional develops coping strategies for sequential exposure to high medical acuity, a high degree of responsibility, intense therapy regimens, and exposure to incredible physical and psychological suffering. For example, caregivers may underemphasize key concerns, such as suffering and emotional labor for patients who fail to respond to aggressive treatments or die from treatment-induced complications [5]. Like their patients, caregivers utilize a wide range of coping mechanisms during extremely stressful times, such as humor, rationalization, and emotional shutdown, which may be difficult to understand to someone outside the SCT team. It should not be surprising that SCT physicians may extrapolate and mix and compare data in ways that are the most positive, not just for the patient, but to sustain themselves. Consequently, it is important to recognize the limiting cultural and professional factors contributing to the lack of attention on the issues of symptoms, death, and dying and the emotional intensity within SCT care settings.

As a consequence of spending weeks to months on the SCT unit and increased dependence on caregivers during the periods of intense treatment, patients and medical providers develop close relationships. This intimate patient–caregiver relationship and the intellectual challenge of caring for complicated patients with potential for cure can be highly rewarding for caregivers. Consequently, it has been reported that SCT staff report high job satisfaction and personal accomplishment from working with transplant patients [6]. Caregivers draw strength by sharing success stories of long-term SCT survivors, including the sickest patients who improved despite all odds ("Lazarus phenomena"). Deaths or less positive outcomes may be framed as "casualties in the war on cancer" as a way to sustain the high commitment to the life-saving potential and the improvement of the modality through research.

Despite the observed commitment to their patients, it has been shown that patients describe significantly more distress from their symptoms than the physicians and nurses caring for them [7,8]. This may be the result of SCT cultural phenomena that focus on potential for a cure despite current suffering. In a survey of physicians' attitudes about quality of life (QOL) issues in hematopoietic stem-cell transplant, 72% of physicians were willing to accept poor QOL for a small chance of cure. Only 28% said that QOL considerations "often" or "almost all the time" enter into patients' decisions about transplantation. This contrasted with the physicians' reported attention to QOL in their discussion with patients [8]. This reported disparity is disturbing, but it is an important clue to SCT culture.

INTEGRATION OF PALLIATIVE CARE IN STEM-CELL TRANSPLANT PROGRAMS

Primary palliative care plays a key role in stem-cell transplant programs as the bulk of day-to-day management of physical, psychological, social, and spiritual symptoms and difficulties rests with the physicians, nurses, social workers, psychologists, pharmacists, and others working on the SCT team. However, given the burden and complexity of symptoms associated with SCT, many patients require specialized or secondary, palliative care expertise. Access to such services is often not extended to SCT patients due to the misperception that palliative care is only applied to patients with terminal illness near the end of life. This is a missed opportunity to relieve patients who are struggling through the arduous process of SCT. Palliative services should be available to all SCT patients who are suffering, regardless of the stage of illness.

Successful integration of palliative care into a transplant program requires attention to several key principles. First, palliative care team members must have an understanding of the SCT process and culture, build relationships with the SCT team, and earn the respect of transplant physicians and nurses. In our experience, the most successful techniques to achieve this include a daily physical presence and availability to assist the SCT team, giving clear and concise symptom intervention recommendations, and remaining focused on the specific reason for the consult. Palliative care consultants should also initially emphasize recommendations on physical symptoms. After trusting relationships are established, this can be expanded to psychosocial and spiritual suffering. Above all, the palliative care team must focus more on its relationship with the treating SCT team than on the outcome of an individual patient. Careful attention to these close relationships with health-care providers will enable future access to SCT patients.

SYMPTOMS

Physical and psychological symptom burden can be defined as the combined impact of all disease- or therapy-related symptoms on the patient's ability to function [9].

In approaching symptom management, the division between physical and psychological symptoms is blurred. Physical symptoms are often interrelated to the patient's emotional status. For example, one study evaluated several biomedical, psychological, and social variables as possible predictors for the intensity of treatment-related mouth pain and anxious mood in 63 patients undergoing SCT prospectively [10]. The results indicated that psychological and social variables were important predictors of mouth pain, besides biomedical variables. The biomedical variables revealed the most predictive power during the second week posttransplant, while psychological predictors were more important during the early and late phases of the treatment.

Physical

Although physical symptoms and the degree to which they are experienced depend on a multitude of factors, in our experience, the following symptoms frequently occur in SCT: pain, nausea, mucositis, diarrhea, and delirium.

GRAFT-VERSUS-HOST

Prior to focusing on individual symptoms, GVHD merits particular mention as it is extremely common and has multiple features. Despite improvements in transplant medicine, GVHD remains a common complication of allogeneic SCT. Acute and chronic GVHD traditionally were defined by time of onset but now are defined by their clinical and pathological features. Acute GVHD is likely mediated by donor T cells that are coinfused with the stem-cell graft and likely involves intricate interactions between cellular and cytokine components of the immune system [11]. Acute GVHD primarily involves the skin, gastrointestinal (GI) tract, and liver. The severity of the GI condition generally parallels that of the skin and liver involvement, although profound GI symptoms can occur without any gross skin or liver changes. Standard treatment for acute GVHD is high-dose corticosteroids and more recently immunosuppressive therapy such as mycophenolate mofetil.

Chronic GVHD affects from 30% to 90% of long-term survivors of allogeneic SCT [12]. The incidence is increasing due to the older age of patients undergoing transplants, the use of peripheral blood SCTs, and the use of mismatched and unrelated donors. Chronic GVHD is recognized as a distinct disorder from acute GVHD whose manifestations often resemble symptoms seen in autoimmune disorders. Diagnostic features of chronic GVHD typically involve the skin and mucosa including poikiloderma (pigmentary and atrophic changes), lichen-planus-like features, sclerosis, vaginal scarring, esophageal web and strictures, and joint contractures to name a few. Typical signs associated with of chronic GVHD include depigmentation, nail loss, alopecia, xerostomia, and myositis [12]. This wide diversity of manifestations of chronic GVHD has hindered its clinical study. Therapy for chronic GVHD also depends on steroids.

PAIN

Pain is a common symptom in patients who undergo a SCT for a hematological malignancy. Treatment of acute pain in hospitalized SCT patients predominantly relies on intravenous (IV) opioids via bolus doses or patient-controlled analgesia (PCA). SCT patients are frequently unable to take oral, subcutaneous, rectal, or transdermal opioids. In fact, the rectal route is contraindicated in the setting of neutropenia. Adjuvant analgesics such as nonsteroidal anti-inflammatory drugs (NSAIDs) and corticosteroids should be avoided due to the risk of bleeding disorders, coexisting renal disease, and peptic ulcer [13]. In general, patients may also describe symptoms of neuropathic pain, of which anticonvulsants and tricyclic antidepressants are used. However, these may not be appropriate options in SCT patients based on limited routes of administration, of which few anticonvulsants and tricyclic antidepressants are available at IV formulations.

ACUTE PAIN

During an acute pain episode, IV opioids should be used judiciously and be dosed, in part, by knowledge of IV opioid pharmacokinetics. As described in detail in prior chapters, the maximum analgesic effect for a dose of an IV opioid generally corresponds with the maximum serum concentration. For most IV opioids, the maximum serum concentration is 5–10 min. If additional doses of the IV opioid are needed, repeat dosing can safely occur 10 min after previous IV opioid administration. This concept is also applicable for PCAs, as the dosing interval is generally every 8–10 min.

DOSE FINDING TO DETERMINE OPTIMAL DOSE FOR PATIENT

Finding an optimal dose for the patient often requires rapid dose escalation. Providers often are conservative with dose escalations due to unwarranted fears of overdosing opioids. Patients do not notice a change in analgesia when dose escalations are less than 25% above the previous dose (e.g., baseline). One suggested formula is to increase opioid doses by 25%–50% for mild to moderate pain and by 50%–100% for moderate to severe pain [14]. In the setting of inadequate pain relief, the IV opioid dose may safely be doubled based on the maximum serum concentration of morphine (5–10 min). Continue to double the dose with carefully monitoring at each serum half-life until the patient experiences adequate analgesia.

CHOOSE THE APPROPRIATE MAINTENANCE DOSE

To determine the maintenance dose for providing sustained pain control, total the amount of opioid that gives the patient relief from the bolus doses administered during the dose-finding period. Then divide the total amount of opioid by 2. Next divide the opioid amount by the known half-life of the opioid to determine a continuous infusion rate (e.g., maintenance dose). The half-life of a drug is the amount of time required for the total amount (e.g., dose) of drug or the serum concentration to decrease by 50%. In summary, determining the appropriate maintenance dose is dependent of completion of a dose-finding period. Incremental changes of the infusion rate without dose finding of the appropriate bolus dose(s) will not provide adequate and prompt pain relief due to lack of achieving steady state blood concentrations.

ABDOMINAL PAIN CRAMPS

Abdominal pain cramps are frequent in patients with bowel GVHD. Anticholinergic, antispasmodic drugs such as dicyclomine may be needed as an adjuvant for abdominal pain cramps. Of note, glycopyrrolate, the only potent quaternary anticholinergic ammonium compound available in the United States, has reduced penetration across the blood–brain barrier and a decreased incidence of unwanted centrally mediated side effects [15].

CHALLENGING PAIN CIRCUMSTANCES

Patients may have physical symptoms exacerbated by their emotional status and poor coping skills. In these particularly challenging patients, addressing anxiety, depression, drug abuse, fear, and prior trauma is essential in order to adequately address and treat the patient's pain [16]. Patients who chemically cope with stressful situations can be expected to continue to chemically cope during the hospital admission. Examples of such behaviors include, but are not limited to, frequent request for a specific IV opioid and frequent request for an opioid administration preference (e.g., IV bolus doses). For members of the SCT team, this can be challenging to treat the patient's pain due to fears of contributing or causing addiction. However, such aberrant behavior probably reflects undertreated pain and not addiction. In the SCT environment, undertreated pain may be due to inappropriate opioid administration (e.g., dose or dosing interval), malabsorption, nausea and vomiting, and pseudoaddiction.

Pseudoaddiction is defined as "an iatrogenic syndrome of abnormal behavior developing as a direct consequence of inadequate pain management" [17]. Treatment strategies must include an establishment of trust between the patient and health-care team and adequate and timely analgesics for achieving pain control. Knowledge and application of opioid pharmacokinetic concepts (e.g., maximum concentration, half-life) is invaluable in achieving appropriate opioid doses and dosing intervals. In addition, patients should be evaluated by psychology/psychiatry and have routine follow-ups by the palliative care team.

NAUSEA AND VOMITING

Nausea is defined as the subjective feeling of the need to vomit, whereas vomiting is the reflex expulsion of gastric contents through the mouth. Nausea may be present in the absence of vomiting and vice versa. For SCT patients, delayed and chronic nausea and vomiting may be experienced during the hospitalization and posttransplant [18,19]. In addition, acute nausea due to opioid use may also be observed in SCT patients. The approach to treating nausea and vomiting should be no different for SCT patients. A review of chemotherapy-induced nausea and vomiting is discussed elsewhere [20]. Identifying possible etiologies and the most likely pathophysiology is crucial to determining appropriate pharmacotherapy.

A detailed patient interview often provides invaluable information regarding the pathophysiology of the patient's nausea and vomiting. For example, if the patient reports brief nausea immediately before vomiting, this is suggestive of hyperperistalsis to overcome a mechanical obstruction in the intestine. If the patient vomits immediately after food intake, this is suggestive of a cortical learned response or anxiety-related response. Delayed gastric emptying may be suspected if a patient vomits about 45 min after eating or if the patient vomits hours after eating, this is suggestive of intestinal or bowel involvement. Other critical pieces of information to obtain from the patient include when nausea and vomiting occurs, if it is acute or chronic, intermittent or constant, associated with specific sights, odors, or events, and if vomiting makes the patient feel better. In addition, patients should be asked what medications (both over the counter [OTC] and prescription) have been used. Often, patient bowel patterns are not assessed, as constipation is a frequent cause of chronic nausea.

A complete physical examination will also aid in the understanding of the patient's nausea and vomiting. Adjusting head position or posture may worsen nausea and is thus suggestive of vestibular apparatus involvement. The absence of bowel sounds during an abdominal examination may suggest obstruction, while an enlarged liver or presence of ascites or stool in the rectal vault may suggest diminished peristalsis. There are also several diagnostic studies that can be considered. Nausea due to increased intracranial pressure may be confirmed by a funduscopic examination. A plain radiograph of the abdomen looking for presence and quantity of stool and evidence of ileus is useful. An abdominal ultrasound (for enlarged liver or ascites assessment), computed tomography scans of the head or abdomen, and motility studies may be useful in selected cases.

MANAGEMENT OF NAUSEA AND VOMITING

The etiology of nausea and vomiting should be determined, if possible, to specifically correct the underlying etiology. Correction of dehydration, hypokalemia, and metabolic alkalosis will sometimes resolve nausea and vomiting. Prior chapters describe in detail the major causes of nausea/vomiting, which are summarized in Table 126.1. This clarification is intended to set the stage for the rational use of the antiemetics, which can be classified by their mechanism of action.

Table 126.1   *Management of nausea/vomiting based on etiology (the 12 M's of emesis)*

Etiology	Pathophysiology	Therapy
Metastases		
Cerebral (increased ICP)	Increased ICP, direct CTZ effect	Steroids, mannitol, anti
Liver	Toxin buildup	anti-DA/Hist
Meningeal irritation	Increased ICP	Steroids
Movement	Vestibular stimulation (may be worse with morphine)	Anti-Ach
Mentation, e.g., anxiety	Cortical	Anxiolytics, e.g., benzodiazepines, THC
Medications		
Opioids	CTZ, vestibular effect, GUT	Anti-DA/Hist, anti-Ach, prokinetic agents, stimulant cathartics
Chemotherapy	CTZ, GUT	Anti-5HT/DA, steroids
Others (NSAIDs; see "Mucosal irritation")	CTZ	Anti-DA/Hist
Mucosal irritation		
NSAIDs	GUT, gastritis	Cytoprotective agents
Hyperacidity, gastroesophageal reflux	GUT, gastritis, duodenitis	Antacids
Mechanical obstruction		
Intraluminal	Constipation, obstipation	Manage constipation
Extraluminal	Tumor, fibrotic stricture	*Reversible*—surgery
		Irreversible—manage fluids, steroids, inhibit secretions with octreotide, scopolamine
Motility		
Opioids, ileus, other medications	GUT, CNS	Prokinetic agents, stimulant laxatives
Metabolic		
Hypercalcemia, hyponatremia, hepatic/renal failure	CTZ	Anti-DA/Hist, rehydration, steroids
Microbes		
Local irritation, e.g., esophagitis, gastritis from *Candida*, *H. pylori*, herpes, CMV	GUT	Antibacterials, antivirals, antifungals, antacids
Systemic sepsis	CTZ	Anti-DA/Hist, antibacterials, antivirals, antifungals
Maternal	Unknown	Pyridoxine (vitamin B6), antihistamines, anti-DA
Myocardial Ischemia		
congestive heart failure	Vagal stimulation, cortical, CTZ	Oxygen, opioids, anti-DA/Hist, anxiolytics

Anti-Ach, acetylcholine antagonists; Anti-DA, dopamine antagonists; Anti-Hist, histamine antagonists; Anti-5HT, serotonin antagonists; CTZ, chemoreceptor trigger zone; GUT, gastrointestinal tract; ICP, intracranial pressure; THC, tetrahydrocannabinol.

Antiemetics can be generally classified as dopamine antagonists, serotonin subtype 3 (5-HT$_3$) antagonists, antihistamines, anticholinergics, and neurokinin one receptor antagonists. Numerous adjunctive medications, while not directly antiemetics, can also treat specific causes of nausea and vomiting such as hyperacidity or gut dysmotility. Empiric treatment generally begins with a single antiemetic medication targeting the presumed mechanism of nausea and vomiting. The dose should be optimized before a second medication is started. It is important that the second medication possess a different mechanism of action than then first medication that was initiated. Sequential antiemetic combination therapy may be required in some patients.

CHEMOTHERAPY-INDUCED NAUSEA/VOMITING

Chemotherapy-induced nausea and vomiting can occur in different phases. Acute chemotherapy-induced nausea and vomiting can occur within the first 24 hours after chemotherapy. These symptoms usually start within 1–2 hours and peaks around 4–6 hours [20]. Delayed chemotherapy-induced nausea and vomiting occurs more than 24 hours after chemotherapy, with symptoms peaking about 2–3 days and lasting 6–7 days [21,22]. Anticipatory nausea and vomiting is a conditioned response in which symptoms occur before chemotherapy starts. This can be challenging to treat as it is a learned response and symptoms are poorly controlled with antiemetic therapies [23,24]. Breakthrough nausea and vomiting can occur if the primary prophylactic antiemetic therapies fail to provide complete symptom relief.

Chemotherapy- and patient-related factors predict the risk of chemotherapy-induced nausea and vomiting. Emetogenicity of the chemotherapy agent is the most predictive factor to cause chemotherapy-induced nausea and vomiting [25–27]. Highly emetogenic chemotherapy is expected to occur on more than 90% of patients and includes chemotherapies such as cisplatin ($\geq$50 mg/m^2), cyclophosphamide ($\geq$100 mg/m^2), and certain combinations. Moderate emetogenic chemotherapy is expected to cause symptoms in 30%–90% of patients, while minimal emetogenic chemotherapy is expected to cause symptoms in 10%–30% of patients. Finally, minimal emetogenic chemotherapy is anticipated to cause symptoms in less than 10% of patients.

OPIOID-INDUCED NAUSEA AND VOMITING

Opioids induce nausea and vomiting by simulating the chemoreceptor trigger zone. A vestibular component is also likely. Opioids have been associated with acute nausea in up to 30% of patients. In high-risk patients, particularly young women, premedication with a dopamine antagonist (e.g., prochlorperazine) can be recommended. Serotonin antagonists, antihistamines, and anticholinergics are also possible options as efficacy has been reported [28,29]. Opioid-induced nausea and vomiting generally subsides within 5–7 days of starting opioid therapy due to development of tolerance. If opioid-induced nausea and vomiting continues after 5–7 days, changing to a different opioid is also a reasonable alternative. Nausea that emerges after chronic opioid use is probably due to diminished gut motility and/or constipation causing pseudoobstruction, which should be managed by increasing gut motility and aggressively treating constipation.

SEROTONIN ANTAGONISTS

5-HT$_3$ antagonists inhibit the activity of serotonin in the GI tract and CNS and thus block transmission of emetic signals to the vomiting center. All of the 5-HT$_3$ antagonists are considered equally effective, with response rates ranging 60%–80% for acute chemotherapy-induced nausea and vomiting [26,27,30,31]. For each drug, there is a plateau in efficacy, meaning that additional dose titration provides little to no improvement of symptoms. The use of 5-HT$_3$ antagonists is appropriate for chemotherapy prophylaxis, radiotherapy prophylaxis to the abdomen (which stimulates serotonin release from the gut lining), and postoperative nausea. They can also be useful for refractory nausea of diverse types but are typically tried only when other medications have failed. 5-HT$_3$ antagonists should be promptly discontinued if they provide little relief of symptoms after a short trial. Medication and dosing options include

- Dolasetron 100 mg or 1.8 mg/kg IV
- Dolasetron 100–200 mg by mouth
- Granisetron 1 mg or 0.01 mg/kg IV
- Granisetron 1–2 mg by mouth
- Ondansetron 8 mg or 0.15 mg/kg IV
- Ondansetron 8 mg by mouth twice to three times daily
- Palonosetron 0.25 mg IV

DOPAMINE ANTAGONISTS

Dopamine antagonists are useful agents for breakthrough nausea and vomiting or for SCT patients who are refractory to other antiemetic agents. These are also appropriate for prevention of chemotherapy-induced nausea and vomiting from low-emetogenic-risk chemotherapies. Dopamine antagonists generally have a lower therapeutic index compared to 5-HT$_3$ antagonists and have a larger side effect profile that limits their use. Sedation and extrapyramidal symptoms such as dystonia and akathisia have been reported with phenothiazine and butyrophenone neuroleptics. Medication dosing options include

- Droperidol 2.5–5 mg IV every 6 hours
- Haloperidol 0.5–2.0 mg by mouth or IV or subcutaneously every 6 hours (may need to titrate dose)
- Metoclopramide 10–20 mg by mouth every 6 hours
- Olanzapine 5–10 mg by mouth once daily
- Perphenazine 2–8 mg by mouth or IV every 6 hours
- Prochlorperazine 10–20 mg by mouth every 6 hours
- Prochlorperazine 25 mg by rectum every 12 hours
- Prochlorperazine 5–10 mg IV every 6 hours
- Promethazine 12.5–25 mg IV
- Promethazine 25 mg by mouth or by rectum every 4–6 hours
- Thiethylperazine 10–20 mg by mouth every 6 hours

NEUROKININ-1 RECEPTOR ANTAGONISTS

Aprepitant was the first-in-class agent approved in 2003 by the U.S. Food and Drug Administration. The neurokinin-1 receptor antagonist is used in combination with a serotonin inhibitor and dexamethasone for prevention of high to moderate emetogenic chemotherapies. Aprepitant is generally administered as a 3-day oral regimen of 125 mg on day 1 and 80 mg on days 2 and 3. Aprepitant is well tolerated with clinical studies reporting diarrhea, fatigue, headache, and hiccups [25,32–34]. Aprepitant is metabolized by cytochrome P450 (CYP)3A and is a mixed CYP3A inhibitor and CYP2C9 inducer. Concomitant administration of medications that are also metabolized by overlapping CYP pathways should be monitored to minimize possible drug–drug interactions.

ANTIHISTAMINES

Nonselective histamine antagonists used to control nausea are likely to cause sedation. In some patients, this expected adverse effect may be beneficial in helping with sleep. Nonselective antihistamines also cause dry eyes, dry mouth, urinary retention, and constipation due to anticholinergic properties. Medication dosing options include

- Diphenhydramine 25–50 mg by mouth every 6 hours
- Hydroxyzine 25–50 mg by mouth every 6 hours
- Meclizine 25–50 mg by mouth every 6 hours

ANTICHOLINERGICS

If a motion-related component is suspected, then involvement of the vestibular apparatus is highly likely. Opioids and anesthetics can also trigger acetylcholine-mediated nausea in the vestibular apparatus. A medication from this class may be added to other antiemetics [35]. Scopolamine is available in various routes of administration and can be administered as scopolamine 0.1–0.4 mg subcutaneous or IV every 4 hours or as a transdermal patch every 72 hours.

PROKINETIC AGENTS

Nausea and vomiting in patients with advanced disease may be due to carcinomatosis, opioid therapy, or other medications resulting in a dyskinetic gut. Pseudoobstruction due to ascites or peritoneal disease can also result in nausea and vomiting. Constipation can be an exacerbating factor. Medication and dosing options include

- Domperidone 10–20 mg by mouth every 6 hours before meals and at bedtime
- Erythromycin 250 mg by mouth every 6 hours before meals and at bedtime
- Metoclopramide 10–20 mg by mouth or IV every 6 hours before meals and at bedtime

ANTACIDS

Hyperacidity, with or without gastroesophageal reflux and/or gastric or duodenal erosions, may result in nausea and vomiting. Medication and dosing options include

- Antacids 1–2 tablespoons by mouth every 2 hours as needed
- H_2 receptor antagonists
  - Cimetidine 800 mg by mouth at bedtime
  - Famotidine 40 mg by mouth at bedtime
  - Ranitidine 150 mg by mouth at bedtime
- Proton pump inhibitors
  - Esomeprazole 20 mg by mouth daily
  - Lansoprazole 30 mg by mouth daily
  - Omeprazole 20 mg by mouth daily
  - Pantoprazole 40 mg by mouth daily

OTHER MEDICATIONS

This heterogeneous class of medications has unclear mechanisms of action but uncontested benefits in some patients [24,36–38]. Medication and dosing options include

- Dexamethasone 6–20 mg by mouth daily
- Lorazepam 0.5–2 mg by mouth or buccal or subcutaneously every 4–6 hours
- Tetrahydrocannabinol 2.5–5 mg by mouth three times daily

MUCOSITIS

The prevalence of mucositis is high in patients who undergo a hematopoietic SCT. The symptoms are short lived, self-limiting, and predictable with onset occurring in 5 days with peak severity in 7–10 days posttherapy in autologous, allogeneic, or matched unrelated donor. Similarly, its resolution is also predictable with an average of 2 weeks [39]. Patients receiving conditioning regimens for total body irradiation, have a body mass index ≥25, not taking multivitamins prior to transplantation, and having methylenetetrahydrofolate reductase 677TT genotype have a higher risk of developing severe oral mucositis [40,41].

Prevention of mucositis with oral evaluation and encouraging appropriate oral hygiene is important. Human keratinocyte growth factors such as palifermin were developed for the use of mucositis prevention. In a study of the use of palifermin with high-dose chemotherapy and radiotherapy for hematological cancers, a lower duration and severity of oral mucositis was observed [42]. Amifostine has shown promise in preventing severe oral mucositis in a retrospective study where patients receiving high dose of melphalan followed by autologous stem-cell transplants received concomitant amifostine [43].

Although the data are scarce, the primary approach in management of mucositis is the use of topical oral formulations including, but not limited to, equal parts lidocaine/diphenhydramine/Mylanta. Some have added dexamethasone, ibuprofen, morphine, and other opioids to the mixture [44–47]. Recently, topical ketamine has shown a trend in improvement of mucositis pain [48]. Based on the available literature, our institution dilutes 20 mg of IV ketamine in 5 mL of artificial saliva or normal saline to be "swished for 1 min and spit" every 3 hours. Gelclair® is a concentrated bioadherent oral gel indicated for the relief and management of pain [49]. Initial results were promising, but due to high cost and lack of sustained efficacy, Gelclair is not used frequently. Interestingly, there is an OCT agent, Rincinol®, that is advertised as "mouth sore rinse" that has the same active ingredient as Gelclair but much less expensive. Usually, the topical agents are not adequate and patients need additional systemic therapy mainly including opioids through PCA [44,50]. Unfortunately, until the mucositis resolves, patients are at high risk for developing infections, respiratory complications when the mucositis is endangering the breathing pathway, and severe morbidity [51,52].

DIARRHEA

The majority of patients will develop diarrhea after a SCT. In a recent study, 66% of SCT patients developed one or more episodes of diarrhea in the first 100 days posttransplant. Allogeneic SCT recipient developed significantly more diarrhea than autologous SCT recipients. Standard of care includes hydration, correction of electrolytes, and then determining etiology. The most common cause of diarrhea in patients receiving SCT is acute GI GVHD followed by other less common causes that include opportunistic infections, medications like mycophenolate required posttransplant, mucosal damaged caused by high-dose chemotherapy and total body irradiation [53], and neutropenic enterocolitis [54]. Patient receiving cord-blood SCT can also develop a culture-negative diarrhea termed cord colitis syndrome [55]. Thus far, the etiology of cord colitis is unknown, but fortunately, it is responsive to antibiotics.

Acute GI GVHD has an onset or continuance of profuse, water diarrhea for 3 weeks following SCT, which is indicative of intestinal acute GVHD. Intestinal acute GVHD involves the small and large intestines, which may result in diarrhea, nausea, vomiting, abdominal pain, intestinal bleeding, and ileus. The amount of high-volume diarrhea generated is an index of the extent and severity of disease activity and extensive GVHD may produce up to 10 L of diarrhea a day. Features that distinguish acute GVHD from the enteritis associated with induction protocols and opportunistic intestinal infections include an erythematous, maculopapular skin rash over the palms, soles, and trunk, as well hyperbilirubinemia (as discussed previously). Protein loss in the stool may be sufficiently severe to lead to profound hypoalbuminemia. The absence of pathogens in the stool is important, but does not necessarily rule out an infection of the GI tract.

Management of intestinal acute GVHD consists of nutritional support, maintenance of fluid and electrolytes, corticosteroids and immunosuppressive treatment, and monitoring for secondary infectious complications. Once infectious causes have been ruled out, patients with severe high-volume diarrhea may find relief from careful titration of loperamide (maximum dose 16 mg daily). Since loperamide is a poorly absorbed opioid, it will not be very effective for patients already receiving opioids for symptom control. Octreotide is an alternative strategy to manage the secretory diarrhea [56]. Starting doses for octreotide are 200–600 mcg daily by subcutaneous or IV bolus or continuous infusion (maximum dose is 900 mcg daily) [57].

ANOREXIA

Most SCT patients experience a decrease in appetite as a consequence of cellular damage related to the high-dose chemotherapy and radiotherapy and marked shifts in cytokines. Pain, mucositis, nausea, GI complications, constipation, diarrhea, and psychosocial issues also frequently contribute to a decreased desire for food. In one series, eating difficulty was noted in 66% of patients at day 50 posttransplant. This was due to poor appetite, dry mouth, altered taste, nausea, and fatigue [58]. Additionally, SCT patients are placed on dietary restrictions due to their immunocompromised state or GVHD that make food less appetizing and preparation cumbersome [59].

The first step in managing transplant-associated anorexia should be to address the root cause; however, this is not always feasible when symptoms are directly related to the treatment and the recovery is slow. Total parenteral nutrition (TPN) is commonly used to supply necessary nutrients, but is not superior to enteral feeding with regard to time to recovery or days spent in the hospital [60]. TPN is also associated with such complications as IV catheter infection, liver dysfunction, and hyperglycemia. Management of anorexia is problematic in this patient population. Although not specifically studied in the SCT setting, approaches utilized in other patient populations, including advanced cancer and HIV/AIDS patients, are worth considering here.

CORTICOSTEROIDS

Dexamethasone, prednisolone, and methylprednisolone have been found to be effective appetite stimulants since the 1970s in patients with advanced cancer [37]. Unfortunately, their effect is time limited, and the appetite stimulus does not correspond to an increase in body mass [61]. Many patients are already taking significant doses of glucocorticoids as part of transplant for prolonged periods, and associated toxicities such as myopathy, infection, and adrenal insufficiency are common in this patient population. These limitations make corticosteroids less useful in SCT patients.

MEGESTROL ACETATE

Megestrol acetate has been demonstrated to improve anorexia and cachexia in AIDS patients. A 2007 Cochrane review of randomized studies on patients with cancer, HIV/AIDS, and other conditions (COPD, cystic fibrosis and elderly) found that megestrol acetate improved appetite and weight gain in patients with cancer, but there was not enough evidence to prove an impact on QOL or for a specific dose recommendation [62]. Doses range from 100 to 1600 mg a day have been recommended [61]. Megestrol acetate can be started at these doses in SCT patients and titrated as necessary, though this has not been demonstrated to be effective. Megestrol acetate should be used with caution in patients with history of thromboembolic disease.

CANNABINOIDS

Dronabinol has been shown to improve appetite and stabilize the body weight in patients with HIV/AIDS [63]. Doses used were 2.5 mg once or twice day. A prospective randomized study comparing megestrol acetate with dronabinol in patients with advanced cancer found that megestrol acetate was significantly more effective than dronabinol for appetite improvement and weight gain [64]. We do not recommend use of cannabinoids for anorexia in SCT.

EICOSAPENTAENOIC ACID

Eicosapentaenoic acid (EPA), an omega-3 fatty acid present in fish oils, has been found in several studies to increase appetite and body weight in cancer patients [64–66]; however, a Cochrane database review found that EPA was no more effective than placebo [67].

DELIRIUM

Delirium is defined as a cognitive disorder with disturbance of consciousness (including inattention) and at least one of the following symptoms: disorganized thinking, disorientation, memory impairment, or perceptual disturbance. The onset is typically acute. Delirium is marked by a fluctuating course and is due to an underlying medical cause. One prospective series found a rate of 50% in the peritransplant period [68], similar to other estimates of delirium in patients with advanced cancer (45%–85%) [69–71]. This mirrors our experience.

Delirium is a serious condition that has clearly been associated with adverse outcomes. A significantly higher mortality rate, with an odds ratio of 14, has been reported in SCT patients who developed delirium [72]. In a cohort of 61 elderly patients with femoral neck fracture, those with delirium had longer hospital stays, were less independent in their activities of daily living, had more medical complications, and were less likely to regain the ability to walk and return to prefracture living accommodation [73]. In a cohort of patients requiring mechanical ventilation, those who developed delirium had higher 6-month mortality rates, longer hospital stays, and a higher incidence of cognitive impairment at hospital discharge [74]. In a study of late-stage cancer patients admitted to a palliative care unit, patients with delirium had a significantly shorter survival, living an average of 21 days compared with 39 days for patients without delirium [75].

Delirium is underdiagnosed in SCT patients. Recognition of delirium remains a major problem, largely because the most common signs and symptoms of delirium in this group differ in some respects from those seen in other patient populations. Fann et al. prospectively followed a cohort of 90 patients from the pretransplant period through their first 30 days after transplant [68]. In patients with delirium, they reported a marked preponderance of hypoactive psychomotor disturbance, rather than hyperactive symptoms, which are commonly seen in other disease states. The hypoactive delirium often manifested as alteration in the sleep–wake cycle and cognitive disturbance (demonstrated by impaired attention and memory). They found that hallucinations and delusions were uncommon in this patient population. The cause of delirium in any individual SCT patient is usually difficult to elucidate and the majority of cases have multiple potential causes. They include organ dysfunction such as of the liver or kidneys and resulting metabolic and electrolyte derangements, respiratory insufficiency and resulting hypoxia, anemia and poor oxygen delivery, sepsis or other serious infection, opioid analgesics, benzodiazepines, anticholinergic drugs, CNS involvement by malignancy, illicit drug use, drug withdrawal, hypovolemia, and nutritional deficiencies [70].

MANAGEMENT

Early recognition is the first step to managing delirium in the transplant setting. It is important to maintain a high level of suspicion in transplant patients when working with this patient population. This should include careful monitoring for sleep–wake disturbance and checks for inattention to simple tasks such as counting backward by serial sevens, or any evidence of even mild confusion.

Once delirium is diagnosed, the ideal solution is to identify and correct the underlying cause. This step is particularly challenging in the SCT population because of the complexity of the clinical scenario and the difficulty of quickly reversing abnormalities as the transplant process moves over several weeks.

Nonpharmacological interventions are frequently helpful. Inouye and colleagues reported a decreased rate of delirium using such techniques in a population of hospitalized elderly patients; interventions included daily orientation, cognitively stimulating activities, nonpharmacological sleep aids (noise reduction, changing times of medications, and relaxation techniques), early mobilization, vision and hearing aids as needed, and attention to volume status [76]. A similar intervention by geriatric consultants evaluating elderly patients admitted with hip fracture also included minimization of high-risk drugs [77]. Although nonpharmacological techniques have not been formally tested in the SCT population, we advocate their use.

There are almost no data to guide the pharmacological management of delirium in the SCT patient population. In a study of 33 hospitalized patients with AIDS who were randomized to receive haloperidol, chlorpromazine, or lorazepam, it was reported that symptoms of delirium improved with both of the neuroleptic agents but not with lorazepam [78]. The data from three trials comparing different neuroleptics were reviewed. No difference was found between haloperidol and the atypical antipsychotics risperidone and olanzapine [79]. Two of these studies included a placebo arm, which had poorer outcomes in both studies. Haloperidol, risperidone, olanzapine, and quetiapine are reasonable choices, and for patients with marked delirium unresponsive to nonpharmacological interventions, we recommend scheduled doses, with additional doses available as needed for agitation. If delirium persists, we recommend titration of the dose of the antipsychotic rather than switching to another agent [80]. Risks of extrapyramidal effects and QT prolongation exist with many of these agents.

Social

Humans are social creatures; a network of relationships sustains them. However, the SCT process isolates patients from their normal social environment, and their usual networks are disrupted. Due to their immunocompromised state and risk of nosocomial infections, patients are often confined to their hospital room and deprived of physical touch, with visits with their loved ones behind gowns and masks, and are frequently unable to interact with children and pets. This kind of deprivation in emotionally resilient patients does not pose a problem, but in emotionally vulnerable patients, it may predispose them to severe psychological impairments.

This isolation adds to disruptions in the patient's social roles. Social roles are expected behavior patterns associated with an individual's function in various social groups and provide a means for social participation and a way to identify with others as in the family unit. The parent, who is now a patient and strongly identifies himself or herself as the primary provider or caregiver in the family, may now become the primary recipient of care within the family unit. This role reversal may be very disorienting for some patients.

PATIENT COPING

Coping is the ability to seek social support, positive reframing, information seeking, problem solving, and emotional expression [81]. Using a life span developmental model, we can assess coping from a chronological age as well as an emotional age. A developmental model of psychosocial functioning is based on the concept that there are sequential developmental tasks at each stage, or age range, that are the building blocks for the subsequent stage [82]. The normal developmental trajectory can be interrupted, or arrested, by emotional trauma [83]. People who have not mastered or completed certain tasks or stages often present special problems for health-care providers. For example, patients caught in a struggle between dependence and independence may develop serious transference problems with their health-care provider, including codependence. Some may find it difficult to make decisions and will want to transfer that responsibility on their health-care provider. They may blur boundaries by seeking advice or friendship in inappropriate ways and exaggerate symptoms in order to get attention. They may schedule frequent appointments to gain the attention and nurturance from their health-care provider, which they did not receive as an infant [82].

Coping can be conceptualized into several types, of which each can be viewed on a continuum from healthy coping to maladaptive coping, acknowledging everyone regresses during times of stress:

- Fighting spirit—The tendency to view the illness as a challenge and to strive to prevent it from overwhelming them. "Is taking a positive attitude something that is difficult or easy for you?"
- Helplessness—The tendency to feel utterly at a loss and unable to do anything about the impact that cancer has on their life. "It's not unusual to feel overwhelmed and helpless. How do you feel about what has happened?"
- Stoic acceptance—The tendency to view things in a passive way and accept things for what they are. "Some people feel they want to leave everything to the doctor. Is that how you feel?"
- Denial—The tendency to show a benign reaction to all that is going on around them. "Would you like to know more about the treatment options?"
- Anxious preoccupation—The tendency to focus on having cancer and allowing the disease to consume the patient's life. "It sounds like you've been seeking a lot of information about your illness. Has this helped or do you think it makes you worry more?"
- Fatalism—The tendency to accept things for what they are and make no attempt to take control. "Are you the sort of person who tends to accept things as they are or do you question what goes on?"
- Cognitive avoidance—The tendency to find ways of avoiding thoughts or blocking off worrying feelings. "Some people find it helps to avoid thinking about things to do with their illness. Are you that sort of person?"

COPING INTERVENTIONS

- Help the patient identify prior successful adaptive coping mechanisms and help them bring that into the present.
- Assist the patient to prioritize needs or problems.
- Encourage the patient to ask for help and if needed demonstrate how to do this.
- Identify a strong support person for the patient.

Psychological

Overall, the literature does not provide definitive evidence for a relationship between psychological variables and survival post-SCT, but there do exist data that select psychosocial variables can affect BMT survival. For example, Hoodin et al. in 2004 identified the SCT patient most likely to survive longest was a young, married, educated, European-American, nonsmoker who was more defiant, better adjusted, and less depressed [84]. Despite factors affecting survival, clearly, SCT is recognized as one of the most stressful treatments in modern cancer care. Caregivers must acknowledge that all patients experience some degree of psychological distress as we all regress to a more immature form of coping during stress. These stressors include changes in social life, treatment side effects, uncertainty regarding outcomes, family-related stress, fear of death, and depressive thoughts [85].

SCT places patients under severe psychological stress. Although SCT studies demonstrate that many patients show long-term improvement in psychosocial well-being, the experience of the transplant process may vary greatly, and a considerable number of transplant recipients require psychosocial support [86]. These data suggest that if the psychological symptoms that the transplant patient experiences are better managed, there will be better long-term outcomes for patients who survive the transplant.

As is observed with physical symptoms, there exists considerable overlap of psychological symptoms. For purposes of this review, we will artificially separate these topics. Based on our experience, we believe it is critical to have the input and evaluation from a psychologist or clinical social worker trained in this specialty. Patients require an accurate diagnosis to be treated properly. For example, depression, demoralization, and grief and loss, at first look, may present similarly but require different interventions. Additionally, if left untreated, psychological symptoms can become a barrier to treatment, treatment compliance, and, when appropriate, transition to end-of-life care.

DEPRESSION AND ANXIETY

Depression is a psychiatric diagnosis and is defined as having five or more symptoms listed in Table 126.2 present in the same 2-week period that interfere with routine daily activities [87]. Optimal treatment of depression requires both pharmacological and nonpharmacological approaches. Typical pharmacological treatment of depression (selective serotonin reuptake inhibitors, tricyclic antidepressants) takes weeks to be

Table 126.2 *Symptoms of depression*

- Persistent sad, anxious, or "empty" mood
- Feelings of hopelessness, pessimism
- Feelings of guilt, worthlessness, helplessness
- Loss of interest or pleasure in hobbies and activities that were once enjoyed, including sex
- Decreased energy, fatigue, being "slowed down"
- Difficulty concentrating, remembering, making decisions
- Insomnia, early morning awakening, or oversleeping
- Appetite and/or weight changes
- Thoughts of death or suicide or suicide attempts

Source: Data from National Institute of Mental Health, Depression and cancer, National Institute of Mental Health, Bethesda, MD, 2009, http://www.nimh.nih.gov/health/publications/depression.

therapeutic and often require three or four different medications in combination since the response rate to an individual drug is only 30% [88]. This time frame may be too long for the severely depressed SCT patient. Some preliminary data suggest that psychostimulants like methylphenidate and modafinil may help decrease depression within days with a response rate of 60% [89]. For example, for the depressed SCT patient, start methylphenidate 5 mg at 9 AM and noon and increase to 10 mg at 9 AM and noon the next day. Depressive symptoms should begin to improve by the third day.

Additionally, nonpharmacological interventions should be instituted. The gold standard treatment for depression is the combination of psychotherapy (particularly cognitive behavioral therapy) and antidepressants [91]. We can further support the patient by empathic listening, bedside presence, reframing negative cognitions/statements, eliciting positive coping strategies, humor, and distraction. Life review, legacy work, relaxation breathing, healing touch, and guided imagery have also been noted to aid in mediating patient suffering. When plausible, behavioral interventions are beneficial, such as going outside into the sunshine or minimal increase in physical activity.

GRIEF AND LOSS

Loss is the condition of being deprived of something or someone. Grief is a healthy response to loss. The purpose of grief is to acknowledge and work through difficult thoughts and feelings associated with a loss until they are diminished and more positive ones become prominent. One way to conceptualize grief is to categorize it as either instrumental or intuitive. Instrumental is more thought oriented where feelings are tempered: disorientation, disorganized thought, and difficulty concentrating may exist. Whereas with intuitive grievers, emotions are more dominant: profoundly painful feelings are expressed with tears to wailing, depressed mood, confusion, anxiety, inability to concentrate, anger, and fatigue [92].

Grief has a temporal variation; the patient may experience good days and bad as opposed to clinical depression, which is unremitting. Much like demoralization, the patient will still enjoy certain activities. A classic example is the woman in her 50s diagnosed with multiple myeloma who may be grieving

the loss of her career and independence but brightens and experiences joy when her grandchildren visit.

In our experience, grief in cancer patients is common. This is particularly true for patients undergoing SCT because these patients can experience distressing, sometimes debilitating, physical symptoms, which can last weeks or months. They experience loss of some hopes and dreams, real or imagined: the loss of career, independence, possibility dignity, vitality, retirement, marriage, children, etc.

Normalizing the grief process and encouraging patients to work through it can be effective. For example, "I work with many patients very much like you and they express similar feelings. This is not uncommon." Acknowledging the loss is the first step. Giving patients reassurance and presence and listening to their story can be helpful. With intuitive grievers eliciting emotions, providing empathy and connecting with others in the same situation may also help. Identifying support systems to help with these processes can be useful, including faith communities, family, friends, and, if needed, professional counselors.

DEMORALIZATION

The definition of demoralization is to deprive a person of spirit, courage, or discipline, to reduce to a state of weakness or disorder. "It is a syndrome of existential distress occurring in patients suffering from … physical illness, specifically ones that threaten life or integrity of being" [93]. The patient no longer has the internal resources to cope with adversity. Demoralization is a normal response under certain circumstances and is most often precipitated by chronic diseases. A patient's mood may be sad, anxious, irritable, demanding, and uncooperative, and his or her thinking pessimistic and even suicidal. Although these phenomena are distressing, they do not constitute a psychiatric disorder and the diagnosis of depression does not fit [83].

Listening for patient comments such as "They keep telling me I'm going to go home then it doesn't happen" and "I just thought I'd be better by now, they said I would" are clues to identifying demoralization. Supporting the patient's own pattern of coping (please see patient coping mentioned earlier) and identifying small, attainable daily goals can engender hope and joy.

Both before and during transplantation, patients must adjust to uncertainty regarding outcome [94]. Although frequently not verbalized, SCT patients fear periods of relapse, rapid fluctuations in medical status, frequent and often life-threatening infections, and even failure of sustained engraftment. SCT patients, at the end of a long hospitalization, will understandably look forward to the planned discharge. When the not uncommon but unexpected complication arises and the discharge is delayed, a patient can become demoralized—hopes are built up and dashed repeatedly. These are the patients who can appear hopeless and helpless [92]. Depressed patients experience anhedonia, the diminished ability to experience pleasure, while demoralized patients primarily experience subjective incompetence and helplessness. A demoralized patient can still experience pleasure and look forward to pleasurable activities; a depressed patient cannot [93].

From our experience, the patient's mood and outlook improves as physical symptoms diminish. One key approach to the demoralized patient is to aggressively treat their physical symptoms; symptomatic relief is pertinent as cognitively based therapies, goal setting, and the scheduling of positive activities [93].

Most importantly is the empathic understanding of the patient. Patients, family, and staff all look to physician for understanding and action [95]. However, it is not unusual for a patient to express their feelings in a linear, logical fashion, which is the preferred communication style of physicians and the medical culture. We have observed that it is not unusual for patients to use the language of medicine (lab values, side effects, diagnosis, treatment, etc.) when communicating about their distress. They may be trying to express their demoralization but lack the self-awareness, vocabulary, or permission by the medical culture to express difficult feelings. They are unable to express their emotions directly, and consequently, the emotional content of what the patient is saying can be easily missed.

Additionally, the preferred intervention for most medical providers with distressed patients is to explain or educate the patient. We have observed that if a patient repeatedly asks the same question, one of two things may be happening. Either we are using language too abstract for them or we are missing the emotional content they are trying to convey. Both instances require a change in how we, the medical team, relate to the patient. A more successful approach may be for the physician to "communicate understanding" or empathy, which validates the patient's experience, diminishes feelings of isolation, and rekindles a sense of hope [95]. A therapeutic response of being present to the emotion, without trying to objectify or "fix" the emotion is a skill that eludes many physicians.

Using "I wish" statements can validate the patient's experience without falling into the trap of having to have an "answer" or "solve" every question asked by the patient:

- "I wish I had better news to give you."
- "This is so hard for you, just when our hopes were so high. I wish things were different."
- "I wish medical science had better treatments for your GVHD, pain, etc."

ANGER

Anger occurs more frequently than recognized in the SCT setting. Patients have plenty to be angry about—isolation, loss of control, complications of treatment, change in body image, disease relapse, and unrealistic expectations of the SCT process. Patients who have a negative experience of the transplantation experience, either during hospitalization or during the posttransplantation outpatient period, often report anger and regret for having undergone the procedure. Although the SCT team assures informed consent before the treatment, it is impossible for the layperson to really conceptualize the entirety of the SCT process.

It is useful to recognize that anger can be a healthy response, particularly to the frequently frustrating complex medical culture the patient may find himself or herself. The response of the inexpert clinician to anger is frequently to retaliate by returning the anger, defending ones actions or to physically or psychologically withdraw [96]. None of these are helpful to the situation or to either the patient's or the provider's emotional well-being. First acknowledge the anger, "I can see you are angry," "I think anyone would be angry in your situation," "Of course you're angry that the treatment didn't work as well as we would have liked."

Second, allow the patient to express his anger. Fear, along with other emotions related to our survival, is processed in the limbic system of the brain. It is very difficult to problem solve, if not impossible, with a person when they are functioning out of their limbic system [97]. Wait until the patient shifts out of the emotional response, which usually takes only a few minutes. They will then be more rational as they transition back to their frontal lobe and are more able to think logically and problem solve.

It is helpful to remember that an expression of anger may actually be a common expression of fear or other more vulnerable underlying feelings. A patient may be unable to express his or her worst fear such as disease relapse. Naming the emotion you think the patient might be expressing has proven to be helpful: "Many of the patients I work with very similar to you tell me they feel scared, worried, anxious, etc., at this point in their treatment. I'm wondering if that might be true for you?" Mirroring back to patients what you think might be going on with them emotionally is an intervention that can help them identify the process of the intense emotions they are feeling. This can be noted when the patient becomes more quiet, less intense, and/or begins to ask questions, not in a rhetorical fashion but in a more direct manner (Table 126.3).

Table 126.3 *Approach to the angry patient*

- Check in with yourself first. Recognize your own feelings and do not participate in the patient's emotion.
- Set the stage. Ensure the proper time and place to respond. Remove yourself from the situation until you can respond in an appropriate positive, professional, and dignified way.
- Know the patient's name in your reply. Addressing the patient with his or her name in a respectful way can ease the situation.
- Avoid rationalizing or problem solving. Emotional patients act out of their limbic system, not their frontal lobe.
- Listen. Let the patient speak without interruption. If you try to solve the problem while they speak, you may fix the problem, but not fix the relationship.
- Remember that expression of anger may be a common expression of fear. A patient unable to express his or her worst fears may present as misdirected anger.
- Name the emotion you think the patient might be expressing.
- Acknowledge the anger and validate it as a normal response.
- Summarize your understanding. "What I hear you saying is...."

Spiritual

Spirituality is what gives meaning to our lives. From the moment a patient hears the diagnosis of cancer, he or she may begin to question the meaning of his or her own existence. A diagnosis of cancer can remain theoretical, or cognitively understood, until a patient begins to physically suffer when it then becomes more real. SCT patients, due to the nature of the process, will experience unpleasant symptoms. This makes the cancer diagnosis more real to the patient; one's meaning, or lack thereof, in life can become sharply in focus at this time. Spiritual pain can be viewed through four basic domains: meaning, hope, forgiveness, and relatedness [98]. Presence and the asking of open-ended questions are at the core of treating spiritual pain. A clinician cannot expect to fix the distress with a specified dose of medication; treatment for spiritual pain is by way of exploring beliefs and feelings and planting seeds. Patients need time to mull over new thoughts and to examine the meaning of their life. Asking key questions, waiting, and showing up again create the impetus for this process:

- "What is the most difficult part of this illness for you?"
- "As you think about what lies ahead, what is most important to you?"
- "When you think of the future, what are you hoping for?"
- "How do you make sense of what is happening to you?"
- "What do you think happens when people die?"
- "What are you most proud of in your life?"

Interventions for spiritual pain include

- Journaling
- Dream work
- Logo therapy (exploring one's purpose or meaning in life)
- Music therapy
- Life review
- Breath work/relaxation breathing
- Meditation or mindfulness
- 12-step exercises
- Religious ritual
- Healing touch

CONCLUSION

As SCT continues to evolve, we will be increasingly challenged to balance potentially life-saving treatments with patient-centered care emphasizing QOL. Ideally, specialized palliative care services are simultaneously integrated into the SCT process at the day of diagnosis. Misconceptions about palliative care often inhibit its full integration. True assimilation requires mutual respect between the palliative care consult team and SCT team, which begins with a sound understanding of the SCT process, recognition of the SCT team's needs, daily presence on rounds, and concise recommendations. Most importantly, the palliative care team must emphasize its relationship with the treating SCT team over that of the individual patient.

REFERENCES

1. Little M, Jordens CFC, McGrath C, Montgomery K, Lipworth W, Kerridge I. Informed consent and medical ordeal: A qualitative study. *Intern Med J.* 2008 August 1;38(8):624–628.
2. Fife BLB, Huster GAG, Cornetta KGK, Kennedy VNV, Akard LPL, Broun ERE. Longitudinal study of adaptation to the stress of bone marrow transplantation. *J Clin Oncol.* 2000 April 1;18(7):1539–1549.
3. Jowsey SG, Taylor ML, Schneekloth TD, Clark MM. Psychosocial challenges in transplantation. *J Psychiatr Pract.* 2001;7(6):404.
4. Goetzmann L, Klaghofer R, Wagner-Huber R, Halter J, Boehler A, Muellhaupt B et al. Psychosocial vulnerability predicts psychosocial outcome after an organ transplant: Results of a prospective study with lung, liver, and bone-marrow patients. *J Psychosom Res.* 2007 January 1;62(1):93–100.
5. Kelly DD, Ross SS, Gray BB, Smith PP. Death, dying and emotional labour: Problematic dimensions of the bone marrow transplant nursing role? *J Adv Nurs.* 2000 October 1;32(4):952–960.
6. Molassiotis AA, Haberman MM. Evaluation of burnout and job satisfaction in marrow transplant nurses. *Cancer Nurs.* 1996 October 1;19(5):360–367.
7. Larsen JJ, Nordström GG, Ljungman PP, Gardulf AA. Symptom occurrence, symptom intensity, and symptom distress in patients undergoing high-dose chemotherapy with stem-cell transplantation. *Cancer Nurs.* 2004 January 1;27(1):55–64.
8. Lee SJS, Joffe SS, Kim HTH, Socie GG, Gilman ALA, Wingard JRJ et al. Physicians' attitudes about quality-of-life issues in hematopoietic stem cell transplantation. *Blood.* 2004 October 1;104(7):2194–2200.
9. Williams LA, Wang XS, Cleeland CS, Mobley G, Giralt S. Assessment of symptoms and symptom burden before and after engraftment during allogeneic blood or marrow transplant (BMT). *Biol Blood Marrow Transplant.* 2006;12(2):135 (Elsevier).
10. Schulz-Kindermann F, Hennings U, Ramm G, Zander AR, Hasenbring M. The role of biomedical and psychosocial factors for the prediction of pain and distress in patients undergoing high-dose therapy and BMT/PBSCT. *Bone Marrow Transplant.* 2002 February 1;29(4):341–351.
11. Ho VT, Cutler C. Current and novel therapies in acute GVHD. *Best Pract Res Clin Haematol.* 2008 June;21(2):223–237.
12. Gilleece MH. Blood and marrow transplant handbook: Comprehensive guide for patient care. *Bone Marrow Transplant.* 2011 December 1;46(12):1590.
13. Niscola P, Tendas A, Scaramucci L, Giovaninni M, Cupelli L, De Sanctis V et al. Pain in malignant hematology. *Expert Rev Hematol.* 2011 February 1;4(1):81–93.
14. Davis MPM, Weissman DED, Arnold RMR. Opioid dose titration for severe cancer pain: A systematic evidence-based review. *J Palliat Med.* 2004 June 1;7(3):462–468.
15. Proakis AG, Harris GB. Comparative penetration of glycopyrrolate and atropine across the blood-brain and placental barriers in anesthetized dogs. *Anesthesiology.* 1978;48(5):339.
16. Modesto-Lowe VV, Girard LL, Chaplin MM. Cancer pain in the opioid-addicted patient: Can we treat it right? *J Opioid Manag.* 2012 May 1;8(3):167–175.
17. Weissman DED, Haddox JDJ. Opioid pseudoaddiction—An iatrogenic syndrome. *Pain.* 1989 March 1;36(3):363–366.
18. Trigg MEM, Inverso DMD. Nausea and vomiting with high-dose chemotherapy and stem cell rescue therapy: A review of antiemetic regimens. *Bone Marrow Transplant.* 2008 October 1;42(8):501–506.

19　Einhorn LHL, Grunberg SMS, Rapoport BB, Rittenberg CC, Feyer PP. Antiemetic therapy for multiple-day chemotherapy and additional topics consisting of rescue antiemetics and high-dose chemotherapy with stem cell transplant: Review and consensus statement. *Support Care Cancer.* 2011 March 1;19(Suppl. 1):S1–S4.

20　Hesketh PJ. Chemotherapy-induced nausea and vomiting. *N Engl J Med.* 2008 June 5;358(23):2482–2494.

21　Kris MG, Gralla RJ, Clark RA, Tyson LB, O'Connell JP, Wertheim MS et al. Incidence, course, and severity of delayed nausea and vomiting following the administration of high-dose cisplatin. *J Clin Oncol.* 1985 October 1;3(10):1379–1384.

22　Tavorath R, Hesketh PJ. Drug treatment of chemotherapy-induced delayed emesis. *Drugs.* 1996 November;52(5):639–648.

23　Morrow GR, Roscoe JA, Kirshner JJ, Hynes HE, Rosenbluth RJ. Anticipatory nausea and vomiting in the era of 5-HT3 antiemetics. *Support Care Cancer.* 1998; 244–247.

24　Roscoe JA, Morrow GR, Aapro MS, Molassiotis A, Olver I. Anticipatory nausea and vomiting. *Support Care Cancer.* 2010 August 30;19(10):1533–1538.

25　Grunberg SM, Warr D, Gralla RJ, Rapoport BL, Hesketh PJ, Jordan K et al. Evaluation of new antiemetic agents and definition of antineoplastic agent emetogenicity—State of the art. *Support Care Cancer.* 2011;19:43–47 (Springer).

26　American Society of Clinical Oncology, Kris MG, Hesketh PJ, Somerfield MR, Feyer P, Clark-Snow R et al. American Society of Clinical Oncology guideline for antiemetics in oncology: Update 2006. *J Clin Oncol.* 2006;24(18):2932–2947.

27　Ettinger DS, Armstrong DK, Barbour S, Berger MJ, Bierman PJ, Bradbury B et al. Antiemesis. *J Natl Compr Canc Netw.* 2012 April;10(4):456–485. jnccn.org.

28　Ferris FDF, Kerr IGI, Sone MM, Marcuzzi MM. Transdermal scopolamine use in the control of narcotic-induced nausea. *J Pain Symptom Manage.* 1991 August 1;6(6):389–393.

29　Laugsand EA, Kaasa S, Klepstad P. Management of opioid-induced nausea and vomiting in cancer patients: Systematic review and evidence-based recommendations. *Palliat Med.* 2011 July;25(5):442–453.

30　Jordan K, Hinke A, Grothey A, Voigt W, Arnold D, Wolf H-H et al. A meta-analysis comparing the efficacy of four 5-HT3-receptor antagonists for acute chemotherapy-induced emesis. *Support Care Cancer.* 2007 September;15(9):1023–1033.

31　Jordan K, Schmoll HJ, Aapro MS. Comparative activity of antiemetic drugs. *Crit Rev Oncol Hematol.* 2007 February 1;61(2):162–175.

32　Chawla SPS, Grunberg SMS, Gralla RJR, Hesketh PJP, Rittenberg CC, Elmer MEM et al. Establishing the dose of the oral NK1 antagonist aprepitant for the prevention of chemotherapy-induced nausea and vomiting. *Cancer.* 2003 May 1;97(9):2290–2300.

33　Hesketh PJP, Grunberg SMS, Gralla RJR, Warr DGD, Roila FF, de Wit RR et al. The oral neurokinin-1 antagonist aprepitant for the prevention of chemotherapy-induced nausea and vomiting: A multinational, randomized, double-blind, placebo-controlled trial in patients receiving high-dose cisplatin—The Aprepitant Protocol 052 Study Group. *J Clin Oncol.* 2003 November 15;21(22):4112–4119.

34　Warr DGD, Hesketh PJP, Gralla RJR, Muss HBH, Herrstedt JJ, Eisenberg PDP et al. Efficacy and tolerability of aprepitant for the prevention of chemotherapy-induced nausea and vomiting in patients with breast cancer after moderately emetogenic chemotherapy. *J Clin Oncol.* 2005 April 20;23(12):2822–2830.

35　Spinks A, Wasiak J. Scopolamine (hyoscine) for preventing and treating motion sickness. *Coch Database Syst Rev.* 2011;(6):CD002851.

36　Bowcock SJS, Stockdale ADA, Bolton JAJ, Kang AAA, Retsas SS. Antiemetic prophylaxis with high dose metoclopramide or lorazepam in vomiting induced by chemotherapy. *BMJ.* 1984 June 23;288(6434):1879.

37　Moertel CG, Schutt AJ, Reitemeier RJ, Hahn RG. Corticosteroid therapy of preterminal gastrointestinal cancer. *Cancer.* 1974 June;33(6):1607–1609.

38　Cotter J. Efficacy of crude marijuana and synthetic delta-9-tetrahydrocannabinol as treatment for chemotherapy-induced nausea and vomiting: A systematic literature review. *Am J Surg.* 2009 May 4;36(3):345–352.

39　Pico JL, Avila-Garavito A, Naccache P. Mucositis: Its occurrence, consequences, and treatment in the oncology setting. *Oncologist.* 1998;3(6):446–451 (Alpha Med Press).

40　Robien K. Predictors of oral mucositis in patients receiving hematopoietic cell transplants for chronic myelogenous leukemia. *Am J Surg.* 2004 February 23;22(7):1268–1275.

41　Blijlevens N, Schwenkglenks M, Bacon P, D'Addio A, Einsele H, Maertens J et al. Prospective oral mucositis audit: Oral mucositis in patients receiving high-dose melphalan or BEAM conditioning chemotherapy—European blood and marrow transplantation mucositis advisory group. *Am J Surg.* 2008 March 20;26(9):1519–1525.

42　Spielberger R, Stiff P, Bensinger W, Gentile T, Weisdorf D, Kewalramani T et al. Palifermin for oral mucositis after intensive therapy for hematologic cancers. *Am J Surg.* 2004 December 16;351(25):2590–2598.

43　Capelli D, Santini G, De Souza C, Poloni A, Marino G, Montanari M et al. Amifostine can reduce mucosal damage after high-dose melphalan conditioning for peripheral blood progenitor cell autotransplant: A retrospective study. *Br J Haematol.* 2000 August;110(2):300–307.

44　Peterson DE, Bensadoun RJ, Roila F. Management of oral and gastrointestinal mucositis: ESMO clinical recommendations. *Ann Oncol.* 2009 May;20(Suppl. 4):174–177.

45　Bellm LAL, Epstein JBJ, Rose-Ped AMA, Fu RR, Martin PJP, Fuchs HJH. Assessment of various topical oral formulations by bone marrow transplant recipients. *Oral Oncol.* 2001 January 1;37(1):42–49.

46　Cerchietti LCA, Navigante AH, Bonomi MR, Zaderajko MA, Menéndez PR, Pogany CE et al. Effect of topical morphine for mucositis-associated pain following concomitant chemoradiotherapy for head and neck carcinoma. *Cancer.* 2002 November 15;95(10):2230–2236.

47　Berger AA, Henderson MM, Nadoolman WW, Duffy VV, Cooper DD, Saberski LL et al. Oral capsaicin provides temporary relief for oral mucositis pain secondary to chemotherapy/radiation therapy. *J Pain Symp Manage.* 1995 April 1;10(3):243–248.

48　Ryan AJ, Lin F, Atayee RS. Ketamine mouthwash for mucositis pain. *J Palliat Med.* 2009 November;12(11):989–991.

49　Hita-Iglesias PP, Torres-Lagares DD, Gutiérrez-Pérez JLJ. Evaluation of the clinical behaviour of a polyvinylpyrrolidone and sodium hyalonurate gel (Gelclair) in patients subjected to surgical treatment with CO_2 laser. *Int J Oral Maxillofac Surg.* 2006 June 1;35(6):514–517.

50　Coda BAB, O'Sullivan BB, Donaldson GG, Bohl SS, Chapman CRC, Shen DDD. Comparative efficacy of patient-controlled administration of morphine, hydromorphone, or sufentanil for the treatment of oral mucositis pain following bone marrow transplantation. *Pain.* 1997 September 1;72(3):333–346.

51　Sonis ST, Oster G, Fuchs H, Bellm L, Bradford WZ, Edelsberg J et al. Oral mucositis and the clinical and economic outcomes of hematopoietic stem-cell transplantation. *J Clin Oncol.* 2001 April 15;19(8):2201–2205.

52　Ruescher TJ, Sodeifi A, Scrivani SJ, Kaban LB, Sonis ST. The impact of mucositis on alpha-hemolytic streptococcal infection in patients undergoing autologous bone marrow transplantation for hematologic malignancies. *Cancer.* 1998 June 1;82(11):2275–2281.

53　Bow EJ, Loewen R, Cheang MS, Shore TB, Rubinger M, Schacter B. Cytotoxic therapy-induced D-xylose malabsorption and invasive infection during remission-induction therapy for acute myeloid leukemia in adults. *J Clin Oncol.* 1997 June;15(6):2254–2261.

54   Davila ML. Neutropenic enterocolitis. *Curr Treat Options Gastroenterol.* 2006 June;9(3):249–255.

55   Herrera AF, Soriano G, Bellizzi AM, Hornick JL, Ho VT, Ballen KK et al. Cord colitis syndrome in cord-blood stem-cell transplantation. *N Engl J Med.* 2011 September 1;365(9):815–824.

56   Ippoliti C, Champlin R, Bugazia N, Przepiorka D, Neumann J, Giralt S et al. Use of octreotide in the symptomatic management of diarrhea induced by graft-versus-host disease in patients with hematologic malignancies. *J Clin Oncol.* 1997 November;15(11):3350–3354.

57   Ripamonti C, Mercadante S. How to use octreotide for malignant bowel obstruction. *J Support Oncol.* 2004;2(4):357–364.

58   Iestra JA, Fibbe We, Zwinderman AH, van Stavern WA, Kromhout D. Body weight recovery, eating difficulties and compliance with dietary advice in the first year after stem cell transplantation: A prospective study. *Bone Marrow Transplant.* 2002;29(5):417–424 (Nature Publishing Group).

59   Henry LL. Immunocompromised patients and nutrition. *Prof Nurse.* 1997 June 1;12(9):655–659.

60   Szeluga DJ, Stuart RK, Brookmeyer R, Utermohlen V, Santos GW. Nutritional support of bone marrow transplant recipients: A prospective, randomized clinical trial comparing total parenteral nutrition to an enteral feeding program. *Cancer Res.* 1987 June 15;47(12):3309–3316. vpn-2.ucsd.edu.

61   Tisdale MJM. Clinical anticachexia treatments. *Nutr Clin Pract.* 2006 April 1;21(2):168–174.

62   Berenstein EG, Ortiz Z. Megestrol acetate for the treatment of anorexia-cachexia syndrome. *Cochrane Database Syst Rev.* 2005;(2):CD004310 (Wiley Online Library).

63   Beal JE, Olson R, Lefkowitz L, Laubenstein L, Bellman P, Yangco B et al. Long-term efficacy and safety of dronabinol for acquired immunodeficiency syndrome-associated anorexia. *J Pain Symptom Manage.* 1997;14(1):7–14 (Elsevier).

64   Jatoi A, Windschitl HE, Loprinzi CL, Sloan JA, Dakhil SR, Mailliard JA et al. Dronabinol versus megestrol acetate versus combination therapy for cancer-associated anorexia: A North Central Cancer Treatment Group study. *J Clin Oncol.* 2002 January 15;20(2):567–573. vpn-2.ucsd.edu.

65   Fearon KCH, Meyenfeldt von MF, Moses AGW, van Geenen R, Roy A, Gouma DJ et al. Effect of a protein and energy dense n-3 fatty acid enriched oral supplement on loss of weight and lean tissue in cancer cachexia: A randomised double blind trial. *Gut.* 2003 October;52(10):1479–1486. vpn-2.ucsd.edu.

66   Moses AWGA, Slater CC, Preston TT, Barber MDM, Fearon KCHK. Reduced total energy expenditure and physical activity in cachectic patients with pancreatic cancer can be modulated by an energy and protein dense oral supplement enriched with n-3 fatty acids. *Br J Cancer.* 2004 March 8;90(5):996–1002.

67   Dewey A, Baughan C, Dean T, Higgins B, Johnson I. Eicosapentaenoic acid (EPA, an omega-3 fatty acid from fish oils) for the treatment of cancer cachexia. *Cochrane Database Syst Rev.* 2007;(1):CD004597.

68   Fann JR, Roth-Roemer S, Burington BE, Katon WJ, Syrjala KL. Delirium in patients undergoing hematopoietic stem cell transplantation. *Cancer.* 2002 November 1;95(9):1971–1981.

69   Massie MJ, Holland J, Glass E. Delirium in terminally ill cancer patients. *Am J Psychiatry.* 1983;140(8):1048–1050.

70   Minagawa HH, Uchitomi YY, Yamawaki SS, Ishitani KK. Psychiatric morbidity in terminally ill cancer patients. A prospective study. *Cancer.* 1996 September 1;78(5):1131–1137.

71   Gagnon P, Allard P, Mâsse B, DeSerres M. Delirium in terminal cancer: A prospective study using daily screening, early diagnosis, and continuous monitoring. *J Pain Symptom Manage.* 2000;19(6):412–426 (Elsevier).

72   Weckmann MT, Gingrich R, Mills JA, Hook L, Beglinger LJ. Risk factors for delirium in patients undergoing hematopoietic stem cell transplantation. *Ann Clin Psychiatry.* 2012 August;24(3):204–214.

73   Olofsson BB, Lundström MM, Borssén BB, Nyberg LL, Gustafson YY. Delirium is associated with poor rehabilitation outcome in elderly patients treated for femoral neck fractures. *Scand J Caring Sci.* 2005 June 1;19(2):119–127.

74   Ely EW, Shintani A, Truman B, Speroff T, Gordon SM, Harrell FE et al. Delirium as a predictor of mortality in mechanically ventilated patients in the intensive care unit. *JAMA.* 2004 April 14;291(14):1753–1762.

75   Caraceni AA, Nanni OO, Maltoni MM, Piva LL, Indelli MM, Arnoldi EE et al. Impact of delirium on the short term prognosis of advanced cancer patients. Italian multicenter study group on palliative care. *Cancer.* 2000 September 1;89(5):1145–1149.

76   Inouye SK, Bogardus ST, Charpentier PA, Leo-Summers L, Acampora D, Holford TR et al. A multicomponent intervention to prevent delirium in hospitalized older patients. *N Engl J Med.* 1999 March 4;340(9):669–676.

77   Marcantonio ER, Flacker JM, Wright RJ, Resnick NM. Reducing delirium after hip fracture: A randomized trial. *J Am Geriatr Soc.* 2001 May 1;49(5):516–522.

78   Breitbart W, Marotta R, Platt MM, Weisman H, Derevenco M, Grau C et al. A double-blind trial of haloperidol, chlorpromazine, and lorazepam in the treatment of delirium in hospitalized AIDS patients. *Am J Psychiatry.* 1996;153(2):231.

79   Lonergan EE, Britton AMA, Luxenberg JJ, Wyller TT. Antipsychotics for delirium. *Cochrane Database Syst Rev.* 2007 January 1;(2):CD005594.

80   Schwartz TL, Masand PS. The role of atypical antipsychotics in the treatment of delirium. *Psychosomatics.* 2002 May;43(3):171–174.

81   Institute of Medicine (U.S.) Committee on Psychosocial Services to Cancer Patients/Families in a Community Setting, Adler NE, Page AE. *Cancer Care for the Whole Patient: Meeting Psychosocial Health Needs.* Washington, DC: National Academies Press, 2008.

82   Kirk HW, Weisbrod JA, Ericson KA. *Psychosocial & Behavioral Aspects of Medicine.* Baltimore, MA: Lippincott Williams & Wilkins, 2003.

83   Kaplan HI, Sadock BJ. *Theories of Personality and Psychopathology Synopsis of Psychiatry* (8th edn.). 1998, pp. 234–239.

84   Hoodin F, Kalbfleisch KR, Thorton J, Ratanatharathorn V. Psychosocial influences on 305 adults' survival after bone marrow transplantation; depression, smoking, and behavioral self-regulation. *J Psychosom Res.* 2004: 57(2): 145–154.

85   Heinonen H, Volin L, Zevon MA, Uutela A, Barrick C, Ruutu T. Stress among allogeneic bone marrow transplantation patients. *Patient Educ Couns.* 2005;56:62–71.

86   Goetzmann L, Ruegg L, Stamm M, Ambuhl P, Boehler A, Halter J et al. Psychosocial profiles after transplantation: A 24-month follow-up of heart, lung, liver, kidney and allogeneic bone-marrow patients. *Transplantation.* 2008; 86(5): 662–668.

87   American Psychiatric Association. *Diagnostic and Statistical Manual of Mental Disorders* (4th edn.), Text Revision. Washington, DC: American Psychiatric Association, 2000.

88   Mann JJ. The medical management of depression. *N Engl J Med.* 2005;353:1819–1834.

89   Hardy SE. Methylphenidate for the treatment of depressive symptoms, including fatigue and apathy, in medically ill older adults and terminally ill adults. *Am J Geriatr Pharmacother.* 2009;7:34–59.

90   National Institute of Mental Health. Depression and cancer. Bethesda, MD: National Institute of Mental Health, 2009. http://www.nimh.nih.gov/health/publications/depression.

91   Ng B. Is there a role for psychostimulants in old age depression and apathy? *Int Psychogeriatrics.* 2009;21:417–418.

92   Martin TL, Doka KJ. *Men Don't Cry...Women Do: Transcending Gender Stereotypes of Grief.* Philadelphia, PA: George H. Buchanan, 2000.

93 Clarke DM, Kissane DW. Demoralization: Its phenomenology and importance. *Aust N Z J Psychiatry.* 2002;36:733–742.

94 Andrykowki MA. Psychiatric and psychological aspects of bone marrow transplantation. *Psychosomatics.* 1994;35:13–24.

95 Slavney, PR. *Psychiatric Dimensions of Medical Malpractice. What Primary-Care Physicians Should Know About Delirium, Demoralization, Suicidal Thinking, and Competence to Refuse Medical Advice.* Baltimore, MA: Johns Hopkins Press, 1998.

96 Burton M, Watson M. *Counselling People with Cancer.* England, U.K.: John Wiley & Sons, 1998.

97 Johnson S. *Mind Wide Open: Your Brain and the Neuroscience of Everyday Life.* New York: Scribner, 2004.

98 Groves RF, Klauser HA. *American Book of Dying.* Berkely, CA: Celestial Arts, 2005.

PART 18

Rehabilitation and survivorship

127

End of therapy: Building the psychosocial and spiritual bridges to survivorship

MARVIN OMAR DELGADO-GUAY, SILVIA TANZI

SURVIVORS: THE DEFINITION

The definition of survivor has evolved with time, when cancer was considered incurable; the term "survivor" was used to describe family members who survived the loss of a loved one to cancer [1]. As knowledge and success in understanding cancer increased, physicians began to use a 5-year time frame to define survivorship. If cancer did not recur in 5 years following either diagnosis or treatment, patients were considered to have become "survivors" [1]. An individual is considered a cancer survivor from the time of cancer diagnosis through the balance of his or her life; family members, friends, and caregivers are also impacted by the survivorship experience and are therefore included in this definition [1–3].

A survivor is one who has been exposed to the possibility of dying or has witnessed the death of others yet remained alive. The responses of survivors vary greatly, depending on the particular encounter with death and on personal traits. But I have found certain psychological patterns to be quite consistent [4].

Survivors struggle with images of death and dying—what I call a "death imprint." They feel a sense of debt to the dead, a need to placate them or carry out their wishes in order to justify their own survival. Survivors embark on an anguished quest for meaning and form [5].

EPIDEMIOLOGY

Currently, in the United States, one in three women and one in two men will develop cancer in his or her lifetime. Increases in the number of individuals diagnosed with cancer each year, due in large part to aging and growth of the population, as well as improving survival rates, have led to an ever-increasing number of cancer survivors. As of January 2008, it is estimated that there are 11.9 million cancer survivors. This represents approximately 4% of the population [4]. Sixty percent of survivors are currently 65 years of age and older. Among today's

survivors, the most common cancer sites represented include female breast (22%), prostate (20%), colorectal (9%), and gynecologic (8%). Today, 67% of adults diagnosed with cancer will be alive in 5 years. Among children, over 75% of childhood cancer survivors will be alive after 10 years. Approximately 15% of the 11.9 million estimated cancer survivors were diagnosed 20 or more years ago [6].

The number of cancer survivors is growing for several reasons: doctors' ability to find cancer earlier, diagnose cancer more accurately, and treat cancer more effectively. Also, better follow-up care after cancer treatment, fewer deaths from other causes, and an aging U.S. population contribute to the large number of cancer survivors. The risk of dying from cancer following diagnosis has steadily decreased over the past several decades. Fewer than half of the people diagnosed with cancer today will die of the disease; in fact, some are completely cured, and many more survive for years because of early diagnosis or treatments that control many types of cancer [2].

Cancer can become a chronic disease that often has long-term effects on a survivor's life. Although many cancers can now be cured or their growth greatly slowed, the impact of diagnosis and complications of treatments will remain with the survivor for years. Because more survivors are living longer, especially those diagnosed with cancer as a child or young adult, there is a need to address long-term issues of survivorship. These can include ongoing physical, psychological, and other types of issues.

NEW NORMAL IN CANCER SURVIVORS: CONSEQUENCES

It is well known that patients undergoing active treatment for cancer experience multiple symptoms, including fatigue, pain, lack of appetite, shortness of breath, constipation, numbness and tingling, and cognitive and sexual dysfunction; these symptoms cause significant distress and they impair posttreatment function and rehabilitation [7]. The physical side effects experienced by cancer patients can be caused by the cancer itself and/or aggressive therapies used to treat it. The patients who have completed primary anticancer treatment, whom we define herein as "cancer survivors," sometimes experience similar symptoms [8–10], many of which persist indefinitely [8].

Physical sequelae

RISK OF DEVELOPING A SECOND MALIGNANCY

Long-term survivors of adult cancer are at a slightly increased risk to develop a new cancer [11,12]. This is most probably due to genetic or environmental risk factors shared with the first tumor [13,14], treatment-related factors that include long-lasting immunosuppression [15], and/or genetic susceptibility [16,17]. Radiotherapy-induced solid tumors are typically diagnosed after a latency of at least 10 years [18], whereas secondary leukemia peaks between 5 and 10 years [19].

In general, the combination of radiotherapy and chemotherapy further increases the incidence rates for second solid tumors [18,20]. The treatment-induced menopause reduces the risk of subsequent breast cancer [21]. Even hormone treatment may be carcinogenic as evidenced by increased risks of endometrial cancer in patients with tamoxifen therapy [22].

CARDIOVASCULAR DISORDERS

Both mediastinal radiotherapy and systemic chemotherapy can induce late cardiovascular adverse effects like myocardiac infarction and cardiac insufficiency. The development of these sequelae typically takes one to two decades [23]. The histological findings of irradiated vessels are compatible with accelerated atherosclerosis [24], which leads to compromised blood flow. These vascular effects add to the radiotherapy-related necrotic and fibrotic changes of the myocardium and the pericardial structures. Long-term postradiotherapy cardiotoxicity has thus been described in ≥5-year survivors after Hodgkin's lymphoma [25,26] and in long-term survivors after testicular [27] and breast [28,29] cancer. These consequences have led to recent modifications in the use of radiotherapy in these patients. Typically, clinical symptoms start 5–10 years after radiotherapy, and the mortality rates increase after the first posttreatment decade [30]. Late cardiovascular adverse effects, such as premature development of hypertension, have to be expected after any treatment, which has reduced the renal function in long-term cancer survivors [31].

GONADAL TOXICITY AND ENDOCRINOLOGICAL DISORDERS

Gonadal toxicity and infertility are frequently feared long-term adverse effects of cancer treatment. Posttreatment infertility and sexual life disturbances have become an increasing problem in men ≥60 years old, as some begin a second marriage with a young partner. The nonsexual long-term side effects of hormonal manipulation such as loss of energy or muscular strength and/or reduction of bone density, abnormal weight gain, and/or hot flushes are often overlooked in daily clinical practice [32–34]. Though new antigonadal therapies reduce some of these risks, other side effects have emerged such as gynecomastia during long-term treatment with oral nonsteroidal antiandrogens [35] and osteoporosis in long-term breast cancer survivors using aromatase inhibitors [36]. In younger individuals, some of these gonadal alterations are reversible after discontinuation of long-term hormone manipulation [37,38].

In male survivors, clinicians should have in mind that chemotherapy may lead to permanently reduced Leydig cell function and subclinical hypogonadism [39]. Long-lasting male hypogonadism may secondarily lead to the development of metabolic syndrome as shown for long-term survivors after testicular cancer [40] and prostate cancer [41]. In women, gonadotoxic chemotherapy may accelerate the age-related physiological loss of oocytes without the possibility of regeneration [42], with the risk of premature menopause [43]. In contrast, in testicular cancer, recovery of spermatogenesis is possible as long as spermatogonial stem cells are preserved, even though repopulation of the seminiferous tubule may take several years [44]. Ovarian irradiation at doses of 8 Gy or greater is frequently followed by permanent ovarian failure, with lower doses required in older patients [45]. Fractionated scattered testicular irradiation (from pelvic or abdominal fields) up to 2 Gy reversibly reduces spermatogenesis dependent on the patient's age and the fractionation pattern. Target doses of ≥4 Gy lead in most men to irreversible azoospermia.

Hypothyroidism is an important and often undetected long-term morbidity after irradiation of the thyroid gland, for example, during mantle field irradiation for Hodgkin's lymphoma [19,25] (particularly females), but it can also be associated with scattered irradiation during adjuvant locoregional radiotherapy of breast cancer [46]. Finally, hypofunction of the pituitary gland has to be considered in long-term cancer survivors after cranial radiotherapy, with multiple endocrinological imbalances and the need for substitution of gonadal, adrenal, and thyroid hormones [47].

GENITOURINARY DISORDERS

Urinary leakage and erectile dysfunction are the most frequent long-term sequelae following cystectomy for bladder cancer. The leakage has been recorded in up to 70% of cases after orthotropic bladder substitution [48] and in 5%–50% after radical prostatectomy [49,50]. Persistent dry ejaculation without erectile dysfunction may develop after any type of pelvic surgery in long-term survivors, for example, for rectal cancer, or after retroperitoneal lymph node dissection, although with reduced incidence after the introduction of nerve-sparing techniques [51].

After high-dose pelvic radiotherapy (for prostate, cervical, or rectal cancer), 6%–8% of long-term survivors complain about irradiation symptoms from the bladder (urgency, hematuria, and dysuria), the frequency and severity dependent on the radiotherapy techniques and the radiation doses applied.

Neurological and neurophysiological long-term sequelae

After whole brain irradiation at doses ≥50 Gy, the following sequelae have been described in 2%–5% of long-term survivors: cognitive deficits, damage to the middle and inner ear and of the visual pathways, and the development of new postradiotherapy meningiomas [52]. MRI-identifiable white matter changes, calcifications, lacunar lesions, and cerebral atrophy with hydrocephalus have also been observed. Such changes are even more frequent if intrathecal chemotherapy is combined with cerebral irradiation [53].

Brachial plexopathy is well-known sequelae after locoregional radiotherapy of breast cancer [54]. The dose-related long-term neurological problems after cisplatin-based chemotherapy consist of ototoxicity (tinnitus, hearing loss at ≥4000 Hz) and peripheral sensory neuropathy in 20%–25% of testicular cancer patients, surviving ≥5 years [55].

GASTROINTESTINAL DISORDERS

Dependent on the target radiation dose, up to 8% of long-term cancer survivors complain about moderate or severe esophageal side effects after radiotherapy [56]. Though most long-term survivors report minimal symptoms after abdominopelvic radiotherapy (bloating, dyspepsia, or slight diarrhea), submucous fibrosis and impaired blood supply may require surgical interventions due to hemorrhagic ulcers or stenotic parts of the gastrointestinal tract [57]. Moderate or severe late gastrointestinal toxicity is also described in up to 10% of survivors after radiotherapy for cervical cancer [58]. In approximately 10%–20% of the long-term patients, high-dose pelvic radiotherapy is followed by a persistent slight degree of diarrhea and dysfunction of the anal sphincter with mucous or hemorrhagic discharge from the rectum [59,60].

PULMONARY LATE EFFECTS

Late postradiotherapy pulmonary sequelae (respiratory failure, cor pulmonale) depend on the radiation dose and the irradiated lung volume receiving at least 20 Gy [52,61]. After high-dose radiotherapy for inoperable lung cancer, about 20% of 18-month survivors display reduced pulmonary function due to lung fibrosis [52]. Multiple cytotoxic drugs are associated with acute pulmonary toxicity, bleomycin being the agent with the highest risk [61]. However, long-term pulmonary toxicity related to chemotherapy alone occurs in few survivors (up to 3%).

OTHER IMPORTANT LATE ADVERSE EFFECTS

After splenectomy or irradiation to the spleen by >30 Gy, the immune defense may be permanently reduced with increased risk of infectious episodes. Regular pneumococcal, meningococcal, and *Haemophilus influenzae* vaccinations have been recommended eventually combined with antibiotic prophylaxis [62,63]. Aseptic bone necrosis should be considered in long-term cancer survivors who after long-lasting corticosteroid treatment complain about increasing pain of the hip [64] and eventually other skeletal regions.

There is increasing evidence for long-term dental problems after cranial radiotherapy and probably also after chemotherapy due to impaired salivation and chronic mucosal inflammation of the oral mucosa [65]. Finally, both cranial radiotherapy and chemotherapy may lead to late adverse effects of the eye, cataract being the most frequent late toxicity after doses of ≥2 Gy to the lens but also after long-lasting treatment with corticosteroids [66]. Thus, cataract was mentioned as a long-term problem in 4% of 3936 cancer survivors, affecting their daily life in 56% of them [67].

PHYSICAL PERFORMANCE LIMITATIONS AND SOCIAL PARTICIPATION RESTRICTIONS

Several population-based studies from the United States have shown that long-term cancer survivors in general have significantly higher rates of physical performance limitations and social participation restrictions compared to those with no cancer history [68,69]. A recent study from Norway documented that common chronic diseases (cardiovascular disorders and/or diabetes) lead to impaired physical and social function in cancer survivors [70]. Fatigue is a common complaint in many cancer survivors and has been described in 20%–30% of survivors after breast cancer [32] and Hodgkin's lymphoma [71,72].

CHRONIC AND LATE-EFFECT HEALTH CONDITIONS IN ADULT SURVIVORS OF CHILDHOOD CANCER

The frequency and severity of post-cancer-treatment chronic conditions have been reviewed by Oeffinger et al. [73], showing that chronic conditions were more common among survivors than their siblings and also the incidence of chronic sequel of treatments increased with time. These sequels are usually associated with chemoradiation regimens and/or with those containing doxorubicin and alkylating agents. Significant issues include development of congestive heart failure, secondary malignant neoplasm, severe cognitive dysfunctions, and coronary artery disease. Significant psychosocial distress has been reported in survivors of childhood sarcoma treated with combined modality therapy [8].

Psychological, social, emotional, and spiritual impacts of cancer survivors

PSYCHOSOCIAL SYMPTOMS

Given the challenges that cancer survivors face, it is not surprising that several studies have suggested that long-term cancer survivors may be at risk for a variety of psychological symptoms, including anxiety, depression, and fatigue [74–78]. The extent of psychological symptoms varies among these studies owing to differences in patient characteristics, survey timing, and study design [74,79–82].

These psychosocial issues are different between different types of cancer, different ethnicity, and also between short- or long-term survivors [74–78,83–85]: nationally, representative sample of adults in the United States to determine the prevalence of serious psychological distress (SPD) among long-term survivors of adult-onset cancer [83] shows that survivors with more comorbid illnesses, difficulty performing IADLs, lower educational attainment, and no spouse or no health insurance were more likely to report SPD. The link between SPD and these sociodemographic factors in cancer survivors is disquieting and highlights the importance of developing accessible and affordable support systems that include psychiatric care for this vulnerable population.

Studies have shown an association between increased psychological symptoms and comorbid illness, functional impairment, lack of health insurance, decreased social support, lower educational attainment, and smoking [86–91]. Survivors are more likely to report SPD because of treatment-related fatigue, an underlying sense of loss for what might have been, or an underlying fear of recurrence and death [86–91].

The most frequent psychological distresses are related to depression, anxiety, and fatigue in cancer survivors and also in their caregivers [80,92–95].

SPIRITUALITY

Spirituality can be defined as "the aspect of humanity that refers to the way individuals seek and express meaning and purpose and the way they experience their connectedness to the moment, to self, to others, to nature, and to the significant or sacred" [96]. Spirituality can be seen as a dimension of personhood, while religion is a construct of human making, which enables the conceptualization and expression of spirituality [97]. Spirituality and religiosity become increasingly important as patients approach the end of life [98]. Patients who report greater religiosity/spirituality also report more adaptive coping styles and a better quality of life [99–103].

Both religious practices and spiritual beliefs are common in the United States [104,105]. Gallup [105] reported in 2000–2001 that religion/spirituality was noted as "very important" by 60% of Americans aged 50–64, 67% of those aged 65–74, and 75% of those aged 75 and older.

In a recent publication, it was described a cohort of advanced cancer patients evaluated in the palliative care outpatient clinic where almost all of them considered themselves spiritual (98%) and religious (98%). The patients also reported spirituality and/or religiosity help them cope with their illness (99%) and serve as a source of strength (100%) and have a positive impact on their physical (69%) and emotional (84%) symptoms [106].

Religiosity and spirituality have been associated with better health-related quality of life [107,108] and general mental health [109] and lower levels of depression [107,110] and traumatic stress in cancer survivors [109]. Similarly, reliance on a benevolent relationship with God is associated with better emotional and interpersonal functioning [111,112]. In addition, enhanced religiosity/spirituality is a common component of posttraumatic growth, or positive benefits of difficult life challenges, in people with cancer [113].

Cancer survivors also report praising and thanking God in prayer [114–117]. African American cancer survivors stated that God provided them with support and healing and lifted their spirits [116,118]. In a sample of middle-aged cancer survivors, participants reported giving God control over uncontrollable aspects of their disease, which strengthened participants' spirituality [119].

Religious and spiritual beliefs and behaviors are often described in qualitative research as helpful and beneficial in the context of cancer. For example, cancer survivors reported receiving support from church members [20,21] and emotional healing from their religious beliefs [119]. Spirituality and religiosity are also involved in making meaning of the cancer [115,119]. In a study of breast cancer survivors, participants viewed the cancer as "part of God's plan" [115]. Survivors of hematological malignancies described their cancer experience as a spiritual journey that happened for a particular reason and included a sense of being chosen, viewing cancer as a challenge and taking responsibility for that challenge [120]. This journey led to increased confidence and assertiveness, greater compassion for others, increased closeness in familial relationships, and emphasis on living life to its fullest. Participants reported feeling fortunate to have undergone this journey due to these positive changes. In other studies, cancer allowed participants to deepen their relationship with God [119] and focus on positive aspects of life [115]. Spiritual growth due to cancer was characterized by reprioritization and greater appreciation of important aspects of life, increased empathy for others, and reductions in self-centeredness [119].

We reported also that caregivers of advanced cancer patients expressed their inner strength and meaning of life in terms of their relationship with the divine in 62%, in terms of their own value as a person in 10%, and in terms of their relationships with family members, friends, and nature and music in 26% [121].

The caregivers of cancer patients often face significant physical, social, and emotional hardships and indicate that they rely heavily on their faith to cope with these burdens [122]. Caregivers who are more religious feel more positively about their role as caregivers [123] and get along better with those they care for [124]. This may be due in part to the fact that faith communities foster belief systems of responsibility and compassion that are likely to help the persons doing the emotionally difficult work of caring for others [125].

Caregivers' age and the stress associated with caregiving are significant predictors of diverse aspects of quality of life in the long-term survivorship and bereavement phases. Current caregivers report worst levels of quality of life. Bereaved caregivers reported lower levels of psychological and spiritual adjustment than former caregivers whose recipients were in remission. In addition, caregivers' age and stress were consistent predictors of quality of life across three caregiver groups at 5-year postdiagnosis [126].

Spiritual struggles are connected with psychological distress not only in cancer patients but also in healthy individuals

[127–129], having poor physical outcomes and higher rates of mortality [130–132]. Spiritual pain may manifest itself as symptoms in any area of a person's experience, including physical, psychological, religious, or social [130,131]; this suffering is experienced by persons, not merely by bodies, that has its own source in challenges that threaten the intactness of the person as a complex psychological and social entity [133,134].

Like the physical pain that is defined as "an unpleasant sensory and emotional experience associated with actual or potential tissue damage and described in terms of such damage" [135] and a subjective experience [136], spiritual pain can be an elusive concept [137], but it can be identified and quantified. In a study of 57 patients with advanced stage cancer in a palliative care setting, Mako et al. [132] briefly defined spiritual pain as "a pain deep in your being that is not physical" and then asked patients (a) to explain in their own words what spiritual pain meant to them, (b) to explain whether they had ever experienced spiritual pain in their lives and whether they were currently experiencing spiritual pain, and (c) to rate their spiritual pain on a 10-point Likert-type scale (0–10, with 10 being the worst symptom). They found that patients framed their spiritual pain in three major categories [138]: spiritual pain in intrapsychic terms (e.g., suffering loss, despair, regret, or anxiety), spiritual pain in relation to the divine (e.g., being without faith and/or religious/spiritual community, feeling abandoned by God), and spiritual pain in relation to the interpersonal dimension (e.g., feeling disconnected from others and unwanted by family). Approximately, 96% of patients reported that they had experienced some type of spiritual pain in their lives, and 61% reported experiencing spiritual pain at the time of the study. Moreover, the average intensity of spiritual pain reported by patients at the time of the study was 4.7.

In the cohort of advanced cancer patients, a prevalence of spiritual pain of 44% was reported [106]. The patients with spiritual pain expressed less spirituality and religiosity, were more likely to report that spiritual pain made their physical/emotional symptoms worse, and had higher levels of anorexia, drowsiness, depression, and anxiety. And also these patients expressed less religious beliefs and worse religious coping strategies and decreased quality of life.

Concerns about spiritual issues also arise in the caregiver population. It has been described that caregivers that are facing significant physical, social, and emotional hardships rely heavily in their faith to cope with these burdens [122].

Spirituality, religiosity, worry, and spiritual pain may affect cancer survivors' symptom expression, coping strategies, and quality of life. Limited research is available to define these concepts in cancer survivors and their caregivers. Identifying the ways in which adults cope with the distress of cancer survivorship will improve our understanding of their experience and inform interventions to reduce their distress.

PSYCHOSOCIAL CONCERNS AND NEEDS OF CAREGIVERS

As the number of cancer patients and survivors of all ages increases, the role of caregivers grows as well. Most caregiving is provided by families and friends, often taking a major toll on them in emotional and economic terms. Most cancer caregivers worldwide are women, although the number of male caregivers is growing especially for older patients [139].

Most of the studies agree about the presence of anxiety and depression in caregivers [140] that changes and arises during illness trajectory and differs between cancer types [141–144], especially after 6–12 months from the end of the treatment. The relationship between caregiver burden, including interference in regular activities, and distress has also been documented [144,140].

With long-term survivors, the things are quite different because most partners or family members of long-term survivors of breast, colorectal, and prostate cancer have similar health status and levels of anxiety and depression to that reported by the general population [145,146].

A commonly reported unmet need was information about familial risk and help managing fears of recurrence [145]. Familial risk could be addressed by the provision of written and verbal information with a referral to genetic counseling services if required. Screening strategies are also currently being developed [147] to identify those with high levels of fear of recurrence so that targeted interventions can be delivered. The other most commonly identified unmet needs relate to the provision of comprehensive and coordinated cancer care.

Supportive care specialists can assist in developing effective strategies for family and friends to ask for help, enjoy aspects of their own lives without feeling guilty, recognize signs of stress and depression, and seek professional help when needed. Supportive cancer care should include making caregivers aware of their country's laws and regulations in matters of employment and leaves of absences and of available support structures in their communities.

Finally, new aspects of caregiving are emerging with regard to the long-term psychosocial repercussions on the families of long-term cancer survivors. These may range from psychological distress to financial issues to different degrees of stigmatization or discrimination [148].

In the long term, the majority of partners put their cancer experience behind them, and they report positive outcomes following their experience [149–151].

FINANCIAL AND LEGAL IMPACTS OF CANCER

Long-term employment and financial concerns are also an issue for many survivors, and return to work may be distressing, with some never returning to work [152–155].

Few people escape the financial repercussions of surviving cancer. For patients who must self-pay, the cost of treatment for the first year alone can exceed $100,000. For patients with leukemia or lymphoma, that amount can reach $200,000 or more in the first year. Even those with good health insurance have reported spending hundreds of dollars in copayments for one cycle of chemotherapy in a treatment regimen that requires six cycles. Out-of-pocket medical expenses for these insured patients can average $35,000. In addition, some insurance companies may not pay for cancer treatments that they consider experimental. Patients who receive treatment outside their hometown or state face the additional costs of travel, lodging, meals, and other living expenses. If the patient is the major wage earner, family income may decrease or even disappear once vacation and sick time are used up. Benefits may be reduced or lost. As a result, survivors and their families can face significant debt.

Financial issues can continue long after treatment has ended. Some survivors are forced into early retirement, which may leave them without health insurance coverage or make it difficult to find another job with health, disability, and life insurance benefits.

While this is an issue that has not been well addressed, here is a list of considerations that may aid survivors in dealing with the economic impacts of survivorship [154,155].

STRATEGIES TO IMPROVE THE CARE OF SURVIVORS

Different kinds of coping and different attitudes between patients can impact on their living survivorships and consequently on their distress. Positive outcomes travel along the negative in the survivors' lives [156].

There are numerous factors associated with good or poor adaptation. Long-term cancer survivors reflect on how cancer has affected or changed them in different ways, probably related to their age, diagnosis, treatment, and their attitudes and beliefs [156,157]. It is important to recognize that each individual sees the diagnosis of cancer and their experience of life in different way. There are some survivors that accept the diagnosis in a matter-of-fact kind of way. These survivors report that cancer is just one of the many issues that they had already faced or would face during life, and they often say that cancer has not changed them much or has changed them less than other experiences, such as divorce or other losses. Other survivors would see their experience as a personal growth, which has helped them to build on their own strengths and to find new strengths and help them to have a spiritual view of their journey or otherwise accept that they are not in control of what life has in store for them. While these survivors might have a positive outcome living their cancer experience, some others experience more distress, and some long-term survivors reflect on their lives stressing their sense of loss, anger, and depression about the effects of cancer and its treatment on them [157].

Emotional and psychosocial dimensions should be addressed in initial encounters with patients [75]. The National Cancer Institute (NCI) Office of Cancer Survivorship recommends that oncology professionals acquire specific education on both immediate treatment decisions and long-term sequelae of cancer treatments [158]. The American College of Physicians and the American Academy of Family Physicians affirm the importance for health professionals to recognize and assess cultural, psychosocial, existential, spiritual, and religious aspects of patients' suffering and learn how to address them as part of their caring for individual patients [159–161].

The posttreatment phase of survivorship is now recognized as a distinct phase in the cancer continuum occurring at the end of primary treatment and encompassing the domains of psychosocial and supportive care, health promotion, surveillance and long-term monitoring, and early intervention for late and long-term effects [162].

Surveillance

First of all with implementation of cancer surveillance (using cancer registries and national surveys), it's possible to direct effective cancer prevention and control program. A comprehensive database system could provide this information on the ongoing health and survivors needs.

Research programs that involve cancer survivors could also help to obtain important data to increase our knowledge of issues related to survivors and help us develop appropriate interventions to decrease distress in these patients and their caregivers.

Survivors and community education

Communication with the general public and policy about these issues aim to accept this growing population and their issues. It's necessary to address issues related to this population as a public health problem at national and community level and in this way to increase legislation, regulation, and ordinances to improve their care and quality of life. If the states, nations, and others recognize this reality and think about effective programs, they can also understand the need of state or local health department to deliver this needed care.

It is fundamental to provide tailored survivors' education according to the stage of survivorship. Patient navigation through different mechanisms (online, print, telephone, fax, etc.) could be a tool directed by health professionals and trained patients. It was recommended that survivors be provided with knowledge regarding the adverse late effects that may occur in the survivorship phase [163], new and persistent symptoms to report without waiting for the next scheduled appointment [163], and clear designation of which care provider to contact for emerging problems. The goal is to enable survivors to participate actively in their care by providing tools and training on how to obtain information, make decisions, solve problems, and communicate more effectively with their health-care provider [164].

Providers' training

It is extremely important to develop programs to train providers on specific medical and psychological needs of survivors to refer them to appropriate services and so enhance quality of their lives. Clinical practice guidelines should be implemented to extend treatment options and therapies to manage side effects and also help survivors to cope with emotional, spiritual, and practical concerns especially from the active to post primary treatment [163,164].

The public health must guarantee access to quality care for specific needs of these patients like pain, fatigue, heart problems, and infertility and also end-of-life care. It must be recognized that survivors will require navigated access to multidisciplinary specialists and other physician specialists depending on emerging or expected late effects (i.e., endocrinologists, cardiac specialists). Currently, access to coordinated interdisciplinary teams that can address the broad range of issues experienced by posttreatment survivors inclusive of psychosocial distress is important but untested.

Little is known about prevention or early detection of these problems. For oncology practitioners, the openness to change—and clear evidence that there is still much room for improvement in the type and level of behaviors being pursued—may create a window of opportunity in which to intervene, to help survivors identify behaviors that put them at risk for poor health outcomes (e.g., smoking, poor dietary practices, lack of exercise, sun exposure), and provide them with the support required to make and adhere to desired lifestyle modifications. The research should be also important in this way. It is important also that national cancer organizations, professional associations, and voluntary organizations expand and coordinate their efforts to provide educational opportunities to healthcare providers to equip them to address the health-care needs and quality-of-life issues facing cancer survivors [164,165].

Four distinct models for follow-up care have been identified including nurse-led, family physician-led, specialist- or oncologist-led, or shared care [165]. More recently, survivor-initiated models of care for follow-up of survivors have also been identified as a possible approach [166].

Although the evidence base is limited, the trials reviewed suggest that nurses and primary care physician follow-up care is equivalent in detecting recurrence when compared to oncologist-led care, and patients are satisfied with this approach [167].

Risk-based models of care are considered most beneficial for populations who are considered high risk for persistent posttreatment problems and recurrence that requires ongoing monitoring and intervention by oncology specialist teams [168].

Given the high prevalence of unmet physical and psychosocial needs in posttreatment cancer survivors, it is extremely important to provide a comprehensive evaluation with an interdisciplinary approach to improve the quality of life of these survivors and their caregivers.

REFERENCES

1 Leigh SA. Defining our destiny. In: Hoffman B (ed.), *A Cancer Survivor's Almanac: Charting the Journey.* Minneapolis, MN: Chromed Publishing; 1996, pp. 261–271.
2 National Cancer Institute (NCI). Cancer control and population sciences: Research findings [online]. Available at: http://dccps.nci.nih.gov/ocs/prevalence/index.html, (last accessed September 10, 2012).
3 Aziz N. Cancer survivorship research: Challenge and opportunity. *J Nutr* 2002;132(11):3494S–3503S.
4 Lifton RJ. *The Future of Immortality: And Other Essays for a Nuclear Age.* New York: Basic Books; 1987, pp. 231–256.
5 Lindemann E. Symptomatology and management of acute grief. *Am J Psychiatry* 1944;101:141–148.
6 Howlader N, Noone AM, Krapcho M et al. (eds.). *SEER Cancer Statistics Review, 1975–2008.* Bethesda, MD: National Cancer Institute; 2011, http://seer.cancer.gov/csr/1975_2008/, based on November 2010 SEER data submission, posted to the SEER web site.
7 Hewitt ME, Greenfield S, Stovall E (eds.). *From Cancer Patient to Cancer Survivor: Lost in Transition.* Washington, DC: National Academies Press; 2005.
8 Aziz NM. Cancer survivorship research: Challenge and opportunity. *J Nutr* 2002;132(11 Suppl.):3494S–3503S.
9 Ganz, PA. Late effects of cancer and its treatment. *Semin Oncol Nurs* 2001;17(4):241–248.
10 Ganz PA. Monitoring the physical health of cancer survivors: A survivorship-focused medical history. *J Clin Oncol* 2006;24(32):5105–5111.
11 Dong C, Hemminki K. Second primary neoplasms in 633,964 cancer patients in Sweden, 1958–1996. *Int J Cancer* 2001;93(2):155–161.
12 Travis LB. The epidemiology of second primary cancers. *Cancer Epidemiol Biomarkers Prev* 2006;15(11):2020–2026.
13 Oosterhuis JW, Looijenga LHJ. Current views on the pathogenesis of testicular germ cell tumours and perspectives for future research: Highlights of the 5th Copenhagen workshop on carcinoma in situ and cancer of the testis. *APMIS* 2003;111(1):280–289.
14 Daly MB, Axilbund JE, Bryant E et al. Genetic/familial high-risk assessment: Breast and ovarian. *J Natl Compr Canc Netw* 2006;4(2):156–176.
15 Ghelani D, Saliba R, de Lima M. Secondary malignancies after hematopoietic stem cell transplantation. *Crit Rev Oncol/Hematol* 2005;56(1):115–126.
16 Allan JM, Travis LB. Mechanisms of therapy-related carcinogenesis. *Nat Rev Cancer* 2005;5(12):943–955.
17 Lillington DM, Micallef IN, Carpenter E, Neat MJ, Amess JA, Matthews J, Foot NJ, Lister TA, Young BD, Rohatiner AZ. Genetic susceptibility to Hodgkin's disease and secondary neoplasm: FISH analysis reveals patients at high risk of developing secondary neoplasm. *Ann Oncol* 2002;13(Suppl. 1):40–43.
18 Travis LB, Fossa SD, Schonfeld SJ et al. Second cancers among 40,576 testicular cancer patients: Focus on long-term survivors. *J Natl Cancer Inst* 2005;97(18):1354–1365.
19 Tichelli A, Socié G. Considerations for adult cancer survivors. *Hematology Am Soc Hematol Educ Program* 2005;516–522.
20 Hodgson DC, Gilbert ES, Dores GM et al. Long-term solid cancer risk among 5-year survivors of Hodgkin's lymphoma. *J Clin Oncol* 2007;25(12):1489–1497.
21 Travis LB, Hill DA, Dores GM et al. Breast cancer following radiotherapy and chemotherapy among young women with Hodgkin disease. *JAMA* 2003;290(4):465–475.
22 Vogel VG, Costantino JP, Wickerham DL et al. Effects of Tamoxifen vs. Raloxifene on the risk of developing invasive breast cancer and other disease outcomes. *JAMA* 2006;295(23):2727–2741.
23 Prosnitz RG, Chen YH, Marks LB. Cardiac toxicity following thoracic radiation. *Semin Oncol* 2005;32(2):71–80.
24 Hooning MJ, Botma A, Aleman BMP, Baaijens MH, Bartelink H, Klijn JG, Taylor CW, van Leeuwen FE. Long-term risk of cardiovascular disease in 10-year survivors of breast cancer. *J Natl Cancer Inst* 2007;99(5):365–375.
25 Stone HB, Coleman CN, Anscher MS, McBride WH. Effects of radiation on normal tissue: Consequences and mechanisms. *Lancet Oncol* 2003;4(9):529–536.
26 Friedman DL, Constine LS. Late effects of treatment for Hodgkin lymphoma. *J Natl Compr Canc Netw* 2006;4(3):249–257.
27 Aleman BMP, van den Belt-Dusebout AW, De Bruin ML et al. Late cardiotoxicity after treatment for Hodgkin lymphoma. *Blood* 2007;109(5):1878–1886.

28 Van den Belt-Dusebout AW, Nuver J, de Wit R et al. Long-term risk of cardiovascular disease in 5-year survivors of testicular cancer. *J Clin Oncol* 2006;24(3):467–475.

29 Dewar JA. Postmastectomy radiotherapy. *Clin Oncol* 2006;18(3):185–190.

30 Fossa SD, Gilbert E, Dores GM et al. Noncancer causes of death in survivors of testicular cancer. *J Natl Cancer Inst* 2007;99(7):533–544.

31 Fossa SD, Aass N, Winderen M, Börmer OP, Olsen DR. Long-term renal function after treatment for malignant germ cell tumours. *Ann Oncol* 2003;13(2):222–228.

32 Bower JE, Ganz PA, Desmond KA et al. Fatigue in long-term breast carcinoma survivors: A longitudinal investigation. *Cancer* 2006;106(4):751–758.

33 Pheilschifter J, Diel IJ. Osteoporosis due to cancer treatment: Pathogenesis and management. *J Clin Oncol* 2000;18(7):1570–1593.

34 Tammela T. Endocrine treatment of prostate cancer. *J Steroid Biochem Mol Biol* 2004;92(4):287–295.

35 Iversen P, Johansson JE, Lodding P et al. Bicalutamide 150 mg in addition to standard care for patients with early non-metastatic prostate cancer: Updated from the Scandinavian Prostate Cancer Period Group-6 Study after a median follow-up period of 7.1 years. *Scand J Urol Nephrol* 2006;40(6):441–452.

36 Lonning PE, Geisler J, Krag LE et al. Effects of exemestane administered for 2 years versus placebo on bone mineral density, bone biomarkers, and plasma lipids in patients with surgically resected early breast cancer. *J Clin Oncol* 2005;23(22):5126–5137.

37 Jonat W. Overview of luteinizing hormone-releasing hormone agonists in early breast cancer-benefits of reversible ovarian ablation. *Breast Cancer Res Treat* 2002;75:23–26.

38 Fridmans A, Chertin B, Koulikov D et al. Reversibility of androgen deprivation therapy in patients with prostate cancer. *J Urol* 2005;173(3):784–789.

39 Howell SJ, Shalet SM. Effect of cancer therapy on pituitary testicular axis. *Int J Androl* 2002;25(5):269–276.

40 Haugnes HS, Aass N, Fossa SD et al. Components of the metabolic syndrome in long-term survivors of testicular cancer. *Ann Oncol* 2007;18(2):241–248.

41 Braga-Basaria M, Dobs AS, Muller DC, Carducci MA, John M, Egan J, Basaria S. Metabolic syndrome in men with prostate cancer undergoing long-term androgen-deprivation therapy. *J Clin Oncol* 2006;24(24):3979–3983.

42 Lobo RA. Potential options for preservation of fertility in women. *N Engl J Med* 2005;353(1):64–73.

43 Haukvik UK, Dieset I, Bjoro T, Holte H, Fossa SD. Treatment related premature ovarian failure as a long-term complication after Hodgkin's lymphoma. *Ann Oncol* 2006;17(9):1428–1433.

44 Magelssen H, Brydoy M, Fossa SD. The effects of cancer and cancer treatments on male reproductive function. *Nat Clin Pract Urol* 2006;3(6):312–322.

45 Wallace WH, Thomson AB, Saran F, Kelsey TW. Predicting age of ovarian failure after radiation to a field that includes the ovaries. *Int J Radiat Oncol Biol Phys* 2005;62(3):738–744.

46 Kumar N, Allen KA, Riccardi D, Bercu BB, Cantor A, Minton S, Balducci L, Jacobsen PB. Fatigue, weight gain, lethargy and amenorrhea in breast cancer patients on chemotherapy: Is subclinical hypothyroidism the culprit? *Breast Cancer Res Treat* 2004;83(2):149–159.

47 Agha A, Sherlock M, Brennan S et al. Hypothalamic–pituitary dysfunction after irradiation of non-pituitary brain tumors in adults. *J Clin Endocrinol Metab* 2005;90(12):6355–6360.

48 Tal R, Baniel J. Sexual function-preserving cystectomy. *Urology* 2005;66(2):235–241.

49 Bianco FJ Jr, Scardino PT, Eastham JA. Radical prostatectomy: Long-term cancer control and recovery of sexual and urinary function ("trifecta"). *Urology* 2005;66(5):83–94.

50 Potosky AL, Davis WW, Hoffman RM, Standford JL, Stephenson RA, Penson DF, Harlan LC. Five-year outcomes after prostatectomy or radiotherapy for prostate cancer: The prostate cancer outcome study. *J Natl Cancer Inst* 2004;96(18):1358–1367.

51 Fossa SD, Magelssen H, Melve K, Jacobsen AB, Langmark F, Skjaerven R. Parenthood in survivors after adulthood cancer and perinatal health in their offspring: A preliminary report. *J Natl Cancer Inst Monographs* 2005;34:77–82.

52 Armstrong CL, Gyato K, Awadalla AW, Lustiq R, Tochner ZA. A critical review of the clinical effects of therapeutic irradiation damage to the brain: The roots of controversy. *Neuropsychol Rev* 2004;14(1):65–86; *J Cancer Surviv* 2008;2:3–11.

53 Gavrilovic IT, Hormigo A, Yahalom J, De Angelis LM, Abrey LE. Long-term follow-up of high-dose Methotrexate-based therapy with and without whole brain irradiation for newly diagnosed primary CNS lymphoma. *J Clin Oncol* 2006;24(28):4570–4574.

54 Galecki J, Hicer-Grzenkowicz J, Grudzien-Kowalska M, Michalska T, Zalucki W. Radiation-induced brachial plexopathy and hypofractionated regimens in adjuvant irradiation of patients with breast cancer—A review. *Acta Oncol* 2006;45(3):280–284.

55 Mykletun A, Dahl AA, Haaland CF, Bremnes R, Dahl O, Klepp O, Wist E, Fossa SD. Side-effects and cancer-related stress determine quality of life in long-term survivors of testicular cancer. *J Clin Oncol* 2005;23(13):3061–3068.

56 Bradley J, Graham MV, Winter K et al. Toxicity and outcome results of RTOG 9311: A phase I–II dose-escalation study using three-dimensional conformal radiotherapy in patients with inoperable non-small-cell lung carcinoma. *Int J Radiat Oncol Biol Phys* 2005;61(2):318–328.

57 Stensvold E, Aass N, Gladhaug I, Stenwig AE, Claussen OP, Fossa SD. Erroneous diagnosis of pancreatic cancer after radiotherapy of testicular cancer. *Eur J Surg Oncol* 2004;30(3):352–355.

58 Maduro JH, Pras E, Willemse PHB, de Vries EGE. Acute and long-term toxicity following radiotherapy alone or in combination with chemotherapy for locally advanced cervical cancer. *Cancer Treat Rev* 2003;29:471–488.

59 Lundby L, Krogh K, Jensen VJ et al. Long-term anorectal dysfunction after postoperative radiotherapy for rectal cancer. *Dis Colon Rectum* 2005;45(7):1343–1349.

60 Dearnaley DP, Sydes MR, Graham JD et al. Escalated-dose versus standard-dose conformal radiotherapy in prostate cancer: First results from the MRC RT01 randomized controlled trial. *Lancet Oncol* 2007;8(6):475–487.

61 Carver JR, Shapiro CL, Ng A, Jacobs L, Schwartz C, Virgo KS, Hagerty KL, Somerfield MR, Vaughn DJ. ASCO cancer survivorship expert panel. *J Clin Oncol* 2007;25(25):3991–4008.

62 Working Party of the British Committee for Standards in Hematology, Clinical Hematology Task Force. Guidelines for prevention and treatment of infection in post splenectomy patients or those with dysfunction spleen. *Br Med J* 1996;312(7028):430–434.

63 Webb CW, Crowell K, Cravens D. Clinical inquiries. Which vaccinations are indicated after splenectomy? *J Fam Pract* 2006;55(8):711–712.

64 Winquist EW, Bauman GS, Balogh J. Nontraumatic osteonecrosis after chemotherapy for testicular cancer: A systematic review. *Am J Clin Oncol* 2001;24(6):603–606.

65 Sciubba JJ, Goldenberg D. Oral complications of radiotherapy. *Lancet Oncol* 2006;7(2):75–83.

66 Gordon KG, Char DH, Sagerman RH. Late effects of radiation on the eye and ocular adnexa. *Int J Radiat Oncol Biol Phys* 1995;31(5):1123–1139.

67   Stava C, Beck M, Vassilopoulou-Sellin R. Cataracts among cancer survivors. *Am J Clin Oncol* 2005;28(6):603–608.

68   Ness KK, Wall MM, Oakes JM, Robinson LL, Gurney JG. Physical performance limitations and participation restrictions among cancer survivors: A population-based study. *Ann Epidemiol* 2006;16(3):197–205.

69   Hewitt M, Rowland JH, Yancik R. Cancer survivors in the United States: Age, health, and disability. *J Gerontol A: Biol Sci Med Sci* 2003;58(1):82–91.

70   Fossa SD, Hess SL, Dahl AA, Hjermstad MJ, Veenstra M. Stability of health-related quality of life in the Norwegian general population and impact of chronic morbidity in individuals with and without a cancer diagnosis. *Acta Oncol* 2007;46(4):452–461.

71   Ruffer JU, Fletchner H, Tralls P, Josting A, Sieber M, Lathan B, Diehl V. Fatigue in long-term survivors of Hodgkin's lymphoma: A report from the German Hodgkin Lymphoma Study Group(GHSG). *Eur J Cancer* 2003;39(15):2179–2186.

72   Hjermstad MJ, Oldervoll L, Fossa SD, Holte H, Jacobsen AB, Loge JH. Quality of life in long-term Hodgkin's disease survivors with chronic fatigue. *Eur J Cancer* 2006;42(3):327–333.

73   Oeffinger KC, Mertens AC, Sklar CA et al. Chronic health conditions in adult survivors of childhood cancer. *N Engl J Med* 2006;355(15):1572–1582.

74   Ganz PA, Greendale GA, Petersen L, Kahn B, Bower JE. Breast cancer in younger women: Reproductive and late health effects of treatment. *J Clin Oncol* 2003;21(22):4184–4193.

75   Ganz PA, Desmond KA, Leedham B, Rowland JH, Meyerowitz BE, Belin TR. Quality of life in long-term, disease-free survivors of breast cancer: A follow-up study. *J Natl Cancer Inst* 2002;94(1):39–49.

76   Casso D, Buist DS, Taplin S. Quality of life of 5–10 year breast cancer survivors diagnosed between age 40 and 49. *Health Qual Life Outcomes* 2004;2:25.

77   Bloom JR, Stewart SL, Chang S, Banks PJ. Then and now: Quality of life of young breast cancer survivors. *Psychooncology* 2004;13(3):147–160.

78   Kornblith AB, Herndon JE II, Weiss RB et al. Long-term adjustment of survivors of early-stage breast carcinoma, 20 years after adjuvant chemotherapy. *Cancer* 2003;98(4):679–689.

79   Helgeson VS, Tomich PL. Surviving cancer: A comparison of 5-year disease free breast cancer survivors with healthy women. *Psychooncology* 2005;14(4):307–317.

80   Loge JH, Abrahamsen AF, Ekeberg O, Kaasa S. Fatigue and psychiatric morbidity among Hodgkin's disease survivors. *J Pain Symptom Manage* 2000;19(2):91–99.

81   Wettergren L, Bjorkholm M, Axdorph U, Langius-Eklof A. Determinants of health related quality of life in long-term survivors of Hodgkin's lymphoma. *Qual Life Res* 2004;13(8):1369–1379.

82   Gil-Fernandez J, Ramos C, Tamayo T et al. Quality of life and psychological wellbeing in Spanish long-term survivors of Hodgkin's disease: Results of a controlled pilot study. *Ann Hematol* 2003;82(1):14–18.

83   Hoffman KE, McCarthy EO, Recklitis CJ et al. Psychological distress in long-term survivors of adult-onset cancer. *Arch Intern Med* 2009;169(14):1274–1281.

84   Carlson LE, Angen M, Cullum J et al. High levels of untreated distress and fatigue in cancer patients. *Br J Cancer* 2004;90(12):2297–2304.

85   Zabora J, Brintzenhofe Szoc K, Curbow B, Hooker C, Piantadosi S. The prevalence of psychological distress by cancer site. *Psychooncology* 2001;10(1):19–28.

86   Pratt L, Dye A, Cohen A. *Characteristics of Adults with Serious Psychological Distress as Measured by the K6 Scale: United States 2001–04.* Hyattsville, MD: National Center for Health Statistics; 2007.

87   Benton T, Staab J, Evans DL. Medical co-morbidity in depressive disorders. *Ann Clin Psychiatry* 2007;19(4):289–303.

88   Candib LM. Obesity and diabetes in vulnerable populations: Reflection on proximal and distal causes. *Ann Fam Med* 2007;5(6):547–556.

89   Champion V, Williams SD, Miller A et al. Quality of life in long-term survivors of ovarian germ cell tumors: A Gynecologic Oncology Group study. *Gynecol Oncol* 2007;105(3):687–694.

90   Fu SS, McFall M, Saxon AJ et al. Post-traumatic stress disorder and smoking: A systematic review. *Nicotine Tob Res* 2007;9(11):1071–1084.

91   McWilliams JM, Meara E, Zaslavsky AM, Ayanian JZ. Health of previously uninsured adults after acquiring Medicare coverage. *JAMA* 2007;298(24):2886–2894.

92   Stanton AL. Psychosocial concerns and interventions for cancer survivors. *J Clin Oncol* 2006;24(32):5132–5137.

93   Dahl AA, Haaland CF, Mykletun A et al. Study of anxiety disorder and depression in long-term survivors of testicular cancer. *J Clin Oncol* 2005;23(10):2389–2395.

94   Deshields T, Tibbs T, Fan MY, Taylor M. Differences in patterns of depression after treatment for breast cancer. *Psychooncology* 2006;15(5):398–406.

95   Lambert SD, Girgis A, Lecathelinais C, Stacey F. Walking a mile in their shoes: Anxiety and depression among partners and caregivers of cancer survivors at 6 and 12 months post-diagnosis. *Support Care Cancer* 2013;21(1):75–85.

96   Puchalski C, Ferrell B, Virani R et al. Improving the quality of spiritual care as a dimension of palliative care: The report of the consensus conference. *J Palliat Med* 2009;12:885–904.

97   Hill PC, Pargament KI. Advances in the conceptualization and measurement of religion and spirituality. Implications for physical and mental health research. *Am Psychol* 2003;58:64–74.

98   Sulmasy DP. Spiritual issues in the care of dying patients: "... it's okay between me and god". *JAMA* 2006;296:1385–1392.

99   Nelson C, Rosenfeld B, Breitbart W et al. Spirituality, religion, and depression in the terminally ill. *Psychosomatics* 2002;43:213–220.

100 Cotton S, Levine E, Fitzpatrick C et al. Exploring the relationships among spiritual well being, quality of life, and psychological adjustment in women with breast cancer. *Psychooncology* 1999;8:429–438.

101 Tarakeshwar N, Vanderwerker L, Paulk E et al. Religious coping is associated with the quality of life of patients with advanced cancer. *J Palliat Med* 2006;9:646–657.

102 Brady M, Peterman A, Fitchett G et al. A case for including spirituality in quality of life measurement in oncology. *Psychooncology* 1999;8:417–428.

103 Simon C, Crowther M. The stage-specific role of spirituality among African American Christian women throughout the breast cancer experience. *Cult Div Ethnic Min Psychol* 2007;13:26–34.

104 Koenig H, George L, Titus P. Religion, spirituality, and health in medically ill hospitalized older patients. *J Am Geriatr Soc* 2004;52:554–562.

105 Gallup G. The religiosity cycle. Gallup Tuesday Briefing, June 2, 2002 [online]. Available at: http://www.gallup.com/poll/6124/Religiosity-Cycle.aspx, (last accessed September 2012).

106 Delgado-Guay MO, Hui D, Parsons HA, Govan K, De la Cruz M, Thorney S, Bruera E. Spirituality, religiosity, and spiritual pain in advanced cancer patients. *J Pain Symptom Manage* 2011;41(6):986–994.

107 Canada LA, Murphy PE, Fitchett G, Peterman AH, Schover LR. A 3-factor model for the FACIT-Sp. *Psychooncology* 2008;17:908–916.

108 Edmondson D, Park CL, Blank TO, Fenster JR, Mills MA. Deconstructing spiritual well-being: Existential well-being and HRQOL in cancer survivors. *Psychooncology* 2008;17:161–169.

109 Purnell JQ, Andersen BL, Wilmot JP. Religious practice and spirituality in the psychological adjustment of survivors of breast cancer. *Couns Values* 2009;53:165–181.

110   Hamilton JB, Crandell JL, Kameron Carter J, Lynn MR. Reliability and validity of the perspectives of Support from God Scale. *Nurs Res* 2010;59:102–109.

111   Agarwal M, Hamilton JB, Crandell JL, Moore CE. Coping strategies of African American head and neck cancer survivors. *J Psychosoc Oncol* 2010;28:526–538.

112   Gall TL. Relationship with God and the quality of life of prostate cancer survivors. *Qual Life Res* 2004;13:1357–1368.

113   Stanton AL, Bower JE, Low CA. Posttraumatic growth after cancer. In: Calhoun LG, Tedeschi RG (eds.), *Handbook of Posttraumatic Growth: Research and Practice*. Mahwah, NJ: Erlbaum Associates; 2006, pp. 121–137.

114   Campesino M. Exploring perceptions of cancer care delivery among older Mexican American adults. *Oncol Nurs Forum* 2009;36:413–420.

115   Gall TL, Cornblat MW. Breast cancer survivors give voice: A qualitative analysis of spiritual factors in long-term adjustment. *Psychooncology* 2002;11:524–535.

116   Hamilton JB, Moore CE, Powe BD, Agarwal M, Martin P. Perceptions of support among older African American cancer survivors. *Oncol Nurs Forum* 2010;37:484–493.

117   Levine, EG, Aviv C, Yoo G, Ewing C, Au A. The benefits of prayer on mood and well-being of breast cancer survivors. *Support Care Cancer* 2009;17:295–306.

118   Holt CL, Caplan L, Schulz E, Blake V, Southward P, Buckner A, Lawrence H. Role of religion in cancer coping among African Americans: A qualitative examination. *J Psychosoc Oncol* 2009;27:248–273.

119   Ardelt M, Ai AL, Eichenberger SE. In search for meaning: The differential role of religion for middle-aged and older persons diagnosed with a life-threatening illness. *J Relig Spiritual Aging* 2008;20:288–312.

120   McGrath P. Reflections on serious illness as spiritual journey by survivors of haematological malignancies. *Eur J Cancer Care* 2004;13:227–237.

121   Delgado-Guay MO, Parsons HA, Hui D et al. *Spirituality: An Expression of Inner Strength and Meaning of Life in Patients with advanced cancer (ACAP) and Their Caregivers in the Palliative Care Setting*. Athens, Greece: Poster Presentation in EAPC; 2011.

122   Weaver AJ, Flannelly KJ. The role of religion/spirituality for cancer patients and their caregivers. *South Med J* 2004;97(12):1210–1214.

123   Picot SJ, Debanne SM, Namazi KH et al. Religiosity and perceived rewards of black and white caregivers. *Gerontologist* 1997;37:89–101.

124   Chang B, Noonan AE, Tennstedt SL. The role of religion/spirituality in coping with caregiving for disabled elders. *Gerontologist* 1998;38:463–470.

125   Koenig HG, Weaver AJ. *Counseling Troubled Older Adults: A Handbook for Pastors and Religious Caregivers*. Nashville, TN: Abingdon Press; 1997.

126   Kim Y, Spillers RL, Hall DL. Quality of life of family caregivers 5 years after a relative's cancer diagnosis: Follow-up of the national quality of life survey for caregivers. *Psychooncology* 2012;21(3):273–281. doi:10.1002/pon.1888.

127   Wilson K, Chochinov H, McPherson C et al. Suffering with advanced cancer. *J Clin Oncol* 2007;25:1691–1697.

128   Krause H, Ingersoll-Dayton B, Ellison C, Wulff K. Aging, religious doubt, and psychological well-being. *Gerontologist* 1999;39:525–533.

129   Exline J, Yali A, Sanderson W. Guilt, discord, and alienation: The role of religious strain in depression and suicidality. *J Clin Psychol* 2000;56:1481–1496.

130   Fitchett G, Rybarczyk B, De Marco G, Nicholas J. The role of religion in medical rehabilitation outcomes: A longitudinal study. *Rehabil Psychol* 1999;44:333–353.

131   Pargament K, Koenig H, Tarakeshwar N, Hahn J. Religious struggle as a predictor of mortality among medically ill elderly patients: A two year longitudinal study. *Arch Intern Med* 2001;161:1881–1885.

132   Mako C, Galek K, Poppito S. Spiritual pain among patients with advanced cancer in palliative care. *J Palliat Med* 2006;9:1106–1113.

133   Millspaugh D. Assessment and response to spiritual pain: Part I. *J Palliat Med* 2005;8:919–923.

134   Cassell E. The nature of suffering and the goals of medicine. *N Engl J Med* 1982;306:639–645.

135   Merskey H, Bogduk N. *Classification of Chronic Pain: Descriptions of Chronic Pain Syndromes and Definitions of Pain Terms*. Seattle, WA: International Association for the Study of Pain; 1994.

136   Turk D, Melzack R (eds.). *Handbook of Pain Assessment*, 2nd edn. New York: Guilford Press; 2001.

137   Chochinov H, Cann B. Interventions to enhance the spiritual aspects of dying. *J Palliat Med* 2005;8:S103–S115.

138   Pargament K, Murray-Swank N, Magyar G, Ano G. Spiritual struggle: A phenomenon of interest to psychology and religion. In: Miller W, Delaney H (eds.), *Psychology and Human Nature*. Washington, DC: APA Press; 2006.

139   Surbone A. The difficult tasks of family care giving in oncology: Exactly which roles do autonomy and gender play? *Support Care Cancer* 2003;11:617–619.

140   Rhee YS, Yun YH, Park S et al. Depression in family caregivers of cancer patients: The feeling of burden as a predictor of depression. *J Clin Oncol* 2008;26:5890–5895.

141   Siminoff LA, Wilson-Genderson M, Baker S. Depressive symptoms in lung cancer patients and their family caregivers and the influence of family environment. *Psychooncology* 2010;19(12):1285–1293.

142   Manne S, Badr H. Intimacy processes and psychological distress among couples coping with head and neck or lung cancers. *Psychooncology* 2010;19(9):941–954.

143   Vickery LE, Latchford G, Hewison J, Bellew M, Feber T. The impact of head and neck cancer and facial disfigurement on the quality of life of patients and their partners. *Head Neck* 2003;25(4):289–296.

144   Pitceathly C, Maguire P. The psychological impact of cancer on patients' partners and other key relatives: A review. *Eur J Cancer* 2003;39(11):1517–1524.

145   Turner D, Adams E, Boulton M et al. Partners and close family members of long-term cancer survivors: Health status, psychosocial well-being and unmet supportive care needs. *Psychooncology* 2013;22(1):12–9. doi:10.1002/pon.2050.

146   Hodgkinson K, Butow P, Hunt GE, Wyse R, Hobbs KM, Wain G. Life after cancer: Couples' and partners; psychological adjustment and supportive care needs. *Support Care Cancer* 2007;15:405–415.

147   Simard S, Savard J. Fear of Cancer Recurrence Inventory: Development and initial validation of a multidimensional measure of fear of cancer recurrence. *Support Care Cancer* 2009;17:241–251.

148   Lewis F. The effects of survivorship on families and caregivers. *Cancer Nurs* 2006;29(2 Suppl.):20–21, 23–25.

149   Hodges LJ, Humphris GM, Macfarlane G. A meta-analytic investigation of the relationship between the psychological distress of cancer patients and their carers. *Soc Sci Med* 2005;60:1–12.

150   Sprangers M, Schwartz C. Integrating response shift into health-related quality of life research: A theoretical model. *Soc Sci Med* 1999;48:1507–1515.

151   Sharpe L, Butow P, Smith C, McConnell D, Clarke S. Changes in quality of life in patients with advanced cancer: Evidence of response shift and response restriction. *J Psychosom Res* 2005;58:497–504.

152   Ell K, Xie B, Wells A, Nedjat-Haiem F, Lee PJ, Vourlekis B. Economic stress among low-income women with cancer: Effects on quality of life. *Cancer* 2008;112(3):616–625.

153 de Boer AG, Taskila T, Ojajarvi A, van Dijk FJ, Verbeek JH. Cancer survivors and unemployment: A meta-analysis and meta-regression. *JAMA* 2009;301(7):753–762.

154 Hoving JL, Broekhuizen ML, Frings-Dresen MH. Return to work of breast cancer survivors: A systematic review of intervention studies. *BMC Cancer* 2009;9:117.

155 Lee MK, Lee KM, Bae JM et al. Employment status and work-related difficulties in stomach cancer survivors compared with the general population. *Br J Cancer* 2008;98(4):708–715.

156 Helgeson VS, Reynolds KA, Tomich PL. A meta-analytic review of benefit finding and growth. *J Consult Clin Psychol* 2006;74:797–816.

157 Foley KL, Farmer DF, Petronis VM et al. A qualitative exploration of the cancer experience among long-term survivors: Comparisons by cancer type, ethnicity, gender, and age. *Psychooncology* 2006;15:248–258.

158 US Department of Health and Human Services, National Institutes of Health. The NCI Strategic Plan for leading the nation to eliminate the suffering and death due to cancer, 2007. Accessible at: http://strategicplan.nci.nih-gov/, (last accessed September 2012).

159 Lo B, Quill T, Tulsky J. Discussing palliative care with patients ACP-ASIM End-of-Life Care Consensus Panel. American College of Physicians. American Society of Internal Medicine. *Ann Intern Med* 1999;130:744–749.

160 Russell-Searight H, Gafford J. Cultural diversity at the end of life: Issues and guidelines for family physicians. *Am Fam Physician* 2005;71:515–522.

161 Ngo-Metzger Q, August KJ, Srinivasan M, Liao S, Meyskens FL Jr. End-of-life care: Guidelines for patient-centered communication. *Am Fam Physician* 2008;77:167–174.

162 Landler W. Survivorship care: Essential components and models of delivery. *Oncology* 2009;23(4 Suppl. Nurse Ed.):46–53.

163 Grunfeld E, Dhesy-Thind S, Levine M, for the Steering Committee on Clinical Practice Guidelines for the Care and Treatment of Breast Cancer. Clinical practice guidelines for the care and treatment of breast cancer: 9. Follow-up after treatment for breast cancer. *CMAJ* 2005;172(10):1319.

164 Hewitt M, Greenfield S, Stovall E (eds.). *From Cancer Patient to Cancer Survivor: Lost in Transition.* Washington, DC: National Academies Press; 2006.

165 Oeffinger KC, McCabe MS. Models for delivering survivorship care. *J Clin Oncol* 2006;24(32):5117–5124.

166 Brown L, Payne S, Royle G. Patient initiated follow up of breast cancer. *Psychooncology* 2002;11:346–355.

167 Howell D, Hack TF, Oliver TK et al. Models of care for post-treatment follow-up of adult cancer survivors: A systematic review and quality appraisal of the evidence. *J Cancer Surviv* 2012;6(4):359–371. doi: 10.1007/s11764-012-0232-z.

168 Hudson MM, Landler W, Ganz PA. Impact of survivorship-based research on defining clinical care guidelines. *Cancer Epidemiol Biomarkers Prev* 2011;20:2085–2092.

128

Rehabilitation in the acute and chronic care setting

BENEDICT KONZEN, YING GUO, KI Y. SHIN

INTRODUCTION

The role of palliative care medicine is a microcosm of the general tenets of medicine. One analyzes the physiologic state of the patient. Where there is a lack of homeostasis, supportive care attempts to define the imbalance, remedy symptoms of disease/distress, and promote—if possible—a return to premorbid function. With astute and diligent care, it is hoped that the patient will regain some degree of his/her level of independent functioning. Restoration of physical and social norms will also, hopefully, resolve in part patient/family/caretaker conflict—often exacerbated by a patient's illness.

In much the same way as supportive care, the field of physical medicine and rehabilitation predicates itself on function. Where human functioning has been lost or altered, the field attempts to restore a patient to the highest level of premorbid activity. Indeed, in some areas of prosthetics and orthotics, we are now able to surpass the human dynamics in terms of gait, running, and weight-lifting. These developments have had to keep pace with human advancements, technologic developments, and societal conflicts.

Both disciplines have traditional roles in the care of acute, subacute, and chronic patients. Dyspnea, fatigue, anorexia, poor sense of well-being, insomnia, and pain are seen frequently in the cancer patient. With similar goals but slightly different approaches to care and symptom management, both symptom management and rehabilitation often work in tandem to treat a chronically ill or dying patient. This collaborative effort also tends to alleviate both patient and family distress.

As noted, the goal of both fields is to promote independent physical and mental functioning with the fewest symptoms—for as long as possible. The point at which we accept the chronicity of a disease state—despite the likelihood of approaching mortality—is what differentiates supportive care and cancer rehabilitation from the more mainstream branches of standard physical medicine.

Additionally, the argument is often made over increased societal and economic costs when caring for the chronically ill or dying patient. New medical studies, technologies, and evolving treatments foster the ongoing hope of cure. Often, patients with nowhere else to turn will seek out nontraditional treatment options—holistic treatment, acupuncture, or diet modification. There may be a sudden increase in spirituality, religiosity, or strict adherence to a code of conduct. Patients may willingly relinquish their prior independence/autonomy and defer to the untested authority of the treating physician and his entourage. The danger in this approach is the potential loss of self-identity, one's convictions, and unquestioned adherence to the health care team's plan. It is important for all treating team members to recognize and incorporate the patient's wishes and autonomy into the decision-making process.

Even with the completion of treatment and the alleviation of symptoms, a physician's role in care does not end. Chronicity of disease and the expectations in end-of-life care imply an ongoing patient/physician relationship predicated on close follow-up.

By placing total faith in the possibility versus probability of cure, patients are often ignorant of the side effects of treatment. In effect, by the time they realize the additive consequences of treatment, they may have experienced marked debility in their physical strength, mobility, and self-care. By extension, this may then affect their family's economic livelihood and ability to interact socially. Indeed, futility in treatment often becomes an ethical concern. At what point do we treat a patient? When do we stop? If we stop care, is this abandonment? If we stop treatment, how do we ensure ongoing supportive care? Are we actually helping or hurting the patient by extending medical treatment?

In rehabilitation medicine, we often need to work with and train both the family and designated caregiver. Those who end up caring for a patient often do not understand the mandated scope of involvement. Even if treatment is deemed successful by the medical community, the patient and his family are often left with financial/economic and social woes.

Premorbid arrangements for end-of-life care (e.g., code status) often are made without the patient's full understanding of the current medical establishment or the physical and mental challenges associated with cancer care. A patient expecting a full recovery may be horrified at intermediate treatment steps, such as placement in a regional extended care center—where the patient's support system of family, friends, and spiritual resources may be restricted. In such instances, a patient is often at the mercy of an unfamiliar caregiver. He has to trust and rely on the care of individuals who really do not know him, and whose care may be simply "their job."

Tenets of physical medicine and rehabilitation

Physical medicine and rehabilitation arose more of out of necessity than as a well-established allied field of medicine. This specialty initially comprised the practice of modalities of medical treatment. By the 1920s, the field dealt with solar therapy/open-air sanitoriums for tubercular patients and spa therapy for arthritic patients. One of the earliest practitioners of physical medicine was Dr. Henry Krusen at the Mayo Clinic—who utilized modalities of treatment as an adjunct to his practice of internal medicine. With the advent of the World Wars, orthopedists were dealing with returning amputees. Advances in physical activity, bracing prosthetics, and schools of physical and occupational therapy began. During World War II, Dr. Howard Rusk developed the concept of the inpatient rehabilitation unit. The two disciplines of physiatry and rehabilitation medicine merged and received specialty status in 1950. Residency schools began in the 1940s in an effort to deal with polio and the returning war veterans.

Currently, the practice of physical medicine and rehabilitation is global. The field arose in an effort to "palliate" symptoms of musculoskeletal and neurologic loss by enhancing sensory and motor restoration. This was done in collaboration with varying treatment modalities—diathermy, heat, cold, desensitization techniques, solar/spa therapies. Today, acupuncture, acupressure, e-stimulation (TENS), iontophoresis, massage, injections, nerve blocks, phenoland botox injections round out the arsenal. Additionally, the field is intimately allied with physical, occupational, and speech therapies as well as orthotic and prosthetic specialists.

As technologies have advanced, so, too, has the need to understand neuropathy, limb and head trauma; recreational/spinal cord injuries; workplace injuries (crush injuries, burns, carpal tunnel syndrome); and cognitive dysfunction (caused by trauma to the brain, stroke, bleeding, and tumor). The field of physical medicine and rehabilitation recognizes the intimate importance of each organ system to human functioning. As such, physical medicine and rehabilitation has had to keep pace and closely allied with fields of orthopedics, neurology, and neurosurgery.

Physiatry has also developed common ground with the supportive care physician. Functioning is not only predicated on an intact neuromuscular, cardiopulmonary, and musculoskeletal system. It is severely limited by homeostatic imbalances—for example, anemia, dyspnea, pain, fatigue, anorexia, poor steep, constipation, and distress. As such, there is an inherent need to master basic principles of internal medicine and its deregulation—diabetes, hypertension, renal insufficiency, respiratory insufficiency, coagulopathy,

thrombosis, neuropathic pain, musculoskeletal pain, spasticity, stroke, insomnia, and constipation.

In free standing rehabilitation facilities, physiatrists are required to manage pain issues (pain pumps, spinal stimulators, TENS units); spasticity (botox and phenol injections); neuromuscular diagnostics (electromyography). Movement disorders (Parkinson's disease, neurodegenerative diseases such as ALS, Eaton-Lambert Syndrome, myasthenia gravis) also come under the realm of general rehabilitation.

In the fast-paced world of recreational drug use, cocaine-induced stroke, drugs of abuse with parkinsonian side effects and alcohol-/motor vehicle-/gunshot-related accidents—stroke, coma, and traumatic brain injury—round out the portfolio of the physiatrist's repertoire.

Similar to the supportive care model of care, rehabilitation medicine requires an interdisciplinary team of physician/nursing, physical and occupational therapies, speech pathology and neuropsychology, social work, case management, and chaplaincy. Every team member must feel unimpeded in contributing their expertise, observations, and input in the care of the patient. This interaction often culminates in a weekly team meeting. In this discussion, the initial goals of care are put forward; progress is noted; goals are revised; family concerns are presented, and future care needs—regarding housing, equipment for self cares, mobility, future therapy needs, clinic follow-up, and disposition planning—are addressed.

TRADITIONAL REHABILITATION

Traditionally, the rehabilitation patient often is referred to a physiatrist in the outpatient setting. These programs may be independently incorporated, managed by hospital-affiliated satellites, or located within a hospital itself. In cases where individuals have been hospitalized—for example, motor vehicle accidents, sustained fractures, sport injuries, trauma, neurologic sequelae (e.g., stroke), or surgery—patients are often seen initially by a rehabilitation consultant. A determination of functional status is made.

If patients have marked loss of physical or cognitive functioning, they may be considered for an inpatient rehabilitation stay—often in a dedicated rehabilitation unit. Unit size varies. Each patient's care, however, should be uniquely tailored to that patient's respective impairment. To offset the potential for disability, the rehabilitation physician must consistently encourage and educate the patient on personal and team goals.

From a rehabilitation perspective, a successful hospitalization focuses on regaining independence with mobility and self-care. There still may be a continued reliance on a caregiver. However, the emphasis should always be on restoring patient autonomy if possible. Independence and advocacy are stressed. Emphasis is placed on both patient and caregiver safety. Once inpatient rehabilitation has been completed, the task at hand evolves into the outpatient arena of care.

TRANSITIONING FROM HOSPITAL-BASED TO COMMUNITY-BASED REHABILITATION

Patients need to function in the real world. In addition to remastery of self-care and household management, many individuals will want to resume their premorbid lives. They want to drive, go back to work, and resume hobbies. Outpatient therapists are often called into action. Patients often require limb strengthening; work on hand dexterity; enhanced mobility (transitioning from rolling walker to cane or provisional prosthesis to the final prosthetic stage). For a stroke patient, this may involve transitioning from level to uneven surfaces (averting potholes in a street, negotiating a curb/street corner); visual modifications secondary to hemianopia/quadrantanopia). From an occupational therapy perspective, a patient may require modification to the workplace (ergonomic keyboard layout and seating; home modifications for kitchen, standing, seating, toileting, bathing). Every premorbid activity will likely need to be scrutinized and potentially adapted. As we evolve with new life technologies—so do the complexities of our "new" environment. An impediment and/or impairment often becomes the necessary catalyst for change, and this is the ultimate challenge of physical medicine.

Given the need to delve into a person's daily functioning, the world of rehabilitation medicine is both personal and invasive in its purview. How people interact with one another physically, intellectually, politically, emotionally, spiritually, and sexually are expressions of their humanity. Any disease state will alter this balance. The rehabilitation team has to be open to these challenges. With great discretion, a physiatrist has to remove himself/herself from cultural biases. Discretion, integrity, honesty, and ethical treatment are paramount in caring for a patient.

The greatest challenge to the field of rehabilitation is its scope. Every medical and surgical specialty benefits from the widespread role played by rehabilitation medicine. Restoration of a person is a difficult process. Despite the myriad of challenges, the field allows for creative expression. Outcomes do not necessarily follow a prescribed course. Rather, each patient, their challenges, and their treatment are unique.

CANCER REHABILITATION

Cancer rehabilitation remains a subspecialization of the field of physical medicine and rehabilitation. The basic infrastructure and goals are similar. The premise is unaltered—that is, restoring a patient's function to the highest premorbid level of activity. Again, this is a coordinated, multidisciplinary effort. Unlike the general rehabilitation patient, the cancer patient's disease state often is uncertain. Patients may respond to treatment. Treatment, however, may induce a host of unexpected new side effects with worsening function. The disease state may become metastatic and involve multiple organ systems irreversibly. Cancer and its treatment often lead to chronic side effects of fatigue, pain, cognitive impairment, and a closer reliance on hospital services, clinics, physicians, nurses, and technical specialists.

Treating a cancer patient requires a sophisticated knowledge of anatomy, physiology, and pathology. Treatment necessitates an understanding of pharmacokinetics, pain medications; the interaction of antidepressants; anxiolytics; modulators of brain chemistry; seizure activity; and delirium.

For the cancer rehabilitation, the physician has to extend his medical knowledge beyond standards of traditional rehabilitation. There needs to be an integral understanding of the body and its disease states—hematopoiesis; endocrinopathies, neuropathies, cardiopulmonary, and renal disease. These disease states indeed need to be effectively managed in order to restore a patient's physical functioning. In traditional rehabilitation, the physician generally anticipates some restoration in function. However, in cancer rehabilitation, restoration in function may be fleeting. Indeed, there is often a vague endpoint.

As there is no cure to cancer at this time, the treatment of cancer and the palliation of symptoms will likely require constant revision. The term "complete cure" continues to be replaced with euphemisms—"no current evidence of disease… lessening of tumor burden…cytoreduction." Chemotherapy, surgery, and/or radiation therapy are understood as the current standards of care. With advancements in diagnosis and treatment, due diligence in care, now, is often equated with a proliferation in new treatment protocols and extensive radiographic studies.

The ultimate goal of a patient, his family, oncologist, and surgeon may be reduction or elimination of a tumor. The ramifications of that treatment from a functioning perspective, however, may be devastating. Additionally, there is often an attached financial hardship. Patients may have to liquidate life-acquired assets and potentially relocate. Individuals who may be older and without significant physical and emotional supports are often overwhelmed in a foreign urban/medical environment. In cases of liquid tumor malignancies, patients may be permanently tied to the hospital-setting secondary to blood product dependency or need for continued antibiotic/antiviral or antifungal management. Side effects in treatment may include transfusion dependency, anorexia, cachexia, marked debility, bedsores, falls with fracture/head trauma, bleeds, deep venous thromboses, and pulmonary emboli. In cases of stem cell transplantations, patients may experience graft-versus-host disease. Patients and their families may no longer be able to extricate themselves from the treatment web of the hospital. Paradoxically, patient may not want to leave the treatment center—but realistically, they may not be able to tolerate additional therapies or the costs incurred. Ultimately, a patient may deteriorate even in spite of ongoing state-of-the-art care/rehabilitation services and the time to return to their former residence is long past.

Generally speaking, the goal of treatment may be altered at any point in treatment/hospitalization. This is dependent on a patient's tolerance to surgery and/or chemoradiation. For example, a seemingly ambulatory individual with prostate cancer that has metastasized to the spine may also demonstrate an impending spinal cord compression. Despite surgery, radiation, or high-dose steroid management, the patient may still progress to paraplegia and a neurogenic bowel and/or bladder. Premorbid mobility may now be replaced by a patient requiring complete assistance of family for self-care, mobility, and financial support.

In these instances, the cancer rehabilitation physician has to process a great deal of information and interact with the oncology specialist, radiation oncologist, medical specialists, and surgeons. Following up on the medical and surgical plan, the cancer rehabilitation physician must also develop a rehabilitation plan that can be realistically and efficiently executed. Often, the time to treat and rehabilitate a patient is finite and short. Urgency and practicality are paramount.

In today's world—where possessions, status, achievement, and financial resources have great importance—we often overlook the value of function until we experience a medical impairment. When this impairment leads to a disability, our attention becomes riveted to preserving the most basic of functions—bowel/bladder functioning and walking.

CONCLUSION

The goal of general rehabilitation is the restoration of function. Similarly, the goal of cancer rehabilitation continues with this quest. The difference, however, is that the rehabilitation physician needs to look at the cancer patient with a sense of urgency. Built into the rehabilitation process is an anticipation that a patient's current functioning may be fleeting. The goal, therefore, is to allow for independence in the home whenever this is possible. To that end, the cancer patient needs to be evaluated on a fairly routine basis. Interventions need to be swift—especially if there has been an acute decline in mobility or

function. When the patient finds himself back in the hospital, the objective is efficient, systemic, spiritual, and ethical care—before returning the patient safely home. This often requires a close integrative "well-greased" machine of therapists and symptom management experts.

TEACHING POINTS

1. Traditional rehabilitation and cancer rehabilitation utilize similar treatment and intervention strategies. The approach to care is multidisciplinary.
2. Cancer rehabilitation is focused on the urgency of functional restoration. Time is limited.
3. Cancer rehabilitation has to dynamically involve symptom management and oncology specialists for a safe return to the home setting.

REFERENCES

Alfano CM, Ganz PA, Rowland JH. Cancer survivorship and cancer rehabilitation: Revitalizing the link. *J Clin Oncol* 2012;30:904–906.

DeLisa JA. A history of cancer rehabilitation. *Cancer Suppl* 2001;92:970–974.

Fu J. The state of cancer rehabilitation. *J Palliative Care Med* 2012;2:1–2.

Gamble GL, Gerber LH, Spill GR. The future of cancer rehabilitation: Emerging subspecialty. *Am J Phys Med Rehabil* 2011;90(Suppl):S83–S94.

Mellette SJ, Parker GG. Future directions in cancer rehabilitation. *Semin Oncol Nurs* 1992;8:219–223.

Paul K, Buschbacher R. Cancer rehabilitation: Increasing awareness and removing barriers. *Am J Phys Med Rehabil* 2011;90(Suppl):S1–S4.

Silver JK. Strategies to overcome cancer survivorship care barriers. *Phys Med Rehabil* 2011;3:503–506.

Vargo MM. The oncology-rehabilitation interface: Better systems needed. *J Clin Oncol* 2009;26:2610–2611.

129

Long-term cognitive function

ASAO OGAWA

INTRODUCTION

In recent years, cancer treatment has progressed remarkably owing to the development of various molecular biological approaches and advances in therapeutic drugs. In the past, surgical excision was the only way of treating cancer. Now, drug therapy, radiotherapy, and surgery are established as the three pillars of cancer treatment. Furthermore, regarding drug therapy, in addition to various cytocidal antineoplastic drugs, hormone therapy and molecularly targeted drugs have been successively developed and introduced into clinical practice. Multidisciplinary treatment combining these approaches is the mainstay of current cancer treatment. As a result, in addition to the maintenance of physical function, patients now have longer life expectancy with cancer treatment.

While the treatment methods have advanced greatly, adverse events (side effects) may be associated with any treatment. Some cancer treatments affect various organs not only because of direct actions but also because of various direct or indirect physical burdens. As for the neurological system, it is reported that drug therapy can cause acute or chronic peripheral nerve disorders and central nervous system disorders such as encephalitis and encephalopathy. These treatment-related cognitive dysfunctions are now collectively referred to as cancer brain. Especially, in recent years, the terminology cancer brain has also been widely used to include the effects of malignant neoplasm per se on the central nervous system. Lowered quality of life due to cancer per se or treatment during healing or follow-up has attracted attention.

This chapter discusses the relationship between cancer and central nervous disorders generally and the effects of cancer and drug therapy in particular.

INTRACRANIAL METASTASIS

Cancer metastatic to brain is the most prevalent complication seen in about 10% of cancer patients [1]. In particular, the frequency of brain metastases has increased in recent years because of a rise in the response rate to systemic chemotherapy and subsequent improvement of life expectancy. The primary diseases responsible for brain metastases include lung cancer (50%–60%), breast cancer (15%–20%), malignant melanoma (5%–10%), and digestive tract tumors (4%–6%) [2].

Generally, brain metastases present with very severe symptoms and the prognosis is very poor, varying according to histological types, metastatic sites, the number and size of the site, neurological symptoms, and accompanying symptoms. Metastatic brain tumor is associated with poor systemic conditions and mortality and is the main cause of approximately one-third of deaths [3]. Patients die of neurological complications within 4 weeks of the detection of brain metastasis if left to its natural course; even when corticosteroid treatment is used to reduce brain edema, the remaining life expectancy is 8 weeks at best. Furthermore, when surgery or radiotherapy is used concomitantly, the remaining life expectancy is 12–20 weeks [1].

METABOLIC CENTRAL NERVOUS SYSTEM DISORDERS

Metabolic disorders are widely observed in cancer patients (Table 129.1). Many of them develop following organ disorders (hepatic metastasis, renal metastasis, etc.) secondary to tumor metastasis, poor nutritional conditions, or infections; however, some of them occur because of the secretion of hormone-related substances from the tumors [4].

Metabolic central nervous system disorders are diagnosed as delirium. Patients who were referred to psychiatric consultation for "altered mental status" or "confusion" accounted for 16% according to a previous follow-up survey. About 30% of metabolic central nervous system disorders are caused by metabolic disorders alone [4].

Although it has been thought that delirium is a temporary state and self-limiting even if it is not treated pharmacologically, delirium may result in long-term cognitive impairment. In a recent study on cognitive trajectory after cardiac surgery, 40% of patients with postoperative delirium had not returned to their preoperative baseline level at 6 months. By comparison, 24% of patients without postoperative delirium had not recovered baseline function [5].

Table 129.1 *Cancer and metabolic central nervous system disorders*

Organ failure	Respiratory failure	Hypoxemia
		Hypercapnia
	Liver	Liver failure (hyperammonemia)
	Kidney	Uremia
Electrolyte abnormality	Hypercalcemia	
	Hyponatremia	
	Other electrolyte abnormalities	
Hypoglycemia	Diabetes mellitus	
	Terminal phase	
	Paraneoplastic syndrome	
	Increased glucose metabolism due to tumor proliferation	
	Drug-induced	
Hyperglycemia	Diabetes mellitus	
	Steroid-induced	
Vitamin deficiency	Vitamin B1	
	Vitamin B12	
Endocrine dysfunction	Adrenal failure	
	Thyroid dysfunction	
Septic encephalopathy		
Drug-induced	Antineoplastic drugs	
	Anticonvulsants	
	Morphine	
	Antianxiety drugs	
	Antipsychotic drugs	
	Antidepressant drugs	

There is a link between delirium and dementia. Cognitive impairment has been consistently demonstrated to be a significant risk factor for delirium. Both dementia and delirium are associated with metabolic changes. Incident delirium has been shown to accelerate the trajectory of cognitive dysfunction in hospitalized patients with Alzheimer's disease. Clinical investigations show that delirium leads to reduced blood flow in subcortical structures. The association between long-term cognitive impairment and episodes of delirium is unknown in cancer treatment. Further research is required to explore whether delirium is associated with the cognitive impairment in cancer.

NEUROTOXICITY DUE TO ANTICANCER DRUGS

Anticancer drugs cause a wide variety of neurotoxicities. The occurrence of neurotoxicity due to anticancer drugs is affected not only by the mode of action of the drugs but also by the method of administration, dose, presence/absence of concomitant therapies, etc.

In particular, leukoencephalopathy is an acute neurotoxicity known to occur in the central nervous system. Leukoencephalopathy is a syndrome that presents with gait disorder, autonomic nerve symptoms, and psychoneurological symptoms including memory disturbance after the administration of anticancer drugs. In addition, the disease can cause disturbance of consciousness. Although the frequency is rare, once the disease develops, the symptoms become serious and can cause irreversible neuropathy. Neurotoxicity occurs after treatment with 5-fluorouracil, methotrexate, cyclophosphamide, carmofur, tegafur, etc.

COGNITIVE DYSFUNCTION DUE TO ANTICANCER DRUGS

In addition to the acute neurotoxicities described earlier, subtle cognitive dysfunction possibly occurs after treatment with anticancer drugs.

Previous studies have shown that patients who received anticancer treatment complained of being unable to concentrate or feeling foggy-headed and dopey. Such case reports have been published since the 1980s, but patient groups voiced their opinions in the 1990s that these reports could be obstacles to their social rehabilitation. Since then, cognitive dysfunction associated with drug treatment has been collectively known as "chemo brain" or "chemo fog" [6]. Follow-up surveys have been conducted since 2000.

Cognitive dysfunction has mainly been investigated in breast cancer patients, but it can occur in patients with other types of cancer [7]. The prevalence of objectively measured cognitive impairment following chemotherapy varies from 15% to 50% of patients with solid tumors [8]. It has been reported that even in cases where cognitive dysfunction was subtle, various symptoms such as deterioration in verbal memory, visual memory, psychomotor speed, or executive function were observed [9].

Recently, reports of meta-analysis summarizing longitudinal studies have been published. Firstly, Anderson-Hanley et al. examined the subitems of cognitive function tests (attention and information processing, verbal memory, visual memory, spatial function, executive function, and motor function) based on 30 research papers on cognitive function in patients who received anticancer drug treatment (most patients had breast cancer, but some had other types of cancer) [10]. Comparison of those patients who received anticancer treatment with those who did not showed that the test results for the former group were lower than those for the latter group in all items. However, when the test results before and after cancer treatment were compared, no significant differences were observed. Psychophysiological symptoms such as insomnia, anxiety, and depression, which are considered to be factors affecting cognitive function, are observed frequently (30%–40%) in cancer patients. Because the effects of these symptoms could not be ruled out, the authors suggested that further studies adjusting for background factors should be conducted.

In 2006, Stewart et al. conducted meta-analysis in which they observed mild to moderate cognitive dysfunction in all items, including attention and concentration, working memory, and short-term memory [11]. Jansen et al. also reported that while subjective symptoms regarding cognitive dysfunction were prominent, cognitive dysfunction detected by neuropsychological examination was generally mild, an outcome in common with other studies [12].

The cognitive dysfunction profile may not yet be clear because of the following reasons:

1. Because of study design, there are very few controlled studies comparing patients before and after anticancer treatment.
2. Because of study characteristics, the sample sizes of most studies are small.
3. Because of the characteristics of neuropsychological examination, learning can affect the results.
4. Because of neuropsychological examinations, many items are tested at the same time, leading to problems caused by multiple testing. Also, these examinations provide the best performance in an ideal situation, and findings may not detect mild cognitive impairment evident in daily life.

In particular, because neuropsychological examinations were originally developed for diseases with defined lesions such as cerebral infarction, whether this evaluation method is suitable for examining conditions where sites of lesions are not identified and where disorders are subtle should be reexamined. As is often discussed in the case of dementia, the brain has residual capacity that is expected to compensate for subtle cognitive dysfunction. If evaluation of conditions where these compensatory functions are mobilized becomes possible, then more appropriate evaluation of the clinical conditions of cognitive function may become possible.

INVESTIGATION OF COGNITIVE FUNCTION AND BACKGROUND FACTORS

Cognitive dysfunction and its background factors associated with chemotherapy have been investigated. Falleti et al. conducted a meta-analysis based on five cross-sectional studies and one longitudinal study and reported that (1) subtle cognitive dysfunction was observed in overall cognitive functions (six areas except attention and concentration), (2) cognitive dysfunction was gradually improved after the completion of treatment, (3) cognitive dysfunction increased with age, and (4) concomitant use of hormone therapy with tamoxifen worsened cognitive dysfunction [13].

PATHOGENIC MECHANISM OF COGNITIVE DYSFUNCTION

Anticancer drugs are administered systemically. Although anticancer drugs are considered to act systemically, historically, attention has not been paid to their effects on the central nervous system. There are two reasons for this: (1) Penetration of anticancer drugs into the central nervous system was considered small due to the blood–brain barrier (BBB) and (2) the effects of anticancer drugs on neurons, which do not undergo cell division, were considered small in view of the mode of action of anticancer drugs, which is to inhibit DNA synthesis or cell division associated with the unlimited proliferation of cancer cells.

Indeed, determining whether anticancer drugs are active against the central nervous system can be difficult. Clinically, a PET study investigating the brain penetrability of paclitaxel has shown that the efficacy of systemic chemotherapy for metastatic brain tumor is low and that the concentration of paclitaxel in the brain was low [14,15]. In contrast, anticancer drugs cause peripheral neuropathy and leukoencephalopathy, which is a condition of acute toxicity in the central nervous system. Thus, the occurrence of adverse events in the central nervous system may depend not only on penetrability into the central nervous system but also on the mode of action and penetrability of drugs.

At the same time, the pathogenic mechanism by which anticancer drugs damage the central nervous system is also important. Ahles et al. summarized the pathogenic mechanisms considered to underlie cognitive dysfunction associated with chemotherapy [16]. By adding currently considered mechanisms to the mechanisms summarized by the authors, their summary of mechanisms are shown as follows:

1. *Direct injury hypothesis*
   Anticancer drugs entering the central nervous system injure the DNA, RNA, or microtubules of neurons directly and induce apoptosis of the neurons.
   Anticancer drugs may injure the surrounding supporting cells such as astrocytes and microglia and cause inflammatory reactions and subsequently injure neurons by a similar mechanism.
2. *Secondary dysfunction hypothesis*
   Systemic administration of anticancer drugs causes systemic inflammatory reactions. Cytokines (IL-6 and/or TNF-α) produced as a result penetrate into the central nervous system, causing secondary dysfunction.
   With regard to similar pathology, the relationship between inflammatory cytokine concentrations and brain volume or cognitive function in a systemic inflammatory disease has been reported.
3. *Indirect injury hypothesis*
   Anticancer drugs act not only on tumors but also on cells throughout the body. In particular, vascular endothelial cells are exposed to high concentrations of drugs and are known to be easily injured, resulting in angiitis. Thus, angiopathy can occur not only in great blood vessels but also in peripheral blood vessels. In the brain in particular, microangiopathy causes ischemia and circulatory disturbance, which lead to dysfunction of the BBB. This causes brain edema and metabolic disorder, which indirectly lead to inflammation in supporting cells, resulting in neuronal injury.

In addition to the injury mechanism, protective factors have also been examined. Similar to other central nervous system disorders, it has been hypothesized that the following may be related to the extent of injury: (1) the effects of protective factors/nutritional factors such as apolipoprotein E (ApoE) gene polymorphism and brain-derived neurotrophic factor (BDNF) gene polymorphism; (2) factors related to the metabolism of neurotransmitters, such as catechol-O-methyltransferase gene polymorphism; and (3) polymorphisms that remove harmful substances from cells and are related to the BBB, such as the multidrug resistance 1 (MDR1) gene encoding P-glycoprotein (P-gp) [16]. Ahles et al. examined the relationship between the extent of injury and ApoE gene polymorphism and reported that after chemotherapy was given, the extent of cognitive dysfunction in cancer patients possessing the ApoE4 gene was greater than that in patients without ApoE4 [17].

INVESTIGATIONS USING ANIMAL MODELS

The pathogenic mechanism of central nervous system injury by anticancer drugs has also been studied, albeit at a slow pace. These studies are performed mainly in rats. One paper reported that methotrexate caused injury in the vascular endothelium of the dentate gyrus [18]; another paper described that 5-fluorouracil induced inflammatory reactions in the brain or caused apoptosis of the vascular endothelium [19]. Furthermore, cyclophosphamide and doxorubicin decreased short-term memory in the avoidance task [20], and methotrexate decreased exploratory behavior or lowered performance in the spatial cognition task and memory task. The effect of anticancer drugs on oxidative stress and on white-matter deficit can also be speculated from animal models [20]. However, the relationship between human and animal pathologies is not clear because single administration is used in most animal experiments (multiple administrations are used mostly in humans) and because the doses used in animals are extremely higher than those used in humans. Future studies should investigate the reproducibility of low-dose repeated administration that mimics the dosage regimen for humans, the effects of intravascular administration (peritoneal administration is used mostly in animal experiments), and evaluation methods that correspond to cognition tasks for humans.

NEUROSCIENTIFIC INVESTIGATION

Other neuroscientific investigations regarding the effect of anticancer drugs are also in progress. With regard to neurophysiological investigations, a decrease in the amplitude of event-related potential P300 or an abnormality in basic rhythm related to attention has been reported [21]. Methods to examine the structure of the brain more closely have also been investigated. Using diffusion tensor imaging, Abraham et al. examined the changes in the orientation of white-matter fibers after adjuvant chemotherapy for breast cancer and reported that anisotropy in the genu of corpus callosum was higher in breast cancer patients than in healthy subjects [22].

Furthermore, a new approach investigating changes in the activated area of the brain undergoing cognition tasks by functional MRI was reported. Silverman et al. measured functional MR images of monozygotic twins, one of whom was a breast cancer patient who received adjuvant chemotherapy for the disease and the other who was healthy and did not receive adjuvant chemotherapy, undergoing cognition tasks, and found that the area of signal change was wider in the breast cancer patient than in the other twin [23]. However, no difference in the performance of the task was observed between the twins, and the authors concluded that the results reflected mobilization of functional compensation.

CANCER BRAIN AND DEPRESSION

As described earlier, the confounding effects of anticancer drugs or neoplasm on the central nervous system have been investigated mainly with regard to cognition dysfunction. On the other hand, the associations between cognitive impairment and emotional distress are discussed. Peppelreuter et al. showed the significant relationships were not significant between the results of the neuropsychological testing and the current affective status or self-reports of attentional deficits in daily life [24]. Subjective cognitive impairment may indicate emotional distress more than objective cognitive dysfunction.

COGNITIVE DYSFUNCTION DUE TO RADIATION THERAPY

Whole-brain radiation therapy

Whole-brain radiation therapy (WBRT) is the standard treatment given for brain metastases, employing external beam, fractionated radiation of approximately 30–36 Gy given over 2 or 3 weeks. WBRT palliates symptoms and improves neurologic function in approximately 60% of patients.

The long-term side effect has to do with deterioration of cognitive function. The most common is with short-term memory loss and decrease in attention, but severe dementia can occur in a small number of cases. In a study published by DeAngelis et al., the incidence of severe dementia was 1.9%–5.1% [25]. Moretti et al. published the paper that compared neurocognitive side effects of patients that received different doses of WBRT [26]. It was found that with doses less than 35 Gy, there were no signs of neurocognitive side effects; between 35 and 45 Gy, there was slowness of executive function and profound alterations of frontal functions (attention, focusing, mentation control, analytical judgment, and insight); and with doses greater than 45 Gy, there was profound cognitive decline.

Prophylactic cranial irradiation

Small-cell lung cancer (SCLC) progresses with distant metastases occurring early in the course of the disease. The brain is an important site of tumor relapse. It has been presumed that the microscopic tumor is protected against systemic chemotherapy by the intact BBB. In fact, about 50% of patients with SCLC have a risk of brain metastases in two years, and numerous studies demonstrated that Prophylactic cranial irradiation (PCI) decreased the risk of brain metastasis and prolonged progression-free survival and overall survival.

On the other hand, PCI has potential long-term side effect, such as leukoencephalopathy and dementia. These effects usually occur about 6 months to a year after radiation. A mild, long-term neurocognitive impairment is recognized in adult cancer patients. Two prospective studies did not show the increased incidence of neuropsychological impairments in the patients with PCI [27,28]; however, others have argued that the small numbers of long-term survivors precluded accurate assessment of the risk of leukoencephalopathy [29].

COGNITIVE DYSFUNCTION IN NONCANCER PATIENTS

Heart failure

Advances in the treatment of ischemic heart disease have increased the survival of an elderly population with chronic heart failure. The prevalence of chronic heart failure is estimated 3%–10% among those over 75. Recently, heart failure has been proposed as a possible cause of cognitive impairment. The reported prevalence of cognitive impairment in heart failure ranged from 25% to 74% [30–32].

The prevention of cognitive impairment is associated with the disease control. About 50% of hospital admission for heart failure are associated with poor adherence with a prescribed management plan. Among patients hospitalized for decompensated chronic heart failure, 42%–80% were noncompliant with medications, and 49%–78% were noncompliant with diet [33]. Several studies showed that decreased heart function, as measured by indices of low cardiac output, is independently associated with poor results in various cognitive domains [34,35].

Several mechanisms that play an important role in induction of cognitive impairment have been identified. These include vascular injury from ischemic stroke, cardiac surgery, and chronic cerebral hypoperfusion.

STROKE

Chronic heart failure is one of the most common conditions leading to stroke and the main causes of heart failure;

dilated cardiomyopathy increases the risk of stroke by twofold to threefold [36]. Most have a cardioembolic mechanism. Especially left ventricular dysfunction can increase diastolic volume and trigger thrombus formation. Multiple subcortical infarctions are clinically silent and have been identified in 34% of patients prior to heart transplantation [37]. Also, atrial fibrillation, complicating chronic heart failure in elderly, is the independent risk factor of cognitive impairment and increases the risk threefold.

CEREBRAL HYPOPERFUSION

In chronic heart failure, cardiac output decreases and the distribution of blood flow is remodeled. Ischemia does not result from heart failure because brain blood flow is maintained at near-normal levels over a wide range of systemic blood pressures (autoregulation). However, long-term decline of cardiac output exhausts the heart and autoregulation is broken down.

Reversibility

Although the studies were limited, cognitive impairment related to cardiac heart failure would be reversible. Some studies reported the cognitive functions improved in the patients with cardiac transplantation [36,38].

CONCLUSION

Cancer-related cognitive impairment is an important clinical problem that negatively impacts quality of life for cancer patients. However, the definition of the cognitive impairment remains at odds and there is a lack of information about the phenomena. Despite these discrepancies, patient perceptions of the cognitive problems in daily life are important. Further research is needed to declare the phenomena and mechanisms of cancer-related cognitive dysfunction.

Key learning points

- Long-term cognitive impairment is an important problem that has a negative influence on the quality of life.

- The prevalence of objectively measured cognitive impairment following chemotherapy varies from 15% to 50% of cancer patients.

- Cognitive dysfunction detected by neuropsychological examination was diffuse and generally mild.

- Subjective cognitive impairment may indicate emotional distress more than objective cognitive dysfunction.

REFERENCES

1 Barnholtz-Sloan JS, Sloan AE, Davis FG, Vigneau FD, Lai P, Sawaya RE. Incidence proportions of brain metastases in patients diagnosed (1973 to 2001) in the Metropolitan Detroit Cancer Surveillance System. *J Clin Oncol.* 2004 July 15;22(14):2865–2872.

◆ 2 Langer CJ, Mehta MP. Current management of brain metastases, with a focus on systemic options. *J Clin Oncol.* 2005 Sept 1;23(25):6207–6219.

3 Bajaj GK, Kleinberg L, Terezakis S. Current concepts and controversies in the treatment of parenchymal brain metastases: Improved outcomes with aggressive management. *Cancer Invest.* 2005;23(4):363–376.

4 Clouston PD, DeAngelis LM, Posner JB. The spectrum of neurological disease in patients with systemic cancer. *Ann Neurol.* 1992 Mar;31(3):268–273.

5 Selnes OA, Gottesman RF, Grega MA, Baumgartner WA, Zeger SL, McKhann GM. Cognitive and neurologic outcomes after coronary-artery bypass surgery. *N Engl J Med.* 2012 Jan 19;366(3):250–257.

6 President's Cancer Panel. 1998. Cancer Care Issues in the United States: Quality of Care, Quality of Life. NCI Web site, http://deainfo.nci.nih.gov/advisory/pcp/archive/index.htm

7 Tannock IF, Ahles TA, Ganz PA, Van Dam FS. Cognitive impairment associated with chemotherapy for cancer: Report of a workshop. *J Clin Oncol.* 2004 June 1;22(11):2233–2239.

◆ 8 Vardy J, Tannock I. Cognitive function after chemotherapy in adults with solid tumours. *Crit Rev Oncol Hematol.* 2007 Sept;63(3):183–202.

9 Vardy J, Wefel JS, Ahles T, Tannock IF, Schagen SB. Cancer and cancer-therapy related cognitive dysfunction: An international perspective from the Venice cognitive workshop. *Ann Oncol.* 2008 Apr;19(4):623–629.

◆ 10 Anderson-Hanley C, Sherman ML, Riggs R, Agocha VB, Compas BE. Neuropsychological effects of treatments for adults with cancer: A meta-analysis and review of the literature. *J Int Neuropsychol Soc.* 2003 Nov;9(7):967–982.

11 Stewart A, Bielajew C, Collins B, Parkinson M, Tomiak E. A meta-analysis of the neuropsychological effects of adjuvant chemotherapy treatment in women treated for breast cancer. *Clin Neuropsychol.* 2006 Feb;20(1):76–89.

◆ 12 Jansen CE, Miaskowski C, Dodd M, Dowling G, Kramer J. A metaanalysis of studies of the effects of cancer chemotherapy on various domains of cognitive function. *Cancer* 2005 Nov 15;104(10):2222–2233.

13 Falleti MG, Sanfilippo A, Maruff P, Weih L, Phillips KA. The nature and severity of cognitive impairment associated with adjuvant chemotherapy in women with breast cancer: A meta-analysis of the current literature. *Brain Cogn.* 2005 Oct;59(1):60–70.

14 Gangloff A, Hsueh WA, Kesner AL, Kiesewetter DO, Pio BS, Pegram MD et al. Estimation of paclitaxel biodistribution and uptake in human-derived xenografts in vivo with (18)F-fluoropaclitaxel. *J Nucl Med.* 2005 Nov;46(11):1866–1871.

15 Hsueh WA, Kesner AL, Gangloff A, Pegram MD, Beryt M, Czernin J et al. Predicting chemotherapy response to paclitaxel with 18F-Fluoropaclitaxel and PET. *J Nucl Med.* 2006 Dec;47(12):1995–1999.

◆ 16 Ahles TA, Saykin AJ. Candidate mechanisms for chemotherapy-induced cognitive changes. *Nat Rev Cancer* 2007 Mar;7(3):192–201.

17 Ahles TA, Saykin AJ, Noll WW, Furstenberg CT, Guerin S, Cole B et al. The relationship of APOE genotype to neuropsychological performance in long-term cancer survivors treated with standard dose chemotherapy. *Psychooncology* 2003 Sept;12(6):612–619.

18 Seigers R, Timmermans J, van der Horn HJ, de Vries EF, Dierckx RA, Visser L et al. Methotrexate reduces hippocampal blood vessel density and activates microglia in rats but does not elevate central cytokine release. *Behav Brain Res.* 2010 Mar 5;207(2):265–272.

19 Han R, Yang YM, Dietrich J, Luebke A, Mayer-Proschel M, Noble M. Systemic 5-fluorouracil treatment causes a syndrome of delayed myelin destruction in the central nervous system. *J Biol.* 2008;7(4):12.

20 Konat GW, Kraszpulski M, James I, Zhang HT, Abraham J. Cognitive dysfunction induced by chronic administration of common cancer chemotherapeutics in rats. *Metab Brain Dis.* 2008 Sept;23(3):325–333.

21 Kreukels BP, Schagen SB, Ridderinkhof KR, Boogerd W, Hamburger HL, van Dam FS. Electrophysiological correlates of information processing in breast-cancer patients treated with adjuvant chemotherapy. *Breast Cancer Res Treat.* 2005 Nov;94(1):53–61.

22 Abraham J, Haut MW, Moran MT, Filburn S, Lemiuex S, Kuwabara H. Adjuvant chemotherapy for breast cancer: Effects on cerebral white matter seen in diffusion tensor imaging. *Clin Breast Cancer* 2008 Feb;8(1):88–91.

23 Silverman DH, Dy CJ, Castellon SA, Lai J, Pio BS, Abraham L et al. Altered frontocortical, cerebellar, and basal ganglia activity in adjuvant-treated breast cancer survivors 5–10 years after chemotherapy. *Breast Cancer Res Treat.* 2007 July;103(3):303–311.

24 Poppelreuter M, Weis J, Kulz AK, Tucha O, Lange KW, Bartsch HH. Cognitive dysfunction and subjective complaints of cancer patients. A cross-sectional study in a cancer rehabilitation centre. *Eur J Cancer* 2004 Jan;40(1):43–49.

25 DeAngelis LM, Delattre JY, Posner JB. Radiation-induced dementia in patients cured of brain metastases. *Neurology* 1989 June;39(6):789–796.

26 Moretti R, Torre P, Antonello RM, Cattaruzza T, Cazzato G, Bava A et al. Neuropsychological evaluation of late-onset post-radiotherapy encephalopathy: A comparison with vascular dementia. *J Neurol Sci.* 2005 Mar 15;229–230:195–200.

27 Arriagada R, Le Chevalier T, Borie F, Riviere A, Chomy P, Monnet I et al. Prophylactic cranial irradiation for patients with small-cell lung cancer in complete remission. *J Natl Cancer Inst.* 1995 Feb 1;87(3):183–190.

28 Gregor A, Cull A, Stephens RJ, Kirkpatrick JA, Yarnold JR, Girling DJ et al. Prophylactic cranial irradiation is indicated following complete response to induction therapy in small cell lung cancer: Results of a multicentre randomised trial. United Kingdom Coordinating Committee for Cancer Research (UKCCCR) and the European Organization for Research and Treatment of Cancer (EORTC). *Eur J Cancer* 1997 Oct;33(11):1752–1758.

29 Bunn PA Jr., Kelly K. Prophylactic cranial irradiation for patients with small-cell lung cancer. *J Natl Cancer Inst.* 1995 Feb 1;87(3):161–162.

30 Grubb NR, Simpson C, Fox KA. Memory function in patients with stable, moderate to severe cardiac failure. *Am Heart J.* 2000 July;140(1):E1–E5.

31 Gorkin L, Norvell NK, Rosen RC, Charles E, Shumaker SA, McIntyre KM et al. Assessment of quality of life as observed from the baseline data of the Studies of Left Ventricular Dysfunction (SOLVD) trial quality-of-life substudy. *Am J Cardiol.* 1993 May 1;71(12):1069–1073.

32 Petrucci RJ, Truesdell KC, Carter A, Goldstein NE, Russell MM, Dilkes D et al. Cognitive dysfunction in advanced heart failure and prospective cardiac assist device patients. *Ann Thorac Surg.* 2006 May;81(5):1738–1744.

33 Evangelista LS, Dracup K. A closer look at compliance research in heart failure patients in the last decade. *Prog Cardiovasc Nurs.* 2000 Summer;15(3):97–103.

34 Trojano L, Antonelli Incalzi R, Acanfora D, Picone C, Mecocci P, Rengo F. Cognitive impairment: A key feature of congestive heart failure in the elderly. *J Neurol.* 2003 Dec;250(12):1456–1463.

35 Bennett SJ, Sauve MJ. Cognitive deficits in patients with heart failure: A review of the literature. *J Cardiovasc Nurs.* 2003 July–Aug;18(3):219–242.

36 Putzke JD, Williams MA, Rayburn BK, Kirklin JK, Boll TJ. The relationship between cardiac function and neuropsychological status among heart transplant candidates. *J Card Fail.* 1998 Dec;4(4):295–303.

37 Siachos T, Vanbakel A, Feldman DS, Uber W, Simpson KN, Pereira NL. Silent strokes in patients with heart failure. *J Card Fail.* 2005 Sept;11(7):485–489.

38 Grimm M, Yeganehfar W, Laufer G, Madl C, Kramer L, Eisenhuber E et al. Cyclosporine may affect improvement of cognitive brain function after successful cardiac transplantation. *Circulation* 1996 Sept 15;94(6):1339–1345.

130

Gonadal functions and reproductive health

KOJI KAWAI, HIROYUKI NISHIYAMA

INTRODUCTION

Recently, gonadal dysfunctions and alterations in reproductive health have been recognized as the most common long-term morbidity in cancer survivors. The clinical manifestations of gonadal dysfunction vary widely by patient age and gender, type of cancer, and treatment modality. A woman who survives cancer may develop menopausal symptoms due to aging regardless of the cancer type or cancer treatment. In addition, as the testosterone level decreases with normal aging, a male patient can suffer from similar symptoms, termed late-onset hypogonadism (LOH). The symptoms of menopause and LOH are wide ranging and nonspecific, and the physician should be aware of these symptoms. In this chapter, we review the current understanding of the roles that sex hormones play in health and quality of life (QoL) separate from, as well as including, sexual function. Also, we briefly discuss the current status and future direction of fertility-preservation technologies for cancer survivors.

PHYSIOLOGICAL REGULATION OF SEX HORMONES

In both men and women, gonadal function is regulated by the hypothalamic–pituitary–gonadal axis (Figure 130.1). The hypothalamus synthesizes and releases gonadotropin-releasing hormone (Gn-RH) into the hypothalamohypophyseal portal circulation in a pulsatile fashion. The Gn-RH stimulates the anterior pituitary gland to secrete two kinds of gonadotropins, luteinizing hormone (LH) and follicle-stimulating hormone (FSH). In men, LH controls testosterone synthesis in Leydig cells of the testes. FSH acts on Sertoli cells and supports spermatogenesis in combination with testosterone [1***]. The ovary is responsible for sex hormone production and gamete formation, but it is a more complex endocrine organ. Both theca cells and granulosa cells are required for ovarian follicles to produce estrogen under the control of LH and FSH [2]. The negative and positive feedbacks of the sex hormones, testosterone and estrogen, occur at the pituitary and hypothalamic levels. The inhibin or activin produced

by Leydig cells and granulosa cells negatively regulate FSH secretion by the anterior pituitary gland.

The primary gonadal damage induced by chemotherapy and radiotherapy results in elevation of LH and FSH levels due to negative feedback of sex hormones and inhibin (hypergonadotropic hypogonadism) [3]. Therefore, the LH and FSH levels are used as indicators of primary gonadal dysfunction. In the setting of secondary gonadal damage due to hypothalamic or pituitary dysfunction, both sex hormones and gonadotropins decrease to below the normal range (hypogonadotropic hypogonadism) [3]. This type of gonadal dysfunction is seen in brain tumor patients after surgery or radiotherapy and prostate cancer patients receiving androgen deprivation therapy (ADT).

It is noteworthy that germinal dysfunction and endocrine dysfunction do not necessarily progress synchronously. Generally, endocrine function is better preserved than germinal function. Among testicular cells, Leydig cells are more resistant to radiation damage than spermatogonia and can retain function after fractionated radiation to the testis of less than 20 Gy [4]. Thus, infertility may occur in patients having normal sexual function with normal sex hormone and gonadotropin levels.

PATHOPHYSIOLOGY OF SEX HORMONE DEFICIENCY IN CANCER SURVIVORS

Women

Most women experience the permanent cessation of menstruation by their mid-50s. Menopause is diagnosed retrospectively after 1 year of amenorrhea. During the perimenopausal period, including that preceding both the menopausal transition and after the postmenopausal transition, some women suffer from a variety of symptoms related to ovarian dysfunction, but others experience few symptoms and some absolutely none.

The multimodality used in cancer treatment including surgery, radiotherapy, chemotherapy, and hormone therapy can result in premature menopause and menopause-related symptoms. In premenopausal breast cancer survivors, chemotherapy-related amenorrhea (CRA) is the most significant long-term

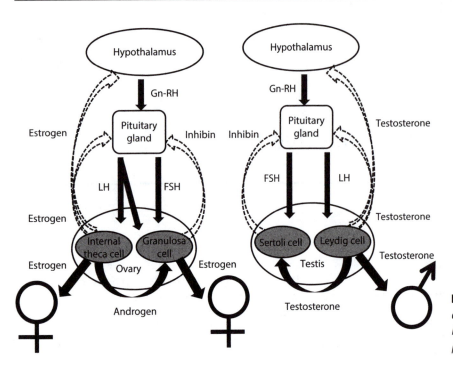

Figure 130.1 *Hypothalamic–pituitary–gonadal axis. The negative and positive feedbacks of the sex hormones, testosterone, and estrogen occur at the pituitary and hypothalamic levels.*

morbidity of adjuvant chemotherapy. Bines et al. reported that CRA rates varied with age, anticancer drugs, and cumulative dose [5*]. The average CRA rate was 68% (range: 20%–80%) in combination chemotherapy with cyclophosphamide, methotrexate, and fluorouracil [5]. Cyclophosphamide, the most widely used drug, is known to affect CRA in a dose-dependent manner. Generally, younger women require a higher dose to produce menopause [6*]. A retrospective review reported that the addition of paclitaxel to the standard anthracycline-based adjuvant chemotherapy did not increase the CRA rates when used to treat breast cancer patients under 40 years old [7*]. As in cases of breast cancer, chemotherapy can damage ovarian function in premenopausal women. Meirow et al. reported that ovarian failure was noted in 34% of young women who received chemotherapy for hematological malignancy or breast cancer [8*]. The risk for developing ovarian failure was highest with alkylating agents, followed by cisplatin.

In gynecological cancer treatment, in addition to chemotherapy, both surgery and radiotherapy can directly induce ovarian damage. Iatrogenic menopause in gynecological cancer patients most often occurs after bilateral oophorectomy, which results in immediate menopause. In these cases, menopausal symptoms are usually more severe than in physiological menopause. It is worth noting that even if an ovary can be partially preserved at surgery, ovarian failure may occur after additional chemotherapy or radiotherapy.

Negative effects on ovarian function are observed after radiotherapy to the abdominal or pelvic region in cases of gynecological cancer, rectal cancer, Hodgkin's lymphoma, and total body irradiation. The estimated dose that induces premature ovarian failure is known to decrease with increasing age at treatment [9*]. Several studies evaluated the risk of infertility and early menopause in female childhood cancer survivors who received abdominal pelvic radiotherapy [10*,11].

The hot flush is the main adverse effect (AE) of administration of tamoxifen, a key drug for hormone-receptor-positive breast cancer patients [12***]. Third-generation aromatase inhibitors (AIs) are also widely used as hormonal therapy for postmenopausal hormone-receptor-positive breast cancer patients. AIs strongly suppress plasma estrogen levels in women, which enhances postmenopausal symptoms. A QoL assessment of breast cancer patients participating in a large randomized study (RCT) revealed that patients treated with anastrozole experienced more vaginal dryness, painful intercourse, and loss of sexual interest than patients treated with tamoxifen [13].

Men

LOH is defined as a clinical and biochemical syndrome associated with advancing age and characterized by typical symptoms and a deficiency in serum testosterone levels [14***]. It may result in significant deterioration in QoL and adversely affect the functions of multiple organ systems [14***]. LOH occurs mainly in the latter half of life, but the prevalence of LOH in the general population is difficult to estimate exactly because the condition is largely underdiagnosed due to its nonspecific presentation. Further, evidence for LOH among male cancer survivors is limited compared to female menopausal symptoms. However, in prostate cancer survivors, where ADT is a widely used treatment modality, decreased libido, erectile dysfunction, and hot flushes are commonly seen AEs [15***]. ADT is the standard management for metastatic prostate cancer and commonly used in an adjuvant setting for locally advanced cases. Although transient flare-ups are noticed, the most frequently used agents, Gn-RH analogues, ultimately decrease the serum testosterone levels to castration levels as effectively as bilateral orchiectomy does.

The nonsteroidal antiandrogens such as bicalutamide, flutamide, and nilutamide, which are competitive inhibitors of androgen binding, show different AE profiles [16], although the nonsteroidal antiandrogens are frequently used in combination with Gn-RH analogues. The testicular germ cell tumor (TGCT) is a representative curable cancer, with recent cure rates reaching over 80% even in metastatic cases with intensive chemotherapy and surgery. Recently, the results of a large population study have revealed the long-term morbidity of TGCT treatment including nephrotoxicity, neurotoxicity, cardiovascular disease, and secondary malignancy [17***]. TGCT patients are known to frequently have hypogonadism before treatment. In addition, as a consequence of multimodality treatment, 12%–16% of TGCT survivors are reported to be classified as having hypogonadal status [18,19]. Although the clinical significance of low-grade hypogonadism in TGTC survivors is less well understood, several studies suggested the association of hypogonadism and development of metabolic syndrome in TGTC survivors [20].

SIGNS AND SYMPTOMS OF SEX HORMONE DEFICIENCY AND OTHER SEXUAL PROBLEMS IN CANCER SURVIVORS

Women

As listed in Table 130.1, a wide range of signs and symptoms are considered to be associated with estrogen withdrawal due to menopause. Some of these symptoms are difficult to distinguish from other age-related changes. Further, it is important to rule out other diseases that may present similar symptoms [21***,22*]. The hot flush, a sudden onset of reddening of the skin over the neck and chest, accompanied by a feeling of warmth, is the most common and bothersome symptom. It may occur several times daily and disrupt the sleep cycle. Vaginal dryness is also a frequent complaint and can be associated with painful intercourse, bleeding, and discharge. In gynecological cancer survivors, these symptoms, along with vaginal stricture and shortening after radical hysterectomy or radiotherapy, can be a major cause of sexual dysfunction. Bergmark et al. reported that persistent vaginal changes compromise sexual activity and result in considerable distress in cervical cancer survivors [23*]. Sleep disturbances may be caused by from menopause itself and confounded by

Table 130.1 *Menopause-related symptoms and signs*

Vasomotor: Hot flush, night sweat
Gynecological: Irregular bleeding, vaginal dryness, dyspareunia
Sleep disturbance
Mood and cognitive function: Anxiety, memory impairment, irritability
Sexual dysfunction
Urinary incontinence
Decrease in bone mineral density
Other somatic symptoms

Table 130.2 *Late-onset hypogonadism-related symptoms and signs*

Sexual dysfunction
Mood and cognitive function: Anxiety, memory impairment, irritability
Sleep disturbance
Decline in muscle mass and strength
Increase in fat mass
Skin and body hair alteration
Decrease in bone mineral density

hot flushes at night [24*]. There is less evidence to show a direct association between ovarian failure and other symptoms, such as mood disturbances, cognitive dysfunction, urinary incontinence, and sexually dysfunction. However, sexual dysfunction is a common morbidity associated with cancer and cancer treatment and is not limited to gynecological cancer [25]. Postmenopausal osteoporosis is a well-known public health issue; physicians should pay attention not only to postmenopausal osteoporosis but also to osteoporosis secondary to treatment-induced gonadal dysfunction.

Men

Sexual dysfunction such as decreased libido and erectile dysfunction are known to be the most common symptoms associated with LOH [14***]. The various symptoms listed in Table 130.2, alterations of mood and cognitive function, sleep disturbance, decline in muscle mass, and others are also associated with hypogonadism in men. As a biochemical assessment of LOH, measurement of serum testosterone levels or serum free testosterone levels is highly recommended [14***], but it is noteworthy that hypogonadism is only one of the multiple factors causing these age-related conditions. It should be kept in mind that the psychiatric symptoms of LOH are not easy to distinguish from those of depression, which requires a psychiatric consultation [26].

Hot flushes affect over half of prostate cancer patients receiving ADT with various severities [27,28]. Most AEs of ADT overlap with those of LOH, but annual bone loss of patients receiving ADT is reported to be more rapid than the age-related decrease [29]. The normocytic, normochromic anemia due to decreased erythropoiesis is commonly seen in ADT and may be responsible for general fatigue.

MANAGEMENT OF SEX HORMONE DEFICIENCY

Women

Strong evidence has shown the efficacy of hormone replace treatment (HRT) with estrogen alone or a combination of estrogen and progestational agents for various menopausal symptoms [21***]. Because unopposed estrogen is a definite risk factor for developing endometrial cancer, the addition of progestational agents to estrogen is recommended in HRT for women with an intact uterus [21***]. Generally, HRT is considered to be contraindicated for patients with estrogen-dependent cancers such as breast cancer, endometrial cancer, and other estrogen-sensitive malignancies [21***]. In contrast, several recent studies suggested the efficacy and safety of HRT in selected breast cancer and endometrial cancer survivors. However, most of these studies are retrospective and comprise insufficient numbers of cases and lengths of observation periods to draw a definitive conclusion [30,31]. Therefore, the physician should discuss the details of the oncological and treatment profile of each patient with the oncologist and inform the patient of the lack of strong evidence when considering HRT for breast cancer and endometrial cancer survivors. It is of note that bothersome menopausal symptoms vary among Asian and Western populations [32*]. Management policy should be tailored to cultural, religious, and also socioeconomic background.

Table 130.3 lists the alternative treatments to HRT for menopausal symptoms. Cigarette smoking and obesity are risk factors for hot flush; therefore, life style changes should be recommended to women who cannot or do not wish to use HRT [33]. The progestational agents megestrol and depot medroxyprogesterone are known to be effective for treatment of hot flushes, but there are limited data to support the safety of long-term progestin use in breast cancer survivors [34]. The efficacy of selective serotonin reuptake inhibitors (SSRIs) for hot flush were shown in RCTs [35**,36**,37**]. The SSRIs are known to inhibit some of the cytochrome P450s. Sterns et al. reported that serum concentrations of endoxifen, a tamoxifen metabolite, was decreased with combined use of tamoxifen and paroxetine [38], although long-term data on oncological outcomes are lacking. Vitamin E is relatively safe but marginally effective treatment for hot flush. A vaginal moisturizer can be used for palliation of vaginal symptoms. If nonhormonal preparations fail to control the symptoms, a low-dose estrogen cream is another option. However, estrogen cream results in some degree of systemic absorption; therefore, the physician should inform the patient of both the benefit and the lack of sufficient data on the safety of the preparation for breast cancer survivors [39].

Table 130.3 *Alternatives to hormone replacement therapy for menopausal symptoms*

Hot flush
Lifestyle modification
Megestrol: 20–40 mg orally/day
Depot medroxyprogesterone: 500 mg intramuscularly every 2 weeks
Selective serotonin reuptake inhibitors (venlafaxine, fluoxetine, paroxetine)
Vitamin E: 800 mg orally/day

Vaginal dryness
Vaginal moisturizer
Vaginal estrogen creams

Osteoporosis
Vitamin D: 400–800 IU orally/day
Calcium: 1000–1500 mg orally/day
Bisphosphonates

Men

Studies have demonstrated improvement of multiple symptoms with HRT using testosterone in patients with biochemical evidence of LOH [14]. The contraindications of HRT in the general population include suspected and diagnosed prostate cancer and breast cancer, polycythemia, sleep apnea, severe heart failure, and severe symptoms of benign prostatic hypertrophy [14]. There are some data to support the use of progestational agents, antidepressants, and gabapentin for palliation of hot flushes induced by ADT [15]. However, several case reports described the progression of prostate cancer after the use of progestational agents, probably due to a mechanism similar to that of nonsteroidal antiandrogen withdrawal syndrome [40*,41].

PRACTICAL MANAGEMENT OF INFERTILITY AFTER CANCER TREATMENT

Infertility is defined as the biological inability to conceive after 1 year of intercourse without contraception. Treatment-induced infertility can be a source of emotional distress to cancer survivors and can significantly affect QoL. Although surgery on the genitourinary tract or radiation of the gonads can damage reproductive function, we will discuss chemotherapy-induced reproductive dysfunction in this chapter. As shown in Table 130.4, the risks of drug-induced hypospermatogenesis differ among anticancer drugs. The risk of infertility varies with the chemotherapy regimen. Because most patients are treated with combination chemotherapy, data concerning the risk of individual drugs are limited. However, the alkylating agents (except dacarbazine) and cisplatin are known to be highly associated with infertility. A high cumulative dose of cyclophosphamide, chlorambucil, procarbazine, and cisplatin can induce prolonged azoospermia [42***]. In TGCT chemotherapy, in which cisplatin is the key drug, infertility is the most important long-term morbidity [43***]. In addition to chemotherapy, over half of TGCT patients have impaired spermatogenesis before treatment [44]. This is possibly due to preexisting testicular dysgenesis syndrome, history of cryptorchidism, human chorionic gonadotropin production by the tumor, and other tumor-related factors. Because some tumor-related factors are eliminated by successful treatment, the reported rates of successful paternity after TGCT chemotherapy are 70%–80% [45,46*]. However, this depends on the number of chemotherapy cycles received, and several authors reported a higher risk of infertility in patients who received more than four cycles of cisplatin-based chemotherapy [44,47]. In combination chemotherapy, an additive effect of each drug is observed. When cyclophosphamide is used with doxorubicin, vincristine, prednisone, and bleomycin (CHOP-Bleo), the standard chemotherapy for non-Hodgkin's lymphoma, the low cumulative dose of cyclophosphamide can induce prolonged sterility [48*]. In Hodgkin's lymphoma, a prospective study showed that the combination of mechlorethamine, vincristine, procarbazine, prednisone (MOPP) induced

Table 130.4 *Common anticancer drugs associated with hypospermatogenesis*

	Agents		
Severe	Cyclophosphamide Procarbazine	Chlorambucil Cisplatin	Busulfan
Moderate	Doxorubicin Etoposide	Dactinomycin D Cytarabine	Vinblastine
Mild	Vincristine 6-Mercaptopurine	Methotrexate	5-Fluorouracil

infertility at significantly higher rates than the alternative regimen using doxorubicin, bleomycin, vinblastine, dacarbazine (ABVD) [49*].

Recent developments of reproductive technology such as in vitro fertilization (IVF) and intracytoplasmic sperm injection (ICSI) make sperm cryopreservation a more important and efficacious procedure for preserving the fertility potential of men treated with chemotherapy. The guidelines recommend that sperm cryopreservation should be considered as early as possible when patients are planning to receive treatment that may render them infertile [42,50***]. Although the efficacy of postchemotherapy microdissection testicular sperm extraction (TESE)-ICSI [51*] was reported recently, it is quite important to inform patients of the potential risk of treatment-induced infertility and the possibility of fertility preservation.

In women also, the treatments carrying a high risk for causing permanent amenorrhea have been identified. A risk of permanent amenorrhea of over 80% is estimated for the hematopoietic stem cell transplantation using high-dose cyclophosphamide or more than six cycles of adjuvant chemotherapy containing cyclophosphamide for breast cancer in women age 40 or over [42]. Cryostoring oocytes, unlike sperm cryopreservation, is still considered to be experimental. However, recently, significant improvement in the clinical effectiveness of oocyte freezing/thawing techniques has been achieved [52***].

REFERENCES

◆ 1 Nieschlag E, Simoni M, Gromoll J, Weinbauer GF. Role of FSH in the regulation of spermatogenesis: Clinical aspects. *Clin Endocrinol (Oxf)* 1999;51:139–146.

2 Young JM, McNeilly AS. Theca: The forgotten cell of the ovarian follicle. *Reproduction* 2010;140:489–504.

3 Isidori AM, Giannetta E, Lenzi A. Male hypogonadism. *Pituitary* 2008;11:171–180.

4 Sklar C. Reproductive physiology and treatment-related loss of sex hormone production. *Med Pediatr Oncol* 1999;33:2–8.

5 Bines J, Oleske DM, Cobleigh MA. Ovarian function in premenopausal women treated with adjuvant chemotherapy for breast cancer. *J Clin Oncol* 1996;14:1718–1729.

6 Koyama H, Wada T, Nishizawa Y et al. Cyclophosphamide-induced ovarian failure and its therapeutic significance in patients with breast cancer. *Cancer* 1977;39:1403–1409.

7 Fornier MN, Modi S, Panageas KS et al. Incidence of chemotherapy-induced, long-term amenorrhea in patients with breast carcinoma age 40 years and younger after adjuvant anthracycline and taxane. *Cancer* 2005;104:1575–1579.

8 Meirow D. Ovarian injury and modern options to preserve fertility in female cancer patients treated with high dose radio-chemotherapy for hemato-oncological neoplasias and other cancers. *Leuk Lymphoma* 1999;33:65–76.

9 Wallace WH, Thomson AB, Saran F, Kelsey TW. Predicting age of ovarian failure after radiation to a field that includes the ovaries. *Int J Radiat Oncol Biol Phys* 2005;62:738–744.

10 Chiarelli AM, Marrett LD, Darlington G. Early menopause and infertility in females after treatment for childhood cancer diagnosed in 1964–1988 in Ontario, Canada. *Am J Epidemiol* 1999;150:245–254.

11 Sudour H, Chastagner P, Claude L et al. Fertility and pregnancy outcome after abdominal irradiation that included or excluded the pelvis in childhood tumor survivors. *Int J Radiat Oncol Biol Phys* 2010;76:867–873.

◆ 12 Mom CH, Buijs C, Willemse PH et al. Hot flushes in breast cancer patients. *Crit Rev Oncol Hematol* 2006;57:63–77.

13 Fallowfield L, Cella D, Cuzick J et al. Quality of life of postmenopausal women in the arimidex, tamoxifen, alone or combination (ATAC) adjuvant breast cancer trial. *J Clin Oncol* 2004;22:4261–4271.

✴ 14 Lunenfeld B, Saad F, Hoesl CE. ISA, ISSAM and EAU recommendations for the investigation, treatment and monitoring of late-onset hypogonadism in males: Scientific background and rationale. *Aging Male* 2005;8:59–74.

◆ 15 Mohile SG, Mustian K, Bylow K et al. Management of complications of androgen deprivation therapy in the older man. *Crit Rev Oncol Hematol* 2009;70:235–255.

16 Iversen P. Antiandrogen monotherapy: Indications and results. *Urology* 2002;60(3 Suppl. 1):64–71.

◆ 17 Travis LB, Beard C, Allan JM et al. Testicular cancer survivorship: Research strategies and recommendations. *J Natl Cancer Inst* 2010;102:1114–1130.

18 Huddart RA, Norman A, Moynihan C et al. Fertility, gonadal and sexual function in survivors of testicular cancer. *Br J Cancer* 2005;93:200–207.

19 Nord C, Bjøro T, Ellingsen D et al. Gonadal hormones in long-term survivors 10 years after treatment for unilateral testicular cancer. *Eur Urol* 2003;44:322–328.

20 Nuver J, Smit AJ, Wolffenbuttel BH et al. The metabolic syndrome and disturbances in hormone levels in long-term survivors of disseminated testicular cancer. *J Clin Oncol* 2005;23:3718–3725.

✴ 21 Cobin RH, Futterweit W, Ginzburg SB et al. American Association of Clinical Endocrinologists medical guidelines for clinical practice for the diagnosis and treatment of menopause. *Endocr Pract* 2006;12:315–337.

22 Gjelsvik B, Rosvold EO, Straand J et al. Symptom prevalence during menopause and factors associated with symptoms and menopausal age. Results from the Norwegian Hordaland Women's Cohort study. *Maturitas* 2011;70:383–390.

23 Bergmark K, Avall-Lundqvist E, Dickman PW et al. Vaginal changes and sexuality in women with a history of cervical cancer. *N Engl J Med* 1999;340:1383–1389.

24 Ensrud KE, Stone KL, Blackwell TL et al. Frequency and severity of hot flashes and sleep disturbance in postmenopausal women with hot flashes. *Menopause* 2009;16:286–292.

25 Kornblith AB, Anderson J, Cella DF et al. Comparison of psychosocial adaptation and sexual function of survivors of advanced Hodgkin disease treated by MOPP, ABVD, or MOPP alternating with ABVD. *Cancer* 1992;70:2508–2516.

26 Sato Y, Tanda H, Kato S et al. Prevalence of major depressive disorder in self-referred patients in a late onset hypogonadism clinic. *Int J Impot Res* 2007;19:407–410.

27 Schow DA, Renfer LG, Rozanski TA, Thompson IM. Prevalence of hot flushes during and after neoadjuvant hormonal therapy for localized prostate cancer. *South Med J* 1998;91:855–857.

28 Karling P, Hammar M, Varenhorst E. Prevalence and duration of hot flushes after surgical or medical castration in men with prostatic carcinoma. *J Urol* 1994;152:1170–1173.

29 Higano CS. Androgen-deprivation-therapy-induced fractures in men with nonmetastatic prostate cancer: What do we really know? *Nat Clin Pract Urol* 2008;5:24–34.

30 King J, Wynne CH, Assersohn L, Jones A. Hormone replacement therapy and women with premature menopause—A cancer survivorship issue. *Eur J Cancer* 2011;47:1623–1632.

31 Ibeanu O, Modesitt SC, Ducie J et al. Hormone replacement therapy in gynecologic cancer survivors: Why not? *Gynecol Oncol* 2011;122:447–454.

32 Huang KE. Menopause perspectives and treatment of Asian women. *Semin Reprod Med* 2010;28:396–403.

33 Fisher TE, Chervenak JL. Lifestyle alterations for the amelioration of hot flashes. *Maturitas* 2012;71:217–220.

34 Bruno D, Feeney KJ. Management of postmenopausal symptoms in breast cancer survivors. *Semin Oncol* 2006;33:696–707.

35 Loprinzi CL, Kugler JW, Sloan JA et al. Venlafaxine in management of hot flashes in survivors of breast cancer: A randomised controlled trial. *Lancet* 2000;356:2059–2063.

36 Stearns V, Beebe KL, Iyengar M, Dube E. Paroxetine controlled release in the treatment of menopausal hot flashes: A randomized controlled trial. *JAMA* 2003;289:2827–2834.

37 Loprinzi CL, Sloan JA, Perez EA et al. Phase III evaluation of fluoxetine for treatment of hot flashes. *J Clin Oncol* 2002;20:1578–1583.

38 Stearns V, Johnson MD, Rae JM et al. Active tamoxifen metabolite plasma concentrations after coadministration of tamoxifen and the selective serotonin reuptake inhibitor paroxetine. *J Natl Cancer Inst* 2003;95:1758–1764.

39 Handa VL, Bachus KE, Johnston WW et al. Vaginal administration of low-dose conjugated estrogens: Systemic absorption and effects on the endometrium. *Obstet Gynecol* 1994;84:215–218.

40 Sekido N, Kawai K, Akaza H, Koiso K. Chlormadinone acetate withdrawal syndrome under combined androgen blockade for advanced prostate cancer. *Jpn J Clin Oncol* 1995;25:164–167.

41 Suzuki H, Akakura K, Komiya A et al. Codon 877 mutation in the androgen receptor gene in advanced prostate cancer: Relation to antiandrogen withdrawal syndrome. *Prostate* 1996;29:153–158.

✶ 42 Lee SJ, Schover LR, Partridge AH et al. American Society of Clinical Oncology recommendations on fertility preservation in cancer patients. *J Clin Oncol* 2006;24:2917–2931.

◆ 43 Abouassaly R, Fossa SD, Giwercman A et al. Sequelae of treatment in long-term survivors of testis cancer. *Eur Urol* 2011;60:516–526.

44 Pont J, Albrecht W. Fertility after chemotherapy for testicular germ cell cancer. *Fertil Steril* 1997;68:1–5.

45 Huyghe E, Matsuda T, Daudin M et al. Fertility after testicular cancer treatments: Results of a large multicenter study. *Cancer* 2004;100:732–737.

46 Brydøy M, Fosså SD, Klepp O et al. Paternity and testicular function among testicular cancer survivors treated with two to four cycles of cisplatin-based chemotherapy. *Eur Urol* 2010;58:134–140.

47 Bokemeyer C, Berger CC, Kuczyk MA, Schmoll HJ. Evaluation of long-term toxicity after chemotherapy for testicular cancer. *J Clin Oncol* 1996;14:2923–2932.

48 Pryzant RM, Meistrich ML, Wilson G et al. Long-term reduction in sperm count after chemotherapy with and without radiation therapy for non-Hodgkin's lymphomas. *J Clin Oncol* 1993;11:239–247.

49 Viviani S, Santoro A, Ragni G et al. Gonadal toxicity after combination chemotherapy for Hodgkin's disease. Comparative results of MOPP vs ABVD. *Eur J Cancer Clin Oncol* 1985;21:601–605.

◆ 50 Sharma V. Sperm storage for cancer patients in the UK: A review of current practice. *Hum Reprod* 2011;26:2935–2943.

51 Hsiao W, Stahl PJ, Osterberg EC et al. Successful treatment of postchemotherapy azoospermia with microsurgical testicular sperm extraction: The Weill Cornell experience. *J Clin Oncol* 2011;29:1607–1611.

◆ 52 Revelli A, Molinari E, Salvagno F et al. Oocyte cryostorage to preserve fertility in oncological patients. *Obstet Gynecol Int* 2012;2012:525896. Epub 2012 Jan 15.

131

Genetic counseling in the palliative care setting

LISA MADLENSKY, ERIC ROELAND, KIM BOWER

WHAT IS GENETIC COUNSELLING?

Genetic counselling is the process of helping people understand and adapt to the medical, psychological, and familial implications of genetic contributions to disease. This process integrates

- Interpretation of family and medical histories to assess the chance of disease occurrence or recurrence
- Education about inheritance, testing, management, prevention, resources, and research
- Counselling to promote informed choices and adaptation to the risk or condition

National Society of Genetic Counselors (2006)[1]

The Human Genetics Programme of the World Health Organization (WHO) notes that while genetic counselling services are generally available throughout developed nations, rural regions and developing nations with limited access to health care often have inadequate or no formal genetic counselling services available for patients. However, under these circumstances, other health-care providers including physicians, nurses, and scientists can provide genetic counselling.

Genetic counsellors and other genetic specialists (typically physician geneticists or advanced practice genetics nurses) have much in common with palliative care specialists. For both specialties, while the clinical focus is on the patient, the patient's family is considered an integral part of the medical evaluation and decision-making process. Many individuals pursue a genetic assessment and/or genetic testing not for themselves, but rather because they have a desire to provide potentially lifesaving information to their children and relatives.

Although there are rapid changes occurring in the genetics and genomics fields, the primary tool of the genetic counsellor is the careful construction of an extended family medical history. The scope of practice for genetic counsellors includes the taking of a four- or five-generation pedigree, verifying the history with medical records (when possible), and evaluating the pattern of inheritance that is seen in the family history. This serves to inform recommendations for genetic testing, the making of an accurate clinical diagnosis, and the identification of potentially at-risk family members.

Genetic counsellors work with the affected patient and family to assess the personal and family history of disease, coordinate genetic testing when appropriate, and provide education, advocacy, and support. This includes linking families to appropriate medical specialists as well as patient support and advocacy organizations. Education for patients and families includes describing the natural history of the disease, what types of medical interventions are indicated, the mode of inheritance, reproductive options, and eligibility for clinical research studies.

Along with providing accurate medical information, genetic counsellors are also trained to attend to the psychosocial needs of patients and families as they go through the genetic counselling process. Discussing the medical history of relatives who have had the same condition as the patient is an inherently emotional undertaking, as is discussing the likelihood that the condition may have been passed on to the patient's children or inherited by other close family members.

LOGISTICAL ISSUES IN GENETIC COUNSELLING

Patient identification

It is important to identify the most appropriate person (or group of people) within a family to test *first* in order to obtain the most accurate and complete information. The process for evaluating genetic risk in a family is most effective and accurate when genetic testing can be first carried out on the most appropriate index patient in the family (i.e., the person in the family most likely to test positive for a genetic syndrome). This reduces the likelihood of a false-negative result. Genetic specialists can help to identify the appropriate patient within a given family to proceed to testing first.

Informed consent

The informed consent process for genetic testing is typically more complex than for other types of medical tests. The concept of "genetic exceptionalism"[2] refers to the unique aspects of genetic information, including the notion that the test result will have implications not only for the patient but also for their blood relatives. This also encompasses the idea that genetic information can uniquely identify an individual and may deserve special treatment in a medical chart. In the informed consent process, issues are discussed including the likelihood that a genetic test will/will not be informative and the implications of a positive/negative/uncertain test result for the patient *and* their family.

Financial concerns

In some countries, genetic counselling and testing is a covered medical benefit by public and/or private health insurers when there is a medical indication. Coverage of genetic testing is highly variable, and part of the genetic testing process is navigating patients through the often complicated process of obtaining insurance authorization, determining "medical necessity," and understanding what, if any, the out-of-pocket costs will be.

Disclosure of test results to family members

A critical component of genetic testing is facilitating the disclosure of relevant test results to family members who could potentially benefit from knowing the information. Typically this involves reviewing the family history in detail to identify specific family members who should be notified, as well as helping patients create personalized letters or email templates that they can provide to their families with accurate information.

Opportunities for research participation, support, and advocacy

Given that many genetic diseases are rare, patients and families may appreciate the opportunity to enrol in a patient registry. Some studies collect information from medical records, others collect patient-reported data (e.g., quality of life or symptom measures), and others collect biospecimens for basic research into the understanding of disease. In addition, many patient-run support, education, and advocacy groups exist in person and online to connect patients facing the same diagnosis so that they can have peer support as well as practical tips for living with a particular condition. Part of the genetic counselling process is to provide patients with current information about research and support opportunities.

GENETIC COUNSELLING IN PALLIATIVE CARE

In the initial assessment of a patient referred to a palliative care service, it is important to acknowledge the possibility of a genetic condition and initiate a genetic assessment if consistent with the patient's goals.[3] As palliative care increasingly expands into a simultaneous care delivery model (see

Chapter 33), we recommend implementing an *early* genetic risk assessment as part of the initial palliative care assessment. The key reason to raise the possibility of genetic assessment when a patient is first referred to palliative care is that this will allow the patient to participate directly if desired. Too often, patients and families delay discussions regarding genetic counselling because they are overwhelmed with diagnosis and treatment. Some patients are referred to genetics services but decline for various reasons including anxiety, fear of results, objections from family members, and perceiving that genetic information is not relevant.[4,5] Delaying genetic counselling discussions may create an urgent situation when a patient's death is imminent, and they can no longer fully engage in the process.

Optimal genetic counselling engages the patient and family when both are able to

- Provide details about their personal and family medical history that may not be known to other relatives or their health-care proxies
- Provide informed consent for genetic testing, where appropriate
- Consider that undergoing a genetic risk assessment (and possible genetic testing) can often provide reassurance for family members that there is *not* likely to be a strong genetic component to the patient's illness
- Consider that alternatively, the genetic risk assessment may reveal a clear hereditary condition important for surviving family members (this allows the patient to actively participate in disclosing information to their relatives, providing a "gift" of health information as part of their legacy)

Leaving this important discussion about the possible heritability of a condition until a patient's last days can cause unnecessary distress for the patient and family, given that there may not be enough time to coordinate the logistical issues that are often needed when genetic testing is being considered, and a sense of "rushing" to get testing completed.[6] If there are no alternatives, DNA banking (See page 1290) can be a less traumatic alternative both emotionally and financially for families.

SOME QUESTIONS TO ASK A NEWLY REFERRED PATIENT ABOUT GENETICS

- Is there any concern that your diagnosis might be genetic or run in the family?
- Have any of your health-care providers recommended genetic counselling or testing?
- Do you have any family members that have also had the same diagnosis?
- Have any family members asked you whether you have had genetic testing?
- Have you already met with a geneticist or genetic counsellor? Have you ever had genetic testing?

GENETIC COUNSELLING IN PEDIATRIC PALLIATIVE CARE

About half of children who die each year in the United States die within the first year of life; and many of these children have a genetic disease or multiple congenital anomalies.[7] One North American multi-institutional study found that 41% of pediatric palliative care patients had a genetic disease or congenital anomaly,[8] so there is clearly a need for genetic specialists to work with palliative care teams to care for young patients and their families. Genetic specialists should be involved as soon as there is suspicion of a genetic condition; involvement frequently occurs as early as the prenatal period. Obtaining an accurate diagnosis for a child with major medical problems in the prenatal period, infancy, or early childhood is critical for several reasons. First, the family can be informed about the natural history, treatment options, and prognosis of the condition. Second, the immediate and extended family members can learn whether there is a risk of future children having the same disease and whether genetic testing is available for subsequent pregnancies.

Often there exists a need for both palliative medicine and genetic medicine concurrently. Clinicians in these two specialties can work together to ensure that whenever possible, there is a coordinated approach to care. Genetic counsellors and other genetic specialists are frequently in the position of working with families very early in the course of the child's treatment, and they can play an important role in identifying and referring patients who would benefit from palliative care services.[9] Genetic counsellors are frequently involved even prior to the birth of the child. In many geographic areas, there are perinatal palliative care programs that are able to partner with genetic counsellors to provide affected families with psychosocial, emotional, and spiritual support, help with decision-making, and provide information about symptom management both before and after the birth of their child. These programs can help ensure that the family's wishes for the care of their baby are clearly communicated to all involved medical providers and are natural partners for genetic specialists. In one qualitative study, parents of children with a newly diagnosed lethal genetic condition reported wanting information about end-of-life care, pain control, and medical decision-making, as well as indicating a desire for genetic counselling.[10]

In pediatric palliative care, it is not uncommon that even after extensive genetic testing, the cause of the child's medical condition is not identified. The uncertainty that is associated with the lack of a firm diagnosis can be quite difficult for families. Some families openly speak about the importance of knowing their child's diagnosis and others do not raise the issue unless it is specifically raised. It is very important that providers of pediatric palliative care are comfortable speaking with families about the options of autopsy and DNA banking (See page 1290) as a way to possibly diagnose the child's medical condition. It is also important that providers feel comfortable in respecting whatever decision the family makes. Just as some families struggle to live with the uncertainty of an undiagnosed condition, others feel very comfortable in not knowing. Each community will have its own set of resources for obtaining autopsy and DNA banking for a child. It is important for palliative care providers to be aware of what is available in their communities. Many children's hospitals will perform autopsies free of charge for patients for whom they have cared. See "Genetic Counselling in Adult Palliative Care" section on autopsy and DNA banking for more details on these subjects.

GENETIC COUNSELLING IN ADULT PALLIATIVE CARE

For adult populations, a clear-cut genetic disease may not be encountered as often as in the neonatal or pediatric palliative setting. However, a substantial subset of palliative care patients are at risk of having a genetic predisposition or syndrome.[11] As genetic testing becomes more commonplace, there may be many palliative care patients who have already had genetic counselling and testing. For these patients, a genetic workup is not likely indicated, but palliative medicine clinicians can use this genetic information in discussions with their patients about creating a legacy for family members.

The few studies describing the role of genetic counselling in palliative care are based in adult-onset cancer. In fact, clinical cancer genetics is considered a subspecialty within the genetic counselling field due to the high prevalence of cancer predisposition syndromes and the growing number of genetic tests used to identify families with an inherited predisposition to cancer.[12] Current oncology guidelines and practice indicators include clear referral recommendations for newly diagnosed cancer patients to help oncologists determine which patients are appropriate for a genetic assessment.[13] Despite these recommendations, many appropriate patients are not referred for early genetic evaluation, while other patients are referred but choose not to pursue genetic counselling. However, patients sometimes reconsider when their disease progresses and later wish to proceed with genetic testing for the benefit of their family members. As a result, the opportunity for the patient to complete the genetic risk assessment and testing process may be missed entirely.[14] Therefore, the responsibility may fall to the palliative care provider who must determine if a genetic workup was ever undertaken and, if not, how to initiate this workup if consistent with the patients goals of care.

GENETIC COUNSELLING IN HOSPICE AND END–OF–LIFE CARE

Genetic counselling in the end-of-life hospice population provides unique challenges and opportunities.[15] One limitation of providing genetic counselling in this setting is funding. Once a patient enters into hospice care, health insurers may not cover the cost of genetic tests since they will not likely alter medical management. Indeed, many authorization requests from private health insurers require that the ordering health-care provider specifically indicate how the genetic test results will inform the treatment of the patient. In countries with public health insurance, there may be restrictions on the use of genetic counselling and testing in hospice care for the same reasons. One available option is DNA banking (See page 1290), which is relatively inexpensive, is available in many countries, and is more frequently done noninvasively through a buccal or saliva sample rather than a blood draw.

GENETIC INFORMATION AND PATIENT LEGACY

Palliative care patients often wonder how they will be remembered after they die; patients want to be remembered and want their lives to make a difference and seek out meaningful ways to accomplish this. Broadly defined, a legacy is what one leaves behind after he or she is gone. The desire to create and leave a legacy of meaning and purpose parallels the belief that we are part of something larger than just our own lifetimes or ourselves. It is a way for patients to live on. Legacy is a process and often requires time to shift from the emotional reaction at time of diagnosis and during treatment to reframing one's thinking to the pragmatic implications for loved ones and the greater good. Legacy may help patients complete relationships, reframe spiritual and religious issues, attend to family, and redefine the meaning of hope.

This is not a new concept. In fact, one of Erik Erikson's eight stages of life specifically focuses on this task—generativity versus stagnation.[16] In this stage, the focus is on the extensional question: How can I make my life count? Strength comes through care of others and production of something that contributes to the betterment of society, which Erikson calls generativity. Generativity is the concern of guiding the next generation. Socially valued work and disciplines are expressions of generativity. The adult stage of generativity has broad application to family, relationships, work, and society. "Generativity, then is primarily the concern in establishing and guiding the next generation…the concept is meant to include…productivity and creativity."[16] For some, legacy can take the form of directly contributing to the medical knowledge of family or more broadly to the international medical community. In genetics, this contribution can take many forms, including help guiding diagnosis and treatment of loved ones or contributing to the greater good by participating in research and clinical trials. Involving patients in genetic counselling often provides an opportunity to actively participate in their own care during a time when they are increasingly dependent on others. Furthermore, patients may express gratitude to their caregivers by participating in genetic research and clinical trials thereby contributing to a growing body of knowledge. This creates opportunities for medical providers to reflect and share with the patient how we have learned and will continue to learn from them.[17]

DNA BANKING, AUTOPSY, AND DONATION OF TISSUES FOR RESEARCH

One option for patients to consider is the banking of a DNA sample for future use by family members. This is an important option to offer select patients[18]:

- Those who are suspected to have a hereditary condition but have had negative genetic testing to date. Genetic and genomic research is progressing at a rapid rate, and new genetic tests are being developed and made available as new disease-causing genes are discovered.
- Those who are suspected to have a hereditary condition but have not previously had any genetic testing.
- Those who have had a positive genetic test for a genetic condition but for which there is a limited understanding of the natural history of the syndrome or a great deal of clinical variability. Banking a DNA sample for future research may be desired by the patient and/or family as a way of contributing to research.

For some very rare genetic conditions, researchers have protocols that allow them to obtain tissue samples shortly after death to facilitate research of the condition. When there is a clear diagnosis, and the patient and their family have expressed an interest in helping researchers learn more about the condition, genetics service providers can help to identify research labs or patient advocacy societies that are soliciting tissue samples. The genetic counsellor (or health-care provider serving in that role) can help coordinate the consent process, as well as the logistics of respectfully obtaining and shipping the samples.[19]

For patients who have not been given a clear diagnosis, a discussion of autopsy may also be important to have with the family, particularly in the neonatal setting if a child has multiple congenital anomalies. Parents can be informed of the benefits of trying to establish a definitive diagnosis to inform decisions about future family planning for themselves and for any other family members who are planning on having children. A definitive diagnosis may enable prenatal or preimplantation genetic testing in future pregnancies if desired.

GAPS IN KNOWLEDGE AND FUTURE RESEARCH

Genetics and palliative care share much in common. Both medical specialties involve an evaluation of the medical and psychosocial needs of the patient and family and treatment approaches based on the goals of care and patient values and require advanced communication skills to describe complex topics in understandable and relevant terms. However, there is surprisingly little empiric research looking at the intersection of these two fields.[11] One of the few studies to date found that palliative medicine specialists do not frequently refer patients for genetic assessment and/or testing, or utilize DNA banking, and self-report low ratings of expertise in genetics topics.[18] Another study surveyed hospice nurses extensively on a variety of topics relating to the perceived level of importance of genetics and the perceived level of confidence in carrying out various tasks related to helping patients access genetics services or undergo a genetic risk assessment.[20] The results for nearly all genetics topics were quite uniform, with nurses rating the issues relating to genetics as very important but rating their level of confidence in handling these issues for their patients as very low. There clearly exists a defined niche of genetic counselling in the palliative care setting as yet to be filled by a formalized dual educational program. There are tremendous opportunities for genetic specialists and palliative care specialists to develop continuing education curricula, create readily accessible patient and provider resources, expand research specific to this intersection, and improve clinical partnerships to provide mutual professional support.

RECOMMENDED RESOURCES

Current clinical information on genetic conditions

GeneReviews.org
Omim.org
Orpha.net

Find a genetic counsellor or genetic specialist

NSGC.org (select "Find a Counselor")
ABGC.net
List of international human genetics societies: www.kumc.edu/gec/prof/soclist.html

DNA testing and banking labs worldwide

Genetests.org
Ncbi.nlm.nih.gov/gtr

REFERENCES

◆ 1 Resta R, Biesecker BB, Bennett RL, Blum S, Hahn SE, Strecker MN et al. A new definition of Genetic Counseling: National Society of Genetic Counselors' Task Force report. *J Genet Couns.* 2006;15(2):77–83.

2 Zimmern RL, Khoury MJ. The impact of genomics on public health practice: The case for change. *Public Health Genomics.* 2012;15(3–4):118–124.

◆ 3 Raudonis BM, Cauble DM. Palliative care in the genomic era. *J Hospice Palliat Nurs.* 2011;13(5):298–308.

4 Riedijk SR, Niermeijer MF, Dooijes D, Tibben A. A decade of genetic counseling in frontotemporal dementia affected families: Few counseling requests and much familial opposition to testing. *J Genet Couns.* 2009;18(4):350–356.

5 Schlich-Bakker KJ, ten Kroode HF, Wárlám-Rodenhuis CC, van den Bout J, Ausems MG. Barriers to participating in genetic counseling and BRCA testing during primary treatment for breast cancer. *Genet Med.* 2007;9(11):766–777.

◆ 6 Lillie AK, Clifford C, Metcalfe A. Caring for families with a family history of cancer: Why concerns about genetic predisposition are missing from the palliative agenda. *Palliat Med.* 2011;25(2):117–124.

7 Kochanek KD, Kirmeyer SE, Martin JA, Strobino DM, Guyer B. Annual summary of vital statistics: 2009. *Pediatrics.* 2012;129(2):338–348.

8 Feudtner C, Kang TI, Hexem KR, Friedrichsdorf SJ, Osenga K, Siden H et al. Pediatric palliative care patients: A prospective multicenter cohort study. *Pediatrics.* 2011;127(6):1094–1101.

9 Arias R, Andrews J, Pandya S, Pettit K, Trout C, Apkon S et al. Palliative care services in families of males with duchenne muscular dystrophy. *Muscle Nerve.* 2011;44(1):93–101.

10 Yuen WY, Duipmans JC, Jonkman MF. The needs of parents with children suffering from lethal epidermolysis bullosa. *Br J Dermatol.* 2012;167(3):613–618.

◆ 11 Quillin JM, Bodurtha JN, Smith TJ. Genetics assessment at the end of life: Suggestions for implementation in clinic and future research. *J Palliat Med.* 2008;11(3):451–458.

12 DeMarco TA, Smith KL, Nusbaum RH, Peshkin BN, Schwartz MD, Isaacs C. Practical aspects of delivering hereditary cancer risk counseling. *Semin Oncol.* 2007;34(5):369–378.

13 Bruinooge SS, ASCO. American Society of Clinical Oncology policy statement update: Genetic testing for cancer susceptibility. *J Clin Oncol.* 2003;21(12):2397–2406.

● 14 Quillin JM, Bodurtha JN, Siminoff LA, Smith TJ. Exploring hereditary cancer among dying cancer patients—A cross-sectional study of hereditary risk and perceived awareness of DNA testing and banking. *J Genet Couns.* 2010;19(5):497–525.

15 Daniels MS, Burzawa JK, Brandt AC, Schmeler KM, Lu KH. A clinical perspective on genetic counseling and testing during end of life care for women with recurrent progressive ovarian cancer: Opportunities and challenges. *Fam Cancer.* 2011;10(2):193–197.

16 Slater C. Generativity versus stagnation: An elaboration of Erikson's adult stage of human development. *J Adult Dev.* 2003;10(1):53–65.

17 Block S, Cohen T. Issues in psychotherapy with terminally ill patients. *Palliat Support Care.* 2004;2(2):181–189.

● 18 Quillin JM, Bodurtha JN, Siminoff LA, Smith TJ. Physicians' current practices and opportunities for DNA banking of dying patients with cancer. *J Oncol Pract/Am Soc Clin Oncol.* 2011;7(3):183–187.

19 Hawkins AK. Biobanks: Importance, implications and opportunities for genetic counselors. *J Genet Couns.* 2010;19(5):423–429.

● 20 Metcalfe A, Pumphrey R, Clifford C. Hospice nurses and genetics: Implications for end-of-life care. *J Clin Nurs.* 2010;19(1–2):192–207.

132

Pulmonary rehabilitation

RYO KOZU

WHAT IS PULMONARY REHABILITATION?

The aims of pulmonary rehabilitation are to reduce symptoms, increase participation in physical and social activities, improve health status, and maximize independence for patients with respiratory disease. According to the American Thoracic Society (ATS) and the European Respiratory Society (ERS) Society Statement, pulmonary rehabilitation is defined as "Pulmonary rehabilitation is an evidence-based, multidisciplinary, and comprehensive intervention for patients with chronic respiratory diseases who are symptomatic and often have decreased daily life activities. Integrated into the individualized treatment of the patient, pulmonary rehabilitation is designed to reduce symptoms, optimize functional status, increase participation, and reduce healthcare costs through stabilizing or reversing systemic manifestations of the disease" [1]. Pulmonary rehabilitation has developed as a nonpharmacological treatment in chronic obstructive pulmonary disease (COPD), one of the leading causes of mortality, disability, and a rise in healthcare costs worldwide, and is positioned one of the most effective interventions. Pulmonary rehabilitation programs (PRP) involve patient assessment, exercise training, physiotherapy, education, psychosocial support, and nutritional intervention [2]. It has been demonstrated to reduce dyspnea, fatigue, anxiety, and depression; improve exercise capacity, emotional function, and health-related quality of life (HRQL); decrease healthcare utilization; and enhance patients' sense of control over their condition [1,2]. Exercise training especially is a single mandatory component and alone has clear benefits.

WHY IS PULMONARY REHABILITATION BENEFICIAL TO THE PATIENTS?

Since chronic respiratory impairment is irreversible and causes shortness of breath on exertion for a long time, these patients become sedentary. The resultant chronic inactivity deconditions skeletal muscle function and general endurance. Much of the disability does not result from respiratory impairment, but from such secondary morbidities due to physical inactivity. Although the pulmonary function of chronic respiratory disease does not change with pulmonary rehabilitation, the dysfunction of muscle often is treatable and patients well respond well to treatment [3]. The benefits of pulmonary rehabilitation are improvement in muscle deconditioning, weakness and dysfunction of peripheral muscles, anxiety and depression, and nutritional state, and so enabling patients to walk farther with less dyspnea [4]. The effects of PRP have been established by many of the randomized controlled trials. Significant reduction in dyspnea and increases in maximal exercise capacity, as well as HRQL, have been observed [5].

Some clinical studies have shown no significant difference in improvement in exercise tolerance or HRQL following pulmonary rehabilitation in COPD versus non-COPD patients [2]. Therefore, it is effective for patients with disability due to any chronic respiratory disease. However, its suitability to the palliative-care setting is not well established.

PATIENT SELECTION AND ASSESSMENT

Although most patients have COPD, the benefits of pulmonary rehabilitation can be applied to all patients with dyspnea from other respiratory diseases, despite optimal medical management. Pulmonary rehabilitation is effective for people with moderate to severe COPD and therefore should be offered to these patients [6]. It is considered that indication is not based on the age, severity of physiologic impairment, and disability. It is not suitable for patients who are unable to walk and who have unstable cardiac diseases or severe orthopedic or neurological impairments. The same principles can be applied to patients with other respiratory diseases, including asthma, bronchiectasis, cystic fibrosis, interstitial lung disease, chest wall disease, lung cancer, and selected neuromuscular diseases.

Comprehensive patient assessment is essential for developing an appropriate, individualized plan of care. It should include medical history, current therapy, symptoms, physical examination, and diagnostic investigations, for example, pulmonary function tests, to determine the severity of respiratory impairment [7]. The physical function involving measurement of peripheral muscle strength, performance of activities of daily living (ADL), health status, cognitive function, emotional and mood state, and nutritional status is necessary to evaluate the patient's disability and handicap. The determination of baseline exercise capacity is essential for formulating the exercise training prescription and in evaluating for hypoxemia and dyspnea during exercise.

WHAT DOES A PULMONARY REHABILITATION PROGRAM INCLUDE?

PRP generally includes exercise training, physiotherapy, education, and psychosocial support. Current position statements recommend that these interventions are provided by a multidisciplinary team that consists of respiratory physician, nurses, physiotherapist, occupational therapists, dietitian, pharmacist, psychologist, and social worker [1]. Although pulmonary rehabilitation is administered in hospital settings, in the community, and in the patient's home, programs are most commonly provided within a hospital outpatient department or community health facility [8].

Exercise training

In addition, dyspnea as a consequence of chronic respiratory disease often limits daily activities and causes exercise intolerance and functional impairment in most patients. People with chronic respiratory disease are less physically active compared with healthy age-matched individuals [9].

A primary goal of pulmonary rehabilitation is to reduce the patient's perception of dyspnea and enable patients to tolerate a higher level of activity. Exercise training is the most effective intervention to reduce dyspnea and improve exercise tolerance and HRQL [2]. Both lower and upper limb endurance and strength training are included. According to the graded evidence-based guidelines [2], the exercise training should especially focus on the lower extremity endurance training such as walking or cycling.

Exercise prescription is composed of duration, frequency, mode, and intensity of exercise. It should be individually assessed based on disease severity, functional status, and initial exercise testing. Lower limb endurance training intensity should usually be targeted at 60%–70% of maximal workload of exercise testing [10]. Exercise intensity has to be recorded and can be gradually increased through the program if appropriate and tolerated. Effects of high-intensity training are to increase physiological improvements such as increased peak VO_2 and oxidative enzyme capacity of muscle, decreased HR, blood lactate levels, and ventilation at isoworkload [10–12]. Because all patients cannot tolerate high-intensity exercise, lower-intensity training or interval training can be used. The benefit obtained from low-intensity exercise has been demonstrated and improved patient exercise tolerance [2,13]. An

interval training regimen consisting of 2–3 min of high-intensity exercise (60%–80% maximal exercise capacity) alternating with equal periods of rest might be a substitute for patients who cannot sustain extended, continuous periods of high-intensity exercise [14]. The frequency and duration of the endurance training involve three to five times a week, of which at least two should be supervised, 20–30 min/session, and extend over a period of 4–12 weeks [1]. Most programs are between 6 and 9 weeks in duration [15,16].

Lower limb, with large muscles, training can improve not only walking ability, balance, and stairs climbing but also exercise tolerance of patients with COPD and other respiratory diseases. Because many ADL involves the use of the upper limb, moderate to severe patients complain of dyspnea during ADLs. Exercise training of the upper extremities is essential for improving arm function. Training of the arms is effective in increasing muscle endurance and strength, reducing metabolic demand associated with arm exercise [2]. Supported arm exercises are usually prescribed with ergometry or unsupported arm exercises by lifting free weights.

Since skeletal muscle dysfunction that is characterized by reductions in muscle mass and strength can significantly contribute to exercise limitation in patients with pulmonary disease [17], strength training is a rational component of exercise training. Lower and upper limb strength training can lead to improvements in muscle strength and dyspnea due to reduction in ventilatory equivalent and increased exercise endurance [2]. Respiratory muscle training improves the strength of the inspiratory muscles in patients with COPD. Because the addition of this training to an exercise training program does not gain additional benefits, it is not recommended as a routine component of a PRP [2]. Respiratory muscle training should be individually considered.

Supplementary oxygen during training should be provided for those patients with hypoxemia during exercise. It is important to optimize bronchodilator and other pharmacotherapy before and during exercise program, if necessary. The Rollator, wheeled walker, can reduce dyspnea during walk [18,19]. While patient uses a Rollator, fixation of the upper limbs allows the accessory muscles to contribute to ventilation, thereby reducing the work of breathing and minimizing dyspnea. Helium-hyperoxia [20], noninvasive positive pressure ventilation [21] are additional strategies to reduce dyspnea during training, and neuromuscular electrical stimulation (NMES) [22,23], can improve muscle strength of lower limb and exercise tolerance.

Physiotherapy

There are controlled breathing techniques (breathing retraining) and airway clearance techniques such as physiotherapy in PRP. The breathing techniques include pursed lip breathing, diaphragmatic breathing, and positioning that is used for postural relief of dyspnea.

The evidence to support these breathing techniques in patients with chronic respiratory disease is limited [24,25]. However, there are some patients with moderate to severe disease who can receive benefits from breathing techniques. The positioning, forward-lean position, especially if this is combined with fixation of the shoulder girdle, often provides some relief from dyspnea [26,27].

Airway clearance techniques are interventions that reduce effort of clearing sputum for people who produces large amount of sputum and/or often have difficulty removing secretion such as cystic fibrosis, bronchiectasis, or COPD. The techniques include coughing, huffing, active cycle of breathing techniques, postural drainage, or positive expiratory pressure and so on.

Education

Education for patient and family is an important part of PRP, encouraging active participation in health care, which leads to a better understanding of the physical and psychological changes that occur with chronic illness.

Traditionally, education in PRP has been presented by a healthcare staff, one-to-one teaching or group classes. It was disease specific but not patient specific. It is currently recommended to use collaborative self-management education [28]. Patients can become more active and skilled by teaching individualized problem-solving methods at collaborative self-management education.

Psychosocial and behavioral intervention

Anxiety, depression, and difficulties in coping with chronic illness are common in respiratory patients [29]. The inability to cope with illness contributes to the handicap of their disease. Psychosocial and behavioral interventions in PRP include regular patient education sessions, or support groups focusing on specific problems are very helpful. Instructions in progressive muscle relaxation, stress reduction, and panic control may help to reduce dyspnea and anxiety. Because of the effects of chronic respiratory disease on the family, participation of family members or friends in PRP support groups is encouraged.

OUTCOME ASSESSMENT

Outcome assessment is an essential component of a PRP. It is used to determine individual patient responses (patient-centered outcomes) and to evaluate the overall effectiveness of the program. These mean that how effective of the intervention was to the patients, and of the program met its quality improvement. Patient-centered outcomes have to be assessed before and after PRP and during follow-up, for example, every 6 and/or 12 months.

The most common measures consist of evaluating symptoms, dyspnea particularly, exercise capacity, and HRQL. Several questionnaires or functional assessment scales for pulmonary rehabilitation can be utilized in clinical setting as follows.

DYSPNEA

Modified Medical Research Council (MMRC) Dyspnea Scale [30] is a simple grading system to assess the effect of breathlessness on daily activities. It comprises five statements that describe almost the entire range of respiratory disability from none (grade 0) to almost complete incapacity (grade 4). It can be self-administered by asking patients to choose a phrase that best describes their condition.

Modified Borg Dyspnea Scale [31] is a categorical scale that assesses the patient's perception of shortness of breath at one specific time point. This score is from 0 to 10, where 0 corresponds to the sensation of normal breathing (absence of dyspnea) and 10 corresponds to the subject's maximum possible sensation of dyspnea.

EXERCISE CAPACITY

The 6-minute walk test (6MWT) [32] is a self-paced endurance assessment of the distance walked during a 6 min period on a level surface. The 6MWT is a useful measure of functional capacity and is widely used for measuring response to pulmonary rehabilitation interventions. The minimal important difference (MID) is estimated to be 25–54 m [8].

The incremental shuttle walking test (ISWT) [33] is a field test that is externally paced and progressive. During ISWT, there is a linear relationship between VO_2 and walking speed, similar to the relationship between VO_2 and work rate in incremental laboratory testing. Singh has reported an improvement of 47.5 m in ISWT indicates that patients with COPD are "slightly better" and an improvement of 78.7 m represents "better" [34].

HRQL

Medical Outcomes Study Short Form 36 (MOS SF 36) [35] was constructed to survey generic health status in the Medical Outcomes Study. The SF-36 consists of eight subscales that assess components of physical and mental health. Scores for each subscale and the component summary scores range from 0 to 100, with a lower score indicating a greater level of impairment.

Chronic Respiratory Disease Questionnaire (CRDQ or CRQ) [36] is a disease-specific HRQL questionnaire. It was developed to measure the impact of COPD and consists of 20 items across four dimensions, dyspnea, fatigue, emotional function, and mastery. These items in each section are scored from 1 (most severe) to 7 (no impairment).

St. George's Respiratory Questionnaire (SGRQ) [37] is also a disease-specific instrument designed to measure impact on overall health, daily life, and perceived well-being in patients with COPD. It consists of 2 parts and 3 components, symptoms, activity, and impacts, and scores range from 0 to 100, with higher scores indicating more limitations.

The COPD Assessment Test (CAT) [38] is a patient-completed instrument that has been designed to provide a simple and reliable measure of health status in COPD. It is designed to measure the impact of COPD (cough, sputum, dyspnea, chest tightness) on health status. The CAT is very simple to administer, because it is composed of 8 items and scaling from 1 to 5, and CAT scores range from 0 to 40. Higher scores denote a more severe impact of COPD on a patient's life.

PULMONARY REHABILITATION AND PALLIATIVE CARE

The goals of pulmonary rehabilitation overlapped with palliative care in terms of management of symptoms and achievement of a sense of well-being. Dyspnea especially is a common and distressing symptom in the advanced stages of malignant and nonmalignant diseases and is the most difficult to treat. Techniques of pulmonary rehabilitation produce significant improvements in dyspnea. Bausewein et al. [39] have analyzed 47 studies (2532 participants) in a Cochrane review; they found that breathing training, walking aids, NMES, and chest wall vibration appear to be effective as nonpharmacological interventions for relieving dyspnea due to advanced stages of cancer, COPD, interstitial lung disease, chronic heart failure, or motor neuron disease. Principles and techniques of pulmonary rehabilitation are applied into palliative-care setting; the care may lead to more success.

REFERENCES

1 Spruit MA, Singh SJ, Garvey C, ZuWallack R, et al. ATS/ERS Task Force on Pulmonary Rehabilitation. An official American Thoracic Society/European Respiratory Society statement: Key concepts and advances in pulmonary rehabilitation. Am J Respir Crit Care Med. 2013;188:e13–64.

2 Ries AL, Bauldoff GS, Carlin BW, Casaburi R, Emery CF et al. Pulmonary rehabilitation: Joint ACCP/AACVPR evidence-based clinical practice guidelines. Chest. 2007;131(5 Suppl.):4S–42S.

3 Troosters T, Gosselink R, Decramer M. Exercise training in COPD: How to distinguish responders from nonresponders. J Cardiopulm Rehabil. 2001;21:10–17.

4 Troosters T, Casaburi R, Gosselink R, Decramer M. Pulmonary rehabilitation in chronic obstructive pulmonary disease. Am J Respir Crit Care Med. 2005;172:19–38.

5 Lacasse Y, Goldstein R, Lasserson TJ, Martin S. Pulmonary rehabilitation for chronic obstructive pulmonary disease. Cochrane Database Syst Rev. 2006;(4):CD003793.

6 British Thoracic Society. Statement on pulmonary rehabilitation. Thorax. 2001;56:827–834.

7 American Association of Cardiovascular and Pulmonary Rehabilitation (ed.). Guidelines for Pulmonary Rehabilitation Programs, 4th edn. Champaign, IL: Human Kinetics; 2010, pp. 9–19.

8 Jenkins S, Hill K, Cecins NM. State of the art: How to set up a pulmonary rehabilitation program. Respirology. 2010;15:1157–1173.

9 Pitta F, Troosters T, Spruit MA, Probst VS, Decramer M et al. Characteristics of physical activities in daily life in chronic obstructive pulmonary disease. Am J Respir Crit Care Med. 2005;171:972–927.

10 Casaburi R, Patessio A, Ioli F, Zanaboni S, Donner CF et al. Reductions in exercise lactic acidosis and ventilation as a result of exercise training in patients with obstructive lung disease. Am Rev Respir Dis. 1991;143:9–18.

11 Maltais F, LeBlanc P, Jobin J, Bérubé C, Bruneau J et al. Intensity of training and physiologic adaptation in patients with chronic obstructive pulmonary disease. Am J Respir Crit Care Med. 1997;155:555–561.

12 Gimenez M, Servera E, Vergara P, Bach JR, Polu JM. Endurance training in patients with chronic obstructive pulmonary disease: A comparison of high versus moderate intensity. Arch Phys Med Rehabil. 2000;81:102–109.

13 Datta D, ZuWallack R. High versus low intensity exercise training in pulmonary rehabilitation: Is more better? Chron Respir Dis. 2004;1:143–149.

14 Beauchamp MK, Nonoyama M, Goldstein RS, Hill K, Dolmage TE et al. Interval versus continuous training in individuals with chronic obstructive pulmonary disease—A systematic review. Thorax. 2010;65:157–164.

15 Yohannes AM, Connolly MJ. Pulmonary rehabilitation programmes in the UK: A national representative survey. Clin Rehabil. 2004;18:444–449.

16 Brooks D, Sottana R, Bell B, Hanna M, Laframboise L et al. Characterization of pulmonary rehabilitation programs in Canada in 2005. Can Respir J. 2007;14:87–92.

17 Gosselink R, Troosters T, Decramer M. Peripheral muscle weakness contributes to exercise limitation in COPD. Am J Respir Crit Care Med. 1996;153:976–980.

18 Solway S, Brooks D, Lau L, Goldstein R. The short-term effect of a rollator on functional exercise capacity among individuals with severe COPD. Chest. 2002;122:56–65.

19 Probst VS, Troosters T, Coosemans I, Spruit MA, Pitta Fde O et al. Mechanisms of improvement in exercise capacity using a rollator in patients with COPD. Chest. 2004;126:1102–1107.

20 Eves ND, Sandmeyer LC, Wong EY, Jones LW, MacDonald GF et al. Helium-hyperoxia: A novel intervention to improve the benefits of pulmonary rehabilitation for patients with COPD. Chest. 2009;135:609–618.

21 van't Hul A, Kwakkel G, Gosselink R. The acute effects of noninvasive ventilatory support during exercise on exercise endurance and dyspnea in patients with chronic obstructive pulmonary disease: A systematic review. J Cardiopulm Rehabil. 2002;22:290–297.

22 Vivodtzev I, Lacasse Y, Maltais F. Neuromuscular electrical stimulation of the lower limbs in patients with chronic obstructive pulmonary disease. J Cardiopulm Rehabil Prev. 2008;28:79–91.

23 Sillen MJ, Speksnijder CM, Eterman RM, Janssen PP, Wagers SS et al. Effects of neuromuscular electrical stimulation of muscles of ambulation in patients with chronic heart failure or COPD: A systematic review of the English-language literature. Chest. 2009;136:44–61.

24 Gosselink R. Breathing techniques in patients with chronic obstructive pulmonary disease (COPD). Chron Respir Dis. 2004;1:163–172.

25 Bott J, Blumenthal S, Buxton M, Ellum S, Falconer C et al. Guidelines for the physiotherapy management of the adult, medical, spontaneously breathing patient. Thorax. 2009;64(Suppl. 1):i1–51.

26 Sharp JT, Drutz WS, Moisan T, Foster J, Machnach W. Postural relief of dyspnea in severe chronic obstructive pulmonary disease. Am Rev Respir Dis. 1980;122:201–211.

27 O'Neill S, McCarthy DS. Postural relief of dyspnoea in severe chronic airflow limitation: Relationship to respiratory muscle strength. Thorax. 1983;38:595–600.

28 Bodenheimer T, Lorig K, Holman H, Grumbach K. Patient self-management of chronic disease in primary care. JAMA. 2002;288:2469–2475.

29 Kunik ME, Roundy K, Veazey C, Souchek J, Richardson P et al. Surprisingly high prevalence of anxiety and depression in chronic breathing disorders. Chest. 2005;127:1205–1211.

30 Ferris BG. Epidemiology standardization project (American Thoracic Society). Am Rev Respir Dis. 1978;118(6 Pt 2):1–120.

31 Borg GA. Psychophysical bases of perceived exertion. *Med Sci Sports Exerc.* 1982;14:377–381.

32 ATS Committee on Proficiency Standards for Clinical Pulmonary Function Laboratories. ATS statement: Guidelines for the six-minute walk test. *Am J Respir Crit Care Med.* 2002;166:111–117.

33 Singh SJ, Morgan MD, Scott S, Walters D, Hardman AE. Development of a shuttle walking test of disability in patients with chronic airways obstruction. *Thorax.* 1992;47:1019–1024.

34 Singh SJ, Jones PW, Evans R, Morgan MD. Minimum clinically important improvement for the incremental shuttle walking test. *Thorax.* 2008;63:775–777.

35 Ware JE Jr, Sherbourne CD. The MOS 36-item short-form health survey (SF-36). I. Conceptual framework and item selection. *Med Care.* 1992;30:473–483.

36 Guyatt GH, Berman LB, Townsend M, Pugsley SO, Chambers LW. A measure of quality of life for clinical trials in chronic lung disease. *Thorax.* 1987;42:773–778.

37 Jones PW, Quirk FH, Baveystock CM, Littlejohns P. A self-complete measure of health status for chronic airflow limitation. The St. George's Respiratory Questionnaire. *Am Rev Respir Dis.* 1992;145(6):1321–1327.

38 Jones PW, Harding G, Berry P, Wiklund I, Chen WH et al. Development and first validation of the COPD Assessment Test. *Eur Respir J.* 2009;34:648–654.

39 Bausewein C, Booth S, Gysels M, Higginson I. Non-pharmacological interventions for breathlessness in advanced stages of malignant and non-malignant diseases. *Cochrane Database Syst Rev.* 2008;(2):CD005623. doi:10.1002/14651858.CD005623.pub2.

Index